MW01154491

# Operative Techniques in Pediatric Orthopaedic Surgery

SECOND EDITION

**Also Available In This Series**

OPERATIVE TECHNIQUES IN FOOT AND ANKLE SURGERY, Second Edition
Editor: **Mark E. Easley**
Editor-in-Chief: **Sam W. Wiesel**

OPERATIVE TECHNIQUES IN ORTHOPAEDIC TRAUMA SURGERY, Second Edition
Editor: **Paul Tornetta III**
Editor-in-Chief: **Sam W. Wiesel**

OPERATIVE TECHNIQUES IN SHOULDER AND ELBOW SURGERY, Second Edition
Editors: **Gerald R. Williams, Jr., Matthew L. Ramsey, & Brent B. Wiesel**
Editor-in-Chief: **Sam W. Wiesel**

OPERATIVE TECHNIQUES IN SPORTS MEDICINE SURGERY, Second Edition
Editor: **Mark D. Miller**
Editor-in-Chief: **Sam W. Wiesel**

OPERATIVE TECHNIQUES IN JOINT RECONSTRUCTION SURGERY, Second Edition
Editors: **Javad Parvizi & Richard H. Rothman**
Editor-in-Chief: **Sam W. Wiesel**

OPERATIVE TECHNIQUES IN HAND, WRIST, AND ELBOW SURGERY, Second Edition
Editor: **Thomas R. Hunt III**
Associate Editor: **Brian D. Adams**
Editor-in-Chief: **Sam W. Wiesel**

OPERATIVE TECHNIQUES IN SPINE SURGERY, Second Edition
Editors: **John M. Rhee & Scott D. Boden**
Editor-in-Chief: **Sam W. Wiesel**

OPERATIVE TECHNIQUES IN ORTHOPAEDIC SURGICAL ONCOLOGY, Second Edition
Editors: **Martin M. Malawer, James C. Wittig, & Jacob Bickels**
Editor-in-Chief: **Sam W. Wiesel**

# Operative Techniques in Pediatric Orthopaedic Surgery

SECOND EDITION

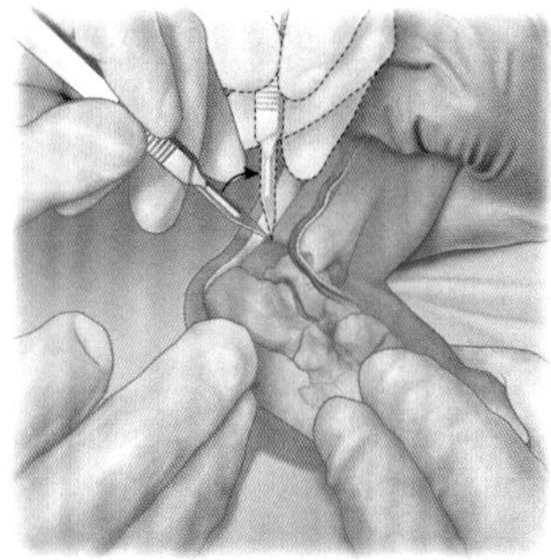

**John M. Flynn, MD**
Chief of Orthopedic Surgery
The Children's Hospital of Philadelphia
Professor of Orthopaedic Surgery
Perelman School of Medicine at the University of Pennsylvania
Philadelphia, Pennsylvania

**Wudbhav N. Sankar, MD**
Director, Young Adult Hip Preservation Program
The Children's Hospital of Philadelphia
Assistant Professor of Orthopedic Surgery
Perelman School of Medicine at the University of Pennsylvania
Philadelphia, Pennsylvania

**Sam W. Wiesel, MD**
EDITOR-IN-CHIEF
Chairman and Professor
Department of Orthopaedic Surgery
Georgetown University Medical School
Washington, DC

**With select chapters from:**

**Adult Reconstruction edited by**
Javad Parvizi, MD
Richard H. Rothman, MD

**Pelvis and Lower Extremity Trauma edited by**
Paul Tornetta III, MD

**Spine edited by**
John M. Rhee, MD
Scott D. Boden, MD

**Hand Wrist and Forearm edited by**
Thomas R. Hunt III, MD, DSc

**Shoulder and Elbow edited by**
Gerald R. Williams, Jr., MD
Matthew L. Ramsey, MD
Brent B. Wiesel, MD

**Sports Medicine edited by**
Mark D. Miller, MD

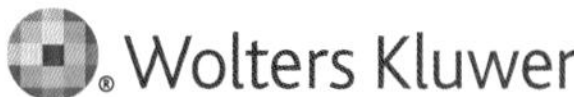


Philadelphia • Baltimore • New York • London
Buenos Aires • Hong Kong • Sydney • Tokyo

*Acquisitions Editor:* Brian Brown
*Product Development Editor:* Dave Murphy
*Marketing Manager:* Daniel Dressler
*Production Project Manager:* Bridgett Dougherty
*Design Coordinator:* Holly McLaughlin
*Manufacturing Coordinator:* Beth Welsh
*Prepress Vendor:* Absolute Service, Inc.

2nd edition



9 8 7 6 5 4 3 2 1

Printed in China

**Library of Congress Cataloging-in-Publication Data**

Names: Flynn, John M., editor. | Sankar, Wudbhav N., editor. | Wiesel, Sam W., editor.
Title: Operative techniques in pediatric orthopaedic surgery / [edited by] John M. Flynn, Wudbhav N. Sankar ; Sam W. Wiesel, editor-in-chief.
Other titles: Operative techniques in orthopaedic pediatric surgery.
Description: Second edition. | Philadelphia : Wolters Kluwer, [2016] | Preceded by Operative techniques in orthopaedic pediatric surgery / [edited by] John M. Flynn ; Sam W. Wiesel, editor-in-chief. c2011. | Contained in Operative techniques in orthopaedic surgery / Sam. W. Wiesel, editor-in-chief. Second edition. 2016. | Includes bibliographical references and index.
Identifiers: LCCN 2015040261 | ISBN 9781451193084 (alk. paper)
Subjects: | MESH: Orthopedic Procedures. | Child.
Classification: LCC RD731 | NLM WS 270 | DDC 617.4/7—dc23 LC record available at http://lccn.loc.gov/2015040261

This work is provided "as is," and the publisher disclaims any and all warranties, express or implied, including any warranties as to accuracy, comprehensiveness, or currency of the content of this work.

This work is no substitute for individual patient assessment based on healthcare professionals' examination of each patient and consideration of, among other things, age, weight, gender, current or prior medical conditions, medication history, laboratory data, and other factors unique to the patient. The publisher does not provide medical advice or guidance, and this work is merely a reference tool. Healthcare professionals, and not the publisher, are solely responsible for the use of this work including all medical judgments and for any resulting diagnosis and treatments.

Given continuous, rapid advances in medical science and health information, independent professional verification of medical diagnoses, indications, appropriate pharmaceutical selections and dosages, and treatment options should be made and healthcare professionals should consult a variety of sources. When prescribing medication, healthcare professionals are advised to consult the product information sheet (the manufacturer's package insert) accompanying each drug to verify, among other things, conditions of use, warnings, and side effects and identify any changes in dosage schedule or contraindications, particularly if the medication to be administered is new, infrequently used, or has a narrow therapeutic range. To the maximum extent permitted under applicable law, no responsibility is assumed by the publisher for any injury and/or damage to persons or property, as a matter of products liability, negligence law or otherwise, or from any reference to or use by any person of this work.

LWW.com

CCS1215

# Dedication

*To my orthopaedic mentors, especially Ed Hanley, John Hall, Jim Kasser, and Peter Waters, who have inspired me to write and teach and give back to orthopaedics, the way they have.*

—JMF

*First and foremost, thanks to my wife and best friend Ariana, and my wonderful children, Isla and Kamran for your patience, support, and understanding. And to my orthopaedic mentors at Children's Hospital of Philadelphia, Children's Hospital Los Angeles, and Boston Children's Hospital—thanks for being my giants.*

—WS

# Contents

## SECTION II **ARTHROSCOPIC AND SPORTS MEDICINE**

# Contributors

**Matthew D. Abbott, MD**
Assistant Clinical Professor
Department of Orthopaedic Surgery
University of Michigan Health System
Ann Arbor, Michigan

**Joshua M. Abzug, MD**
Assistant Professor
Department of Orthopaedics
University of Maryland School of Medicine
Baltimore, Maryland

**Farshad Adib, MD**
Assistant Professor
Department of Orthopaedics
University of Maryland School of Medicine
Baltimore, Maryland

**Animesh Agarwal, MD**
Professor
Division of Orthopaedic Trauma
UT Health Science Center San Antonio
Department of Orthopaedics
Traumatologist Orthopaedic
University Hospital
San Antonio, Texas

**Laith M. Al-Shihabi, MD**
Resident
Department of Orthopedic Surgery
Rush University Medical Center
Chicago, Illinois

**Jay C. Albright, MD**
Assistant Professor
Surgical Director of Sports Medicine
Children's Hospital Colorado
Aurora, Colorado

**Alexandre Arkader, MD**
Assistant Professor of Orthopaedic Surgery
Keck School of Medicine of the University of Southern California
University of Southern California
Director, Musculoskeletal Tumor Program
Children's Orthopaedic Center
Children's Hospital Los Angeles
Los Angles, California

**Donald S. Bae, MD**
Associate Professor
Department of Orthopaedic Surgery
Harvard Medical School
Attending Physician
Department of Orthopedic Surgery
Boston Children's Hospital
Boston, Massachusetts

**Carla Baldrighi, MD**
Department of Reconstructive Microsurgery
Ospedale CTO
Azienda Ospedaliero-Universitaria Careggi
Florence, Italy

**Keith D. Baldwin, MD, MSPT, MPH**
Assistant Professor
Neuromuscular Orthopedic and Orthopedic Trauma
Division of Orthopedics
The Children's Hospital of Philadelphia
Philadelphia, Pennsylvania

**Asheesh Bedi, MD**
Harold and Helen W. Gehring Early Career Professor of Orthopaedic Surgery
Assistant Professor of Sports Medicine and Shoulder Surgery
Department of Orthopaedic Surgery
University of Michigan
Ann Arbor, Michigan

**Robert M. Bernstein, MD**
Medical Director
Cedars-Sinai Orthopaedic Center
Cedars-Sinai Medical Center
Los Angeles, California

**Diana Bitar, MD**
Orthopaedic Surgeon
Research Fellow
Rothman Institute
Thomas Jefferson University Hospital
Philadelphia, Pennsylvania

**Arkady Blyakher, MD**
Department of Orthopedic Surgery
Hospital for Special Surgery
New York, New York

**J. Richard Bowen, MD**
Nemours Professor of Orthopaedic Education and Research
Department of Orthopedics
Nemours/Alfred I. duPont Hospital for Children
Wilmington, Delaware

**Richard E. Bowen, MD**
Clinical Professor
Department of Orthopaedic Surgery
David Geffen School of Medicine at UCLA
Director of Medical Education
Department of Pediatric Orthopaedics
Orthopaedic Institute for Children
Los Angeles, California

**Jaysson T. Brooks, MD**
Resident Physician
Department of Orthopaedic Surgery
Johns Hopkins Medicine
Baltimore, Maryland

**Michelle S. Caird, MD**
Assistant Professor
Department of Orthopaedic Surgery
University of Michigan Health System
Ann Arbor, Michigan

**Robert M. Campbell, Jr., MD**
Director
Division of Orthopedics
Center for Thoracic Insufficiency Syndrome
The Children's Hospital of Philadelphia
Philadelphia, Pennsylvania

**Robert Carrigan, MD**
Assistant Professor of Clinical Orthopaedic Surgery
Perelman School of Medicine at the University of Pennsylvania
Attending Orthopaedic Surgeon
Division of Orthopedics
The Children's Hospital of Philadelphia
Philadelphia, Pennsylvania

**Paul D. Choi, MD**
Assistant Professor
Department of Orthopaedic Surgery
University of Southern California
Faculty
Children's Orthopaedic Center
Children's Hospital Los Angeles
Los Angeles, California

**Michael P. Clare, MD**
Director of Fellowship Education
Foot and Ankle Fellowship
Florida Orthopaedic Institute
Tampa, Florida

**Dino Colo, MD**
Research Fellow
Division of Orthopedics
The Children's Hospital of Philadelphia
Philadelphia, Pennsylvania

**Roger Cornwall, MD**
Associate Professor
Department of Orthopaedic Surgery
University of Cincinnati College of Medicine
Clinical Director of Pediatric Orthopaedics
Department of Orthopaedic Surgery
Cincinnati Children's Hospital Medical Center
Cincinnati, Ohio

**Andrew J. Cosgarea, MD**
Professor
Department of Orthopaedic Surgery
Director
Division of Sports Medicine
Head Team Physician
Johns Hopkins University
Baltimore, Maryland

**Lindsay Crawford, MD**
Assistant Professor
Department of Orthopaedic Surgery
The University of Texas Health Science
Center at Houston
Pediatric Orthopedic Surgeon
Department of Pediatric Orthopedic Surgery
Children's Memorial Hermann Hospital
Houston, Texas

**Brett Crist, MD**
Associate Professor
Department of Orthopaedic Surgery
University of Missouri
Columbia, Missouri

**Anna V. Cuomo, MD**
Assistant Clinical Professor
Department of Orthopaedic Surgery
David Geffen School of Medicine at UCLA
University of California, Los Angeles
Staff Orthopedic Surgeon
Department of Orthopedic Surgery
Shriners Hospitals for Children—Los Angeles
Los Angeles, California

**Kirk W. Dabney, MD**
Pediatric Orthopedic Surgeon
Codirector, Cerebral Palsy Program
Division of Orthopedics
Nemours/Alfred I. duPont Hospital for Children
Wilmington, Delaware
Assistant Professor of Orthopaedic Surgery
Jefferson Medical College
Thomas Jefferson University
Philadelphia, Pennsylvania

**Jon R. Davids, MD**
Professor
Department of Orthopaedic Surgery
UC Davis Health System
Assistant Chief
Department of Orthopaedic Surgery
Shriners Hospitals for Children—Northern
California
Sacramento, California

**Richard S. Davidson, MD**
Clinical Professor of Orthopaedic Surgery
Perelman School of Medicine at the University
of Pennsylvania
Attending Surgeon
The Children's Hospital of Philadelphia
Philadelphia, Pennsylvania

**John R. Dawson, MD**
Assistant Professor
Chief of Orthopedics, Ben Taub General
Hospital
Joseph Barnhart Department of Orthopedic
Surgery
Baylor College of Medicine
Houston, Texas

**Mark T. Dillon, MD**
Department of Orthopaedic Surgery
Kaiser Permanente
Sacramento Medical Center
Sacramento, California

**Matthew B. Dobbs, MD**
Professor
Department of Orthopedic Surgery
Washington University School of Medicine
St. Louis Children's Hospital and Shriners
Hospitals for Children—St. Louis
St. Louis, Missouri

**Emily R. Dodwell, MD**
Assistant Attending Pediatric Orthopedic
Surgeon
Hospital for Special Surgery
Assistant Attending Pediatric Orthopedic
Surgeon
New York Presbyterian Hospital
Attending Pediatric Orthopedic Surgeon
New York Hospital Queens
Assistant Professor of Orthopaedic Surgery
Weill Cornell Medical College
New York, New York

**John P. Dormans, MD**
Professor
Department of Orthopaedic Surgery
Perelman School of Medicine at the University
of Pennsylvania
Division Chief
Department of Surgery
Division of Orthopedics
The Children's Hospital of Philadelphia
Philadelphia, Pennsylvania

**Denis S. Drummond, MD**
Emeritus Professor of Orthopaedic Surgery
Perelman School of Medicine at the University
of Pennsylvania
Research Physician
Former Chief
Division of Orthopedics
The Children's Hospital of Philadelphia
Philadelphia, Pennsylvania

**Jonathan G. Eastman, MD**
Assistant Professor
Department of Orthopaedic Surgery
University of California, Davis
Sacramento, California

**Craig P. Eberson, MD**
Associate Professor
Department of Orthopaedics
Warren Alpert Medical School of Brown
University
Chief, Division of Pediatric Orthopedics
Department of Orthopedics
Hasbro Children's Hospital
Providence, Rhode Island

**Eric W. Edmonds, MD**
Director, Orthopaedic Research
Codirector, 360 Sports Medicine
Pediatric Orthopedic & Scoliosis Center
Rady Children's Hospital—San Diego
Assistant Clinical Professor
Department of Orthopaedic Surgery
UC San Diego School of Medicine
San Diego, California

**Kenneth A. Egol, MD**
Professor and Vice Chairman
Orthopaedic Surgery
Hospital for Joint Diseases
NYU Langone Medical Center
New York, New York

**Howard R. Epps, MD**
Medical Director
Pediatric Orthopedic Surgery
Texas Children's Hospital
Associate Professor
Pediatric Orthopedic Surgery
Baylor College of Medicine
Houston, Texas

**Paul W. Esposito, MD**
Professor
Department of Pediatric Surgery
University of Nebraska Medical Center
Clinical Service Chief
Department of Orthopaedic Surgery
Children's Hospital & Medical Center
Omaha, Nebraska

**Marybeth Ezaki, MD**
Professor of Orthopaedic Surgery
Department of Orthopaedic Surgery
UT Southwestern Medical Center
Director of Hand Surgery
Texas Scottish Rite Hospital for Children
Dallas, Texas

**François Fassier, MD**
Associate Professor
Department of Pediatric Surgery
McGill University
Chief of Staff Emeritus
Department of Surgery
Shriners Hospitals for Children—Canada
Montreal, Quebec, Canada

**John J. Fernandez, MD**
Assistant Professor
Rush University Medical Center
Chicago, Illinois

**John M. Flynn, MD**
Chief of Orthopedic Surgery
The Children's Hospital of Philadelphia
Professor of Orthopaedic Surgery
Perelman School of Medicine at the University of Pennsylvania
Philadelphia, Pennsylvania

**John P. Fulkerson, MD**
Orthopedic Associates of Hartford, PC
Clinical Professor of Orthopedic Surgery
University of Connecticut
Farmington, Connecticut

**Andrew Furey, MSc, MD, FRCSC**
Assistant Professor
Department of Surgery
Memorial University of Newfoundland
St. John's, Newfoundland, Canada

**Theodore J. Ganley, MD**
Associate Professor
Department of Orthopaedic Surgery
Perelman School of Medicine at the University of Pennsylvania
Director Sports Medicine
Orthopedic Surgery
The Children's Hospital of Philadelphia
Philadelphia, Pennsylvania

**Itai Gans, MD**
Benjamin Fox Orthopedic Research Fellow
Division of Orthopedics
The Children's Hospital of Philadelphia
Philadelphia, Pennsylvania

**Matthew J. Garberina, MD**
Department of Orthopaedics/Sports Medicine
Summit Medical Group
Berkeley Heights, New Jersey

**Matthew R. Garner, MD**
Resident
Department of Orthopedic Surgery
Hospital for Special Surgery
New York, New York

**Charles L. Getz, MD**
Associate Professor
Thomas Jefferson University Hospital
Rothman Institute
Philadelphia, Pennsylvania

**Purushottam A. Gholve, MD, MBMS, MRCS**
Assistant Professor
Department of Orthopaedic Surgery
Tufts University School of Medicine
Boston, Massachusetts

**Mohit Gilotra, MD**
Assistant Professor of Orthopaedics
Department of Orthopaedic Surgery
University of Maryland Medical Center
Baltimore, Maryland

**David L. Glaser, MD**
Chief, Shoulder and Elbow Service
Associate Professor of Orthopaedic Surgery
Hospital of the University of Pennsylvania
Philadelphia, Pennsylvania

**Michael P. Glotzbecker, MD**
Instructor
Department of Orthopaedic Surgery
Harvard Medical School
Boston Children's Hospital
Boston, Massachusetts

**Jonathan A. Godin, MD, MBA**
Resident Physician
Department of Orthopaedic Surgery
Duke University Medical Center
Durham, North Carolina

**Jaime A. Gomez, MD**
Pediatric Orthopedic Fellow
Department of Pediatric Orthopedic Surgery
Boston Children's Hospital/Harvard Medical School
Boston, Massachusetts

**Christine M. Goodbody, MD**
The Children's Hospital of Philadelphia
Perelman School of Medicine at the University of Pennsylvania
Philadelphia, Pennsylvania

**J. Eric Gordon, MD**
Professor
Department of Orthopedic Surgery
Washington University School of Medicine
Cochief
Department of Orthopaedic Surgery
St. Louis Children's Hospital
St. Louis, Missouri

**Daniel Grant, MD**
Assistant Professor
Department of Orthopaedics
West Virginia University
Morgantown, West Virginia

**Nathan L. Grimm, MD**
Orthopaedic Surgeon
Department of Orthopaedic Surgery
Duke University Medical Center
Durham, North Carolina

**Yung Han, MD**
Orthopaedic Surgeon
Kerlan-Jobe Orthopaedic Clinic
Los Angeles, California

**Christopher D. Harner, MD**
Professor
Department of Orthopaedic Surgery
University of Pittsburgh
Pittsburgh, Pennsylvania

**Nanjundappa S. Harshavardhana, MD**
Clinical Fellow
Division of Orthopedics
The Children's Hospital of Philadelphia
Philadelphia, Pennsylvania

**George Frederick Hatch III, MD**
Assistant Professor of Orthopaedic Surgery
Department of Orthopaedic Surgery
Keck School of Medicine of the University of Southern California
Los Angeles, California

**Daniel J. Hedequist, MD**
Instructor
Department of Orthopedic Surgery
Boston Children's Hospital
Boston, Massachusetts

**Martin J. Herman, MD**
Professor of Orthopaedic Surgery and Pediatrics
Drexel University College of Medicine
St. Christopher's Hospital for Children
Philadelphia, Pennsylvania

**Levi Hinkelman, MD**
Orthopedic Surgery Resident
Grand Rapids Medical Education Partners
Michigan State University College of Human Medicine
Grand Rapids, Michigan

**B. David Horn, MD**
Assistant Professor Clinical Orthopaedic Surgery
Department of Orthopaedic Surgery
Perelman School of Medicine at the University of Pennsylvania
Philadelphia, Pennsylvania

**Asif M. Ilyas, MD, FACS**
Program Director of Hand and Upper Extremity Surgery Fellowship
Rothman Institute
Associate Professor of Orthopaedic Surgery
Thomas Jefferson University
Philadelphia, Pennsylvania

**John M. Itamura, MD**
Associate Professor
Clinical Professor of Orthopaedic Surgery
Keck School of Medicine of the University of Southern California
Orthopaedic Surgeon
Kerlan-Jobe Orthopaedic Clinic
Los Angeles California

**Jesse B. Jupiter, MD**
Hansjorg Wyss/AO Professor of Orthopaedic Surgery
Harvard Medical School
Massachusetts General Hospital
Boston, Massachusetts

**Lori A. Karol, MD**
Professor
Department of Orthopaedic Surgery
UT Southwestern Medical Center
Texas Scottish Rite Hospital for Children
Dallas, Texas

**Robert M. Kay, MD**
Professor
Department of Orthopaedic Surgery
Keck School of Medicine of the University of Southern California
Vice Chief
Children's Orthopaedic Center
Children's Hospital Los Angeles
Los Angeles, California

**Simon P. Kelley, MBChB, FRCS**
Assistant Professor
Department of Surgery
University of Toronto
Orthopaedic Surgeon
Division of Orthopaedics
The Hospital for Sick Children
Toronto, Ontario, Canada

**Michael P. Kelly, MD**
Assistant Professor of Orthopedic Surgery
Assistant Professor of Neurological Surgery
Washington University School of Medicine
St. Louis, Missouri

**Young-Jo Kim, MD**
Associate Professor of Orthopaedic Surgery
Department of Orthopaedic Surgery
Harvard Medical School
Boston Children's Hospital
Boston, Massachusetts

**Mininder S. Kocher, MD, MPH**
Professor of Orthopaedic Surgery
Department of Orthopaedic Surgery
Harvard Medical School
Associate Director
Division of Sports Medicine
Boston Children's Hospital
Boston, Massachusetts

**Sanjit R. Konda, MD**
Assistant Professor
Associate Director of Trauma
Jamaica Hospital Medical Center
Department of Orthopaedic Surgery
NYU Hospital for Joint Diseases
NYU Langone School of Medicine
New York, New York

**Scott H. Kozin, MD**
Chief of Staff
Shriners Hospitals for Children—Philadelphia
Clinical Professor
Department of Orthopaedic Surgery
Temple University School of Medicine
Philadelphia, Pennsylvania

**Leok-Lim Lau, MD**
Consultant
Divisions of Spine and Paediatric Orthopaedics Surgery
University Orthopaedics, Hand and Reconstructive Microsurgery Cluster
National University Health System
Singapore

**J. Todd R. Lawrence, MD**
Assistant Professor
Department of Orthopaedic Surgery
University of Pennsylvania
Attending Surgeon
Division of Orthopedics
The Children's Hospital of Philadelphia
Philadelphia, Pennsylvania

**Peter J.L. Jebson, MD**
Associate Professor
Michigan State College of Human Medicine
Clinical Instructor
Grand Rapids Medical Education Partners
Department of Orthopaedic Surgery
Spectrum Health Medical Group
Grand Rapids, Michigan

**Mark A. Lee, MD**
Associate Professor
Director, Orthopaedic Trauma Fellowship
Department of Orthopaedic Surgery
UC Davis Health System
Sacramento, California

**R. Jay Lee, MD**
Assistant Professor of Orthopaedic Surgery
The Johns Hopkins Hospital
Baltimore, Maryland

**Lawrence G. Lenke, MD**
The Jerome J. Gilden Distinguished Professor of Orthopaedic Surgery
Professor of Neurological Surgery
Chief
Spine Surgery
Codirector
Spinal Deformity Service
Director
Advanced Deformity Fellowship (ADF)
Washington University School of Medicine
St. Louis, Missouri

**L. Scott Levin, MD FACS**
Paul B. Magnuson Professor and Chairman of the Department of Orthopaedic Surgery
Professor of Surgery (Plastic Surgery)
Perelman School of Medicine at the University of Pennsylvania
Philadelphia, Pennsylvania

**David M. Lutton, MD**
Orthopaedic Surgeon
Washington Circle Orthopaedic Associates, P.C.
Washington, DC

**Jeffrey E. Martus, MD**
Assistant Professor of Orthopaedics Surgery and Rehabilitation
Assistant Professor of Pediatrics
Vanderbilt University Medical Center
Nashville, Tennessee

**Travis H. Matheney, MD**
Assistant Professor
Department of Orthopaedic Surgery
Harvard Medical School
Staff Physician
Department of Orthopedic Surgery
Boston Children's Hospital
Boston, Massachusetts

**Craig S. Mauro, MD**
Clinical Assistant Professor
University of Pittsburgh Medical Center
Burke and Bradley Orthopedics
Pittsburgh, Pennsylvania

**James J. McCarthy, MD**
Professor
Department of Orthopaedic Surgery
University of Cincinnati College of Medicine
Director
Pediatric Orthopaedic Surgery
Cincinnati Children's Hospital Medical Center
Cincinnati, Ohio

**Richard E. McCarthy, MD**
Professor
Department of Orthopedic & Neurosurgery
University of Arkansas for Medical Sciences
Chief of Spinal Deformities
Department of Orthopaedics
Arkansas Children's Hospital
Little Rock, Arkansas

**Janay E. Mckie, MD**
Staff
Shriners Hospitals for Children—Shreveport
Shreveport, Louisiana

**Charles T. Mehlman, DO, MPH**
Professor, Pediatric Orthopaedics
University of Cincinnati College of Medicine
Director
Pediatric Musculoskeletal Outcomes Research
Pediatric Orthopaedic Resident Education
Cincinnati Children's Hospital Medical Center
Cincinnati, Ohio

**Chris Mellano, MD**
Clinical Fellow
Department of Sports Medicine
Rush University Medical Center
Chicago, Illinois

**Gokce Mik, MD**
Operator Doctor
Istanbul Surgery Hospital
Istanbul, Turkey

**Freeman Miller, MD**
Director of the Cerebral Palsy Program
Department of Orthopedics
Nemours/Alfred I. duPont Hospital for Children
Wilmington, Delaware

**Michael B. Millis, MD**
Professor of Orthopaedic Surgery
Harvard Medical School
Boston Children's Hospital
Boston, Massachusetts

**R. Justin Mistovich, MD**
Fellow
Division of Orthopedics
The Children's Hospital of Philadelphia
Philadelphia, Pennsylvania

**Ronald Mitchell, MD**
Orthopaedic Resident
Houston Methodist Hospital
Houston, Texas

**Claude T. Moorman III, MD**
Professor and Vice Chairman, Orthopaedic Surgery
Professor, Evolutionary Anthropology
Director, Duke Sports Medicine
Head Team Physician, Duke Athletics
Duke University Medical Center
Durham, North Carolina

**Vincent S. Mosca, MD**
Professor of Pediatrics
Department of Orthopedics
University of Washington School of Medicine
Pediatric Orthopedic Surgeon
Department of Orthopedics
Seattle Children's Hospital
Seattle, Washington

**Scott J. Mubarak, MD**
Clinical Professor
Department of Orthopaedic Surgery
UC San Diego School of Medicine
Vice Chair of Division of Pediatric Orthopedics
Department of Orthopedics
Rady Children's Hospital—San Diego
San Diego, California

**Ryan D. Muchow, MD**
Assistant Professor
Department of Orthopaedic Surgery
University of Kentucky
Staff Orthopedic Surgeon
Department of Orthopaedic Surgery
Shriners Hospital for Children—Lexington
Lexington, Kentucky

**Afamefuna M. Nduaguba, BS**
Division of Orthopedics
The Children's Hospital of Philadelphia
Philadelphia, Pennsylvania

**Blaise Nemeth, MD**
Associate Professor
Department of Orthopedics and Rehabilitation
University of Wisconsin School of Medicine and Public Health
Madison, Wisconsin

**Peter O. Newton, MD**
Chief
Division of Orthopedics & Scoliosis
Rady Children's Hospital—San Diego
Clinical Professor
UC San Diego School of Medicine
San Diego, California

**Kenneth J. Noonan, MD**
Associate Professor
Department of Orthopedics and Rehabilitation
University of Wisconsin School of Medicine and Public Health
Madison, Wisconsin

**Tom F. Novacheck, MD**
Adjunct Associate Professor
Department of Orthopaedic Surgery
University of Minnesota
Minneapolis, Minnesota
Director
James R. Gage Center for Gait and Motion Analysis
Gillette Children's Specialty Healthcare
St. Paul, Minnesota

**Scott N. Oishi, MD**
Associate Professor
Department of Plastic Surgery
Department of Orthopaedic Surgery
UT Southwestern Medical Center
Head Surgeon
Hand Surgery Department
Texas Scottish Rite Hospital for Children
Dallas, Texas

**Brad Olney, MD**
Professor
Department of Orthopaedic Surgery
University of Missouri—Kansas City
Chief
Department of Orthopaedic Surgery
Children's Mercy Hospital
Kansas City, Missouri

**Robert Ostrum, MD**
Professor
Department of Orthopaedic Surgery
University of North Carolina at Chapel Hill
Chapel Hill, North Carolina

**Robert V. O'Toole, MD**
Associate Professor
Department of Orthopaedic Surgery
University of Maryland School of Medicine
Baltimore, Maryland

**Norman Y. Otsuka, MD**
Joseph E. Milgram Professor of Orthopaedic Surgery
Department of Orthopaedic Surgery
New York University
Director
Center for Children
NYU Langone Medical Center Hospital for Joint Diseases
New York, New York

**Dror Paley, MD**
Director
Paley Advanced Limb Lengthening Institute
St. Mary's Medical Center
West Palm Beach, Florida

**Bradford O. Parsons, MD**
Associate Professor
Department of Orthopaedics
Mount Sinai Hospital
New York, New York

**George Partal, MD**
Orthopaedic Trauma Surgery
Eastern Maine Medical Center
Bangor, Maine

**Javad Parvizi, MD**
James Edwards Professor of Orthopaedic Surgery
Sidney Kimmel School of Medicine
Rothman Institute at Thomas Jefferson University
Philadelphia, Pennsylvania

**Andrew T. Pennock, MD**
Assistant Clinical Professor
Department of Orthopaedic Surgery
UC San Diego School of Medicine
Department of Orthopedic Surgery
Rady Children's Hospital—San Diego
San Diego, California

**Jonathan H. Phillips, MD**
Assistant Professor of Orthopaedic Surgery
College of Medicine
University of Central Florida
Attending
Arnold Palmer Hospital Center for Orthopedics
Orlando Health
Orlando, Florida

**Kristan A. Pierz, MD**
Assistant Professor
Department of Pediatric Orthopaedics
Medical Director, Center for Motion Analysis
Connecticut Children's Medical Center
Hartford, Connecticut

**John Polousky, MD**
Surgical Director, Sports Medicine
Department of Orthopedic Surgery
The Rocky Mountain Hospital for Children
Denver, Colorado

**Anish G. R. Potty, MD**
Clinical Fellow
Division of Orthopedics
The Children's Hospital of Philadelphia
Philadelphia, Pennsylvania

**Maya E. Pring, MD**
Associate Professor
Department of Orthopaedic Surgery
UC San Diego School of Medicine
Vice Chair of Department of Orthopedic Surgery
Department of Pediatric Orthopedic Surgery
Rady Children's Hospital—San Diego
San Diego, California

**Michael Quackenbush, DO**
Assistant Professor
Department of Orthopaedics
Division of Orthopaedic Trauma
Wexner Medical Center at The Ohio State University
Columbus, Ohio

**Lee M. Reichel, MD**
Assistant Professor
Joseph Barnhart Department of Orthopedic Surgery
Baylor College of Medicine
Houston, Texas

**Benjamin F. Ricciardi, MD**
Resident
Department of Orthopedic Surgery
Hospital for Special Surgery
New York, New York

**Margaret M. Rich, MD**
Assistant Chief of Staff
Shriners Hospitals for Children—St. Louis
St. Louis, Missouri

**Michael Rivlin, MD**
Orthopaedic Surgeon
Department of Orthopaedic Surgery
Thomas Jefferson University Hospital
Rothman Institute
Philadelphia, Pennsylvania

**Anthony A. Romeo, MD**
Professor
Department of Orthopedic Surgery
Program Director
Shoulder and Elbow Fellowship
Section Head, Shoulder and Elbow Surgery
Division of Sports Medicine
Rush University Medical Center
Team Physician, Chicago White Sox and Bulls
Chief Medical Editor, Orthopedics Today
Chicago, Illinois

**John P. Salvo, MD**
Clinical Associate Professor
Orthopaedic Surgery
Rothman Institute
Thomas Jefferson University Hospital
Philadelphia, Pennsylvania

**James O. Sanders, MD**
Professor of Orthopaedics
Pediatric Orthopaedics and Scoliosis
University of Rochester Medical Center
Chief of Pediatric Orthopaedic Division
URMC Orthopaedics and Rehabilitation
Strong Memorial Hospital
Rochester, New York

**Roy W. Sanders, MD**
Professor and Chairman
Department of Orthopaedic Surgery
University of South Florida
Director of Orthopaedic Trauma Services
President
Florida Orthopaedic Institute
Editor-in-Chief
*Journal of Orthopaedic Trauma*
Tampa, Florida

**Wudbhav N. Sankar, MD**
Assistant Professor of Orthopaedic Surgery
Director
Young Adult Hip Preservation Program
The Children's Hospital of Philadelphia
Assistant Professor of Orthopaedic Surgery
Perelman School of Medicine at the University of Pennsylvania
Philadelphia, Pennsylvania

**Anthony Scaduto, MD**
Executive Vice Chair
Department of Orthopaedic Surgery
University of California, Los Angeles
Charles LeRoy Lowman Professor
Department of Orthopaedic Surgery
Orthopaedic Institute for Children
Los Angeles, California

**David Scher, MD**
Associate Professor of Clinical Orthopaedic Surgery
Weill Cornell Medical College
Associate Attending Orthopedic Surgeon
Department of Orthopedic Surgery
Hospital for Special Surgery
New York, New York

**Perry L. Schoenecker, MD**
Chief of Staff
Shriners Hospitals for Children—St. Louis
Professor of Orthopedic Surgery
Department of Orthopedic Surgery
Washington University School of Medicine
St. Louis, Missouri

**Tim Schrader, MD**
Staff Surgeon
Children's Orthopaedics of Atlanta
Medical Director, Hip Program
Children's Healthcare of Atlanta
Atlanta, Georgia

**Richard M. Schwend, MD**
Professor of Orthopaedics and Pediatrics
Department of Orthopaedics
University of Missouri School of Medicine
Columbia, Missouri
Director of Orthopaedic Research
Division of Orthopaedics
Children's Mercy Hospital
Kansas City, Missouri

**Noah Archibald-Seiffer, BS**
Clinical Research Associate
Department of Orthopedic Surgery
St. Luke's Regional Medical Center
Boise, Idaho

**Apurva S. Shah, MD**
Assistant Professor
Department of Orthopaedics and Rehabilitation
University of Iowa
University of Iowa Hospitals & Clinics
Iowa City, Iowa

**Suken A. Shah, MD**
Associate Professor
Department of Orthopaedic Surgery and Pediatrics
Jefferson Medical College of Thomas Jefferson University
Philadelphia, Pennsylvania
Division Chief, Spine and Scoliosis Center
Department of Orthopaedics
Nemours/Alfred I. duPont Hospital for Children
Wilmington, Delaware

**Kevin G. Shea, MD**
University of Utah
Adjunct Associate Clinical Faculty
Department of Orthopaedics
Salt Lake City, Utah
Department of Orthopedics
St. Lukes Health System
Boise, Idaho

**Ernest L. Sink, MD**
Associate Professor
Department of Orthopedic Surgery
Hospital for Special Surgery
New York, New York

**David L. Skaggs, MD**
Professor
Department of Orthopaedic Surgery
Keck School of Medicine of the University of Southern California
Chief of Orthopaedic Surgery
Department of Orthopaedic Surgery
Children's Hospital Los Angeles
Los Angeles, California

**Nathan W. Skelley, MD**
Resident Physician
Department of Orthopaedic Surgery
Washington University School of Medicine
Barnes-Jewish Hospital
St. Louis, Missouri

**Brian G. Smith, MD**
Professor
Department of Orthopedics
Yale University
Director
Pediatric Orthopedics
Yale-New Haven Children's Hospital
New Haven, Connecticut

**June C. Smith, MPH**
Research Coordinator
Department of Orthopedics
Washington University Orthopedics
St. Louis, Missouri

**Brian Snyder, MD**
Associate Professor
Department of Orthopaedic Surgery
Harvard Medical School
Attending Orthopedic Surgery
Department of Orthopedic Surgery
Boston Children's Hospital
Boston, Massachusetts

**David A. Spiegel, MD**
Associate Professor of Orthopaedic Surgery
Department of Orthopaedic Surgery
Perelman School of Medicine at the University of Pennsylvania
Pediatric Orthopedic Surgeon
Division of Orthopedics
The Children's Hospital of Philadelphia
Philadelphia, Pennsylvania

**Andrea M. Spiker, MD**
Department of Orthopaedics
Johns Hopkins University
Baltimore, Maryland

**Paul D. Sponseller, MD, MBA**
Professor and Head, Pediatric Orthopaedics
Johns Hopkins Children's Center
Baltimore, Maryland

**Anthony A. Stans, MD**
Assistant Professor
Department of Orthopedic Surgery
Mayo Clinic
Rochester, Minnesota

**Sarah R. Steward, MD**
Fellow
Department of Orthopaedics
Cincinnati Children's Hospital Medical Center
Cincinnati, Ohio

**Philipp N. Streubel, MD**
Assistant Professor
Hand and Upper Extremity Surgery
Shoulder and Elbow Surgery
Department of Orthopaedic Surgery and Rehabilitation
University of Nebraska College of Medicine
Omaha, Nebraska

**Daniel J. Sucato, MD, MS**
Professor
Department of Orthopaedic Surgery
UT Southwestern Medical Center
Chief of Staff
Department of Orthopedic
Texas Scottish Rite Hospital for Children
Dallas, Texas

**Stephen Torres, MD**
Resident
Department of Orthopaedics
Perelman School of Medicine at the University of Pennsylvania
Philadelphia, Pennsylvania

**Vidyadhar V. Upasani, MD**
Assistant Clinical Professor
Department of Orthopedic Surgery
UC San Diego School of Medicine
Rady Children's Hospital—San Diego
San Diego, California

**Ann E. Van Heest, MD**
Professor
Department of Orthopaedic Surgery
University of Minnesota Medical Center
Active Staff
Department of Orthopaedic Surgery
Shriners Hospitals for Children—Twin Cities
University of Minnesota Fairview
Minneapolis, Minnesota
Active Staff
Department of Orthopaedic Surgery
Gillette Children's Specialty Hospital
St. Paul, Minnesota

**Carley Vuillermin, MBSS, FRACS**
Orthopedic Surgery Department
Boston Children's Hospital
Boston, Massachusetts

**Thanapong Waitayawinyu, MD**
Associate Professor
Nonthavej Hospital
Nonthaburi, Thailand

**Eric J. Wall, MD**
Professor
Department of Orthopaedic Surgery
University of Cincinnati College of Medicine
Director, Orthopaedic Sports Medicine
Pediatric Orthopaedic Surgery
Cincinnati Children's Hospital Medical Center
Cincinnati, Ohio

**W. Timothy Ward, MD**
Professor
Department of Orthopaedics
University of Pittsburgh
Chief
Department of Pediatric Orthopaedics
Children's Hospital of Pittsburgh of UPMC
Pittsburgh, Pennsylvania

**Peter M. Waters, MD**
John E. Hall Professor
Department of Orthopaedic Surgery
Harvard Medical School
Surgeon-in-Chief
Department of Orthopedic Surgery
Boston Children's Hospital
Boston, Massachusetts

**J. Tracy Watson, MD**
Professor and Chief
Orthopaedic Trauma Service
Department of Orthopaedic Surgery
St. Louis University School of Medicine
St. Louis, Missouri

**John H. Wedge, OC, MD, FRCSC**
Professor
Department of Surgery
University of Toronto
Orthopaedic Surgeon
Department of Surgery
The Hospital for Sick Children
Toronto, Ontario, Canada

**Bradley K. Weiner, MD**
Professor
Vice Chairman and Chief of Spinal Surgery
Department of Orthopaedic Surgery
Houston Methodist Hospital
Houston, Texas

**Amanda L. Weller, MD**
Sports Medicine Fellow
Department of Orthopaedic Surgery
University of Pittsburgh
Pittsburgh, Pennsylvania

**Dennis R. Wenger, MD**
Clinical Professor
Department of Orthopedic Surgery
UC San Diego School Of Medicine
Director, Orthopedic Training Program
Department of Orthopedics
Rady Children's Hospital—San Diego
San Diego, California

**Roger F. Widmann, MD**
Chief of Pediatric Orthopedic Surgery
Hospital for Special Surgery
Professor of Clinical Orthopaedic Surgery
Weill Cornell Medical College
New York, New York

**Carl H. Wierks, MD**
Private Practice
Holland, Michigan

**Jocelyn R. Wittstein, MD**
Director of Research
Bassett Shoulder & Sports Medicine Research Institute
Attending Surgeon
Bassett Healthcare Network
Oneonta, New York

**Daniel P. Woods, MD**
Orthopedic Sports Medicine Fellow
Rothman Institute
Thomas Jefferson University Hospital
Philadelphia, Pennsylvania

**Robert W. Wysocki, MD**
Assistant Professor
Department of Orthopedic Surgery
Rush University Medical Center
Chicago, Illinois

**Yi-Meng Yen, MD, PhD**
Assistant Professor
Department of Orthopaedic Surgery
Harvard Medical School
Boston Children's Hospital
Boston, Massachusetts

**Lukas P. Zebala, MD**
Assistant Professor of Medicine
Department of Orthopaedic Surgery
Washington University School of Medicine in St. Louis
St. Louis, Missouri

# Preface

The purpose of the second edition of *Operative Techniques in Orthopaedic Surgery* remains the same as the first: to describe in a detailed, step-by-step manner the technical parts of "how to do" the majority of orthopaedic procedures.

It is assumed that the surgeon understands the "why" and the "when," although this information is covered in outline form at the beginning of each procedure.

Each of the nine major sections has been carefully reviewed and updated in both its content and artwork. The second edition has given each section editor the ability to include additional procedures and has also placed more emphasis in creating online content which is easily accessible and fully searchable.

The section editors and chapter authors have done an excellent job. Each has specific expertise and experience in their area and has given their time and effort most generously. It has again been stimulating to interact with these wonderful and talented people, and I am honored to have been able to play a part in this rewarding experience.

I also would like to thank all of the people at Wolters Kluwer. Dave Murphy has been especially helpful and had a great deal of input into this edition, as with the first edition. I would like, as well, to acknowledge Bob Hurley, who was a driving force for the first edition and has been a great resource for this second one as well.

Finally, special thanks goes to Brian Brown, the new acquisitions editor. It has been a wonderful experience to work with Brian who has done an excellent job of bringing this text to completion.

Sam W. Wiesel, MD
Washington, DC
January 2, 2015

# Preface
## *to the First Edition*

When a surgeon contemplates performing a procedure, there are three major questions to consider: Why is the surgery being done? When in the course of a disease process should it be performed? And, finally, what are the technical steps involved? The purpose of this text is to describe in a detailed, step-by-step manner the "how to do it" of the vast majority of orthopaedic procedures. The "why" and "when" are covered in outline form at the beginning of each procedure. However, it is assumed that the surgeon understands the basics of "why" and "when," and has made the definitive decision to undertake a specific case. This text is designed to review and make clear the detailed steps of the anticipated operation.

*Operative Techniques in Pediatric Orthopaedic Surgery* differs from other books because it is mainly visual. Each procedure is described in a systematic way that makes liberal use of focused, original artwork. It is hoped that the surgeon will be able to visualize each significant step of a procedure as it unfolds during a case.

Each chapter has been edited by a specialist who has specific expertise and experience in the discipline. It has taken a tremendous amount of work for each editor to enlist talented authors for each procedure and then review the final work. It has been very stimulating to work with all of these wonderful and talented people, and I am honored to have taken part in this rewarding experience.

Finally, I would like to thank everyone who has contributed to the development of this book. Specifically, Grace Caputo at Dovetail Content Solutions, and Dave Murphy and Eileen Wolfberg at Lippincott Williams & Wilkins, who have been very helpful and generous with their input. Special thanks, as well, goes to Bob Hurley at LWW, who has adeptly guided this textbook from original concept to publication.

SWW
January 1, 2010

*Trauma*

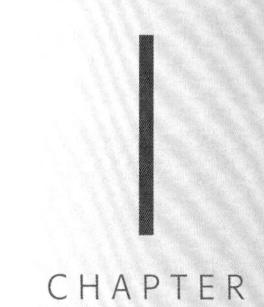


# Volar Plating of Distal Radius Fractures

John J. Fernandez and Philipp N. Streubel

## DEFINITION

- Distal radius fractures are defined by their involvement of the metaphysis of the distal radius.
- They are assessed on the basis of fracture pattern, alignment, and stability:
  - Articular versus nonarticular
  - Reducible versus irreducible
  - Stable versus unstable
- Irreducible or unstable fractures require surgical reduction and stable fixation.
- Volar plating historically has been the method of choice for volar shear-type fractures.
  - Fixed-angle plates have become the preferred method of fixation for most types of distal radius fractures.

## ANATOMY

- The distal radius serves as a buttress for the proximal carpus, transmitting 75% to 80% of its forces into the forearm.
  - The remaining 20% to 25% of force is transmitted through the distal ulna and the triangular fibrocartilage complex (TFCC).
- Thickness of distal radius articular cartilage is 1 mm or less.[16]
- Dorsally
  - The distal radius is the origin for the dorsal radiocarpal ligament.
  - It is the floor of the fibro-osseous extensor tendon compartments and includes Lister tubercle, assisting in extensor pollicis longus function (**FIG 1A**).
  - The extensor tendons are in immediate contact with the dorsal surface of the distal radius.
- Volarly
  - The distal radius is the origin for volar extrinsic ligaments of the wrist, including the radioscaphocapitate ligament and long and short radiolunate ligaments.
  - It also is the origin of the pronator quadratus.
  - The flexor tendons are separated from the distal radius by the pronator quadratus.
- Ulnarly
  - The distal radius is the origin for the triangular fibrocartilage (see **FIG 1A**).
  - It also contains the sigmoid notch, which articulates with the head of the distal ulna, allowing forearm rotation.
- Distally
  - The surface is divided into a triangular scaphoid fossa and a square lunate fossa articulating with each respective carpal bone (**FIG 1B**).
- The distal articular surface is inclined approximately 22 degrees ulnarly in the coronal plane and 11 degrees volarly in the sagittal plane (**FIG 1C,D**).
- The metaphysis is defined by the distal radius within a length of the articular surface that is equivalent to the widest portion of the entire wrist.
- The dorsal cortical bone is less substantial than the volar cortical bone, contributing to the characteristic dorsal bending fracture pattern of distal radius fractures.

## PATHOGENESIS

- The mechanism of injury in a distal radius fracture is an axial force across the wrist, with the pattern of injury determined by bone density, the position of the wrist, and the magnitude and direction of force.
- Most distal radius fractures result from falls with the wrist extended and pronated, which places a dorsal bending moment across the distal radius.
  - Relatively weaker, thinner dorsal bone collapses under compression, whereas stronger volar bone fails under tension, resulting in a characteristic "triangle" of bone comminution with the apex volar and greater comminution dorsal.
- Other possible mechanisms form a basis for some fracture classifications such as the one proposed by Jupiter and Fernandez.[6]
  - Bending
  - Axial compression
  - Shear
  - Avulsion
  - Combinations
- Articular involvement and its severity are the basis of some fracture classifications, such as the AO Orthopaedic Trauma Association (AO/OTA)[10] and Melone[12] classifications.
- Articular involvement splits the distal radius into distinct fragments separate from the radius shaft (**FIG 2**):
  - Scaphoid fossa fragment
  - Lunate fossa fragment. With comminution of this fragment may be separated into two impacted articular fragments, involving the dorsal ulnar corner and the volar rim.[11]

## NATURAL HISTORY

- Clinical outcome usually, but not always, correlates with deformity.
  - Variable residual deformity can be tolerated best by individuals with fewer functional demands.
- As wrist deformity increases, physiologic function is progressively altered.
  - Intra-articular displacement of 1 to 2 mm results in an increased risk of osteoarthritis.[3,7]
  - Radial shortening of 3 to 5 mm or more results in increased loading of the ulnar complex.[1,15]

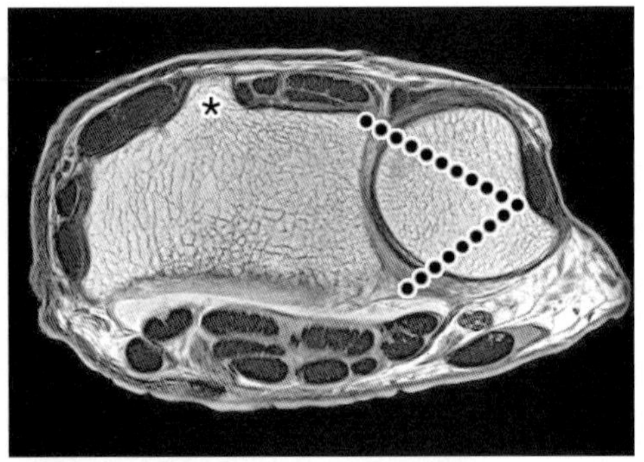
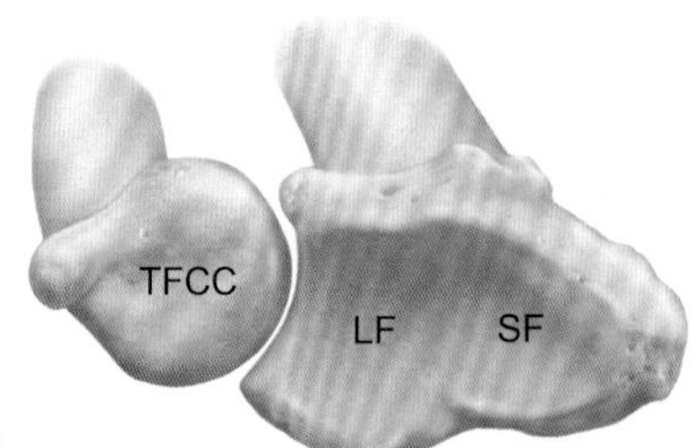

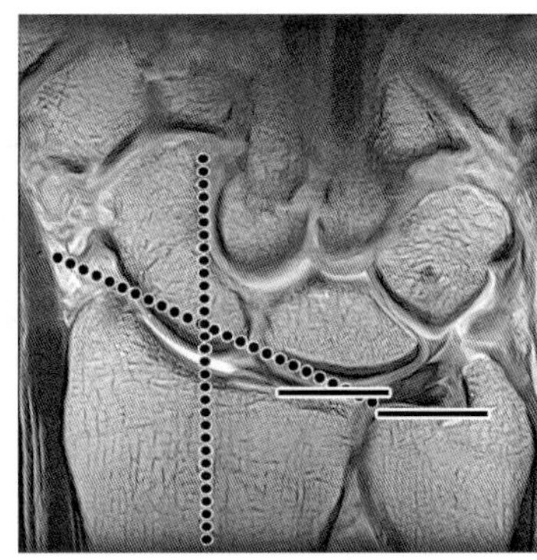
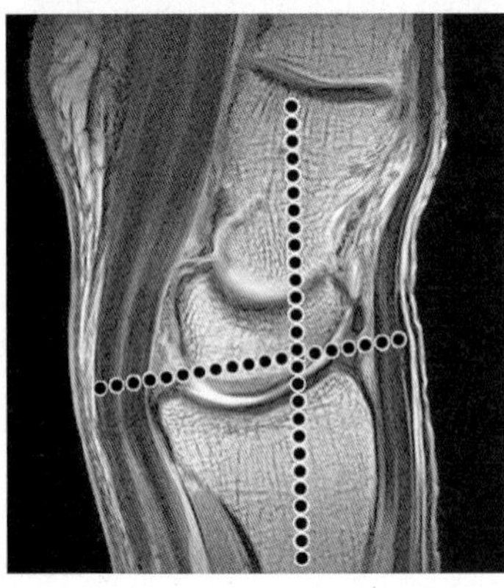

**FIG 1** • **A.** Axial magnetic resonance (MR) image of the wrist at the level of the distal radius. Lister tubercle is marked with an *asterisk*. *Dotted lines* represent dorsal and volar borders of the triangular fibrocartilage that helps stabilize the distal radioulnar joint. The dorsal distal radius acts as an attachment for dorsal extensor compartment sheaths. **B.** The distal articular surface of the radius is divided into a triangularly shaped scaphoid fossa (*SF*) and a square-shaped lunate fossa (*LF*). The distal ulna and the *TFCC* act as ulnar buttresses for the wrist. **C.** MR coronal cut of the distal radius. The articular surface of the distal radius is inclined about 22 degrees relative to the forearm axis (*dotted lines*). The ulnar aspect of the distal radius (ie, the lunate fossa) usually is distal to the end of the distal ulna (ie, negative ulnar variance). Note the *solid lines* marking ulnar variance. **D.** MR sagittal cut of the distal radius. The articular surface of the distal radius is inclined approximately 11-degree palmar relative to the forearm axis (*dotted lines*). Proximally, there exists relatively thinner dorsal cortical bone versus the thicker volar bone.

- Dorsal angulation greater than 10 degrees shifts contact forces to the dorsal scaphoid fossa and the ulnar complex, causing increased disability.[17,20]
- The incidence of associated intracarpal injuries increases with fracture severity. Such injuries can account for poor outcomes. These injuries often are not recognized at first, leading to delayed treatment.[4,18]
  - TFCC tears
  - Scapholunate and lunotriquetral ligament tears
  - Chondral injuries involving the carpal surfaces
  - Distal radioulnar joint injury
  - Distal ulnar fractures

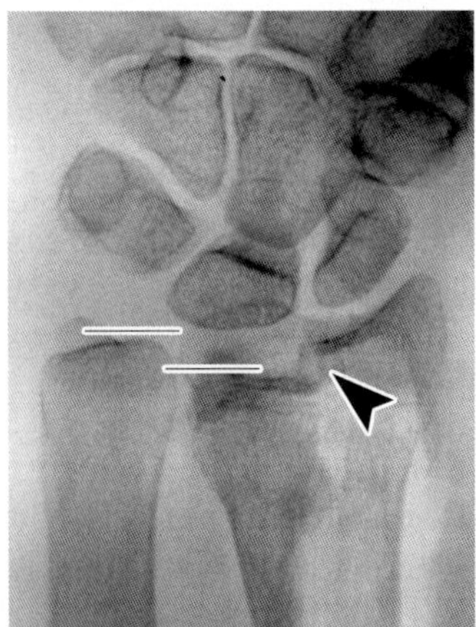

**FIG 2** • The *arrowhead* points to the articular split. Articular displacement of the scaphoid fossa fragment radially and the lunate fossa fragment ulnarly is apparent, as is significant shortening (ulnar positive variance) as outlined by the *lines*.

- By predicting the stability of a distal radius fracture, deformity and its complications can be minimized. Several risk factors have been suggested by LaFontaine et al[8] and others. The presence of three or more indicates instability:
  - Dorsal (or volar apex) angulation greater than 20 degrees
  - Dorsal comminution
  - Intra-articular extension
  - Associated ulnar fracture
  - Patient age older than 60 years

## PATIENT HISTORY AND PHYSICAL FINDINGS

- The mechanism of injury should be sought to assist in assessing the energy and level of trauma.
- Associated injuries are not uncommon and should be carefully ruled out.
  - Injuries to the hand, carpus, and proximal arm, including other fractures or dislocations
  - Injuries to other extremities or the head, neck, and torso
- Establish the patient's functional and occupational demands.
- Document coexisting medical conditions that may affect healing such as smoking or diabetes.
- Determine possible risk factors for anesthesia and surgery, such as cardiac disease.
- The physical examination should document the following:
  - Condition of surrounding soft tissues (ie, skin and subcutaneous tissues)
  - Quality of vascular perfusion and pulses
  - Integrity of nerve function
  - Sensory two-point discrimination or threshold sensory testing
  - Motor function of intrinsic muscles, including thenar and hypothenar muscles, of the hand

- Examination of the distal ulna, TFCC, and distal radioulnar joint should rule out disruption and instability.
- Reliable physical examination of the carpus often is difficult, making radiographic review even more critical and follow-up examinations important.

## IMAGING AND OTHER DIAGNOSTIC STUDIES

- Imaging establishes fracture severity, helps determine stability, and guides the operative approach and choice of fixation.
- Plain radiographs should be obtained before and after reduction: posteroanterior (PA) (with the forearm in neutral rotation), lateral, and two separate oblique views.
  - Oblique views, in particular, help evaluate articular involvement, particularly the lunate fossa fragment (**FIG 3A,B**).
  - The lateral view should be modified with the forearm inclined 15 to 20 degrees to best visualize the articular surface (**FIG 3C**; see **TECH FIG 5B,C**).
- Fluoroscopic evaluation can be useful because it gives a complete circumferential view of the wrist and, with traction applied, can help evaluate injuries of the carpus.
- Computed tomography (CT) helps define intra-articular involvement and helps detect small or impacted fragments, which may not be apparent on plain radiographs, particularly those involving the central portion of the distal radius (**FIG 3D,E**).

## DIFFERENTIAL DIAGNOSIS

- Diagnosis is directly confirmed by radiographs.
- Associated and contributory injuries should always be considered.
  - Pathologic fracture (eg, related to tumor, infection)
  - Associated injuries to the carpus (eg, scaphoid fracture, scapholunate ligament injury)

## NONOPERATIVE MANAGEMENT

- Nonoperative treatment is reserved for distal radius fractures that are reducible and stable based on the criteria previously discussed.
- The goal of nonoperative treatment is to immobilize the wrist while maintaining acceptable alignment until the fracture is healed.

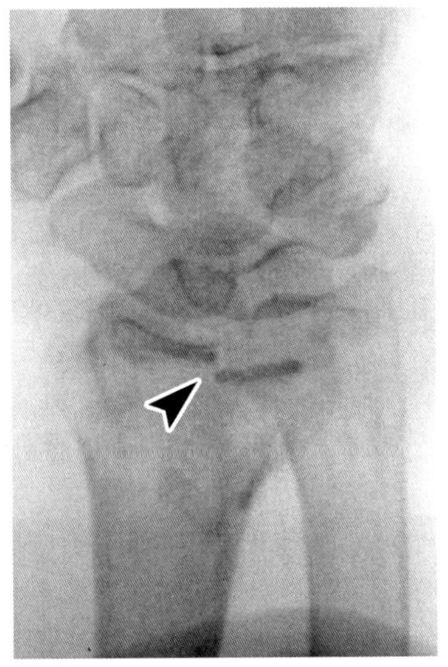
A

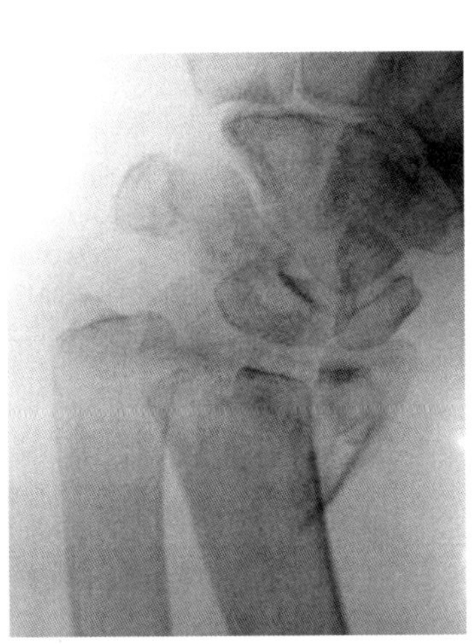
B

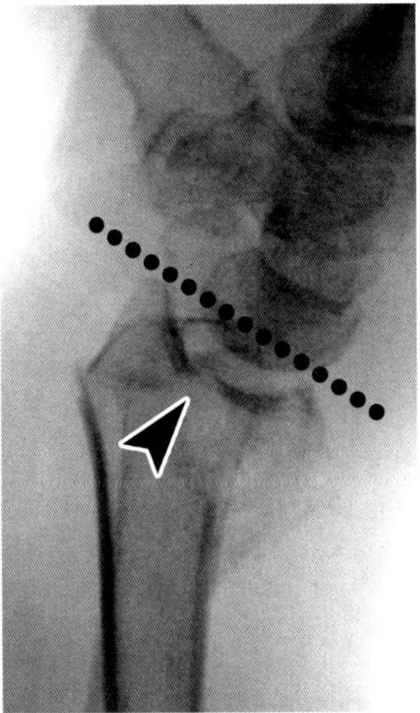
C

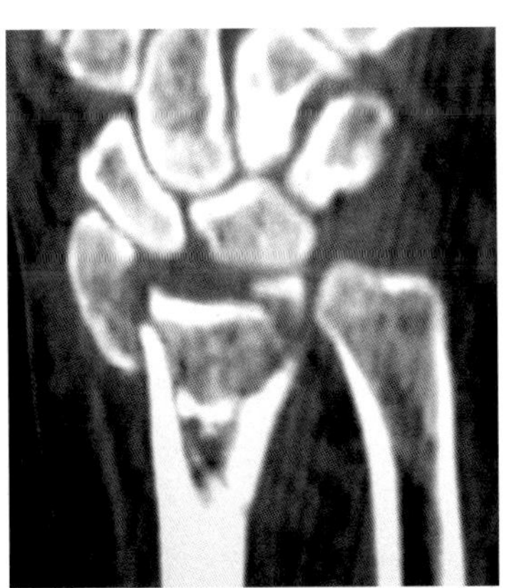
D

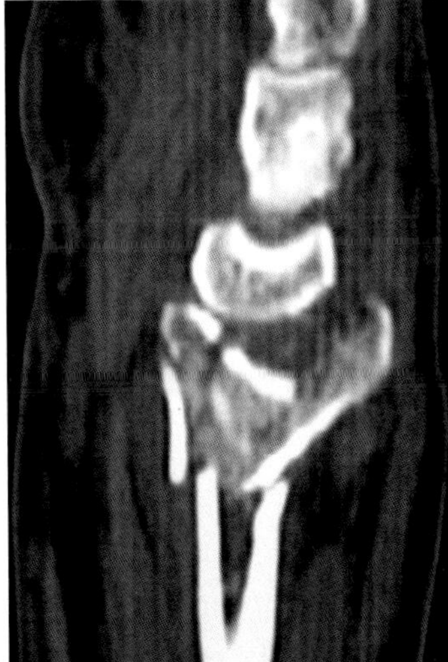
E

**FIG 3** • **A.** This pronated view accentuates the dorsal articular surface irregularity (*arrowhead*) and the displaced fragment. **B.** This supinated view accentuates the displaced radial styloid fragment. **C.** On this lateral radiograph, the *arrowhead* points to the articular split and the displacement of the lunate fossa fragment. Note the dorsal angulation and collapse (*dotted line*). Observe the significantly thicker volar cortical bone in comparison to the dorsal bone. **D,E.** AP and lateral cuts taken from CT images of a distal radius fracture revealing the extent of comminution and central impaction, which are not easily appreciated on plain radiographs.

- Goals for treatment[9]
  - Radial inclination greater than 10 degrees
  - Ulnar variance less than 3-mm positive
  - Palmar tilt less than 10 degrees dorsal or 20 degrees volar
  - Articular congruity with less than a 2-mm gap or step-off
- Patients are immobilized in a short-arm cast for 6 weeks. Radiographic follow-up is performed on a weekly basis for the first 2 to 3 weeks to identify fracture displacement that may warrant reduction.

## SURGICAL MANAGEMENT

- The goal of operative treatment is to achieve acceptable alignment and stable fixation.
- Various methods of fixation are available: pins, external fixators, intramedullary devices, and plates (volar, dorsal, fragment specific).

### Preoperative Planning

- Preoperative medical and anesthesia evaluation are performed as required.
- Discontinue blood-thinning medications (anticoagulants and nonsteroidal anti-inflammatory drugs, especially acetylsalicylic acid).
- Request necessary equipment, including fluoroscopic and power equipment.
- Confirm the plate fixation system to be used, and check the equipment before beginning surgery for completeness (ie, all appropriate drills, plates, and screws).
- Have a contingency plan or additional fixation (external fixator, bone graft, or bone graft substitute).
- Review and have previous radiographic studies available.
- Consider use of a regional anesthetic for postoperative pain control.

### Positioning

- Place the patient in the supine position with the affected extremity on an arm table.
- Apply an upper arm tourniquet, preferably within the sterile field.
- Incorporate weights or a traction system to apply distraction across the fracture (**FIG 4**).
- The surgeon is seated so that the elbow is pointing toward the patient's torso and the dominant hand works toward the fingers of the patients.
- The assistant is seated opposite the surgeon.
- The fluoroscopy unit is brought in from the end or corner of the table.

### Approach

- Dorsal exposure allows for direct visualization of the articular surface when necessary.

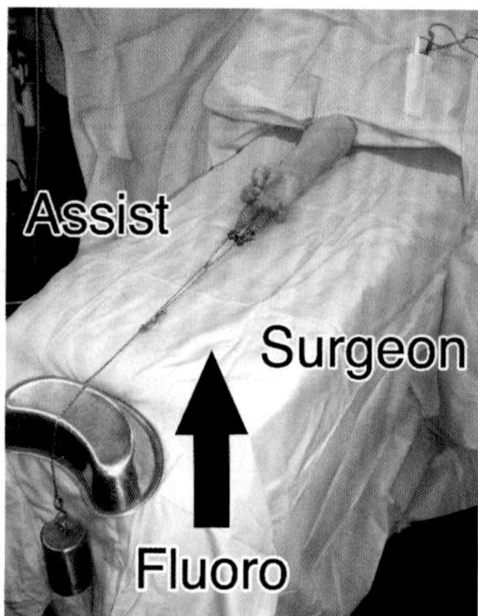


**FIG 4** • Traction is applied over the arm table with finger traps and hanging weights. The surgeon sits on the volar side and the assistant on the dorsal side. Fluoroscopy can be brought in from any direction but preferably from the side adjacent or the opposite surgeon.

- Fracture comminution is more severe dorsally, making overall alignment more difficult to judge.
- The thicker volar cortex is less comminuted, allowing for more precise reduction and buttressing of bone fragments.
- Sometimes, both dorsal and volar exposures may be necessary to achieve articular congruency and volar reduction and fixation, respectively.
- An extended volar ulnar exposure may be necessary to manage isolated volar fractures of the lunate facet or to perform a simultaneous carpal tunnel release if indicated.
- The techniques described in this chapter use the volar approach to distal radius, as described by Henry (**FIG 5**).

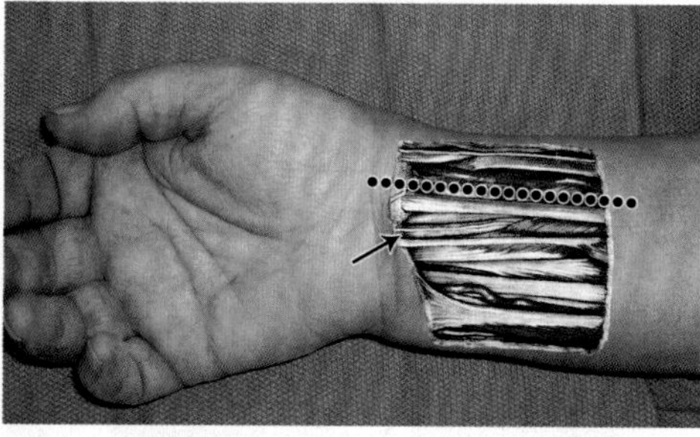

**FIG 5** • The volar incision is represented by the *dotted line* just proximal to the wrist flexion creases and radial to the flexor carpi radialis longus. Care is exercised to avoid dissection from ulnar to the flexor carpi radialis because the palmar cutaneous nerve branch of the median nerve (*arrow*) is at risk.

## Volar Fixed-Angle Plate Fixation of the Distal Radius

### Incision and Dissection

- Make a 4- to 8-cm longitudinal incision from the proximal wrist flexion crease proximally, along the radial border of the flexor carpi radialis tendon.
  - Use a zigzag incision to cross the wrist flexion creases if required.
- Carefully avoid the palmar cutaneous branch of the median nerve which arises within 10 cm of the wrist flexion crease and travels along the ulnar side of the flexor carpi radialis tendon.
  - Branches of the dorsal radial sensory nerve and lateral antebrachial cutaneous nerve may appear along the path of the incision and also need to be protected.
- At the distal end of the incision, protect the palmar branch of the radial artery to the deep palmar arch.
  - It usually is not necessary to dissect out the radial artery (**TECH FIG 1A**).
- Incise the anterior sheath of the flexor carpi radialis tendon and retract the tendon ulnarly to help protect the median nerve (**TECH FIG 1B**).
- Incise the posterior sheath of the flexor carpi radialis tendon.
  - The deep tissues likely will bulge out from the pressure of swelling and fracture hematoma.
  - The median nerve is at risk lying within the subcutaneous tissues along the ulnar portion of the wound (**TECH FIG 1C,D**).
  - The flexor pollicis longus tendon sits along the radial margin of the wound.
- Using blunt dissection with a gauze-covered finger, sweep the tendons and the nerve ulnarly.
  - A self-retaining retractor is carefully placed just deep to the radial artery radially and the tendons and median nerve ulnarly.
  - The pronator quadratus is now visualized on the floor of the wound.
- Incise the pronator quadratus at its radial insertion, leaving fascial tissue on either side to aid in closure. Also, determine the proximal and distal extent of the muscle, and make horizontal incisions at both of those points (**TECH FIG 1E**).
  - The distal margin of the pronator quadratus attaches along the distal volar lip of the distal radius, along the "teardrop" and the watershed line.
  - The radial margin is in proximity to the tendons of the first dorsal compartment and the brachioradialis.

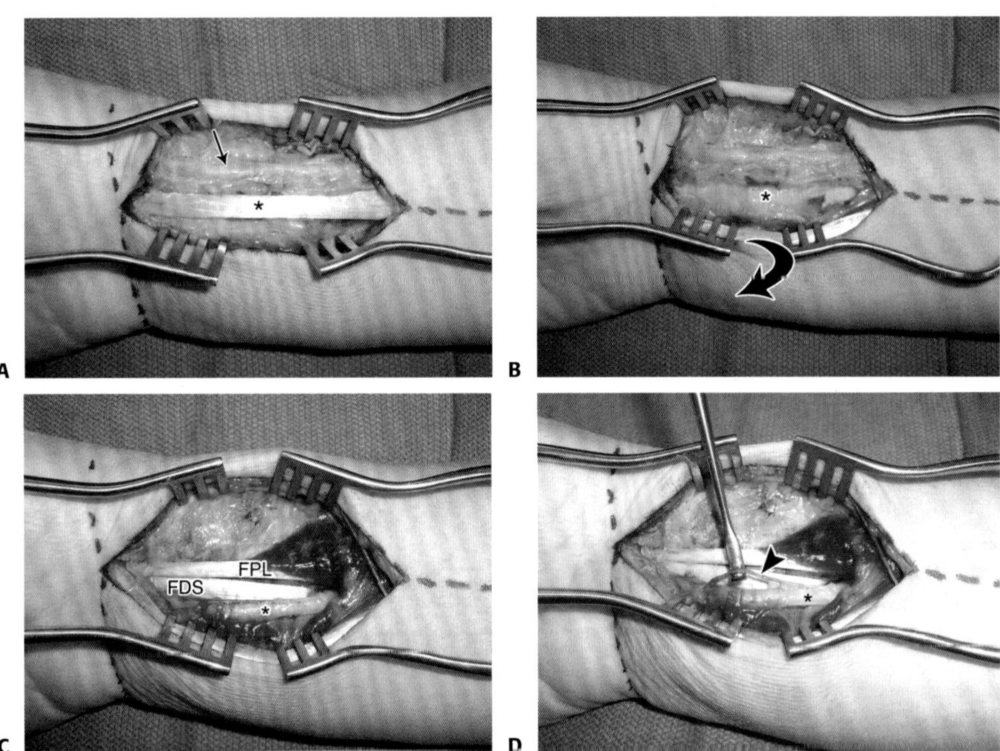


**TECH FIG 1** • **A.** The interval between the radial artery (*arrow*) and the flexor carpi radialis tendon (*asterisk*) is seen. **B.** The posterior sheath (*asterisk*) of the flexor carpi radialis is visible after retracting the flexor carpi radialis ulnarly (*arrow*). Be careful during deeper dissection because swelling and hematoma may distort the position of the median nerve beneath the sheath. **C.** Following incision in the flexor carpi radialis posterior sheath, the deep tendons are visible, including the flexor pollicis longus (*FPL*) and the flexor digitorum superficialis (*FDS*) of the index finger. The median nerve also is visible (*asterisk*). **D.** The palmar cutaneous nerve branches of the median nerve (*arrowhead*) and median nerve (*asterisk*) are both at risk for injury during this approach. Be careful regarding placement of retractors and during dissection and plate placement. *(continued)*

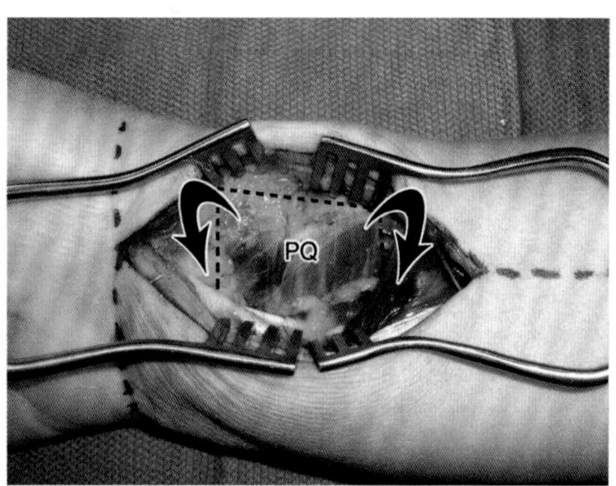


E

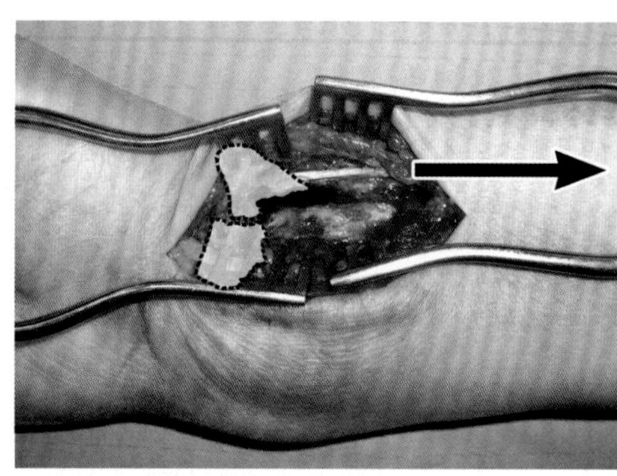

F

**TECH FIG 1** • *(continued)* **E.** The pronator quadratus (*PQ*) is incised distally, radially, and proximally and then reflected ulnarly after dissection off the volar distal radius. **F.** The brachioradialis (*arrow*) can be a deforming force, especially in comminuted fractures and in those for which treatment has been delayed. This tendon can be released if necessary.

- Subperiosteally, dissect the pronator quadratus off the volar surface of the distal radius as an ulnarly based flap with a knife or elevator.
- Retract the pronator ulnarly with the flexor tendons and median nerve.
- Particularly, if significant shortening of radial-sided fracture fragments has occurred, incise the broad insertion of the brachioradialis to eliminate the deforming force (**TECH FIG 1F**).
  - Release the first dorsal compartment and retract the tendons before releasing the brachioradialis.
  - Alternatively, Z-lengthen the brachioradialis tendon to allow for repair at the completion of the case.

## Fracture Reduction and Provisional Fixation

- Apply a lobster claw clamp around the radius shaft at a perpendicular angle to the volar surface at the most proximal portion of the wound (**TECH FIG 2A**).
  - This allows for excellent control of the proximal shaft for rotation and translation, providing an excellent counterforce when correcting the dorsal angulation collapse.
  - It also aids in soft tissue retraction.
- With the fracture now exposed, apply traction distally to distract and disimpact the fragments.
- Carefully clean the fracture of any interposed muscle, fascia, hematoma, or callus while maintaining the bony contours.
- In the case of significant volar comminution, reduce and provisionally stabilize the fragments with K-wires.
  - Take plate positioning into account when placing these K-wires.
- The articular surface is first reduced, if necessary.
- Under fluoroscopic guidance, manipulate the articular fragments through the fracture with a periosteal elevator, osteotome, or K-wires (**TECH FIG 2B,C**).
  - Longitudinal traction is important during this reduction phase. It can be performed by an assistant or using cross-table weights and finger traps.
  - A dorsal exposure is performed at this stage if there is significant articular impaction, particularly centrally, that cannot be corrected using the extra-articular technique described here.
- Place K-wires from the radial styloid fragment into the lunate fossa fragment to maintain the articular reduction (**TECH FIG 2D**).
  - The K-wires should be placed as close as possible to subchondral bone (**TECH FIG 2E,F**).
- Once the distal articular reduction is complete, reduce the distal radius as a single unit to the radius shaft.
- Insert K-wires as required to maintain the provisional reduction between the distal fragments and the proximal shaft fragment.
  - If radial collapse and translation are prominent, a large K-wire can be introduced into the radial portion of the fracture. By advancing it proximally and ulnarly, it behaves like an intrafocal pin, providing a radial buttress by pushing the distal fragment ulnarly.
  - A similar technique can be applied through the dorsal fracture to assist in maintaining palmar tilt correction.

## Plate Application

- Apply a fixed-angle volar plate to the volar surface of the distal radius and shaft. Position the plate to accommodate for the unique design characteristics of the plating system as well as the location of the fracture fragments.
  - Each plating system has unique characteristics that determine its optimal placement.
  - Ideally, the plate should be placed as close to the articular margin as possible without the distal locking pegs or screws penetrating the joint.
  - If the fracture has not yet been fully reduced, this must be taken into account when placing the device.
  - Plate placement distal to the watershed line should be avoided as this increases the risk for flexor tendon rupture.
- Clamp the previously applied lobster claw to the proximal portion of the plate to keep the plate centralized on the radius shaft.
- Place provisional K-wires through the plate to maintain position (**TECH FIG 3**). Then fluoroscopically confirm proper plate position in both the distal proximal and radioulnar directions.
  - Proper alignment of the plate can be determined only using a true anteroposterior (AP) image in which the distal radioulnar joint is well visualized.
  - The K-wires allow for fine adjustment in plate position before committing to insertion of a screw.

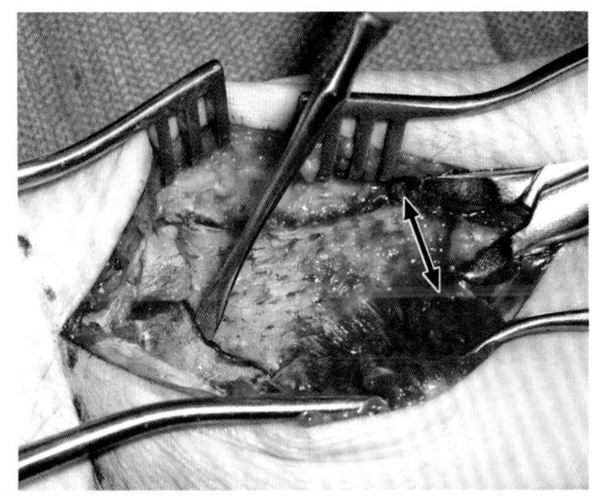

A

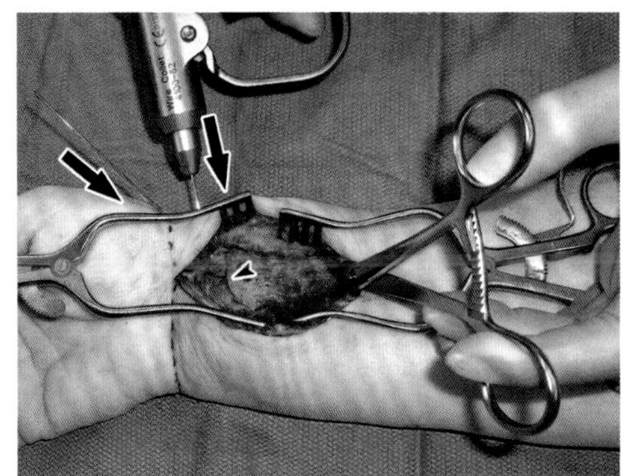

D

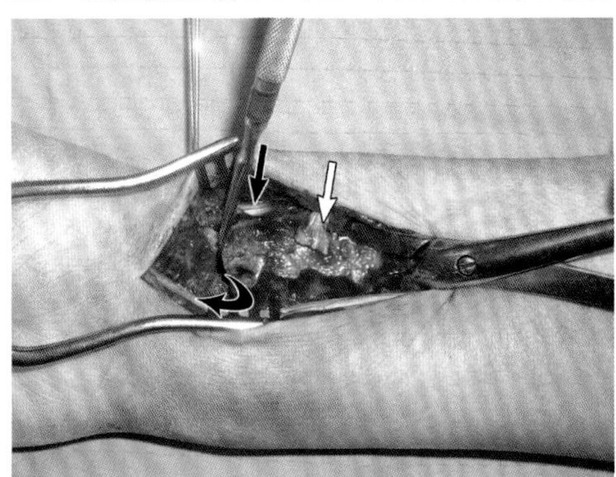

B

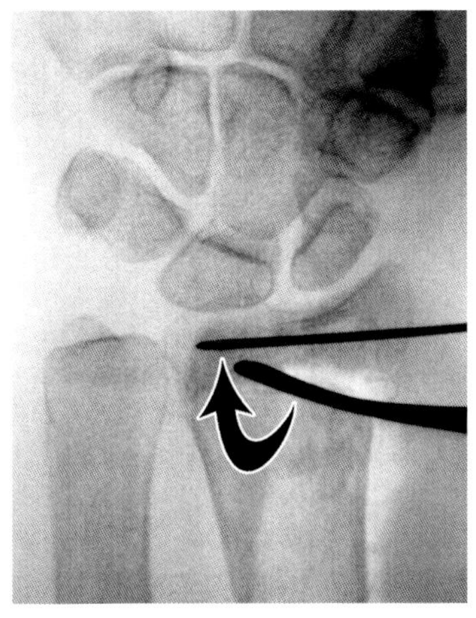

E

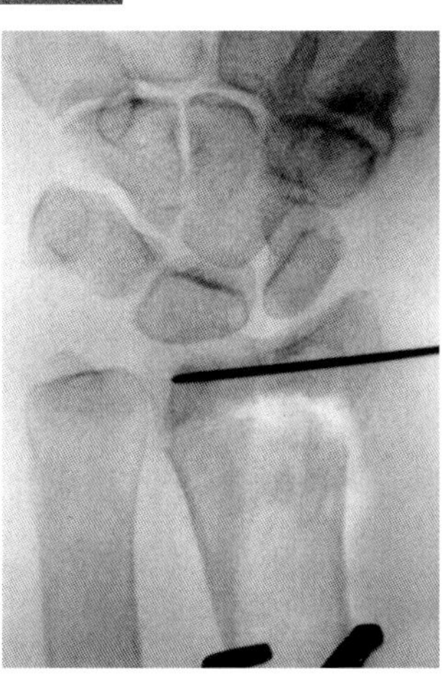

F

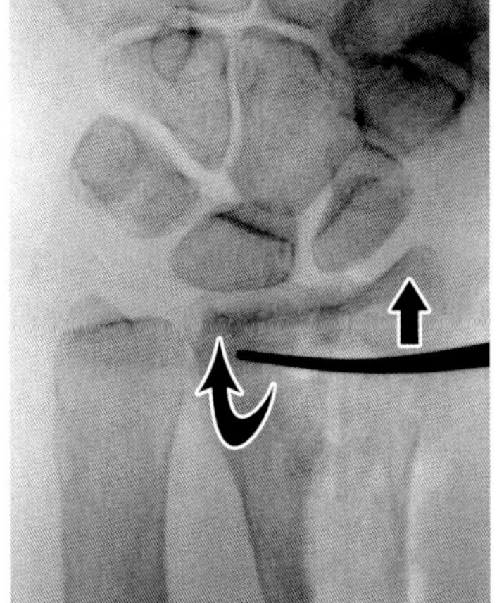

C

**TECH FIG 2** ● **A.** A lobster claw clamp (*double arrow*) is applied to the radius shaft well proximal to the fracture. This instrument helps the surgeon control the radius during reduction and define the lateral margins of the radius. A Freer elevator is inserted into the fracture to help disimpact the fragments and assist in their reduction. **B.** The brachioradialis (*white arrow*) is released, and the first compartment extensor tendons are visible in the background (*black arrow*). An instrument can now be placed to assist in the reduction (*arrow*). **C.** The Freer elevator is used to reduce the fragments. In this case, the intra-articular step-off is being corrected, and the radial length and inclination are being restored. **D.** K-wires are placed across the radial styloid into the reduced ulna fossa fragment. An assistant usually applies traction, and the lobster claw clamp can be used for powerful leverage. If there is no articular involvement, this K-wire can be placed into the radius metaphysis or diaphysis proximally. **E.** The K-wire should be placed as close as possible to the subchondral bone, avoiding areas of comminution. **F.** The K-wire should maintain the articular reduction without any support.

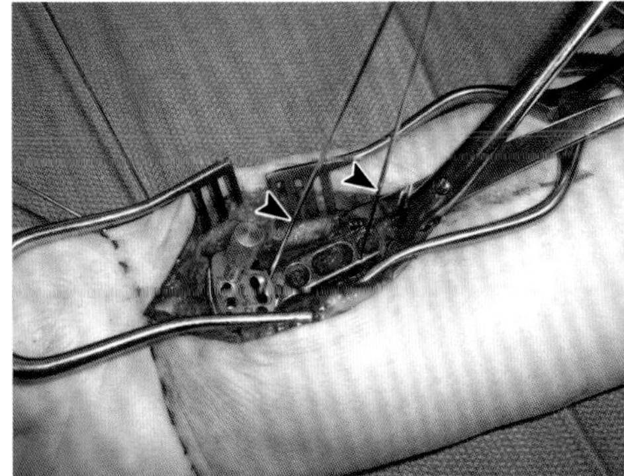

**TECH FIG 3** ● Keep the plate centered on the radius and as distal as possible. The lobster claw clamp helps keep the plate centered. K-wires (*arrowheads*) are helpful as provision fixation until alignment can be confirmed radiographically and screws placed.

- Drill and insert a provisional screw in the oblong hole in the plate.
  - If the bone is osteopenic, a screw longer than the initial measurement should be placed to ensure that both cortices are engaged. Otherwise, the plate may not be held securely, and reduction will be compromised. After the remaining screws have been secured, this screw can be replaced with one of appropriate length.
- Insert at least one additional proximal screw and remove the provisional K-wires holding the plate in place.

## Distal Fragment Reduction

- Once the plate has been secured proximally, execute any additionally needed reduction.
  - A well-designed plate serves as an excellent buttress for correction of palmar tilt (**TECH FIG 4A**).

- Apply counterforce through the lobster claw clamp in a dorsal direction while the distal hand and wrist are translated palmarly and flexed (**TECH FIG 4B**).
  - This maneuver reduces the distal radius to the plate, effectively restoring volar tilt by pushing the lunate against the volar lip of the distal radius (**TECH FIG 4C,D**).
- Additional distraction and ulnar deviation correct radial collapse and loss of radial inclination.

## Plate Fixation

- While the reduction is held, drill the holes in the distal plate segment (**TECH FIG 5A**).
  - Some plate systems allow for provisional fixation using K-wires placed through the distal plate segment.
  - Do not penetrate the dorsal distal radius with the drill, thereby avoiding injury to the dorsal extensor tendons.
- Drill and place the distal ulnar screws first and then proceed radially and proximally.
- Accurate screw placement using the same inclination of the drill is required to avoid cross-threading into the plate and lessening stability.
- Judge the placement of all distal screws or pegs precisely using fluoroscopic imaging in multiple planes.
  - In order to confirm extra-articular placement of distal screws, perform a "true" lateral view of the wrist with the x-ray beam at a 20-degree angle to the radius shaft (**TECH FIG 5B,C**). This is facilitated by lifting the wrist off the table with the elbow maintained on the table and the forearm at a 20-degree angle to the table (**TECH FIG 5D,E**).
  - The extensor pollicis longus is at greatest risk of injury from a protruding screw.
  - Because of the prominence of Lister tubercle and the triangular configuration of the distal radius, the lateral view of the wrist may not accurately rule out dorsal screw protrusion.
  - The dorsal horizon view can aid in assessing adequate screw length dorsally. It is obtained by wrist hyperflexion and aiming the beam of the image intensifier along the long axis of the radius.[5]
- Sequentially insert the remaining distal screws or pegs, followed by the remaining proximal plate screws (**TECH FIG 5F**).
- If necessary, add bone graft or bone graft substitute around the plate into the fracture site or through a small dorsal incision.
- Precisely assess the stability of the construct after the plate has been applied. If appropriate, remove the provisional K-wires.
  - If the K-wires are deemed critical for fracture stability, they can be left in place and removed 4 to 8 weeks later.
  - If residual instability exists, add additional fixation with K-wires, an external fixator, a dorsal plate, or a combination.

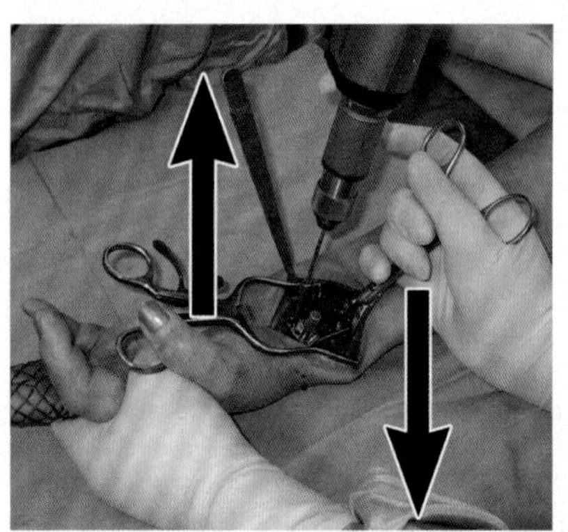
A

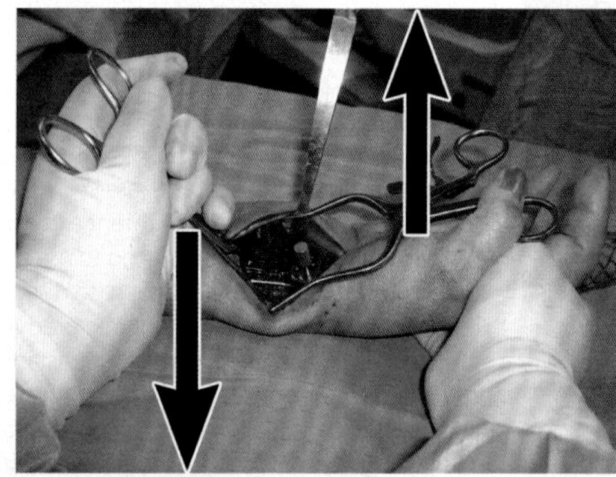
B

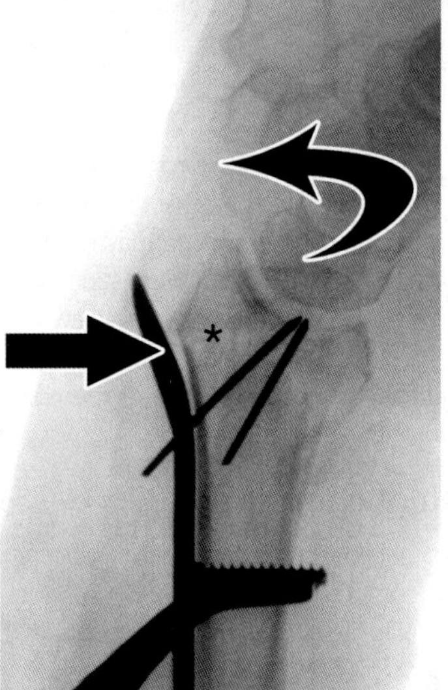

C

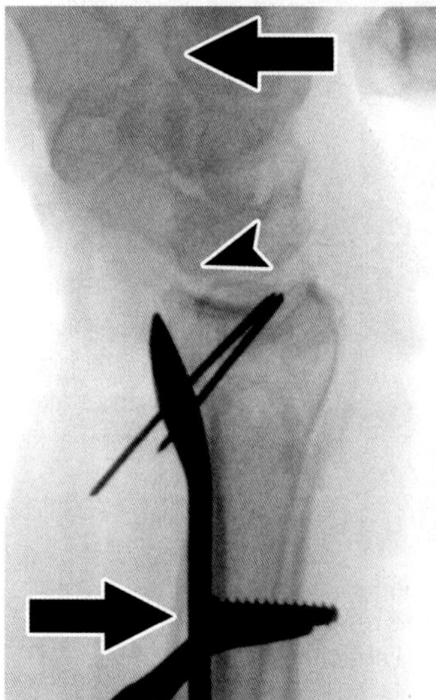
D

**TECH FIG 4** • **A.** The final reduction is performed with traction on the hand and with the radius held proximally with a clamp. Once the reduction is confirmed radiographically, the assistant places the distal screws or K-wires. **B.** The hand is translated (not appreciably flexed) palmarly while the radius shaft is held with the clamp. Prereduction (**C**) and postreduction (**D**) radiographs demonstrating the palmar translation reduction maneuver. The volar plate acts as a strong buttress (*arrows*), allowing the translated lunate to push on the volar radius (*asterisk*) and correct the dorsal angulation deformity.

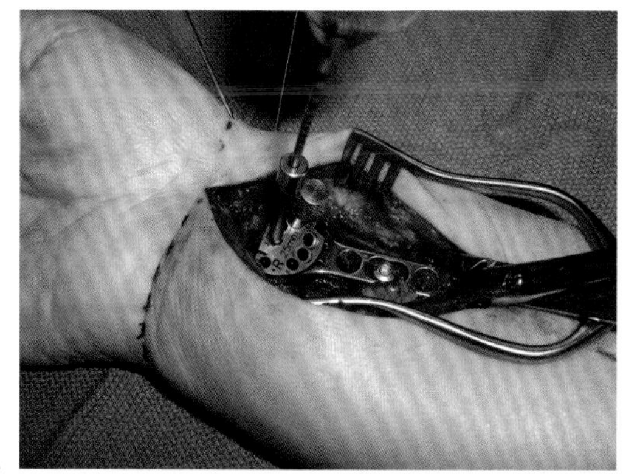
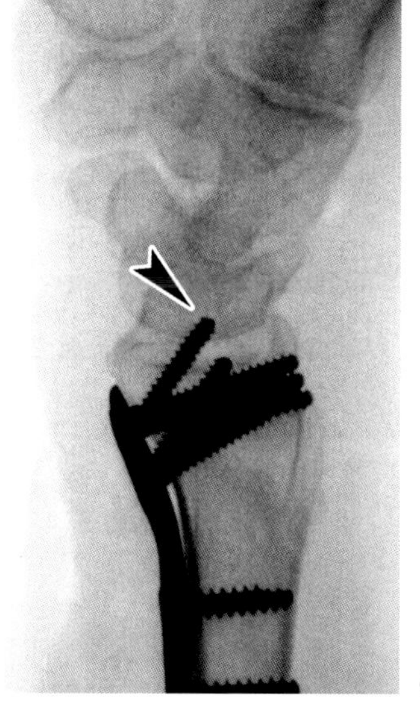
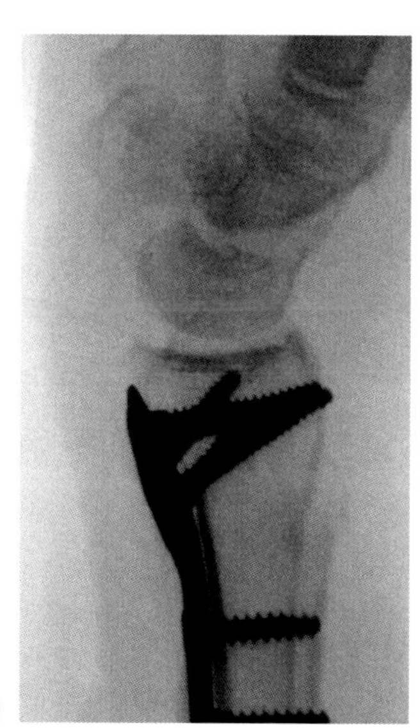
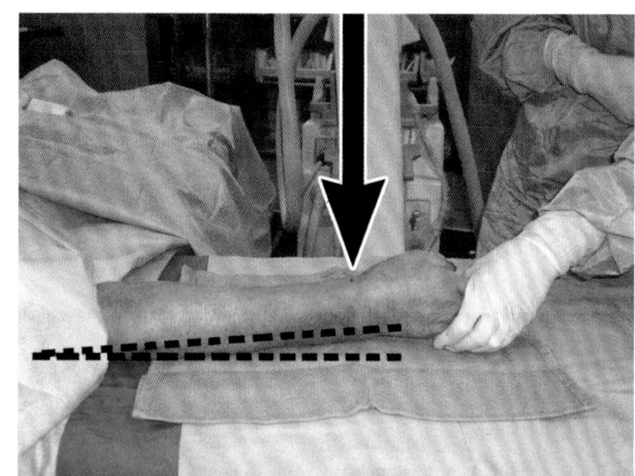
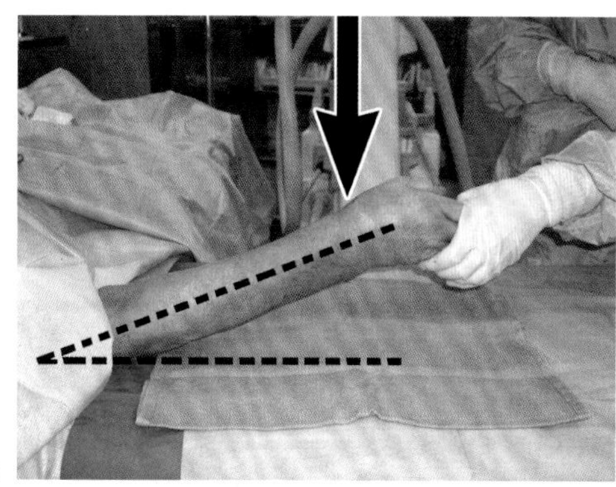
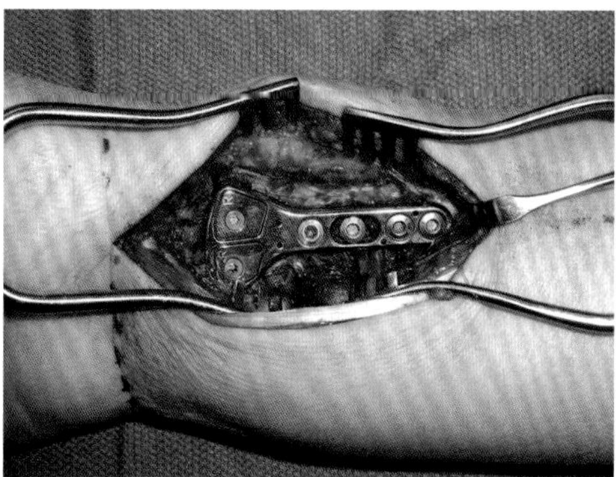

**TECH FIG 5** • **A.** The remaining holes can now be drilled and screws placed where needed. **B.** This screw (*arrowhead*) looks as though it has penetrated the joint, when in reality, it is simply the angle of the radiographic beam that throws its projection into the joint. **C.** A true lateral view of the distal radius is necessary to judge placement of the radial screws. **D.** A radiograph is being taken with the wrist perpendicular to the x-ray beam (*arrow*). This is not a true lateral image because the distal surface of the radius is inclined 20 degrees radially. **E.** By lifting the hand and wrist 20 degrees off the table, a true lateral image can be achieved. The x-ray beam is now perpendicular to the joint (*arrow*). **F.** The remaining screws have been placed.

## Closure

- Repair the pronator quadratus to its insertion site with a series of 3-0 absorbable horizontal mattress sutures (**TECH FIG 6A**).
  - In many cases, it is impossible to repair the pronator quadratus because the muscle and fascia are extremely thin or the muscle is damaged. In this situation, the muscle can be débrided or simply left in place.
- Before skin closure, obtain final radiographs (**TECH FIG 6B,C**) and assess the stability of the distal radioulnar joint.
- Place a drain only if excessive bleeding is anticipated.
- Consider methods to minimize postoperative pain.
  - Percutaneous placement of a pain pump catheter
  - Injection of a long-acting local anesthetic
- Close the subcutaneous tissues with a 4-0 braided absorbable suture and reapproximate the skin with interrupted 4-0 or 5-0 nylon sutures or a running subcuticular stitch.
- Place two layers of gauze and a nonadherent gauze over the wound, wrap the wrist and forearm with thick Webril (Kendall, Mansfield, MA), and apply a below-elbow splint in a neutral wrist position, leaving the metacarpophalangeal joints free for range of motion (ROM) (**TECH FIG 6D**).
  - If there is injury to the ulnar wrist (eg, ulnar styloid fracture, distal radioulnar joint injury), immobilize the forearm in slight supination with an above-elbow or sugar-tong (Munster) splint.

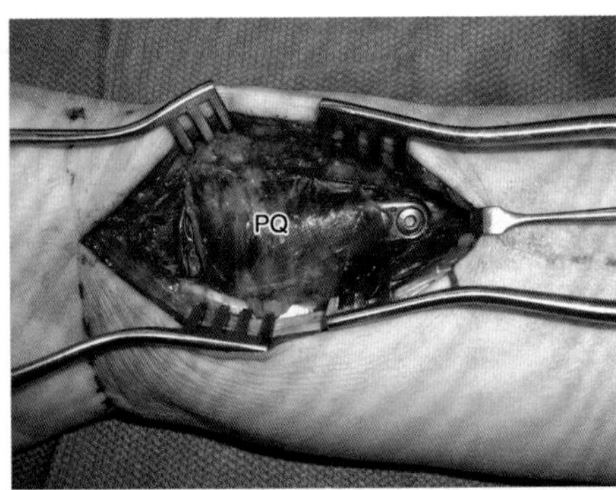


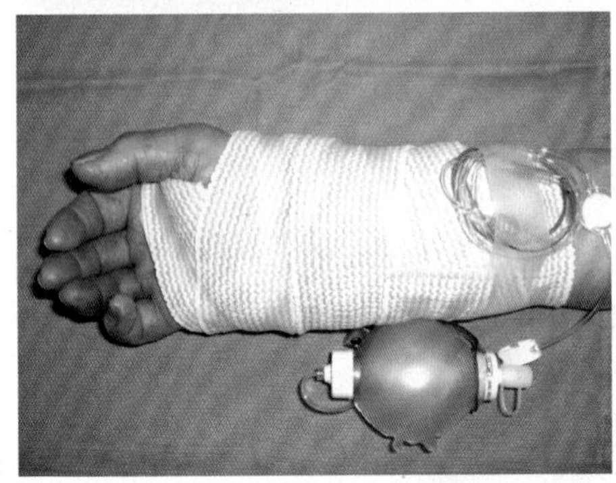

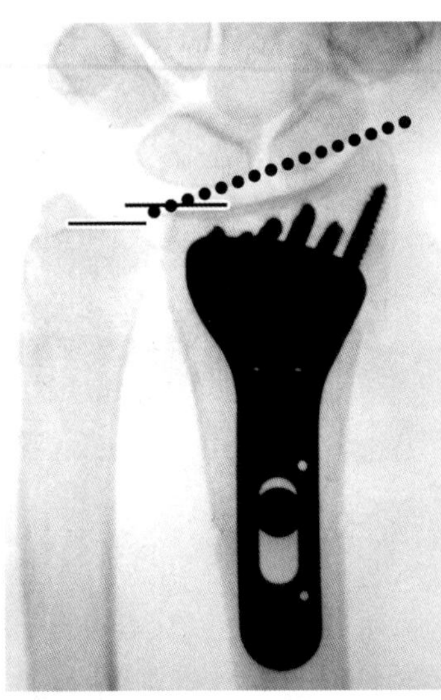

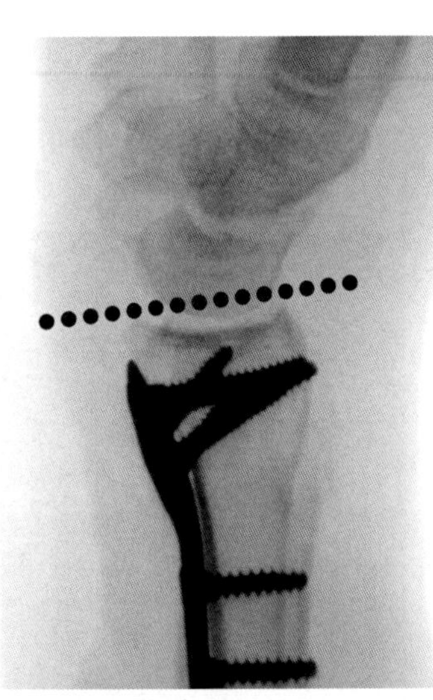

**TECH FIG 6** • **A.** The pronator quadratus (*PQ*) has been repaired. **B.** AP radiograph demonstrating correction of the articular surface, radial height (*lines*), and radial inclination (*dotted line*). **C.** Lateral radiograph demonstrating correction of the palmar tilt (*dotted line*). **D.** A bulky dressing is applied with a volar splint holding the wrist in a neutral position. A pain pump catheter has been inserted for additional pain control.

## Volar Fixed-Angle Plate Using the Plate as Reduction Tool

- We do not recommend use of the volar fixed-angle plate as a reduction tool in the acute setting. It is best employed (if at all) for a malunion or perhaps for a fracture with minimal articular comminution.
  - This technique is difficult because the plate must be applied accounting for the coronal, sagittal, and translational deformities associated with the fracture fragments before the reduction has been achieved.
- Perform the surgical approach as previously described.
- Address first any distal articular involvement with reduction and K-wire fixation.
- Affix the plate to the distal fragment, accounting for where the plate will sit on the radius shaft once the reduction is completed.
- Place the screws so that they are parallel to the articular surface on the lateral x-ray view (**TECH FIG 7A,B**).
- On the AP radiograph, align the plate with the perpendicular of the radial inclination of the distal radius (20 degrees; **TECH FIG 7C,D**).
- Once distal fixation is complete, secure the proximal plate to the radius shaft, thereby completing the reduction.
- Close and splint as described previously.

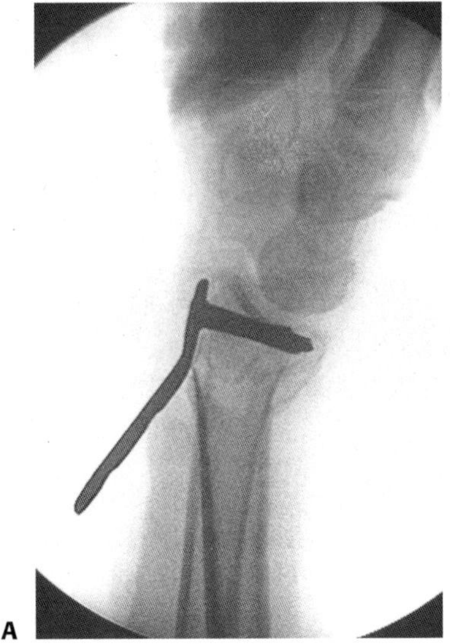

**TECH FIG 7** • **A.** The volar plate is applied with the distal screws placed first (parallel to distal articular surface). *(continued)*

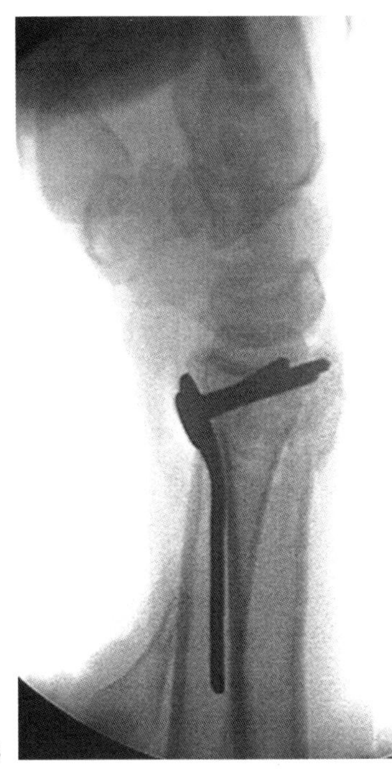

B

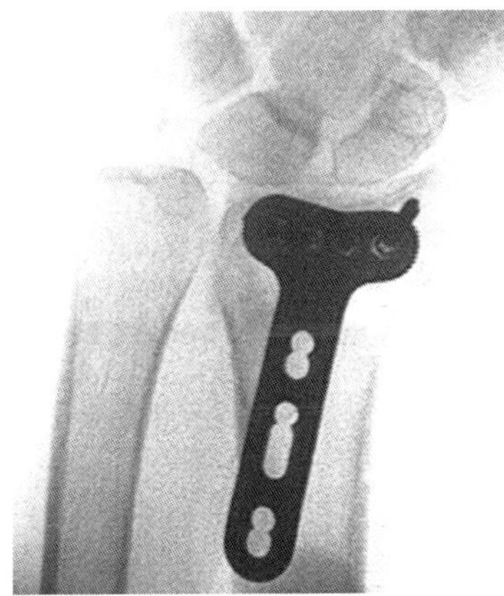

C

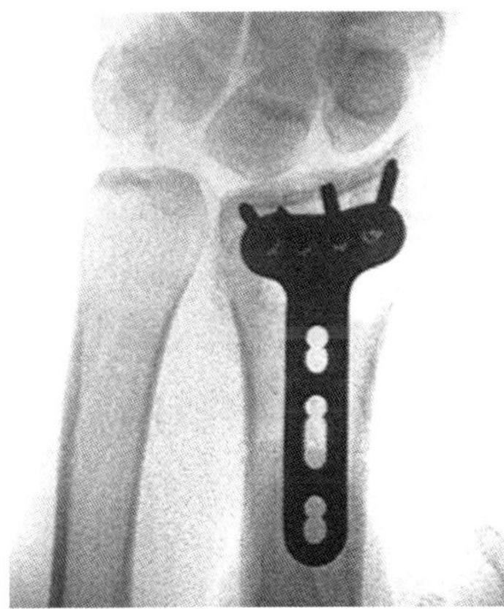

D

**TECH FIG 7 •** *(continued)* **B.** Reducing the plate to the diaphysis proximally accomplishes the reduction. **C.** The plate is applied at approximately a 20-degree angle relative to the distal articular surface or to the amount of angulation that is estimated. **D.** By reducing the plate to the diaphysis, the distal angulation is corrected.

## PEARLS AND PITFALLS

| | |
|---|---|
| **Preoperative planning** | ■ Obtain multiple radiographs in different positions (eg, several oblique views), especially in the setting of comminution or articular involvement.<br>■ Obtain a CT scan if assessing the pattern of fracture when radiographs alone are difficult or uncertain. |
| **Surgical approach** | ■ Avoid crossing the distal flexion creases of the wrist.<br>■ Avoid ulnar exposure to the midline of the flexor carpi radialis.<br>■ Use extra care with deep dissection in the presence of hematoma or significant swelling. |
| **Fracture reduction** | ■ Employ traction across the wrist with a device or weights.<br>■ Use a lobster claw clamp on the proximal radius shaft for control of the forearm and as a reference for the lateral margins.<br>■ Use instruments to disimpact and reduce articular fragments through the fracture itself, either volarly, dorsally, or both.<br>■ Employ a temporary K-wire to stabilize the reduction before placement of the plate. |
| **Plate alignment** | ■ Confirm appropriate radial–ulnar positioning of the proximal plate using a true AP radiograph (ie, forearm in supination with open view of the distal radioulnar joint).<br>■ Confirm proper distal plate position on a true lateral view (ie, forearm 20 degrees off the table).<br>■ Place the plate as distal as possible, up to the volar teardrop (watershed line) of the distal radius, if possible.<br>■ Evaluate the screws for possible joint penetration using 360-degree fluoroscopic images. |
| **Plate fixation** | ■ Use K-wires to fix the plate provisionally to the proximal radius.<br>■ The initial "oblong hole" screw should be slightly longer than the measured length to ensure better initial fixation. |
| **Postoperative** | ■ Closure of the pronator quadratus is not critical and should be reserved for more substantial muscles with limited trauma.<br>■ Begin immediate ROM to digits with edema. |

## POSTOPERATIVE CARE

- The wrist is splinted in a neutral position, leaving the digits free.
  - If the fracture is particularly tenuous or there is injury to the ulnar wrist, a long-arm or sugar-tong (Munster) splint is applied.
- Vitamin C 500 to 1500 mg per day for 6 weeks is recommended to reduce the incidence of complex regional pain syndrome.[22]
- The patient is instructed to perform active ROM exercises for the digits every hour and to engage in strict elevation for at least 3 days.
  - It is critical to emphasize edema prevention and immediate ROM of the digits.
- At 1 week postoperatively, the splint is removed and the wound is examined.
- If swelling permits, the therapist fabricates a molded Orthoplast splint (Johnson & Johnson Orthopedics, New Brunswick, NJ) to be worn at all times.
- Active ROM exercises of the wrist are implemented 1 week postoperatively.
- At 4 to 6 weeks, putty and grip exercises are added.
- At 6 to 8 weeks, the splint is discontinued, and progressive strengthening exercises are advanced.
- If necessary, progressive passive ROM can begin, including use of dynamic splints.
- At 10 to 12 weeks, the patient usually can be discharged to all activities as tolerated.
- Elderly patients with distal radius fractures are at increased risk of sustaining other osteoporosis-related fractures. A referral to an osteoporosis clinic is advised.

## OUTCOMES

- Overall good to excellent results can be expected in over 80% of patients with ROM, strength, and outcomes scoring.[13,14,19,21]
- Studies comparing volar fixation to other forms of fixation (eg, external fixators, pins, and dorsal plating) have revealed similar if not superior results.
  - Results appear to be superior in the early recovery period, with the final outcome yielding equivalent results among all fixation groups.
  - Some studies suggest better maintenance in overall reduction compared to other forms of fixation.

## COMPLICATIONS

- Complication rates as high as 27% have been reported.
- Complications can be categorized into those involving hardware, fracture, soft tissues, nerves, and tendons.[2]
- Failures of hardware, such as plate or screw breakage, can occur but are rare. Usually, such failures are an indication of other problems, such as nonunion.
- The hardware becomes unacceptably prominent in a minority of patients.
  - This complication may become evident only after some time has elapsed, as swelling of fibrous tissue subsides and bone remodels.
  - The most common sites include the dorsal wrist, when screws have been inserted, and the radial wrist, when a plate has been used.
  - It can be avoided with careful screw and plate placement and radiographic verification of their position.
- Nonunion and delayed union are unusual. Consider a diagnosis of osteomyelitis or other risk factors such as smoking.
- Loss of fracture reduction and fixation can occur and is most common in patients with osteopenic bone or comminuted and articular fractures.
  - This can be avoided with frequent and early follow-up with repeat radiographs.
  - If instability is suspected, the fracture can be casted.
  - In the operating room, if instability is suspected, additional fixation should be considered (eg, external fixator, pins, bone graft).
- Soft tissue complications are proportional to the energy of the initial injury.
- Open wounds usually can be addressed with local measures.
- Significant swelling must be addressed with early and aggressive modalities. Swelling can lead to other complications, such as joint stiffness and tendon adhesions.
- Nerve injuries can be the result of initial trauma or subsequent surgical trauma.
  - Assess and document neurologic status before surgery.
  - Avoid further injury to nerves with careful placement of retractors.
  - The palmar cutaneous branch of the median nerve can be injured during incision and exposure.
  - Postoperative neuromas can cause pain and sensitivity along scar.
  - Avoid the nerve with a well-placed incision radial to the flexor carpi radialis and careful deep dissection.
- Postoperative swelling also can lead to median neuropathy. Carpal tunnel release should be performed if there is any suspected compression neuropathy or if this is to be anticipated as a result of postoperative swelling.
- Tendon complications include adhesions and ruptures.
- Most tendon adhesions involve the dorsal extensor tendons resulting in extrinsic extensor tightness.
- Flexor tendon adhesions are uncommon and involve primarily the flexor pollicis longus.
- Tendon ruptures have been described, especially involving the flexor pollicis longus and the extensor pollicis longus, as a result of plate and screw prominence, respectively.
  - The distal screws must not be left prominent, and caution must be applied when drilling.
  - The sagittal and coronal profiles of the plate being used must be taken into consideration—some plates are very prominent and extend far radially.

## REFERENCES


1. Aro HT, Koivunen T. Minor axial shortening of the radius affects outcome of Colles' fracture treatment. J Hand Surg Am 1991;16(3):392–398.
2. Arora R, Lutz M, Hennerbichler A, et al. Complications following internal fixation of unstable distal radius fracture with a palmar locking-plate. J Orthop Trauma 2007;21(5):316–322.
3. Fernandez JJ, Gruen GS, Herndon JH. Outcome of distal radius fractures using the short form 36 health survey. Clin Orthop Relat Res 1997;(341):36–41.
4. Geissler WB, Freeland AE, Savoie FH, et al. Intracarpal soft-tissue lesions associated with an intra-articular fracture of the distal end of the radius. J Bone Joint Surg Am 1996;78(3):357–365.
5. Joseph SJ, Harvey JN. The dorsal horizon view: detecting screw protrusion at the distal radius. J Hand Surg Am 2011;36(10):1691–1693.
6. Jupiter JB, Fernandez DL. Comparative classification for fractures of the distal end of the radius. J Hand Surg Am 1997;22(4):563–571.

7. Knirk JL, Jupiter JB. Intra-articular fractures of the distal end of the radius in young adults. J Bone Joint Surg Am 1986;68(5):647–659.
8. Lafontaine M, Hardy D, Delince P. Stability assessment of distal radius fractures. Injury 1989;20(4):208–210.
9. Lichtman DM, Bindra RR, Boyer MI, et al. American Academy of Orthopaedic Surgeons clinical practice guideline on: the treatment of distal radius fractures. J Bone Joint Surg Am 2011;93(8):775–778.
10. Marsh JL, Slongo TF, Agel J, et al. Fracture and dislocation classification compendium–2007: Orthopaedic Trauma Association classification, database and outcomes committee. J Orthop Trauma 2007;21 (10 suppl):S1–S133.
11. Medoff RJ. Essential radiographic evaluation for distal radius fractures. Hand Clin 2005;21(3):279–288.
12. Melone CP Jr. Articular fractures of the distal radius. Orthop Clin North Am 1984;15(2):217–236.
13. Musgrave DS, Idler RS. Volar fixation of dorsally displaced distal radius fractures using the 2.4-mm locking compression plates. J Hand Surg Am 2005;30(4):743–749.
14. Orbay JL, Fernandez DL. Volar fixed-angle plate fixation for unstable distal radius fractures in the elderly patient. J Hand Surg Am 2004;29(1):96–102.
15. Pogue DJ, Viegas SF, Patterson RM, et al. Effects of distal radius fracture malunion on wrist joint mechanics. J Hand Surg Am 1990;15(5):721–727.
16. Pollock J, O'Toole RV, Nowicki SD, et al. Articular cartilage thickness at the distal radius: a cadaveric study. J Hand Surg Am 2013;38(8):1477–1481.
17. Porter M, Stockley I. Fractures of the distal radius. Intermediate and end results in relation to radiologic parameters. Clin Orthop Relat Res 1987;(220):241–252.
18. Richards RS, Bennett JD, Roth JH, et al. Arthroscopic diagnosis of intra-articular soft tissue injuries associated with distal radial fractures. J Hand Surg Am 1997;22(5):772–776.
19. Rozental TD, Blazar PE, Franko OI, et al. Functional outcomes for unstable distal radial fractures treated with open reduction and internal fixation or closed reduction and percutaneous fixation. A prospective randomized trial. J Bone Joint Surg Am 2009;91(8): 1837–1846.
20. Short WH, Palmer AK, Werner FW, et al. A biomechanical study of distal radial fractures. J Hand Surg Am 1987;12(4): 529–534.
21. Wright TW, Horodyski M, Smith DW. Functional outcome of unstable distal radius fractures: ORIF with a volar fixed-angle tine plate versus external fixation. J Hand Surg Am 2005;30(2):289–299.
22. Zollinger PE, Tuinebreijer WE, Breederveld RS, et al. Can vitamin C prevent complex regional pain syndrome in patients with wrist fractures? A randomized, controlled, multicenter dose-response study. J Bone Joint Surg Am 2007;89(7):1424–1431.

# Open Reduction and Internal Fixation of Scaphoid Fractures

**Asheesh Bedi, Peter J.L. Jebson, and Levi Hinkelman**

## DEFINITION

- The scaphoid is the most commonly fractured carpal bone, accounting for 1 in every 100,000 emergency department visits.[15]
- Scaphoid fractures typically result from a fall on an outstretched hand or less commonly following forced palmar flexion of the wrist[20] or axial loading of the flexed wrist such as in punching.[12]
- Scaphoid nonunion or proximal pole avascular necrosis (AVN) after a fracture has been associated with considerable morbidity and a predictable pattern of wrist arthritis.[18,21,25]
- The complex anatomy and tenuous blood supply to the scaphoid make operative management of these fractures technically challenging.[25]

## ANATOMY

- The scaphoid has a complex three-dimensional geometry that has been likened to a "twisted peanut." It can be divided into three regions: proximal pole, waist, and distal pole.
- The scaphoid functions as the primary link between the forearm and the distal carpal row and therefore plays a critical role in maintaining normal carpal kinematics.
- Articulating with the scaphoid fossa of the radius, the lunate, capitate, trapezium, and trapezoid, more than 70% of the scaphoid is covered with articular cartilage.
- Gelberman and Menon[8] have described the vascular supply of the scaphoid. The main arterial supply is from the radial artery; it enters the scaphoid via two main branches:
  - A dorsal branch, entering through the dorsal ridge, is the primary supply and provides 70% to 80% of the vascularity, including the entire proximal pole via retrograde endosteal branches.
  - A volar branch, entering through the tubercle, supplies the remaining 20% to 30%, predominantly the distal pole and tuberosity.
- The proximal pole is at increased risk for AVN secondary to disruption of its tenuous retrograde blood supply after a fracture of the scaphoid waist or proximal pole.
- Due to its tenuous vascular supply, the scaphoid heals almost entirely by primary bone healing, resulting in minimal callus formation.
- The size and shape of the scaphoid, in combination with its precarious blood supply, demands attention to detail and accurate implantation of fixation devices during fracture fixation. Scaphoid dimensions vary between genders; the male scaphoid is usually longer and wider than the females. In addition, the diameter of most commercially available standard screws are larger than the proximal pole of the female scaphoid.[11]

## PATHOGENESIS

- Scaphoid fractures are most commonly seen in young, active males.[15]
- With the wrist dorsiflexed greater than 95 degrees, in combination with 10 degrees or more of radial deviation, the distal radius abuts the scaphoid and precipitates a fracture.[15]
- The scaphoid can also be fractured with forced palmar flexion of the wrist[20] or axial loading of the flexed wrist.[12]
- Most of these fractures occur at the waist region, although 10% to 20% occur in the proximal pole.
- Proximal pole fractures are associated with an increased risk of nonunion, delayed union, and AVN.
- In children, scaphoid fractures are less common and are most frequently seen in the distal pole.

## NATURAL HISTORY

- An untreated or inadequately treated scaphoid fracture has a higher likelihood of nonunion. The overall incidence of nonunion is estimated at 5% to 10%, but the risk is significantly increased with nonoperative treatment of a displaced waist or proximal pole fracture.
- The natural history of scaphoid nonunions is controversial, but they are believed to result in a predictable pattern of progressive radiocarpal and midcarpal arthritis.[8,9,14,17,18,21,25]
- In an established scaphoid nonunion, the distal portion of the scaphoid may flex, producing a "humpback" deformity of the scaphoid. The loss of scaphoid integrity can result in carpal instability and abnormal carpal kinematics, most frequently manifesting as a dorsal intercalated segment instability (DISI) pattern.
  - The pattern of carpal instability and secondary arthrosis due to an unstable scaphoid nonunion has been termed an *SNAC wrist* (scaphoid nonunion advanced collapse pattern of wrist arthritis).[14,21]
  - In the SNAC wrist, there is a loss of carpal height with proximal capitate migration, flexion and pronation of the scaphoid, and secondary midcarpal arthritis.[21]
- Factors associated with the development of a scaphoid fracture nonunion include the following[17]:
  - Delayed diagnosis or treatment
  - Inadequate immobilization

- Proximal fracture
- Initial and progressive fracture displacement
- Fracture comminution
- Presence of associated carpal injuries (ie, perilunate injury)

## PATIENT HISTORY AND PHYSICAL FINDINGS

- Scaphoid fractures classically occur in the active, young adult population. Patients present with radial-sided wrist pain.
- Classic physical examination findings include the following:
  - Swelling over the dorsoradial aspect of the wrist
  - Tenderness to palpation in the "anatomic snuffbox"
  - Tenderness with palpation volarly over the distal tubercle
  - Pain with axial compression of the wrist (scaphoid compression test)
- Scaphoid fractures can be part of a greater arc injury.
  - The physician should examine the entire wrist carefully for areas of tenderness and swelling.
  - Plain radiographs are scrutinized for an associated ligamentous injury or disruption of the midcarpal joint as seen in the transscaphoid perilunate fracture-dislocation.

## IMAGING AND OTHER DIAGNOSTIC STUDIES

- The following plain radiographs should routinely be ordered in the patient with a suspected scaphoid fracture: posteroanterior (PA), oblique, lateral, and dedicated scaphoid views.
  - The PA view allows visualization of the proximal pole of the scaphoid.
  - The semipronated oblique view provides the best visualization of the waist and distal pole regions.
  - The semisupinated oblique view provides the best visualization of the dorsal ridge.
  - The lateral view permits an assessment of fracture angulation, carpal alignment, and carpal instability.
  - The dedicated scaphoid view is a PA view with the wrist in ulnar deviation. This results in scaphoid extension, allowing visualization of the scaphoid in profile (**FIG 1A**).
- The following criteria define a displaced or unstable fracture as noted on plain radiographs[2,9,17]:
  - At least 1 mm of displacement
  - More than 10 degrees of angular displacement
  - Fracture comminution
  - Radiolunate angle of more than 15 degrees
  - Scapholunate angle of more than 60 degrees
  - Intrascaphoid angle of more than 35 degrees
- Computed tomography (CT) with reconstruction images in multiple planes is used to identify an acute fracture not detected on plain radiographs and to determine the amount of displacement and comminution (**FIG 1B,C**).
  - CT is most useful in evaluating an established scaphoid nonunion or malunion.[6]
  - Because plain radiographs are often unreliable, CT is preferred for confirming union after a scaphoid fracture particularly before permitting a return to contact sports.
- Magnetic resonance imaging (MRI) may be indicated in the evaluation of a suspected scaphoid fracture not detected on plain radiographs (**FIG 1D,E**). MRI is highly sensitive, with

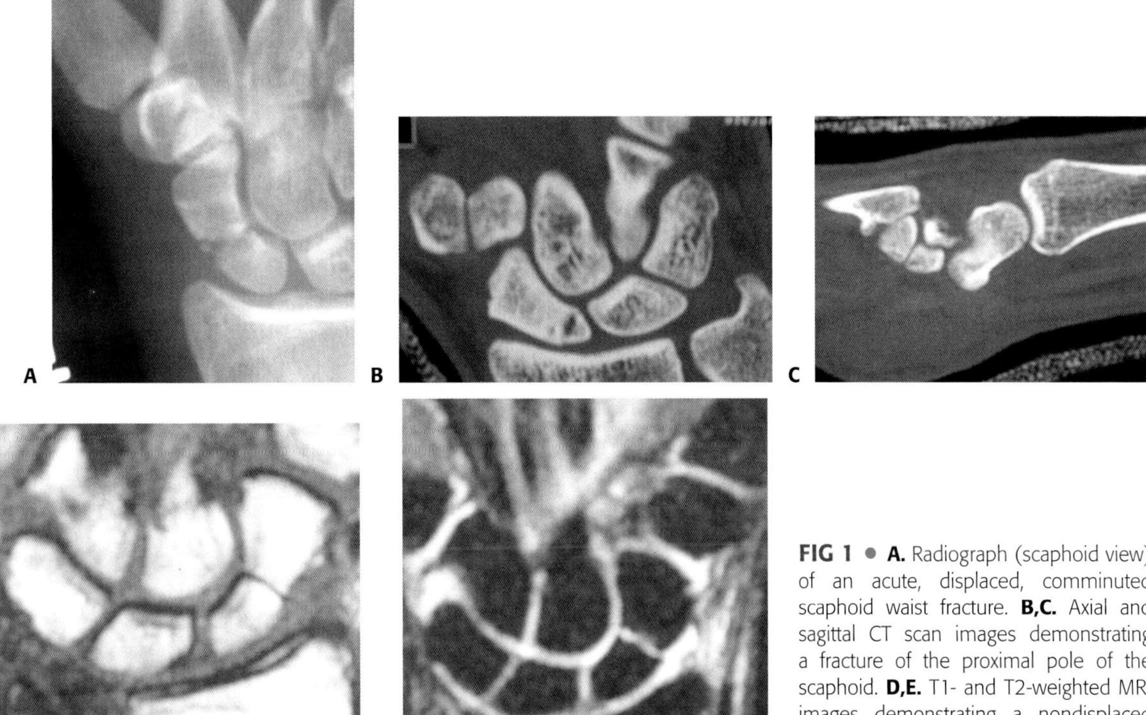

**FIG 1** • **A.** Radiograph (scaphoid view) of an acute, displaced, comminuted scaphoid waist fracture. **B,C.** Axial and sagittal CT scan images demonstrating a fracture of the proximal pole of the scaphoid. **D,E.** T1- and T2-weighted MRI images demonstrating a nondisplaced scaphoid waist fracture. (Copyright Peter J.L. Jebson, MD.)

a specificity approaching 100% when performed within 48 hours of injury.[16]

- Bone bruising without a fracture detected on MRI can lead to an occult fracture in 2% of cases.[23]
- MRI with intravenous gadolinium contrast is helpful in assessing the vascularity of the proximal pole, particularly in the patient with an established nonunion.

- A technetium bone scan has been shown to be up to 100% sensitive in identifying an occult fracture.[27] Unfortunately, it is also associated with a low specificity and often will not be positive immediately after the fracture.

## DIFFERENTIAL DIAGNOSIS

- Scapholunate injury
- Wrist sprain
- Wrist contusion
- Fracture of other carpal bone
- Greater arc injury
- Distal radius fracture

## NONOPERATIVE MANAGEMENT

- Nonoperative management is indicated for a nondisplaced, stable scaphoid waist or distal pole fracture.
  - Unstable fractures and nondisplaced fractures of the proximal pole are indications for internal fixation based on studies that have demonstrated a poor outcome with nonoperative treatment.[2,4,17]
- The appropriate type and duration of cast immobilization remain controversial and none has proven to be superior. Our preference is a short-arm thumb spica cast until the clinical examination and radiologic studies (usually a CT scan) confirm fracture union. If there are concerns for patient compliance, we prefer an initial period (4 to 6 weeks) of long-arm thumb spica cast immobilization.
  - Clinical studies have failed to demonstrate any benefit from including the thumb or fingers in the cast.[2,4]
  - Similarly, wrist position has not been proven to improve scaphoid fracture healing.
  - Numerous studies have revealed no difference in union rates for a long-arm versus short-arm cast; however, a randomized prospective study by Gellman et al[10] documented a shorter time to union and fewer nonunions and delayed unions with initial use of a long-arm cast.
- The morbidity of a nonoperative approach, specifically cast immobilization, has become of increasing concern. A prolonged duration of immobilization is often required for waist fractures, and this can be accompanied by muscle atrophy, stiffness, reduced grip strength, and residual pain. In addition, cast immobilization can cause significant inconvenience for the patient and interference with activities of daily living. The prolonged duration of immobilization is of particular concern in the young laborer, athlete, or military personnel, who typically desire expedient functional recovery.[5,19,29]
- If the clinical history and physical examination are suggestive of a scaphoid fracture but initial radiographs are negative, the wrist should be immobilized for 2 weeks. Repeat radiographs are then obtained. If a fracture is present, resorption at the fracture may be noted. If wrist pain and "snuffbox" tenderness persist but radiographs are negative, an MRI or CT scan may be obtained.[16,27]
- Alternatively, if there is a high index of suspicion at initial presentation with "normal" radiographs or if there is a need to know the status of the scaphoid, such as in the elite athlete, we prefer MRI.

## SURGICAL MANAGEMENT

- Indications for open reduction and internal fixation (ORIF) of scaphoid fractures include the following[2,17]:
  - Proximal pole fracture
  - A displaced, unstable fracture of the scaphoid waist
  - Associated carpal instability or perilunate instability
  - Associated distal radius fracture
  - Delayed presentation (more than 3 to 4 weeks) with no prior treatment
  - A nondisplaced, stable scaphoid waist fracture in a patient who wishes to avoid the morbidity of cast immobilization. In this clinical scenario, operative treatment should occur only after an explanation of the rationale for, and the risks and benefits of, operative treatment versus cast immobilization.

### Preoperative Planning

- All imaging studies should be reviewed to accurately define the fracture pattern.
- Required equipment are as follows:
  - Portable mini-fluoroscopy unit
  - Kirschner wires
  - Cannulated headless compression screw system. We prefer to use the Acutrak 2 or mini-Acutrak 2 screw system (Acumed, Beaverton, OR), but any cannulated screw system that permits screw insertion beneath the articular surface may be used.

### Positioning

- General or regional anesthesia may be used.
- The patient is positioned supine on the operating table with a radiolucent hand table at the shoulder level.
- The fluoroscopy unit is draped and positioned at the end of the hand table.
- A pneumatic tourniquet is carefully applied to the proximal arm.
- An intravenous antibiotic is provided before inflation of the tourniquet as prophylaxis for infection.
- The limb is prepared and draped, followed by exsanguination of the limb with an Esmarch bandage and tourniquet inflation, usually to a pressure of 250 mm Hg.

### Approach

- ORIF of scaphoid fractures can be performed through either a dorsal or volar approach.
- The specific approaches that will be described include the following:
  - Open dorsal approach[19]
  - Open volar approach

## Open Dorsal Approach (Authors' Preferred Approach)

### Exposure

- Pronate the forearm and make a longitudinal skin incision, about 2 to 3 cm long, beginning at the proximal aspect of the tubercle of Lister and extending distally along the axis of the third metacarpal (**TECH FIG 1A**).
  - If the fracture is nondisplaced, a smaller skin incision and limited capsulotomy may be used.
- Raise skin flaps at the level of the extensor retinaculum.
- Incise the extensor retinaculum overlying the third compartment immediately distal to the tubercle of Lister and carefully release the fascia overlying the extensor pollicis longus (EPL) tendon, permitting gentle retraction of the EPL radially. Similarly, incise the dorsal hand fascia longitudinally.
  - Gently retract the extensor digitorum communis (EDC) tendons ulnarly while retracting the extensor carpi radialis brevis (ECRB) and extensor carpi radialis longus (ECRL) tendons radially with the EPL, thus exposing the underlying radiocarpal joint capsule (**TECH FIG 1B**).
- For nondisplaced fractures, make a limited transverse capsulotomy just distal to the dorsal rim of the radius.
  - Evacuate fracture hematoma.
  - Inspect the scapholunate ligament complex for associated injury.[13,22,24,28]
- If the fracture is displaced, it is often helpful to create an inverted T-shaped capsulotomy with the longitudinal limb directly over the scapholunate ligament complex (**TECH FIG 1C**). Extend the longitudinal limb of the capsulotomy to expose the scaphocapitate articulation and the radial aspect of the midcarpal joint.
  - The tubercle of Lister is helpful in locating the scapholunate articulation.
- Carefully elevate the capsular flaps from the proximal pole of the scaphoid and lunate. Avoid damaging the important dorsal component of the scapholunate ligament.
  - Especially when elevating the radial flap, take care to avoid stripping the dorsal ridge vessels entering at the scaphoid waist region.

### Fracture Reduction and Provisional Fixation

- Distract the carpus manually via longitudinal traction on the index and long fingers.
- If the fracture is displaced, insert 0.045-inch Kirschner wire joysticks perpendicularly into the proximal and distal scaphoid fragments to assist in the reduction (**TECH FIG 2A**).
  - The accuracy of the reduction can be determined by assessing congruency of the radioscaphoid and scaphocapitate articulations.
- When a satisfactory reduction has been achieved, obtain provisional fixation with parallel derotational 0.045-inch Kirschner wires.
  - The first wire is inserted dorsal and ulnar to the central axis of the scaphoid, into the trapezium for enhanced stability.
  - The second derotational wire may be inserted volar and radial to the anticipated central axis insertion site if more fixation is needed.
  - The derotational wires must be placed such that they will not interfere with central axis guidewire placement, reaming, and screw insertion (**TECH FIG 2B**).

### Guidewire Placement

- The starting position for guidewire is at the membranous portion of the scapholunate ligament origin (**TECH FIG 3A,B**).
  - In very proximal fractures, the starting point for the guidewire is as far proximally in the scaphoid as possible, at the mid-aspect of the membranous portion of the scapholunate ligament complex. This point is critical to avoid propagation of the fracture into the proximal scaphoid during insertion of the screw.
- With the wrist flexed over a bolster, insert the guidewire down the central axis of the scaphoid in line with the thumb metacarpal.
  - Be very patient with this important step; proceed with reaming and screw insertion only after central placement has been confirmed on the PA, lateral, and 30-degree pronated lateral views (**TECH FIG 3C**).
  - It is critical to insert the wire in the optimal position in all three views to avoid violating the midcarpal joint or the volar surface of the scaphoid.
  - Take care to avoid bending the guidewire.
- Advance the wire up to but not into the scaphotrapezial joint.

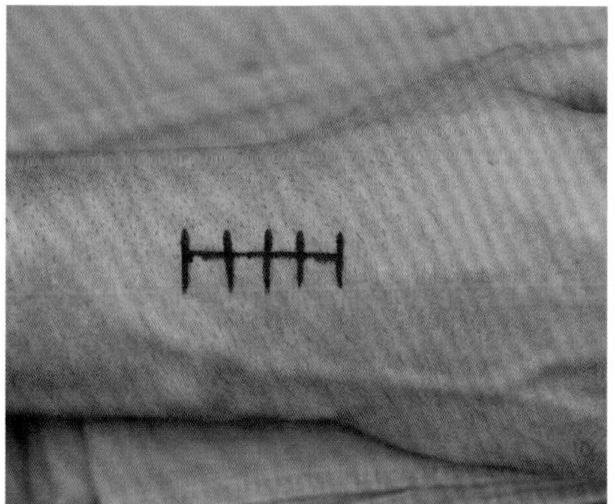

A

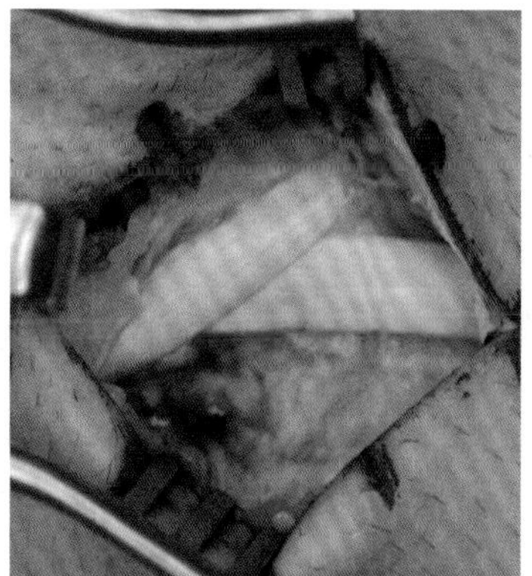

B

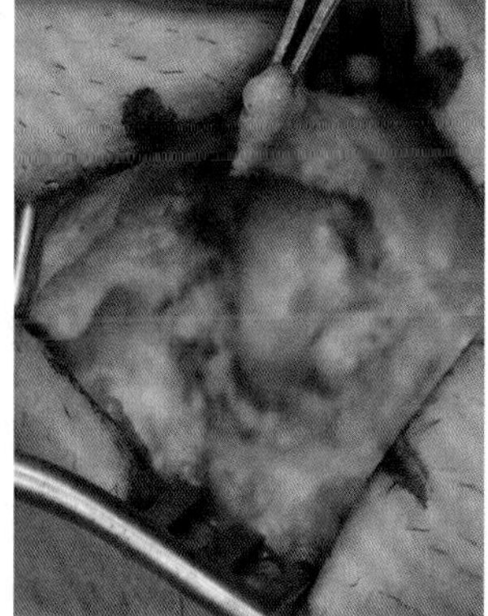

C

**TECH FIG 1** • **A.** Skin incision used for ORIF of scaphoid fractures via the dorsal approach. **B.** Retracting the thumb and wrist extensor tendons radially and the finger extensor tendons ulnarly facilitates exposure of the underlying capsule. **C.** A limited capsulotomy should be performed to expose the proximal scaphoid and scapholunate ligament. (Copyright of Peter J.L. Jebson, MD.)

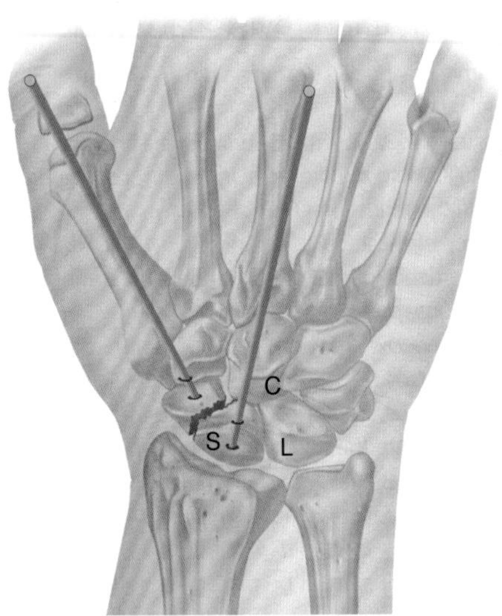


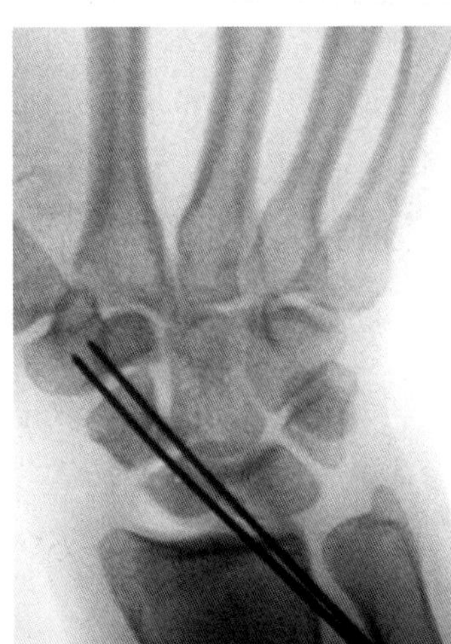

**TECH FIG 2** • **A.** Percutaneous insertion of Kirschner wires into the proximal and distal scaphoid (*S*) fragments is helpful to facilitate manual reduction of a displaced fracture. *C*, capitate; *L*, lunate. **B.** A displaced scaphoid waist fracture has been stabilized with a derotational Kirschner wire placed dorsally and ulnarly to the guidewire. The derotational Kirschner wire does not interfere with insertion of the screw in the central axis. (Radiograph Copyright Peter J.L. Jebson, MD.)

## Screw Insertion

- Determine screw length by measuring the guidewire (**TECH FIG 4A**).
  - In the case of minimal fragment separation, subtract 4 mm from the measured length of the wire to allow recession of the proximal screw beneath the articular surface.
  - If fragments are more displaced, consider compression and choose an even shorter screw. The common mistake is placement of a screw that is too long.
- Advance the wire into the trapezium to avoid loss of position during drilling.
- Use the cannulated drill to open up the proximal cortex (**TECH FIG 4B**) and manually insert the screw (**TECH FIG 4C,D**).
  - We use the larger Acutrak 2 screw when feasible, but the mini-Acutrak 2 system may be necessary in patients with a small scaphoid or if the fracture is located proximally such that insertion of an Acutrak 2 screw may result in inadvertent propagation of the fracture to the insertion site with fragmentation of the proximal scaphoid. Any cannulated, headless compression screw may be used but size is critical.
- Remove the guidewire and assess screw position via fluoroscopy using the same views.
  - If the fracture is highly unstable or the quality of fixation is less than ideal, two micro-Acutrak 2 screws (or equivalent screws) may be carefully inserted for enhanced stability.
  - If a limited capsulotomy is used, it does not need to be repaired. Capsule repair is recommended with the larger T-shaped capsulotomy.

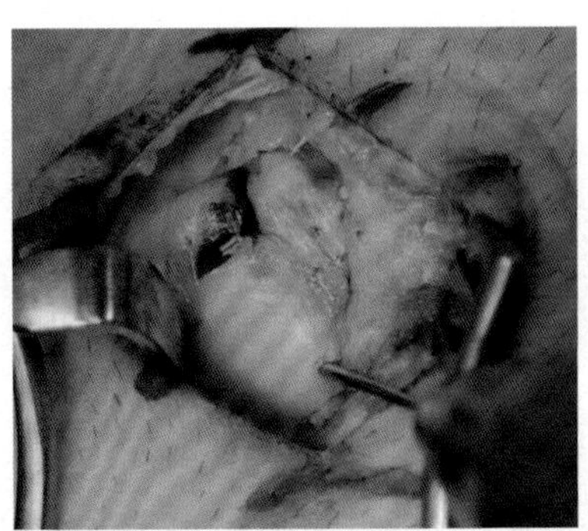

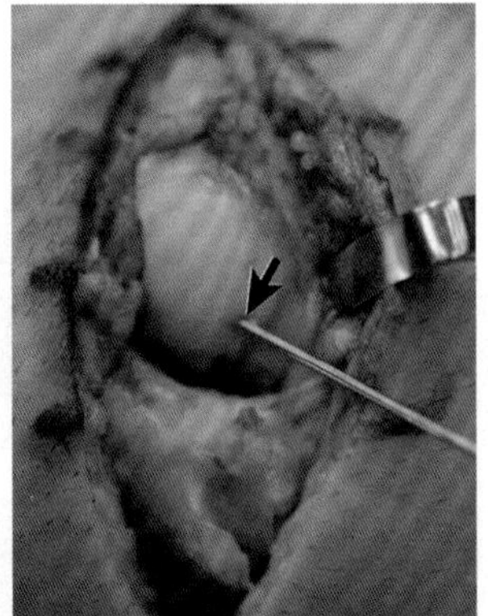

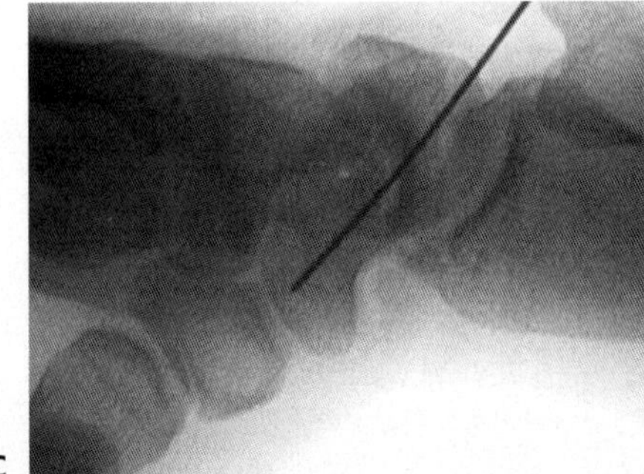

**TECH FIG 3** • **A,B.** Note the starting point at the membranous portion of the scapholunate ligament (*arrow*). **C.** The 30-degree pronated oblique view demonstrating guidewire placement down the central axis of the scaphoid. **A:** Top is distal, bottom is proximal, left is radial, and right is ulnar. (Copyright Peter J.L. Jebson, MD.)

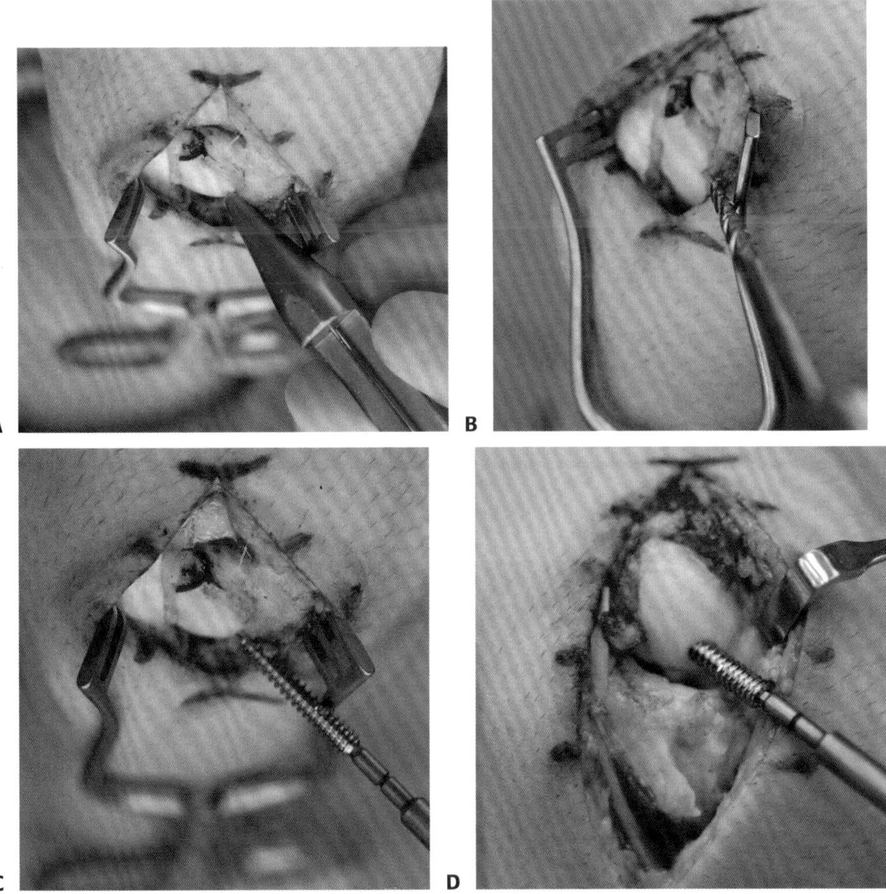

**TECH FIG 4** • **A.** Determining the appropriate screw length. **B.** Reaming with the cannulated reamer. **C,D.** Insertion of the screw. **A–D:** Top is distal, bottom is proximal, left is radial, and right is ulnar. (Copyright Peter J.L. Jebson, MD.)

## Open Volar Approach

### Exposure

- Radially, deviate the wrist and palpate the scaphoid tubercle.
- Make a 3- to 4-cm incision centered over the scaphoid tubercle, directed distally toward the base of the thumb and proximally over the flexor carpi radialis (FCR) tendon sheath. If the superficial volar branch of the radial artery is encountered, cauterize it at the level of the wrist flexion crease.
- Open the FCR sheath, and retract the tendon ulnarly. Open the floor of the sheath distally to expose the underlying volar wrist capsule.
- Distally, develop the interval by splitting the origin of the thenar muscles in line with their fibers over the distal scaphoid and trapezium.
- Incise the capsule longitudinally, taking care to avoid damage to the underlying articular cartilage.
  - Proximally, divide the thickened radiolunate and radioscaphocapitate ligaments to allow exposure of the proximal scaphoid pole.
- Identify the scaphotrapezial joint with a Freer elevator and bluntly expose it.
  - Dissection over the radial aspect of the scaphoid is limited to avoid injury to the dorsal ridge vessel.
- Define and clear the fracture site by irrigation, sharp excision of periosteal flaps, and curetting of debris and hematoma.
  - Assess the instability of the fracture by wrist manipulation.
  - It is critical to identify any bone loss, as compression during screw placement can result in an iatrogenic malunion.

### Fracture Reduction and Fixation

- Obtain correct fracture alignment through longitudinal traction, followed by wrist manipulation.
  - An anatomic reduction may also be achieved by direct manipulation of the fragments with a dental pick, pointed reduction forceps, or joystick Kirschner wires.
- Place a provisional 0.045-inch Kirschner wire to secure the reduction. Insert the wire in a retrograde manner from volar distal to dorsal proximal, gaining fixation in the proximal pole.
  - It is critical to place this wire such that it does not interfere with subsequent screw placement which should be placed in the central axis of the scaphoid.
- The central axis guidewire is placed, taking into consideration all the factors detailed previously.
- To gain the needed dorsal starting position in the distal scaphoid pole, displace the trapezium dorsally with an elevator or resect a small portion of the proximal volar trapezium with a rongeur (**TECH FIG 5**).

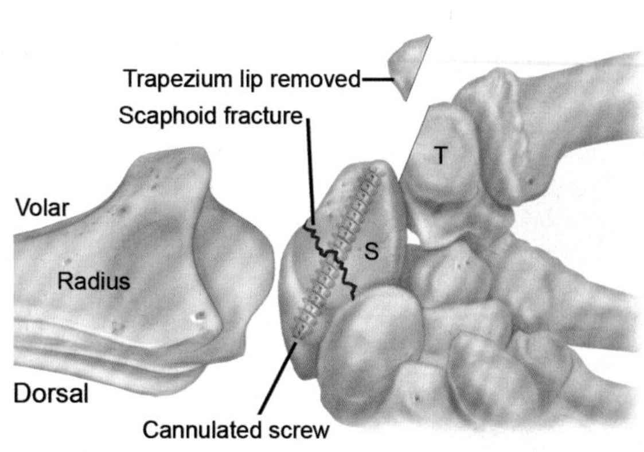


- The cannulated compression screw may be inserted using a freehand technique or a commercial device, which simultaneously facilitates fracture reduction and guidewire positioning.
  - Fluoroscopy is invaluable during wire and screw insertion and to confirm accurate placement and fracture reduction as described earlier.
- Precisely repair the volar wrist capsule and radiolunate and radioscaphocapitate ligaments with permanent suture.

**TECH FIG 5** • Accurate insertion of a screw via the volar approach usually requires partial resection or dorsal displacement of the volar trapezium to expose the distal scaphoid.

## PEARLS AND PITFALLS

| | |
|---|---|
| **Injury to the scaphoid blood supply** | ■ Meticulous limited dissection of the capsule. Avoid any dissection on the dorsal ridge of the scaphoid. |
| **Malpositioning of guidewire** | ■ Pronate and flex wrist during the dorsal approach to allow appropriate trajectory. Confirm position on multiple views to ensure insertion in the central axis of the scaphoid. |
| **Screw position** | ■ Select a screw that is 4 mm shorter than measured length unless fracture fragments are separated; in that case, choose a shorter screw. |
| **Reduction of an unstable fracture** | ■ Perpendicular Kirschner wire joysticks inserted into the proximal and distal scaphoid fragments are useful to obtain a reduction.<br>■ Provisional derotational Kirschner wires placed before screw insertion can be used to stabilize fragments during screw insertion.<br>■ Recognize comminution and bone loss to avoid inadvertent shortening or malreduction with screw compression. |
| **Small proximal pole fracture** | ■ Use of a small screw (ie, mini-Acutrak 2) may be necessary to prevent comminution of the proximal fragment.<br>■ Confirm central axis screw position, especially in the proximal pole. |

## POSTOPERATIVE CARE

- The patient is immobilized in a below-elbow volar splint and discharged to home with instructions on strict limb elevation and frequent digital range-of-motion exercises.
- At 2 weeks, the patient returns for suture removal. Range-of-motion exercises are begun, and a removable forearm-based thumb splint is worn. The splint is discontinued at 6 weeks postoperatively.
  - If the fracture involves the proximal pole or if significant comminution was noted at surgery and there is concern regarding stability of the fixation, immobilization in a short-arm cast for 6 to 10 weeks is indicated. Typically, such fractures take longer to achieve union.
- After cast removal, a formal supervised therapy program is initiated to achieve satisfactory range of motion, strength, and function.
- Fracture healing is assessed at 2, 6, and 12 weeks postoperatively with plain radiography. Fracture union is defined as progressive obliteration of the fracture and clear trabeculation across the fracture site (**FIG 2**).
- If there is any question regarding fracture union, a CT scan is obtained at 3 months postoperatively or before the patient is allowed to return to unrestricted sporting activities.

## OUTCOMES

- Surgical fixation of unstable, displaced scaphoid fractures has been increasingly advocated, given the unsatisfactory outcomes that have been reported with nonoperative management.[2,4,17] Rigid internal fixation allows for early physiotherapy throughout the healing phase, a more rapid time to union, improved range of motion, and rapid functional recovery.[5,10,19,29] Several studies have reported a high rate of union and excellent clinical outcome with minimal morbidity using both limited open and percutaneous techniques.[1,3,5,10,26,29]
- Clinical and biomechanical studies have also recently documented the importance of screw position after fixation of

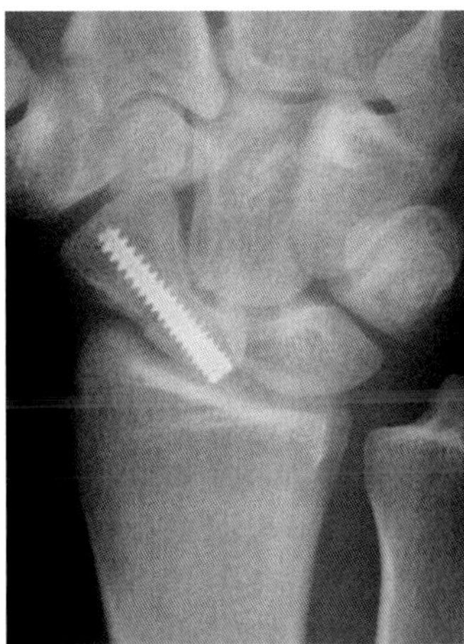

**FIG 2** • A healed scaphoid waist fracture after ORIF via the dorsal approach. Although the screw may appear slightly long, both the proximal scaphoid and distal scaphoid are covered with hyaline cartilage not detected on diagnostic imaging. (Copyright Peter J.L. Jebson, MD.)

scaphoid fractures.[7,25] Central placement of the screw is biomechanically advantageous, with greater stiffness and load to failure.[7] Trumble et al[25] demonstrated more rapid progression to union with central screw position in cases of scaphoid nonunion.

- A volar approach has traditionally been used for screw insertion. However, recent studies have raised potential concerns regarding eccentric screw placement and damage to the scaphotrapezial articulation with this approach.[29]
- Our preferred technique for fixation of a scaphoid proximal pole or waist region fracture involves a limited dorsal approach with compression screw fixation.[19] The technique is simple and permits visualization of a reliable starting point for screw placement within the central axis of the scaphoid, offering a significant potential advantage over the volar approach. We recently reported our clinical experience in a consecutive series of nondisplaced scaphoid waist fractures.[3]

## COMPLICATIONS

- Postoperative wound infections are rare and can be prevented with routine preoperative antibiotic prophylaxis, thorough wound irrigation, and appropriate soft tissue management.
- Intraoperative technical problems
  - Inadvertent bending or breakage of the guidewire can occur if the wrist is dorsiflexed with the wire in position or during drilling before screw insertion.
  - Care should be taken to confirm that the screw is fully seated beneath the articular cartilage to avoid prominence and erosion of the distal radius articular surface. Similarly, failure to carefully judge accurate screw length intraoperatively can result in prominence within the scaphotrapezial articulation.
- Nonunion with or without AVN can occur despite compression screw fixation, particularly with a proximal pole or displaced waist fracture. Stripping of the dorsal ridge vasculature should be avoided. Supplemental cancellous bone graft from the distal radius may be used at the time of fixation of a displaced or comminuted fracture if desired.
- Other potential but rare complications
  - Hypertrophic scar
  - Injury to the dorsal branches of the superficial radial nerve
  - Damage to the scaphotrapezial articulation
  - Proximal pole fragment comminution

## REFERENCES

1. Adams BD, Blair WF, Reagan DS, et al. Technical factors related to Herbert screw fixation. J Hand Surg Am 1988;13(6):893–899.
2. Amadio PC, Moran SL. Fractures of the carpal bones. In: Green D, Hotchkiss R, Pederson WC, eds. Green's Operative Hand Surgery, ed 5. Philadelphia: Churchill Livingstone, 2005:711–740.
3. Bedi A, Jebson PJ, Hayden RJ, et al. Internal fixation of acute, non-displaced scaphoid waist fractures via a limited dorsal approach: an assessment of radiographic and functional outcomes. J Hand Surg Am 2007;32(3):326–333.
4. Burge P. Closed cast treatment of scaphoid fractures. Hand Clin 2001;17:541–552.
5. Chen AC, Chao EK, Hung SS, et al. Percutaneous screw fixation for unstable scaphoid fractures. J Trauma 2005;59:184–187.
6. Dias JJ, Taylor M, Thompson J, et al. Radiographic signs of union of scaphoid fractures. An analysis of inter-observer agreement and reproducibility. J Bone Joint Surg Br 1988;70(2):299–301.
7. Dodds SD, Panjabi MM, Slade JF III. Screw fixation of scaphoid fractures: a biomechanical assessment of screw length and screw augmentation. J Hand Surg Am 2006;31(3):405–413.
8. Gelberman RH, Menon J. The vascularity of the scaphoid bone. J Hand Surg Am 1980;5(5):508–513.
9. Gelberman RH, Wolock BS, Siegel DB. Fractures and non-unions of the carpal scaphoid. J Bone Joint Surg Am 1989;71A:1560–1565.
10. Gellman H, Caputo RJ, Carter V, et al. Comparison of short and long thumb-spica casts for non-displaced fractures of the carpal scaphoid. J Bone Joint Surg Am 1989;71(3):354–357.
11. Heinzelmann AD, Archer G, Bindra RR. Anthropometry of the human scaphoid. J Hand Surg Am 2007;32(7):1005–1008.
12. Horii E, Nakamura R, Watanabe K, et al. Scaphoid fracture as a "puncher's fracture." J Orthop Trauma 1994;8:107–110.
13. Jørgsholm P, Thomsen NO, Björkman A, et al. The incidence of intrinsic and extrinsic ligament injuries in scaphoid waist fractures. J Hand Surg Am 2010;35(3):368–374.
14. Kerluke L, McCabe SJ. Nonunion of the scaphoid: a critical analysis of recent natural history studies. J Hand Surg Am 1993;18(1):1–3.
15. Kozin SH. Incidence, mechanism, and natural history of scaphoid fractures. Hand Clin 2001;17:515–524.
16. Kukla C, Gaebler C, Breitenseher MJ, et al. Occult fractures of the scaphoid. The diagnostic usefulness and indirect economic repercussions of radiography versus magnetic resonance scanning. J Hand Surg Br 1997;22(6):810–813.
17. Leslie IJ, Dickson RA. The fractured carpal scaphoid. Natural history and factors influencing outcome. J Bone Joint Surg Br 1981; 63-B(2):225–230.
18. Mack GR, Bosse MJ, Gelberman RH, et al. The natural history of scaphoid nonunion. J Bone Joint Surg Am 1984;66(4):504–509.
19. Martus J, Bedi A, Jebson PJL. Cannulated variable pitch compression screw fixation of scaphoid fractures using a limited dorsal approach. Tech Hand Up Extrem Surg 2005;9:202–206.
20. Ritchie JV, Munter DW. Emergency department evaluation and treatment of wrist injuries. Emerg Med Clin North Am 1999;17: 823–842.
21. Ruby LK, Stinson J, Belsky MR. The natural history of scaphoid non-union. A review of fifty-five cases. J Bone Joint Surg Am 1985;67(3):428–432.
22. Schädel-Höpfner M, Junge A, Böhringer G. Scapholunate ligament injury occurring with scaphoid fracture—a rare coincidence? J Hand Surg Br 2005;30:137–142.
23. Thavarajah D, Syed T, Shah Y, et al. Does scaphoid bone bruising lead to occult fractures? A prospective study of 50 patients. Injury 2011;42:1303–1306.

24. Thomsen L, Falcone MO. Lesions of the scapholunate ligament associated with minimally displaced or non-displaced fractures of the scaphoid waist. Which incidence? Chir Main 2012;31:234–238.
25. Trumble TE, Clarke T, Kreder HJ. Non-union of the scaphoid: treatment with cannulated screws compared with treatment with Herbert screws. J Bone Joint Surg Am 1996;78(12):1829–1837.
26. Trumble TE, Gilbert M, Murray LW, et al. Displaced scaphoid fractures treated with open reduction and internal fixation with a cannulated screw. J Bone Joint Surg Am 2000;82(5):633–641.
27. Waizenegger M, Wastie ML, Barton NJ, et al. Scintigraphy in the evaluation of the "clinical" scaphoid fracture. J Hand Surg Br 1994;19(6):750–753.
28. Wong TC, Yip TH, Wu WC. Carpal ligament injuries with acute scaphoid fractures: a combined wrist injury. J Hand Surg Br 2005;30:415–418.
29. Yip HS, Wu WC, Chang RY, et al. Percutaneous cannulated screw fixation of acute scaphoid waist fracture. J Hand Surg Br 2002;27(1):42–46.

# Intramedullary Fixation of Forearm Shaft Fractures

3
CHAPTER

Charles T. Mehlman

## DEFINITION

- Forearm shaft fractures represent the third most common fracture encountered in the pediatric population.[5]
- Closed fracture care is successful in the large majority of children who sustain forearm shaft fractures (especially the common greenstick fracture pattern).[4]
- For children who are 8 to 10 years of age and older with complete fracture patterns, the limits of acceptable displacement (angulation, rotation, and translation) become more strict and the likelihood of surgical intervention increases.[1,13]

## ANATOMY

- The forearm represents a largely nonsynovial, two bone joint with a high-amplitude range of motion (roughly 180 degrees). In the fully supinated anteroposterior (AP) plane, the radius bows naturally out and away from the relatively straight ulna, whereas both bones are predominantly straight in the lateral plane.
- Anatomically, the shaft of the radius extends from the most proximal aspect of the tubercle of Lister (which approximates the distal metaphyseal–diaphyseal junction) to the proximal base of the bicipital tuberosity. The shaft of the ulna corresponds to these same points on the radius (**FIG 1**).[11,13]
- In unfractured bones, the normal orientation of the radial styloid and bicipital tuberosity is slightly less than 180 degrees from one another, whereas the ulnar styloid and coronoid process come closer to a true 180-degree relationship.
- Classically, forearm shaft fractures are divided into distal third (pronator quadratus region), central third (pronator teres region), and proximal third (biceps and supinator region). These anatomic relationships offer insight into the deforming forces acting on the fractured forearm (**FIG 2**).

## PATHOGENESIS

- Forearm shaft fractures most commonly occur secondary to a fall on an outstretched arm and usually involve both bones. Forward falls tend to involve a pronated forearm, and backward falls involve a supinated forearm.
- Single-bone forearm shaft fractures should raise significant suspicion regarding the presence of a Galeazzi or Monteggia-type injury (see Chap. 9).
- Mechanisms of injury that involve little rotational force result in forearm fractures at nearly the same levels, whereas greater rotational force results in fractures at rather different levels.

## NATURAL HISTORY

- The remodeling potential of the pediatric forearm shaft has been well documented and is considered to be most predictable in children younger than about 8 to 10 years of age.
- Spontaneous correction and improvement of malaligned shaft fractures are considered to occur in young children via three mechanisms:
  - Adjacent physes produce "straight bone" via normal growth.
  - Physeal orientation tends to "right its horizon" via the Hueter-Volkmann law.[12]
  - True shaft remodeling occurs via Wolff law.[15]

## PATIENT HISTORY AND PHYSICAL FINDINGS

- The clinician should gather as much pertinent information as possible regarding the mechanism of injury (eg, a fall from the bottom step of the playground sliding board may be much different from a fall from the top step of the same sliding board).
- The clinician should determine whether the patient has any other complaints of pain beyond the forearm shaft region (eg, wrist or elbow tenderness). Any perceived deformity or pain to palpation should trigger dedicated radiographs of the problematic region.
- The clinician should elicit any past history of fracture or bone disease in the patient or the patient's family.
- Physical examination of the skin of the child's forearm should be performed to rule out the presence of an open fracture. Any wound, no matter how small or seemingly superficial, should be carefully evaluated. Persistent bleeding or oozing from a small suspicious wound should be considered an open fracture until proven otherwise.
- The environment of the injury has special significance for open fracture management. For instance, farm-related injuries may alter the treatment regimen for the patient.
- Multiple trauma or high-energy trauma scenarios dictate that a screening orthopaedic examination be performed to help rule out injuries to the other extremities as well as the spine.
- Brachial, radial, and ulnar pulses should be palpated, and distal capillary refill should be assessed.
- Sensory examination should include, at minimum, light touch sensation testing (or pinprick testing if necessary)

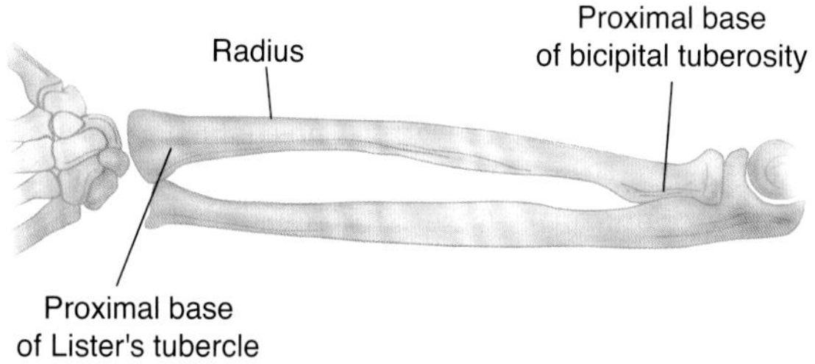


**FIG 1** • The radial diaphysis extends from the most proximal aspect of the tubercle of Lister to the proximal base of the bicipital tuberosity. The ulnar diaphysis corresponds to these same points on the radius.

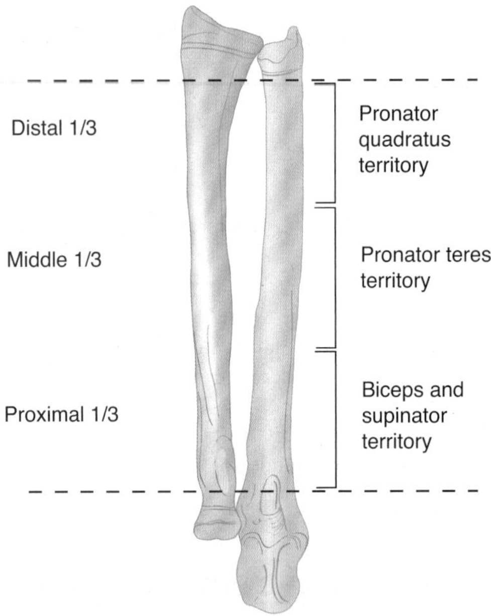


**FIG 2** • Forearm shaft fractures are divided into distal third (pronator quadratus region), central third (pronator teres region), and proximal third (biceps and supinator region).

of the autonomous zones of the radial, ulnar, and median nerves. Older children may be able to comply with formal two-point discrimination testing.

- It has been said that you need only a thumb to test the motor function of all three major nerves: radial nerve = extensor pollicis longus, ulnar nerve = adductor pollicis, median nerve = opponens pollicis.
- Peripheral nerves in the fractured extremity are assessed with the "rock–paper–scissors" method.
  - The radial nerve (really the posterior interosseous nerve in the forearm) is tested with "paper"—extension of the fingers and wrist well above a zero-degree wrist position. The autonomous zone is the dorsal web space between the thumb and index finger. There is a risk of iatrogenic injury during surgical exposure of the proximal radial shaft.
  - The ulnar nerve is tested with "scissors"—adducted thumb, abducted fingers, and flexor digitorum profundus function to ring and pinky. The autonomous zone is palmar tip pinky finger. This is the most common iatrogenic nerve injury after internal fixation of forearm shaft fractures.
  - The median nerve is tested with "rock." The autonomous zone is palmar tip index finger. The median is the most commonly injured nerve after closed or open forearm shaft fractures.
- The anterior interosseous nerve is tested with the "okay" sign. Flexion of the distal interphalangeal of the index finger and the interphalangeal of the thumb herald flexor digitorum profundus and flexor pollicis longus function of these digits. This is a motor branch only (it has no cutaneous innervation, only articular). Isolated palsy has been reported secondary to constrictive dressings and after proximal ulnar fracture.

## IMAGING AND OTHER DIAGNOSTIC STUDIES

- AP and lateral radiographs (two orthogonal views) that include the entire radius and ulna are essential for proper diagnosis of forearm shaft fractures in children (**FIG 3**). If suspicion exists for compromise of the distal or proximal radioulnar joints (Galeazzi or Monteggia injuries), dedicated wrist and elbow radiographs are also indicated.
- If fracture angulation is noted on both orthogonal forearm views, the true fracture angulation exceeds that measured on either individual view (**FIG 4**).
- The radiographs should be used to classify the forearm fracture in a practical fashion with respect to two bones, three

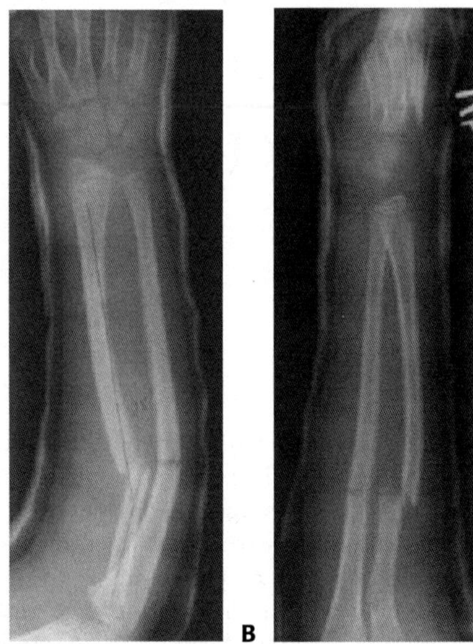


**FIG 3** • AP (**A**) and lateral (**B**) radiographs of a boy age 9 years and 11 months with a forearm shaft fracture.

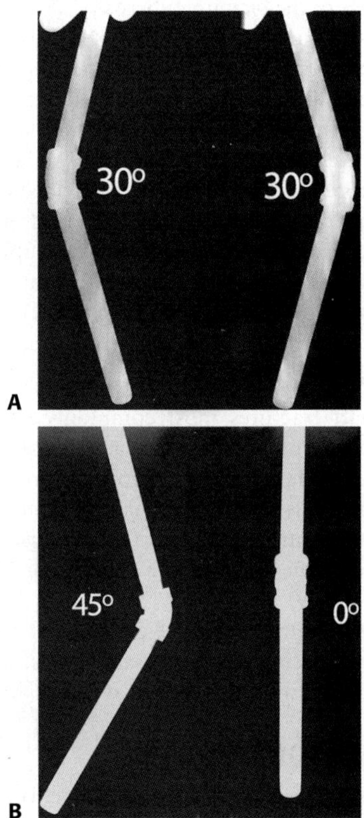


**FIG 4** • **A.** Out-of-plane AP and lateral views of a 45-degree angulated iron pipe. **B.** True AP and lateral views of the same pipe.

**Table 1 Practical Classification of Forearm Shaft Fractures**

**Bones:** Single-bone fractures occur but both-bone injuries predominate.
- Radius
- Ulna

**Level:** Fracture level has bearing on nonoperative versus operative decision making.
- Distal third
- Middle third
- Proximal third

**Pattern:** Fracture pattern has bearing on nonoperative versus operative decision making.
- Bow (also known as *plastic deformation*)
- Greenstick
- Complete
- Comminuted

levels, four fracture patterns (Table 1). This is akin to describing bone tumors in terms of matrix, margins, and so forth.

## DIFFERENTIAL DIAGNOSIS

- Galeazzi injury (concomitant distal radioulnar joint disruption)
- Monteggia injury (concomitant proximal radioulnar joint disruption)
- Coexisting distal humeral fracture (eg, supracondylar humeral fracture, also known as *floating elbow*)
- Open fracture (the clinician must be beware of small, innocuous-appearing wounds)
- Compartment syndrome (more common in setting of floating elbow and extended efforts at indirect reduction of difficult to reduce fractures)[3]

## NONOPERATIVE MANAGEMENT

- Nonoperative (closed) fracture management is used in the vast majority of pediatric forearm shaft fractures.[4]
- Successful nonoperative treatment requires an eclectic mix of anatomic knowledge, skillful application of reduction techniques, appreciation for remodeling potential, and respect for the character of the soft tissue envelope.
- Greenstick fracture patterns retain a degree of inherent stability; intentional completion of these fractures is *not* recommended. Davis and Green[7] reported a 10% loss of reduction rate with greenstick fractures and a 25% rate with complete fractures.
- Greenstick fracture patterns often involve variable amounts of rotational deformity such that when the forearm is appropriately derotated, reduction of angulation occurs simultaneously.
- Apex volar greenstick fractures are considered to represent supination injuries that require a relative degree of pronation to effect reduction.
- Apex dorsal greenstick fractures are considered to be pronation injuries that require supination to aid reduction.
- Classic finger-trap and traction reduction techniques are probably best reserved for complete both-bone fracture patterns. When dealing with complete both-bone shaft fractures, respect should be paid to the level of the fractures when choosing a relatively neutral, pronated, or supinated forearm position.
- Price et al[14] has suggested that estimated rotational malalignment should not exceed 45 degrees. The related concepts of maintenance of an appropriate amount of radial bow and interosseous space on the AP radiograph must also not be forgotten, but precise criteria do not exist at this time.
- Initial above-elbow cast immobilization is the rule for all forearm shaft fractures, as this appropriately controls pronation–supination as well as obeying the orthopaedic maxim of immobilizing the joints above and below the fracture. An extra benefit of above-elbow immobilization relates to the activity limitation it imposes; in some instances, this may increase the chances of maintaining a satisfactory reduction in an otherwise very active customer.

## SURGICAL MANAGEMENT

- Flexible intramedullary nail treatment of pediatric forearm shaft fractures focuses predominantly on displaced complete fractures, many of which may have minor comminution (butterfly fragments usually <25% of a shaft diameter).
- When efforts at closed fracture management do not achieve and maintain fracture reduction within accepted guidelines, surgical treatment is indicated.
- When complete fractures occur in children younger than about 8 to 10 years of age with angulation of at least 20 degrees in the distal third, 15 degrees in the central third, or 10 degrees in the proximal third, risk–benefit discussions are appropriate regarding further efforts at fracture reduction and possible internal fixation.[8,17]
- Lesser measured angulation associated with significant forearm deformity (as defined in a discussion between the orthopaedic surgeon and the parents) may also prompt intervention in selected children.
- Complete forearm shaft fractures in children older than 8 to 10 years of age should be evaluated very critically with the intention to accept no more than 10 degrees of angulation at any level.[8,17] Compromise (loss) of interosseous space should also be considered as well as rotational malalignment (difficult to assess precisely) when debating the merits of continued cast treatment versus flexible intramedullary nail fixation.
- Single bone fixation of pediatric forearm shaft fractures has been described by some authors but is *not* advocated due to increased risk of redisplacement.[6]

### Preoperative Planning

- Rotational alignment of the radius and ulna should be assessed and estimated using the guidelines mentioned in the Anatomy section. Concern is increased if greater than 45 degrees of rotational malalignment is judged to be present.
- Measurement of the narrowest canal diameter of the radius (usually midshaft) and ulna (usually distal third) will aid in the selection of appropriately sized intramedullary nails. Implants 2 mm in diameter or smaller are commonly used, and the same-sized nail is used in each bone. It is far worse to select implants that are too big rather than too small.
- Assessment of existing or impending comminution is prudent. Significant comminution may lead the surgeon to choose plate fixation over intramedullary fixation for one or both bones.
- Assessment of the soft tissue envelope of the forearm is important. Tense swelling of the forearm certainly increases suspicion for compartment syndrome, and the surgeon should be prepared to measure compartment pressures accordingly.

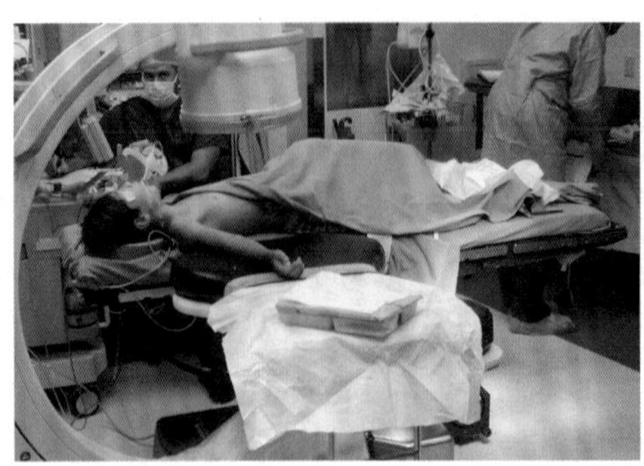

**FIG 5** ● My preferred operating room setup, with the injured arm on the radiolucent hand table and the C-arm properly positioned.

## Positioning

- The patient is placed in a supine position on the operating room table with the involved extremity positioned on a sturdy hand table to allow easy, unobstructed radiographic visualization of the entire forearm (**FIG 5**).
- In general, the monitor for the portable fluoroscopy unit should be positioned near the end of the operating table, opposite the imaging unit (C-arm).
- A nonsterile tourniquet may be applied about the upper arm (near the axilla) before preparation and draping, but it is *not* routinely inflated.
- The limb is appropriately prepared and draped, with care being taken to ensure that the first layer is a sterile impervious one (eg, blue plastic U-drape). The C-arm is also appropriately protected with a C-arm sterile plastic drape and an additional sterile skirt (usually a sterile paper half-sheet). Without this sterile skirt, certain limb positions and certain surgical maneuvers occur far too close to nonsterile territory.

## Approach

- Physeal-sparing distal radial entry is routinely obtained via the floor of the first dorsal compartment (alternately, the interval between the second and third dorsal compartments near the proximal base of the tubercle of Lister may be used).
- Physeal-sparing proximal ulnar entry is typically achieved via an anconeus starting point just off the posterolateral ridge of the olecranon. The true tip of the olecranon is avoided as an entry point because it needlessly violates an apophyseal growth plate, and a subcutaneous nail in this region often leads to painful olecranon bursitis.
- In complete both-bone fractures, the radius is routinely approached first, as it is considered to be the more difficult bone to reduce.
- No power instruments are required for completion of the procedure. Key instruments are a stout sharp-tipped awl and T-handled chucks that achieve a firm grip on the flexible nail such that it can be rotated as needed (**FIG 6**).

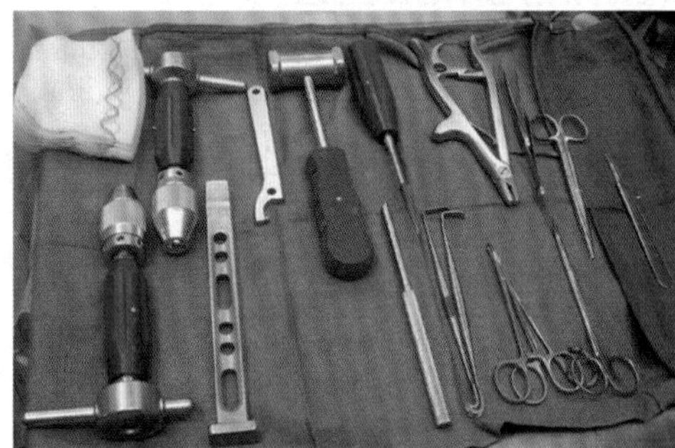

**FIG 6** ● Valuable tools for intramedullary nailing of pediatric forearm fractures.

TECHNIQUES

## Distal Radial Entry Point (Physeal Sparing)

- Using fluoroscopy (C-arm), a physeal-sparing distal radial incision is fashioned overlying the first dorsal compartment (**TECH FIG 1A**).
- Care is taken to protect branches of the superficial radial nerve. A short portion of the first dorsal compartment is opened.
- The tendons within the first dorsal compartment are retracted and protected before the awl engages the distal radius (**TECH FIG 1B**).

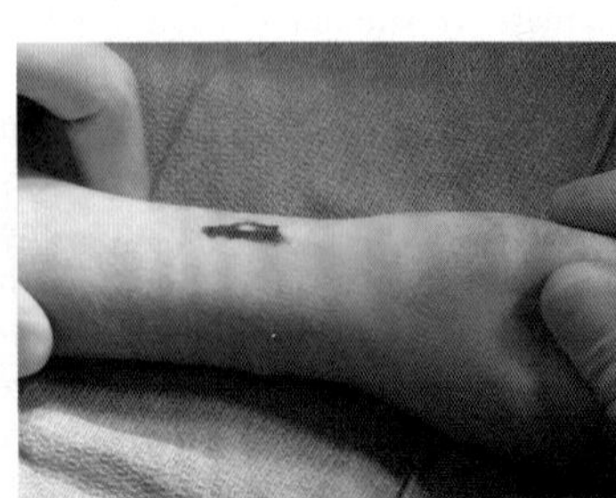

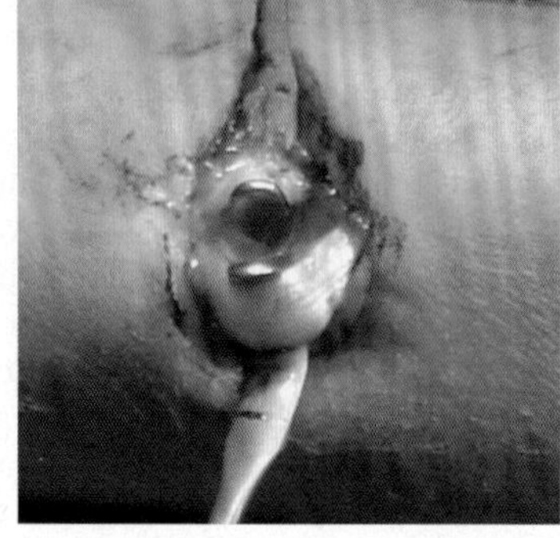

**TECH FIG 1** ● Repair of forearm fracture of the patient in **FIG 3**. **A.** Physeal-sparing incision fashioned with fluoroscopic assistance. **B.** The surgeon must identify and protect the abductor pollicis longus and extensor pollicis brevis. *(continued)*

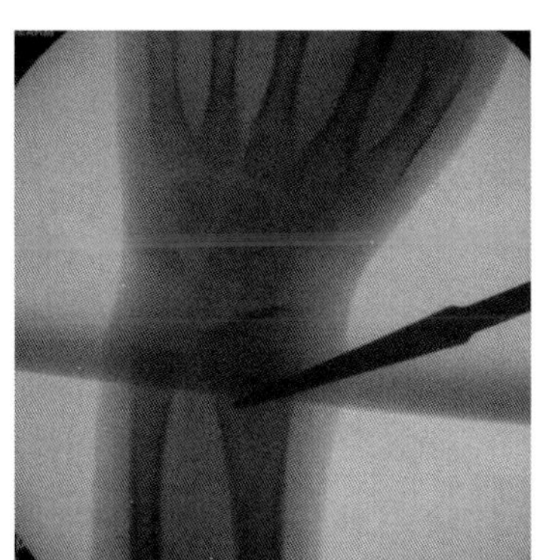

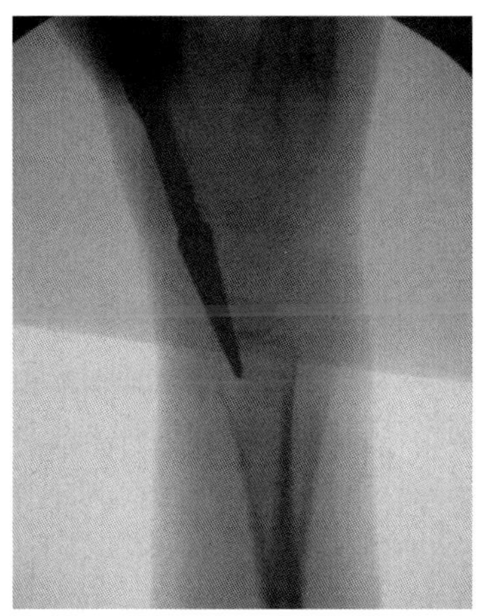

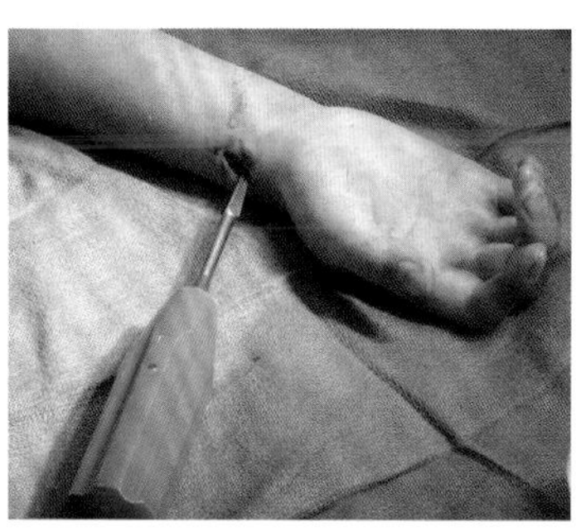

**TECH FIG 1** • *(continued)* **C,D.** AP and lateral fluoroscopic confirmation of entry point. **E.** Well-seated and slightly angulated awl.

- After fluoroscopic confirmation of starting awl position, partial right and left rotations (not full turns) are used to gain satisfactory distal radial entry. A two-handed awl technique is used.
- Satisfactory intramedullary awl position is confirmed by a gentle "bounce" against the far cortex as well as fluoroscopic AP and lateral projections (**TECH FIG 1C–E**).
- The awl is temporarily left in its intraosseous position before insertion of the radial flexible intramedullary nail. Thus, the surgeon's ability to judge both the portal location and the angle of nail entry will be facilitated by immediate sequential awl removal and nail tip insertion.

## Reduction and Nail Passage within the Radius

- The flexible nail for the radius is contoured such that it will reestablish appropriate radial bow. Nail contouring is gradual, smooth, and substantial. Acute bends in the nail should *not* be apparent (**TECH FIG 2A–C**).
- Entry into the distal radius entry site should be directly visualized, and the feel of the nail within the intramedullary canal offers distinct tactile feedback called scrape. Entry is further confirmed fluoroscopically (**TECH FIG 2D**).
- The radial nail is gently advanced up to the level of the fracture. Reduction is achieved via a combination of longitudinal traction and judicious use of AP compression with a radiolucent tool such as a vinyl Meyerding mallet (**TECH FIG 2E**).
- The nail is rotated to optimize nail passage across the fracture site (**TECH FIG 2F–H**), and then it is advanced to an appropriate depth within the proximal fragment (**TECH FIG 2I**).

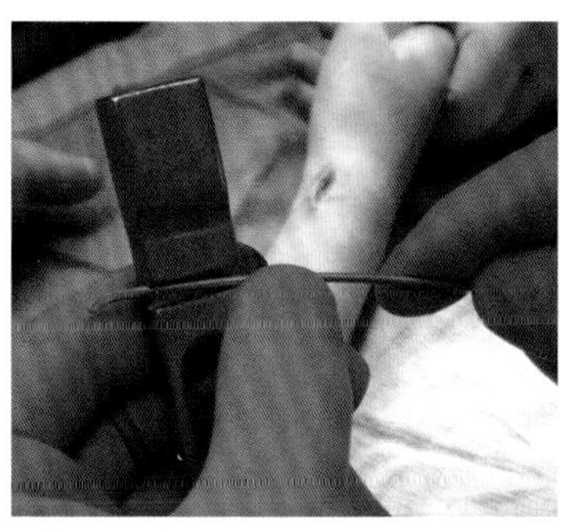

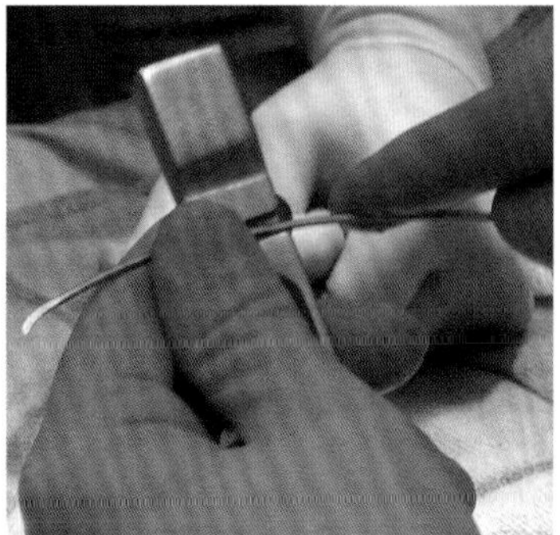

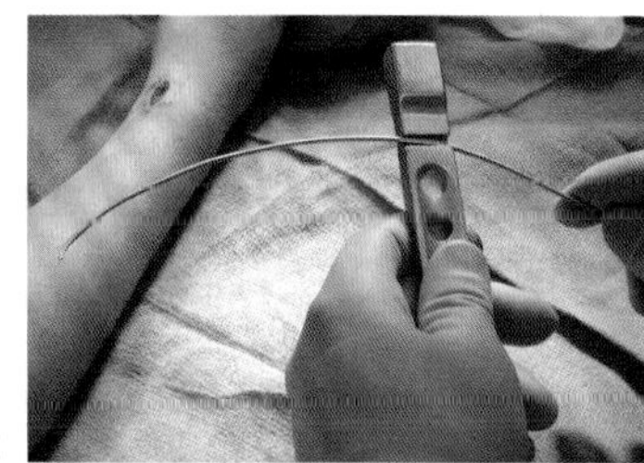

**TECH FIG 2** • Insertion and passing of the radial nail. **A.** Gentle contouring of the distal aspect of the radial nail is important, as overbending effectively increases the diameter of the implant and may lead to nail incarceration. **B.** The "channel bender" is an effective tool for creating a properly contoured radial nail. **C.** The apex of the contoured nail should be placed so as to recreate appropriate radial bow (slightly distal of midshaft radius). *(continued)*

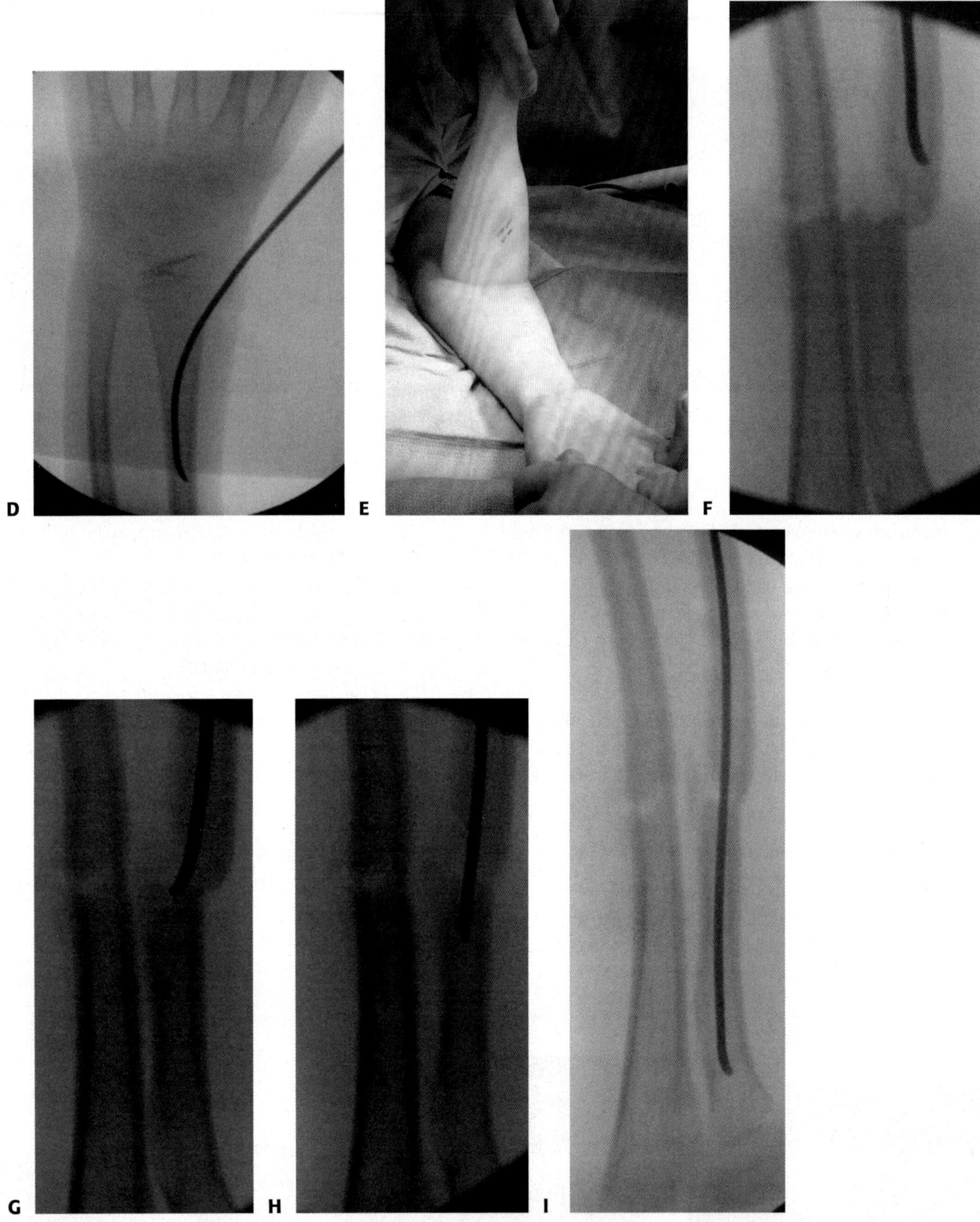

**TECH FIG 2 •** *(continued)* **D.** Under direct visualization, the contoured radial nail is manually inserted into the previously prepared entry point. Distinctive intramedullary tactile feedback (scrape) should be detected, and the implant advanced as far as possible using only the surgeon's hands. Note the trajectory of the nail (tip points radially), as this nail orientation should be maintained during most of the procedure. **E.** Appropriate longitudinal traction needs to be applied by an assistant as well as supplemental reduction forces such as that provided by the broad flat surface of a vinyl Meyerding mallet. **F.** The bent tip of the nail (the "fang") approaches the fracture site after being advanced as far as possible without using a hammer. "Manual forces only" should be used as much as possible to advance the nail within the canal using a properly tightened T handle or similar chuck. **G.** As the fang crosses the fracture site, proximal fragment intramedullary canal entry is often facilitated by nail rotation. At this point, finesse is much, much more important than brute strength. **H.** Once the nail properly enters the proximal fragment, the position is radiographically confirmed, and the nail is rotated back toward its "entry trajectory." **I.** The nail is advanced to an appropriate level in the region of the radial neck and rotated so as to properly recreate radial bow. Restoration of radial bow can be quite striking when visualized under live C-arm imaging. When radial nail contouring is preserved during the insertion process, the nail should be rotated 180 degrees such that the fang points in an ulnar direction. If this position does *not* optimize radial bow, then live C-arm imaging will allow the surgeon to choose the nail rotation that does.

## Proximal Ulna Entry Point (Physeal-Sparing)

- An entry point is selected on the lateral edge of the subcutaneous border of the proximal ulna. The skin is touched but not pierced by the awl (**TECH FIG 3A**).
- Once correct position is confirmed fluoroscopically, the awl is used to gain percutaneous entry to the intramedullary canal of the proximal ulna (**TECH FIG 3B**).
- A mildly contoured (ie, nearly straight) flexible nail is inserted into the proximal ulna intramedullary canal (**TECH FIG 3C**).
- Proper position within the proximal ulna is confirmed fluoroscopically (**TECH FIG 3D**).

### Reduction and Nail Passage within the Ulna

- The ulna is reduced, and the nail is passed across the fracture site in a manner similar to the radius. If open reduction becomes necessary, a simple Müller (AO-type) approach to the ulna is used (exploiting the interval between the extensor carpi ulnaris and the flexor carpi ulnaris).
- The ulnar nail is cut such that it is subcutaneous yet easily palpable.

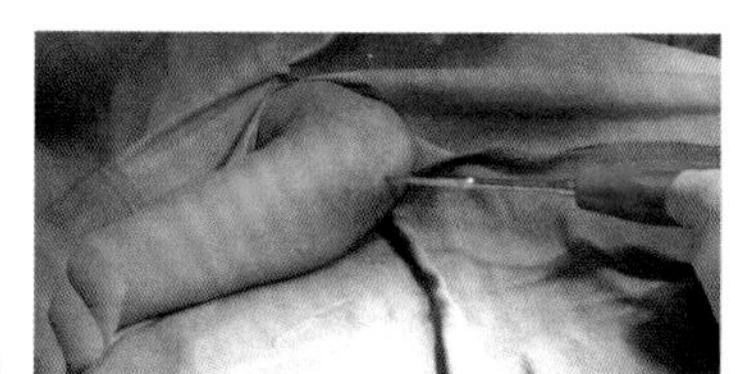
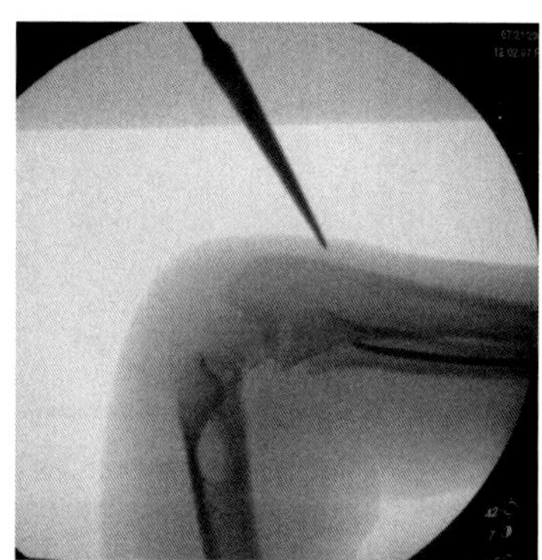
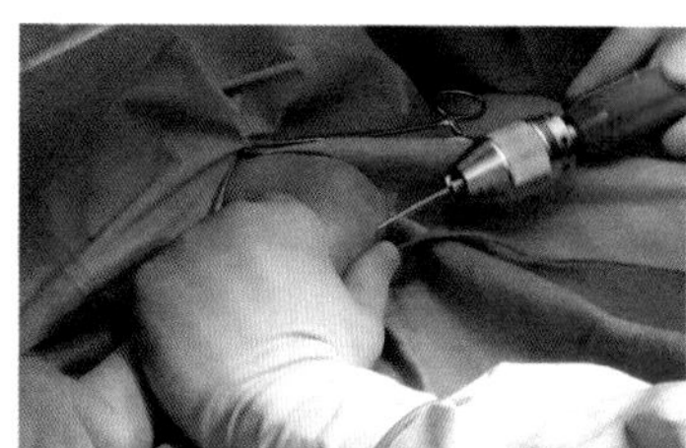
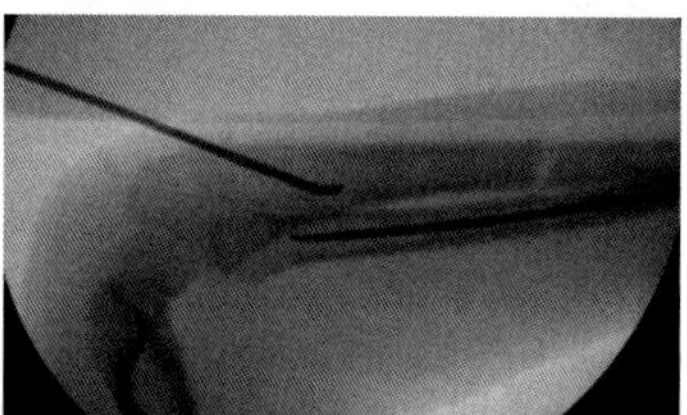

**TECH FIG 3** • Insertion and passing of the ulnar nail. **A.** As opposed to the radial entry point where a true incision is very important to allow protection of nerves and tendons, true percutaneous entry is an option for the anconeus starting point (distal to olecranon physis and just lateral off the ridge of the ulna). **B.** Radiographic confirmation of an acceptable awl entry point as well as awl trajectory is necessary. Anconeus entry is preferred over true tip-of-the-olecranon entry for two reasons: the anconeus entry point avoids unnecessary physeal injury and also decreases the likelihood of large painful olecranon bursae. **C.** The ulnar nail is contoured in a far more gentle fashion, as the ulna is a predominantly straight bone compared to the radius. After manual nail entry, the ulnar nail is advanced with the use of a chuck. Note the 90-degree flexed position of the elbow and the 90-degree external rotation of the shoulder. **D.** Similar nail advancement technique is used for the ulna, with the exception of any dramatic nail rotation maneuver at the end of nail insertion.

## Final Rotation and Cutting of the Radial Nail

- The precontoured radial nail is rotated so as to optimize and normalize the anatomic bow of the radial shaft. This step is most dramatic when performed under several seconds of live fluoroscopic imaging.
- Appropriate full-length forearm imaging must be performed at the end of the case to ensure an acceptable rotational relationship between the radial styloid and the bicipital tuberosity as well as the ulnar styloid and the coronoid process.
- Care must be taken when cutting the radial nail. If the nail is too short, removal will be difficult, and dorsal compartment tendons adjacent to a sharp nail edge will be at risk. Thus, the nail should be cut to protrude beyond the tendons while still remaining subcutaneous.

## Closure, Dressing, Splinting, and Aftercare

- Closure of the radial entry site is performed with absorbable subcutaneous and subcuticular suture and Steri-Strips. Care is taken to protect branches of the superficial branch of the radial nerve (**TECH FIG 4A,B**).
- Light Xeroform, sterile gauze, and Tegaderm dressings are applied to the surgical sites (**TECH FIG 4C–E**).
- A removable forearm fracture brace may also be applied to increase patient comfort (**TECH FIG 4F**).

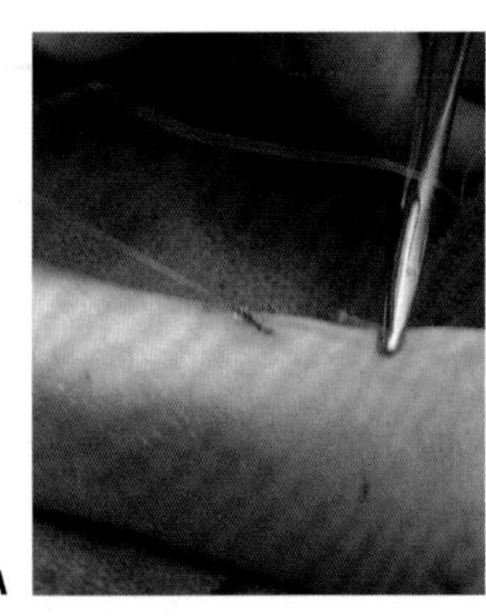
A

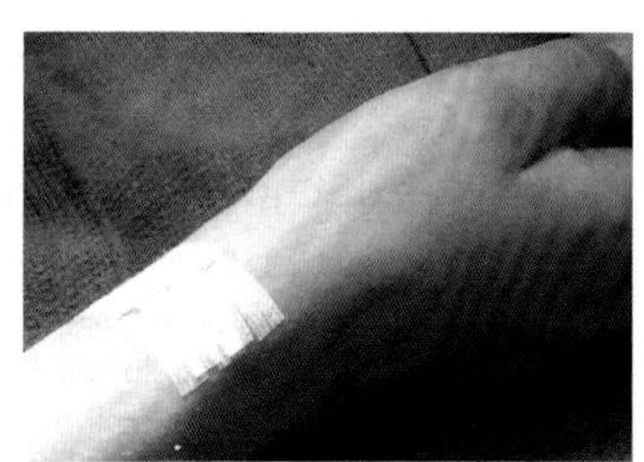
B

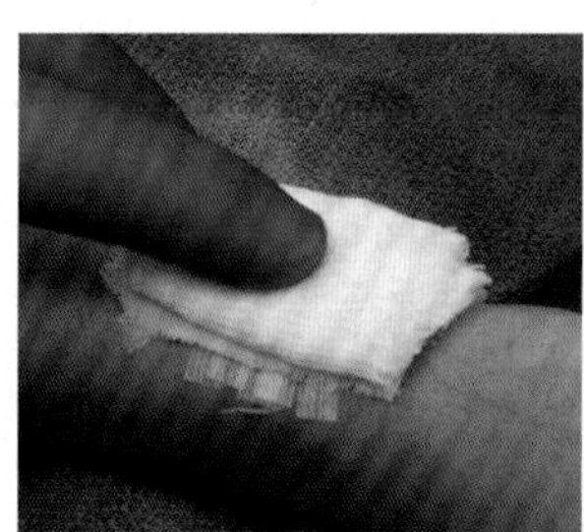
C

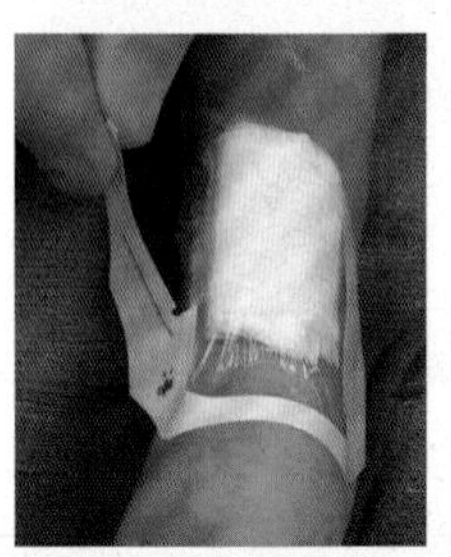
D

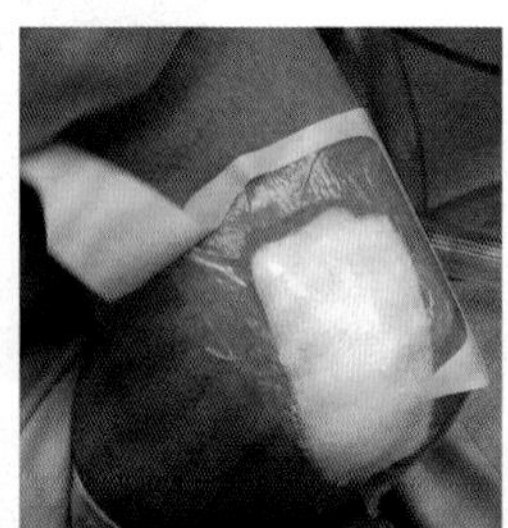
E

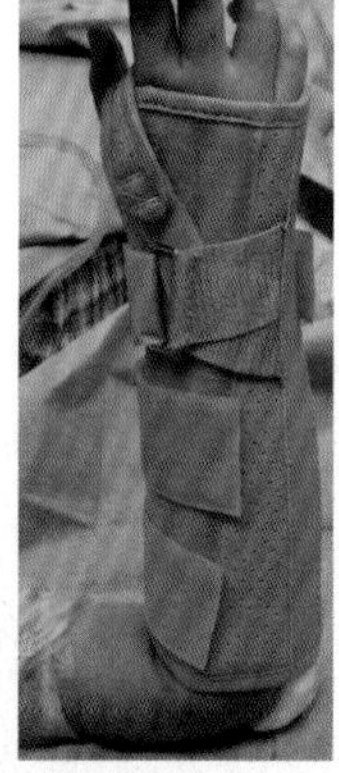
F

**TECH FIG 4** • My preferred closure, dressing, and splinting technique. **A.** Several interrupted absorbable sutures (typically 3-0 Vicryl) are used for closure of the subcutaneous and subcuticular portion of the radial wound. Steri-Strips are added for final wound closure (**B**), followed by Xeroform and sterile gauze (**C**), and a Tegaderm dressing (**D**). **E.** A similar dressing consisting of Xeroform, sterile gauze, and Tegaderm is applied to the proximal ulnar wound. **F.** A removable Velcro forearm fracture brace is applied at the end of the procedure.

## PEARLS AND PITFALLS

| | |
|---|---|
| Which bone to reduce and fix first? | ▪ Once one bone is successfully reduced and stabilized via indirect techniques, achieving the same for the second bone will be more difficult. Thus, the radius should be stabilized first, as it is "deeper." Then, if required, exposure of the nearly subcutaneous ulna is relatively easy. |
| How much flexible nail should be left extruding from the bone? | ▪ If it is too long, soft tissue adjacent to sharp nail edges is at risk. If it is too short, nail removal will be needlessly difficult. |
| At what point should efforts at closed reduction be abandoned in favor of a limited open reduction? | ▪ The author use the "three strikes and you're out" rule (three low-amplitude shots at crossing the fracture site) or the "11-minute rule." Once either or both are violated, the author convert the case to an open reduction. Remember, cases of forearm compartment syndrome have been attributed to extended efforts at indirect reduction. |
| What if an intramedullary nail seems to become incarcerated after crossing the fracture site? | ▪ The surgeon should remove the nail and convert to one of a smaller diameter before creating new comminution or distracting the fracture site. Distracted fracture fragments may lead to nonunion. |
| What if sterile intraoperative radiographs suggest malrotation of one or both of the forearm bones? | ▪ The surgeon should back the offending nail up a bit and see if improved rotational alignment of the fracture fragments can be obtained via forearm rotation and T-handle chuck manipulation. The surgeon then readvances the nail to hold position. If this does not work, the surgeon should consider switching to a smaller diameter nail, as intramedullary interference fit may be excessive. |
| When should the flexible nails be removed? | ▪ The originators of this technique suggest nail removal by about the sixth postoperative month. Forearm shaft fractures have the highest refracture rate (about 12%) of all pediatric fractures. |

## POSTOPERATIVE CARE

- Other than patients with open fracture, flexible nailing of the forearm can be performed as an outpatient procedure so long as there are absolutely no concerns about swelling or compartment syndrome.
- Oral prophylactic antibiotics may be continued for several doses postoperatively if desired, but usually, an appropriately administered preoperative intravenous antibiotic (within 2 hours of the surgical incision) is all that is required.
- The patient is allowed immediate active elbow and hand motion. Concerns about rotational stability after flexible nail stabilization seem to have been vastly overstated, and above-elbow immobilization is not required.
- As there are no sutures to remove, outpatient follow-up may occur in 4 to 6 weeks (**FIG 7A,B**).
- The originators of this procedure have suggested that the nails be removed by about the sixth postoperative month (**FIG 7C,D**).

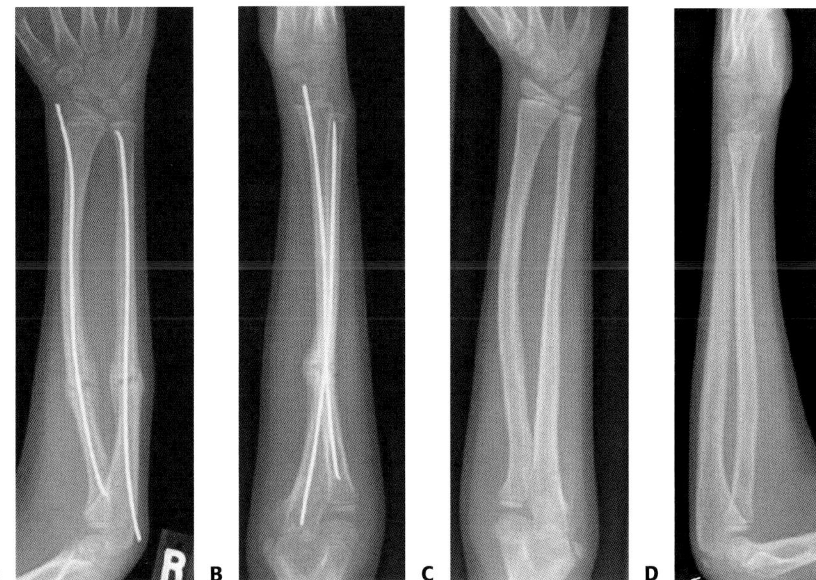


**FIG 7** • Postoperative AP and lateral radiographs at 4 weeks (**A,B**) and 1 year (**C,D**) of the patient in **FIG 3** and all techniques figures.

## OUTCOMES

- At this time, no randomized trials comparing flexible intramedullary nailing of forearm shaft fractures versus cast treatment have been conducted.
- A systematic review of English-language reports comparing flexible nailing to cast treatment found a significantly lower risk of forearm stiffness with nailing (25% stiffness with casting vs. 5% with flexible nailing). This comes at the price of a higher rate of minor complications (21%) with surgery versus casting (6%).[13]
- One of the largest published series[4] of pediatric forearm shaft fractures treated using flexible intramedullary nailing showed 92% excellent results with full range of motion at an average of 3.5 years of follow-up.[10]

## COMPLICATIONS

- Sensory neurapraxia (usually the superficial branch of the radial nerve) occurs at a rate of at least 2% after flexible intramedullary nailing. These deficits are almost always temporary, resolving over weeks to months. The branching pattern of this nerve is such that it presents itself throughout the region of the first, second, and third extensor compartments (**FIG 8**).[2]
- The deep infection rate (osteomyelitis) after flexible intramedullary nailing of pediatric forearm shaft fractures is less than 0.5%; this can be compared to the reported 5% rate of osteomyelitis after plate fixation of similar fractures.[13]
- Extensor tendon injury (especially the extensor pollicis longus) has been reported by multiple authors and may occur during nail insertion or nail removal as well as when tendons repetitively glide past a sharp nail tip (slowly sawing the tendon in two). Radial entry through the floor of the first compartment may minimize this complication (vs. entry between the second and third compartments).[9,16]
- In the clinical setting of forearm shaft fractures coexisting with ipsilateral humeral fracture (floating elbow), the incidence of compartment syndrome may be as high as 33%. When longer operative times are required (about 2 hours), a 7.5% rate of compartment syndrome has also been reported.[18]

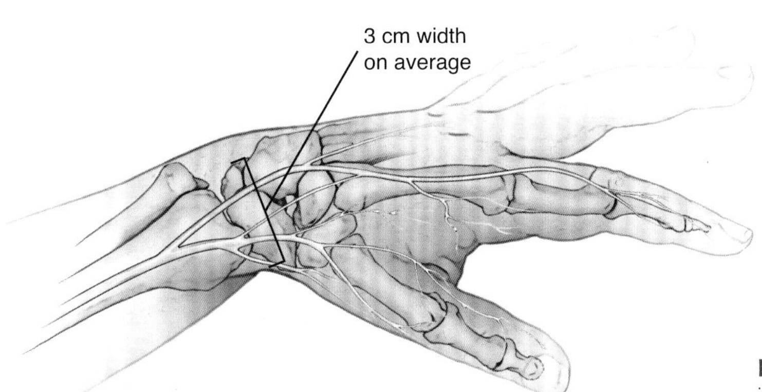


**FIG 8** • Relevant anatomy of superficial branch of the radial nerve in the region of the first, second, and third extensor compartments.

- Delayed union and nonunion are decidedly rare after flexible intramedullary nailing of pediatric forearm fractures. If either delayed union or nonunion occurs, there is usually some explanation, such as a technical error (eg, too large an intramedullary implant distracting the ulnar fracture site), infection, or neurofibromatosis.
- There should be a 5% or less chance of long-term forearm stiffness (defined as exceeding a 20 degree loss of pronation or supination) after flexible intramedullary forearm shaft fixation.[1]

## REFERENCES

1. Antabak A, Luetic T, Ivo S, et al. Treatment outcomes of both-bone diaphyseal paediatric forearm fractures. Injury 2013;44(suppl 3):S11–S15.
2. Auerbach DM, Collins ED, Kunkle KL, et al. The radial sensory nerve. An anatomic study. Clin Orthop Rel Res 1994;(308):241–249.
3. Blackman AJ, Wall LB, Keeler KA, et al. Acute compartment syndrome after intramedullary nailing of isolated radius and ulna fractures in children. J Pediatr Orthop 2014;34(1):50–54.
4. Bowman EN, Mehlman CT, Lindsell CJ, et al. Nonoperative treatment of both-bone forearm shaft fractures in children: predictors of early radiographic failure. J Pediatr Orthop 2011;31:23–32.
5. Cheng JC, Ng BK, Ying SY, et al. A 10-year study of the changes in the pattern and treatment of 6,493 fractures. J Pediatr Orthop 1999;19:344–350.
6. Colaris J, Reijman M, Allerma JH, et al. Single-bone intramedullary fixation of unstable both-bone diaphyseal forearm fractures in children leads to increased re-displacement: a multicenter randomized controlled trial. Arch Orthop Trauma Surg 2013;133:1079–1087.
7. Davis DR, Green DP. Forearm fractures in children: pitfalls and complications. Clin Orthop Relat Res 1976;(120):172–183.
8. Johari AN, Sinha M. Remodeling of forearm fractures in children. J Pediatr Orthop B 1999;8:84–87.
9. Kravel T, Sher-Lurie N, Ganel A. Extensor pollicis longus rupture after fixation of radius and ulna fracture with titanium elastic nail (TEN) in a child: a case report. J Trauma 2007;63:1169–1170.
10. Lascombes P, Prevot J, Ligier JN, et al. Elastic stable intramedullary nailing in forearm shaft fractures in children: 85 cases. J Pediatr Orthop 1990;10:167–171.
11. Mehlman CT. Fractures of the forearm, wrist, and hand. Orthopaedic Knowledge Update 9. Rosemont, IL: AAOS, 2008.
12. Mehlman CT, Araghi A, Roy DR. Hyphenated history: the Hueter-Volkmann law. Am J Orthop 1997;26:798–800.
13. Mehlman CT, Wall EJ. Injuries to the shafts of the radius and ulna. In: Beaty JH, Kasser JR, eds. Rockwood and Wilkins' Fractures in Children, ed 6. Philadelphia: Lippincott Williams & Wilkins, 2006:399–441.
14. Price CT, Scott DS, Kurzner ME, et al. Malunited forearm fractures in children. J Pediatr Orthop 1990;10:705–712.
15. Schock CC. The crooked straight: distal radial remodeling. J Ark Med Soc 1987;84:97–100.
16. Sproule JA, Roche SJ, Murthy EG. Attritional rupture of extensor pollicis longus tendon: a rare complication following elastic stable intramedullary nailing of a paediatric radial fracture. Hand Surg 2011;16:69–72.
17. Younger AS, Tredwell SJ, Mackenzie WG, et al. Accurate prediction of outcome after pediatric forearm fracture. J Pediatr Orthop 1994;14:200–206.
18. Yuan PS, Pring ME, Gaynor TP, et al. Compartment syndrome following fixation of pediatric forearm fractures. J Pediatr Orthop 2004;24:370–375.

# Open Reduction and Internal Fixation of Diaphyseal Forearm Fractures

CHAPTER 4

Lee M. Reichel and John R. Dawson

## DEFINITION

- Diaphyseal forearm fractures include isolated or combined radial and ulnar fractures ("both-bone fractures"). They occur distal to the elbow joint and proximal to the wrist joint.
- It is critical to evaluate the distal radioulnar joint (DRUJ) and radiocapitellar joint preoperatively, intraoperatively, and postoperatively to avoid missing Galeazzi- and Monteggia-type injuries.
- Fixation techniques should be tailored to the age of the patient and the location and pattern of fracture.
- Excellent functional results and union rates can be obtained when skeletal length and alignment are restored with stable internal fixation.

## ANATOMY

- Complete knowledge of neural, vascular, and muscular anatomy is expected. Neural anatomy is particularly important, as a nerve injury in the forearm rarely completely recovers. Nerve injuries result in disabling, temporary or permanent, motor and sensory dysfunction in the hand.
- Injury
  - Radial, posterior interosseous (PIN), median, anterior interosseous (AIN), and ulnar nerve injuries can all occur, although their incidence is not frequent. Preoperative nerve assessment is best performed by measurement of static two-point discrimination. Acutely, motor examinations are difficult secondary to pain. If a nerve injury is suspected preoperatively, that nerve must be explored within the zone of injury. Although the majority of nerves are found to be in continuity, the surgeon should be prepared to repair the nerve either primarily or with nerve cable grafts following bony stabilization.
  - Unless injured preoperatively, the radial, median, and ulnar nerves are not typically encountered. If they are encountered, this should alert the surgeon that he or she might be in the wrong dissection interval.
  - Muscle injury may be significant following fracture. It is typically not clinically significant except for injury to the flexor pollicis longus, which may even be nonfunctioning in severe injuries. This can be difficult to differentiate preoperatively from a partial AIN injury.
- Approaches to the radius (**FIG 1**)
  - Five muscles cover the radius (supinator, flexor digitorum superficialis, pronator teres, flexor pollicis longus, pronator quadratus). When the soft tissue injury is significant, muscle size, fiber orientation, and tendinous insertions (particularly the pronator teres) help orient the surgeon. The supinator muscle is especially important to identify in both volar and posterior approaches to the radius to avoid injury to the PIN. Its fibers are obliquely oriented to the longitudinally oriented flexor and extensor muscles.
  - During the volar, or anterior, approach, the lateral antebrachial cutaneous nerve, superficial radial sensory nerve, AIN, and PIN are usually encountered. The lateral antebrachial cutaneous nerve is sometimes encountered during blunt scissor dissection through the subcutaneous fat following the skin incision. Proximally, the superficial radial nerve lies deep to the brachioradialis. One must avoid placing self-retaining retractors on it.
  - The radial artery is encountered in every anterior approach to the radius. It is found deep to the brachioradialis in the proximal one-third of the forearm and visualized just beneath the forearm fascia exiting near the divergence of the brachioradialis and flexor carpi radialis muscle bellies in the midforearm. In very proximal volar approaches, near the bicipital tuberosity, crossing veins and the recurrent radial artery can be visualized.
  - Superficial veins of the volar and dorsal forearm can be large and contribute to significant bleeding. Formal suture ligation may be needed for large veins.
  - During the dorsal, or posterior, approach to the radius, the PIN and possibly the superficial radial sensory nerve may be encountered.
- Approaches to the ulna (see **FIG 1**)
  - The dorsal ulnar cutaneous nerve is most commonly visualized passing in a volar to dorsal direction through the subcutaneous tissue, distal to the ulnar styloid. However, rarely, variations do exist where this nerve crosses the ulna more proximally. Therefore, blunt dissection through the subcutaneous fat in the distal one-third of the forearm is safest for preventing inadvertent nerve injury.
  - The entire ulna is a subcutaneous bone, and subperiosteal dissection provides extensile exposure. Flexor carpi ulnaris and flexor carpi radialis border the volar and dorsal sides of the ulna. These muscles converge in the middle third of the ulna, requiring only shallow intramuscular dissection to expose the ulnar shaft.
- Fixation
  - Both the AIN and PIN lay millimeters away from the radius in anterior and posterior approaches. Reduction clamps inadvertently placed around them when affixing a plate to the bone or reducing fracture fragments can damage them. Additionally, avoid using monopolar cautery on the ulnar aspect of the radius. When bleeding is

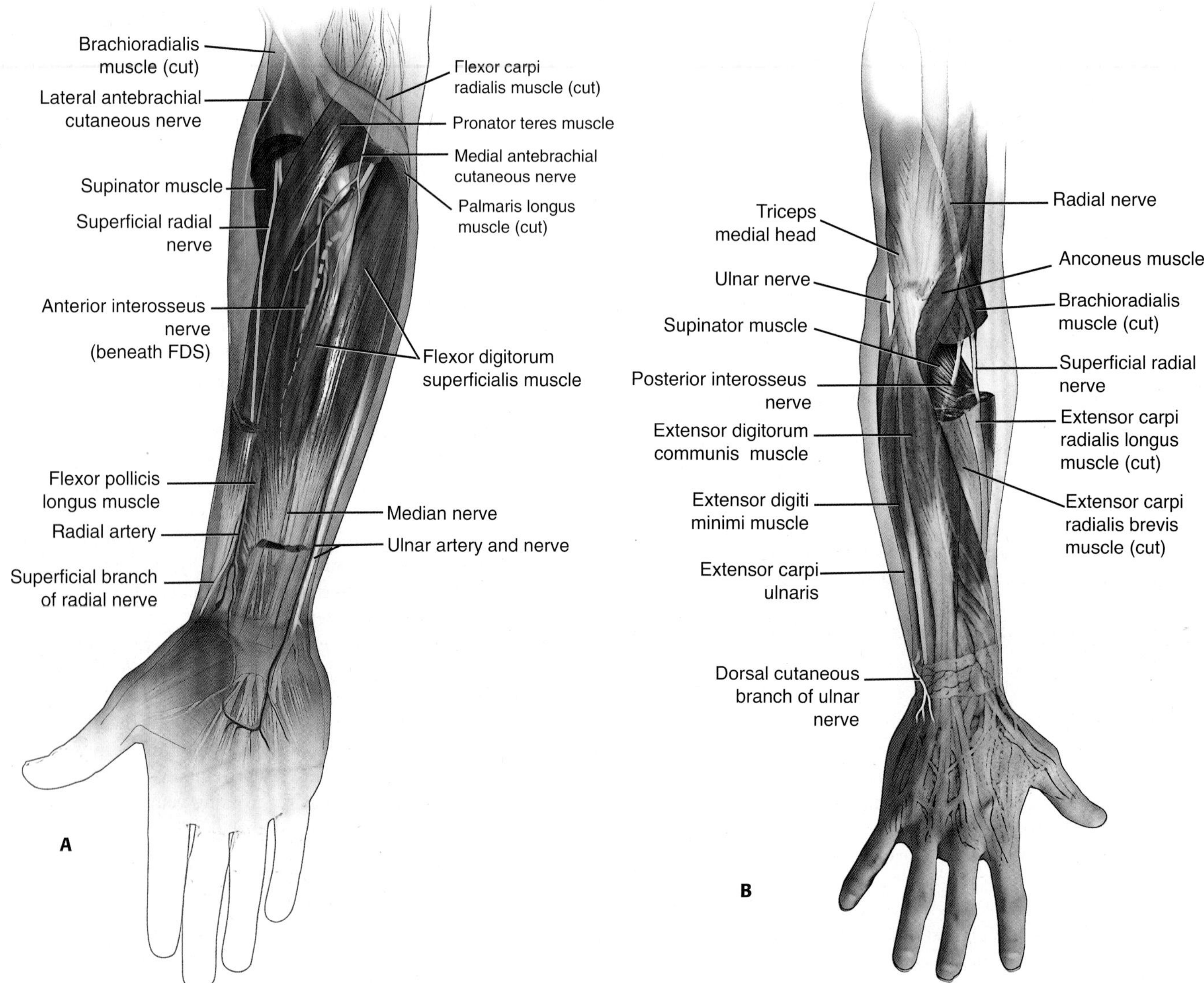


**FIG 1** ● Muscular and neurovascular anatomy of the forearm. **A.** During a volar approach to the forearm, the radial artery, superficial radial nerve, anterior interosseus neurovascular structures, and posterior interosseous nerve may all be encountered. Detailed knowledge of their location and ability to visually identify these structures are critical to avoiding injury when their anatomic location is disrupted by injury. **B.** Dorsal approaches must demand identification of the posterior interosseious nerve proximally and superficial radlal nerve branches distally. During distal third ulnar approaches, the dorsal cutaneous branch of the ulnar nerve may be encountered notably when anatomy is aberrant.

encountered from the anterior interosseous vessels, they must be dissected away from the nerve prior to obtaining hemostasis to avoid nerve injury. Bleeding is stopped with bipolar cautery or small vascular clips.

- Osteology
  - The radius has a complex osteology with both a radial and sagittal bow. The radial bow has an arc of approximately 10 degrees and lies in the coronal midshaft, whereas the sagittal bow has an approximately 5 degree arc and lies in the proximal third of the radius.[9] Contouring of anteriorly placed plates on the proximal radius accommodates the sagittal bow. Anatomic plates are available to accommodate the radial bow.
  - The ulna is generally flat in the sagittal plane and curved in the coronal plane (with the exception of the proximal ulna which in some patients has a slight apex posterior curvature at the olecranon).[8] In the middle and distal thirds of the forearm, plate fixation can be placed anteriorly or posteriorly to avoid symptomatic hardware. In proximal ulnar shaft fractures, plate placement along the subcutaneous border, although possibly more symptomatic, obviates the need for plate contouring to the ulnar coronal bow. This placement also helps resist the forces generated during elbow flexion and extension from the long lever arm of the forearm.

## PATHOGENESIS

- Direct trauma (guarding face against direct blow, gunshot wound)
- Indirect trauma (motor vehicle collision, falls)
- The incidence of associated injuries in patients presenting to a trauma center with a both-bone forearm fracture is significant. In one series of 87 patients presenting to a regional

trauma center, 40% had multiple injuries (25% with closed head injury, 26% associated major injuries in the same extremity).[3]

## NATURAL HISTORY

- Closed treatment of radius or both-bone forearm fractures generally yields unacceptable results.[1]
- Plate fixation using 3.5-mm compression plates of radial and ulnar fractures is the standard of care yielding good or excellent functional results and union rates greater than 95%.[3]
- Restoration of forearm rotation depends on obtaining proper skeletal length and axial and rotational alignment.[11]

## PATIENT HISTORY AND PHYSICAL FINDINGS

- Evaluate for life-threatening injuries first.
- When there is obvious injury to the forearm, it should be examined last so that satisfaction of search does not result in missed injuries.
- Examination begins at the neck and shoulder girdle away from the injured area. In an awake, cooperative patient, palpation of each bony structure will typically reveal injury for which imaging should be obtained. In an uncooperative or intubated patient, a very low threshold for obtaining imaging is needed.
- It is particularly important to palpate the radial head, collateral ligaments of the elbow, distal radius and ulna, and triangular fibrocartilage complex to avoid missing soft tissue, Monteggia, or Galeazzi injuries. If a ligamentous or tendinous injury is suspected in the setting of a stable joint, a magnetic resonance imaging (MRI) scan is ordered to make the diagnosis and allow for early repair if indicated.
- Usually, obvious gross deformity is present when both the radius and ulna are fractured, but isolated radius or ulna fractures are easily missed especially in a polytrauma, intubated, or noncommunicative patient.
- It is critical that the forearm compartments be visualized in their entirety and palpated to assess for compartment syndrome. All splints and dressings must be removed so the skin can be examined circumferentially. The signs and symptoms of compartment syndrome should be checked and documented even when they are "negative."
- The neurovascular examination at a minimum should include an assessment of radial and ulnar pulses and a detailed documented examination of the sensorimotor function of the median, radial, and ulnar nerves. Preoperative AIN function should be documented as well.

## IMAGING AND OTHER DIAGNOSTIC STUDIES

- Anteroposterior and lateral radiographs of the forearm, wrist, and elbow generally suffice.
- Careful scrutiny of the DRUJ and radiocapitellar joint alignment are performed on wrist and elbow radiographs.
- In comminuted fractures, contralateral imaging of the uninjured forearm and wrist is helpful to determine the patient's native bony alignment and ulnar variance.

## DIFFERENTIAL DIAGNOSIS

- Radial shaft fracture with DRUJ injury (Galeazzi fracture)
- Ulnar fracture with radiocapitellar dislocation (Monteggia fracture)
- Compartment syndrome

## NONOPERATIVE MANAGEMENT

- Nonoperative care is reserved for middle or distal third isolated ulnar fractures with no associated injury to the proximal radioulnar joint (PRUJ) or DRUJ. Proximal fractures are rarely treated nonoperatively.
  - Generally, greater than 50% of bony overlap and less than 15 degrees of angulation are appropriate for nonoperative management.
  - Distal fractures can be maintained in a fracture brace or short-arm cast. Midshaft fractures can be immobilized in "Munster cast" as described earlier or in a fracture brace.
  - The duration of immobilization is until pain subsides and the patient can tolerate mobilization. Weight bearing through the extremity is avoided until there is clinical and radiographic evidence of fracture union. Early mobilization may lead to more rapid union.[2]
- Rarely, stable isolated nondisplaced radius shaft fractures can be treated in a cast or functional brace that allows elbow flexion and extension but no forearm rotation.
- Radiographic union can be expected between 8 and 10 weeks.

## SURGICAL MANAGEMENT

- The two primary goals of treatment are to obtain union and restore function. The primary surgical aim is the stable restoration of length, angular alignment, and rotational alignment.
- Approach
  - Separate approaches are needed for the radius and ulna to minimize the risk of synostosis.
  - Radius fixation is performed through an anterior or a posterior approach. Anterior fixation minimizes but does not eliminate the possibility for symptomatic hardware. Anterior fixation is straightforward for middle-third and distal-third radius fractures but is more difficult in proximal-third fractures. The posterior approach has traditionally been recommended for the middle-third radius fracture but is rarely used. The posterior approach is most helpful during proximal radius exposure but care needs to be taken to protect the PIN.
  - The entire ulna can be exposed through a subcutaneous approach. Plate fixation can be on the subcutaneous surface, anterior surface, or dorsal surface.
- Internal fixation
  - The order of operation in both-bone forearm fractures depends on the degree of comminution of each bone. Typically, the less comminuted bone is fixed first so as to have the most precise restoration of length.
  - Radius fractures are stabilized with the arm extended, whereas the ulna is typically stabilized with elbow flexed 90 degrees. Therefore, if indicated, radius fixation first allows a stable forearm during elbow flexion for ulnar fixation.
  - 3.5-mm compression plates with six cortices of fixation on either side of the fracture are the standard of care. Anatomic and straight plates are available with locking and nonlocking screw options. Comminuted fractures may require bridge plating. Anatomic plates are very helpful for restoring the radial bow.
  - In osteoporotic fractures, the use of locking screws is indicated.

- Locked plates are also indicated when bridging a defect or when one segment is very short and six cortices of fixation cannot be achieved.
- Care must be taken to ensure plates and screws placed on the both the distal ulna and the proximal radius does not impinge in each respective radioulnar joint. Locked unicortical screws must sometimes be used to avoid screw tip prominence in the joint. Live intraoperative fluoroscopic examination is used to assessing screw placement near the DRUJ or PRUJ. Additionally, it is critical to pronosupinate the forearm to ensure there is no plate impingement in these joints.

- Bone grafting
  - Controversy exists regarding the role of acute autologous bone grafting. Use in the setting of comminuted segments of devascularized bone may be one indication.[6,7]
- Closure
  - The tourniquet must always be taken down and meticulous hemostasis obtained.
  - Fascia is left open and only skin and subcutaneous tissues are approximated.
  - When there is significant swelling that results in a tight closure, skin should be left open, and a delayed primary closure is usually obtainable after 72 hours.
  - Soft well-padded dressings with no tight circumferential wrapping minimize the risk of postoperative compartment syndrome.
- Special circumstances
  - If the patient presents with signs and symptoms of compartment syndrome, they should be taken STAT to the operating room for decompressive fasciotomy of the forearm and carpal tunnel at a minimum. Typically, a single volar incision fasciotomy with release of superficial and deep fascial structures will suffice in decompressing the forearm compartments. Mobile wad and dorsal extensor compartments and hand compartments need to be critically evaluated following volar fasciotomy. They should be released if any suspicion exists for compartment syndrome of these compartments.
  - When large areas of bone loss are present, bridge plating is useful to keep the forearm bones out to the proper length. Consider using stainless steel plates, rather than titanium, because of their greater strength.
    - Dissection should be kept at a minimum in anticipation of further reconstruction, and if a vascularized bone graft is anticipated, no unnecessary vascular dissection should be performed in order to protect recipient arteries and veins needed for final reconstruction.

## Preoperative Planning

- Preoperatively, the surgeon needs to decide the approach and the type of fixation required.
- Approach
  - Middle- and distal-third radius fractures are stabilized through a volar approach.
  - Proximal-third fractures can be stabilized through either a volar or posterior approach. Proximal-third fractures requiring exposure of the radial neck are approached dorsally.
- Internal fixation
  - Plate selection for radius fractures depends on a variety of factors including the location of the fracture, fracture pattern, bone defects, quality of the bone, patient compliance, and size of the patient.
  - In proximal radius fractures, fixation of the proximal segment is frequently limited to two screws. The bone of the proximal radius near the radial tuberosity is more cancellous than cortical in nature, limiting screw purchase. Therefore, the use of locking plates and screws in the proximal segment can provide more reliable, stable internal fixation when the number of screws is limited. Additionally, when placed on the anterior radius surface, pronation must be evaluated for plate impingement between the ulna and biceps tendon at this level. A palpable clunk may be noted during pronation. If so, plate placement may need to be revised, but this can be difficult secondary to limited bone stock.
  - For simple pattern midshaft fractures, straight, small fragmentary 3.5-mm compression-type plates suffice with six cortices of fixation on each side of the fracture. A seven-hole plate is typically chosen with an open hole left over the fracture site (unless an interfragmentary screw can be placed through this hole).
  - Distal-third radius fractures can be stabilized with long periarticular volar locking plates, some of which incorporate a radial bow. Alternatively, small fragmentary 3.5-mm compression plates can be contoured distally to match the anterior metaphyseal curvature of the distal radius. Additionally, screw purchase in the cancellous distal radius may be poor, and placement of locking screws is sometimes helpful.

## Positioning

- The patient is placed supine with the injured arm out on a radiolucent arm table. A nonsterile pneumatic tourniquet is placed on the upper arm protected by a stockinette or padding. If acute autologous bone grafting is considered, the ipsilateral anterior iliac crest should be included in the surgical field.

## Approach

- For radius fractures, an anterior approach as described by Henry[5] or posterior approach as described by Thompson[10] may be used.
- All radius fractures, except those extending to the radial neck and head, can be stabilized through a volar approach. One should consider the following when choosing an approach to the proximal radius:
  - In proximal fractures, there is more depth in the volar approach than the posterior approach, sometimes limiting visualization.
  - The volar approach is between the flexor mass as it comes to its confluence at the medial humerus and the biceps tendon insertion on the radial tuberosity. This limits the soft tissue mobility significantly again, sometimes limiting visualization.
  - Large caliber vascular structures and a network of tortuous veins make wide exposure of the bone more difficult in the volar approach.
  - After identification and protection of the PIN, the posterior approach provides wide exposure of the tension side of the radius. Unfortunately, the PIN crosses the radius in proximal fractures, which make hardware placement more tedious and hardware removal, if needed, challenging.

## Anterior (Volar) Approach to the Radius

- Light exsanguination is performed by elevation or loose wrapping with a sterile Ace wrap and the tourniquet is inflated.
- The incision is drawn centered on the fracture from the lateral edge of the biceps tendon to the radial styloid. Length depends on the degree of comminution but in general will comprise approximately one-third of the forearm length (**TECH FIG 1A**).
- An incision is made through the skin only, followed by blunt dissection down to the fascia. Attention is paid to visualization of the lateral antebrachial cutaneous nerve (**TECH FIG 1B**). (We generally score the skin with our knife blade then deepen the incision with a needle tip cautery through the dermis to aid in hemostasis at the skin level.)
  - Small branches of the lateral antebrachial cutaneous nerve if encountered are sacrificed to mobilize the main nerve out of the field of dissection.
- A sponge can be used to sweep away the deep fat off the fascia if needed.
- The fascia is incised and released with scissors.
- The radial artery and venae comitantes must be identified and mobilized. In the proximal third of the forearm, the radial artery lies deep to the brachioradialis muscle belly, which at this level nears the midline of the anterior forearm.
- Bipolar cauterization of perforators to the brachioradialis muscle allows mobilization of the radial artery medially.
- In the middle third of the forearm, the radial artery is more superficial—often in a layer of fat just beneath the fascia—as it exits the interval between brachioradialis muscle belly and flexor carpi radialis muscle belly (**TECH FIG 1C**). Again, the artery is mobilized medially.
- In the distal third of the forearm, it is sometimes safer to mobilize the radial artery laterally, and in the very distal forearm, the approach can be made through the floor of the flexor carpi radialis, thereby avoiding the radial artery completely.
- In the proximal forearm, the muscular envelope is deep, and dissection proceeds along the medial edge of brachioradialis.
- The superficial radial nerve is identified, and care is taken not to place retractors directly on the nerve.
- The supinator will be identified by the oblique muscle fiber orientation, and the surgeon must be mindful that the PIN runs proximal-medial to distal-lateral, entering 90 degrees to the orientation of the muscle fibers and fascia.
  - With the radius broken, it is difficult to effectively supinate the proximal forearm in order to protect the PIN.
  - If the bone is exposed distal to the supinator, a reduction forceps can be placed on the bone and the assistant can supinate the proximal radius. This allows the muscle to be peeled with a freer elevator or knife in a medial to lateral direction, safely keeping the PIN laterally.
  - Alternatively, the PIN can be identified, although this is usually not necessary.
- When dissecting near the biceps tuberosity, usually, a small amount of clear, thick fluid from the biceps bursae will be released as dissection nears the biceps insertion. This burst of fluid is helpful in orienting the surgeon to their location. Just proximal to this, there are typically multiple crossing vessels that need not be disturbed. They can be retracted en masse with a blunt retractor if necessary.

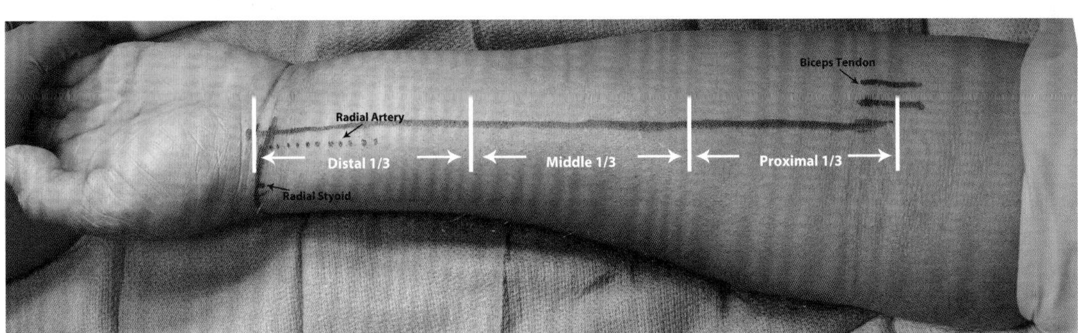


A

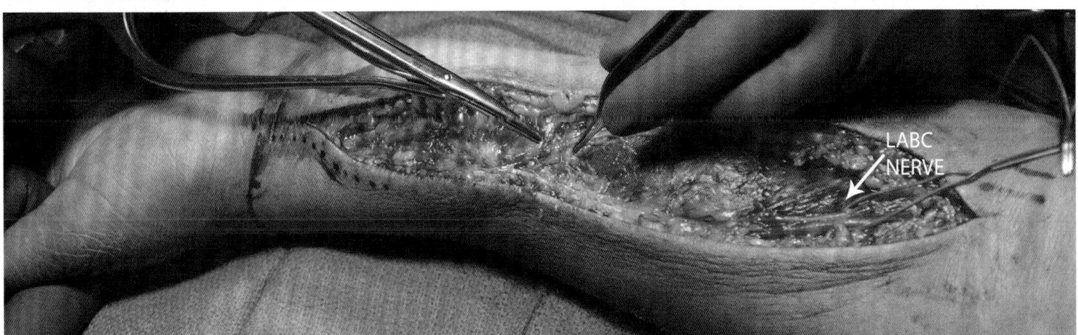


B

**TECH FIG 1** • Anterior approach to the radius. **A.** The forearm is mentally divided in thirds. Each third has unique anatomic structures that must be recognized during the approach. Extensile exposure extends from the biceps tendon to the radial styloid. Distal-third fractures can alternatively be approached through the floor of the flexor carpi radialis (FCR) tendon. **B.** Blunt dissection is performed superficially, and the main trunk of the lateral antebrachial cutaneous nerve (LABC) is identified and protected. *(continued)*

- The most efficient dissection to the middle and distal thirds of the radius proceeds down to its lateral border. Proximally, where the supinator lies the dissection on the medial radius avoids the PIN.
  - In the middle third of the radius, the flexor digitorum profundus and pronator teres can be sharply released from lateral to medial.
  - The pronator teres can be Z-lengthened or taken off the bone in a subperiosteal fashion. Alternatively, if only a limited amount of exposure is needed, its muscle fibers can be dissected off the tendinous portion for a short distance, leaving the tendon intact. If taken off the radius, it can be sutured back down to the plate (**TECH FIG 1D**). Our preference is the latter during extensile exposures.
  - Distally, the flexor pollicis longus and pronator quadratus are taken off the radius laterally to medially with a knife.
- Bone fixation techniques are then performed as described in the following text (**TECH FIG 1G**).
- The tourniquet is always taken down. If a meticulous dissection has been performed with liberal use of bipolar cautery, little bleeding is encountered.
- Fascia is not closed, but inverted interrupted absorbable monofilament suture is used as needed to reapproximate the subcutaneous tissues followed by 3-0 nylon suture for the skin.

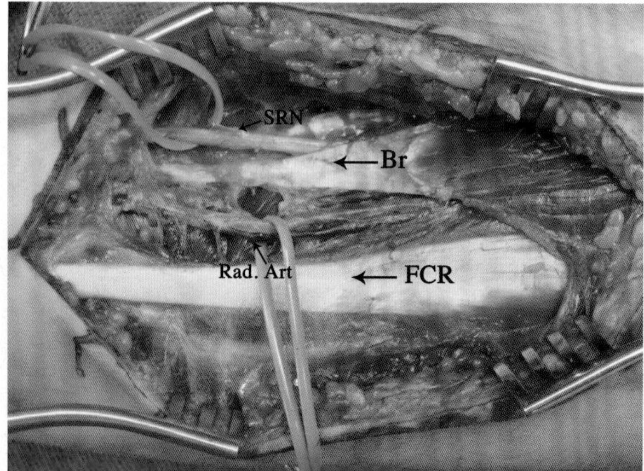


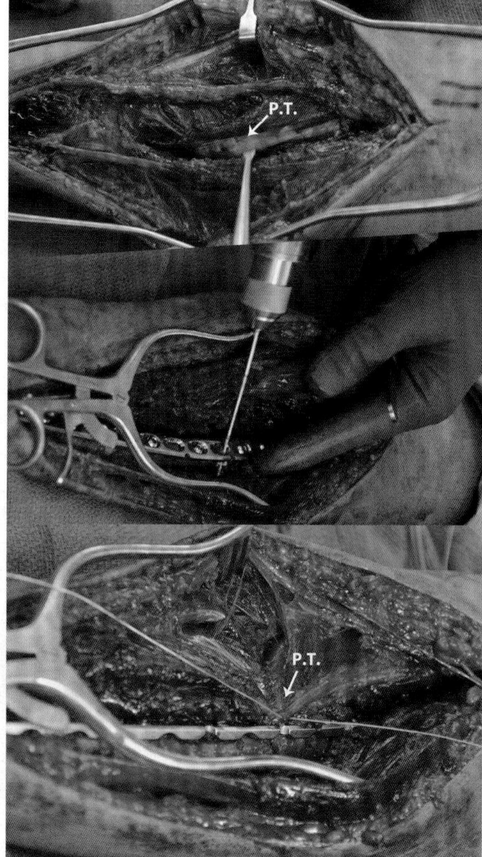


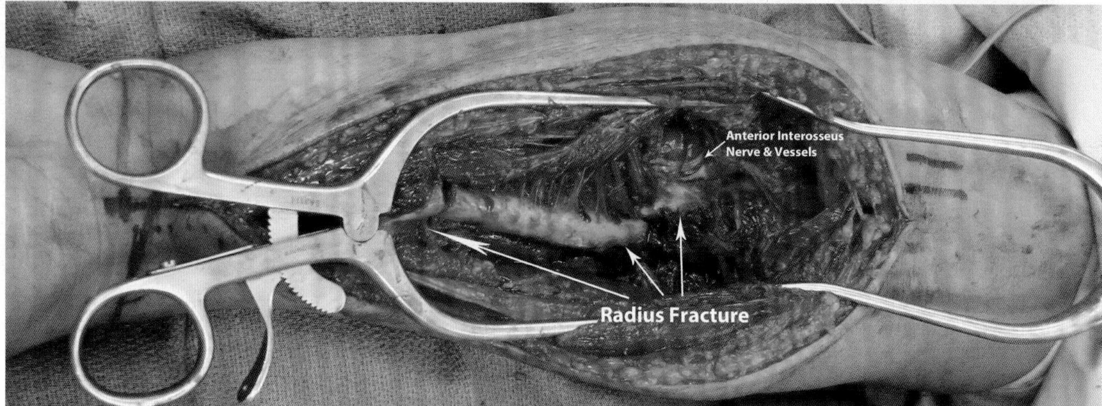


**TECH FIG 1** • *(continued)* **C.** In the middle third, the radial artery (*Rad. Art*) and venae comitantes are identified exiting between brachioradialis (*Br*) and flexor carpi radialis (*FCR*). Light exsanguination assists in identifying vascular structures. The superficial radial nerve (*SRN*) is seen coursing between Br and FCR. **D.** The *upper* images demonstrate the pronator teres (*P.T.*) insertion on the radius. *Middle* image demonstrates drill hole placed through plate hole and radius for reattachment of P.T. (*lower* image). **E.** A segmental radius fracture and the AIN and vessel closely approximated to the proximal fragment. *(continued)*

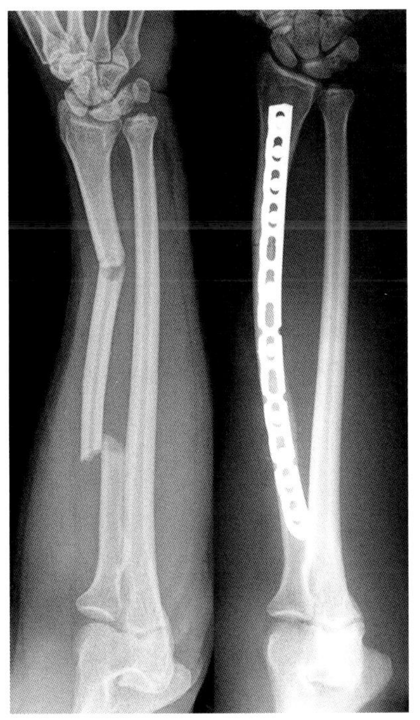

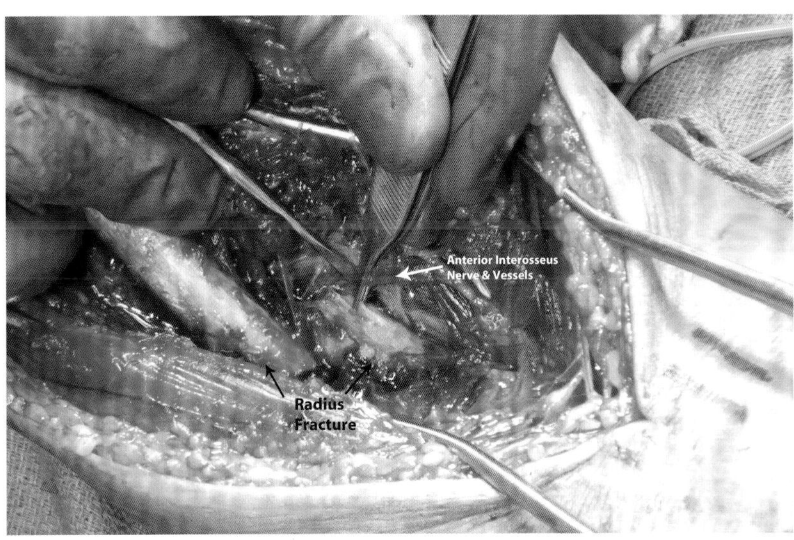


**TECH FIG 1** • *(continued)* **F.** Retraction of vessels with a Freer, allowing safe exposure of radius. **G.** Anatomic plate fixation of the segmental radius fracture with restoration of the radial bow.

## Posterior Approach to the Radius

- The posterior approach is typically used for proximal- or middle-third radius shaft fractures. Extensile exposure of the entire proximal and middle thirds of the radius is described in the following text.
- An incision is drawn from the lateral epicondyle of the humerus to Lister tubercle and centered on the fracture.
  - The incision length typically approximates one-third the length of the radius centered at the fracture (**TECH FIG 2A**).
  - Blunt dissection is performed down to the level of the fascia, and small fasciocutaneous flaps are elevated. Perforating fasciocutaneous vessels can usually be seen and cauterized with a needle-tip cautery.
  - Proximally, the interval lies between the white, thick tendinous band of the extensor digitorum communis tendon at the confluence of the extensor mass and the muscle belly of the extensor carpi radialis brevis just anterior to it (**TECH FIG 2B**).
  - It is important to identify the tendinous origin of the extensor digitorum communis, as the radial portion of the lateral collateral ligament complex of the elbow lies directly deep to it.
  - The fascia is incised just anterior to the white, thick tendinous band, and a Freer elevator is used to elevate the muscle fibers off the septum.
  - The deep facial layer is then carefully opened with scissors in a distal to proximal direction revealing the supinator muscle, identified by the changing direction of muscle fibers proximal/posterior to distal/anterior (**TECH FIG 2C**).
  - The PIN enters the supinator approximately 90 degrees to the orientation of its muscle fibers. By lifting the radial wrist extensors and brachioradialis off of the supinator with a blunt retractor, one can frequently identify the PIN entering the supinator.
  - Alternatively, the PIN is identified distally and traced proximally through the supinator (**TECH FIG 2D,E**).
- In the middle third of the radius, the abductor pollicis longus and extensor pollicis brevis are identified and elevated off the radius sharply for exposure.

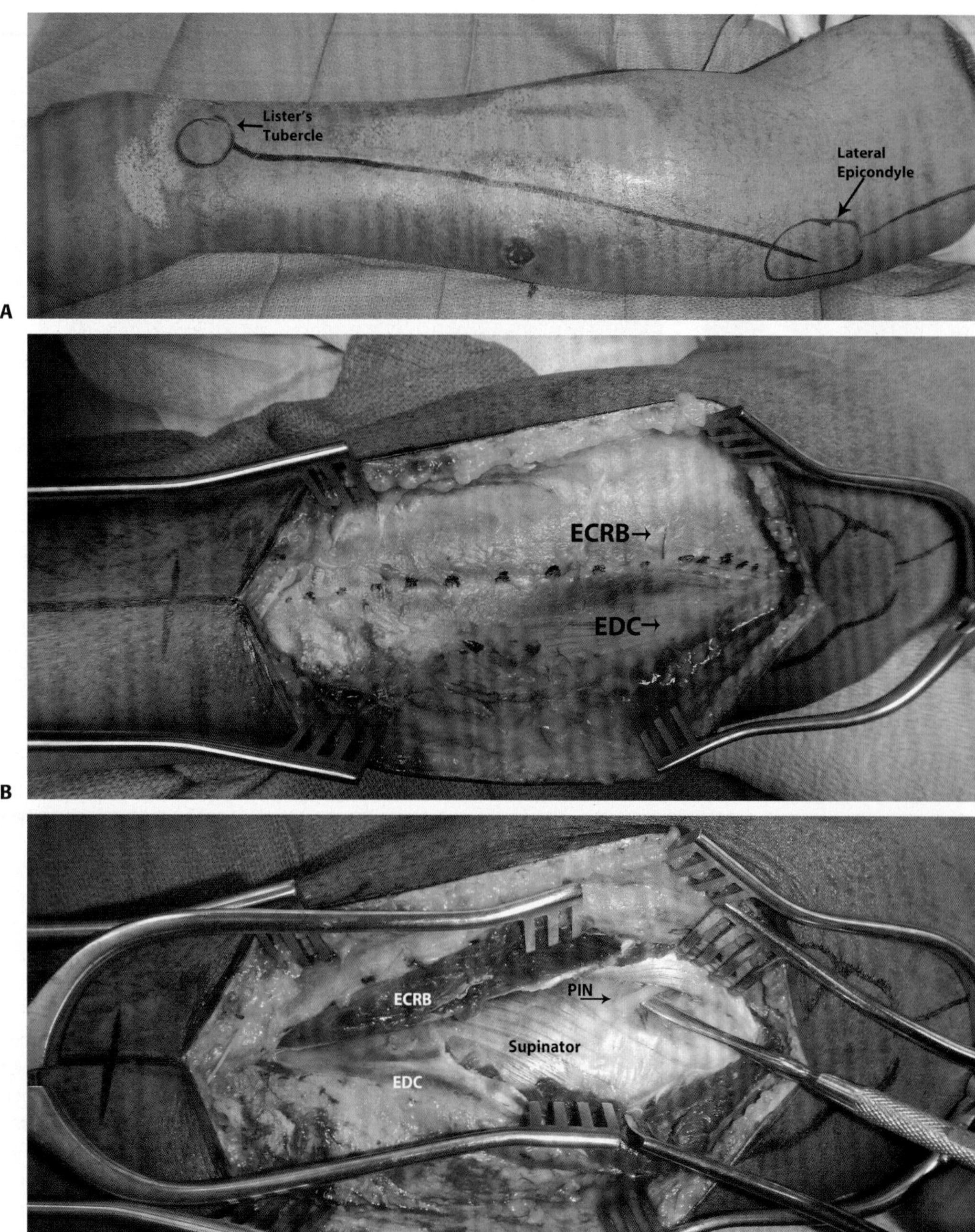


**TECH FIG 2** • Posterior approach to the radius. **A.** Extensile exposure (lateral humeral epicondyle to Lister tubercle). **B.** Proximal interval is located between extensor digitorum communis (*EDC*) and extensor carpi radialis brevis (*ECRB*). **C.** The deep fascia of ECRB and EDC has been divided, and the oblique fibers of the supinator are now visualized. The posterior interosseous nerve (PIN) can be seen entering supinator perpendicular to its fibers. *(continued)*

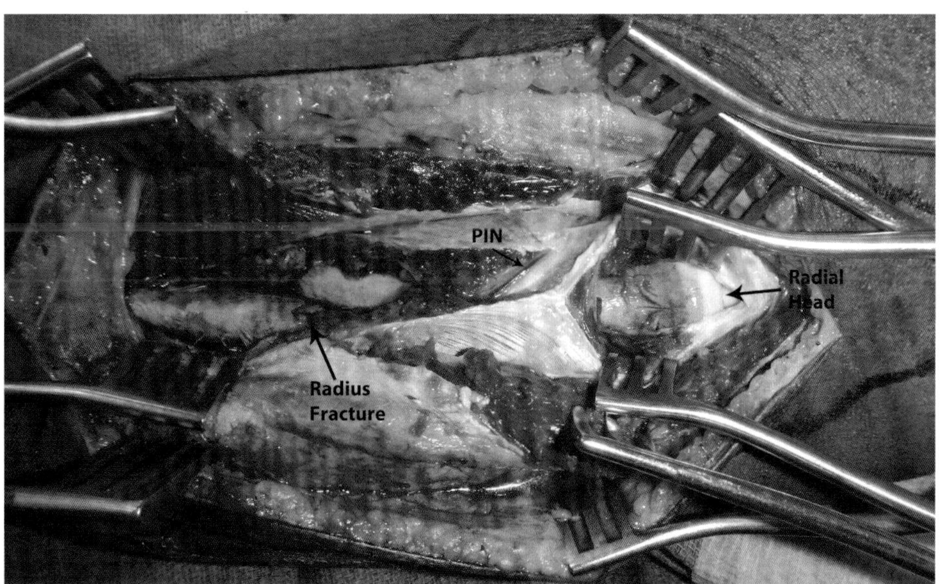


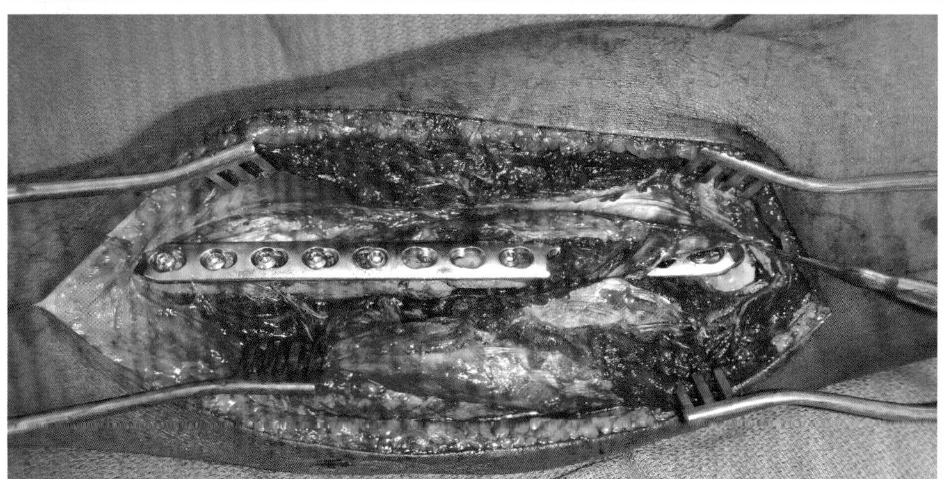


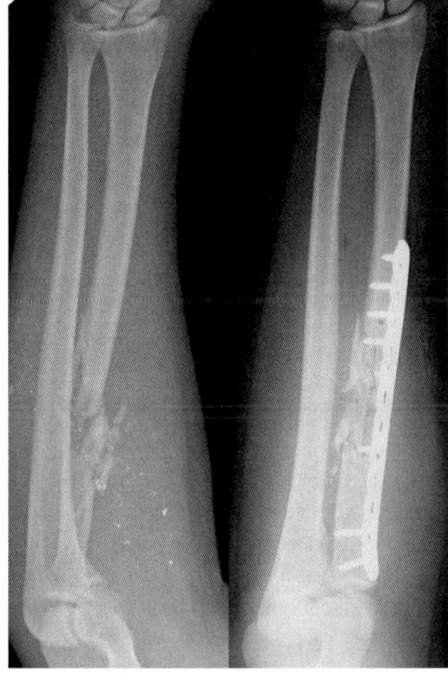


**TECH FIG 2** • *(continued)* **D.** The supinator has been partially divided to reveal the PIN coursing through its substance. The radial head is seen proximally and the radius fracture is seen distally. **E.** A 3.5-mm locking compression plate has been applied to the proximal radius. In this case, only two screws of proximal fixation were available, therefore locking screws were used. **F.** Pre and postoperative radiographs demonstrating bridge plating of this comminuted proximal radius fracture. A 3.5-mm locking plate was utilized. Proximally, the plate placement must be scrutinized to avoid impingement during forearm pronosupination. In our experience, this fracture is at significant risk for infection and nonunion. Acute bone grafting was not performed secondary to concern for infection.

## Approach to the Ulna

- The incision is drawn from the olecranon to the ulnar styloid centered on the fracture.
- After incision, blunt dissection down to the ulnar shaft is performed (**TECH FIG 3A**).
- In the distal third of the ulna, care must be taken not to injure the dorsal ulnar cutaneous nerve branch, which is typically found in the subcutaneous tissues just distal to the ulnar styloid, passing obliquely in a proximal-volar to distal-dorsal direction, obliquely to the dorsum of the hand. Rarely, it crosses the ulna more proximally.
- Once the ulna has been identified, sharp dissection readily exposes bone needed for fracture reduction and stabilization as previously described (**TECH FIG 3B,C**).

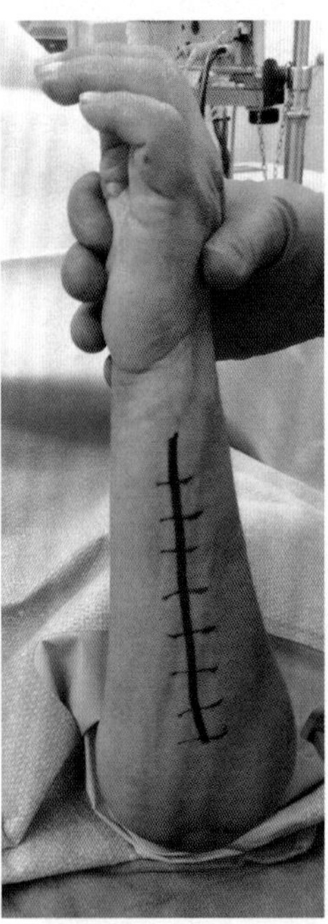
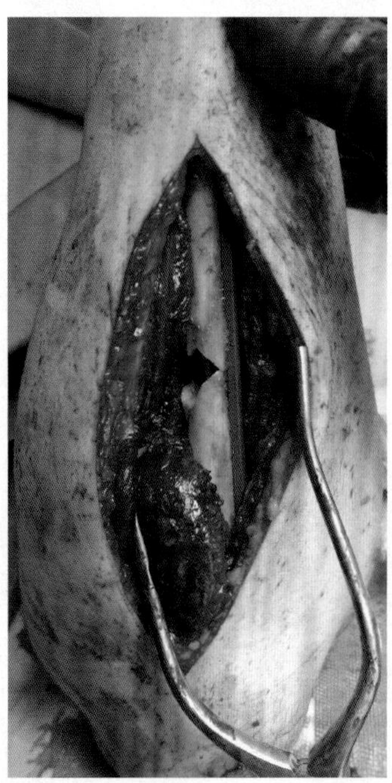
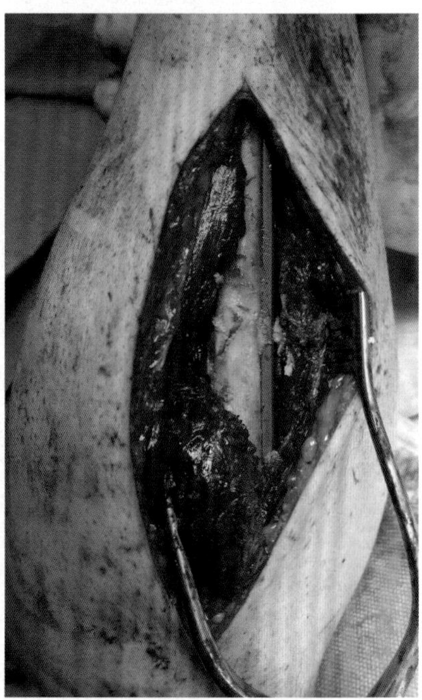

**TECH FIG 3** • Approach to the ulna. **A.** Incision drawn along the ulnar subcutaneous border. **B.** Open reduction and internal fixation (ORIF) of the ulna with comminuted butterfly fragment with dorsal plate. **C.** Comminuted butterfly fragment and supplemental allograft bone graft fills the defect. (Autograft bone grafting for this type of defect may be preferred. This can be performed acutely in closed fractures if necessary.)

## Fracture Reduction

- To stabilize transverse or short oblique fractures, the plate is applied on the distal fragment first affixing a far hole and then a near hole centered on the bony fragment.
  - Next, the proximal fragment is reduced and held reduced with reduction forceps while standard compression screws are placed.
  - A seven-hole, 3.5-mm compression plate with the open hole over the fracture site is typically used with three bicortical nonlocking screws placed on each side of the fracture.
  - Consider overbending the plate slightly into a concave configuration to compress the side of the fracture opposite the plate.
- For transverse fractures with a butterfly fragment, our preference is to reduce and stabilize the butterfly fragment with a free screw outside the plate. Often, this screw may be a 2.4-mm cortical screw.
  - Typically, a lag technique is not used unless the butterfly piece is large enough to accommodate two screws. The butterfly fragment is held reduced with a pointed reduction clamp and a bicortical screw is placed. A bicortical rather than lag screw is used to allow greater fixation in a small piece of bone that is already compressed using the clamp. If lag screw fixation is attempted and fails, it is usually impossible to affix the butterfly fragment.
  - This turns a three-part fracture into a two-part fracture, which is stabilized as earlier except aggressive compression is avoided so as to not displace the previously fixed butterfly fragment.
  - In our experience, even devascularized butterfly fragments typically unite when well fixed.
- Bridge plating using an anatomic plate is performed for comminuted fractures.
- Again, the plate is centered and fixed to the radius on one side of the comminuted segment. The assistant applies manual traction through the hand, and fluoroscopy is used until the desired length is achieved. The plate is then fixed to the other side of the comminuted segment.
  - If pulling the traction and affixing the plate is too cumbersome, the radius and ulna are pinned together with a 1.6-mm or 2-mm smooth stainless steel pin near the DRUJ to maintain the desired ulnar variance while plate fixation to the distal segment is applied.

- Full-length forearm or wrist films of the uninjured forearm in supination are very helpful in determining the correct bone length (intraoperative fluoroscopic imaging of the uninjured forearm and wrist can be used is preoperative imaging is not available). Ulnar variance is used a comparative marker of length.
- Long anatomic distal radius plates can be helpful for distal radial shaft fractures, particularly when bone quality is poor and more plate length is desired.
  - If 3.5-mm compression plates are used on the volar distal radial shaft, the distal segment of the plate should be contoured to match the slope of the distal radius.
  - Distally, the bone is cancellous in nature and cancellous-type screws may be preferred to gain better screw purchase.
- Despite the possibility of symptomatic hardware, proximal ulnar fractures are plated on the subcutaneous surface.
  - This surface has minimal sagittal bow and better resists angular stresses of elbow flexion and extension.
- Middle- and distal-third ulnar fractures can be plated anteriorly or posteriorly.
- Again, the plate is typically affixed first to the more narrow fragment of the fracture. Next, the fracture is reduced and the other fragment is fixed using compression technique.
- Combination plates (3.5-mm dynamic tubular plate [DCP]–one-third tubular) are helpful in balancing fixation plate strength and prominent hardware concerns in distal-third ulnar fractures. In very distal ulnar fractures, 90-90 fixation with locking hand modular plates, 2.5 mm or larger, may be helpful.
- When longer plate constructs are used on the radius (as in bridge plating or in the presence of a butterfly fragment), care must be taken to restore the radial bow to ensure the recovery of normal forearm rotation.
  - This may require either contouring of the plate chosen or use of an anatomic plate.

## PEARLS AND PITFALLS

| | |
|---|---|
| **Compartment syndrome** | ▪ Strictly avoid regional anesthetic when bony stabilization is done within the first several days from injury or when there is any significant swelling to avoid masking a compartment syndrome.<br>▪ Never close the forearm fascia. Discuss preoperatively that the skin may need to be left open with planned delayed closure 2–3 days later.<br>▪ If presenting with compartment syndrome, proceed with STAT decompressive fasciotomy, plating, primary closure of the ulnar wound, and delayed closure of the volar forearm wound. |
| **Light exsanguination** | ▪ Light exsanguination allows easy identification of vessels for mobilization and cauterization minimizing the risk of postoperative bleeding (see **TECH FIG 1C,E**). |
| **Transverse fractures** | ▪ This fracture pattern is difficult to hold reduced with clamps: First, fix plate to one side of the fracture using the hole farthest from the fracture and then fix the plate using the hole closest to the fracture. Last, reduce the other fractured segment and continue with compression plating. |
| **Oblique fractures with butterfly fragments** | ▪ Fix butterfly fragment to one side of fracture first to create a two-part fracture from a three-part fracture. If the fracture dictates that interfragmentary screws are best placed on the same surface of the bone as the plate, place them through the plate as to not interfere with plate placement on the bone. |
| **Comminuted fractures** | ▪ Obtain contralateral x-rays to evaluate "normal" bony architecture and ulnar variance. Strongly consider anatomic plates to aid in fracture reduction and restoration of radial bow. |
| **Osteoporotic fractures** | ▪ Consider longer than typical plate selection and liberal use of locking screws after compression is obtained. |
| **Restoring radial bow in posterior approaches** | ▪ If anatomic plating is needed during a posterior approach, a straight compression plate can be manually contoured to the edge of an unused anatomic anterior plate to prior to its placement to obtain the proper bow. |

## POSTOPERATIVE CARE

- Bulky, soft fan-folded dressings; loosely placed circumferential cast padding; and a sling are placed.
- Active range of motion of the shoulder, elbow, forearm, wrist, and hand is encouraged. Supervised therapy is recommended with a focus on pronosupination, which is the most difficult motion to recover.
- In patients with a lower pain tolerance, a long posterior splint that stabilizes the forearm in neutral but leaves the fingers free is placed. At the first postoperative visit, all immobilization is discontinued.
- Supervised therapy is recommended for patients not demonstrating improvement with self-directed range-of-motion exercises.

## OUTCOMES

- Classically, Anderson and colleagues[1] defined an excellent result as fracture union with less than a 10 degree loss of wrist or elbow motion and less than 25% loss of forearm rotation. They reported 54% excellent results in compression plating of 106 both-bone fractures.[1] Using the same criteria, Chapman and colleagues[3] reported 86% excellent results in the treatment of both-bone fractures.

- Recently, Goldfarb and colleagues[4] used the Disability of the Arm, Shoulder, and Hand (DASH) and the musculoskeletal functional attachment (MFA) validated outcome measures to assess functional outcomes of both-bone forearm fractures treated with 3.5-mm compression plates.
  - They reported that pronation was significantly reduced compared to the uninjured limb.
  - Additionally, the outcome questionnaires found a subjective decrease in function when the range of motion of the forearm and wrist were less than the contralateral limb. Overall, outcomes based on DASH and MFA were considered good.[4]

## COMPLICATIONS

- Larger series demonstrate an approximate 2% rate of postoperative infection.[3]
- Other postoperative complications include compartment syndrome, nerve injury, radioulnar synostosis, failure of fixation, and symptomatic hardware. Use of 4.5-mm compression plates has been associated with a higher incidence of refracture following plate removal presumable from the larger holes.[3]
- Nonunion is rare in simple pattern radius and ulnar shaft fracture. Those with segmental defects may go onto nonunion and need to be followed closely postoperatively. Smoking cessation and metabolic optimization may minimize nonunion development.
- Rotational malunion of radius fractures will significantly limit pronosupination, which is very difficult to correct.
- Superficial radial nerve parasthesias and dysthesias are not infrequent following radial shaft fracture fixation. These typically resolve and likely related to overretraction during anterior exposure.
- Iatrogenic AIN injury can occur with the use of monopolar cautery along the ulnar border of the radius (bipolar cautery should be used).
  - Additionally, the nerve can be injured by the placement of reduction clamps around the radius if care is not taken to stay close to bone with the clamp.
- Proximally placed volar radius plates can impinge between the radius, ulna, and biceps tendon. This may be discovered during intraoperative pronosupination testing.
  - Unfortunately, due to the limited bone stock, repositioning the plate once placed may not be possible. Planned hardware removal may be considered in these circumstances.
- When distal periarticular plates are used, especially long plates, it is imperative the plate fully contact the bone because it can irritate the flexor tendons if it is off bone.
- With no exceptions, the tourniquet must be taken down and meticulous hemostasis obtained.
  - Compartment syndrome can result from a bleeding subcutaneous vein even when the fascia is left open.

## REFERENCES


1. Anderson LD, Sisk TD, Tooms RE, et al. Compression-plate fixation in acute diaphyseal fractures of the radius and ulna. J Bone Joint Surg Am 1975;57(3):287–297.
2. Cai XZ, Yan SG, Giddins G. A systematic review of the non-operative treatment of nightstick fractures of the ulna. J Bone Joint Surg Br 2013;95-B(7):952–959.
3. Chapman MW, Gordon JE, Zissimos AG. Compression-plate fixation of acute fractures of the diaphysis of the radius and ulna. J Bone Joint Surg Am 1989;71(2):159–169.
4. Goldfarb CA, Ricci WM, Tull F, et al. Functional outcome after fracture of both bones of the forearm. J Bone Joint Surg Br 2005; 87(3):374–379.
5. Henry AK. Extensile Exposure, ed 2. Baltimore: Williams & Wilkins, 1970.
6. Moed BR, Kellam JF, Foster RJ, et al. Immediate internal fixation of open fractures of the diaphysis of the forearm. J Bone Joint Surg Am 1986;68(7):1008–1017.
7. Ring D, Rhim R, Carpenter C, et al. Comminuted diaphyseal fractures of the radius and ulna: does bone grafting affect nonunion rate? J Trauma 2005;59:438–441.
8. Rouleau DM, Faber KJ, Athwal GS. The proximal ulna dorsal angulation: a radiographic study. J Shoulder Elbow Surg 2010;19(1):26–30.
9. Rupasinghe SL, Poon PC. Radius morphology and its effects on rotation with contoured and noncontoured plating of the proximal radius. J Shoulder Elbow Surg 2012;21:568–573.
10. Thompson JE. Anatomical methods of approach in operations on the long bones of the extremities. Ann Surg 1918;68:309–329.
11. Trousdale RT, Linscheid RL. Operative treatment of malunited fractures of the forearm. J Bone Joint Surg Am 1995;77(6):894–902.

# Open Reduction and Internal Fixation of Displaced Lateral Condyle Fractures of the Humerus

5 CHAPTER

Kristan A. Pierz and Brian G. Smith

## DEFINITION

- Lateral condyle fractures refer to fractures of the outer (lateral) aspect of the distal humerus and may involve any or all of the following: metaphysis, physis, epiphysis, and articular surface.
- Fractures of the lateral condyle of the distal humerus account for 10% to 15% of all pediatric elbow fractures, second in frequency only to supracondylar distal humerus fractures.[6]
- Nondisplaced fractures may hinge on the articular cartilage, making them more stable than their unstable, displaced counterparts.

## ANATOMY

- Proximally, lateral condyle fractures almost always include some portion of the posterolateral metaphysis and then propagate along the physis before exiting through or around the ossification center of the capitellum.
- The articular cartilage may or may not be violated.
- The extensor carpi radialis longus and brevis muscles and lateral collateral ligament typically remain attached to the distal fragment.
- Anterior and posterior portions of the elbow joint capsule may be torn if there is significant displacement.
- Milch[11] classified lateral condyle fractures based on the distal portion of the fracture line (**FIG 1**).
  - Milch type I fractures (the less common) traverse the metaphysis and physis as well as extend across the ossification center of the lateral condyle.
  - Milch type II fractures (the more common) extend from the metaphysis, through the physis, and exit in the unossified trochlea, medial to the capitellum ossification center. Displacement of the trochlear crista allows lateral translation of the forearm and increases the instability of this pattern.

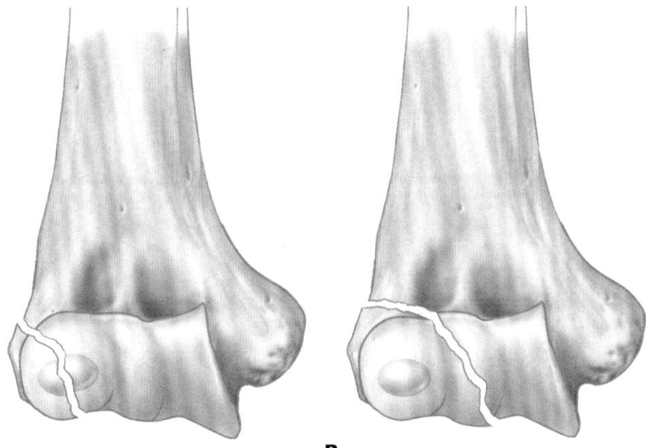


**FIG 1** • Milch classification of lateral condyle fractures is based on location. **A.** Type I fracture line passes through the ossific nucleus of the capitellum. **B.** Type II fracture line passes medial to the capitellar ossific nucleus into the trochlear groove.

- It is difficult to apply the Salter-Harris classification system to lateral condyle fractures because portions of the distal humeral epiphysis may not yet be ossified.
  - A fracture propagating from the metaphysis through the physis and then through the capitellum ossification center (Milch I) is analogous to a Salter-Harris type IV fracture.
  - A fracture that extends from the metaphysis through the physis and exits through the unossified trochlea medial to the capitellar ossification center (Milch II) may appear radiographically analogous to a Salter-Harris type II fracture, but its involvement of the articular cartilage is analogous to Salter-Harris types III and IV.
- A numeric classification system identifies fractures based on displacement.[8,13]
  - Stage I fractures involve the metaphysis and physis but often do not violate the articular cartilage, thus limiting their ability to displace. Displacement is less than 2 mm.
  - Stage II fractures cross the articular surface but are minimally displaced. Displacement is 2 to 4 mm.
  - Stage III fractures are displaced fractures that cross the metaphysis, physis, and articular surface, frequently resulting in rotation of the distal fragment (**FIG 2**).

## PATHOGENESIS

- The typical mechanism for a lateral condyle fracture is a fall on an outstretched hand.
- Adduction of a supinated forearm with the elbow extended can result in avulsion of the lateral condyle.
- Axial load of the forearm combined with valgus force can also propagate a fracture through the lateral condyle.
- Lateral condyle fractures usually occur as isolated injuries, although elbow joint subluxation and radial head or olecranon fractures may be associated.

## NATURAL HISTORY

- The natural history of lateral condyle fractures depends on the fracture displacement as well as the long-term viability of the growing physis.[5]
- Completely nondisplaced lateral condyle fractures may heal regardless of treatment.
- Nondisplaced fractures can displace over time if the articular cartilage is violated or if there is significant associated soft tissue injury.
- Delayed union can occur even in nondisplaced fractures and may be due to poor metaphyseal circulation, bathing of the

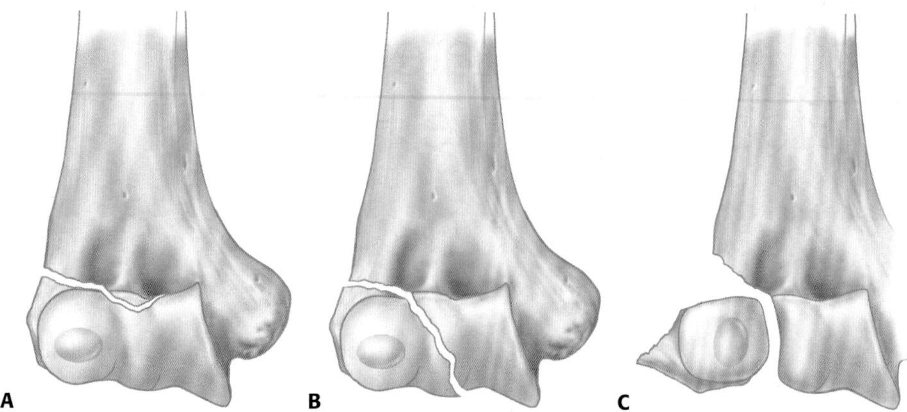


**FIG 2** • Numeric classification of lateral condyle fractures is based on displacement. **A.** Stage I fractures are nondisplaced and do not violate the articular surface. **B.** Stage II fractures violate the articular surface but are minimally displaced (0 to 2 mm). **C.** Stage III fractures are displaced more than 2 mm and may be rotated.

fracture in synovial fluid, or tension on the condylar fragment by attached muscles.

- Fractures that heal in near-anatomic alignment can yield excellent functional and cosmetic outcomes.
- Lateral condyle fractures associated with lateral physeal arrest can result in valgus deformity and tardy ulnar nerve palsy.
- Lateral condyle fractures associated with central physeal arrest can result in a "fishtail" deformity due to continued growth medially and laterally but limited growth in between.

## PATIENT HISTORY AND PHYSICAL FINDINGS

- Most patients report a fall, either on an outstretched hand or from some height, resulting in pain and inability to fully move the elbow.
- It may be difficult to obtain a history from a young child; therefore, parents or caregivers may need to be questioned.
- The clinician should be patient during the physical examination. Young children may be very fearful. The clinician should ask the child to point to what hurts most, and this part should be examined last. This allows the clinician to establish the patient's trust and rule out other associated injuries.
- The clinician should look for obvious deformity, swelling, ecchymosis, and open wounds about the elbow.
- The clinician should assess for pulses and capillary refill.
- Sensation is assessed by comparison with the uninvolved side. Rather than stroking a finger and asking a young child, "Do you feel this?", the clinician can rub the same site on both hands and ask, "Does it feel the same or different?"
- Motor function is assessed by observing for spontaneous movement during the entire encounter. A scared child may refuse to move when asked by a physician but may demonstrate voluntary movement when asked by a parent or sibling. Being playful during the examination can help. For example, when testing for ulnar nerve function, asking a 5-year-old to show you how old he or she is may be more rewarding than asking the child to spread his or her fingers.
- The wrist and shoulder are palpated before touching the elbow.
- A single finger is used to gently palpate the olecranon, medial epicondyle, posterior humerus, lateral condyle, and radial head to try to localize the specific site of injury. Crepitus suggests displacement and instability of the fracture fragment.
- Increased motion during varus stress testing suggests instability of the fracture. Due to pain, however, this test can rarely be done on an awake child. It is often reserved for intraoperative assessment rather than preoperative diagnosis.

## IMAGING AND OTHER DIAGNOSTIC STUDIES

- Radiographs of a suspected lateral condyle fracture should include anteroposterior (AP), lateral, and internal oblique views (**FIG 3A–C**).
- Valgus and varus stress radiographs can provide information about the stability of the fracture. Because such films are poorly tolerated in an awake child, they are rarely obtained outside of the operating room.
- For nondisplaced or minimally displaced fractures, magnetic resonance imaging (MRI) can be used to determine whether the articular surface is violated[7] (**FIG 3D**).
  - Such studies, however, are expensive, are rarely needed for surgical decision making, and frequently require sedation in young children, so they are not obtained routinely.
- Arthrograms can provide detail about the articular congruity of lateral condyle fractures but are typically reserved for intraoperative assessment[10] (**FIG 3E**).

## DIFFERENTIAL DIAGNOSIS

- Contusion
- Lateral collateral ligament strain or sprain
- Radial head or neck fracture
- Supracondylar distal humerus fracture
- Transphyseal fractures
- Medial condyle fractures
- Proximal ulnar or Monteggia fractures
- Elbow dislocation
- Child abuse

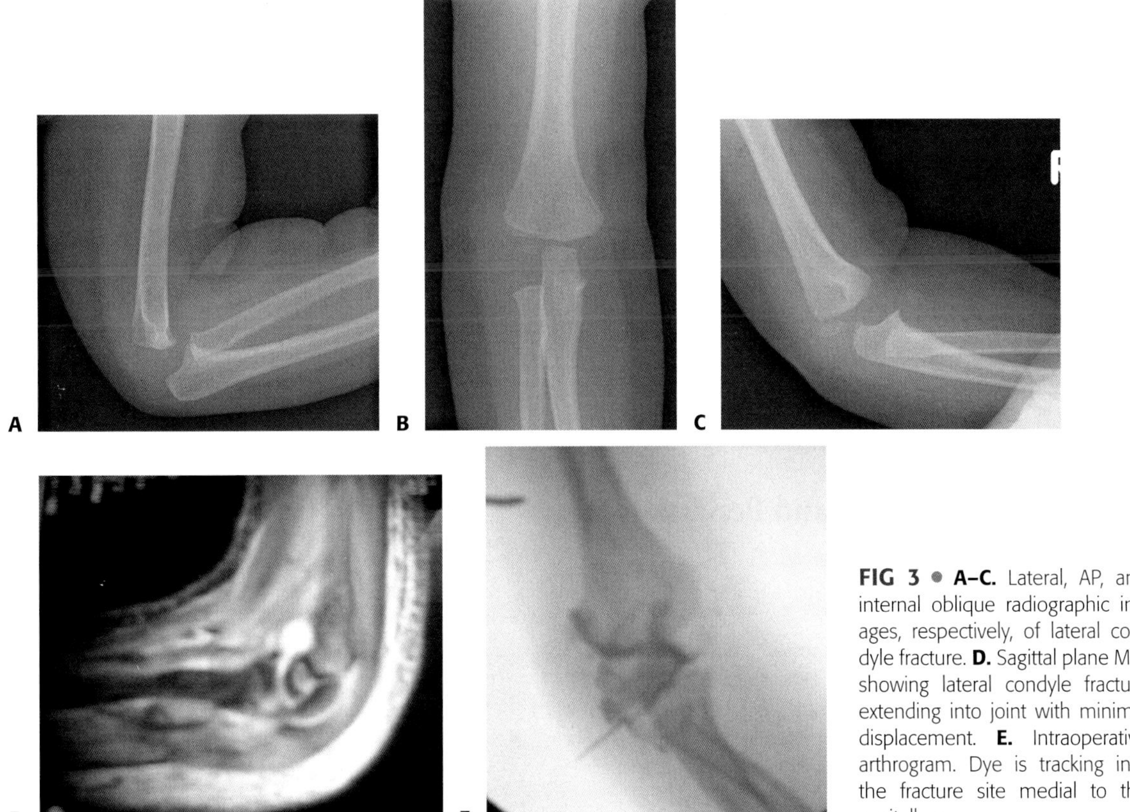

**FIG 3 • A–C.** Lateral, AP, and internal oblique radiographic images, respectively, of lateral condyle fracture. **D.** Sagittal plane MRI showing lateral condyle fracture extending into joint with minimal displacement. **E.** Intraoperative arthrogram. Dye is tracking into the fracture site medial to the capitellum.

## NONOPERATIVE MANAGEMENT

- Nonoperative management of lateral condyle fractures is typically reserved for nondisplaced or minimally displaced (<2 mm) fractures.
- The upper extremity is immobilized in a long-arm splint or cast with the elbow flexed 90 degrees and the forearm in neutral.
  - Casts that are excessively heavy or short on the upper arm tend to slide down, thus increasing the risk of later displacement.
- Follow-up radiographs should be obtained in 3 to 5 days to assess for further displacement.
- If displacement occurs, operative treatment is indicated.
- If the fracture remains nondisplaced, long-arm casting is continued for another week, and then repeat radiographs are obtained.
  - If still nondisplaced, the fracture is maintained in a long-arm cast until there is radiographic evidence of fracture union, typically at 4 to 6 weeks.
- Delayed union may occur, requiring up to 12 weeks of immobilization. Poor vascularization of the fracture fragment and bathing of the fragment in articular fluid may contribute to this phenomenon.

## SURGICAL MANAGEMENT

- Surgery is recommended for lateral condyle fractures with more than 2 mm of displacement or rotational deformity that occurs acutely or during the early follow-up period of nonoperative treatment.[1]
- Closed techniques with percutaneous pinning are reserved for minimally displaced fractures, with a congruous articular surface confirmed by arthrography.
- Open surgery is required for displaced fractures.

### Preoperative Planning

- Preoperatively, a careful neurovascular examination should be performed and documented. Fortunately, unlike supracondylar fractures, isolated lateral condyle fractures rarely have any associated neurovascular injury.
- Plain radiographs, including AP, lateral, and internal oblique views, should be adequate to make the decision to operate.
  - Displacement of more than 2 mm indicates the need for surgical intervention.
- Displacement of more than 2 mm on two or more views suggests instability and often requires open treatment.
- Displacement of more than 2 mm on only one view suggests that the fracture may be hinging on intact articular cartilage and may be treatable by percutaneous techniques.
- Fractures with borderline displacement (2 to 3 mm) may be better assessed under anesthesia, where stress radiographs or an arthrogram can guide treatment.

### Positioning

- The patient is placed in the supine position on the operating table, and general anesthesia is induced.
- The child should be brought to the edge of the operating table to facilitate fluoroscopic imaging of the operative limb (**FIG 4**).

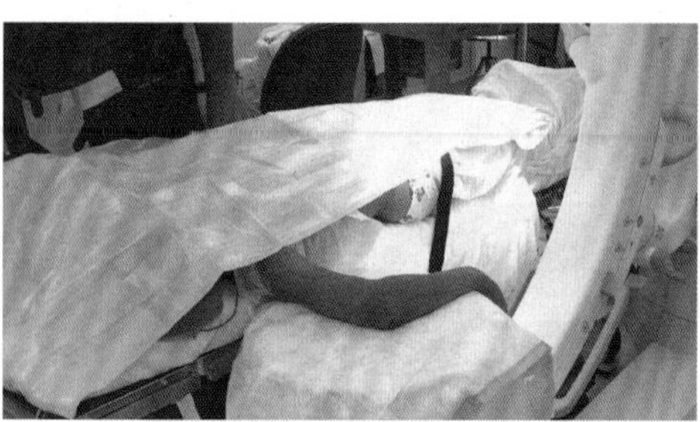

**FIG 4** • Positioning the patient on the edge of the table allows easy access for fluoroscopy. The base of the unit may be used as an arm table.

- Care must be taken to prevent the patient's head from rolling off the table's edge. Placing a foam doughnut under the head can provide stability. Additionally, a small arm board may be attached to the proximal side of the operating table to help support the head.
- The receiving end of a standard fluoroscopy unit can be used as the operative table for the involved limb. Bringing the fluoroscopy unit up from the foot of the bed allows room for the surgeon and assistant to access the lateral side of the elbow.
  - Alternatively, a hand table may be used, and the fluoroscopy unit can be brought in after draping.
- For open cases, a sterile tourniquet is recommended to allow full access to the elbow after draping.



## Closed Reduction and Percutaneous Pinning

- This technique is reserved for minimally displaced (2 to 4 mm) fractures.
- Fracture stability should be assessed under anesthesia with varus stress radiographs and/or arthrography.
- Two divergent smooth pins are recommended. Although 0.062-inch Kirschner wires are usually adequate, 5/64-inch Steinmann pins may be used in larger children.
- The first wire is placed through the skin into the lateral condyle to engage the metaphyseal fragment distally (bicortical purchase).
  - The wire should be directed from distal lateral to proximal medial, penetrating the cortex medially.
- A second wire is then placed in a similar manner, diverging at the fracture site.
  - Increasing the distance between the wires at the fracture site increases stability[2] (**TECH FIG 1A**).
- Wires may cross the ossification center of the capitellum to improve divergence (**TECH FIG 1B,C**).

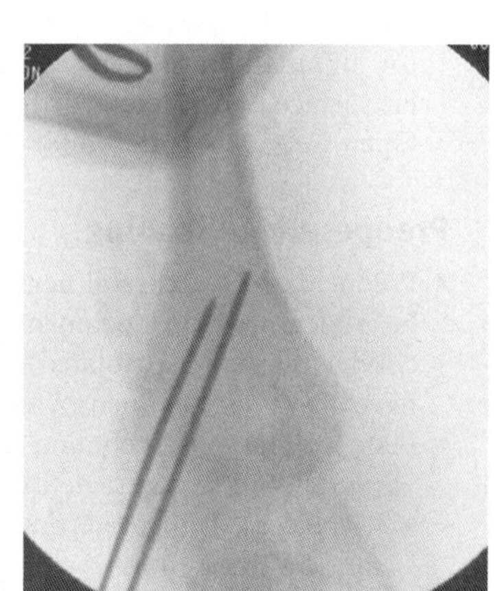
A

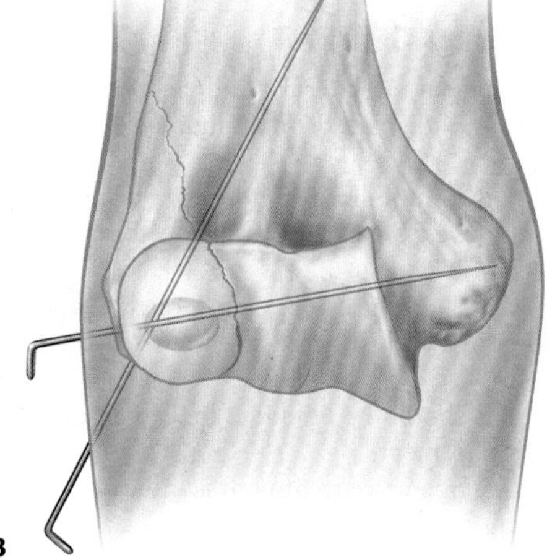
B

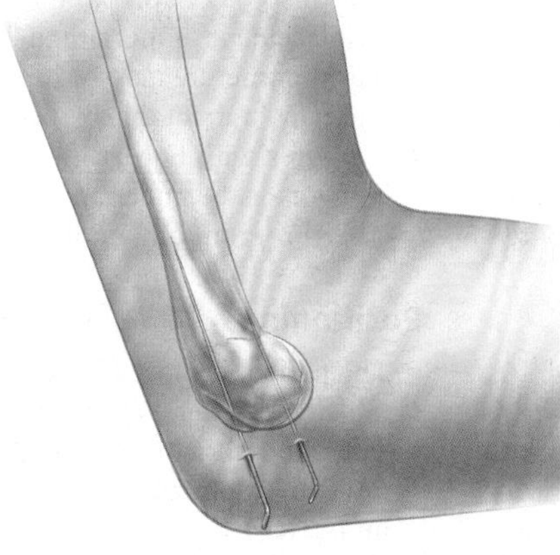
C

**TECH FIG 1** • **A.** Intraoperative fluoroscopic image showing two percutaneously placed Kirschner wires stabilizing a lateral condyle fracture. **B,C.** AP and lateral views of fracture treated with two divergent Kirschner wires.

- Occasionally, a third wire is needed. This wire is added if, after placing the first two wires, there is still motion at the fracture site when the elbow is varus stressed under fluoroscopy.
- The wires can be cut and bent 90 degrees outside of the skin.
- Wrapping gauze around the pin as it exits the skin may limit pin migration and provide a protective barrier. Sterile felt can also be placed between the skin and the cut end of the wire. This helps prevent the cut end of the wire from digging into the skin during the postoperative swelling phase.

## Open Reduction and Internal Fixation

- Unstable fractures usually require open treatment. This includes acutely displaced fractures as well as originally nondisplaced fractures that displace during early follow-up.[9] Although one can attempt a closed reduction of an unstable fracture, open reduction should be performed if any displacement persists.[14]

### Exposure

- The lateral Kocher approach is used, although the dissection is typically facilitated by the rent in the brachioradialis that leads directly to the lateral condyle.
- A 5- to 6-cm curvilinear incision is used, with two-thirds of the incision proximal and one-third distal to the elbow joint (**TECH FIG 2A**).
- The interval is between the brachioradialis and the triceps down to the lateral humeral condyle. The anterior articular surface of the elbow joint is exposed by working from proximal to distal and retracting the soft tissues of the antecubital fossa anteriorly.[15]
  - Although the fracture hematoma can obscure distinct muscular planes, a tear in the aponeurosis of the brachioradialis may lead directly to the fracture site.
- Dissection is kept anteriorly. Care should be taken to avoid stripping any of the soft tissues from the posterior aspect of the fracture fragment while the soft tissues are elevated off the anterior distal humerus because this contains the blood supply to the lateral condyle epiphysis[18] (**TECH FIG 2B**).
- Exposure is complete when the trochlear or medial extent of the fracture can be assessed anteriorly.

### Fracture Reduction

- The goal of reduction is to achieve a congruent articular surface without any step-off.
- Lifting the anterior soft tissues with a Zenker retractor or similar instrument can allow direct visualization and inspection of the articular surface.
  - A Zenker retractor is narrow and angled, which makes it useful for lifting and retracting the anterior soft tissues without unnecessary stretch (**TECH FIG 3A**).

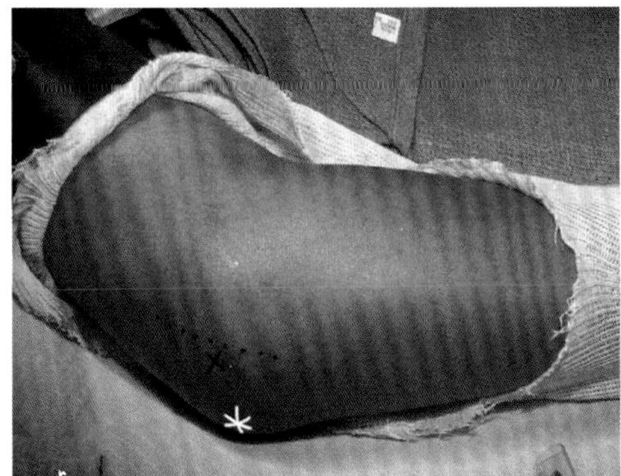


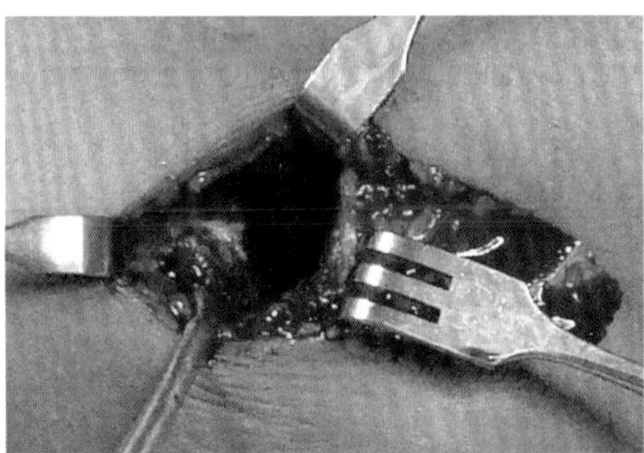


**TECH FIG 2** • **A.** Kocher-type lateral incision is marked by *dotted line*. *X* marks lateral condyle. The *asterisk* marks olecranon. **B.** Dissection is carried out anteriorly to expose the articular surface.

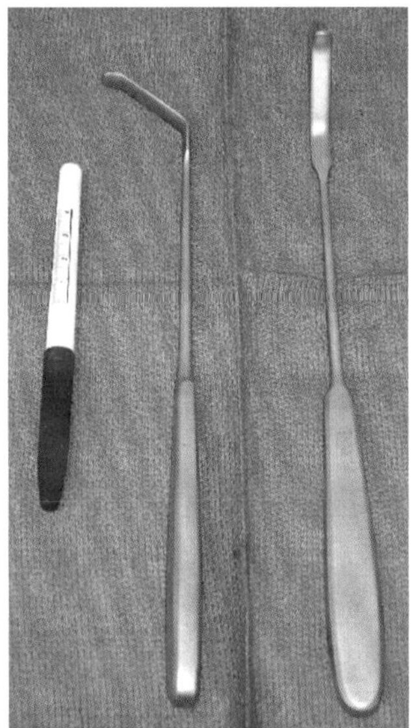


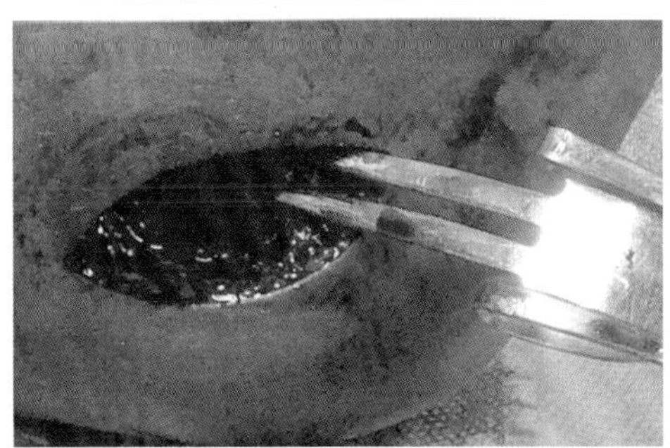


**TECH FIG 3** • **A.** The Zenker retractor is narrow and angled, making it ideal to elevate the anterior soft tissues. A pen is shown for reference. **B.** A sterilized standard kitchen fork can be a useful reduction tool.

- A small finger or elevator can be placed into the anterior elbow joint to palpate the trochlear–capitellar junction.
- A sterilized common kitchen fork can be a useful instrument in this case.
  - Bending the outer tines back decreases the width of the fork and allows the central tines to fit into a small wound.
  - The central tines can be used to engage the distal fragment, which is then rotated and pushed into position.
- Gaps between the tines allow room for placement of Kirschner wires (**TECH FIG 3B**).
- Alternatively, a Kirschner wire can be placed into the distal fragment and used as a joystick to help control the reduction.

## Fixation

- Once the fragment is reduced, a smooth Kirschner wire is advanced from the metaphyseal portion of the distal fragment, across the fracture site, and into the medial cortex proximal to the fracture.
- A second Kirschner wire (or the original joystick wire) can now be advanced across the fracture site into the medial cortex.
- The wires can be cut and bent 90 degrees outside the skin to facilitate easy removal in the office in about 4 weeks (3 to 6 weeks depending on appearance of healing on radiographs).[3,17]
  - Alternatively, they can be cut very short and bent under the skin. This technique has not been proven to decrease the risk of deep infections, and it requires a return to the operating room for removal; hence, it may not be as cost effective as leaving the pins exposed[4] (**TECH FIG 4**).
- If the wires are to be cut and bent outside the skin, the wires enter the skin through a separate stab site posterior to the incision.
  - If a wire needs to be placed through the incision, it can be cut and the posterior skin can be pulled up and over the sharp cut end before closure.
- Increasing the space between the wires at the fracture site increases rotational control.
  - Recently, bioresorbable implants have been tried, but long-term results are limited.[16]
- In older children with a larger metaphyseal fragment, a compression screw can be used rather than wires.
  - The screw head may be prominent under the skin and symptomatic after healing, however, thus requiring a return to the operating room for removal.
  - Compressive threads across immature cartilage can potentially impede growth in younger children.
  - This technique, therefore, is usually reserved for older patients or delayed unions or nonunions.
- In many cases, closure of the lateral periosteum may be possible with sutures. Such closure may lessen the chance of lateral spur formation, add stability, and speed healing.

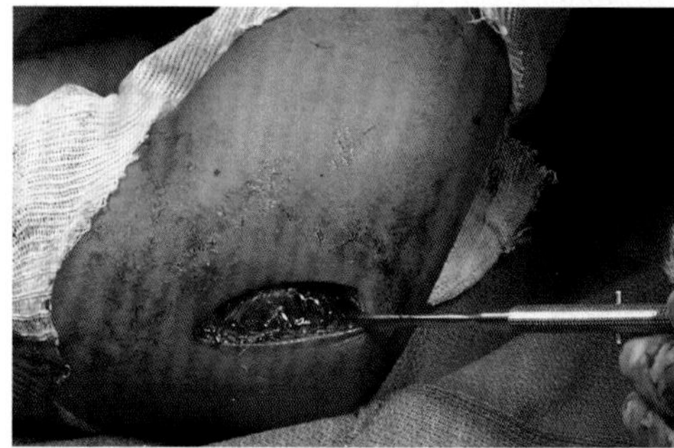

**TECH FIG 4** • After reduction and pinning, Kirschner wires may be cut and bent. Here, they are to be buried under the skin.

## PEARLS AND PITFALLS

| | |
|---|---|
| **Nonoperative management** | ▪ Follow-up radiographs should be obtained within 3 to 5 days.<br>▪ Any loss of reduction suggests instability and prompts the need for operative intervention. |
| **Postoperative bone spur** | ▪ A posterior or posterolateral metaphyseal bone spur frequently forms postoperatively. This is best seen on lateral radiographs. The bony prominence may give the clinical appearance of cubitus varus. Fortunately, this tends to improve over time and rarely requires intervention. Warning the parents initially of the probability of the occurrence can reduce anxiety later. |
| **Postoperative swelling** | ▪ Placing felt over the cut, bend ends of the wires onto the skin decreases the risk of skin swelling over or pressing into their sharp tips while in the cast.<br>▪ Bivalving the cast decreases the risk of postoperative compartment syndrome. |
| **Delayed union and nonunion** | ▪ This occurs more commonly in fractures treated nonoperatively.<br>▪ Prolonged casting of up to 12 weeks may be needed.<br>▪ If the fracture does not heal, open reduction with bone grafting may be necessary. |
| **Cubitus valgus and tardy ulnar nerve palsy** | ▪ Premature closure of the lateral physis may lead to gradual deformity as the medial side continues to grow.<br>▪ Anatomic reduction decreases the risk.<br>▪ Follow-up radiographs can reveal the deformity.<br>▪ Nerve symptoms can take years to develop; therefore, patients should be counseled about signs and symptoms of ulnar nerve stretch. |
| **Cubitus varus** | ▪ Unstable fractures treated nonoperatively can displace proximally and laterally, allowing the elbow to drift into a varus position.<br>▪ Doing careful early follow-up and fixing unstable fractures should prevent this. |

## POSTOPERATIVE CARE

- The arm is placed in a long-arm cast with the elbow flexed 90 degrees and the forearm in neutral to slight pronation.
- If there is significant swelling, the cast can be bivalved in the operating room and overwrapped the following week.
- Radiographs are obtained in 1 week to look for any loss of reduction.
- Wires can usually be pulled in 4 weeks.
  - Authors have debated the exact timing. Although some have shown adequate healing by 3 weeks, a period of 4 to 6 weeks is generally required; the decision should be based on radiographic evidence of early callus.
- Gentle early active range of motion is encouraged after wire removal.
- A removable posterior splint can be made for children who will not comply with activity modifications.
- Physical or occupational therapy is rarely needed in children but may be recommended for those who fail to show improved range of motion.

## OUTCOMES

- Patients who are treated quickly and whose fractures heal in an anatomic position with no subsequent growth arrest can expect excellent (90%) function and range of motion. Approximately, 10% have minor loss of extension (10 to 15 degrees) at 1 to 2 years.[17]
  - Complications are three times as likely to occur in fractures with displaced articular cartilage than in those with an intact articular surface.[19]
- Outcome studies following patients into adulthood are lacking.
- Patients who are treated with open reduction at 3 or more weeks after fracture are at greater risk for loss of range of motion (about 34 degrees), premature physeal closure, valgus deformity, tardy ulnar nerve palsy, and avascular necrosis, thus emphasizing the need for early treatment.[8]

## COMPLICATIONS

- Pin tract infections can occur but usually resolve after wire removal and oral antibiotics.
- Posterior or posterolateral metaphyseal bone spurs frequently form postoperatively and are best seen on lateral radiographs (**FIG 5**). The size of the spur has been associated with the initial fracture displacement.[12] Fortunately, these tend to smooth over time and are rarely symptomatic; thus, they usually require no treatment.
- Delayed union and nonunion are more common with nonoperative treatment than with surgical treatment.
- Malunion may occur in unstable fractures treated nonoperatively or in those with premature growth arrest.
- Avascular necrosis is more common after operative treatment than nonoperative management and is likely due to excessive posterior stripping that disrupts the epiphyseal blood supply.
- Tardy ulnar nerve palsy can develop slowly with progressive valgus deformity following premature growth arrest or nonunion.

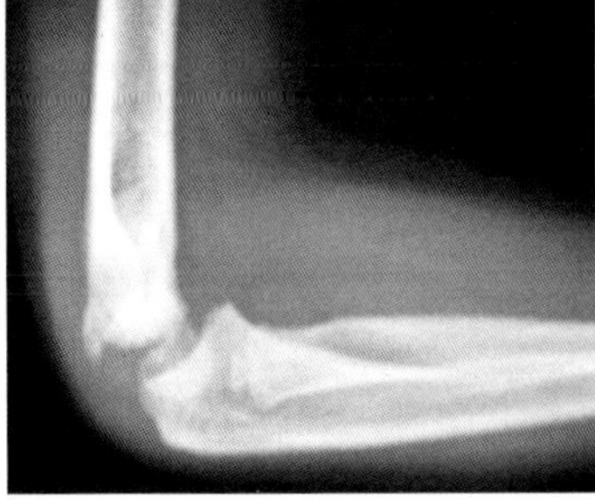

**FIG 5** • Lateral radiograph showing postoperative bone spur projecting from posterior metaphysis.

## REFERENCES


1. Bhandari M, Tornetta P, Swiontkowski MF. Displaced lateral condyle fractures of the distal humerus. J Orthop Trauma 2003;17:306–308.
2. Bloom T, Chen LY, Sabharwal S. Biomechanical analysis of lateral humeral condyle fracture pinning. J Pediatr Orthop 2011;31:130–137.
3. Cardona JI, Riddle E, Kumar SJ. Displaced fractures of the lateral humeral condyle: criteria for implant removal. J Pediatr Orthop 2002;22:194–197.
4. Das De S, Bae DS, Waters PM. Displaced humeral lateral condyle fractures in children: should we bury the pins? J Pediatr Orthop 2012;32:573–578.
5. Flynn JC, Richards JF Jr, Saltzman RI. Prevention and treatment of nonunion of slightly displaced fractures of the lateral humeral condyle in children. An end-result study. J Bone Joint Surg Am 1975;57(8):1087–1092.
6. Gorgola GR. Pediatric humeral condyle fractures. Hand Clin 2006;22:77–85.
7. Horn BD, Herman MJ, Crisci K, et al. Fractures of the lateral humeral condyle: role of the articular hinge in fracture stability. J Pediatr Orthop 2002;22:8–11.
8. Jakob R, Fowles JV, Rang M, et al. Observations concerning fractures of the lateral humeral condyle in children. J Bone Joint Surg Br 1975;57:430–436.
9. Launay F, Leet AI, Jacopin S, et al. Lateral humeral condyle fractures in children: a comparison of two approaches to treatment. J Pediatr Orthop 2004;24:385–391.
10. Marzo JM, D'Amato C, Strong M, et al. Usefulness and accuracy of arthrography in management of lateral humeral condyle fractures in children. J Pediatr Orthop 1990;10:317–321.
11. Milch H. Fractures and fracture-dislocations of the humeral condyles. J Trauma 1964;4:592–607.
12. Pribaz JR, Bernthal NM, Wong TC, et al. Lateral spurring (overgrowth) after pediatric lateral condyle fractres. J Pediatr Orthop 2012;32:456–460.
13. Rutherford A. Fractures of the lateral humeral condyle in children. J Bone Joint Surg Am 1985;67:851–856.
14. Song KS, Kang CH, Min BW, et al. Closed reduction and internal fixation of displaced unstable lateral condylar fractures of the humerus in children. J Bone Joint Surg Am 2008;90:2673–2681.
15. Sullivan JA. Fractures of the lateral condyle of the humerus. J Am Acad Orthop Surg 2006;14:58–62.
16. Takada N, Otsuka T, Suzuki H, et al. Pediatric displaced fractures of the lateral condyle of the humerus treated using high strength, bioactive, bioresorbable F-u-HA/PLLA pins: a case report of 8 patients with at least 3 years of follow-up. J Orthop Trauma 2013;27(5):281–284.
17. Thomas DP, Howard AW, Cole WG, et al. Three weeks of Kirschner wire fixation for displaced lateral condylar fractures of the humerus in children. J Pediatr Orthop 2001;21:565–569.
18. Wattenbarger JM, Gerardi J, Johnston CE. Late open reduction internal fixation of lateral condyle fractures. J Pediatr Orthop 2002;22:394–398.
19. Weiss JM, Graves S, Yang S, et al. A new classification system predictive of complications in surgically treated pediatric humeral lateral condyle fractures. J Pediatr Orthop 2009;29:602–605.

CHAPTER

# Open Reduction and Internal Fixation of Fractures of the Medial Epicondyle

**Brian G. Smith and Kristan A. Pierz**

## DEFINITION

- Trauma to the medial aspect of the elbow may cause a medial epicondyle fracture, which is an injury to the apophysis of the medial epicondyle.

## ANATOMY

- Medial epicondylar fractures involve the medial epicondylar apophysis on the posteromedial aspect of the elbow.
- The flexor–pronator muscle mass arises from this apophysis, including the palmaris longus, the flexor carpi ulnaris and radialis, the flexor digitorum superficialis, and one part of the pronator teres and the ulnar collateral ligament (**FIG 1**).[3]

## PATHOGENESIS

- A direct blow to the medial aspect of the elbow may cause a fracture to the medial epicondyle, but this is rare.
- More commonly, a fall on an outstretched arm causes an avulsion of the medical epicondyle via tension generated by stretch of the muscles attaching to it. Elbow dislocation is frequently associated with a medial epicondyle fracture and may occur with spontaneous reduction at the time of the injury (**FIG 2**).
- Considerable force applied to the arm may cause elbow dislocation and associated disruption of the ulnar collateral ligament. This ligament, the principal stabilizing ligament of the elbow, can avulse the medial epicondyle, and the apophyseal fragment may sometimes become lodged in the elbow joint.[3]
- Overuse may cause a chronic stress-type injury or an apophysitis, an example of which would be Little League elbow.

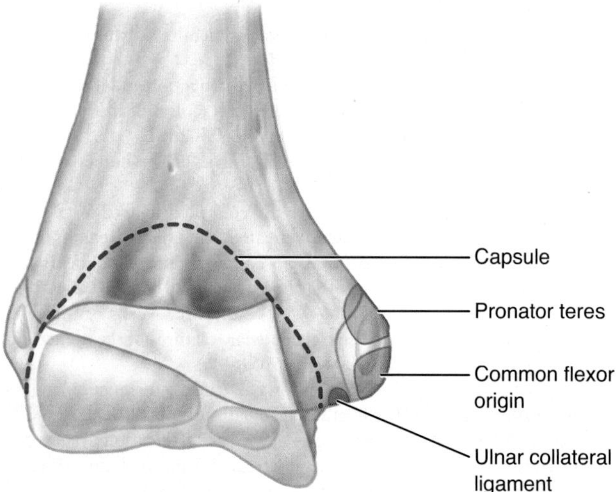


**FIG 1** • Anatomic landmarks and site of muscle and ligament attachments on medial epicondyle.

## NATURAL HISTORY

- The outcome of medial epicondyle fractures is related to the amount of fracture displacement and also the demands placed on the elbow by the patient.
- Minimally displaced fractures treated nonoperatively generally do well, especially if the patient is not an athlete or if the fracture involves the patient's nondominant arm.
- Untreated displaced fractures may lead to chronic medial elbow instability and even recurrent elbow dislocations.
  - Throwing athletes may have significant impairment in their sports activities.[9]

## PATIENT HISTORY AND PHYSICAL FINDINGS

- For any elbow injury, the mechanism of injury should be sought, with particular attention to the details of a fall. In children, this may be difficult to elicit, but often, a witness may be available. Medial epicondyle fractures frequently arise from a fall.
- The two most important issues in the physical examination are to document neurovascular status and to assess for elbow stability. Determination of stability includes determination of whether the elbow is dislocated, which can be assessed clinically and confirmed radiographically.

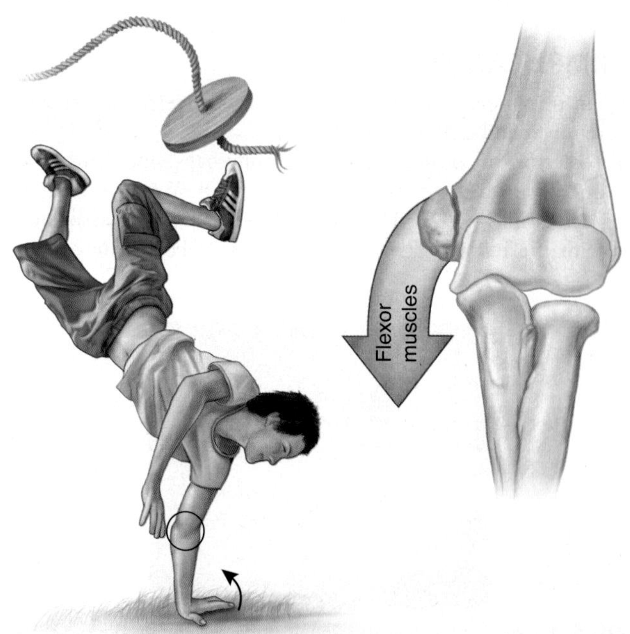


**FIG 2** • A common mechanism of injury: a fall on an outstretched arm causing either a "pull-off" or a "push-off" avulsion of the medial epicondyle.

- Assessment of medial elbow stability is often important in determining treatment.
- A positive valgus stress test confirms medial elbow instability. Persistence of medial elbow instability may cause significant elbow disability in athletes or those doing heavy labor.

## IMAGING AND OTHER DIAGNOSTIC STUDIES

- Standard anteroposterior (AP) and lateral radiographs of the elbow are required, but oblique views are often helpful to visualize the medial epicondyle, which is on the posteromedial aspect of the distal humerus.
- Widening of the apophysis may be the only sign of injury, so comparison views of the unaffected elbow are often helpful to assess and determine subtle degrees of displacement.
- If there is radiographic absence of the medial epicondyle and suspected joint incarceration, an arthrogram, computed tomography (CT) scan, or magnetic resonance imaging (MRI) may occasionally be needed.

## DIFFERENTIAL DIAGNOSIS

- Medial condylar fractures
- Supracondylar fractures
- Elbow dislocation

## NONOPERATIVE MANAGEMENT

- Smith in 1950 became a strong advocate of nonoperative management of this injury, pointing out that the fracture involved an apophysis rather than a physis and thus future growth was not compromised. He also documented that imperfect reduction or even nonunion was not automatically associated with a poor outcome in terms of elbow function and strength.[3]
- A more recent study from Sweden where all patients were treated nonoperatively showed 96% good to excellent results. Over 60% of the patients had a fibrous union or nonunion.[3]
- Two studies have compared nonoperative and operative treatment. Bede and associates[1] found that nonoperative treatment had better outcomes than operative treatment.
  - Farsetti and coworkers[5] demonstrated similar results of nonoperative treatment and open reduction and internal fixation (ORIF) with Kirschner wires in displaced fractures.
- Indications for nonoperative management of medial epicondyle fractures include patients who do not place high physical demands on their elbows and most nondominant elbows.
- Nonoperative treatment encompasses splinting for 5 to 7 days or until acute soft tissue swelling resolves and then early active range of motion starting as soon as possible after the injury.
  - Physical therapy may be required if range of motion is slow to return, but passive stretch may cause more injury and should be avoided.

## SURGICAL MANAGEMENT

- Absolute indications
  - Incarceration of the medical epicondylar fragment in the joint
  - Associated elbow dislocation with ulnar nerve dysfunction
- Relative indications
  - Elbow dislocation in a high-demand patient
  - A displaced fracture with medial elbow instability in a high-demand patient

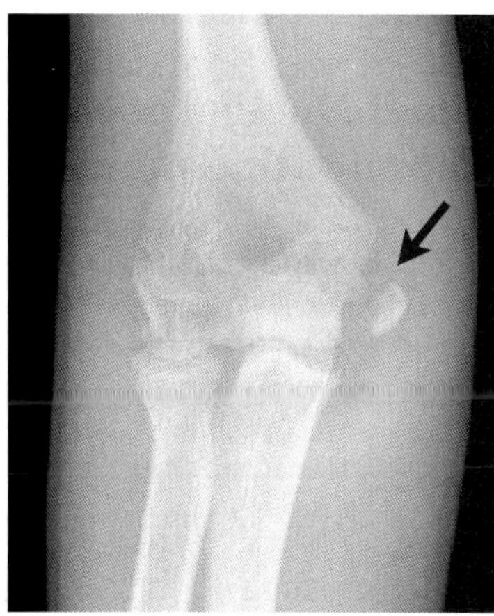

**FIG 3** • Injury film. The medial epicondylar fragment is displaced and located in the joint.

## PREOPERATIVE PLANNING

- Careful review of radiographs is done to assess the elbow joint for reduction and to assess the amount of displacement of the medical epicondylar fracture (**FIG 3**). Recent research indicates plain radiography may underestimate the actual displacement of medical epicondyle fractures based on imaging by CT scans.[4]
- A complete assessment of neurovascular status of the upper extremity is performed, with particular attention to the ulnar nerve examination.
- A valgus stress test is performed to assess for medial elbow instability, typically under sedation or anesthesia.

### Positioning

- The patient is placed supine on the operating table with the arm abducted 90 degrees at the shoulder and placed on a radiolucent hand table. The arm is externally rotated such that the medial aspect of the elbow is accessible (**FIG 4**).
- Alternatively, a C-arm image intensifier base may serve as the operating table for a smaller child or based on the surgeon's preference.
- The surgeon should be positioned in the patient's axilla for surgery.
  - Another option for positioning for the patient has been proposed: Placing the patient prone with the shoulder internally rotated has been advocated as a means of relaxing the flexor–pronator group and facilitating reduction of the fracture.[6]

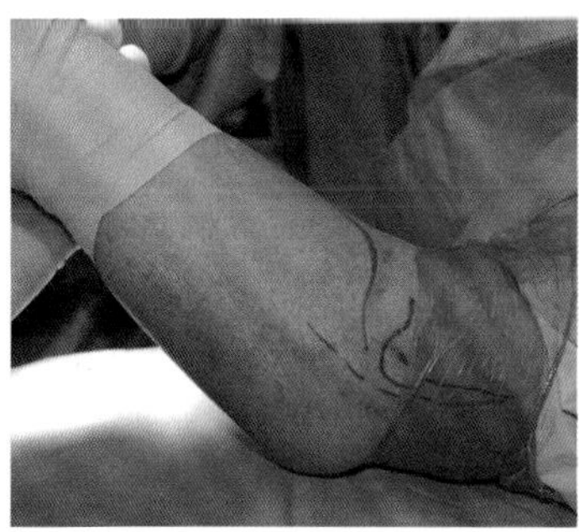

**FIG 4** • Arm positioning and approach to the medial epicondyle, with the ulnar nerve course marked out.

## Open Reduction and Internal Fixation with Cannulated Screw

- A skin incision about 4 cm long is made centered over the medial epicondyle after exsanguination of the limb and inflation of a tourniquet on the upper arm (**TECH FIG 1A**). Often with displaced injuries, the fractured fragment is just subcutaneous and little dissection is required.
- The ulnar nerve should be identified and carefully protected. Most experts do not recommend routine mobilization or transposition of the nerve.
- The fracture is identified, and any organized hematoma is removed (**TECH FIG 1B**).
- The fracture is reduced with a towel clip. Elbow flexion, forearm pronation, and wrist flexion aid in reducing the fracture.
- Some surgeons suggest curettage of the apophyseal cartilage to expedite healing of the fracture, which may persist as a healed apophysis if this is not done. This tip may be especially advantageous in the throwing athlete who is eager to return to sports as soon as possible.
- The fracture is stabilized with one or two guide pins from the 4.0-mm cannulated screw set. An 18-gauge needle may even be used as the second pin.[7]
- An alternative method of placing the pin is to drill from the inside of the medial epicondyle fracture fragment out, cut the pin to achieve a beveled edge at the fracture margin, and use it as a joystick to help reduce the fragment back to the humeral metaphysis and drill it into place.[7] Some surgeons will even predrill the metaphyseal side of the humerus to make fracture reduction easier.
- Radiographs are checked to assess reduction and pin placement.
- The pin selected for overdrilling should not be in the olecranon fossa. The second pin provides rotational stability of the fragment during drilling and screw placement.
- An appropriate-length screw is selected and inserted over the guide pin, stabilizing the fracture.
  - A washer may be used to provide a wide surface area of fixation and prevent screw head migration.
- AP and lateral intraoperative radiographs should confirm reduction and screw placement position (**TECH FIG 1C–G**).
- Elbow stability should be checked and full range of motion confirmed before closure.
- Standard skin closure is carried out, and the arm is splinted or casted at 90 degrees of elbow flexion.

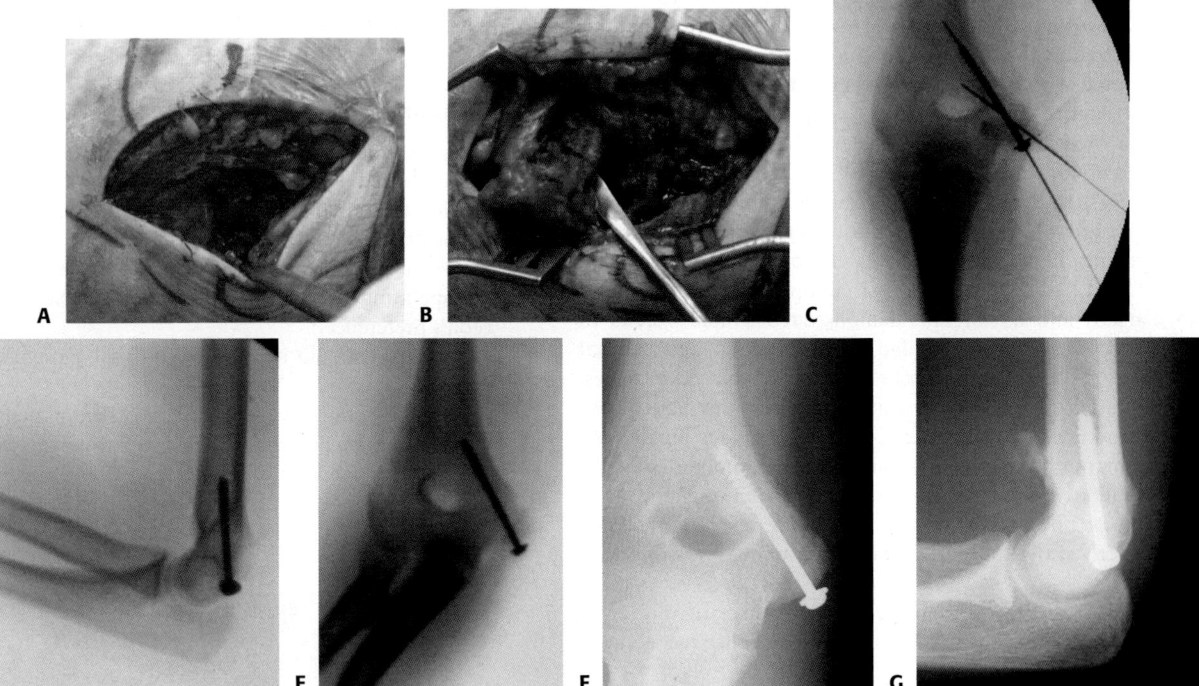

**TECH FIG 1** • **A.** Incision with ulnar nerve identified. **B.** The fracture fragment is mobilized. **C.** Fluoroscopic image showing two pins spanning the fracture fragment for rotational stability. **D,E.** Cannulated screw fixation shown fluoroscopically. **F,G.** Radiographs showing healed fracture. Heterotopic bone formation anteriorly can be seen on the lateral radiograph.

## Suture or K-Wire Fixation

- Should the fracture cause comminution of the medial epicondyle, repair with sutures may be warranted in a high-demand patient or one with medial instability.
- This would involve sutures placed directly in the tendinous tissue and secured to the periosteum adjacent to the bed from which the epicondyle was avulsed.
- K-wires may be used as a means of fixation in the presence of comminution or if the epicondyle fragment is too small for a screw (**TECH FIG 2**).

A 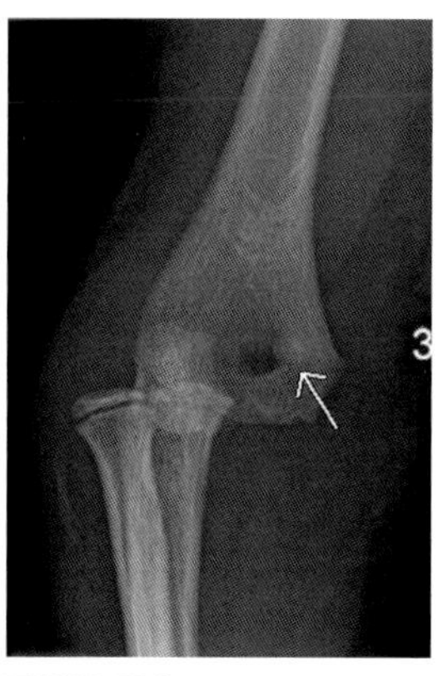
B 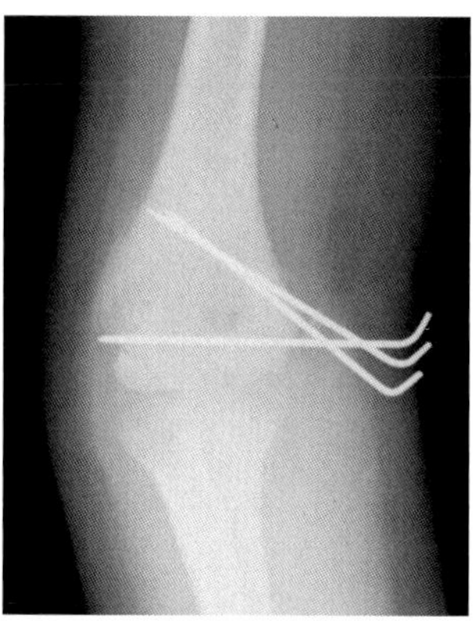
C 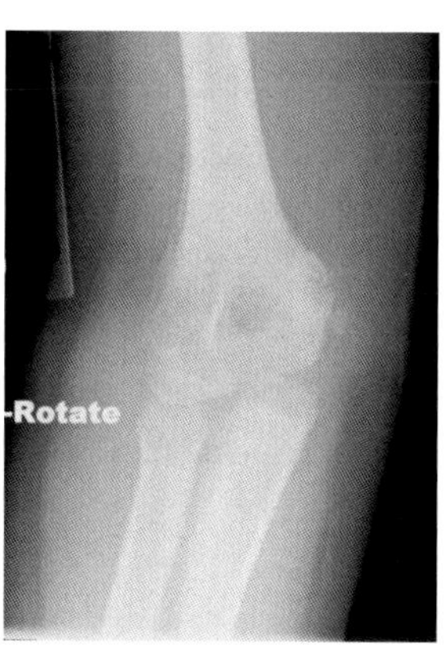


**TECH FIG 2** • **A.** AP radiograph of an almost 8-year-old boy with an elbow fracture-dislocation and a displaced medial epicondyle fracture; *arrow* identifies the fracture fragment. **B.** Because of the small size of the fragment, K-wire fixation was selected to stabilize the fracture fragment. **C.** Follow-up radiograph at 7 weeks postoperatively. (Courtesy of Felicity Fishman, MD.)

## Extraction of Medial Epicondyle from Elbow Joint: Roberts Technique

- A valgus stress is applied to the elbow with the forearm supinated.
- The wrist and fingers are dorsiflexed.
- As the position is reached, the fragment should be dislodged from the joint.
- This technique is most effective in the first 24 hours after the injury, before much muscle spasm occurs.[3]

## PEARLS AND PITFALLS

| | |
|---|---|
| **Postoperative stiffness** | ▪ Medial epicondyle fracture fragment should be fixed with a cannulated screw if possible rather than pins to have rigid fixation permitting early motion. Elbow motion is encouraged as soon as possible. |
| **Recognition** | ▪ The surgeon must beware of a medial epicondyle that is absent on radiography: It may be trapped in the joint. |
| **Loss of extension** | ▪ The surgeon must document radiographically that the internal fixation is not in the olecranon fossa, where it may block elbow extension. |

## POSTOPERATIVE CARE

- Postoperative management after open reduction of medial epicondyle fractures depends on the type and stability of the fixation of the epicondylar fragment.
- For ORIF with screws, initial splinting for 3 to 5 days in about 50 to 60 degrees of flexion is recommended, followed by early active range of motion.
- Some authors recommend a removable brace preventing valgus stress but permitting full flexion and extension for 4 weeks.[2]
- In one recent series on young athletes with this injury repaired with screw fixation, active range of motion out of the brace continued from weeks 5 to 8 postoperatively. At 8 weeks, noncontact sports were allowed, and return to full activity was possible at 12 weeks after surgery.[2]

## OUTCOMES

- Eight adolescent athletes undergoing ORIF with screw fixation for this fracture had excellent results with no residual valgus instability and full return to all sports. One patient had a loss of 5 degrees of hyperextension, but all other patients had recovery of full range of motion.[2]
- In another series, 21 of 23 patients treated operatively had recovery of full movement, whereas only 14 of 20 patients treated nonoperatively had full range of motion.[10]
- A recent series of operative treatment and early motion in 25 patients with displaced fractures showed good to excellent results in all patients.[9]
- Similarly, another study of competitive athletes found excellent results in 20 patients, 6 treated nonoperatively and 14 operatively. All overhead athletes were able to return to their sport.[7,8]

## COMPLICATIONS

- Failure to diagnose joint entrapment of the medial epicondyle fracture
- Ulnar nerve dysfunction
- Loss of range of motion
- Nonunion
- Myositis ossificans

## REFERENCES

1. Bede WB, Lefebvre AR, Rosman MA. Fractures of the medial humeral epicondyle in children. Can J Surg 1975;18:137–142.
2. Case SL, Hennrikus WL. Surgical treatment of displaced medial epicondyle fractures in adolescent athletes. Am J Sports Med 1997;25:682–686.
3. Chambers HG, Wilkins KE. Medial apophyseal fractures. In: Rockwood CA, Wilkins KE, Beaty JH, eds. Fractures in Children, ed 6. Philadelphia: Lippincott-Raven, 1996:800–819.
4. Edmonds EW. How displaced are "nondisplaced" fractures of the medial humeral epicondyle in children? Results of a three-dimensional computed tomography analysis. J Bone Joint Surg Am 2010;92(17):2785–2791.
5. Farsetti P, Potenza V, Caterini R, et al. Long-term results of treatment of fractures of the medial humeral epicondyle in children. J Bone Joint Surg Am 2001;83-A(9):1299–1305.
6. Glotzbecker MP, Shore B, Matheney T, et al. Alternative technique for open reduction and fixation of displaced pediatric medial epicondyle fractures. J Child Orthop 2012;6:105–109.
7. Gottschalk HP, Eisner E, Hosalkar, HS. Medial epicondyle fractures in the pediatric population. J Am Acad Orthop Surg 2012;20:223–232.
8. Lawrence JT, Patel NM, Macknin MD, et al. Return to competitive sports after medial epicondyle fractures in adolescent athletes. Am J Sports Med 2013;41:1152–1157.
9. Lee HH, Shen HC, Chang JH, et al. Operative treatment of displaced medial epicondyle fractures in children and adolescents. J Shoulder Elbow Surg 2005;14:178–185.
10. Wilson NI, Ingram R, Rymaszewski L, et al. Treatment of fractures of the medial epicondyle of the humerus. Injury 1988;19:342–344.

# Open Reduction of Supracondylar Fractures of the Humerus

Christine M. Goodbody and John M. Flynn

## DEFINITION

- A supracondylar fracture that requires open reduction is one that cannot be treated with closed reduction and percutaneous pinning.

## ANATOMY

- The neurovascular anatomy to consider for an open reduction includes the following:
  - The ulnar nerve passes behind the medial epicondyle.
  - The radial nerve courses from posterior to anterior just above the olecranon fossa.
  - The brachial artery and median nerve pass through the antecubital fossa and are often immediately subcutaneous anteriorly because of fracture displacement, putting them at risk during the skin incision.

## PATIENT HISTORY AND PHYSICAL FINDINGS

- The patient history is the same for supracondylar fractures being treated by closed methods.
- A careful neurovascular examination must also be performed.

## SURGICAL MANAGEMENT

- Indications for open treatment of a supracondylar fracture include an open fracture, a fracture that proves irreducible by closed techniques, and a compromised vascular supply to the hand that does not reconstitute with closed reduction.
- The timing for surgical intervention has been a matter of debate. Many surgeons believe that prompt reduction is optimal. Other studies show no significant increase in complication rates with delayed treatment.[2,3]

### Preoperative Planning

- For children with a severe, potentially irreducible fracture, it is helpful to make a provisional attempt at fracture reduction immediately after the induction of anesthesia.
- After milking the fracture from its entrapment in the brachialis muscle, standard reduction maneuvers are performed to reduce the distal fragment into generally good alignment.
- Although time should not be spent perfecting the reduction (which will likely be lost during prepping and draping), this provisional reduction of severe fractures after induction can alert the surgical team that open reduction may be necessary, allowing time to gather equipment (such as a sterile tourniquet) and to obtain and place a radiolucent table to facilitate open reduction.

### Positioning

- The patient is placed supine on the operating table. A hand table attachment is valuable when open reduction is needed.
- A sterile tourniquet is placed on the child's arm after preparation and draping.
- The surgeon should make sure that the portable image intensifier can be moved easily into and out of the operative field to assist with pinning of the fracture.

### Approach

- In general, a transverse anterior incision through the antecubital fossa is the most useful and cosmetic.
- If more visualization is needed, this incision can be extended medially or laterally based on displacement, but this is rarely necessary.
- Extension of the incision on the opposite side of the displacement of the distal fragment allows for removal of soft tissue obstacles to reduction.
- If there is a suspicion of neurovascular compromise, the anterior approach provides the best extensile exposure to explore these structures.
- An inability to reduce the fracture may indicate that the proximal fragment has buttonholed through the brachialis muscle. Again, an anterior approach provides the most useful exposure to reduce this deformity.

## Open Reduction through an Anterior Approach

### Incision and Dissection

- Once the patient has been prepared and draped, the tourniquet is inflated.
- A transverse incision is made across the antecubital fossa (**TECH FIG 1A**). Care must be taken in dissecting, as the neurovascular bundle may be in a nonanatomic location—typically immediately subcutaneous and at risk for damage during the initial dissection (**TECH FIG 1B**).
- Dissection proceeds until the metaphyseal spike is encountered. It is often covered by a small amount of tissue and parts of the brachialis muscle that may be torn (**TECH FIG 1C**).
- It is at this point that the neurovascular bundle should be located, if it has not yet been identified. This usually involves dissecting across the anterior aspect of the metaphyseal spike. This step should not be omitted even if there is no vascular compromise. Once the vessels are identified, they should be retracted out of the field.

### Fracture Reduction

- Defining the outline of the distal fragment can be the most challenging aspect of the procedure. It is usually posterior and lateral, and the periosteum is folded over its surface (**TECH FIG 2**).
- Reduction is obtained by reaching into the fracture site with a hemostat and getting hold of the cut edge of the periosteum. This cut edge is extended with scissors to increase the size of the buttonhole and to help free up the distal fragment. The distal fragment is then brought anteriorly and reduced to the shaft fragment, which is maneuvered back through the buttonhole into its resting position posterior to the brachialis muscle.
- Alternatively, the surgeon can hold his or her thumb on the proximal fragment and push downward while an assistant applies traction to the forearm with the elbow flexed at 90 degrees.[1] A periosteal elevator can be used as a lever to assist the reduction.

### Pinning

- Once a reduction has been obtained, the fracture is fixed with smooth Kirschner wires. This is accomplished in the same manner as closed reduction with percutaneous pinning.
- Three divergent, lateral entry pins are placed as described in Chapter 8.

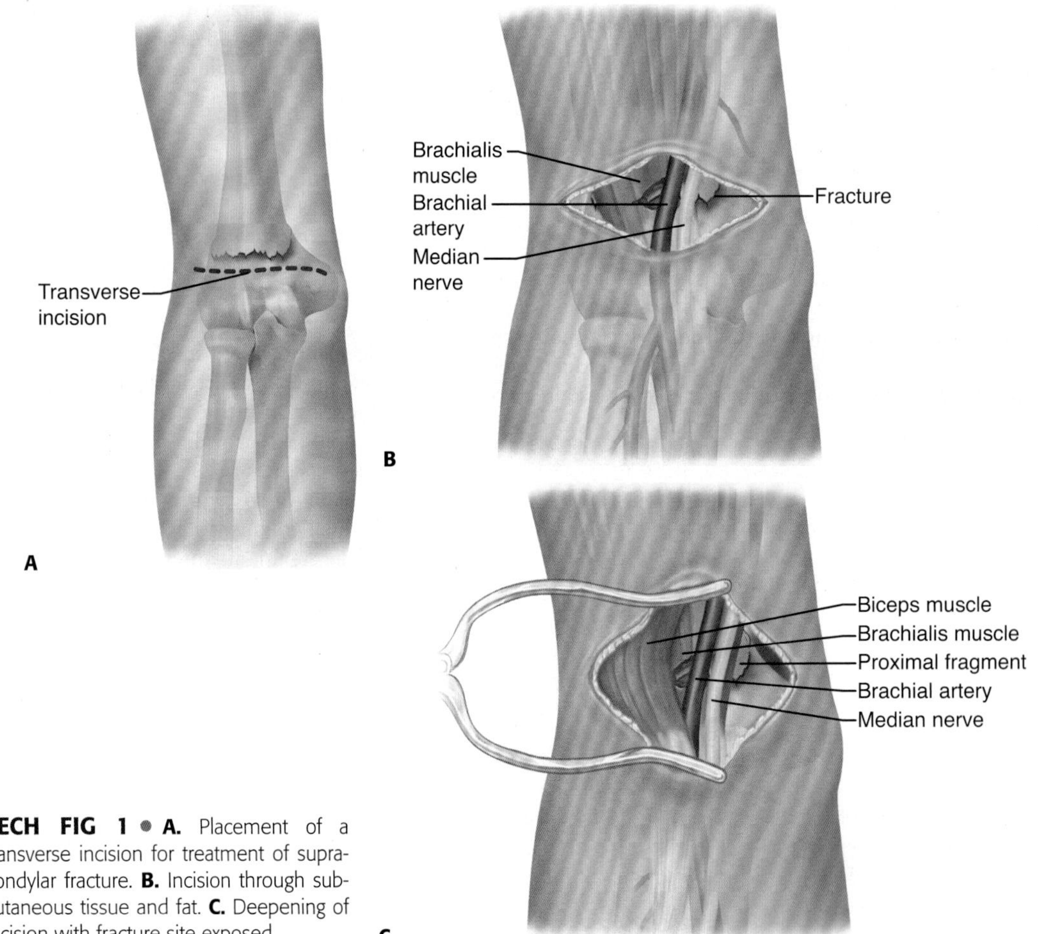


**TECH FIG 1** • **A.** Placement of a transverse incision for treatment of supracondylar fracture. **B.** Incision through subcutaneous tissue and fat. **C.** Deepening of incision with fracture site exposed.

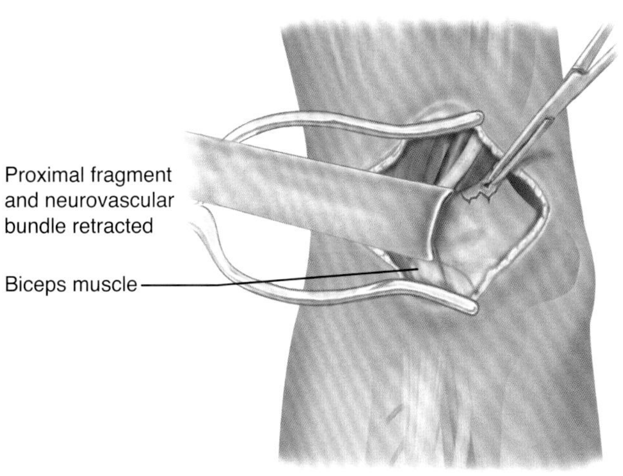


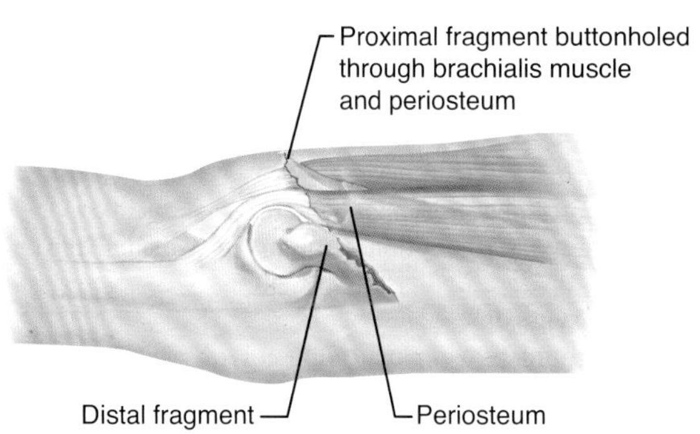


**TECH FIG 2** • **A.** Proximal fragment is retracted to expose distal fragment. **B.** Sagittal view of fracture with proximal fragment shown buttonholing muscle and periosteum.

- Alternatively, a cross-pinning strategy can be used with medial and lateral entry pins. Ideally, both the medial and lateral pins should cross proximal to the fracture site. The surgeon must be sure to engage both the medial and lateral columns of the distal fragment.
- The surgeon checks pin placement and reduction with fluoroscopy. If acceptable, the pins are bent, cut, and left out of the skin. Once healed, they can easily be removed in the office.
- The incision is closed with absorbable sutures.

## PEARLS AND PITFALLS

| | |
|---|---|
| **Indications** | ■ The primary indications for an open reduction are interposed tissue in the fracture site preventing closed reduction and vascular compromise that does not improve with closed reduction and percutaneous pinning. |
| **Neurovascular structures** | ■ The neurovascular bundle can be located anywhere within the operative field and must be identified even if there is no suspicion of compromise. |
| **Reduction of the fracture** | ■ The distal fragment often can be palpated but not seen, as it is hidden by the overlying periosteum. The surgeon should expand the buttonhole through the periosteum for better visualization. |
| **Fracture pinning** | ■ Pins should be maximally separated at the fracture site if three lateral pins are used. Convergent pins are not stable. If medial and lateral pins are used, the surgeon should engage the medial and lateral columns of the distal fragment. |

## POSTOPERATIVE CARE

- Sterile dressings are applied over the incision.
- A strip of Xeroform dressing is wrapped around the pins, followed by soft dressings.
- The elbow is splinted in 60 to 90 degrees of flexion with a neutral forearm.
- The patient is admitted overnight for observation. Often, a long-arm cast can be placed safely the next day, with the arm flexed about 80 degrees. This cast can be maintained until the pins are removed 3 or 4 weeks after surgery.
  - Supracondylar fractures in children reliably heal in 3 weeks, but when open reduction is used, healing may be delayed by an additional week. It is wise to get an x-ray with the cast off but the pins still in at 3 weeks after injury. If the fracture is not completely healed, cast protection for an additional week is recommended.
- The patient can then be placed back into a sling and started on gentle range-of-motion exercises out of the sling for another 2 weeks.
- The child can then start to use the arm normally.
- Formal physical therapy is usually not necessary.

## OUTCOMES

- It is generally agreed that prompt attention to reduction and stabilization of supracondylar fractures results in better outcomes and fewer complications.[4,5]
- Postoperative loss of reduction is uncommon.[7] However, children with supracondylar fractures that have been treated with open reduction generally take longer to regain their elbow motion than children treated with closed pinning. Families should be advised about this longer period of elbow stiffness in the immediate postoperative period.
- A 2001 study of 862 supracondylar fractures, 65 of which were treated with open reduction, found 55% excellent results, 24% good results, 9% fair results, and 12% poor results 5.8 months after injury in those treated with open reduction.[6]

## COMPLICATIONS

- Complications can result from the injury itself or from surgery.
- The risk of infection is decreased with the use of perioperative antibiotics.
- Iatrogenic neurovascular injury
  - Identification of neurovascular structures is crucial.
  - The ulnar nerve is susceptible to injury if a medial pin is used.
- Compartment syndrome
  - The child should be kept overnight for observation, and the surgeon should make sure that serial neurovascular examinations are performed.
  - The first sign of compartment syndrome in a child is usually increased pain or increased pain medication requirements.
  - The children most at risk are those who had compromised blood flow to the hand immediately after injury.
  - Children who have compartment syndrome in the setting of a median nerve injury often do not complain of pain because of the sensory deficit.
- Loss of motion
  - Although rare, some loss of full extension has been reported.
  - If there is excessive posterior angulation at the time of healing, some loss of full flexion can occur.
- Cubitus valgus and cubitus varus
  - Varus angulation is mostly cosmetic.
  - Valgus deformity can cause loss of full elbow extension and can result in tardy ulnar nerve palsy.
- Myositis ossificans is rare and should resolve in 1 to 2 years.

## REFERENCES

1. Ay S, Akinci M, Kamiloglu S, et al. Open reduction of displaced supracondylar humeral fractures through the anterior cubital approach. J Pediatr Orthop 2005;25:149–153.
2. Leet AI, Frisancho J, Ebramzadeh E. Delayed treatment of type 3 supracondylar humerus fractures in children. J Pediatr Orthop 2002;22:203–207.
3. Mehlman CT, Strub WM, Roy DR, et al. The effect of surgical timing on the perioperative complications of treatment of supracondylar humeral fractures in children. J Bone Joint Surg Am 2001;83-A(3):323–327.
4. Morrisy RT, Weinstein SL. Open reduction of supracondylar fractures of the humerus. In: Atlas of Pediatric Orthopaedic Surgery, ed 3. Philadelphia: Lippincott Williams & Wilkins, 2001:63–67.
5. Otsuka NY, Kasser JR. Supracondylar fractures of the humerus in children. J Am Acad Orthop Surg 1997;5:19–26.
6. Reitman RD, Waters P, Millis M. Open reduction and internal fixation for supracondylar humerus fractures in children. J Pediatr Orthop 2001;21:157–161.
7. Sankar WN, Hebela NM, Skaggs DL, et al. Loss of pin fixation in displaced supracondylar humeral fractures in children: causes and prevention. J Bone Joint Surg Am 2007;89(4):713–717.

# Closed Reduction and Percutaneous Pinning of Supracondylar Fractures of the Humerus

CHAPTER 8

Paul D. Choi and David L. Skaggs

## DEFINITION

- Supracondylar fractures of the humerus are common injuries in children. As many as 67% of children hospitalized with elbow injuries have supracondylar fractures; supracondylar fractures of the humerus represent 3% to 17% of all childhood fractures.[7,10,11] The annual incidence of supracondylar fractures has been estimated at 177.3 per 100,000.[9]
- The peak age at fracture is 5 to 7 years.
- The cause of injury is most commonly trauma to the elbow, most often resulting from a fall from height (70%) or related to sports activities.
- Nearly all (98%) supracondylar fractures of the humerus are of the extension type.[1] Flexion-type injuries also occur.
- Open injuries occur in 1% of cases. Concurrent fractures, most commonly involving the distal radius, scaphoid, and proximal humerus, occur in 1% of cases. Associated neurovascular injuries can occur, with nerve injury existing in 11% of cases and vascular insufficiency present in up to 20% of cases.[1,2,10] Anterior interosseous nerve injury is the most common nerve injury associated with extension-type supracondylar fractures of the humerus.

## ANATOMY

- The periosteum most commonly fails anteriorly with extension-type supracondylar fractures of the humerus.
  - With posteromedial displacement, the periosteum also fails laterally.
    - Therefore, with posteromedially displaced fractures, forearm pronation can aid in the reduction (**FIG 1**).
  - With posterolateral displacement, the periosteum also fails medially.
    - Forearm supination usually aids in the reduction of these posterolaterally displaced fractures.
- The direction of displacement has implications for which neurovascular structures are at risk from the penetrating injury of the proximal metaphyseal fragment (**FIG 2**).
  - Medial displacement of the distal fragment places the radial nerve at risk.
  - Lateral displacement of the distal fragment places the median nerve and brachial artery at risk.
- The ulnar nerve courses through the cubital tunnel posterior to the medial epicondyle. It is at particular risk with flexion-type fractures or when a medial pin is placed for fracture fixation.
  - The ulnar nerve subluxates anteriorly as the elbow is flexed. Therefore, the elbow should be relatively extended if a medial pin is placed for fracture fixation.

## PATHOGENESIS

- Supracondylar fractures of the humerus generally occur as a result of a fall onto an outstretched hand with the elbow in full extension.
- The distal humerus is very thin at the supracondylar region, a critical factor in producing a consistent injury pattern and failure in the supracondylar humeral region.
  - During a fall with the elbow in full extension, the olecranon in its fossa acts as a fulcrum.
  - The capsule, as it inserts distal to the olecranon fossa and proximal to the physis, transmits an extension force to this region, resulting in failure and fracture.
- With the elbow in full extension and the elbow becoming tightly interlocked, bending forces are concentrated in the distal humeral region.
- Increased ligamentous laxity, leading to hyperextension of the elbow, may be a contributing factor to this injury pattern.

## NATURAL HISTORY

- The physis of the distal humerus contributes little to the overall growth of the humerus (20% of the humerus); therefore,

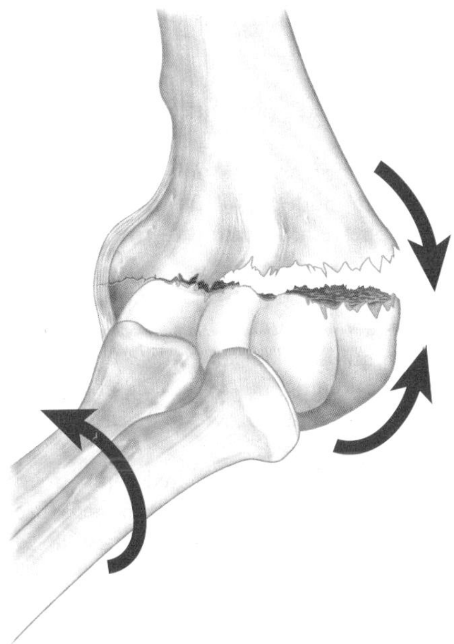

**FIG 1** • Reduction of a posteromedially displaced supracondylar fracture of the humerus. Pronation of the forearm closes the hinge and aids in reduction.

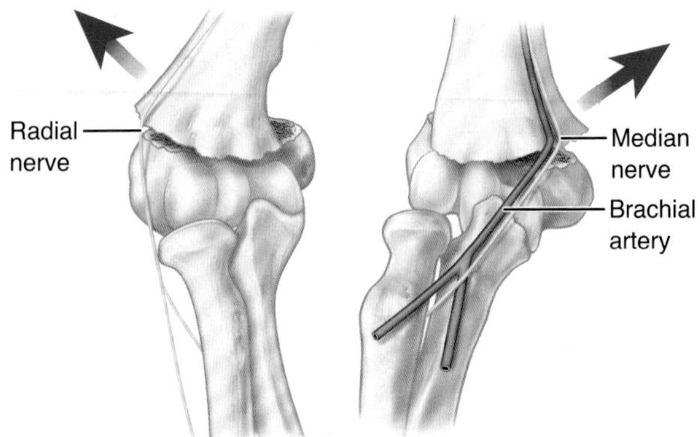


**FIG 2** • Relationship to neurovascular structures. The proximal metaphyseal spike penetrates laterally with posteromedially displaced fractures and places the radial nerve at risk. With posterolaterally displaced fractures, the spike penetrates medially and places the median nerve and brachial artery at risk.

the remodeling capacity of supracondylar fractures of the humerus is limited. Near-anatomic reduction of these fractures is important.

- The majority of supracondylar fractures of the humerus (other than extension type I fractures) are unstable; therefore, stabilization in the form of cast immobilization or, preferably, operative fixation is usually necessary.

## PATIENT HISTORY AND PHYSICAL FINDINGS

- Evaluation of the child with an elbow injury must include an overall assessment to look for associated trauma (especially in the proximal humerus and distal radius regions) as well as associated neurovascular injury.
- The physical examination may reveal swelling, tenderness, ecchymosis, and deformity. The pucker sign, which occurs as a result of the proximal fracture fragment spike penetrating through the brachialis and anterior fascia into the subcutaneous tissue, may be present.
- Thorough neurologic examination of the involved extremity is critical. Physical examinations to perform include the following:
  - Assessing for potential associated injury to the ulnar nerve. Finger abduction and adduction (interossei) strength are tested. Sensation in the palmar little finger is tested.
  - Assessing for potential associated injury to the radial nerve. Finger, wrist, and thumb extension (extensor digitorum communis, extensor indicis proprius, extensor carpi radialis longus and brevis, extensor carpi ulnaris, extensor pollicis longus) are tested. Sensation in the dorsal first web space is tested.
  - Assessing for potential associated injury to the median nerve. Thenar strength (abductor pollicis brevis, flexor pollicis brevis, opponens pollicis) is tested. Sensation in the palmar index finger is tested.
  - Assessing for potential associated injury to the anterior interosseous nerve. Index distal interphalangeal flexion (flexor digitorum profundus index) and thumb interphalangeal flexion (flexor pollicis longus) are tested.
- Accurate vascular assessment of the involved extremity is also critical. Examinations to perform include the following:
  - Palpation of distal radial pulse
  - General evaluation of perfusion: capillary refill, skin temperature and color
  - The role of modalities like Doppler ultrasonography and pulse oximetry is still unclear.
  - Preoperative angiography is not usually warranted.

## IMAGING AND OTHER DIAGNOSTIC STUDIES

- Initial imaging studies should include plain radiographs of the elbow—anteroposterior (AP), lateral, and sometimes oblique views.
- Comparison views of the contralateral elbow are sometimes helpful.
  - The fat pad sign, particularly posterior, represents an intra-articular effusion and can be associated with a supracondylar fracture of the humerus (53% of the time) (**FIG 3A**).[10]
  - On the AP view, the Baumann angle correlates with the carrying angle and should be 70 to 78 degrees or symmetric with the contralateral elbow (**FIG 3B**).
  - On the lateral view, the anterior humeral line (line drawn along the anterior aspect of the humerus) should intersect the capitellum (**FIG 3C**).
    - This line crosses the middle third of the capitellum in most healthy children older than 4 years.
    - In children younger than 4 years, this line may cross the anterior one-third of the capitellum.[1]
- The most commonly used classification system, the Gartland classification, is based on plain radiographic appearance:
  - Extension type I: nondisplaced
  - Extension type II: capitellum displaced posterior to anterior humeral line with variable amount of extension and angulation; posterior cortex of the humerus is intact
  - Extension type III: completely displaced with no cortex intact
  - A multidirectionally unstable type IV fracture has more recently been described. These fractures are unstable in both flexion and extension because of complete circumferential loss of a periosteal hinge.[1,10]
  - Flexion type

## DIFFERENTIAL DIAGNOSIS

- Fracture of elbow (other than involving the supracondylar humeral region)
  - Salter-Harris fractures involving the elbow
- Nursemaid's elbow
- Infection

## NONOPERATIVE MANAGEMENT

- Recent clinical practice guidelines by the American Academy of Orthopaedic Surgeons (AAOS) recommend nonsurgical immobilization of the injured limb for nondisplaced fractures (type I) meeting the following criteria[4,9]:
  - The anterior humeral line transects the capitellum on the lateral radiograph.
  - The Baumann angle is greater than 10 degrees or equal to the other side.
  - The olecranon fossa and medial and lateral cortices are intact.

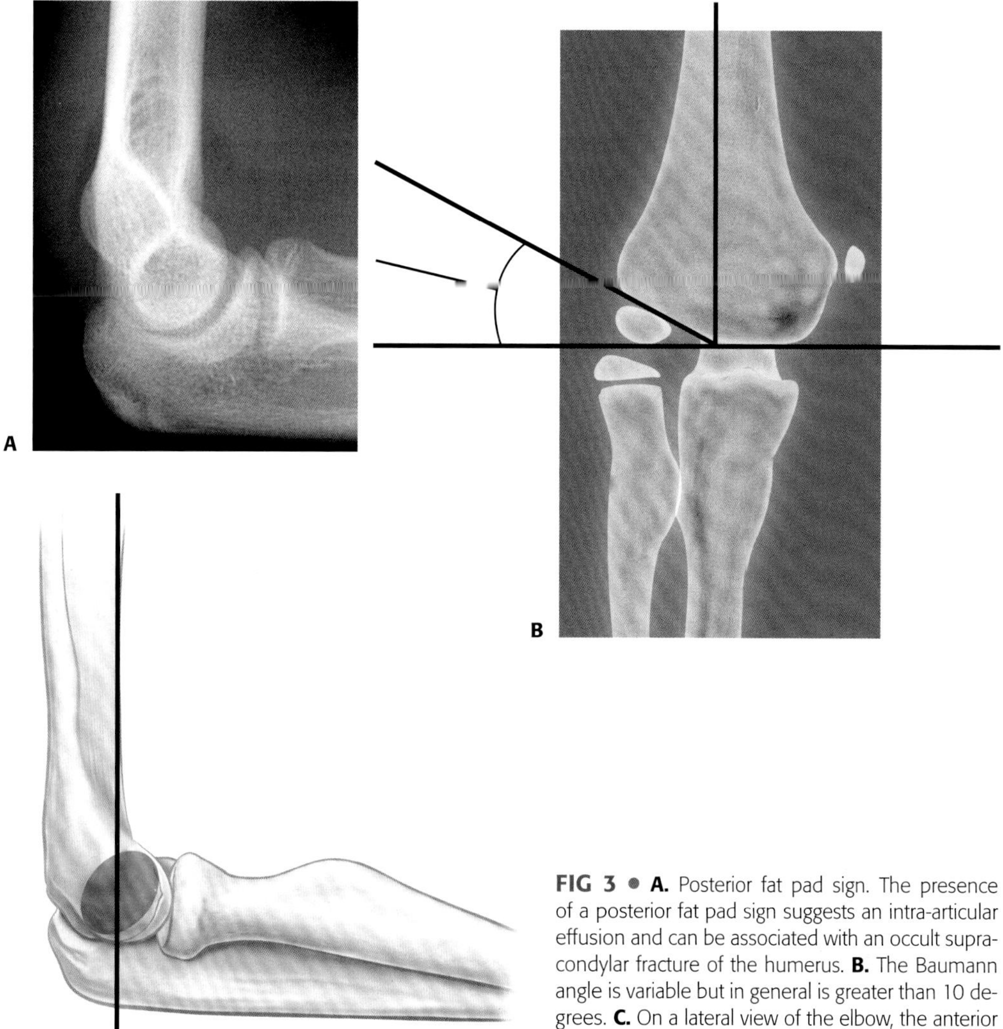


**FIG 3** • **A.** Posterior fat pad sign. The presence of a posterior fat pad sign suggests an intra-articular effusion and can be associated with an occult supracondylar fracture of the humerus. **B.** The Baumann angle is variable but in general is greater than 10 degrees. **C.** On a lateral view of the elbow, the anterior humeral line should intersect the capitellum.

- Nonoperative management consists of immobilization of the elbow in no more than 90 degrees of flexion in a splint or cast.
  - As the brachial artery becomes compressed with increasing flexion of the elbow, the clinician must ensure that the distal radial pulse is intact and that there is adequate perfusion distally.

## SURGICAL MANAGEMENT

- Clinical practice guidelines by the AAOS advocate closed reduction and percutaneous pin fixation for most displaced supracondylar fractures of the humerus.[9]
- The two main options for percutaneous pin fixation are the lateral entry pin and crossed-pin techniques.
- Most fractures can be stabilized successfully by the lateral entry pin technique.[5,9,12]
  - Two pins are usually adequate for type II fractures; three pins are recommended for type III fractures.
- Biomechanical studies have revealed comparable stability in the lateral entry and crossed-pin techniques.
- An advantage of the lateral entry pin technique is the significantly lower risk of iatrogenic nerve injury. The ulnar nerve is at risk when pins are inserted medially (5% to 6% risk).
- The crossed-pin technique may be indicated if persistent instability is noted intraoperatively after placement of three lateral entry pins.

### Preoperative Planning

- Displaced supracondylar fractures of the humerus (including Gartland type II and III) require reduction. Usually, reduction can be achieved by closed means. The preferred method for fixation is percutaneous pinning.
- Indications for open reduction of supracondylar fractures of the humerus are limited but include open injuries, fractures irreducible by closed means, and fractures associated with persistent vascular compromise even after adequate closed reduction.
  - One may consider open reduction and early antecubital fossa exploration in the setting of displaced supracondylar fractures of the humerus with vascular compromise and median nerve injury—as higher risk of nerve and/or vascular entrapment at the fracture site has been reported.[6]
- All imaging studies are reviewed. A high index of suspicion for associated fractures, especially of the forearm, is important; if present, there is an increased risk of compartment syndrome.

- Complete preoperative neurologic and vascular examination is performed and documented.
- The contralateral arm should be examined, and the carrying angle of the contralateral arm should be noted.
- The timing of surgery remains controversial. Recent retrospective evidence suggests that a delay in treatment of some supracondylar fractures may be acceptable.[1,3,8]
- Fractures with "red flags" usually require urgent treatment.
  - Significant swelling
  - Antecubital skin tenting, puckering, or ecchymosis
  - Neurologic or vascular compromise (except an isolated anterior interosseous nerve injury)
  - Concern for compartment syndrome (firm compartments, increasing analgesic requirements, increased anxiety, associated forearm fracture ["floating elbow"])

## Positioning

- The patient is positioned supine on the operating room table.
- The fractured elbow is placed on a radiolucent arm board (**FIG 4A**). The arm should be far enough onto the arm board to allow for complete visualization of the elbow and distal humerus. In smaller children, the child's shoulder and head may need to rest on the arm board as well.
  - The wide end of a fluoroscopy unit is sometimes used as a table.
  - In cases of severe instability of the fracture, use of the fluoroscopy unit as an arm board is suboptimal because reduction of the fracture is frequently lost with rotation of the arm, which is needed for AP and lateral views of the elbow.
  - The fluoroscopy monitor is placed opposite to the surgeon for ease of viewing (**FIG 4B**).

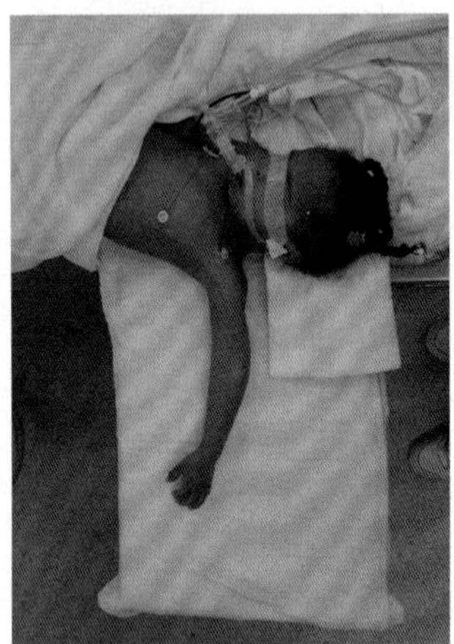
A

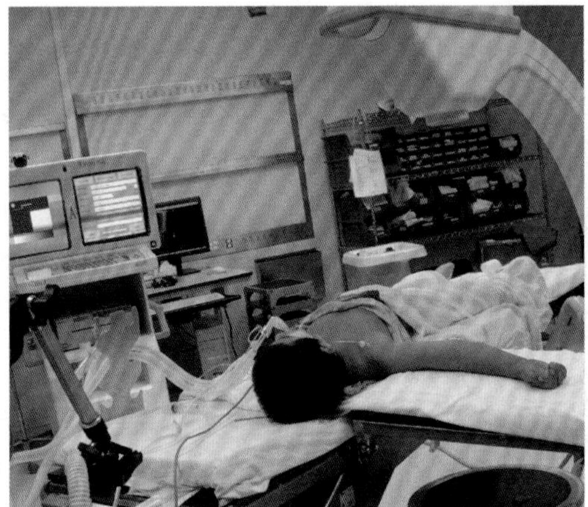
B

**FIG 4** • **A.** Positioning of patient. The injured elbow is positioned on a radiolucent arm board. In smaller children, the child's shoulder and head may also need to rest on the arm board to allow full views of the elbow and distal humerus. **B.** Positioning the fluoroscopy monitor on the opposite side of the bed allows the surgeon to see the images easily while operating.

TECHNIQUES

## Closed Reduction

- Traction is applied with the elbow in 20 to 30 degrees of flexion (**TECH FIG 1A**) to prevent tethering of the neurovascular structures over the anteriorly displaced proximal fragment.
- For severely displaced fractures, where the proximal fragment is entrapped in the brachialis muscle, the "milking maneuver" is performed (**TECH FIG 1B**).
  - The soft tissue overlying the fracture is manipulated in a proximal to distal direction.
- Once length is restored, the medial and lateral columns are realigned on the AP image.
  - Varus and valgus angular alignment is restored.
  - Medial and lateral translation is also corrected.
- For the majority of fractures (ie, extension type), the flexion reduction maneuver is performed next (**TECH FIG 1C**).
  - The elbow is gradually flexed while applying anteriorly directed pressure on the olecranon (and distal condyles of the humerus) with the thumbs.
- The elbow is held in hyperflexion as the reduction is assessed by fluoroscopy.
- Reduction is adequate if the following criteria are fulfilled:
  - The anterior humeral line crosses the capitellum.
  - The Baumann angle is greater than 10 degrees or comparable to the contralateral side.
  - Oblique views show intact medial and lateral columns.
- The forearm is held in pronation for posteromedial fractures.
- The forearm is held in supination for posterolateral fractures.
- For unstable fractures, the fluoroscopy machine instead of the arm is rotated to obtain lateral views of the elbow (**TECH FIG 1D**).

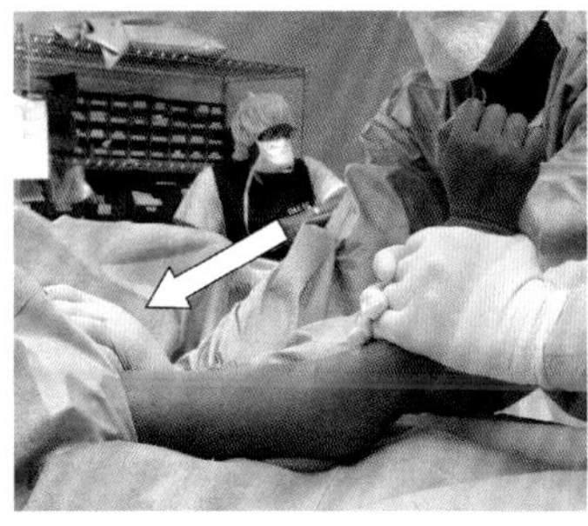
A

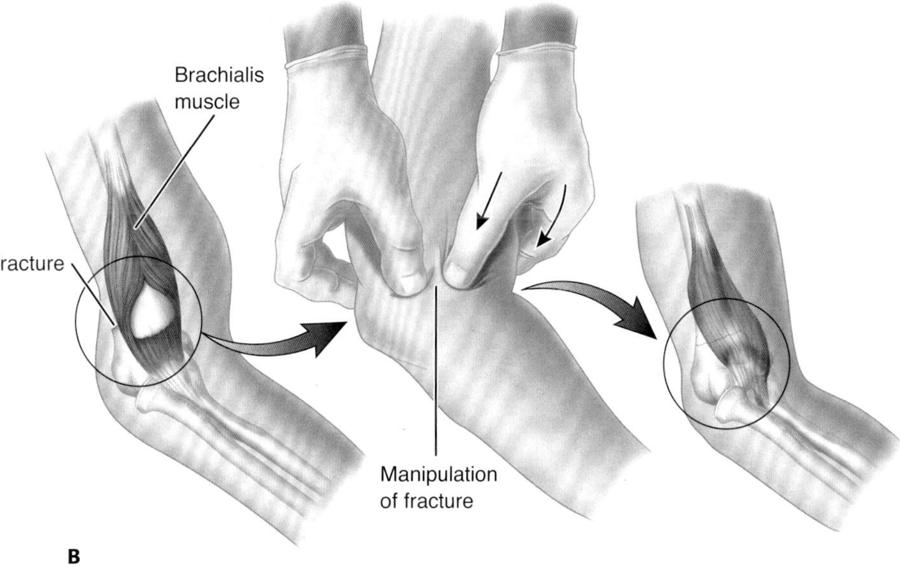

B

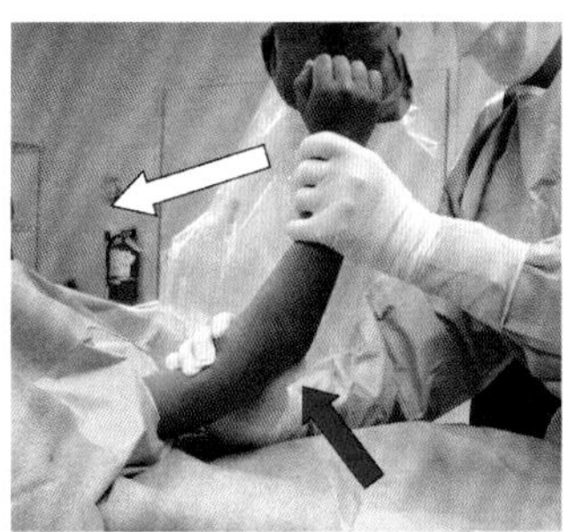
C

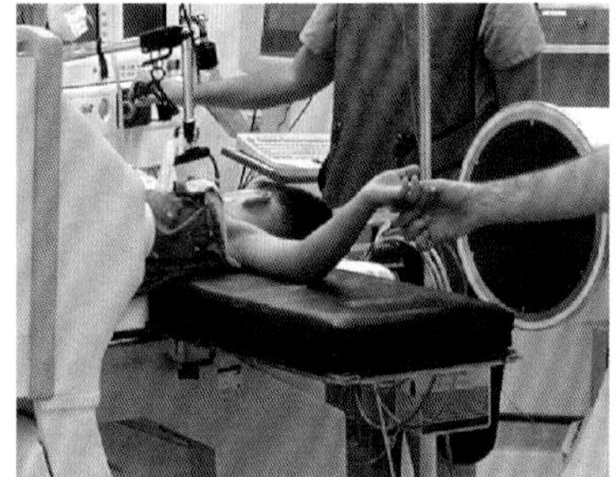
D

**TECH FIG 1** • **A.** Reduction. Traction is applied with the elbow flexed 20 to 30 degrees. Countertraction should be provided by the assistant with pressure applied to the axilla. **B.** If the fracture is difficult to reduce, the proximal fracture fragment may be interposed in the brachialis muscle. The milking maneuver is performed to free the fracture from the overlying soft tissue. **C.** The elbow is flexed while pushing anteriorly on the olecranon with the thumbs. **D.** For unstable fractures, the fluoroscopy unit instead of the arm is rotated to obtain lateral views of the elbow.

## Lateral Entry Pin Technique

- Once satisfactory reduction is obtained, K-wires can be inserted percutaneously for fracture stabilization.
  - A 0.062-inch smooth K-wires are commonly used.
  - Smaller or larger sizes may be used depending on the size of the child.
- The goals of the lateral entry pin technique are to maximally separate the pins at the fracture site and to engage both the medial and lateral columns (**TECH FIG 2A–C**).
  - The pins can be divergent or parallel.
  - Sufficient bone must be engaged in the proximal and distal fragments.
  - Pins may cross the olecranon fossa.
- As a general rule, two pins are adequate for type II fractures; three pins are recommended for type III fractures.
- The K-wire is positioned against the lateral condyle without piercing the skin (**TECH FIG 2D**).
  - The starting point is assessed under AP fluoroscopic guidance.
  - The K-wire is held freehand to allow maximum control.
- Once a satisfactory starting point and trajectory are confirmed, the K-wire is pushed through the skin and into the cartilage.
  - The cartilage of the distal lateral condyle functions as a pincushion.
- The starting point and trajectory are assessed by AP and lateral fluoroscopic guidance.
- When satisfactory starting point and trajectory are confirmed, the pin is advanced with a drill until at least two cortices are engaged.
- At this point, the reduction is again assessed.
  - The reduction must appear satisfactory on AP, lateral, and two oblique views.
  - The elbow is rotated to allow for oblique views of the medial and lateral columns.
- Additional pins are inserted (**TECH FIG 2E–H**).
- The elbow is stressed under live fluoroscopy in both the AP and lateral planes.
- Once satisfactory reduction and stability are confirmed, the vascular status is again assessed.
- Upon completion, the pins can be bent and cut approximately 1 to 2 cm off the skin.

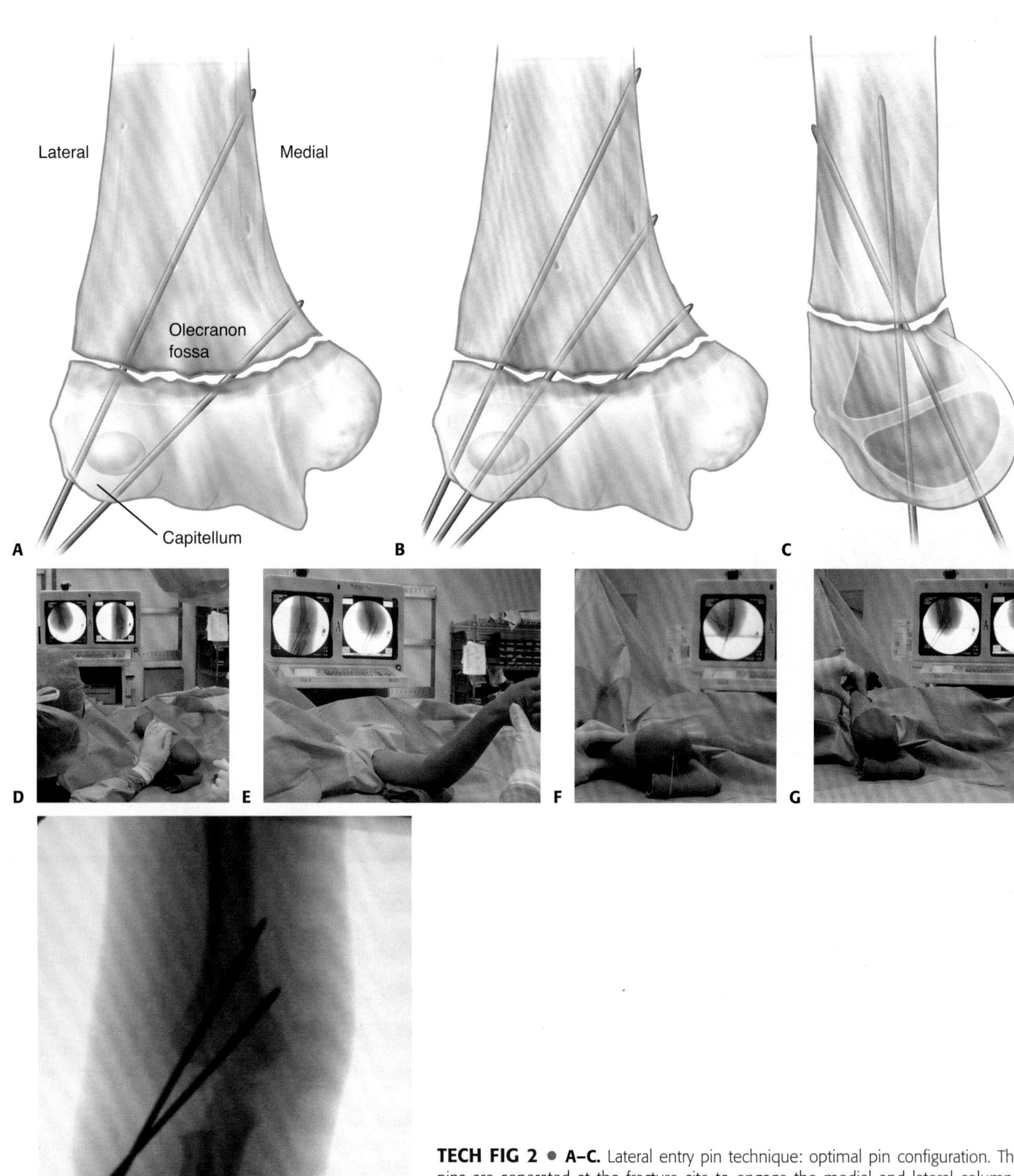


**TECH FIG 2** • **A–C.** Lateral entry pin technique: optimal pin configuration. The pins are separated at the fracture site to engage the medial and lateral columns. **A.** Optimal pin configuration for two pins (AP view). **B.** Optimal pin configuration for three pins (AP view). **C.** Optimal pin configuration (lateral view). **D.** The pin is held freehand. Once starting point and trajectory are confirmed under fluoroscopic guidance, the pin is pushed through the skin and into the cartilage. **E,F.** Assessment of coronal alignment on AP and lateral views. **G.** Externally and internally rotated oblique views are used to assess the medial and lateral columns. **H.** Stress fracture. The elbow should be stressed under live fluoroscopy to confirm adequate stability.

## Crossed-Pin Technique

- If satisfactory stability cannot be achieved by lateral entry pins or if the surgeon is more comfortable with lateral and medial entry pins, the crossed-pin technique can be performed.
- The lateral entry pins are inserted first: This will allow the elbow to be extended when placing the medial entry pins.
  - The ulnar nerve subluxates anteriorly with increasing flexion of the elbow; therefore, the ulnar nerve may be at risk when medial entry pins are placed with the elbow in 90 degrees or more of flexion.
- After insertion of the lateral entry pins, the elbow is extended to 20 to 30 degrees of flexion (**TECH FIG 3A**).
- A small incision is made over the medial epicondyle.
- Blunt dissection is performed down to the level of the medial epicondyle.
- A pin is positioned on the medial epicondyle (**TECH FIG 3B**).
- The starting position and trajectory are assessed under fluoroscopic guidance.
- When a satisfactory starting point and trajectory are confirmed, the pin is advanced with a drill until at least two cortices are engaged (**TECH FIG 3C,D**). The medial column should be engaged.
  - Ideally, the pin should be separated from the other pins maximally at the fracture site.
- The reduction and stability of the fracture are assessed just as with the lateral entry pin technique. The vascular status is similarly evaluated.

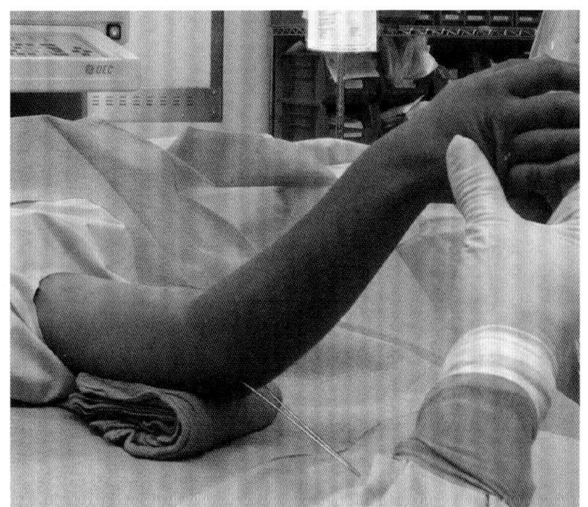

A

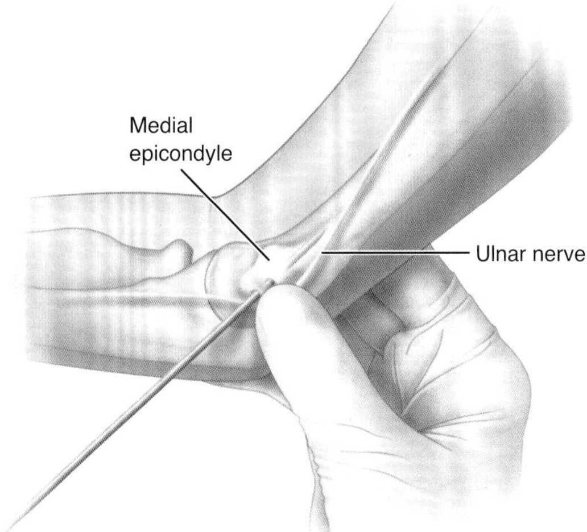


B

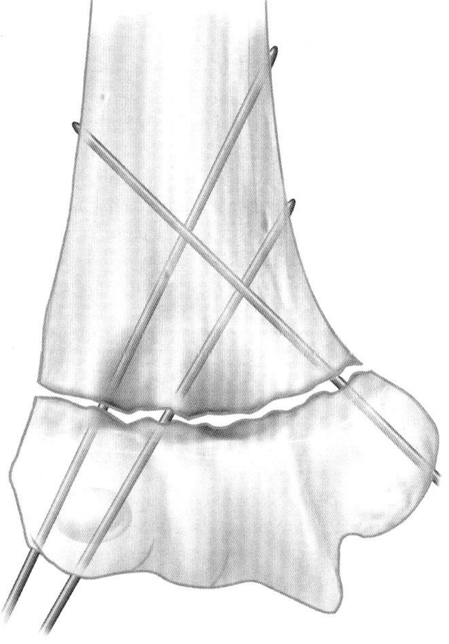

C

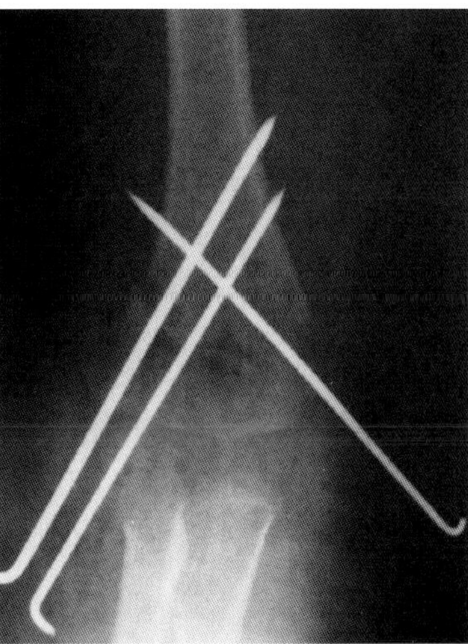

D

**TECH FIG 3** • Crossed-pin technique. **A.** To minimize risk of iatrogenic injury to the ulnar nerve, the elbow is extended to 20 to 30 degrees of flexion before the pins are inserted medially. **B.** The starting point is on the medial epicondyle. **C,D.** The medial pin should engage the medial column and at least two cortices.

## PEARLS AND PITFALLS

| | |
|---|---|
| **Clinical examination** | ■ A thorough preoperative neurologic and vascular examination should be performed and documented.<br>■ The surgeon should look for red flags such as ecchymosis, excessive swelling, puckering of skin, and associated fractures, which may be indications for an urgent reduction. |
| **Indications** | ■ Nondisplaced (type I) fractures can be treated nonoperatively with splint or cast immobilization.<br>■ Fractures with medial comminution or impaction should be treated operatively to avoid cubitus varus.<br>■ Displaced fractures require reduction (usually closed) and operative fixation (usually percutaneous pinning). |
| **Reduction** | ■ Traction is applied with the elbow in 20–30 degrees of flexion. |
| **Lateral entry pin placement** | ■ Maximal pin separation at the fracture site to engage the medial and lateral columns is the goal.<br>■ For type II fractures, two pins are usually adequate; for type III fractures, additional fixation with a third pin is usually indicated. |
| **Medial entry pin placement** | ■ Lateral entry pins are inserted first so that the elbow can be extended to 20–30 degrees of flexion, allowing for safer insertion of medial entry pins. |

## POSTOPERATIVE CARE

- The arm is immobilized, preferably in a cast (sometimes a splint), with the elbow in 45 to 60 degrees of flexion.
  - Flexing the elbow to 90 degrees, as is used for most other casting, is not recommended because it will increase the risk of compartment syndrome. Moreover, flexion to 90 degrees is not needed since the fracture reduction is stabilized by the pins, not the cast.
  - Sterile foam may be directly applied to the skin before cast application to allow for postoperative swelling.
- The arm is immobilized for 3 to 4 weeks, with follow-up evaluations at 1 and 3 (or 4) weeks. Postoperative radiographs (AP and lateral views) are obtained.
- Pins are usually discontinued at 3 to 4 weeks postoperatively.
- Range-of-motion exercises are initiated shortly after pins and immobilization are discontinued.
- Return to full activity typically occurs by 6 to 8 weeks postoperatively.

## OUTCOMES

- The AAOS has reported improved outcomes (radiographic, clinical, and functional) following closed reduction and percutaneous pin fixation of most displaced supracondylar fractures of the humerus (type 2, type 3, flexion).[4,9]
- Multiple studies have reported on the efficacy and high safety profile of the lateral entry pin technique.[4,5,9,12,13]
  - No significant difference in loss of reduction between lateral entry and crossed-pin techniques
  - No significant difference in radiographic outcome (Baumann angle, Baumann angle change)
  - Significantly lower risk of iatrogenic nerve injury (ulnar) with lateral entry technique
- Studies have suggested that treatment of some supracondylar fractures may be delayed without significant added risk in appropriately selected patients.[1,3,8]

## COMPLICATIONS

- Elbow stiffness
- Infection
- Vascular injury
- Neurologic injury
- Malunion
- Nonunion
- Avascular necrosis
- Myositis ossificans

## REFERENCES


1. Abzug JM, Herman MJ. Management of supracondylar humerus fractures in children: current concepts. J Am Acad Orthop Surg 2012;20(2):69–77.
2. Franklin CC, Skaggs DL. Approach to the pediatric supracondylar humeral fracture with neurovascular compromise. Instr Course Lect 2013;62:429–433.
3. Gupta N, Kay RM, Leitch K, et al. Effect of surgical delay on perioperative complications and need for open reduction in supracondylar humerus fractures in children. J Pediatr Orthop 2004;24(3):245–248.
4. Howard A, Mulpuri K, Abel MF, et al. The treatment of pediatric supracondylar humerus fractures. J Am Acad Orthop Surg 2012;20(5):320–327.
5. Kocher MS, Kasser JR, Waters PM, et al. Lateral entry compared with medial and lateral entry pin fixation for completely displaced supracondylar humeral fractures in children. A randomized clinical trial. J Bone Joint Surg Am 2007;89(4):706–712.
6. Mangat KS, Martin AG, Bache CE. The "pulseless pink" hand after supracondylar fracture of the humerus in children: the predictive value of nerve palsy. J Bone Joint Surg Br 2009;91(11):1521–1525.
7. Mangwani J, Nadarajah R, Paterson JM. Supracondylar humeral fractures in children: ten years' experience in a teaching hospital. J Bone Joint Surg Br 2006;88(3):362–365.
8. Mehlman CT, Strub WM, Roy DR, et al. The effect of surgical timing on the perioperative complications of treatment of supracondylar humeral fractures in children. J Bone Joint Surg Am 2001;83-A(3):323–327.
9. Mulpuri K, Wilkins K. The treatment of displaced supracondylar humerus fractures: evidence-based guideline. J Pediatr Orthop 2012;32(suppl 2):S143–S152.
10. Omid R, Choi PD, Skaggs DL. Supracondylar humeral fractures in children. J Bone Joint Surg Am 2008;90(5):1121–1132.
11. Otsuka NY, Kasser JR. Supracondylar fractures of the humerus in children. J Am Acad Orthop Surg 1997;5(1):19–26.
12. Skaggs DL, Cluck MW, Mostofi A, et al. Lateral-entry pin fixation in the management of supracondylar fractures in children. J Bone Joint Surg Am 2004;86-A(4):702–707.
13. Woratanarat P, Angsanuntsukh C, Rattanasiri S, et al. Meta-analysis of pinning in supracondylar fracture of the humerus in children. J Orthop Trauma 2012;26(1):48–53.

# Reconstruction for Missed Monteggia Lesion

9

CHAPTER

Apurva S. Shah and Peter M. Waters

## DEFINITION

- Monteggia fracture-dislocations are rare complex traumatic upper limb injuries defined by fracture of the ulna associated with proximal radioulnar joint dissociation and radiocapitellar joint dislocation. These injuries typically affect patients between 4 and 10 years of age.[19]
- The diagnosis of an acute Monteggia fracture-dislocation is often missed by skilled radiologists, emergency room physicians, pediatricians, and orthopaedic surgeons.[4,21]
- Late presentation of a previously undetected traumatic dislocation of the radial head occurs.
  - In children with a seemingly isolated dislocation of the radial head, scrutiny of forearm radiographs often demonstrates plastic deformation or fracture malunion of the ulna (**FIG 1**). The combination of these radiographic findings establishes the diagnosis of a chronic Monteggia fracture-dislocation or chronic Monteggia lesion, as opposed to a congenital dislocation of the radial head.[4]
- Patients with chronic Monteggia lesions can present for evaluation at a variety of time points.[21]
  - In some children, radial head dislocation is first noted several weeks after initiating treatment for a misdiagnosed, isolated ulnar fracture.
  - In other patients, the diagnosis may not be established for months to years following injury due to the development of pain, loss of motion, and/or valgus malalignment.
- Even a few weeks after injury, treatment of a Monteggia lesion is much more complicated than acute recognition and treatment.[21]
  - Nonetheless, due to pain, restriction of motion, and functional disability, most patients with chronic Monteggia lesions are offered surgical correction.

## ANATOMY

- Understanding the anatomy of the radiocapitellar joint and proximal radioulnar joint is crucial for understanding safe and appropriate treatment of chronic Monteggia lesions.
- The bony architecture, joint contour, and periarticular ligaments all contribute to stability of radial head and congruity of the radiocapitellar and proximal radioulnar joints.
- The radial head exhibits an asymmetric cylindrical shape with a concavity in the midportion to accommodate its articulation with the convex capitellum.
  - The radial head also articulates with the lesser sigmoid or radial notch of the proximal ulna. This complex pair of articulations permits forearm rotation in addition to elbow flexion and extension.
- The annular ligament is the principal stabilizer of the radial head during forearm rotation. The annular ligament originates on the anterior margin of the lesser sigmoid notch of the proximal ulna and encircles the radial neck before inserting on or adjacent to the posterior margin of the lesser sigmoid notch (**FIG 2**).[16]
  - The annular ligament occupies 80% of the fibro-osseous ring.[16]
  - The annular ligament is one component of the Y-shaped lateral ligamentous complex and maintains the radial head in contact with the ulna at the proximal radioulnar joint (**FIG 3**).

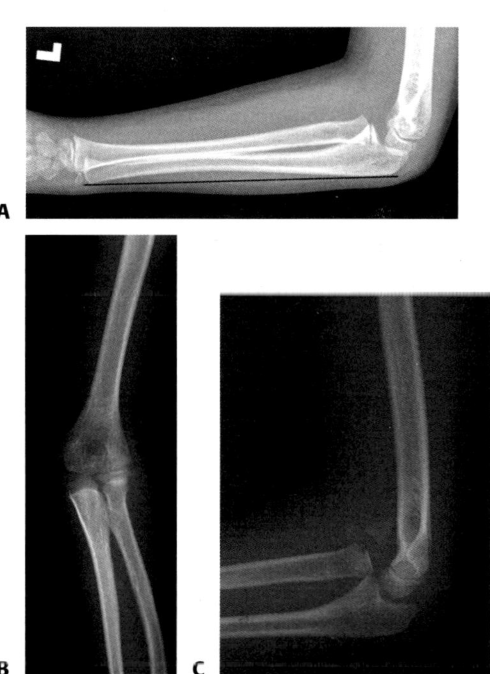


**FIG 1** • Chronic Monteggia lesion in a 7-year-old girl with a 5-week history of elbow pain and loss of motion following trauma. **A.** Initial lateral forearm radiograph demonstrates an abnormal ulnar bow line, or deviation of the ulna from its normally straight dorsal border, and is suggestive of plastic deformation. Anterior dislocation of the radial head is also noted. These findings were not detected in the emergency department where dedicated elbow films were not obtained, and the child was diagnosed with an elbow sprain. **B.** AP elbow radiograph 5 weeks after injury demonstrates a normal radiocapitellar line with a poorly characterized calcification overlying the lateral aspect of the capitellum. On the AP view, the radiocapitellar line is often normal in acute or chronic Bado type I Monteggia lesions. **C.** Lateral elbow radiograph 5 weeks after injury demonstrates disruption of the radiocapitellar line and anterior translation of the radial head. There is calcification of the displaced annular ligament and anterior elbow capsule, which can be mistaken for heterotopic ossification.

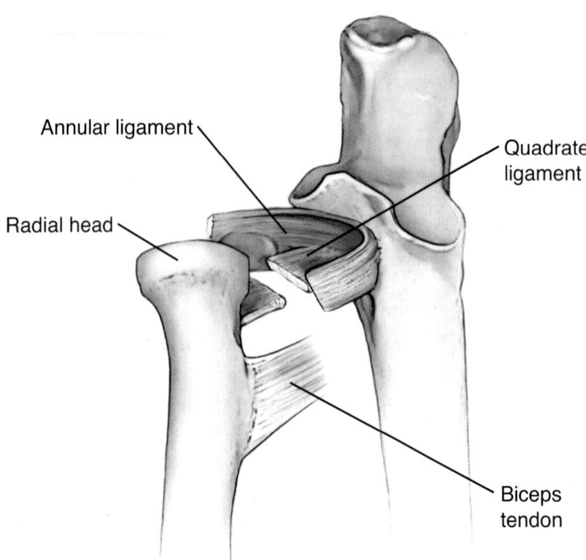


**FIG 2** • Ligamentous anatomy of the proximal radioulnar joint. The annular ligament is the principal stabilizer of the radial head during forearm rotation. In supination, the annular and quadrate ligaments are taught and increase stability of the proximal radioulnar joint.

- Because the radial head is not perfectly cylindrical, the annular ligament has been found to tighten anteriorly in forearm supination and posteriorly in forearm pronation.[16]
- The quadrate ligament lies just distal to the annular ligament and connects the proximal ulna and the radial neck (see **FIG 2**).
  - The anterior portion of the quadrate ligament is stronger and denser than the posterior portion, whereas the central portion is relatively thin.
  - The anterior portion stabilizes the proximal radioulnar joint in maximum supination and the weaker posterior portion stabilizes the joint in maximum pronation.[24]
- The oblique cord is a small, inconsistent fibrous bundle that originates from the lateral side of the ulna just distal to the lesser sigmoid notch and inserts just distal to the bicipital tuberosity of the radius.[27] The oblique cord progressively tightens in supination and also stabilizes the proximal radioulnar joint. This structure is not thought to be clinically relevant.[27]
- The radial head is most stable with the forearm in a position of supination.[24] Although the bony architecture provides little inherent stability to the proximal radioulnar joint, the elliptical shape of the radial head contributes to ligament function. In forearm supination, the long axis of the radial head is perpendicular to the lesser sigmoid notch, causing the annular ligament and the anterior segment of the quadrate ligament to tighten (**FIG 4**).
- The posterior interosseous nerve passes under the arcade of Frohse and through the supinator (**FIG 5**). The proximity of

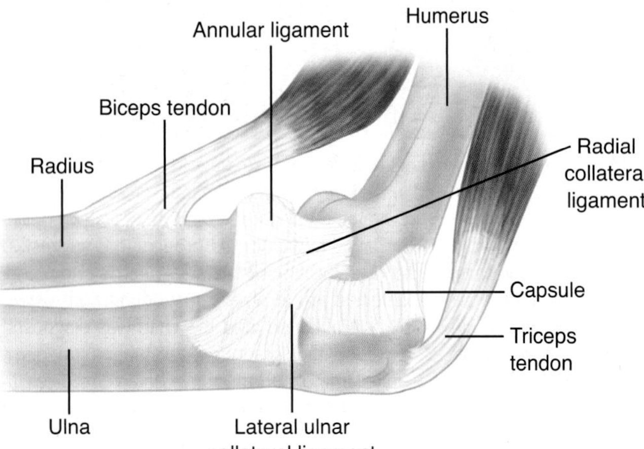


**FIG 3** • The Y-shaped lateral ligamentous complex of the elbow consists of the radial collateral ligament, the lateral ulnar collateral ligament, and the annular ligament.

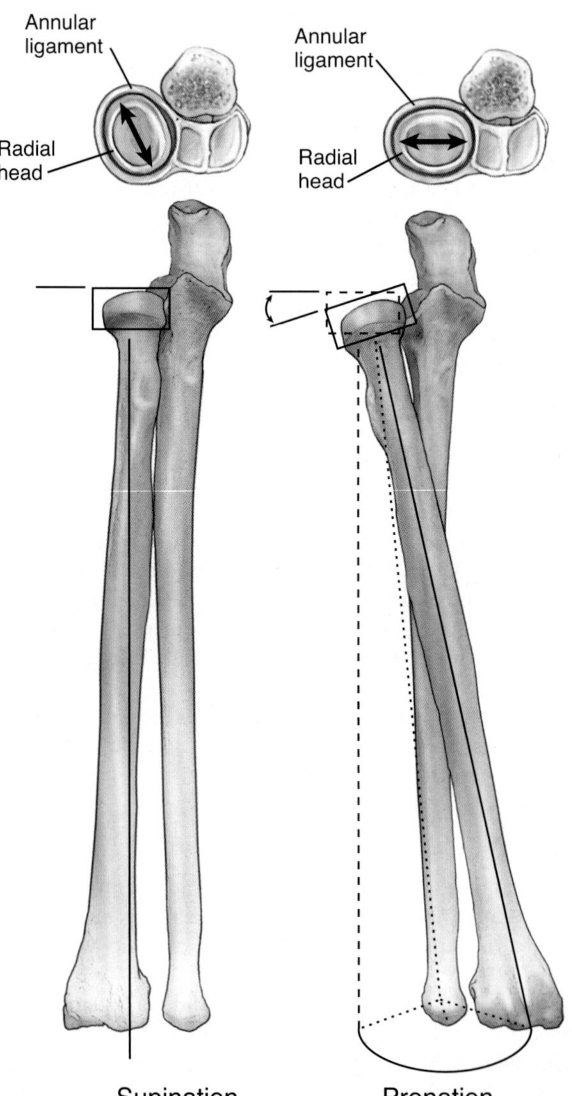


**FIG 4** • The radial head is most stable with the forearm in a position of supination. The radial head is elliptical and is stabilized at the proximal radioulnar joint by the annular ligament. In forearm supination, the long axis of the radial head is perpendicular to the lesser sigmoid notch, causing the annular ligament and the anterior segment of the quadrate ligament to tighten and maximize stability.

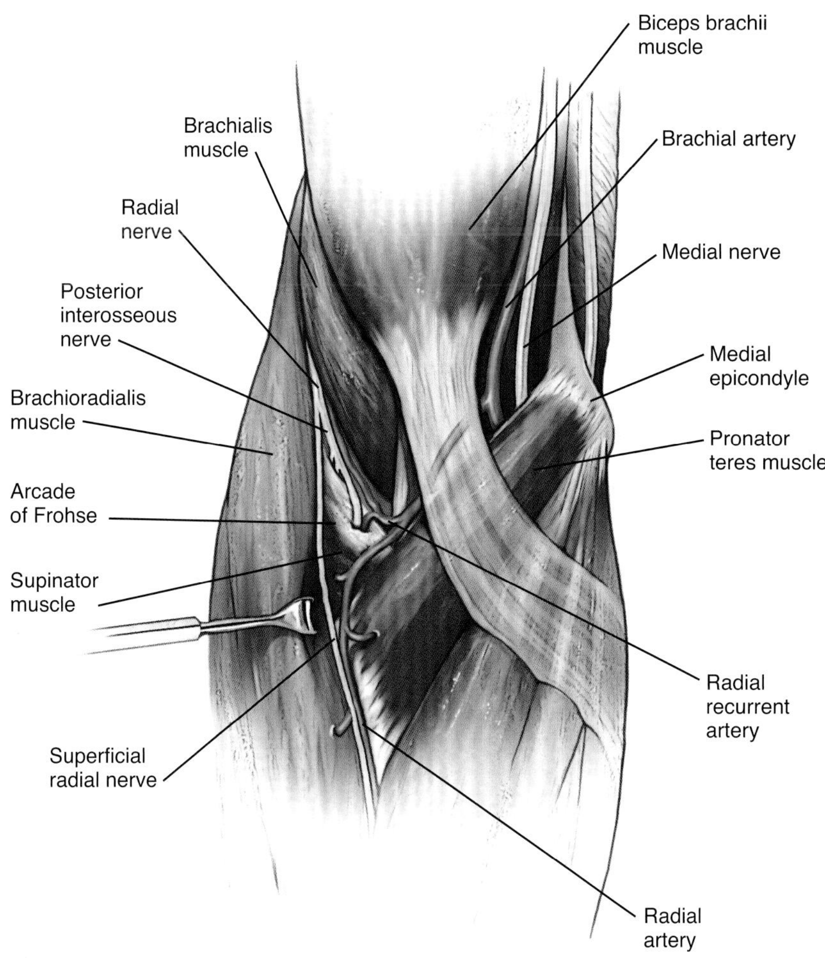


**FIG 5** • Diagram of the anterior elbow. The radial nerve emerges above the elbow in the interval between the brachioradialis and the brachialis. The radial nerve divides into the superficial sensory branch and the posterior interosseous branch. The posterior interosseous nerve passes under the arcade of Frohse and through the supinator. The proximity of the posterior interosseous nerve to the radial head and neck makes the nerve susceptible to injury during reconstruction of a chronic Monteggia lesion.

the posterior interosseous nerve to the radial head and neck makes the nerve susceptible to injury during reconstruction of a chronic Monteggia lesion. The posterior interosseous nerve is often adherent to a chronically dislocated radial head/neck and rarely can be entrapped in the radiocapitellar joint.[21] Identification of the nerve during the reconstruction is critical for avoidance of iatrogenic injury.

## PATHOGENESIS

- There are multiple patterns of Monteggia fracture-dislocations in children.
- Bado's original classification of Monteggia lesions is well recognized and had undergone minimal modification other than the description of various Monteggia equivalent lesions (**FIG 6**).[1] The scheme is based on the direction of the radial head dislocation and ulnar fracture angulation.
  - Bado type I lesions represent anterior dislocations of the radial head associated with an apex anterior ulnar diaphyseal fracture or plastic deformation. This pattern is the most common in children and represents approximately 70% to 75% of all injuries.[19]
    - Type I lesions can occur secondary to direct blow, hyperpronation, or hyperextension.
    - The most common mechanism is fall on an outstretched hand that forces the elbow into maximal extension with the forearm in relative pronation.[26] Due to the laxity of

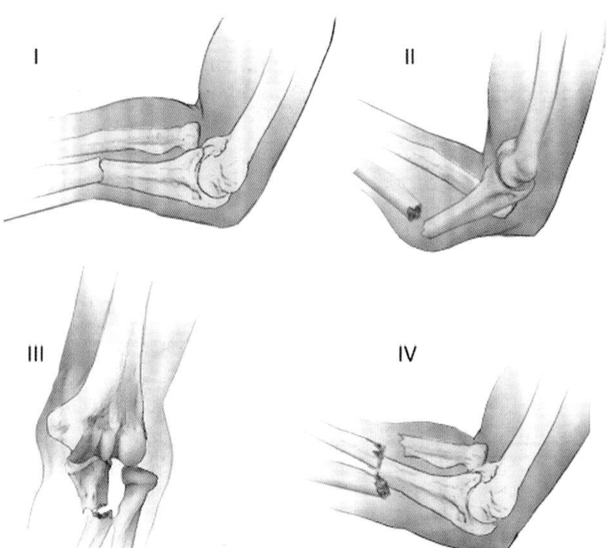


**FIG 6** • Schematic diagram of the Bado classification of Monteggia fracture-dislocations, which is based on the direction of the radial head dislocation and the ulnar fracture. Type I, anterior dislocation, is the most common pattern in children. Type II is posterior dislocation. Type III, lateral dislocation, is the second most common Monteggia lesion in children. Type IV is anterior dislocation with radial shaft fracture distal to the associated ulnar fracture.

the annular and quadrate ligaments in pronation, the stability of the radial head is tenuous and the anterior bending force combined with reflexive contraction of the biceps brachii results in anterior dislocation of the radial head. Due to the continued bending moment, the ulna undergoes plastic deformation or tension failure of the anterior cortex.
  - Bado type II lesions are characterized by posterior or posterolateral dislocation of the radial ahead associated with a posterior ulnar diaphyseal or metaphyseal fracture. This is the most common pattern in adults but represents approximately 5% of Monteggia lesions in children.[19]
  - Bado type III lesions demonstrate lateral dislocation of the radial head and are associated with an apex lateral (varus) fracture of the proximal ulna. This is the second most common Monteggia lesion in children and represents nearly 30% of all pediatric injuries.[19]
  - Bado type IV lesions are characterized by anterior dislocation of the radial head and fractures of both the radius and ulna. Type IV lesions are rare in children.
- The initial diagnosis of a Monteggia fracture-dislocation is often missed by qualified physicians.[4,21] Because the ulna heals rapidly in children, a chronic Monteggia lesion can develop over a period of 3 to 4 weeks. Due to the frequency of Bado type I lesions, most chronic Monteggia lesions in children are characterized by anterior dislocation of the radial head and apex anterior ulnar fracture malunion or plastic deformation.[13,21]
- Suboptimal treatment of the ulnar fracture in an acute Monteggia lesion can also result in unrecognized or late subluxation or dislocation of the radial head, resulting in a chronic Monteggia lesion.[19]
  - In general, only plastic and greenstick ulnar fractures should be treated with closed reduction and casting. All complete fractures should be treated surgically to avoid late instability.[20]
  - Transverse or short oblique ulnar fractures should be treated with intramedullary pin fixation and long oblique or comminuted fractures should be treated with open reduction and plate fixation.[20]
  - Always obtain dedicated elbow radiographs to evaluate congruency of the radiocapitellar reduction following reduction of the ulnar fracture.
- Chronic Monteggia lesions can result in substantial loss of function and are far more complex than acute injuries in terms of surgical decision making and management.[21]

## NATURAL HISTORY

- Initial reports on chronic Monteggia fracture-dislocations suggested that the natural history of the untreated lesion was not problematic. In these reports, results from late surgical reconstruction were complicated by scarring, arthrosis, and loss of motion. For these reasons, the classic treatment was neglect and radial head excision at skeletal maturity if necessary.
- More recent data suggests that most chronic Monteggia lesions are not tolerated well over time.[6,21] Patients can develop pain, arthrosis and loss of motion, functional impairment, progressive cubitus valgus, and late neuropathy even if initial symptoms are mild.[2,6,21] Loss of elbow flexion and forearm pronation can occur.[21] The best treatment for this problem remains preventative.
- Tardy ulnar, median, and posterior interosseous nerve palsy have been reported secondary to cubitus valgus and radial head dislocation in the setting of chronic Monteggia lesions.[3,11]

## PATIENT HISTORY AND PHYSICAL FINDINGS

- Most patients presenting with a chronic Monteggia lesion note a distinct history of trauma. The traumatic episode often involves significant force and is frequently characterized by a fall on to an outstretched hand with the elbow in extension and the forearm in pronation.
  - A history of trauma aids in distinguishing a traumatic radial head dislocation form a congenital radial head dislocation.
  - A history of acute elbow pain and temporary loss of motion in a child younger than 4 years of age secondary to minor trauma should prompt consideration of radial head subluxation or nursemaid's elbow. Radiographs will reveal an aligned radial head and no ulnar fracture or deformity. Children with a nursemaid's elbow usually have prompt resolution of discomfort and restoration of movement following closed reduction maneuvers.
- The timing of the injury and nature of prior medical treatment should be clarified. Patients presenting within 2 weeks of injury may still be candidates for standard treatment strategies for acute Monteggia fracture-dislocations.
- Physical examination may reveal cubitus valgus as well as loss of forearm rotation and elbow flexion. Nerve functional testing should be performed.
  - On inspection, anterior fullness in the cubital fossa may be detected. This corresponds to a palpable anterior dislocation of the radial head. The dislocated radiocapitellar joint should be palpated during forearm rotation to detect crepitation or other signs of elbow arthrosis.
  - The elbow carrying angle should be evaluated. The carrying angle in normal children increases with age and averages 9.3 degrees in males and 11.5 degrees in females.[7] Patients with chronic Monteggia lesions frequently demonstrate cubitus valgus and can present with carrying angles that exceed 30 degrees.[21] For some patients and families, this represents a significant aesthetic concern.
  - Elbow motion and forearm rotation should be precisely assessed. Normal elbow motion varies by child and averages 4 degrees of hyperextension to 145 degrees of flexion.[7] Loss of elbow motion is common, particularly in chronic Bado type I Monteggia lesions where anterior dislocation of radial head results in abutment against the humerus.[21] Elbow flexion is limited in the majority of patients with chronic Bado type I lesions and averages 110 degrees.[13] Terminal elbow flexion may be associated with visible discomfort. Loss of forearm rotation, particularly pronation, is also common.[21] Many children with chronic Monteggia lesions demonstrate compensatory radiocarpal and midcarpal rotation which can obscure assessment of true forearm rotation. In order to careful track true forearm rotation, the examiner must assess rotation of the radial styloid relative to the axis of the ulna.

- A detailed neurologic examination should be performed to assess peripheral nerve function, including the ulnar nerve, median nerve, and posterior interosseous nerve (see Exam Table at the end of the book). Sensibility can be assessed subjectively with light touch or objectively with two-point discrimination in a cooperative child older than 5 years of age. Hand and wrist strength is tested.
  - In tardy ulnar nerve palsy, patients may demonstrate diminished sensibility at the volar pad of the small finger (autonomous zone). Patients may also present with intrinsic muscle atrophy, clawing of the small finger and ring finger, diminished digital abduction strength, a positive Froment sign, or a positive Wartenberg sign.[3]
  - Patients with a tardy posterior interosseous nerve palsy will demonstrate weakness with finger metacarpophalangeal joint extension and thumb retropulsion.[11] Because the extensor carpi radialis longus is innervated by the radial nerve, patients may demonstrate preserved wrist extension with a tendency toward radial deviation. Sensation at the first dorsal web space is typically normal.

## IMAGING AND OTHER DIAGNOSTIC STUDIES

- The standard evaluation of a suspected chronic Monteggia lesion includes anteroposterior (AP) and lateral radiographs of the forearm and elbow.
  - Any disruption of the ulna, including subtle ulnar bowing, should alert the clinician to scrutinize the radiocapitellar joint (see **FIG 1A**). As noted, radial head subluxation or dislocation is often missed in the acute setting, particularly when the ulnar plastic deformation or greenstick fracture.[4]
  - Forearm radiographs are not a substitute for dedicated elbow radiographs when attempting to precisely characterize radiocapitellar alignment.
- Radiocapitellar alignment should be carefully scrutinized on the AP and lateral elbow radiographs.
  - In a chronic Bado type I Monteggia lesion, the radiocapitellar alignment may appear normal on an AP radiograph (see **FIG 1B**) despite demonstrating obvious anterior translation of the radial head on the lateral radiograph (see **FIG 1C**).
  - In a chronic Bado type III Monteggia lesion, the radiocapitellar alignment may appear normal on a lateral radiograph despite demonstrating obvious lateral or anterolateral translation of the radial head on the AP radiograph.
  - Radiocapitellar alignment can be assessed through marking of the radiocapitellar line on both the lateral (**FIG 7**) and AP radiograph. A line drawn through the center of the radial neck and head passes through the capitellum in 95% of normal elbows.[15] However, in contrast to early reports, the radiocapitellar line does not reliably interest the middle third of the capitellum and measurement can be affected by clinician bias, patient age, and forearm rotation.[15] For this reason, disruption of the radiocapitellar line suggests, but is not pathognomonic, for subluxation or dislocation of the radial head. Contralateral radiographs are often useful for comparison. Despite limitations, the radiocapitellar line should be used as a tool for evaluating radiocapitellar alignment. If subtle radiocapitellar subluxation is suspected, magnetic resonance imaging (MRI) should be obtained to visualize cartilaginous articular congruity.

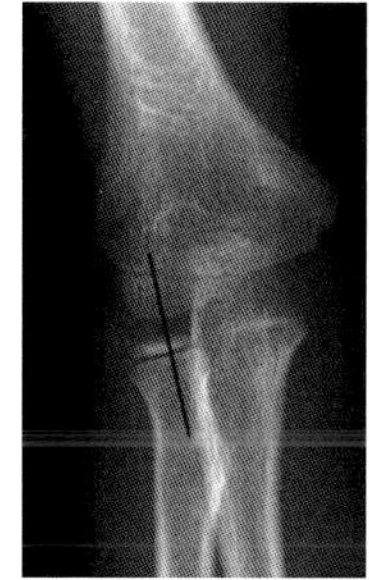
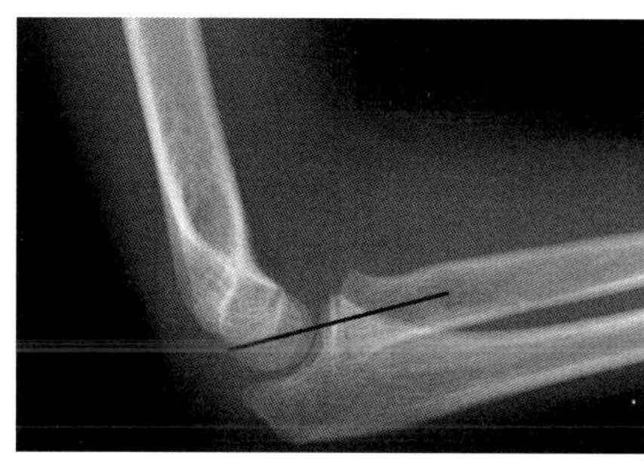

**FIG 7** • In a normal elbow, the radiocapitellar line generally bisects the capitellum. A disruption of the radiocapitellar line is concerning for radial head subluxation or dislocation but due to variation in the normal pediatric population is not pathognomonic for a Monteggia lesion. **A.** AP elbow radiograph in a 7-year-old girl demonstrating a normal radiocapitellar line. **B.** Lateral elbow radiograph in a 7-year-old girl demonstrating a normal radiocapitellar line.

- With late presentation of a chronic Monteggia lesion, congruency of the radial head and capitellum should be evaluated on plain radiographs and, if necessary, MRI. If the radial head is no longer centrally concave or the capitellum appears irregularly convex, joint congruity may not be achievable with surgical reduction.
- Elbow radiographs may demonstrate calcification of the displaced annular ligament or anterior elbow capsule and can be misinterpreted as heterotopic ossification (see **FIG 1**). This calcification may appear within weeks of the initial trauma and its presence is not a contraindication to surgical reconstruction.
- Distinguishing traumatic and congenital radial head dislocations can be difficult (**FIG 8**). When there is clear disruption of

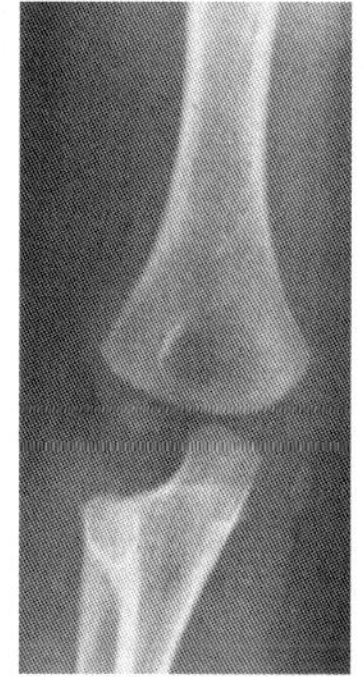
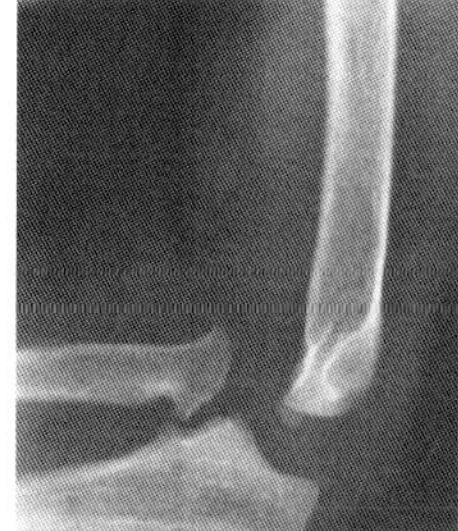

**FIG 8** • Congenital dislocation of the radial head in a 7-year-old boy with limited forearm rotation. **A.** AP radiograph demonstrates an abnormal radiocapitellar line. **B.** Lateral elbow radiograph also demonstrates an abnormal radiocapitellar line with anterior dislocation of the radial head. The dysplasia of the radial head and hypoplastic appearance of the capitellum are consistent with a congenital etiology despite the anterior radial head dislocation which is more frequently seen following trauma. (From Shah AS, Waters PM. Monteggia fracture-dislocation in children. In: Rockwood and Wilkins' Fractures in Children, ed 8. Philadelphia: Lippincott Williams & Wilkins. In press.)

radiocapitellar alignment on plain radiographs, it is important to inspect the shape of the radial head and capitellum. Hypoplasia of the capitellum and convex deformity of the radial head are usually indicative of a congenital radial head dislocation. Congenital radial head dislocation can be associated with ulnar dysplasia, radioulnar synostosis, and a variety of syndromes including nail patella syndrome. Congenital radial head dislocations are frequently posterior and may be bilateral. If there is no history of trauma or the force of described trauma seems minimal, a congenital etiology should be considered. Chronic anterior dislocations of the radial head are most frequently associated with a traumatic etiology.

## DIFFERENTIAL DIAGNOSIS

- Congenital radial head dislocation (see **FIG 8**)
- Nursemaid's elbow (pulled elbow, radial head subluxation)
- Isolated traumatic radial head dislocation
- Traumatic elbow dislocation

## NONOPERATIVE MANAGEMENT

- The indications for reconstruction of a chronic Monteggia lesion are not well defined in the literature.
- Nonoperative management can be considered in an asymptomatic child, but yearly clinical and radiographic follow-up is recommended.
- There are important contraindications for chronic Monteggia reconstruction. Some surgeons have advocated patient age (before age 12 years) or time from injury (<3 years) as discriminating factors for surgical consideration,[10,17] but it is more important to consider the morphology of the radial head and the capitellum.[18,22,25] In older patients or more chronic lesions, MRI can be obtained to further delineate cartilage quality and potential joint congruity. Patients with radial head enlargement or deformity, flattening of the capitellum, or joint arthrosis are not candidates for reconstruction.[10,22,25] In these patients, radial head excision can be considered if pain does not resolve with nonoperative means but does place the patient at risk of developing wrist pain or progressive cubitus valgus.

## SURGICAL MANAGEMENT

- At present, there is limited evidence and conflicting retrospective literature on the management of chronic Monteggia lesions. Evidence regarding management of chronic Monteggia lesions is limited to small, single-center retrospective case series.
- Unless there is concern regarding the morphology of the radial head or capitellum, we believe that symptomatic patients with chronic Monteggia lesions are candidates for surgical reconstruction.
- Descriptions of surgical reconstructions for patients with chronic Monteggia lesions include annular ligament repair or reconstruction alone,[2,8,12,13,21,22] ulnar osteotomy alone,[5,9,10,12,14,21,23] combined ulnar osteotomy and annular ligament repair/reconstruction,[8,12–14,17,21,22,25,28] and radial osteotomy.[12,13,25] The relative merit of each surgical technique has not been well elucidated and is likely to vary by patient and lesion. However, almost every series advocates for an ulnar realignment osteotomy when reconstructing a chronic Monteggia lesion. The principal controversy revolves around whether an annular ligament reconstruction should be performed in addition to the ulnar osteotomy.
- The technique for open reduction of the radial head and annular ligament reconstruction in the setting of a chronic Monteggia fracture-dislocation is attributed to Bell Tawse.[2] This technique for radiocapitellar reduction in chronic Monteggia lesions employed the Boyd approach and reconstructed the annular ligament by turning down a strip of triceps fascia.
- Our overall approach for surgical treatment of chronic Monteggia lesions includes an open osteotomy of the ulna with plate fixation, open reduction of radiocapitellar joint, and repair or reconstruction of the annular ligament.
  - To avoid potential complications of posterior interosseous nerve injury and compartment syndrome, the reconstruction is performed via an extensile posterior approach that permits identification and protection of the posterior interosseous nerve and prophylactic forearm fasciotomies.
- There are surgeons who advocate extra-articular osteotomy of the ulna alone, including use of external or intramedullary fixation of the ulna.

### Preoperative Planning

- The morphology of the radial head and capitellum should be evaluated on plain radiographs and, if necessary, on MRI to define the concavity of the radial head and the reducibility of the proximal radioulnar joint and radiocapitellar joints. A normal concave radial head articular surface and normal convex capitellar articular surface are requirements for reconstruction. Three-dimensional imaging in children with radial head dislocation more than 3 years from injury can reveal flattening of the radial head and even development of a dome-shaped deformity.[18] Corresponding flattening of the lesser sigmoid notch can also be observed.[18]
- Preoperative elbow flexion–extension and forearm supination–pronation should be measured and recorded.

### Positioning

- General anesthesia is preferred over a regional block to allow postoperative assessment of peripheral nerve function and compartment syndrome.
- The patient is placed in a supine position on the operating table with the elbow, forearm, and hand outstretched onto a hand table. The entire upper limb including the axilla should be included in the surgical field.
- A sterile pneumatic tourniquet is employed to maximize access to the upper arm, which is required for the extensile surgical approach.

### Approach

- One of two surgical intervals, the Boyd (extensile posterior) or the Kocher (posterolateral), can be employed for open reduction of the radiocapitellar joint and repair or reconstruction of the annular ligament (**FIG 9**).
  - Either approach can be extended distally along the subcutaneous border of the ulna which can be exposed in the interval between the extensor carpi ulnaris and the flexor carpi ulnaris.

- Either approach can also be extended proximally to help identify the radial nerve and expose the triceps fascia if required for reconstruction of the annular ligament.
- The Boyd or extensile posterior approach to the elbow requires development of an interval between the anconeus and the ulna and permits excellent visualization of the radiocapitellar joint.
- The Kocher or posterior approach to the elbow is developed between the anconeus and the extensor carpi ulnaris.

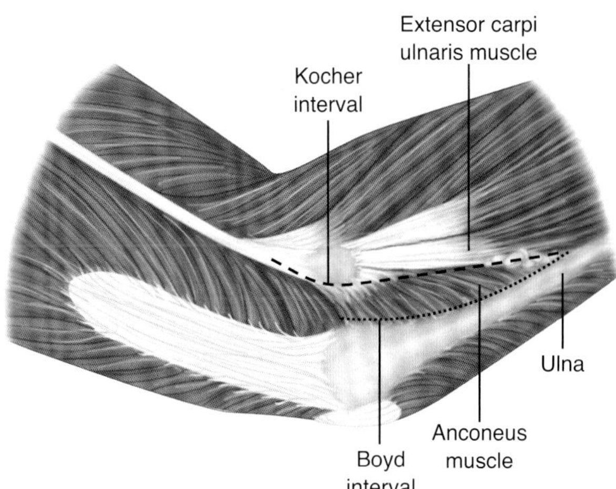


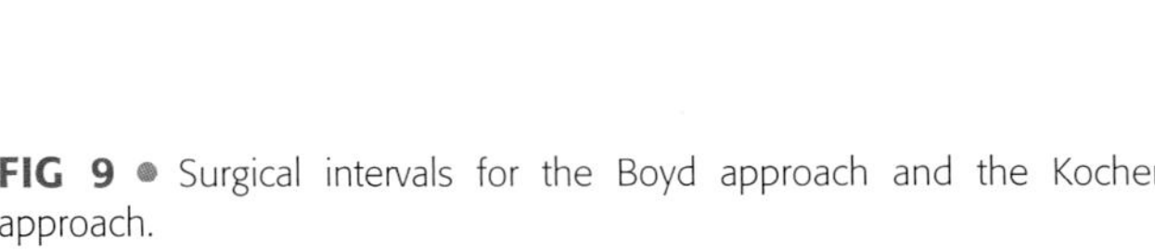

**FIG 9** • Surgical intervals for the Boyd approach and the Kocher approach.



## Extensile Posterolateral Approach

- An extensile curvilinear posterolateral incision is planned (**TECH FIG 1A**).
- The midportion of the incision permits access to the radiocapitellar joint through the Kocher interval, defined as the interval between the anconeus and the extensor carpi ulnaris.
- The incision can be extended proximally which allows identification and decompression of the radial nerve and harvesting of the triceps fascia if required for annular ligament reconstruction.
- The incision can be extended distally toward the subcutaneous border of the ulna for the ulnar opening wedge osteotomy. The ulna is exposed between the extensor carpi ulnaris and the flexor carpi ulnaris.
- Initially, only the proximal and midportion of the incision is opened.
  - The radial nerve should be identified between the brachioradialis and the brachialis and can be traced distally as it bifurcates into its sensory and motor (posterior interosseous) branches (**TECH FIG 1B**).
  - As noted earlier, the posterior intraosseous nerve can be adherent to the anterior elbow joint capsule which itself is distorted by the dislocated radial head.
  - Identification of the posterior interosseous nerve allows for its protection during joint reduction and annular ligament repair/reconstruction.
- In the midportion of the incision, the interval between the anconeus and the extensor carpi ulnaris is then developed (**TECH FIG 1C**).
  - If necessary for visualization, the extensor–supinator mass can be elevated off of the anterior lateral epicondyle and lateral supracondylar ridge as a single soft tissue sleeve.
  - Placement of marking sutures will facilitate anatomic repair of the extensor–supinator origin during closure.
  - The elbow capsule is incised anterior to the lateral ulnar collateral ligament to preserve the integrity of lateral ligamentous complex and ulnohumeral stability.

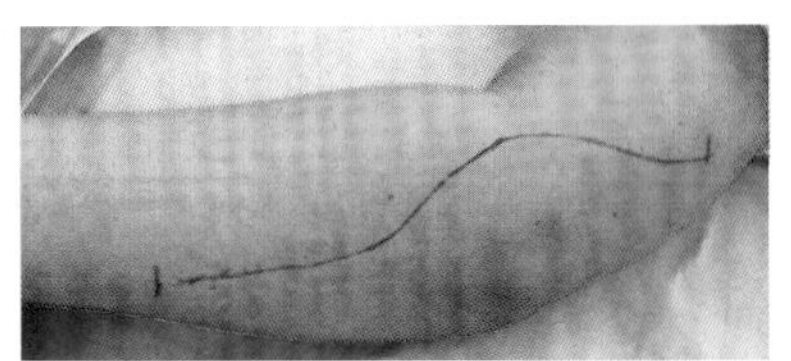
A

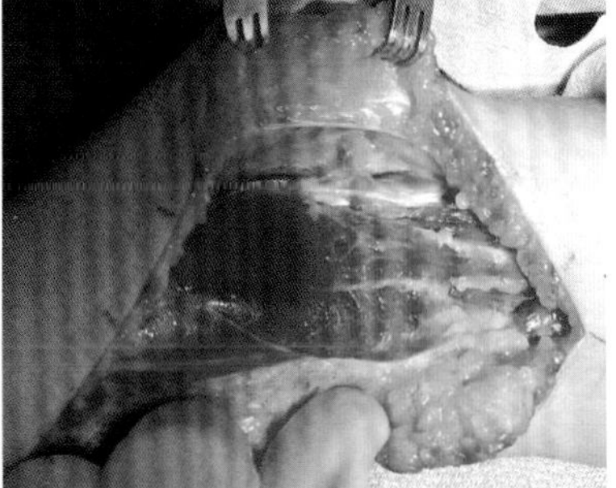
B

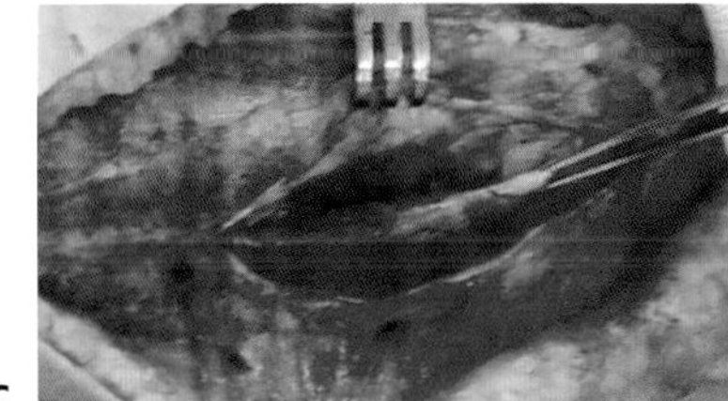
C

**TECH FIG 1** • Surgical exposure for reconstruction of a chronic Monteggia lesion. **A.** A curvilinear posterolateral approach to the elbow is planned. The proximal and distal extent of the incision is used as necessary. **B.** The posterior interosseous nerve should be identified at its bifurcation from the radial nerve and traced distally. The posterior interosseous nerve should be carefully dissected off of the anterior elbow capsule to avoid iatrogenic injury during radiocapitellar reduction. **C.** The interval between the anconeus and the extensor carpi ulnaris is used to access the radiocapitellar joint. (© COSF, Boston. From Flynn J, ed. Pediatric Hand and Upper Limb Surgery. Philadelphia: Lippincott Williams & Wilkins, 2012.)

## Open Reduction of the Radiocapitellar Joint

- Inspection of the radiocapitellar joint is initially obscured by fibrosis and synovitis. The radial head is typically dislocated anteriorly with a wall of anterior capsule and annular ligament blocking reduction.
- Pulvinar and synovitis are carefully débrided from the radiocapitellar joint to permit visualization of the radial head, annular ligament, and capitellum (**TECH FIG 2**). The lesser sigmoid notch should also be thoroughly débrided to permit reduction of the proximal radioulnar joint. Thorough débridement of this region is critical to anatomic joint reduction and stabilization.
- Protection of the posterior interosseous nerve is necessary during joint débridement.
- Although tedious, the annular ligament can generally be identified. The central aperture of the annular ligament may not be readily appreciated, but careful dissection and dilation of its aperture allows reconstitution of its typical ring shape.
  - Dilation is performed by making small radial incisions extending from the center toward the periphery.
  - At this stage, a decision must be made about whether the native annular ligament can be salvaged. The native ligament is generally usable.
- If the annular ligament cannot be reduced over the radial head, the ligament may be incised along its posterior insertion (at or adjacent to the posterior rim of the lesser sigmoid notch) and repaired following reduction of the radial head.
  - If necessary, repair of the annular ligament is completed through ulnar periosteal tunnels with braided 2-0 polyester suture (Ethibond, Ethicon, Inc., Somerville, NJ).
- If the annular ligament can be salvaged, the reduction of the radial head is evaluated with fluoroscopy.
- If there is anatomic restoration of radiocapitellar alignment, annular ligament repair (or reconstruction) alone may be sufficient.
  - This is very unusual, and typically, ulnar osteotomy is required.
- If the annular ligament cannot be salvaged, its remnant is sharply excised in preparation for subsequent annular ligament reconstruction, usually with a strip of triceps or extensor–supinator fascia.

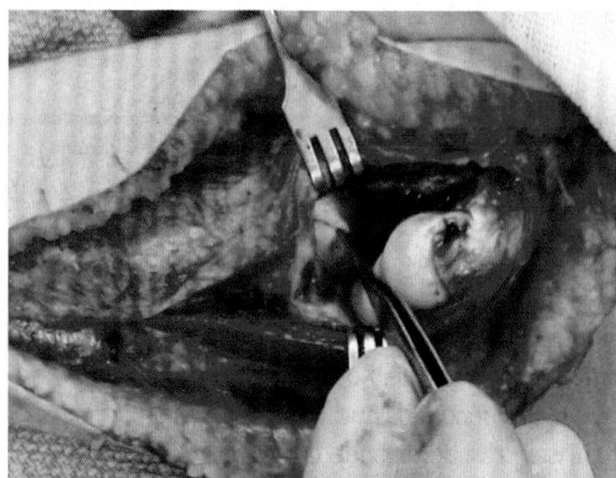

**TECH FIG 2** • The dislocated radial head and the collapsed annular ligament are identified. (© COSF, Boston. From Flynn J, ed. Pediatric Hand and Upper Limb Surgery. Philadelphia: Lippincott Williams & Wilkins, 2012.)

## Ulnar Osteotomy

- In general, annular ligament repair or reconstruction alone does not result in a congruent, stable radiocapitellar reduction due to the deforming force created by concomitant ulnar malunion.
- An opening wedge osteotomy of the ulna is normally required. Some surgeons only perform an extra-articular reconstruction with ulnar osteotomy and do not routinely obtain an open reduction of the radiocapitellar joint or perform an annular ligament reconstruction.
- The ulna is exposed in the extensor carpi ulnaris–flexor carpi ulnaris interval. Osteotomy of the ulna is planned at the apex of the malunion (**TECH FIG 3A**).
  - When the ulnar injury is characterized by plastic deformation, the osteotomy can be made proximal to the apex and closer to the elbow to more effectively correct of radiocapitellar malalignment.
  - Fluoroscopy is used to localize the site of the intended osteotomy, and a subperiosteal exposure is obtained.
- An oscillating saw is used to create an osteotomy with preservation of the far cortex. Copious irrigation with saline is used to minimize thermal necrosis. A laminar spreader is used to create an opening wedge. Partial overcorrection of the ulna is suggested to avoid late radial head dislocation.[14]
- Temporary pinning of the radiocapitellar joint can help determine the size of the opening wedge osteotomy. In this technique, the radiocapitellar and proximal radioulnar joints are anatomically reduced. A smooth 0.045- to 0.062-inch Kirschner wire is temporarily inserted across the radiocapitellar joint to stabilize the reduction.
  - Anatomic reduction of the radial head allows the ulnar osteotomy to open the necessary amount to maintain the reduction.
- When the radial head is anatomically reduced, the ulnar osteotomy is provisionally stabilized with appropriately contoured plate and screw fixation (**TECH FIG 3B**). We typically use double-stacked one-third tubular plates in younger patients and a 3.5-mm dynamic compression plate in larger patients (Synthes, West Chester, PA).
  - Other options include external fixation or intramedullary fixation.

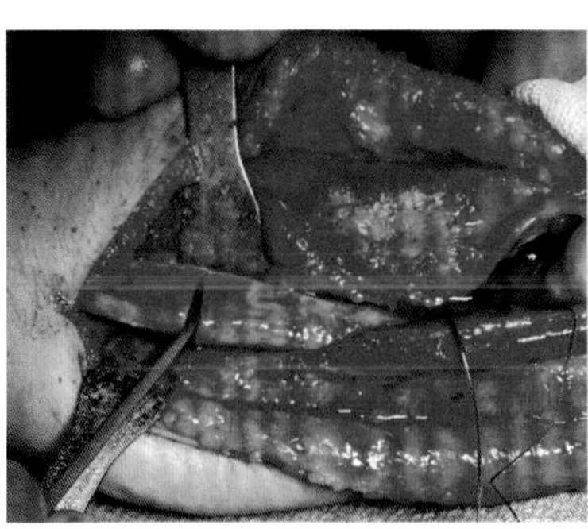
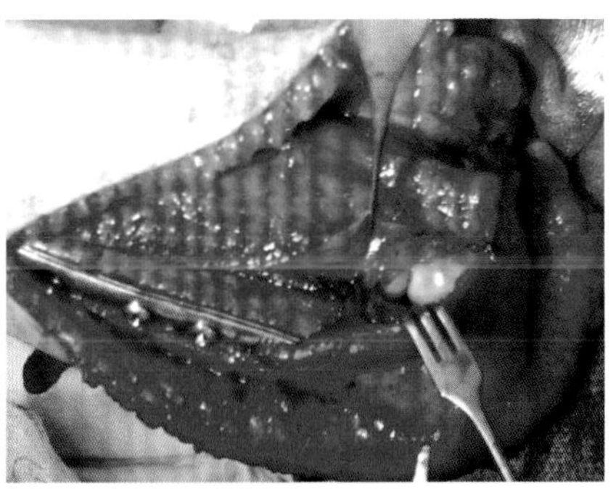
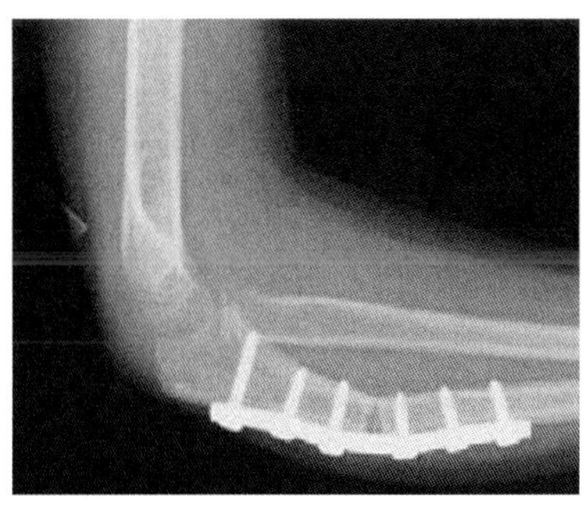

**TECH FIG 3** • Ulnar osteotomy. **A.** An osteotomy of the ulna is performed at the apex of the malunion using an oscillating saw. **B.** The ulnar osteotomy is stabilized with appropriately contoured plate and screw fixation. In younger children, double-stacked one-third tubular plates are employed as illustrated in this case. **C.** Four to six cortices of fixation should be obtained on either side of the ulnar osteotomy. Overcorrection of the ulna, as illustrated here, can help avoid late subluxation of the radial head. (© COSF, Boston. **A,B:** From Flynn J, ed. Pediatric Hand and Upper Limb Surgery. Philadelphia: Lippincott Williams & Wilkins, 2012; **C:** From Shah AS, Waters PM. Monteggia fracture-dislocation in children. In: Rockwood and Wilkins' Fractures in Children, ed 8. Philadelphia: Lippincott Williams & Wilkins. In press.)

- The temporary Kirschner wire is removed. Further testing under direct visualization and fluoroscopy is performed to confirm that the correct angle and degree of osteotomy was selected for maintenance of radiocapitellar and proximal radioulnar joint alignment.
  - If correct, the fixation is completed. Four to six cortices of fixation should be achieved proximal and distal to the osteotomy site (**TECH FIG 3C**).
- If available at the malunion site, fracture callous and periosteal bone can be used for local graft after completion of the osteotomy. Periosteal repair is performed to expedite bone healing.
- As mentioned, an alternative to plate and screw fixation is external fixation.[5,9] External fixation can be used with an acute opening wedge osteotomy[9] or by gradual lengthening and angulation.[5]

## Annular Ligament Reconstruction

- In our opinion, annular ligament repair or reconstruction is indicated. This involves either suture repair of the reduced annular ligament to the proximal ulna or, if an annular ligament repair is not feasible, use of local fascia for reconstruction.
  - Although this is supported by many surgeons, several investigators report success with isolated ulnar osteotomy. Sufficient evidence does not exist to demonstrate a clear advantage to either approach.
- A strip of triceps fascia may be used to perform an annular ligament reconstruction. While preserving its attachment to the olecranon, an 8-cm strip of the central triceps fascia is elevated off the muscle in a proximal to distal fashion, all the way to the level of the radial neck. The extensor–supinator fascia may be used as an alternative.
- Careful dissection is required to avoid inadvertent amputation of the triceps fascia from olecranon apophysis.
- The fascial strip is then passed around the radial neck in order to recreate the annular ligament.
- The reconstructed ligament can be passed through drill holes created in the ulna or reapproximated to the ulnar periosteum using braided 2-0 polyester suture.
  - Often, periosteal repair is sufficient in the young child.
- Seel and Peterson[22] advocate use of two crossing drill holes in the proximal ulna placed at the anterior and posterior margins of the lesser sigmoid notch. Although this procedure increases the technical difficulty, the resulting reconstruction may prevent the more posteriorly directed force that can occur with the Bell Tawse technique (**TECH FIG 4**).[2,22]
  - To facilitate annular ligament reconstruction using the Seel and Peterson technique, we recommend provisionally suturing the triceps fascia and using a wire loop for suture passage.
- Overtensioning of the reconstruction should be avoided in order to prevent notching of the radial neck in the long term.

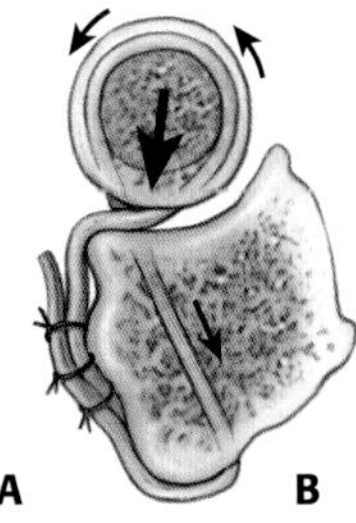
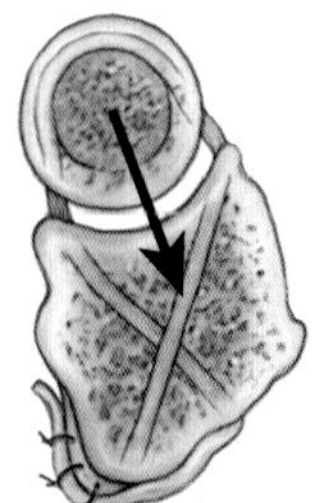

**TECH FIG 4** • Schematic representation of annular ligament reconstruction techniques. **A.** The Bell Tawse reconstruction which results in a posteriorly directed force.[2] **B.** The technique suggested by Seel and Peterson. In this technique, crossing drill holes are created at the anterior and posterior rim of the lesser sigmoid notch. The resulting reconstruction may improve stability of the radial head.[22] (Adapted from Seel MJ, Peterson HA. Management of chronic posttraumatic radial head dislocation in children. J Pediatr Orthop 1999;19:306–312.)

## Prophylactic Forearm Fasciotomies

- Under direct visualization, limited prophylactic fasciotomies of the volar and dorsal compartments are performed to minimize risk of postoperative compartment syndrome.
- Prophylactic fasciotomies have the secondary advantage of facilitating periosteal closure.

## Final Evaluation of Reduction and Wound Closure

- Final orthogonal fluoroscopy images should be obtained to verify stable reduction of the radiocapitellar and proximal radio-ulnar joints.
- Continued wire fixation of the radiocapitellar joint is rarely needed if the ulnar osteotomy and annular ligament repair/reconstruction are performed correctly.
  - In our experience, this has been occasionally necessary in revision reconstruction of a chronic Monteggia lesion where reconstructive options are more limited.
  - In this case, a wire of sufficient size is mandatory to avoid fatigue and breakage. As always, a smooth wire should be used to avoid physeal injury. The wire is typically removed 3 to 4 weeks postoperatively.
- Following radiocapitellar reduction, annular ligament repair or reconstruction, and ulnar osteotomy, a layered wound closure is performed. The periosteum overlying the ulna is repaired to expedite bone healing.
- The capsule is repaired and the extensor–supinator origin is reattached to the lateral epicondyle and lateral supracondylar ridge of the humerus. Intermuscular intervals are reapproximated, and the wound is closed over a Jackson-Pratt drain.

## PEARLS AND PITFALLS

| | |
|---|---|
| **Distinguish congenital and traumatic dislocation of the radial head** | ▪ Hypoplasia of the capitellum and convex deformity of the radial head is indicative of a congenital radial head dislocation. |
| **Avoidance of compartment syndrome** | ▪ Avoid preoperative regional block to monitor the child following reconstruction.<br>▪ Prophylactic volar and dorsal forearm fasciotomies can be performed to minimize risk of postoperative compartment syndrome.<br>▪ Wounds should be closed over a drain if there is a concern for hemostasis. |
| **Protection of the posterior interosseous nerve** | ▪ When planning an intra-articular reconstruction of a long-standing lesion or in the presence of a preoperative radial neuropathy, the radial nerve should be identified in the brachioradialis–brachialis interval and then followed distally as it branches into the superficial radial nerve and the posterior interosseous nerve.<br>▪ The posterior interosseous nerve can be adherent to the joint capsule and displaced radial head or incarcerated at the radiocapitellar joint. Careful identification and protection of the posterior interosseous nerve during surgical exposure can help avoid iatrogenic injury during the reconstruction. |
| **Late subluxation of the radial head** | ▪ Combined annular ligament reconstruction and ulnar osteotomy is advocated.<br>▪ After completion of the ulnar osteotomy, setting the radiocapitellar alignment first is helpful as this determines the amount of ulnar correction needed to maintain a stable reduction.<br>▪ Overcorrection of the ulna is often required for stable reduction of the radial head.<br>▪ Carefully scrutinize the reduction with intraoperative fluoroscopy, and do not accept subtle malalignment.<br>▪ Serial radiographs should be obtained 2–6 weeks after surgical intervention in order to detect unexpected loss of reduction early. |
| **Ulnar nonunion** | ▪ If an oscillating saw is used for the osteotomy, copious irrigation should be employed to minimize thermal necrosis.<br>▪ Plate fixation is mandatory to avoid loss of fixation.<br>▪ Fracture callous and periosteal bone at the site of the malunion can be used as local bone graft after completion of the osteotomy.<br>▪ If needed, allograft bone is added to the osteotomy site. |

## POSTOPERATIVE CARE

- Following wound closure, a bivalved long-arm cast is applied, typically with the elbow in 80 to 90 degrees of flexion and the forearm in 60 to 90 degrees of supination to maximize stability of the radiocapitellar and proximal radioulnar joints.
- All children should be admitted overnight for pain control and neurovascular monitoring.
- Casting is discontinued 4 to 6 weeks after surgical reconstruction and children are transitioned to a protective long-arm splint for an additional 3 to 4 weeks. Splint removal for active motion, particularly forearm rotation, is important. Formal rehabilitation is initiated and maximal recovery is anticipated at 6 months. Elbow flexion and extension return more rapidly than forearm rotation.

## OUTCOMES

- Data on outcomes following reconstruction of chronic Monteggia lesions is limited to small, retrospective case series. Most reports lack long-term follow-up and fail to report validated functional outcome measures.
- Nakamura et al[17] reported long-term clinical and radiographic outcomes in 22 children that underwent combined ulnar osteotomy and annular ligament reconstruction, at an average follow-up of 84 months.
  - The radial head remained stable in nearly 80% of patients and was subluxated (but not frankly dislocated) in approximately 20% of patients, which is representative of other results reported in the literature.[8,12,21,23]
  - Postoperative functional outcomes (Mayo Elbow Performance Index) reliably improved, with the vast majority of patients experiencing excellent (19 of 22) or good (2 of 22) results.
  - Average elbow flexion improved from 124 to 138 degrees. Average postoperative forearm pronation exceeded 65 degrees. Improvement in elbow motion is reliable and similar results have been described by other investigators. Loss of some forearm rotation, particularly pronation, can be expected.[8,12,13,21,23]
- The complication rate for chronic Monteggia reconstruction is high and includes late radial head subluxation, notching of the radial neck, osteoarthritis, delayed ulnar union, ulnar nonunion, compartment syndrome, peripheral nerve injury, and stiffness, amongst others.[17,21]
- Good results can more reliably be obtained in children younger than 12 years of age or within 3 years of injury.[17]

## COMPLICATIONS

- Restricted elbow or forearm motion, particularly pronation
- Postoperative compartment syndrome can occur. Routine perioperative neurovascular monitoring is recommended for early detection. Pain out of proportion to examination or increasing narcotic requirements represent early signs of compartment syndrome and should prompt immediate evaluation. Prophylactic intraoperative forearm fasciotomies are advocated to lessen the risk.
- Posterior interosseous nerve palsy can occur following reconstruction. If the nerve was identified and protected during surgery, expectant management is recommended. Serial clinical examination will demonstrate an advancing Tinel sign and progressive return of motor function. Failure of recognizable clinical recovery by 6 months is a relative indication for surgical exploration.
- Ulnar nerve palsy can occur with extensive lengthening of the ulna and may be an indication for decompression.
- Recurrent subluxation or dislocation of the radial head does occur and negates the original purpose for surgical reconstruction. This is not an operation for the uninitiated.
- Notching of the radial neck if the annular ligament reconstruction is too taut.[17]
- Ulnar nonunion can occur. An incomplete hinged osteotomy, supplemental bone grafting, stable fixation, and periosteal repair lessen the risk.

## REFERENCES


1. Bado JL. The Monteggia lesion. Clin Orthop Relat Res 1967;50:71–86.
2. Bell Tawse AJ. The treatment of malunited anterior Monteggia fractures in children. J Bone Joint Surg Br 1965;47:718–723.
3. Chen WS. Late neuropathy in chronic dislocation of the radial head. Report of two cases. Acta Orthop Scand 1992;63:343–344.
4. Dormans JP, Rang M. The problem of Monteggia fracture-dislocations in children. Orthop Clin North Am 1990;21:251–256.
5. Exner GU. Missed chronic anterior Monteggia lesion. Closed reduction by gradual lengthening and angulation of the ulna. J Bone Joint Surg Br 2001;83:547–550.
6. Fahey JJ. Fractures of the elbow in children. Instr Course Lect 1960;17:13–46.
7. Golden DW, Jhee JT, Gilpin SP, et al. Elbow range of motion and clinical carrying angle in a healthy pediatric population. J Pediatr Orthop B 2007;16:144–149.
8. Gyr BM, Stevens PM, Smith JT. Chronic Monteggia fractures in children: outcome after treatment with the Bell-Tawse procedure. J Pediatr Orthop B 2004;13:402–406.
9. Hasler CC, Von Laer L, Hell AK. Open reduction, ulnar osteotomy and external fixation for chronic anterior dislocation of the head of the radius. J Bone Joint Surg Br 2005;87:88–94.
10. Hirayama T, Takemitsu Y, Yagihara K, et al. Operation for chronic dislocation of the radial head in children. Reduction by osteotomy of the ulna. J Bone Joint Surg Br 1987;69:639–642.
11. Holst-Nielsen F, Jensen V. Tardy posterior interosseous nerve palsy as a result of an unreduced radial head dislocation in Monteggia fractures: a report of two cases. J Hand Surg Am 1984;9:572–575.
12. Horii E, Nakamura R, Koh S, et al. Surgical treatment for chronic radial head dislocation. J Bone Joint Surg Am 2002;84-A(7):1183–1188.
13. Hui JH, Sulaiman AR, Lee HC, et al. Open reduction and annular ligament reconstruction with fascia of the forearm in chronic monteggia lesions in children. J Pediatr Orthop 2005;25:501–506.
14. Inoue G, Shionoya K. Corrective ulnar osteotomy for malunited anterior Monteggia lesions in children. 12 patients followed for 1-12 years. Acta Orthop Scand 1998;69:73–76.
15. Kunkel S, Cornwall R, Little K, et al. Limitations of the radiocapitellar line for assessment of pediatric elbow radiographs. J Pediatr Orthop 2011;31:628–632.
16. Martin BF. The annular ligament of the superior radio-ulnar joint. J Anat 1958;92:473–482.
17. Nakamura K, Hirachi K, Uchiyama S, et al. Long-term clinical and radiographic outcomes after open reduction for missed Monteggia fracture-dislocations in children. J Bone Joint Surg Am 2009;91:1394–1404.
18. Oka K, Murase T, Moritomo H, et al. Morphologic evaluation of chronic radial head dislocation: three-dimensional and quantitative analyses. Clin Orthop Relat Res 2010;468:2410–2418.
19. Ramski DE, Hennrikus WP, Bae DS, et al. Pediatric Monteggia fractures: a multicenter examination of treatment strategy and early clinical and radiographic results. J Pediatr Orthop 2015;35(2):115–120.
20. Ring D, Waters PM. Operative fixation of Monteggia fractures in children. J Bone Joint Surg Br 1996;78:734–739.

21. Rodgers WB, Waters PM, Hall JE. Chronic Monteggia lesions in children. Complications and results of reconstruction. J Bone Joint Surg Am 1996;78:1322–1329.
22. Seel MJ, Peterson HA. Management of chronic posttraumatic radial head dislocation in children. J Pediatr Orthop 1999;19:306–312.
23. Song KS, Ramnani K, Bae KC, et al. Indirect reduction of the radial head in children with chronic Monteggia lesions. J Orthop Trauma 2012;26:597–601.
24. Spinner M, Kaplan EB. The quadrate ligament of the elbow—its relationship to the stability of the proximal radio-ulnar joint. Acta Orthop Scand 1970;41:632–647.
25. Stoll TM, Willis RB, Paterson DC. Treatment of the missed Monteggia fracture in the child. J Bone Joint Surg Br 1992;74:436–440.
26. Tompkins DG. The anterior Monteggia fracture: observations on etiology and treatment. J Bone Joint Surg Am 1971;53:1109–1114.
27. Tubbs RS, O'Neil JT Jr, Key CD, et al. The oblique cord of the forearm in man. Clin Anat 2007;20:411–415.
28. Wang MN, Chang WN. Chronic posttraumatic anterior dislocation of the radial head in children: thirteen cases treated by open reduction, ulnar osteotomy, and annular ligament reconstruction through a Boyd incision. J Orthop Trauma 2006;20:1–5.

# Closed, Percutaneous, Intramedullary, and Open Reduction of Radial Head and Neck Fractures

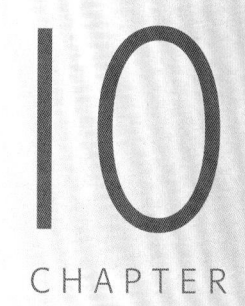


Roger Cornwall

## DEFINITION

- Radial neck fractures are extra-articular fractures of the radius proximal to the bicipital tuberosity.
- Radial neck fractures are most common in children 9 to 12 years old and represent 14% of elbow fractures in children.[17] The physis is typically involved as a Salter-Harris I or II pattern (**FIG 1**), yet Salter-Harris III and IV patterns also occur. Alternatively, the fracture can be extraphyseal through the metaphysis.[1,33]
- Intra-articular radial head fractures are less common elbow injuries in patients with open physes than in skeletally mature patients (7% vs. 52%).[18]
- The Wilkins classification of radial head and neck fractures is based on the mechanism of injury and the pattern of the fracture, specifically whether there is physeal or articular involvement[34]:
  - Type I: valgus injury
    - A: physeal injury—Salter-Harris I or II
    - B: intra-articular—Salter-Harris III or IV
    - C: metaphyseal fracture
  - Type II: elbow dislocation
    - D: fracture occurred during reduction
    - E: fracture occurred during dislocation
- The O'Brien and Judet classifications of radial neck fractures are based on degree of angulation.
  - O'Brien classification[22]
    - Type I: less than 30 degrees
    - Type II: 30 to 60 degrees
    - Type III: more than 60 degrees
  - Judet classification[14] (**FIG 2**)
    - Type I: undisplaced
    - Type II: less than 30 degrees
    - Type III: 30 to 60 degrees
    - Type IVa: 60 to 80 degrees
    - Type IVb: more than 80 degrees

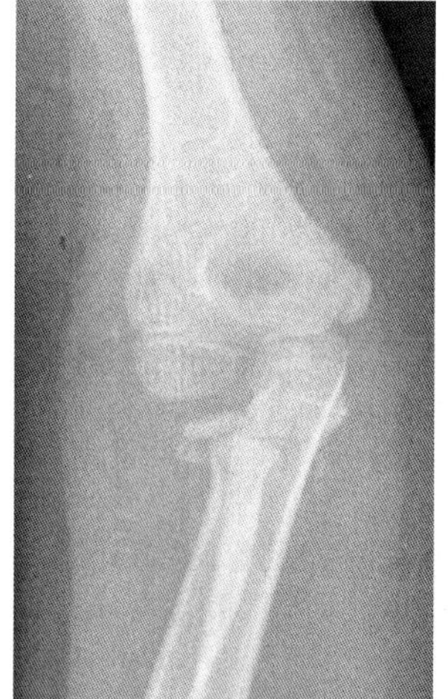
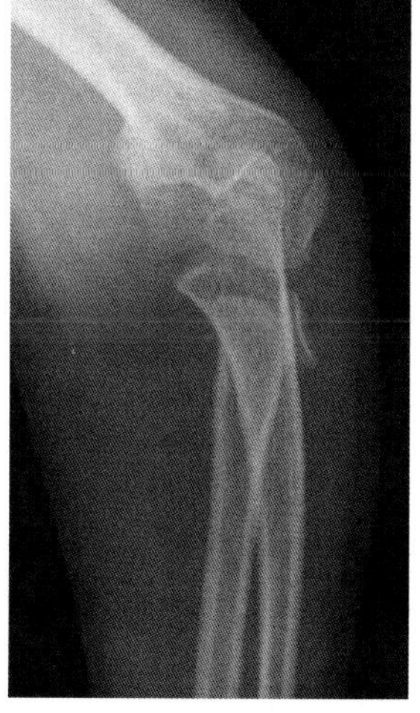

**FIG 1** • Displaced radial neck fractures. **A.** Salter-Harris type II. **B.** Salter-Harris type I.

## ANATOMY

- The radial head articulates with the capitellum and the radial notch of the ulna. The radial neck is extra-articular and has a normal 15 degrees of angulation on anteroposterior (AP) and 5 degrees on lateral radiographic views. The radial head ossific nucleus appears at about 4 years of age.
- Ossification of the proximal radial epiphysis (radial head) occurs by 4 years of age, at which time the radial head and neck have assumed their adult shape. The proximal radial physis closes at 14 years in girls and 17 years in boys.
- The proximal radioulnar joint is stabilized by the annular ligament and the accessory collateral ligament.
- There are no muscular attachments to the radial neck. The blood supply is derived from the adjacent periosteum.
- The radial nerve gives rise to the superficial radial nerve and the posterior interosseous nerve at the level of the lateral condyle. The posterior interosseous nerve travels distally anterior to the radial head and neck, enters the arcade of Frohse 2.6 cm distal to the radial head (**FIG 3**), and submerges between the superficial and deep fibers of the supinator 6.7 cm distal to the radial head.[5] The radial recurrent artery originates from the radial artery and travels toward the lateral epicondyle in the opposite direction along the path of the radial nerve on the anteromedial surface of the supinator.

## PATHOGENESIS

- The most common mechanism of radial neck fractures is a valgus and axial force to the elbow caused by a fall on an outstretched hand. This mechanism results in a lateral compression and a medial traction injury. The actual plane of maximal radial head angulation depends on the forearm position of supination or pronation at the time of impact.[12]
- The other mechanism of injury is an elbow dislocation where the fracture occurs either during the dislocation (radial head anterior) or during the elbow reduction (radial head posterior).[12]
- Associated injuries, such as medial collateral ligament rupture or occult elbow dislocation, occur in 30% to 50% of radial neck fractures.[28]

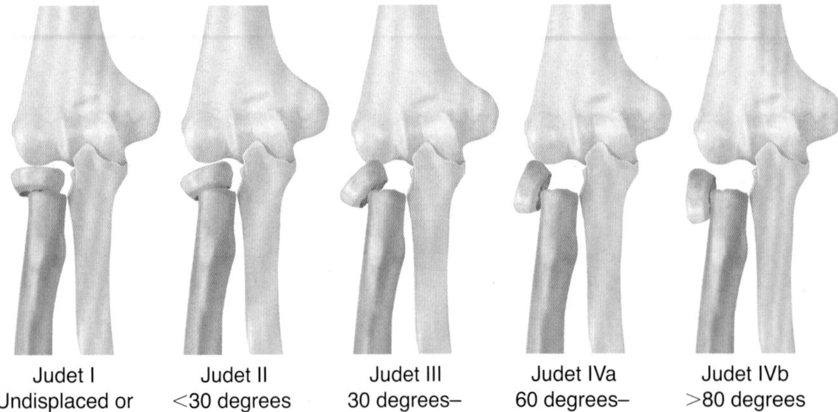


**FIG 2** • Judet classification of radial neck fractures in children.

- A posteriorly displaced radial neck fracture can occur during the spontaneous reduction of a posterior elbow dislocation.[11]
- Alternatively, an unrecognized (undisplaced) radial neck fracture can be displaced posteriorly during the manipulative reduction of a posterior elbow dislocation. During the reduction maneuver, if the elbow is flexed, the distal humerus (lateral condyle) strikes the radial head, knocking it posteriorly off the metaphysis (**FIG 4**).
- Chronic stress fractures of the radial head and neck can occur with repetitive valgus loading, such as overhead throwing.

## NATURAL HISTORY

- The prognosis for radial neck fractures depends on the energy of injury, the amount of displacement, and the presence of any associated injuries.
- Most radial neck fractures are minimally displaced or undisplaced. These heal uneventfully.
- The greater the degree of angulation or translation, the greater the disruption in the relationship of the radiocapitellar joint, which may be associated with a decrease in the range of pronation and supination.[3]
- The upper limit of acceptable angulation (0 to 60 degrees) is unclear and may be age-dependent.[24] Most believe that angulation less than 30 degrees is unlikely to cause a clinically (functionally) significant loss of motion.
- Other reported consequences include avascular necrosis of the radial head, heterotopic ossification, radioulnar synostosis, and premature physeal closure, which may result in pain, crepitus, and valgus deformity and stiffness.[3,13,24,26,27]
  - These outcomes may be associated with age, severity of displacement, presence of associated injuries, or delay in treatment.
- Some of these might be a complication of the treatment (poor reduction, open treatment, or internal fixation) rather than the natural history.
- Overall, poor results have been reported in up to 15% to 33% of all radial neck fractures in children.[7,10,13,27,30]

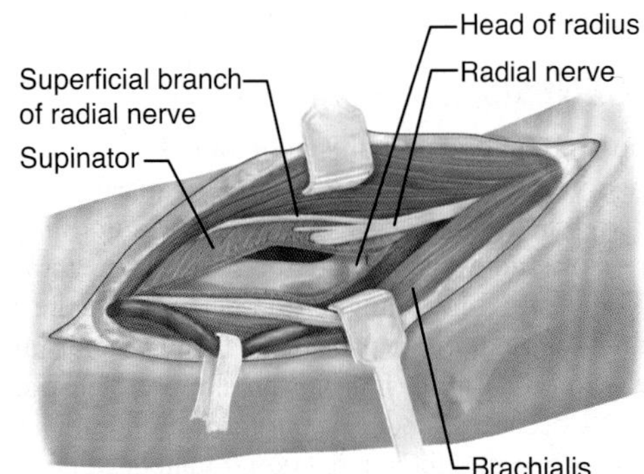


**FIG 3** • The posterior interosseous nerve courses volarly to the radial head and neck and enters the arcade of Frohse about 2.6 cm distal to the articular surface of the radial head.

## PATIENT HISTORY AND PHYSICAL FINDINGS

- Elucidating the mechanism of injury is important to truly understand the personality of the fracture, which can help in directing treatment. Higher energy mechanisms are more likely to be associated with concomitant injuries. Elbow dislocations that have reduced before presentation are not uncommon, so it is helpful to ask the patient and family whether a marked deformity was noted at the time of injury.
- Carefully palpating each anatomic area in the elbow to find the points of maximal tenderness helps diagnose the fracture as well as additional injuries. Associated injuries include medial collateral ligament tears, medial epicondyle fractures, ulnar fractures, and supracondylar humerus fractures. A neurologic evaluation assesses distal radial, medial, and ulnar nerve motor and sensory function.
- Assessing elbow stability and range of motion can help determine the need for treatment.
  - Valgus instability indicates a medial elbow injury in addition to an unstable radial neck fracture.
  - Blocks in forearm rotation, in particular pronation, are typically due to loss of congruity of the radioulnar joint and indicate a need for reduction.
  - Stability and range-of-motion assessment may necessitate either an intra-articular anesthetic injection or an examination under anesthesia.

## IMAGING AND OTHER DIAGNOSTIC STUDIES

- AP, lateral, and oblique radiographs often show radial neck fractures well (**FIG 5A,B**). However, the true extent of fracture angulation can be underestimated on plain radiographs, as orthogonal views may fail to capture the true plane of angulation.

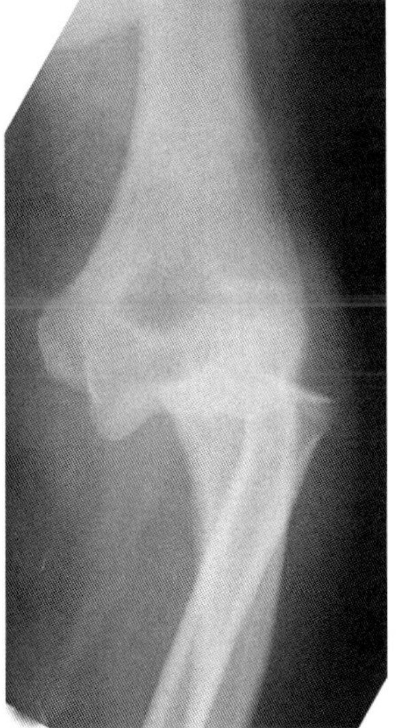
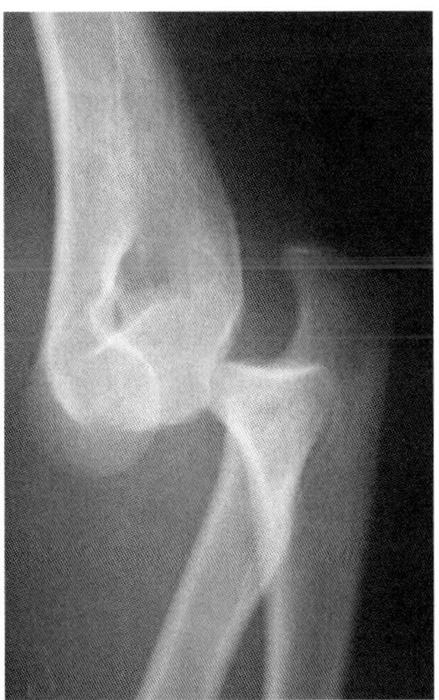
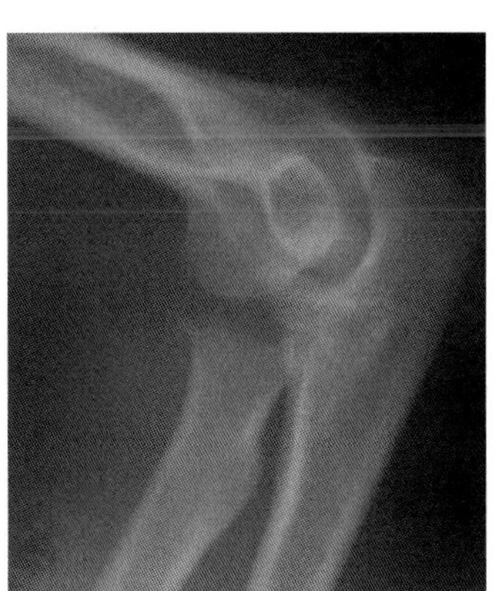
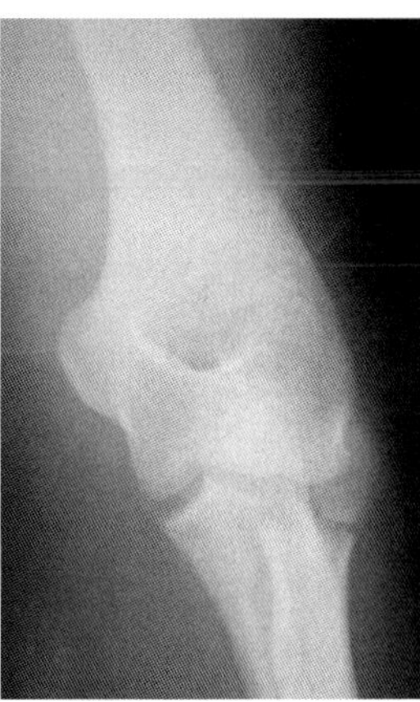

**FIG 4** • Posteriorly displaced radial neck fracture produced during the reduction of a posterior elbow dislocation. **A,B.** AP and lateral views of the elbow dislocation. **C.** The radial head is no longer visible on the lateral view after elbow reduction. **D.** Displaced radial head apparent on AP view.

- The clinician should carefully rule out associated injuries such as fractures of the olecranon (intra-articular) (**FIG 5C,D**), proximal ulna, medial epicondyle, or lateral condyle or elbow dislocation.
- In posterior elbow dislocations, the clinician should carefully examine the radial neck for an occult fracture that is at risk for displacement during the reduction maneuver.
- Radial neck fractures can occur before the ossification of the radial head, without clear evidence of fracture on plain radiographs.
  - Ultrasound, magnetic resonance imaging (MRI) (**FIG 5E**), and arthrography (**FIG 5F,G**) are useful for diagnosing and evaluating radial neck fractures in young patients with nonossified radial heads.
  - In the operating room, arthrography is useful in outlining the nonossified radial head when monitoring and verifying reduction.

## DIFFERENTIAL DIAGNOSIS

- The diagnosis of a radial neck fracture is usually easily made with appropriate imaging. However, the presence or absence of the following associated injuries should be ascertained:
  - Medial collateral ligament rupture
  - Medial epicondyle fracture
  - Olecranon fracture
  - Monteggia equivalent type IV fracture

## NONOPERATIVE MANAGEMENT

- Ultimately, the objective is to obtain and maintain a congruent joint with restored elbow range of motion in all planes. Most consider up to 30 degrees of angulation and 3 mm of translation as limits of an acceptable reduction.

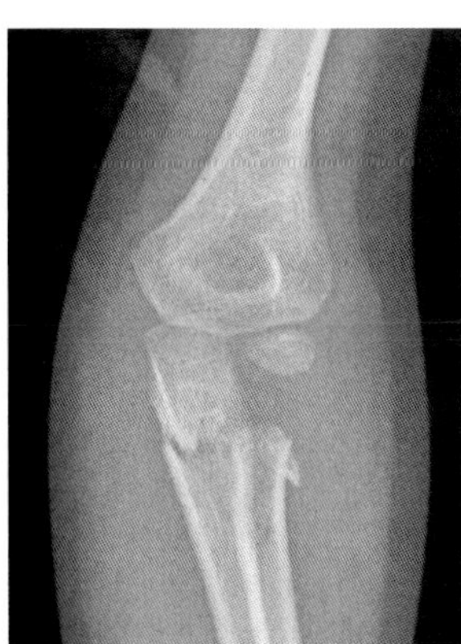
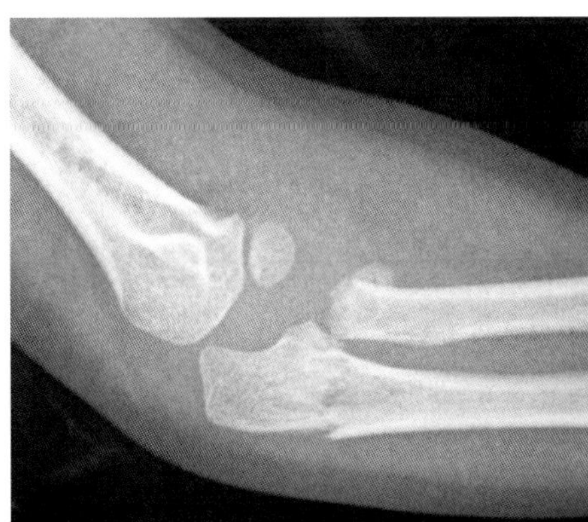
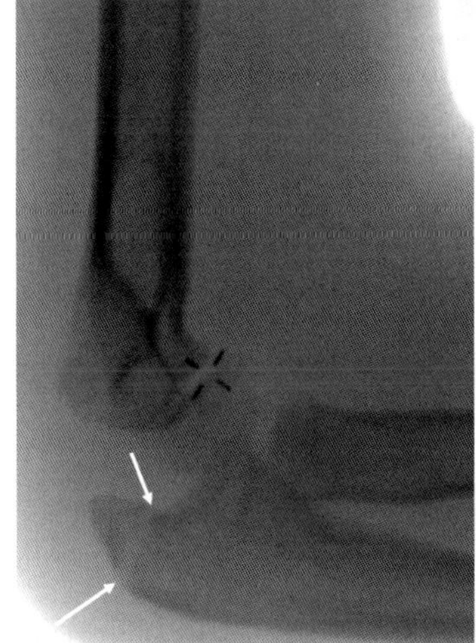

**FIG 5** • **A,B.** AP and lateral radiographs demonstrate an ulnar fracture and radial neck fracture in a 3-year-old child with a nonossified radial head. However, it is difficult to discern the degree of angulation on plain radiographs. MRI is useful when evaluating radial neck fractures in children with nonossified radial heads. **C.** Radial neck fracture with associated intra-articular fracture of the olecranon. Olecranon fracture (*arrows*) appears minimally displaced on lateral view. *(continued)*

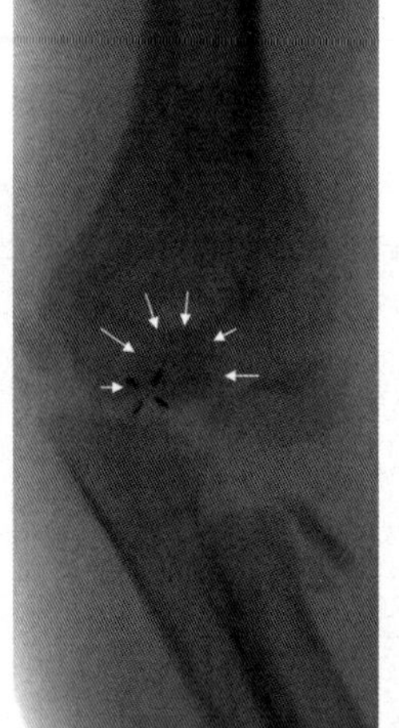
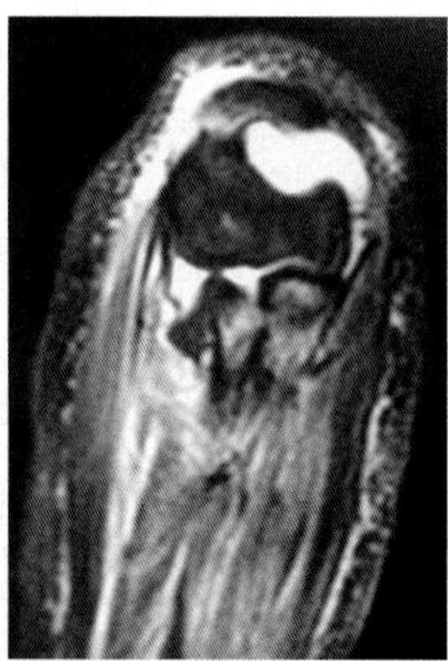
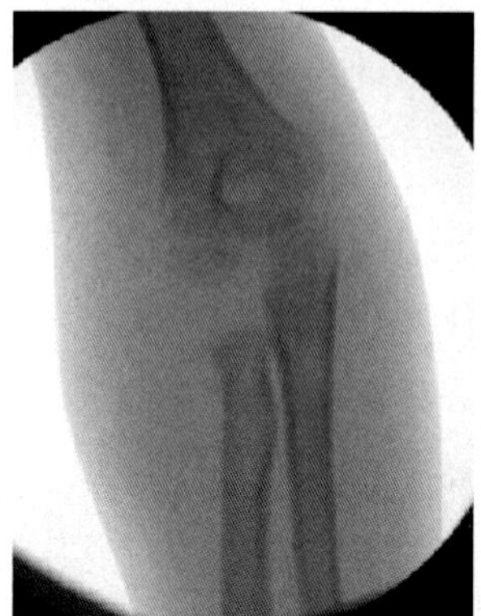
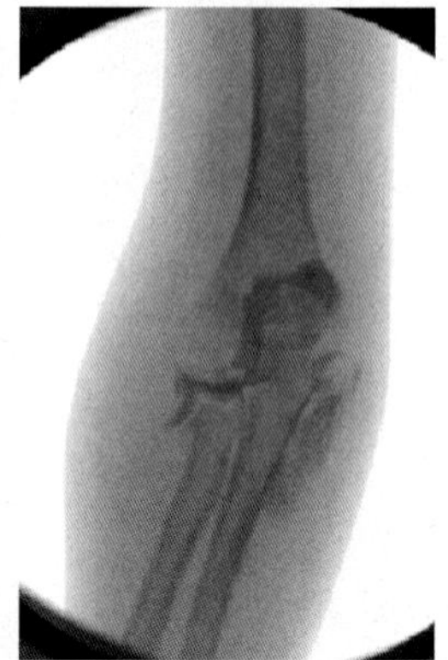
D E F G

**FIG 5** • *(continued)* **D.** Significant displacement of the proximal olecron fragment (*arrows*) is seen on AP view. **E.** MRI from patient in **A** and **B** clearly shows the 60-degree radial neck angulation not defined on plain films. **F,G.** Arthrography demonstrates a 90-degree displaced radial neck fracture not seen on plain films. It is also useful to monitor and verify reduction intraoperatively.

Controversy exists regarding the exact numbers, however, with reported acceptable angulation ranging from 20 to 60 degrees.[1,3,15,21,26,30–34]

- Two things partially account for the controversy:
  - The accuracy of the radiographic measurement is variable and depends on whether the radiographic beam is perpendicular to the true plane of the fracture.
  - Twenty-five degrees of fracture angulation can have variable effects on the congruity of the radioulnar joint, depending on the direction of angulation.
- It is therefore important to base the decision of treatment on the functional effects of the angulation rather than a specific number. Any block of pronation or supination warrants a reduction of the fracture, no matter what the radiographic angulation is.

- As remodeling potential decreases with advancing skeletal maturity, less residual angulation is acceptable (15 to 20 degrees).[9,32]
- Closed reduction is recommended if there is more than 30 degrees of angulation or 3 mm of translation or if there is any block to range of motion. Reduction can be done either with sedation in the emergency room or in the operating room. The advantage of the latter is the immediate ability to proceed to a percutaneous reduction technique should the closed techniques fail, which is more likely in cases with severe displacement.
- The nature and duration of immobilization depend on the fracture pattern, the presumed stability, and the maturity of the patient. For example, a 17-year-old reliable patient with a nondisplaced stable radial neck fracture can be treated with a sling and early range of motion. Physeal fractures, fractures needing reduction, and fractures in young patients usually need immobilization in a cast for 3 weeks, however.
  - When clinical and radiographic signs of healing are lacking, the cast may remain for an additional 2 weeks, followed by a reevaluation of the healing progress.

## SURGICAL MANAGEMENT

- If closed reduction fails, the next step is to proceed to a percutaneous reduction technique. Techniques using a Steinmann pin to push or lever are described in detail in the Techniques section.
- Every attempt to achieve a closed or percutaneous reduction is made, as the rates of complications, including avascular necrosis, heterotopic ossification, and nonunion, are higher with an open approach.[3,21,36]
- The markedly displaced floating fragments associated with elbow dislocations often require an open approach, whereas most angulated radial head fractures can be reduced by a combination of closed and percutaneous techniques.

### Preoperative Planning

- It is essential to obtain proper elbow and forearm radiographs and diagnose all injuries before proceeding to the operating room.
- Familiarity with all of the closed and percutaneous reduction techniques described in the Techniques section is useful, as each fracture behaves and responds differently to different techniques.
- It is prudent to advise both the parents and the operating room staff that a range of techniques from closed to open may be employed to obtain reduction. Doing so eliminates any element of surprise. The surgeon should ensure the availability of elastic titanium nails, Kirschner wires, and Steinmann pins if needed.
- Elbow range of motion and stability are assessed under anesthesia. The elbow is then pronated and supinated under fluoroscopy to find the maximum plane of angulation before reduction (**FIG 6**).
- Several different techniques of closed and percutaneous reduction make up the "reduction ladder" covered in the Techniques section, much like the plastic surgeon's reconstructive ladder. These tools may be used in stepwise progression or in conjunction as needed.

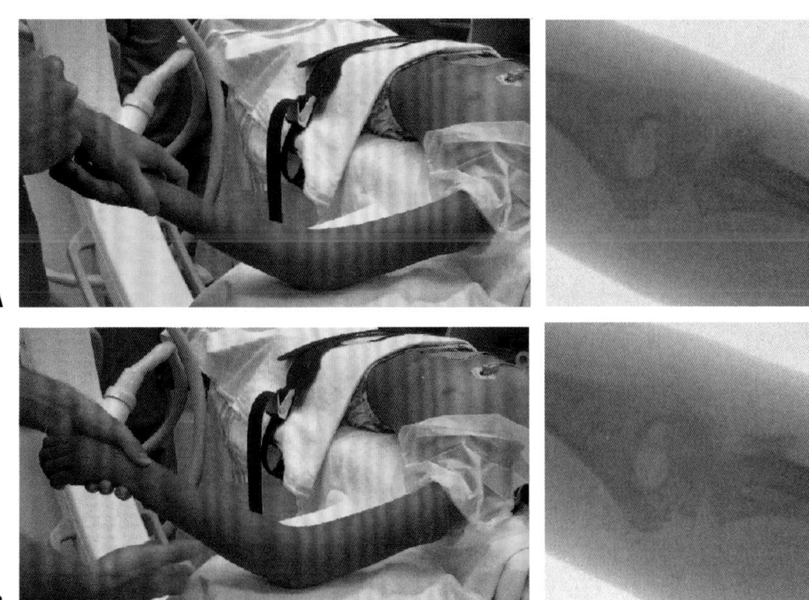

FIG 6 • The maximal angle of displacement is found with fluoroscopy imaging through the ranges of full supination (**A**) to pronation (**B**). In this case, maximal angulation is noted with 50 degrees of pronation.

## Positioning

- The patient is positioned supine on the operating room table, with the elbow on the fluoroscopy C-arm and the arm positioned on the collimator of the C-arm (**FIG 7**).
- The imaging monitor is placed at the opposite side of the bed for easy visualization.
- Alternatively, the patient may be positioned supine with the injured arm positioned over a radiolucent arm board and the image intensifier positioned parallel to the operating table to allow the C-arm to be moved freely from the AP to lateral position.

## Approach

- The posterolateral Kocher approach is used for open reduction of severely displaced floating fragments. The approach is further described in the Techniques section.

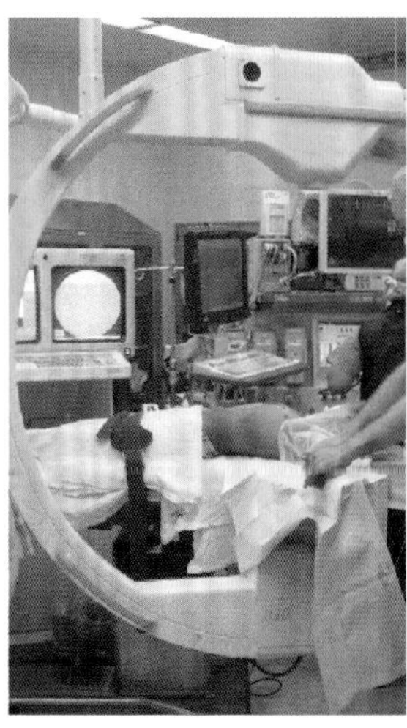

FIG 7 • After sterile preparation, the arm is draped out using the C-arm as an operating table. The imaging monitor is placed for easy visualization on the other side of the bed.

TECHNIQUES

# Closed Reduction

## Israeli or Kaufman Technique

- Kaufman et al[15] described a closed reduction technique with the elbow flexed 90 degrees.
- Fluoroscopy is used to establish the forearm position demonstrating maximal angulation (see **FIG 6**).
- One hand is used to control forearm rotation, and the other hand is used to provide lateral pressure to the displaced radial head with the thumb (**TECH FIG 1A–C**).
- After reduction, fracture stability and range of motion are assessed (**TECH FIG 1D–G**).

## Patterson Technique

- With the elbow extended and forearm supinated, varus stress is applied to the elbow by an assistant. The surgeon reduces the fragment with lateral digital pressure (**TECH FIG 2**).
- Drawbacks of this technique include the need for a knowledgeable assistant providing countertraction and varus stress and the potential difficulty in palpating the radial head in this position.

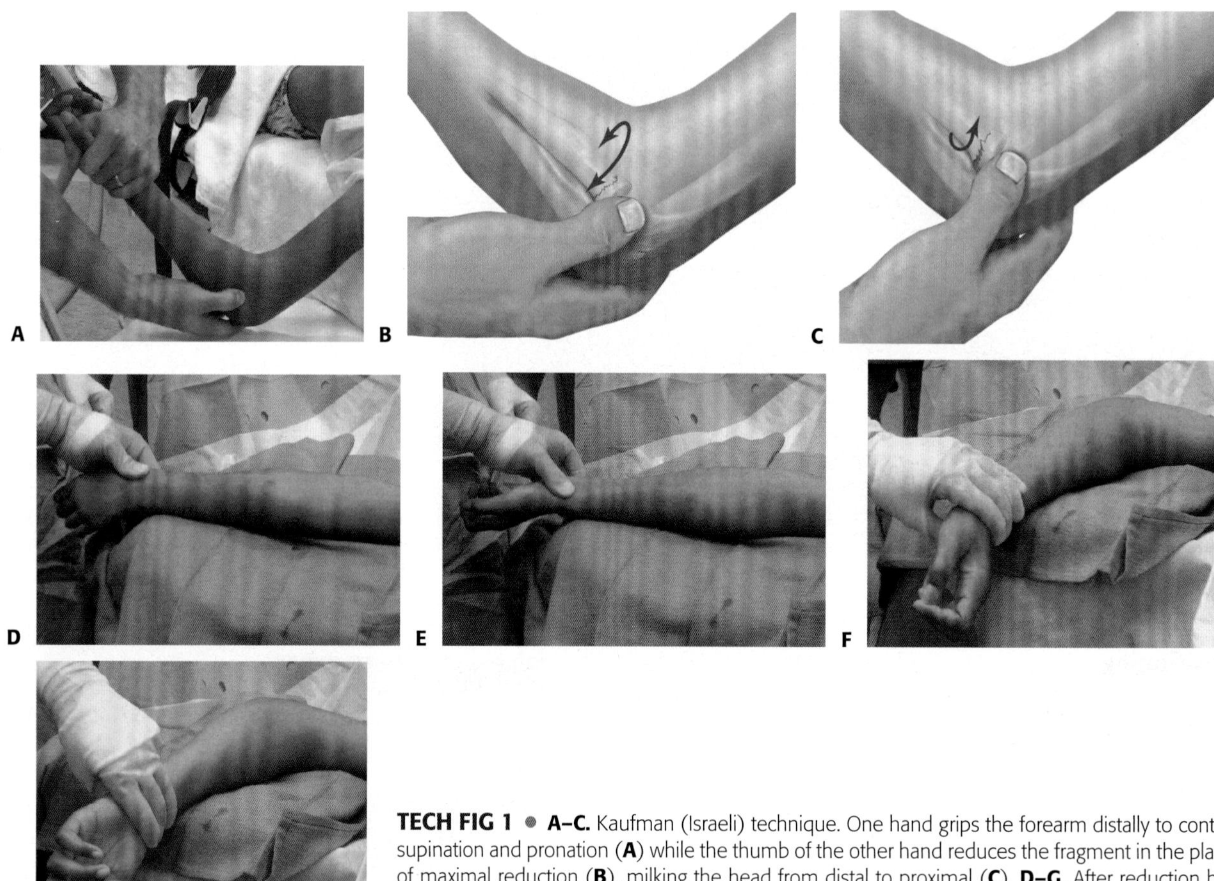

**TECH FIG 1** • **A–C.** Kaufman (Israeli) technique. One hand grips the forearm distally to control supination and pronation (**A**) while the thumb of the other hand reduces the fragment in the plane of maximal reduction (**B**), milking the head from distal to proximal (**C**). **D–G.** After reduction has been obtained, the stability and range of motion (pronation–supination) are assessed in extension and 90 degrees of flexion.

**TECH FIG 2** • Patterson technique. **A.** The assistant helps with positioning the elbow in extension, applying a varus force while holding the forearm in supination. **B,C.** Digital pressure from the thumb is applied to the radial head to achieve reduction.

## Percutaneous Reduction with a Kirschner Wire or Steinmann Pin

- If closed reduction fails, a Kirschner wire or a Steinmann pin can be used to directly push or lever the radial head into anatomic position.
- The surgeon must beware of the posterior interosseous nerve coursing volarly and distally over the radial head. The radial head can be protected by pronating the forearm and by using a posterolateral pin approach (**TECH FIG 3**).
- The forearm is rotated using fluoroscopic guidance so that the plane of maximal angulation is visualized.

### Push Technique

- The blunt end of a larger Kirschner wire, 0.062 inch or larger, is percutaneously inserted through the skin distal to the fracture and just off the lateral border of the ulna (**TECH FIG 4A,B**) through a 2-mm incision.
- With fluoroscopic guidance, the pin is placed against the posterolateral aspect of the proximal fragment, and the radial head is pushed into place (**TECH FIG 4C,D**).
- Axial traction and rotation of the forearm can dislodge an impacted fracture and assist in the reduction.

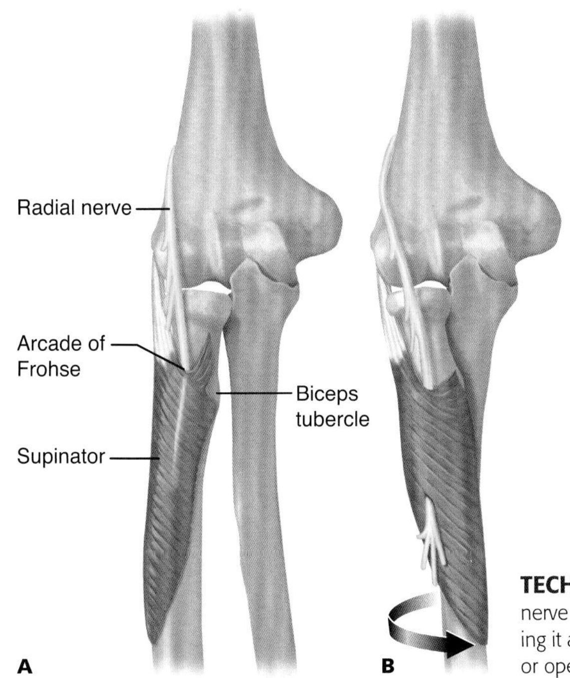


**TECH FIG 3** • **A,B.** The posterior interosseous nerve moves volarly and medially with pronation, moving it away from the working area during percutaneous or open treatment of radial head and neck fractures.

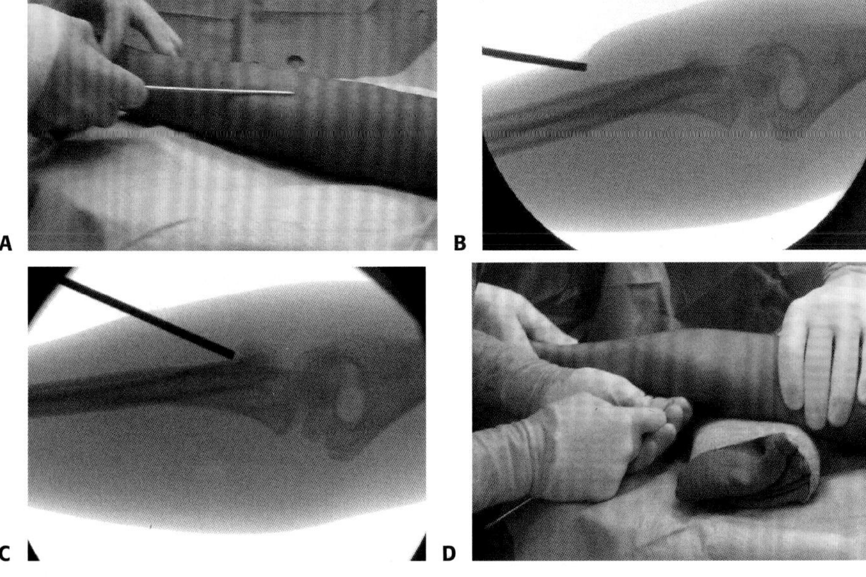


**TECH FIG 4** • Push technique for percutaneous reduction of radial neck fracture. **A,B.** Imaging is used to plan the trajectory of the push pin. The pin is inserted posterolaterally, avoiding the volar posterior interosseous nerve. **C,D.** Using imaging as guidance, the radial head fragment is pushed into reduction.

## Lever Technique

- Alternatively, the pin (or a Freer elevator) can be used as a lever. When doing so, the skin entry site of the pin must be placed more proximally, however, at the level of the fracture site (**TECH FIG 5A**).
- With the pin just through the skin, the pin is pulled distally (applying tension to the skin) to allow a retrograde approach to the fracture.
- The deeper soft tissues are then pierced, the fracture site is entered (**TECH FIG 5B**), and the proximal fragment is levered proximally to correct the angulation while translation is corrected with simultaneous lateral digital pressure. During the levering maneuver, the tensioned skin relaxes, thus making the reduction easier (**TECH FIG 5C**).
  - If the skin instead were entered distally for the lever maneuver, however, the skin tension during the reduction maneuver would make the reduction substantially more difficult.
- After percutaneous reduction, fracture stability in all planes is assessed. If unstable, pin fixation of the fragment is recommended.

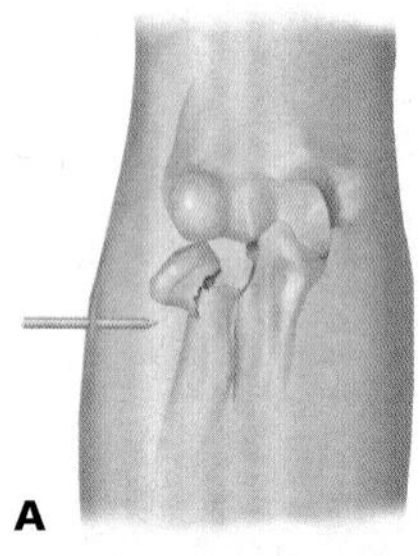
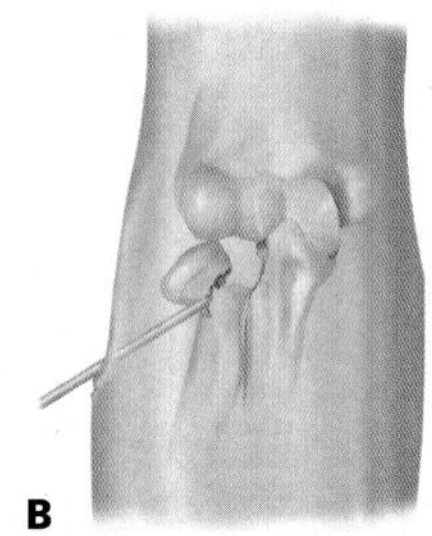
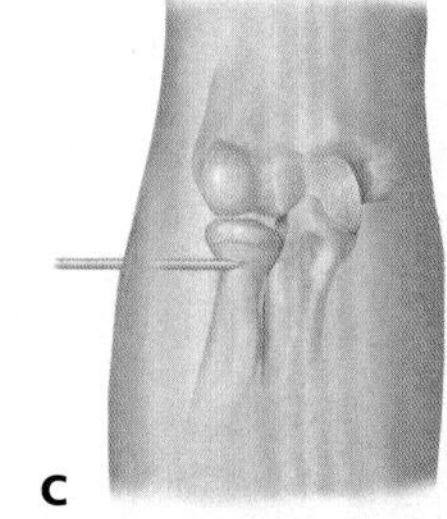

**TECH FIG 5** • Lever technique. **A.** The lever pin is inserted at the level of the fracture through the skin. **B.** The pin is then pushed distally, applying tension to the skin before approaching the physeal side of the fracture and (**C**) levering the fragment into place, allowing the built-up tension of the skin to aid in the reduction.

# Closed Intramedullary Reduction and Fixation (Metaizeau Technique)

## Description

- Metaizeau described an intramedullary reduction and fixation technique for the treatment of displaced radial neck fractures[9] that has been widely adopted.[4,6,8,16,20,23,25,29]
- The intramedullary manipulation of the radial head can be accomplished by an elastic titanium nail or a Kirschner wire of sufficient length, the tip of which is bent about 30 degrees.
- The diameter of the elastic nail or Kirschner wire is usually 2 mm. A 2.5-mm nail may be suitable in some children older than 10 years. The curved nail tip can be bent additionally.
- The entry point for the nail can either be a radial or dorsal site on the radius as described for radial shaft fracture flexible intramedullary nailing. On the dorsal side, the entry site is immediately proximal to Lister tubercle between the second and third extensor compartments. The bare cortical area can be reliably identified between these compartments by avoiding retraction of the tendons in these compartments. The alternative radial entry site is 1.5 to 2 cm proximal to the physis, taking care to avoid injury to the sensory branch of the radial nerve (**TECH FIG 6**). Through either approach, the cortex is entered with an awl, taking care to avoid penetration of the far cortex of the radius.

## Engaging the Fragment

- The elastic nail is attached to a T-handle and advanced proximally through the medullary canal under fluoroscopic guidance (**TECH FIG 7A–C**).
  - The forearm is rotated until the plane of maximum deformity is visualized.
- The curved tip of the nail or the Kirschner wire is directed toward the displaced proximal fragment and gently advanced across the fracture until the tip engages the epiphyseal fragment without penetrating the articular surface (**TECH FIG 7D–F**).
- AP and lateral radiographs are obtained to confirm the position of the nail tip in the epiphyseal fragment.

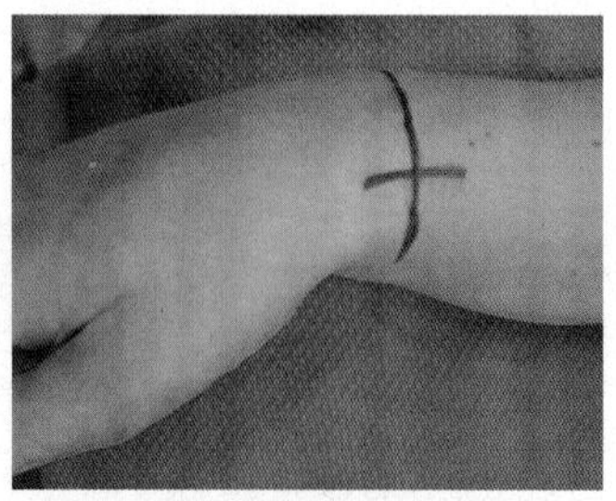
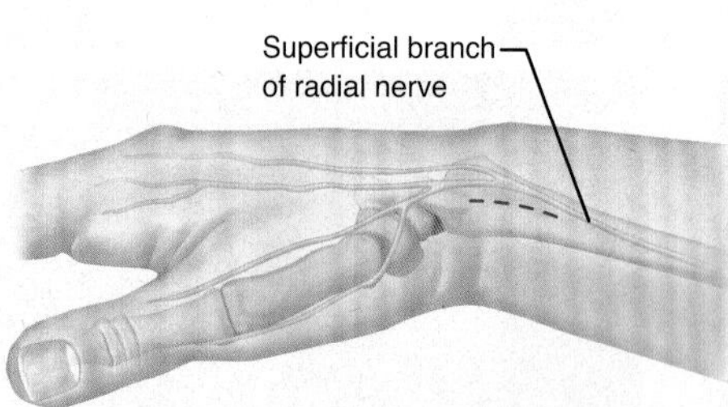

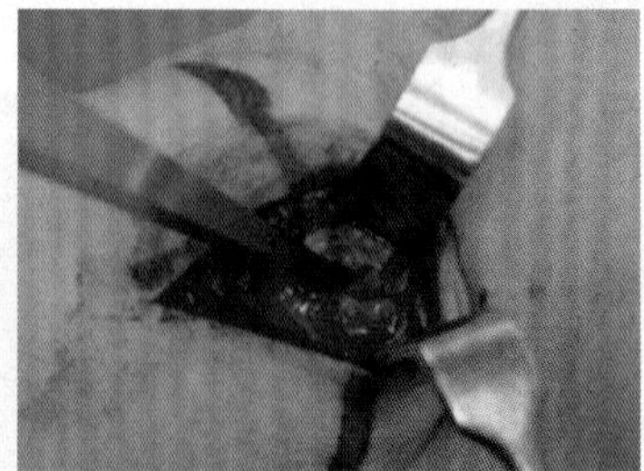

**TECH FIG 6** • **A–F.** Radial-side entry point for elastic nail for centromedullary reduction technique. **A.** Incision centered over the distal radial physis. **B.** The surgeon should avoid injury to the superficial branch of the radial nerve. **C.** Entry point is 1.5 cm proximal to the distal radial physis. *(continued)*

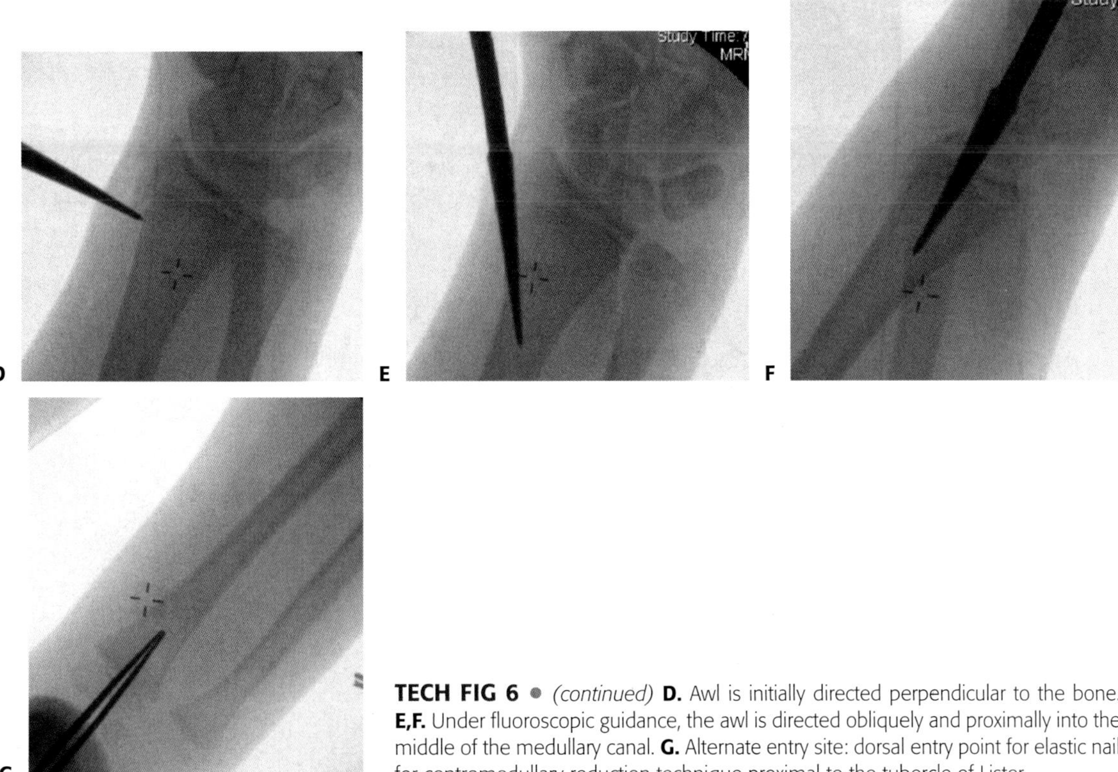

**TECH FIG 6** • *(continued)* **D.** Awl is initially directed perpendicular to the bone. **E,F.** Under fluoroscopic guidance, the awl is directed obliquely and proximally into the middle of the medullary canal. **G.** Alternate entry site: dorsal entry point for elastic nail for centromedullary reduction technique proximal to the tubercle of Lister.

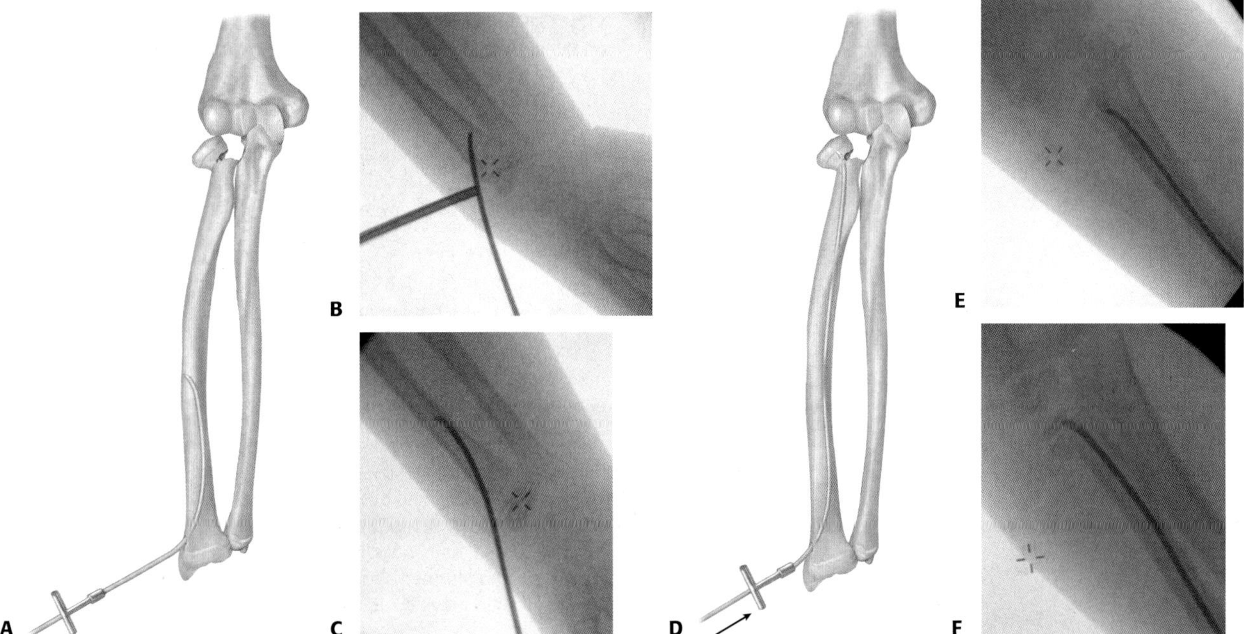

**TECH FIG 7** • Closed intramedullary reduction and fixation technique of Metaizeau with an elastic nail. **A–C.** Proximal advancement of elastic nail through the medullary canal. **D–F.** The curved tip is directed toward and advanced into the displaced epiphyseal fragment.

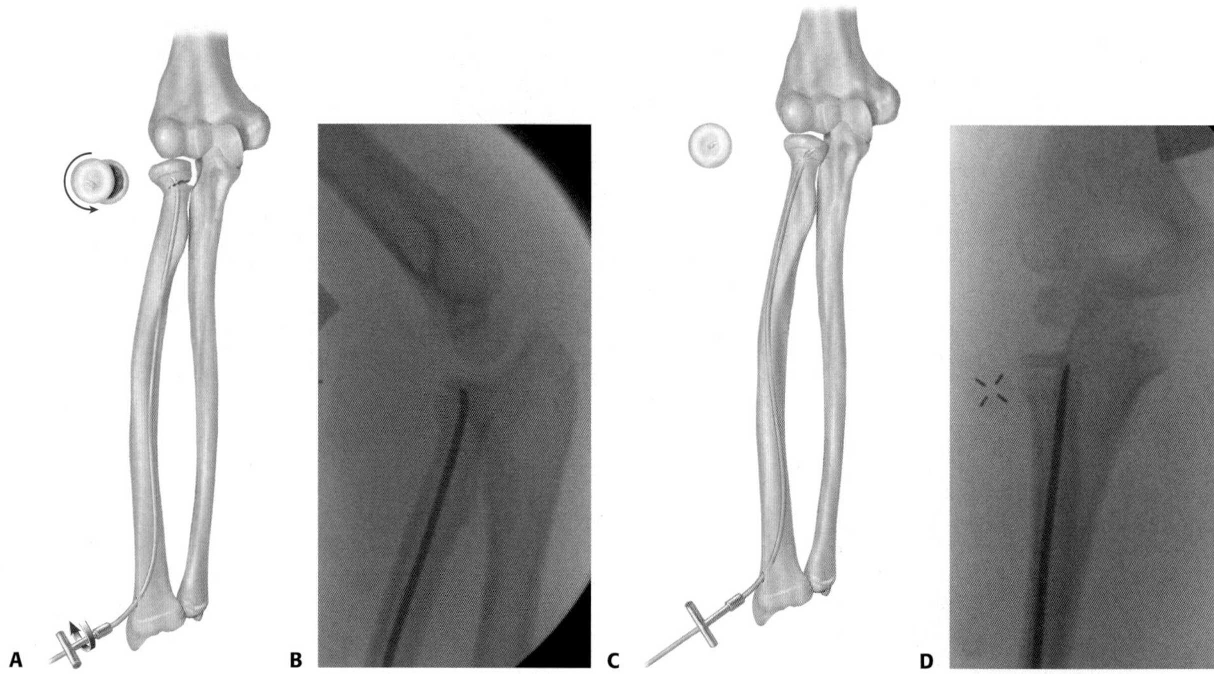


**TECH FIG 8** • **A–D.** The elastic nail is rotated anteriorly and medially to reduce the radial head.

## Rotating the Fragment into Place

- The nail tip is used to elevate the fragment to reduce the tilt anchoring the proximal fragment against the lateral condyle.
- The T-handle is then used to rotate the nail or Kirschner wire typically anteriorly and medially, thereby reducing the lateral or posterolaterally displaced radial head back to its normal location (**TECH FIG 8**).
  - If the epiphysis is displaced anterolaterally, the nail is rotated posteriorly and medially.
- The intact periosteum prevents overcorrection of the fragment medially.

## Completing the Procedure

- The reduction maneuver may be facilitated with a prior or concurrent closed reduction. In severely displaced radial neck fractures, the percutaneous technique described earlier may be performed concurrently to facilitate the intramedullary reduction (**TECH FIG 9A**).
- With the nail tip engaged in the epiphysis and the reduction complete, the stability of the fracture is assessed, and the nail is left in situ.
- The nail is trimmed 1 cm proud of the bone at the entry site (**TECH FIG 9B**).
- If the dorsal approach is used, the nail can be bent 90 degrees dorsally and trimmed just above the plane of the extensor pollicis longus tendon to ensure that the end of the nail does not abrade the tendon (**TECH FIG 9C**).

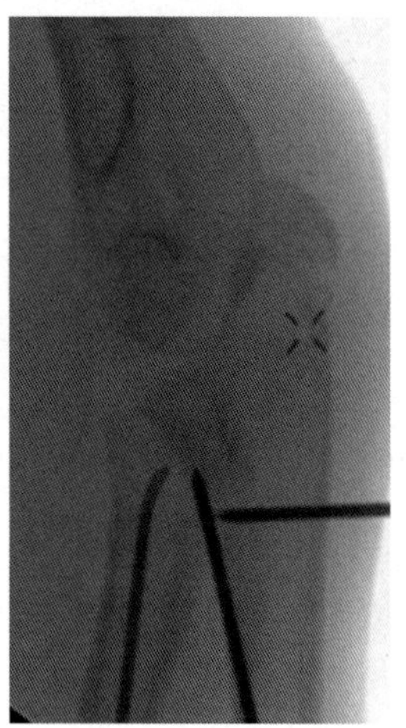


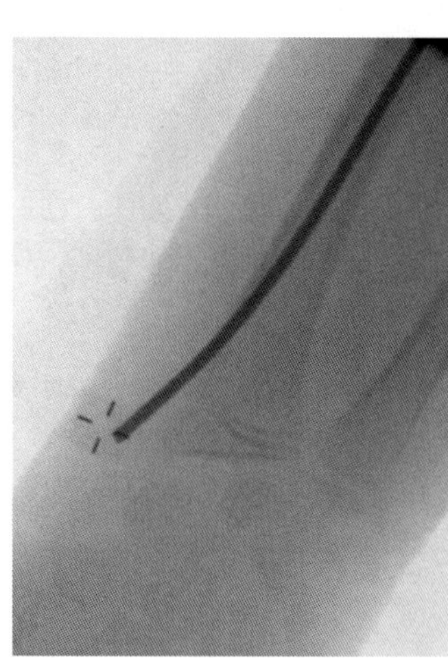


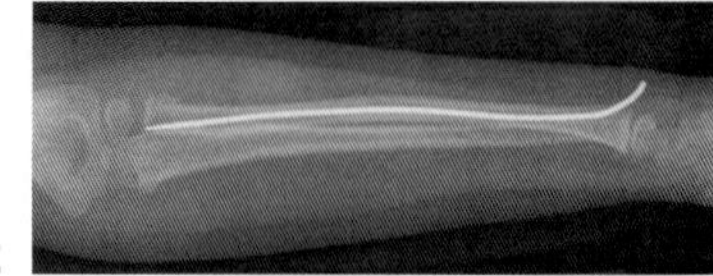


**TECH FIG 9** • **A.** Intramedullary reduction can be facilitated by concurrent percutaneous pin reduction technique. **B.** The end of the nail is left proud off the entry site to facilitate removal. **C.** If a dorsal entry point is used, the end of the nail is trimmed above the level of the tendons to prevent rupture.

## Open Reduction

- Kocher posterolateral approach to the radial head is used. Pronating the forearm brings the posterior interosseous nerve further anteromedially, away from the surgical field.
- A skin incision about 5 cm long is made, centered over the posterolateral aspect of the radial head (**TECH FIG 10A**). The interval between the anconeus (radial nerve) and the extensor carpi ulnaris (posterior interosseous nerve) is developed (**TECH FIG 10B**).
- A longitudinal incision is made along the capsule, unless the capsule has not already been torn open by the injury causing trauma (**TECH FIG 10C**).
- The proximal fragment is identified and reduced under direct visualization and fluoroscopic guidance. If the annular ligament has been injured, it should be repaired.
- Occasionally, the fracture is widely displaced anteromedially, necessitating further exposure before identification. In such a case, a more extensile approach is recommended as well as a formal proximal identification of the radial nerve and posterior interosseous nerve.
- If the fracture requires open reduction, internal fixation is recommended.
  - A retrospective review of radial neck nonunions noted that they were commonly associated with an early loss of fixation, related to either displacement or premature removal of pins.[33]
  - Options for internal fixation include pins placed obliquely through the radial head in an ice cream cone pattern throughout the safe zone. Absorbable pins can also be used. Radial head fixation can be achieved with epiphyseal–metaphyseal interrupted, circumferentially placed absorbable sutures.[2] For skeletally mature children, headless screws or a T-plate in the safe zone can be used.
  - Although seldom indicated, Leung and Tse[19] described a lateral mini-plate buttress technique for the open physis. The plate is anchored distally in the radial neck with 2-mm screws and left unattached proximally, providing a buttress preventing lateral dislocation of the radial head.
  - Transcapitellar pin fixation has been described, but it provides poor distal fixation and is associated with pin breakage at the radiocapitellar joint.[3]

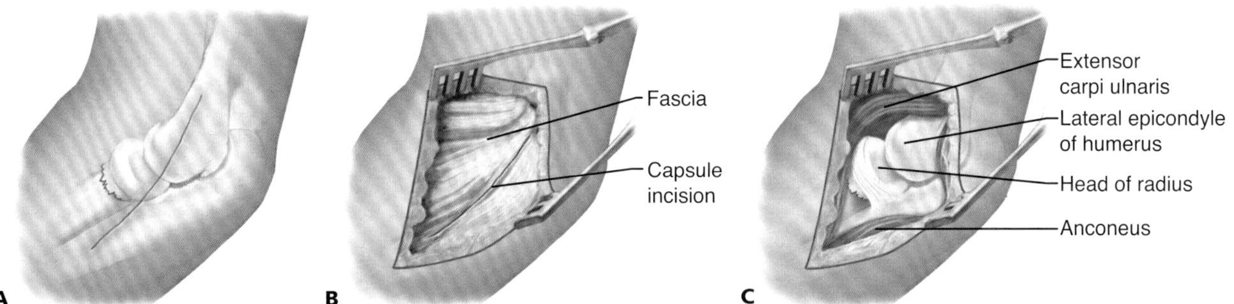


**TECH FIG 10** • **A.** The Kocher posterolateral approach to the elbow uses the interval between the anconeus and the extensor carpi ulnaris. **B.** The capsule is incised longitudinally. **C.** The radial head fragment may be readily visualized after exposure, unless medially or posteriorly displaced.

## PEARLS AND PITFALLS

| | |
|---|---|
| **Indications** | ■ The surgeon should have a discussion with the family and alert the operating room staff regarding the "reduction ladder" and the various techniques that may be employed. |
| **Operative technique** | ■ Although percutaneous reduction can be a tedious and time-consuming procedure, open reduction should be avoided if at all possible.<br>■ A mini-open approach using a Freer elevator as a shoehorn can sometimes reduce the fragment when percutaneous Steinmann pin reduction is unsuccessful.<br>■ For intramedullary reduction and fixation, in the radial approach, the surgeon should avoid injury to the sensory branch of the radial nerve. If the dorsal approach is used, the nail is bent away from Lister tubercle and trimmed above the dorsal aspect of the extensor tendons so as not to abrade it.<br>■ If an open reduction is necessary, fixation is necessary.<br>■ Transarticular pins should be avoided, as they may break at the joint.<br>■ Radial head excision is contraindicated in children because of valgus elbow deformity, longitudinal forearm instability, and high incidence of overgrowth. |
| **Imaging** | ■ After achieving reduction, the surgeon should verify improved range of motion and make sure that the reduction is a true change in alignment and not simply a radiograph taken out of the plane with maximal angulation.<br>■ The surgeon should beware of reversal of radial head position during radial head reductions and should make sure on plain radiographs that the radial head is properly reduced and not flipped 180 degrees.[35] |
| **Follow-up** | ■ Clinical or radiographic signs of fracture healing should be present before removing pin fixation. The period of pin fixation or immobilization should be longer for unstable, high-energy injuries. |

## POSTOPERATIVE CARE

- After reduction, the elbow is immobilized in 90 degrees of flexion in the position of supination–pronation that is most stable for 3 weeks.
- If a splint is used postoperatively because of swelling, it is changed to a cast at 1 week.
- At follow-up, the cast is removed for radiographic and clinical examination. If healing is inadequate (which is more likely in higher energy injuries in older children), the cast (and the pins if used) is continued for 2 more weeks, after which patient is reevaluated for healing.
- If pin fixation is used, no elbow motion is allowed until pins are removed.
- Graduated range-of-motion exercises begin when the cast is removed.

## OUTCOMES

- Many series have shown a good to excellent outcome in 76% to 94% of children with radial neck fractures.[1,3,26,28,30]
  - Indicators for a favorable prognosis include younger age (younger than 10 years), isolated low-energy injury, closed reduction, early treatment, less than 30 degrees of initial angulation, less than 3 mm of initial translation, and reduction within parameters discussed earlier.[3,21,28]
- Poor outcomes, such as limitations in range of motion, have been reported in 6% to 33% of patients, usually after a severely displaced radial neck fracture.
  - Risk factors for a poor outcome include severe displacement, associated injuries, delayed treatment, poor reductions, old age, fractures needing open treatment and internal fixation, and intra-articular fractures in patients with an open physis.[18,21,26,28,33,36]
  - Poor outcomes that have been noted with open procedures are partially due to a selection bias, where patients needing open procedures are more likely to have had high-energy injuries with additional vascular and soft tissue trauma.

## COMPLICATIONS

- Loss of joint congruity, fibrous adhesions, and radial head overgrowth result in a loss of elbow motion. In order of decreasing frequency, pronation, supination, extension, and flexion are affected.[28]
- Radial head overgrowth is observed in 20% to 40% of cases due to presumed increased vascularity stimulating the physis. Premature physeal closure can occur and is seldom symptomatic, but it can accentuate a valgus deformity. Delayed appearance of the ossific nucleus is possible after a fracture occurring before ossification.
- Avascular necrosis of the radial head occurs in 10% to 20% of patients.[3,21] Seventy percent of cases occur in cases of open reduction.[3]
- Radial neck nonunions are rare but have been reported and are often associated with premature loss of fixation.[33]
- Posttraumatic radioulnar synostosis occurs in 0% to 10% of cases,[3,21,26] typically in association with open reductions, extensive dissection, residual displacement, and concurrent ulnar fracture. Exostectomy of synostosis is a technically demanding procedure with a variable success rate.
- Heterotopic ossification (6% to 25% of cases)[3,21] can occur as myositis ossificans in the supinator or as ossification within the capsule. Surgical treatment is rarely indicated.

## REFERENCES


1. Bernstein SM, McKeever P, Bernstein L. Percutaneous reduction of displaced radial neck fractures in children. J Pediatr Orthop 1993; 13:85–88.
2. Chotel F, Vallese P, Parot R, et al. Complete dislocation of the radial head following fracture of the radial neck in children: the Jeffery type II lesion. J Pediatr Orthop B 2004;13:268–274.
3. D'Souza S, Vaishya R, Klenerman L. Management of radial neck fractures in children: a retrospective analysis of one hundred patients. J Pediatr Orthop 1993;13:232–238.
4. Eberl R, Singer G, Fruhmann J, et al. Intramedullary nailing for the treatment of dislocated pediatric radial neck fractures. Eur J Pediatr Surg 2010;20:250–252.
5. Ebraheim NA, Jin F, Pulisetti D, et al. Quantitative anatomical study of the posterior interosseous nerve. Am J Orthop 2000;29:702–704.
6. Endele SM, Wirth T, Eberhardt O, et al. The treatment of radial neck fractures in children according to Metaizeau. J Pediatr Orthop B 2010;19:246–255.
7. Fowles JV, Kassab MT. Observations concerning radial neck fractures in children. J Pediatr Orthop 1986;6:51–57.
8. González-Herranz P, Alvarez-Romera A, Burgos J, et al. Displaced radial neck fractures in children treated by closed intramedullary pinning (Metaizeau technique). J Pediatr Orthop 1997;17:325–331.
9. Green NE. Fractures and dislocations of the elbow. In: Green NE, Swiontkowski MF, eds. Skeletal Trauma in Children. Philadelphia: Saunders, 2003.
10. Henrikson B. Isolated fractures of the proximal end of the radius in children epidemiology, treatment and prognosis. Acta Orthop Scand 1969;40:246–260.
11. Jeffery CC. Fractures of the head of the radius in children. J Bone Joint Surg Br 1950;32-B:314–324.
12. Jeffery CC. Fractures of the neck of the radius in children. Mechanism of causation. J Bone Joint Surg Br 1972;54:717–719.
13. Jones ER, Esah M. Displaced fractures of the neck of the radius in children. J Bone Joint Surg Br 1971;53:429–439.
14. Judet H, Judet J. Fractures et Orthopedique de L'enfant. Paris: Maloine, 1974.
15. Kaufman B, Rinott MG, Tanzman M. Closed reduction of fractures of the proximal radius in children. J Bone Joint Surg Br 1989;71:66–67.
16. Klitscher D, Richter S, Bodenschatz K, et al. Evaluation of severely displaced radial neck fractures in children treated with elastic stable intramedullary nailing. J Pediatr Orthop 2009;29:698–703.
17. Landin LA, Danielsson LG. Elbow fractures in children. An epidemiological analysis of 589 cases. Acta Orthop Scand 1986;57:309–312.
18. Leung AG, Peterson HA. Fractures of the proximal radial head and neck in children with emphasis on those that involve the articular cartilage. J Pediatr Orthop 2000;20:7–14.
19. Leung KS, Tse PY. A new method of fixing radial neck fractures: brief report. J Bone Joint Surg Br 1989;71:326–327.
20. Metaizeau JP, Lascombes P, Lemelle JL, et al. Reduction and fixation of displaced radial neck fractures by closed intramedullary pinning. J Pediatr Orthop 1993;13:355–360.
21. Newman JH. Displaced radial neck fractures in children. Injury 1977;9:114–121.
22. O'Brien PI. Injuries involving the proximal radial epiphysis. Clin Orthop Relat Res 1965;41:51–58.
23. Prathapkumar KR, Garg NK, Bruce CE. Elastic stable intramedullary nail fixation for severely displaced fractures of the neck of the radius in children. J Bone Joint Surg Br 2006;88:358–361.
24. Radomisli TE, Rosen AL. Controversies regarding radial neck fractures in children. Clin Orthop Relat Res 1998;(353):30–39.

25. Schmittenbecher PP, Haevernick B, Herold A, et al. Treatment decision, method of osteosynthesis, and outcome in radial neck fractures in children: a multicenter study. J Pediatr Orthop 2005;25:45–50.
26. Steele JA, Graham HK. Angulated radial neck fractures in children. A prospective study of percutaneous reduction. J Bone Joint Surg Br 1992;74:760–764.
27. Steinberg EL, Golomb D, Salama R, et al. Radial head and neck fractures in children. J Pediatr Orthop 1988;8:35–40.
28. Tibone JE, Stoltz M. Fractures of the radial head and neck in children. J Bone Joint Surg Am 1981;63:100–106.
29. Ugutmen E, Ozkan K, Ozkan FU, et al. Reduction and fixation of radius neck fractures in children with intramedullary pin. J Pediatr Orthop B 2010;19:289–293.
30. Vahvanen V, Gripenberg L. Fracture of the radial neck in children. A long-term follow-up study of 43 cases. Acta Orthop Scand 1978;49:32–38.
31. Vocke AK, Von Laer L. Displaced fractures of the radial neck in children: long-term results and prognosis of conservative treatment. J Pediatr Orthop B 1998;7:217–222.
32. Waters PM. Injuries of the shoulder, elbow and forearm. In: Abel MF, ed. Orthopaedic Knowledge Update: Pediatrics 3. Rosemont, IL: American Academy of Orthopaedic Surgeons, 2006.
33. Waters PM, Stewart SL. Radial neck fracture nonunion in children. J Pediatr Orthop 2001;21:570–576.
34. Wilkins KE. Fractures of the neck and head of the radius. In: Rockwood CA, Wilkins KE, King RE, eds. Fractures in Children. Philadelphia: Lippincott, 1984.
35. Wood SK. Reversal of the radial head during reduction of fracture of the neck of the radius in children. J Bone Joint Surg Br 1969;51:707–710.
36. Zimmerman RM, Kalish LA, Hresko MT, et al. Surgical management of pediatric radial neck fractures. J Bone Joint Surg Am 2013;95:1825–1832.

# Open Reduction and Internal Fixation of Radial Head and Neck Fractures

Yung Han, George Frederick Hatch III, and John M. Itamura

## DEFINITION

- Radial head and neck fractures are the most common elbow fractures in adults representing 33% of elbow fractures.
- They may occur in isolation or with concurrent osseous, osteochondral, and/or ligamentous injuries.
- Management (which involves nonoperative, open reduction internal fixation [ORIF], fragment excision, radial head excision, or radial head replacement) is aimed at restoring motion or both motion and stability to the elbow and forearm, depending on the pattern of injury. This chapter focuses on the decision-making principles and operative techniques for ORIF of radial head and neck fractures.

## ANATOMY AND BIOMECHANICS

- The radial head is entirely intra-articular with two articulations: (1) radiocapitellar joint and (2) proximal radioulnar joint (PRUJ).
  - The radiocapitellar joint has a saddle-shaped articulation allowing flexion, extension, and forearm rotation.
  - The PRUJ, constrained by the annular ligament, allows rotation of the radial head in the lesser sigmoid notch of the proximal ulna.
    - To avoid creating a mechanical block to pronation and supination, implants must be limited to a 90-degree arc (the "safe zone") outside the PRUJ (**FIG 1**).[7]
- There is considerable variability in the shape of the radial head, from nearly round to elliptical, as well as variability in the offset of the head from the neck.[14]
- Blood supply to the radial head is tenuous with a major contribution from a single branch of the radial recurrent artery in the safe zone and minor contributions from both the radial and interosseous recurrent arteries which penetrate the capsule at its insertion into the neck (**FIG 2**).[26]
- The anterior band of the medial collateral ligament (MCL) is the primary stabilizer to valgus stress. The radial head, a secondary stabilizer, maintains up to 30% of valgus resistance in the native elbow. Therefore, in cases where the MCL is ruptured:
  - A radial head that is not reparable should be replaced with a prosthesis and not excised given its biomechanical importance.
  - It may be prudent to protect a repaired radial head from high valgus stress during early range of motion.
- The radial head also functions in the transmission of axial load, transmitting 60% of the load from the wrist to the elbow.[21] This is a crucial consideration when the interosseous membrane is disrupted in the Essex-Lopresti lesion.[9] Resection of the radial head in this setting results in devastating longitudinal radioulnar instability, proximal migration of the radius, and possible ulnar–carpal impingement.

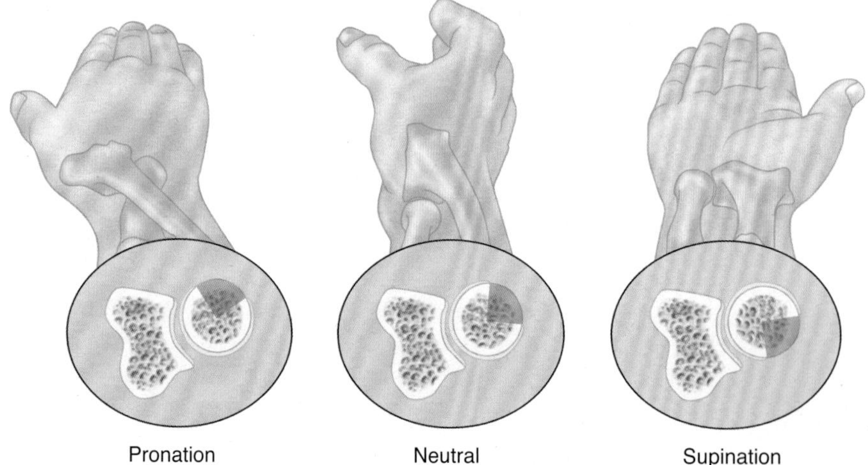


**FIG 1** • The safe zone is a roughly 90-degree arc of the radial head that does not articulate with the ulna in the PRUJ with full supination and pronation. With the wrist in neutral rotation, the safe zone is anterolateral.

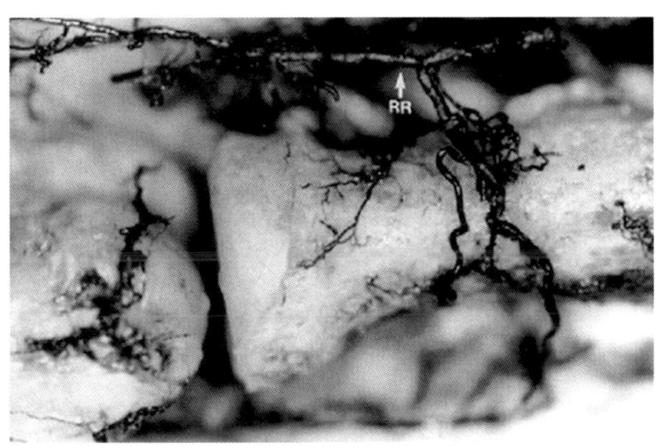

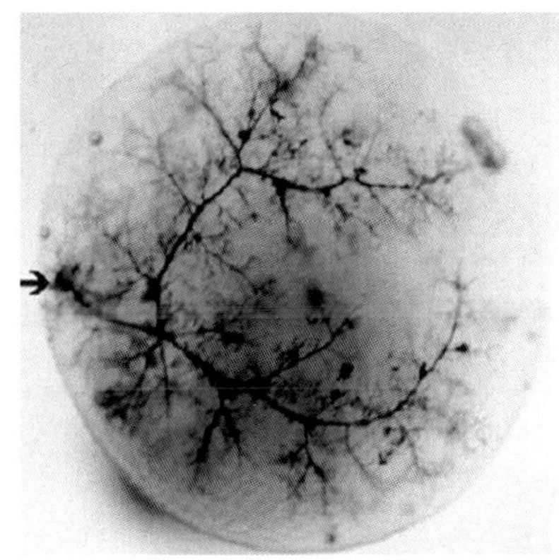

**FIG 2** • **A.** The radial recurrent artery, a branch of the radial artery, provides the main blood supply to the radial head. **B.** In most cadaveric specimens, a branch of the radial recurrent penetrates the radial head in the safe zone. (From Yamaguchi K, Sweet FA, Bindra R, et al. The extraosseous and intraosseous arterial anatomy of the adult elbow. J Bone Joint Surg Am 1997;79[11]:1653–1662.)

## PATHOGENESIS

- Radial head fractures result from trauma. A fall on an outstretched hand with the elbow in extension and the forearm in pronation produces an axial or valgus load (or both) driving the radial head into the capitellum, fracturing the relatively osteopenic radial head.[2]
- Nondisplaced or minimally displaced injuries do not usually have associated injuries. However, displaced, comminuted, or unstable fractures have a high association of soft tissue injuries (**FIG 3**) that can lead to considerable complications, including pain, arthrosis, instability, and disability:
  - Capitellar cartilage defects, capitellar bone bruises, and/or posterior dislocation can occur with radial head fractures.
- Axial loading may also rupture the interosseous membrane causing longitudinal radioulnar instability with dislocation of the distal radioulnar joint (DRUJ) (Essex-Lopresti fracture). An impacted radial neck or depressed radial head fracture should be highly suspicious of a concomitant interosseous membrane and DRUJ injury (**FIG 4**).
- The "terrible triad" injury results from valgus loading of the elbow, disrupting the MCL or lateral ulnar collateral ligament, and fracturing the radial head and coronoid process.
- Radial head fractures can also occur with proximal ulnar fractures (Monteggia fracture) (**FIG 5**).

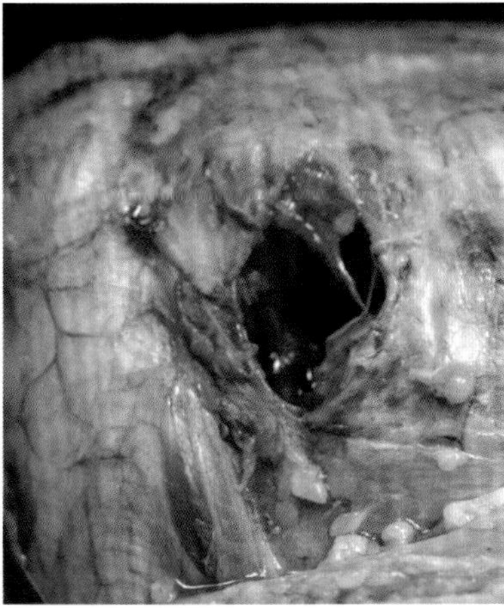
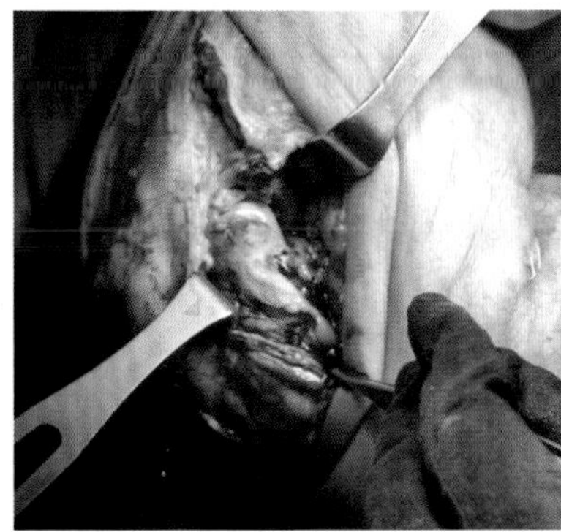

**FIG 3** • Soft tissue injuries occur with unstable radial head fractures. Sample pictures showing (**A**) large capsular rupture and (**B**) avulsion of the lateral collateral ligament (LCL) and common extensor tendons from the lateral epicondyle.

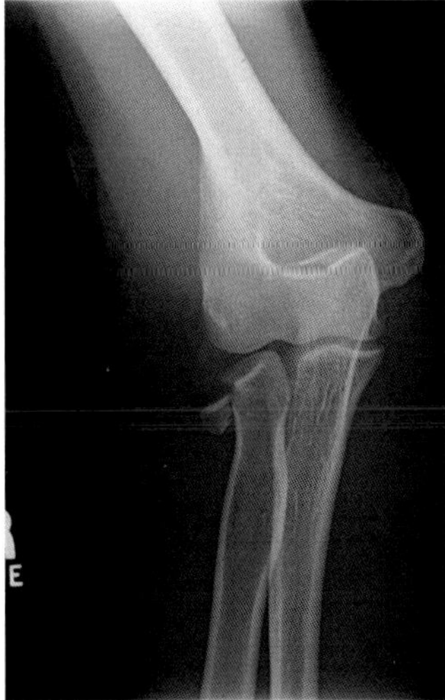

**FIG 4** • AP x-ray showing a depressed articular fracture with impaction at the radial neck. This fracture pattern is highly suspicious for an Essex-Lopresti fracture. Radial head replacement is recommended. If ORIF is performed, the DRUJ should be stabilized to prevent instability.

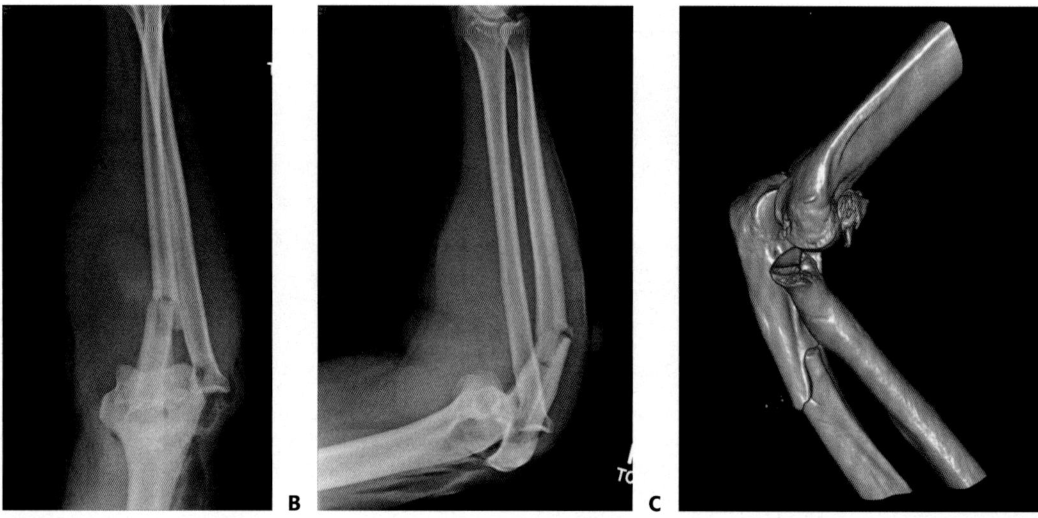


**FIG 5** • **A,B.** AP and lateral x-ray showing a type II Monteggia fracture—posterior dislocation of radial head (or fracture) and proximal ulnar fracture with posterior angulation. **C.** CT scan clearly showing impaction fracture of the radial head that may not be appreciable on x-ray.

## NATURAL HISTORY

- The original Mason classification was modified by Johnson, and then Morrey. Hotchkiss proposed that the classification system be used to provide guidance for treatment. It has poor intraobserver and interobserver reliability (**FIG 6**).[9]

### Type I Fractures

- Nondisplaced and offer no block to pronation and supination on examination
- Represents approximately 82% of radial head fractures[18]
- Nonoperative treatment generally results in good to excellent outcomes with minimal loss of motion or resultant arthrosis.[1,3,8,12]
- Stiffness due to capsular contracture is the main reason for a poor outcome; however, it can often be managed successfully with physical therapy.

### Type II Fractures

- Displaced marginal segments that can block normal forearm rotation. According to Broberg and Morrey,[6] the fragment should be greater than or equal to 30% of the articular surface and be displaced greater than or equal to 2 mm. We only include fractures with three or fewer articular fragments, which meet criteria for fractures that can be operatively reduced and fixed with reproducibly good results.
- Represents approximately 14% of radial head fractures[18]
- Earlier studies suggested nonoperative treatment or radial head excision as the standard treatment,[13,19,20,23] but as knowledge and technology advanced, optimal treatment has become more controversial.
- Greater than 2 mm of displacement has often been cited as an indication for ORIF, but good results have been obtained in studies treating 2 to 5 mm of displacement nonoperatively.[1,12]
- A mechanical block is the only clear indication for surgery.
- A recent meta-analysis[16] found successful nonoperative treatment in 80% compared to successful ORIF treatment in 93% for stable Mason type II fractures; however, the authors concluded that there was insufficient evidence to recommend optimal treatment.
- Complications from nonoperative treatment such as painful clicking, nonunion, and arthrosis can be treated with radial head excision or arthroplasty; however, it is considered with modest increase in function. It has shown 23% fair or poor results at 15 years of follow-up.[5]

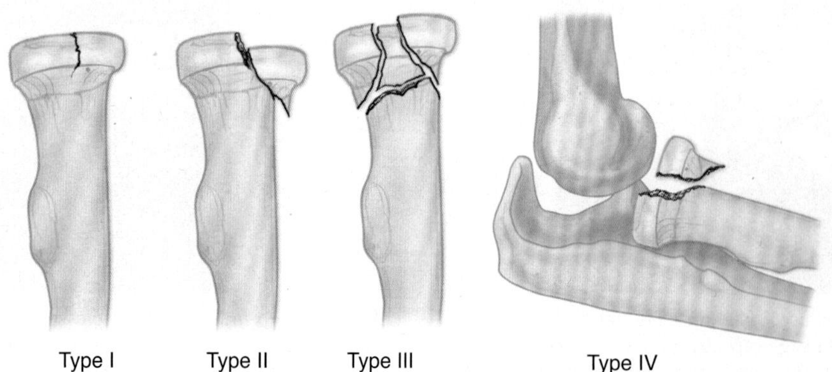


**FIG 6** • The modified Mason classification for radial head fractures.

- Delayed excision of the radial head after failed nonoperative management may be considered with modest increase in function; it has shown 23% fair or poor results at 15 years of follow-up.[5] Other studies suggested that there is no difference between delayed and primary excision.[11]

### Type III Fractures

- Comminuted or impacted articular fractures (see **FIG 4**) are optimally managed with prosthetic replacement.
- Represents approximately 3% of radial head fractures[18]
- Radial head arthroplasty or excision is considered when satisfactory reduction or stable fixation is not obtained or in comminuted fractures because fixation of a radial head with more than three articular fragments is fraught with poor results.[22]
- Results of excision are poor in patients with concomitant MCL, coronoid, or interosseous membrane injury.
- Radial head resection should be reserved for patients with low functional demands, limited life expectancy, or in the presence of infection, and when the surgeon has excluded elbow instability with a fluoroscopic examination.
- Radiographic, but usually clinically silent, degenerative changes such as cysts, sclerosis, and osteophytes occur radiographically in about 75% of elbows after radial head excision.
- There is also a demonstrable increase in ulnar variance at the wrist and increased carrying angle and a 10% to 20% loss of strength is expected.
- Radial head arthroplasty can provide radiocapitellar contact similar to the native radial head and thus resists valgus and posterior instability. Additionally, it resists proximal migration of the radius in response to axial loading. It facilitates uneventful healing of the MCL, interosseous ligaments, and DRUJ.

### Type IV Fractures

- Radial head fractures associated with elbow instability. The radial head should never be resected in the acute setting.
- Represents approximately 1% of radial head fractures[18]
- Treatment involves immediate reduction of the elbow joint and treatment of the radial head fracture and associated bony injuries. Whether the radial head is fixed or replaced, it must be capable of bearing load immediately. If the radial head can be fixed, repair of the torn ligaments and application of a hinged fixator to protect the repaired radial head may be considered. Otherwise, satisfactory results have been obtained with radial head replacement without ligamentous repair.[10]

## PATIENT HISTORY AND PHYSICAL FINDINGS

### History

- The history typically involves a fall on an outstretched hand followed by pain and edema over the lateral elbow, accompanied by limited range of motion.
- The mechanism of the injury should be determined to add information about associated elbow injuries or injuries to the shoulder or hand.
- The examiner should note the patient's activity level and profession.

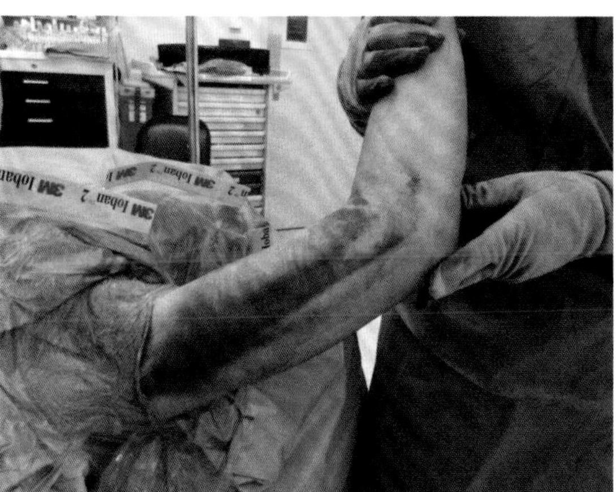

**FIG 7** • MCL injury with extensive medial ecchymosis.

### Physical Examination

- Physical examination should include neurovascular status, examination of the joint above (shoulder) and below (wrist), and examination of the skin to look for medial ecchymosis (**FIG 7**), which may suggest injury to the MCL.
  - A detailed examination of the elbow must include bony palpation of the medial and lateral epicondyles, olecranon process, DRUJ, and radial head as well as the squeeze test of the interosseous membrane and DRUJ to screen for potential longitudinal instability.
  - Varus and valgus stress testing, with or without fluoroscopy, can indicate injury to the anterior band of the MCL or to the lateral ulnar collateral ligament, respectively.
- Range-of-motion and stress examinations are vital to proper decision making and may obviate the need for advanced imaging if performed correctly with adequate anesthesia. If omitted, this will lead to undiagnosed associated injuries and may result in flawed decision making.
  - In the emergency department or office, adequate anesthesia may be obtained by aspirating hematoma, then injecting the elbow joint with 5 mL of local anesthetic and examining the elbow under fluoroscopy. This may be performed by the traditional lateral injection in the "soft spot" or posteriorly into the olecranon fossa (**FIG 8**).[25] A mechanical block is an indication for operative intervention.
  - If operative intervention is clearly indicated, this examination can be performed under a general anesthetic, provided the surgeon and patient are prepared for a change in operative plan as dictated by the examination.
  - Normal values are 0 to 145 degrees of flexion–extension, 85 degrees of supination, and 80 degrees of pronation. The examiner should check for a bony block to motion.

## DIAGNOSTIC STUDIES

### Radiography

- Anteroposterior (AP), lateral, and oblique views are the standard of care, but they may underestimate or overestimate joint impaction and degree of comminution.
  - A radiocapitellar view with forearm in neutral and at 45 degrees of flexion gives an improved view of the articular surfaces.
  - A sailboat sign can provide suspicion to an occult radial neck fracture.

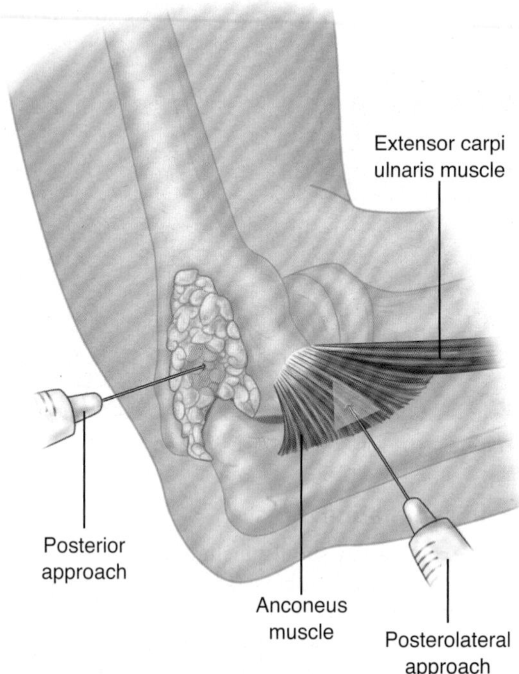


**FIG 8** • The elbow joint can be aspirated and injected through the posterior and posterolateral approaches. They are equally effective and should be used based on soft tissue injury.

- If the examination reveals wrist or forearm tenderness, the examiner should have a low threshold for obtaining bilateral wrist posteroanterior (PA) views to rule out an Essex-Lopresti lesion. Alternatively, this can be done with a one cassette view to minimize radiation exposure (**FIG 9**).

### Magnetic Resonance Imaging

- Magnetic resonance imaging (MRI) is a useful adjunct to physical examination for evaluating associated injuries such as collateral ligament tears, chondral defects, and loose bodies,[15] but it is not routinely indicated. Most of the associated injuries found on MRI at the time of injury have been found to be not clinically significant.[15,17]

### Computed Tomography

- If decision is made for operative treatment, we routinely obtain a computed tomography (CT) scan to better understand the fracture pattern for preoperative planning, so that operative time is efficient and to minimize intraoperative surprises. Three-dimensional reconstructions provide further information not always easily appreciated on routine CT scans.

## DIFFERENTIAL DIAGNOSIS

- Simple elbow dislocation
- Distal humerus fracture
- Olecranon fracture
- Septic elbow

## NONOPERATIVE MANAGEMENT

- The standard protocol for treating radial head fractures is shown in **FIG 10**.
- Conservative management, with a week of sling immobilization followed by range of motion once the acute pain resolves, is the treatment of choice in nondisplaced radial head fractures, where universally good and excellent results have been reported.
- Nonoperative management is also the treatment of choice in fractures with less than 2 mm of displacement, with minor head involvement, and without bony blockage to range of motion.
  - A 7-day period of cast or splint immobilization is followed by aggressive motion after the inflammatory phase.
- Our current practice for fractures that are more than 2 mm displaced is to determine whether there is a blockage of motion on fluoroscopic examination.
  - If there is maintenance of at least 50 degrees of both pronation and supination, we typically recommend conservative treatment.

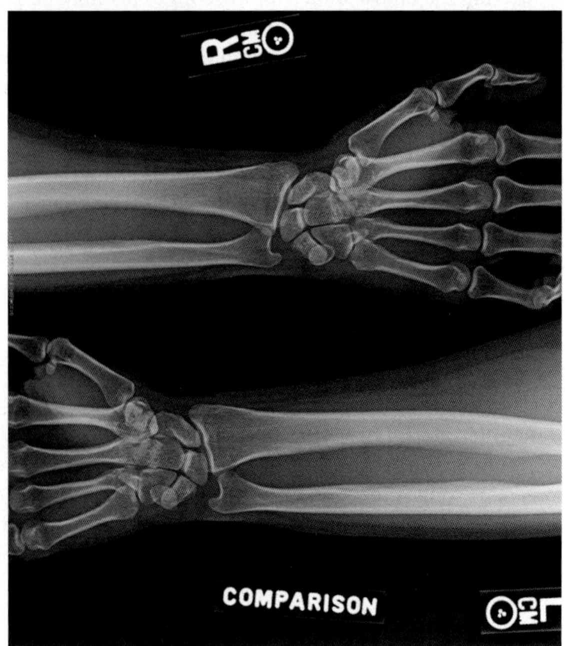


A

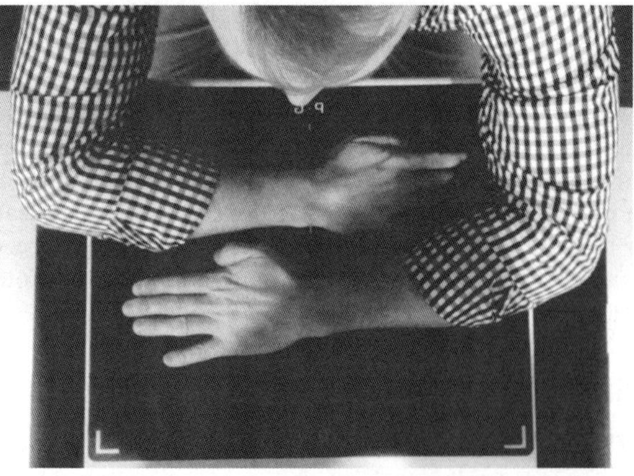

B

**FIG 9** • **A.** A positive *Itamura simultaneous DRUJ view* showing negative ulnar variance of the uninjured left DRUJ compared with neutral ulnar variance of the right injured DRUJ suggesting interosseous membrane disruption. Patient had a right radial head fracture and proximal migration of the radius respective to the ulna (Essex-Lopresti fracture). **B.** Image is taken with 90-degree shoulder flexion, 90-degree elbow flexion, and 90-degree forearm pronation.

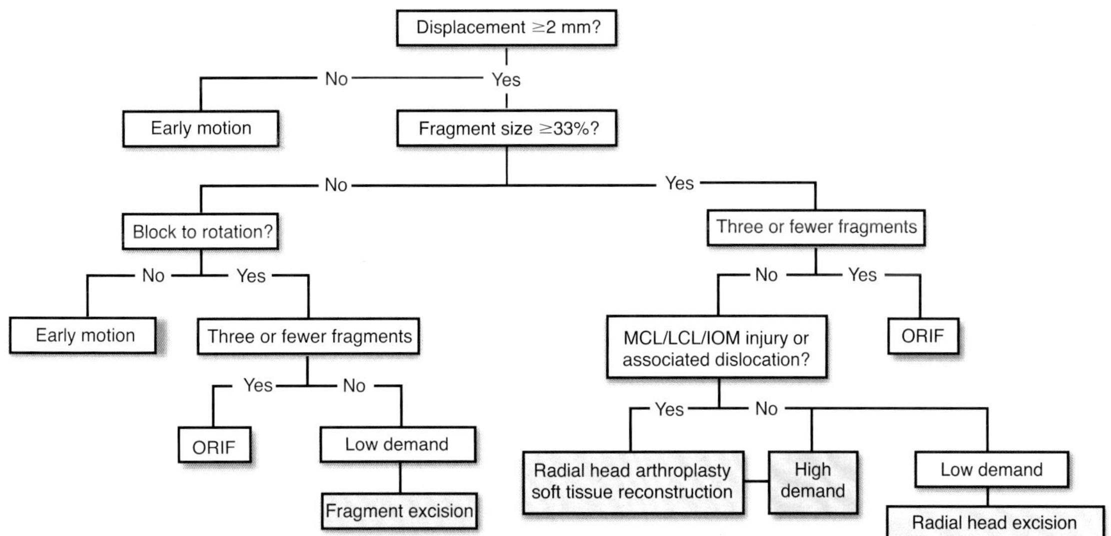


**FIG 10** • Treatment algorithm for radial head fractures.

- If there is a blockage or instability, excision, fixation, or arthroplasty is recommended based on patient factors and instability.
- A recent report regarding the long-term results of nonoperative management (similar to that described) of 49 patients with radial head fractures encompassing over 30% of the joint surface and displaced 2 to 5 mm revealed that 81% of patients had no subjective complaints and minimal loss of motion versus the uninjured extremity. Only one patient had daily pain.[1]

## SURGICAL MANAGEMENT

### Preoperative Planning

- It is essential to review all imaging and perform thorough history, physical, and fluoroscopic examinations before making an incision.
  - The presence of instability or associated fractures warrants a more extensile approach.

### Positioning

- Positioning depends on the planned approach and the surgeon's preference.
  - We prefer the patient supine with the affected extremity brought across the chest over a bump to allow access to the posterolateral elbow.
  - A sterile tourniquet is placed high on the arm.

### Approach

- The posterolateral (Kocher) approach has traditionally been presented to approach radial head fractures; however, we prefer a modified Wrightington approach[24] which is a modified posterior (Boyd) approach[4] between the interval between the ulna and anconeus for the following reasons: (**FIG 11**).
  - It offers superior visualization of the radial head and neck which is important in ORIF.
  - It is also the only approach that allows visualization of the radioulnar, radiohumeral, and ulnohumeral joint spaces which is essential in selecting the appropriate radial head implant size if arthroplasty is warranted.
- The approach is extensile and can allow the surgeon to address ligamentous injuries in addition to the radial head fracture with less risk of neuroma formation and neurologic injury.

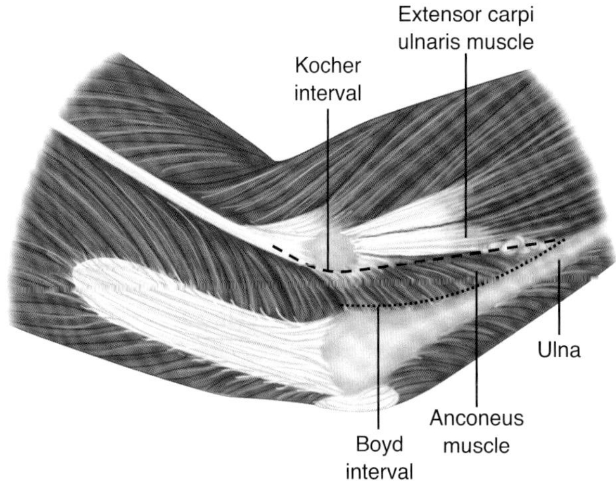


**FIG 11** • Surgical intervals for the Boyd approach and the Kocher approach.

## Kocher Approach

- The traditional posterolateral (Kocher) approach between the anconeus and extensor carpi ulnaris is cosmetic and spares the lateral ulnar collateral ligament.
  - We recommend not using an Esmarch tourniquet to allow visualization of penetrating veins that help identify the interval.
- A 5-cm oblique incision is made from the posterolateral aspect of the lateral epicondyle obliquely to a point three fingerbreadths below the tip of the olecranon in line with the radial neck (**TECH FIG 1A**).
- The radial head and epicondyle are palpated, and the fascia is divided in line with the skin incision.
- The Kocher interval is identified distally by small penetrating veins and bluntly developed, revealing the lateral ligament complex and joint capsule (**TECH FIG 1B**).
- The anconeus is reflected posteriorly and the extensor carpi ulnaris origin anteriorly. The capsule is incised obliquely anterior to the lateral ulnar collateral ligament (**TECH FIG 1C,D**).
- The proximal edge of the annular ligament may also be divided and tagged, with care taken not to proceed distally and damage the posterior interosseous nerve.

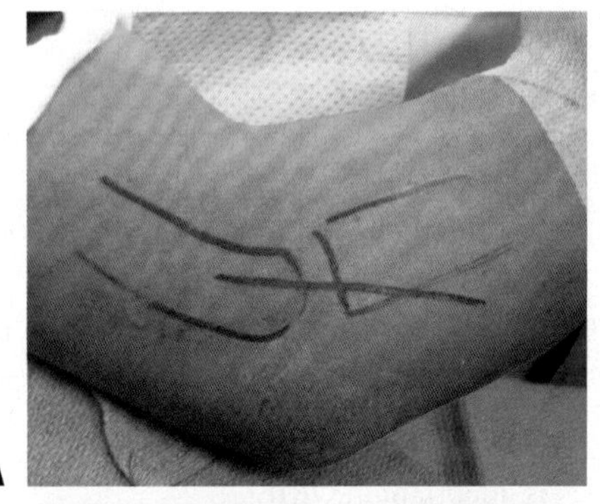
A

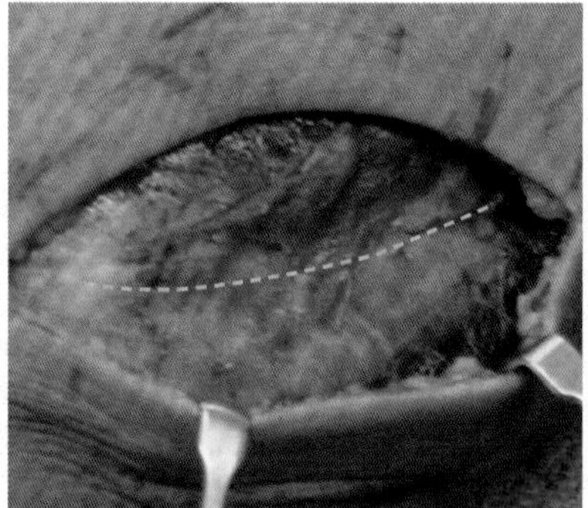
B

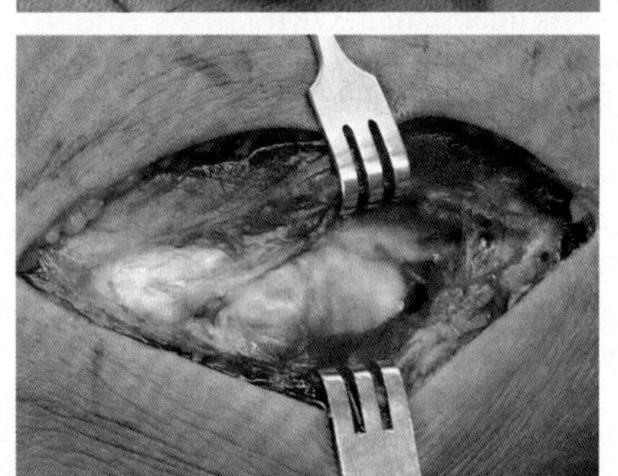
C

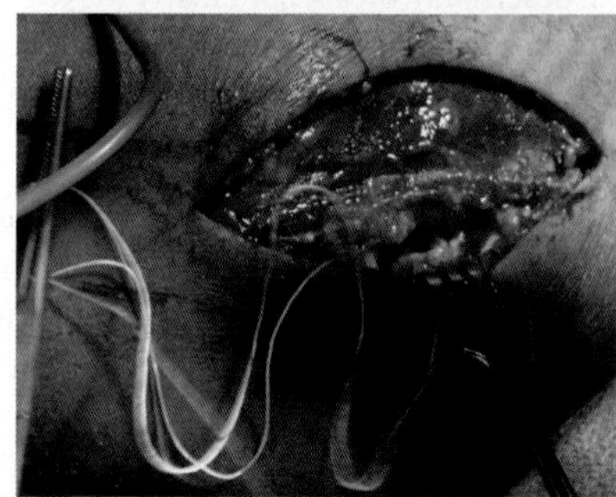
D

**TECH FIG 1** • Kocher approach. **A.** The skin incision proceeds distally from the posterolateral aspect of the lateral epicondyle to the posterior aspect of the proximal radius. **B.** Full-thickness flaps are made and the fascial interval between the extensor carpi ulnaris and anconeus muscles is identified. **C.** With longitudinal incision of the fascia and blunt division of the muscles, the joint capsule is evident. **D.** The capsule is longitudinally incised, and the fascia is tagged with figure-8 stitches for later anatomic repair.

## Modified Wrightington Approach

- An 8-cm straight longitudinal incision is made just lateral to the olecranon (**TECH FIG 2A**).
- Full-thickness skin flaps are developed bluntly over the fascia.
- The fascia is longitudinally incised in the interval between the anconeus and ulna (**TECH FIG 2B**).
- The anconeus is dissected off the ulna, elevating proximal to distal to preserve the distal vascular pedicle. Great care is taken not to violate the joint capsule or lateral ulnar collateral ligament by using blunt fashion (**TECH FIG 2C**).
- The lateral ulnar collateral ligament and annular ligament complex are sharply divided and tagged from their insertion on the crista supinatoris of the ulna. The radial head and its articulation with the capitellum are now evident (**TECH FIG 2D**).
- After repair or replacement, the ligaments are repaired to their insertion with suture anchors.

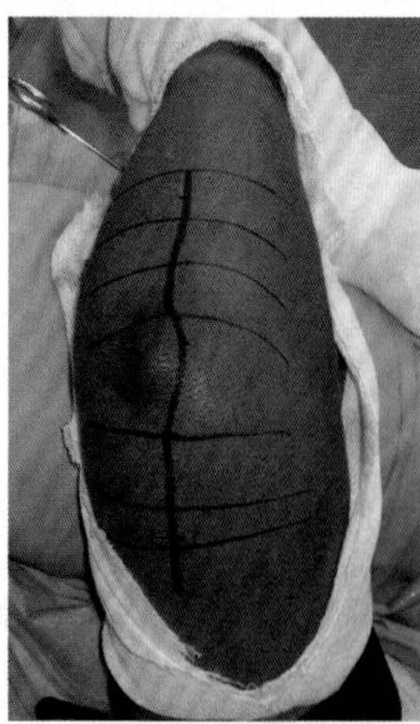
A

**TECH FIG 2** • Modified Wrightington approach. **A.** Make an 8-cm longitudinal incision at the junction of the ulna and anconeus starting about four fingerbreadths distal to the olecranon and extending 2 cm proximal to the olecranon. *(continued)*

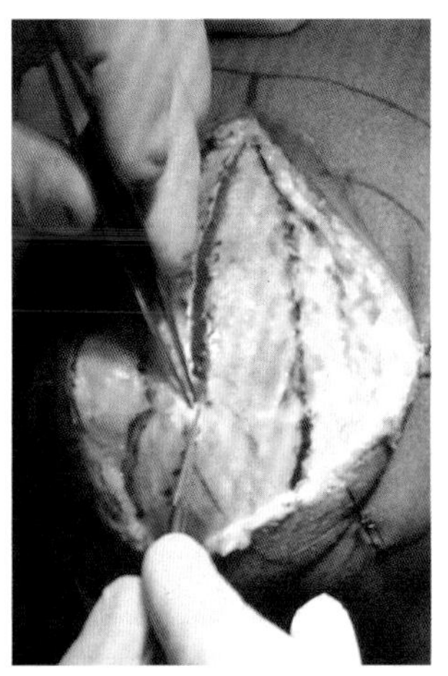

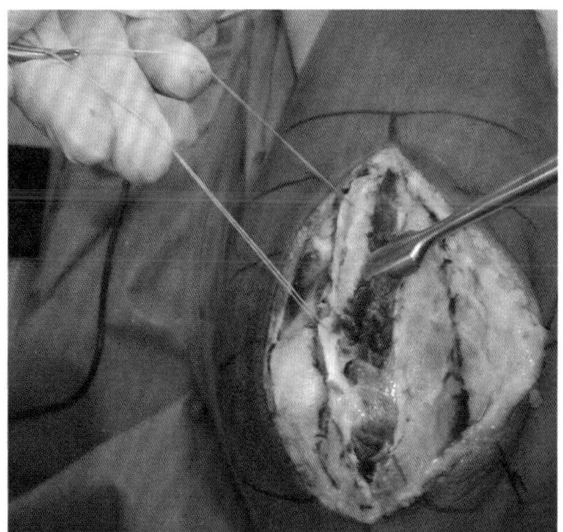

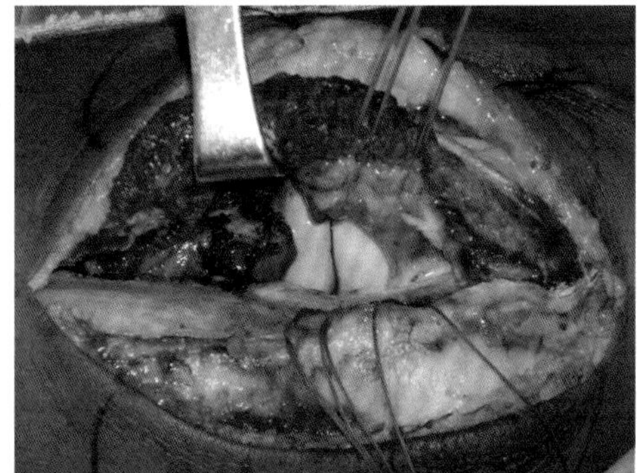

**TECH FIG 2** • *(continued)* **B.** The interval between the ulna and anconeus is incised sharply, with care taken not to violate the periosteum or muscle to minimize the risk of proximal radioulnar synostosis. **C.** Blunt elevation of the anconeus is crucial to avoid damaging the capsule or lateral ligament complex. **D.** The capsule and lateral ligament complex are tagged during the approach to facilitate final repair with suture anchors.

## Fracture Inspection and Preparation

- The fracture is now completely visible along with full visualization of the radial head by posteriorly subluxing the radial head out of the joint (**TECH FIG 3**).
- The wound is irrigated, and loose bodies are removed.
- The forearm is rotated to obtain a circumferential view of the fracture and appreciate the safe zone for hardware placement.
- If comminution (more than three pieces) is evident at this step or significant impaction with a DRUJ injury, we elect to replace the radial head.

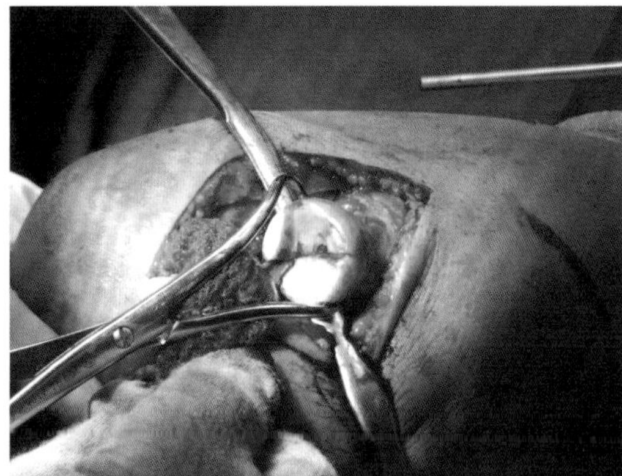

**TECH FIG 3** • The modified Wrightington approach allows for full visualization of the radial head and fracture by subluxing the radial head posteriorly out of the joint.

## Reduction and Provisional Fixation

- Any joint impaction is elevated and the void filed with local cancellous graft from the lateral epicondyle.
- The fragments are reduced provisionally with a tenaculum and held with small Kirschner wires placed out of the zone where definitive fixation is planned.
- It is acceptable to place this temporary fixation in the safe zone.

## Fixation

- There are many options for definitive fixation[7]:
  - One or two countersunk 2.0- or 2.7-mm AO cortical screws perpendicular to the fracture
  - Mini-plates
  - Small headless screws
  - Polyglycolide pins
  - Poly-L-lactic acid screws
  - Small threaded wires
- We prefer to use two parallel Biotrak screws (Acumed, Hillsboro, Oregon), which are cannulated, headless, resorbable, and variable pitched for isolated head fractures (**TECH FIG 4**). For fractures with neck extension, we prefer AO 2.0- or 2.7-mm mini-plates along the safe zone.

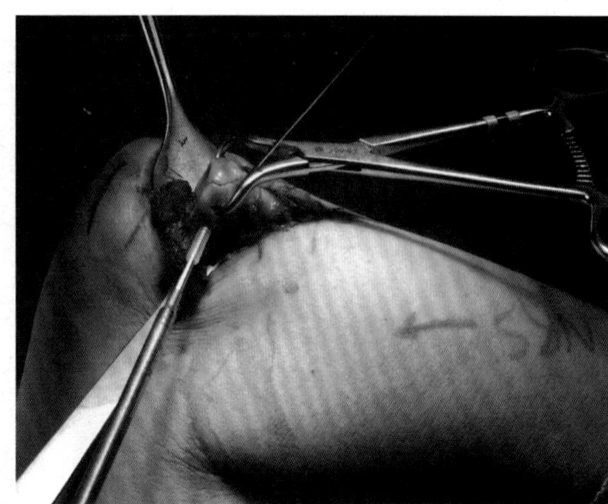

**TECH FIG 4** • Tenaculum clamps and 0.062-inch Kirschner wires are placed outside the zone of planned definitive fixation to provisionally hold the reduction. Two Biotrak screws are inserted for definitive fixation while the fracture is held reduced.

## Closure

- Any releases or injury to the annular ligament or lateral ulnar collateral ligament must be repaired anatomically. Drill holes with transosseous sutures are a proven method, but most authors now use suture anchors with reproducible results.
- Skin closure is performed in standard fashion with drains at the surgeon's discretion.

## PEARLS AND PITFALLS

| | |
|---|---|
| **Protection of the posterior interosseous nerve** | ■ Pronation of the forearm moves the posterior interosseous nerve away from the operative field during posterior approaches.<br>■ Dissection should remain subperiosteally. |
| **Comminution** | ■ We have a low threshold for excision or arthroplasty in the setting of comminution. |
| **Fluoroscopy** | ■ A fluoroscopy unit should be available for examination under anesthesia before sterile preparation. |
| **Hardware** | ■ Prosthetic radial head replacement should be discussed with the patient as an option and should be available in the room should the fracture prove to be comminuted.<br>■ A hinged external fixator should be available if instability may be an issue. |
| **Examination** | ■ A thorough fluoroscopic examination is the most important factor in deciding what treatment is appropriate. To obtain a true lateral view, we recommend abducting the arm and externally rotating the shoulder while placing the elbow on the image intensifier. |

## POSTOPERATIVE CARE

- The elbow is immobilized in a splint for 7 to 10 days.
- Serial x-rays are obtained to detect any loss of reduction at immediate postoperative, 2 weeks, 6 weeks, and 3 months, until healing is achieved (**FIG 12**).
- Active range of motion is allowed as soon as tolerable. Supervised therapy may be considered if the patient is not making adequate progress.
- Associated injuries may call for more protected range of motion.
- Light activities of daily living are allowed at 2 weeks, with increased weight bearing at 6 weeks.

## OUTCOMES

- The results of ORIF depend both on host factors such as the type of fracture, smoking, compliance, level of physical demand as well as surgical and rehabilitation protocols.
  - In uncomplicated fractures, over 90% satisfactory results can be expected.
  - Complications and resultant secondary procedures will be more likely in cases with undiagnosed instability and associated injury.

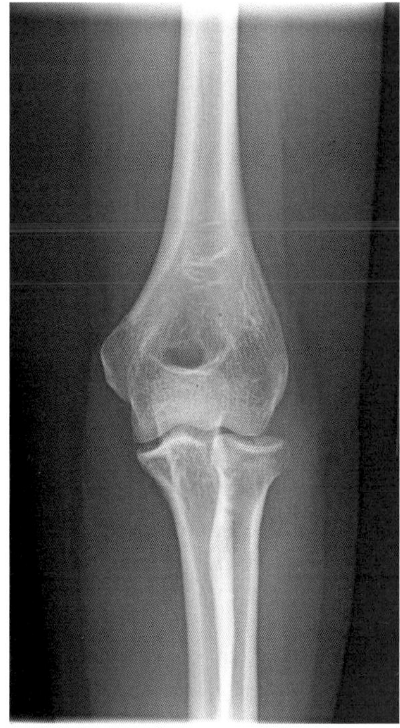

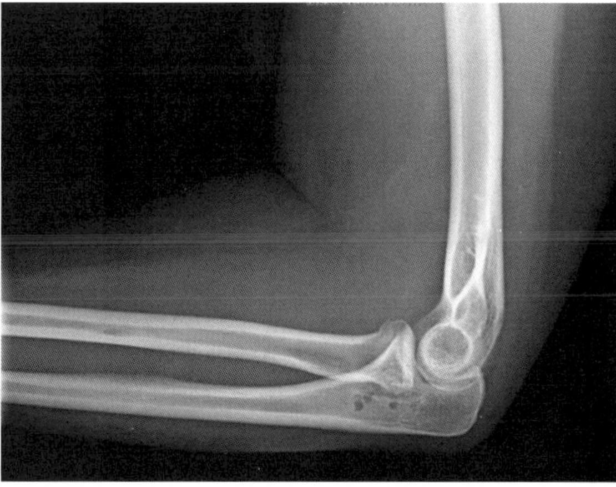

**FIG 12** • Postoperative x-rays showing anatomic reduction of the radial head fracture. The Biotrak screws are radiolucent. Note that anchor holes are seen at the crista supinatoris where the lateral ulnar collateral ligament (LUCL) and annular ligament complex are repaired.

## COMPLICATIONS

- Stiffness is the most common complication, with loss of terminal extension, supination, and pronation being most evident.
- Arthritis of the radiocapitellar joint or PRUJ
- Heterotopic ossification
- Symptomatic hardware may require secondary removal (**FIG 13**).
- Infection
- Early and late instability from missed or failed treatment of associated injuries
- The rate of avascular necrosis is about 10%, significantly higher in displaced fractures. This is expected given that the radial recurrent artery inserts in the safe zone where hardware is placed. This is generally clinically silent.
- Loss of reduction
- Nonunion (**FIG 14**)

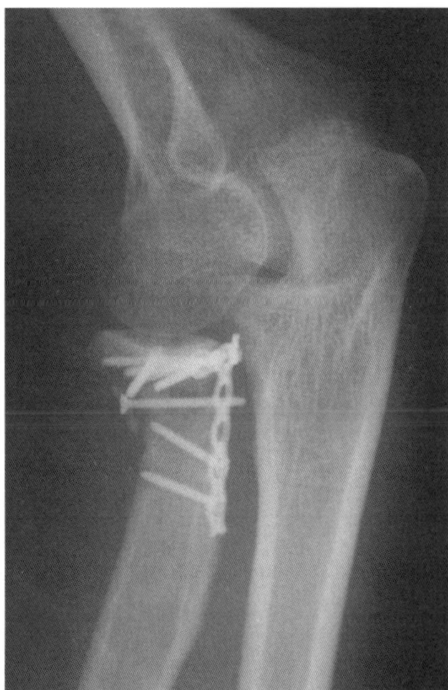
A

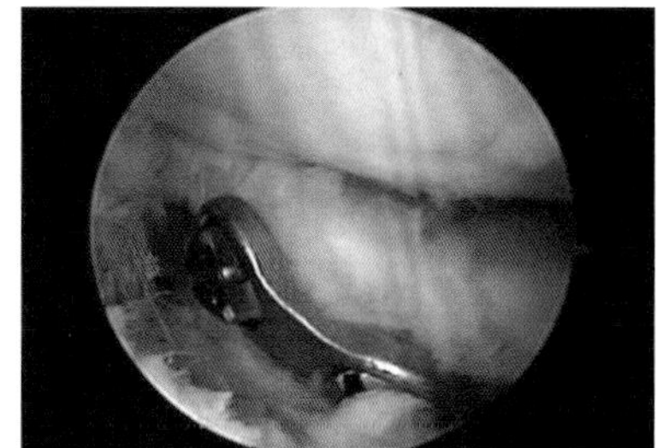
B

**FIG 13** • **A.** Oblique radiograph demonstrating prominent hardware limiting forearm rotation. **B.** Arthroscopic view in the lateral gutter demonstrating hardware impingement at the PRUJ.

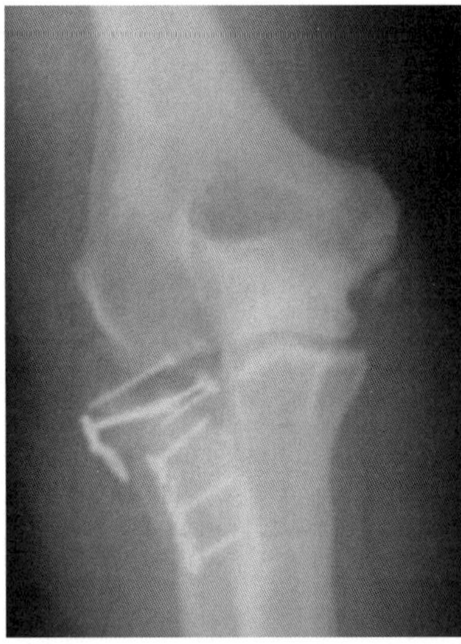
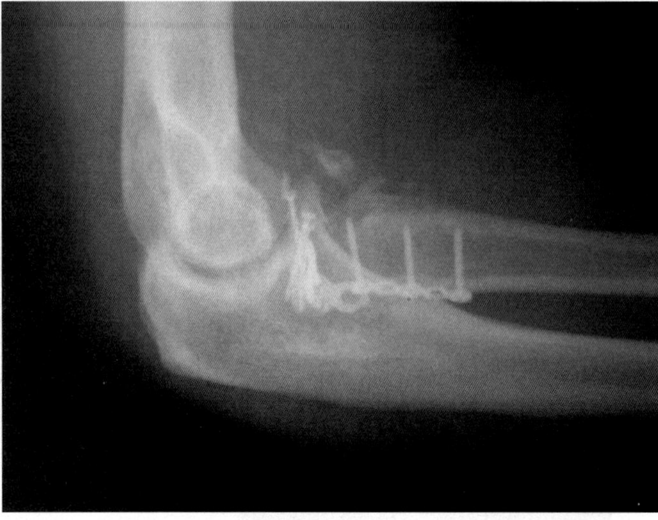

**FIG 14** • ORIF of radial neck fracture that went on to nonunion and avascular necrosis.

## REFERENCES


1. Akesson T, Herbertsson P, Josefsson PO, et al. Primary nonoperative treatment of moderately displaced two-part fractures of the radial head. J Bone Joint Surg Am 2006;88(9):1909–1914.
2. Amis AA, Miller JH. The mechanisms of elbow fractures: an investigation using impact tests in vitro. Injury 1995;26:163–168.
3. Antuna SA, Sánchez-Márquez JM, Barco R. Long-term results of radial head resection following isolated radial head fractures in patients younger than forty years old. J Bone Joint Surg Am 2010;92:558–566.
4. Boyd HB. Surgical exposure of the ulna and proximal third of the radius through one incision. Surg Gynecol Obstet 1940;71:86–88.
5. Broberg MA, Morrey BF. Results of delayed excision of the radial head after fracture. J Bone Joint Surg Am 1986;68(5):669–674.
6. Broberg MA, Morrey BF. Results of treatment of fracture-elbow dislocations of the elbow and intraarticular fractures. Clin Orthop Relat Res 1989;246:126–130.
7. Caputo AE, Mazzocca AD, Sontoro VM. The nonarticulating portion of the radial head: anatomic and clinical correlations for internal fixation. J Hand Surg Am 1998;23(6):1082–1090.
8. Esser RD, Davis S, Taavao T. Fractures of the radial head treated by internal fixation: late results in 26 cases. J Orthop Trauma 1995;9:318–323.
9. Essex-Lopresti P. Fractures of the radial head with distal radioulnar dislocation. J Bone Joint Surg Br 1951;33(2):244–250.
10. Harrington IJ, Tountas AA. Replacement of the radial head in the treatment of unstable elbow fractures. Injury 1981;12(5):405–412.
11. Herbertsson P, Josefsson PO, Hasserius R, et al. Fractures of the radial head and neck treated with radial head excision. J Bone Joint Surg Am 2004;86-A(9):1925–1930.
12. Herbertsson P, Josefsson PO, Hasserius R, et al. Uncomplicated Mason type-II and III fractures of the radial head and neck in adults. A long-term follow-up study. J Bone Joint Surg Am 2004;86-A(3):569–574.
13. Hotchkiss RN. Fractures and dislocations of the elbow. In: Rockwood CA Jr, Green DP, eds. Fractures in Adults, ed 4. Philadelphia: Lippincott-Raven, 1996:929–1024.
14. Itamura JM, Roidis NT, Chong AK, et al. Computed tomography study of radial head morphology. J Shoulder Elbow Surg 2008;17(2):347–354.
15. Itamura J, Roidis N, Mirzayan R, et al. Radial head fractures: MRI evaluation of associated injuries. J Shoulder Elbow Surg 2005;14(4):421–424.
16. Kaas L, Struijs PA, Ring D, et al. Treatment of Mason type II radial head fractures without associated fractures or elbow dislocation: a systematic review. J Hand Surg Am 2012;37(7):1416–1421.
17. Kaas L, van Riet RP, Turkenburg JL, et al. Magnetic resonance imaging in radial head fractures: most associated injuries are not clinically relevant. J Shoulder Elbow Surg 2011;20(8):1282–1288.
18. Kovar FM, Jaindl M, Thalhammer G, et al. Incidence and analysis of radial head and neck fractures. World J Orthop 2013;4(2):80–84.
19. McKee MD, Jupiter JB. Trauma to the adult elbow and fractures of the distal humerus. In: Browner BD, Jupiter JR, Levine AM, et al, eds. Skeletal Trauma, ed 2. Philadelphia: WB Saunders, 1998:1455–1522.
20. Morrey BF. Radial head fracture. In: Morrey BF, ed. The Elbow and Its Disorders, ed 3. Philadelphia: WB Saunders, 2000:341–364.
21. Morrey BF, An KN, Stormont TJ. Force transmission through the radial head. J Bone Joint Surg Am 1988;70(2):250–256.
22. Ring D, Quintero J, Jupiter JB. Open reduction and internal fixation of fractures of the radial head. J Bone Joint Surg Am 2002;84-A(10):1811–1815.
23. Roidis NT, Papadakis SA, Rigopoulos N, et al. Current concepts and controversies in the management of radial head fractures. Orthopedics 2006;29(10):904–916.
24. Stanley JK, Penn DS, Wasseem M. Exposure of the head of the radius using the Wrightington approach. J Bone Joint Surg Br 2006;88(9):1178–1182.
25. Tang CW, Skaggs DL, Kay RM. Elbow aspiration and arthrogram: an alternative method. Am J Orthop 2001;30:256.
26. Yamaguchi K, Sweet FA, Bindra R, et al. The extraosseous and intraosseous arterial anatomy of the adult elbow. J Bone Joint Surg Am 1997;79(11):1653–1662.

# Management of Simple Elbow Dislocation

12

CHAPTER

Bradford O. Parsons and David M. Lutton

## DEFINITION

- Simple elbow dislocation is a dislocation of the ulnohumeral joint without concomitant fracture.
- Complex instability denotes the presence of a fracture associated with dislocation.
- The elbow is the second most commonly dislocated large joint.

## PATHOANATOMY

- Elbow stability is conferred by highly constrained osseous anatomy and the ligamentous anatomy.
- Essentially, there are three primary stabilizers of the elbow.[9,12]
  - The osseous architecture of the ulnohumeral joint, including the coronoid process and greater sigmoid notch of the ulna, and the trochlea of the humerus
  - The anterior band of the medial collateral ligament (aMCL) resists valgus stress. The aMCL originates on the anterior inferior face of the medial epicondyle and inserts on the sublime tubercle of the ulna.
  - The lateral ulnar collateral ligament (LUCL) resists varus stress. The LUCL originates from an isometric point on the lateral supracondylar column and traverses across the inferior aspect of the radial head, inserting on the supinator crest of the ulna.[8] Unlike the aMCL, the LUCL originates in the precise center of rotation of the elbow; this is important when reconstructing the ligament.
- Secondary stabilizers include the radial head and dynamic constraints such as the flexor and extensor muscles of the forearm.
  - When the elbow is extended, the anterior joint capsule contributes about 15% of varus–valgus stability.[9]
  - The radial head does not resist physiologic valgus stress in the presence of an intact aMCL; however, it plays a major role in the presence of aMCL insufficiency.
- O'Driscoll has described the term *ring of disability* to describe series of pathologic events that result in ulnohumeral dislocation.
  - A simple elbow dislocation begins with an extension varus stress that disrupts the LUCL and progresses medially with tearing of the anterior and posterior capsules. This allows the ulna to "perch" on the distal humerus. Further soft tissue or osseous injury results in dislocation[13] (**FIG 1A**).
    - Most traumatic injuries to the LUCL result in avulsion of the ligament from the lateral humerus (**FIG 1B**).
  - As forces continue from lateral to medial across the joint, the anterior and posterior capsular tissues and eventually the medial collateral ligament (MCL) may be disrupted; however, it is theoretically possible to dislocate the ulnohumeral joint with disruption of the LUCL and preservation of the aMCL.[12]
- O'Driscoll et al[12] has proposed the term *posterolateral rotatory instability* (PLRI) to describe the condition of chronic LUCL insufficiency resulting in rotatory recurrent ulnohumeral instability.
- Fractures may occur with elbow dislocations, and the risk of recurrent instability increases significantly with complex dislocations. These fractures commonly include radial head or neck and coronoid fractures, although any fracture about the elbow may be observed.
  - Radial head fractures are usually readily apparent on plain radiographs.
  - Coronoid fractures may be subtle, and even a "fleck" of coronoid is often a hallmark of a more significant injury (eg, "terrible triad" injury), and its importance should not be underestimated.
  - Recently, a variant of elbow instability termed *posteromedial rotatory instability* (PMRI) has been described. PMRI is the sequela of a LUCL injury and a medial coronoid facet fracture. This injury pattern is most commonly observed without radial head fracture, making it potentially very subtle on plain radiographs. A computed tomography (CT) scan can delineate this injury in detail and should be obtained if any suspicion exists (**FIG 1C–E**).[2,11]

## ETIOLOGY AND CLASSIFICATION

- Most elbow dislocations occur with a fall on an outstretched arm.
- Forces of valgus, extension, supination, and axial compression across the joint can result in the ulna rotating away from the humerus, disrupting lateral anterior soft tissues initially, and dislocating the elbow.
- Simple elbow dislocations are classified by the direction of displacement of the ulna in reference to the humerus, with posterolateral dislocation the most common.
  - Less common variants include anterior, medial, or lateral dislocations.

## PATIENT HISTORY AND PHYSICAL FINDINGS

- History is aimed at determining the timeline and mechanism of injury, frequency of dislocations, and previous treatment.
- Unlike the shoulder, recurrent instability of the elbow is rare after an initial simple dislocation that was treated expediently.
  - Recurrent instability is more common in association with fractures (eg, the terrible triad injury).
  - Chronic instability, although rare in the United States, does occasionally occur, and management often requires reconstructive surgery or elbow replacement. Closed treatment is rarely successful in these patients.

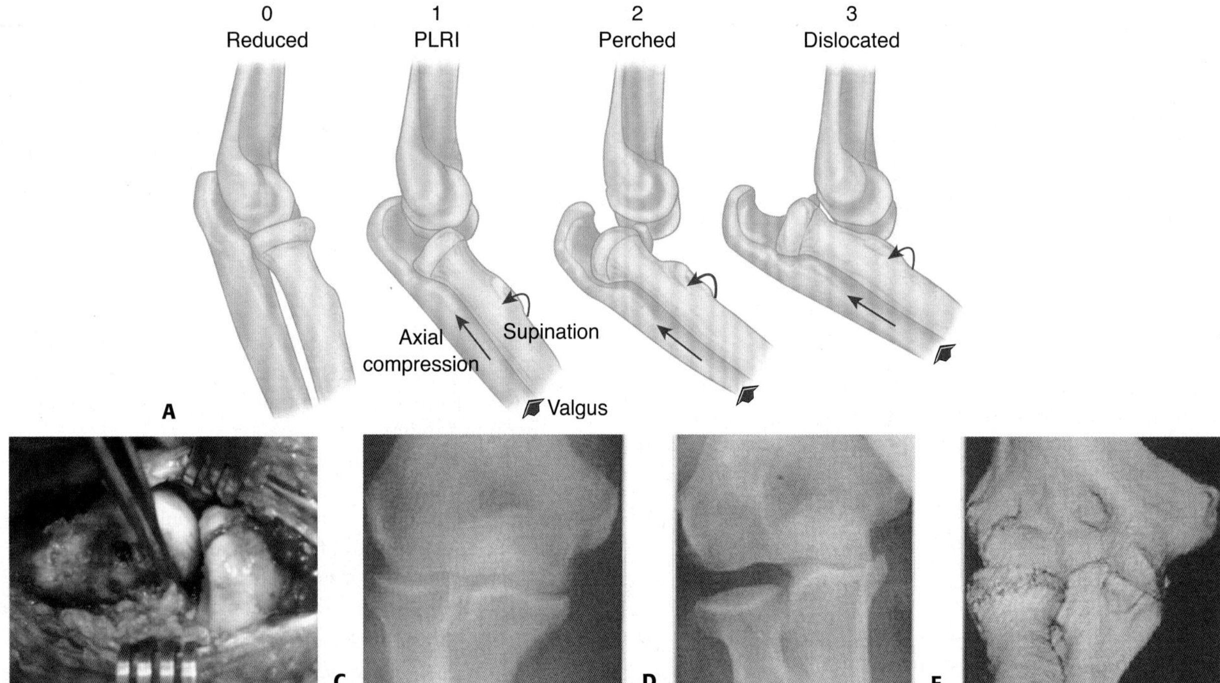


**FIG 1** • **A.** PLRI follows a typical progression of disruption, allowing the joint to become perched and then dislocate as soft tissue injury progresses. **B.** Intraoperative photograph demonstrating avulsion of the origin of the LUCL after traumatic dislocation of the elbow. The origin of the LUCL and the extensor muscles are avulsed as one layer, held by the forceps. **C–E.** PMRI is a variant of elbow instability in which the elbow dislocates, rupturing the LUCL, and the medial coronoid sustains an impaction fracture. **C,D.** In this injury pattern, the radial head remains intact, making appropriate diagnosis of the severity of the injury difficult on standard radiographs. CT scans help better delineate the injury pattern. **E.** Impaction fracture can be seen on the 3-D CT reconstruction. (**A:** Adapted from O'Driscoll SW, Morrey BF, Korinek S, et al. Elbow subluxation and dislocation: a spectrum of instability. Clin Orthop Relat Res 1982;280:194; **C–E:** Copyright the Mayo Foundation, Rochester, MN.)

- Iatrogenic injury of the LUCL (during procedures such as open tennis elbow release or radial head fracture management) is a known cause of recurrent PLRI. However, these patients often complain of subtle lateral elbow pain due to subluxation of the joint with activities, such as rising from a chair, but rarely have recurrent dislocation.
- Examination at the time of injury requires attention to the neurovascular anatomy.
  - Nerve injury can occur after elbow dislocation, and a thorough neurologic examination of the extremity is mandatory before any treatment of the dislocation.
    - Most nerve injuries are neurapraxia that often resolve.
    - The ulnar nerve is most frequently involved, although median or radial nerve injury may also occur.[14]
- The dislocated elbow has obvious deformity, with the elbow typically held in a varus position and the forearm supinated.
- After initial reduction, the neurovascular status of the limb is reevaluated. Loss of neurologic function after closed reduction is rare but can be an indication for surgical exploration to rule out an entrapped nerve.
- Stability of the joint is assessed based on the amount of extension obtainable and association of pronation or supination with instability.
  - It is helpful to evaluate the stability throughout the elbow range of motion while the patient is still anesthetized, as this may guide treatment (examination under anesthesia).
  - Stressing of the lateral soft tissues is performed with the lateral pivot shift maneuver, which can be performed under anesthesia and with fluoroscopic imaging[12] (**FIG 2**).
    - This test can be used to assess the degree of PLRI and may aid in determining treatment.
- Medial ecchymosis may be a sign of an aMCL injury and often is apparent 3 to 5 days after dislocation when the MCL has been injured.

## IMAGING AND OTHER DIAGNOSTIC STUDIES

- Standard orthogonal radiographs of the elbow are obtained before and after reduction to assess for fracture and confirm relocation of the joint.
  - Congruency of the trochlea–ulna and radial head–capitellum is assessed.
  - Slight widing of the ulnohumeral joint (drop sign) or posterior displacement of the radial head relative to the capitellum should be noted.
- Valgus stress views, once the joint is reduced, may help demonstrate an aMCL injury.
  - With the elbow flexed 30 degrees and the forearm in pronation, a valgus stress is placed under fluoroscopic evaluation to see if the medial ulnohumeral joint opens compared to the resting state.
- Varus stress views are often not helpful.
- CT scans with three-dimensional (3-D) reconstructions are obtained in any situation where a fracture may be

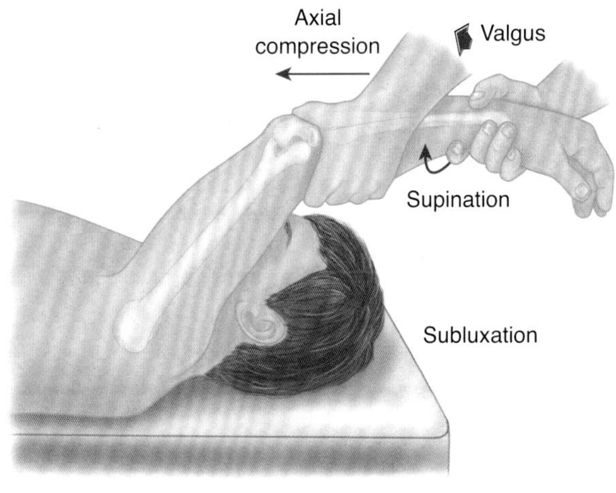


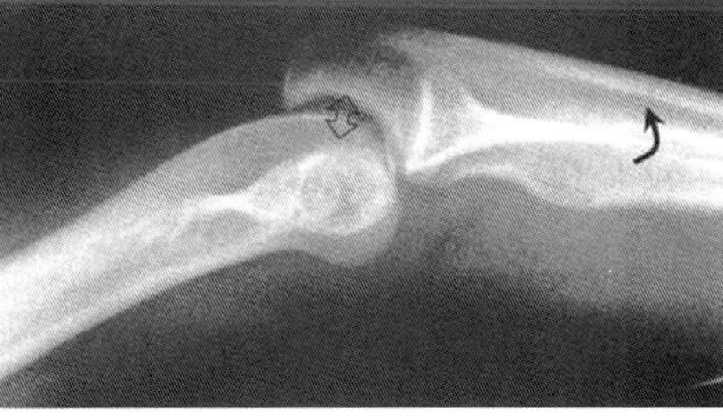


**FIG 2** • **A.** The lateral pivot shift maneuver is performed with the patient's arm positioned overhead, and a supination valgus stress is applied. As the elbow is brought into flexion, the joint reduces, often with a clunk. **B.** When performed under fluoroscopy, subluxation of the radial head posterior to the capitellum can be observed, consistent with PLRI. (**B:** From O'Driscoll SW, Bell DF, Morrey BF. Posterolateral rotatory instability of the elbow. J Bone Joint Surg Am 1991;73[3]:440–446.)

suspected, as it is critical to identify PMRI variants or subtle coronoid fractures, which may be an indication for surgical management.

- Magnetic resonance imaging (MRI) is usually not necessary in the management of acute simple dislocation; however, it can be useful in the case of recurrent PLRI.

## NONOPERATIVE MANAGEMENT

- Most simple dislocations may be managed nonoperatively with splinting or bracing, guided by the degree of instability determined during the examination under anesthesia after reduction.[12]
- Once reduced, elbow stability is assessed during flexion–extension in neutral forearm rotation.
  - If the elbow is stable throughout an arc of motion, it is immobilized in a sling or splint for 3 to 5 days for comfort and then range-of-motion exercises are initiated.
  - If instability is present in less than 30 degrees of flexion, the forearm is pronated and stability is reassessed.
    - If pronation confers stability, then a hinged orthosis that maintains forearm pronation is used, after 3 to 5 days of splinting, to allow protected range of motion.
- Elbows that sublux (confirmed by fluoroscopic imaging) in less than 30 degrees of flexion and pronation of the forearm are managed with a brief period of splinting, followed by a hinged orthosis that controls rotation of the forearm and has an extension block.
- Elbow instability above 30 degrees of flexion can be an indication for surgical stabilization.
- Hinged bracing is maintained for 6 weeks, with progressive advancement of extension and rotation, as allowed by stability of the joint.
  - Weekly radiographs are needed to ensure maintenance of a congruent joint during the first 4 to 6 weeks.
- After 6 weeks, bracing is discontinued, and terminal stretching to regain motion is used if flexion contractures exist.

## SURGICAL MANAGEMENT

### Indications

- Surgical management is indicated in elbows that are unstable, even when placed in flexion (more than 30 degrees) and pronation, elbows that recurrently subluxate or dislocate during the treatment protocol, or those with associated fractures ("complex" instability).
- Management of simple dislocation requires repair or reconstruction of the ligamentous structures leading to the instability. By definition, simple dislocation occurs without fracture.
- An algorithmic approach to ligament repair is used to stabilize the elbow. LUCL insufficiency is felt to be the primary lesion with simple dislocations and is therefore addressed first.
- The LUCL usually avulses from the humerus and can be repaired in the acute setting.
  - Repair may be performed via bone tunnels in the humerus or with suture anchors, depending on the surgeon's preference.
  - Reconstruction of the LUCL is rarely needed in acute management but is often needed in chronic instability. Reconstruction is performed with autograft (either palmaris or gracilis) or allograft.
    - Repair or reconstruction of the LUCL typically confers stability, even in the face of MCL injury, as the intact radial head is a secondary stabilizer to valgus instability.
- Persistent instability after LUCL repair is rare and is more commonly observed with fracture-dislocations or chronic instability.
  - If persistent instability exists, the MCL is repaired or reconstructed. A hinged external fixator may be placed to protect the repair.

### Preoperative Planning

- Planning should include preparing for the possibility of reconstruction of the LUCL which requires either autograft or allograft tendon.
  - If autograft is to be harvested, a tendon stripper is needed.
  - For allograft, we routinely use semitendinosus tendon.

- A hinged external fixator should be available in the rare case that the elbow remains unstable after ligamentous repair or reconstruction.
- A 2.0- and 3.2-mm drill bits or burrs are used to make bone tunnels for LUCL repair or reconstruction.
  - Some surgeons prefer suture anchor repair of ligament avulsions; if desired, these should be available.
- Fluoroscopy is useful for confirming reduction and is required for placement of a hinged external fixator.
- A sterile tourniquet is used to provide a bloodless surgical field.

## Patient Positioning

- Patients are positioned supine with the arm on a radiolucent hand table.
- A small bump is placed under the scapula to aid in arm positioning.
- The forequarter is draped free to ensure the entire brachium is kept in the surgical field.
- If hamstring autograft is to be used for LUCL, the leg should be draped free, and a bump is placed under the hemipelvis to aid in exposure.



# Lateral Ulnar Collateral Ligament Repair

## Surgical Approach and Arthrotomy

- Tourniquet control is used during this procedure.
- A fluoroscopic examination under anesthesia is performed to allow for an accurate assessment of the instability pattern
- Two different surgical approaches may be used to manage elbow instability.
- A posterior midline skin incision is versatile and can be used to gain access to both the medial and lateral aspects of the joint.
  - Alternatively, a "column" incision, centered over the lateral epicondyle, may be used (**TECH FIG 1A**). If medial-sided exposure is needed, a similar column incision may be made over the medial epicondyle to gain access.
  - There are benefits to both approaches, and currently, no data exist delineating which approach is better.
    - For simple dislocation, we routinely use a lateral column approach.
- After skin incision, skin flaps are raised anteroposterior at the level of the deep fascia.
- In the acute setting, the lateral soft tissues are usually avulsed off the epicondyle, exposing the joint. Occasionally, however, the extensor origin is intact with an underlying ligament injury.
  - If the extensor muscles are intact, the interval between the extensor carpi ulnaris (ECU) and anconeus (the Kocher approach), which directly overlies the LUCL, is used. This interval is often readily identified by the presence of a "fat stripe" in the deep fascia (**TECH FIG 1B**). The anconeus is reflected posteriorly, and the ECU is reflected anteriorly to expose the capsuloligamentous complex.
- The elbow joint is then exposed by incising the proximal capsule along the lateral column of the humerus, continuing distally along the radial neck (through the supinator muscle and underling capsule) in line with the ECU–anconeus interval.
  - The posterior interosseous nerve (PIN) is at risk with this exposure, and therefore, the forearm is kept in pronation to protect the PIN.
- The radiocapitellar joint and coronoid are inspected to confirm no fractures are present and that no soft tissue is interposed in the joint, preventing reduction.
- Once the joint is clear of debris, the ability to obtain a concentric reduction is confirmed with fluoroscopy.

## Ligament Repair

- The origin of the LUCL is identified.
  - Often, the LUCL is avulsed from the isometric point on the lateral capitellum, and the origin can be identified by a "fold" of tissue on the deep surface of the capsule (**TECH FIG 2A**).
- Starting at the origin, a running no. 2 nonabsorbable Krackow locking suture is placed along the anterior and posterior aspect of the ligament. Once placed, the suture–ligament construct is tensioned to confirm the integrity of the insertion onto the ulna.
  - A common mistake is to start the repair at the level of the proximal origin of the superficial tissue, which is not the origin of the LUCL but part of the extensor origin.

A
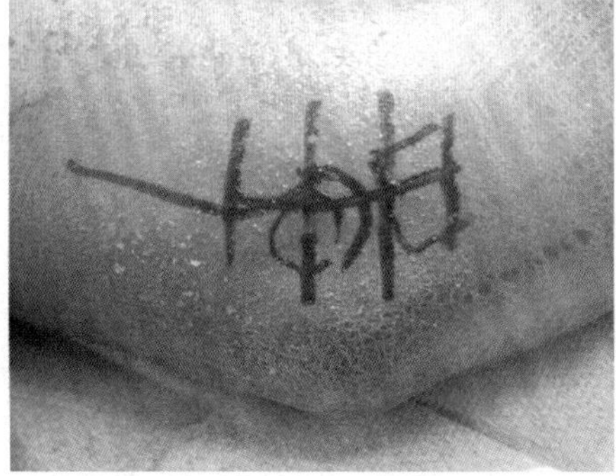

B
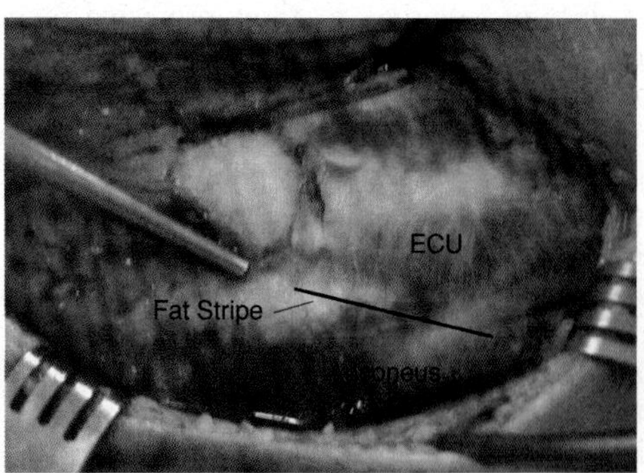


**TECH FIG 1** • **A.** Lateral column skin incision. The lateral incision is centered over the epicondyle and radiocapitellar joint and is often the primary incision, as the LUCL rupture is thought to be the primary injury in simple dislocations. **B.** The deep interval between the ECU and anconeus is used to gain exposure to the joint. This is often identified by a fat stripe in the fascia. Care should be taken not to violate the LUCL, which traverses in line with this interval deep to the fascia and supinator muscle.

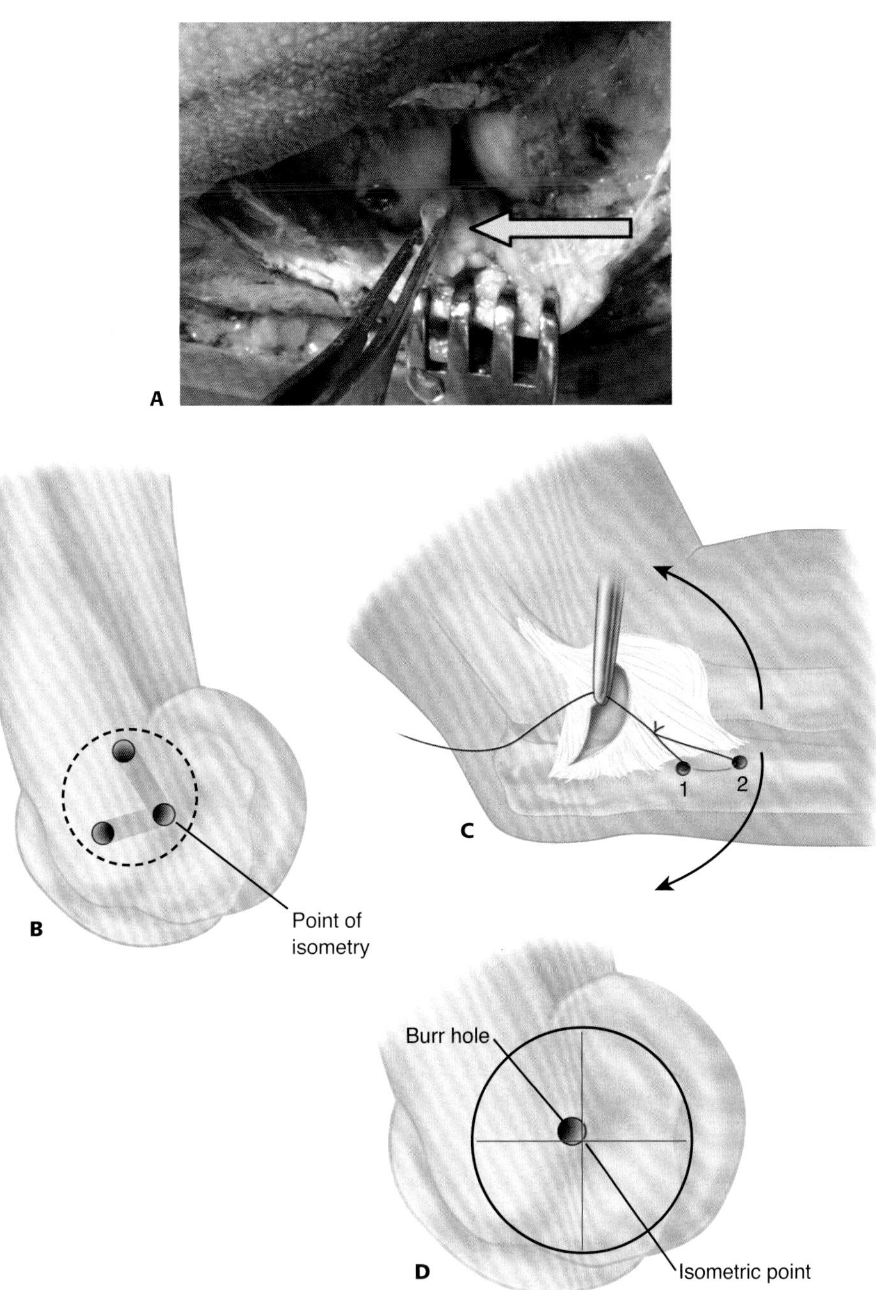


**TECH FIG 2 • A.** The origin of the LUCL, which often avulses during elbow dislocation, is identified by a fold of tissue on the deep surface of the capsule. The isometric point of the joint is in the center of rotation of the capitellum (**B**), and confirmation is made using the previously placed sutures in the ligament remnant to ensure that an isometric repair will be obtained (**C**). **D.** It is important to make the humeral tunnel so that the most anterior aspect of the tunnel is placed at the isometric point. Exit holes for the humeral tunnel are made anterior and posterior to the lateral supracondylar ridge (**B**).

- The isometric origin on the humerus is then identified in the center of the capitellum, not the lateral epicondyle (**TECH FIG 2B,C**).
  - Confirmation of the isometric point is made by clamping the limbs of the running suture at the point of isometry and then flexing and extending the elbow to confirm proper placement.
- A 2.0-mm burr is used to make a humeral bone tunnel.
  - It is critical to make the most anterior aspect of the bone tunnel at the isometric point, not the center of the tunnel, as this small translation can result in a lax LUCL repair (**TECH FIG 2D**).
- Two "exit" tunnels (in a Y configuration), one anterior and one posterior to the lateral column, are then made with a 2.0-mm

drill bit or burr, connected to the distal humeral tunnel at the isometric point.

- Once the humeral tunnels are completed, the limbs of the running suture are passed through the humeral tunnels.
- The joint is concentrically reduced with fluoroscopic confirmation, and the LUCL repair sutures are then tied with the joint reduced and the elbow in 30 degrees of flexion and neutral rotation.
- The elbow is ranged through an arc of motion to assess stability, with careful attention placed on the radial head's articulation with the capitellum, looking for posterior sag in extension, indicating either a lax LUCL or a nonisometric repair.
- If the elbow is stable through an arc of motion, the extensor origin is repaired with interrupted, heavy (no. 0) nonabsorbable suture, and the skin is closed in layers.

## Lateral Ulnar Collateral Ligament Reconstruction

- Occasionally, the native LUCL is damaged beyond repair (more often with iatrogenic PLRI than with primary instability) or attenuated after recurrent or chronic elbow instability, and reconstruction is necessary.
- Autograft palmaris, autograft gracilis, or allograft may be used.
- Autograft and allograft options should be discussed with the patient and decisions made preoperatively. We routinely use semitendinosus allograft unless the patient desires autograft.

### Bone Tunnel Preparation

- We use a "docking" technique, similar to those described for MCL reconstruction,[1] for LUCL reconstruction.
- The insertion of the LUCL is at the supinator crest of the ulna, and reconstruction begins with creation of the ulnar tunnels at the supinator crest.
- Reflecting the supinator origin from the ulna posterior to the radial head exposes the supinator crest.
  - The forearm is held in pronation to protect the PIN.
- Once the crest is exposed, the ulnar tunnel is made at the level of the radial head using two 3.4-mm burr holes placed 1 cm apart. Care is taken to connect the holes using small curettes or awls without fracturing the roof of the tunnel (**TECH FIG 3**).
- Once the ulnar tunnel is made, a suture is placed in the tunnel to aid in graft passage and to help identify the isometric point on the humerus, similar to the technique described with ligament repair.
- Once the isometric origin on the humerus is confirmed, humeral bone tunnels are made as mentioned in the LUCL Repair section.
  - With LUCL reconstruction, the isometric tunnel is deepened to about 1 cm to allow graft docking.
  - Furthermore, the docking tunnel is widened using a 3.4-mm burr to be able to accept both limbs of the graft.
  - It is important to widen the docking hole anterior and proximal to the isometric point, as the most posterior aspect of the tunnel needs to be at the isometric point.

### Graft Preparation

- One end of the graft is freshened and tubularized using a no. 2 nonabsorbable suture in a running Krackow fashion.
- The graft is then passed through the ulnar bone tunnels using the passage suture previously placed.
- The limb of the graft with locking suture is then fully docked into the humeral origin, and the joint is reduced.
- The final length of the graft is determined by tensioning the graft and identifying the point at which the free limb of the graft meets the isometric origin. This point is marked on the graft.
  - Care should be taken to ensure appropriate graft tension and length by fully docking the first limb and then marking the free limb at the point of initial contact with the humerus, thereby allowing some overlap of graft limbs in the humeral tunnel but minimizing the likelihood of slack in the final construct.
- The marked graft end is then freshened and tubularized in an identical fashion as the other limb.

### Final Reconstruction

- Once the graft is placed and ready for final tensioning and fixation, the capsule and remnant of the LUCL is repaired back to the humerus in an effort to make the ligament reconstruction extra-articular, if possible.
- Each limb of the graft is then placed into the isometric docking tunnel on the humerus with corresponding limbs from each locking suture exiting the proximal humeral tunnels.
  - Both limbs of locking suture from one end of the graft are passed through one proximal tunnel in the humerus, followed by the limbs from the other end of the graft through the second proximal tunnel.

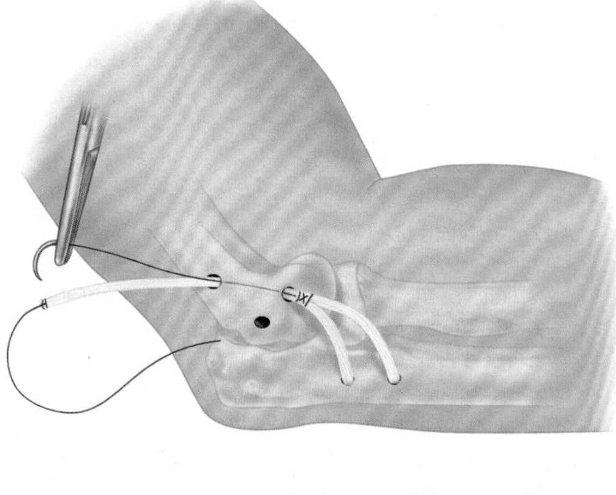

**TECH FIG 3** • The insertion of the LUCL is the supinator crest of the ulna. Reconstruction uses an ulnar tunnel in the supinator crest made at the level of the radial head. Holes are made about 1 cm apart and connected to form a tunnel.

- The joint is then reduced, and the graft is finally tensioned to ensure there is no slack and neither graft end has "bottomed out" in the humeral docking tunnel.
- The locking sutures are then tied together over the lateral column of the distal humerus with the joint concentrically reduced in 30 degrees of flexion and neutral rotation.
- The joint is then ranged and stability assessed. If the joint is stable, no further reconstruction is necessary, and the extensor muscles are repaired using a nonabsorbable interrupted stitch, followed by skin closure.

## Hinged External Fixation

- A hinged fixator may be necessary in chronic dislocations, some fracture-dislocations, or rarely in patients with persistent instability after LUCL repair or reconstruction for simple dislocation.[4,16]
- Once any soft tissue blocking reduction is removed and a concentric reduction can be obtained, the fixator is placed.
- All hinged elbow fixators are constructed around the axis or rotation of the elbow to allow range of motion to occur while maintaining a concentric reduction.
  - Most implants are built around an axis pin, placed in this center of rotation.
  - The center of rotation is identified as the center of the capitellum on a lateral aspect of the elbow, and on the medial side, it is just anteroinferior to the medial epicondyle, in the center of curvature of the trochlea (**TECH FIG 4**).
  - The axis pin is placed through both of these points, parallel to the joint surface, and the position is confirmed by fluoroscopy.
- After placement of the axis pin, the humeral and ulnar pins are placed after confirmation of concentric reduction of the elbow is made.
- Once the external fixator is fully constructed, the elbow is taken through an arc of motion, and maintenance of reduction is confirmed.
- Fixators are kept on for 6 to 8 weeks.
- Meticulous pin care is necessary to minimize pin tract infections or loosening.

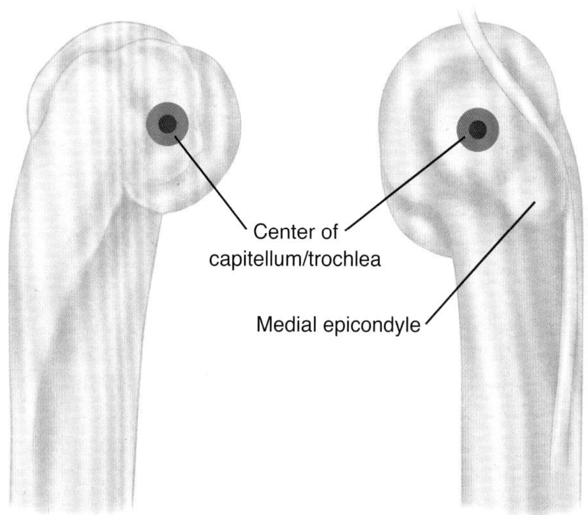


**TECH FIG 4** • The center of rotation of the elbow, along which an axis pin for hinged fixators is placed, is identified by the center of the capitellum and just anteroinferior to the medial epicondyle.

## PEARLS AND PITFALLS

- LUCL avulsion is the primary ligamentous injury in most simple dislocations of the elbow.
- If the radial head and coronoid are intact (as is the case in a simple dislocation), the MCL rarely needs to be repaired or reconstructed, as the radial head acts as a secondary stabilizer in the elbow with a repaired lateral ligament complex.
- The LUCL origin can be identified by a capsular fold of tissue. This is the point at which repair sutures should be placed, not at the origin of the more superficial extensor tendons.
- The isometric origin of the LUCL is in the center of the capitellum, as projected onto the lateral column, and repair or reconstruction needs to be brought to this point to have an isometric ligament.
- Bone tunnels in the humerus for repair or reconstruction are made so the anteroinferior aspect of the tunnel is at the isometric origin.
- A hinged external fixator may be necessary in management of elbow dislocation, especially chronic or recurrent situations, and should be available.
- All hinged fixators are constructed around the axis of rotation of the elbow, identified by a line between the isometric point on the lateral capitellum, and the center of rotation of the trochlea on the medial aspect of the joint.
- Stiffness is the most common adverse sequela of elbow dislocation, and therefore, range of motion should be started as soon as soft tissue and skin healing allows, with care taken to avoid varus or valgus stress.

## POSTOPERATIVE CARE

- After operative stabilization without external fixation, the elbow is splinted in 90 degrees of flexion for 3 to 5 days to allow wound healing.
- Range-of-motion exercises are then begun in flexion, extension, and rotation, with care taken to avoid varus or valgus stress.
  - A hinged orthosis can be helpful in protecting the ligament repair or reconstruction.
- Active and passive motion is continued for 6 weeks, when strengthening is added.
- Residual contractures, often loss of extension, can be managed with static splinting and terminal stretching.
- Most patients return to full activity by 4 to 6 months.

## OUTCOMES

- Most series have reported the results of closed management of simple dislocation.
  - Mehlhoff and colleagues[7] reported the results of 52 simple dislocations managed, with most patients having normal elbows. Length of immobilization, especially greater than 3 weeks, was found to be more likely to result in persistent loss of extension.
  - Similarly, Eygendaal and colleagues[3] reported the long-term results of 50 patients after closed management of simple dislocations. Sixty-two percent of patients described their elbow function as good or excellent, and 24 of 50 (48%) patients had loss of extension of 5 to 10 degrees.
- Some series have examined the surgical management of PLRI, often as a result of recurrent instability after traumatic dislocation.
  - Nestor and colleagues[10] reported the results of 11 patients with recurrent PLRI managed with either repair or reconstruction of the LUCL. Ten of 11 (91%) remained stable and 7 of 11 (64%) had an excellent result.
  - More recently, Sanchez-Sotelo and colleagues[15] reported the results of 44 patients treated for recurrent PLRI (9 occurred after simple dislocation). Thirty-two (75%) of the patients had an excellent result by Mayo score.
  - Lee and Teo[5] found that in patients with chronic PLRI, reconstruction offered more predictable outcomes than repair.

## COMPLICATIONS

- Stiffness[3,7]
- Heterotopic ossification[6]
- Neurovascular injury[14]
- Recurrent instability[3,7]
- Compartment syndrome
- Hematoma or infection

## REFERENCES

1. Dodson CC, Thomas A, Dines JS, et al. Medial ulnar collateral ligament reconstruction of the elbow in throwing athletes. Am J Sports Med 2006;34:1926–1932.
2. Doornberg JN, Ring DC. Fracture of the anteromedial facet of the coronoid process. J Bone Joint Surg Am 2006;88(10):2216–2224.
3. Eygendaal D, Verdegaal SH, Obermann WR, et al. Posterolateral dislocation of the elbow joint. Relationship to medial instability. J Bone Joint Surg Am 2000;82(4):555–560.
4. Jupiter JB, Ring D. Treatment of unreduced elbow dislocations with hinged external fixation. J Bone Joint Surg Am 2002;84-A(9):1630–1635.
5. Lee BP, Teo LH. Surgical reconstruction for posterolateral rotatory instability of the elbow. J Shoulder Elbow Surg 2003;12:476–479.
6. Linscheid RL, Wheeler DK. Elbow dislocations. JAMA 1965;194:1171–1176.
7. Mehlhoff TL, Noble PC, Bennett JB, et al. Simple dislocation of the elbow in the adult. Results after closed treatment. J Bone Joint Surg Am 1988;70(2):244–249.
8. Morrey BF, An KN. Functional anatomy of the ligaments of the elbow. Clin Orthop Relat Res 1985;(201):84–90.
9. Morrey BF, Tanaka S, An KN. Valgus stability of the elbow. A definition of primary and secondary constraints. Clin Orthop Relat Res 1991;(265):187–195.
10. Nestor BJ, O'Driscoll SW, Morrey BF. Ligamentous reconstruction for posterolateral rotatory instability of the elbow. J Bone Joint Surg Am 1992;74(8):1235–1241.
11. O'Driscoll SW. Acute, recurrent, and chronic elbow instabilities. In: Norris TR, ed. Orthopaedic Knowledge Update: Shoulder and Elbow 2. Rosemont: American Academy of Orthopaedic Surgeons, 2002:313–323.
12. O'Driscoll SW, Bell DF, Morrey BF. Posterolateral rotatory instability of the elbow. J Bone Joint Surg Am 1991;73(3):440–446.
13. O'Driscoll SW, Morrey BF, Korinek S, et al. Elbow subluxation and dislocation. A spectrum of instability. Clin Orthop Relat Res 1992;(280):186–197.
14. Rana NA, Kenwright J, Taylor RG, et al. Complete lesion of the median nerve associated with dislocation of the elbow joint. Acta Orthop Scand 1974;45:365–369.
15. Sanchez-Sotelo J, Morrey BF, O'Driscoll SW. Ligamentous repair and reconstruction for posterolateral rotatory instability of the elbow. J Bone Joint Surg Br 2005;87(1):54–61.
16. Tan V, Daluiski A, Capo J, et al. Hinged elbow external fixators: indications and uses. J Am Acad Orthop Surg 2005;13:503–514.

# Open Reduction and Internal Fixation of Pediatric T-Condylar Fractures

13

CHAPTER

Keith D. Baldwin and John M. Flynn

## DEFINITION

- T-condylar fractures of the distal humerus in children and adolescents are relatively rare occurrences. They are thought to represent 2% of all pediatric elbow fractures.[5]
- The proposed mechanism is similar to that of pediatric supracondylar fractures but with a higher energy mechanism of injury.[6]
- The olecranon acts as a wedge during hyperextension and creates a Y- or T-shaped fracture with the center in the olecranon fossa.
- These fractures are less likely to be comminuted than in adults.
- In younger children, an acceptable result can often be obtained with closed reduction and pinning, although this is generally not as straightforward as in a standard supracondylar humerus fracture (**FIG 1**).

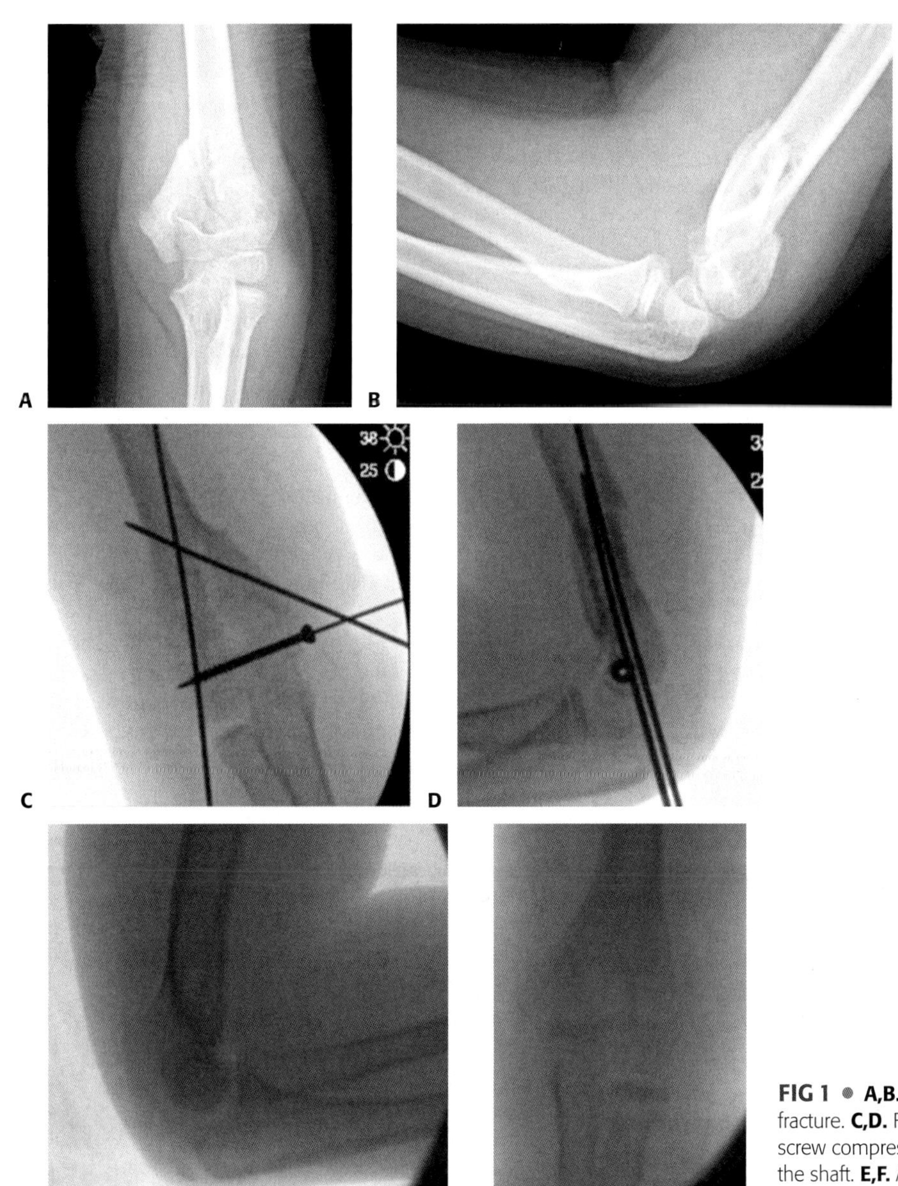

**FIG 1** • **A,B.** An 8-year-old boy with T-condylar distal humerus fracture. **C,D.** Fixed with mini-open reduction with intercondylar screw compression and K-wire fixation of the distal humerus to the shaft. **E,F.** After hardware removal, the patient had 0 to 140 degrees range of motion with no pain.

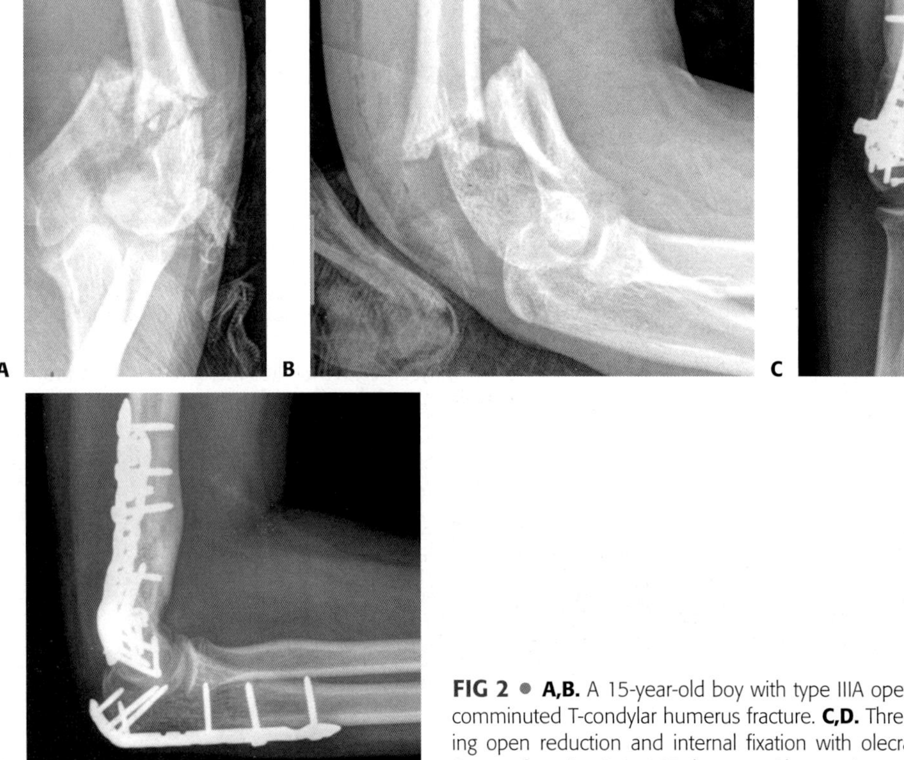

**FIG 2 • A,B.** A 15-year-old boy with type IIIA open distal humerus comminuted T-condylar humerus fracture. **C,D.** Three months following open reduction and internal fixation with olecranon osteotomy. Range of motion 0 to 140 degrees with no pain.

- Older children and young adolescents will often require an open approach.
- Comminution in the fossa may necessitate an olecranon osteotomy (**FIG 2**).
- Generally, pediatric fractures are less comminuted than adult fractures and may not require a full osteotomy.
  - A Morrey slide approach is used in such a case where the triceps and ulnar periosteum are elevated off the ulna medially to expose the distal humerus without performing an osteotomy.[3]
  - It was originally described to avoid olecranon osteotomies in cases where total elbow replacement would be a salvage operation.
  - It can be useful in adolescents because the fractures are not as comminuted, but excellent visualization of the joint is desirable to provide anatomic reduction and restoration of elbow function.

## ANATOMY

- The distal humerus is a complex articulation.
- The ulnohumeral articulation is the articulation which needs to be reconstructed in this type of fracture. Occasionally, the radiocapitellar joint is also damaged with capitellar comminution (**FIG 3A**).
- The remainder of the limb should be carefully examined. Coexisting wrist fractures can increase the risk of compartment syndrome and other soft tissue complications (**FIG 3B**).
- Conceptually, the distal humerus is a hinge which contains a medial and a lateral column connected by a middle hinge.

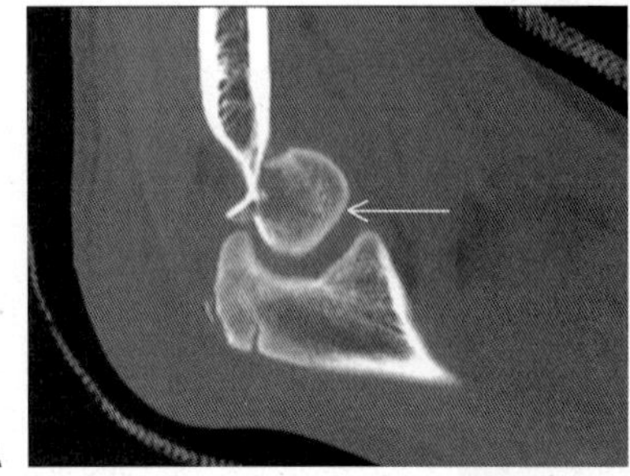

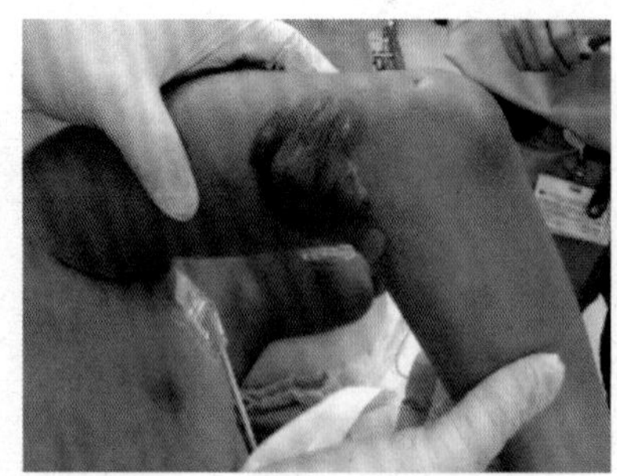

**FIG 3 • A.** A 13-year-old boy with a T-condylar humerus fracture with coronal split of the capitellum. **B.** Fracture blisters result from severe soft tissue injury.

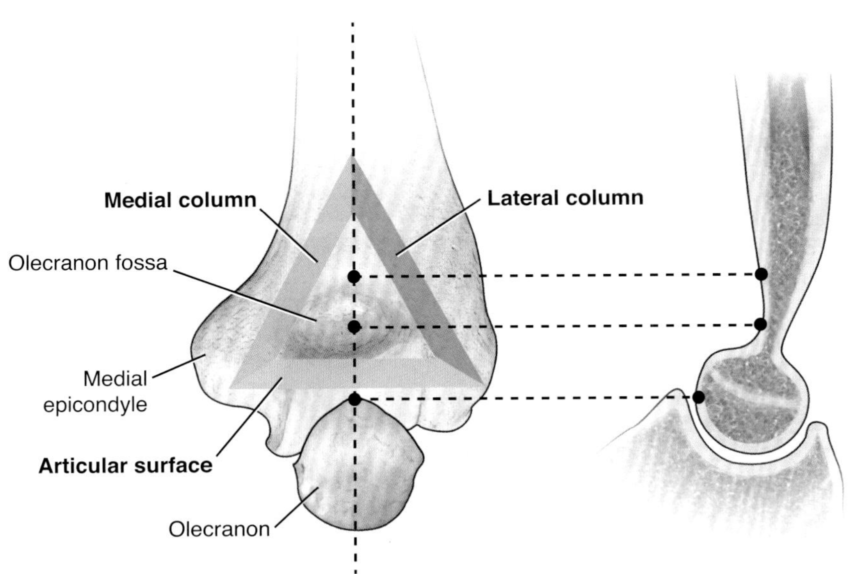


**FIG 4** • Triangle of stability concept. The mechanical properties of the distal humerus are based on a triangle of stability, comprising the medial and lateral columns and the articular surface. (Adapted from Bonczar MR, Rikli D, Ring D. Distal humerus 13-C1 open reduction; perpendicular [biplanar] plating. AO Foundation Web site. Available at: http://bit.ly/1wEegQS. Published June 21, 2007. Accessed November 1, 2013.)

This creates a "triangle of stability," which must be recreated in order for fixation to be successful in T-condylar humerus fractures.[2] Regardless of the fixation strategy, this concept must be followed (**FIG 4**).

- Posteromedially, the ulnar nerve travels through a groove in the distal humerus called the *cubital tunnel*. The nerve must be exposed along the medial border of the triceps down to the first motor branch, which pierces the flexor carpi ulnaris.
- The triceps covers the distal humerus and attaches to the proximal ulna at the olecranon process.
- The olecranon obscures the view of the distal humerus articular surface, with the elbow in extension.
- To visualize the fracture line with the Morrey slide, the elbow must be flexed past 90 degrees.
- Also important, the distal fracture fragments typically rotate with the apex anteriorly, which is important to remember when reducing the joint surface.

## PATHOGENESIS

- The mechanism of injury is a direct impact of the semilunar notch or coronoid process of the olecranon. Either of these structures can wedge into the trochlea, causing a split in the condyles.
- This most frequently occurs with a fall of the flexed elbow.

## NATURAL HISTORY

- The natural history of this fracture without anatomic restoration is characterized by stiffness, varus malunion, and chronic elbow dysfunction.

## PATIENT HISTORY AND PHYSICAL FINDINGS

- Mechanism of injury is important to obtain, higher energy injuries suggest an increased risk for compartment syndrome
- A careful neurovascular examination should be performed, with particular attention to the median, ulnar, and radial nerves.
- The limb should be inspected for open wounds. High-energy T-condylar fractures are often open injuries.

## IMAGING AND OTHER DIAGNOSTIC STUDIES

- Quality anteroposterior (AP) internal and external oblique views can be useful if the diagnosis is in question.
- Traction views can often be useful in fractures where shortening is present, although children and adolescents will often tolerate these poorly.
- Computed tomography (CT) can be useful, but the coronal and sagittal reconstructions must be rendered in the plane of the joint or perpendicular to it (normal AP and lateral planes); otherwise, the information obtained will be difficult to interpret.
- Coronal fragments may be missed if high-quality imaging is not obtained (see **FIG 3A**).

## DIFFERENTIAL DIAGNOSIS

- T-condylar fractures must be differentiated from other fractures of the distal humerus in children and adolescents because the treatment will differ.
- High-quality radiographs are generally sufficient to make this diagnosis.
- A CT or traction views can be helpful if the diagnosis is in question or if a coronal shear fragment is suspected on plain radiographs.

## NONOPERATIVE MANAGEMENT

- Initial management includes a well-padded splint following adequate physical examination.
- If the injury is open, an intravenous (IV) first-generation cephalosporin should be administered as soon as the injury is identified. If there is excessive contamination, comminution, or soft tissue injury, IV gentamicin is also recommended.
- There is limited value in nonsurgical management with the exception of patients with nonfunctional upper limbs at baseline.

## SURGICAL MANAGEMENT

- Open injuries should be addressed surgically within 24 hours; closed injuries may be addressed semielectively.
- Attention is given to the distal radius; "floating elbows," in which both the distal humerus and distal radius and/or ulna are affected, are not uncommon. These injuries should be identified early, as they are at increased risk for compartment syndrome.
- The soft tissue envelope is an important consideration. Fracture blisters (see **FIG 3B**) can be present, which can compromise the sterility and the closure of the procedure.
- The vast majority of T-condylar humerus fractures require operative treatment.
- In younger children, a percutaneous or mini-open approach may be possible.
- In older children and adolescents, an open posterior approach offers direct visualization and anatomic reduction and fixation of fracture fragments.

### Preoperative Planning

- High-quality AP and lateral radiographs are mandatory prior to surgery.
- Internal and external oblique views may be useful in identifying columnar comminution.
- CT scan can be useful in identifying coronal shear fragments.
- Method of fixation should be chosen by patient age, degree of displacement, and amount of comminution.
  - Specialized distal humeral plating systems are available from several different manufacturers to allow either bicolumn or "90:90" plating.

### Positioning

- We prefer positioning in a lateral position.
- The patient is intubated supine and then flipped to a lateral position over a beanbag.
- The bony prominences of the lateral malleolus and fibular head are carefully padded. A pillow is placed between the legs.
- The beanbag is inflated holding the patient in lateral decubitus, and an axillary roll is placed.

A

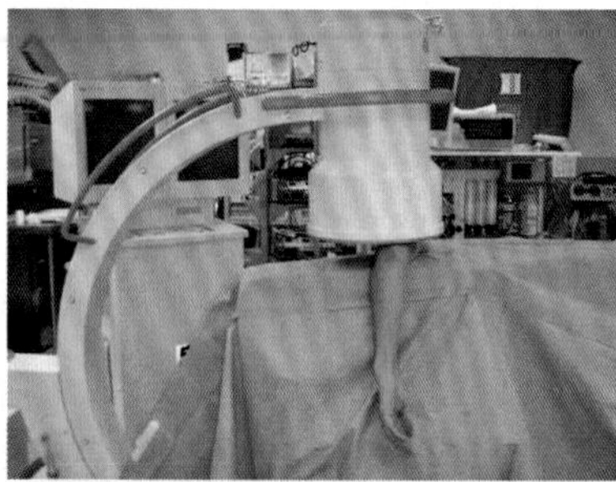

B

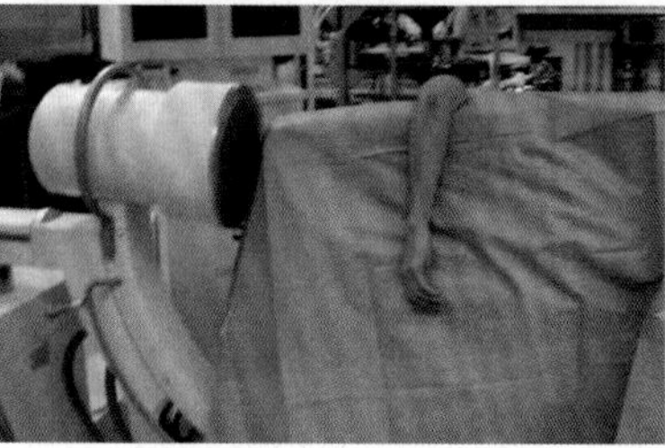

**FIG 5 • A,B.** Patient positioning for distal humerus fractures. (Courtesy of Samir Mehta, MD.)

- The contralateral arm is flexed at the shoulder and elbow to 90 degrees and placed on an arm board that is rotated so it is flush with the bed. This arm is then secured to the arm board.
- The operative arm is laid over a radiolucent arm board or paint roller so that the elbow is flexed 90 degrees (**FIG 5**).
- C-arm is brought in to assure that AP and lateral x-rays are adequate.
- The arm is then prepped and draped sterilely.
- A sterile tourniquet is used if one is desired.
- A "brain bag" is placed under the arm to be used to catch any blood or irrigant that comes from the field.
- The Bovie and suction are also placed in this bag for use.

### Approach

- As described in the following text. A posterior incision is used.

TECHNIQUES

## Exposure

- In highly comminuted fractures, an olecranon osteotomy is recommended for full joint visualization and reduction of comminuted pieces.
- A long posterior midline incision is used, the skin incision curves medially around the olecranon and then proceeds along the posterior border of the ulna. The incision is around 7 cm distal to the olecranon and 9 cm proximal as originally described.
- Then the dissection is carried deeply until the fascia is identified.

## Morrey Slide

- The fascia is then divided and the ulnar nerve identified proximally in the perineural fat adjacent to the medial head of the triceps. The ulnar nerve is then dissected free of the cubital tunnel and traced back distally to its first motor branch.
- After identification of the ulnar nerve, the superficial fascia of the forearm is incised to the distal extent of the incision. The periosteum of the medial ulna is incised 6 cm below the tip of the olecranon (**TECH FIG 1A**).
- The periosteum and fascia are preserved together as a unit and reflected in a subperiosteal fashion off the bone (**TECH FIG 1B**).
- At the insertion of the triceps, Sharpey fibers connect the triceps to the olecranon (**TECH FIG 1C**). A modification of the Morrey technique exists in which a small wafer of bone is detached with

the periosteal sleeve at this point in order to have bone-to-bone healing and not to risk disconnecting the tendon altogether (**TECH FIG 1D**).

- If the bone wafer technique is not employed, the arm should be extended to 20 to 30 degrees to relieve tension and allow safe release of the entire triceps mechanism with the periosteal sleeve.
- Following release of the triceps, the remainder of the periosteum/fascial sleeve is slid laterally.
- This allows for visualization of the elbow joint. If access to the radial head is desired for capitellar comminution, the anconeus can be elevated off of the lateral ulna. The tip of the olecranon can also be excised if joint exposure is insufficient (**TECH FIG 1E**).

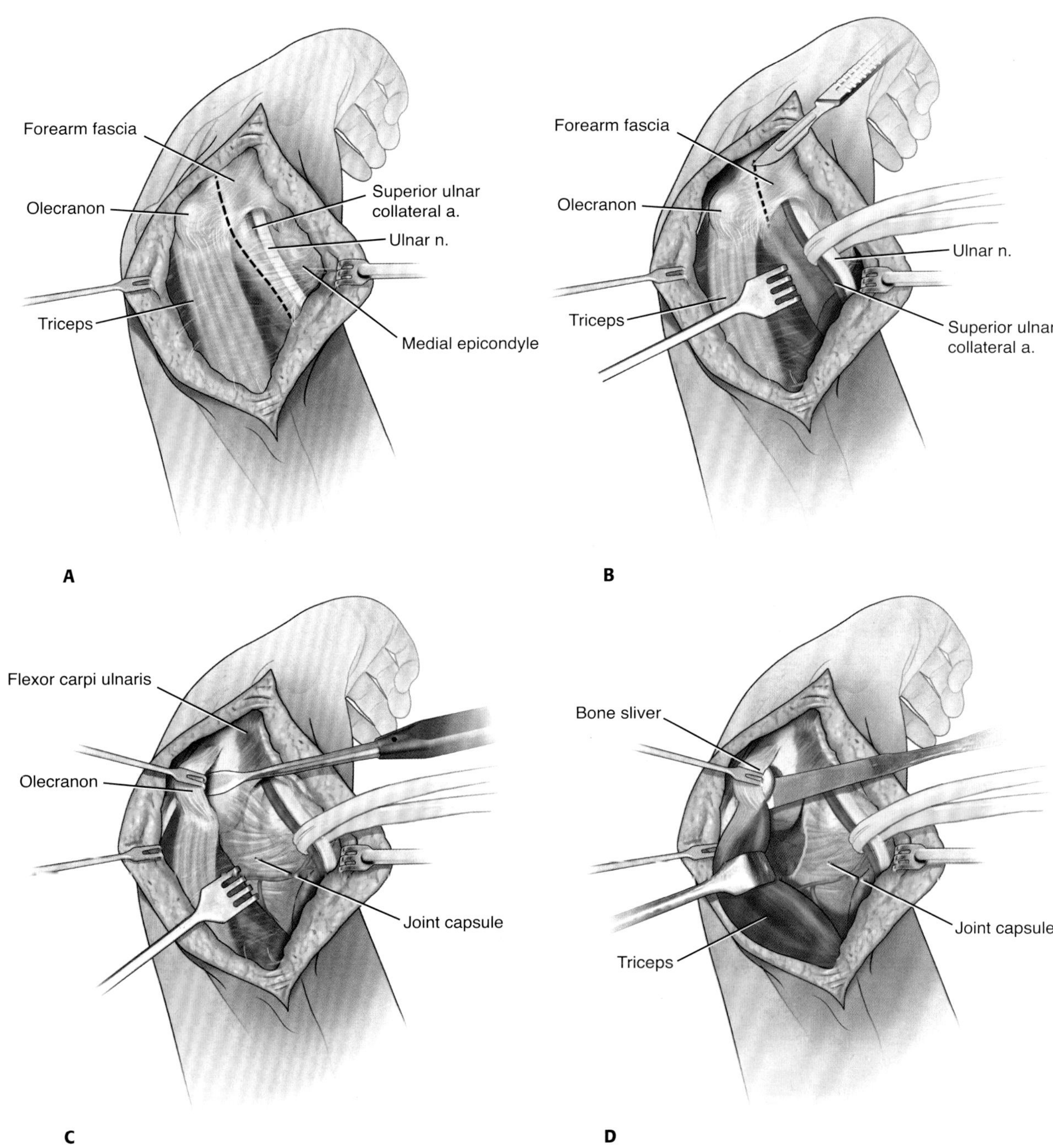


**TECH FIG 1** • **A.** Superficial exposure. **B.** Elevation of the triceps off of the ulna. **C.** Medial periosteal flap being created. **D.** Morrey slide technique with bone wafer modification. *(continued)*

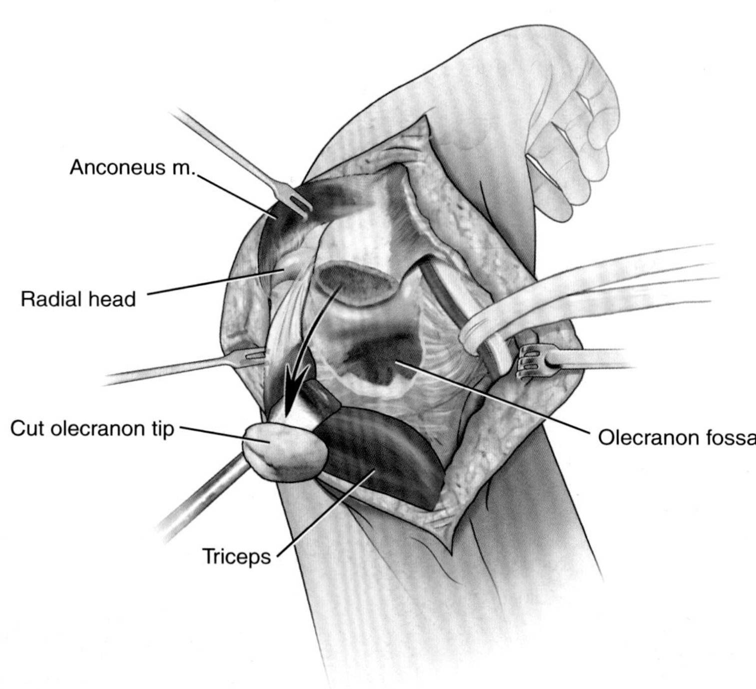


**TECH FIG 1** • *(continued)* **E.** The tip of the olecranon can be resected if more joint visualization is required. Additionally, the anconeus can be subperiosteally reflected if access to the radial head is necessary in the case of a coronal capitellar split. (Adapted from Bryan RS, Morrey BF. Extensive posterior exposure of the elbow: a triceps-sparing approach. Clin Orthop Relat Res 1982;[166]:188–192.)

## Reduction and Fixation

- Articular reduction must be accomplished first. In adolescent T-condylar fractures, there tend to be three large fragments, the medial condyle, the lateral condyle, and the shaft. Occasionally, coronal splits or comminution exist. These will occasionally necessitate an olecranon osteotomy approach.
- The condyles tend to be rotated toward each other in the axial plane toward the midline (**TECH FIG 2A**). A large reduction clamp can be placed on each epicondyle and used to reduce and compress the condyles. The condyles are then provisionally fixed with Kirschner wires.
- If comminution exists, generally the joint is provisionally reconstructed in an anterior to posterior direction.[4]
- The shaft is then reduced to the now intact and provisionally fixed joint. The joint is generally flexed and anteriorly translated with respect to the shaft. The distal arm is translated posteriorly and the elbow flexed and extended until an anatomic reduction is obtained.
- A 5/64 or 7/32 Kirschner wires are then placed in a cross-pin configuration in such a way that they are out of the way of the final fixation (usually dual plates in adolescents). When the provisional fixation is in place, a medial and lateral plate are selected that are most appropriate for the patient's bone.
- Of note, 2.7-mm precontoured plates are now available from various vendors that allow for the smaller sizes needed in pediatric-sized elbows.
- The plates are provisionally fixed on the bone in one of the distal screw holes (traditionally hole 2 from distal to proximal). A proximal screw is then placed in the slotted hole of the more proximal portion of the plate but not fully tightened (**TECH FIG 2B**).
- Fluoroscopic shots are obtained at this point to assure that the provisional reduction is adequate.
- A large bone clamp is then used to compress the bone between the plates (ie, placed from the medial to the lateral plate).
- Two distal screws (one medial and one lateral) are then placed using the locking towers. These screws should engage the opposite column of bone.[4]
- Following this, the proximal screws are placed with the condyles in compression with a large clamp (**TECH FIG 2C,D**).
- The remaining distal locking screws are then placed.
- Final intraoperative image intensifier shots are then obtained after provisional fixation is removed.

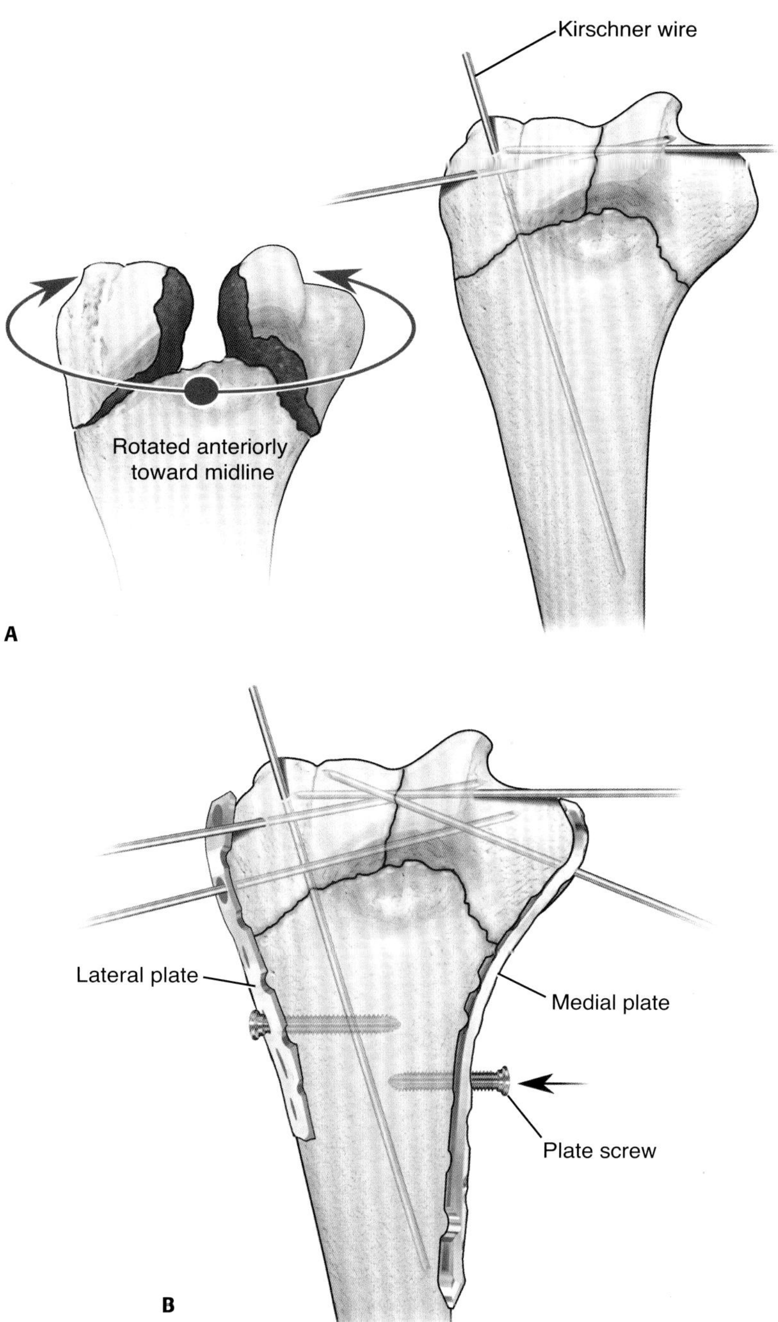


**TECH FIG 2** • **A.** Fragments tend to be rotated anteriorly toward the midline. **B.** Plates are provisionally held on with Kirschner wires and shaft screws. *(continued)*

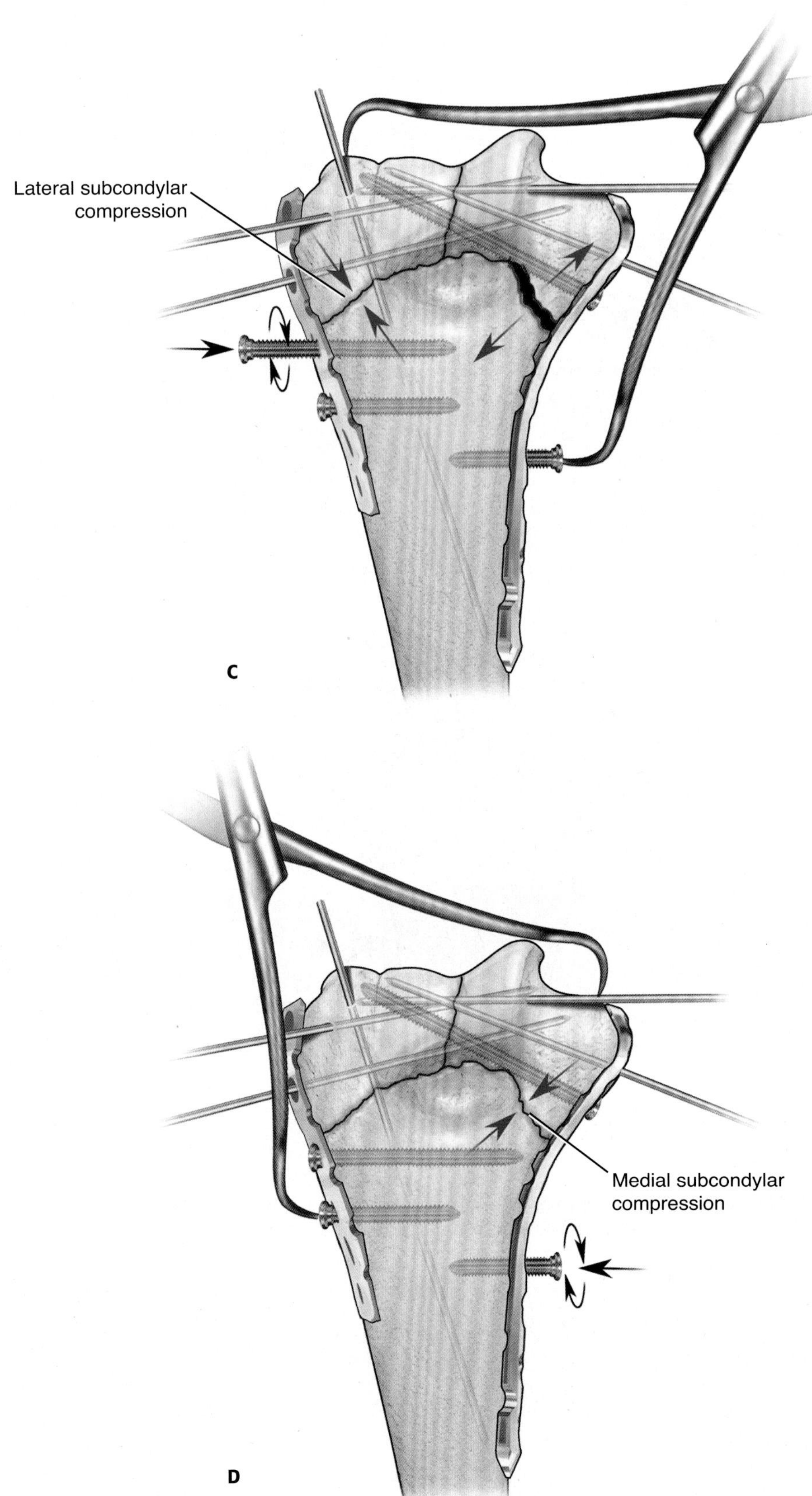


**TECH FIG 2** • *(continued)* Supracondylar compression is accomplished first laterally (**C**) then medially (**D**). (Adapted from O'Driscoll SW. Green's Operative Hand Surgery, ed 4. New York: Churchill Livingstone, 1999:339.)

## Closure

- The surgical field is carefully irrigated with 3 L of normal saline solution.
- If the bone wafer technique is used, the wafer is replaced anatomically using heavy, transosseous nonabsorbable suture. If the elevation is used, the triceps is repaired to the bone through transosseous sutures (**TECH FIG 3**).
- The ulnar nerve is not routinely transposed unless there appears to be pressure on the nerve from the plate.
- The fascia/periosteum layer is carefully repaired to itself using heavy Vicryl suture.
- A 10F Jackson-Pratt drain is routinely placed.
- A subcutaneous loose closure of 2-0 Vicryl is then used.
- Last, the skin is closed with simple nylon stitches if the closure appears to be complex or if it is simple and loose, absorbable monofilament simple stitches may be placed, although the patient should be advised that they take several months to reabsorb and fall off.

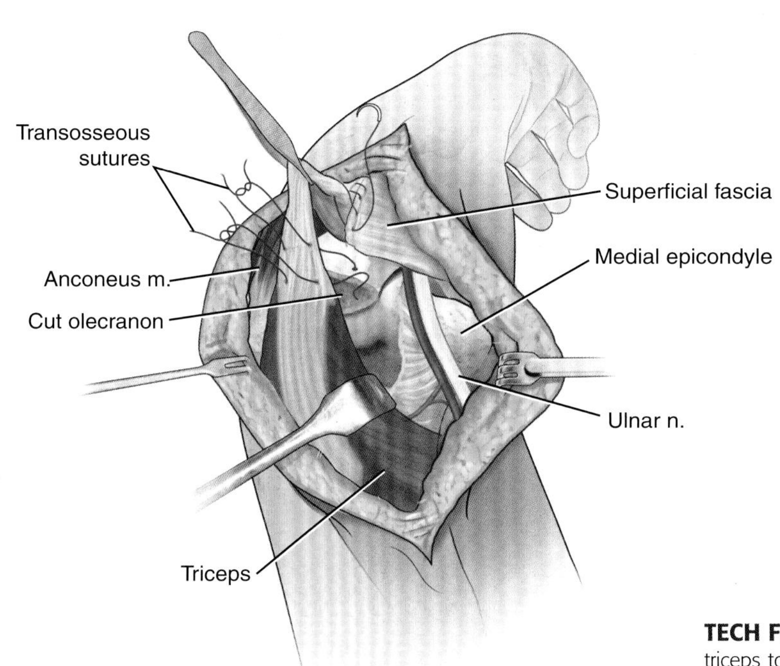


**TECH FIG 3** • Transosseous sutures are used to repair the triceps to the olecranon. The defect in the fascia/periosteum unit is then repaired. (Adapted from Bryan RS, Morrey BF. Extensive posterior exposure of the elbow: a triceps-sparing approach. Clin Orthop Relat Res 1982;[166]:188–192.)

## PEARLS AND PITFALLS

| | |
|---|---|
| **Visualizing the fracture** | ■ The C-arm should be brought in prior to draping to assure that adequate imaging can be obtained intraoperatively. A radiolucent arm board is quite helpful in this regard. |
| **Preoperative planning** | ■ A CT scan or traction x-rays can be helpful preoperatively to assess the degree of comminution or presence of coronal split fracture lines which could impede reduction at the time of surgery. |
| **Obtaining the reduction** | ■ The articular block should be reconstructed first; in adolescents, there is generally less comminution than in adults, so this block can generally be reconstructed into one large fragment. After this fragment is reduced, the articular block can be reduced to the shaft segment. |
| **Preventing stiffness** | ■ The goal of surgery is to provide a stable enough construct that immediate motion or, at the very least, motion within 3 weeks is possible. Often, adolescents are nonadherent to self-therapy regimens, and frequent follow-up is necessary to prevent elbow stiffness or need for arthrolysis. Consider a continuous passive motion (CPM) postoperatively. Patients should be advised that usually 10 degrees of extension loss can be expected. |
| **Closure** | ■ Closure with staples or nylon stitches is advised; remove every other day at 10–14 days. These will allow for wound care with early motion. |
| **Follow-up** | ■ Follow-up once a week for 4–6 weeks for motion checks. Multiple x-rays are unnecessary, but monitoring the early motion is essential. |

## POSTOPERATIVE CARE

- A well-padded posterior splint in about 70 degrees of flexion is placed, and a sling applied.
- The patient is kept in house for 24 to 48 hours; the drain is pulled when less than 20 mL of drainage per shift is recorded.
- In open fractures, antibiotics are given for 48 hours. In closed fractures, antibiotics are stopped after 24 hours.
- Patients are sent home in a posterior splint which is removed five times a day for active and active-assisted range of motion (30 repetitions each session). They may also shower at this point.
- The patient is seen back in 2 weeks for a wound check.
- At 6 weeks, all immobilization is removed, and the patient is started on home low load prolonged stretching exercises and formal physical therapy.
- No gym or sports are allowed for 3 months or until the maximum range of motion (or full range of motion) has occurred and physical therapy has cleared the patient for activity.

## OUTCOMES

- Re et al[6] reported a series of T-condylar humerus fractures in children and adolescents and reported that the Bernard Morrey approach resulted in significantly better motion than the more traditional triceps-splitting approach. This group also reported that early motion resulted in better final flexion and earlier functional range of motion than when range of motion was delayed.
- Beck et al[1] reported on 26 children and adolescents who had T-condylar fractures who were operatively treated. Approximately, one-third had elbow stiffness at final follow-up. Early range of motion resulted in earlier return to motion.

## COMPLICATIONS

- Stiffness is quite common in T-condylar humerus fractures; preventing stiffness can be achieved by adequate stabilization to allow early motion.
- Symptomatic hardware is common; in adolescents, we do not routinely remove hardware unless the patient complains of it.
- Infection is more common in open injuries but still quite rare.
- Nerve injuries are generally neurapraxias and resolve spontaneously in 3 to 6 months.

## REFERENCES

1. Beck NA, Ganley TJ, McKay S, et al. T-condylar fractures of the distal humerus in children: does early motion affect final range of motion? J Child Orthop 2014;8:161–165.
2. Bonczar MR, Rikli D, Ring D. Distal humerus 13-C1 Open reduction; perpendicular (biplanar) plating. AO Foundation Web site. Available at: http://bit.ly/1wEegQS. Published June 21, 2007. Accessed November 11, 2013.
3. Bryan RS, Morrey BF. Extensive posterior exposure of the elbow. A triceps-sparing approach. Clin Orthop Relat Res 1982;(166):188–192.
4. Green DP, Hotchkiss RN, Pederson WC; Dr. D. Sergeant Pepper Memorial Fund. Green's Operative Hand Surgery, ed 4. New York: Churchill Livingstone, 1999.
5. Maylahn DJ, Fahey JJ. Fractures of the elbow in children: review of three hundred consecutive cases. J Am Med Assoc 1958;166:220–228.
6. Re PR, Waters PM, Hresko T. T-condylar fractures of the distal humerus in children and adolescents. J Pediatr Orthop 1999;19:313–318.

# Open Reduction and Internal Fixation of Capitellum and Capitellar–Trochlear Shear Fractures

14 CHAPTER

Asif M. Ilyas, Michael Rivlin, and Jesse B. Jupiter

## DEFINITION

- Capitellar fractures are uncommon, accounting for less than 1% of all elbow fractures and 6% of all distal humerus fractures.[4]
- They often are associated with radial head fractures and posterior elbow dislocations.
- A classification system for capitellar fractures has been proposed by Bryan and Morrey[4] and modified by McKee:
  - Type 1: complete fractures of the capitellum[14]
  - Type 2: superficial subchondral fractures of the capitellar articular surface[29]
  - Type 3: comminuted fractures[2]
  - Type 4: coronal shear fractures that include a portion of the trochlea as well as the capitellum as one piece[21] (**FIG 1**)
- Ring et al[25] have proposed a new classification, expanding on the growing understanding that isolated capitellum fractures are rare and often are involved as part of articular shear fractures of the distal humerus. The classification includes five anatomic components, with type 1 articular injuries encompassing the capitellum and capitellar–trochlear shear patterns (**FIG 2**):
  - Type 1: capitellum and lateral aspect of the trochlea
  - Type 2: lateral epicondyle
  - Type 3: posterior aspect of the lateral column
  - Type 4: posterior aspect of the trochlea
  - Type 5: medial epicondyle
- More recently, Dubberley and colleagues[8] introduced a classification system based on radiographic pattern of injury taking posterior comminution into account.
  - Type 1: fracture of the capitellum (with or without trochlear ridge involvement)
  - Type 2: capitellum and trochlea fracture that remain as one fragment
  - Type 3: capitellum and trochlea as separate fragments
  - Type A: no posterior condyle comminution
  - Type B: posterior condyle comminution present

## ANATOMY

- The two condyles of the distal humerus diverge from the humeral shaft to form the lateral and medial columns, which support the trochlea between them. The anterior aspect of the lateral column is covered with articular cartilage, forming the capitellum. Distally, these two condyles can be visualized as forming a triangle at the end of the humerus.
- The capitellum is the first epiphyseal center of the elbow to ossify

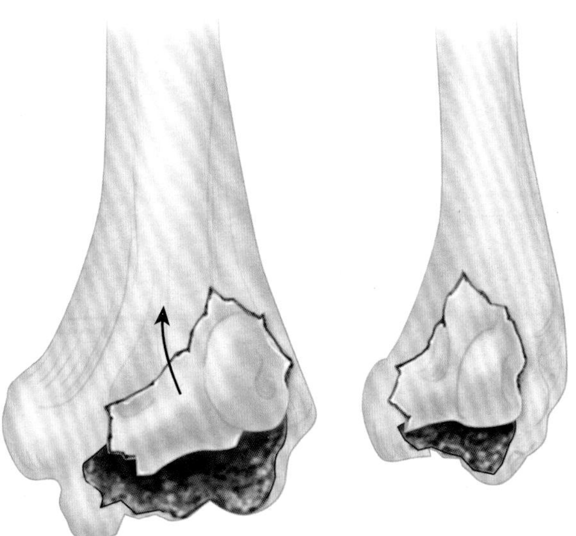

**FIG 1** • Type 4 coronal shear fractures of the distal humerus. (Adapted from McKee MD, Jupiter JB, Bamberger HB, et al. Coronal shear fractures of the distal end of the humerus. J Bone Joint Surg Am 1996;78[1]:49–54.)

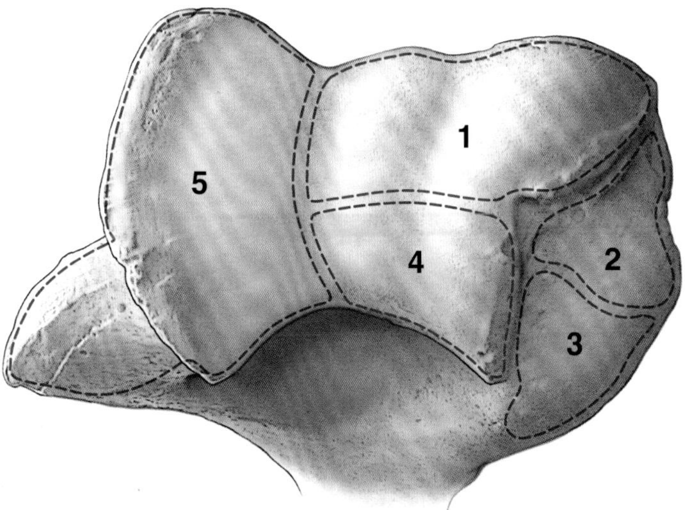


**FIG 2** • Articular fractures of the distal part of the humerus, including type 1 fractures that encompass capitellum and capitellar–trochlear shear fractures. (Adapted from Ring D, Jupiter JB, Gulotta L. Articular fractures of the distal part of the humerus. J Bone Joint Surg Am 2003;85-A[2]:232–238.)

- It is covered by articular surface anteriorly but devoid of it posteriorly.
- The capitellum is directed distally and anteriorly at an angle of 30 degrees to the long axis of the humerus.
- The radial head rotates on the anterior surface of the capitellum in elbow flexion and articulates with its inferior surface in elbow extension.
- The lateral collateral ligament inserts next to the lateral margin of the capitellum.
- The blood supply of the capitellum is derived posteriorly. It arises from the lateral arcade, which is the anastomosis of the radial collateral arteries of the profunda brachii and the radial recurrent artery.[30]

## PATHOGENESIS

- Capitellum and capitellar–trochlear shear fractures involve impaction of the radial head against the lateral column of the distal humerus in a partially extended position, resulting in shearing of the articular cartilage of the distal humerus.
- Fracture fragments vary in size and displace superiorly and anteriorly into the radial fossa, resulting in impingement with elbow flexion.
- Associated injuries include proximal and distal radial as well as carpal fractures; ligamentous injuries include collateral ligament (lateral more common than medial) and triceps ruptures.[8]

## NATURAL HISTORY

- Capitellar fractures occur almost exclusively in adults. These fractures do not occur in children because in that age group, the capitellum is largely cartilaginous, and a similar mechanism of injury would instead cause a supracondylar or lateral condyle fracture.
- Capitellar fractures are more common in females, a finding that can be attributed to the increased carrying angle of the female elbow.
- Displaced fractures that go untreated can be expected to have a poor outcome owing to the progressive loss of motion from the mechanical block to flexion, potential longitudinal instability of the forearm, and the likely development of subsequent posttraumatic arthrosis from the residual articular incongruity.
- Capitellar and trochlear fractures are prone to nonunion if multiple articular fragments are present or the posterior column is involved.[3]

## PATIENT HISTORY AND PHYSICAL FINDINGS

- Symptoms of capitellar fractures are similar to those of radial head fractures, including pain and swelling along the lateral elbow and pain with elbow motion.
- Although there may be variable loss of forearm rotation, loss of flexion and extension is most common, often accompanied by crepitus and pain.
- The association of concomitant radial head fractures and ligamentous injuries with capitellar fractures is high.[22]
- The shoulder and wrist should also be examined for concomitant injury.

## IMAGING AND OTHER DIAGNOSTIC STUDIES

- Standard radiographs are often inadequate for accurate assessment of capitellar fractures.
- Lateral radiographs are best for obtaining an initial evaluation of capitellar fractures.
- Anteroposterior views do not reliably show the fracture because the outline of the distal humerus is not consistently affected.
- The radial head–capitellum view can help identify fractures of the capitellum. This view is a lateral oblique projection taken with the x-ray beam pointing 45 degrees dorsoventrally, thereby eliminating the ulno- and radiohumeral articulation shadows.[13]
  - A type 1 fracture appears as a semilunar fragment sitting superiorly with its articular surface pointing up and away from the radial head in most cases.
  - Type 2 fractures are more difficult to diagnose, depending on the amount of subchondral bone accompanying the articular fragment. They may appear as a loose body lying in the superior part of the joint.
  - Type 3 fractures display variable amounts of comminution.
  - Coronal shear fractures show a characteristic "double arc" sign on lateral radiographic views (**FIG 3A**).
- Computed tomography (CT) scans can provide excellent characterization of the fracture, and we subsequently recommend routine use of it for preoperative planning.
  - CT scanning of the elbow should be done at 1- to 2-mm intervals using axial or transverse cuts.

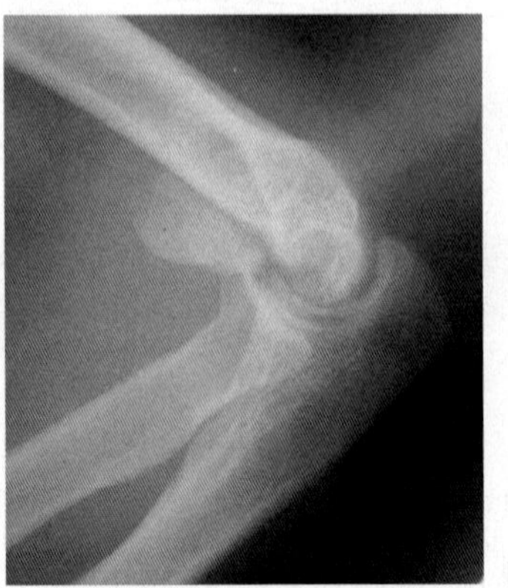
A

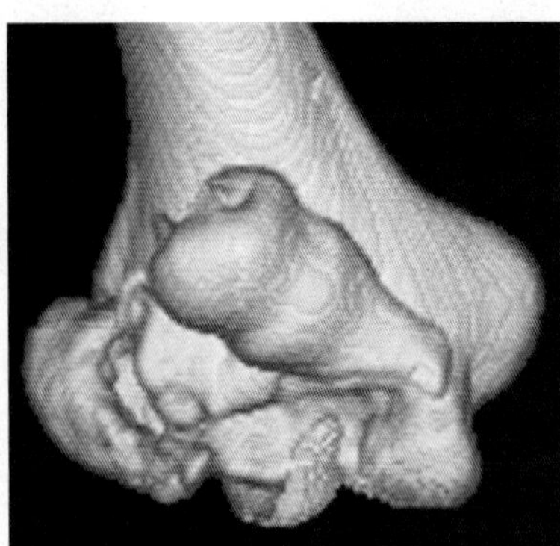
B

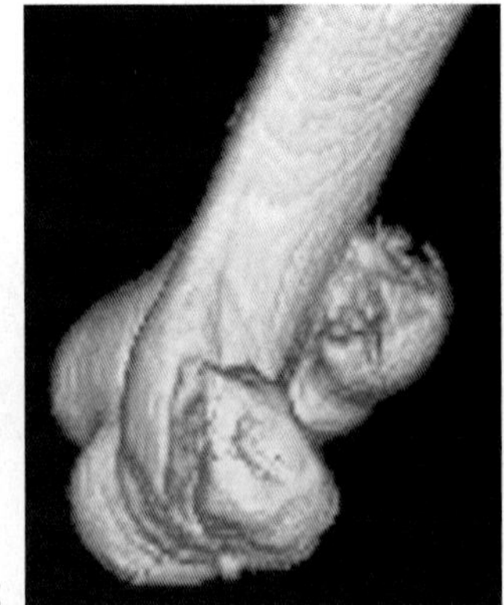
C

**FIG 3** • **A.** Characteristic double arc sign on lateral radiographs of coronal shear fractures. **B,C.** 3-D CT reconstructions of a coronal shear fracture of the distal humerus.

- Three-dimensional (3-D) CT reconstructions provide the best detail and ability to appreciate the anatomic orientation of the fracture patterns and should be considered if 3-D imaging is available (**FIG 3B,C**).

## DIFFERENTIAL DIAGNOSIS

- Radial head fracture
- Distal humeral lateral condyle fracture
- Elbow dislocation

## NONOPERATIVE MANAGEMENT

- We recommend operative management for capitellum and capitellar–trochlear shear fractures.
- Truly nondisplaced and isolated capitellum fractures can be splinted for 3 weeks, followed by protected motion. However, close supervision is required, as this fracture is inherently unstable and prone to displacement.
- Closed reduction techniques, which have been described in the literature, should be performed with caution, and only complete anatomic reduction should be accepted for nonoperative management.[5,23]
- Capitellar–trochlear shear fractures should not be treated nonoperatively because of their inherent instability and the expectant loss of motion and posttraumatic arthrosis from residual articular incongruity.

## SURGICAL MANAGEMENT

- The short-term goal of surgery is anatomic reduction and stable fixation of the fracture to allow for early motion without mechanical block.
- The long-term goals of surgery are a pain-free elbow with maximal motion, minimal stiffness, and avoidance of posttraumatic arthrosis.
- Capitellar fractures are uncommon, and the wide array of treatment options presented in the literature is based on relatively small series.
  - Treatment options include closed reduction,[5,23] open excision,[1,10,20] open reduction and internal fixation (ORIF), and arthroplasty.[6,11]
- With the improvement in techniques for fixation of small fragments and management of articular surfaces, ORIF has become the mainstay of treatment.
  - Advantages of ORIF include restoration of the native anatomy and function.
  - Disadvantages include stiffness and possible failure of fixation.
- In elderly patients, we do consider total elbow arthroplasty for complex intra-articular distal humerus fractures.[15,17]
  - Advantages include early return to function and motion.
  - Disadvantages include functional limitations.

### Preoperative Planning

- Before proceeding with surgery, a thorough understanding of the fracture and its orientation should be obtained with the help of a CT scan, and if possible, 3-D reconstructions.
- The timing of surgery is important. Fractures preferably should be approached within 2 weeks, before osseous healing sets in, but after swelling has diminished.
- Ensure that the necessary implants and hardware are available.
- Reduction and fixation of the fracture will require minimum K wires, articular or headless screws, and small fragment AO screws.
- Additional implants to consider include lateral column periarticular locking plates.
- An image intensifier should be used during surgery to confirm reduction of the fracture and proper positioning of implanted hardware.

### Positioning

- General anesthesia is recommended for maximum soft tissue relaxation.
- The patient usually is positioned supine on the operating table, with the arm extended onto a radiolucent hand table, facilitating the lateral approach.
- Alternatively, a lateral or prone position can be considered, with the anterior surface of the elbow supported by a padded bolster if a posterior approach is planned.

### Approach

- Either a lateral or posterior midline incision should be used.
- A lateral incision allows for direct visualization to a lateral approach to the elbow.
- A posterior incision also allows for access to the lateral approach to the elbow but also facilitates access to the posterior and medial approaches to the elbow, if necessary.
- Multiple intervals can be used in the lateral approach to the elbow, including the Kocher, Hotchkiss, and Wagner approaches.
  - We advocate the Wagner approach, which uses the interval between the extensor carpi radialis longus (ECRL) and the extensor digitorum communis (EDC), as it provides ready access to the anterolateral aspect of the radiocapitellar joint while protecting the insertion of the lateral collateral ligament complex.
  - To increase exposure, the lateral collateral ligament complex can be raised posteriorly sharply with a scalpel or osteotomized with a wedge of lateral epicondyle for subsequent suture anchor repair or internal fixation, respectively.
- Alternatively, the Kocher approach, which uses the interval between the extensor carpi ulnaris (ECU) and the anconeus can provide access to the capitellum while affording greater protection of the posterior interosseous nerve.
- In many cases, a capsular violation has occurred. This can be exploited and used as the interval to expose the fracture, thereby avoiding the need to cause an additional soft tissue defect.

## Capitellar Fractures

### Exposure

- The incision should begin 2 cm proximal to the lateral epicondyle and extend 3 to 4 cm distally toward the radial neck.
- If no large soft tissue or capsular defect is present, a direct lateral Wagner approach between the ECRL and EDC interval is recommended.
- The remaining common extensor origin is sharply raised off the lateral epicondyle and reflected anteriorly to expose the anterolateral elbow joint.
    - The capitellar fracture will most likely be found displaced anteriorly and proximally.
    - Care must be taken to avoid excessive proximal dissection and injury to the radial nerve traveling between the brachialis and brachioradialis.
    - Care must also be taken to avoid excessive distal dissection and injury to the posterior interosseous nerve by limiting dissection to only the radial neck. In addition, the forearm should be kept pronated, and no retractors should be placed anteriorly around the radial neck.
- Often, the lateral ligamentous complex will be avulsed from the distal aspect of the humerus, with or without some aspect of the lateral epicondyle.
    - This ligamentous violation can be exploited to improve exposure by hinging open the joint on the medial collateral ligament with a varus stress.
- The capitellar fracture fragment will typically be displaced anteriorly and proximally (**TECH FIG 1**).
- The fracture fragment will also typically be devoid of any soft tissue attachments and therefore prone to displacing out of the joint with excessive manipulation. Hence, care must be taken to avoid losing the fragment off the surgical field.

### Reduction and Fixation

- The fragment is reduced under direct visualization, held with reduction tenaculums, and provisionally fixed with 0.045-inch K-wires. Alternatively, the guidewires that will be used for cannulated screw fixation can be used for provisional fixation as well.
- Internal fixation options include fixation with (1) headless compression screws from either an anterior or posterior direction, (2) cancellous screws from a posterior direction, (3) posterolateral column locking plate fixation, or (4) a hybrid construct using any or all of these techniques.
- Headless compression screws allow for guidewire-directed placement, direct fracture reduction, and maximal compression of the fracture fragment. Similarly, headless compression screws may be particularly useful in cases with fragments with less subchondral bone, such as type 2 and small type 1 fracture fragments (**TECH FIG 2A**). However, anterior screw placement can be challenging due to the thick anterior soft tissue envelope that will be present with an intact lateral collateral ligament complex. Alternatively, headless compression screws can be placed retrograde from a posterior direction to ease hardware placement (**TECH FIG 2B**). However, this direction does not achieve maximum fracture compression and can risk fracture distraction.
- Cancellous screws are best for fracture fragments with a large subchondral component as with type 1 fracture fragments. However, extending the dissection posteriorly around the lateral column

A
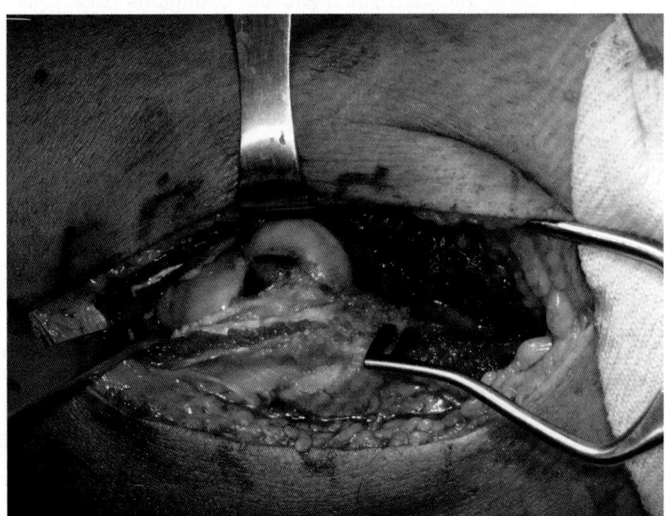

B
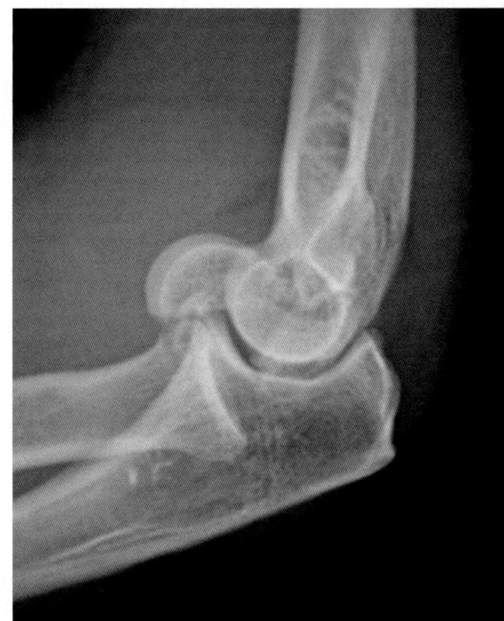

**TECH FIG 1** • **A,B.** The displaced capitellar fracture fragment will typically be displaced anteriorly and proximally and will be devoid of any soft tissue attachments.

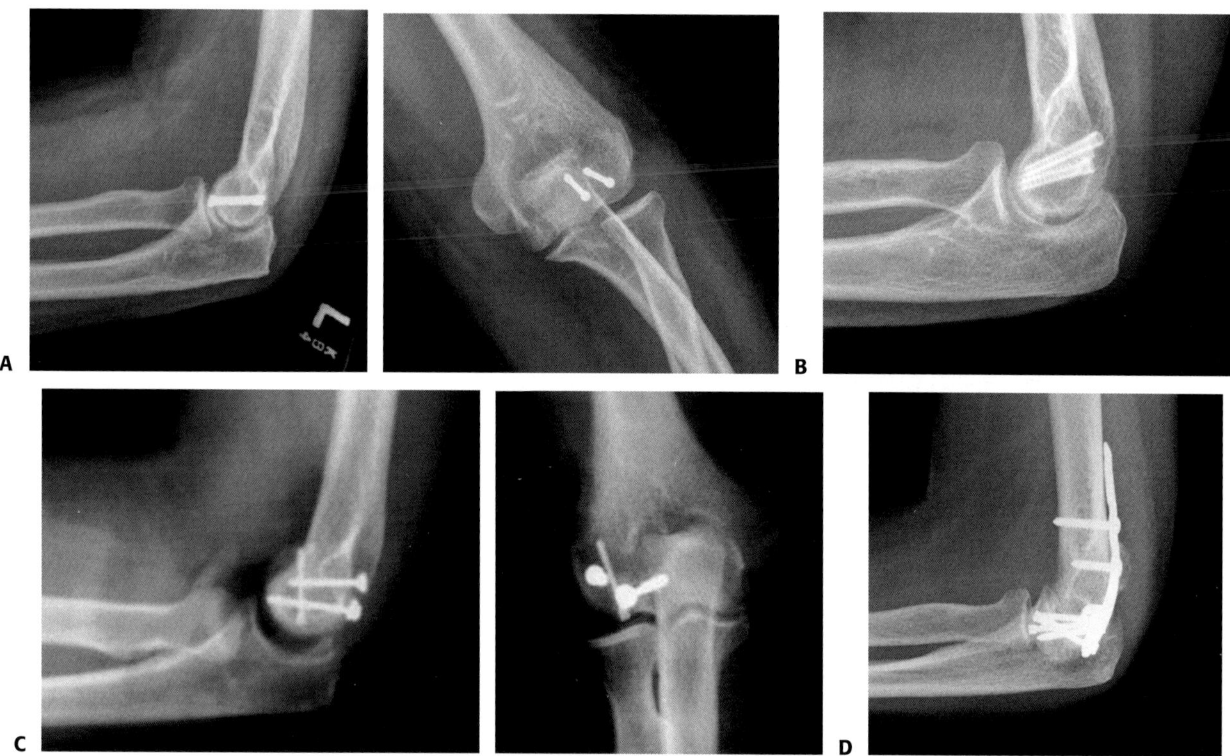

**TECH FIG 2** • Fixation of capitellar fractures with (**A**) anteriorly placed headless compression screws, (**B**) posteriorly placed headless compression screws, (**C**) combination of a headless screw anteriorly and cancellous screws posteriorly, and (**D**) hybrid fixation using anteriorly placed headless compression screws followed by neutralization of the fracture with a locked periarticular plate applied posteriorly.

theoretically increases the risk of osteonecrosis (**TECH FIG 2C**). We recommend using partially threaded cannulated screw to optimize fracture reduction, screw placement, and fracture compression.

- Use of a periarticular locking plate alone or in a hybrid construct with headless compression screws can be of value to improve the stability of the construct (**TECH FIG 2D**). This technique will require greater posterior dissection, therefore increasing the theoretical risk of osteonecrosis. However, application of a posterolateral plate can provide posterior stability in cases with posterior cortical extension or comminution.
- Excision of fracture fragments can be considered in type 2 fractures with small, thin articular pieces and type 3 comminuted fractures where the fragments are not amenable to internal fixation.
- Fragment reduction and hardware position should be confirmed by image intensifier.
- Unrestricted forearm rotation and elbow flexion–extension without mechanical block or catching should be confirmed intraoperatively.
- If the lateral collateral ligament complex is found to be avulsed, it should be repaired back to the lateral epicondyle with drill holes and heavy nonabsorbable sutures or suture anchors.
- The capsule should be closed.
- The retracted extensor origin should be relaxed and closed to the surrounding soft tissue.

## Capitellar–Trochlear Shear Fractures

### Exposure

- A posterior midline incision should be used, but initially, a lateral approach to the joint will be performed.
  - A posterior incision provides extensile exposure, access to both sides of the elbow, and ease of osteotomy, if necessary (**TECH FIG 3A**).
- A direct lateral Wagner approach between the ECRL and EDC interval is recommended.
- The remaining common extensor origin is sharply raised off the lateral epicondyle and reflected anteriorly to expose the anterolateral elbow joint. Alternatively, a capsular violation may be present that can be exploited (**TECH FIG 3B**).
- The capitellar–trochlear shear fracture will most likely be found displaced anteriorly and proximally.
  - Care must be taken to avoid excessive proximal dissection and injury to the radial nerve traveling between the brachialis and brachioradialis.
  - Care must also be taken to avoid excessive distal dissection and injury to the posterior interosseous nerve by limiting dissection to only the radial neck. In addition, the forearm should be kept pronated, and no retractors should be placed anteriorly around the radial neck.

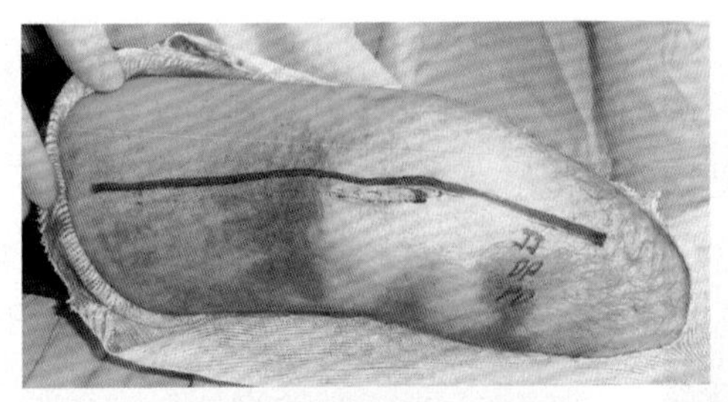

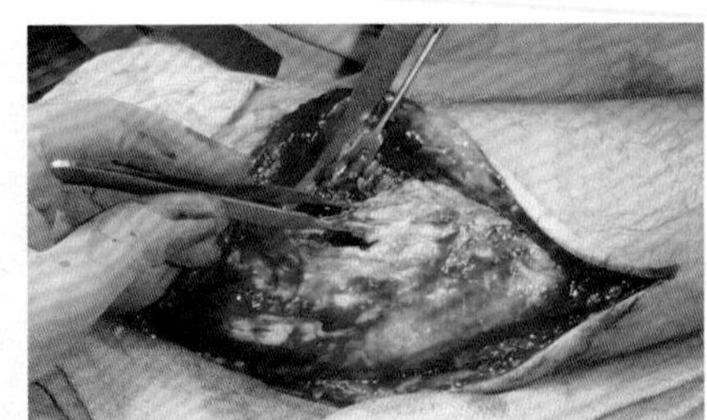

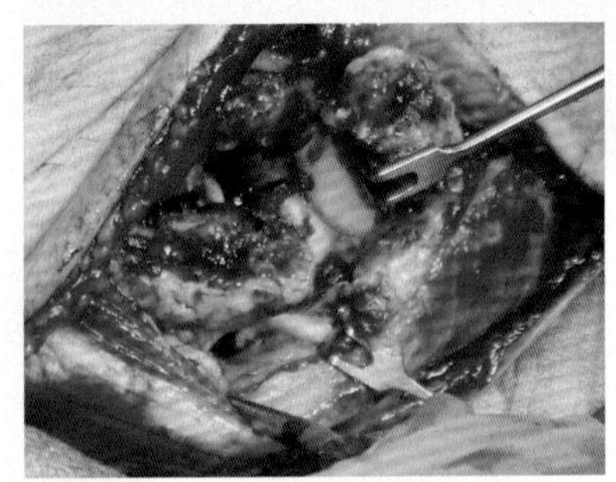

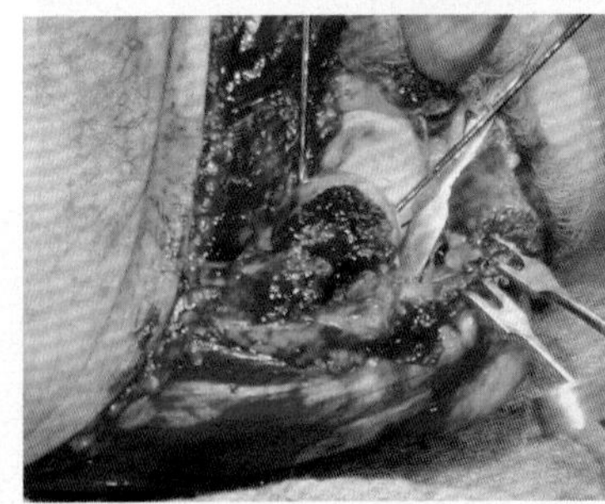

**TECH FIG 3** • **A.** Posterior midline incision used for capitellar–trochlear shear fractures. **B.** Deep lateral approach to the elbow using the capsular violation to enter the radiocapitellar joint. **C.** The fracture fragments tend to displace proximally and internally rotate. Note, avulsion of the lateral epicondyle with subsequent retraction allowing for excellent visualization. **D.** The fracture is reduced and provisionally pinned with 0.045-inch K-wires.

- Often, the lateral ligamentous complex will be avulsed from the distal aspect of the humerus, with or without some aspect of the lateral epicondyle.
  - This ligamentous violation can be exploited to improve exposure by hinging open the joint on the medial collateral ligament with a varus stress.
  - Alternatively, a formal lateral epicondyle osteotomy can be performed to enhance visualization while maintaining the integrity of the lateral ligamentous complex.
  - Additionally, a formal olecranon osteotomy may be performed to improve visualization and fixation of fractures extending medially and posteriorly.
- The fracture fragments should now be visualized and accounted for. They are most commonly displaced proximally and internally rotated (**TECH FIG 3C**).

## Reduction and Fixation

- The fragment is reduced under direct visualization, held with reduction tenaculums, and provisionally fixed with 0.045-inch K-wires (**TECH FIG 3D**).
- Inability to reduce the fracture anatomically may represent fracture impaction, requiring either disimpaction or bone grafting, or both.
- Internal fixation options include fixation with (1) headless compression screws from either an anterior or posterior direction, (2) cancellous screws from a posterior direction, (3) posterolateral column locking plate fixation, or (4) a hybrid construct using any or all of these techniques.
- Headless compression screws allow for guidewire-directed placement, direct fracture reduction, and maximal compression of the fracture fragment (**TECH FIG 4A**). Similarly, headless

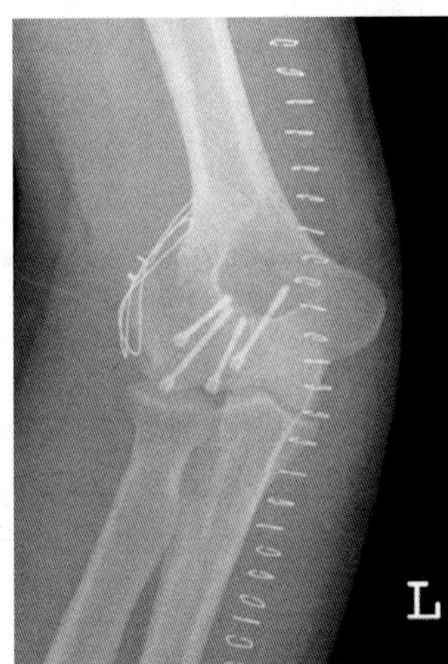


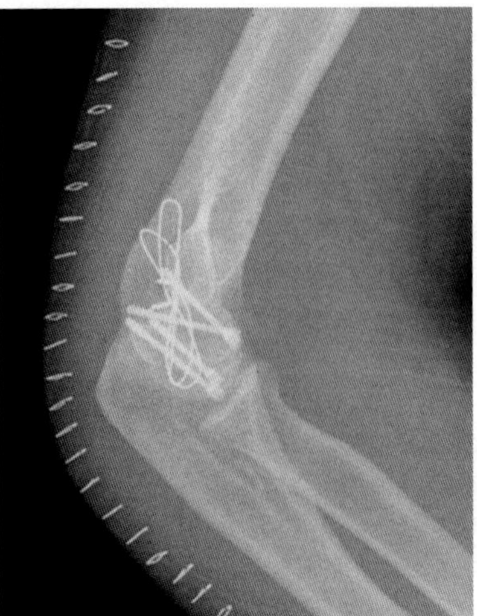

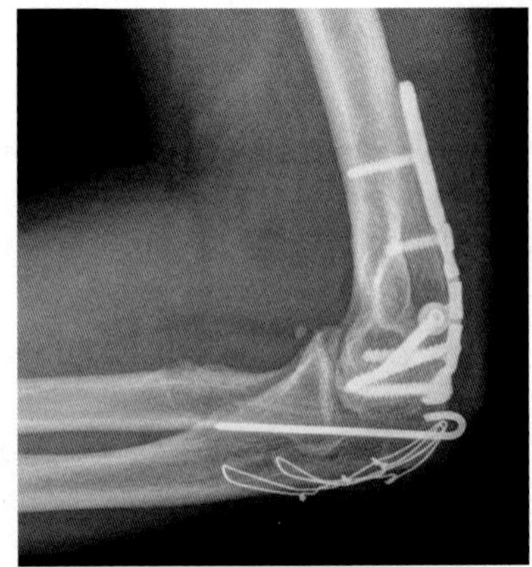

**TECH FIG 4** • Postoperative radiographs illustrating (**A**) repair of the lateral epicondyle and anterior fixation of a capitellar–trochlear shear fracture with multiple headless compression screws. Alternatively, (**B**) note repair of a different capitellar–trochlear shear fracture using a periarticular locking plate applied to the posterolateral aspect of the distal humerus, facilitated with an olecranon osteotomy.

compression screws may be particularly useful in cases with fragments with less subchondral bone, such as type 2 and small type 1 fracture fragments.

- Cancellous screws are best for fracture fragments with a large subchondral component as with type 1 fracture fragments. However, extending the dissection posteriorly around the lateral column theoretically increases the risk of osteonecrosis. We recommend using partially threaded cannulated screw to optimize fracture reduction, screw placement, and fracture compression.
- Use of a periarticular locking plate alone or in a hybrid construct with headless compression screws can be of value to improve the stability of the construct (**TECH FIG 4B**). This technique will require greater posterior dissection, therefore increasing the theoretical risk of osteonecrosis. However, application of a posterolateral plate can provide posterior stability in cases with posterior cortical extension or comminution.
- Fragment reduction and hardware position should be confirmed by image intensifier.
- Unrestricted forearm rotation and elbow flexion–extension without mechanical block or catching should be confirmed intraoperatively.
- The lateral epicondyle, if avulsed or osteotomized, should be repaired with a tension band technique or plate and screws.
- The capsule should be closed.
- The interval and released extensor origin should be relaxed and closed to the surrounding soft tissue.

## PEARLS AND PITFALLS

| | |
|---|---|
| **Diagnosis** | ▪ Diligence should be paid to identifying concomitant injuries such as elbow dislocations, radial head fractures, and ligamentous instability. |
| **Imaging** | ▪ Plain radiographs are insufficient, and a CT scan should be considered routinely.<br>▪ Order 3-D reconstructions if possible. |
| **Nonoperative management** | ▪ Nonoperative management should be chosen cautiously. Anatomic and stable reduction of the fracture is necessary. Otherwise, a painful elbow with restricted motion may result.<br>▪ We do not recommend nonoperative management of any capitellar–trochlear shear fractures. |
| **Surgical management** | ▪ Lateral epicondyle osteotomy can enhance exposure.<br>▪ A posterior skin incision will afford access to both sides of the joint and an olecranon osteotomy, if necessary.<br>▪ Inability to reduce the fracture anatomically may represent impaction of the lateral column and require disimpaction or bone grafting.<br>▪ Excision of small comminuted fragments that cannot be fixed internally is preferred over nonanatomic reduction and malunion.<br>▪ Concomitant fractures and ligamentous injuries should be treated simultaneously to optimize outcomes. |
| **Postoperative management** | ▪ Stable fixation should be sought to facilitate early motion.<br>▪ Heterotopic ossification is common after elbow fractures, and prophylaxis with nonsteroidal anti-inflammatory drugs should be considered. |

## POSTOPERATIVE CARE

- If secure fixation has been obtained, immediate mobilization can be initiated postoperatively.
- If fixation is tenuous, splint or cast the elbow for 3 to 4 weeks, followed by active and assisted range-of-motion exercises. Some advocate the use of hinged external fixator for complex articular fractures or with severe ligamentous injuries.[12]

## OUTCOMES

- Focusing initially on outcomes after ORIF of types 1 and 2 capitellar fractures, multiple small series have shown good results using Herbert screws in an anterior to posterior direction.[7,16,18,24]
- More recently, Mahirogullari et al[19] reported on 11 cases of type 1 capitellum fractures treated with Herbert screws, which yielded 8 excellent and 3 good results. They recommended fixation in a posterior to anterior direction with at least two Herbert screws.
- Reported outcomes on type 4 capitellar–trochlear shear fractures are limited. McKee et al[21] originally described this pattern and reported on 6 cases.
  - Each case involved an extended lateral Kocher approach and fixation with Herbert screws from an anterior to posterior direction. Good or excellent results were achieved in all cases, with average elbow motion of 15 to 141 degrees, and forearm rotation of 83 degrees pronation, and 84 degrees supination.
- Ring and Jupiter examined 21 cases of articular fractures of the distal humerus treated with Herbert screw fixation and found 4 excellent results, 12 good results, and 5 fair results.
  - All of the fractures healed and had an average range of motion of 96 degrees. No ulnohumeral instability, arthrosis, or osteonecrosis was reported.
- The authors stressed the importance of proper evaluation of these fractures and awareness that apparent capitellum fractures often are complex articular fractures of the distal humerus.[25]

- Dubberley et al[8] further subclassified type 4 fractures in their series of 28 cases. They achieved an average range of motion of flexion–extension of 25 degrees less than the contralateral elbow and 4 degrees of supination–pronation less than the contralateral elbow.
  - Two comminuted cases required conversion to a total elbow arthroplasty.
  - Varied fixation methods were used, including Herbert screws, cancellous screws, absorbable pins, and supplementation with K-wires.
- Ruchelsman and colleagues[26,27] reported a case series of 16 patients that were treated with ORIF.
- All patients achieved full forearm rotation and all but two had functional arc of elbow range of motion.
- They reported 15 good to excellent results and one fair result.
- The authors did not find association between concomitant radial head fracture and worse outcomes.
- Sen and colleagues[28] reported internal fixation of isolated trochlear fractures with promising results in a small case series.
- Comminuted fractures (Dubberley type B) have been shown to be more prone to inferior outcomes complicated by avascular necrosis, degenerative arthritis, and heterotopic ossification.[9]

## COMPLICATIONS

- The most common complication of capitellar fractures is loss of elbow motion and residual pain. The compromised motion most commonly is manifested in loss of flexion and extension.
- Ulnar neuropathy has been noted after ORIF, and some recommend routine ulnar nerve decompression.[25] This is especially important in capitellar–trochlear shear fractures, as hinging of the elbow on the medial side increases the risk of ulnar nerve compression.
- Osteonecrosis may occur from the initial fracture displacement or surgical exposure. Blood is supplied to the capitellum from a posterior to anterior direction and may be compromised by surgical dissection.
  - In symptomatic cases in which revascularization after fixation has not occurred, delayed excision is indicated.
- Malunions may occur when the patient has delayed seeking treatment, when inadequate reduction or loss of closed reduction occurs, or after ORIF. Malunions result in loss of motion and may require excision of the fragment and soft tissue releases.
- Nonunions may occur, although this is uncommon. They most likely result secondary to inadequate reduction or lack of revascularization of the fragment.

## REFERENCES


1. Alvarez E, Patel M, Nimberg P, et al. Fractures of the capitulum humeri. J Bone Joint Surg Am 1975;57(8):1093–1096.
2. Broberg MA, Morrey BF. Results of delayed excision of the radial head after fracture. J Bone Joint Surg Am 1986;68(5):669–674.
3. Brouwer KM, Jupiter JB, Ring D. Nonunion of operatively treated capitellum and trochlear fractures. J Hand Surg Am 2011;36(5):804–807.
4. Bryan RS, Morrey BF. Fractures of the distal humerus. In: Morrey BF, ed. The Elbow and Its Disorders. Philadelphia: WB Saunders, 1985:302–399.
5. Christopher F, Bushnell L. Conservative treatment of fractures of the capitellum. J Bone Joint Surg 1935;17:489–492.
6. Cobb TK, Morrey BF. Total elbow arthroplasty as primary treatment for distal humerus fractures in elderly patients. J Bone Joint Surg Am 1997;79(6):826–832.
7. Collert S. Surgical management of fracture of the capitulum humeri. Acta Orthop Scand 1977;48:603–606.
8. Dubberley JH, Faber KJ, Macdermid JC, et al. Outcome after open reduction and internal fixation of capitellar and trochlear fractures. J Bone Joint Surg Am 2006;88(1):46–54.
9. Durakbasa MO, Gumussuyu G, Gungor M, et al. Distal humeral coronal plane fractures: management, complications and outcome. J Shoulder Elbow Surg 2013;22(4):560–566.
10. Fowles JV, Kassab MT. Fracture of the capitulum humeri. Treatment by excision. J Bone Joint Surg Am 1975;56(4):794–798.
11. Garcia JA, Mykula R, Stanley D. Complex fractures of the distal humerus in the elderly. The role of total elbow replacement as primary treatment. J Bone Joint Surg Br 2002;84(6):812–816.
12. Giannicola G, Sacchetti FM, Greco A, et al. Open reduction and internal fixation combined with hinged elbow fixator in capitellum and trochlea fractures. Acta Orthop 2010;81(2):228–233.
13. Greenspan A, Norman A. The radial head, capitellum view: useful technique in elbow trauma. AJR Am J Roentgenol 1982;138:1186–1188.
14. Hahn NF. Fall von einer besonderes Varietat der Frakturen des Ellenbogens. Z Wund Geburt 1853;6:185.
15. Kamineni S, Morrey BF. Distal humeral fractures treated with noncustom total elbow replacement. Surgical technique. J Bone Joint Surg Am 2005;87(suppl 1)(pt 1):41–50.
16. Lansinger O, Mare K. Fracture of the capitulum humeri. Acta Orthop Scand 1981;52:39–44.
17. Lee JJ, Lawton JN. Coronal shear fractures of the distal humerus. J Hand Surg Am 2012;37(11):2412–2417.
18. Liberman N, Katz T, Howard CV, et al. Fixation of capitellar fractures with Herbert screws. Arch Orthop Trauma Surg 1991;110:155–157.
19. Mahirogullari M, Kiral A, Solakoglu C, et al. Treatment of fractures of the humeral capitellum using Herbert screws. J Hand Surg Br 2006;31:320–325.
20. Mazel MS. Fracture of the capitellum. J Bone Joint Surg 1935;17:483–488.
21. McKee MD, Jupiter JB, Bamberger HB. Coronal shear fractures of the distal end of the humerus. J Bone Joint Surg Am 1996;78(1):49–54.
22. Milch H. Fractures and fracture-dislocations of the humeral condyles. J Trauma 1964;13:882–886.
23. Ochner RS, Bloom H, Palumbo RC, et al. Closed reduction of coronal fractures of the capitellum. J Trauma 1996;40:199–203.
24. Richards RR, Khoury GW, Burke FD, et al. Internal fixation of capitellar fractures using Herbert screw: a report of four cases. Can J Surg 1987;30:188–191.
25. Ring D, Jupiter JB, Gulotta L. Articular fractures of the distal part of the humerus. J Bone Joint Surg Am 2003;85-A(2):232–238.
26. Ruchelsman DE, Tejwani NC, Kwon YW, et al. Open reduction and internal fixation of capitellar fractures with headless screws. J Bone Joint Surg Am 2008;90(6):1321–1329.
27. Ruchelsman DE, Tejwani NC, Kwon YW, et al. Open reduction and internal fixation of capitellar fractures with headless screws. Surgical technique. J Bone Joint Surg Am 2009;91(suppl 2, pt 1):38–49.
28. Sen RK, Tripahty SK, Goyal T, et al. Coronal shear fracture of the humeral trochlea. J Orthop Surg 2013;21(1):82–86.
29. Steinthal D. Die isolirte Fraktur der eminentia Capetala in Ellengogelenk. Zentralk Chir 1898;15:17.
30. Yamaguchi K, Sweet FA, Bindra R, et al. The extraosseous and intraosseous arterial anatomy of the adult elbow. J Bone Joint Surg Am 1997;79(11):1653–1662.

# Supracondylar Humeral Osteotomy for Correction of Cubitus Varus

15

CHAPTER

Yi-Meng Yen, Richard E. Bowen, and Norman Y. Otsuka

## DEFINITION

- Cubitus varus is a deformity of the distal humerus that results in a change in the carrying angle from physiologic valgus alignment between the upper arm and forearm.
- Historically, before modern pinning techniques, cubitus varus was the most common complication following supracondylar humerus fracture, with an average reported frequency of 30%, with rates as high as 60%.
- The appearance of the deformity is the major concern for the parents and patient, as there is little functional deficit.[4]

## ANATOMY

- Bone
  - The distal humerus consists of two structural columns of bone medially and laterally.
  - The olecranon and coronoid fossae separate the two structural columns.
  - The cortices of the distal humerus are thinner in the child than the adult, and the anteroposterior (AP) diameter of the distal humerus is decreased in children.
- Neurovascular
  - The median nerve and brachial artery run along the medial border of the biceps brachii muscle in the upper arm and come to lie anterior and slightly medial in the cubital fossa.
  - The radial nerve enters the anterior compartment of the arm in the distal third of the upper arm and travels between the brachialis and brachioradialis over the anterolateral distal humerus before it enters the supinator muscle in the proximal forearm. There have been reports of the radial nerve enclosed within the callus of a supracondylar fracture.

## PATHOGENESIS

- Cubitus varus occurs predominantly because of a malunited supracondylar humerus fracture. Unequal growth of the distal humerus can cause cubitus varus, particularly medial physeal growth arrest.
- The primary cause is coronal varus angulation of the distal humeral metaphysis.
- Varus angulation can be caused by medial column comminution, causing the fracture to collapse into varus. Varus angulation can rarely be caused by lateral gaping at the fracture site.
- Other coexisting deformities can exist with cubitus varus, including extension and internal rotation of the distal fragment.[7]

## NATURAL HISTORY

- The deformity is usually static and does not evolve with time, unless caused by a medial physeal disturbance.
- The deformity is often not appreciated until several months after the fracture heals and the elbow flexion contracture that results from casting resolves.
- Tardy ulnar nerve palsy may occur, owing to compression by chronic malpositioning of the triceps muscle due to a shift of the olecranon in the olecranon fossa.
- Significant cubitus varus may contribute to elbow discomfort and posterolateral rotatory instability.
- There may be a slight increased risk of subsequent lateral condyle fractures in children with cubitus varus.[1]

## PATIENT HISTORY AND PHYSICAL FINDINGS

- A detailed history is essential to understand parental and patient expectations of treatment in cubitus varus.
- Physical findings include a varus change in the carrying angle when compared to the opposite, unaffected side.
- Elbow and forearm range of motion should be documented.
- A thorough examination of nerve function to the forearm and hand should be performed.
- Hyperextension of the elbow indicates coexisting extension deformity at the malunion site.
- A loss of external rotation can be due to shoulder pathology or due to an internal rotation malunion at the distal humerus.
- The difference in carrying angle between the affected and unaffected side is the amount of cubitus varus.

## IMAGING AND OTHER DIAGNOSTIC STUDIES

- Plain AP and lateral radiographs of the affected elbow should be obtained (**FIG 1**).
- Additionally, an AP radiograph of the affected and unaffected elbow in full extension and supination that includes the distal humerus, forearm, and wrist should be obtained. This is used to plan the amount of surgical correction desired.
- Advanced imaging (magnetic resonance imaging [MRI] of the elbow) may be of value in young children where distal humeral growth disturbance is suspected.[3]

## DIFFERENTIAL DIAGNOSIS

- Medial humeral condylar or trochlear growth disturbance
- Malunited lateral humeral condyle fracture
- Congenital dislocation of the radial head
- Malunited fracture/separation of the distal humeral physis

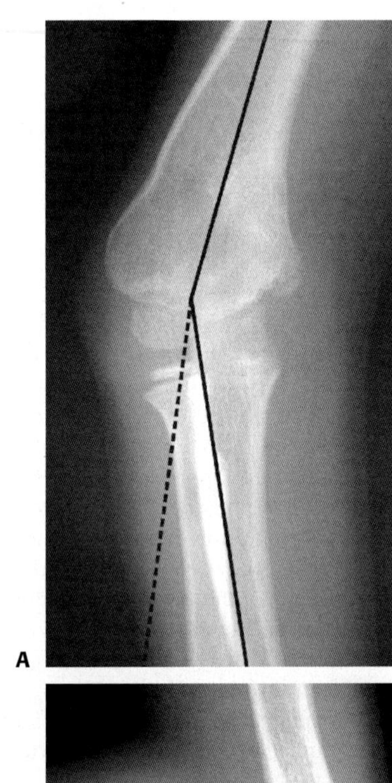

FIG 1 • A,B. AP and lateral radiographs obtained preoperatively for a patient with cubitus varus.

## NONOPERATIVE MANAGEMENT

- Nonoperative management does not affect the appearance of cubitus varus.
- If correction is contemplated, surgery should be undertaken at least 1 year after injury to ensure that there is no evidence of distal humeral avascular necrosis.

## SURGICAL MANAGEMENT

- Indications
  - Skeletally immature child with posttraumatic cubitus varus
  - Full elbow extension and flexion to at least 130 degrees
  - Child and family unaccepting of the appearance of the elbow
  - At least 1 year after initial injury
- Goals
  - Correction of the carrying angle to equal the contralateral side[7]
  - In our experience, rotational deformity less than 45 degrees is well compensated for by shoulder and forearm rotation and does not need to be addressed in the osteotomy.

### Preoperative Planning

- Preoperative AP radiographs of both elbows should be taken in full extension and supination.
  - The angle of Baumann and the humeral-elbow-wrist angle should be determined for both sides.
  - A tracing of the normal arm on tracing paper is reversed and superimposed on the radiograph of the operative arm (**FIG 2A–C**).
  - By adding the humeral-elbow-wrist angles, the amount of planned correction can be estimated (**FIG 2D**).[5] Alternatively, attempting to match the Baumann angle of the contralateral side can help estimate the amount of correction needed.
- The distal osteotomy cut is just proximal to the olecranon fossa.
- The osteotomy is planned with equal lengths of the proximal and distal limbs; this diminishes the tendency for a lateral condylar prominence.[5]

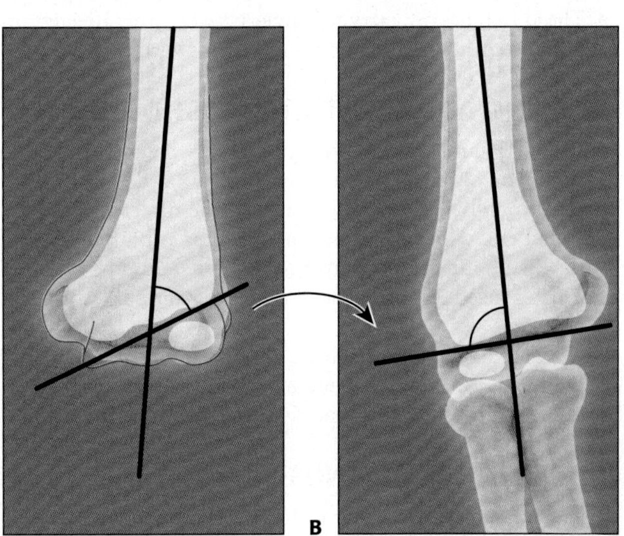

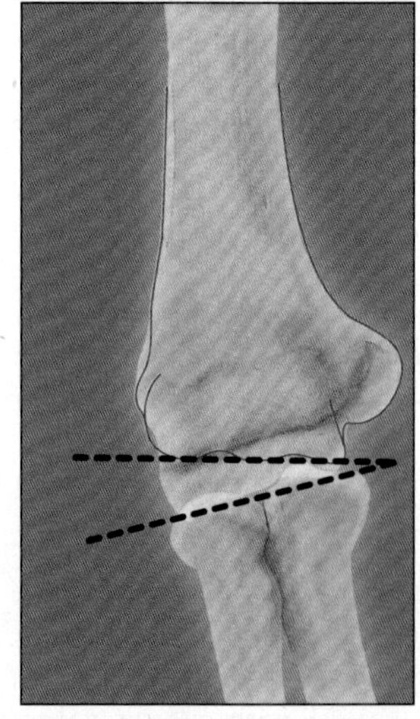

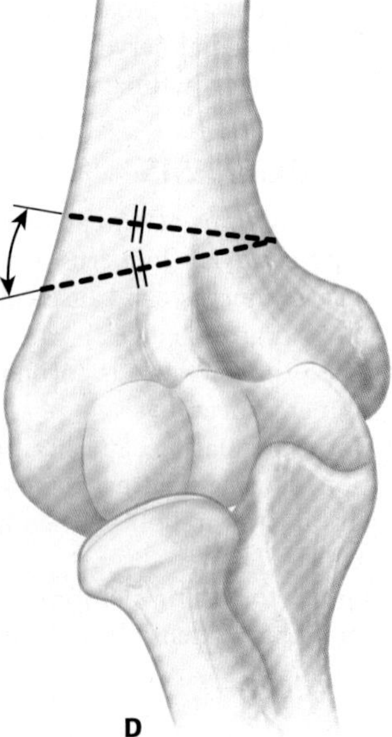

**FIG 2** • Preoperative templating for the osteotomy. **A–C.** Preoperative assessment using radiographs of the affected and nonaffected sides. A tracing of the nonaffected side is reversed and placed over a radiograph of the affected side to estimate the amount of correction. **D.** Planning of equal limb lengths for the osteotomy. *(continued)*

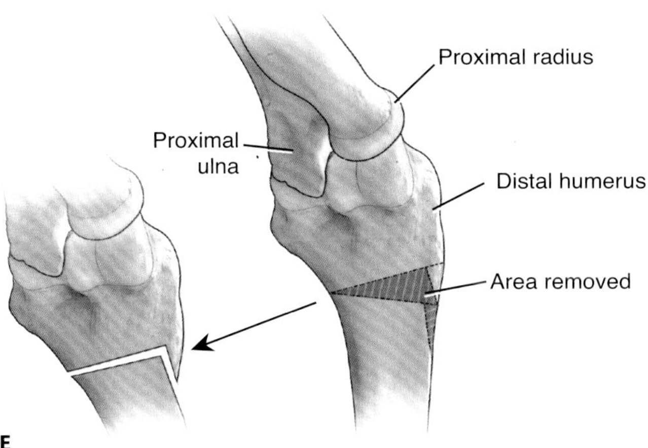


**FIG 2** • *(continued)* **E.** Example of a step cut osteotomy. Shaded areas show bone that will be removed.

- The angle of the wedge to be removed is the same as the angle of desired correction.
- Because the osteotomy is performed proximal to the deformity apex and hinges medially, there is a lateral shift of the forearm axis that will make the lateral condyle more prominent than in the normal arm, even with equal osteotomy limbs.
  - This appearance is more accentuated in patients with neutral humeral-elbow-wrist angles.
  - In these cases, a complete osteotomy with medial translation of the distal fragment should be planned, or a translation step cut osteotomy can be performed (**FIG 2E**).

## Positioning

- The patient is placed supine with the arm on a radiolucent extremity table. A sterile upper arm tourniquet is used; this facilitates complete intraoperative visualization of the upper arm.



## Exposure

- The lateral approach to the distal humerus is used between the lateral head of the triceps muscle and the extensor carpi radialis longus muscles (**TECH FIG 1A**). A posterior approach can be used as well, if cosmetic appearance is of paramount importance; however, the lateral approach is technically simpler.
- The distal humerus is subperiosteally exposed both anteriorly and posteriorly, and small Hohmann retractors are placed (**TECH FIG 1B**).
- The proximal and distal osteotomy cuts are made with a small oscillating saw as per the preoperative template. Kirschner wires inserted under image intensifier can be used to mark the osteotomy sites.
- The distal osteotomy is performed proximal to the olecranon fossa. The proximal osteotomy meets the distal osteotomy at the medial cortex, leaving it intact.

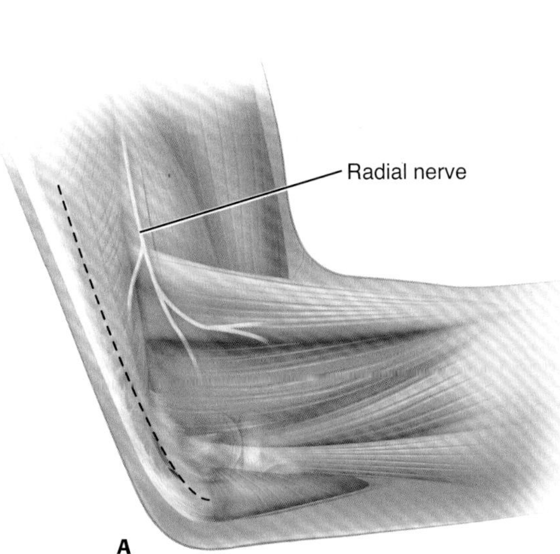


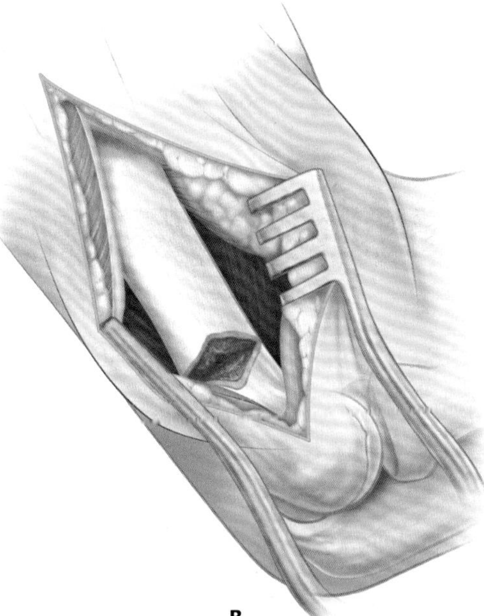


**TECH FIG 1** • **A.** Lateral approach to the elbow between the lateral head of the triceps and the extensor carpi radialis longus. Incision is placed posterior to the epicondylar ridge. **B.** The incision is carried down to the epicondylar ridge with the triceps posterior and the extensor carpi radialis longus anterior. The dissection is continued subperiosteally both anterior and posterior completely to the medial side. The osteotomy is then performed with an oscillating saw.

TECHNIQUES

## Osteotomy Closure and Fixation

- With the elbow extended, a valgus force is placed on the elbow, closing the osteotomy by creating a greenstick fracture at the medial cortex.
- A single distal lateral to proximal medial Kirschner wire is placed percutaneously (not through the incision) to hold the osteotomy apposed.
- The osteotomy site is tested for stability with real-time fluoroscopy. If the osteotomy is unstable, a second distal medial to proximal lateral Kirschner wire is used to supplement fixation (**TECH FIG 2**).
- If there is a lateral condylar prominence after performing the greenstick osteotomy, the Kirschner wire is removed, the medial cortex is cut, and the distal fragment is translated medially to remove the prominence. In this situation, routine medial and lateral Kirschner wire fixation is used.
- The medial Kirschner wire is inserted with the elbow relatively extended.
  - The thumb is used to hold the ulnar nerve posterior to the medial epicondyle within the cubital tunnel.
  - A small skin incision is made over the medial epicondyle, and a hemostat is used to spread the subcutaneous tissue to the underlying bone.

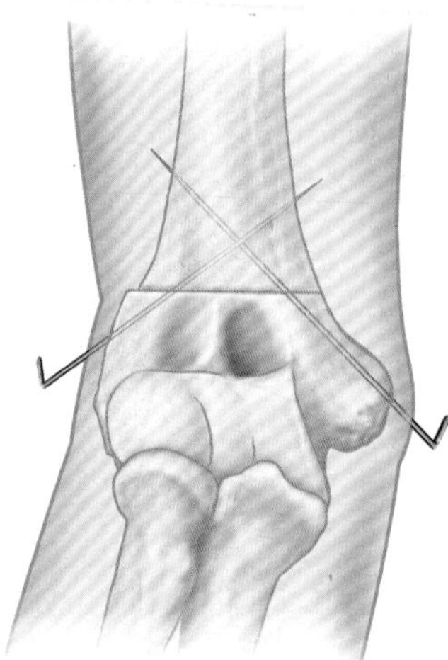

**TECH FIG 2** • Fixation with medial and lateral Kirschner wires above the physis.

- Care is taken to prevent the wires from crossing at the osteotomy site.
- Fixation is evaluated with biplanar fluoroscopy to ensure proper pin placement before wound closure.

## Closure

- The wound is irrigated and closed in layers in the standard fashion.
- The Kirschner wires are left protruding from the skin and are bent to prevent migration of the pins underneath the skin.
- A long-arm cast or splint is applied with the elbow in 90 degrees of flexion and the forearm in slight pronation. The patient should be closely monitored in the early postoperative period for swelling.
- If a splint is used, it is converted to a long-arm cast after swelling has subsided.

## PEARLS AND PITFALLS

| | |
|---|---|
| **Patient selection** | ▪ Parents and patients should understand the goal of the surgery, which is to improve the appearance of the elbow. |
| **Diagnosis** | ▪ Patients with other conditions, such as growth disturbance of the distal humerus, should be identified preoperatively.<br>▪ These patients often have a progressive deformity and are better treated at skeletal maturity using other fixation methods. |
| **Preoperative planning** | ▪ Before operating, the surgeon must know the normal humeral-elbow-wrist angle for each particular patient as well as the amount of deformity. |
| **Performing the osteotomy** | ▪ Subperiosteal exposure in the distal humerus is essential.<br>▪ An intact medial cortex greatly enhances osteotomy stability. |
| **Lateral condylar prominence** | ▪ The osteotomy should be assessed with the elbow extended after closing the osteotomy.<br>▪ Patients with a neutral contralateral carrying angle should have complete osteotomy with translation of the distal fragment. |
| **Fixation problems** | ▪ Stability of fixation should be tested intraoperatively with fluoroscopy, and additional fixation is added as necessary. |

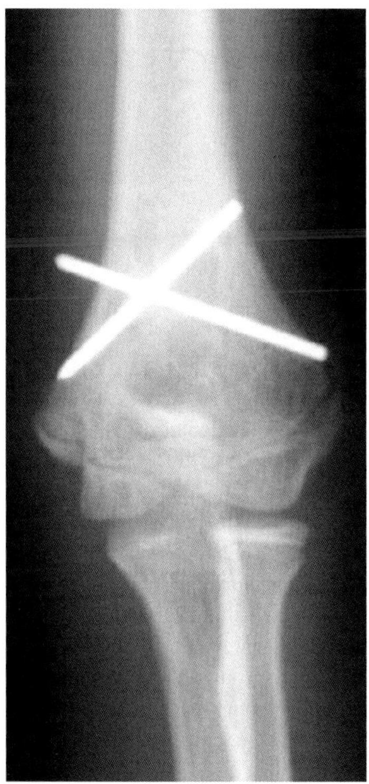
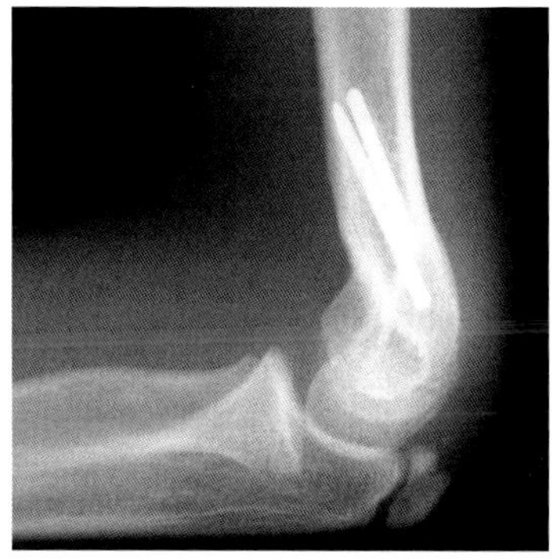

**FIG 3** • **A,B.** Postoperative AP and lateral radiographs.

## POSTOPERATIVE CARE

- With the technique described, patients are immobilized in a long-arm cast for 4 to 6 weeks. When radiographs show callus formation at the osteotomy site, the percutaneous Kirschner wires can be removed (**FIG 3**).
- The patient is then given a sling, and active range-of-motion exercises are initiated.
- Once radiographic union is achieved, the sling is discontinued, and the patient can begin full activities once range of motion is restored.

## OUTCOMES

- Patient outcomes after supracondylar humeral osteotomy are good to excellent in most cases, with retention of range of motion and improved appearance of the elbow as the major outcome measures.
- Loss of fixation, persistent lateral condyle prominence or undercorrection, and hypertrophic scar negatively impact outcome.[6]

## COMPLICATIONS

- Persistent lateral condylar prominence[6]
- Nonunion
- Refracture[6]
- Hypertrophic lateral scar[6]
- Loss of fixation[2]
- Recurrent deformity
- Radial or ulnar nerve palsy
- Infection

## REFERENCES


1. Davids JR, Maguire MF, Mubarak SJ, et al. Lateral condylar fracture of the humerus following posttraumatic cubitus varus. J Pediatr Orthop 1994;14:466–470.
2. Hernandez MA III, Roach JW. Corrective osteotomy for cubitus varus deformity. J Pediatr Orthop 1994;14:487–491.
3. Ippolito E, Moneta MR, D'Arrigo C. Post-traumatic cubitus varus. Long-term follow-up of corrective supracondylar humeral osteotomy in children. J Bone Joint Surg Am 1990;72(5):757–765.
4. Labelle H, Bunnell WP, Duhaime M, et al. Cubitus varus deformity following supracondylar fractures of the humerus in children. J Pediatr Orthop 1982;2:539–546.
5. Oppenheim WL, Clader TJ, Smith C, et al. Supracondylar humeral osteotomy for traumatic childhood cubitus varus deformity. Clin Orthop Relat Res 1984;(188):34–39.
6. Voss FR, Kasser JR, Trepman E, et al. Uniplanar supracondylar humeral osteotomy with preset Kirschner wires for posttraumatic cubitus varus. J Pediatr Orthop 1994;14:471–478.
7. Wong HK, Balasubramanian P. Humeral torsional deformity after supracondylar osteotomy for cubitus varus: its influence on the postosteotomy carrying angle. J Pediatr Orthop 1992;12:490–493.

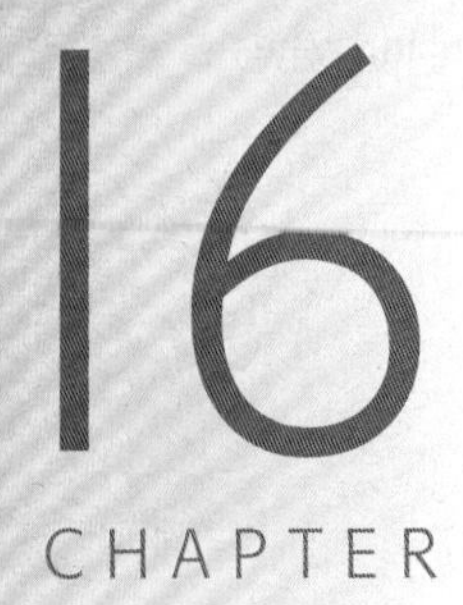

CHAPTER 16

# Humeral Shaft Fracture Stabilization with Elastic Nails

Nathan W. Skelley and J. Eric Gordon

## DEFINITION

- Humeral shaft fractures comprise approximately 2.5% of all traumatic fractures in children.[11]
- Nearly all humeral diaphyseal fractures in children can commonly be treated nonoperatively with bracing and sling support.[9,10]
- Titanium elastic nails can be used to stabilize selected humeral shaft fractures in children and adolescents from the distal metaphysis to the proximal humeral physis.

## ANATOMY

- Proximally, the neurovascular bundles are located near the axilla, however, distally, the ulnar nerve and radial nerve pass in proximity to the medial epicondyle and lateral condyle, respectively (**FIG 1**).
- If antegrade nails are to be used, the course of the axillary nerve is important as it passes lateral to the proximal humerus from posterior to anterior approximately 3.5 cm distal to the greater tuberosity in adults.[5]

## PATHOGENESIS

- The humerus is initially made of woven bone that is gradually replaced by stronger lamellar bone during childhood.
- This developmental transition makes the bone prone to fracture with direct impact and falls on outstretched arms.
- An increasingly active pediatric population and the increased prevalence of motorized sports has led to an increase in humeral shaft fractures.[1,3,6,11]
- Clinical examination and radiographs can assist in characterizing the injury mechanism.

## NATURAL HISTORY

- Most humeral shaft fractures are amenable to nonoperative treatment.
- In young children, moderate shortening (<3 cm) is well tolerated as is angulation up to 30 degrees for fractures in the proximal third, 25 degrees in the middle third, and 20 degrees in the distal third.[3,6]
- Fractures in the distal one-fourth humeral metaphysis are more sensitive to angulation and should be maintained within 10 degrees of anatomic alignment.

## PATIENT HISTORY AND PHYSICAL FINDINGS

- Most humeral shaft fractures are identified by the common complaints of pain, discomfort, or disuse. In pediatrics, the patients may not clearly verbalize the pain. Therefore, discomfort or disuse of the extremity should encourage further evaluation.
- High-energy trauma is commonly associated with shortening and angulation of the upper extremity. Soft tissue injuries are also common findings (**FIG 2**).
- Humeral shaft fractures are commonly the result of mild trauma in the presence of pathologic lesions such as unicameral bone cysts.[8]
- A complete distal neurologic and vascular examinations should be performed and documented to verify the patient is neurovascularly intact. In younger children, a careful motor examination is essential, as the sensory examination can be unreliable.
- Examination with careful palpation of the remainder of the extremity should be performed because ipsilateral forearm, wrist, or shoulder injuries are not unusual (see **FIG 2**).

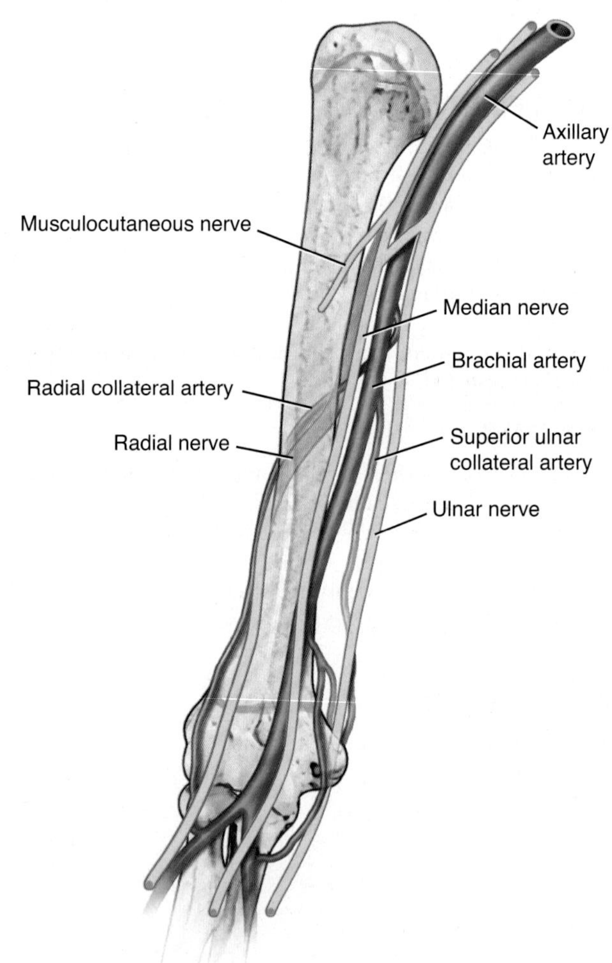


**FIG 1** • Anatomy of the humerus with important neurovascular structures shown.

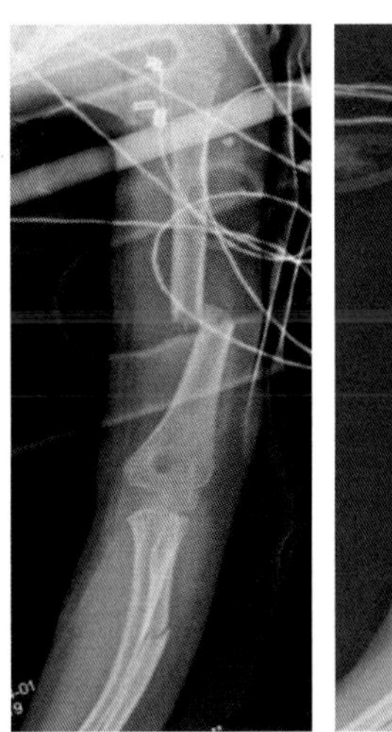
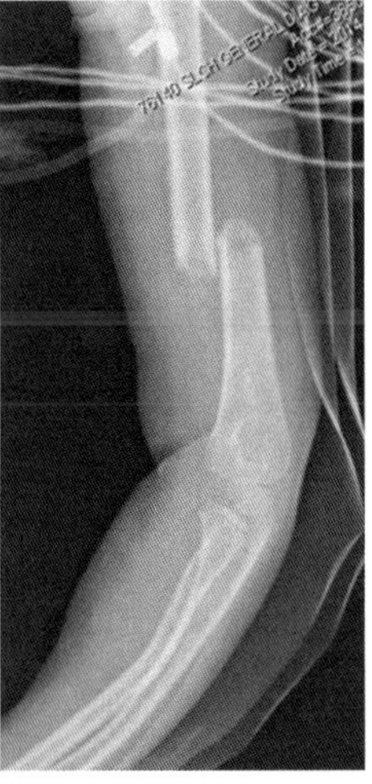

**FIG 2** • Anteroposterior and lateral radiographs of the humerus in a 6-year-old girl demonstrating a displaced diaphyseal fracture sustained in a rollover motor vehicle accident. The patient also sustained an ipsilateral radius fracture, multiple head injuries, and ipsilateral tibia fracture.

- Plain radiography is usually adequate to make a definitive diagnosis, although magnetic resonance imaging (MRI) can be occasionally helpful in distinguishing pathologic fractures through benign and malignant lesions.

## IMAGING AND OTHER DIAGNOSTIC STUDIES

- Two views (internally and externally rotated) of the humerus are usually sufficient to diagnose a humeral shaft fracture.
- The joint above and below should be clearly visualized.
- Concern on physical examination for injuries to the shoulder, forearm, or wrist should be evaluated by appropriate radiographs.

## DIFFERENTIAL DIAGNOSIS

- Pathologic fracture
- Benign or malignant tumor

## NONOPERATIVE MANAGEMENT

- Humeral shaft fractures commonly do well functionally and cosmetically from nonoperative treatment.
- Functional bracing, coaptation splints, hanging arm casts, or sling immobilization are common treatments.
- Younger children have profound remodeling potential and can successfully remodel fractures with significant angulation up to 45 degrees.
- Authors have recommended that older children should be reduced to less than 30 degrees for proximal third, less than 20 degrees for middle third, and less than 15 degrees for distal third shaft fractures before proceeding with nonoperative treatment.[3,6]

## SURGICAL MANAGEMENT

- Surgical stabilization of humeral shaft fractures is indicated in certain scenarios including the following:
  - Open fracture
  - Inability to maintain adequate alignment by closed mean
  - Ipsilateral forearm fractures (floating elbow)
  - Closed head injuries to simplify nursing care
  - Polytraumatized patients, particularly with lower extremity fractures to facilitate mobilization out of bed by allowing upper extremity weight bearing[6]
- The main goal of elastic nailing in humeral shaft fractures is to create a biomechanical stable reduction with axial, angular, translational, and rotational stability.
- This is typically accomplished with two nails inserted through the metaphysis using a three-point application about the diaphyseal fracture site.
- The nails are contoured by hand or with a plate-bending press to place the apex of the nail at the fracture site.
- Elastic nailing is ideal for transverse and minimally comminuted fractures. Oblique diaphyseal fractures and unstable comminuted fractures can also be treated with flexible nailing because mild to moderate shortening rarely causes clinical problems.
- Plate fixation requires a large incision, extensive dissection, and often requires exposure of neurovascular structures.

### Preoperative Planning

- A decision should be made between antegrade and retrograde nailing techniques.
- Most fractures are treated with retrograde nailing. This technique allows stabilization of distal, midshaft, and proximal fractures with excellent stability.
- The primary indication for antegrade nailing is soft tissue injury about the elbow requiring secondary procedures to obtain coverage.
- Fractures in the distal and middle thirds of the humerus are best stabilized using retrograde nails placed from the medial and lateral sides of the elbow. Fractures in the proximal third of the humerus can be stabilized using two nails placed from the lateral side of the elbow, obviating the risk of ulnar nerve injury. **FIG 3** shows incision sites and nail starting points.
- A fluoroscopic image intensifier with a radiolucent hand table is necessary to follow nail progression in the humerus and to confirm reduction with both antegrade and retrograde techniques.
- The nail selected for fixation is commonly about 40% of the narrowest diameter (isthmus) of the humerus. Most fractures can be stabilized with either 3.0- or 3.5-mm nails. If increased rigidity is needed, stainless steel nails can be used.
- As in other applications of flexible nails, if two nails are being placed, the same size should be used for both nails to prevent asymmetric forces.

### Positioning

- The patient is placed supine on a radiolucent table with an arm table on the affected side (**FIG 4**).
- The affected upper extremity is abducted approximately 90 degrees.
- The upper extremity is draped free. The shoulder area should be squared off using towels leaving as much of the shoulder surgically accessible as possible to facilitate changes in operative approach from retrograde to antegrade approaches in the event of intraoperative problems.
- A tourniquet is not typically needed for elastic nailing. If an open reduction of the fracture is necessary, a sterile tourniquet can be used.

### Approach

- Placement of retrograde nails can be nearly percutaneous.

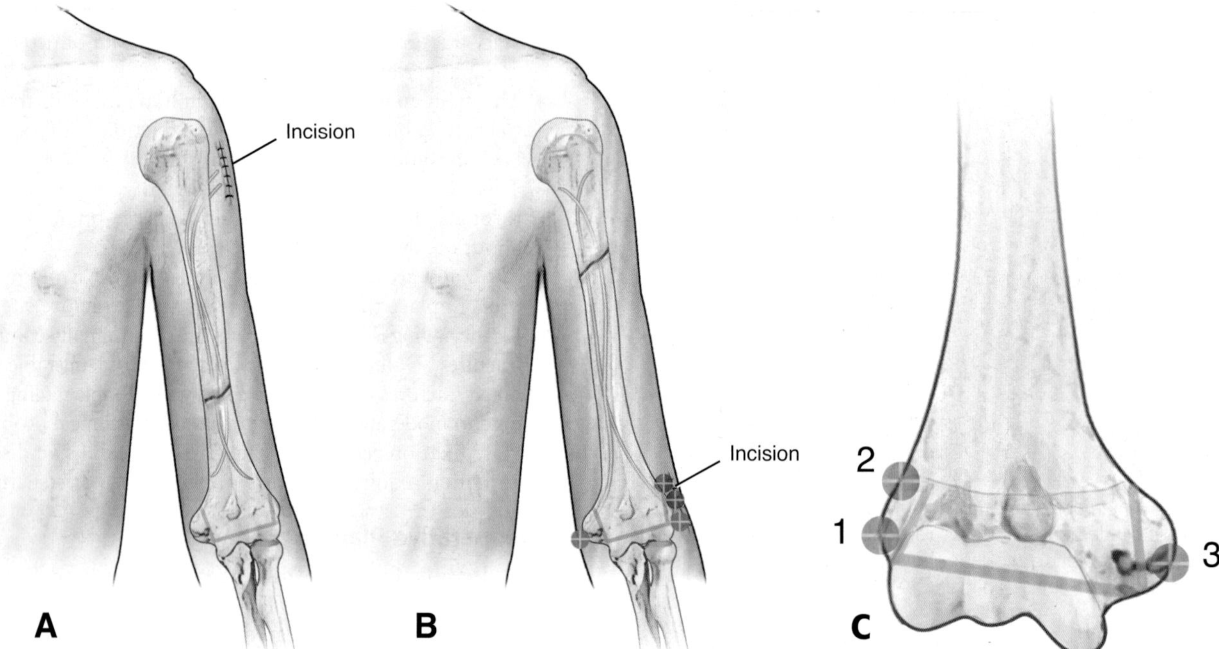


**FIG 3** • **A,B.** Incision locations are shown for antegrade (**A**) and retrograde (**B**) approaches for humeral nailing. **C.** The crosshairs mark the general starting points for either antegrade (*1*) or retrograde (*2*) humeral nails.

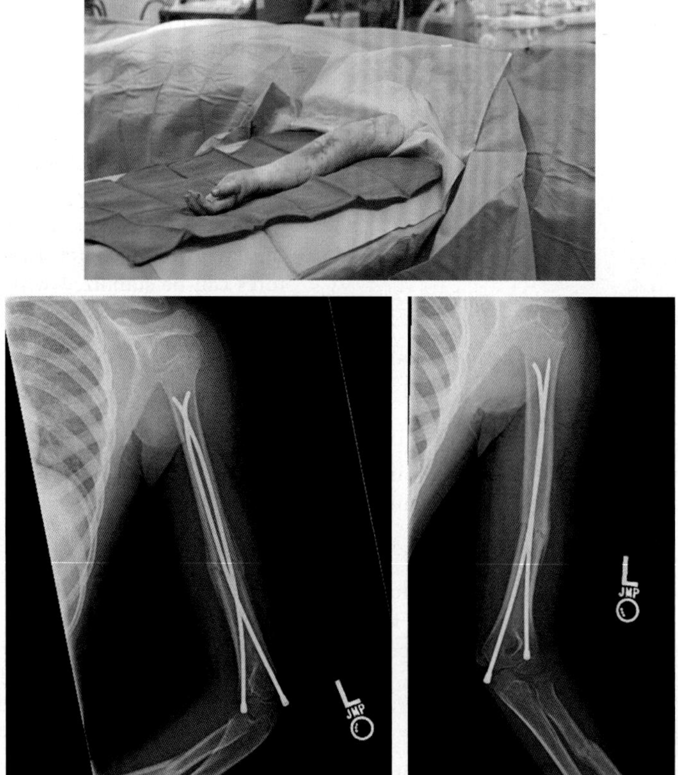


**FIG 4** • Patient prepped and draped in the supine position and with the arm on a radiolucent hand table.

## Antegrade Flexible Intramedullary Nailing

### Exposure and Drilling

- Fluoroscopy is used to localize the starting point and incision.
- A 1- to 2-cm longitudinal incision is made laterally over the shoulder just distal to the lateral edge of the acromion.
- Dissection is performed with tenotomy scissors or electrocautery down to the level of the humeral metaphysis, incising the deltoid and the rotator cuff longitudinally in line with their fibers.
- The metaphysis is entered with a 3.2- or 4.5-mm drill approximately 2 cm lateral to the glenohumeral joint articular surface. Alternatively, an awl can be used to create a cortical opening for the nail.
- Once the cortex is breached, the drill or awl should be angled obliquely to the fracture site to facilitate nail entry into the canal.

### Nail Placement

- The implants are selected and the first nail is prebent and passed down the intramedullary canal to the fracture site. Use the image intensifier periodically to verify correct nail placement in the canal.
- The nail is passed by attaching the nail inserter 5 to 10 cm from the skin to provide for better control during impaction with a hammer. When the inserter is close to the skin, the device should be released, moved back on the nail, tightened again, and impacted. This process is repeated until the nail is in an appropriate position.
  - The nail should pass easily in the intramedullary canal when hammering. If the nail does not pass easily, consider these common issues: nail orientation in the canal, insufficient contour of the nail tip, poor choice of nail diameter, and cancellous or cortical blockage.
- The fracture is most often reduced closed, and the nail is driven across the fracture site and into the distal portion of the humerus. The nail is impacted into the supracondylar region either medially or laterally.
- A second nail of the same size is then selected and prebent.
  - To avoid producing angulation at the fracture site, it is important to choose nails of the same diameter.
  - Again, a drill is used to enter the proximal humeral metaphysis adjacent to the initial starting point. The nail is passed down the medullary canal, across the fracture site, and impacted into the distal humerus opposite the first nail.
- An alternative acceptable technique preferred by some surgeons is to pass both nails to the fracture site, then reduce the fracture and pass both nails across the fracture site and advance them distally together into final position.

## Retrograde Flexible Intramedullary Nailing

### Exposure

- A 1- to 2-cm longitudinal incision is made over the lateral epicondyle of the distal humerus. Dissection is carried out down to the epicondyle bluntly (**TECH FIG 1**).

### Drilling

- The bone is entered with a 3.2- or 4.5-mm drill at the level of the epicondyle.
- Under image intensification, the drill is passed up through the lateral column of the humerus and into the medullary canal.
  - It is important to pass the drill fully through the lateral column and into the medullary canal, as the bone in the lateral column is very dense, and if the drill is not passed completely into the medullary canal, passing the nail can be extremely difficult (**TECH FIG 2**).
- It is essential that frequent anteroposterior and lateral images of the elbow be obtained while drilling, as perforation of the cortex with the drill leading to inability to pass the nail can happen easily.

### First Nail Placement

- A nail is then selected, prebent, and passed up the lateral distal humerus to the fracture site (**TECH FIG 3**). The fracture site is reduced manually and maintained with traction.
- The nail is passed across the fracture with a hammer impacting the nail inserter device. The nail may need to be advanced and retracted several times to successfully pass the fracture site and remain in the intramedullary canal. Use the image intensifier to confirm placement.
- The nail is impacted into the proximal humeral metaphysis either laterally or medially.

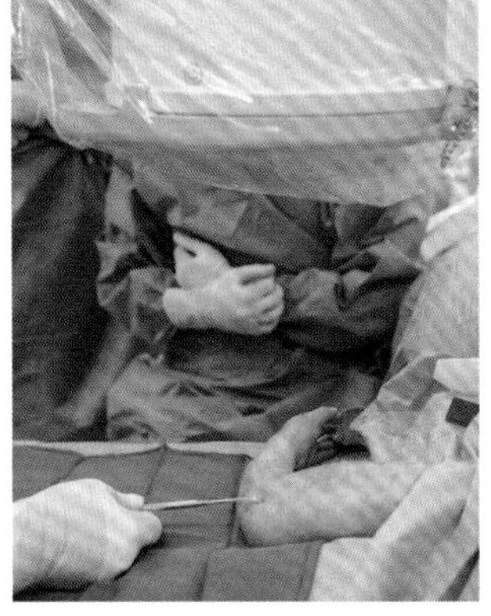
A

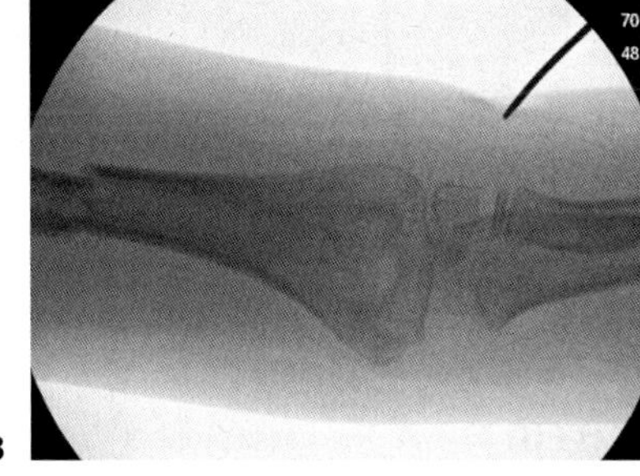
B

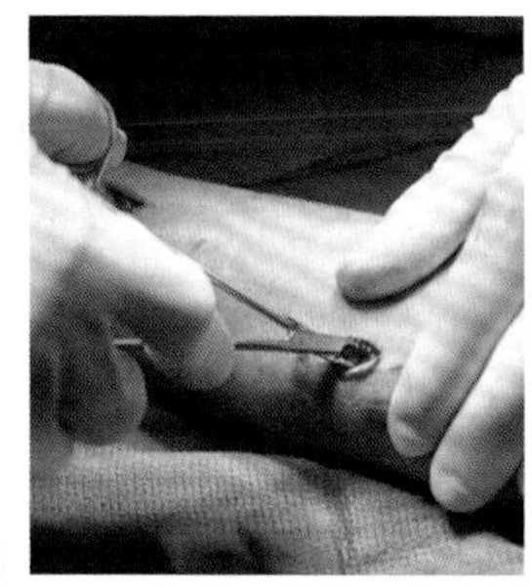
C

**TECH FIG 1** • **A,B.** Fluoroscopy is used to localize the starting point and incision. **C.** The subcutaneous tissues are gently spread until contact is made with the humerus.

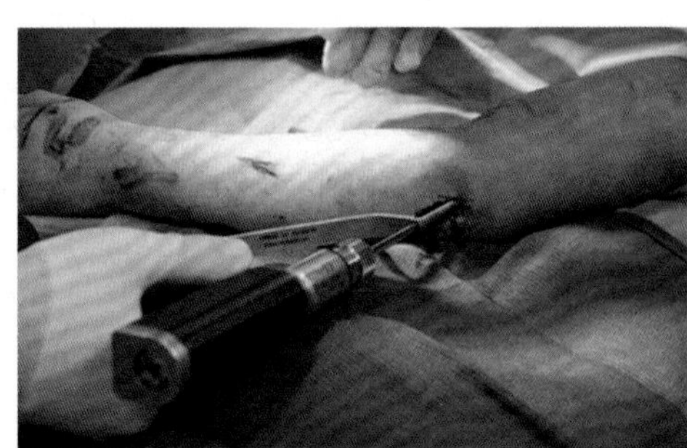
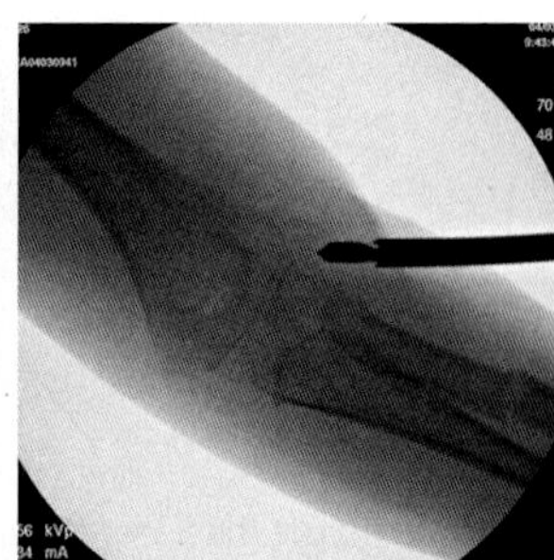
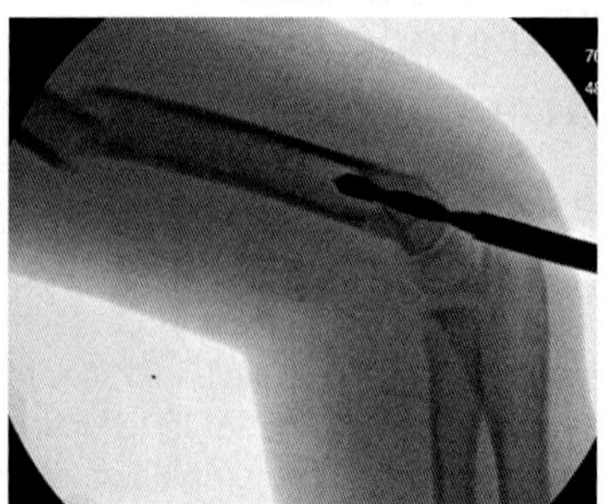

**TECH FIG 2** • Fluoroscopy is used to find the starting point and confirm drill placement within the medullary canal.

## Second Nail Placement

- The second nail can be placed either laterally or medially depending on the location of the fracture. Usually, a lateral placement is selected if the fracture is in the proximal third of the humerus.
- If a second lateral nail is to be placed, a second entry into the distal humerus is made 3 to 5 mm proximal to the initial starting point, and again, the drill is passed up the lateral humeral column into the medullary canal.
- A medial placement is selected if the fracture is in the middle or distal third of the humerus to enhance construct stability.
- If a medial nail is required, placement is through the medial epicondyle.
- Ulnar nerve subluxation with the elbow in flexion should be assumed because of the high rate of subluxation in children and adolescents.[2] Therefore, the elbow should be kept extended throughout the process of entering the medial epicondyle.
- With the elbow extended, a 1- to 2-cm incision is made over the medial epicondyle and the ulnar nerve is visualized. It is not necessary to dissect the nerve free as long as it can be visualized and protected during drilling and nail placement (**TECH FIG 4**).
- A 3.2- or 4.5-mm drill is passed up the medial column of the humerus into the medullary canal. Again, frequent imaging checks of the elbow are necessary to assure appropriate drilling of the medial column.
- A nail the same size as the initial nail is then selected and passed through the entry site, either laterally or medially. The nail is driven across the fracture site and impacted into the proximal humeral metaphysis opposite the initial nail.
- As with the antegrade technique, an alternative acceptable technique preferred by some surgeons is to pass both nails to the fracture site, then reduce the fracture and pass both nails across the fracture site and advance them together proximally into final position.

## Completion

- The nails are then cut off, capped, and impacted into the bone. End caps are particularly helpful in this area to minimize

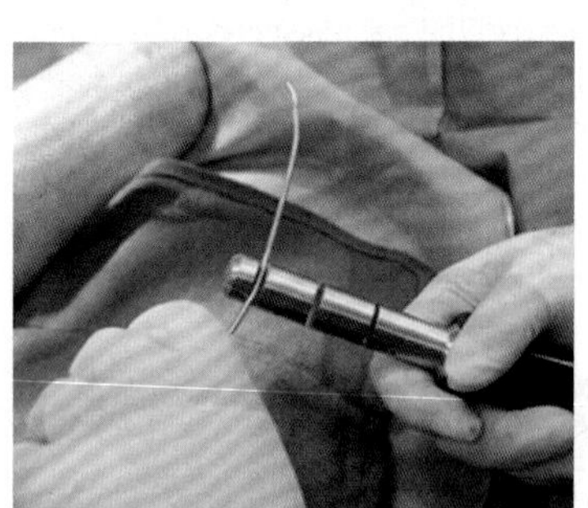
A

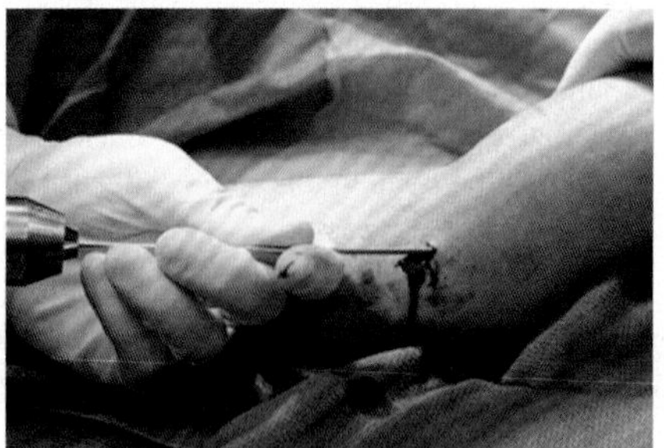
B

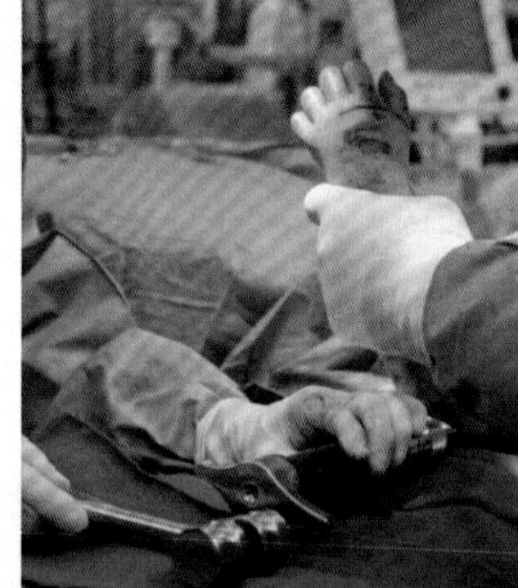
C

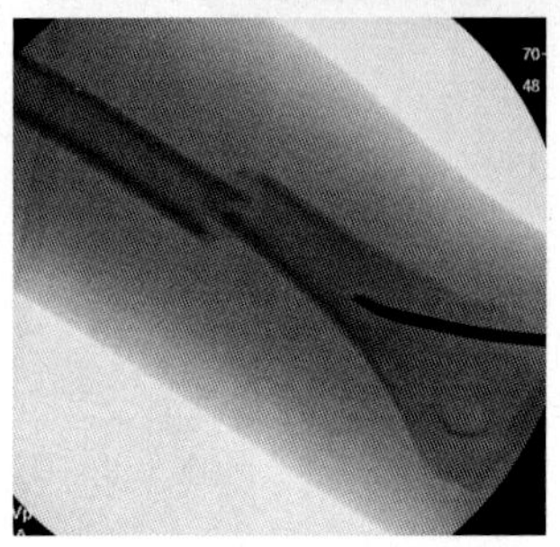
D

**TECH FIG 3** • **A.** The nail is prebent to assist with placement. **B,C.** The nail is secured with nail inserter device and placed in the drilled site. The nail inserter device is hammered through the humerus while the fracture site is reduced with manual traction. **D.** The passage of the nail should be monitored and corrected on fluoroscopy to properly reduce the fracture. The nail should be partially removed and redirected if proper reduction is not obtained.

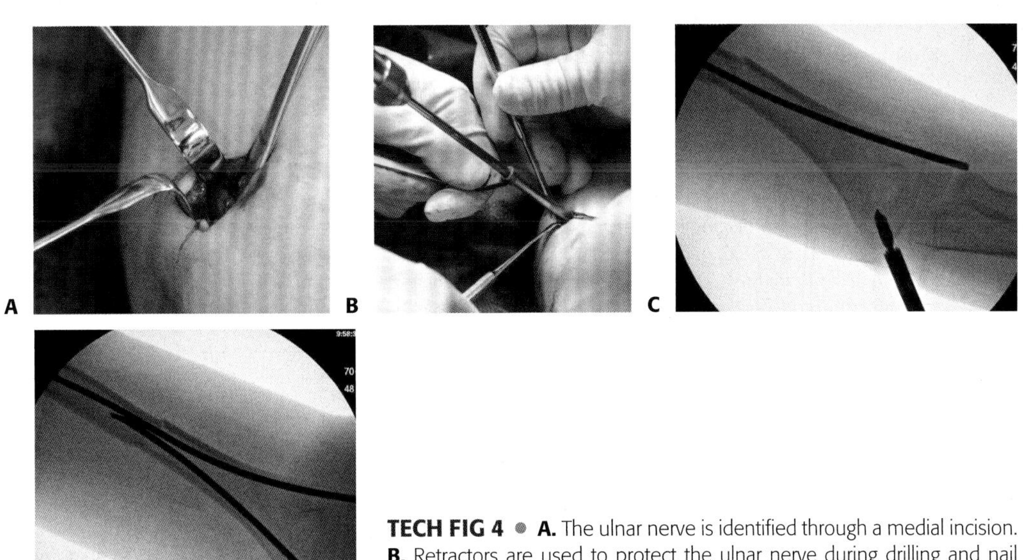

**TECH FIG 4** ● **A.** The ulnar nerve is identified through a medial incision. **B.** Retractors are used to protect the ulnar nerve during drilling and nail placement. **C,D.** Fluoroscopy is used to confirm correct nail placement and fracture reduction.

discomfort with elbow motion and if used should be placed prior to impacting the nails into the bone (**TECH FIG 5**).

- Once the nails have been placed into position, final images should be taken with the image intensifier. The fracture site is also checked to ensure that the fracture site is not distracted.
  - If distraction is present, the elbow can be gently impacted with the palm of the hand to compress the fracture site. If this is done, it is important to check the nails for prominence prior to closure.
- The incisions are irrigated with normal saline, and a standard layered closure is performed.
  - We use 2-0 absorbable sutures for the deep dermal layer and 3-0 absorbable sutures for the subcutaneous closure.
  - A dermal adhesive or Steri-Strips can be used to support the skin closure.

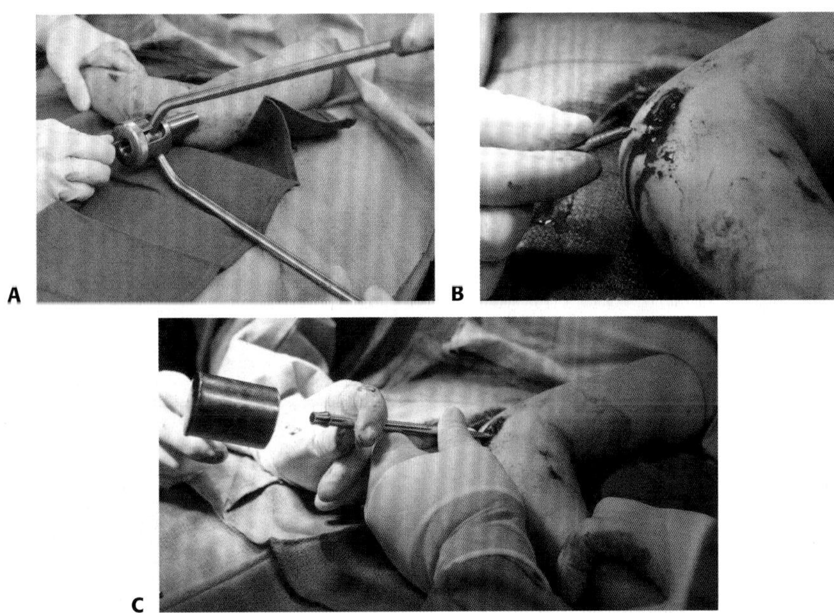

**TECH FIG 5** ● **A.** The excess nail is cut near the skin. **B.** The end cap has been placed after bending the delivery device to break off the end cap. End caps are placed to prevent soft tissue injury from the cut nail. **C.** The end cap and nail are tapped under the soft tissues.

## PEARLS AND PITFALLS

| | |
|---|---|
| **Indications** | ■ Most humeral shaft fractures can be treated nonoperatively.<br>■ Open fractures, unacceptable alignment, and polytraumatized patients are some indications to fix humeral shaft fractures with elastic nails. |
| **Approach** | ■ Placement of a medial retrograde nail requires the surgeon to be aware of the proximity of the ulnar nerve. All dissection and manipulation around this entry site requires awareness of the nerve and protection from damage during the procedure.<br>■ It is important when placing the nails in a retrograde fashion to drill completely up both columns of the humerus into the medullary canal and to use an adequate drill bit size. Even when placing 3.0-mm nails, we have used a 4.5-mm drill bit to allow adequate space to place the prebent nail. Attempts to drive the nails through the columns without completely drilling are difficult because of the dense bone and incompletely developed medullary canal in the distal portions of the humerus. |
| **Fracture fixation** | ■ Remember, if the nail ceases to advance, rotation of the nail often will facilitate passage and prevent a cortical breach during impaction. |
| **Difficulty in reduction** | ■ The humerus commonly reduces easily with manual traction.<br>■ If the fracture cannot be reduced closed, a small open approach to the fracture site allows removal of tissue preventing reduction. |
| **Skin irritation** | ■ Skin irritation is decreased with nails that are flush with the metaphysis. This is facilitated by using a larger drill than might otherwise be anticipated. Except in very small patients, a 4.5-mm drill is used to open the medullary canal during both antegrade and retrograde applications.<br>■ When the nails are cut off, care should be taken to impact these well into the bone without distracting the fracture site. |

## POSTOPERATIVE CARE

- A long-arm posterior splint or cast is often applied for comfort in the immediate postoperative setting. This is removed in the first 1 to 2 weeks postoperatively.
- Weight bearing can be started immediately if necessary in length-stable fractures. A platform type walker or crutch is often helpful for the patient.
- If appropriate for ipsilateral injuries, motion may be started 10 days postoperatively. A sling may be used for comfort during the first 10 to 14 days.
- If additional protection is desired, a fracture brace can be used to add additional stability.
- Patients should be followed for at least 6 months postoperatively until solid bony union and then as needed.

## OUTCOMES

- Patients with humeral fractures requiring stabilization at our institution have ranged from 4 to 16 years of age at the time of surgery. All of these fractures have gone on to union in acceptable alignment (**FIG 5**).[6]
- Retrograde nailing has been used in most patients (84%) and antegrade nailing was used in patients with significant soft tissue trauma about the elbow. Some of these patients had severe trauma with a number (23%) having open Gustilo class III fractures.[6,7]
- Nearly all patients have regained normal motion at the shoulder and elbow.
- The technique of nail placement is familiar to most surgeons who frequently treat pediatric fractures and requires little

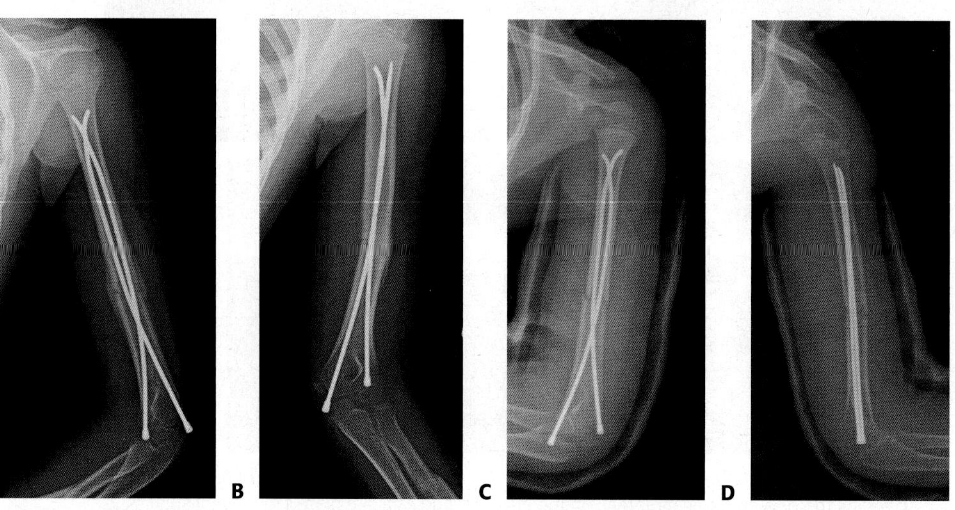


**FIG 5** ● **A,B.** Radiographs at 6 weeks postoperatively demonstrate final nail fixation, improved alignment, and fracture healing in the patient in all the technique figures. **C,D.** Postoperative radiographs of the patient in **FIG 2** show humeral nailing with elastic nails.

special equipment, but there are treatment details that are unique to the humerus.

- Collapse at the fracture site can cause nail migration and nail prominence under the skin.
- Stainless steel nails have demonstrated satisfactory results with humeral fixation and provide increased rigidity. They may result in a lower incidence of migration.[4]

## COMPLICATIONS

- Nail migration caused by fracture shortening in the first 6 weeks postoperatively has been the most frequent complication.[6]
- There have been no postoperative wound infections, delayed unions, refractures, or malunions reported to our knowledge.
- Motion deficits postoperatively are rare and have not caused functional deficit in any patients.

## REFERENCES

1. Beaty JH. Fractures of the proximal humerus and shaft in children. Instr Course Lect 1992;41:369–372.
2. Calfee RP, Manske PR, Gelberman RH, et al. Clinical Assessment of the ulnar nerve at the elbow: reliability of instability testing and the association of hypermobility with clinical symptoms. J Bone Joint Surg Am 2010;92(17):2801–2808. doi:10.2106/JBJS.J.00097.
3. Caviglia H, Garrido CP, Palazzi FF, et al. Pediatric fractures of the humerus. Clin Orthop Relat Res 2005;(432):49–56.
4. Chitgopkar SD. Flexible nailing of fractures in children using stainless steel Kirschner wires. J Pediatr Orthop B 2008;17(5):251–255. doi:10.1097/BPB.0b013e328306898d.
5. Gardner MJ, Griffith MH, Dines JS, et al. The extended anterolateral acromial approach allows minimally invasive access to the proximal humerus. Clin Orthop Relat Res 2005;(434):123–129.
6. Gordon JE, Garg S. Pediatric humerus fractures: indications and technique for flexible titanium intramedullary nailing. J Pediatr Orthop 2010;30:S73–S76. doi:10.1097/BPO.0b013e3181bbf19a.
7. Gustilo RB. Interobserver agreement in the classification of open fractures of the tibia. The results of a survey of two hundred and forty-five orthopaedic surgeons. J Bone Joint Surg Am 1995;77(8):1291–1292.
8. Knorr P, Schmittenbecher PP, Dietz HG. Elastic stable intramedullary nailing for the treatment of complicated juvenile bone cysts of the humerus. Eur J Pediatr Surg 2003;13(1):44–49. doi:10.1055/s-2003-38288.
9. Sarmiento A, Kinman PB, Galvin EG, et al. Functional bracing of fractures of the shaft of the humerus. J Bone Joint Surg Am 1977;59(5):596–601.
10. Sarmiento A, Latta L. The evolution of functional bracing of fractures. J Bone Joint Surg Br 2006;88(2):141–148. doi:10.1302/0301-620X.88B2.16381.
11. Shrader MW. Proximal humerus and humeral shaft fractures in children. Hand Clin 2007;23(4):431–435, vi. doi:10.1016/j.hcl.2007.09.002.

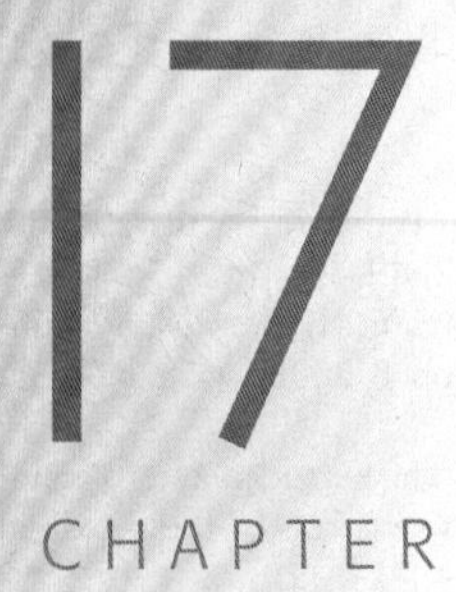

CHAPTER 17

# Plate Fixation of Humeral Shaft Fractures

Matthew J. Garberina and Charles L. Getz

## DEFINITION

- Humeral shaft fractures, which account for about 3% of adult fractures, usually result from a direct blow or indirect twisting injury to the brachium.
- These injuries are most commonly treated nonoperatively with a prefabricated fracture brace. The humerus is the most freely movable long bone, and anatomic reduction is not required.
- Patients often can tolerate up to 20 degrees of anterior angulation, 30 degrees of varus angulation, and 3 cm of shortening without significant functional loss.
- There are, however, several indications for surgical treatment of humeral shaft fractures:
  - Open fracture
  - Bilateral humeral shaft fractures or polytrauma; floating elbow
  - Segmental fracture
  - Inability to maintain acceptable alignment with closed treatment (ie, angulation >20 degrees, complete or near complete fracture displacement with lack of bony contact)—seen more commonly with transverse fractures (**FIG 1**)
  - Humeral shaft nonunion
  - Pathologic fractures
  - Arterial or brachial plexus injury
- Open reduction with internal plate fixation requires extensive dissection and operative skill. However, it offers advantages over intramedullary fixation because the rotator cuff is not violated, which leads to improved postoperative shoulder function.[3]

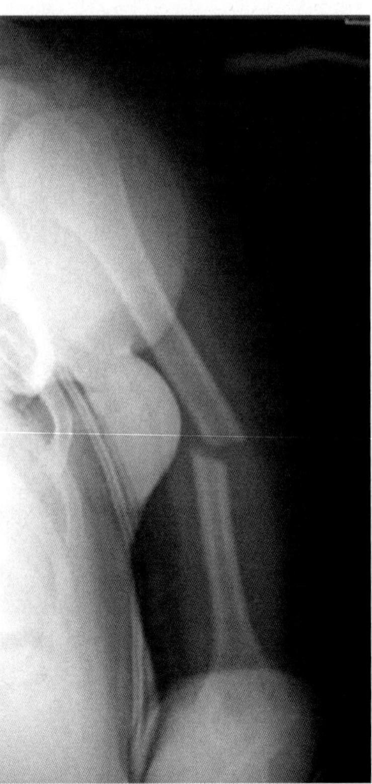

**FIG 1** • X-ray of an unstable transverse humeral shaft fracture.

## ANATOMY

- The humeral shaft is defined using key landmarks: the area between the upper margin of the pectoralis major tendon and the supracondylar ridge.[5]
- The blood supply of the humeral shaft comes from the posterior humeral circumflex vessels and branches of the brachial and profunda brachial arteries.
- The radial nerve and profunda brachial artery pass through the triangular interval (bordered superiorly by the teres major, medially by the medial head of the triceps, and laterally by the humeral shaft). The nerve then transverses from medial to lateral behind the humeral shaft and travels distally to a location between the brachialis and brachioradialis muscles (**FIG 2**).
- The musculocutaneous nerve lies on the undersurface of the biceps muscle and terminates distally as the lateral antebrachial cutaneous nerve.
- The humeral shaft has anteromedial, anterolateral, and posterior surfaces. Proximal and midshaft fractures are more amenable to plating on the anterolateral surface, whereas distal fractures often require posterior plate fixation.

## PATHOGENESIS

- Humeral shaft fractures occur after both direct and indirect injuries. Direct blows to the brachium can fracture the humeral shaft in a transverse pattern, often with a butterfly fragment. Injuries with high degrees of energy often result in a greater degree of fracture comminution.
- Indirect injuries, such as those that can occur with activities such as arm wrestling, often involve a twisting mechanism and result in a spiral fracture pattern. Higher energy injuries may result in muscle interposition between the fracture fragments, which can inhibit reduction and healing.
- A study of 240 humeral shaft fractures revealed radial nerve palsies in 42 patients, for an overall rate of 18% (17% in closed injuries). Fractures in the midshaft were more likely to have concomitant radial nerve palsy. Twenty five of these patients had complete recovery in a range of 1 day to 10 months. Ten patients did not have radial nerve recovery. Median and ulnar nerve palsies were seen very rarely in patients with open fractures.[7]
- Concomitant vascular injuries are present in about 3% of patients with humeral shaft fractures.

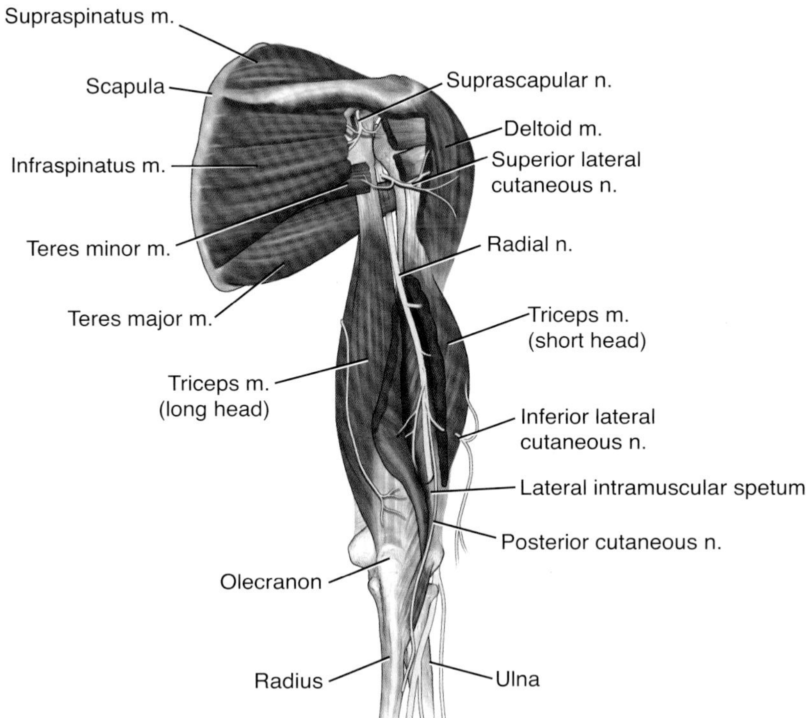


**FIG 2** • The course of the radial nerve along the position humerus is illustrated.

## NATURAL HISTORY

- Most humeral shaft fractures heal with nonoperative management. The most common treatment method is initial splinting from shoulder to wrist, followed by application of a prefabricated fracture brace when the patient is comfortable, usually within 2 weeks of the injury.
- Studies by Sarmiento and coauthors[10,11] have shown the effectiveness of functional bracing in the treatment of humeral shaft fractures. Nonunion rates with this method of treatment are in the 4% range, lower than seen when treating with external fixators, plates, or intramedullary nails.
- Closed fractures with initial radial nerve palsy can be observed, with expected recovery over a period of 3 to 6 months. Late-developing radial nerve palsies require surgical exploration.
- Angulation of the humeral shaft after fracture healing is expected and is well tolerated when it is less than 20 degrees. Varus deformity is most common.[10]
- Adjacent joint stiffness of the shoulder and elbow also is common. If the situation dictates treatment, physical therapy reliably restores joint motion in these patients.
- Relative contraindications to closed treatment include bilateral humeral shaft fractures or patients with polytrauma who require an intact brachium to ambulate. Transverse fractures and those with significant muscle imposition also are more amenable to operative fixation.[11]

## PATIENT HISTORY AND PHYSICAL FINDINGS

- The examining physician must perform a complete examination of the affected limb to rule out concomitant injuries.
- The skin should be thoroughly evaluated for evidence of an open fracture. This includes examination of the axilla. Entry and exit wounds are sought in gunshot victims. Swelling is common, and the patient may have an obvious deformity.
- The patient often braces the affected limb to his or her side, making evaluation of shoulder and elbow range of motion difficult. Bony prominences should be gently palpated to evaluate for other injuries, such as an olecranon fracture.
- Evaluate the appearance and skeletal stability of the forearm to rule out the presence of a coexisting both-bone forearm fracture ("floating elbow"). This finding necessitates operative fixation of humeral, radial, and ulnar fractures.
- Determine the vascular status of the upper extremity by palpating the radial and ulnar pulses at the wrist. Compare these findings with the unaffected limb. Selected cases may require Doppler arterial examination.[2]
- A complete neurologic assessment is necessary, with particular attention focused on the status of the radial nerve. This structure is at risk proximally, as it passes posteriorly to the humeral shaft after emerging from the triangular interval, as well as distally, as it lies adjacent to the supracondylar ridge (near the location of the Holstein-Lewis distal one-third spiral humeral shaft fracture).
- Examine sensory function in the first dorsal web space, wrist extension, and thumb interphalangeal joint extension to determine the functional status of the radial nerve.

## IMAGING AND OTHER DIAGNOSTIC STUDIES

- At least two plain radiographs at 90-degree angles to each other are necessary to evaluate the displacement, shortening, and comminution of the humeral shaft fracture.
- Radiographic views of the shoulder and elbow are necessary to rule out proximal extension of the shaft fracture or

concomitant elbow injury (ie, olecranon fracture). This is especially important in high-energy injuries.
- If swelling or evidence of skeletal instability about the forearm is present, dedicated forearm radiographs can determine the presence of a floating elbow (ie, ipsilateral humeral shaft fracture plus both-bone forearm fractures).

## DIFFERENTIAL DIAGNOSIS

- Distal humerus fracture
- Proximal humerus fracture
- Elbow dislocation
- Shoulder dislocation

## NONOPERATIVE MANAGEMENT

- Most isolated humeral shaft fractures can be treated nonoperatively. Initial treatment can vary with fracture location and involves splinting in either a posterior elbow or coaptation splint. The elbow is positioned in 90 degrees of flexion. An isolated humeral shaft fracture rarely necessitates an overnight hospital stay.
- In the past, definitive nonoperative treatment involved coaptation splinting or the use of hanging arm casts. Currently, functional fracture bracing provides adequate bony alignment, whereas local muscle compression and fracture motion promote osteogenesis. These braces provide soft tissue compression and allow functional use of the extremity.[11]
- Timing of brace application depends on the degree of swelling and patient discomfort. On average, the brace is applied about 2 weeks after the injury. A collar and cuff help with initial patient comfort and should be worn during recumbency until the fracture heals.
- The brace often requires frequent retightening over the first 2 weeks as swelling subsides. Elbow and wrist range-of-motion exercises out of the sling are encouraged.
- Functional bracing requires that the patient be able to sit erect, and weight bearing on the humerus is not allowed. The level of humeral shaft fracture does not preclude the use of functional bracing, even if the fracture line extends above or below the brace.
- Anatomic alignment of the humerus rarely is achieved, with varus deformity most common. However, patients often are able to tolerate the bony angulation and still perform activities of daily living after injury. A cosmetic deformity rarely exists.
- Pendulum exercises are encouraged as soon as possible postinjury. Active elevation and abduction are avoided until bony healing has occurred to prevent fracture angulation. The surgeon obtains radiographs after brace application and again 1 week later. If alignment is acceptable, repeat radiographs are obtained at 3- to 4- week intervals until fracture healing occurs.[10,11]

## SURGICAL MANAGEMENT

- Certain humeral shaft fractures are not amenable to conservative treatment. Open fractures or high-energy injuries with significant axial distraction are treated with open reduction and internal fixation. Patients with polytrauma, bilateral humeral shaft fractures, vascular injury, or an inability to sit erect are best treated with operative fixation. Unacceptable fracture alignment requires abandonment of nonoperative treatment. Finally, humeral shaft nonunion is a clear indication for open reduction and internal fixation with bone grafting.[4,9]

### Preoperative Planning

- The surgeon must review all radiographic images and must rule out ipsilateral elbow or shoulder injury.[1]
- Preoperative radiographs help the surgeon estimate the required plate length. Higher energy injuries with comminution may benefit from plating and supplemental bone grafting. The surgeon must plan for various scenarios based on these studies: Moderate comminution or bone loss can be addressed with cancellous allograft or autograft bone, whereas more extensive bone defects may require strut grafting.
- Proximal and middle-third humeral shaft fractures are addressed using an anterolateral approach. Distal-third humeral shaft fractures often are treated via a posterior approach because the distal humeral shaft is flat posteriorly, making it an ideal location for plate placement.
- Fracture patterns with extension into the proximal humerus can be exposed with a deltopectoral extension to the anterolateral humeral dissection. Often, a long, anatomic proximal humeral locking plate is helpful to ensure adequate superior fixation (**FIG 3**).

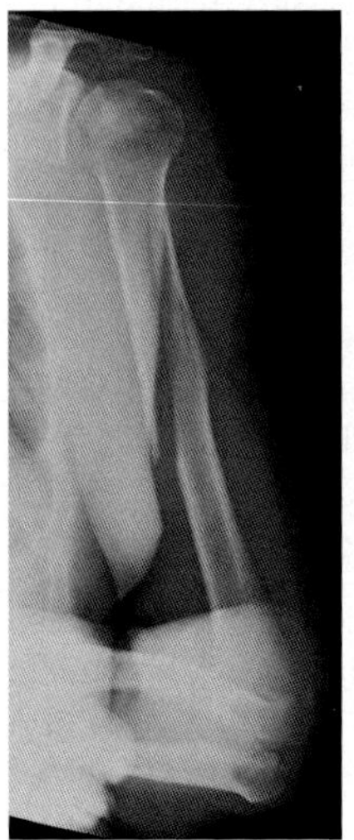
A

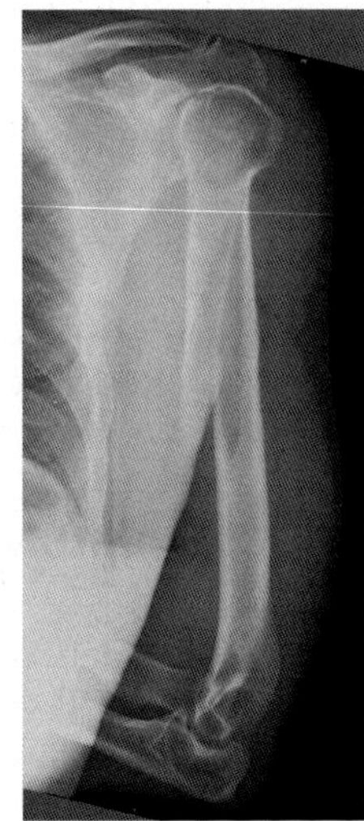
B

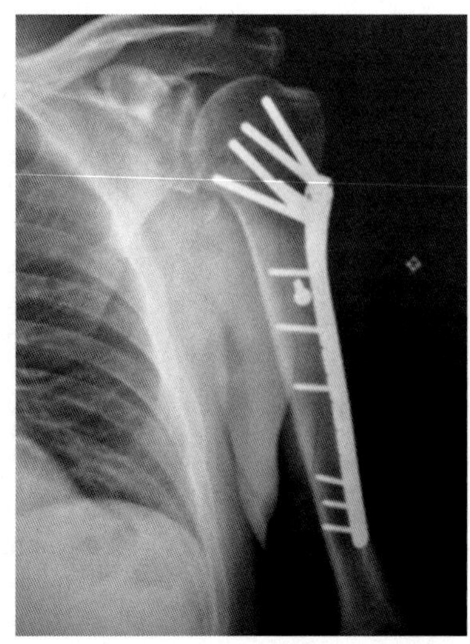
C

**FIG 3** • **A.** Anteroposterior (AP) and (**B**) lateral views of a humeral shaft fracture with proximal extension. **C.** A deltopectoral approach extended distally into an anterolateral approach allows proper exposure and placement of a long proximal humeral locking plate.

- The surgeon notes any preexisting scars that may affect the desired surgical approach, and neurovascular status is documented, with particular attention to radial nerve function.

## Positioning

- Positioning depends on the intended surgical approach. For an anterolateral or medial approach, the patient is brought to the edge of the bed in the supine position. A hand table is attached to the bed, and the patient's injured arm is placed on the hand table in slight abduction (**FIG 4A**).
- For a posterior approach, the patient can be placed prone or in the lateral decubitus position. A stack of pillows can support the brachium during the procedure (**FIG 4B**).

## Approach

- The approach depends on fracture location and the presence of any previous surgical incisions. The anterolateral and posterior approaches to the humerus are used most commonly, for proximal two-thirds and distal-third fractures, respectively.
- In patients who have already undergone multiple procedures to the affected extremity, Jupiter[6] recommends consideration of a medial approach to take advantage of virgin tissue planes.

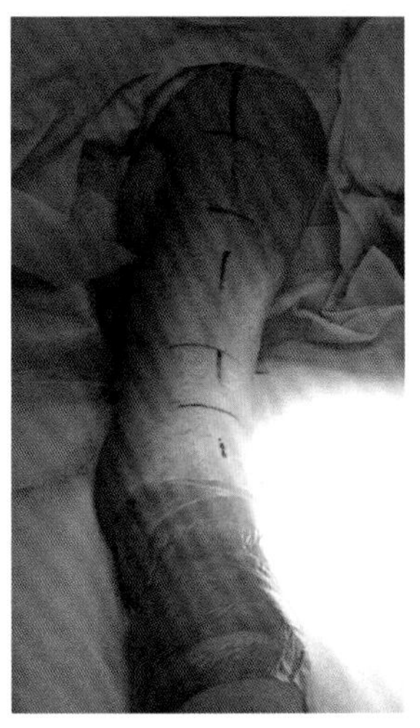
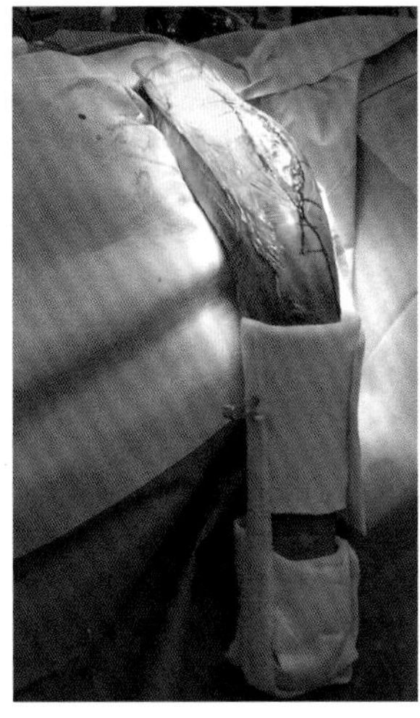

**FIG 4** • **A.** Positioning for the anterolateral approach to the humeral shaft with the shoulder abducted and the arm on a hand table. **B.** Positioning for the posterior approach to the humeral shaft with the patient in the lateral decubitus position.

TECHNIQUES

## Anterolateral Approach to the Humerus

- The incision courses over the lateral aspect of the biceps, beginning proximally at the deltoid tubercle and terminating just proximal to the antecubital crease (**TECH FIG 1A**). For more proximal fractures, the incision may extend proximally toward the coracoid to allow deltopectoral exposure.
- A tourniquet rarely is used because it often limits proximal exposure. The biceps fascia is incised in line with the incision to expose the underlying biceps muscle (**TECH FIG 1B**).
- The lateral antebrachial cutaneous nerve lies in the distal aspect of the incision and must be protected if exposure extends far distally.
- Bluntly enter the interval between the biceps and brachialis by sweeping a finger from proximal to distal and lateral to medial.
- At the level of the midhumerus, identify the musculocutaneous nerve on the undersurface of the biceps muscle (**TECH FIG 1C**). Trace this nerve out distally to protect its terminal branch, which forms the lateral antebrachial cutaneous nerve.
- Distally, the interval between the brachialis and brachioradialis is dissected to expose the radial nerve (**TECH FIG 1D**). Protect the radial nerve with a vessel loop so that it can be identified at all times.
- The brachialis is split in line with its fibers between the medial two-thirds and lateral one-third. This is an internervous plane between the radial nerve medially and the musculocutaneous nerve laterally (**TECH FIG 1E**).
- Identify the fracture site and remove any hematoma. Sharply remove fragments of periosteum off of the fracture ends to aid in reduction (**TECH FIG 1F**).

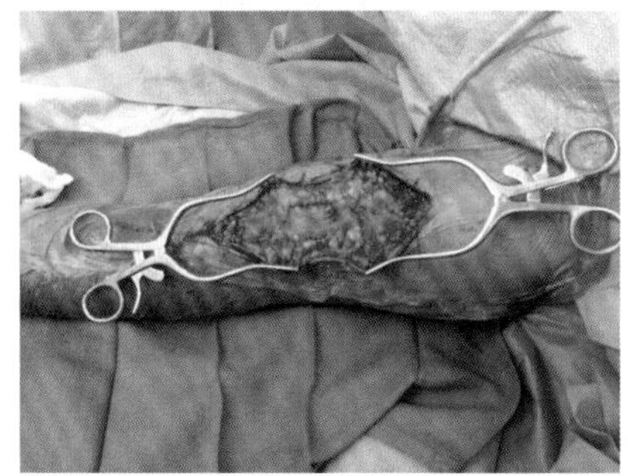
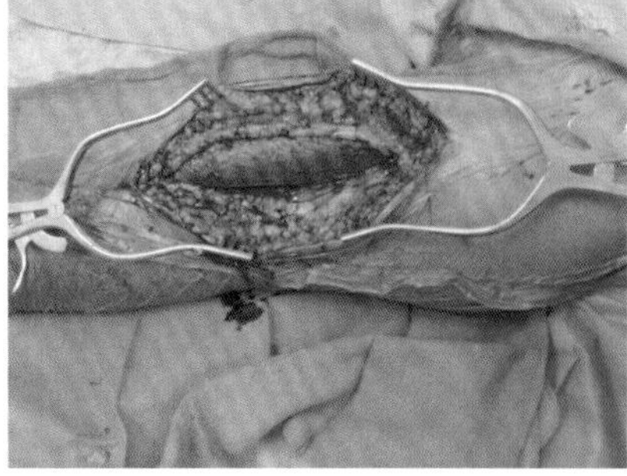

**TECH FIG 1** • **A.** Initial incision along the anterolateral brachium with exposure of the biceps fascia. **B.** The biceps fascia is incised in line with the skin incision exposing the underlying biceps muscle. *(continued)*

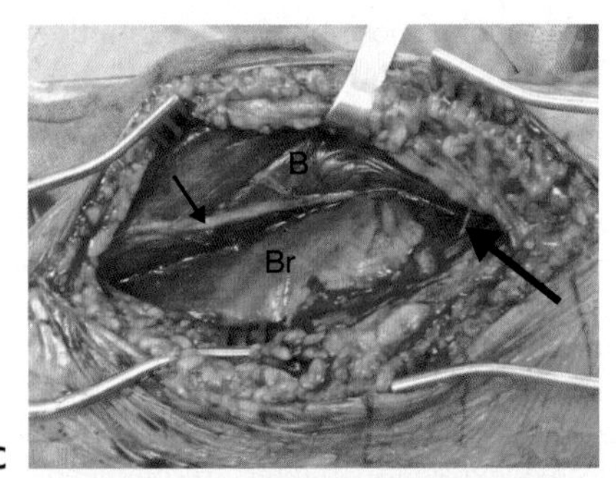


C

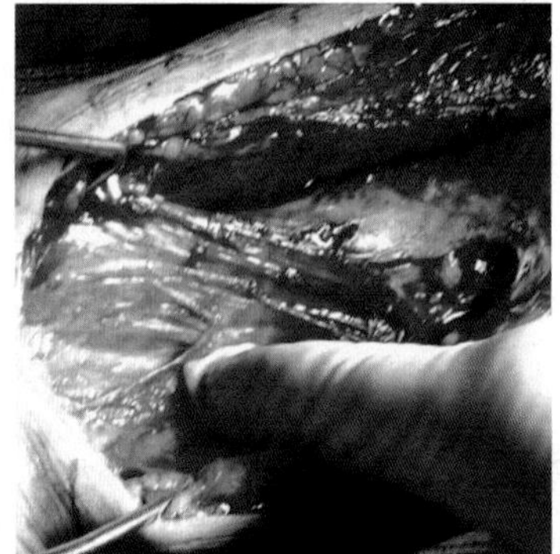

D

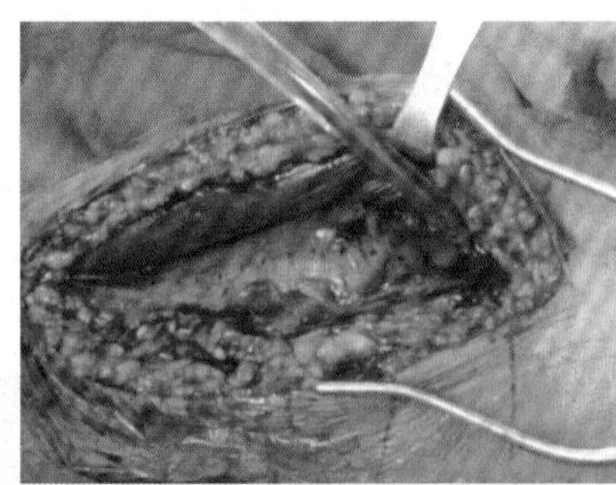

E

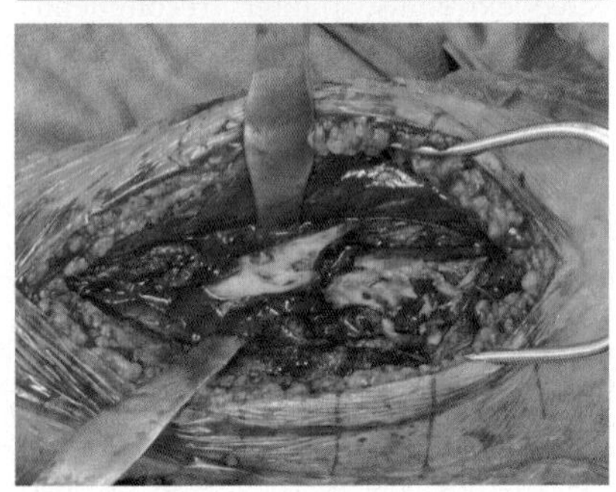

F

**TECH FIG 1** • *(continued)* **C.** The biceps (*B*) is bluntly lifted up exposing the underlying musculocutaneous nerve (*small arrow*), brachialis muscle (*Br*), and proximal vascular leash (*large arrow*). **D.** Radial nerve in interval between brachialis and brachioradialis. **E.** The brachialis is incised at the interval between its lateral and middle thirds. **F.** The fracture is well visualized through the brachialis split.

## Exposure of Fracture Nonunion

- Exposure of the radial nerve is more challenging, but it is very important in this situation. In many cases, it is best to dissect out the nerve distally in the interval between the brachialis and brachioradialis and proximally medial to the spiral groove. The nerve is then carefully dissected free from the nonunion site.
- Pinpoint the exact location of the nonunion with a no. 15 scalpel.
- The ends of the nonunion can be brought out through the wound, and all fibrous material is extracted.
- After thorough fracture débridement, the amount of bone loss becomes clear. The surgeon can now determine whether standard cancellous bone grafting or strut grafting is necessary.

## Posterior Approach to the Humerus

- Make a generous incision over the midline of the posterior arm extending to the olecranon fossa (**TECH FIG 2**).
- Identify the interval between the long and lateral heads of the triceps proximally. Bluntly dissect this interval, taking the long head medially and the lateral head laterally.
- Distally, several blood vessels cross this plane; they require coagulation before transection.
- Identify the radial nerve proximal to the medial head of the triceps in the spiral groove. Protect the radial nerve throughout the case.
- Split the medial head of the triceps in its midline from proximal to distal to expose the fracture site.

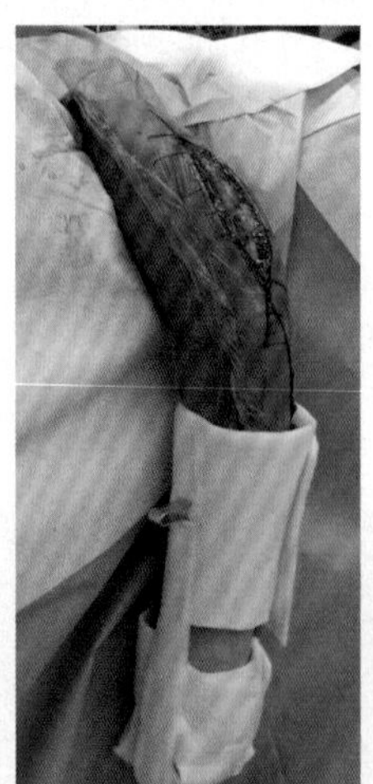

A

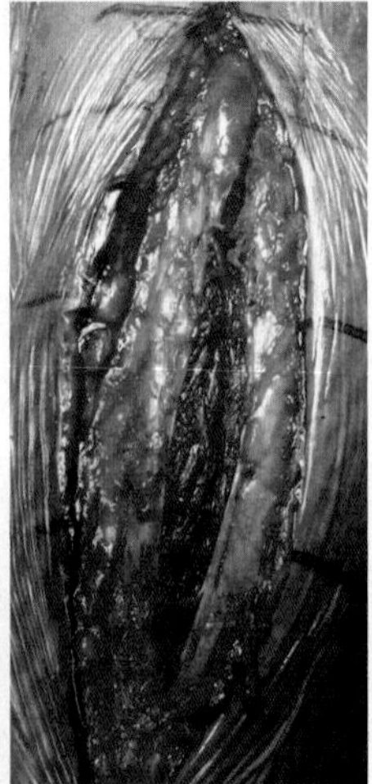

B

**TECH FIG 2** • **A.** Incision for posterior approach. **B.** Superficial triceps split. *(continued)*

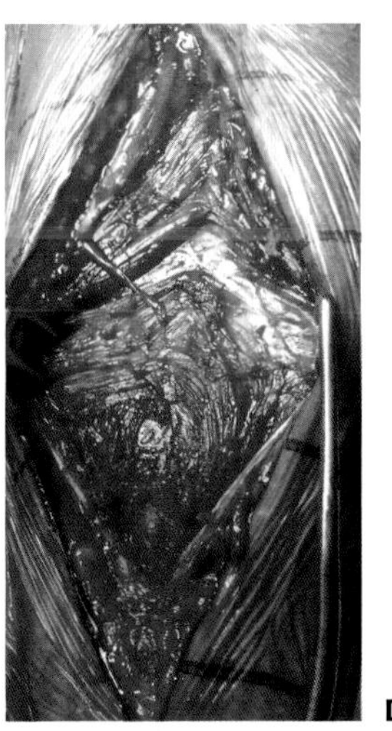

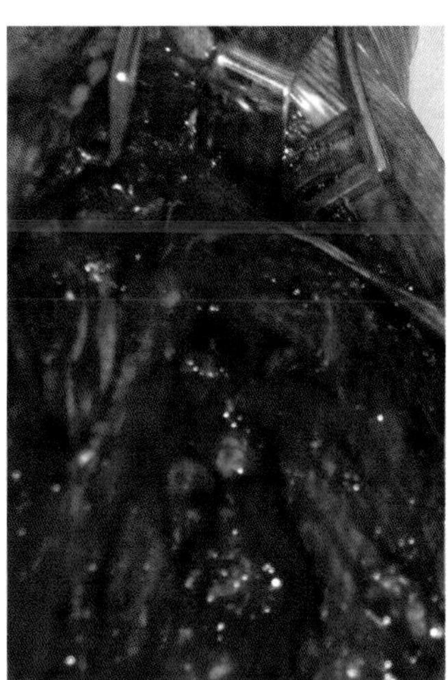

**TECH FIG 2** • *(continued)* **C.** Deep triceps split. **D.** The probe points to the radial nerve as it exits the spiral groove from medial to lateral; the fracture site is seen distally.

## Medial Approach

- Positioning is similar to the anterolateral approach.
- Make an incision over the medial intermuscular septum from the axilla to 5 cm proximal to the medial epicondyle (**TECH FIG 3**).
- Mobilize the ulnar nerve.
- Resect the medial intermuscular septum; identify and coagulate the adjacent venous plexus with bipolar electrocautery.
- Mobilize the triceps posteriorly and the biceps/brachialis anteriorly.
- Expose the fracture site.
- The axillary incision raises concern for infection; there is also concern that the ulnar nerve can scar to the plate.

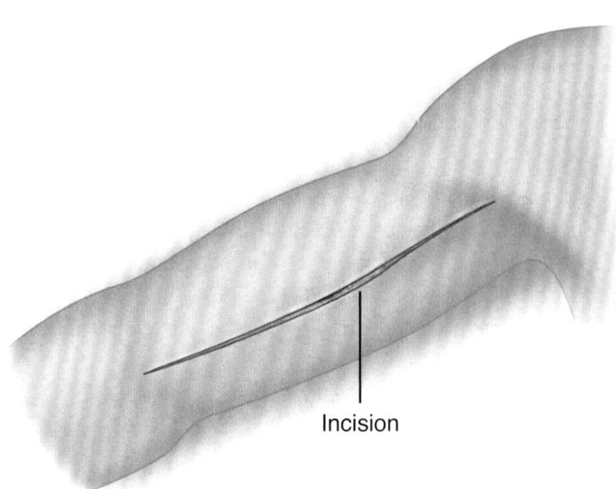


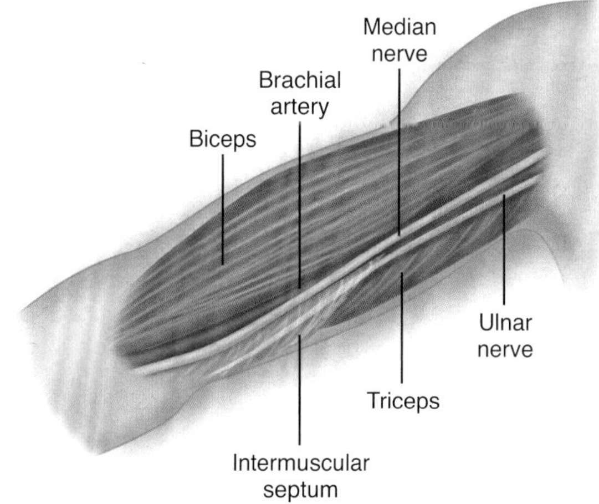


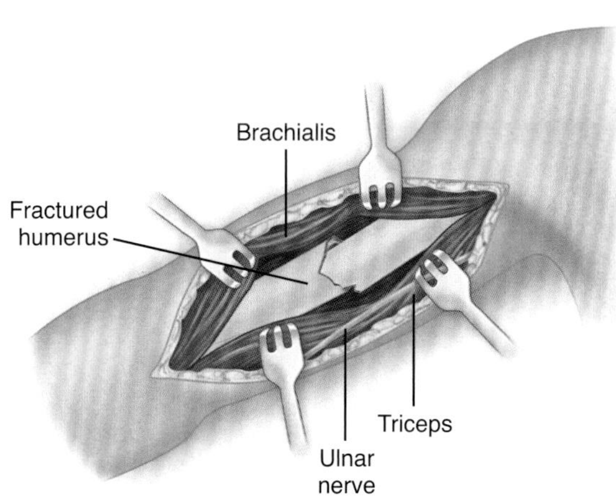


**TECH FIG 3** • **A.** Incision for the medial approach. **B,C.** The brachialis and biceps are raised anteriorly, and the triceps is raised posteriorly for fracture exposure.

## Fracture Reduction

- Sharp periosteal dissection exposes the fracture site. Evaluate the degree, if any, of comminution.
- Limit periosteal stripping to adequately expose the fracture. Make every attempt to leave some soft tissue attached to each fragment so as not to devascularize the fragments.
- Gentle traction and rotation often can bring the fracture fragments into better alignment.
- Anatomically reduce the fracture with one or more reduction clamps. It is advisable to reduce the fracture completely before definitive fixation, and this often requires the use of multiple reduction clamps (**TECH FIG 4A**).
- After the fracture is reduced, 3.5- or 4.5-mm interfragmentary screws can be used to hold the fracture aligned until plate fixation. Temporary Kirschner wires may also be used in this capacity.
- Alternatively, fractures with minimal comminution often can be directly reduced with the plate and Faberge clamps (**TECH FIG 4B,C**).

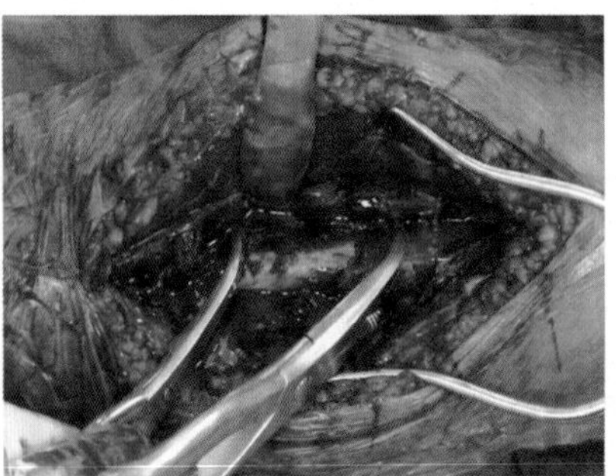
A

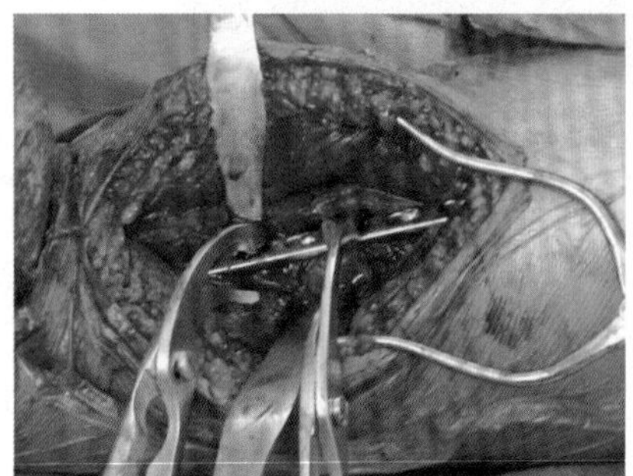
B

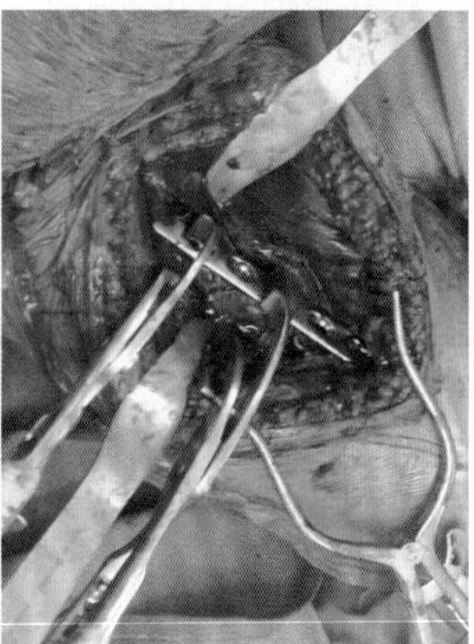
C

**TECH FIG 4 • A.** Bone reduction clamps help realign the fracture ends. **B,C.** Verbrugge clamps can hold plate and fracture alignment intact prior to drilling and placement of cortical screws.

## Plate Application

- After fracture reduction, the plate length is determined.
- Humeral shaft fractures require at least six cortices of fixation above and below the fracture site (**TECH FIG 5A**).
- In larger bones, a broad 4.5-mm dynamic compression plate can provide optimal fixation. In smaller bones, a 4.5-mm limited contour dynamic compression plate often provides a better fit.
- Provisionally, place the plate on a flat surface of the humerus and hold it in place with a plate-holding clamp.
- A 4.5-mm cortical screws are placed through the plate holes proximal and distal to the fracture. Compression techniques can be used where appropriate (**TECH FIG 5B**).
- Ensure that no soft tissue, especially nerve, is trapped between the plate and the bone.
- Make sure to obtain screw purchase in at least six cortices above and below the fracture (**TECH FIG 5C**).
- Cerclage wiring over the plate can add supplemental fixation, especially in weak bone (**TECH FIG 5D**).
- Rotate the arm and flex and extend the elbow to evaluate fracture stability.
- Apply cancellous bone graft into defects as needed.
- Close the brachialis over the plate (**TECH FIG 6**).

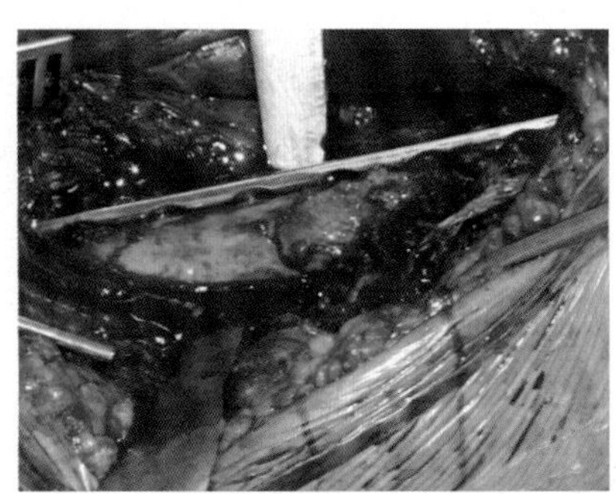
A

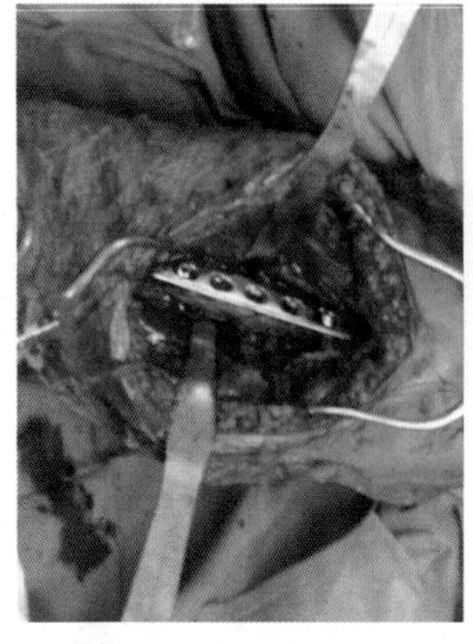
B

**TECH FIG 5 • A.** Stable fixation requires six cortices of fixation above and below the fracture. **B.** A 4.5-mm cortical screws are placed in compression mode proximal and distal to the fracture. *(continued)*

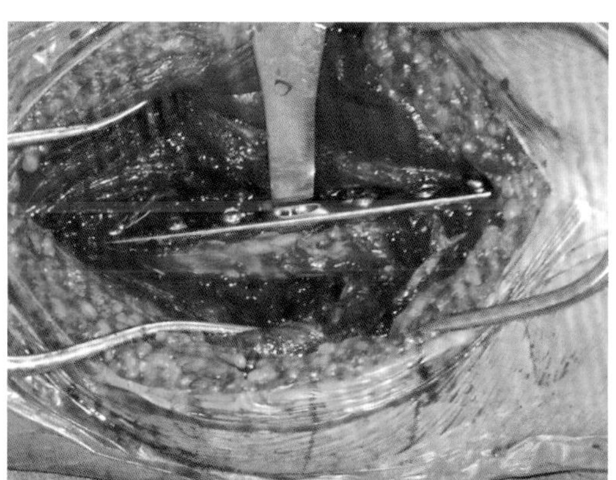

C

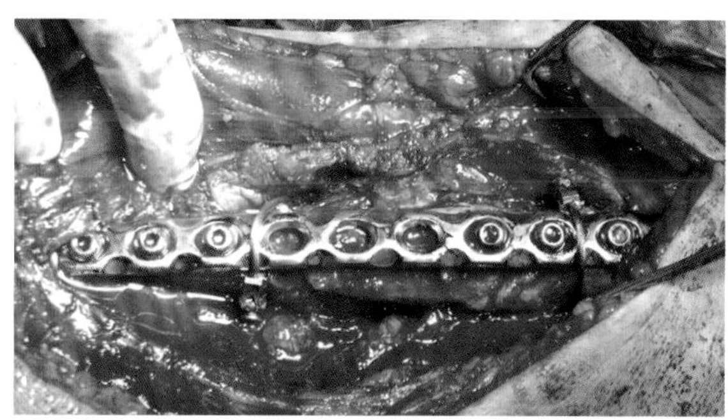

D

**TECH FIG 5** • *(continued)* **C.** Six cortices of fixation proximal and distal to the fracture site. **D.** Supplemental cerclage wire fixation can augment stability in weak bone.

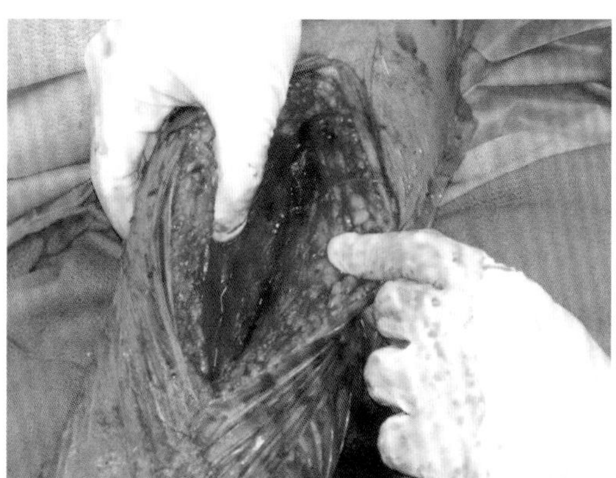

**TECH FIG 6** • Close the brachialis interval after definitive fracture fixation.

## PEARLS AND PITFALLS

| | |
|---|---|
| **Indications** | ■ Operative treatment is reserved for open fractures, patients with multiple fractures, and fractures with inadequate reduction. |
| **Preoperative planning** | ■ Review all radiographs and determine the best surgical approach.<br>■ Estimate potential plate length and prepare for possible bone grafting. |
| **Surgical exposure** | ■ Locate and protect the radial nerve.<br>■ Expose and reduce fracture fragments and temporarily hold them in place with pins or clamps.<br>■ Alternatively, fix larger fragments with interfragmentary screws. |
| **Plate fixation** | ■ Ensure that plate length allows six cortices of fixation proximal and distal to the fracture.<br>■ Use 4.5-mm dynamic compression plates or limited contact dynamic compression plates.<br>■ Use compressive techniques when indicated. |
| **Radial nerve function** | ■ Preoperatively, document a detailed neurovascular examination.<br>■ Ensure that the radial nerve is not trapped within the plate before closure. |

## POSTOPERATIVE CARE

- Postoperative radiographs ensure proper fracture alignment and plate placement (**FIG 5**).
- Initially, the patient can be placed in a sling or posterior elbow splint. This is removed and range-of-motion exercises are started when patient comfort allows (usually 1 to 2 days postoperative).
- Weight bearing on the affected upper extremity is allowed based on patient comfort.[12]
- Initial therapy consists of elbow range-of-motion, shoulder pendulum, and passive self-assisted exercises.
- The patient can come out of the sling after 2 weeks and start waist-level activities with the operative arm.

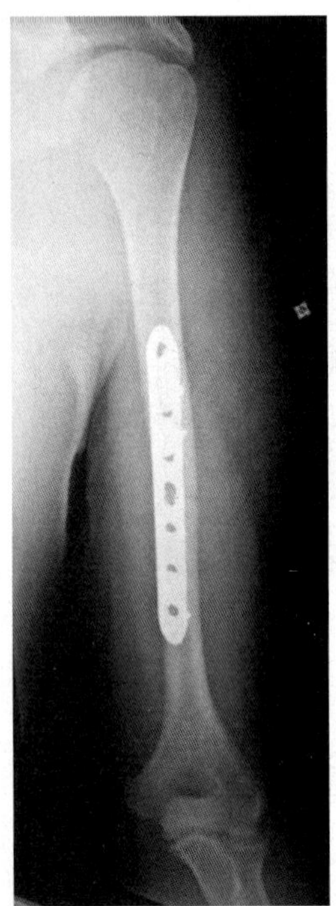

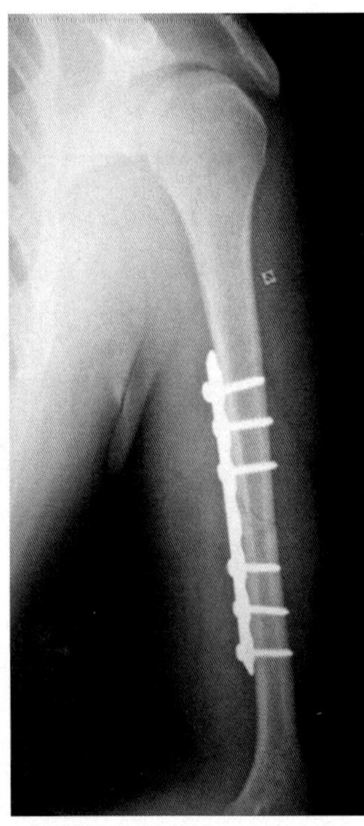

**FIG 5** ● **A,B.** AP and lateral radiographs after humeral shaft fixation with a 4.5-mm dynamic and compression (DC) plate and screws.

- At 6 weeks, elbow motion should be near normal range, and shoulder strengthening is added to the patient's physical therapy.
- At 3 months, radiographs should reveal some callus formation. If no callus is evident, radiographs are repeated every 6 weeks until evidence of healing appears.

## OUTCOMES

- Plate fixation leads to union in 90% to 98% of cases.
- Plating offers decreased complication rates compared to intramedullary nailing, especially in terms of shoulder dysfunction.[8]
- Iatrogenic radial nerve palsy occurs in about 2% to 5% of cases and usually resolves in 3 to 6 months. Electromyography helps monitor return of nerve function in patients with prolonged palsy. Radial nerve exploration is indicated when no nerve function returns by 6 months.
- Elbow and shoulder range of motion usually return to normal postoperatively.

## COMPLICATIONS

- Infection
- Nonunion
- Malunion
- Hardware failure
- Radial nerve palsy
- Shoulder impingement
- Elbow stiffness

## REFERENCES

1. Garberina MJ, Getz CL, Beredjiklian P, et al. Open reduction and internal fixation of humeral shaft nonunions. Tech Shoulder Elbow Surg 2006;7:131–138.
2. Gregory PR. Fractures of the shaft of the humerus. In: Bucholz RW, Heckman JD, eds. Rockwood and Green's Fractures in Adults, ed 5, vol 1. Philadelphia: Lippincott Williams & Wilkins, 2001: 973–996.
3. Gregory PR, Sanders RW. Compression plating versus intramedullary fixation of humeral shaft fractures. J Am Acad Orthop Surg 1997;5:215–223.
4. Healy WL, White GM, Mick CA, et al. Nonunion of the humeral shaft. Clin Orthop Relat Res 1987;(219):206–213.
5. Hoppenfeld S, deBoer P. Surgical Exposures in Orthopaedics: The Anatomic Approach. Philadelphia: Lippincott Williams & Wilkins, 1994:51–82.
6. Jupiter JB. Complex non-union of the humeral diaphysis. Treatment with a medial approach, an anterior plate, and a vascularized fibular graft. J Bone Joint Surg Am 1990;72(5):701–707.
7. Mast JW, Spiegel PG, Harvey JP Jr, et al. Fractures of the humeral shaft: a retrospective study of 240 adult fractures. Clin Orthop Relat Res 1975;(112):254–262.
8. McCormack RG, Brien D, Buckley RE, et al. Fixation of fractures of the shaft of the humerus by dynamic compression plate or intramedullary nail. A prospective, randomised trial. J Bone Joint Surg Br 2000;82(3):336–339.
9. Ring D, Perey BH, Jupiter JB. The functional outcome of operative treatment of ununited fractures of the humeral diaphysis in older patients. J Bone Joint Surg Am 1999;81(2):177–190.
10. Sarmiento A, Latta LL. Functional fracture bracing. J Am Acad Orthop Surg 1999;7:66–75.
11. Sarmiento A, Waddell JP, Latta LL. Diaphyseal humeral fractures: treatment options. J Bone Joint Surg Am 2001;83A:1566–1579.
12. Tingstad EM, Wolinsky PR, Shyr Y, et al. Effect of immediate weightbearing on plated fractures of the humeral shaft. J Trauma 2000;49:278–280.

# Pediatric Proximal Humerus Fractures

Craig P. Eberson

18 CHAPTER

## DEFINITION

- Proximal humerus fractures (physeal and metaphyseal) are common in the pediatric population.
- Most of these injuries can be treated nonoperatively because of the significant remodeling potential.
- Certain fractures will require operative treatment, however, due to decreased remodeling capacity in the older child or fractures with open or threatened skin.
- Opinion varies on the need for surgical repair, although most do well treated nonoperatively.[2,5]
- Aggressive surgical treatment for these injuries is rarely indicated for most children.

## ANATOMY

- The proximal humeral physis is responsible for 80% of humeral growth. It remains open usually until age 14 to 17 years in girls and age 18 years in boys.
  - A major portion of the physis is extracapsular and vulnerable to injury.
  - The anterior periosteum is usually thinner than the posterior, often leading to hinging of the fragments posteriorly and possible entrapment of the periosteum anteriorly.
- The proximal humerus lies in close proximity to the brachial plexus and axillary vessels. Care should be taken to document function of the innervated musculature before initiating treatment (**FIG 1**).

## PATHOGENESIS

- Injuries to the proximal humerus occur from either a direct blow to the region or indirect trauma, such as a fall onto the outstretched hand.

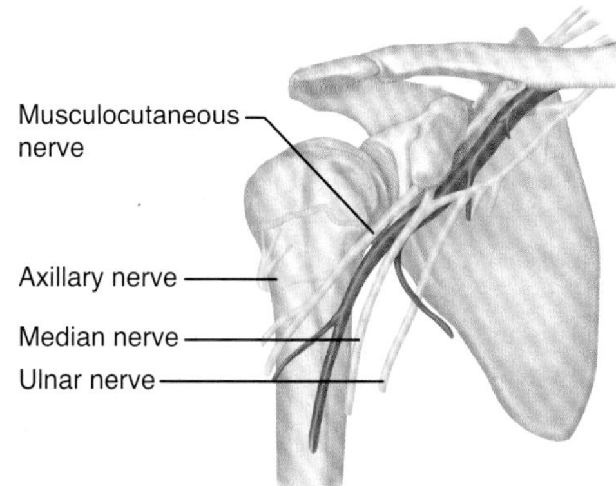


**FIG 1** • Relationship of the brachial plexus and axillary artery to the proximal humerus. The axillary nerve wraps around the humerus to insert into the deltoid, roughly 5 cm distal to the acromion.

  - In cases of pathologic fractures through bone cysts, throwing a ball or reaching overhead can precipitate an injury.

## NATURAL HISTORY

- Because of the significant remodeling potential in young children, most patients will heal without sequelae from fractures of the proximal humerus or clavicle.
- Morbidity from associated injuries, however, may be significant and thus a thorough evaluation is of paramount importance.
- General guidelines are available to define acceptable healing alignment for proximal humeral fractures (Table 1).
  - Examples of complete or near-complete remodeling are readily found in the literature for even completely displaced fractures in children younger than 15 years old, however, so a clear understanding of the goals of the procedure and its associated risks is crucial.[1,4]

## PATIENT HISTORY AND PHYSICAL FINDINGS

- History should include mechanism of injury, antecedent pain, and neurologic symptoms in the hand and arm.
- A high-energy injury should also prompt a full trauma workup using standard Advanced Trauma Life Support protocols.
- Physical examination begins with a thorough assessment of the skin for areas of compromise, particularly with associated clavicle fractures.
- A neurologic examination to include the brachial plexus distribution, as well as a vascular examination of the arm, is necessary.
  - Neurologic injury in conjunction with fracture may signify ongoing compression (ie, sternoclavicular dislocation) and may affect prognosis.
  - A high suspicion for vascular injury is important in preventing late sequelae.

**Table 1 Acceptable Angulation for Proximal Humeral Fractures**

| Patient Age (y) | Maximum Acceptable Degrees of Angulation |
|---|---|
| <7 | 70 |
| 8–12 | 60 |
| >12 | 45 |

Modified from Dobbs MB, Luhmann SL, Gordon JE, et al. Severely displaced proximal humeral epiphyseal fractures. J Pediatr Orthop 2003;23:208–215.

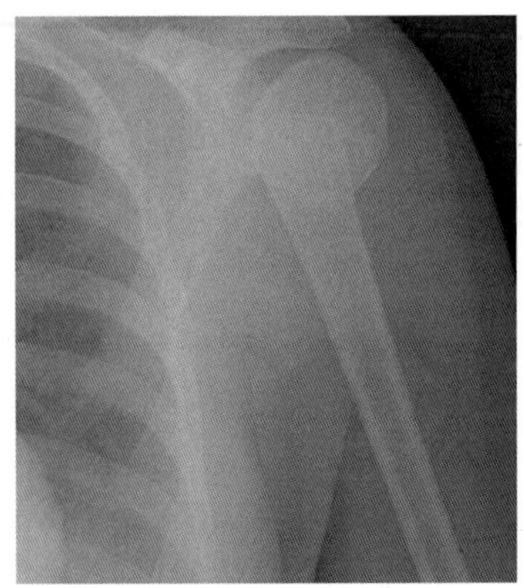

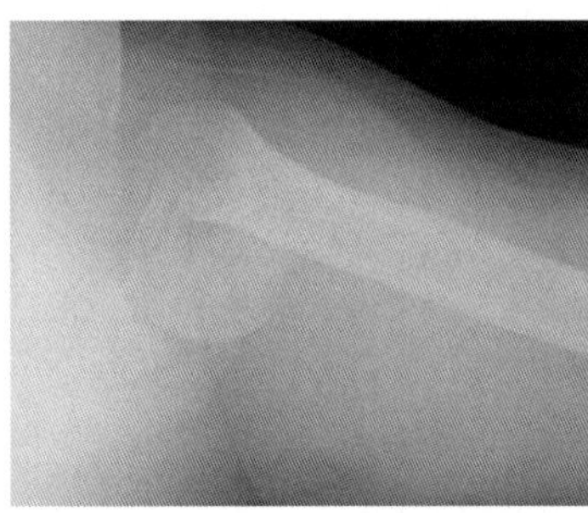

**FIG 2 • A,B.** Preoperative AP and lateral radiographs of a Salter-Harris type II fracture of the proximal humerus in a 15-year-old girl show mild valgus angulation and complete displacement with 90 degrees of angulation on the lateral view.

## IMAGING AND OTHER DIAGNOSTIC STUDIES

- Standard initial views of the shoulder should include a true anteroposterior (AP) view, a "shoot-through" lateral, and an axillary lateral view (**FIG 2**).

## DIFFERENTIAL DIAGNOSIS

- Proximal humerus metaphyseal fracture
- Proximal humerus physeal injury
- Shoulder dislocation
- Acromioclavicular fracture-dislocation
- Sternoclavicular fracture-dislocation
- Child abuse

## NONOPERATIVE MANAGEMENT

- Most of these injuries can be treated nonoperatively.
- For proximal humeral fractures with acceptable alignment, treatment consists of sling management for comfort for several weeks, followed by a home range-of-motion program and return to activities in 6 to 8 weeks.

## SURGICAL MANAGEMENT

- For physeal or metaphyseal fractures of the proximal humerus, operative treatment should be considered for fractures with unacceptable residual displacement.
- Closed reduction is often unstable and fixation is desirable.
- Because of open growth plates, standard plate fixation techniques are rarely indicated.
- Threaded wire fixation provides sufficient temporary fixation to allow healing.
  - Intramedullary elastic nailing is another option for these fractures.
- Failure to obtain a satisfactory closed reduction may require an open reduction, and surgeons should be familiar with this technique as well.
- Interposition of the biceps tendon has been noted to be the most common cause of a failed closed reduction,[3] but other authors disagree.[4]

## PREOPERATIVE PLANNING

- Good-quality radiographs of the shoulder should be available.
- It is important to rule out concomitant glenoid fracture or dislocation before surgery.

### Positioning

#### *Proximal Humerus Fractures*

- For proximal humeral fractures, the patient is positioned in a modified beach-chair position, with the back elevated roughly 30 degrees.
- The imaging machine is then brought in from the head of the table. It can be tilted "over the top" to get an AP view and rotated to get an axillary lateral view (**FIG 3**).
  - If the table is too upright, the AP view may be difficult to obtain because of limited excursion of the C-arm past neutral.
- A vacuum positioning device (beanbag) is positioned under the patient's head, neck, and upper torso. This allows the patient to be slid slightly over the edge of the table to allow full access to the shoulder girdle.
- A chest pad attached to the table prevents the patient from being pulled off the table inadvertently when traction is applied to the arm.
  - Alternately, a sheet can be wrapped around the torso and secured by an assistant on the opposite side of the table.

### Approach

#### *Proximal Humeral Fractures*

- Reduction of proximal humeral fractures is, generally speaking, a closed procedure.
- Interposed tissue may require an open approach, which is through the deltopectoral interval (**FIG 4**).

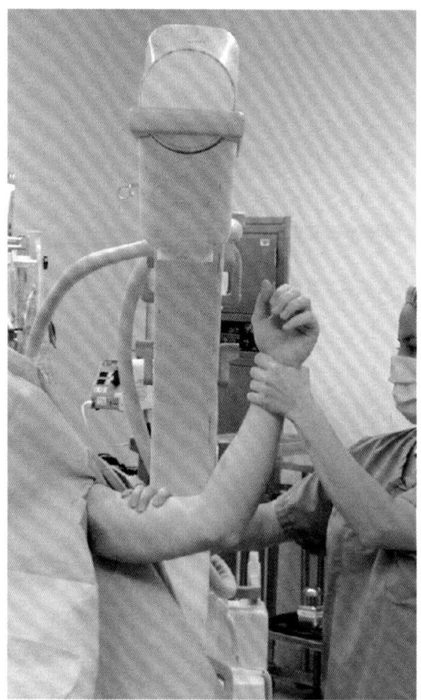

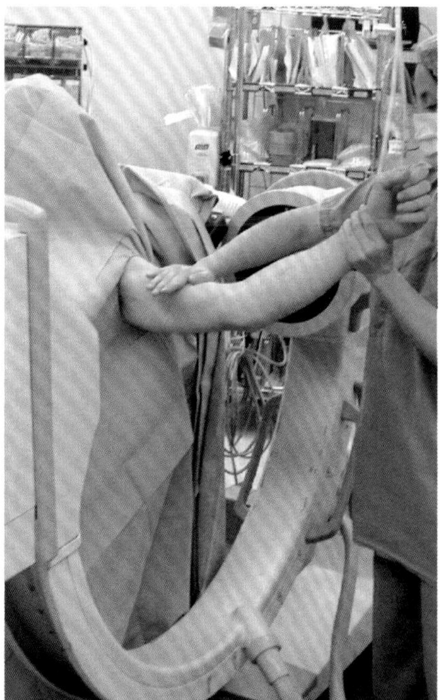

**FIG 3** • Intraoperative positioning for reduction. **A.** The patient is over the edge of the table with the entire arm exposed. The imaging machine is brought in from the head of the table. It is tilted into the over-the-top position to obtain a true AP view of the shoulder. Note the surgeon's hands; traction is applied with the left hand while the right helps to correct the adduction of the distal shaft fragment. **B.** Without moving the arm, the image can be rotated to obtain an axillary lateral view. In this simulated figure, the fluoroscopy unit is not draped for clarity; in practice, it is brought up beneath the drapes to maintain the sterile field. The surgeon is applying pressure to reduce the apex anterior angulation while maintaining traction with the left hand. Under the drapes, a chest pad prevents the patient from being pulled off the table with traction; a sheet wrapped around the torso and held by an assistant would accomplish the same purpose.

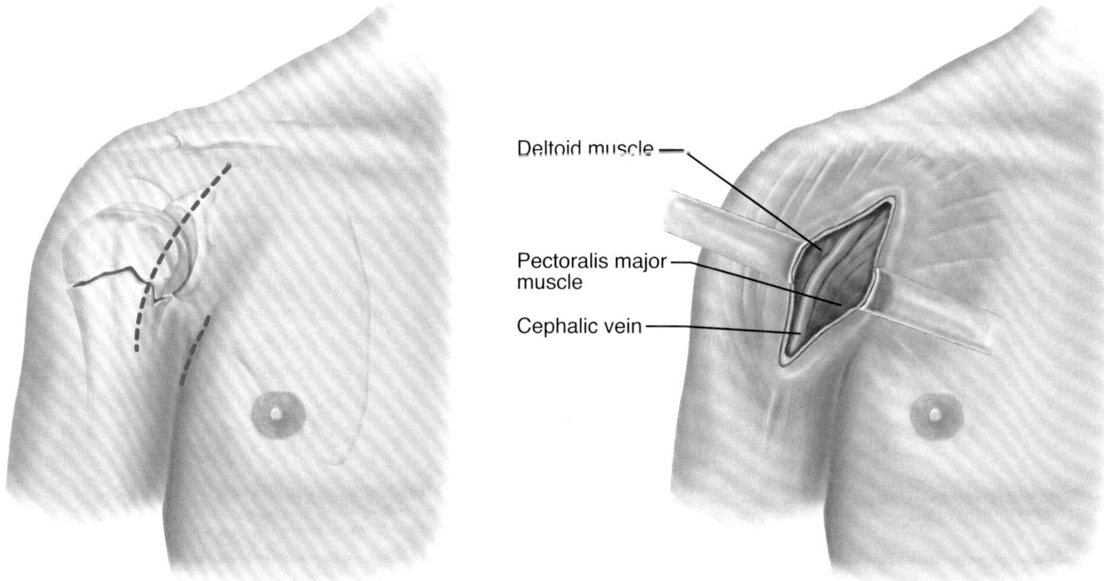


**FIG 4** • Approach for open reduction. **A.** One of two possible incisions is made: the standard incision made in the deltopectoral interval, which is helpful for wide displacement, or a more cosmetic incision in the axilla. In the latter incision, the skin is then undermined to perform the same deep dissection. **B.** The cephalic vein is identified as the marker for the interval. It is dissected free and the interval entered. *(continued)*

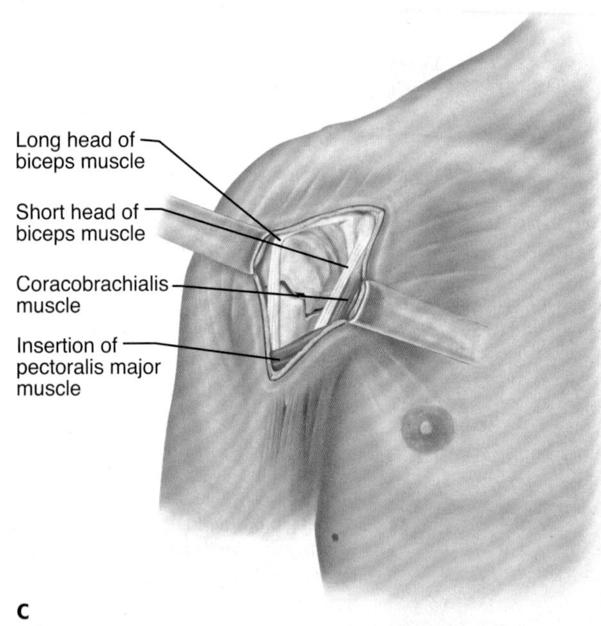


**FIG 4 •** *(continued)* **C.** The obstacles to reduction can now be cleared. Interposed biceps tendon, interposed periosteum, and buttonholing of the shaft through the deltoid are possible causes of inability to obtain a reduction.

TECHNIQUES

## Closed Reduction

- To reduce the fracture, the forces acting on the humerus need to be understood. The proximal fragment tends to be abducted and externally rotated due to the pull of the rotator cuff musculature, whereas the shaft is adducted from the pull of the pectoralis major muscle. To correct this, the first step is usually abduction and external rotation of the arm.
- Traction is then applied to disengage the fragments. It is helpful to have an assistant stabilize the torso.
- Usually, the shaft can be manipulated in line with the head at this point.
  - The typical angulation to be corrected is varus and apex anterior angulation.
  - It is often helpful to think about pushing down on the proximal end of the shaft to correct the angulation while maintaining abduction to correct the varus.
- In smaller, thin patients, it is possible to grasp the head through the axilla to assist with the reduction.
- Once reduced, stabilization ensues (see the following text).

## Open Reduction

- In rare cases, a closed reduction cannot be successfully achieved. A common cause is entrapment of periosteum or biceps tendon.
- In these cases, a small deltopectoral incision can be made.
  - This is a limited approach, not the wide extensile exposure needed for open reduction and internal fixation. In this approach, the skin can be opened in the axilla and then retracted upward. The interval can be bluntly divided until the fracture is exposed and any soft tissue cleared (ie, periosteum, biceps tendon). The fracture is then reduced and pinned in the standard fashion.
  - A finger can usually be inserted through a small opening to allow clearance of obstructing soft tissue.
- Fixation then ensues (see the following text).

## Percutaneous Pin Fixation

- Once reduced, the fracture is then stabilized.
- Threaded-tip pins, such as the 2.5-mm guide pins found in most cannulated hip screw systems, are ideal for pediatric use and are my first choice, although they are potentially unsuitable for use in osteoporotic adult bone. Fully threaded pins can also be used.
- It is important to understand the relationship of the important neurologic structures to the proximal humerus.
  - The axillary nerve lies in the deltoid muscle 5 cm (in an adult, less in a child) from the tip of the acromion laterally.
  - More anteriorly, the musculocutaneous nerve is at risk.
- Pins are placed through small stab incisions using a tissue protection sleeve after a hemostat has been used to spread the tissue down to the bone.
- Often, the reduction is stable enough to allow the arm to be placed down at the patient's side and internally rotated, which is the position of postoperative immobilization.
  - If not, the pin can be inserted in the abducted position, but on moving the arm down, the skin will then be tented by the pin.
  - A relaxing incision can be made, or the first pin put in provisionally, the arm moved to the patient's side, and the first pin removed after additional fixation has been obtained.

- The easiest pin to place first is usually from distal lateral to proximal medial (**TECH FIG 1A**).
  - The pin is started perpendicular to the shaft, and the surgeon's hand is then dropped to the correct angle.
  - It is important to make the initial approach down to the bone along the final angle of pin insertion to avoid skin tension problems later.
  - The pin is advanced into the head, stopping several millimeters below the subchondral bone.
- A second pin is then added (**TECH FIG 1B**).
  - I usually prefer to place this pin starting more proximally and anteriorly to the first pin.
  - If the first pin is aimed at the inferior portion of the head, the second can be aimed more superiorly for greater pin divergence across the fracture (**TECH FIG 1C**).
- If needed, a third pin can be added from the greater tuberosity downward into the shaft.
  - This is helpful in small patients for better purchase in the head, but I usually avoid this pin because of a higher rate of soft tissue complications.
- After fixation is complete, an "approach–withdrawal" test is performed (**TECH FIG 1D**), similar to that done for a slipped capital femoral epiphysis.
  - The shoulder is rotated, and the tips of the pins should appear to approach the joint surface and then withdraw with continued rotation.
  - Pins that appear too long should be pulled back.
- In larger patients near or at skeletal maturity with sufficient bone stock, cannulated screws can be inserted over a wire in the same fashion as described for threaded pins.
  - I have found this technique rarely necessary, but it does avoid the issue of pin management (see next technique).

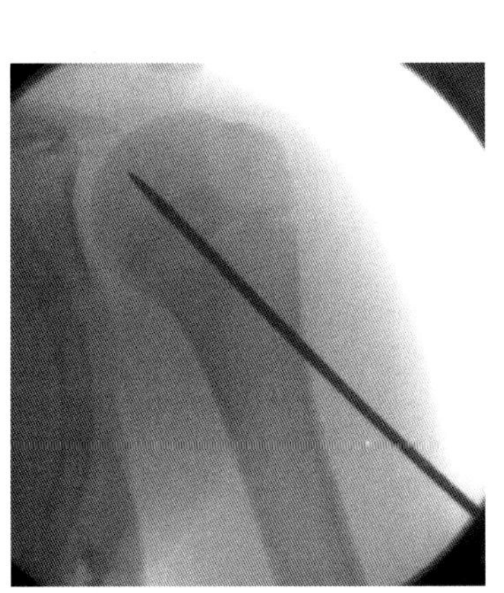
A

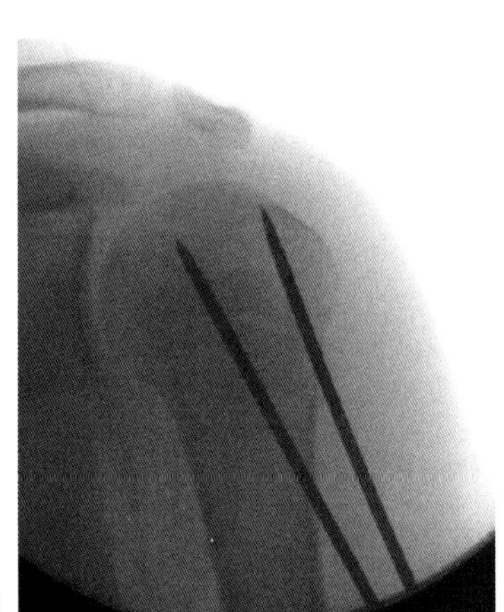
B

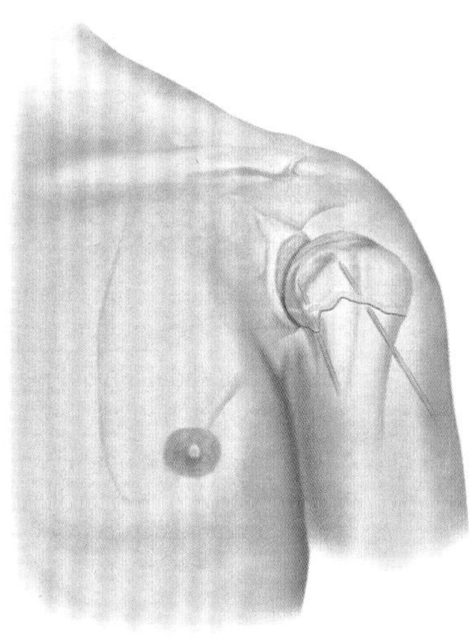
C

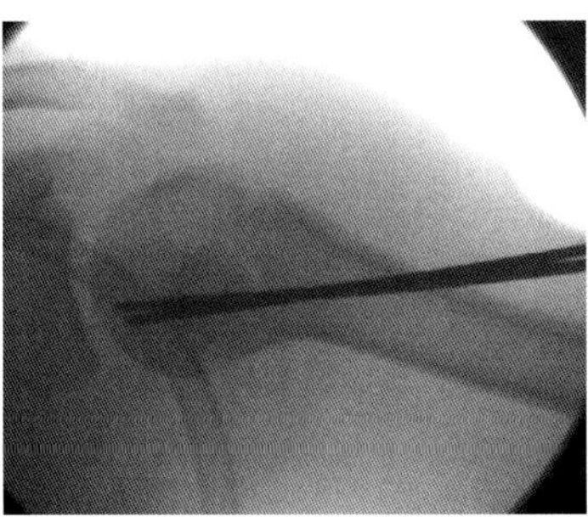
D

**TECH FIG 1** • Pinning of a proximal humeral fracture in the patient in **FIG 2A,B** with a Salter-Harris type II humeral fracture. **A.** After reduction, the first pin is placed. **B.** A second pin is then placed, starting more anteriorly and proximally. **C.** The pins are placed in a divergent fashion. The stab incisions (not shown) should be well distal to the pin–bone interface to prevent soft tissue tension. **D.** An "approach–withdrawal" test is performed under live fluoroscopy to confirm stability as well as the extra-articular nature of the pins.

## Elastic Intramedullary Nail Fixation

- The patient is positioned in a similar fashion as is used for percutaneous pinning.
- A reduction is performed as described for percutaneous pinning.
- An incision is made over the palpable lateral ridge of the distal humerus.
- Care is taken to avoid branches of the lateral antebrachial cutaneous nerve.
- A drill is used to breach the lateral cortex of the humerus, initially perpendicular to the bone, and subsequently angled more vertically parallel with the lateral column.
- The nail is bent and advanced to the fracture site. The curved tip is rotated to effect a reduction and then turned laterally to counteract the tendency of the fracture to go into varus (**TECH FIG 2**).
- The distal end is cut to lie under the skin with about 1 cm left out of the bone.
- A soft dressing and sling are applied.

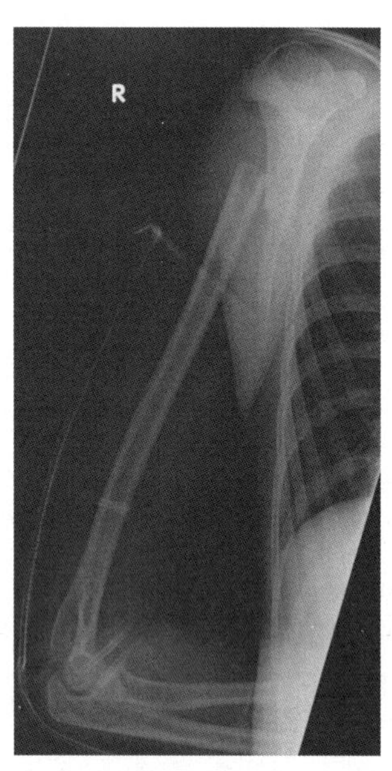

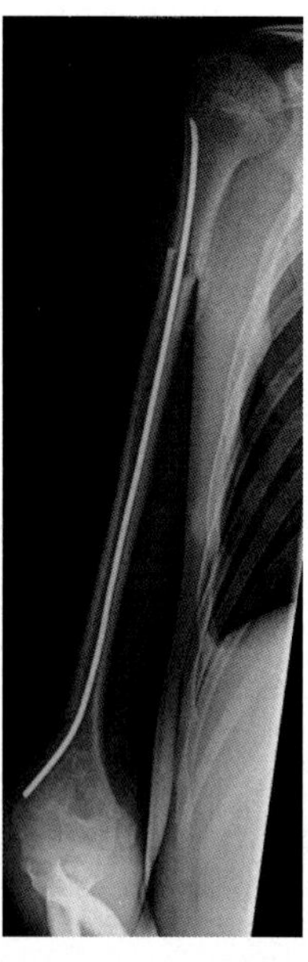

**TECH FIG 2 • A.** Radiograph of a 15-year-old boy who sustained this injury in a motor vehicle injury. His contralateral side sustained a brachial plexus injury at birth and was nonfunctional. Surgical stabilization was elected. **B.** Appearance after lateral insertion of an elastic nail.

## PEARLS AND PITFALLS

| | |
|---|---|
| **Reduction** | ■ The arm should be fully abducted to allow reduction of the shaft onto the head. Gapping at the fracture may signify interposed tissue, and the preparation should allow open exposure if required. |
| **Pinning** | ■ The surgeon should avoid placing the pins in the region of the axillary and musculocutaneous nerve. The skin should be handled carefully and multiple punctures avoided to minimize soft tissue complications. |
| **Indications** | ■ A large remodeling potential exists. The surgeon should carefully consider patient age and remodeling capacity before proceeding with surgery. The surgeon should accept less-than-perfect reduction in lieu of open reduction if possible to avoid the complications associated with an open approach. |

## POSTOPERATIVE CARE

- Aftercare of the pins is controversial. I prefer to leave the pins out of the skin for removal in the office.
  - This is usually easily accomplished at 3 to 4 weeks, when the fracture has gained sufficient stability from healing (**FIG 5**).
  - A battery-powered hand drill is helpful for securely grasping the pins and backing them out, as the tips are threaded.
  - The pins are wrapped in iodine-soaked gauze and covered.
  - They can be checked and redressed if concern exists, and pin care with half-strength peroxide is helpful.
- In obese patients, or in young patients who may have difficulty with activity restriction in the sling, soft tissue movement around the pins may lead to infection.
  - In these patients, the pins should be cut beneath the skin.
  - Removal then requires an additional trip to the operating room, usually at 4 to 6 weeks after surgery.
- After pin removal, the patients are instructed to begin gentle active-assisted shoulder range of motion.
  - Once healing is complete radiographically, formal physical therapy can be initiated to gain any additional mobility and strength.
  - Most children do well, however, by gradually resuming activities at their own pace.
- After elastic nailing, a soft dressing and sling are applied.
- Gentle range of motion is initiated when early callus forms, about 2 weeks. Healing is expected by 6 to 8 weeks.
- For children with more than 2 years of growth remaining, it is my preference to remove the nails 1 year after insertion.

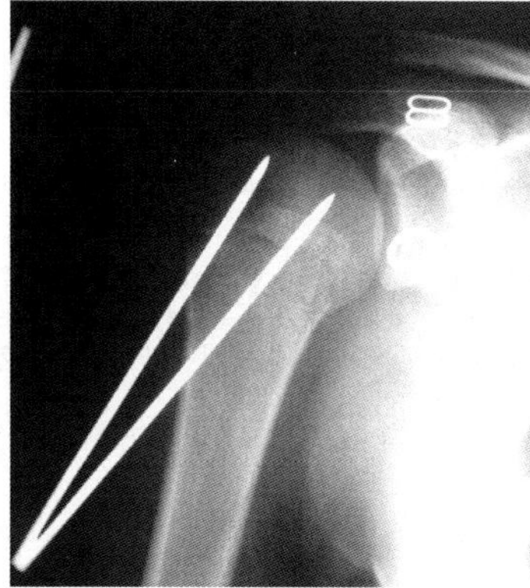

**FIG 5 •** Radiograph taken 4 weeks after surgery of the patient in **TECH FIG 1** before pin removal. Medial sclerosis indicates healing.

## OUTCOMES

- Most patients with proximal humeral fractures will do well regardless of the treatment method chosen.
- Younger patients, particularly younger than 15 years of age, will do well with closed treatment in the absence of neurovascular injury or open fracture.
- Operative treatment usually results in satisfactory healing, although several reports note a high rate of complications from operative treatment, including late fracture through a pin hole and late osteomyelitis.[1]

## COMPLICATIONS

- Nerve injury
- Pin tract infection or osteomyelitis
- Persistent stiffness
- Growth disturbance
- Fracture through pin hole in cortex

## REFERENCES

1. Beringer D, Weiner DS, Noble JS, et al. Severely displaced proximal humerus epiphyseal fractures: a follow-up study. J Pediatr Orthop 1998;18:31–37.
2. Bishop JY, Flatow EL. Pediatric shoulder trauma. Clin Orthop 2005;(432):41–48.
3. Dobbs MB, Luhmann SL, Gordon JE, et al. Severely displaced proximal humeral epiphyseal fractures. J Pediatr Orthop 2003;23:208–215.
4. Kwon Y, Sarwark JF. Proximal humerus, clavicle, and scapula. In: Beatty JH, Kasser JR, eds. Rockwood and Wilkins' Fractures in Children, ed 5. Philadelphia: Lippincott Williams & Wilkins, 2001:741–806.
5. Wilkins KE. Principles of fracture remodelling in children. Injury 2005;36(suppl 1):A3–A11.

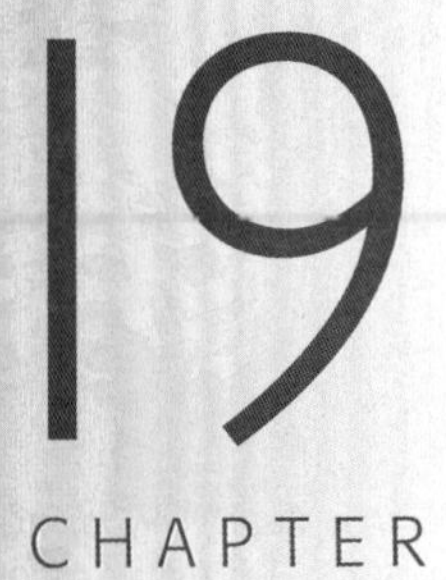

# Open Reduction and Internal Fixation of Proximal Humerus Fractures

Mark T. Dillon, Stephen Torres, Mohit Gilotra, and David L. Glaser

## DEFINITION

- Proximal humerus fractures may involve the surgical neck, the greater tuberosity, and/or the lesser tuberosity.
- The Neer classification, which is most commonly used, categorizes fractures based on the number of displaced parts (**FIG 1**). This classification system involves four segments: the articular surface, the greater tuberosity, the lesser tuberosity, and the humeral shaft. Fracture fragments displaced 1 cm or angulated 45 degrees are considered a displaced part.[22,23]
- The AO/ASIF (Arbeitsgemeinschaft für Osteosynthesefragen–Association for the Study of Internal Fixation) broadly classifies fractures into three types: type 1, unifocal extra-articular; type 2, bifocal extra-articular; and type 3, intra-articular.
  - Each type is then further divided into groups and subgroups.[21]
  - This system places more emphasis on the vascular supply to the humerus, with intra-articular fracture patterns having the highest risk of avascular necrosis.[31]
- Studies have demonstrated that interobserver reliability for both classification systems is not high.[1,28,29]
- Although not included in Neer's original classification, valgus impacted fractures are a unique entity that is important to recognize.
  - Four-part fractures in which the humeral articular surface is impacted on the shaft segment in a valgus position, leading to an increase in the angle between the humeral shaft and the articular surface
  - Often minimally displaced owing to an intact rotator cuff[5]
  - Have a lower incidence of avascular necrosis because the blood supply to the head is less likely to be disrupted

## ANATOMY

- The osseous anatomy of the proximal humerus consists of the greater tuberosity, the lesser tuberosity, and the articular surface.
  - The subscapularis inserts onto the lesser tuberosity, whereas the supraspinatus, infraspinatus, and teres minor insert onto the greater tuberosity.

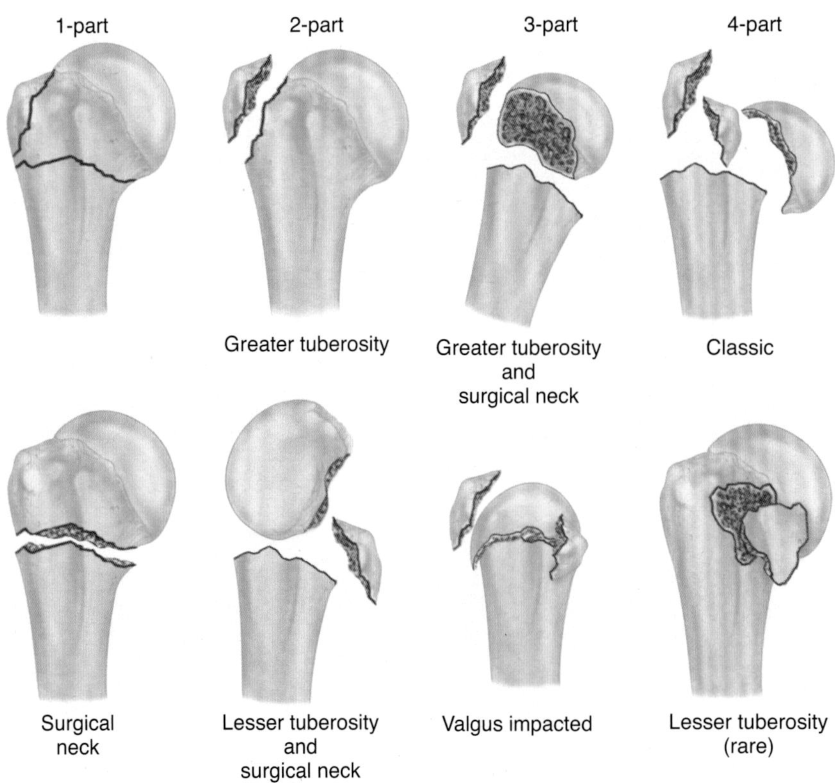


**FIG 1** • Neer classification for fractures of the proximal humerus.

- Knowledge of deforming forces associated with humerus fracture allows the surgeon to better treat proximal humerus fractures by both operative and nonoperative means.
  - In a two-part surgical neck fracture, the pectoralis major pulls the humeral shaft anteromedial.
  - In a two-part greater tuberosity fracture, the pull of the supraspinatus, infraspinatus, and teres minor tendons displaces the greater tuberosity superiorly and/or posteriorly.
  - With a three-part fracture involving the lesser tuberosity, the attachment site of these tendons into the greater tuberosity is intact, and the articular surface of the humeral head rotates externally to face anteriorly.
  - Three-part fractures involving the greater tuberosity result in unopposed subscapularis function, and the humeral articular surface rotates posteriorly.
  - Four-part fractures result in displacement of the shaft and both tuberosities, leaving a free head fragment with little soft tissue attachment.
- An understanding of the vascular anatomy is crucial to treat fractures of the proximal humerus effectively and to predict potential risk of avascular necrosis.
- The proximal humerus receives its blood supply from two branches of the axillary artery: the anterior and posterior circumflex humeral arteries.
- Historically, the main blood supply to the humeral head has been thought to be the anterolateral ascending (arcuate) branch of the anterior circumflex artery[10]; however, there is new evidence to suggest the primary supply is from the posterior circumflex humeral artery.[12]
- The arcuate branch runs just lateral to the tendon of the long head of the biceps in the bicipital groove, enters the humeral head, and becomes interosseous proximally at the transition between the bicipital groove and greater tuberosity and supplies the medial aspect of the humeral head.[12]
- The posterior circumflex humeral artery branches from the axillary artery, travels through the quadrangular space with the axillary nerve, winds superolaterally around the posterior aspect of the humerus, and supplies the superior, lateral, and inferior aspects of the humeral head.[12]
  - The relationship of the arteries to the humerus is important when assessing risk of avascular necrosis as certain fracture patterns put these vessels at increased risk. Fractures with extension into the dorsomedial metaphysis and disruption of the medial calcar have significantly higher rates of ischemia then those that leave these areas intact.[11]

## PATHOGENESIS

- In older patients, proximal humerus fractures usually result from a ground-level, low-energy fall.
- In contrast, younger patients sustain proximal humerus fractures as the result of higher energy mechanisms such as an automobile collision or a sports-related injury (eg, extreme sports).
- The presence of an associated glenohumeral dislocation can also be present and must be determined at the time of initial evaluation.

## PATIENT HISTORY AND PHYSICAL FINDINGS

- History should include the mechanism of injury, social situation, and preexisting shoulder symptoms, which could indicate rotator cuff pathology or arthritis.
- On presentation, patients with proximal humerus fractures complain of pain in the shoulder that is made worse with attempted movement.
- Visual inspection can reveal ecchymosis and swelling of the arm and palpation generally elicits diffuse pain.
- Assessment of the range of motion (ROM) may be difficult due to pain but is important to help determine the stability of the fracture. If the shaft and the proximal portion move as a unit when taken through internal and external rotation, the fracture usually is stable. If however, they do not and crepitus is felt, the fracture is unstable.
- If there is an associated dislocation, it may be possible to palpate the humeral head as an anterior fullness.
- A thorough neurovascular examination is performed to determine the presence of associated injuries.
- Patients younger than 50 years are more prone to nerve injuries. One study demonstrated nerve injury, usually of the axillary nerve, in nearly 40% of patients in this age group who sustained shoulder dislocations or surgical neck fractures.[2]
  - Major vascular injury is very rare in these fractures; however, a high index of suspicion should be present when evaluating fractures with significant medial displacement. The axillary artery can be injured in these instances and diminished radial and ulnar pulses should alert the surgeon to this possibility.[13]

## IMAGING AND OTHER DIAGNOSTIC STUDIES

- Initial imaging studies consist of anteroposterior, scapular Y, and axillary views.
  - Additional views also may include internal and external rotation views if the fracture pattern is stable. Internal rotation views help to visualize the lesser tuberosity, whereas external rotation shows the greater tuberosity. West Point axillary view may be useful for fracture of the anterior glenoid rim and a Stryker notch view for a Hill-Sachs lesion.
  - Traction views also may prove helpful if tolerated by the patient.
- A computed tomography (CT) scan may be helpful if radiographs do not demonstrate the fracture pattern adequately.
- Studies have shown that the addition of a CT scan improves intraobserver reproducibility only minimally and does not affect interobserver reliability.[1]
- However, CT scanning may prove valuable in determining the method of fixation as well as identifying associated injuries such as Hill-Sachs fractures and bony Bankart lesions.
- Indications for magnetic resonance imaging (MRI) are limited, although it may prove useful if there is any concern regarding soft tissue injuries, including the glenoid labrum and rotator cuff.

## DIFFERENTIAL DIAGNOSIS

- Glenohumeral dislocation
- Scapula fracture
- Clavicle fracture
- Humeral shaft fracture
- Neurovascular injury
- Neuropathic arthropathy

## NONOPERATIVE MANAGEMENT

- Historically, conservative treatment usually is recommended for fractures with less than 1 cm of displacement and 45 degrees of angulation.[22] About 85% of proximal humerus fractures can be treated nonoperatively.[20] With newer fixation devices, however, indications for surgical management have been expanded.
- There is less tolerance for displacement in isolated greater tuberosity fractures. It has been suggested that more than 5 mm of displacement leads to poor functional results.[19]
  - Neer's original description called for fixation of greater tuberosity fractures when there was more than 1 cm of displacement.[22]
  - Some authors believe that greater tuberosity displacement of greater than 5 mm may lead to impingement.
    - McLaughlin[19] first suggested that patients in whom a greater tuberosity healed with residual displacement of more than 5 mm had long-standing pain with poor function. Displacement of less than 5 mm does not appear to warrant surgery.
    - Platzer et al[26] looked at minimally displaced fractures of the greater tuberosity and found no statistical significance with varying degrees of displacement less than 5 mm.
- For proximal humerus fractures not involving the humeral shaft, patients initially are immobilized in a simple sling.
- When pain improves and the fracture moves as a unit, passive ROM is started. Patients begin with pendulum exercises, usually 2 to 3 weeks after injury, then progress to ROM in all planes.
- Between 6 and 10 weeks, the fracture usually has healed enough that strengthening exercises may be started.[18]
- When treating proximal humerus fractures conservatively, physical therapy is important to initiate as soon as possible. Koval et al[15] showed significant improvement with one-part fractures when physical therapy was initiated before 2 weeks.
- Several studies have shown that nonoperative management can lead to acceptable results with proximal humerus fractures.[27,30,32]
- Studies comparing patients treated surgically and nonsurgically have shown no difference in outcome with two-part surgical neck fractures[4] and displaced three- and four-part fractures,[33] although these studies were done before the advent of periarticular locked proximal humeral plating.

## SURGICAL MANAGEMENT

- It is imperative that patients have reasonable expectations of their outcome following surgery. A "good" outcome is dependent on these expectations. A functional ROM with minimal pain are the goals. It is often impossible to completely restore the patients preoperative ROM.

### Preoperative Planning

- Acceptable imaging studies, either plain radiographs or a CT scan, are necessary before proceeding to surgery.
- Each proximal humerus fracture is unique, and, in most cases, a planned method of fixation is chosen before entering the operating room. However, the definitive choice of fixation is not made until the fracture is visualized at surgery. Consequently, the surgeon should be prepared with an arsenal of different fixation techniques.
  - If the fracture is not deemed suitable for internal fixation intraoperatively, the surgeon must be prepared to perform a hemiarthroplasty or a reverse shoulder arthroplasty.
- Multiple techniques can be employed for surgical fixation of the proximal humerus. In this chapter, we describe several current techniques. Choice of fixation should be based on the individual patient, the fracture pattern, and the surgeon's own comfort level.

### Positioning

- The techniques discussed in this section are easiest to perform with the patient in the beach-chair position. With the patient nearly seated, the hips and knees are flexed. The patient is moved as far laterally as possible on the table to allow full ROM of the shoulder. A lateral buttress is used to help keep the patient in position on the table.
- C-arm fluoroscopy is helpful in determining the quality of reduction. The C-arm is best positioned with the intensifier posterior to the shoulder and the arm over the patient (**FIG 2**).
- A fluoroscopic image is obtained prior to prepping to ensure that the entire fracture can be visualized without obstruction.

### Approach

- The approach depends on the surgical technique to be used and is discussed further in the Techniques section.
- The deltopectoral approach is most commonly employed. A deltoid split may be performed in select fractures.

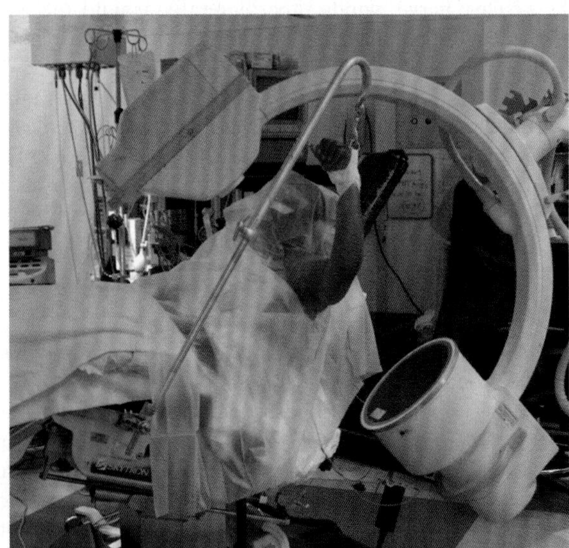

**FIG 2** • Positioning of the patient in the beach-chair position with fluoroscopic imaging. The C-arm intensifier should be posterior to allow for ideal visualization.

## Fixation of Isolated Tuberosity Fractures

- The patient is placed in the beach-chair position.
- A deltoid split or a deltopectoral approach may be used.
- Deltoid split: An incision is made from the anterolateral tip of the acromion extending laterally down the arm.
  - Alternatively, an incision can be made parallel to the lateral border of the acromion, as used in open rotator cuff repair.
- Skin flaps are then raised.
- The deltoid is split in line with its fibers, and the anterior portion of the deltoid may be detached from the acromion.
  - The deltoid fibers should not be split further than 5 cm below the acromion to prevent damage to the axillary nerve. A suture at the distal aspect of the split can help prevent inadvertent extension.[14]
- As with all open procedures described in this chapter, the fracture should be cleaned of hematoma to facilitate reduction.
- The greater tuberosity usually is displaced posteriorly or superiorly. Abducting and externally rotating the shoulder will take tension off the posterosuperior rotator cuff, allowing the greater tuberosity fragment to be more easily reduced.
  - Traction sutures in the rotator cuff may prove valuable in obtaining reduction.
  - Provisional fixation can then be obtained with K-wires (**TECH FIG 1A,B**).
- Cannulated screws placed over the wires may then be used for definitive fixation if the wires are placed in an acceptable location.
  - Screws should be of the appropriate length to gain adequate purchase (**TECH FIG 1C,D**) but not so long that they are symptomatic.
  - The use of washers may prove beneficial in patients with poor bone quality.

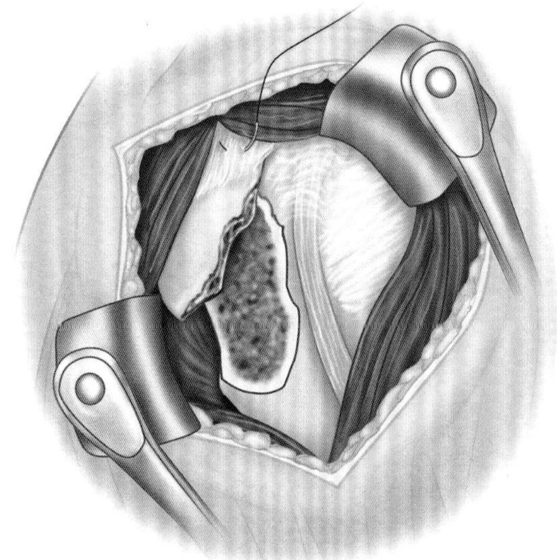
A

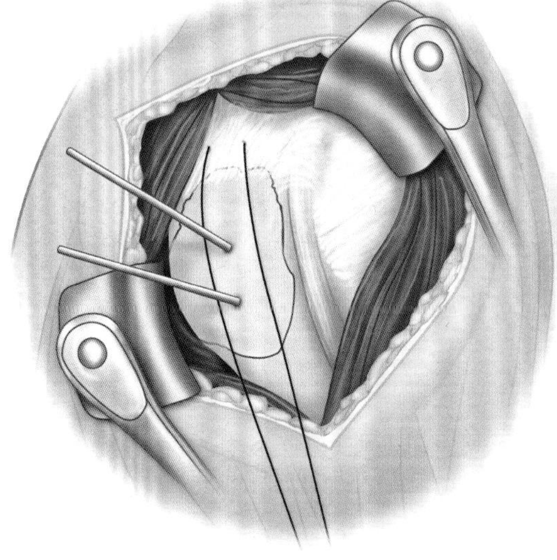
B

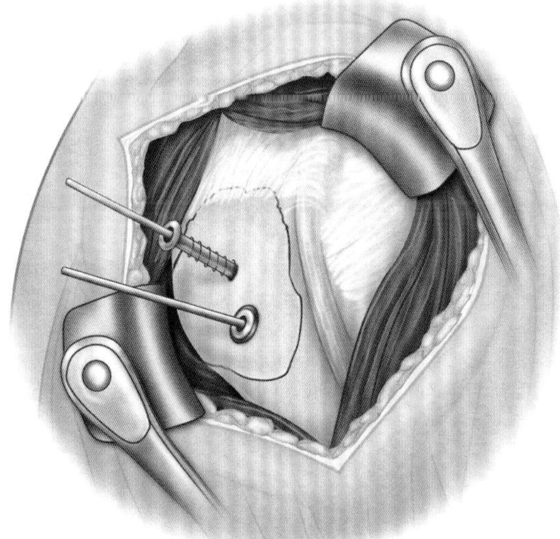
C

**TECH FIG 1** ● **A.** Traction sutures are placed through the rotator cuff tendon to aid in reduction of the displaced greater tuberosity. **B.** Wires may be used to maintain reduction of the tuberosity. **C.** Screw fixation with 4.5-mm cannulated screws. *(continued)*

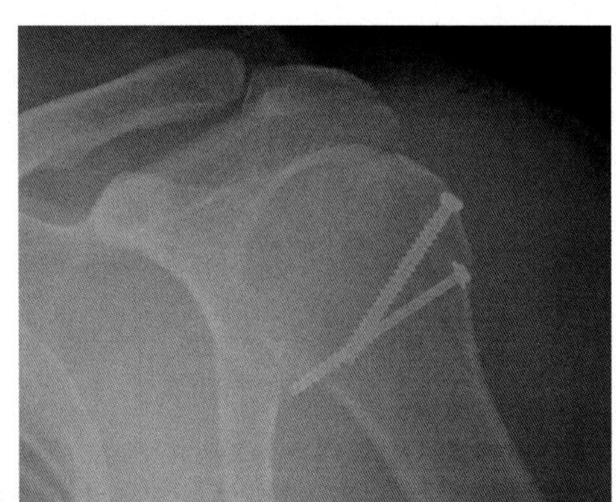

**TECH FIG 1** • *(continued)* **D.** Final fixation. Screws should obtain purchase in the far cortex, but they must not be long enough to damage the axillary nerve. **E.** Placement of suture anchors into the fracture bed. **F.** Reduced fracture with sutures tied over the greater tuberosity.

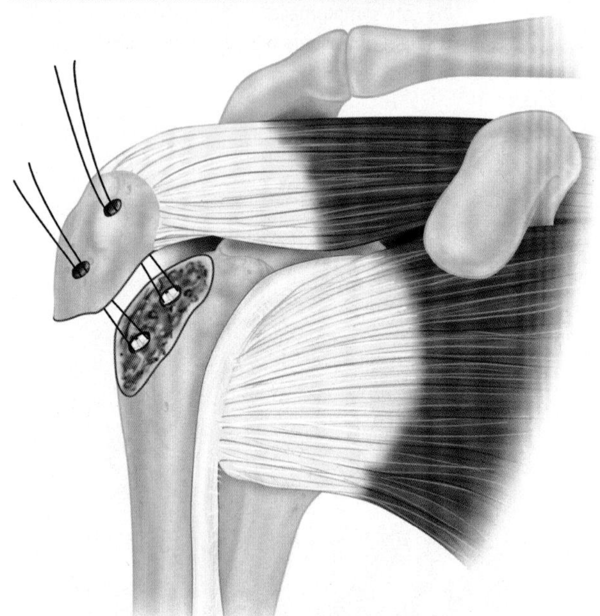

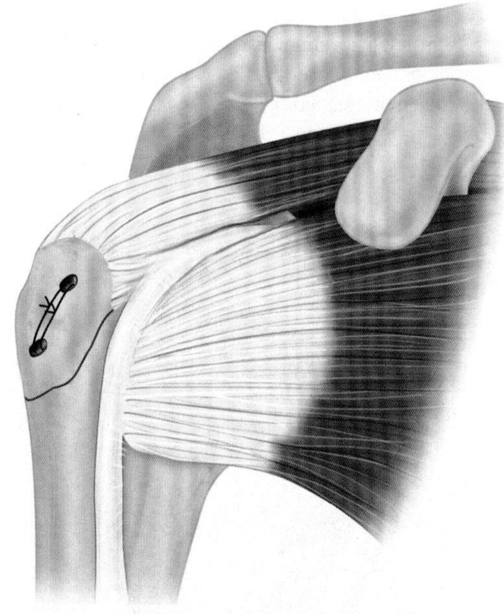

- Alternatively, suture fixation of the greater tuberosity back to the humerus may provide better fixation than cannulated screws in those patients with poor bone quality.
  - This can be accomplished by placing two suture anchors into the fracture bed (**TECH FIG 1E**).
  - Both limbs of each anchor can then be brought through drill holes in the fragment and tied over the top (**TECH FIG 1F**).
  - Suture also can be placed at the bone–tendon interface of the tuberosity fragment and then through bone tunnels in the shaft, as discussed later in this section.
- If the anterior deltoid was detached during the approach, it must be repaired back to the acromion using nonabsorbable sutures.

## Open Reduction and Internal Fixation of Three- or Four-Part Fractures Using Suture

- The patient is placed in the beach-chair position and approached through a deltopectoral interval.
- The rotator interval tissue may be incised. This "interval split" allows visualization of the humeral head articular surface, if needed, in the setting of intact tuberosities and rotator cuff, as with head split patterns.
- Multiple sutures are placed through the tendons of the rotator cuff, preferably no. 5 nonabsorbable sutures or 1-mm tapes.
  - Both the subscapularis tendon and the posterosuperior cuff tendons should be incorporated[25] (**TECH FIG 2A**).
- Drill holes should be placed distal to the fracture site. The bone on either side of the bicipital groove is of excellent quality and should hold sutures well (**TECH FIG 2B,C**).
- In most cases, anatomic reduction is desired.
- With three-part fractures involving the greater tuberosity, the head fragment should first be secured to the shaft followed by reduction of the greater tuberosity.[25]
- For high surgical neck fractures, sutures should be placed into any remaining tuberosity on the head fragment to help maintain fixation.

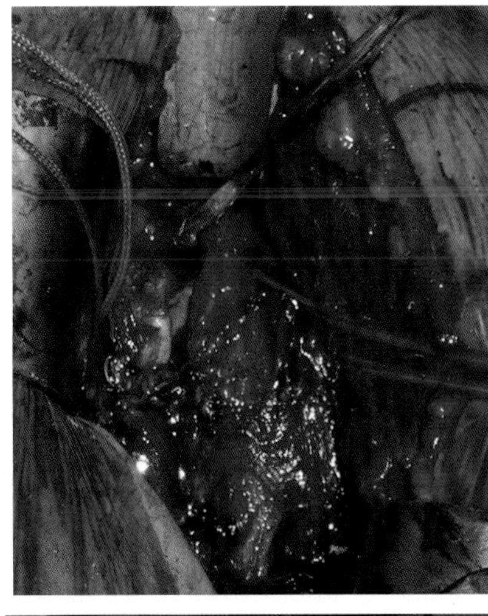

A

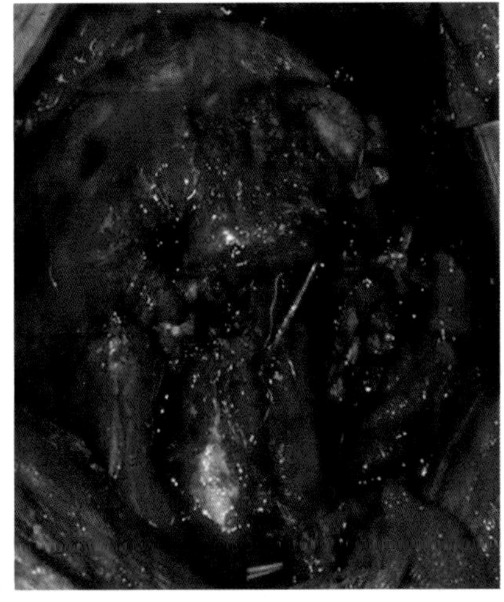

B

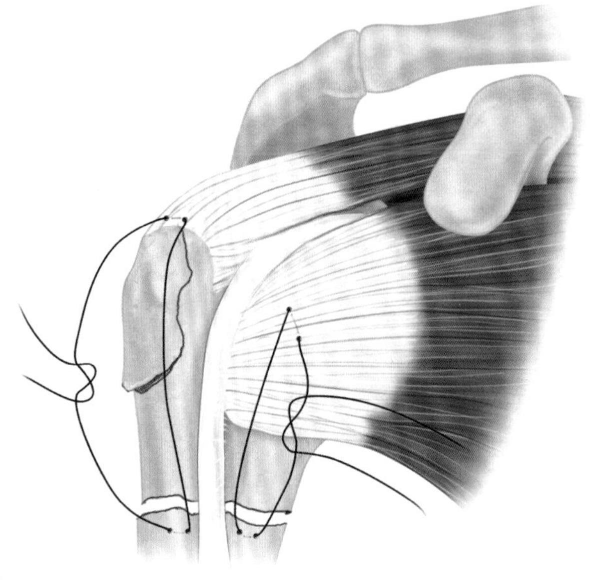

C

**TECH FIG 2** • **A.** Sutures are placed through the subscapularis as well as the posterosuperior rotator cuff tendons at the muscle tendon junction. **B.** Suture is placed through drill holes in the proximal shaft fragment. **C.** Proximal fragment fixed to the shaft with 1-mm tape through the drill holes.

## Open Reduction and Internal Fixation Using Anatomic Plating

### Exposure

- Anatomic plating of the proximal humerus commonly is performed through the deltopectoral interval.
- With the patient in the beach-chair position, an incision is made starting from above the coracoid process and extending distally as needed along the deltopectoral groove (**TECH FIG 3A**).
- The plane between the deltoid and pectoralis major is developed, mobilizing the cephalic vein.
  - Cobb elevators can be used to develop this plane, making it easier for the surgeon to identify and ligate branches of the cephalic vein (**TECH FIG 3B,C**).
- The underlying clavipectoral fascia is identified and incised laterally to the conjoined tendon.[14]
  - The conjoined tendon is carefully retracted medially with the pectoralis major while the deltoid is retracted laterally.

### Reduction

- The fracture and rotator cuff are now visible. With fractures involving displaced tuberosities, we recommend obtaining control of the tuberosities with sutures placed at the bone–tendon interface (**TECH FIG 4A**).
  - Heavy sutures may be placed through the insertions of the cuff tendons and later used as supplemental fixation if necessary.
  - For fractures with minimally displaced tuberosities, sutures may not be needed before a reduction maneuver.
- A Cobb elevator placed in the fracture site will aid in reducing the fracture (**TECH FIG 4B**).
  - The pectoralis major insertion is elevated in a subperiosteal fashion if necessary. The plate should be placed lateral to the biceps tendon so as not to disrupt the blood supply to the humeral head (**TECH FIG 4C**).
  - Often, it may be necessary to release a small portion of the anterior deltoid insertion before placing the plate.

### Plate Fixation

- Fluoroscopy should be used to confirm the reduction and plate placement, especially in regard to plate height, which is specific to each particular plate.
  - A plate positioned too high or a fracture fixed in varus may result in the plate impinging on the undersurface of the acromion.

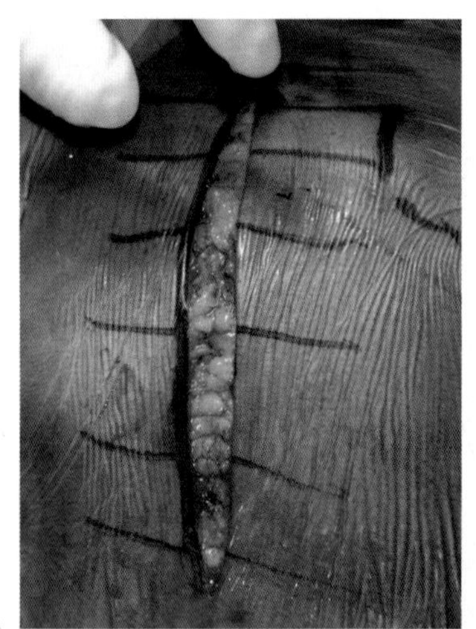

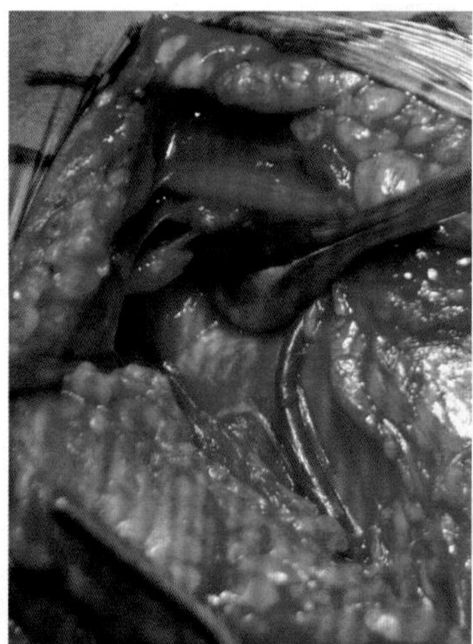

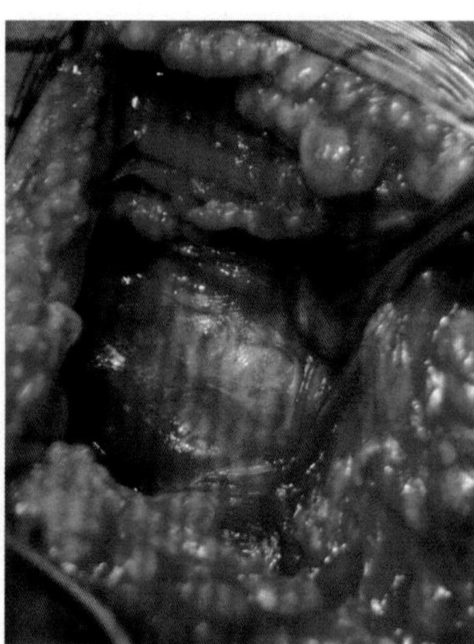

**TECH FIG 3 • A.** The incision is made extending from the coracoid process distally along the deltopectoral groove. **B.** Identifying the interval between the deltoid and pectoralis major. **C.** Using two Cobb elevators to develop the interval, bringing the cephalic vein laterally.

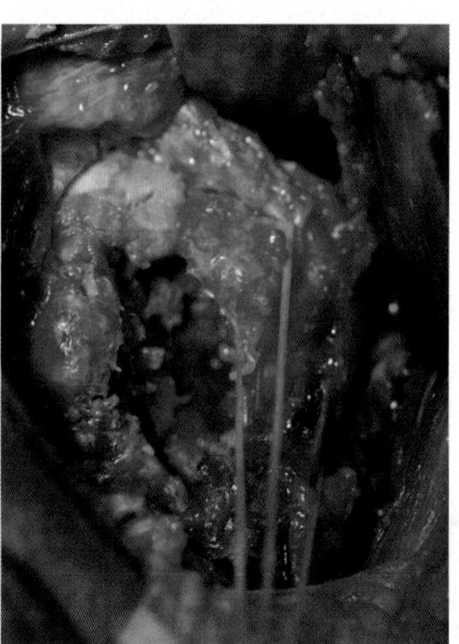

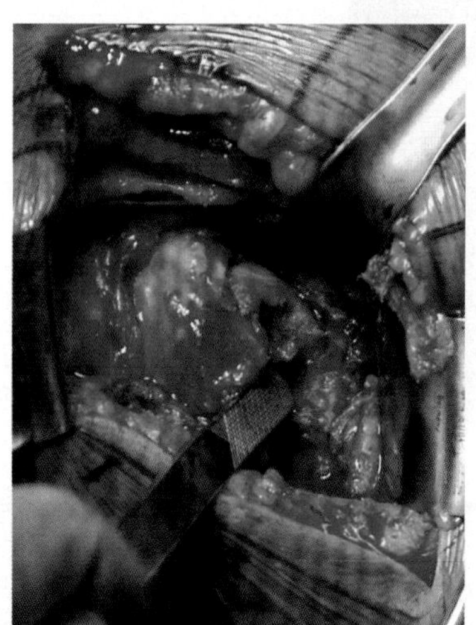

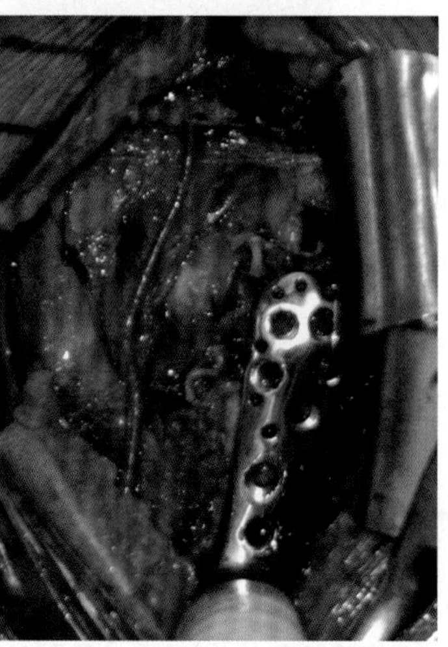

**TECH FIG 4 • A.** Traction sutures through the tendinous attachments of the rotator cuff may be helpful in correcting varus deformity. **B.** Reducing the fracture by elevating the proximal fragment. **C.** Correct placement of the plate is lateral to the biceps tendon (not seen here). Suture fixation has been used to help maintain fixation and supplement the plate.

  - K-wires may be used to temporarily maintain fixation proximally and distally.
  - Alternatively, multiple guidewires may be placed into drill sleeves (**TECH FIG 5A**). Confirm plate location again, both proximally and distally, before placing screws.
- Locking screws usually are placed proximally into the head first, and multiple configurations of screws are possible.
- Once the head is secured to the shaft, distal screws can be placed (**TECH FIG 5B**).
  - The placement of a superiorly directed inferomedial screw to the calcar has been shown to maintain reduction and decrease the risk of postoperative varus collapse.[9]
- Final plate placement should be confirmed fluoroscopically and the lengths of all screws closely assessed by taking the shoulder through multiple planes of motion (**TECH FIG 5C,D**).
- Sutures placed through the cuff tendons also are secured to the plate, shaft, or other tuberosity. These sutures may be preloaded through the plate prior to fixation.
  - At the completion of the procedure, the pectoralis major may be secured with sutures through holes in the plate.
- In osteoporotic bone, the tuberosities can first be attached to the shaft with sutures followed by plate application.
- Fixation of displaced two-part proximal humerus fractures also can be performed using a locking plate in a percutaneous fashion. With this technique, great care must be taken to prevent injury to the axillary nerve.
  - A recent cadaveric study[8] demonstrated that the axillary nerve was an average of 3 mm from the second most proximal diaphyseal screw hole and an average of 7 mm from the third most proximal screw hole. All other screw holes were more than 1 cm from the nerve.

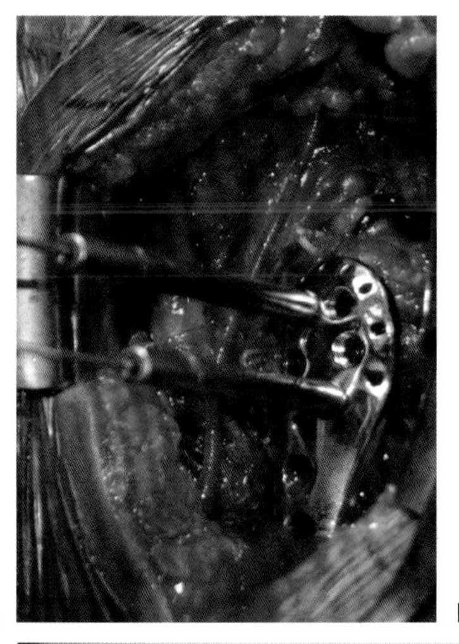
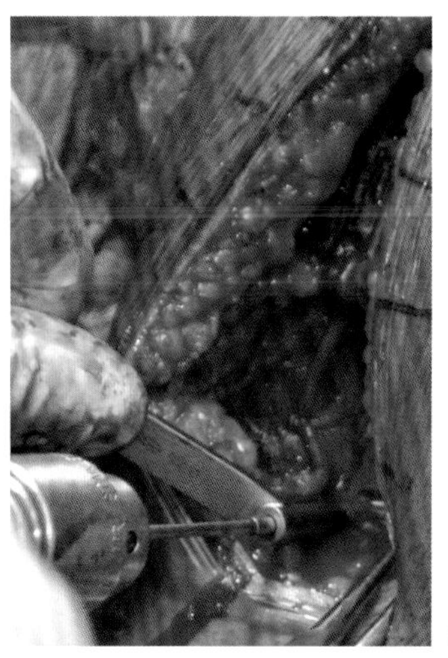
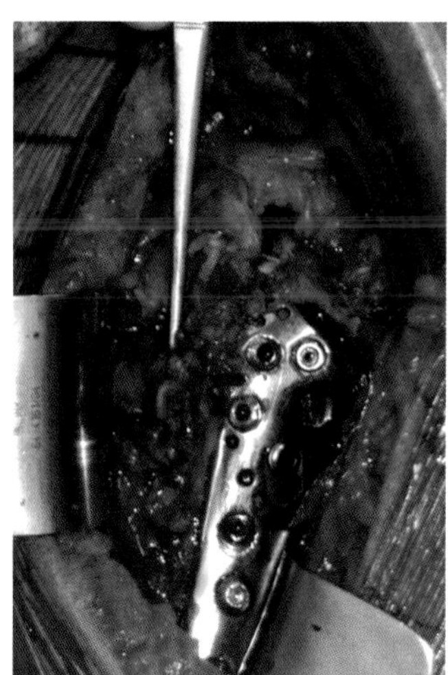
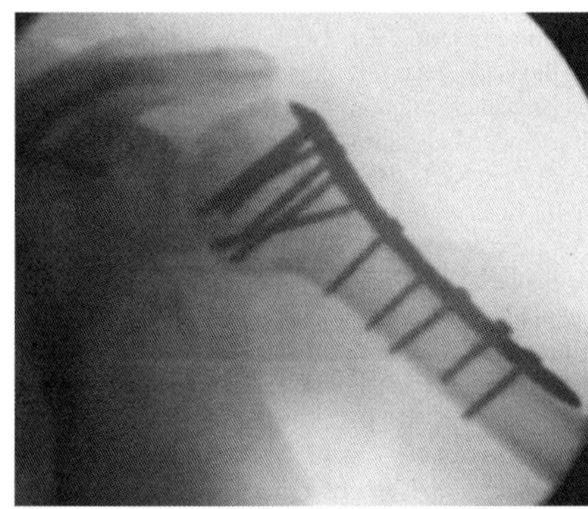

**TECH FIG 5** • **A.** K-wires through drill sleeves are used to maintain plate fixation. Note the position of the superior aspect of the plate in relation to the top of the tuberosity. **B.** Once the head is secured to the plate, distal screws may be placed. **C.** Final plate fixation. **D.** Fluoroscopic image showing screw placement.

## PEARLS AND PITFALLS

| | |
|---|---|
| **Indications** | ■ An understanding of the neurovascular anatomy as well as the deforming forces present in proximal humerus fractures is vital to treating these injuries effectively and understanding which fractures require operative treatment. |
| **Exposure** | ■ Avoid devascularizing fracture fragments by minimizing soft tissue of the pieces during exposure and reduction.<br>■ Development of the interval split aids in fracture visualization and reduction and does not require detachment of the rotator cuff tendons. This is especially helpful when trying to fix a head-splitting fracture in a young patient. |
| **Maintaining fixation** | ■ K-wires are useful for maintaining initial fixation.<br>■ With suture fixation, the strong bone along the bicipital groove of the distal fragment will hold sutures the best. |
| **Poor bone quality** | ■ With osteoporotic three-part fractures, consider suture fixation first followed by a proximal humeral locking plate.<br>■ Anatomic plating is very helpful when medial comminution is present. |
| **Superior impingement** | ■ Avoid placing the locking plate too high on greater tuberosity. |
| **Screw penetration** | ■ Check the lengths of screws in multiple planes to avoid intraoperative screw perforation of the humeral head. |

## POSTOPERATIVE CARE

- Stable fixation must be obtained to allow for immediate ROM.
- A physical therapy regimen should be established based on the stability of fixation, the fracture pattern, the quality of the bone, and individual patient factors.
- Ideally, the fixation should allow physical therapy consisting of pendulum exercises, 130 degrees of passive forward flexion, and 30 degrees of passive external rotation on the first postoperative day.
- Between 4 and 6 weeks after surgery, an overhead pulley can be added, with stretching and active motion added at 6 to 8 weeks.
- Formal strengthening with elastic bands is not started until 10 to 12 weeks after surgery.[3]
- As with nonoperative treatment, participation in physical therapy is key to a successful outcome.

- In a recent study looking at fixation of two- and three-part fractures, the only patients with unsatisfactory outcomes were those who were noncompliant with physical therapy.[25]

## OUTCOMES

- Flatow et al[7] had excellent or good results in 12 of 16 patients with fixation of greater tuberosity fractures displaced more than 1 cm. Forward elevation averaged 170 degrees, and external rotation averaged 63 degrees.
- Open reduction with suture or wire fixation can achieve acceptable fixation, especially in older patients with osteoporotic bone. The technique can be used reliably in two- and three-part fractures.
  - One study showed nearly 80% excellent results with average motion of 155 degrees of average forward flexion, 46 degrees average external rotation, and internal rotation to T11. Furthermore, there were no reported cases of osteonecrosis of the humeral head.[25]
- Early open reduction and internal fixation with a laterally placed T-plate failed to yield consistently good results, especially for four-part fractures.[17,24] Other early osteosynthesis techniques include the cloverleaf and the blade plate, but the current trend is toward anatomic plating technology.
  - Recent studies show promise with the use of such locking plates, although this technique is not without complications.[6]

## COMPLICATIONS

- Infection
- Stiffness/adhesive capsulitis
- Nonunion
- Malunion
- Avascular necrosis
- Nerve injury
- Impingement secondary to fixation or residual tuberosity displacement
- Screw perforation of the humeral head (either by incorrect length placed at the time of surgery or following varus collapse)[16]
- Failure of fixation, including varus malposition and plate fracture following anatomic plating of proximal humerus fractures[6]

## REFERENCES


1. Bernstein J, Adler LM, Blank JE, et al. Evaluation of the Neer system of classification of proximal humeral fractures with computed tomographic scans and plain radiographs. J Bone Joint Surg Am 1996;78A:1371–1375.
2. Blom S, Dahlback LO. Nerve injuries in dislocations of the shoulder joint and fractures of the neck of the humerus. Acta Chir Scand 1970;136:461–466.
3. Cameron BD, Williams GR. Operative fixation of three-part proximal humerus fractures. Tech Shoulder Elbow Surg 2002;3:111–123.
4. Court-Brown CM, Garg A, McQueen MM. The translated two-part fracture of the proximal humerus: epidemiology and outcome in the older patient. J Bone Joint Surg Br 2001;83B:799–804.
5. DeFranco MJ, Brems JJ, Williams GR Jr, et al. Evaluation and management of valgus impacted four-part proximal humerus fractures. Clin Orthop Relat Res 2006;442:109–114.
6. Fankhauser F, Boldin C, Schippinger G, et al. A new locking plate for unstable fractures of the proximal humerus. Clin Orthop Relat Res 2005;430:176–181.
7. Flatow EL, Cuomo F, Maday MG, et al. Open reduction and internal fixation of two-part displaced fractures of the greater tuberosity of the proximal part of the humerus. J Bone Joint Surg Am 1991;73A:1213–1218.
8. Gallo RA, Altman GT. A cadaveric study to evaluate the safety of percutaneous plating of the proximal humerus. Presented at Pennsylvania Orthopaedic Society 2006 Spring Scientific Meeting, Paradise Island, The Bahamas, May 4–6, 2006.
9. Gardner MJ, Weil Y, Barker JU, et al. The importance of medial support in locked plating of proximal humerus fractures. J Orthop Trauma 2007;21(3):185–191.
10. Gerber C, Schneeberger AG, Vinh T. The arterial vascularization of the humeral head. J Bone Joint Surg Am 1990;72A:1486–1494.
11. Hertel R, Hempfing A, Stiehler M, et al. Predictors of humeral head ischemia after intracapsular fracture of the proximal humerus. J Shoulder Elbow Surg 2004;13(4):427–433.
12. Hettrich CM, Boraiah S, Dyke JP, et al. Quantitative assessment of the vascularity of the proximal part of the humerus. J Bone Joint Surg Am 2010;92(4):943–948.
13. Hofman M, Grommes J, Krombach GA, et al. Vascular injury accompanying displaced proximal humeral fractures: two cases and a review of the literature. Emerg Med Int 2011;2011:742870.
14. Hoppenfeld S, deBoer P. Surgical Exposures in Orthopaedics, ed 3. Philadelphia: Lippincott Williams & Wilkins, 2003.
15. Koval KJ, Gallagher MA, Marsicano JG, et al. Functional outcome after minimally displaced fractures of the proximal part of the humerus. J Bone Joint Surg Am 1997;79A:203–207.
16. Konrad G, Bayer J, Hepp P, et al. Open reduction and internal fixation of proximal humeral fractures with use of the locking proximal humerus plate. Surgical technique. J Bone Joint Surg Am 2010;92(suppl 1, pt 1):85–95.
17. Kristiansen B, Christensen SW. Plate fixation of proximal humeral fractures. Acta Orthop Scand 1986;57:320–323.
18. McKoy BE, Bensen CV, Hartsock LA. Fractures about the shoulder: conservative management. Orthop Clin North Am 2000;31:205–216.
19. McLaughlin HL. Dislocation of the shoulder with tuberosity fractures. Surg Clin North Am 1963;43:1615–1620.
20. Moriber LA, Patterson RL Jr. Fractures of the proximal end of the humerus. J Bone Joint Surg Am 1967;49A:1018.
21. Muller ME, Nazarian S, Koch P, et al. The Comprehensive Classification of Fractures of Long Bones. Berlin: Springer-Verlag, 1990.
22. Neer CS II. Displaced proximal humeral fractures. Part I. Classification and evaluation. J Bone Joint Surg Am 1970;52A:1077–1089.
23. Neer CS II. Displaced proximal humeral fractures. Part II. Treatment of three-part and four-part displacement. J Bone Joint Surg Am 1970; 52A:1090–1103.
24. Paavolainen P, Bjorkenheim J, Slatis P, et al. Operative treatment of severe proximal humeral fractures. Acta Orthop Scand 1983;54: 374–379.
25. Park MC, Murthi AM, Roth NS, et al. Two-part and three-part fractures of the proximal humerus treated with suture fixation. J Orthop Trauma 2003;17:319–325.
26. Platzer P, Kutscha-Lissberg F, Lehr S, et al. The influence of displacement on shoulder function in patients with minimally displaced fractures of the greater tuberosity. Injury 2005;36:1185–1189.
27. Rasmussen S, Hvass I, Dalsgaard J, et al. Displaced proximal humeral fractures: results of conservative treatment. Injury 1992;23:41–43.
28. Sidor ML, Zuckerman JD, Lyon T, et al. The Neer Classification system for proximal humeral fractures. J Bone Joint Surg Am 1993;75A: 1745–1750.
29. Siebenrock KA, Gerber C. The reproducibility of classification of fractures of the proximal end of the humerus. J Bone Joint Surg Am 1993;75A:1751–1755.
30. Young TB, Wallace WA. Conservative treatment of fractures and fracture-dislocations of the upper end of the humerus. J Bone Joint Surg Br 1985;67B:373–377.
31. Zuckerman JD, Checroun AJ. Fractures of the proximal humerus: diagnosis and management. In: Iannotti JP, Williams JR, eds. Disorders of the Shoulder: Diagnosis and Management. Philadelphia: Lippincott Williams & Wilkins, 1999;639–685.
32. Zyto K. Non-operative treatment of comminuted fractures of the proximal humerus in elderly patients. Injury 1998;29:349–352.
33. Zyto K, Ahrengart L, Sperber A, et al. Treatment of displaced proximal humeral fractures in elderly patients. J Bone Joint Surg Br 1997;79B:412–417.

# Open Reduction and Internal Fixation of Clavicular Fractures

20

CHAPTER

J. Todd R. Lawrence and R. Justin Mistovich

## DEFINITION

- The clavicle, from the Latin *clavicula*, which means "little branch," is possibly named for the similarly bent hoopstick Roman children used to trundle a hoop.
- Pediatric clavicle fractures are one of the most common childhood injuries and the most common obstetric fracture.[10,13,15]
- Clavicle fractures are classified by anatomic region: proximal third, middle third, and distal third.
- Pediatric clavicle fractures can also be physeal injuries, involving the medial or lateral physis. These injuries are the pediatric equivalent to adult acromioclavicular and sternoclavicular dislocations.[9,11]

## ANATOMY

- The clavicle forms through intramembranous ossification laterally and endochondral ossification medially.
- Ossification begins at 4 to 6 weeks of gestation.
- The medial secondary ossification center appears at 18 to 20 years of age and does not fuse until approximately 25 years of age.[4]
- Thus, the clavicle is the first bone to ossify and the last bone to fuse.
- The middle third of the clavicle is the thinnest portion of the bone and subsequently is most likely to fracture.[3]
- The platysma muscle covers the clavicle.
- The subclavius, sternocleidomastoid, and pectoralis major insert onto the medial end of the clavicle, whereas the trapezius and deltoid insert onto the lateral end.
- The acromioclavicular, coracoclavicular, costoclavicular, and sternoclavicular ligaments stabilize the clavicle and assist in its role as a strut connecting the axial and appendicular skeleton.
- The supraclavicular nerves are deep to the platysma, providing sensation to the anterior chest wall.
- The subclavian artery, subclavian vein, and brachial plexus are intimately associated with the inferior aspect of the medial clavicle.

## PATHOGENESIS

- Clavicle fractures most often result from a direct impact to the apex of the shoulder causing a lateral to medial compression.[4]
- Because both the thinnest part of the bone and the change in shape from convex to concave occur in the middle third of the clavicle, fractures occur most commonly at this location.[3]
- Obstetric-related fractures result from axial compression during birth and are correlated with higher birth weight and forceps delivery.[7]

## NATURAL HISTORY

- Controversy remains in the literature regarding nonoperative treatment versus operative fixation of displaced midshaft clavicle fractures in the adolescent patient with studies supporting both modalities.[2,4–6,8,10,12,14,16]
  - Adult studies have demonstrated measurable shoulder dysfunction associated with shortening greater than 15 to 20 mm.
  - Some studies in adolescents have demonstrated no nonunions and no significant negative clinical results from nonoperative treatment even with greater than 2 cm of shortening.
  - Other studies in adolescents, however, have demonstrated negative effects on overall satisfaction, functional, and cosmetic scores when patients with shortened fractures were treated nonoperatively.
- The risks and benefits as well as the most current literature should be discussed with patients and their families to reach a consensus regarding preferred treatment.
- Nonoperative treatment may result in a bump at the site of union. This typically remodels over the subsequent 1 or 2 years but may remain prominent in some cases (FIG 1).
- Significant malunions may result in brachial plexopathy secondary to compression.

## PATIENT HISTORY AND PHYSICAL FINDINGS

- Children with clavicle fractures will often use the contralateral arm to support the affected arm.
- To minimize posterosuperior displacement by the sternocleidomastoid and trapezius, children may tilt their heads toward the fracture.

A

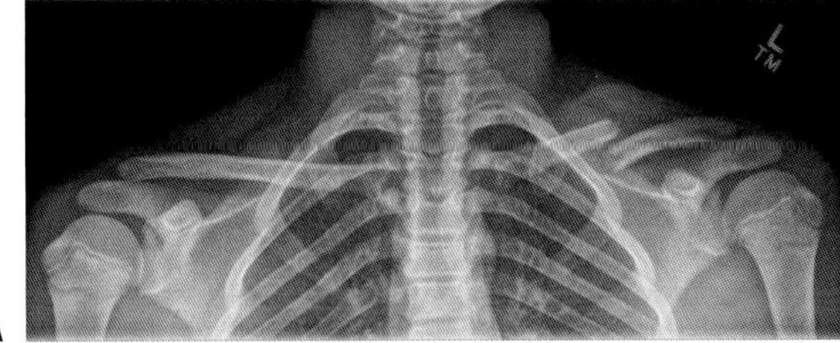

B

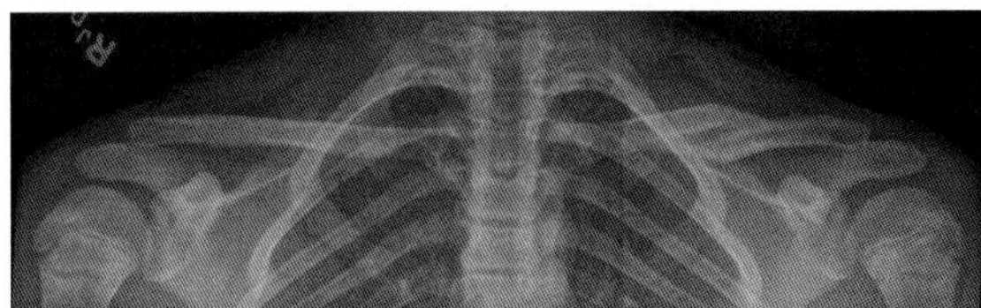

**FIG 1** • **A.** Radiograph of a shortened, displaced midshaft clavicle fracture that was treated nonoperatively in an adolescent. **B.** In a radiograph made at 2 months after initial injury, the patient has an exuberant healing response with callus and a resultant bump at the site of the fracture.

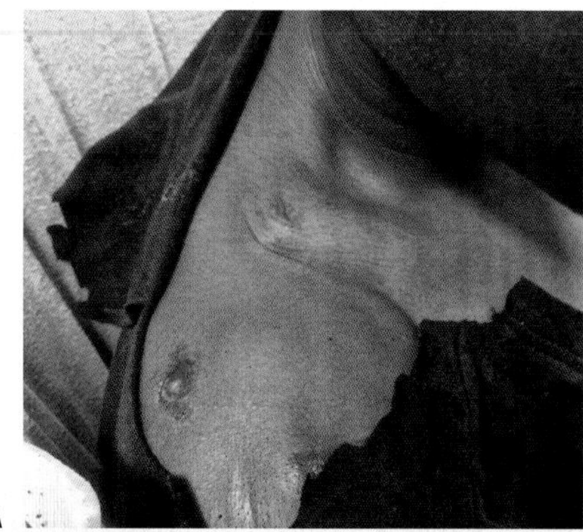
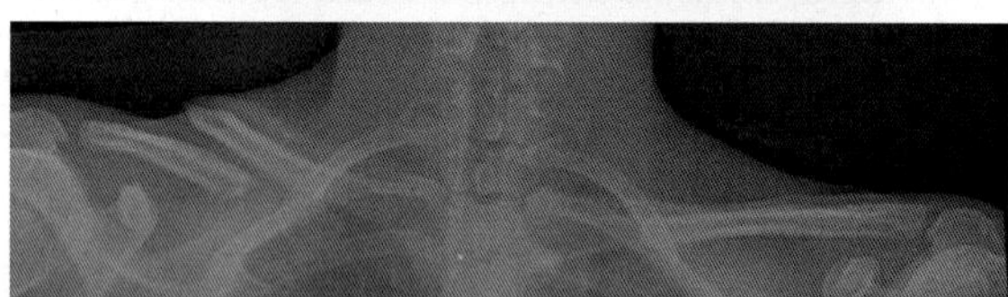
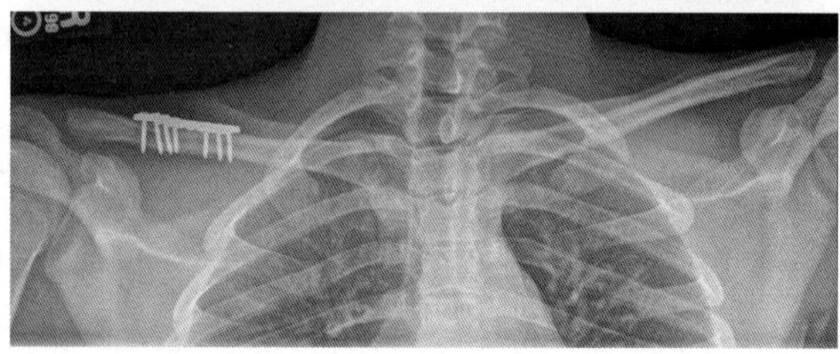

**FIG 2** ● Patient with right clavicle fracture. **A.** Skin contusion with puckering and tenting and thus threatened pressure necrosis. **B.** Radiograph demonstrating the displaced, shortened middle-third clavicle fracture with the medial fragment spike approaching the skin. **C.** Radiograph after fixation and healing.

- Carefully examine the skin for tenting or puncture (**FIG 2**).
- Perform a full neurologic and vascular assessment of the involved limb to rule out brachial plexopathy or vascular injury.
- Clavicle fractures in the neonate may present as a pseudoparalysis of the involved limb due to the pain associated with movement.

## IMAGING AND OTHER DIAGNOSTIC STUDIES

- An anteroposterior (AP) radiograph may not identify subtle fractures.
- The modified Garth apical oblique view, obtained with 20-degree cephalic tilt and 45 degrees of chest rotation away from the film cassette, can be more effective at detecting nondisplaced middle-third fractures.
- Rockwood's serendipity view, taken with 40-degree cephalic tilt, is helpful for visualization of medial third fractures.
- The Zanca view, obtained with half-normal penetration and 15-degree cephalic tilt, is helpful to identify lateral physeal fractures.
- Radiographs obtained with 45 degrees of caudal tilt can help identify AP displacement.
- A radiograph of the bilateral clavicles can be helpful in estimating the degree of shortening as well as providing a comparison view for subtle deformities.
- Although often not necessary to obtain a diagnosis, a computed tomography (CT) scan, if obtained as a component of a trauma workup, can help with understanding the three-dimensional nature of the deformity and may also demonstrate potential vascular compression.

## DIFFERENTIAL DIAGNOSIS

- Congenital pseudarthrosis of the clavicle: Almost all cases are on the right side unless situs inversus is present.
- Cleidocranial dysostosis
- Acromioclavicular or sternoclavicular sprain or dislocation

## NONOPERATIVE MANAGEMENT

- Over 200 nonoperative protocols have been described for clavicle fractures, but when nonoperative indications are met, a simple sling results in typically excellent outcomes.[1]
- There is no benefit to a figure-of-eight brace over a sling.
- A closed reduction should not be attempted, as there is no closed means to reliably maintain a reduction in addition to the potential for neurovascular injury.

## SURGICAL MANAGEMENT

- Although controversy remains regarding the proper modality of treatment with respect to displaced midshaft fractures, absolute indications for operative treatment include the following:
  - Open fractures
  - Threatened skin necrosis
  - Multitrauma patients who would benefit from fixation for their ambulatory and transfer needs
- Multiple methods have been described for operative fixation of clavicle fractures, including intramedullary pin or screw fixation, flexible intramedullary rod fixation, and superior and anterior plating.
- Because of the small diameter of the medullary canal in the pediatric clavicle, intramedullary fixation can be technically difficult in the pediatric patient.
- The authors' preferred technique in pediatric clavicle fracture fixation is plate fixation. The plate can either be placed superiorly or anteriorly.

### Preoperative Planning

- Review imaging studies to understand the fracture pattern and deformity.
- Note that the pediatric clavicle may be too small to use standard precontoured clavicle locking plates. Reconstruction plates contoured to the specific patient are an excellent option. Measure appropriate dimensions on radiographs and ensure that a backup fixation system is available.

### Positioning

- The patient can be positioned either supine or in the beach-chair position. The authors prefer the beach-chair position for ease of obtaining imaging.
- A rolled small towel can be placed between the shoulder blades to assist with obtaining the reduction and correct shortening.
- The fracture is directly visualized, and C-arm should not be needed for reduction aid. Confirmatory C-arm imaging can be used during the case, and a flat plate x-ray can be obtained at the conclusion of the case if desired.

## Exposure

- Make an incision in line with the long axis of the clavicle. This should be slightly anterior or inferior to the clavicle to avoid having the incision directly over the fixation hardware.
- Incise the platysma, leaving clean margins to repair and cover the plate.
- Identify and preserve the medial and lateral supraclavicular nerves. These branches will run perpendicular to the clavicle, just deep to the platysma.
- Expose the fracture and enough of the preferred plating surface (anterior or superior) while taking care to preserve as much periosteum and soft tissue attachments as possible.

## Fracture Reduction and Plating

- Taking care to avoid damage to inferior structures, reduction clamps may be used to facilitate reduction.
- If the fracture pattern permits, a lag screw can be used for both holding reduction and improving the overall stability of the construct.
- A plate can be fitted either anteriorly or superiorly.
  - Superior plating puts the inferior neurovascular structures at greater risk of potential injury with drilling screw holes (**TECH FIG 1A,B**).
  - Anterior plating requires partial detachment of the pectoralis major and deltoid origins and greater overall soft tissue stripping but may provide advantages with decreased hardware prominence (**TECH FIG 1C,D**).
- Pediatric hardware considerations are as follows:
  - 2.7-mm screws may be a better match than 3.5-mm screws for the size of the pediatric bone.
  - A rule of thumb is that the screw should not exceed 33% to 40% of the width of the bone.
- There should be at least six cortices of fixation on either side of the fracture. Given the relative good quality of pediatric bone, locking screws are not usually necessary.

A
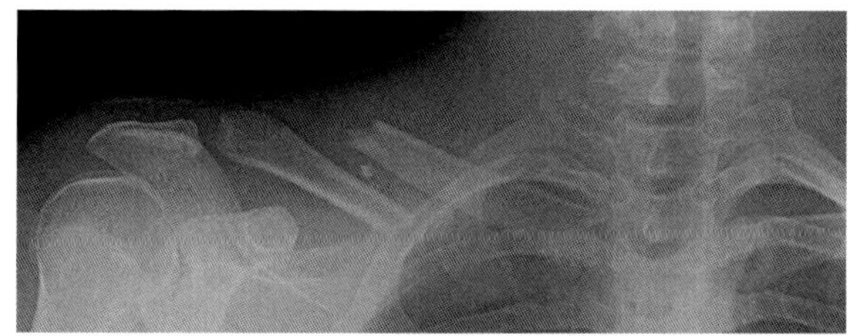

B
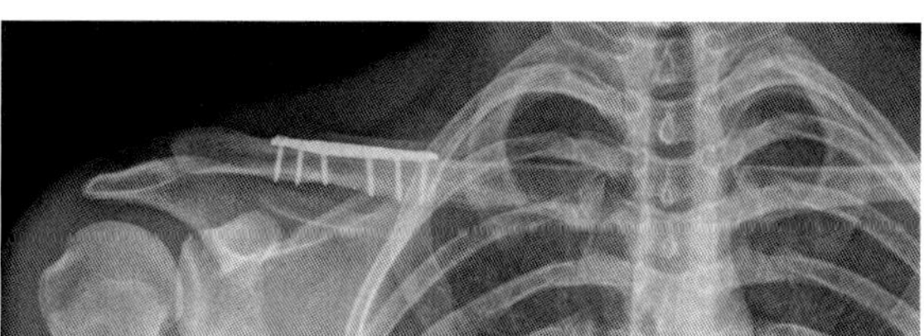

C
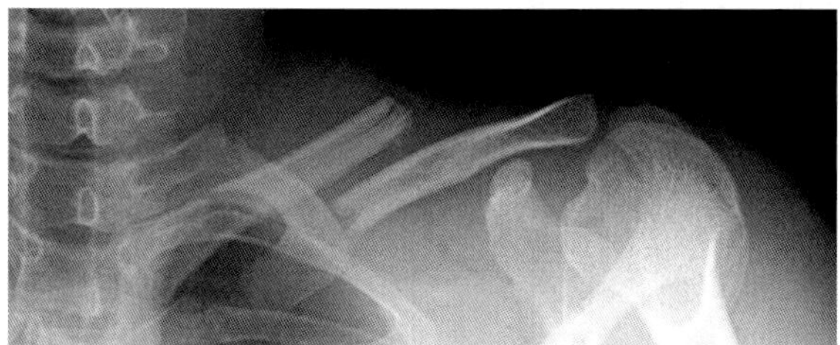

D
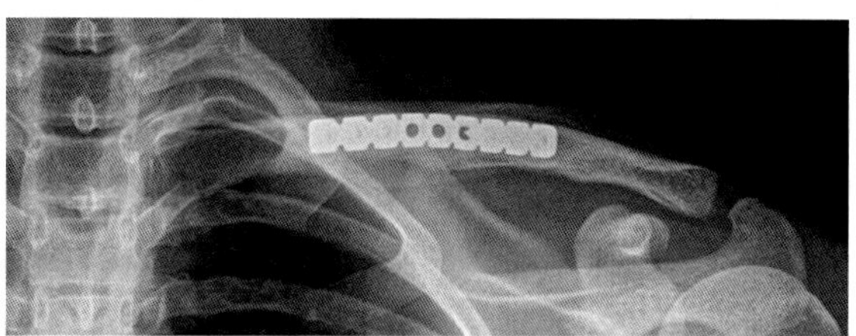

**TECH FIG 1** ● **A.** Radiograph of a shortened, displaced midshaft clavicle fracture. **B.** Postoperative radiograph demonstrating good healing following precontoured superior plate fixation. **C.** Radiograph of a shortened, displaced midshaft clavicle fracture in a different patient. **D.** Postoperative radiograph demonstrating good healing following anterior plate fixation.

## Closure

- Close the platysma over the plate.
- Close the subcutaneous tissue and skin in layers.
- We recommend a running subcuticular closure with an absorbable stitch for cosmesis as well as ease of postoperative office management in the pediatric patient.

## PEARLS AND PITFALLS

| | |
|---|---|
| **Chest wall hypoesthesia** | ▪ Attempt to preserve the supraclavicular nerves. |
| **Painful, prominent hardware** | ▪ Anterior plating may result in better cosmesis and less palpable hardware, especially in patients with a smaller soft tissue envelope. |
| **Neurologic risks** | ▪ Use gentle reduction maneuvers to avoid brachial plexus neurapraxia. |
| **Vascular risks** | ▪ Maintain steady control of the drill, avoid plunging when drilling screw holes, and protect the inferior aspect of the clavicle with a retractor, especially medially. |

## POSTOPERATIVE CARE

- A sterile dressing is placed. Patients are placed in a simple sling.
- Patients remove the sling several times daily for gentle elbow, wrist, and hand range-of-motion exercises.
- The sling is discontinued at 4 weeks. Patients may begin gentle shoulder range-of-motion exercises at 4 to 6 weeks.
- Patients remain restricted from heavy contact activities, repetitive overhead activities, or any pursuit that puts them at risk for a hard fall for at least 3 months, until full clinical and radiographic healing has been observed.
- Hardware removal is not required but can be offered to symptomatic patients at 1 year postoperatively.

## OUTCOMES

- Multiple authors have recorded excellent clinical outcomes in the pediatric population with high satisfaction rate and return to prior level of athletic performance.[10,12]
- These operative outcomes, however, must be viewed in the light of recent studies that report minimal functional deficits even in clavicle fractures with significant shortening and resulting malunion that were treated nonoperatively.[2,16]

## COMPLICATIONS

- Prominent and symptomatic hardware, especially with backpack use or other shoulder straps is common following operative treatment and is often a reason for hardware removal.
- Infection is rare and can be minimized with preoperative antibiotics, wound irrigation prior to closure, and meticulous soft tissue handling and closure.
- Skin breakdown is a risk with the subcutaneous nature of the clavicle. Consider making the incision somewhat anterior and inferior so the healing wound is not directly over the prominence of the plate.
- Neurovascular complications, although anatomically possible, are rare with gentle reduction and cautious drilling and screw placement.
- Patients should be counseled preoperatively regarding the risk of chest wall numbness from injury to the supraclavicular nerves.
- Nonunion is rare in the pediatric population. The clinical significance of malunion, especially as it relates to the results of nonoperative treatment, continues to be debated in the literature.

## REFERENCES


1. Andersen K, Jensen PO, Lauritzen J. Treatment of clavicular fractures. Figure-of-eight bandage versus a simple sling. Acta Orthop Scand 1987;58(1):71–74.
2. Bae DS, Shah AS, Kalish LA, et al. Shoulder motion, strength, and functional outcomes in children with established malunion of the clavicle. J Pediatr Orthop 2013;33(5):544–550.
3. Browner BD, Jupiter J, Levine A, et al. Skeletal Trauma: Basic Science, Management, and Reconstruction, ed 3, vol 1. Philadelphia: Saunders, 2003.
4. Caird MS. Clavicle shaft fractures: are children little adults? J Pediatr Orthop 2012;32(suppl 1):S1–S4.
5. Canadian Orthopaedic Trauma Society. Nonoperative treatment compared with plate fixation of displaced midshaft clavicular fractures. A multicenter, randomized clinical trial. J Bone Joint Surg Am 2007;89(1):1–10.
6. Carry PM, Koonce R, Pan Z, et al. A survey of physician opinion: adolescent midshaft clavicle fracture treatment preferences among POSNA members. J Pediatr Orthop 2011;31(1):44–49.
7. Cohen AW, Otto SR. Obstetric clavicular fractures. A three-year analysis. J Reprod Med 1980;25(3):119–122.
8. Hill JM, McGuire MH, Crosby LA. Closed treatment of displaced middle-third fractures of the clavicle gives poor results. J Bone Joint Surg 1997;79(4):537–539.
9. Koch MJ, Wells L. Proximal clavicle physeal fracture with posterior displacement: diagnosis, treatment, and prevention. Orthopedics 2012;35(1):e108–111.
10. Namdari S, Ganley TJ, Baldwin K, et al. Fixation of displaced midshaft clavicle fractures in skeletally immature patients. J Pediatr Orthop 2011;31(5):507–511.
11. Ogden JA. Distal clavicular physeal injury. Clin Orthop Relat Res 1984;(188):68–73.
12. Pandya NK, Namdari S, Hosalkar HS. Displaced clavicle fractures in adolescents: facts, controversies, and current trends. J Am Acad Orthop Surg 2012;20(8):498–505.
13. Park MS, Chung CY, Choi IH, et al. Incidence patterns of pediatric and adolescent orthopaedic fractures according to age groups and seasons in South Korea: a population-based study. Clin Orthop Surg 2013;5(3):161–166.
14. Randsborg PH, Fuglesang HF, Røtterud JH, et al. Long-term patient-reported outcome after fractures of the clavicle in patients aged 10 to 18 years. J Pediatr Orthop 2014;34(4):393–399.
15. Rubin A. Birth injuries: incidence, mechanisms, and end results. Obstet Gynecol 1964;23:218–221.
16. Schulz J, Moor M, Roocroft J, et al. Functional and radiographic outcomes of nonoperative treatment of displaced adolescent clavicle fractures. J Bone Joint Surg Am 2013;95(13):1159–1165.

# Sternoclavicular Fracture Injury

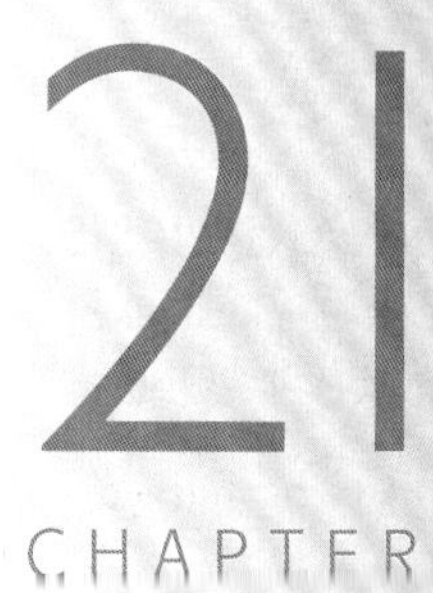


**R. Jay Lee, Afamefuna M. Nduaguba, and David A. Spiegel**

## DEFINITION

- Sternoclavicular fracture-dislocation is an injury to the only bony articulation between the upper extremity and the axial skeleton.
- Sternoclavicular fracture-dislocation is reported to be only 3% of upper extremity dislocations, 1% of all joint dislocations.[5]
- Anterior fracture-dislocations are more common, but posterior fracture-dislocations can be associated with life-threatening complications and should be diagnosed promptly.
- The majority of the existing literature concerns the adult population, and there are a limited number of studies, mostly case reports, concerning the management in children and adolescents.

## ANATOMY

- Sternoclavicular joint
  - The clavicle is the first bone to ossify at intrauterine week 5. However, the medial epiphysis does not ossify until 18 to 20 years of age and does not fuse until 22 to 25 years of age.[22]
  - The sternoclavicular joint is formed by the sternal end of the clavicle, the clavicular notch of the manubrium, and the cartilage of the first rib. Only a small portion of the medial end of the clavicle is covered by articular cartilage, anteriorly and inferiorly, and the majority of the articulation between the medial clavicle and the manubrium is fibrous.[19]
  - The primary stabilizers to anterior and posterior translation are the posterior and anterior capsule. The posterior capsule provides the most restraint to both anterior and posterior translation, whereas the anterior capsule provides additional restraint to anterior translation.[18] There is minimal, if any, bony constraint to motion at this articulation.[18]
  - The costoclavicular and interclavicular ligaments do little to limit anterior and posterior translation.[18]
- Mediastinal structures
  - Important mediastinal structures lie in close proximity to the sternoclavicular joint: the trachea, lungs, esophagus, brachiocephalic vein, subclavian artery, and brachial plexus (**FIG 1**).

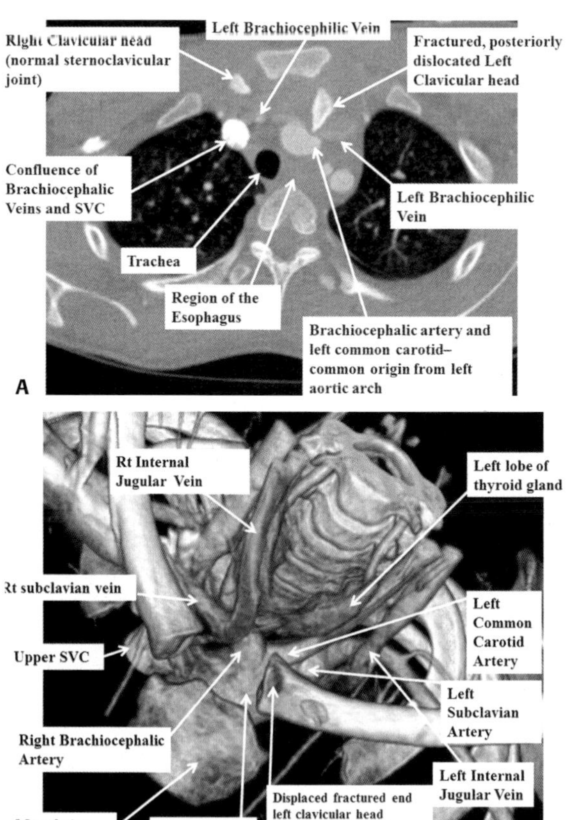


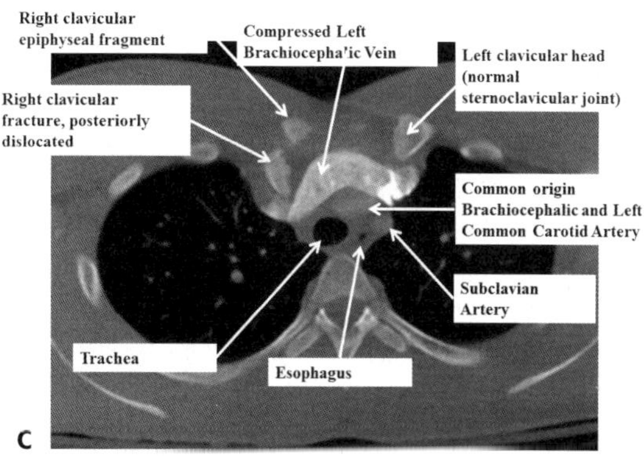


**FIG 1** • **A.** This preoperative CT that was obtained in the case of a left posterior sternoclavicular fracture-dislocation, note the compression of the branches originating from the aortic arch. **B.** The three-dimensional (3-D) reconstruction for the same patient. Note the proximity of the underlying neurovascular structures. **C.** This preoperative CT that was obtained in the case of a right posterior sternoclavicular fracture-dislocation, note the compression on right brachiocephalic vein.

## PATHOGENESIS

- Sternoclavicular fracture-dislocations can result from direct or indirect force.
  - A direct anteromedial force usually results in the clavicle being pushed posteriorly into the sternum and into the mediastinum.
  - An indirect lateral force transmitted along the axis of the clavicle can cause either an anterior or posterior fracture-dislocation, depending on the position of the shoulder relative to the manubrium.[12]
- These injuries are often physeal fractures in children rather than pure dislocations. However, these are difficult to distinguish on imaging studies, as the medial epiphysis does not ossify until age 18 to 20 years (**FIG 2**).

## NATURAL HISTORY

- Posteriorly displaced fractures or dislocations can result in life-threatening and other complications:
  - Obstruction of the trachea can result in acute airway compromise (**FIG 3**), and obstruction of the esophagus can result in dysphagia. If untreated, tracheoesophageal fistulas can result.[20]
  - Obstruction of the underlying brachiocephalic vein or subclavian artery can result in compromised perfusion. If untreated, erosion of the vessels can result.[6]
  - Impingement of underlying structures can lead to brachial plexopathy[17] and thoracic outlet syndrome.[7]
  - Puncture of the underlying structures can cause pneumomediastinum,[13] pneumothorax,[20] bleeding, or death.[14]

## PATIENT HISTORY AND PHYSICAL FINDINGS

- A careful history and physical examination is crucial for identifying this injury. The patient should describe the mechanism of injury and should be asked to point to where the area of maximal discomfort is.
- As with all traumas in the acute setting, airway, breathing, and circulation (ABCs) should be assessed first, as posterior sternoclavicular fracture-dislocation can compromise any of them.
- A careful history may elicit symptoms consistent with obstruction such as dyspnea or dysphagia.
- Physical examination should include the neck, thorax, and shoulder girdles, with particular attention to the neurovascular examination.
- In contrast to anterior fracture-dislocations, where pain and sternoclavicular prominence coincide, posterior fracture-dislocations present with pain contralateral to the "prominent" appearing joint.

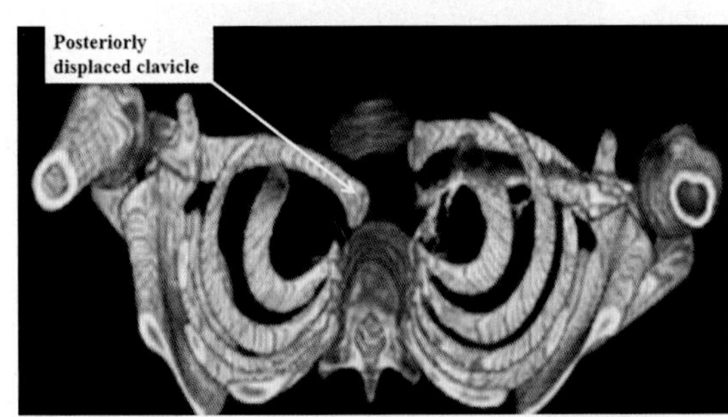


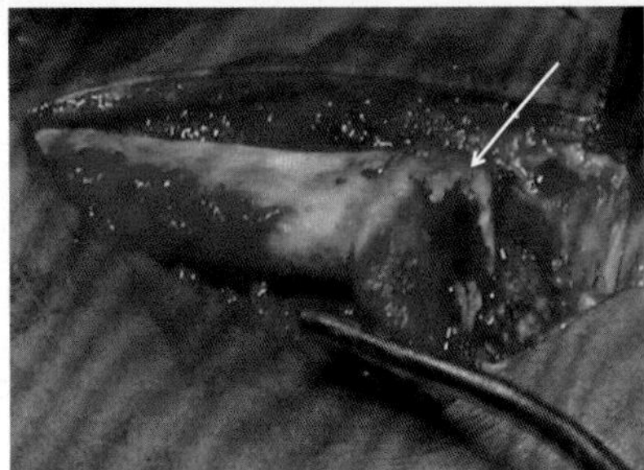


**FIG 2** • **A.** The preoperative CT with three-dimensional (3-D) reconstruction suggests that this injury was a pure sternoclavicular dislocation. **B.** Intraoperatively, direct inspection demonstrated that it was in fact a physeal fracture of the clavicle.

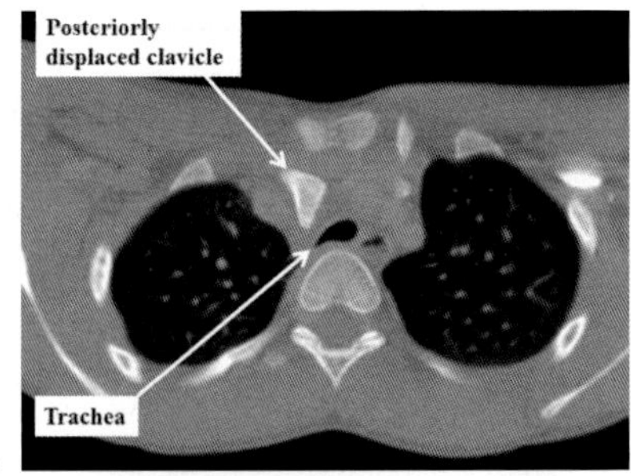


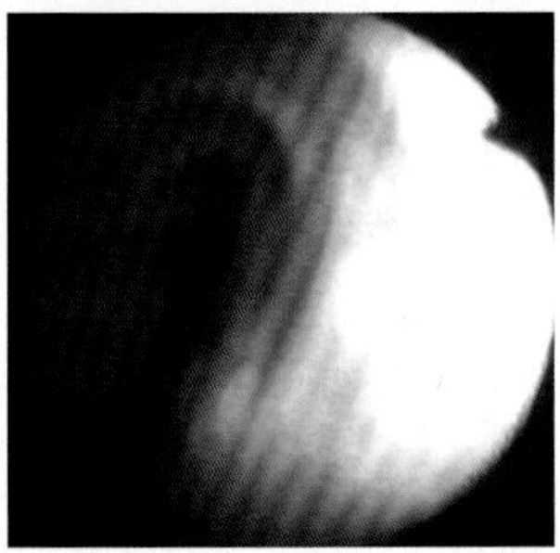


**FIG 3** • **A,B.** The preoperative CT of the same patient as in **FIG 2** shows tracheal compression, which in the endoscopic view is reflected in a narrowed trachea.

## IMAGING AND OTHER DIAGNOSTIC STUDIES

- Sternoclavicular injuries may be missed on standard radiographs. Serendipity views, where the beam centered on the manubrium is aimed 40-degree cephalad, may aid in the diagnosis.
- Computed tomography (CT) is perhaps the best imaging modality to evaluate the sternoclavicular articulation. Strong consideration should be given to obtain the study with intravenous contrast when such injuries are suspected.
- Magnetic resonance imaging (MRI) can also demonstrate the pathology well, can provide greater soft tissue detail, and also differentiate between a fracture and a true dislocation. However, obtaining an MRI may not be practical or achievable in the acute setting. We do not routinely obtain MRI's in our practice.

## DIFFERENTIAL DIAGNOSIS

- Clavicular or sternal fracture
- Sepsis of the sternoclavicular joint

- Sprain of the sternoclavicular joint or surrounding musculature
- Atraumatic sternoclavicular instability in the setting of generalized laxity

## NONOPERATIVE MANAGEMENT

- Nonoperative treatment may be warranted if fracture displacement or joint subluxation is minimal, and there is no compression of any neurovascular structures.

## SURGICAL MANAGEMENT

- Reduction is suggested for those posterior sternoclavicular fractures which are displaced and also those with a true dislocation.
- Options for reduction include closed and open techniques. Indications for open reduction include fractures or dislocations unable to be reduced by closed means or the inability to maintain a reduction.
- Given that routine postreduction axial imaging has not been routinely practiced, and the results of a single study in children in which CT scans following closed reduction demonstrated that resubluxation occurred in 3 out of 3 patients initially treated with closed reduction,[21] we generally prefer open reduction and internal fixation.
- Following reduction, especially if an open technique is required, some clinicians prefer to surgically stabilize the fracture or the articulation. Our personal preference has been to perform open reduction and fixation for all displaced posterior fractures and dislocations.

### Preoperative Planning

- A careful neurovascular assessment should be documented as a baseline reference.
- The available literature suggests the importance of having cardiac or thoracic surgical consultants on "standby" during the procedure, in the highly unlikely event that a vascular injury is identified during the reduction.
  - The term *standby* has not been clearly defined, and it is likely that practice patterns vary between individuals and institutions.
  - We recognize that the likelihood of catastrophic bleeding during reduction or fixation is extremely low, based on just a few anecdotal cases, and that each individual and institution must define how to approach these cases.
- In our practice, the cardiothoracic surgical service is consulted in advance, and we review the details of the case including the imaging.
  - The consulting team—including the cardiothoracic surgeon and the cardiac anesthesia attending, nursing, and perfusion teams that support the surgeon—is available at the time of the procedure and is generally in the operating room or just outside when the reduction is performed.
  - If clinical circumstances allow, the patient is admitted and monitored closely and the case scheduled electively to allow for the necessary planning and coordination.
  - The patient has two large bore intravenous catheters placed; several units of blood and a sternotomy tray are kept available in the room.
  - The patient is prepped and draped to allow access for bypass if necessary, and the cardiopulmonary bypass machine is readied outside the room.
  - Thus, at our institution, a "team" of individuals is sequestered during a limited period of time around the open reduction, and this does require advanced planning. We have not had the occasion to perform a truly emergent open reduction and have thus far had the time to coordinate these efforts.

### Positioning

- The patient is supine on a radiolucent table.
- A 3- to 4-inch bump is placed between shoulders.
- A Foley catheter may be placed for fluid monitoring.
- We prefer to prep and drape the involved upper extremity as well as the entire chest, abdomen, and both groin regions to allow the cardiothoracic team easy access if emergent intervention is required (**FIG 4**).

### Approach

- A direct anterior approach is taken to the clavicle.

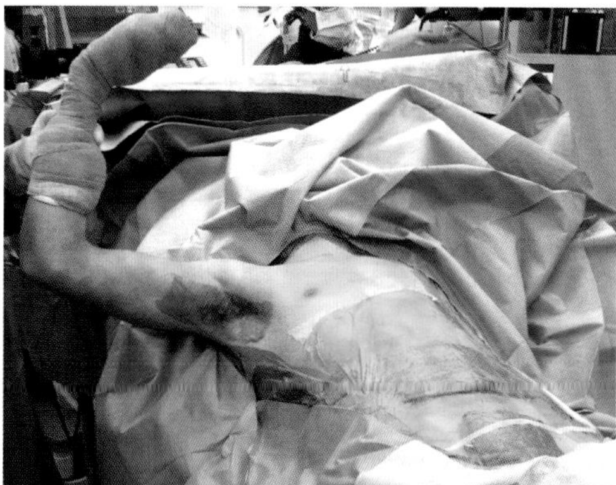

**FIG 4** • Draping the patient with access for both orthopaedic and cardiothoracic intervention, with the involved upper extremity, as well as the entire chest, abdomen, and both groin regions in the field.

## Closed Reduction

- The patient is positioned supine, with the shoulder of the injured side near the edge of the table for accessibility.
- A bump, 3 or 4 inches thick, is placed between the shoulders. This serves to position the shoulders posterior to the manubrium to aid in reduction.
- The ipsilateral shoulder is abducted and extended.
- Lateral traction is then applied while an assistant places countertraction to stabilize the patient.
- The shoulder is gradually brought back into extension.[10]
- An alternative method is caudal traction of the adducted shoulder while posterior pressure is applied to the shoulder.[4]
- Both of these reduction methods can be supplemented by manipulation of the clavicle with percutaneous insertion of a towel clip to aid with control of the clavicle.

## Open Reduction

### Exposure

- Mark out a transverse incision starting laterally over the medial most area of the clavicle that is palpable. Extend this medially across the sternoclavicular joint and onto the manubrium.
  - Alternatively, the incision can be made just superior to this to avoid placing the scar over a prominent area on the skin.
- An incision of the skin is followed by cautery dissection of the subcutaneous tissue, down to the platysma.
  - Care should be taken during dissection, recognizing the underlying structures may be more anterior than normal, relative to the posteriorly displaced clavicle.
- The platysma should be incised in line with skin incision, allowing identification of the periosteum overlying the clavicle.

### Mobilizing the Clavicle

- The clavicle is first identified laterally, outside the zone of injury, where the anatomy is more undisturbed and the periosteum incised (go from "known to unknown").
- The subperiosteal exposure is continued more medially where the soft tissue anatomy is more distorted, although the periosteum may have already been disrupted by the injury (**TECH FIG 1**).

### Reduction

- The lateral portion of the exposed clavicle is grasped with a non-pointed or blunt bone-holding clamp, and the medial end is extracted cautiously.
- Typically, lateral translation either directly through the clamp or indirectly through manipulation of the ipsilateral arm is required initially to "clear" the epiphyseal fragment (or manubrium in the case of a dislocation) before anterior translation of the medial clavicle to complete the reduction (**TECH FIG 2**).
- Direct inspection aids in determining whether the injury is a physeal fracture or a dislocation, which will later dictate method of fixation.
- The adequacy of reduction is assessed.
  - This is easier in the case of a fracture, in which the exposed surface is brought in line with the surface of the epiphyseal fragment. In a dislocation, be mindful that the clavicle sits slightly superiorly and anteriorly relative to the manubrium.[19]
  - It is useful to compare the surface anatomy with the contralateral joint because this area has been prepped and is available for inspection.

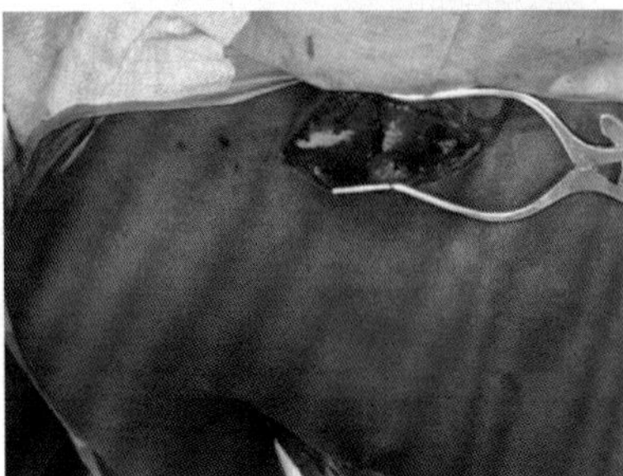

**TECH FIG 1** ● A direct anterior approach, with a subperiosteal exposure of the clavicle.

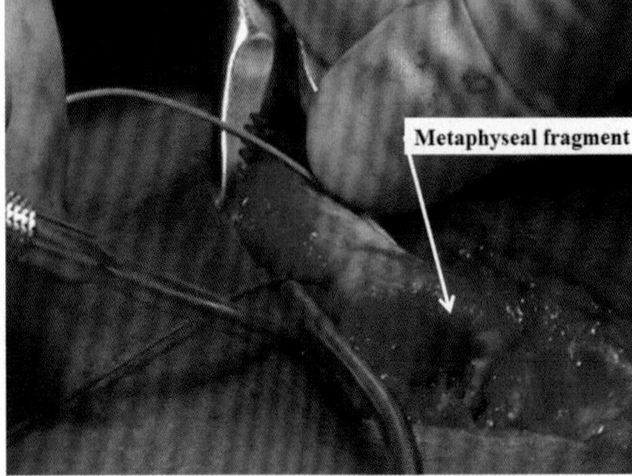


**TECH FIG 2** ● Lateral placement of the clamp and provisional suture passage in anticipation of placing a figure-of-eight stitch.

### Fixation

- Many different techniques have been described for stabilizing the sternoclavicular joint, in the setting of both acute and chronic instability, in both pediatric and adult patients. These include suture repair, stabilization with suture anchors,[1] allograft reconstruction, and stabilization with a plate and screws.[11] We prefer the use of a larger gauge nonabsorbable suture (no. 1 or 2).
- During drilling and passage of sutures, carefully protect the underlying structures against posterior penetration by using a malleable retractor blunt instrument.
- For a physeal fracture, the medial metaphysis of the clavicle may be sutured to the epiphyseal fragment in a figure-of-eight fashion. Unicortical drill holes are placed anteriorly into the

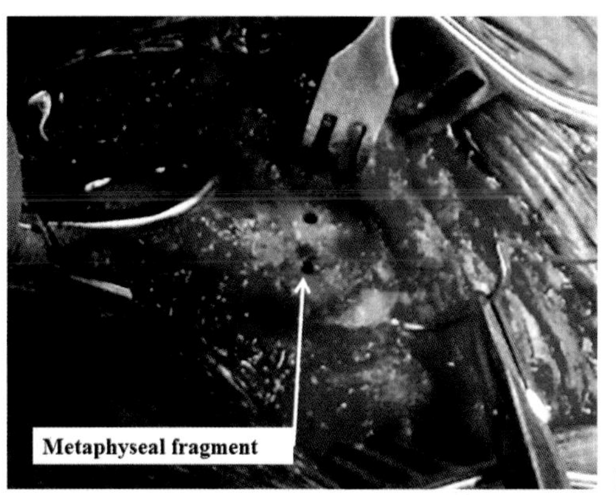


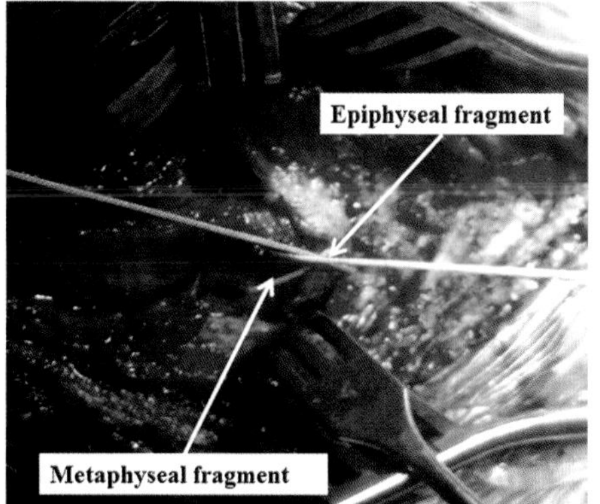


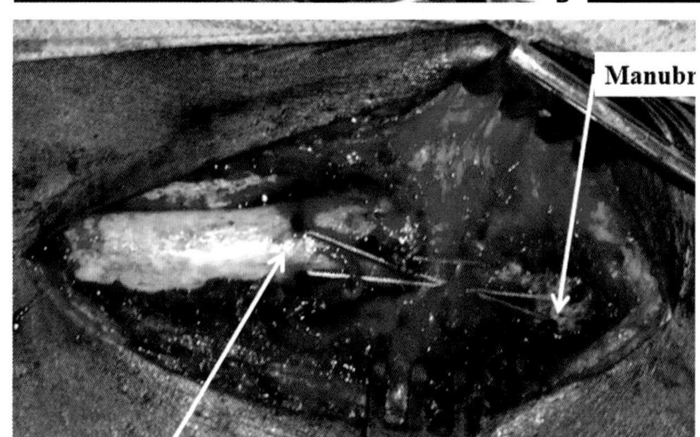


**TECH FIG 3** • **A.** In a sternoclavicular fracture, anterior unicortical drill holes are placed into the medial metaphysis for suture passage while an assistant holds the reduction with the clamp placed laterally. **B.** A figure-of-eight stitch placed through the metaphyseal and epiphyseal fragments. **C.** A figure-of-eight stitch placed through unicortical anterior drill holes in the medial clavicle (*arrow at left*) and manubrium in this case supplementing a suture from the metaphysis through the epiphysis.

metaphyseal and epiphyseal fragments to allow passage of suture (**TECH FIG 3A,B**)

- For a pure dislocation, the end of the clavicle may be sutured to the manubrium using a figure-of-eight technique.
  - Two anterior drill holes are placed in the medial clavicle, and two unicortical drill holes are placed in anterior cortex of the manubrium (**TECH FIG 3C**).
  - This fixation is not rigid, and the goal is to prevent posterior translation during the healing process.
  - It may be desirable to slightly overreduce the fragment when tying down the suture as slight posterior settling can be seen.

## Closure

- The stability of the reconstruction is verified with gentle stress.
- Irrigation of the surgical site is followed by reapproximation of the periosteal sleeve and the accessible capsule and ligaments.
- Sequentially, the platysma, subcutaneous tissues, and skin are closed.

## PEARLS AND PITFALLS

| | |
|---|---|
| **Diagnosis** | ■ A careful history and physical examination is crucial for identifying this injury.<br>■ On x-ray, a sternoclavicular fracture or dislocation may be missed or difficult to interpret. A CT with intravenous contrast better evaluates the articulation and compression of the underlying structures. |
| **Preoperative planning** | ■ Prior consultation and having cardiac or thoracic surgical consultants on standby during the procedure may be beneficial in unlikely event that a vascular injury is identified during the reduction. |
| **Exposure** | ■ The local anatomy may be distorted in the zone of injury. Work lateral to medial, from the known to the unknown. |
| **Reduction** | ■ Remember that the distal fragment will be medially translated in addition to being posteriorly displaced, and that translation must be corrected before bringing the clavicle anteriorly in order to clear the manubrium and/or the epiphysis. |
| **Fixation** | ■ Heavy gauge nonabsorbable sutures through drill holes |

## POSTOPERATIVE CARE

- We generally admit the patients overnight for observation.
- Our preference is to keep the patient in a shoulder immobilizer for 6 weeks, followed by a course of physical therapy. We allow our patients to return to all activities 3 months after surgery if they are asymptomatic.
- Others have reported an immobilizer for 4 to 8 weeks, or a sling for 2 weeks, followed by physical therapy at 6 to 12 weeks, and typically 12 weeks of activity restriction.[10,21]

## OUTCOMES

- Outcomes studies specific to the pediatric population are limited.
- Early closed reduction of both anterior and posterior dislocations is successful in 50% to 88% of cases,[9,15,16] and when closed reduction is successful, there has been favorable outcomes for both posterior and anterior dislocations. In a systematic review, Glass et al[9] reported no functional limitations in the patients who had successful closed reduction for posterior dislocation and limitations in only 15% of anterior dislocations at 45 months follow-up.
- Open reduction is generally successful for (92% to 100%) both anterior and posterior dislocations.[8,9,21] Waters et al[21] reviewed 13 children treated with open reduction for posterior dislocations and reported full return to activities in all patients at 22 months follow-up.

## COMPLICATIONS

- Respiratory compromise
- Hemorrhage which can be life threatening
- Injury to mediastinal structures including the great vessels, esophagus, and trachea
- Loss of reduction
- Persistent instability or malalignment
- Intrathoracic migration if wires and pins are used[2,3]
- Sternoclavicular arthritis[10]

## ACKNOWLEDGMENT

- We thank Ammie M. White, MD, for her assistance in creating the radiographic images for this chapter.

## REFERENCES

1. Abiddin Z, Sinopidis C, Grocock CJ, et al. Suture anchors for treatment of sternoclavicular joint instability. J Shoulder Elbow Surg 2006;15(3):315–318.
2. Aikawa H, Mori H, Miyake H, et al. Percutaneous retrieval of intracardiopulmonary artery metallic needle (Kirschner's wire): a case report. Radiat Med 1996;14(6):335–338.
3. Boutbaoucht M, Nejmi H, Arib S, et al. Postoperative respiratory distress complicating the pin treatment of a sternoclavicular dislocation [in French]. Ann Fr Anesth Reanim 2011;30(1):88–89.
4. Buckerfield CT, Castle ME. Acute traumatic retrosternal dislocation of the clavicle. J Bone Joint Surg Am 1984;66(3):379–385.
5. Cave E. Shoulder girdle injuries. In: Fractures and Other Injuries. Chicago: Yearbook Medical Publishers, 1958:258–259.
6. Ecke H. Late lesions following luxation of the sternoclavicular joint [in German]. Hefte Unfallheilkd 1984;170:52–55.
7. Gangahar DM, Flogaites T. Retrosternal dislocation of the clavicle producing thoracic outlet syndrome. J Trauma 1978;18(5):369–372.
8. Gardeniers JW, Burgemeester J, Luttjeboer J, et al. Surgical technique: results of stabilization of sternoclavicular joint luxations using a polydioxanone envelope plasty. Clin Orthop Relat Res 2013;471(7):2225–2230.
9. Glass ER, Thompson JD, Cole PA, et al. Treatment of sternoclavicular joint dislocations: a systematic review of 251 dislocations in 24 case series. J Trauma 2011;70(5):1294–1298.
10. Groh GI, Wirth MA. Management of traumatic sternoclavicular joint injuries. J Am Acad Orthop Surg 2011;19(1):1–7.
11. Hecox SE, Wood GW II. Ledge plating technique for unstable posterior sternoclavicular dislocation. J Orthop Trauma 2010;24(4):255–257.
12. Jaggard MK, Gupte CM, Gulati V, Reilly P. A comprehensive review of trauma and disruption to the sternoclavicular joint with the proposal of a new classification system. J Trauma 2009;66(2):576–584.
13. Jougon JB, Lepront DJ, Dromer CE. Posterior dislocation of the sternoclavicular joint leading to mediastinal compression. Ann Thorac Surg 1996;61(2):711–713.
14. Kennedy JC. Retrosternal dislocation of the clavicle. J Bone Joint Surg Br 1949;31B(1):74.
15. Laffosse JM, Espié A, Bonnevialle N, et al. Posterior dislocation of the sternoclavicular joint and epiphyseal disruption of the medial clavicle with posterior displacement in sports participants. J Bone Joint Surg Br 2010;92(1):103–109.
16. Nettles JL, Linscheid RL. Sternoclavicular dislocations. J Trauma 1968;8(2):158–164.
17. Noda M, Shiraishi H, Mizuno K. Chronic posterior sternoclavicular dislocation causing compression of a subclavian artery. J Shoulder Elbow Surg 1997;6(6):564–569.
18. Spencer EE Jr, Kuhn JE. Biomechanical analysis of reconstructions for sternoclavicular joint instability. J Bone Joint Surg Am2004;86-A(1):98–105.
19. Van Tongel A, MacDonald P, Leiter J, et al. A cadaveric study of the structural anatomy of the sternoclavicular joint. Clin Anat 2012;25(7):903–910.
20. Wasylenko MJ, Busse EF. Posterior dislocation of the clavicle causing fatal tracheoesophageal fistula. Can J Surg 1981;24(6):626–627.
21. Waters PM, Bae DS, Kadiyala RK. Short-term outcomes after surgical treatment of traumatic posterior sternoclavicular fracture-dislocations in children and adolescents. J Pediatr Orthop 2003;23(4):464–469.
22. Webb PAO, Suchey JM. Epiphyseal union of the anterior iliac crest and medial clavicle in a modern multiracial sample of American males and females. Am J Phys Anthropol 1985;68(4):457–466.

# Pediatric Hip Fractures

Ernest L. Sink and Benjamin F. Ricciardi

22

CHAPTER

## DEFINITION

- Pediatric hip fractures comprise less than 1% of all pediatric fractures; however, appropriate management of these injuries is essential to avoid proximal femoral deformity and maintain hip joint integrity.[14]

## ANATOMY

- Pediatric hip fractures can occur through the physis, but more commonly, they occur through the femoral neck or intertrochanteric region. Therefore, they may be intra-articular or extra-articular (**FIG 1**).
- The femoral head is composed of the capital femoral epiphysis, the subcapital physis, and the most proximal portion of the femoral neck
- The capital femoral epiphysis begins to ossify at around 6 months in boys and 4 months in girls. The trochanteric apophysis center of ossification appears at 4 years of age in both sexes. The proximal femoral physis and trochanteric apophysis fuse at age 14 years for females and 16 years for males.
- Vascular anatomy: Metaphyseal blood supply to the femoral head persists until approximately 4 years of age with primary contributions from both medial and lateral circumflex femoral branches. After 4 years of age, the lateral epiphyseal vessels, derived primarily from posteroinferior and posterosuperior branches of the medial circumflex femoral artery, are the predominant blood supply to the epiphysis of the developing hip.[12]
- The lesser trochanter is an apophysis in the child and the insertion for the iliopsoas.
- Much of the greater trochanter is apophyseal and is the insertion for many of the abductors.
- Classification: Pediatric hip fractures are generally classified as described by Delbet[5] into type I (transphyseal), type II (transcervical), type III (cervicotrochanteric), and type IV (intertrochanteric) (**FIG 2**). Subtrochanteric fractures are not described by this classification system.

## NATURAL HISTORY

- Pediatric hip fractures are rare injuries in children and account for less than 1% of all pediatric fractures.[2]
- Pediatric hip fractures tend to result from high-energy trauma such as motor vehicle accident or fall from height. High rates of concomitant injury have been reported with these injuries.[8]
- Low-energy mechanisms of injury should raise suspicion for pathologic fracture due to underlying metabolic bone disease, benign or malignant lesions, or prior trauma.[15]

## PATIENT HISTORY AND PHYSICAL FINDINGS

- History should include age, mechanism of injury (rule out child abuse in patients younger than 2 years old), locations of pain to rule out concomitant injury, and relevant medical history or family history especially in low-energy mechanism fractures suspicious for underlying pathology.
- Physical examination reveals shortening and rotational deformity of the affected extremity with painful range of motion.
- Infants and newborns can be challenging patients to diagnose with hip fractures due to limited ossification of the proximal

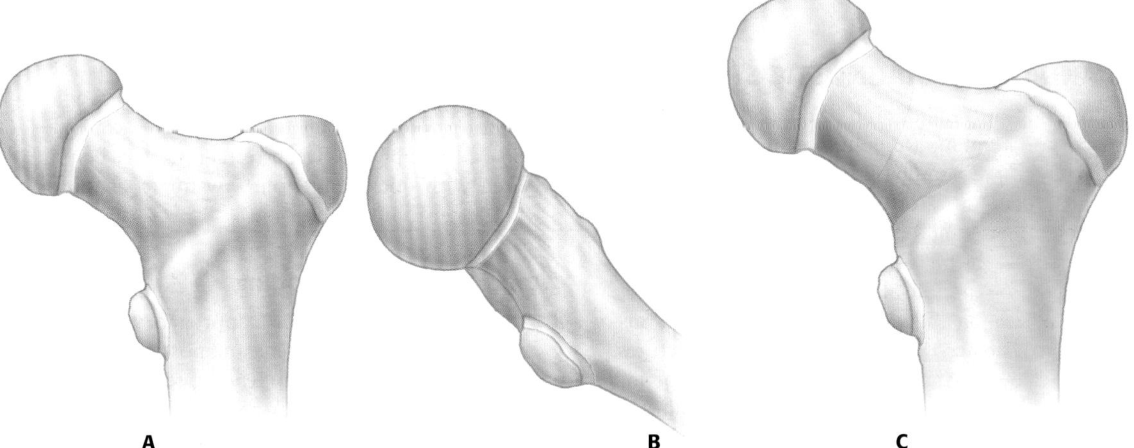


**FIG 1** • **A.** Diagram of the hip from the front. There are growth plates beneath the capital femoral epiphysis, the greater trochanteric apophysis, and the lesser trochanteric apophysis. **B.** Diagram of the hip viewed from the side. The lesser trochanter protrudes posteriorly. **C.** Femoral regions where hips fracture: intracapsular neck (*green*), extracapsular neck (*blue*), and intertrochanteric–subtrochanteric area (*red*).

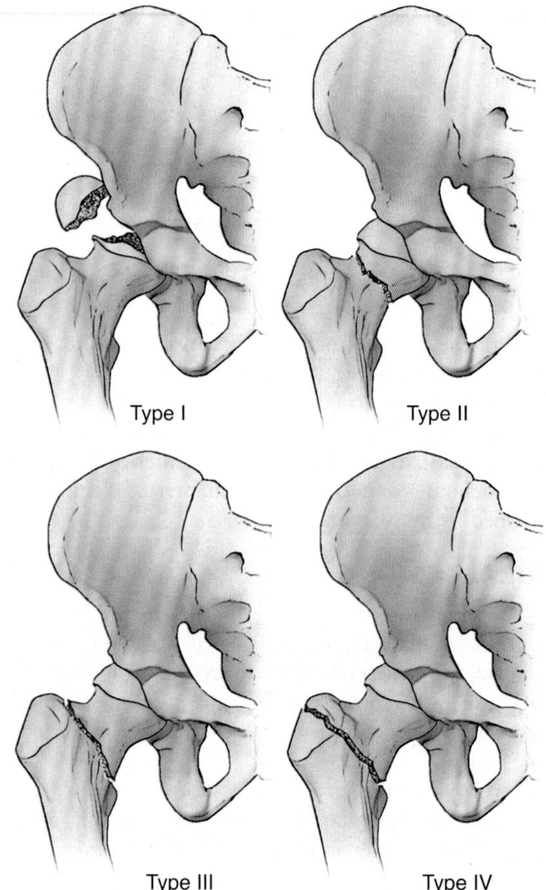


**FIG 2** • Delbet classification of pediatric femoral neck fractures: type I, transphyseal; type II, transcervical; type III, cervicotrochanteric; and type IV, intertrochanteric.

femur, and differential diagnosis may include infection and congenital dislocation of the hip. After excluding infectious etiologies, pseudoparalysis and shortening in this age group should increase suspicion of a fracture.

- Concomitant injury should be ruled out because pediatric hip fractures usually represent high-energy injuries in many cases and can be associated with neurologic, visceral, and other musculoskeletal trauma.

## IMAGING AND OTHER DIAGNOSTIC STUDIES

- An anteroposterior (AP) radiograph of the pelvis provides a view of the contralateral hip for comparison.
- A cross-table lateral radiograph of the injured side should be considered to avoid further displacement and unnecessary discomfort from an attempt at a frog-leg lateral view.
  - Any break or offset of the bony trabeculae near Ward triangle is evidence of a nondisplaced or impacted fracture.
- Magnetic resonance imaging (MRI) can be useful in suspected minimally displaced fractures, pathologic fractures, or stress fractures due to their improved delineation of soft tissue structures, fluid within the hip joint, and ability to assess bone marrow edema signal for nondisplaced fractures or avascular necrosis (AVN).
- Ultrasound can be used to detect epiphyseal separation in infants. Additionally, it can also evaluate for a hip joint effusion in cases of suspected infection and allow concomitant aspiration.
- In a patient with posttraumatic hip pain without evidence of a fracture, complete blood count, erythrocyte sedimentation rate, C-reactive protein, and temperature are helpful to evaluate for infection.

## NONOPERATIVE MANAGEMENT

- For patients younger than 1 year old with nondisplaced or minimally displaced fractures, management can consist of Pavlik harness or abduction brace.
- For children younger than 5 years old with nondisplaced type II or III fractures, spica casting extended distal to the knee can be considered.
- Contraindications
  - All displaced fractures
  - Type I fractures in children older than 2 years old
  - Type II or III fractures in children older than 5 years old. In children older than 5 years even without fracture displacement, internal fixation will help prevent nonunion and fracture displacement.

## SURGICAL MANAGEMENT

- Early operative anatomic reduction with stable internal fixation and selective use of external immobilization (spica casting) is the treatment of choice for pediatric hip fractures in the majority of patients in order to minimize rates of AVN, nonunion, and coxa vara, which are more likely to occur with nonoperative treatments.[1,3,6,7,10,14]
- Open reduction with stable internal fixation should be performed for any residual displacement after attempted closed reduction in order to minimize nonunion, malunion, and AVN.[1,3,4,6,7,11,13–15]
- Urgent (<24 hours) reduction and decompressive capsulotomy with successful closed reductions may help reduce rates of AVN.[4,6,11,13,14]

### Preoperative Planning

- Operating room (OR) table: radiolucent table to assist with reduction and placement of internal fixation. Traction table may aid reduction in older children and adolescents.
- Approaches: Closed versus open reduction; anterior (Smith-Petersen) approach, anterolateral (Watson-Jones) approach, and surgical hip dislocation
- Fluoroscopy: Opposite side from surgeon is usually most helpful. Two C-arm technique may aid in placing internal fixation when possible.
- Special equipment: Deep retractors may help in older children with open reduction; saw for trochanteric osteotomy for surgical hip dislocation.

### Approach and Positioning

- Anterior (Smith-Petersen) approach: supine with support under thoracolumbar spine and posterior superior iliac spine
- Anterolateral (Watson-Jones) approach: partial lateral with support of posterior back and pelvis
- Surgical hip dislocation: full lateral position with axillary roll
- Percutaneous fixation: Positioning on a fracture table with one or two C-arms will facilitate treatment of nondisplaced fractures.

## Exposure and Open Reduction and Internal Fixation

### Anterior (Smith-Petersen) Approach

- A longitudinal incision distal and lateral to the anterior superior iliac spine or bikini approach can be used, with care taken to protect the lateral femoral cutaneous nerve.
- The fascia over the tensor fascia muscle is split longitudinally.
- Blunt dissection is performed on the medial border of the tensor fascia muscle as far proximal as the iliac crest which will expose the rectus femoris muscle.
- The lateral fascia of the rectus muscle is incised and the rectus is retracted medially.
- The fascia underneath the rectus is incised longitudinally and the lateral iliocapsularis is elevated off the hip capsule in a medial direction. The gluteal muscles can be retracted laterally.
- A longitudinal capsulotomy is made along the anterosuperior femoral neck. Retractors can be placed medially and inferiorly around the femoral neck once the capsule is incised, taking care to avoid damage to the femoral neurovascular bundle and medial femoral circumflex artery, respectively.
- After open reduction, internal fixation must be passed percutaneously or through a small separate lateral incision because the lateral greater trochanter is not exposed through this approach.

### Anterolateral (Watson-Jones) Approach

- An incision is made laterally over the proximal femur just anterior to greater trochanter.
- After identification and division of the fascia lata, the tensor muscle is reflected anteriorly taking care not to injure branches of the superior gluteal nerve 2 to 5 cm above the greater trochanter.
- The plane between the gluteus medius and tensor muscle is developed, and the anterior hip capsule is exposed. The anterior aspect of the gluteus medius is retracted, and a small portion of the tendon may be incised to increase mobilization.
- A longitudinal capsulotomy is made along the anterior femoral neck. This can be extended along the acetabulum or intertrochanteric line for wider exposure.
- After open reduction, internal fixation can be passed perpendicular to the fracture along the femoral neck from the base of the greater trochanter (**TECH FIG 1**).

### Surgical Hip Dislocation

- An incision is made laterally over proximal femur centered on anterior third of greater trochanter, extending proximally to midpoint between greater trochanter and iliac crest.
- The tensor fascia is incised in the anterior third of the greater trochanter and along the anterior border of the gluteus maximus muscle.
- The femur is positioned in slight extension and internal rotation for visualization, and the piriformis muscle is identified deep to the gluteus medius. Using gentle retraction of the tendon, the inferior fascia of the gluteus minimus is gently lifted in an anterosuperior direction off the hip capsule.
- A greater trochanteric osteotomy is performed anterior to the tip of the greater trochanter to the posterior border of the vastus lateralis ridge, obtaining a width of 10 to 15 mm in children.
- The gluteus minimus, gluteus medius, osteotomized greater trochanter, vastus lateralis, and vastus intermedius are elevated sharply off the hip capsule in an anterosuperior direction. Flexion and external rotation of the operative hip will facilitate the muscle dissection.
  - The piriformis tendon remains intact to the nonosteotomized portion of the greater trochanter in order to protect the retinacular branches of the medial circumflex artery.
- The hip capsule is opened in a Z-shaped fashion with the longitudinal limb along the axis of the femoral neck in line with the iliofemoral ligament.
  - The distal limb remains proximal but in line with the intertrochanteric ridge.
  - The proximal limb of the capsule is opened in the capsular recess of the acetabulum as far posterior as the piriformis tendon.
- If hip dislocation is warranted, temporary fixation of the fracture with a threaded K-wire is recommended to avoid damage to retinacular vessels.
- The leg is flexed and externally rotated and placed in a sterile leg bag. The hip is subluxated with a bone hook, and curved large scissors are used to transect the ligamentum teres.
- After fracture fixation, the hip capsule is loosely approximated. The greater trochanter is reduced and fixation with two or three 3.5-mm screws is performed.

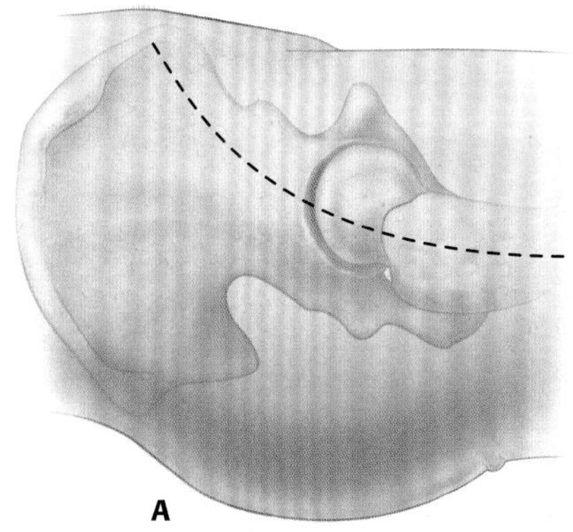


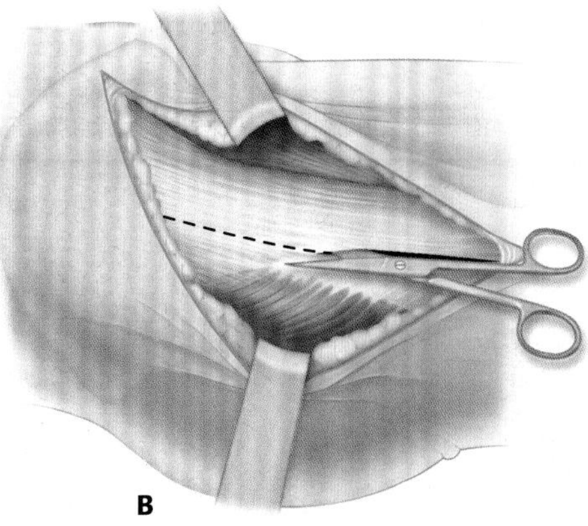


**TECH FIG 1** • Open reduction and internal fixation (ORIF) of intra-articular femoral neck fracture. **A.** Incision is made for Watson-Jones approach. **B.** The fascia lata is split longitudinally. *(continued)*

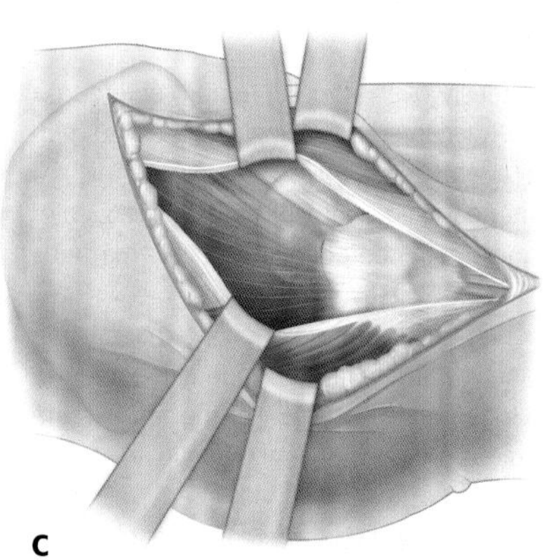
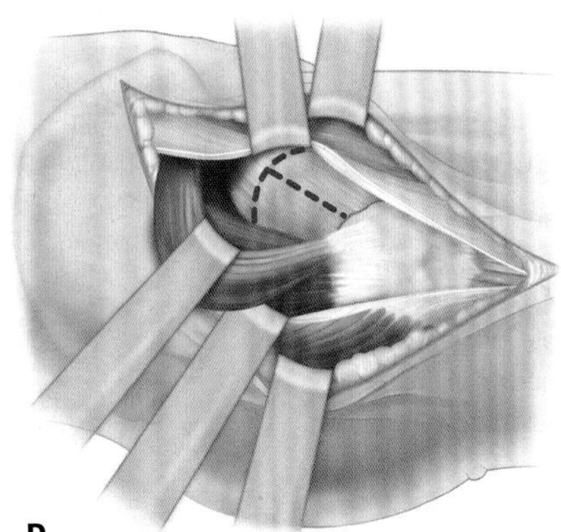
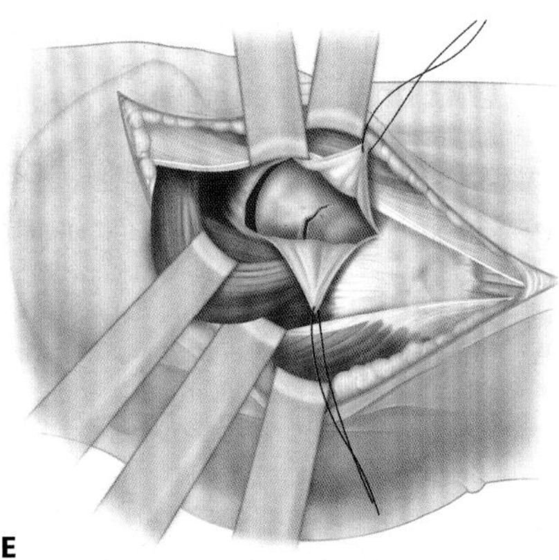

**TECH FIG 1** • *(continued)* **C.** The anterior capsule is exposed. **D.** A T incision is made in the capsule. **E.** The fracture is reduced under direct vision. Pins or screws are placed.

## Type I Fractures

- Nondisplaced or minimally displaced fractures in infants younger than 2 years can be treated with spica casting without internal fixation. Limb is immobilized in abduction and neutral rotation.
- Displaced fractures in infants younger than 2 years and all fractures in children older than 2 years should be anatomically reduced and stabilized with internal fixation.
- A gentle attempted closed reduction is performed. After successful closed reduction, a decompressive capsulotomy can be performed through a limited lateral approach, with access to the hip capsule through the anterior fibers of the gluteus medius muscle.
- If anatomic reduction is not achieved, open reduction is indicated. The approach for open reduction is dictated by the position of the displaced fracture fragments and surgeon preference.
- In small children, 2-mm smooth Kirschner wires (K-wires) can be used for internal fixation, inserted from a lateral position across the physis (two or three wires total). These should be cut off and bent below the skin for later retrieval.
  - Spica casting is performed and immobilization continues for 6 weeks.
- In larger children, 4.0- to 7.3-mm cannulated screws can be used. The decision to have screw fixation cross the physis depends on the size of the child and the location of the fracture (**TECH FIG 2**).
  - In a young child with a lot of growth remaining, the surgeon should stop distal to the physis unless the fracture is more proximal; then, fixation is required to cross the physis to achieve union.

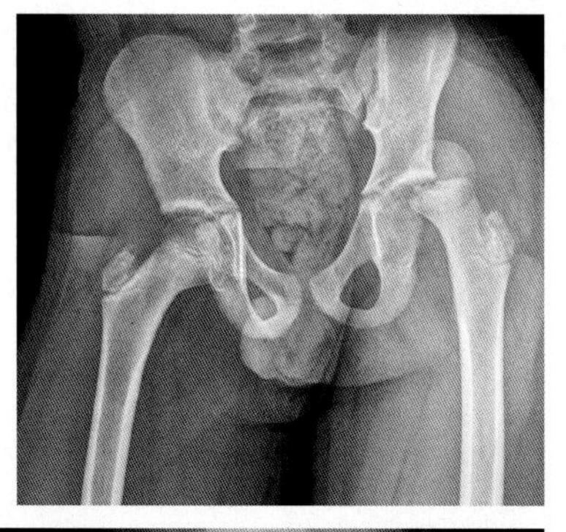
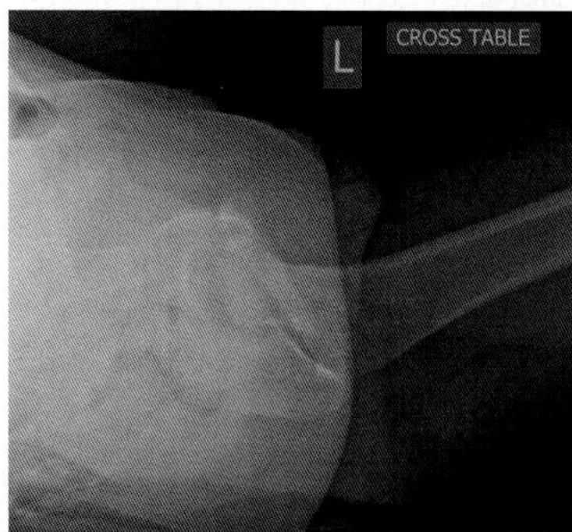

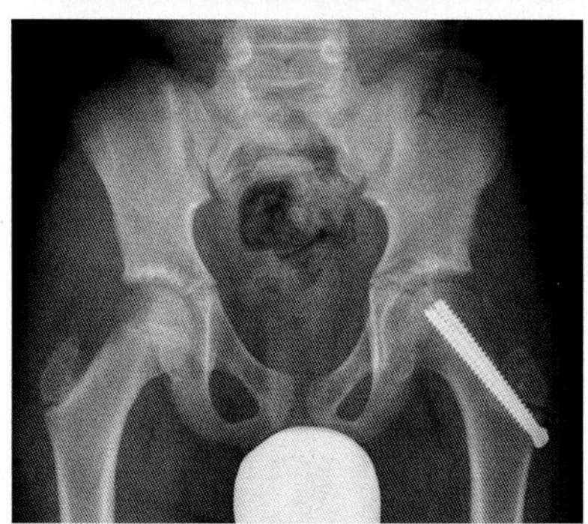
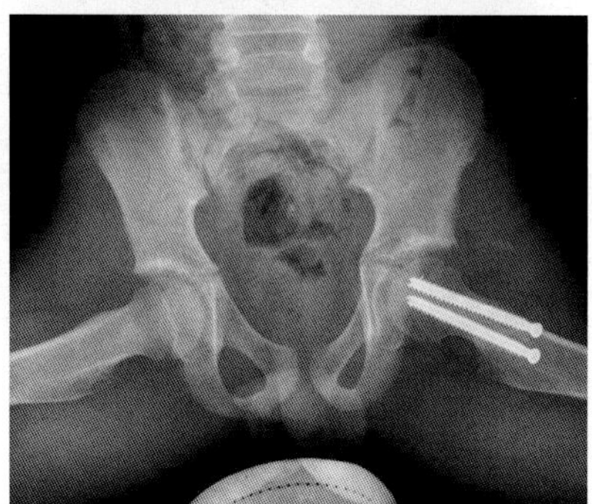

**TECH FIG 2** • **A,B.** AP and lateral radiographs, respectively, of a 10-year-old boy who sustained a type 1 fracture-dislocation playing football. **C,D.** AP and frog-leg lateral radiographs, respectively, 1 year after open reduction and internal fixation (ORIF). For stability, it is necessary for the screws to cross the physis. More follow-up is required because of the possibility of AVN. (Courtesy of W. Sankar, MD; Children's Hospital of Philadelphia.)

- As mentioned, smooth K-wires may be used in younger children but in older children stable fixation should be a primary goal and this may necessitate crossing the physis.
- Guidewires for cannulated screws are inserted across the physis through a small incision over the lateral femur, parallel to the femoral neck on fluoroscopy. The wires are overdrilled to the level of the physis but not across to minimize damage.

- If patient compliance or fracture stability is in question, older children can be placed in spica cast for postoperative immobilization for 6 weeks.

## Types II and III Fractures

- Nondisplaced fractures in children younger than 5 years of age can be managed with spica casting with close radiographic follow-up for displacement.
- All displaced fractures should be treated with an attempted closed reduction. If anatomic reduction is not achieved, then open reduction is indicated. The approach chosen for open reduction typically depends on surgeon preference and experience.
- Internal fixation with two or three 4.0- to 4.5-mm cannulated screws is appropriate for small children up to age 8 years (**TECH FIG 3**). For older children, fixation with 6.5- or 7.3-mm cannulated screws is appropriate with ultimate size dictated by the width of the femoral neck. Similar to type I fractures, internal fixation can be placed over guidewires inserted through the lateral femur in line with the femoral neck.
  - For type II fractures, we attempt to avoid crossing the physis, although this is not always possible with this fracture pattern. Achieving stable fixation is paramount.
  - For type III fractures, it may be possible to achieve stable fixation without crossing the physis, and this would be our preference when possible to avoid growth disturbance.
- We believe that if the physis is not crossed with implants, supplementary spica casting should be performed to prevent malunion or nonunion.

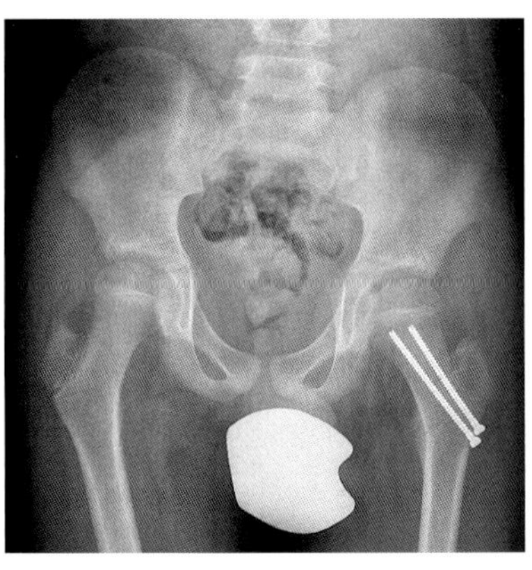

**TECH FIG 3** • AP radiograph of a 10-year-old boy who sustained a nondisplaced femoral neck fracture from a fall. A capsulotomy was performed at the time of surgery and the implants were able to provide enough stability without crossing the physis.

## Type IV Fractures

- Nondisplaced fractures in children younger than 3 to 4 years can be managed in a spica cast without internal fixation. Close radiographic follow-up is necessary to identify lateral displacement.
- Displaced fractures should be treated with attempted closed reduction. This is achieved by a combination of longitudinal traction and internal rotation of the affected limb.
- If anatomic reduction is not achieved, an open reduction is indicated.
- Internal fixation using a pediatric or juvenile compression hip screw or pediatric locking hip plate is our preference. A guide wire is placed parallel to the femoral neck, stopping distal to the physis to avoid penetration. A derotational wire is necessary before drilling and tapping the neck for the dynamic hip screw to avoid fracture displacement (**TECH FIG 4**).
- Spica casting is not typically necessary in older children postoperatively in this fracture pattern with the use of internal fixation.

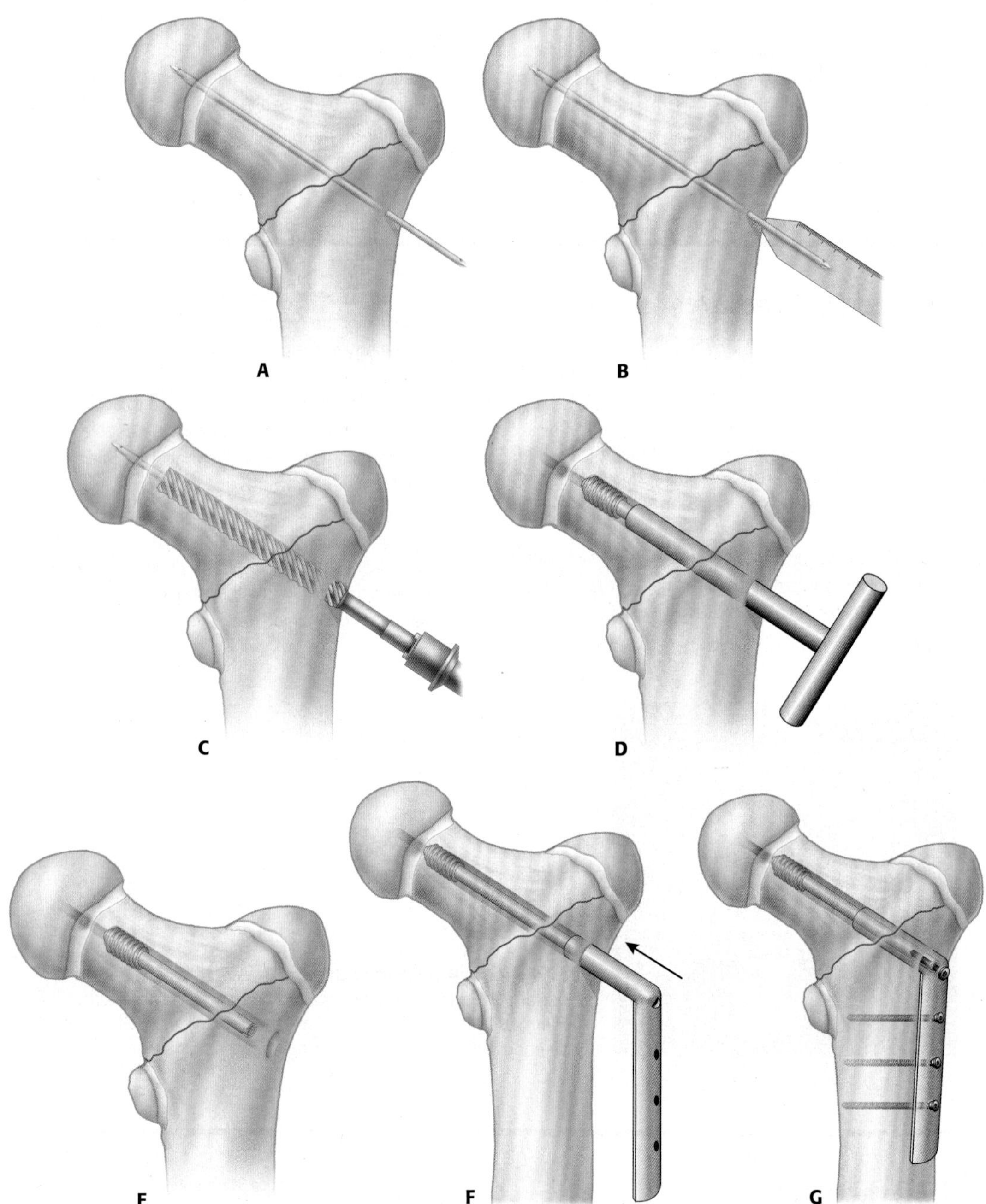


**TECH FIG 4** • Internal fixation of extra-articular hip fracture. **A.** After fracture reduction, a guidewire is inserted from the lateral femoral cortex up the femoral neck. The angle the wire makes with the lateral cortex should match the angle of the fixation device (usually 135 degrees). **B.** The length of the intended lag screw is measured from the protruding guidewire. The lag screw should stop short of the physis. **C.** Reaming is accomplished over the guidewire to accommodate the lag screw and the barrel of the side plate. **D.** The channel is tapped because a child's bone is usually quite hard. **E.** The lag screw is inserted. **F.** The side plate is placed. **G.** The plate is secured to the femur with cortical screws, and the compression screw locks the lag screw in the side plate.

## PEARLS AND PITFALLS

| | |
|---|---|
| **Nonunion** | ■ Anatomic reduction is critical: if unable to achieve anatomic closed reduction, then open reduction is indicated.<br>■ Stable internal fixation<br>■ Supplement with spica cast if younger child (younger than 10 years) or any concerns about fracture stability. |
| **Avascular necrosis** | ■ Urgent reduction (<24 hours) may reduce rates of AVN.<br>■ Achieve an anatomic reduction, open if necessary.<br>■ Supplement anatomic closed reduction with capsulotomy. |
| **Physeal arrest** | ■ Avoid fixation crossing physis if possible (although do not compromise stability). |

## POSTOPERATIVE CARE

- Spica casting
  - All type I fractures except for adolescents with two or three large-diameter cannulated screws into epiphysis
  - Children younger than 10 years old with type II or III fractures
  - All cases in which compliance or fracture stability is in question.
  - For children older than 12 years of age, transphyseal fixation will have less consequences on growth and may avoid the need for spica casting.
- All fractures are followed closely with serial radiographs to assess for late displacement and union.
- Patients are non–weight bearing for at least 6 weeks or until evidence of fracture healing is seen on plain radiographs. Progressive weight bearing and physical therapy as necessary can be prescribed at that time.

## OUTCOMES

- Poor outcomes are associated with the development of complications such as AVN, nonunion, and growth abnormalities of the proximal femur, and patients who avoid these complications generally return to full function.[1,3,6,7,9,10,14,16]

## COMPLICATIONS

- AVN is the most serious complication of pediatric hip fractures. A meta-analysis by Moon and Mehlman[9] found that both fracture classification and patient age were predictive factors for development of AVN.[9] The incidence of AVN in type I through type IV fractures was 38%, 28%, 18%, and 5%, respectively.[9] Early (under 24 hours) fracture reduction, anatomic reduction, stable fixation, and decompressive capsulotomy may all help reduce the rate of AVN.[4,6,11,14]
- Nonunion results from nonanatomic reduction or loss of stable fixation. Increased use of internal fixation and increased recognition of the value of anatomic reduction has helped reduce the incidence of nonunion in more recent series.[1,4,6,14]
- Coxa vara is the second most common reported complication after pediatric hip fractures next to AVN historically. It can result from malunion due to nonanatomic reduction, loss of reduction, and physeal injury. Severe coxa vara increases the height of the greater trochanter in relation to the femoral head, resulting in abductor inefficiency. Remodeling of an established malunion may occur if the child is younger than 8 years of age or with a neck–shaft angle greater than 110 degrees. The use of internal fixation and improved efforts to achieve anatomic reduction have also reduced its incidence.
- Physeal arrest can result from hardware penetration of the physis, AVN, or type I fractures. The contribution of the capital femoral physis is only 13% of total extremity growth; therefore, it only results in significant (>2.5 cm) limb length discrepancies in young children.

## REFERENCES


1. Bali K, Sudesh P, Patel S, et al. Pediatric femoral neck fractures: our 10 years of experience. Clin Orthop Surg 2011;3:302–308.
2. Boardman MJ, Herman MJ, Buck B, et al. Hip fractures in children. J Am Acad Orthop Surg 2009;17:162–173.
3. Canale ST, Bourland WL. Fracture of the neck and intertrochanteric region of the femur in children. J Bone Joint Surg Am 1977;59:431–443.
4. Cheng JC, Tang N. Decompression and stable internal fixation of femoral neck fractures in children can affect the outcome. J Pediatr Orthop 1999;19:338–343.
5. Delbet MP. Fractures du col de femur. Bull Mem Soc Chir 1907;35:387–389.
6. Flynn JM, Wong KL, Yeh GL, et al. Displaced fractures of the hip in children. Management by early operation and immobilisation in a hip spica cast. J Bone Joint Surg Br 2002;84:108–112.
7. Heiser JM, Oppenheim WL. Fractures of the hip in children: a review of forty cases. Clin Orthop Relat Res 1980;(149):177–184.
8. Mirdad T. Fractures of the neck of the femur in children: an experience at the Aseer Central Hospital, Abha, Saudi Arabia. Injury 2002;33:823–827.
9. Moon ES, Mehlman CT. Risk factors for avascular necrosis after femoral neck fractures in children: 25 Cincinnati cases and meta-analysis of 360 cases. J Orthop Trauma 2006;20:323–9.
10. Morsy HA. Complications of fracture of the neck of the femur in children. A long-term follow-up study. Injury 2001;32:45–51.
11. Ng GP, Cole WG. Effect of early hip decompression on the frequency of avascular necrosis in children with fractures of the neck of the femur. Injury 1996;27:419–421.
12. Ogden JA. Changing patterns of proximal femoral vascularity. J Bone Joint Surg Am 1974;56:941–950.
13. Pförringer W, Rosemeyer B. Fractures of the hip in children and adolescents. Acta Orthop Scand 1980;51:91–108.
14. Shrader MW, Jacofsky DJ, Stans AA, et al. Femoral neck fractures in pediatric patients: 30 years experience at a level 1 trauma center. Clin Orthop Relat Res 2007;454:169–173.
15. Swiontkowski MF, Winquist RA. Displaced hip fractures in children and adolescents. J Trauma 1986;26:384–388.
16. Togrul E, Bayram H, Gulsen M, et al. Fractures of the femoral neck in children: long-term follow-up in 62 hip fractures. Injury 2005;36:123–130.

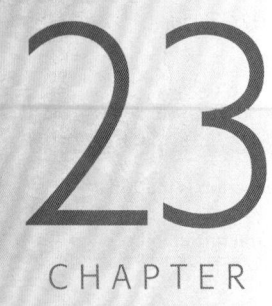

# Closed Reduction and Spica Casting of Femur Fractures

Howard R. Epps, Matthew R. Garner, and John M. Flynn

## DEFINITION

- Femoral shaft fractures in children occur with an incidence of 20 per 100,000.[2,6,14] They constitute 2% of all pediatric fractures.[1,9]
- In the very young child who presents with a femoral shaft fracture, child abuse must be considered, especially if the child is not yet walking.
- In the child who has a history of multiple fractures, osteogenesis imperfecta might be the underlying cause and is often mistaken for child abuse in the young child.
- In children who sustain multiple traumatic injuries, the nature and severity of each injury must be considered to optimize treatment.

## ANATOMY

- The limb bud develops at about 4 weeks age of gestation, with the femoral shaft serving as the primary ossification center. The proximal ossification center is seen by 6 months, and the distal femoral ossification center appears at 7 months.
- The femur is initially composed of weaker woven bone, which is gradually replaced with lamellar bone during childhood.
- Both endosteal circulation and periosteal circulation supply the femur. The profunda femoris artery gives rise to four perforating arteries, which enter the femur posteromedially. The majority of the blood is supplied by endosteal circulation. During fracture healing, however, the majority of the blood is supplied by the periosteal circulation.
- The femoral shaft flares distally, forming the supracondylar area of the femur.

## PATHOGENESIS

- Age is an important factor to consider in terms of the pathogenesis of the injury. The degree of trauma required to cause injury increases exponentially, as the character of the bone changes and gradually becomes stronger and larger from infancy to adolescence. Low-energy injuries resulting in fractures may point to a pathologic nature of the condition, except in toddlers, in whom low-energy femur fractures are common.
- The radiographic appearance of the fracture usually reflects the mechanism of injury and the force applied. High-velocity injuries usually present with more complex, comminuted patterns.
- The position of the fracture fragments after the injury depends on the level of the fracture and reflects the soft tissue and muscle forces acting on the femur.

## PATIENT HISTORY AND PHYSICAL FINDINGS

- In most cases, there is a history of a traumatic event.
- The clinician inspects the lower extremity and looks for open wounds, bruising, or obvious deformity.
  - In the setting of an isolated femur fracture, the thigh appears swollen with minor bruises and abrasions. Shortening may also be present.
  - Open wounds may change the management of this injury; obvious deformity helps in the initial diagnosis.
- The clinician palpates the length of the lower extremity, feeling for bony deformity and checking compartments carefully for tension. Tense compartments may indicate current or developing compartment syndrome.
- The affected extremity should be checked to ensure that there is no vascular or neurologic injury.
  - The clinicians should check carefully for femoral, popliteal, dorsalis pedis, and posterior tibial pulses. Diminished pulses may indicate vascular compromise or compartment syndrome. If diminished, they should be rechecked with Doppler.
  - Sensation to light touch is tested along the length of the entire lower extremity. Decreased sensation in the lower extremity may indicate nerve damage.
- Motor examination may be difficult because of injury. Ankle dorsiflexion and plantarflexion are tested. Diminished strength may indicate nerve damage or compartment syndrome or may also be secondary to pain.
- Examining reflexes may also be difficult. The clinician strikes the patellar and Achilles tendons with a reflex hammer and looks for contraction of the quadriceps and gastrocnemius, respectively. Diminished knee or ankle reflexes may indicate femoral or sciatic nerve injury or may also be secondary to guarding.
- In cases of high-energy trauma, concomitant injuries to the skin and soft tissue as well as other organ systems are usually present.
- The knee is examined to ensure that no ligamentous injury is present. This examination may be performed under anesthesia.

## IMAGING AND OTHER DIAGNOSTIC STUDIES

- Standard high-quality anteroposterior (AP) and lateral radiographs of the femur are usually all that is needed to define the extent and severity of the injury (**FIG 1**).
  - Radiographs should include the joints above and below the fracture site to avoid missing any concomitant injuries.
- Rarely, a computed tomography (CT) scan may be helpful in assessing more complex injury patterns. It also helps in revealing subtle injuries that may not be apparent on radiographs, such as stress fractures, and aids in characterizing intra-articular injuries.

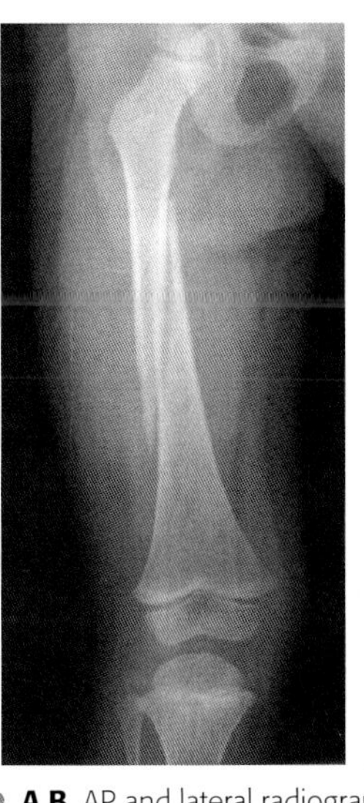
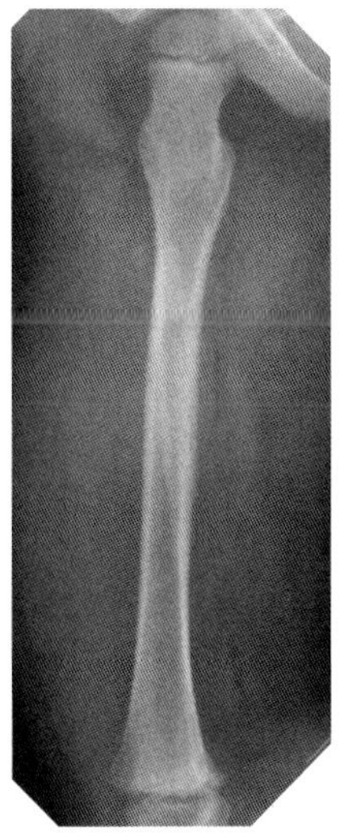

**FIG 1** • **A,B.** AP and lateral radiographs of an oblique diaphyseal femur fracture in a child 4 years and 2 months of age.

## DIFFERENTIAL DIAGNOSIS

- Soft tissue trauma
- Stress fracture
- Tumor
- Metabolic conditions

## NONOPERATIVE MANAGEMENT

- Management of femoral shaft fractures depends on the age of the patient.
- In infants, stable femoral shaft fractures can be treated in a Pavlik harness or a splint.
- In children younger than 6 years, closed reduction and casting is used in the vast majority of cases.
- Immediate spica casting in the emergency department without the use of general anesthesia has been shown to be effective, provided there are no other indications for hospital admission.[3,12]

## SURGICAL MANAGEMENT

- In children younger than 6 years, closed reduction and casting is successful for most femoral shaft fractures.[8]
- For older children and adolescents, 3 weeks of skeletal traction followed by spica casting was once common but has been replaced by internal or external fixation in most cases.

### Preoperative Planning

- A detailed review of the clinical findings and all appropriate imaging studies is performed before the procedure.
- Shortening should be determined to be less than 25 mm using a lateral radiograph,[11] although some suggest spica casting can be performed regardless of shortening.[4,7]
- If the mechanism of injury is considered low energy, a single-leg "walking spica" should be considered, as evidence has shown equivalent outcomes compared to traditional spica casting while significantly decreasing the burden of care on the family.[5,11]
- The presence of concomitant injuries should be considered as well as factors that may hinder or complicate treatment.

### Positioning

- The child is taken to the operating room or sedation unit and placed in the supine position on the table. Cast application in the operating room or the emergency department under sedation has been shown to yield equal results.[12]
- The injured extremity is casted first, and then the patient is transferred to a spica table.

TECHNIQUES

## Traditional Spica Casting

- A long-leg cast is placed with the knee and ankle flexed at 90 degrees (**TECH FIG 1A**). Because of reports of compartment syndrome of the leg after spica casting for pediatric femur fractures,[10,13] many centers (ours included) have been using less hip and knee flexion and not including the foot in the cast of the injured leg.
- Extra padding in the popliteal fossa is applied. To avoid vascular compromise, care must be taken not to flex the knee once the padding is in place.
- A valgus mold at the fracture site is used to prevent varus deformity (**TECH FIG 1B**).
- The patient is transferred to a spica table, where the weight of the legs is supported with manual traction.
- The hip is placed at 90 degrees of flexion and 30 degrees of abduction. Fifteen degrees of external rotation at the hip is used to allow alignment of the proximal and distal fragments (**TECH FIG 1C,D**).
- The remainder of the spica cast is placed while holding the fracture out to length.
- Care should be taken to avoid excessive traction, which increases the risk of compartment syndrome and skin sloughing.
- New AP and lateral radiographs are taken to ensure acceptable anatomic alignment.
- Gore-Tex liners are used at some institutions to prevent diaper rash and superficial infections.

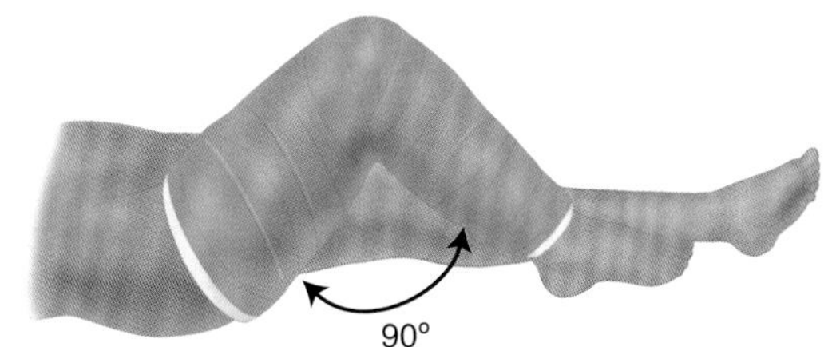


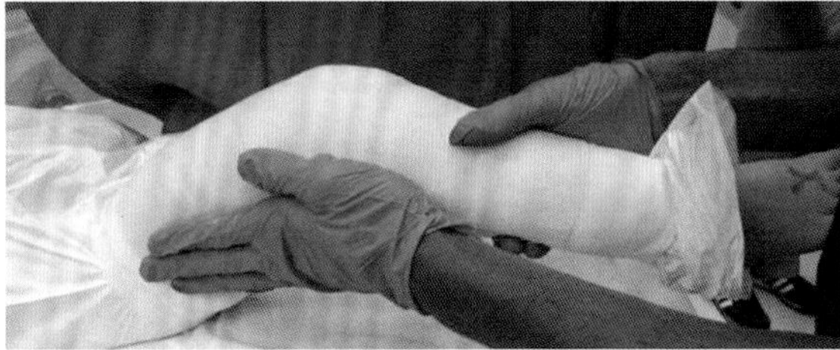

**TECH FIG 1** • **A.** Cylinder cast with 90 degrees of knee flexion for traditional spica casting. **B.** Valgus molding technique to prevent varus deformity in early postcasting period. *(continued)*

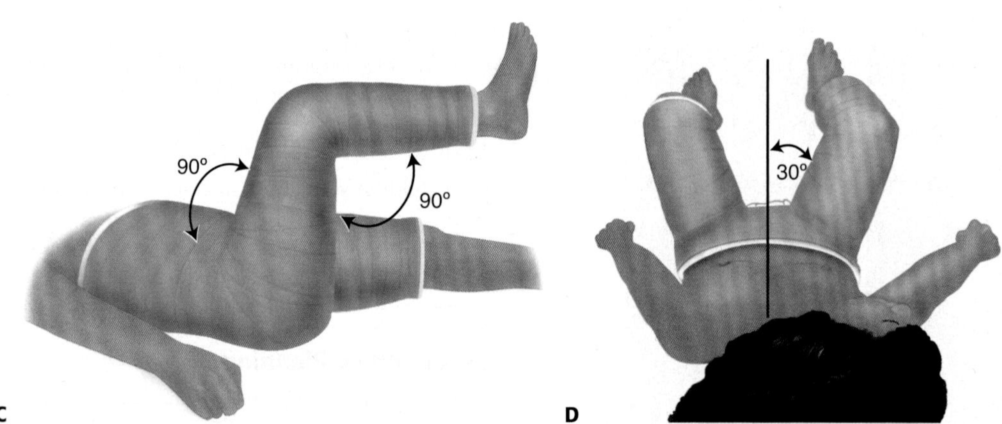


**TECH FIG 1** • *(continued)* **C,D.** Traditional spica casting with 90 degrees of hip flexion, 30 degrees of abduction, and 15 degrees of external rotation.

## Walking Spica Casting

- A walking spica is becoming a popular choice for low-energy femur fractures.
- The cylinder cast should be applied with about 50 degrees of knee flexion.
- The foot remains uncovered with the cast stopping in the supramalleolar area, which is protected with extra padding.
- Before the remainder of the cast is applied, the hip is flexed to 45 degrees and remains abducted to 30 degrees with 15 degrees of external rotation (**TECH FIG 2A,B**).
- The pelvic band is applied with multiple layers of stockinette folded on the abdomen to prevent abdominal compression from the casting. These folded layers of stockinette are removed after the pelvic band is placed (**TECH FIG 2C**).
  - For children who still wear diapers, avoid excessive abdominal padding. The diaper becomes difficult to anchor, and the cast becomes easy to soil.
- It is important to reinforce the cast on the injured side anteriorly at the hip. Seven or eight layers of folded fiberglass are placed in the inter-hip crease to decrease the risk of the cast breaking, whereas a wide pelvic band is needed to immobilize the hip as well as possible.
- Reinforce the anterior aspect of the knee so the cast does not wear out from the child crawling.

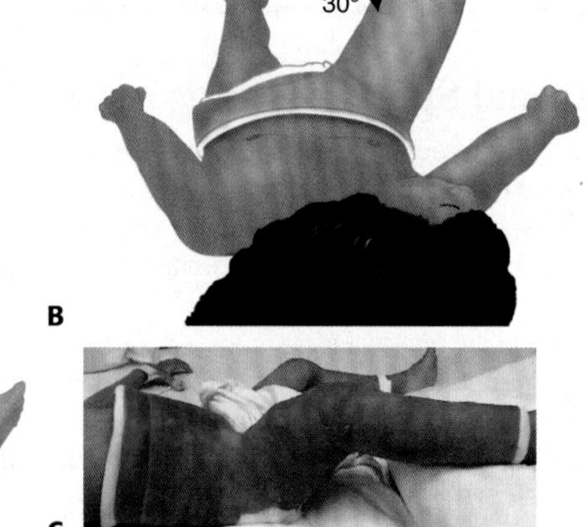


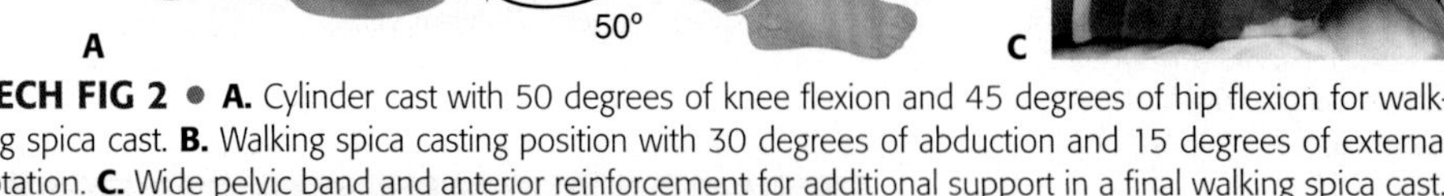


**TECH FIG 2** • **A.** Cylinder cast with 50 degrees of knee flexion and 45 degrees of hip flexion for walking spica cast. **B.** Walking spica casting position with 30 degrees of abduction and 15 degrees of external rotation. **C.** Wide pelvic band and anterior reinforcement for additional support in a final walking spica cast.

## PEARLS AND PITFALLS

| | |
|---|---|
| **Indications** | ■ Spica casting is best used for children 1–6 years old with isolated femoral shaft fractures. |
| **Contraindications** | ■ Shortening of more than 2.5 cm (controversial)<br>■ Massive swelling of the thigh<br>■ Associated injury or skin compromise that precludes cast treatment |
| **Walking spica** | ■ Effective for low-energy isolated femur fractures<br>■ Toddlers typically pull to stand and begin walking in 2–3 weeks. |
| **Reasons for cast change or intervention** | ■ Excessive angulation (more than 15 degrees)<br>■ Shortening (more than 2.5 cm)<br>■ Excessive soiling of the cast |
| **Other complications** | ■ Need for valgus wedge adjustment (angulation <15 degrees)<br>■ Skin irritation, including diaper rash and superficial infections<br>■ Compartment syndrome—may be associated with use of short-leg cast to apply traction during application of 90/90 spica cast[13] |

## POSTOPERATIVE CARE

- A significant burden of care is placed on the family of a child with a spica cast, including cast care, travel difficulties, and loss of time at work.
- We counsel the family, immediately after reduction in casting, that wedging of the cast may be necessary at about 10 to 14 days after injury.
- We schedule the family to return 1 or 2 weeks after injury; at that time, true AP and lateral radiographs are obtained of the injured femur in the cast. If there is unsatisfactory alignment or either angulation or shortening, we will wedge the cast at the clinic and repeat radiographs. This frequently avoids unnecessary trips back to the operating room in the postoperative period for loss of reduction.
- Prior to callus formation, if shortening of more than 2 cm occurs, one of three options may be required: cast change, traction, or external fixation.
- Shortening of more than 2 cm once callus has formed may be treated with osteoclasis and lengthening techniques at a pace of 1 mm per day.
- At union, acceptable angulation and shortening varies by age (Table 1).

## OUTCOMES

- Typically, the spica cast is worn for 4 to 8 weeks, depending on the extent of the injury.
- Infant fractures heal in 3 to 4 weeks.

**Table 1 Acceptable Angulation of the Femur**

| Age | Varus–Valgus | Anteroposterior | Shortening |
|---|---|---|---|
| Birth to 2 y | 30 degrees | 30 degrees | 15 mm |
| 2–5 y | 15 degrees | 20 degrees | 20 mm |
| 6–10 y | 10 degrees | 15 degrees | 15 mm |
| 11 y to maturity | 5 degrees | 10 degrees | 10 mm |

From Beaty JH, Kasser JR, eds. Rockwood and Wilkins' Fractures in Children, ed 7. Philadelphia: Wolters Kluwer/Lippincott Williams & Wilkins, 2010.

- Toddler fractures heal in 6 weeks.
- On removal of the cast, children are encouraged to stand up and walk as soon as they are comfortable.
- Illgen and colleagues[7] found that standard spica casting was successful (without cast change or wedging) about 86% of the time.
- Immediate spica casting in the emergency department under conscious sedation and discharge has been shown to have similar rates of complication and rereduction as "early" spica casting.[3,12]
- Single-leg walking spica casts have been shown to be a safe and effective way to manage low-energy isolated femoral shaft fractures.[4,5,11]

## COMPLICATIONS

- Nonunion
- Delayed union
- Malunion (angular and rotational deformity)
- Leg length discrepancy (shortening and overgrowth)
- Compartment syndrome
- Neurovascular injury

## REFERENCES


1. Beaty JH. Femoral-shaft fractures in children and adolescents. J Am Acad Orthop Surg 1995;3:207–217.
2. Bridgman S, Wilson R. Epidemiology of femoral fractures in children in the West Midlands region of England 1991 to 2001. J Bone Joint Surg Br 2004;86(8):1152–1157.
3. Cassinelli EH, Young B, Vogt M, et al. Spica cast application in the emergency room for select pediatric femur fractures. J Orthop Trauma 2005;19:709–716.
4. Epps HR, Molenaar E, O'Connor DP. Immediate single-leg spica cast for pediatric femoral diaphysis fractures. J Pediatr Orthop 2006;26: 491–496.
5. Flynn JM, Garner MR, Jones KJ, et al. The treatment of low-energy femoral shaft fractures: a prospective study comparing the "walking spica" with the traditional spica cast. J Bone Joint Surg Am 2011;93: 2196–2202.
6. Hinton RY, Lincoln A, Crockett MM, et al. Fractures of the femoral shaft in children. Incidence, mechanisms, and sociodemographic risk factors. J Bone Joint Surg Am 1999;81(4):500–509.
7. Illgen R II, Rodgers WB, Hresko MT, et al. Femur fractures in children: treatment with early sitting spica casting. J Pediatr Orthop 1998;18:481–487.

8. Jauquier N, Doerfler M, Haecker F, et al. Immediate hip spica is as effective as, but more efficient than, flexible intramedullary nailing for femoral shaft fractures in pre-school children. J Child Orthop 2010;4:461–465.
9. Landin LA. Epidemiology of children's fractures. J Pediatr Orthop 1997;6:79–83.
10. Large TM, Frick SL. Compartment syndrome of the leg after treatment of a femoral fracture with an early sitting spica cast. A report of two cases. J Bone Joint Surg Am 2003;85-A(11):2207–2210.
11. Leu D, Sargent MC, Ain MC, et al. Spica casting for pediatric femoral fractures: a prospective, randomized controlled study of single leg versus double-leg spica casts. J Bone Joint Surg Am 2012;94;1259–1264.
12. Mansour AA III, Wilmoth JC, Mansour AS, et al. Immediate spica casting of pediatric femoral fractures in the operating room versus the emergency department: comparison of reduction, complications, and hospital charges. J Pediatr Orthop 2010;8: 813–817.
13. Mubarak SJ, Frick S, Sink E, et al. Volkmann contracture and compartment syndromes after femur fractures in children treated with 90/90 spica casts. J Pediatr Orthop 2006;26:567–572.
14. Rewers A, Hedegaard H, Lezotte D, et al. Childhood femur fractures, associated injuries, and sociodemographic risk factors: a population-based study. Pediatrics 2005;115:e543–e552.

# Closed Reduction and External Fixation of Femoral Shaft Fractures

24

CHAPTER

Afamefuna M. Nduaguba and John M. Flynn

## DEFINITION

- Femoral shaft fractures occur in children with a bimodal age distribution peaking at ages 2 and 12 years.[1]
- The peak in age distribution at age 2 years is due to relative weakness of primarily woven bone at a time when ambulation increases the risk of fall-related trauma.

## ANATOMY

- Muscular deforming forces, if severe, increase the need for surgical fixation. In proximal and midshaft femoral shaft fractures, the proximal fragment tends to be forced into abduction and external rotation. This is more significant in proximal fractures than in midshaft fractures.
- Fractures of the distal third of the femoral shaft tend not to deform greatly, whereas supracondylar femoral fractures are often forced into apex posterior angulation.

## PATHOGENESIS

- In toddlers, these injuries tend to be low energy and occur during normal activity. In adolescents, they tend to be higher energy injuries that may result from motor vehicle, biking, or high-speed sporting accidents.
- Abuse should be considered in the infant or toddler with a femur fracture, especially if the child is nonambulatory.

## PATIENT HISTORY AND PHYSICAL FINDINGS

- In an unconscious patient or a patient with an insensate lower extremity, deformity, erythema, crepitance, and swelling might indicate the presence of a femoral fracture.
- If child abuse is suspected, a skeletal survey should be obtained and Child Protective Services should be notified. Infants are more likely than toddlers to be the victims of child abuse in the setting of a femoral fracture.

## IMAGING AND OTHER DIAGNOSTIC STUDIES

- Anteroposterior (AP) and lateral radiographs of pelvis and femur are obtained. The hip and knee should be visualized as well to evaluate for possible associated injuries (**FIG 1**).
- Radiographs should be evaluated for fracture pattern, location, displacement, angulation, and shortening.

## SURGICAL MANAGEMENT

- Operative management of femoral shaft fractures should be considered in any femur fracture in a child older than 5 years of age. In younger children, polytrauma, head injury, high-energy trauma, open fracture, severe comminution, or body habitus incompatible with spica cast care are relative indications for operative management.
- Surgical options include flexible nailing, plating, rigid intramedullary nailing, and external fixation.
- Indications specifically for external fixation include polytrauma, concomitant head injury, open fracture with severe soft tissue damage or contamination, severe comminution, and very proximal subtrochanteric or distal fractures at the diaphyseal–metaphyseal junction.
- Midshaft transverse fractures are at a higher risk of refracture when treated with external fixation compared to other methods of stabilization.

## PREOPERATIVE PLANNING

- The surgeon should determine where pins will be placed before surgery.
- In each fragment, there must be at least 2 cm of intervening bone between the physis and the outermost pin and at least 2 cm between the fracture and the innermost pin.
- The appropriate pin size varies according to the device. The AO/Synthes device guide recommends 4.0-mm Schanz screws be used, whereas the EBI device guide recommends screws not larger than one-third of the bone diameter.

### Positioning

- The patient should be placed on either a radiolucent operating table or a fracture table. The latter is useful if preoperative reduction is desired.

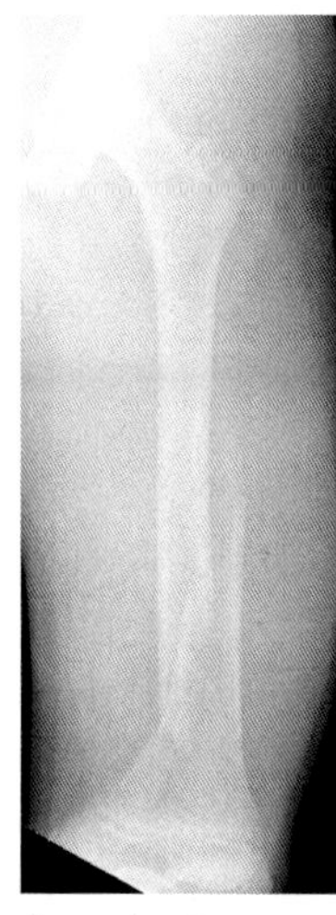

**FIG 1** • Preoperative radiograph of a 12-year-old boy who sustained a distal femoral shaft fracture.

## Biomet DFS XS Fixator Technique

### Pin and Screw Placement

- The first pin inserted should go into the shorter or more difficult bone fragment.
- After making a stab incision over the first pin site, the surgeon dissects bluntly to the near cortex.
- The trocar is inserted into the soft tissue guide and seated onto the femur perpendicular to its long axis. The trocar is removed, and the soft tissue guide is impacted gently to prevent slippage.
- The appropriate drill guide (based on the chosen screw size) is inserted through the soft tissue guide down to bone.
- After attaching a drill stop onto the appropriate bit, the surgeon drills through the near cortex, using the drill guide to keep the pilot hole perpendicular to the long axis of the bone. Drilling should stop once the near cortex is penetrated.
- The surgeon slides the bit up to the far cortex without drilling. The drill stop is adjusted so that the drill can be advanced no more than 5 mm (**TECH FIG 1A**). The surgeon then drills through the far cortex.
- The drill bit and the drill guide are removed without unseating the soft tissue guide.
- The appropriate screw is inserted into the pilot hole, and the screw is advanced using the T-wrench until it protrudes 2 mm beyond the far cortex. The screw cannot be backed out of bone without losing grip because of its conical shape.
- Any tented skin is released with a scalpel.
- The surgeon slides the telescoping arm of the assembled fixator onto the screw in the appropriate position. The clamp bolt is not tightened.
- The soft tissue guide is inserted into another clamp position on the same telescoping arm. Again, the clamp bolt should be loose enough to allow translation of the soft tissue cover through the arm.
- Once the soft tissue guide has been seated on the near cortex, the clamp bolt is tightened to prevent loss of alignment. Repeating the previously mentioned steps, a second screw is inserted in the position now occupied by the soft tissue guide (**TECH FIG 1B**).
- Once both screws have been placed in the first fragment, the previously mentioned steps are repeated on the second fragment (**TECH FIG 1C**).
- The telescoping arm clamp bolts are tightened before final reduction.

### Final Reduction

- The final reduction is made with a variety of adjustments.
- Length can be adjusted on each telescoping arm by either loosening the telescoping set screw and adjusting length manually or by loosening the compression–distraction screw and using this feature to adjust length (**TECH FIG 2A**).
- The locking connector bolts can be loosened for the correction of angular deformity (**TECH FIG 2B**).
- Each telescoping arm can also be rotated using the rotational set screw on the central body of the fixator (**TECH FIG 2C**). These can be loosened simultaneously to rotate the central body of the fixator to bring the central locking joints into the plane of correction (**TECH FIG 2D**).
- Each telescoping arm is able to extend up to 2 cm. If more length is needed, a 4-cm arm may be used. This is especially useful when one arm is occupied by the T-clamp, which has no telescoping feature.

### Alternative T-Clamp Technique

- If desired, the T-clamp can be used when the fracture pattern precludes placement of screws longitudinally in one of the bone fragments.
- The T-clamp is applied before the telescoping arm using the screw insertion technique described.
- After the T-clamp is in place, the screws for the telescoping arm are placed in the other fragment as in the standard configuration described earlier.

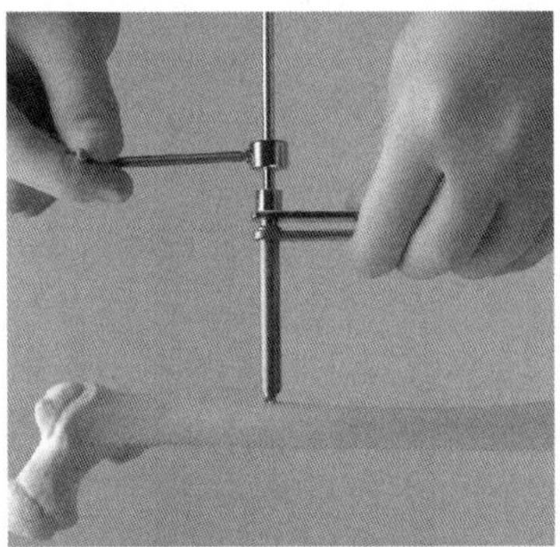
A

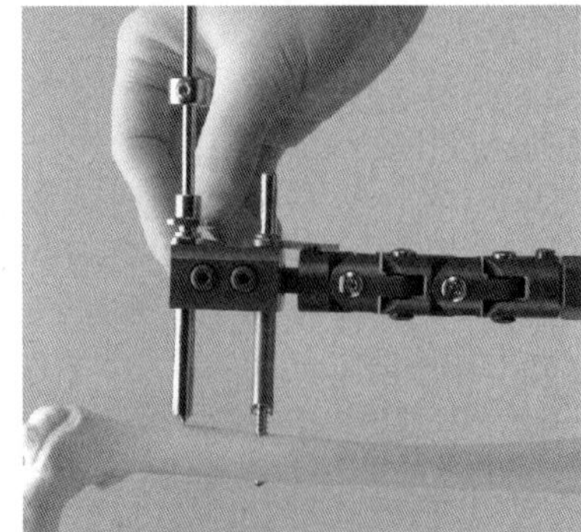
B

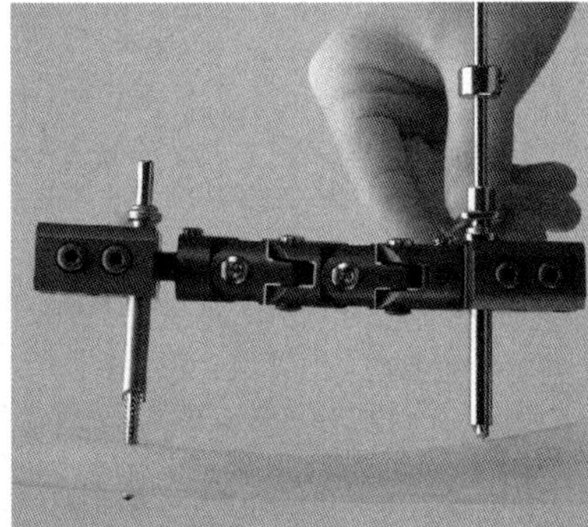
C

**TECH FIG 1** • **A.** Repositioning of drill stop about 5 mm from the base of the drill guide. **B.** Insertion of a second bone screw into the same bone screw cluster using the identical technique as previously described. **C.** Insertion of a second bone screw into the opposite bone screw cluster using the identical technique as previously described. (Courtesy of Biomet Trauma, Copyright 2009. All rights reserved.)

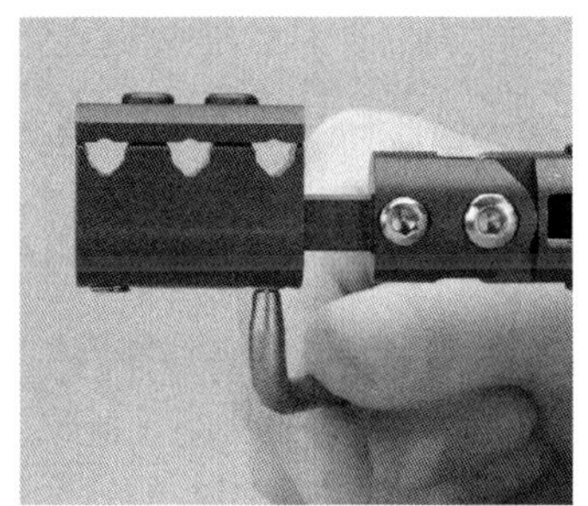
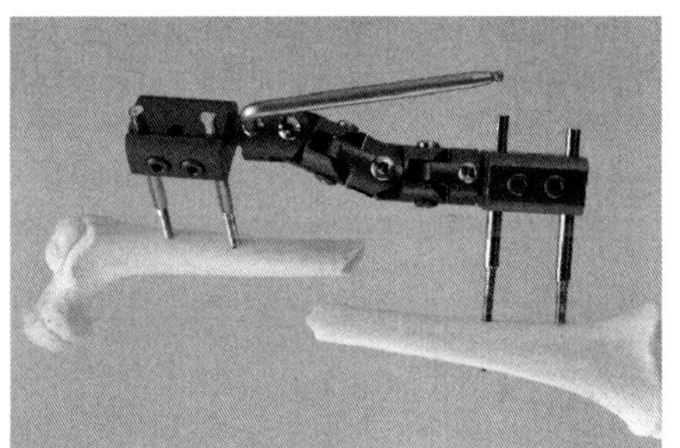
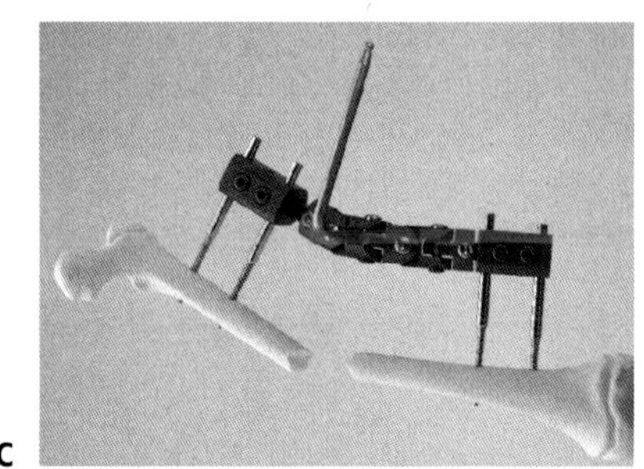
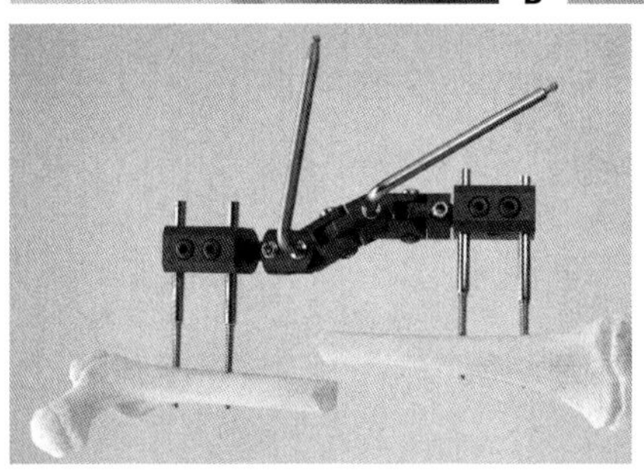

**TECH FIG 2** • **A.** Manual length adjustment. **B.** Each of the locking joints will provide angular adjustments in a plane relative to fixator position as applied to the bone. **C.** Rotation about the axis of the fixator may be achieved by releasing the rotational set screw on either end of the central body component. **D.** Translational adjustments are performed by releasing two locking joints in the same plane as the desired correction. (Courtesy of Biomet Trauma, Copyright 2009. All rights reserved.)

## AO/Synthes Technique Using Pediatric Femoral Shaft Frame with Combination Clamps

### Construct Application

- Note: All Schanz screws must be coplanar if double stacking (for increased rigidity) or dynamization is desired.
- The most proximal screw and the most distal screw are inserted before inserting the inner pins. Screws should be placed with at least 2 cm of bone between the screw and the physis.
- The screw is inserted in the following manner.
  - A stab incision is made.
  - The trocar with protective sleeve is seated onto the femur by passing it through the incision.
  - The trocar is removed, the screw is inserted into the protective sleeve, and the surgeon drills until the screw is embedded in the far cortex.
  - If preferred, a power drill is used until the near cortex is penetrated; then the surgeon can drill into the far cortex by hand.
- After inserting the outermost (most distal and most proximal) Schanz screws, the surgeon attaches a medium combination clamp to each screw.
- The carbon rod is attached to each clamp. The construct should now consist of two screws, two clamps, and one carbon rod.
- The fracture is reduced, and the clamp bolts are tightened.
- Two additional clamps are attached to the carbon rod. These will attach the inner screws to the carbon rod.
- The two inner screws are inserted in the same fashion as the outer screws. There should be at least 2 cm of bone between the screw and the fracture. These screws are attached to the inner combination clamps, and the bolts are tightened.
  - The construct now consists of four screws, four clamps, and one carbon rod (**TECH FIG 3A**).
- A second carbon rod may be added if additional stiffness is desired, and all screws are coplanar. The rod is secured to each screw with a combination clamp.
  - If this step is completed, the construct will consist of four screws, eight clamps, and two rods (**TECH FIG 3B**).

### Dynamization

- Dynamization can be accomplished only in a double-stacked construct. To dynamize the fixator, the outer bolts on the proximal pins and the inner bolts on the distal pins will be adjusted as follows. The bolt is loosened, a dynamization clip is inserted

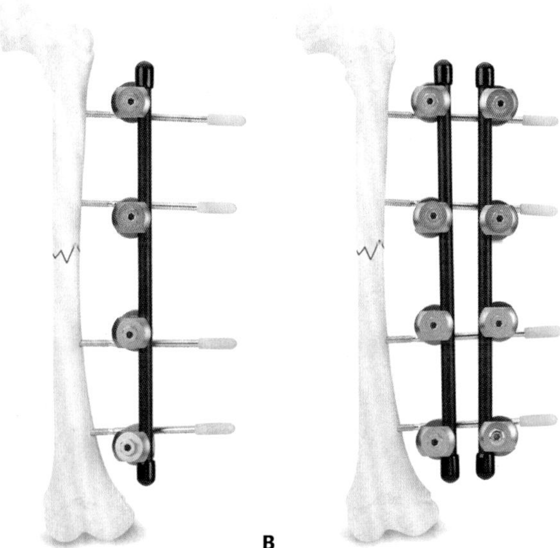

**TECH FIG 3** • **A.** Completed construct with four combination clamps, four Schanz screws, and one carbon rod. **B.** A second rod is added to the frame to increase stiffness. The rod is attached to each Schanz screw using a medium combination clamp. (Copyright Synthes, Inc., or its affiliates. All rights reserved.)

between the rod vise plates, and the bolt is retightened. This procedure is repeated for all four appropriate bolts (**TECH FIG 4A**).

- The dynamization clips can be used in the postoperative setting to increase axial loading across the fracture site or intraoperatively for compression or distraction of the fracture.
- Intraoperative distraction or compression is achieved by dynamizing the fixator, attaching the distractor device adjacent to a dynamized clamp (**TECH FIG 4B**), turning the distractor adjustment ring to either distract or compress, removing the dynamization clips after dynamization or compression, and retightening the clamps.

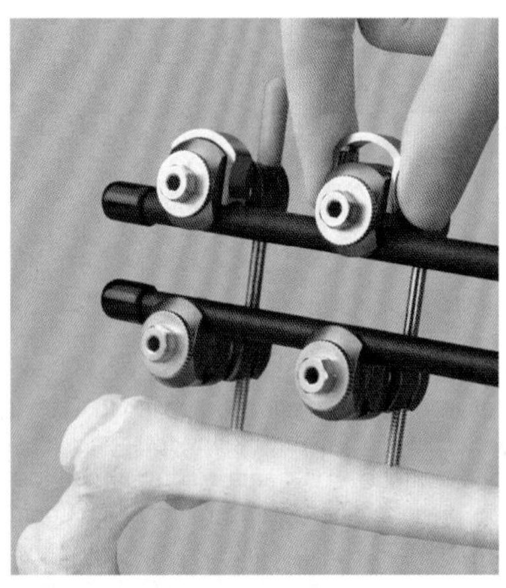
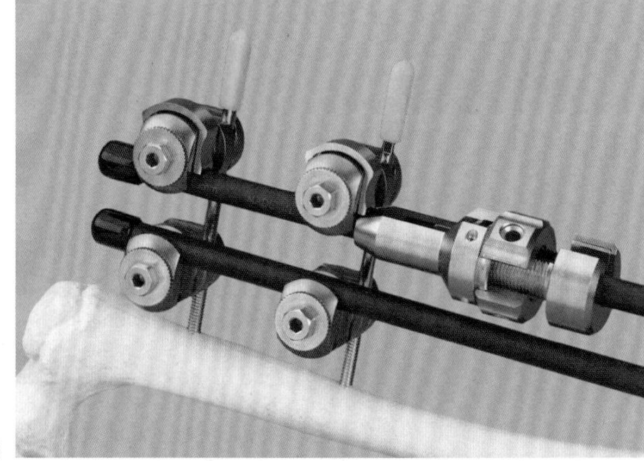

**TECH FIG 4** • **A.** Dynamization technique. Insertion of dynamization clips between rod vise plates. **B.** Distraction–compression technique. Placement of the distractor. (Copyright Synthes, Inc., or its affiliates. All rights reserved.)

## AO/Synthes Technique Using Pediatric Femoral Shaft Frame with Multipin Clamps

- Assembly of this fixator requires screw insertion of one bone fragment to be completed before inserting screws in the other fragment. Therefore, Schanz screws will not be inserted in the outside-to-inside fashion used for the combination clamps.
- The first Schanz screw should be an outer screw, inserted with at least 2 cm of bone between the screw and the physis. A multipin clamp is attached to this first screw and the screw is drilled into the femur. The clamp may be held parallel to the femoral shaft to ensure that the screw enters the femur perpendicularly.
- The second Schanz screw is inserted through the opposite end of the clamp, with at least 2 cm of bone between the screw and the fracture site. This screw and all subsequent screws should be inserted as described earlier, with a stab incision, protective sleeve seating, and screw guidance with the sleeve (**TECH FIG 5A**).

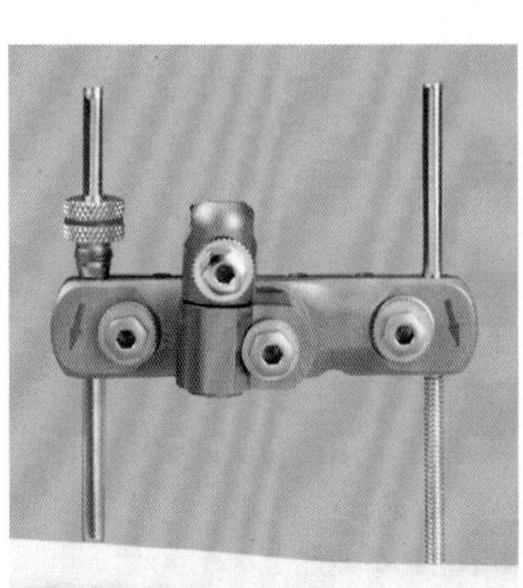
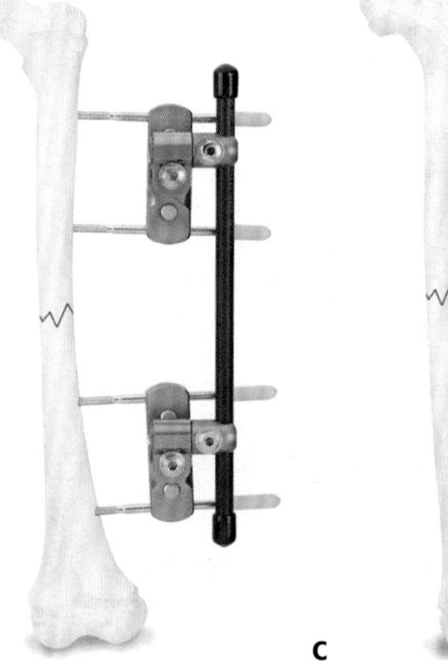
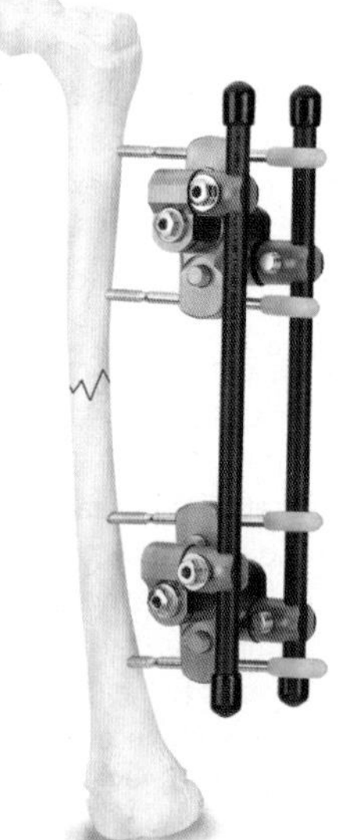

**TECH FIG 5** • **A.** Insertion of Schanz screws through multipin clamp. The screws must be perpendicular to the bone while the clamp is parallel to it. **B.** Completed construct with two multipin clamps with two Schanz screws each and one carbon rod. **C.** Completed construct with double-rod frame. (Copyright Synthes, Inc., or its affiliates. All rights reserved.)

- Up to two additional Schanz screws may be inserted through the multipin clamp if necessary. This completes assembly of the hemifixator.
- These steps are repeated for the other bone fragment.
- The multipin clamp vise plate bolts are tightened on each hemifixator.
- The carbon rod is attached to each multipin clamp.
- The fracture is reduced, and the rod clamping bolt and rod attachment bolt are tightened (**TECH FIG 5B**).
- A second rod may be added to the construct to increase the stiffness of the fixator. This is accomplished with two rod attachment devices (**TECH FIG 5C**).



## AO/Synthes Technique Using Modular Frame

- Modular frame constructs may be created if the fracture pattern precludes coplanar insertion of Schanz screws. This is accomplished by sequential assembly of modules that are then connected by a spanning carbon rod.
- The first screw, which should be an outer screw, is inserted with at least 2 cm of bone between the screw and the physis.
- The second screw, an inner screw, is inserted into the same fragment. There should be at least 2 cm of intervening bone between the screw and the fracture. This screw need not be coplanar with the first screw. This screw and subsequent screws should be inserted as described earlier, with a stab incision, protective sleeve seating, and screw guidance with the sleeve.
- Combination clamps are attached to each screw and the bolts are tightened.
- A carbon rod is connected to each combination clamp. This completes the assembly of the first module.
- The second module is built in the same fashion as the first: The outer screw is inserted, then the inner screw; combination clamps are attached to the screws; and then the clamps are connected with a carbon rod. Each module should consist of two Schanz screws, two combination clamps, and a carbon rod.
- Once each module has been constructed, a combination clamp is attached to each carbon rod. The placement of these clamps should be as follows:
  - The first clamp is placed on the proximal module distal to the most distal screw, and the second clamp is placed proximal to the most proximal screw.
  - These combination clamps are connected to a third carbon rod.
  - If the spanning clamps are placed correctly, the fixator will have a Z formation (**TECH FIG 6A**). If not, the fixator will have an I formation.
- The fracture is reduced before tightening the spanning rod clamps.
- The spanning rod combination clamps are tightened once adequate reduction is obtained.
- To increase the stiffness of the fixator and add rotational stability, a second spanning rod is added. The placement of the second set of spanning clamps should be as follows:
  - The first clamp is placed on the proximal module proximal to the most proximal screw, and the second clamp is placed on the distal rod distal to the most distal screw.
  - These combination clamps are connected to a fourth carbon rod.
  - If this second set of spanning clamps have been placed correctly, the modular rods and the spanning rods will have an hourglass configuration (**TECH FIG 6B**).

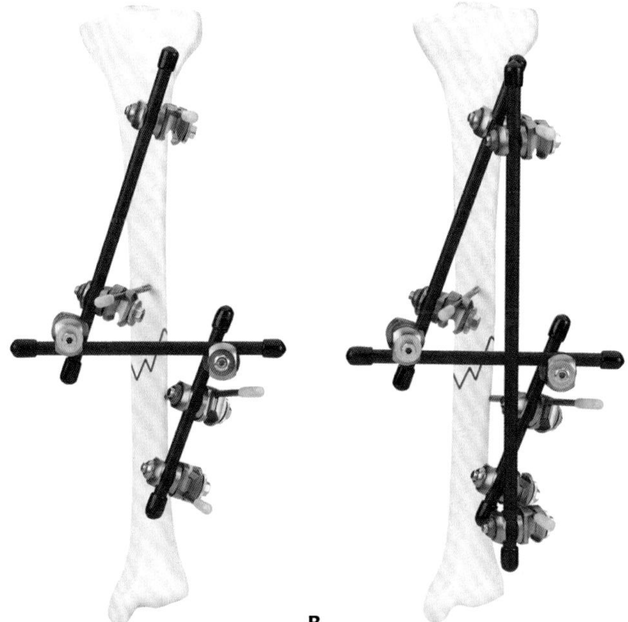


**TECH FIG 6** • **A.** Basic modular frame with connected modules. **B.** Fourth bar is added to frame configuration to increase stiffness and rotational stability. The fourth bar should span the length of the frame, connecting the first and second modules. (Copyright Synthes, Inc., or its affiliates. All rights reserved.)

## PEARLS AND PITFALLS

| | |
|---|---|
| **Indications** | ■ External fixation is best used in cases of polytrauma with concomitant head injuries, open fractures with severe soft tissue damage and contamination, and severe comminution. |
| **Evaluation** | ■ Although many pediatric femur fractures are isolated injuries, high-energy fractures are often associated with head, chest, or abdominal trauma.<br>■ The injured extremity must be thoroughly evaluated for associated trauma.<br>■ Femoral shortening across the fracture site is best visualized with a lateral femur radiograph before traction is applied.<br>■ Corner fractures and bucket-handle fractures are more specific than spiral fractures for nonaccidental injury. |
| **Fixation** | ■ Remodeling potential declines significantly after age 10 years.<br>■ Angulation across the fracture site is better tolerated proximally than distally and better in the sagittal plane than in the coronal plane. |
| **Medicolegal** | ■ Closed treatment of femoral fractures is a common source of malpractice litigation in the field of pediatric orthopaedics. |

## POSTOPERATIVE CARE

- Pin care is essential in avoiding pin tract infection. This skill must be taught in the postoperative setting and reviewed at each office visit.
- Antibiotics with adequate coverage of skin flora should be prescribed at the first sign of pin tract infection.
- Some advocate removal of the external fixator as soon as bridging callus is seen, with subsequent casting if necessary. Others believe that the fixator should be left in place until three of four cortices are bridged by callus.
- A typical radiographic evolution of this injury when treated with external fixation is shown in **FIG 2**.

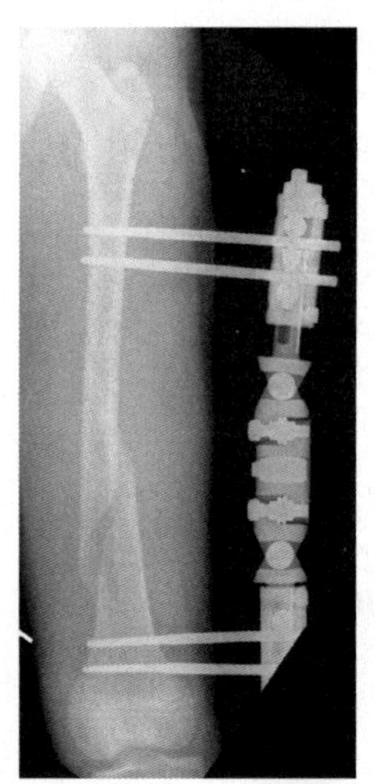
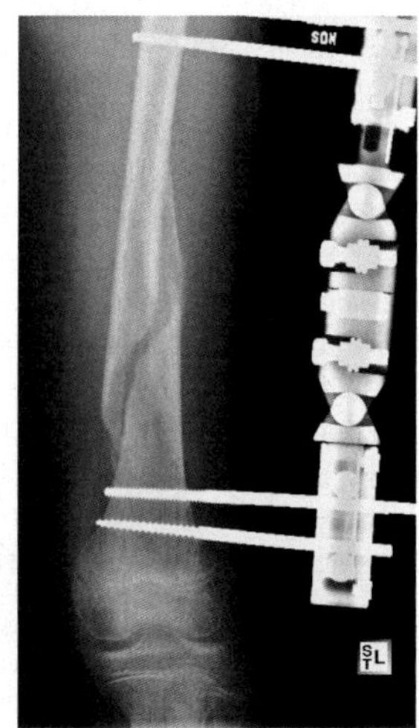
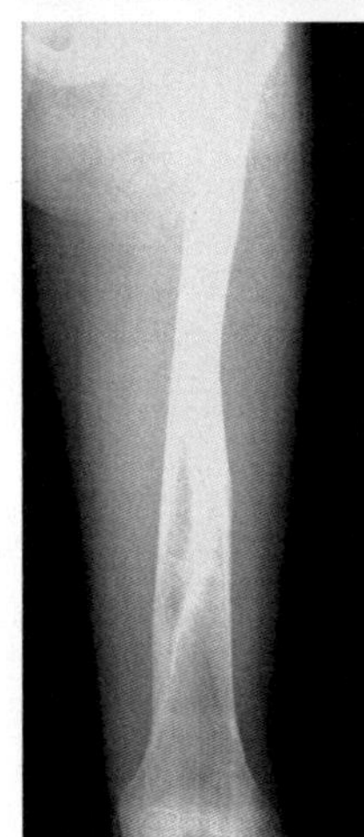

**FIG 2** • Postoperative radiographs from the patient in **FIG 1** on postoperative day 1 (**A**), before external fixator removal on postoperative day 63 (**B**), and at last follow-up on postoperative day 217 (**C**).

## OUTCOMES

- In one series of 37 femur fractures treated with external fixation, the average duration of fixation was 3 to 4 months (range 2 to 5 months). In all but one case, union was achieved at the time of fixator removal.[3]
- Risk of refracture may be as high as 20% after fixator removal.[2,3]
- Pin tract infections occur in about 65% of cases. These can almost always be managed successfully with oral antibiotics; fixator removal is rarely required.
- Although clinically insignificant malunion is often seen, malunion requiring surgical correction is rare.

## COMPLICATIONS

- Pin tract infection
- Deep infection
- Knee stiffness
- Unsightly thigh scars
- Delayed union
- Refracture
- Malunion
- Leg length discrepancy

## REFERENCES


1. Flynn JM, Schwend RM. Management of pediatric femoral shaft fractures. J Am Acad Orthop Surg 2004;12:347–359.
2. Gregory P, Pevny T, Teague D. Early complications with external fixation of pediatric femoral shaft fractures. J Orthop Trauma 1996;10:191–198.
3. Miner T, Carroll KL. Outcomes of external fixation of pediatric femoral shaft fractures. J Pediatr Orthop 2000;20:405–410.

# Flexible Intramedullary Nailing of Femoral Shaft Fractures

25

CHAPTER

Christine M. Goodbody and John M. Flynn

## DEFINITION

- Femoral shaft fractures in children occur with an incidence of 20 per 100,000.[3,9,14] They constitute 2% of all pediatric fractures.[11]
- In a very young child who presents with a femoral shaft fracture, child abuse must be considered, especially if the child is not yet walking.[2] In the young child who has a history of multiple fractures or fracture after minimal trauma, osteogenesis imperfecta might be the underlying cause and is often mistaken for child abuse.
- In children who sustain multiple traumatic injuries, the nature and severity of each injury must be considered in order to prioritize and optimize treatment.

## ANATOMY

- During childhood, the femur is initially composed of weaker woven bone, which is gradually replaced with lamellar bone.
- The profunda femoris artery gives rise to four perforating arteries, which enter the femur posteromedially. The majority of the blood is supplied by the endosteal circulation. During fracture healing, however, the majority of the blood is supplied by the periosteal circulation.
- The femoral shaft flares distally, forming the supracondylar area of the femur. This area serves as the entry point for retrograde nailing with flexible intramedullary nails. Surgeons should maintain an awareness of the nearby distal femoral physis, which can be injured during nail insertion.

## PATHOGENESIS

- Age is an important factor to consider in terms of the pathogenesis of the injury. The degree of trauma required to cause injury increases exponentially, as the character of the bone changes and gradually becomes stronger and larger from infancy to adolescence. Low-energy injuries resulting in fractures may point to a pathologic nature of the condition.
- The radiographic appearance of the fracture usually reflects the mechanism of injury and the force applied. High-velocity injuries usually present with more complex, comminuted patterns.
- The position of the fracture fragments after the injury depends on the level of the fracture and reflects the soft tissue and muscle forces acting on the femur.

## PATIENT HISTORY AND PHYSICAL FINDINGS

- In most cases, there is a history of a traumatic event.
- In an isolated femur fracture, the thigh appears swollen, with minor bruises and abrasions. Shortening may also be present.
- The affected extremity should be checked to ensure that no vascular or neurologic injury is present.
- In cases of high-energy trauma, concomitant injuries to the skin and soft tissue as well as other organ systems are usually present.
- An examination of the knee should be performed to ensure that no ligamentous injury is present. This may be performed under anesthesia.

## IMAGING AND OTHER DIAGNOSTIC STUDIES

- Standard high-quality anteroposterior (AP) and lateral radiographs of the femur are usually all that is needed to define the extent and severity of the injury (**FIG 1**).
  - Radiographs should include the joints above and below the fracture site to avoid missing any concomitant injuries.

## DIFFERENTIAL DIAGNOSIS

- Acute traumatic fracture in normal bone
- Stress fracture
- Pathologic fracture

## SURGICAL MANAGEMENT

- Elastic nailing of the femoral shaft is the optimal treatment for most femur fractures in children 5 to 12 years old.
- In rare cases in the 5- to 12-year-old age group, children with very length-unstable fractures, or older children who are very

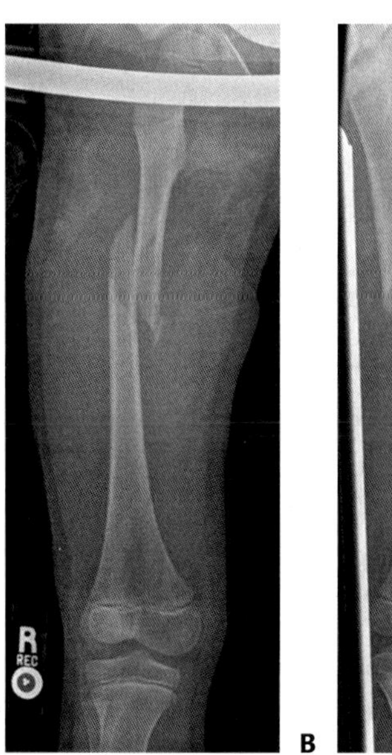


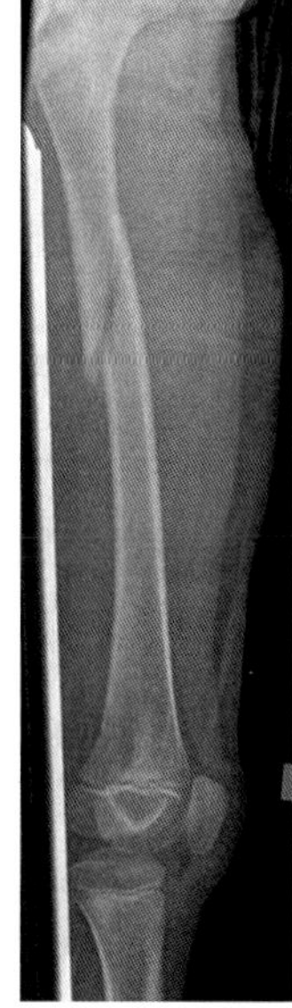


**FIG 1** • Preoperative AP (**A**) and lateral (**B**) radiographs of a 6-year-old girl who sustained a spiral diaphyseal femoral shaft fracture while playing soccer. This injury was treated with titanium elastic nails.

heavy, are best treated with another method (submuscular plating, external fixation, or trochanteric entry nailing, described in other chapters).

- Elastic nailing can be used in skeletally immature adolescents, especially for length stable fractures in children less than 50 kg, although there is a slightly higher rate of loss of alignment, delayed healing, and poor results than in younger children.
- In very rare circumstances, elastic nailing can be used in children 3 to 5 years old. Possible indications include very high energy injury, soft tissue injury that makes casting risky, very obese preschool children, or polytrauma.

## Preoperative Planning

- The diameter of the nails is predetermined by measuring the isthmus of the femoral shaft. The nail size to be used is usually 40% of the narrowest diameter. For instance, if the isthmus measures 1 cm, two 4-mm nails are used.
- The presence of concomitant injuries should be considered as well as factors that may hinder or complicate treatment.

## Positioning

- The patient is positioned in the supine position. We prefer using a fracture table (**FIG 2**), although a radiolucent table may be used as well.
- The groin area is adequately padded before application of the post.
- The affected extremity is abducted 15 to 30 degrees to allow room for nail placement. The uninjured leg can be held by the ankle (the well-foot holder) and "scissored" with extension of the hip so that it does not block the lateral radiographic view.
  - We generally avoid the well-leg holder that places the hip and knee flexed high above the rest of the patient. Compartment syndrome has been associated with this positioning for femoral shaft fracture treatment.
- A distraction force is applied to the affected extremity through the foot using a foot holder. If there is significant soft tissue injury to the leg, the distraction force may be applied through a traction pin. However, this is rarely necessary in children.
- Ideally, the fracture should be brought out to length and reduced to as near an anatomic position as possible before prepping and draping. Time spent optimizing alignment in the unprepped patient generally pays large dividends in time saved struggling with the fracture reduction just before the nail is passed across the fracture site.
- The extremity is then prepared and draped.

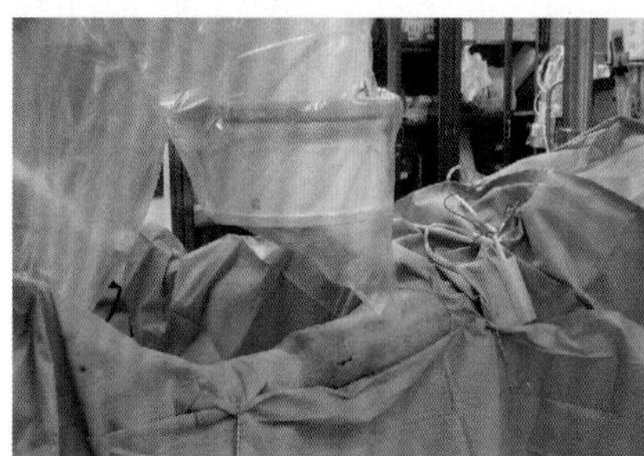

**FIG 2** • The patient is properly positioned in the fracture table, the landmarks are identified fluoroscopically, and the proper incision sites are marked.

TECHNIQUES

## Retrograde Flexible Intramedullary Nailing

### Nail Introduction and Fracture Reduction

- The nail entry sites, which are located on the medial and lateral aspects of the distal femoral metaphysis, are identified using an image intensifier.
- The distal femoral physis is identified, and this position is marked on the skin to remind the surgical team to avoid the dissection in this area.
- A 2-cm incision is made beginning at the level where the nail will enter the femoral metaphysis and extending distally. Incisions proximal to the entry site in the distal femur do not aid in nail placement.
- The incision is made and carried through the fascia and quadriceps muscle; spreading with a hemostat can facilitate exposure down to bone.
- A drill is placed (with a soft tissue protector) through the incision site against the distal femoral metaphysis. The starting point is the midpoint of the femoral shaft in the AP plane (**TECH FIG 1A**).
- The size of the drill bit used is largely dependent on the size of the nail; the drill bit should be slightly larger than the nail (eg, a 4.5-mm drill bit is used when using a 4.0-mm nail).
- The drill is inserted, and once the femoral cortex has been breached, the drill is angled to a very oblique orientation to facilitate nail passage (**TECH FIG 1B**).
- The nails are prebent into a gentle C shape before insertion (**TECH FIG 1C**).
- The first nail is inserted into the entry site and gently tapped into the femur. The position of the nail is checked under fluoroscopy in both the AP and lateral views to ensure proper nail placement (**TECH FIG 1D**).
- Once the tip of the nail has reached the fracture site, the fracture reduction is perfected and documented in both the AP and lateral planes. The "F" tool can be used to maintain alignment if necessary. The tool was constructed from radiolucent fiberglass bars that are available on most sets.
- Once the reduction is ensured, the first nail is passed across the fracture site, advancing 1 or 2 cm into the proximal fragment (just enough so that it will hold the reduction but not so much that it will begin to alter the alignment between the two fragments at the fracture site).
- Once the first nail has crossed the fracture line, the same steps for insertion are followed for introduction of the second nail (**TECH FIG 1E**).

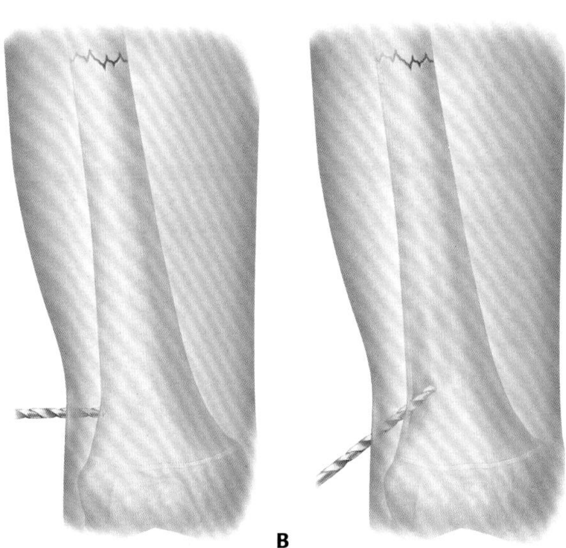

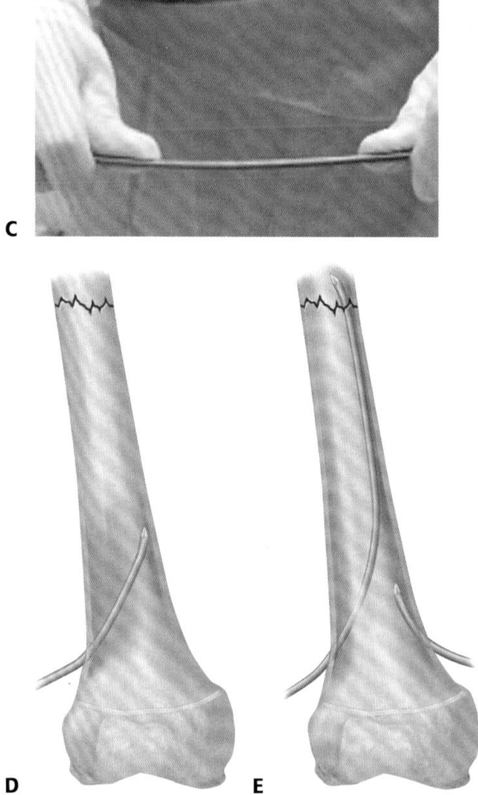

**TECH FIG 1** • **A.** Once the incision has been made, the entry point for the nail is identified 2 cm superior to the growth plate at the midpoint of the femur anteroposteriorly. A 4.5-mm drill bit is used to make the starting point. **B.** Once the cortex has been entered, the drill is angled obliquely to fashion a tract. **C.** The nail is prebent in a gentle C shape before insertion. **D.** The first nail is inserted until it reaches the fracture line. **E.** Once the first nail has reached the fracture line, the second nail is inserted in the same fashion.

## Final Nail Placement

- When reduction has been confirmed and both nails have sufficiently crossed the fracture line (**TECH FIG 2A–C**), both nails are advanced a few millimeters and their position is checked with the image intensifier in both the AP and lateral planes (**TECH FIG 2D**).
- Once the position of both nails has been confirmed, they are gradually advanced to their final proximal point (**TECH FIG 2E**).
- The lateral nail (nail entering through the lateral cortex of the femur) should end at the apophysis of the greater trochanter. The medial nail should come to rest at the medial end side of the calcar at the level of the hip.
- The final position of the nails should be so that only about 1 to 2 cm of each nail is outside its cortical entry site (**TECH FIG 2F,G**). After their final position has been confirmed, the nails are backed out a few centimeters, cut to the proper length, and gently tapped back into their final position with the ends resting flush against the femur and just enough of the nail exposed in order to facilitate later removal. Bending the end of the nails will cause undue irritation of the skin and soft tissue.
- The final fracture configuration is checked (**TECH FIG 2H–J**). If there is a significant gap between the fracture fragments, the distraction is released and the surgeon gently impacts the fracture fragments together.
- A layered closure is performed.
- Rotational alignment of the extremity is evaluated, and any malrotation is corrected before extubation.

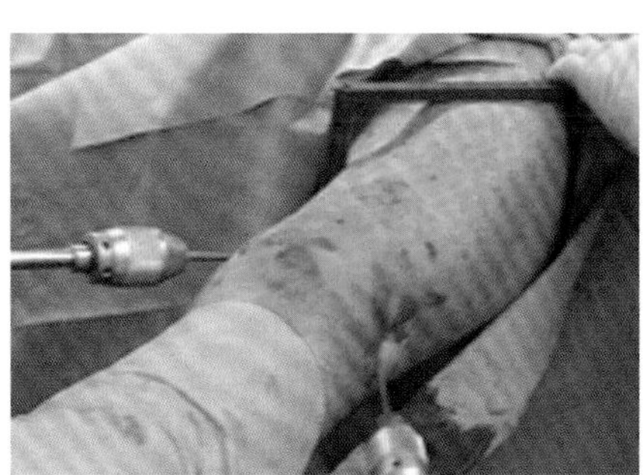

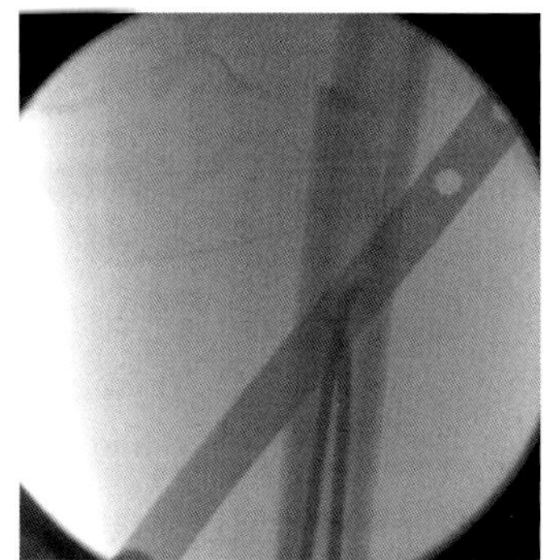

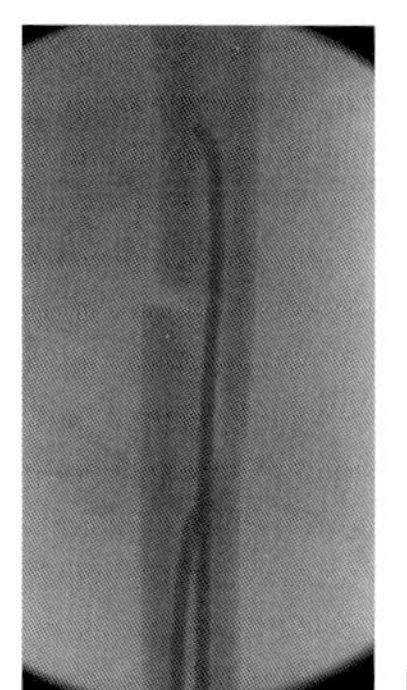

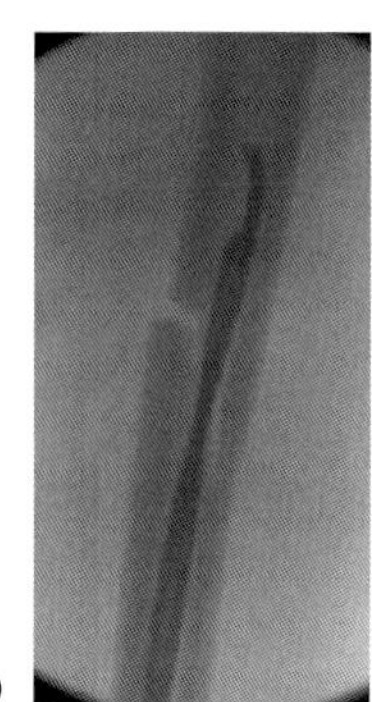

**TECH FIG 2** • **A.** Once both nails have reached the fracture line, reduction of the fracture is checked. The F tool can be used to aid in attaining and maintaining reduction. **B.** The reduction is checked fluoroscopically. **C,D.** Once the reduction is checked, the nails are passed across the fracture line and advanced until they reach their final end point. *(continued)*

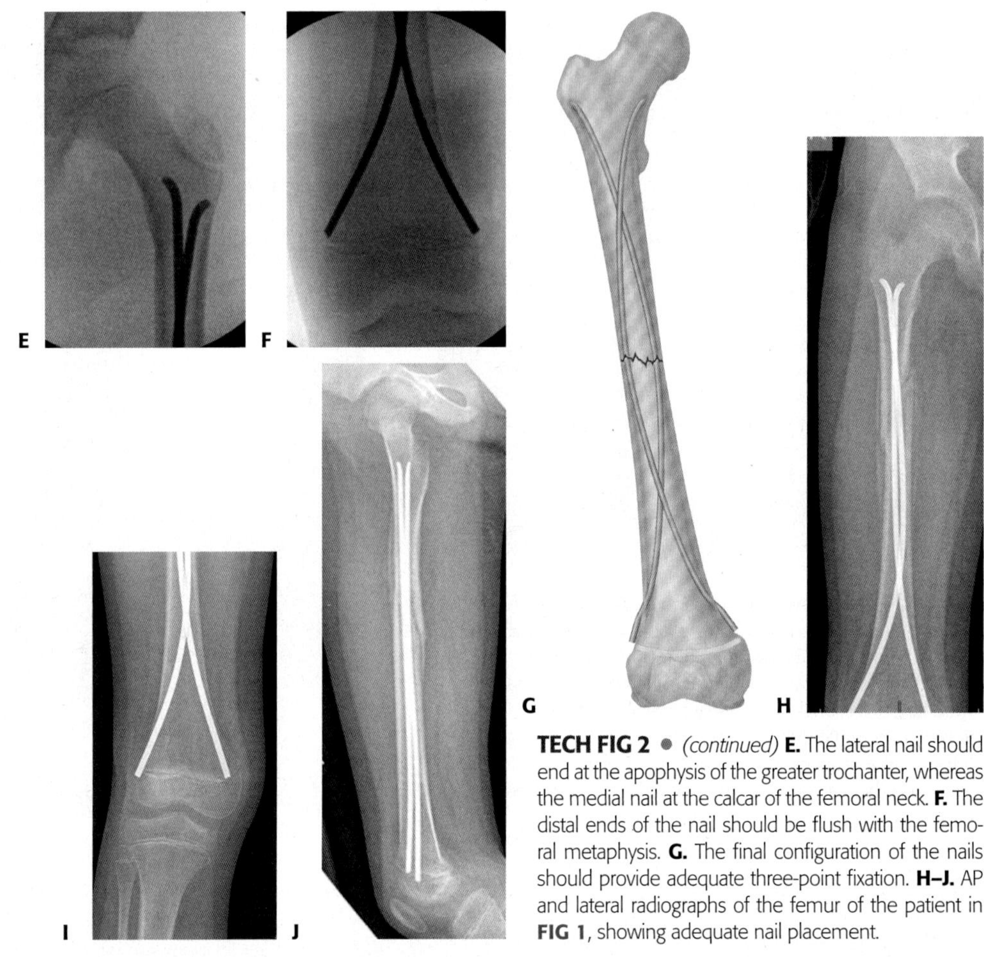

**TECH FIG 2 •** *(continued)* **E.** The lateral nail should end at the apophysis of the greater trochanter, whereas the medial nail at the calcar of the femoral neck. **F.** The distal ends of the nail should be flush with the femoral metaphysis. **G.** The final configuration of the nails should provide adequate three-point fixation. **H–J.** AP and lateral radiographs of the femur of the patient in **FIG 1**, showing adequate nail placement.

## PEARLS AND PITFALLS

| | |
|---|---|
| **Indications** | ▪ The flexible nailing technique is most successful for children ages 5–12 years, weighing less than 50 kg, with length-stable fractures. Skeletally immature adolescents and very proximal, distal, or length-unstable fractures can be treated with flexible nailing, but the complication rate is higher. |
| **Preoperative planning** | ▪ Proper selection and preparation of the nails are crucial, as is proper patient selection. The nail sizes and the entry points should be symmetric. |
| **Fracture fixation** | ▪ Proper nail configuration must be achieved to obtain three-point fixation. The nails should be gently curved before insertion to ensure maximum cortical contact. If insertion or nail passage proves difficult, or the entry site is complicated by soft tissue injury, an anterograde method of insertion through the greater trochanter may be used for one or both nails. |
| **Difficulty in reduction** | ▪ An instrument referred to as the *F tool* is a great aid to reduction. |
| **Skin irritation** | ▪ To avoid skin irritation, the nails should be cut so that they lie flush with the metaphysis of the distal femur, with only about 1–2 cm of the nail outside the cortical entry site. |

## POSTOPERATIVE CARE

- We prefer a knee immobilizer in the immediate postoperative period to reduce the incidence of soft tissue irritation of the knee and to increase the child's comfort.
- Weight bearing is instituted immediately after surgery as tolerated.
- Postoperative analgesics are maintained for continued pain relief and to maximize the rehabilitation period.

## OUTCOMES

- Multiple studies have reported good to excellent outcomes in femoral shaft fractures treated with flexible intramedullary nails.[1,4,5,8,10,15]

- Flynn and coworkers,[6] in a multicenter trial, reported excellent results in 67% (39) of cases and satisfactory results in 31% (18); there was 1 poor result due to malrotation.
- Mehlman and associates[12] showed in a biomechanical study that if an acceptable starting point is achieved, retrograde nailing, as opposed to antegrade nailing, is more stable for fractures of the distal third of the femoral diaphysis.
- Flynn and associates[7] reviewed their first 50 cases and found that insertion site irritation was the most common problem encountered (18% of cases). Very proximal fractures were more challenging to treat, and older, larger children were best managed with additional periods of adjunctive immobilization.
- Moroz and colleagues,[13] in a review of 234 femur fractures in 229 children, found excellent results in 150 (65%), satisfactory in 57 (25%), and poor in 23 (10%). The poor outcomes were secondary to leg length discrepancy in 5 cases, unacceptable angulation in 17, and failure of fixation in 1. They likewise reported a correlation with poor outcome in older children (older than 11 years) and in children who weighed more than 49 kg.
- A systematic review of the available literature on elastic nailing for pediatric femoral shaft fractures by Baldwin and coworkers[1] found that, although most complications were minor, some series reported complication rates upward of 50%. However, functional outcomes were excellent or satisfactory in greater than 88% of patients in each of four studies that reported them.
  - Symptomatic hardware was reported as a complication in 23.4% of all patients.
  - Although nonunion and refracture were uncommon, malunion and malalignment were. The latter occurred with an incidence of 15.1%.
  - Leg length discrepancy was also not unusual but generally not severe.
  - Noted benefits of elastic nailing included decreased length of hospital stay, early return to activity, and high rate of fracture union (99.5%).

## COMPLICATIONS

- Nail irritation at the nail entry site
- Nonunion or delayed union
- Malunion (angular and rotational deformity)
- Leg length discrepancy (shortening and overgrowth)
- Compartment syndrome
- Neurovascular injury
- Implant-related complications

## REFERENCES

1. Baldwin K, Hsu JE, Wenger DR, et al. Treatment of femur fractures in school-aged children using elastic stable intramedullary nailing: a systematic review. J Pediatr Orthop B 2011;20(5):303–308.
2. Beaty JH. Femoral-shaft fractures in children and adolescents. J Am Acad Orthop Surg 1995;3:207–217.
3. Bridgman S, Wilson R. Epidemiology of femoral fractures in children in the West Midlands region of England 1991 to 2001. J Bone Joint Surg Br 2004;86(8):1152–1157.
4. Carey TP, Galpin RD. Flexible intramedullary nail fixation of pediatric femoral fractures. Clin Orthop Relat Res 1996;(332):110–118.
5. Cramer KE, Tornetta P III, Spero CR, et al. Ender rod fixation of femoral shaft fractures in children. Clin Orthop Relat Res 2000;(376):119–123.
6. Flynn JM, Hresko T, Reynolds RA, et al. Titanium elastic nails for pediatric femur fractures: a multicenter study of early results with analysis of complications. J Pediatr Orthop 2001;21:4–8.
7. Flynn JM, Luedtke L, Ganley TJ, et al. Titanium elastic nails for pediatric femur fractures: lessons from the learning curve. Am J Orthop 2002;31:71–74.
8. Heinrich SD, Drvaric DM, Darr K, et al. The operative stabilization of pediatric diaphyseal femur fractures with flexible intramedullary nails: a prospective analysis. J Pediatr Orthop 1994;14:501–507.
9. Hinton RY, Lincoln A, Crockett MM, et al. Fractures of the femoral shaft in children. Incidence, mechanisms, and sociodemographic risk factors. J Bone Joint Surg Am 1999;81(4):500–509.
10. Ho CA, Skaggs DL, Tang CW, et al. Use of flexible intramedullary nails in pediatric femur fractures. J Pediatr Orthop 2006;26:497–504.
11. Landin LA. Epidemiology of children's fractures. J Pediatr Orthop B 1997;6:79–83.
12. Mehlman CT, Nemeth NM, Glos DL. Antegrade versus retrograde titanium elastic nail fixation of pediatric distal-third femoral-shaft fractures: a mechanical study. J Orthop Trauma 2006;20:608–612.
13. Moroz LA, Launay F, Kocher MS, et al. Titanium elastic nailing of fractures of the femur in children: predictors of complications and poor outcome. J Bone Joint Surg Br 2006;88(10):1361–1366.
14. Rewers A, Hedegaard H, Lezotte D, et al. Childhood femur fractures, associated injuries, and sociodemographic risk factors: a population-based study. Pediatrics 2005;115:e543–e552.
15. Saikia K, Bhuyan S, Bhattacharya T, et al. Titanium elastic nailing in femoral diaphyseal fractures of children in 6-16 years of age. Indian J Orthop 2007;41:381–385.

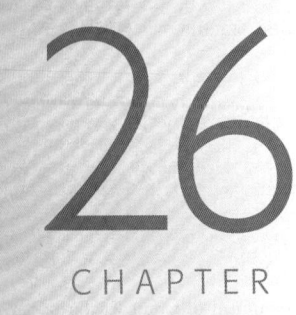

# Submuscular Plating of Pediatric Femur Fractures

Ernest L. Sink and Benjamin F. Ricciardi

## DEFINITION

- Submuscular bridge plating is a minimally invasive, soft tissue preserving approach that provides relative stability for length-unstable pediatric diaphyseal femur fractures.

## ANATOMY

- The distal margin of the vastus lateralis is deep to the iliotibial fascia in line with the proximal pole of the patella.
- The fibers of the distal vastus lateralis are oblique, and the muscle is not attached to the bone, providing a plane between the muscle and lateral periosteum of the femur for plate insertion.

## PATHOGENESIS

- Falls or motor vehicle accidents are the most common mechanisms of injury, representing approximately two-thirds of all pediatric femur fractures.[6]
- Child abuse should be ruled out in pediatric patients with femur fractures, particularly in patients younger than 2 years old.[6]

## NATURAL HISTORY/BACKGROUND

- Femur fractures are the most common cause of hospital admission due to orthopaedic trauma for pediatric patients.[6]
- Male patients are more commonly affected relative to female patients, and there is a bimodal age distribution with peaks in young (younger than 4 years old) patients and adolescent patients.
- Fracture of the femoral diaphysis is more common than trochanteric or distal femoral locations.

## PATIENT HISTORY AND PHYSICAL FINDINGS

- History should include age, mechanism of injury (rule out child abuse in patients younger than 2 years old), other locations of pain to rule out concomitant injury, and relevant medical or family history (eg, cerebral palsy and osteogenesis imperfecta increase the risk of low-energy femur fractures).
- Physical examination reveals shortening and rotational deformity of the affected extremity with painful range of motion. Neurovascular examination, skin integrity, signs of compartment syndrome should all be carefully assessed.
- Concomitant injury should be ruled out because pediatric femur fractures represent high-energy injuries in many cases and can be associated with neurologic, visceral, and other musculoskeletal trauma.

## IMAGING AND OTHER DIAGNOSTIC STUDIES

- An anteroposterior (AP) and lateral view of the injured femur will diagnose the fractured femur. Imaging should include radiographs of the ipsilateral hip and knee to rule out secondary injuries to the femoral neck or knee joint.

## SURGICAL MANAGEMENT

- Operative stabilization is the treatment of choice for pediatric femur fractures in most children 5 years and older through skeletal maturity. Flexible elastic nailing is successful for the majority of diaphyseal femur fractures.[1,3] Factors such as comminution, long oblique length-unstable fractures, and children older than the age of 10 years have resulted in increased complication rates in some series with flexible elastic nailing.[7,10] Therefore, alternative means of stabilization have been suggested for fractures with these characteristics.
- Plate osteosynthesis is a proven method to stabilize pediatric fractures. The use of submuscular bridge plating for comminuted femur fractures allows for rigid stabilization, minimally invasive techniques, avoidance of avascular necrosis (AVN) of the femoral head, and stabilization of the diaphyseal/metaphyseal junction.
- The procedure is indicated for patients 5 years old to skeletal maturity. The fracture patterns most amenable to bridge plating are comminuted or long oblique length-unstable fractures. Older or heavier children with femoral canals unable to accommodate an intramedullary (IM) nail would also be appropriate candidates (**FIG 1**).
- Submuscular plating is also a reliable option for proximal or distal one-third femur fractures.[1] For these fractures, there needs to be room for two to three screws in the proximal or distal diaphyseal region.
- It has a relative contraindication in patients that have transverse fractures. We prefer flexible IM nails to bridge plating for transverse or short oblique mid-diaphyseal fractures.

### Preoperative Planning

- All patients should be carefully evaluated for other injuries including knee or hip injuries.
- An operating room equipped with traction bed and fluoroscopy is critical.
- No preoperative templating is required, as the plate length and contour are chosen under sterile conditions.
- It is important to have the long plates available and the appropriate screw set.
- Finally, evaluating the natural rotation of the contralateral leg is useful as a reference prior to draping.

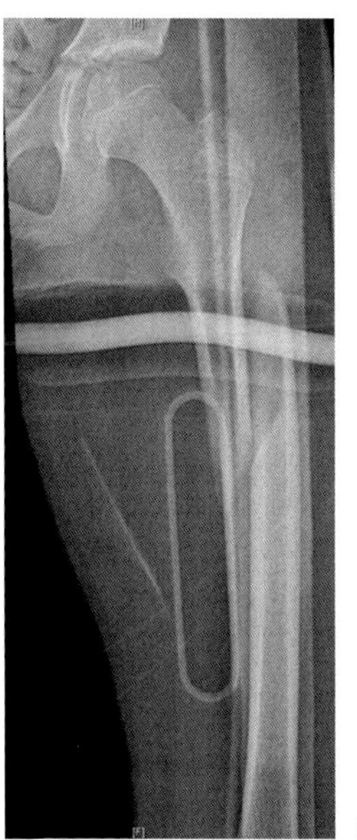
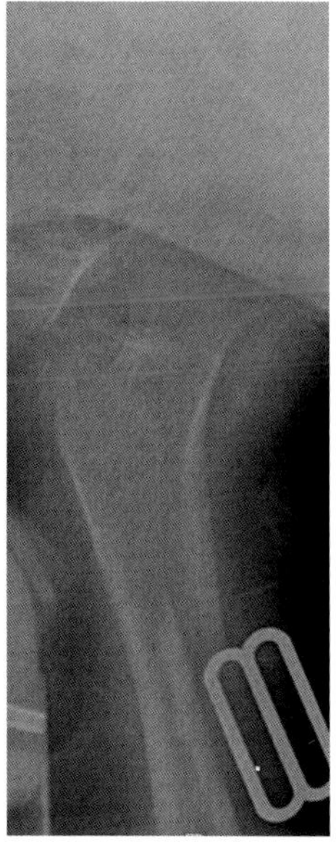
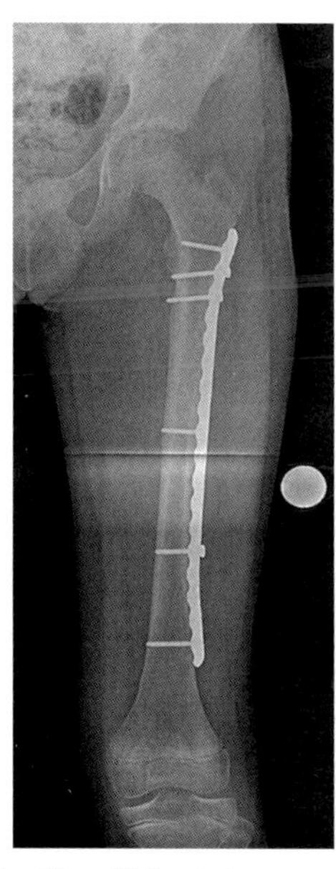
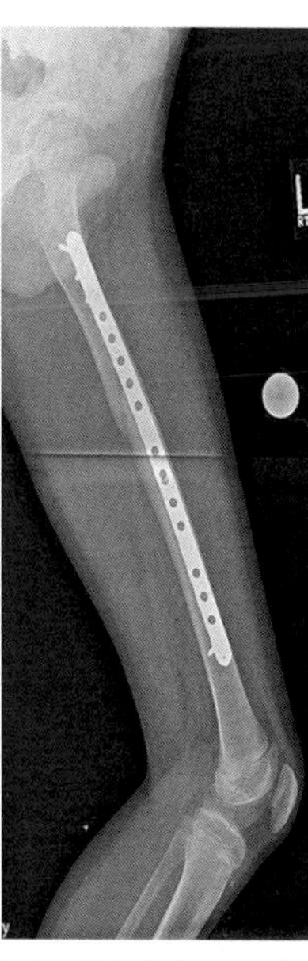

**FIG 1** • **A,B.** Displaced pediatric diaphyseal femur fracture in AP and lateral planes, respectively. **C,D.** Submuscular bridge plating shows appropriate fracture reduction and restoration of length in in AP and lateral planes, respectively.

- A narrow 4.5-mm plate is most often used.
  - This plate is readily available, easy to contour, and percutaneous screw placement is forgiving.
- Many of the currently available implants have the locking or nonlocking screw option.
  - Although nonlocking screws have been successful, locking screws may have some benefit in osteopenic patients or very proximal or distal fractures, where there is little available room for screws.
  - In our experience, nonlocking screws achieve enough stability in this age group and allow easier percutaneous screw placement compared with locking screws.
  - If a locking plate is used, a combination of locking and nonlocking screws are needed to reduce the femur to the plate.
  - It may be easier to place the locking screws with direct plate exposure rather than percutaneous exposure.
- Self-tapping screws are essential for easier percutaneous insertion.
- In smaller children, a long, narrow 3.5-mm plate may be used if absolutely necessary, but a 4.5-mm plate will fit most femurs even in the younger children.
- The plate length chosen is usually 10 to 16 holes, depending on fracture location and patient size.
  - The plate commonly spans from just below the greater trochanteric apophysis to the metaphysis of the distal femur.
  - If possible, the plate length should allow six screw holes proximal and distal to the fracture.

## Positioning

- Patients are positioned supine on a fracture table.
- The normal contralateral leg is extended and slightly abducted to allow a true lateral fluoroscopic image of the fractured femur.
  - Alternatively, a "well-leg" holder may also be used.
- Provisional reduction restoring femoral length and rotation is obtained with boot traction and verified fluoroscopically.
- Final alignment is performed with plate fixation as described later.

TECHNIQUES

## Exposure

- A small (4 to 7 mm) incision is made at the distal lateral thigh.
- The exposure is advanced through the tensor fascia to expose the distal oblique fibers of the vastus lateralis muscle.
- Blunt dissection is performed deep to the distal muscle fibers to enter the plane between the vastus lateralis and lateral femur periosteum. This plane is easily entered and allows proximal plate advancement with minimal force.

## Plate Contouring

- A table top plate bender contours the plate similar to the lateral femur with a slight bend proximally and distally to accommodate the proximal and distal metaphysis.
- The final femoral varus/valgus alignment is that of the plate so it is important to contour the plate as close to anatomic as possible.
- The usual practice is to place the precontoured plate on the anterior thigh and use the AP view on the C-arm to shadow the plate with the lateral femur cortex checking the plate contour (**TECH FIG 1**).
- In our experience, there has been no significant (>5 degrees) misalignment as a result of incorrect contouring.

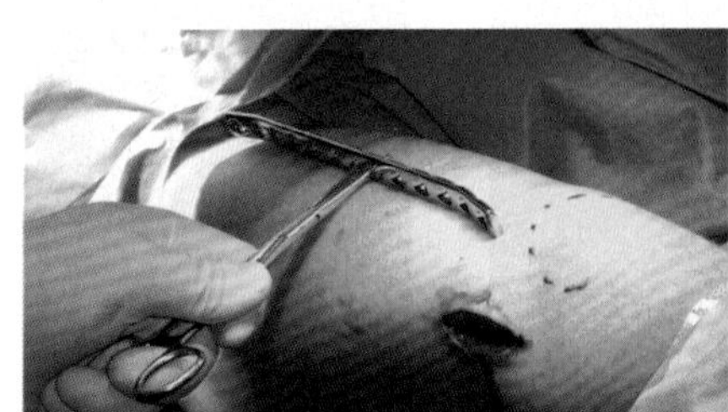

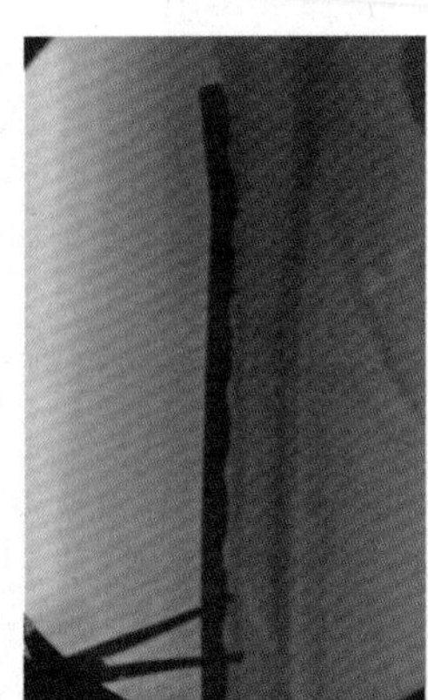

**TECH FIG 1** ● **A.** Plate contour is established using the AP view on the C-arm. **B.** The plate is aligned with the lateral femur cortex.

## Plate Advancement

- Blunt dissection is performed deep to the distal muscle fibers to enter the plane between the vastus lateralis and lateral femur periosteum. This plane allows proximal plate advancement with minimal force.
- The plate is then slowly tunneled proximally in this plane. A plate-holding clamp may be used to grasp the distal aspect of the plate for guidance.
- Care must be taken to keep the plate on the lateral femur, as it is advanced proximally past the fracture to the region of the greater trochanteric apophysis.
- The plate may be more difficult to pass along the lateral femur past the fracture. The surgeon may correct this by pulling the plate back and redirecting it.
- Fluoroscopy may also aid the surgeon in plate advancement.

## Provisional Plate Fixation

- Once the plate is fully advanced, it sits comfortably on the lateral femur; AP and lateral images are obtained to make sure the plate is in a good position in both planes, and the femoral length is restored (**TECH FIG 2**).
- The plate is provisionally fixed to the femur with a Kirschner wire placed in the most proximal and distal screw holes.
- If the fracture is "sagging" posteriorly, the femur can be lifted in an anterior direction while a K-wire is placed through the plate to engage the femur in this region.

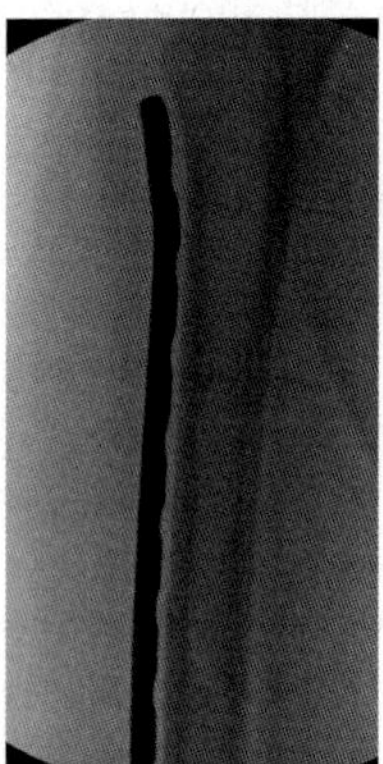

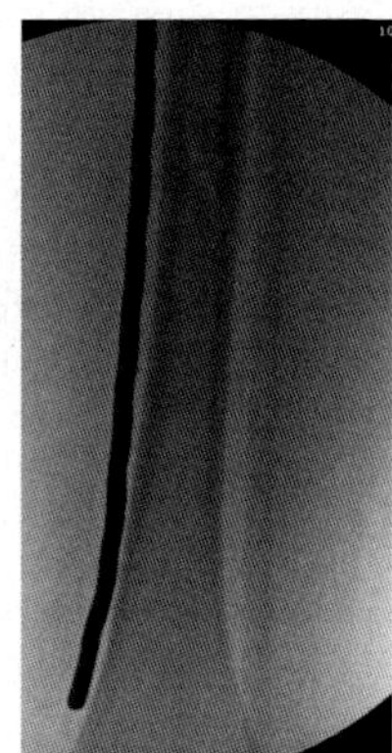

**TECH FIG 2** ● Once the plate is fully advanced, AP (**A**) and lateral (**B**) images are obtained to make sure the plate is in a good position on the lateral femoral cortex in both planes. Femoral length is restored.

## Plate Fixation with Percutaneous Screws

- A long plate and correct screw placement is important for construct stability.
- A screw should be placed in close proximity to the proximal and distal extent of the fracture.
- The remaining screws are placed as far apart as possible. Obtaining maximal screw spread with a long plate will improve construct stability, as there is a long working length of the plate.
    - Three screws proximal and three screws distal to the fracture are optimal.
- The first screw placed should be near the proximal or distal extent of the fracture, where the femur is furthest from the plate.

A screw in this area will reduce the femur to the plate and act as a "reduction screw."
  - As the screw engages the far cortex, the femur will be reduced to the precontoured plate (**TECH FIG 3A,B**).
  - The fracture is "bridged," and no attempt is made to place a screw to lag the fracture fragments.
- The technical aspects of percutaneous screw placement are as follows:
  - Screws are placed using "perfect circles" technique (**TECH FIG 3C**).
  - Using the fluoroscopic image in the lateral plane, a no. 15 blade scalpel is placed on the skin over the hole, then rotated horizontal to the beam through the skin, tensor fascia, and vastus fascia.
  - Using freehand technique, a 3.2-mm drill is placed in this small incision, and its location in the desired hole is confirmed with fluoroscopy.
  - The hole is then drilled through both cortices (**TECH FIG 3D**).
  - The length of the screw is approximated by placing the depth gauge on the anterior thigh as the image is rotated to the AP view.
  - A 0 Vicryl suture is tied around the 4.5-mm fully threaded cortical screw head so it will not be lost in the soft tissue if the screw inadvertently disengages from the screwdriver (**TECH FIG 3E**).
  - The screw is then placed though the plate and across the femur (**TECH FIG 3F,G**). The Vicryl ties are cut, and the incisions are closed with absorbable subcuticular sutures after all screws are placed.

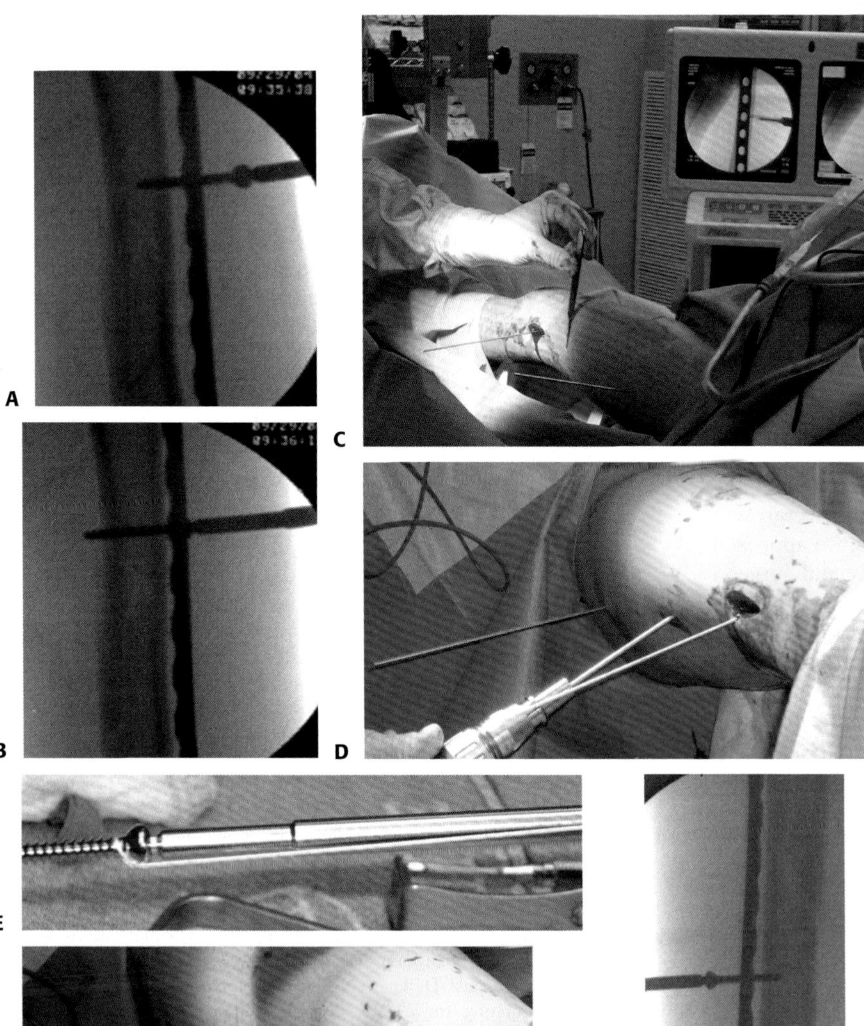

**TECH FIG 3** • **A,B.** As the screw engages the far cortex, the femur will be reduced to the precontoured plate. **C.** Screws are placed using "perfect circles" technique. Using the fluoroscopic image in the lateral plane, a no. 15 blade scalpel is placed on the skin over the hole, then rotated horizontal to the beam through the skin, tensor fascia, and vastus fascia. **D.** Using freehand technique, a 3.2-mm drill is placed in the incision, and its location in the desired hole is confirmed with fluoroscopy. The hole is then drilled through both cortices. **E.** A 0 Vicryl suture is tied around the 4.5-mm fully threaded cortical screw head so it will not be lost in the soft tissue if the screw inadvertently disengages from the screwdriver. The screw is then advanced percutaneously through the plate (**F**), with fluoroscopy confirmation (**G**).

## PEARLS AND PITFALLS

| | |
|---|---|
| **Plate selection** | ▪ Narrow 4.5 mm most common; can include locking options if osteopenic or very proximal/distal fracture; extend from greater trochanteric apophysis to distal metaphysis (10–16 holes) |
| **Plate contouring** | ▪ Bend proximally and distally to accommodate proximal and distal metaphyses. Should be anatomic to avoid varus/valgus malalignment. Fluoroscopy prior to insertion helps refine plate contour. |
| **Plate advancement** | ▪ Insert between plane of femoral periosteum and vastus lateralis. Remain on bone to avoid anterior/posterior plate malalignment. |
| **Provisional fixation** | ▪ K-wires help fix and align plate provisionally. Cortical screws help reduce plate to bone. |
| **Percutaneous screw placement** | ▪ Placed using fluoroscopy and perfect circle technique. Try to obtain six cortices on either side of the fracture. Bridge technique (no lag screws across fracture). |

## POSTOPERATIVE CARE

- A soft dressing is applied. We often place the patients in a knee immobilizer for early comfort with mobilization. No casting is required in the early postoperative period.
- Active knee range of motion is encouraged as comfort allows.
- Patients are kept non–weight bearing or touch-down weight bearing until bridging callus is seen usually at 6 to 10 weeks. Progressive weight bearing is then encouraged.
- Once bridging callus is apparent on three or four cortices, activity as tolerated and sports is allowed in a graded manner. This is usually between 10 and 14 weeks.
- The plate is removed in most patients around 6 months.
  - Later removal may require a larger incision due to tissue and bone ingrowth.
  - There are no clear indications for plate removal, although implant prominence, family preference, younger age, and surgeon preference may all influence this decision.[8]
  - We are more aggressive with offering plate removal in the younger children, as they have more bony overgrowth and leg growth potential. With adolescents, we approach removal on an individual basis, and family and surgeon preference are factors for removal.
- The screws are removed using image guidance, and a dull Cobb elevator is slid along the outer part of the plate to free up surrounding tissue. Then the Cobb with the sharp end directed away from the bone is advanced between the plate and bone freeing up the plate.
  - Once the plate is completely freed, it can be removed from the distal incision where it was advanced.
- Patients are then allowed weight bearing as tolerated and kept from running or sports for 6 weeks.

## OUTCOMES

- Many series report very high rates of fracture union with low rates of clinically evident malrotation, angulation, or shortening even in heavier patients and comminuted fracture patterns.[1,5,9,11]

## COMPLICATIONS

- Reported complications are rare.
- Plate failures are rare, and use of a 4.5-mm plate should minimize this complication from occurring.[2,5]
- Malunion is possible and can be potentially avoided with appropriate plate contouring.
- Patients may be at increased risk of postoperative distal femoral valgus deformity, particularly in fractures extending close to the physis, and this may require longitudinal follow-up.[4]
- Nonunion has not been reported, as this technique is best applied in closed comminuted fractures where the fracture region is bridged.
- Attention to rotation is important prior to screw placement.
- We use the opposite extremity and fracture geometry appearance with fluoroscopy with initial traction setup.
- Asymptomatic leg length discrepancies may be present but rarely require any further management.[1,5,9,11]
- Symptomatic hardware may require plate removal in some patients.

## REFERENCES


1. Abdelgawad AA, Sieg RN, Laughlin MD, et al. Submuscular bridge plating for complex pediatric femur fractures is reliable. Clin Orthop Relat Res 2013;471:2797–2807.
2. Becker T, Weigl D, Mercado E, et al. Fractures and refractures after femoral locking compression plate fixation in children and adolescents. J Pediatr Orthop 2012;32:e40–e46.
3. Flynn JM, Hresko T, Reynolds RA, et al. Titanium elastic nails for pediatric femur fractures: a multicenter study of early results with analysis of complications. J Pediatr Orthop 2001;21:4–8.
4. Heyworth BE, Hedequist DJ, Nasreddine AY, et al. Distal femoral valgus deformity following plate fixation of pediatric femoral shaft fractures. J Bone Joint Surg Am 2013;95:526–533.
5. Kanlic EM, Anglen JO, Smith DG, et al. Advantages of submuscular bridge plating for complex pediatric femur fractures. Clin Orthop Relat Res 2004;(426):244–251.
6. Loder RT, O'Donnell PW, Feinberg JR. Epidemiology and mechanisms of femur fractures in children. J Pediatr Orthop 2006;26:561–566.
7. Moroz LA, Launay F, Kocher MS, et al. Titanium elastic nailing of fractures of the femur in children. Predictors of complications and poor outcome. J Bone Joint Surg Br 2006;88:1361–1366.
8. Pate O, Hedequist D, Leong N, et al. Implant removal after submuscular plating for pediatric femur fractures. J Pediatr Orthop 2009;29:709–712.
9. Sink EL, Faro F, Polousky J, et al. Decreased complications of pediatric femur fractures with a change in management. J Pediatr Orthop 2010;30:633–637.
10. Sink EL, Gralla J, Repine M. Complications of pediatric femur fractures treated with titanium elastic nails: a comparison of fracture types. J Pediatr Orthop 2005;25:577–580.
11. Sink EL, Hedequist D, Morgan SJ, et al. Results and technique of unstable pediatric femoral fractures treated with submuscular bridge plating. J Pediatr Orthop 2006;26:177–181.

# Trochanteric Entry Nailing for Pediatric Femoral Shaft Fractures

27
CHAPTER

J. Eric Gordon and June C. Smith

## DEFINITION

- Fractures of the femoral shaft are characterized by acute, nonpathologic fractures of the femur in which the primary portion of the fracture is at least 5 cm distal to the lesser trochanter and at least as far proximal to the distal femoral physis as the width of the physis.

## ANATOMY

- Understanding of the bony and vascular anatomy of the proximal femur is essential to the successful insertion of lateral trochanteric entry nails.
- The proximal femur originates from a single proximal femoral epiphysis that develops two separate ossification centers that lead to the femoral head and greater trochanter.
- Although the bony portion of the epiphysis is separate at age 8 years, a remnant of the proximal femoral epiphysis lies along the lateral aspect of the femoral neck allowing the femoral neck to increase in diameter (**FIG 1**).[15]
- After age 8 years, injury to the lateral aspect of the greater trochanteric physis has no effect on the ultimate shape of the femoral neck.[3] Injury to the medial aspect of this physis can lead to proximal femoral valgus and femoral neck narrowing (**FIG 2A**).
- The medial femoral circumflex artery originates from the profunda femoris artery and courses medially to the femoral neck, passing adjacent to the piriformis fossa and forming the extracapsular arterial ring which lies at the base of the femoral neck, then anastomosing with branches of the lateral femoral circumflex artery.[12,16]
- Branches of the extracapsular ring give off the ascending cervical branches, which lie along the lateral femoral neck and enter the posterolateral epiphysis of the femoral head (see **FIG 1**).
- Injury to the medial circumflex artery or the external ring can produce avascular necrosis (AVN) of the femoral head (**FIG 2B**).

## PATHOGENESIS

- Fracture of the femoral shaft can result from a direct blow, which can produce a transverse or oblique fracture with or without comminution.
- Fracture of the femoral shaft can also result from rotational stresses or a twisting injury, often seen during sports injuries, leading to a spiral-type fracture.

## NATURAL HISTORY

- Muscle forces following fracture of the femoral shaft produce flexion and external rotation of the proximal fragment.
- Muscle forces on the distal fragment produce shortening of the fracture with varus alignment.
- These muscle forces produce shortening, procurvatum, varus, and an internal rotation deformity in the untreated fracture.

## PATIENT HISTORY AND PHYSICAL FINDINGS

- Fractures of the femoral shaft in adolescents can be produced by either sporting activities or more commonly high-energy trauma.
- Examination usually reveals tenderness at the midthigh area with swelling present. The limb may have obvious deformity and shortening and may show ecchymosis or open wounds in the case of an open fracture.
- A careful neurovascular examination should also be performed—palpating distal pulses and evaluating both motor and sensory neurologic function.

## IMAGING AND OTHER DIAGNOSTIC STUDIES

- Good-quality anteroposterior and lateral radiographs of the femur should be obtained that allow visualization of the entire femur including the hip and knee.
- If any question of a potential femoral neck fracture arises, anteroposterior and lateral views of the hip should be performed.
- Patients with femoral shaft fractures secondary to high-energy trauma should have a separate anteroposterior radiograph of the pelvis to rule out concomitant injury.

## DIFFERENTIAL DIAGNOSIS

- Pathologic femoral shaft fracture due to benign or malignant tumor

## NONOPERATIVE MANAGEMENT

- Nonoperative management of older children with femur fractures consists of skeletal traction for 2 to 3 weeks followed by application of either a spica cast or a cast brace for an additional 6 to 8 weeks.
- Nonoperative management of adolescents with femur fractures historically has consisted of skeletal traction for 3 to 4 weeks followed by application of a spica cast or cast brace for an additional 8 to 12 weeks.

## SURGICAL MANAGEMENT

- Children younger than the age of 12 years and up to 50 kg with femoral shaft fractures can be surgically treated by flexible intramedullary nailing.[2]
- Children older than the age of 8 years can be treated by lateral trochanteric nailing using either reamed or unreamed rigid nails.[5,6]

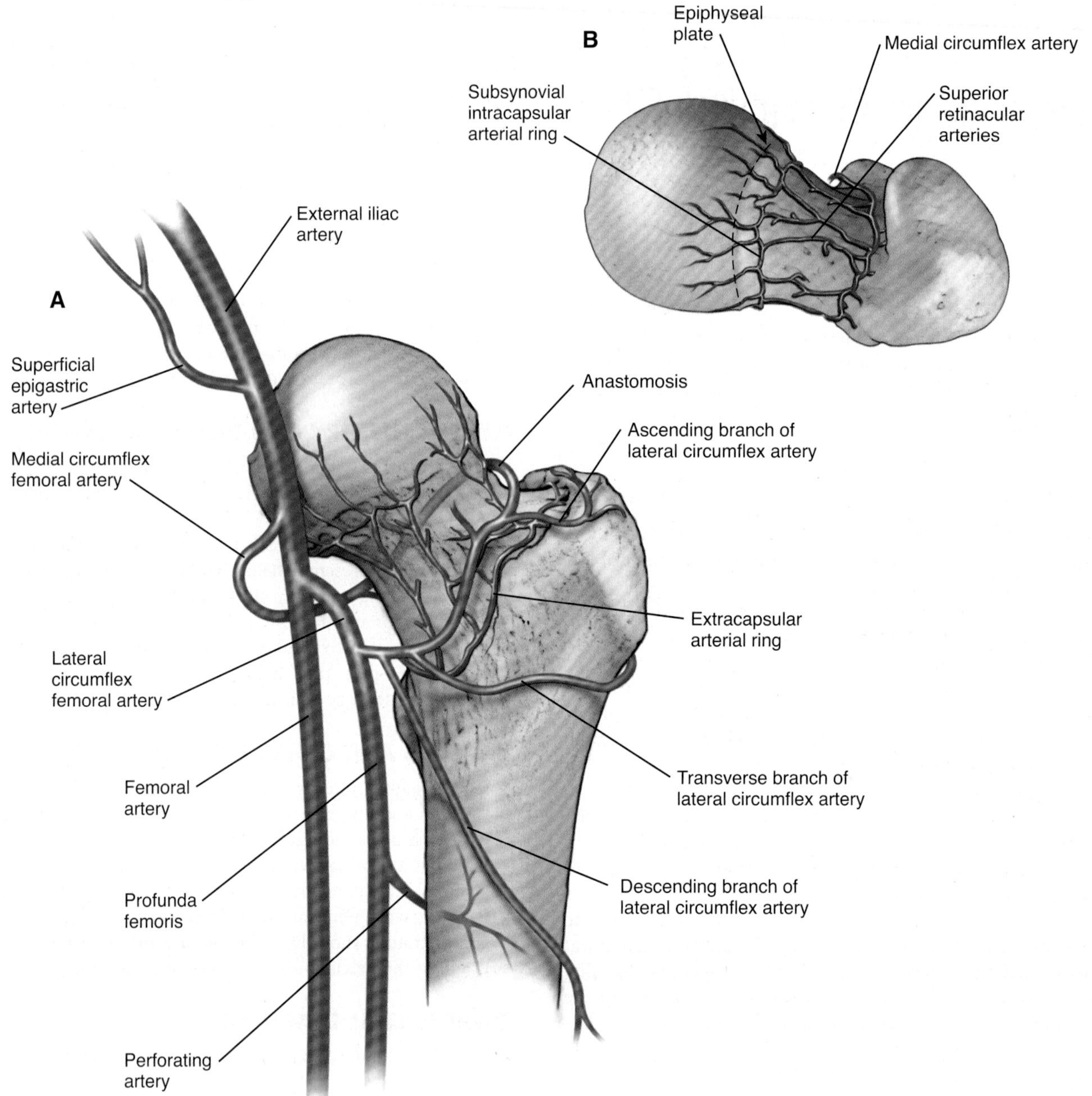


**FIG 1** • **A.** Anteroposterior view of the bony and vascular anatomy of the proximal femur. **B.** Superoinferior view of the bony and vascular anatomy of the proximal femur.

- Lateral trochanteric nails are particularly indicated in children 12 years of age or older or who weigh 50 kg or more up to skeletal maturity.[7,8]
- Lateral trochanteric nailing is also indicated in children age 8 years or older who have length-unstable fractures.

## Preoperative Planning

- Measurement of the femur from the greater trochanter to the distal femoral physis as well as measurement of the diameter of the medullary canal of the femur at the isthmus should be performed preoperatively in order to ensure that appropriately sized implants are available.

## Positioning and Prepping

- The patient is positioned supine on a fracture table.
- The contralateral limb is flexed and abducted away from the injured limb.
- The ipsilateral upper extremity should be positioned across the chest and padded and secured.
- The perineal post should be padded well.
- Traction is applied through a well-padded boot placed on the injured limb.
- Prior to draping, the image intensifier should be used to ensure that the hip and entire femur can be visualized and that adequate traction has been applied through the boot to bring the fracture out to length (**FIG 3A**).

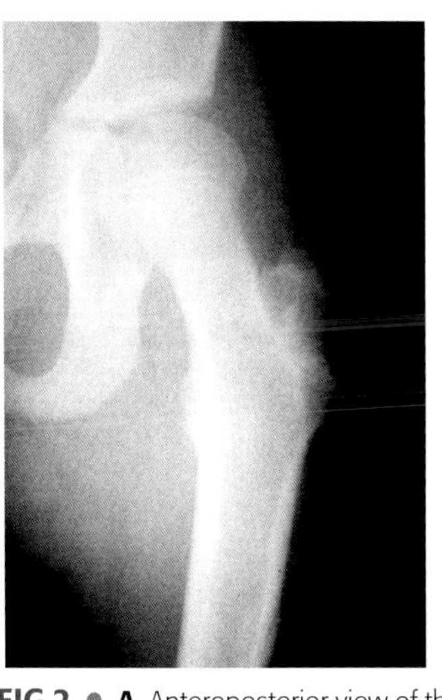

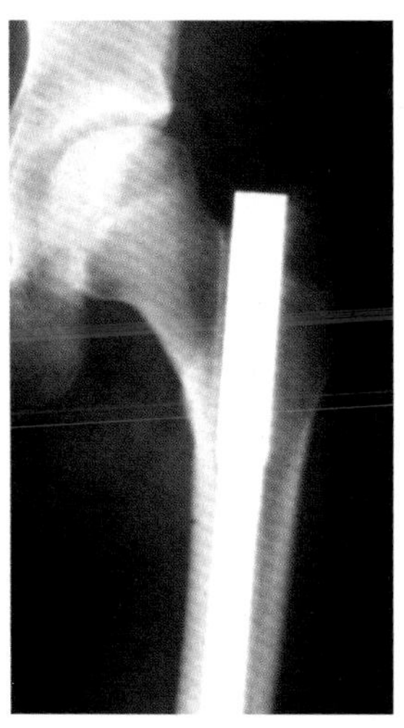

**FIG 2** • **A.** Anteroposterior view of the left hip in a patient with proximal femoral valgus and neck narrowing following nailing through the tip of the trochanter. **B.** Anteroposterior view of the left hip in an adolescent with AVN of the femoral head following intramedullary nailing through the piriformis fossa.

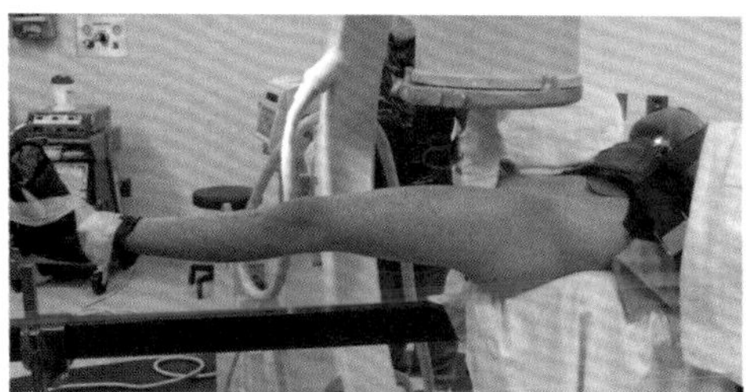

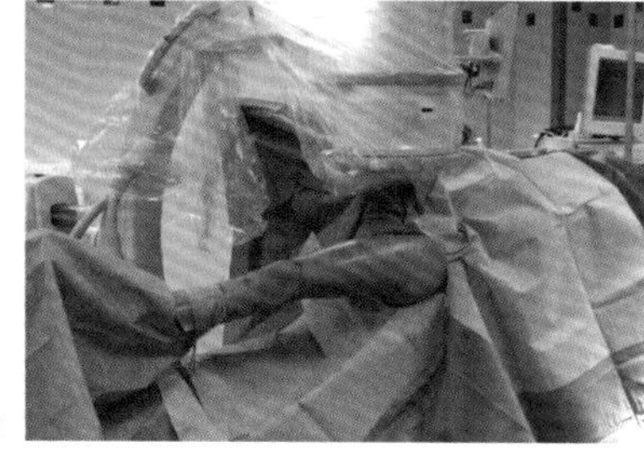

**FIG 3** • **A.** Supine positioning of a patient on a fracture table prior to intramedullary nailing of the femur. **B.** Supine positioning of the patient after draping.

- The patient's skin should be prepared from above the hip at least 10 cm proximal to the tip of the greater trochanter to the midtibia circumferentially.
- Sterile split sheets should be used to drape the patient allowing access to the femur in order to reduce the fracture via manual manipulation or open reduction if necessary.
- The image intensifier should be draped sterilely as well (**FIG 3B**).

## Approach

- The preferred approach is percutaneously to the lateral aspect of the greater trochanter.
- Insertion of the nail can also be performed through a lateral open approach.

## Guide Pin Placement

- The image intensifier should be used to visualize the hip. Because the proximal fragment usually externally rotates, the image intensifier may need to be arced past perpendicular (overrotated) to obtain a good anteroposterior image of the proximal femur (**TECH FIG 1A,B**).
- The guide pin should be placed on the skin proximal to the greater trochanter and the image intensifier used to align the pin

TECHNIQUES

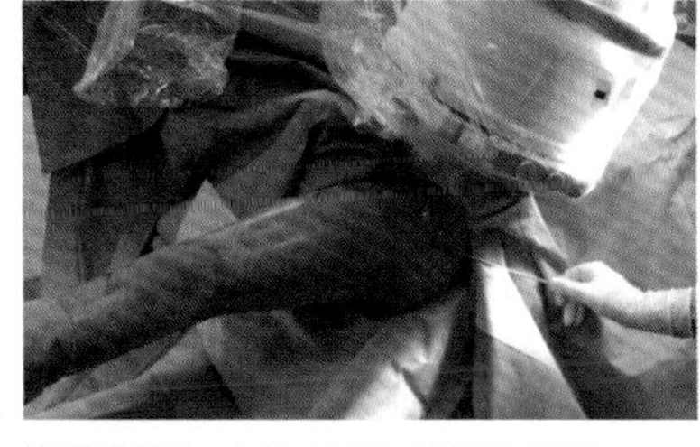

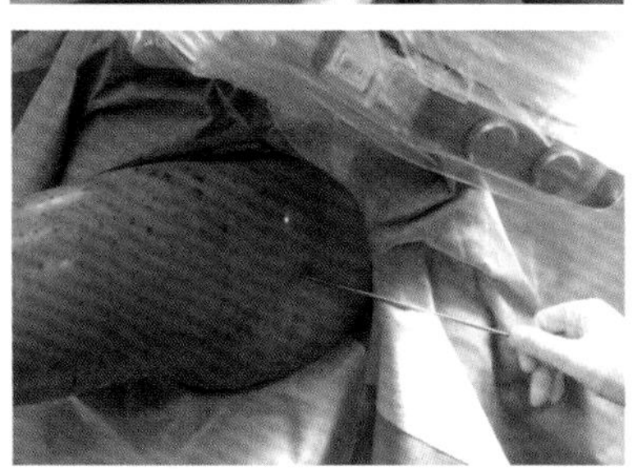

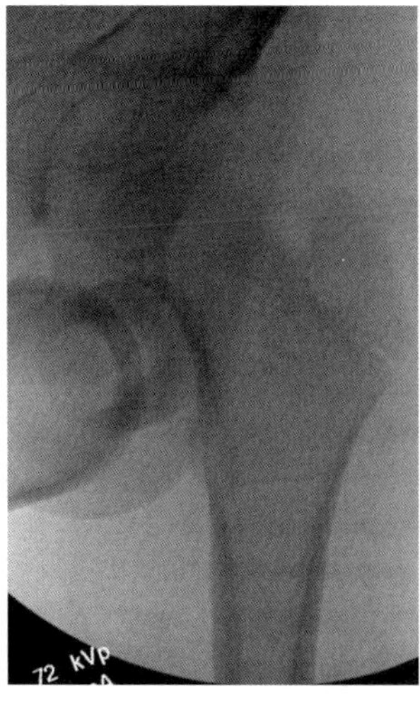


**TECH FIG 1** • **A.** Draped patient with image intensifier oriented to obtain a clear anteroposterior view of the proximal femur. **B.** Anteroposterior image of the proximal femur obtained by the image intensifier. **C.** Marking the entry site of the guide pin. *(continued)*

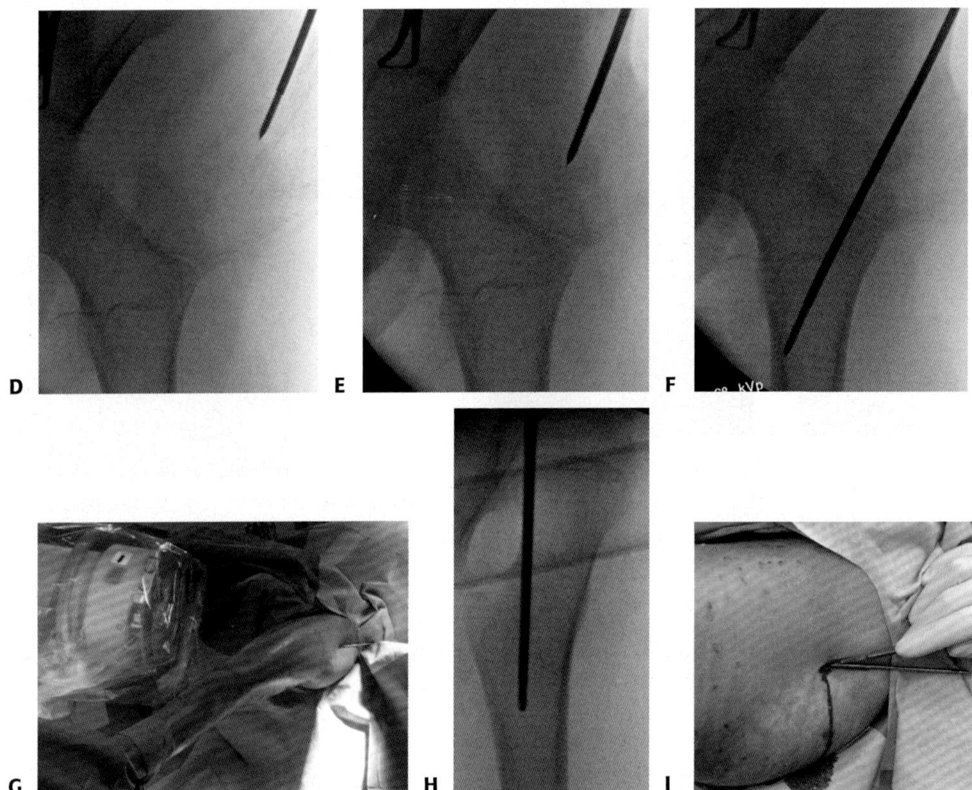

**TECH FIG 1** • *(continued)* **D.** Image of the proximal femur showing the guide pin on the skin oriented to push onto the lateral aspect of the proximal femur. **E.** AP view showing the guide pin placed in the appropriate entry point oriented to a point 1 to 2 cm distal to the inferior edge of the lesser trochanter. **F.** AP view showing the guide pin placed in the appropriate entry point driven to a point 1 to 2 cm distal to the lesser trochanter. **G.** Photograph of the image intensifier oriented to obtain a lateral of the guide pin after placement into the proximal femur. **H.** Lateral view of the proximal femur showing the guide pin placed in the appropriate entry point oriented and placed centered in the femoral canal. **I.** Incising the skin at the site of the guide pin.

so that the entry point allows placement onto the midportion of the lateral aspect of the greater trochanter and allows the pin to be driven in an angle that allows the trajectory of the pin to impact the medial cortex 1 to 2 cm distal to the lower edge of the lesser trochanter (**TECH FIG 1C,D**).

- The pin is then pushed down onto the greater trochanter and aligned (**TECH FIG 1E**).
- After the pin is driven into the proximal femur (**TECH FIG 1F**), a lateral image is obtained by arcing the image intensifier back to obtain an image perpendicular to the anteroposterior image (**TECH FIG 1G,H**).
- Following this, the skin is incised approximately 15 mm proximally from the guide pin, and the scalpel is passed down along the wire through the fascia (**TECH FIG 1I**).

## Reaming and Guidewire Placement

- A soft tissue protector is placed, and a rigid cannulated reamer is then used to enter the greater trochanter (**TECH FIG 2A–C**) and is driven down into the medullary canal beyond the greater trochanteric physis.
- The reamer is then withdrawn, leaving the guide pin in place. If necessary, the obturator is used to keep the guide pin in place.
- Place the short exchange tube over the guide pin down into the medullary canal (**TECH FIG 2D,E**).
- Remove the guide pin, and place the ball-tipped guidewire down into the canal (**TECH FIG 2F**).
- Orient the tip of the guidewire so that it passes distally down to the fracture site (**TECH FIG 2G**).
- Reduce the fracture fragments using direct pressure (**TECH FIG 2H**).
  - If necessary, a guide pin can be placed from anterior to posterior through the quadriceps muscle down onto the anterior aspect of the proximal fragment in order to aid reduction.
- When the fragments are aligned, pass the guidewire across the fracture site into the distal fragment (**TECH FIG 2H,I**).
  - Occasionally, it is helpful to put a small bend in the tip of the ball-tipped guidewire to facilitate nail passage across the fracture site.

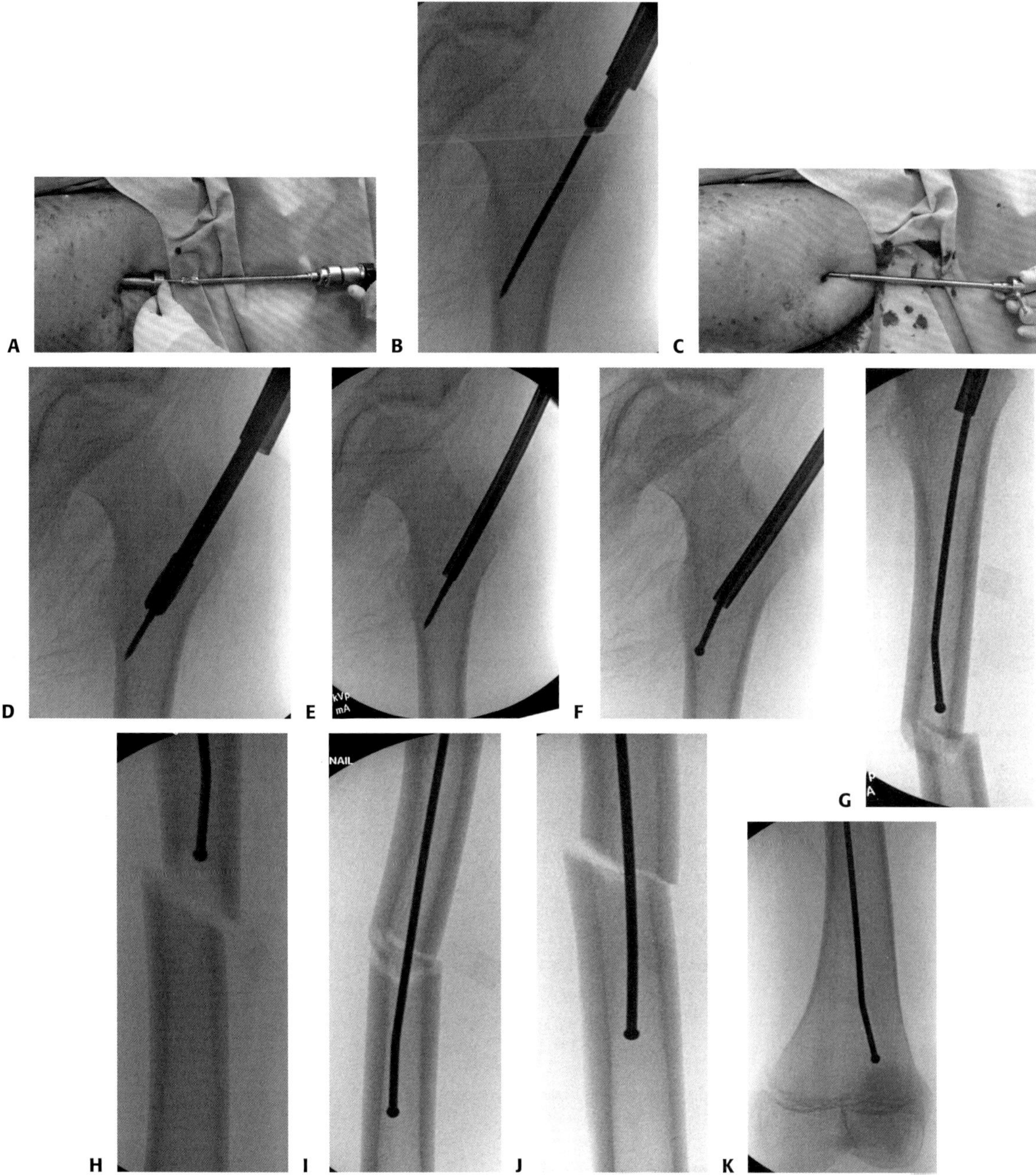


**TECH FIG 2** • **A.** Insertion of the rigid reamer over the guide pin. **B.** Intraoperative image showing rigid reamer insertion onto the greater trochanter. **C.** Intraoperative image of the rigid reamer after entering the medullary canal. **D.** Placing of the rigid exchange tube over the guide pin. **E.** Intraoperative image showing rigid exchange tube in canal with the guide pin. **F.** Intraoperative image obtained after removal of the guide pin showing the ball-tipped guidewire being placed though the rigid exchange tube with the bend in the wire oriented so that the wire is passing down the femoral canal. **G.** Intraoperative anteroposterior image showing guidewire at the fracture site. **H.** Intraoperative lateral image showing guidewire at the fracture site showing reduction of the fracture. **I.** Intraoperative anteroposterior image showing guidewire across the reduced fracture site. **J.** Intraoperative lateral image showing guidewire across the reduced fracture site. **K.** Intraoperative anteroposterior radiograph showing guidewire positioned in the lateral distal femur approximately 1 cm proximal to the distal femoral physis.

- Position of the guidewire must be checked on both the anteroposterior and lateral views to confirm (**TECH FIG 2J**).
- The guidewire is then passed down into the distal femur and positioned in the lateral aspect of the metaphysis (if the nail has a distal bend at the tip to facilitate the lateral trochanteric entry).
  - The ball-tipped guidewire should be left approximately 1 cm proximal to the distal femoral physis (**TECH FIG 2K**).

## Measuring Nail Length and Diameter

- The measuring guide is then passed over the ball-tipped guidewire and into the incision down to the lateral aspect of the greater trochanter (**TECH FIG 3A**).
  - This position is confirmed using the image intensifier (**TECH FIG 3B**).
- The nail length is read from the end of the measuring guide (**TECH FIG 3C**). The nail length will allow placement of one to three potential nail diameters. The nail diameter is selected based on the patient weight and the clinical situation.
  - In a typical patient, an 8-mm diameter nail is planned. Very small patients use a 7-mm diameter nail. Larger patients or patients in which an abnormally long healing time is anticipated will often require a 9-mm nail. Ten millimeter nails are reserved for the largest patients.

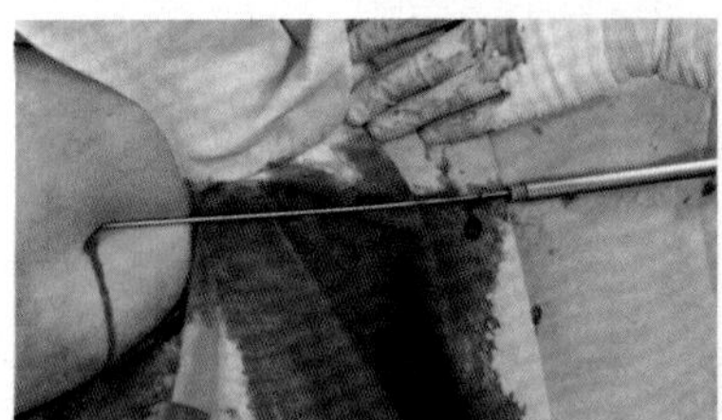

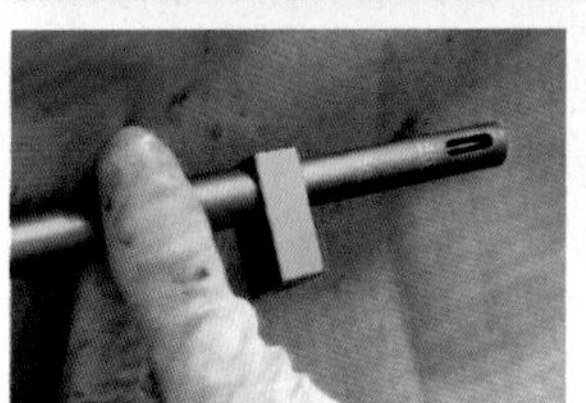

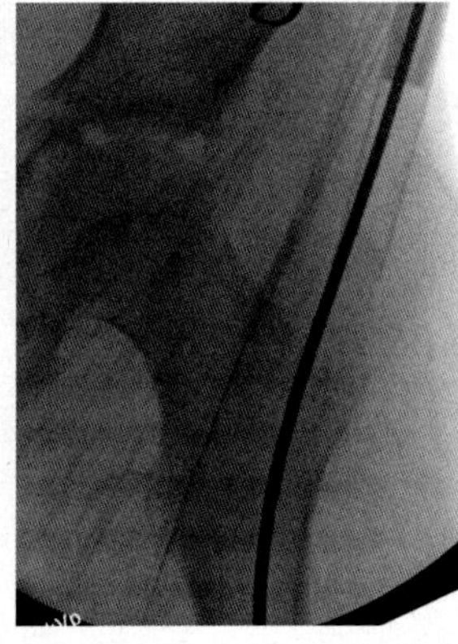

**TECH FIG 3 • A.** Placing of the nail gauge over the guidewire. **B.** Intraoperative anteroposterior image showing the nail measuring guide advanced over the guidewire down to the lateral trochanteric entry site. **C.** Reading of the nail measuring gauge.

## Canal Reaming

- The canal is then reamed using a flexible reamer (**TECH FIG 4A,B**).
- Except in situations where the canal is exceptionally small, the initial reamer should be 8.0 to 8.5 mm in diameter.
- The reamer should be passed down over the guidewire but not beyond the bend in the distal tip of the guidewire.
  - Reamer diameter should be increased in 0.5 to 1.0 mm increments until a reamer diameter 1.5 to 2.0 mm larger than the proposed nail diameter is reached.
- If necessary, an exchange tube is then passed down over the ball-tipped guidewire beyond the fracture site to maintain the reduction (**TECH FIG 4C**).
- The ball-tipped guidewire is removed, and a smooth guidewire is passed down the exchange tube into the distal femur.
- The exchange tube is then removed, leaving the smooth guidewire in place.

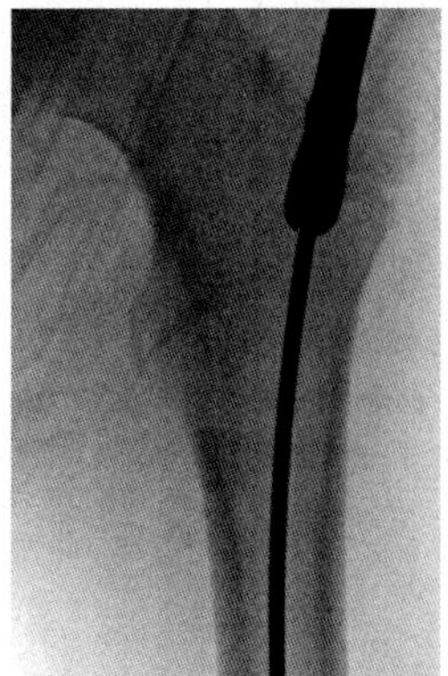

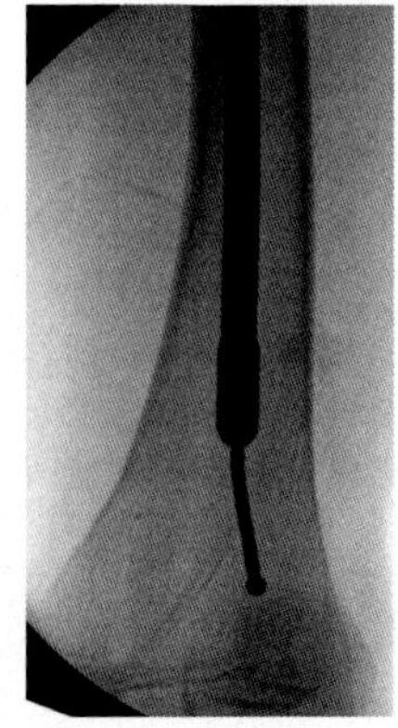

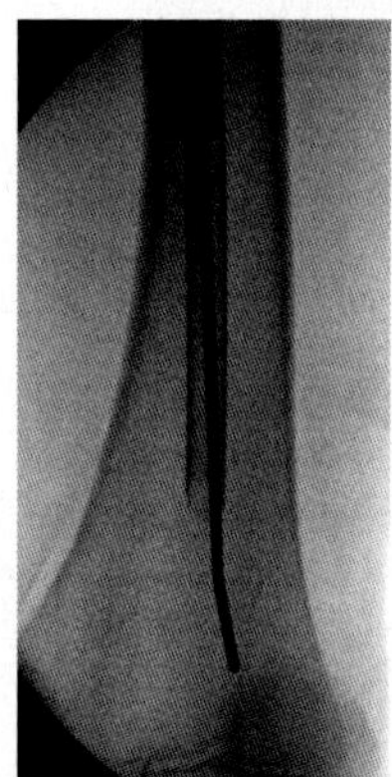

**TECH FIG 4 • A.** Intraoperative image showing the flexible reamer advancing into the proximal femur. **B.** Intraoperative image showing the flexible reamer advancing to the bend in the guidewire. It is important that the reamer not be advanced beyond this bend as the reamer will bind up on the guidewire. **C.** Intraoperative image showing exchange tube in place after insertion of the smooth guidewire in the distal femur.

## Nail Insertion

- The nail is mounted and secured on the inserter ensuring the proper orientation of the nail and checking that the appropriate nail laterality, diameter, and length has been mounted.
- A final check is done to ensure proper mounting of the nail is to place a drill guide through the insertion guide to make sure that when placed, the drill guide aligns with the interlocking hole.
- The nail is then passed down over the guidewire (**TECH FIG 5A**).
  - It is initially advanced by hand, leaving the inserter in a horizontal position. When the nail cannot be advanced further by hand, a mallet is used to advance the nail to the fracture site.
  - The alignment is then checked and the fracture realigned if necessary.
  - The nail is then driven across the fracture site down into the distal fragment (**TECH FIG 5B**).
- When the fracture is stable, the guidewire is removed and the nail impacted into place.
  - The nail should be advanced to a position 1 to 2 cm proximal to the distal femoral physis, and the proximal tip of the nail should be placed just below the bony surface of the greater trochanter (**TECH FIG 5C**).
- The screw securing the nail to the proximal interlocking guide is then tightened to ensure accurate targeting of the proximal interlocking screws.

A 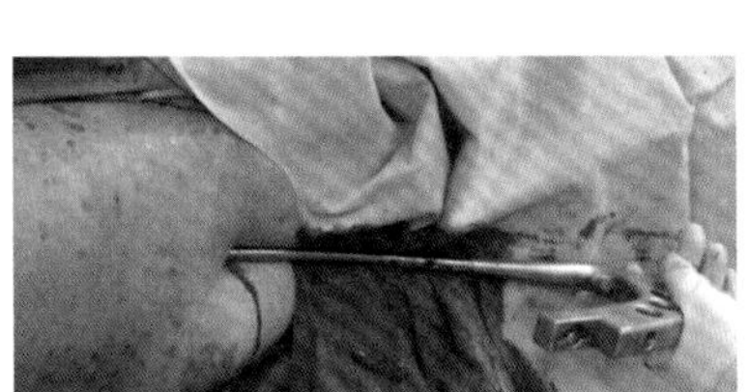

B 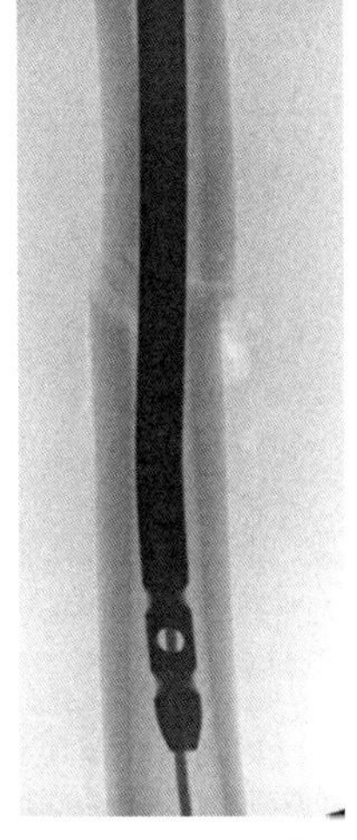

C 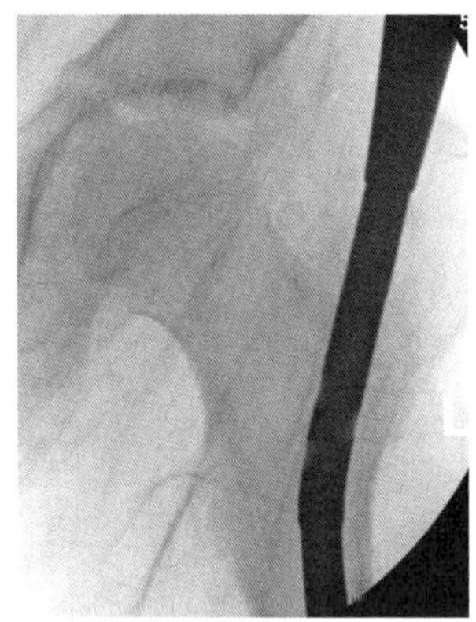

**TECH FIG 5** ● **A.** Insertion of the nail. **B.** Intraoperative image showing nail across fracture site. **C.** Intraoperative image of the nail with the inserter still in place. Careful examination of the image reveals the junction of the nail and inserter to be just below the bony surface of the greater trochanter.

## Placing Interlock Screws (Proximal and Distal)

- The guide sleeves are placed together with the sharp trocar and are placed through the appropriate interlocking hole(s).
  - The sleeves are advanced to the skin, and a 1 cm incision is made through the skin and fascia.
  - The sleeves and trocar are then advanced down to bone and the lateral cortex scored by the trocar to prevent the drill bit from "skating" along the cortex.
  - The trocar is then removed and the drill advanced under image intensification through the lateral cortex, through the interlocking hole in the nail, and up to the medial cortex.
- At this point, the gauge on the drill is used to estimate the screw length and the drill is then advanced through the medial cortex.
  - The drill is withdrawn along with the drill sleeve, leaving the outer sleeve in place.
- The screw is then mounted on the screwdriver, and the screw is placed through the outer sleeve and is driven into the bone through the interlocking hole in the nail (**TECH FIG 6A,B**).
- After proximal interlocking, the alignment of the limb is checked, and the fracture site configuration is evaluated to make sure that rotation is appropriate.
  - When examining the fracture site, the alignment of the fracture line on the proximal and distal fragments is checked.
  - In addition, the relative diameter of the femur above and below the fracture can be used as clues to rotational alignment.
- A decision is made by the surgeon as to how many distal interlocking screws are appropriate for the fracture distally.
  - Typically, a single interlocking screw is appropriate for stable isthmic or proximal fractures.
  - Distal fractures or fractures that are length unstable often require two or three screws.
- The distal interlocking hole is first visualized using the image intensifier.
  - The orientation of the intensifier is changed until a "perfect circle" is observed (**TECH FIG 6C**).

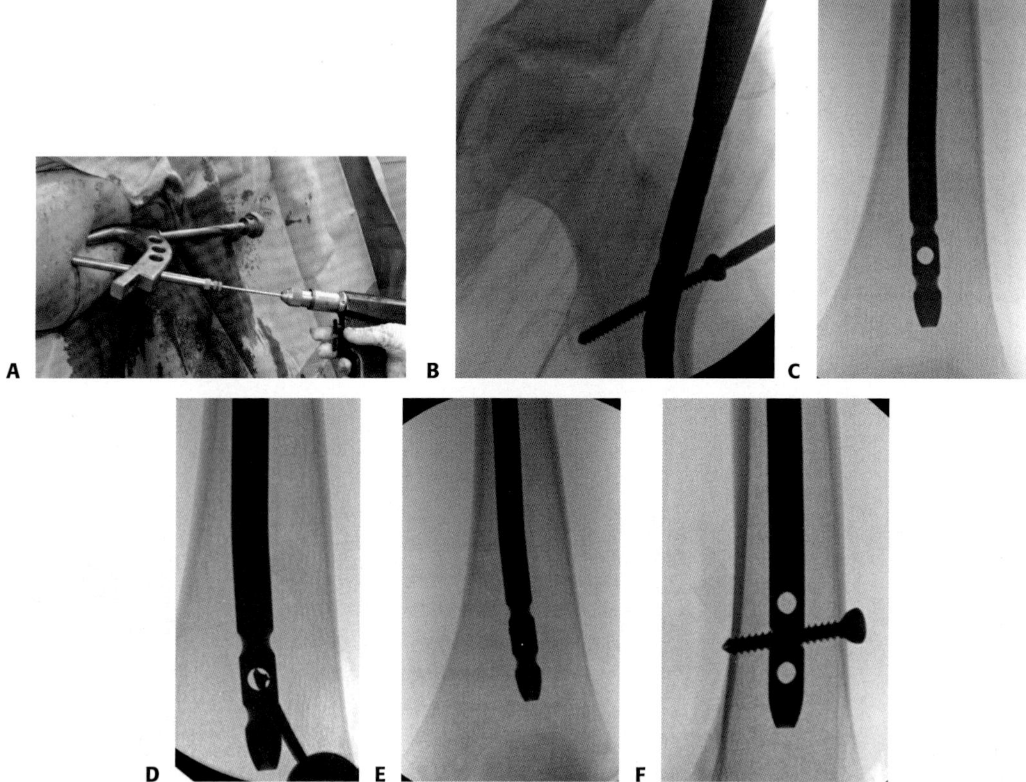

**TECH FIG 6** • **A.** Drilling for the proximal interlocking screw with the guide tubes in place. **B.** Intraoperative image showing the proximal interlocking screw being tightened into position. **C.** Anteroposterior image of the distal femur showing a perfect circle prior to insertion of an anteroposterior interlocking screw. **D.** The drill has been positioned with the tip directly over the distal interlocking hole prior to drilling. **E.** Anteroposterior view of the distal femur showing obscuration of the interlocking hole without extension outside the limits of the nail indicating placement of the screw through the distal interlocking hole. **F.** Lateral view of the distal femur showing good position of the distal interlocking screw with the tip engaging the posterior cortex.

- The position of the intensifier is then locked, and a 1-cm incision is made over the hole.
  - If the screw is anterior to posterior, the incision should be carried down longitudinally though the quadriceps tendon.
  - If the hole is lateral to medial, the incision should be carried down through the iliotibial band laterally.
- A drill is placed down onto the center of the hole as projected with the image intensifier (**TECH FIG 6D**) and advanced through the near cortex and through the interlocking hole.
  - The drill is removed from the drill bit, leaving the drill bit in the bone.
  - A check is made to ensure that the drill is through the interlocking hole.
  - The drill is reconnected to the drill bit and the drill passed through the far cortex.
  - The drill is withdrawn and either a depth gauge used to measure the screw length or the preoperative radiograph measured at the appropriate site to select a screw length.
- Finally, the screw is placed and secured, with screw placement and length confirmed using the image intensifier (**TECH FIG 6E,F**).
- This process is then repeated for any additional screws.

## Closure

- Final radiographic images are then made to confirm appropriate nail placement and reduction of the fracture (**TECH FIG 7A,B**).
- Wounds are closed in layers, closing fascia where appropriate with absorbable suture. The skin can be closed with absorbable monofilament suture, skin staples, or nonabsorbable suture at the surgeon's preference (**TECH FIG 7C,D**).
- Sterile dressings are applied over each wound (**TECH FIG 7E**).
- Drainage is often most significant at the incision for the nail entry site. Typically, minimal drainage is encountered at the interlocking screw sites.

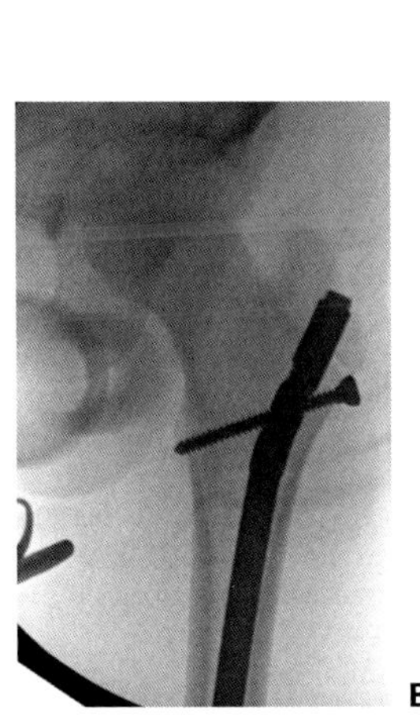
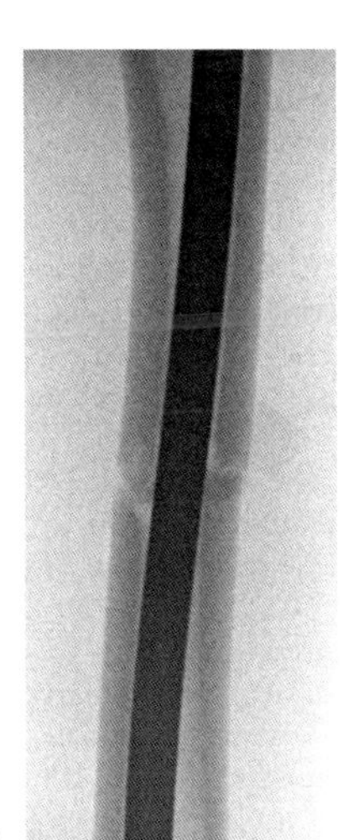
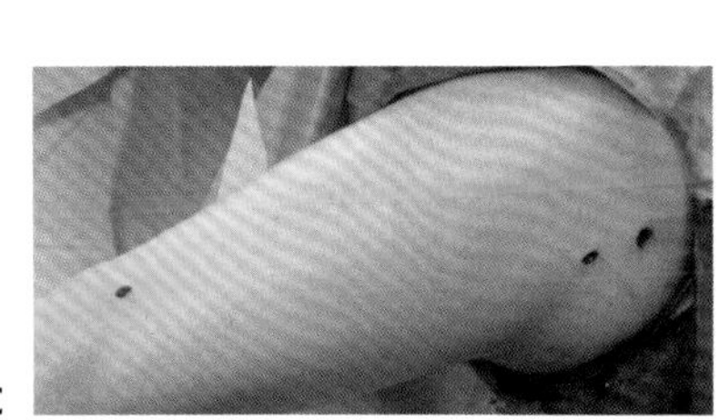
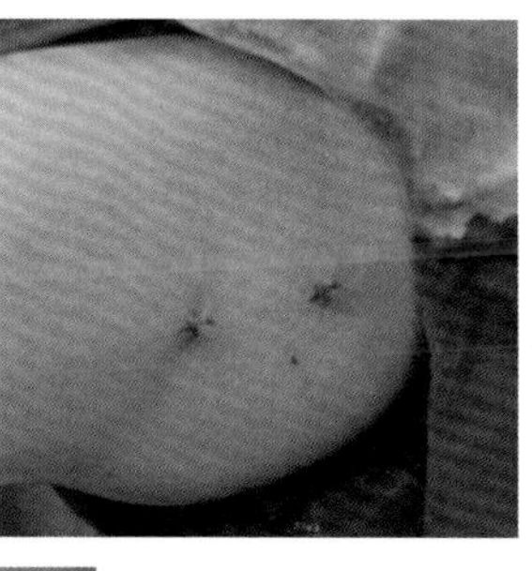
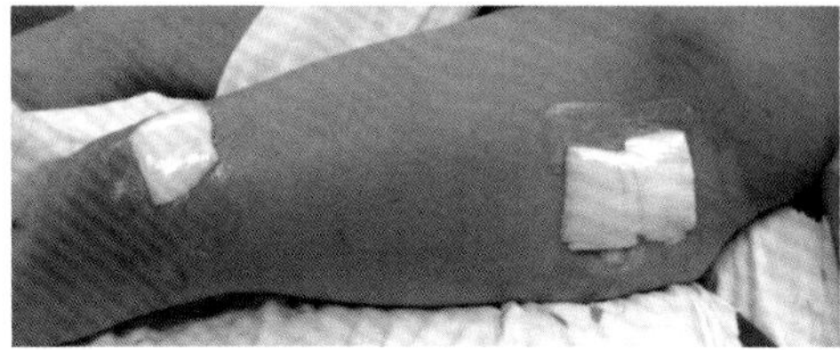

**TECH FIG 7** • **A.** Final intraoperative radiographic AP of the hip to confirm correct position of the nail and proximal interlocking screw. **B.** Final intraoperative anteroposterior view of the fracture site showing near-anatomic reduction. **C.** Incisions prior to closure. **D.** Proximal incisions closed with absorbable suture. **E.** Dressed incisions.

## PEARLS AND PITFALLS

| | |
|---|---|
| Entry point of nail at lateral trochanter | ▪ The guide pin must be inserted at the midportion of the lateral aspect of the greater trochanter.<br>▪ Insertion of the nail too close to the tip of the trochanter risks reaming into the blood supply to the proximal femur and producing AVN of the femoral head.<br>▪ Placement too laterally and too close to the greater trochanteric physis risks a difficult entry with subsequent reaming through the lateral cortex of the femur and subsequent lack of proximal femoral stability. |
| The guide pin should be directed from the midportion of the lateral aspect of the greater trochanter to a point 1–2 cm distal to the lower edge of the lesser trochanter. | ▪ If the guide pin is directed too transversely, at the lesser trochanter or more proximally, the ball-tipped guidewire will be curved significantly, leading to difficulty passing the reamer along the curved guidewire and potentially leading to cutting the guidewire with the reamer. |
| The ball-tipped guidewire should be placed into the lateral aspect of the femoral metaphysis or the center depending on the configuration of the nail. | ▪ Lateral trochanteric nails can have either a straight tip or a bend in the tip to allow easier placement from a lateral trochanteric entry point, reducing the risk of comminuting the medial cortex of the proximal fragment.<br>▪ If the nail has a distal bend, the guidewire should be placed into the lateral aspect of the distal femoral metaphysis.<br>▪ If the guidewire is placed centrally when using one of these nails in a femur with a fracture distal to the isthmus, valgus alignment can potentially be produced. |
| Visualize the guidewire while reaming. | ▪ If the guidewire is not visualized during reaming, migration can occur with the guidewire advancing distally across the physis leading to potential damage or the guidewire being pulled back across the fracture site with resultant loss of fracture reduction. |
| The nail diameter selected should be appropriate for the patient size. | ▪ The tendency for the surgeon is to select the largest diameter nail possible to "fill" the canal.<br>▪ In pediatric and adolescent femur fractures, this is usually not necessary.<br>▪ In adult applications, intramedullary nails are placed, and the diameter selected when the reamer starts to ream the cortical bone as revealed by "chatter."<br>▪ Pediatric fractures heal much more quickly, and there is no need to select very large-diameter nails to maintain stability during a 4–6 month period of healing.<br>▪ Selecting larger diameter nails has a drawback in that passage of an intramedullary nail from a lateral trochanteric entry point requires the nail to flex somewhat as the tip of the nail impacts the medial cortex of the proximal fragment as it passes down the canal.<br>▪ Larger nails have less ability to elastically deform and a greater likelihood of comminuting the medial cortex. |

## POSTOPERATIVE CARE

- Postoperatively, the patient is allowed weight bearing as tolerated in most situations.
- Weight bearing can be limited in situations where healing will be slow, such as severely comminuted fractures or open fractures with bone loss.
- The patient is mobilized postoperatively as soon as practical (usually postoperative day 1) on crutches.
- Dressings are maintained 3 to 4 days postoperatively and then removed. If clean and dry, bathing and showering are then allowed.
- Physical therapy can be instituted for knee and hip range of motion and strengthening beginning at the end of postoperative week 2.
- Consolidation is usually observed within 6 weeks of surgery.

## OUTCOMES

- Union rate with good alignment has been reported in excess of 99%.[7,8]

## COMPLICATIONS

- AVN of the femoral head has not been reported after lateral trochanteric nailing of the femur. The rate of AVN has been reported to be 1.4% after nailing through the tip of the trochanter and 2.0% following nailing through the piriformis fossa in children and adolescents.[1,9–11,13]
- Femoral neck valgus and narrowing of the femoral neck can result from placement of an intramedullary nail through the piriformis fossa or tip of the trochanter, damaging the cartilaginous proximal femoral epiphysis that lies along the lateral aspect of the femoral neck in younger patients.[4,14]

## REFERENCES


1. Astion DJ, Wilbe JH, Scole PV. Avascular necrosis of the capital femoral epiphysis after intramedullary nailing for a fracture of the femoral shaft. A case report. J Bone Joint Surg Am 1995;77(7):1092–1094.
2. Flynn JM, Hresko T, Reynolds RA, et al. Titanium elastic nails for pediatric femur fractures: a multicenter study of early results with analysis of complications. J Pediatr Orthop 2001;21(1):4–8.
3. Gage JR, Cary JM. The effects of trochanteric epiphyseodesis on growth of the proximal end of the femur following necrosis of the capital femoral epiphysis. J Bone Joint Surg Am 1980;62(5):785–794.
4. González-Herranz P, Burgos-Flore J, Rapariz JM, et al. Intramedullary nailing of the femur in children. Effects on its proximal end. J Bone Joint Surg Br 1995;77(2):262–266.
5. Gordon JE, Khanna N, Luhmann SJ, et al. Intramedullary nailing of femoral fractures in children through the lateral aspect of the greater trochanter using a modified rigid humeral intramedullary nail: preliminary results of a new technique in 15 children. J Orthop Trauma 2004;18(7):416–422.
6. Gordon JE, Swenning TA, Burd TA, et al. Proximal femoral changes after lateral transtrochanteric intramedullary nail placement in children: a radiographic analysis. J Bone Joint Surg Am 2003;85:1295–1301.
7. Jencikova-Celerin L, Phillips JH, Werk LN, et al. Flexible interlocked nailing of pediatric femoral fractures: experience with a new flexible interlocking intramedullary nail compared with other fixation procedures. J Pediatr Orthop 2008;28(8):864–873.
8. Keeler KA, Dart B, Luhmann SJ, et al. Antegrade intramedullary nailing of pediatric femoral fractures using an interlocking pediatric femoral nail and a lateral trochanteric entry point. J Pediatr Orthop 2009;29(4):345–351.
9. Macneil JA, Franci A, El-Hawary R. A systematic review of rigid, locked, intramedullary nail insertion sites and avascular necrosis of the femoral head in the skeletally immature. J Pediatr Orthop 2011;31(4):377–380.
10. Mileski RA, Garvin KL, Crosby LA. Avascular necrosis of the femoral head in an adolescent following intramedullary nailing of the femur: a case report. J Bone Joint Surg Am 1994;76(11):1706–1708.
11. Mileski RA, Garvin KL, Huurman WW. Avascular necrosis of the femoral head after closed intramedullary shortening in an adolescent. J Pediatr Orthop 1995;15:24–26.
12. Ogden JA. Changing patterns of proximal femoral vascularity. J Bone Joint Surg Am 1974;56(5):941–950.
13. O'Malley DE, Mazur JM, Cummings RJ. Femoral head avascular necrosis associated with intramedullary nailing in an adolescent. J Pediatr Orthop 1995;15:21–23.
14. Raney EM, Ogden JA, Grogan DP. Premature greater trochanteric epiphysiodesis secondary to intramedullary femoral rodding. J Pediatr Orthop 1993;13:516–520.
15. Siffert RS. Patterns of deformity of the developing hip. Clin Orthop Relat Res 1981;(160):14–29.
16. Trueta J. The normal vascular anatomy of the human femoral head during growth. J Bone Joint Surg Br 1957;39:358–394.

# Distal Femoral Physeal Fractures

Martin J. Herman

28

CHAPTER

## DEFINITION

- Fractures of the distal femoral physis are those that involve the physis or growth plate of the distal femur.
- These fractures occur most commonly in older children and adolescents from falls or sports activities.
- Physeal fractures of the distal femur are best categorized by the Salter-Harris (SH) classification. The vast majority of these fractures are SH type I and II fractures, which are extra-articular. SH III and IV fractures, which are uncommon, are intra-articular (**FIG 1**).[3]
- The goals of treatment for these fractures are healing of the fracture in acceptable alignment and anatomic restoration of the physis and joint line to reduce the risk of growth arrest and premature arthritis of the knee.

## ANATOMY

- The distal femoral physis accounts for 40% of the longitudinal growth of the lower extremity, growing approximately 9 mm per year until skeletal maturity.
- Morphologically, this growth plate is not flat but instead has undulations across its surface which add to the stability of the physis but also make it more prone to damage when fractures of the physis occur.
- The medial and lateral collateral ligaments originate from the distal femoral epiphysis distal to the physis. The anterior and posterior cruciate ligaments originate from the intercondylar notch, also distal to the physis (**FIG 2**).
- The popliteal artery courses along the posterior surface of the distal femur as its traverses the popliteal space. The sciatic nerve divides into the peroneal and posterior tibial branches just proximal to the physis. Anterior displacement of the distal fragment is associated with popliteal artery injury, and medial displacement is associated with peroneal nerve injury.

## PATHOGENESIS

- Physeal fractures generally cleave through the zone of hypertrophic calcification then go either proximal (SH I and II) or distal to this zone (SH III and IV). In distal femoral physeal fractures, however, the fracture cleaves not only through the hypertrophic zone but also crosses other zones including the germinal zone of the growth plate because of its undulating morphology, making growth disturbance likely even after SH I and II fractures.
- These fractures result most commonly from medial or lateral forces applied to the knee, resulting in varus (medial) or valgus (lateral) displacement, respectively.
- Knee hyperextension injuries lead to anteriorly displaced fractures while direct forces applied to the flexed knee, such as a dashboard strike during a motor vehicle crash, commonly cause intra-articular SH III and IV fractures.

## NATURAL HISTORY

- The distal femoral physis has tremendous healing and remodeling potential in children with at least 2 years of growth remaining. In this age group, fractures with anatomic realignment of the joint surface that are realigned with less than 10 degrees of deformity in the anteroposterior (AP) and lateral planes heal with restoration of normal function in most patients who do *not* develop a growth arrest.
- For patients who develop a growth arrest, however, the results are variable. The growth disturbance is the result of either injury to the germinal cells of the physis from the trauma of the initial injury or subsequent reduction, from malreduction with physeal bar formation, or from iatrogenic injury from screws that cross the physis.[1,2,6]
- The resulting problems related to growth disturbance are angular deformities from incomplete arrest or limb length discrepancy from complete physeal closure.

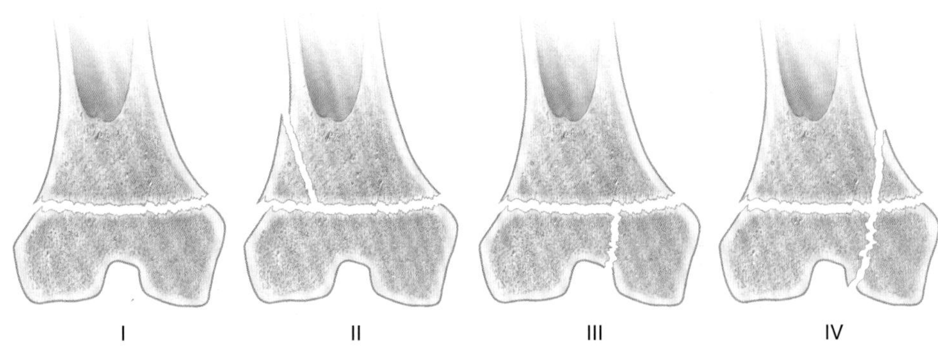


**FIG 1** • Patterns of distal femoral physeal fractures based on the SH classification.

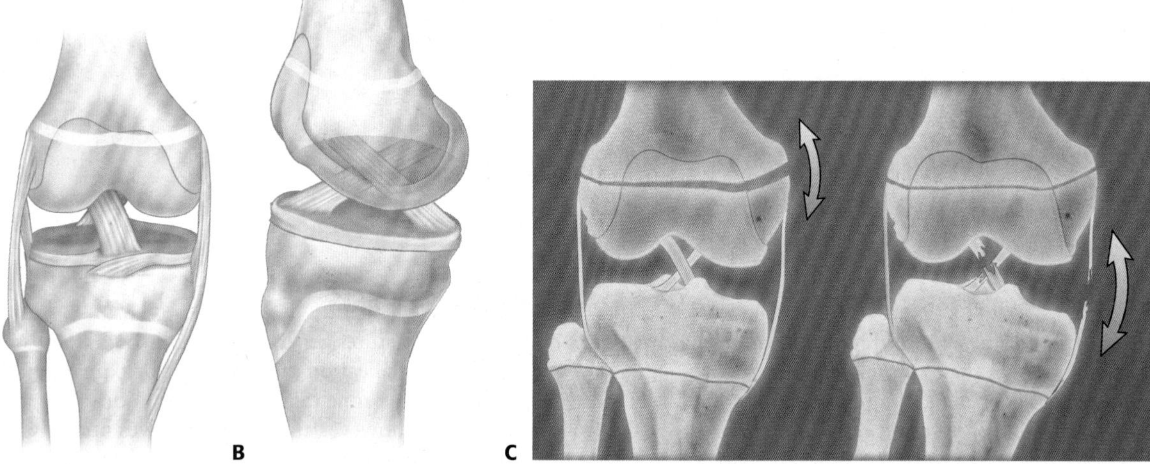

**FIG 2** ● AP (**A**) and lateral (**B**) diagrams of the ligaments of the knee. The collateral and cruciate ligaments have their origins distal to the distal femoral physis. **C.** In a child with an open physis, laxity with valgus stress testing occurs through a physeal fracture more commonly than through a medial collateral ligament tear.

- Because of the high risk of growth-related problems, patients and their families must be counseled at the time of initial treatment about the potential for complications.

## PATIENT HISTORY AND PHYSICAL EXAMINATION

- A complete history includes an inquiry about the precise mechanism of injury and when it occurred, questions about changes in motor or sensory function of the affected limb, and any significant medical history.
- A complete physical examination begins with inspection of the limb for deformity, swelling, knee joint effusion, excessive bleeding from an open injury, and any other defects of the soft tissue such as lacerations or abrasions. The entire limb is then palpated to identify focal areas of tenderness about the knee and any associated injuries proximal and distal to it.
- A motor and sensory examination is necessary to identify neurologic deficits of the peroneal and posterior tibial nerves. The vascular status of the limb is assessed by assessing the distal pulses and other signs of limb perfusion including the capillary refill of the toes and the temperature of the limb.
- In patients without obvious deformity but with a history and examination that is otherwise suspicious for a distal physeal fracture, gentle varus–valgus and anterior drawer or Lachman stress testing may allow the examiner to differentiate between a physeal injury and a ligament injury.

## IMAGING

- High-quality AP and lateral radiographs of the entire extremity are necessary to fully assess these injuries as well as the overall alignment of the limb and other associated fractures (**FIG 3**). Dedicated views of the knee, with comparison views of the uninjured side if necessary, are useful to precisely define the fracture pattern, especially when the fracture is nondisplaced.
- Computed tomography (CT) of the knee is indicated for most intra-articular fractures (SH types III and IV) to define the fracture pattern and the degree of displacement as well as to aid in planning of fixation (**FIG 4**).[5]
- Magnetic resonance imaging (MRI) is used to confirm occult fractures when the radiographs are normal but the examination is suspicious for a fracture as well as to diagnose other knee pathology such as meniscus tears, ligament tears, and osteochondral injuries.[4]

## DIFFERENTIAL DIAGNOSIS

- Distal femoral metaphyseal fracture
- Knee (tibiofemoral) dislocation
- Patellar dislocation
- Proximal tibial fracture
- Collateral ligament tears (vs. nondisplaced fracture)

## NONOPERATIVE TREATMENT

- Long-leg cast immobilization for 4 to 6 weeks is indicated only for fractures which are nondisplaced.
- Fractures which require reduction to achieve satisfactory alignment are generally unstable and are best treated with fixation.

## SURGICAL MANAGEMENT

### Indications

- Surgical reduction and fixation are indicated for all displaced distal femoral physeal fractures.
- Surgical fixation is indicated for some nondisplaced fractures that are at high risk for displacement, such as SH III and IV fractures or those that are associated with severe soft tissue injury or neurovascular abnormalities. Other indications are obesity that inhibits effective long-leg cast immobilization and behavioral or intellectual problems that preclude cooperation with non–weight-bearing instructions.

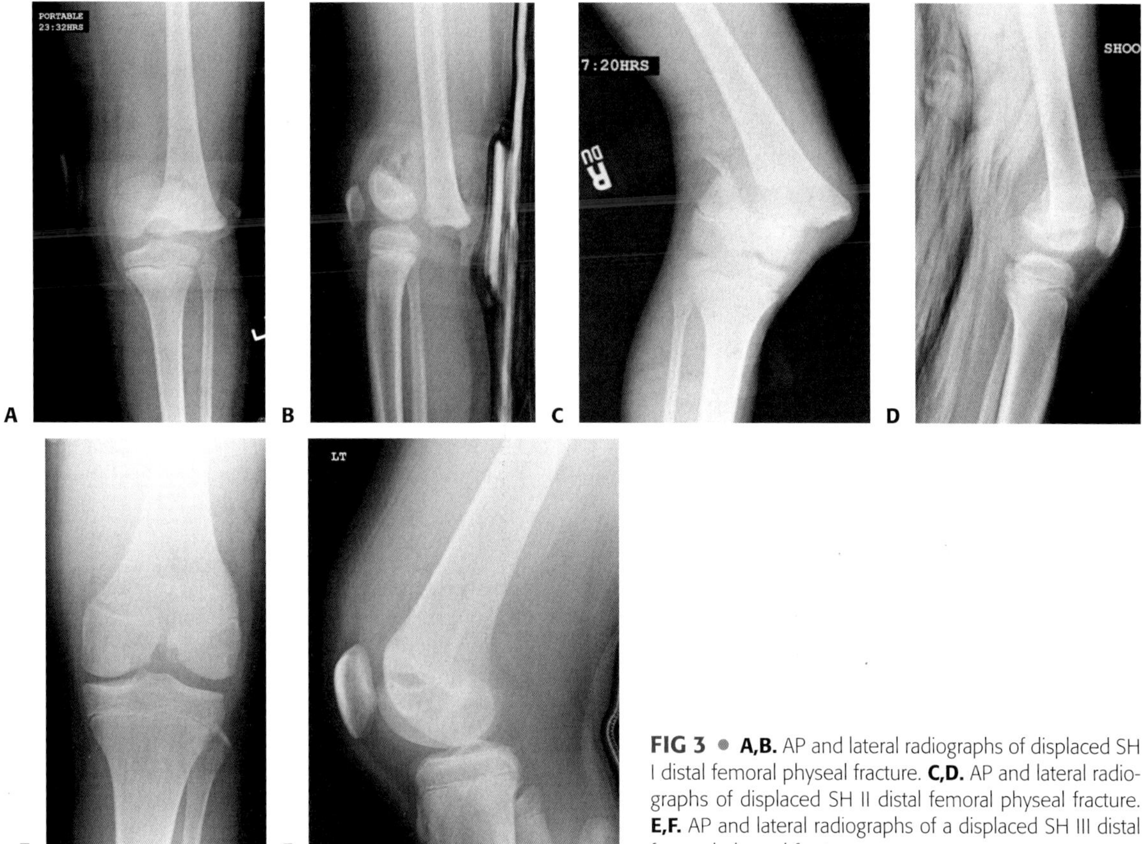


**FIG 3** • **A,B.** AP and lateral radiographs of displaced SH I distal femoral physeal fracture. **C,D.** AP and lateral radiographs of displaced SH II distal femoral physeal fracture. **E,F.** AP and lateral radiographs of a displaced SH III distal femoral physeal fracture.

## Preoperative Planning

- A vascular consultation is best called prior to going to the operating room for those patients with diminished pulses or no limb perfusion, so no intraoperative delay occurs if blood flow does not return after reduction and fixation.
- The surgeon should request muscle relaxation from the anesthesia provider after induction to facilitate reduction.
- The implants necessary to perform the operation include cannulated screws (4.5 to 7.3 mm in diameter), smooth wires (5/64 inch and larger in diameter), and, in rare cases, a distal femoral plating system. Other essential equipment includes instruments to perform an open reduction and a traction bow if the need arises to place a proximal tibial traction pin for achieving length.

## Patient Positioning

- We typically perform the procedure supine on a radiolucent operating table that permits AP and lateral fluoroscopic views with the leg held in extension or with the knee flexed over a bolster or bump (**FIG 5**).
- Alternatively, the patient may be positioned on a fracture table with the affected limb placed in a traction boot.

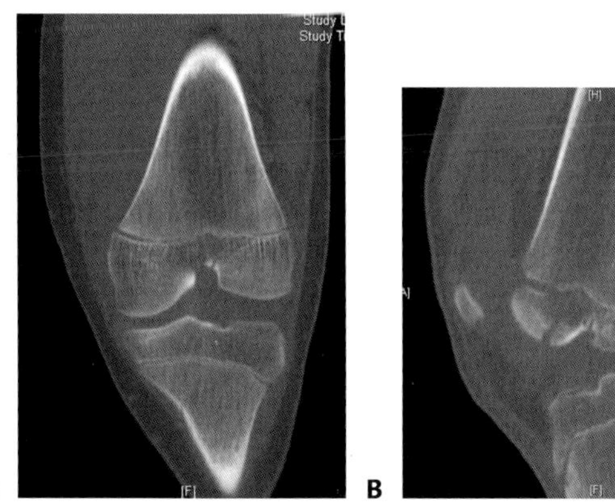


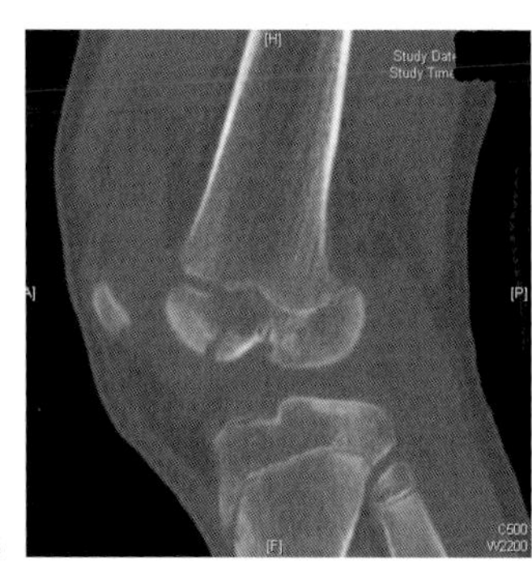


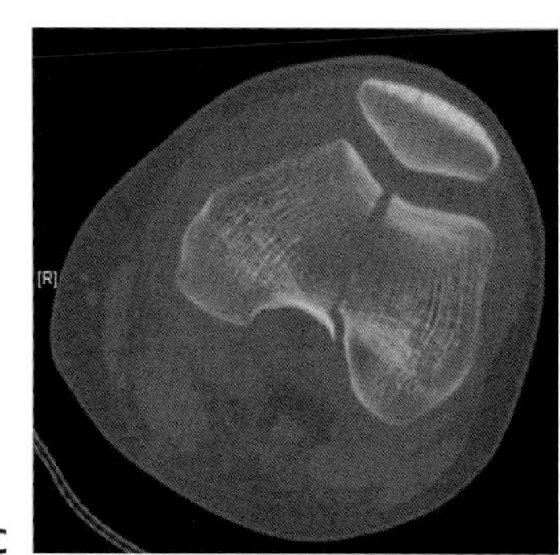


**FIG 4** • CT images (**A**, coronal; **B**, sagittal; **C**, axial) of a displaced SH III fracture.

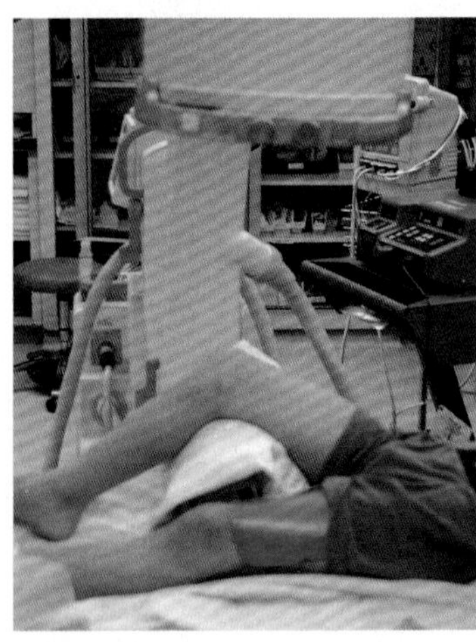
A

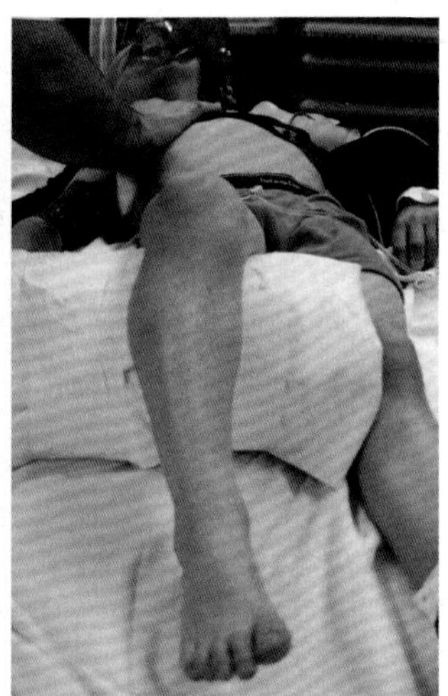
B

**FIG 5** • Views of side (**A**) and foot (**B**) of operating table showing the patient's knee flexed over a bump and the C-arm overhead.

## Surgical Approach

### *SH I and II Fractures*

- Most fractures can be realigned by closed reduction alone. The reduction maneuver entails primarily application of traction to disimpact the physis from the metaphysis and to prevent "scraping" of the two fragments together during reduction, which may exacerbate the physeal damage.
- After traction is applied, appropriate translational forces are then used to achieve a gentle closed reduction. Varus or valgus forces applied to the knee reduce valgus and varus deformities, respectively. Anterior displacement is reduced by flexing the knee, whereas posterior displacement, an uncommon direction of deformity, is reduced by knee extension.
- Crossed transphyseal smooth wires placed either retrograde or antegrade are best for stabilizing SH I fractures and those SH II fractures with a small Thurston-Holland fragment. Transverse metaphyseal screws that capture larger Thurston-Holland fragment are best for stabilizing SH II fractures.
- Open reduction, if necessary, is performed through a longitudinal incision made at the apex of the deformity, typically at the distal end of the proximal fragment. Care must be taken to minimize physeal injury. Entrapped periosteum and soft tissue are impediments to reduction.

### *SH III and IV Fractures*

- Minimally displaced fractures may be reduced with a large reduction forceps or a stout wire used as a "joystick."
- Open reduction performed via an arthrotomy can be done either medially or laterally depending on the location of fracture extension into the joint. Anatomic realignment of the physis and the joint line are the goals of open reduction.
- Stable fixation with epiphyseal screws or transphyseal smooth wires is used to stabilize these fractures.



## Closed Reduction and Percutaneous Wire Fixation

### Fracture Reduction

- Reduction is done emergently for neurovascular compromise, skin tenting, and open fractures. Otherwise, the reduction may be done the next day but no longer than 7 to 10 days after injury.
- Anesthesia with muscle relaxation makes reduction easier and less traumatic to the physis.
- Laterally displaced fractures are reduced by applying traction, then a medially directed force on the distal tibia while stabilizing the limb with a lateral force at the distal femur (**TECH FIG 1A**).
- Anteriorly displaced fractures are reduced by applying traction to disimpact the physis and flexion of the knee (**TECH FIG 1B**).
- The opposite forces are used for posterior and medial fracture displacement.

### Fixation

- Smooth Kirschner wires (larger than 2 mm in diameter) are used for fixation of SH I fractures and SH II fractures with small Thurston-Holland fragments. A crossed-pin configuration is commonly employed.
- Wires may be placed retrograde, starting in the epiphysis and advanced across the physis into the proximal metaphyseal cortices, or antegrade, starting in the proximal metaphyseal cortices and advanced across the physis into the epiphysis.
- Wires left protruding from the joint are at high risk for causing septic arthritis of the knee. Wires should either be cut short and buried beneath the skin within the joint or advanced proximally until the wire ends are proximal to the joint cartilage but fixed in the epiphysis, making it possible to bend and cut them outside the skin adjacent to the metaphyses (**TECH FIG 2**). Buried wires are removed in the operating room, whereas percutaneous wires are removed in the office.
- After fixation, the limb is immobilized in a long-leg bent knee cast or splint.

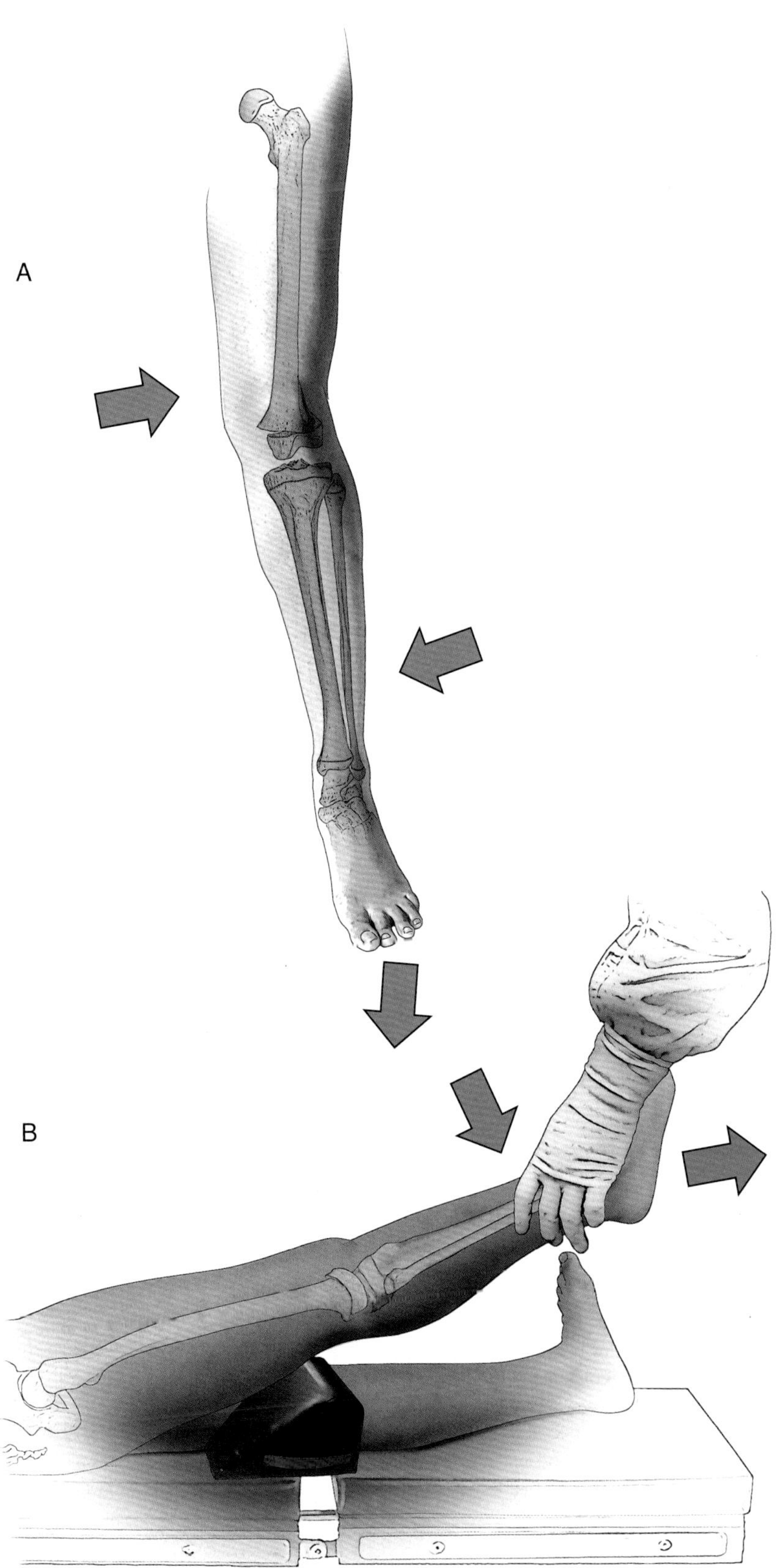


**TECH FIG 1** • Coronal (**A**) and sagittal (**B**) views of an anteriorly and laterally displaced SH II fractures and the forces necessary to achieve reduction.

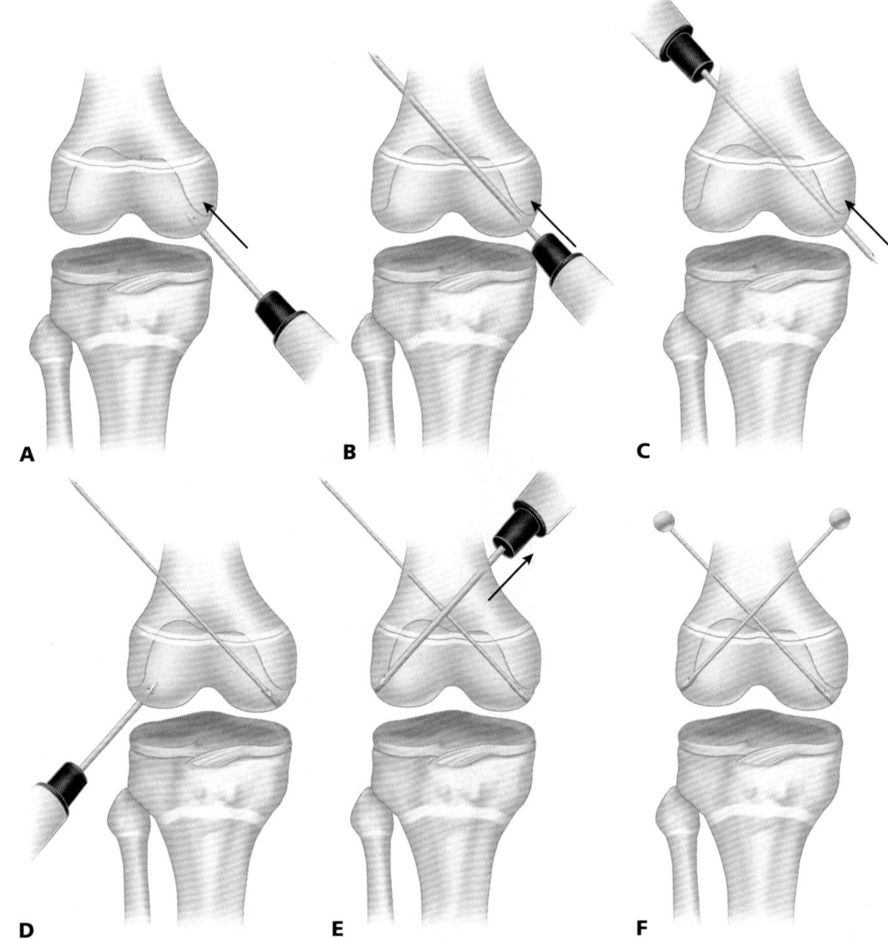


**TECH FIG 2** • AP diagrams. **A.** Wire starting in medial femoral condyle drilled retrograde. **B.** Wire starting in medial femoral condyle drilled retrograde across proximal contralateral metaphysis and out skin. **C.** Wire drilled retrograde from proximal until distal end of wire is buried in the epiphysis. **D.** Wire starting in lateral femoral condyle drilled retrograde across proximal contralateral metaphysis and out skin. **E.** Drilled retrograde across proximal contralateral metaphysis and out skin. **F.** Wire cut and left outside the skin proximally.

## Closed Reduction and Percutaneous Screw Fixation

- Cannulated screws that *do not* cross the physis are most commonly used to stabilize SH II fractures with a large Thurston-Holland fragment and SH III and IV fractures.
- Alternatively, smooth wires can also be used and can be placed across the physis if necessary.
- Although closed reduction and percutaneous fixation is used routinely for SH II fractures, only SH III and IV fractures with minimal separation or rotation are amenable to this technique.

### SH II Fractures

- After closed reduction, two guidewires are placed parallel to the physis, engaging the Thurston-Holland fragment so that short-thread cannulated screws can be placed to compress across the fracture site (**TECH FIGS 3** and **4**).
- Once adequate reduction and guidewire placement are confirmed with biplanar fluoroscopic views, the screws are placed sequentially, first overdrilling the outer cortex before placing the screw.
- Additional fixation may be added if the fracture is unstable when stressed under fluoroscopy.
- The addition of a stout wire transphyseal is often my preference at this point.

### Minimally Displaced SH III and IV

- A large bone forceps can be used to compress across epiphyseal fragments that are separated but otherwise nondisplaced prior to guidewire placement.
- For those with some rotation, the guidewire can also be used to manipulate the fragments prior to drilling the guidewire (**TECH FIG 5**).
- If anatomic alignment of the physis and joint line cannot be achieved, then open reduction is required.
- After fixation, the limb is immobilized in a long-leg bent knee cast or splint.

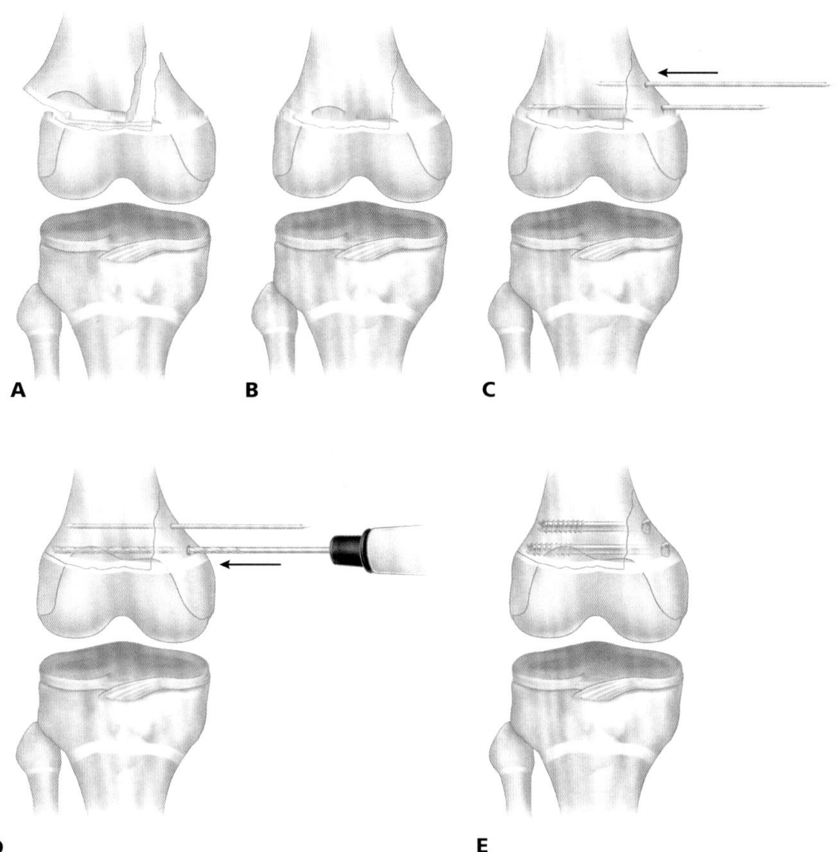


**TECH FIG 3** • AP diagrams. **A.** Displaced SH type II fracture of distal femur. **B.** Reduced SH type II fracture of distal femur. **C.** Guidewires placed across Thurston-Holland fragment, parallel to physis. **D.** Drill over guidewires. **E.** Lag screws in place.

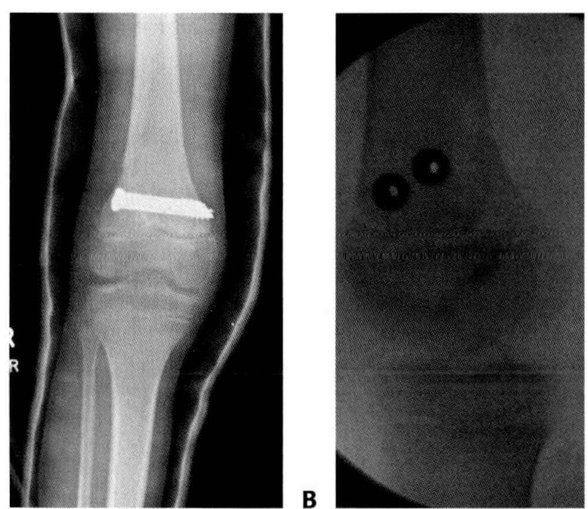


**TECH FIG 4** • AP (**A**) and lateral (**B**) radiographs of the patient in **FIG 3C,D** after closed reduction and fixation with 7.3-mm cannulated screws.

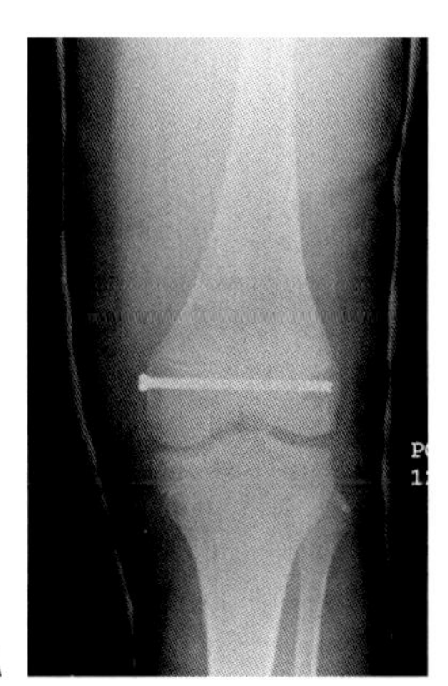
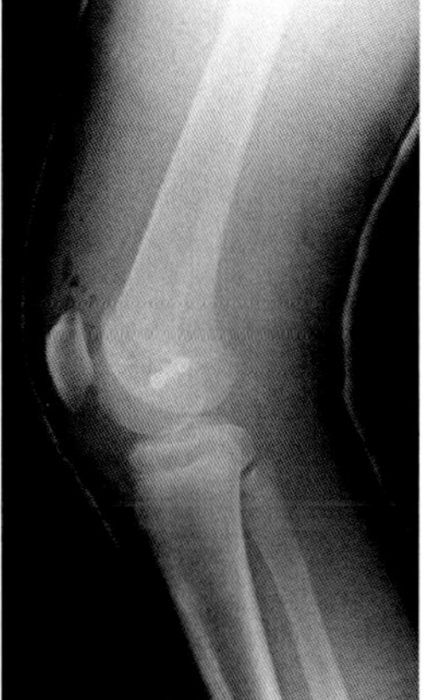


**TECH FIG 5** • AP (**A**) and lateral (**B**) radiographs of the patient in **FIG 3E,F** after closed reduction and percutaneous screw fixation.

## Open Reduction and Internal Fixation

### SH I and II Fractures

- Unacceptable closed reduction parameters vary to some degree by age of the child. For those with more than 2 years of growth remaining, less than 5 to 10 degrees of deformity in either plane with minimal translation or gapping open of the physis is acceptable. Failure to achieve a near-anatomic closed reduction, however, may indicate periosteal interposition, a risk factor for growth arrest, and is an indication in many cases to perform open reduction. Children near skeletal maturity should be reduced anatomically.
- Open reduction is performed under tourniquet. The incision is made either medially or laterally at the site of periosteal disruption, that is, at the apex of the deformity.
- Care must be taken to remove the interposed periosteum and soft tissue (**TECH FIG 6**) and reduce the fracture without causing further damage to the physis.
- Fixation is performed, as described earlier, based on the fracture pattern (**TECH FIG 7**).
- After fixation, the limb is immobilized in a long-leg bent knee cast or splint.

### SH III and IV Fractures

- Open reduction is indicated for all displaced fractures that cannot be closed reduced or have complex fracture patterns.
- Open reduction is performed under tourniquet. The fracture is approached through a parapatellar arthrotomy made on the side of the intra-articular fracture line.
- After evacuation of the hemarthrosis, careful open reduction and fixation is performed, taking care to avoid further damage to the joint cartilage and physis.
- Fixation is performed with cannulated screws placed in the epiphysis or smooth wires placed transphyseal if necessary (**TECH FIG 8**).
- After fixation, the limb is immobilized in a long-leg bent knee cast or splint.

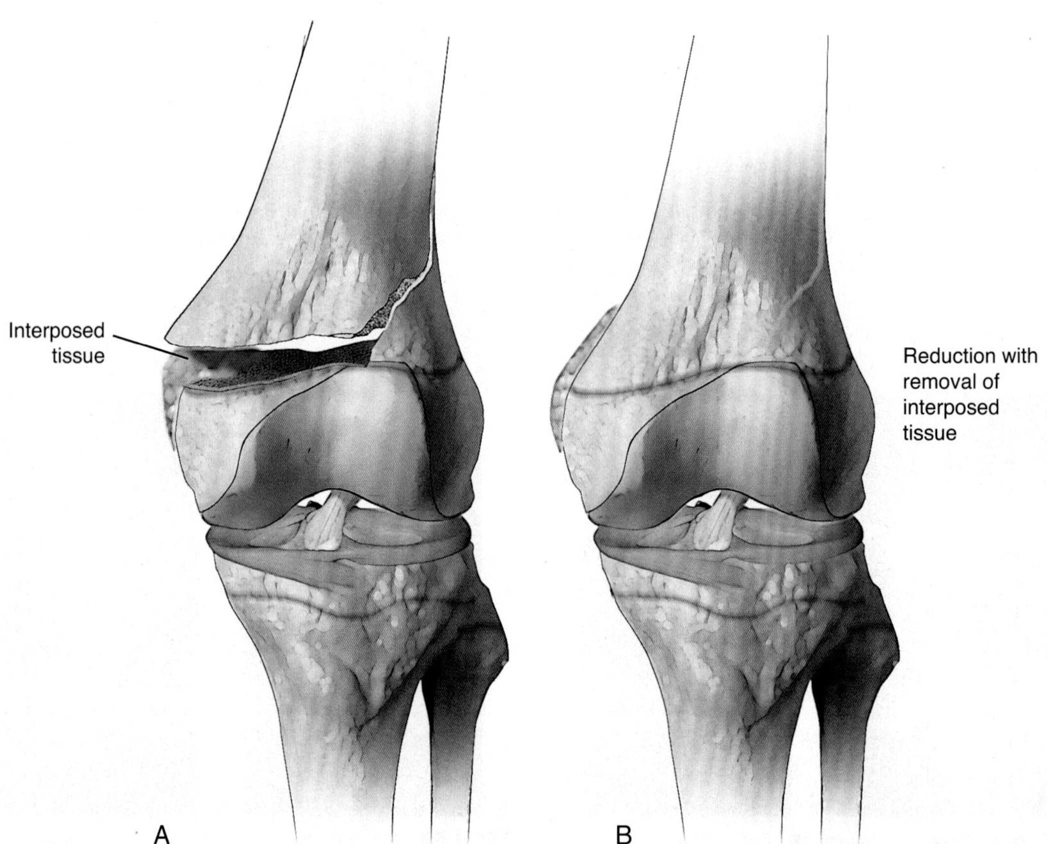


**TECH FIG 6** • AP diagrams of displaced SH type II fracture. **A.** Interposed soft tissue. **B.** Reduction with removal of interposed tissue.

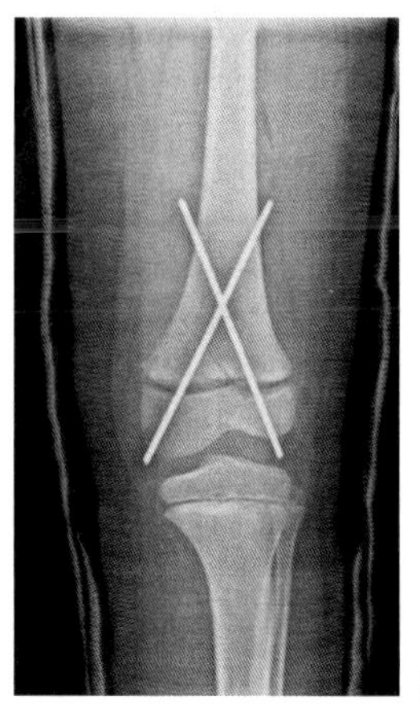
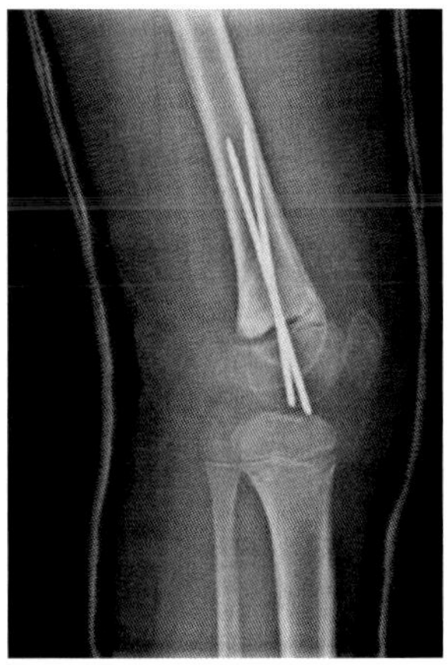

**TECH FIG 7** • AP (**A**) and lateral (**B**) radiographs of the patient in **FIG 3A,B** after open reduction and fixation with smooth wires.

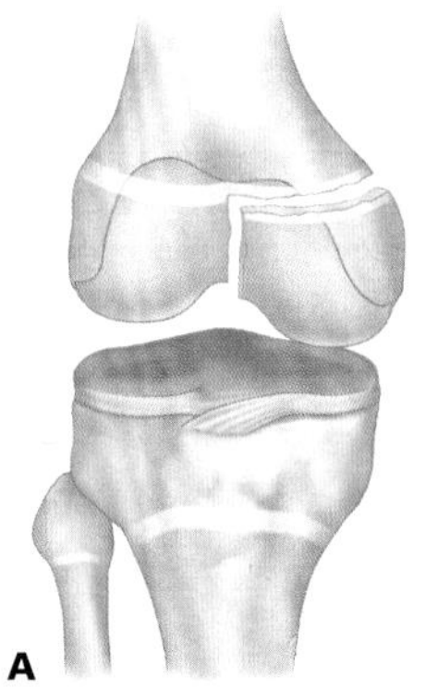
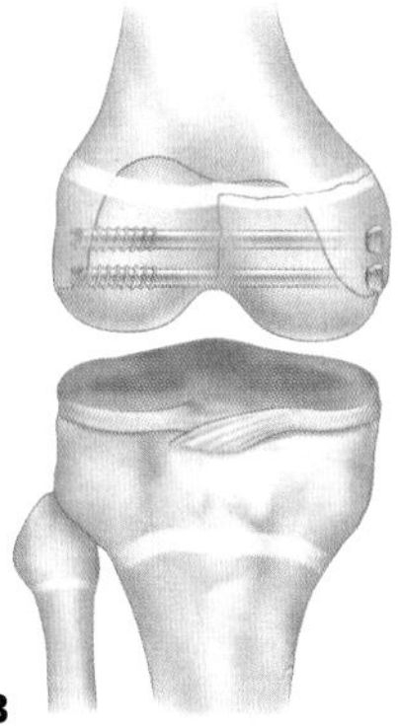

**TECH FIG 8** • AP diagrams of a displaced SH type III fracture (**A**) that has been lagged together (**B**).

## PEARLS AND PITFALLS

| | |
|---|---|
| **Indications** | ▪ Fractures that present later than 7–10 days after injury are best treated without reduction and surgery and instead are allowed to heal. Late manipulation increases the risk of growth arrest. |
| **Examination** | ▪ A careful and thorough neurovascular examination is mandatory before manipulation to identify vascular injury or neurapraxias, especially for severely displaced fractures. |
| **Surgical technique** | ▪ Fracture reduction requires longitudinal traction initially, followed by translational maneuvers to prevent physeal damage.<br>▪ Transphyseal screws inhibit growth and should not be used to stabilize distal femoral physeal fractures.<br>▪ Tension on the skin around pins cut outside the skin should be relieved by extending the incision around the pin to prevent skin necrosis, which increases the risk of infection of the pins. |
| **Follow-up** | ▪ High-quality radiographs of the knee and a lower extremity scanogram done at 6 month intervals after injury are the best ways to identify signs of early growth disturbance. |

## POSTOPERATIVE CARE

- After fixation, the limb is immobilized in a cast or a locked hinged knee brace for 4 to 6 weeks, and instructions are given for non–weight bearing on crutches or a walker.
- Knee range of motion, strengthening exercises, and progressive weight bearing is initiated after the period of immobilization, typically under the direction of a physical therapist.
- All smooth wires are removed either in the clinic within 4 to 6 weeks of surgery for those cut outside the skin or in the operating room for those buried subcutaneously. Screws are removed only for irritation or to improve the quality of imaging with CT or MRI for those with potential complications such as growth arrest and knee ligament or cartilage injuries.

## OUTCOMES

- For children with fractures that heal without complications and have no associated knee injuries, full return of activities and resumption of normal growth is expected.
- As many as 40% to 50% of children with distal femoral physeal fractures will have a complication that requires further care or surgery to manage the complication.

## COMPLICATIONS

- Knee stiffness after rehabilitation is uncommon but may require prolonged therapy, manipulation, and in rare cases, knee arthroscopy and soft tissue releases.
- As many as 40% of patients have associated knee injuries. Anterior cruciate ligament tear is most common and occurs most frequently after SH III and IV fractures that involve the medial condyle.
- Neurovascular injuries are rare. Popliteal artery injury is associated with severely displaced fractures with anterior displacement. Peroneal nerve injury is associated with fractures that are displaced medially (varus deformity).
- Growth disturbance occurs in about one-half of children with distal femoral physeal fractures.[2] Careful follow-up at 4 to 6 months intervals until skeletal maturity is recommended.

## ACKNOWLEDGMENT

- I acknowledge the contribution of R. Dale Blasier, the author of this chapter for the first edition.

## REFERENCES

1. Arkader A, Warner WC Jr, Horn BD, et al. Predicting the outcome of physeal fractures of the distal femur. J Pediatr Orthop 2007;27:703–708
2. Basener CJ, Mehlman CT, DiPasquale TG. Growth disturbance after distal femoral growth plate fractures in children: a meta-analysis. J Orthop Trauma 2009;23(9):663–667.
3. Beaty JH, Kumar A. Fractures about the knee in children. J Bone Joint Surg Am 1994;76(12):1870–1880.
4. Bertin KC, Goble EM. Ligament injuries associated with physeal fractures about the knee. Clin Orthop Relat Res 1983;(177): 188–195.
5. Lippert WC, Owens RF, Wall EJ. Salter-Harris type III fractures of the distal femur: plain radiographs can be deceptive. J Pediatr Orthop 2010;30(6):598–605.
6. Thomson JD, Stricker SJ, Williams MM. Fractures of the distal femoral epiphyseal plate. J Pediatr Orthop 1995;15:474–478.

# Open Reduction and Internal Fixation of the Distal Femur

29 CHAPTER

Animesh Agarwal

## DEFINITION

- Distal femur fractures are difficult, complex injuries that can result in devastating outcomes.
- The distal part of the femur is considered the most distal 9 to 15 cm of the femur and can involve the articular surface. The intra-articular injury can vary from a simple split to extensive comminution.
- Articular involvement can lead to posttraumatic arthritis.
- These fractures constitute 4% to 7% of all femur fractures.
  - If the hip is excluded, they represent nearly one-third of all femur fractures.
  - There is a bimodal distribution defined by the mechanism of injury (see the following discussion).

## ANATOMY

- The supracondylar area of the femur is the zone between the femoral condyles and the metaphyseal–diaphyseal junction.
- The metaphyseal bone has some important structural characteristics.
  - The predominant bone is cancellous.
  - The cortices are especially thin.
  - There is a wide intramedullary canal.
- It is also important to understand the unique bony architecture of the distal femur (**FIG 1**).
  - It is trapezoidal in shape, and hence the posterior aspect is wider than the anterior aspect. There is a gradual decrease by 25% in the width from posterior to anterior.
  - The medial femoral condyle has a larger anterior to posterior dimension than the lateral side and extends farther distally.
  - The shaft is in line with the anterior half of the distal femoral condyles.
- The normal mechanical and anatomic axes of the lower limb must be understood so that the alignment of the limb can be reestablished (**FIG 2**).
  - The mechanical femoral axis, which is from the center of the femoral head to the center of the knee, is 3 degrees off the vertical. The mechanical axis of the entire limb continues to the center of the ankle.
  - The anatomic femoral axis differs from the mechanical femoral axis in that there is 9 degrees of valgus at the knee. This results in an anatomic femoral axis of the lateral distal femur of 81 degrees or an anatomic femoral axis of the medial distal femur of 99 degrees.
  - The mechanical and anatomic axes of the tibia are for practical purposes identical, going from the center of the knee to the center of the ankle.
- The treatment of distal femur fractures can be complicated by the various muscle attachments, which can impede or hamper proper fracture reduction.
  - The quadriceps and hamstrings result in fracture shortening; thus, excellent muscle paralysis must be obtained for proper reduction.
  - The medial and lateral gastrocnemius results in posterior angulation and displacement of the distal segment. The distal femur "extends," resulting in an apex posterior deformity. If an intercondylar extension is present, rotational deformities of the individual condyles can occur (**FIG 3A,B**).
  - The adductors, specifically the adductor magnus, which inserts onto the adductor tubercle of the medial femoral condyle, can lead to a varus deformity of the distal segment (**FIG 3C**).

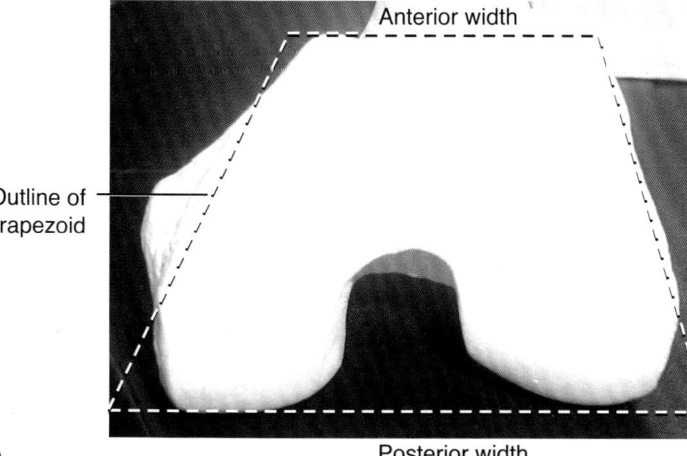


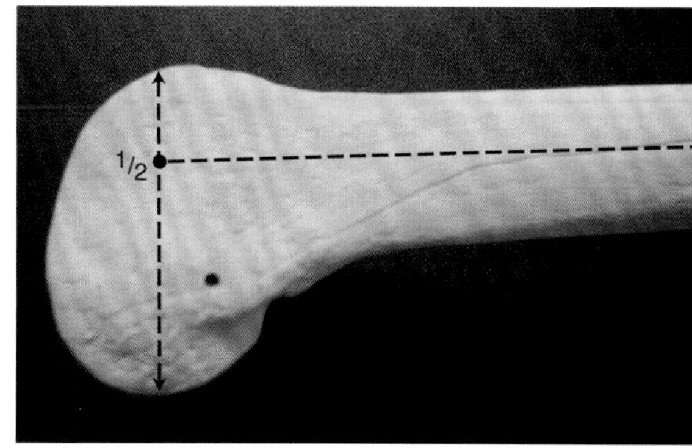


**FIG 1** ● **A.** View of the distal femur showing the wider posterior aspect and trapezoidal shape. **B.** Lateral view of the distal femur; the shaft is in line with the anterior half of the distal femoral condyles.

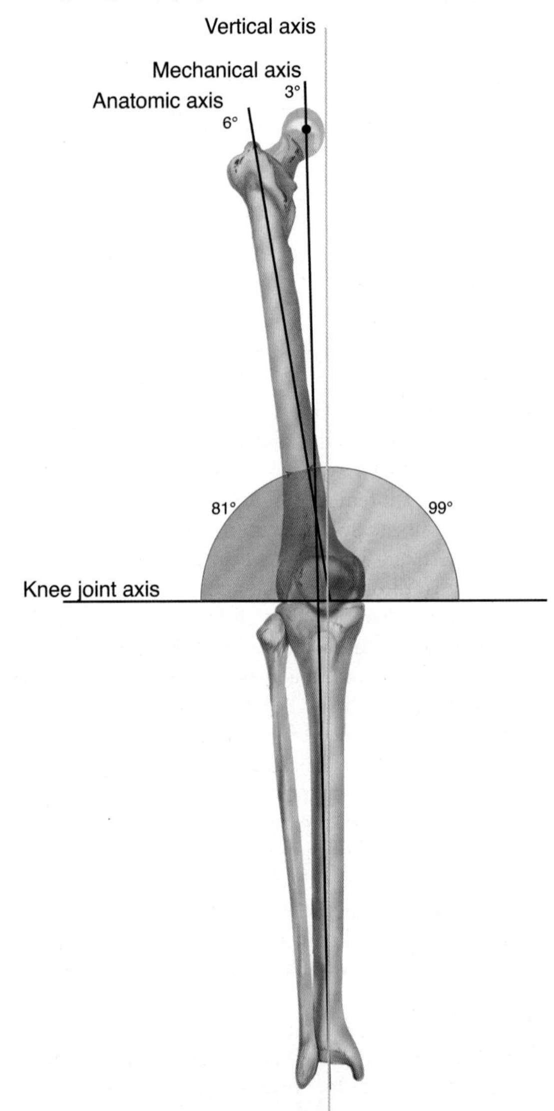


**FIG 2** • Mechanical and anatomic axes of the lower extremity; the 9 degrees of valgus at the knee is noted.

- The neurovascular structures about the knee are at risk when an injury of the distal femur occurs.
  - At the canal of Hunter, roughly 10 cm proximal to the knee on the medial side, the superficial femoral artery enters the popliteal fossa (see **FIG 3C**).
  - Posterior to the knee, both the popliteal artery and the tibial nerve are at risk at the fracture site (**FIG 3D**).

## PATHOGENESIS

- As mentioned, there is a bimodal distribution in terms of age in the epidemiology of distal femur fractures. This relates to the mechanism of injury.
- High-energy and low-energy injuries occur.
  - High-energy injuries usually are from motor vehicle accidents and occur in the young patient. There is a direct impact onto the flexed knee, such as from the dashboard. These patients often have associated injuries such as a hip fracture or dislocation or vascular or nerve injury. These high-energy injuries generally result in comminuted fractures, mostly of the metaphyseal region. The comminution can be articular as well.
  - Low-energy injuries usually occur in the elderly patient who falls from a standing height. The axial loading is accompanied by either varus or valgus with or without rotation. The osteoporotic bone in these individuals leads to fracture. The fracture pattern can vary from the most simple extra-articular type to the most complex intra-articular injury. Owing to the gastrocnemius complex, an apex posterior deformity of the condyles occurs as the fragments are flexed because of the muscle attachment.

## NATURAL HISTORY

- Fractures of the distal femur that have intra-articular displacement can lead to severe posttraumatic arthritis if left untreated.
- Operative treatment has led to a 32% decrease in poor outcomes.[19]

## PATIENT HISTORY AND PHYSICAL FINDINGS

- Direct physical examination of the knee with a distal femur fracture is limited primarily because of pain and the obvious nature of the injury.
  - The patient presents with a swollen and tender knee after either a fall or some high-energy trauma (motor vehicle or motorcycle accident).
  - A large hemarthrosis is present.
  - Any attempts at range of motion result in severe pain, and significant crepitus is usually noted with palpation.
- If there is concern for an open knee joint, the joint can be injected after a sterile preparation to see whether the knee joint communicates with any wound.
- The physical examination is directed primarily at ascertaining the neurovascular status of the lower limb and determining whether any associated injuries exist, especially the hip.
  - If there are any small wounds or tenting of the skin anteriorly, the fracture should be considered as being open.
  - It is important to check for pulses.
    - If diminished or absent, pulses should be assessed with Doppler.
    - The ankle–brachial indices should be obtained if there is a concern for arterial injury.
    - Any side-to-side difference or value less than 0.9 warrants an arteriogram.
    - Computed tomography (CT) arteriogram has been used with increasing frequency as well in cases where there is concern (**FIG 4**).
  - Nerve function should be checked. Sensation and both active dorsiflexion and plantarflexion must be assessed.

## IMAGING AND OTHER DIAGNOSTIC STUDIES

- The initial imaging study is always plain radiographs. Anteroposterior (AP) and lateral radiographs of the knee should be obtained initially.
  - Traction films should be obtained if there is severe comminution of either the metaphysis or articular surface. This aids in the preoperative planning.

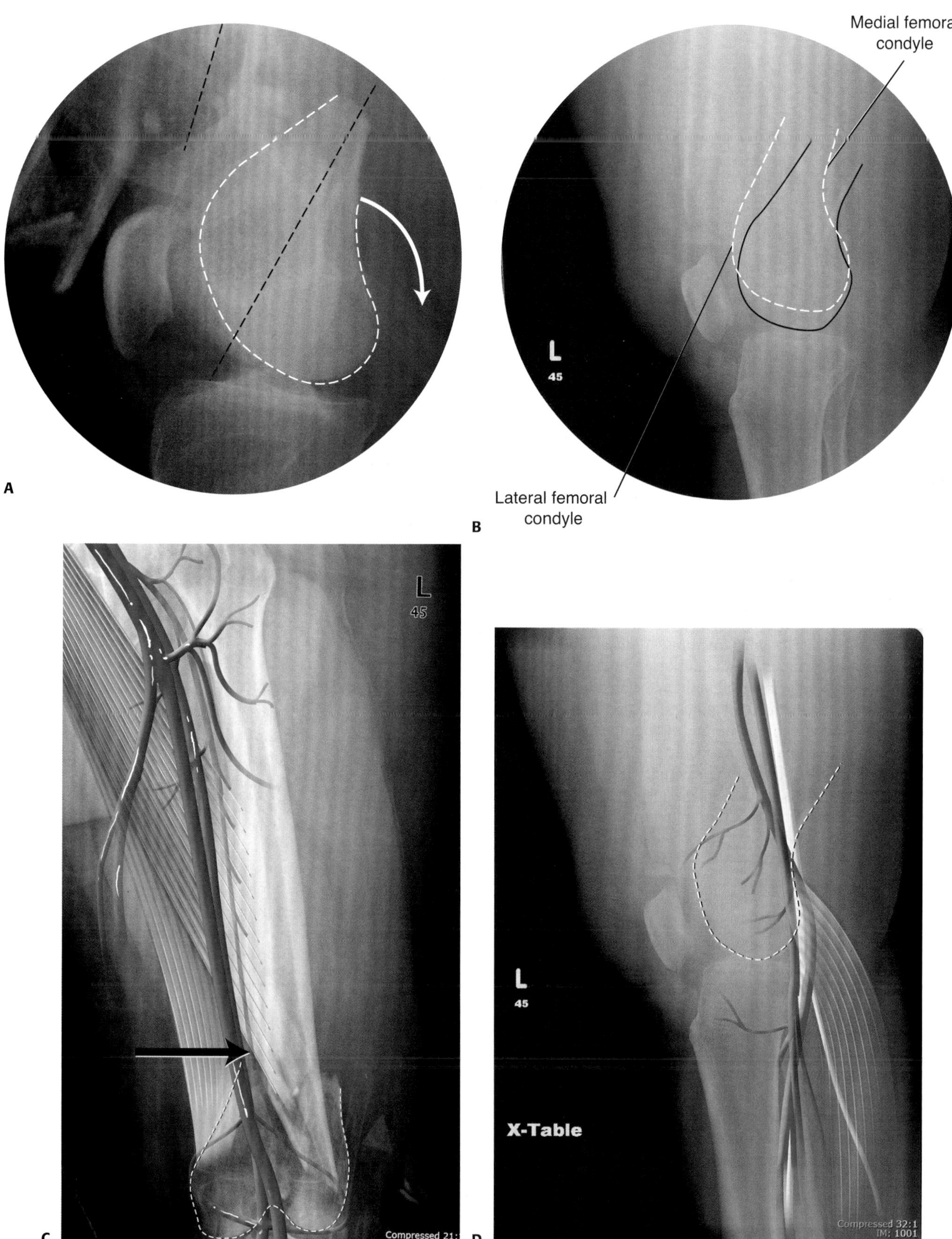


**FIG 3** • **A.** Patient with a grade IIIA open distal femur with extruded fragment; the "extension" of the femoral condyles is outlined. **B.** Patient with a distal femur fracture with intercondylar extension showing the subtle rotational deformities of the individual condyles. **C.** The muscle forces are shown on the distal femur, as is the femoral artery and vein entering the canal of Hunter (*arrow*). The adductor magnus inserts on the adductor tubercle, leading to a varus deformity of the distal segment. **D.** A lateral image of the same patient with the popliteal artery and tibial nerve drawn in to show the relative proximity to the fracture ends.

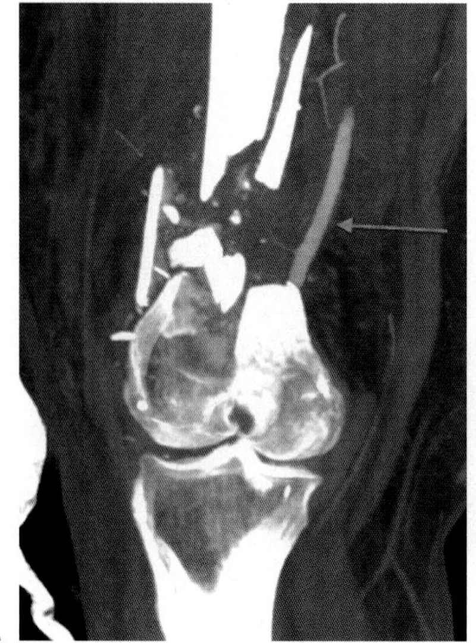

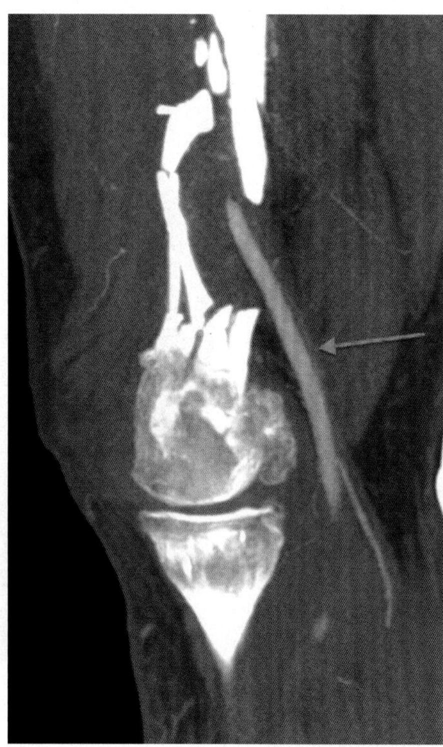

**FIG 4 • A,B.** Coronal and sagittal CT angiography images showing intact femoral artery in a severely comminuted distal femur fracture (*red arrows*).

- Dedicated knee films should always be obtained in the assessment of distal femur fractures. Additionally, the entire femur, to include the hip and knee, should be imaged to look for possible extension and associated injuries and to allow for preoperative planning (**FIG 5**).
  - In cases of severe comminution, radiographs of the contralateral knee can aid in preoperative planning as well.
- A dedicated CT scan is an important adjunct to the preoperative planning when there is articular involvement (**FIG 6**).
- Generally, extra-articular distal femur fractures do not require a CT scan. However, it has been shown that coronal fractures may be missed on plain films, and thus there is a low threshold for obtaining a CT scan for fractures of the distal femur.[11]
  - If the fracture pattern warrants a temporary bridging external fixator, it is best to obtain the CT scan after placement of such a fixator for better definition.
  - Coronal and sagittal reconstructions should be requested.
  - Three-dimensional images can be created from most CT scans. This can also aid in the preoperative planning (**FIG 7A,B**).
  - Subtle sagittal plane rotational malalignment between condyles can be assessed (**FIG 7C**).
- If associated soft tissue injury is suspected, such as ligamentous tears or tendon ruptures, then magnetic resonance imaging (MRI) may be indicated. Routine use of MRI, however, is not needed.

## DIFFERENTIAL DIAGNOSIS

- Proximal tibia fracture
- Femoral shaft fracture
- Septic knee
- Patella fracture
- Anterior cruciate ligament rupture
- Knee dislocation

## NONOPERATIVE MANAGEMENT

- There are few relative indications for nonoperative management of distal femur fractures:
  - Poor overall medical condition
    - Patient has severe comorbidities and is too sick for surgery.
    - Patient has extremely poor bone stock.
  - Spinal cord injury (paraplegia or quadriplegia)
  - Some special situations may warrant nonoperative care on case-by-case basis.
    - Nondisplaced or minimally displaced fracture
    - Select gunshot wounds with incomplete fractures
    - Extra-articular and stable
    - Unreconstructable
    - Lack of experience by the available surgeon or lack of equipment or appropriate facility to adequately treat the injury. Transfer is indicated in these situations; otherwise, nonoperative treatment may be the only option.
- There are several methods for nonoperative treatment.
  - Skeletal traction
  - Cast bracing
  - Knee immobilizer
  - Long-leg cast
- There are acceptable limits for nonoperative management:
  - Seven degrees of varus or valgus
  - Ten degrees of anterior or posterior angulation. A flexion deformity is less well tolerated than an extension deformity.
  - Up to 1 to 1.5 cm of shortening
  - Two to 3 mm of step-off at the joint surface

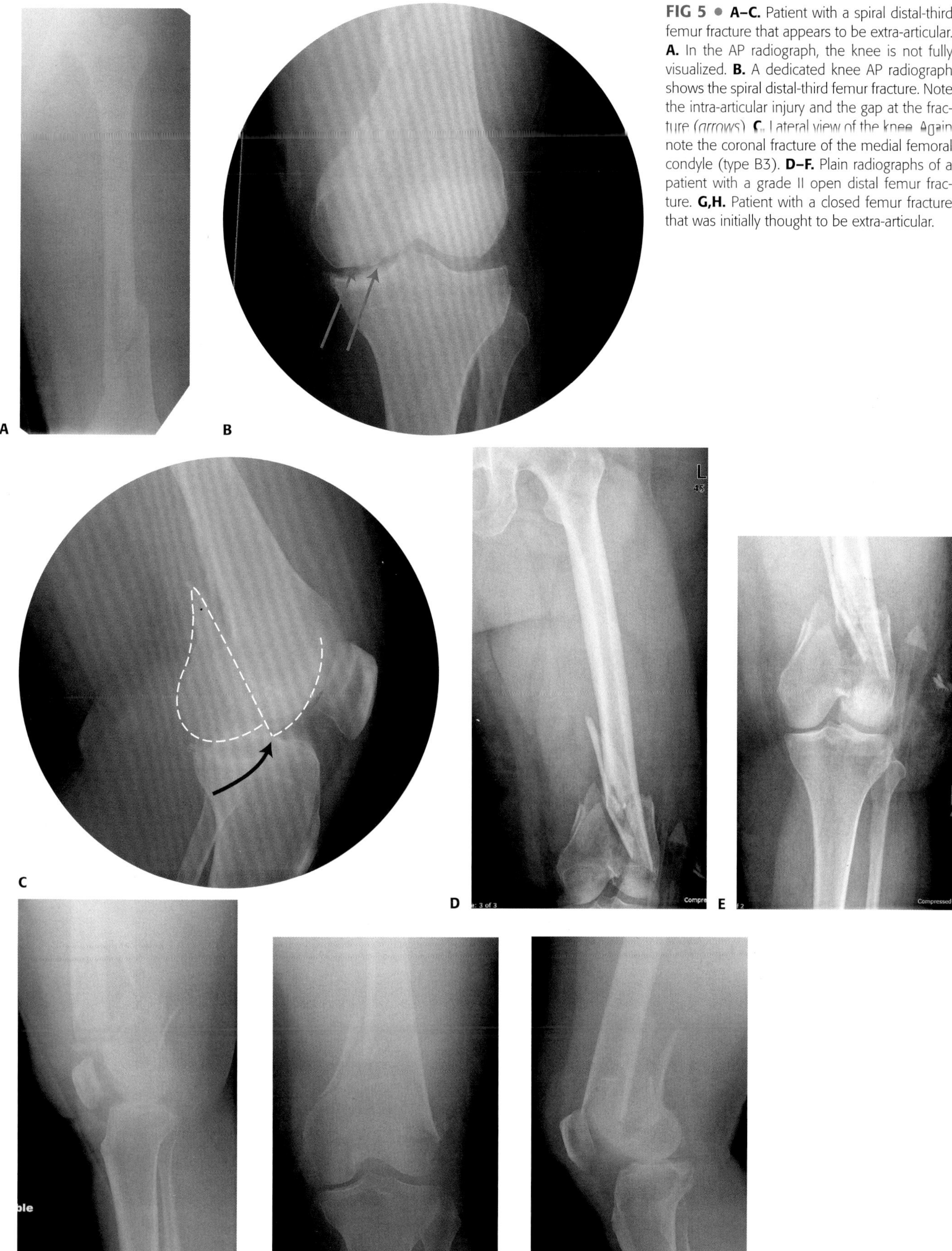


**FIG 5** • **A–C.** Patient with a spiral distal-third femur fracture that appears to be extra-articular. **A.** In the AP radiograph, the knee is not fully visualized. **B.** A dedicated knee AP radiograph shows the spiral distal-third femur fracture. Note the intra-articular injury and the gap at the fracture (*arrows*). **C.** Lateral view of the knee. Again note the coronal fracture of the medial femoral condyle (type B3). **D–F.** Plain radiographs of a patient with a grade II open distal femur fracture. **G,H.** Patient with a closed femur fracture that was initially thought to be extra-articular.

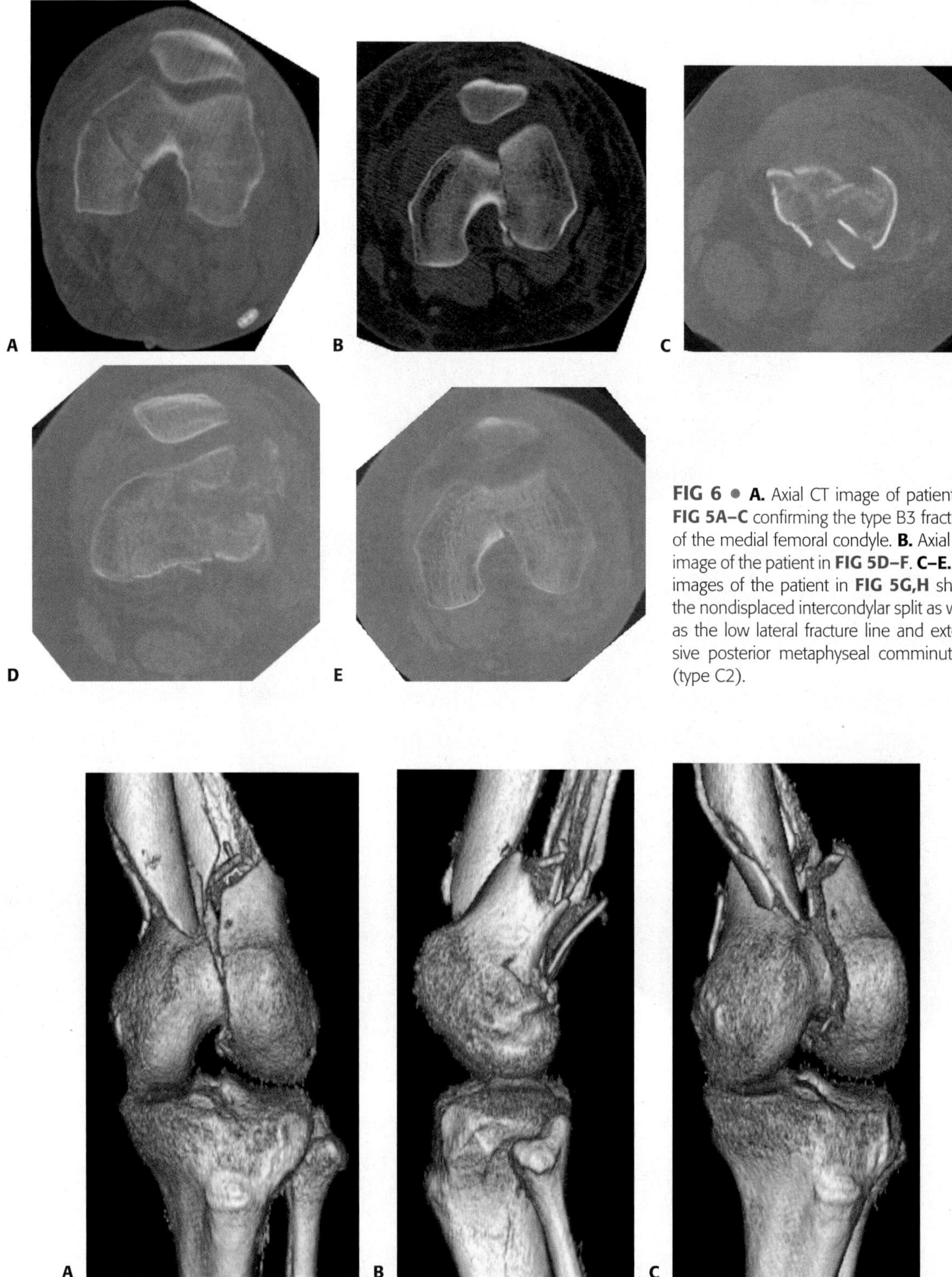

**FIG 6** • **A.** Axial CT image of patient in **FIG 5A–C** confirming the type B3 fracture of the medial femoral condyle. **B.** Axial CT image of the patient in **FIG 5D–F**. **C–E.** CT images of the patient in **FIG 5G,H** show the nondisplaced intercondylar split as well as the low lateral fracture line and extensive posterior metaphyseal comminution (type C2).

**FIG 7** • AP (**A**) and lateral (**B**) views of a three-dimensional (3-D) CT reconstruction of the patient in **FIG 3B** with a distal femur fracture. The fracture is well defined. **C.** An oblique 3-D CT reconstruction view showing the same patient and the rotational malalignment between condyles.

## SURGICAL MANAGEMENT

- The goal of any treatment, nonoperative or operative, is to maintain or restore the congruity of the articular surface and restore the length and alignment of the femur and, subsequently, the limb.
- Once surgery is deemed appropriate for the patient and the particular injury, the surgical technique options available are determined by the particular fracture pattern.
- Distal femur fractures have been classified several ways.
  - The OTA/AO classification is probably the most widely accepted classification system and allows some guidance on which techniques are best (**FIG 8**; Table 1).
- Treatment also must be determined based on factors other than the classification alone.
  - The degree of comminution and injury to both the articular surface and bone
  - The amount of fracture displacement
  - The soft tissue injury
  - Associated injuries, other fractures, and injury to neurovascular structures

**Table 1 OTA/AO Classification of Femoral Fractures**

| Classification | Description |
|---|---|
| Type A | Extra-articular |
| A1 | Simple or two-part fracture |
| A2 | Metaphyseal butterfly or wedge fracture |
| A3 | Metaphysis is comminuted |
| Type B | Partial articular |
| B1 | Sagittal plane fracture of the lateral femoral condyle |
| B2 | Sagittal plane fracture of the medial femoral condyle |
| B3 | Any frontal or coronal plane fracture of the condyle (Hoffa type) |
| Type C | Intra-articular |
| C1 | Simple articular split and metaphyseal injury (T or Y fracture configuration) |
| C2 | Simple articular split with comminuted metaphyseal injury |
| C3 | Comminuted articular with varying metaphyseal injury |

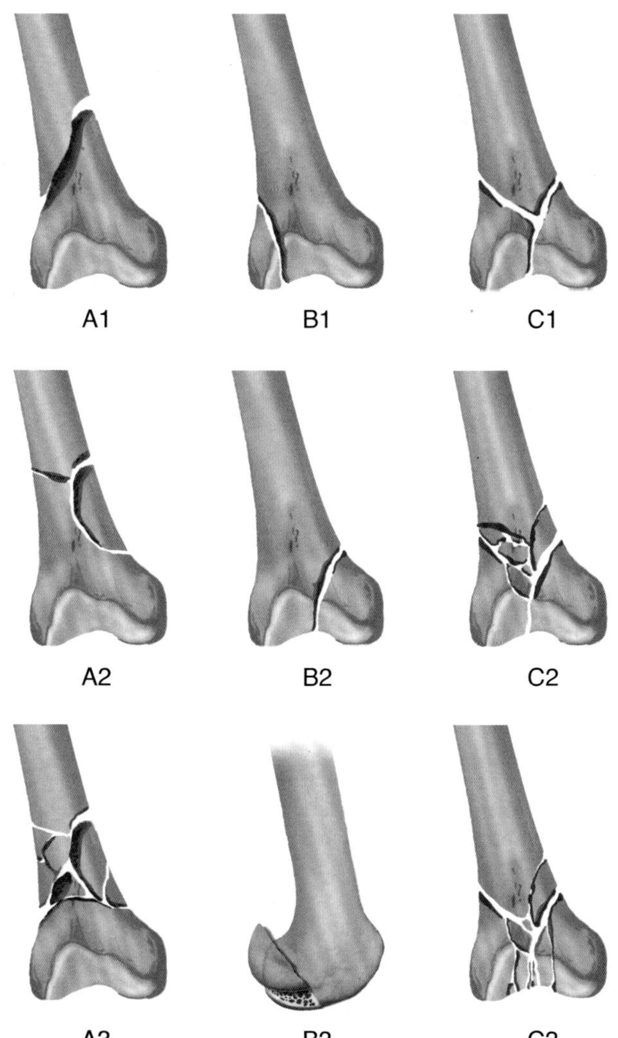


**FIG 8** • OTA/AO classification for distal femur fractures (types 33A, B, and C).

  - Patient's overall condition and injury to other organ systems. This may affect the timing of surgery or the positioning of the patient.
- There are several principles for the surgical management of distal femur fractures.
  - The articular surface must be reduced anatomically, which usually requires direct visualization through an open exposure (arthrotomy). Simple intra-articular splits may be treated with closed reduction and percutaneous fixation.
  - The extra-articular injury should be dealt with using indirect reduction techniques as much as possible to maintain a biologic soft tissue envelope. Avoidance of stripping of the tissues, especially on the medial side, is ideal.
  - The surgeon must reestablish the length, rotation, and alignment of the femur and the limb.
  - The soft tissue injury and bone quality may dictate treatment decisions.

### Fixation Choices

- External fixation
  - A temporary bridging external fixator across the knee joint can be used if temporary stabilization is required before definitive fixation. This is usually the case where definitive open reduction and internal fixation (ORIF) is planned. This could be in cases where the soft tissues prevent immediate fixation.
  - Definitive management with bridging or nonbridging external fixation can be used for nonreconstructible joints, very severe soft tissue injuries, or severe osteopenia.
  - Bridging external fixation can be used when definitive ORIF is problematic in certain patient populations, such as Jehovah's witnesses, where additional blood loss can lead to increased morbidity or mortality. This can be done temporarily until the patient's condition improves or until healing (**FIG 9**).
- Intramedullary nailing
  - This can be performed fairly acutely; temporary bridging external fixation is not necessary.

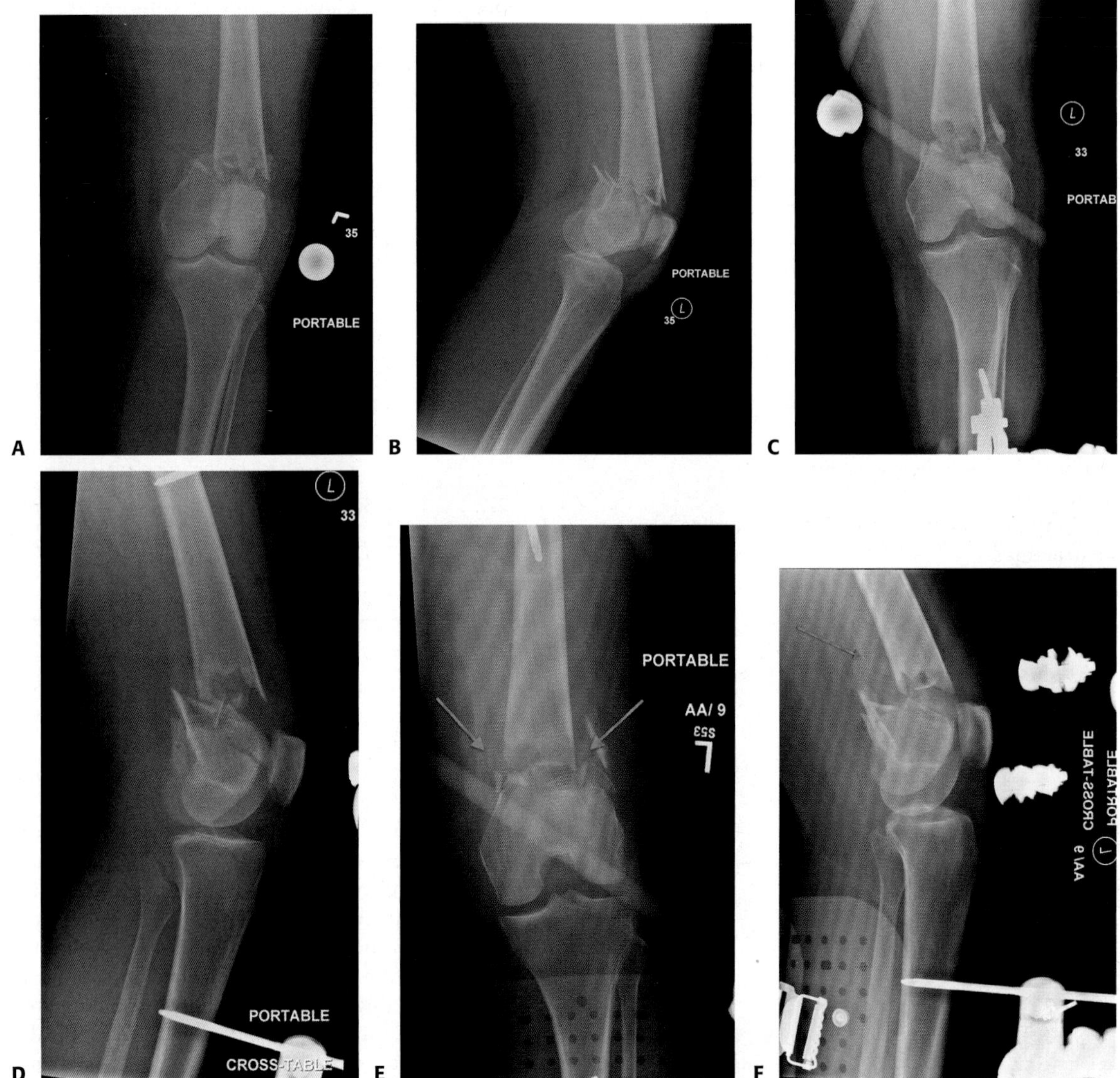


**FIG 9** ● Critically ill elderly polytrauma Jehovah's witness patient with left C1 distal femur fracture. **A,B.** Initial injury AP and lateral views. **C,D.** Due to extremely low hematocrit, external fixation was the only surgical option allowed to minimize blood loss. Radiographs in bridging external fixation. The AP shows excellent alignment but the lateral shows the expected extension deformity secondary to pull of gastrocsoleus complex. **E,F.** After 5 weeks in an external fixator, AP and lateral radiographs show callus formation (*red arrows*). Patient is now cleared for definitive surgical intervention.

- Antegrade intramedullary nailing has been described and can be used for distal fractures with a large enough distal segment to allow for two locking screws. Malalignment has been a problem, as has adequate fixation.[4,8]
- Retrograde intramedullary nailing can be used in the following cases (**FIG 10**):
  - All extra-articular type A fractures greater than 4 cm from the joint. This minimal length of the distal femur allows for multiplanar interlocking in the distal fragment.
  - Type C1 or C2 fractures where the articular fracture can be anatomically reduced closed or with limited exposure. Percutaneous screws are used for the articular injury.
  - Periprosthetic fractures around a total knee arthroplasty with an "open box" femoral component
  - Most surgeons prefer to use a long nail, but short supracondylar nails are available as well. Multiple-hole short supracondylar nails have fallen out of favor.
- Plate fixation
  - ORIF with plates can be used for all types A and C fractures but is ideal for the following injuries:
    - Very distal type A fractures within 4 cm of the knee joint
    - All articular type C fractures, but always for C3 types
    - Periprosthetic fractures about a "closed box" femoral component of a total knee arthroplasty
    - The partial articular type B1 or B2 if an antiglide plate is needed
- Plate options (preferred to least preferred; fixed-angle devices preferred)
  - Fixed-angle locking plates (percutaneous jigs are advantageous and allow for minimally invasive techniques)
  - Variable-angle (polyaxial) locking plates—allow for "fixed variable locking" within a defined range. It is useful for distal fractures and allows for increased screw

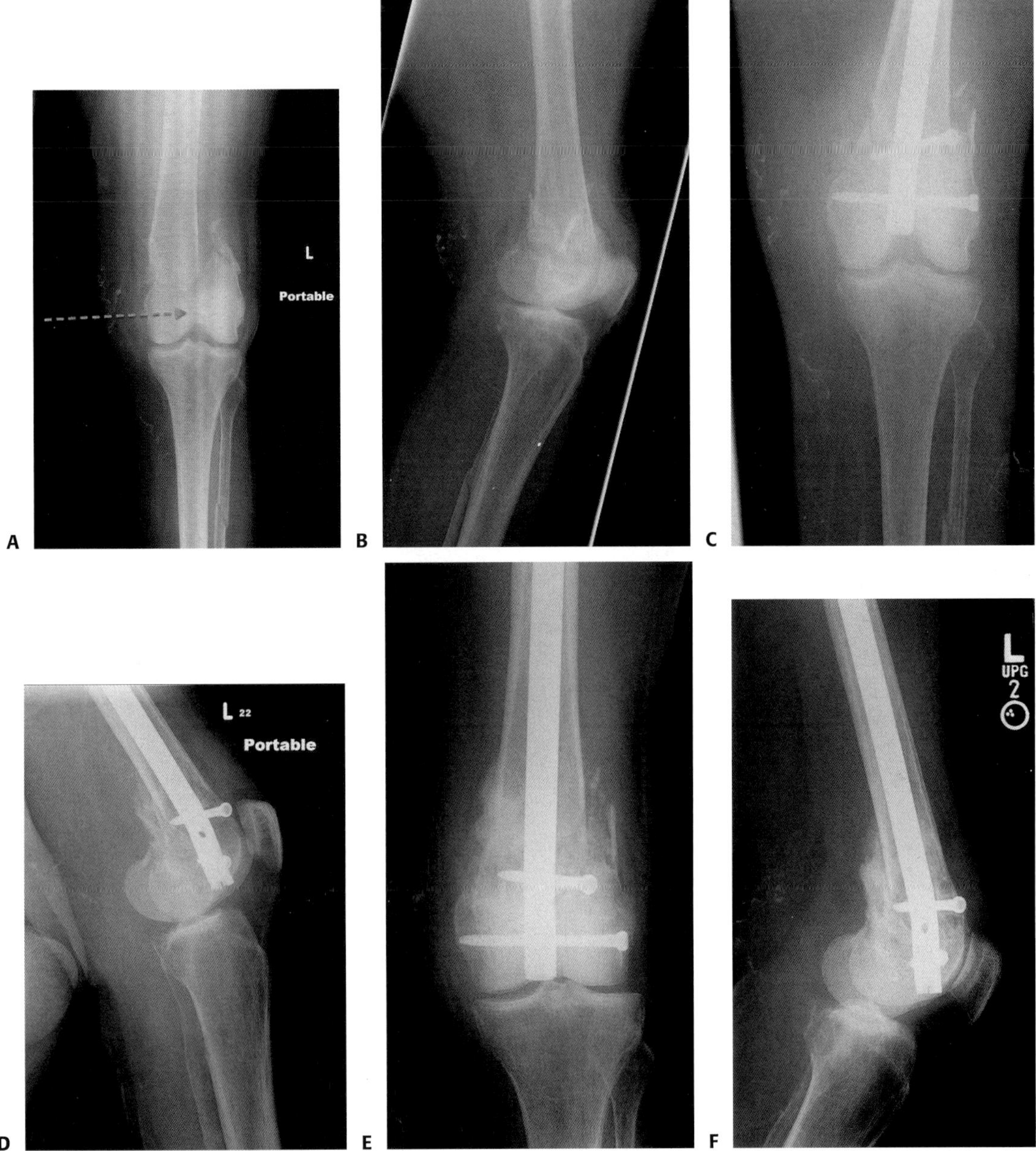


**FIG 10** • **A,B.** AP and lateral radiographs of an elderly patient with multiple comorbidities with an extra-articular distal femur fracture (AO type A; an incomplete intercondylar split—*red dashed arrow*). **C,D.** Postoperative radiographs showing stabilization with retrograde intramedullary nail. **E,F.** One-year postoperative radiographs showing a healed fracture with some subsidence of the metaphyseal region and mild protrusion of hardware through the notch.

trajectories to gain additional locked fixation in short segments, which may not be feasible with fixed-angle trajectory plates (**FIG 11**).
  - Ninety-five–degree condylar screw
  - Ninety-five–degree blade plate
  - Nonlocking plates with or without medial support (medial plate or external fixation)
- Limited internal fixation
  - Limited fixation with screws only can be used for partial articular type B, especially type B3.
  - The amount of open reduction required depends on the adequacy of closed reduction techniques and obtaining an anatomic reduction of the joint surface.
  - Headless screws are useful for type B3 fractures in which the screws have to penetrate the joint surface (**FIG 12**).
  - Countersinking the screw heads can also be performed.
- Biomechanics of fixation: implant considerations
  - There has been concern that the newer locking plate constructs are too stiff, resulting in inconsistent and asymmetric callus formation.[9]
  - Some clinical evidence show less callus formation with stainless steel plates versus titanium plates.[9]
  - Conversely, a biomechanical study has not shown a significant difference mechanically between constructs of stainless steel LISS plates with bicortical screws or titanium LISS plate with unicortical screws.[1]

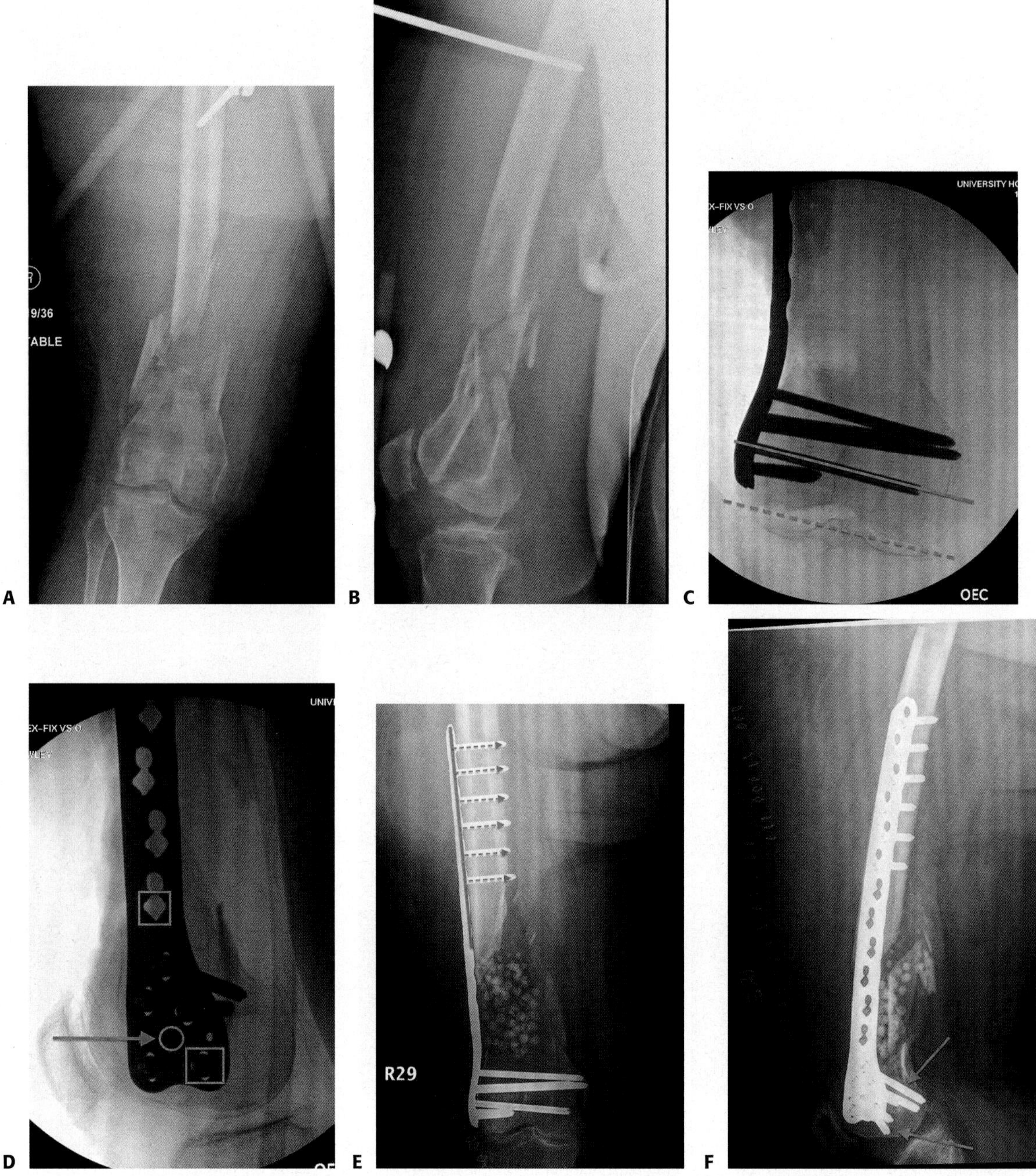


**FIG 11** • Morbidly obese female with a severely comminuted and open right distal C3 femur fracture. **A,B.** AP and lateral radiographs showing the amount of comminution, bone loss, and distal nature of the injury after the initial irrigation, débridement, and bridging external fixation. **C,D.** Intraoperative fluoroscopic images during application of a variable-angle locking plate. The AP shows the "central screw" to aid in reestablishment of the anatomic axis of the femur (*parallel lines solid*, screw; *dashed*, joint line). The lateral view shows the central screw, which is a fixed-angle hole (*arrow* and *circle*), as opposed to the variable-angle holes (*red box*; both for the combination holes and isolated variable-angle screws). **E,F.** Two-week postoperative radiographs. The AP view shows the proximal screws placed perpendicular (*dashed arrows*) to the plate even through the variable-angle portion of the combination holes, which was facilitated by the targeting device. Both views demonstrate the advantage of the variable-angle locking holes distally to allow for additional fixation in this short distal segment with a more posterior and distal trajectory (*solid arrows* on lateral view). The bone substitute placed for the bone defect (*white pellets*) are also clearly visualized. *(continued)*

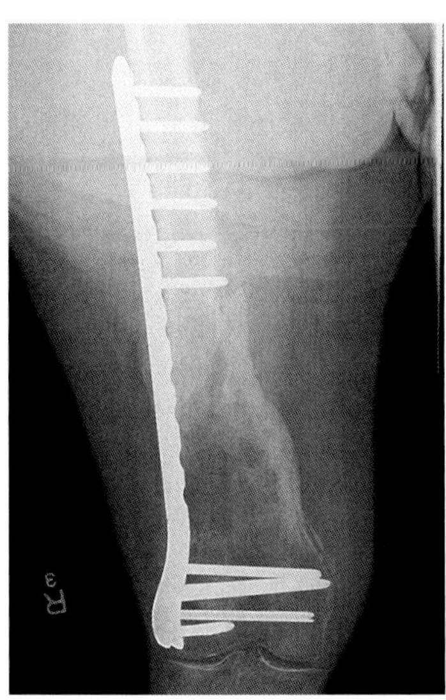

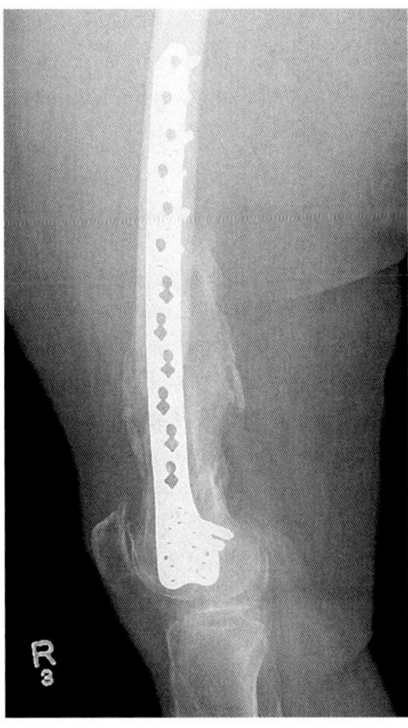

**FIG 11** • *(continued)* **G,H.** Five-month follow-up films showing replacement of the calcium sulfate beads with successful consolidation of the metaphyseal comminution.

- The flexibility of fixation constructs can be increased by the use of a technique referred to as *far cortical locking*. Specialized screws are used, in which the screw locks into the plate and only engages the far cortex. This has been thought to improve fracture healing.[5]
- The "polyaxial" locking plates have been shown to be biomechanically sound in the management of supracondylar femur fractures.[12,18]

## Preoperative Planning

- Surgical timing can be affected by the following:
  - Soft tissue issues
  - Medical condition of the patient
  - Adequacy of available operative team
  - Availability of implants
- The approach must take the following issues into consideration:
  - The ability to incorporate lacerations in open fractures into the incision (**FIG 13**) can be useful and should be considered. However, this is not always necessary or possible.
  - Soft tissue dissection should be limited.
  - Adequate exposure is important to anatomically restore the articular surface.
- Restoration of limb "anatomy" must be accomplished and allow early range of motion.
  - Stable internal fixation and length and sizes of implants should be templated. Radiographs of the injury can be templated with implant templates to ensure that proper lengths are available. A tentative plan of the fixation construct can be drawn on the image. Additionally, "preop planning" of the operating room should be performed; this includes a discussion with the operative team about the positioning and equipment needed for the procedure.
  - The need for bone grafting or the use of bone graft substitutes should be assessed.
  - Fracture fragments and the anticipated fixation construct should be templated.
  - The surgeon should check for coronal plane fractures of the condyles (also known as *Hoffa fragments*) (see **FIGS 5C** and **6**).

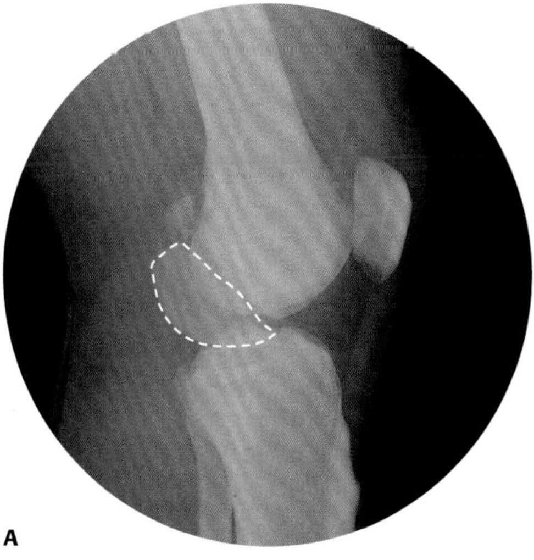

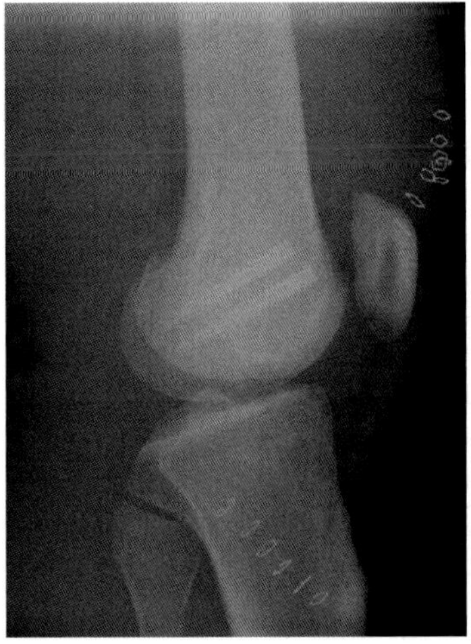

**FIG 12** • **A.** Lateral radiograph of patient with a grade II open distal medial femoral condyle fracture (type B3). The Hoffa fragment is outlined. **B.** Postoperative radiograph after fixation with headless screws, buried underneath the subchondral bone.

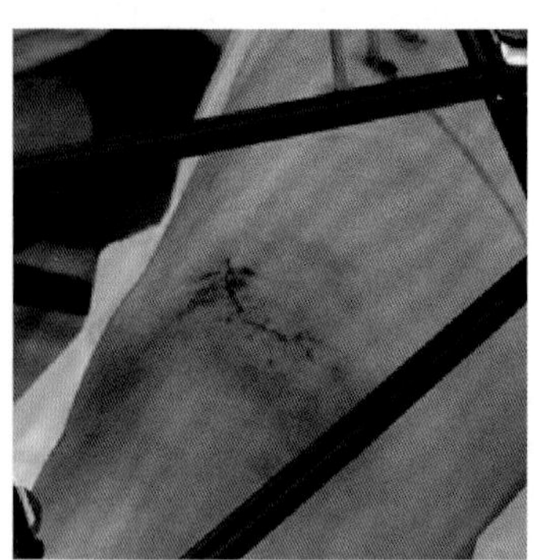

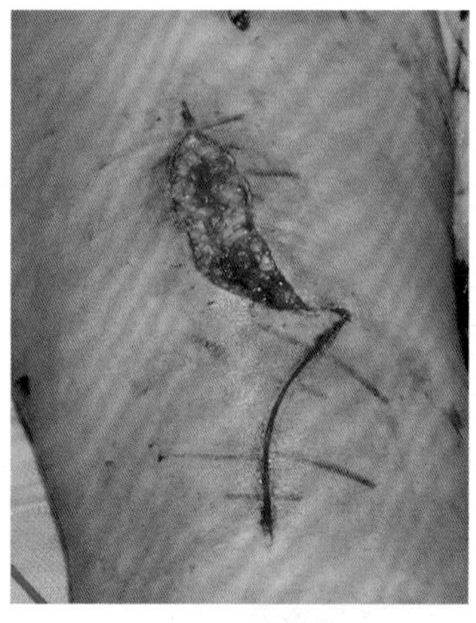

**FIG 13** • **A.** Patient with open distal femur fracture and traumatic oblique laceration after débridement, bridging external fixation, and closure. **B.** Incorporation of the laceration into a modified midline approach.

- Associated injuries may affect the treatment options.
  - An ipsilateral hip or more proximal shaft fracture may alter the implant choice. A longer plate may be needed to address both injuries, or consideration to overlap implants may be warranted to avoid a stress riser.
  - An associated proximal tibia fracture may alter the approach used. A more lateral incision incorporating a lazy S incision for the proximal tibia injury may be required.
  - Critically ill patients may require delayed fixation after temporary stabilization via bridging external fixation methods (**FIG 14**).

## Positioning

- A radiolucent table should be used to allow adequate visualization with a C-arm.
- The patient is placed supine with a hip bump.
  - The rotation of the proximal segment of the fracture (hip) should be aligned before patient preparation.
    - Using the C-arm, the profile of the lesser trochanter with the corresponding knee (patella) straight up is determined on the uninjured side (**FIG 15A,B**).
    - The injured hip is imaged and internally rotated by the hip bump so that duplication of the profile of the normal side is achieved. The size of the bump may be adjusted as needed for the amount of rotation required.
    - The injured knee is placed in the patella-up position to confirm rotation.
    - This technique is helpful in comminuted metaphyseal fractures where the rotation is difficult to assess or in cases where the metaphyseal component will not be directly visualized.
    - Even though the distal segment is not in "fixed" rotation, this technique is useful to minimize the chance of a malrotation during definitive fixation.
- A sterile tourniquet is used unless a temporary fixator prevents its placement.
- A large bump or a sterile triangle is used under the knee.
  - This allows for knee flexion, relaxing the gastrocsoleus complex and facilitating the reduction.
  - A sterile and removable one is most useful.
- The C-arm is brought in from the opposite side.
  - It should be angled so that it is parallel with the femoral shaft.

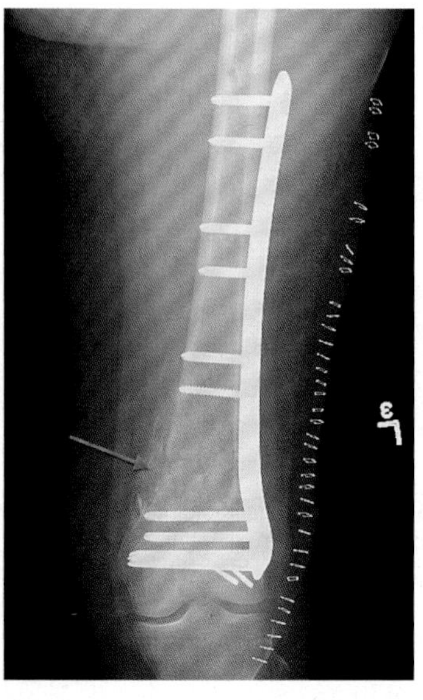

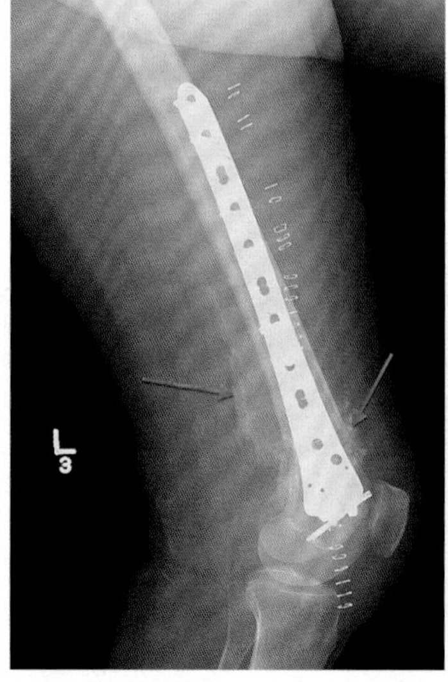

**FIG 14** • **A,B.** Two-week postoperative radiographs of patient from **FIG 9** who underwent delayed ORIF at 5 weeks post injury. These radiographs exhibit the abundant amount of callus present (*red arrows*) after successful ORIF with reestablishment of length, alignment, and rotation was accomplished with takedown of the callus.

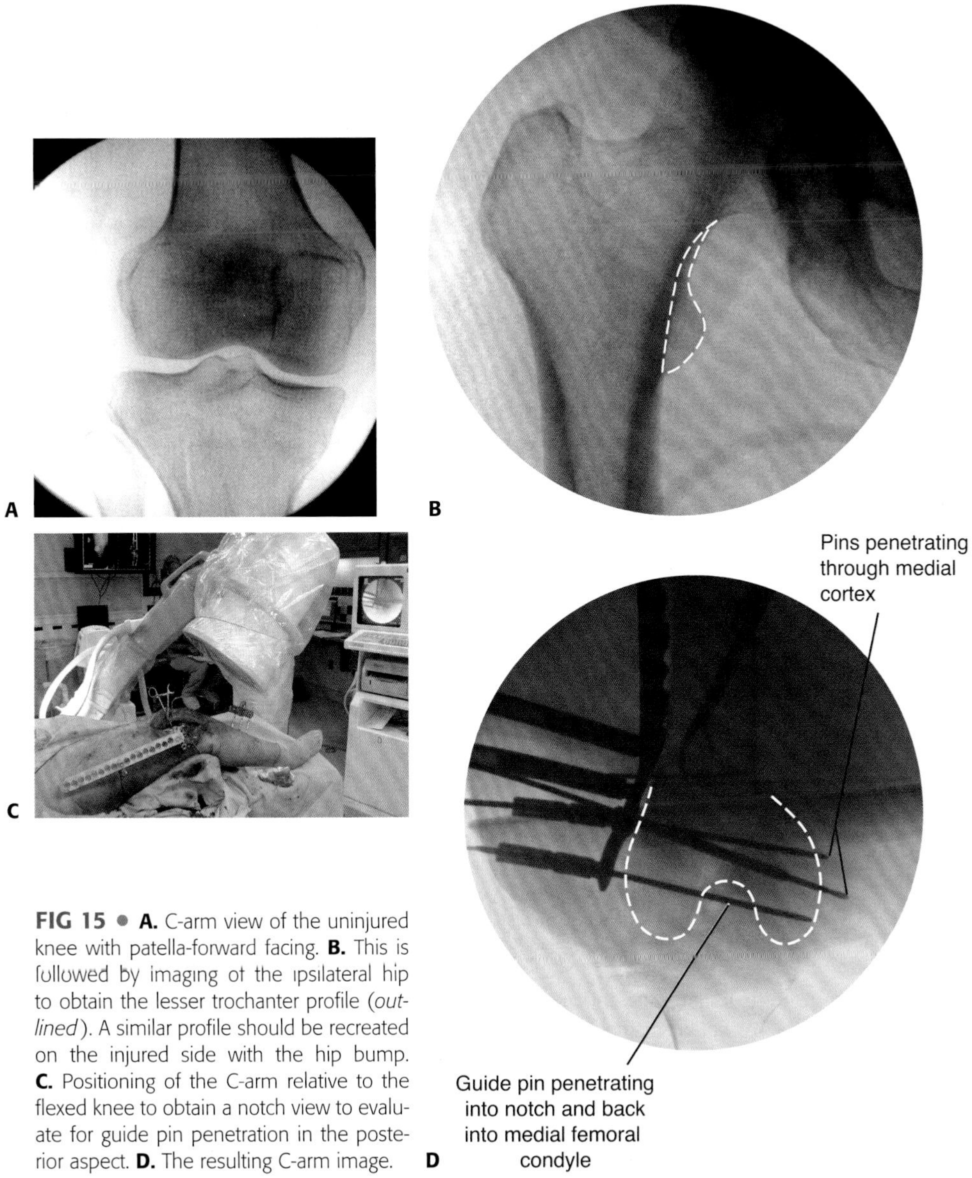

Pins penetrating through medial cortex

Guide pin penetrating into notch and back into medial femoral condyle

**FIG 15** ● **A.** C-arm view of the uninjured knee with patella-forward facing. **B.** This is followed by imaging of the ipsilateral hip to obtain the lesser trochanter profile (*outlined*). A similar profile should be recreated on the injured side with the hip bump. **C.** Positioning of the C-arm relative to the flexed knee to obtain a notch view to evaluate for guide pin penetration in the posterior aspect. **D.** The resulting C-arm image.

- A notch view is useful for screw trajectories in the distal femur. This is achieved by the C-arm angled roughly around 30 to 45 degrees directed cephalad and visualization will depend on the concurrent amount of knee flexion (**FIG 15C,D**).

## Approach

- The best-known approach for the treatment of distal femur fractures has been the straight lateral approach (**FIG 16**).
  - This is suitable for all fracture types, mostly types A and C1.
  - The incision may curve distally toward the tibial tubercle, and osteotomy may be performed.
  - Newer approaches include a lateral inverted U to allow better access to the joint and to allow for plate placement.
- The minimally invasive lateral approach can be used for certain fractures and implants.
  - The joint must be visualized, reduced, and stabilized.
  - The placement of the plate on the shaft is done submuscularly, and reduction and fixation are done percutaneously under fluoroscopic guidance.
  - This is ideal for the LISS plate or plating system with targeting devices for the screws in the plate.
- A modified anterior approach (the swashbuckler) has been described by Starr et al.[16]
  - This involves a midline incision.
  - A lateral parapatellar arthrotomy is done with elevation of the vastus lateralis as in the lateral approach.

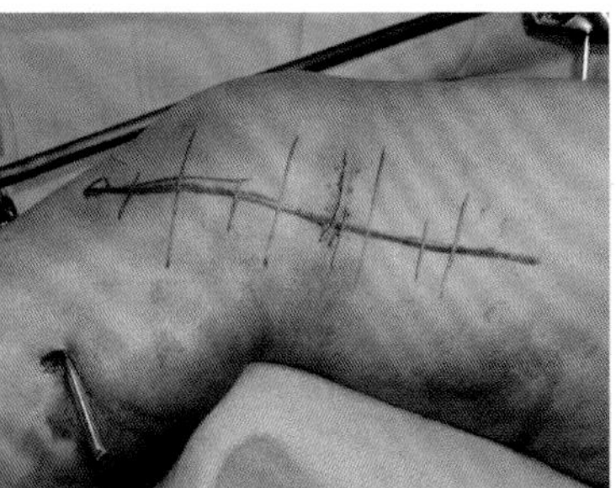

**FIG 16** ● Skin incision for a lateral approach.

- A medial parapatellar arthrotomy can be used for retrograde intramedullary nailing or limited screw fixation.
  - Miniarthrotomy is used for the retrograde nail.
  - Type B injuries may require a formal arthrotomy.
- A medial approach has been described.
  - This is appropriate for types B2 and B3 fractures.
  - It can be used in type C3 fractures if a second plate is being used (in conjunction with a lateral approach).
- A total knee approach has been described by Schatzker.[15]
  - This is extremely helpful for type C2 or C3 fractures.
  - It is used for plates but can be used for retrograde intramedullary nailing once the articular surface is reconstructed.
  - A midline approach is used.
  - An extended medial parapatellar arthrotomy is done.
  - This allows exposure of the condyles for articular reduction.
- A midline incision with a lateral parapatellar arthrotomy is my preferred exposure for type C2 or C3 fractures.
  - A midline approach is used.
  - A lateral parapatellar arthrotomy is done.
  - Proximal extension is made into the quadriceps tendon, enough to repair to itself.
  - Medial dislocation of patella is done.
  - This allows exposure of the condyles for articular reduction and easier lateral plate insertion.

TECHNIQUES

## Temporary Bridging External Fixation

- A large external fixation system is used.
- A small bump is placed under the knee to place the knee in slight flexion.
- The injured extremity is brought out to length with manual traction.
- Two or three 5-mm Schanz pins are placed in the tibia in an anterior to posterior direction just medial to the crest to ensure intramedullary placement.
- Two or three 5-mm Schanz pins are placed in the femoral shaft in an anterior to posterior direction.
  - These should be placed out of the zone of soft tissue injury if possible.
  - The pins are placed while the limb is out to length so that the quadriceps is not "skewered" in a shortened position.
  - The pins can be placed outside of the anticipated plate location. This, however, has not been empirically found to be a problem. In my experience, plates have often overlapped with pin sites, and there has not been an associated problem with infections.
- Pin placement in the tibia may be altered if additional uses of such pins are needed, such as traction for an associated acetabular fracture (**TECH FIG 1A**).
- The bars can be configured in many ways, all of which provide temporary stabilization across the knee joint. I prefer a diamond configuration (**TECH FIG 1B**).

### Reduction of the Metaphyseal Component

- Gross reduction of the metaphyseal component of the fracture should be performed with traction and manipulation of the pins.
- The fracture should be brought out to length.
  - Intraoperatively, the opposite leg can be used to help determine length.
  - Postoperatively, a scanogram can be used to determine whether the length has been regained before definitive

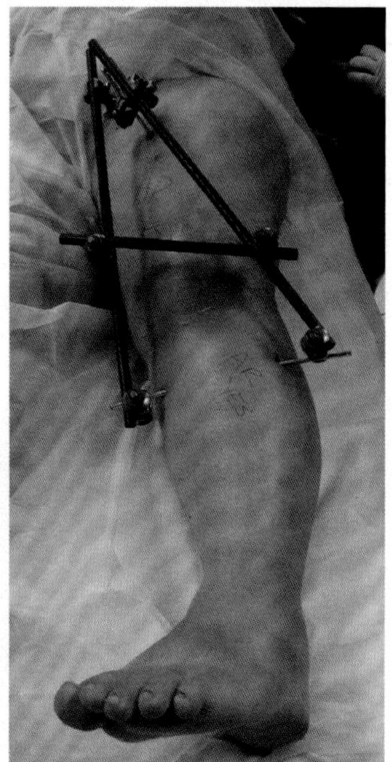

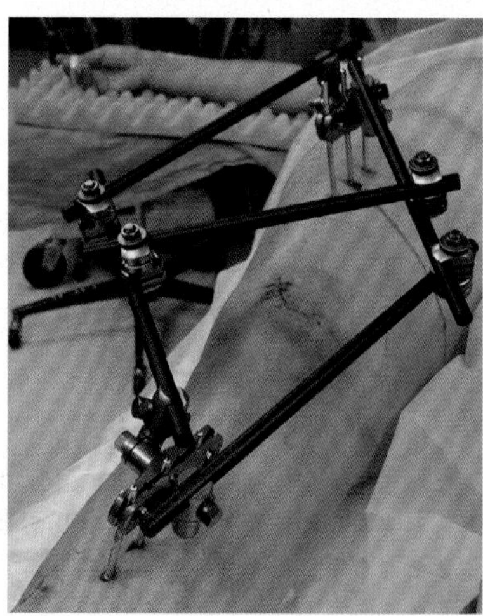

**TECH FIG 1** • **A.** Bridging knee external fixation in patient with associated acetabular fracture; the tibial pin was used for traction purposes as well. **B.** A diamond configuration for bridging knee external fixation.

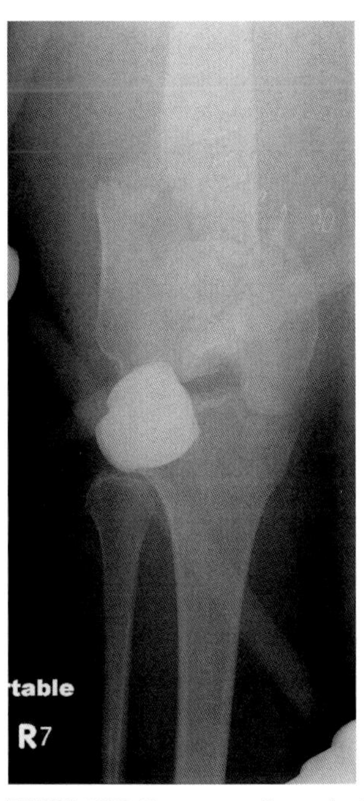


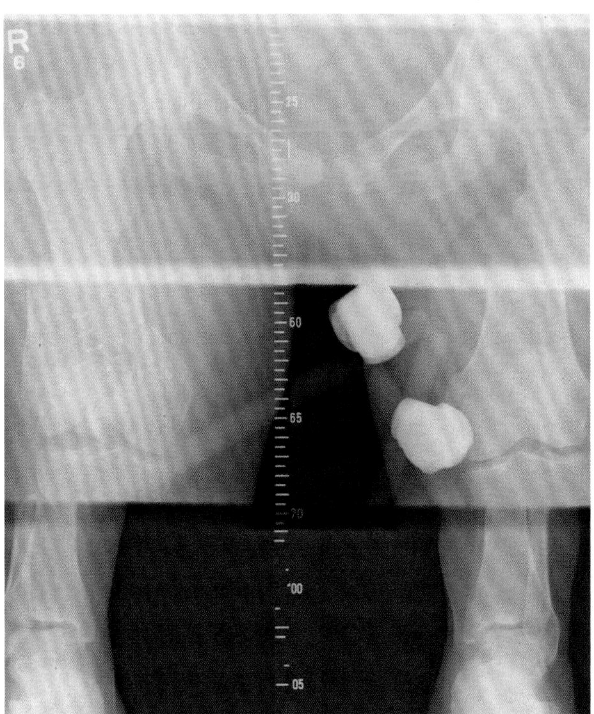

**TECH FIG 2** • AP radiograph (**A**) and scanogram (**B**) showing that length was reestablished with the external fixator.

fixation if there is extensive comminution, but this is not always needed (**TECH FIG 2**). Although the knee may be somewhat flexed, the scanogram can still be obtained and the femoral length determined as opposed to the entire leg length.

- The rotation should be checked once again before locking the external fixator construct, as described earlier under Positioning. The same technique should be performed under sterile conditions.
- Varus–valgus alignment should be assessed before final tightening as well.
  - This can be done by using the Bovie cord intraoperatively and assessing the mechanical axis of the limb by fluoroscopically evaluating from the hip to the ankle with the cord centered at the femoral head all the way to the ankle.
  - The point at which the cord crosses the knee allows one to judge the varus–valgus alignment.

## Open Reduction and Internal Fixation of the Distal Femur with Locking Plates (Type C Fractures)

- This technique can be used regardless of the locking plate system used. Each system's technique guide should be reviewed before use as each system has its own idiosyncrasies. Variations in plate application as well as reduction tools and techniques are unique to each system.
- The temporary external fixator is prepared using a "double-double" technique.
  - The fixator is first prepared with a Betadine "scrub" (7.5% povidone-iodine) solution followed by a Betadine "paint" (10% povidone-iodine) solution (Beta–Beta preparation), followed by the extremity with a second Beta–Beta preparation.
  - The surgeon then does an alcohol preparation, followed by iodine for the fixator, followed by alcohol and iodine on the skin.
  - This has been successful in our practice and allows for maintenance of traction during the preparation and aids in the actual surgery, functioning as a femoral distractor. (Chlorhexidine is used in iodine-allergic patients.)
  - An alternative is to completely remove the fixator components, except the pins, and wash, sterilize, and then reassemble the fixator on the patient after the leg has been prepared.
- If there is no temporary bridging external fixator, the metaphyseal component of the fracture can be reduced and brought out to length with a femoral distractor, a temporary simple external fixator, or manual traction if adequate help is available.
  - Rotation of the proximal segment can be manipulated with the device used.

## Midline Approach with an Extended Lateral Parapatellar Arthrotomy

- A straight incision is made directly anterior about 5 cm proximal to the superior pole of the patella and distally to the level of the tibia tubercle (**TECH FIG 3A**).
- The lateral skin flap is developed to allow for a lateral parapatellar arthrotomy (**TECH FIG 3B**).
- The arthrotomy is performed, ensuring a cuff of tissue on the lateral aspect of the patella for repair as well as medially on the quadriceps (**TECH FIG 3C**).
- The patella can be subluxed medially or inverted with knee flexion to allow exposure of the condyles (**TECH FIG 3D**).
  - Additionally, a blunt Hohmann retractor can be placed on the medial side at the level of the condyle to retract the patella.
- The capsule is subperiosteally elevated off the lateral femoral condyle to allow for placement of the plate.
  - The lateral collateral ligament is preserved because the dissection is limited to the anterior two-thirds of the lateral femoral condyle and plate placement is usually proximal to the lateral epicondyle.
  - The medial side in the metaphyseal region is left undisturbed as much as possible.

## Reduction of the Articular Surface

- The joint is evaluated to determine comminution.
- Joint reconstruction is then performed with direct reduction. Each condyle is fully assessed first for smaller fracture fragments, with the goal of restoring each condyle anatomically. Small-diameter screws (<3.0 mm) may be used and can be countersunk underneath the articular surface.
- Large coronal fracture fragments are best treated with countersunk 3.5- to 4.5-mm lag-type screws. We use headless screws.
- Once each condyle is thought to be restored, or if a simple fracture pattern is present, the condyles should be reduced to each other using a large, pointed reduction forceps (**TECH FIG 4A–C**).
- Each fragment can be rotated relative to another; this must be addressed as discussed before.
  - The best way to assess this is under direct visualization and evaluating the reduction at the trochlear region of the patellofemoral joint.
  - Additionally, preoperative evaluation assessing the lateral radiograph can guide the surgeon. Intraoperative fluoroscopy to reassess the lateral view is also useful.
- Temporary Kirschner wires or the guide pins for the locking screws for the plate can be used for additional stabilization of the two condyles (**TECH FIG 4D**).

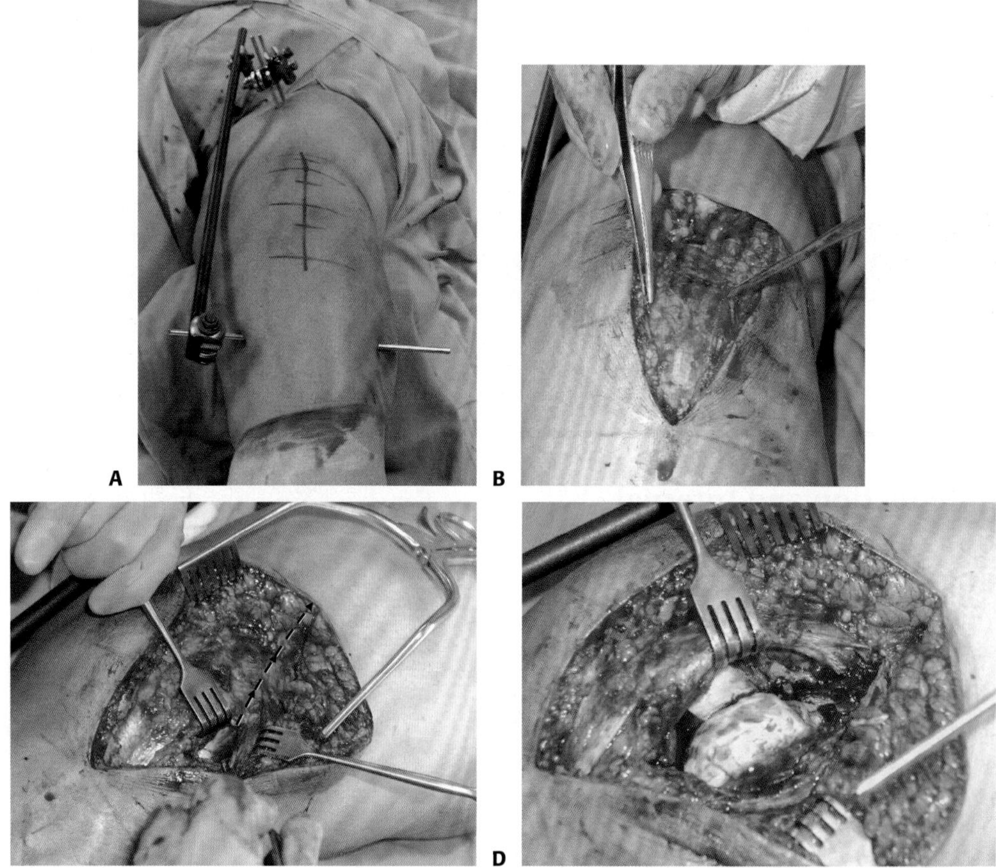


**TECH FIG 3** • Patient with grade II open distal femur fracture (also shown in **FIGS 5D–F**, **6B**, and **7**). **A.** Straight midline incision. **B.** Lateral skin flap is developed. **C.** Arthrotomy is started and then extended proximally into the quad tendon (*dashed line*). **D.** The arthrotomy is completed and the condyles are visualized with medial subluxation of the patella.

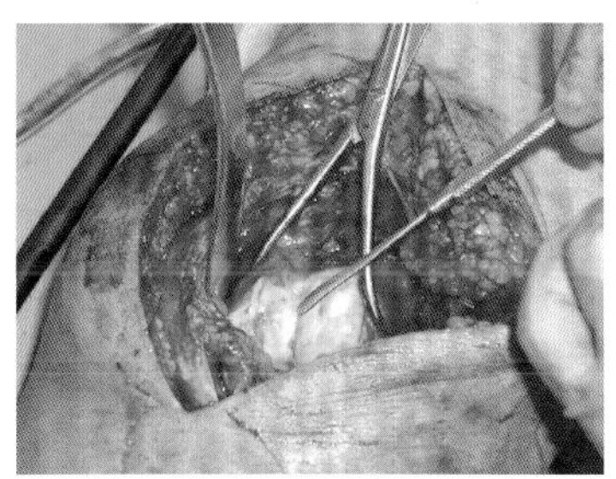

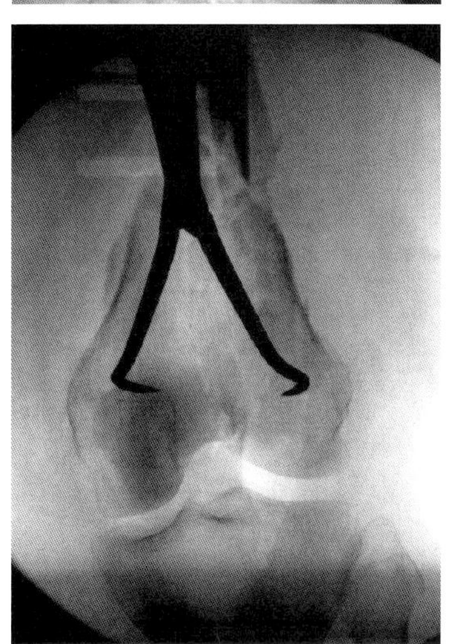

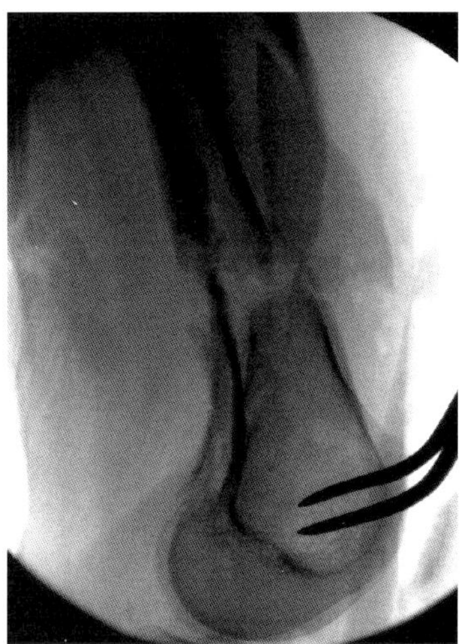

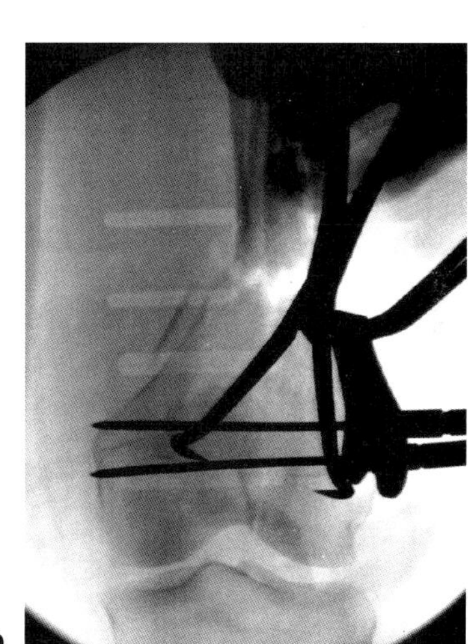

**TECH FIG 4** • The condyles are reduced under direct visualization (**A**) and confirmed with AP (**B**) and lateral (**C**) intraoperative fluoroscopic images. **D.** Guide pins through the plate template or screw trajectory guide are used to temporarily stabilize the intercondylar split.

## Definitive Fixation of the Condyles

- This can be accomplished outside the plate first and supplemented with screws through the plate. The area around the proposed plate, the "periphery," can be used for the screw placement to avoid interference with the plate placement itself.
    - If this is done, then the metaphyseal fracture does not necessarily have to be properly reduced before initial screw placement.
- Screws can also be placed from medial to lateral to avoid interference with the plate.
- Definitive fixation can be accomplished through the plate also (see next section on Screw Placement).
    - If this is done, the metaphyseal component should be reduced to ensure the proper flexion–extension alignment of the shaft with the condyles.
    - This will ensure that the plate is collinear with the shaft once fixed to the distal segment. Otherwise, a malreduction in the sagittal plane will occur.
    - The temporary Kirschner wires can be left in place to stabilize the joint.

## Reduction of the Shaft to the Distal Segment

- Once the articular surface is temporarily stabilized or reduced, the reduction of the shaft to the distal segment should be performed before plate application.
- This can be temporarily stabilized with Kirschner wires or Steinmann pins.
- Alternatively, precisely placed bumps underneath the distal segment can be used to correct the extension of the distal segment and align it with the shaft.
- Adjustment or loosening of the temporary external fixator can aid in reduction if needed.
- The plate can then be placed submuscularly.

## Placement of the Plate

- Each fixed-angle plating system is designed to help reestablish the valgus alignment of the distal femur.
    - The screws in the distal portion of the plate are designed to be parallel to the joint surface.
    - Thus, the initial guidewires for these screws should be placed parallel and confirmed by fluoroscopy.
        - A distal "joint wire" can be placed to better evaluate this (**TECH FIG 5A**).
    - Placing the distal screws parallel to the joint will help ensure that when the shaft is brought to the plate, the anatomic axis of the femur is restored.
    - With the variable-angle locking plates, the same technique should be employed to ensure that the plate is applied in a way to restore the anatomic axis of the femur. A fixed-angle central screw hole still exists in these plates to aid in plate application (**FIG 11C**, parallel lines; **FIG 11D**, red arrow/red circle).
- A distal screw trajectory guide is provided for some systems (**TECH FIG 5B**). This can be used to help ensure accurate placement of the plate distally, and initial guidewires can be placed through this.
    - Once the wires are placed, the guide can be removed and replaced with the plate using the wires as a guide.
    - However, the shaft portion of the plate requires submuscular insertion, and thus the plate cannot be brought to an appropriate position to allow this to occur.

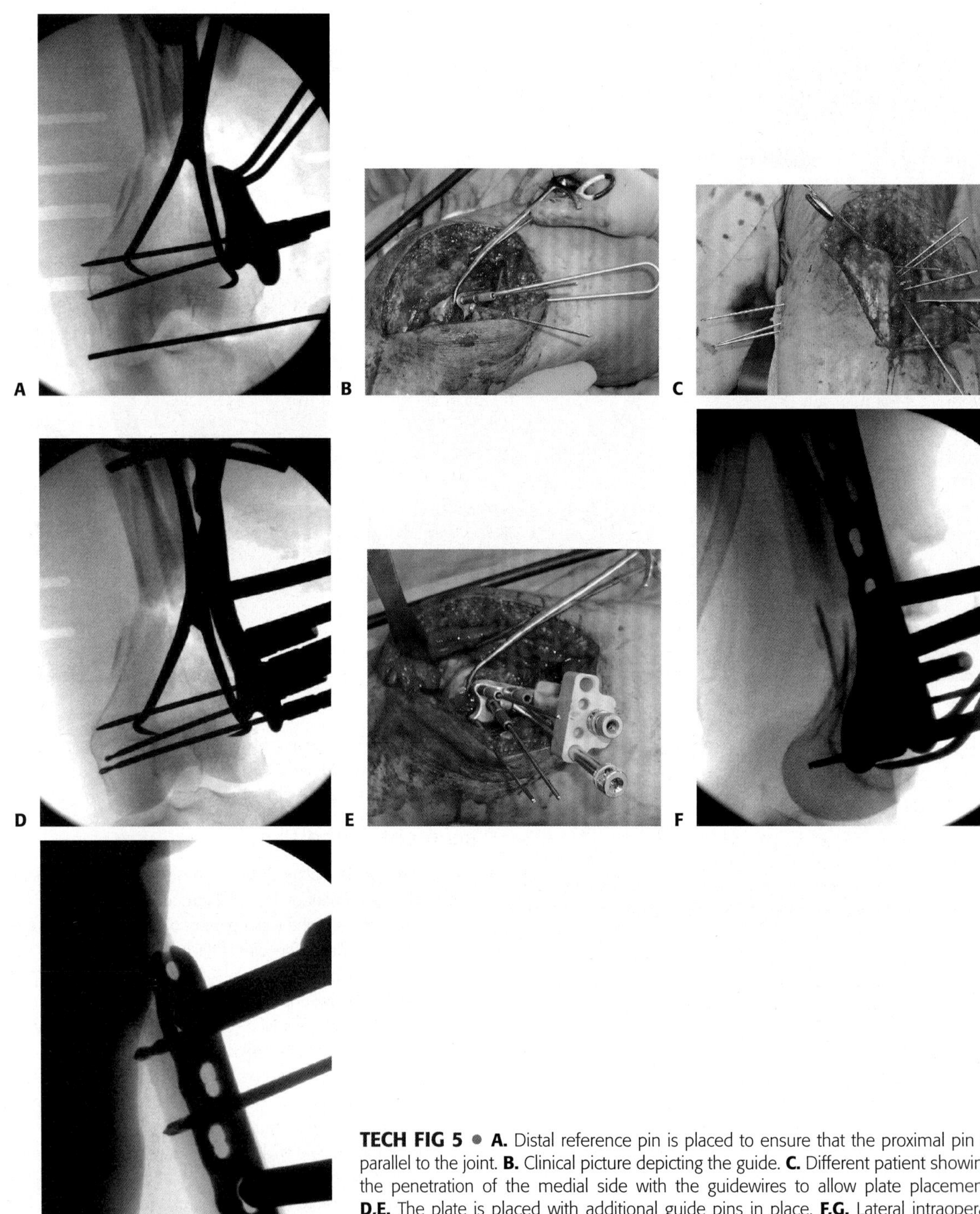

**TECH FIG 5 • A.** Distal reference pin is placed to ensure that the proximal pin is parallel to the joint. **B.** Clinical picture depicting the guide. **C.** Different patient showing the penetration of the medial side with the guidewires to allow plate placement. **D,E.** The plate is placed with additional guide pins in place. **F,G.** Lateral intraoperative fluoroscopic images ensure proper plate placement on the femur before screw insertion.

- To solve this, the guidewires can be driven through the medial side of the knee, which is distal enough to be safe (**TECH FIG 5C**).
- The plate can then be inserted submuscularly and the guidewires driven back through the plate laterally, thus aligning the plate to the distal segment and ensuring proper screw trajectory and plate placement (**TECH FIG 5D,E**).
- A single guidewire in a central hole will still allow flexion–extension placement of the plate if this needs to be adjusted.

- After placing the initial guidewire parallel to the joint distally, and ensuring the fracture is reduced, the surgeon should obtain fluoroscopic visualization of the plate proximally on the shaft to ensure that the plate is on the bone (**TECH FIG 5F,G**).
  - To ensure placement of the plate on the bone both proximally and distally, it is best to stabilize the plate distally

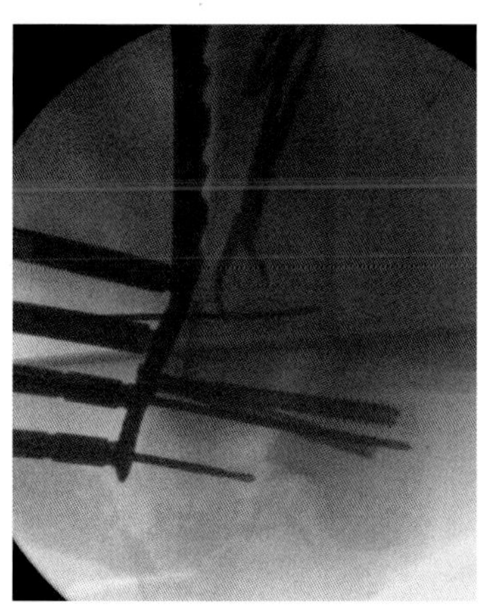


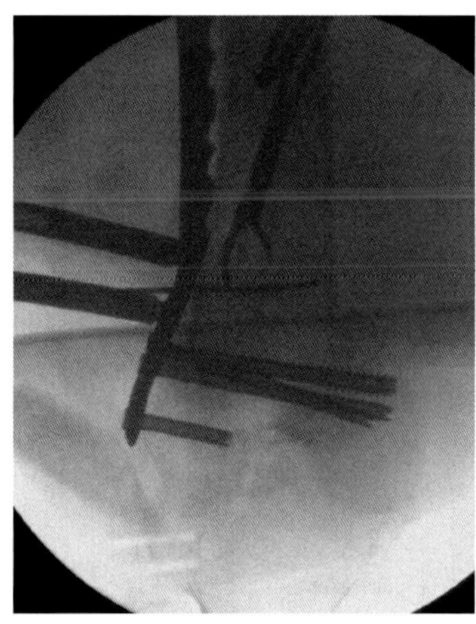


**TECH FIG 6 • A,B.** Patient seen in **FIG 15C,D**, with the guidewire now pulled back and an appropriately sized screw placed.

(where exposure is) using a guidewire in the center hole. This allows for a pivot point around which the AP positioning of the plate can be manipulated for the shaft. Fluoroscopy to image the lateral is then used to ensure placement.

  - Once the AP position is obtained, the plate is stabilized proximally.
- The plate should be temporarily stabilized to the bone proximally.
  - Before the temporary stabilization, the length and rotation must be checked. Ideally, if the temporary fixator is in place, these two parameters have been maintained during the course of the operation.
  - If no screw targeting guide is present, a percutaneous provisional fixation pin can be used to stabilize the plate.
  - If a targeting guide is used, then a soft tissue guide for the most proximal hole is placed percutaneously and a drill bit or guidewire is used to stabilize the plate.
  - The variable-angle locking plates also have proximal shaft targeting devices; however, variable locking trajectories can only be accomplished outside the targeting device and can be cumbersome. Generally, variable-angle locking is not necessary in the shaft and locking screws collinear with the hole can be placed through the targeting device. (**FIG 11E**, red arrows showing perpendicular nature of locking screws; **FIG 11F**, variable-angle locking screws in the shaft are useful in cases where there is a preexisting hip replacement with a femoral component.)
  - Again, the flexion–extension reduction should be checked.
  - This procedure creates our "box" construct, which aids in the placement of screws through the targeting device (if used) and in temporary stabilization of the fracture construct.

## Screw Placement

- If the intercondylar split is going to be stabilized by screws through the plate, partially threaded screws or overdrilled fully threaded screws should be used first to provide interfragmentary compression.
  - Specially designed conical screws for certain systems exist, or large partially threaded screws can be used (>4.5 mm). This also compresses the plate to the bone.
- Once the articular injury is addressed, at least two additional locking screws should be placed into the distal segment to secure the plate and the alignment.
  - The trajectory of distal locking screws can be assessed on the notch view to ensure that penetration through the intercondylar notch does not occur (**TECH FIG 6**; see **FIG 15C** for C-arm setup and position for this image).
  - Before placing the locking screws, the length, rotation, and alignment must be checked again if no fixator or distractor is in place holding the fracture alignment.
  - The plate can be locked to the distal segment and then used to manipulate the distal segment relative to the shaft for the flexion–extension reduction.
    - This, however, is predicated on proper distal alignment of the plate. Otherwise, once the plate is fixed to the distal segment in a malposition and the fracture reduced, the plate may be anterior or posterior on the shaft.
    - The distal screws in a variable-angle locking plate are noncircular to allow for the variable-angle locking mechanism. Screws can be placed directly collinear or with a "variability" of 15 degrees in any direction depending on the system used (see **FIG 11D**, square outline).

## Attaching the Distal Segment to the Shaft

- The distal segment is now fixed and can be attached to the shaft.
- If there is malalignment in the coronal plane but the sagittal plane alignment is reduced, the shaft can be "pulled" to the plate by means of various threaded devices or a nonlocking screw that can be placed freehand under fluoroscopic guidance or through a targeting jig (**TECH FIG 7**).

## Placement of Additional Screws

- Once proper reduction of the fracture is temporarily achieved and the plate is in proper position, additional screws can be placed.
- If the targeting screw guide is used, percutaneous locking screws can be placed through the soft tissue drill or screw guides (**TECH FIG 8A–C**).
- If no targeting guide is available, fluoroscopic guidance and a percutaneous method can be used freehand.

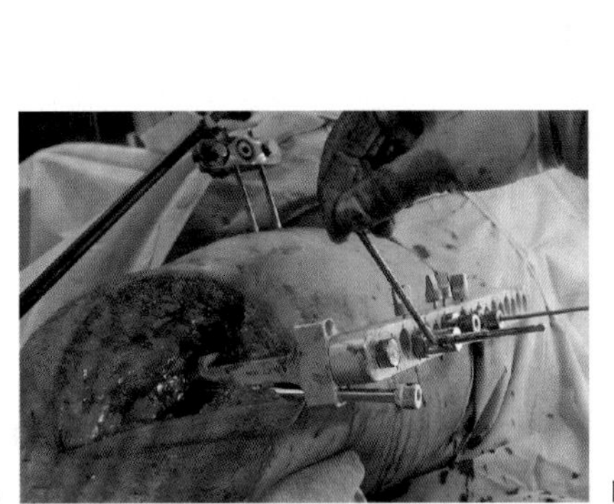

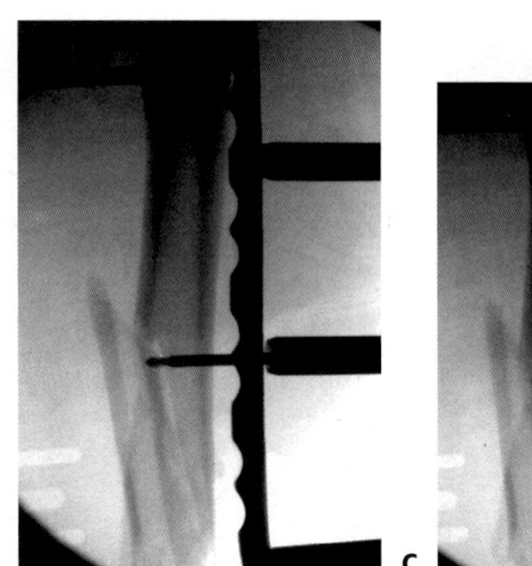

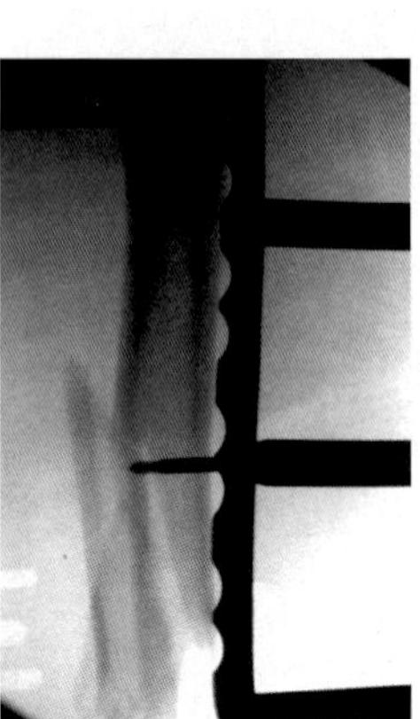

**TECH FIG 7** • **A–C.** The "whirlybird" device is tightened and the bone pulled to the plate.

- Depending on the system, locking drill guides can be placed freehand to ensure proper trajectory of the drill so that locking screws can be used.
- If that is not the case, nonlocking screws should be placed.
  - Experience is required for the freehand percutaneous method; otherwise, an open approach to the shaft should be performed.
  - The final construct should be checked with fluoroscopy on the lateral aspect as well (**TECH FIG 8D,E**).
  - The restoration of the mechanical axis can be checked intraoperatively after temporary stabilization (preferred) or definitive stabilization using the Bovie cord.
  - **TECH FIG 8F–H** show the repair after definitive stabilization.

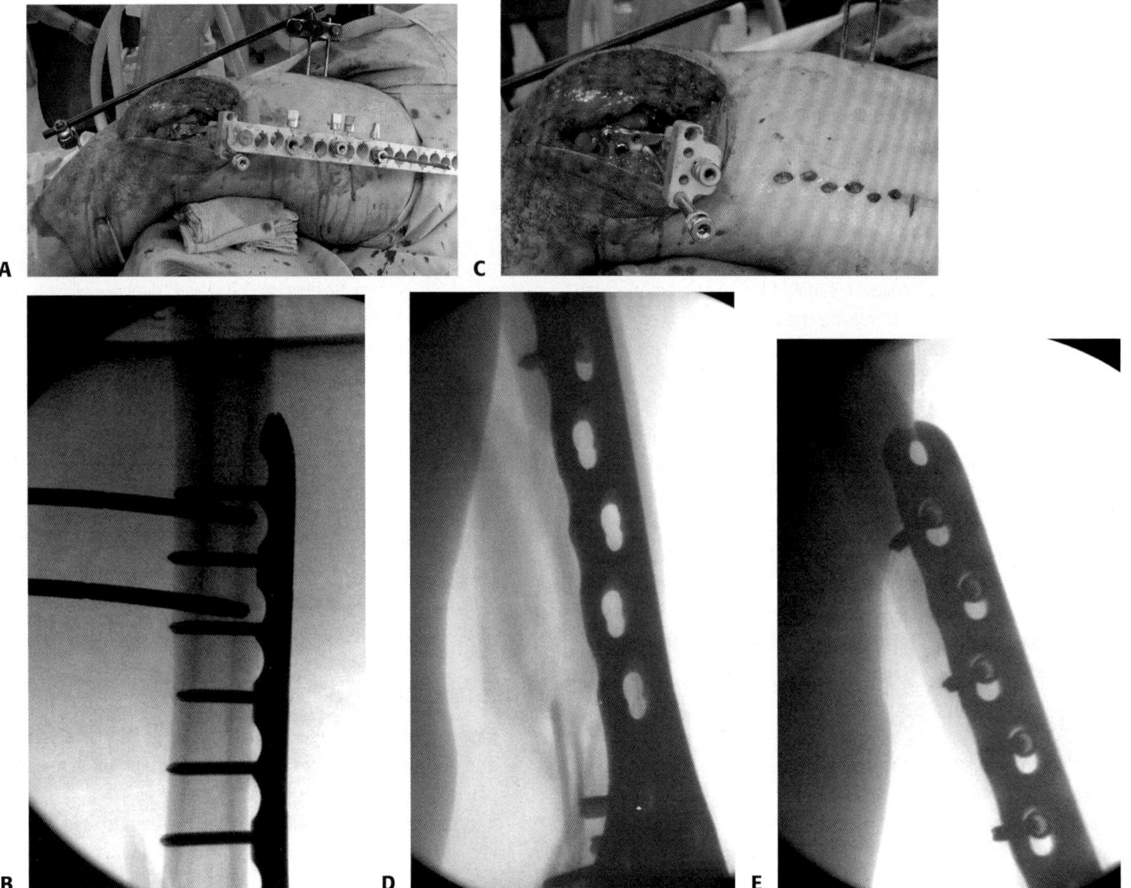

**TECH FIG 8** • **A.** Targeting guide for proximal screws. **B.** C-arm image of screws placed. **C.** Stab incisions used for percutaneous method. **D,E.** Plate placement on the lateral aspect is confirmed. *(continued)*

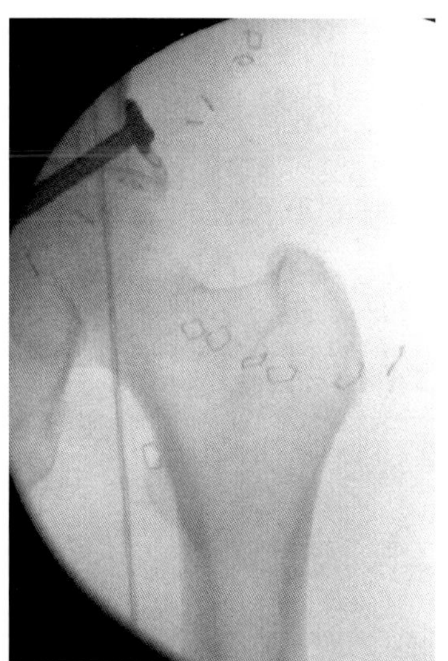
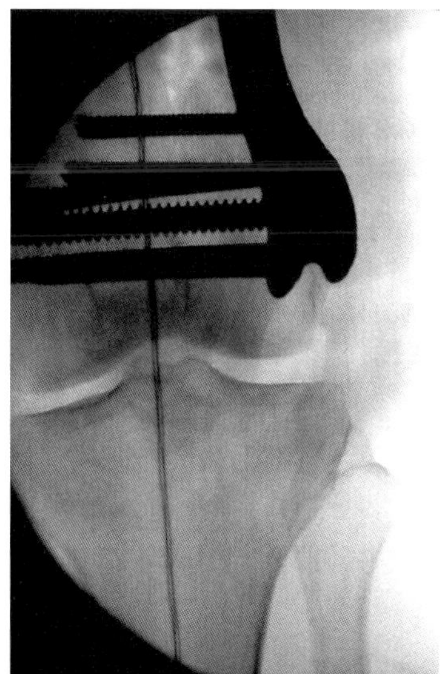
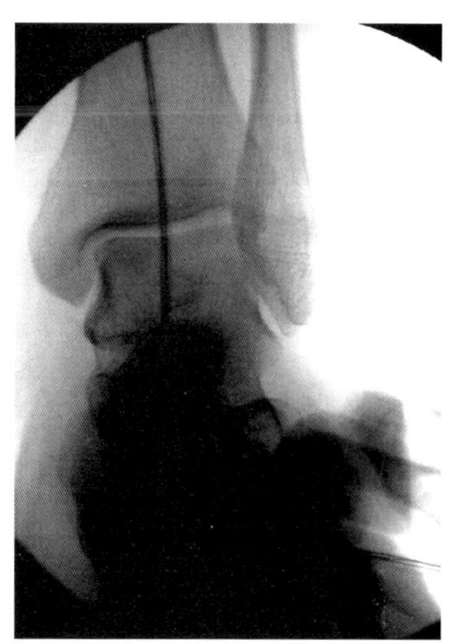

**TECH FIG 8** • *(continued)* **F–H.** Alignment is checked intraoperatively with the Bovie cord. The mechanical axis from the center of the femoral head through the middle of the knee to the middle of the ankle is confirmed.

- The exact number of screws in each fragment has yet to be determined in the literature, but our preference has been to have at least five screws in each fragment if possible at the end of fixation.
  - A longer working length in the shaft should be used, and not all holes need to be filled.
  - Plate longer than nine holes with eight holes being proximal to the fracture has been recommended to avoid complications with hardware failure or healing.[14]
  - There is evidence that in young patients with good bone, no locking screws are needed in the diaphysis.
  - Multiple locking screws are used in the epiphysis because of the short length of these distal fragments.
  - The largest screws available for the epiphysis should be used.

## Bone Grafting

- The metaphyseal comminution may require bone grafting or the use of bone substitutes in cases of open fractures with bone loss.
  - The exact type and need vary and should be based on the surgeon's experience (**TECH FIG 9**).
  - In closed fractures, avoiding stripping of the medial soft tissues often allows for healing without bone grafting.

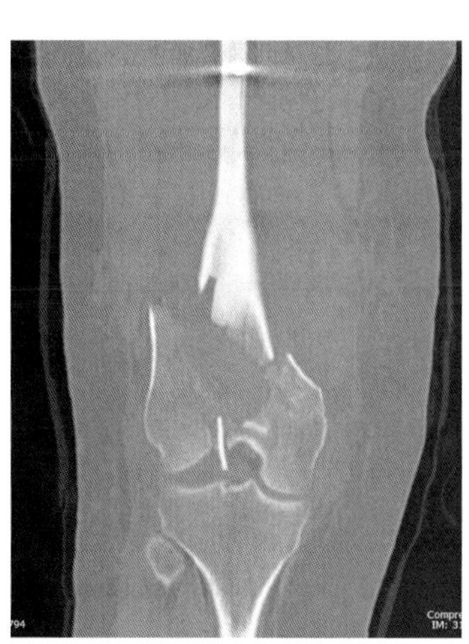
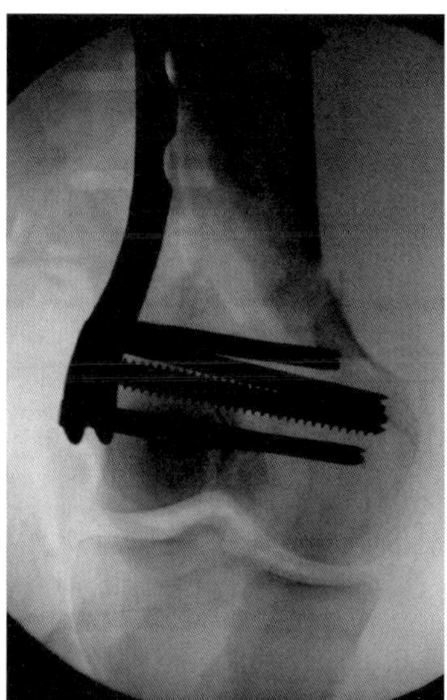
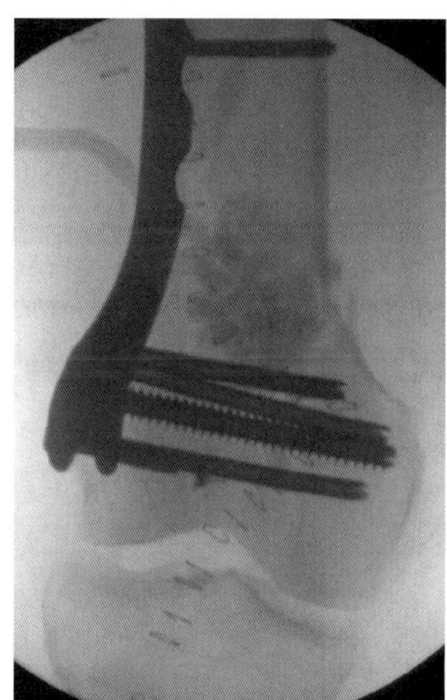

**TECH FIG 9** • **A.** Patient with significant metaphyseal bone loss from an open injury shown on CT scan. **B.** The postfixation radiograph shows the void. **C.** Placement of OsteoSet beads impregnated with vancomycin (off-label use) to fill the void and provide osteoconductive material for healing.

  - In open fractures with significant bone loss, we have had good success with the use of bone substitutes such as calcium sulfate (+/− antibiotics mixed in; off-label use), avoiding the need for later grafting (see **FIG 11A–H**).
- Hemostasis is achieved throughout the procedure or after the tourniquet is released. A tourniquet can be used to help minimize bleeding and improve visualization, especially for articular reconstruction. Often, a sterile tourniquet is used because of the temporary bridging external fixator that is in place.
- After adequate irrigation (before bone graft or substitute placement if used), a drain is placed in the knee joint and brought out laterally.

## Standard Wound Closure

- Closure of the arthrotomy is performed with figure-8 0 Vicryl sutures. This is reinforced by a running 2-0 FiberWire (Arthrex, Inc., Naples, FL) or Ethibond suture (**TECH FIG 10A**).
- The subcutaneous tissue is closed with 2-0 Vicryl.
- The skin is closed with staples, as are the percutaneous stab incisions.
- The knee is flexed and extended fully to ensure restoration of motion as well as to break any adhesions in the quadriceps that may have formed while the temporary bridging external fixator had been in place (**TECH FIG 10B,C**).
- The final radiographs are taken in the operating room (**TECH FIG 10D,E**).

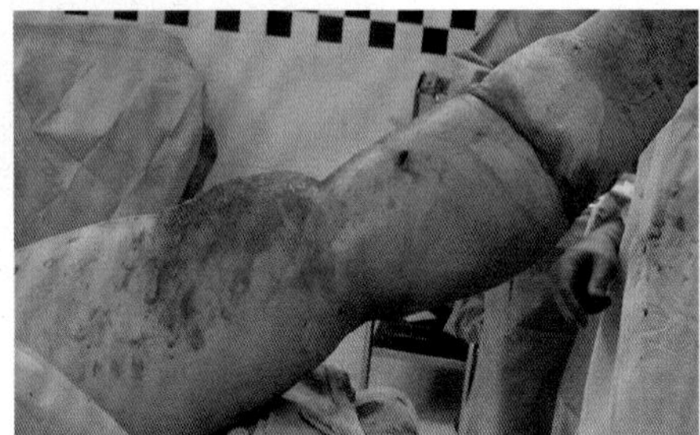
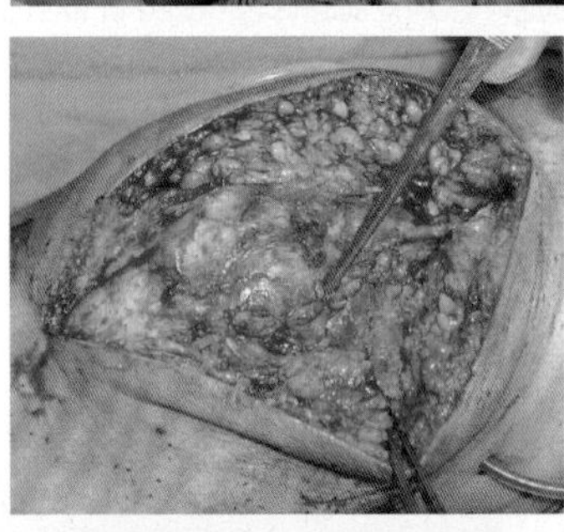
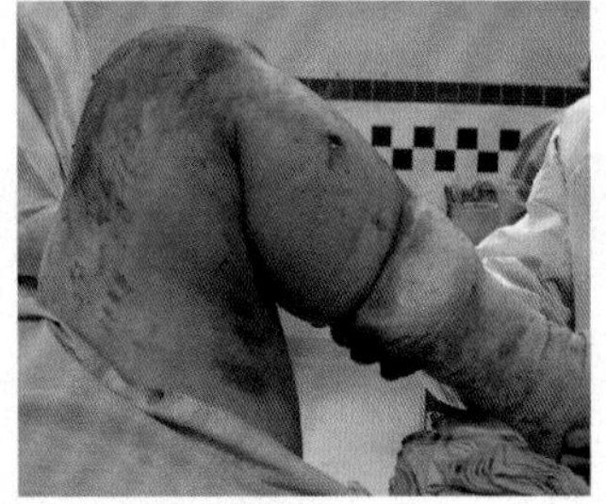
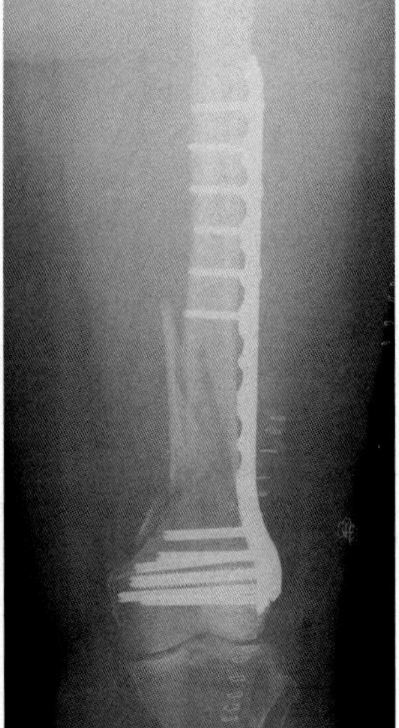
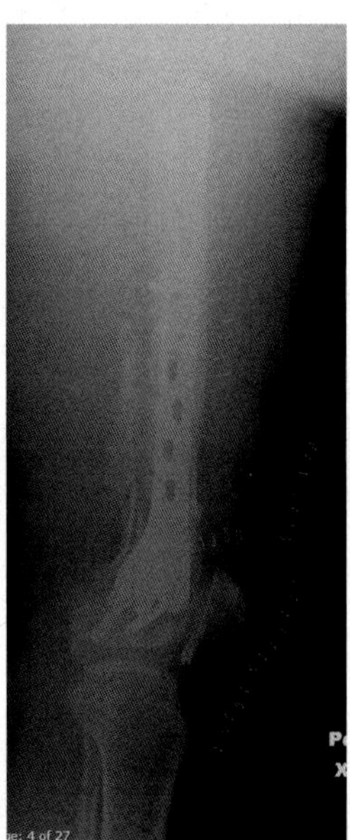

**TECH FIG 10** • **A.** Closure of the arthrotomy. **B,C.** Full flexion and extension of the knee after definitive fixation and closure. As seen in final AP (**D**) and lateral (**E**) radiographs, the metaphyseal comminution is bridged and left undisturbed.

# Open Reduction and Internal Fixation of the Distal Femur with Locking Plates (Type A or Nondisplaced Type C1 or C2)

- This technique can be used regardless of the locking plate system used. Each system's technique guide should be reviewed before use as each system has its own idiosyncrasies. Variations in plate application as well as reduction tools and techniques are unique to each system.
- See comments earlier regarding temporary use of an external fixator or distractor.

## Limited Lateral Approach

- A lateral incision measuring about 5 to 6 cm is made starting at the level of the joint and extending proximally in line with the shaft. The distal extent is curved slightly toward the tibial tubercle, as in the lateral approach (**TECH FIG 11A,B**).
- The iliotibial band is incised in line with the skin incision (**TECH FIG 11C**).
- The dissection is carried down to the lateral femoral condyle. The lateral aspect is exposed enough for plate placement (**TECH FIG 11D**).
- A Cobb elevator is used to create a plane submuscularly up the lateral shaft of the femur for placement of the plate.

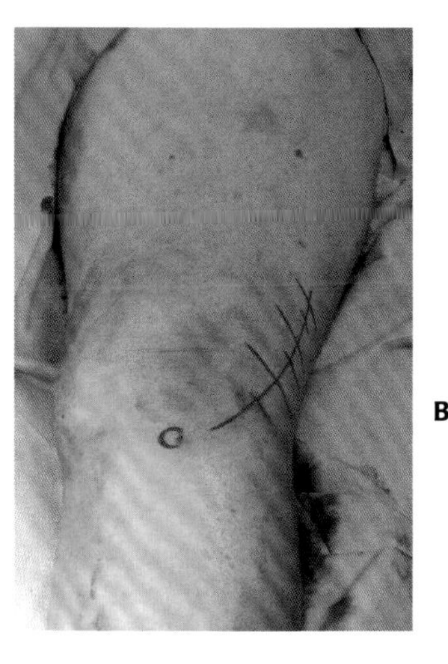

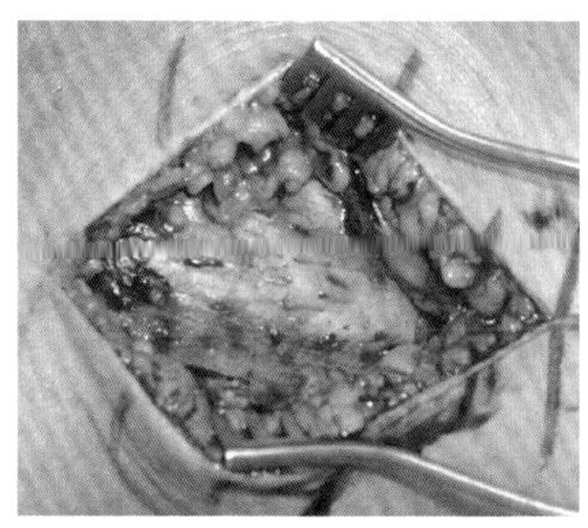

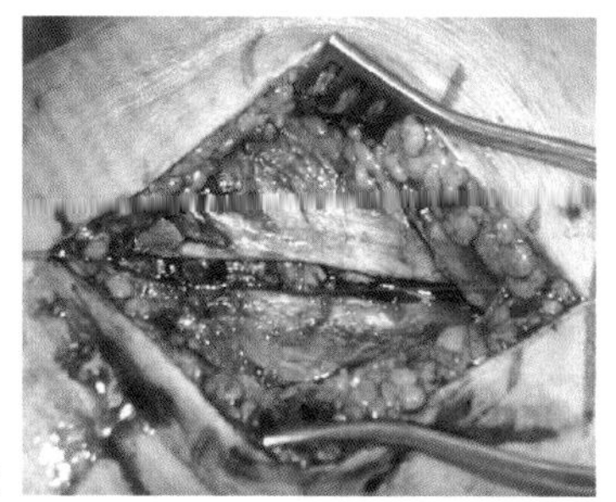

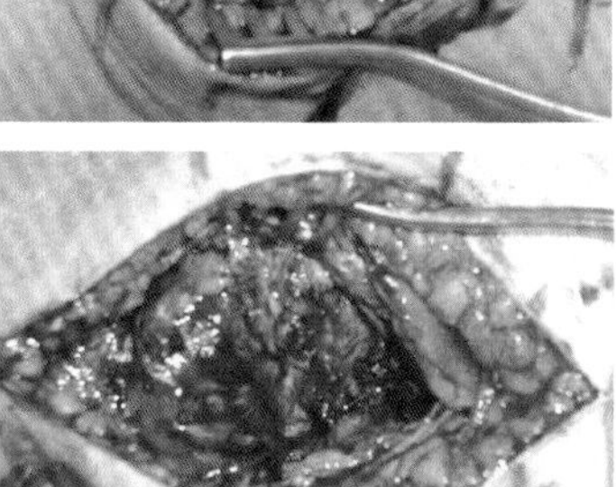

**TECH FIG 11** • Patient with closed distal femur fracture (also shown in **FIG 5G,H** and **6C–E**). **A.** Limited lateral incision, with the tibial tubercle marked. **B.** Skin incision showing the iliotibial band. **C.** Incision of the iliotibial band. **D.** Exposure of the lateral aspect of the femur.

## Stabilizing the Articular Surface

- For nondisplaced type C1 or C2 fractures, the first priority is to stabilize the articular surface.
- Visualization of the joint may be accomplished with placement of a blunt Hohmann retractor (or similar Z retractor) (**TECH FIG 12A**).
- A reduction forceps is placed anteriorly to hold the reduction (**TECH FIG 12B**).
- Temporary Kirschner wires or guidewires from a cannulated system can be placed for additional stability (**TECH FIG 12C,D**).
- All clamps, Kirschner wires, or guidewires should be placed outside the zone of plate application (**TECH FIG 12E,F**).

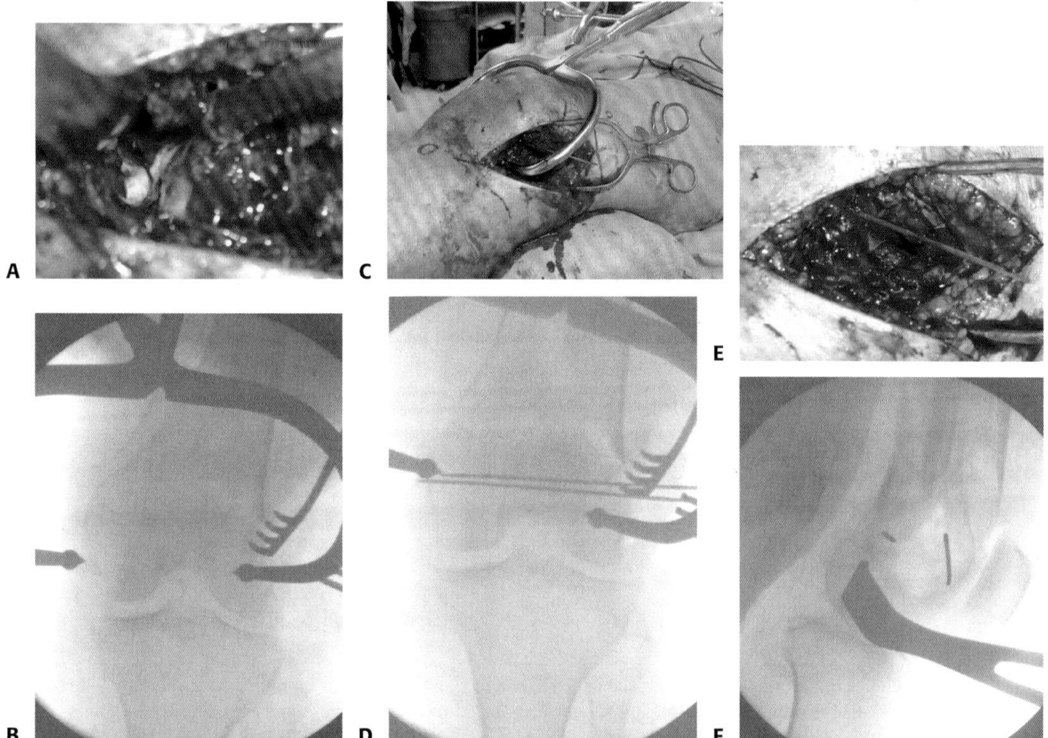

**TECH FIG 12** • **A.** Visualization of the joint for articular reduction. **B.** C-arm image of reduction forceps holding the intercondylar split reduced. **C,D.** Clinical photographs with forceps followed by guidewires for screw placement. **E,F.** Lateral views showing pins and wires outside the zone for either plate application or intramedullary nail. The anterior and posterior placement of the pins is seen. *(continued)*

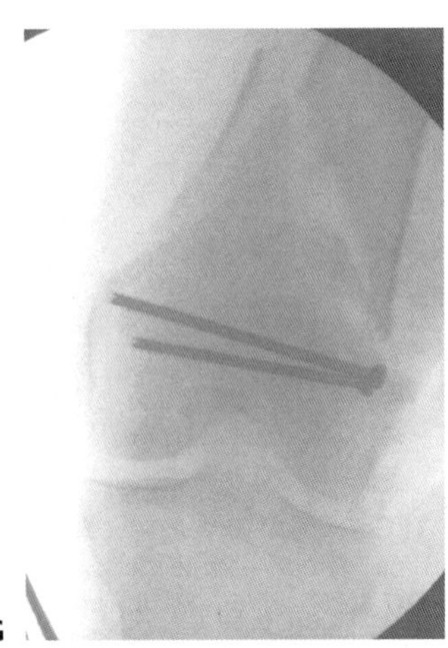

**TECH FIG 12** ● *(continued)* **G.** Definitive fixation of the condyles with 4.5-mm partially threaded cannulated screws.

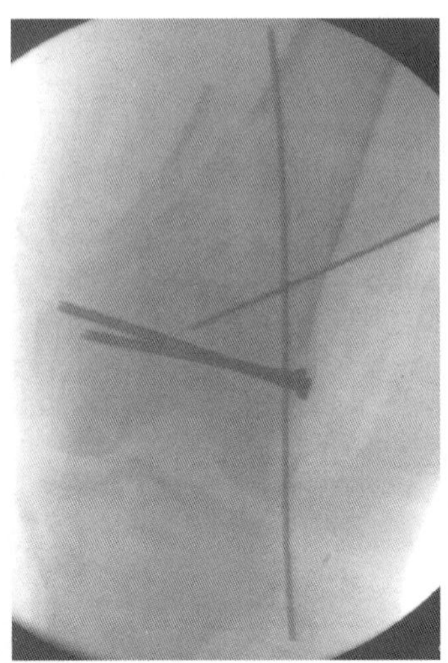

**TECH FIG 13** ● Adjunctive temporary fixation with Steinmann pins to reduce the shaft to the distal construct; pins again are placed outside of the area for plate application.

- Definitive fixation of the condyles should be performed (see technique description earlier) (**TECH FIG 12G**).

## Reduction of the Distal Segment and Plate Placement

- Reduction of the distal segment to the shaft can be performed using temporary Steinmann pins (**TECH FIG 13**).
- The plate can now be applied in a submuscular fashion (see Placement of the Plate section earlier).

## Wound Closure

- Final radiographs are taken in the operating room (**TECH FIG 14**).
- Standard wound closure is undertaken, as described in the previous section.

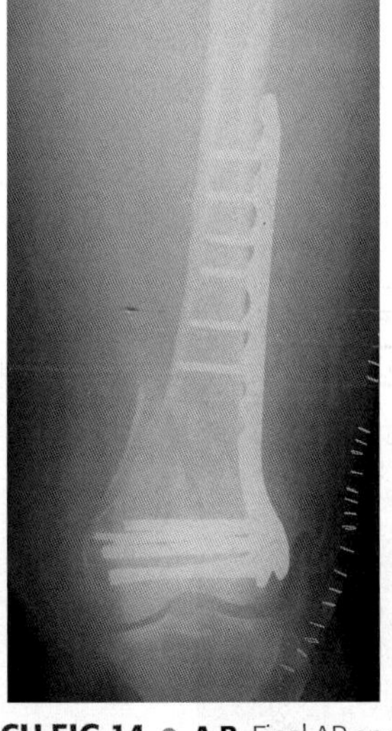

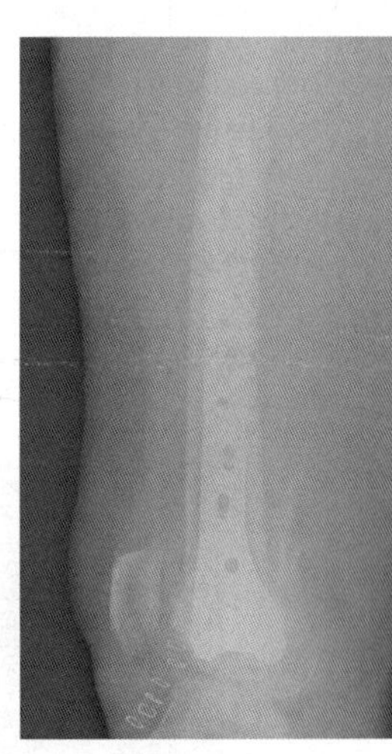

**TECH FIG 14** ● **A,B.** Final AP and lateral radiographs reveal that the posterior and medial metaphyseal comminution is left undisturbed.

## PEARLS AND PITFALLS

| | |
|---|---|
| **Articular reduction** | ■ Direct open reduction should be used.<br>■ Fixation can be outside the plate or through the plate.<br>■ If outside the plate, screws should be out of the way of the plate to maximize fixation points through the plate.<br>■ If a nail is being used with an articular split, the screws should be placed anterior and/or posterior to the proposed nail trajectory. |
| **Plate application** | ■ The initial guidewire through the central hole in the plate should be parallel to the joint. Ninety-five degrees is built into the plate. If locking screws are placed parallel to the joint, then once the plate is reduced to the shaft, the proper alignment is restored.<br>■ Rotation must be continually assessed.<br>■ The fracture should be reduced in the sagittal plane before temporary fixation or creation of a "box construct" with the plate. |

| | |
|---|---|
| | ■ In comminuted cases, a scanogram or opposite-side femur film with a ruler can be obtained to help determine the length.<br>■ Use of a long plate greater than nine holes in overall length with at least eight holes proximal to the fracture has been recommended.[14]<br>■ Anterior plate application on the shaft is linked to compromised fixation and early failure.[3]<br>■ Anterior plate application distally leads to hardware prominence and pain.[3] |
| **Soft tissue handling** | ■ The surgeon should avoid stripping the soft tissues medially. This will obviate the need for bone grafting especially in closed fractures.<br>■ The plate should be placed submuscularly. |
| **Temporary bridging external fixator** | ■ Any construct can be used.<br>■ The pins and bars should be placed in a manner such that the fixator could be used intraoperatively as a femoral distractor to hold the reduction, allowing the plating to occur.<br>■ The fixator pins in the femur should be placed while traction is applied to the limb so as to maximize the length of the quadriceps. This will ensure that difficulty regaining length is not associated with "skewering" of the quadriceps. |
| **Periprosthetic fractures** | ■ The surgeon should ensure that the femoral component will allow an intramedullary nail to be placed (eg, the femoral box is open).<br>■ If the component is stemmed, then the surgeon should make sure that cables are available to help supplement plate fixation; unicortical locked screws may not be sufficient for fixation.<br>■ The new variable-angle (polyaxial) locking plates may allow for screw fixation around the stemmed components and bicortical locked fixation. |
| **Deformity prevention**<br>**Valgus deformity** | ■ Placing the initial guidewire through the "central" hole for plate fixation parallel to the joint ensures proper alignment of the plate relative to the shaft. The plates are designed to recreate the normal anatomic relationship of the distal femur to the shaft. Additionally, a clamp can be placed on the distal fragment and held in the proper position as the plate is applied while adhering to the same principle as outlined earlier. |
| **Varus deformity** | ■ In a similar fashion, a varus deformity can be prevented by the same technique; however, once the plate is fixed to the distal segment in its proper alignment to the distal segment, a nonlocking screw can be used in the shaft to "suck" the plate to the bone, resulting in correction of the varus. |
| **Extension deformity** | ■ Because of the pull of the gastrocnemius complex, the distal fragment tends to flex downward, resulting in a relative "extension" deformity at the metaphysis. To prevent this, the knee is flexed as much as feasible to allow for operative fixation, and a bump directly underneath the apex of the deformity can help prevent the deforming forces. |
| **"Golf-club" deformity[3]** | ■ Placement of the plate too posteriorly on the distal aspect will medialize the distal segment.<br>■ Placement of the plate too distal on the femur can also medialize the distal segment.<br>■ Perfect lateral fluoroscopic visualization to ensure proper placement of the plate on the lateral aspect of the femur is paramount. |

## POSTOPERATIVE CARE

- The goal of stable fixation is to allow early range of motion. My preference is a hinged knee brace locked in extension for 2 weeks, at which time the wound is healed and full motion is then started.
- A continuous passive motion machine can be used.
- Cold therapy products can be used.
- A drain is used for 48 hours postoperatively.
- Deep vein thrombosis prophylaxis may be indicated for certain patients:
  - Obese
  - Multiply injured
  - History of previous deep vein thrombosis
  - Patient who may not be mobile enough despite an isolated injury
  - Length of prophylaxis
    - In cases of an isolated injury to the femur, we prescribe 2 weeks of deep vein thrombosis prophylaxis for these patients and then reassess in terms of mobility.
    - In patients who have additional significant risk factors for deep vein thrombosis and in the polytrauma patient, 6 to 12 weeks is prescribed.
  - Low-molecular-weight heparin is our preferred chemoprophylaxis.
  - Inferior vena cava filter may need to be considered in those multiply injured patients who cannot be anticoagulated.
- Early protected weight bearing
  - Toe-touch weight bearing for at least 6 to 8 weeks for plate fixation
  - Followed by partial weight bearing for 4 to 6 weeks for plate fixation
  - Followed by full weight bearing
  - Immediate weight bearing can be indicated for fixation of type A fractures, with intramedullary nailing if the fracture pattern is stable and not comminuted.
  - For type C fractures treated with intramedullary nailing and screw fixation for the articular component, toe-touch weight bearing or non–weight bearing for 6 to 8 weeks is adequate, followed by full weight bearing.
  - The aforementioned time frames are purely guidelines. The time to weight bearing is based on the fracture pattern, comminution, bone quality, patient body mass index (BMI), and on radiographic evidence of healing.
- Patients are prescribed physical therapy for range of motion and strengthening at 2 weeks.

## OUTCOMES

- Results are good to excellent in 50% to 96% of cases.[10,13,19]
  - Average range of motion is about 110 to 120 degrees.
  - About 70% to 80% of patients can walk without aids.
  - Elderly patients continue to have a higher perioperative risk of dying in the hospital from such injuries, along with poor functional long-term outcomes.[7]
- It is difficult to compare the results of studies in the literature.[19]
  - There is no universally accepted classification.
  - There are varying indications.
  - Different grading systems are used.
  - Not all authors adhere to the same principles.

## COMPLICATIONS

- Locking plates have become useful, but despite this newer plate technology, care must be taken to avoid common pitfalls; complications are still problematic, with overall healing problem reported as high as 32%.[3,6]
- It has been suggested that the use of a longer plate (longer than nine holes in length with eight holes proximal to the fracture) can minimize failures of fixation.[14]
- Neurovascular injuries
  - Can occur from initial trauma
  - Rare after surgery
- Infection
  - 0% to 10% rate after ORIF
  - Predisposing factors
    - High-energy injuries
    - Open fractures
    - Extensive dissection
    - Prolonged operative time
    - Inadequate fixation
- Nonunion
  - 0% to 19% rate after ORIF
  - Predisposing factors
    - Bone loss or defect (**FIG 17A**)
    - High-energy injuries

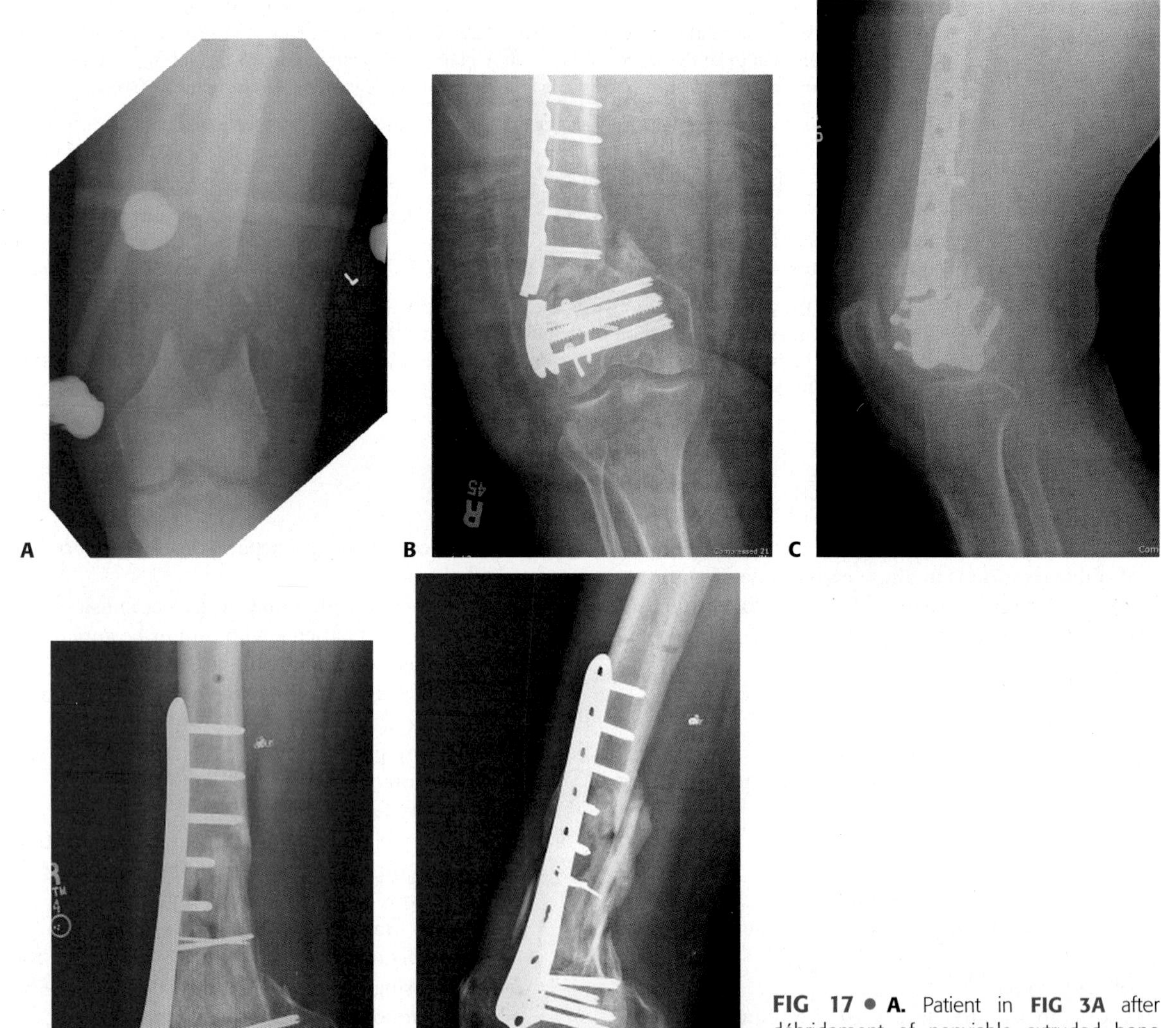

**FIG 17** • **A.** Patient in **FIG 3A** after débridement of nonviable extruded bone and placement of external fixator. The segmental bone loss is seen. **B,C.** Nonunion of a C3 distal femur fracture with subsequent hardware (plate) failure. **D,E.** Early hardware failure at 3 months (screws) in a C1 distal femur fracture.

- Soft tissue stripping
- Loss of osseous vascularity
- Inadequate stabilization
- No bone graft
- Infection

- Malunion
  - More common with nonsurgical treatment, which results in varus and recurvatum
  - Operative treatment with newer locking plates can result in valgus.
  - Malrotation has been reported as high as 38.5%.[2]
  - Treatment required to restore mechanical axis
    - Supracondylar osteotomy
    - Stable fixation
    - Early range of motion
- Hardware failure occurs in 0% to 13% of cases (**FIG 17B,C**, plate; **D,E**, screws).[14,17]
  - Predisposing factors
    - Comminution of metaphyseal area
    - Older age
    - Very distal fracture
    - Premature loading or weight bearing
    - Open fractures
    - Smoking
    - Increased BMI
    - Shorter plates (less than nine holes of overall length)
    - Diabetes
    - Nonunion
    - Infection
- Knee stiffness: Almost all patients exhibit some loss of motion.
  - Protruding hardware (see **FIG 10E,F**)
  - Articular malreduction
  - Adhesions
    - Intra-articular
    - Ligamentous–capsular contractures
    - Muscle scarring
  - Treatment may consist of any or combination of the following:
    - Manipulation
    - Arthroscopic lysis
    - Formal quadricepsplasty
- Posttraumatic arthritis occurs in 0% to 30% of cases.
  - Predisposing factors
    - Severe articular comminution
    - Cartilage loss
    - Cartilage impaction or damage
  - Surgical factors
    - Failure of anatomic reduction
    - Malalignment of fracture

## REFERENCES


1. Beingessner D, Moon E, Barei D, et al. Biomechanical analysis of the less invasive stabilization system for mechanically unstable fractures of the distal femur: comparison of titanium versus stainless steel and bicortical versus unicortical fixation. J Trauma 2011;71(3):620–624.
2. Buckley R, Mohanty K, Malish D. Lower limb malrotation following MIPO technique of distal femoral and proximal tibial fractures. Injury 2011;42(2):194–199.
3. Collinge CA, Gardner MJ, Crist BD. Pitfalls in the application of distal femur plates for fractures. J Orthop Trauma 2011;25(11):695–706.
4. Dominguez I, Rodrigez EM, De Pedro Moro JA, et al. Antegrade nailing for fractures of the distal femur. Clin Orthop Relat Res 1998;350:74–79.
5. Doornink J, Fitzpatrick DC, Madey SM, et al. Far cortical locking enables flexible fixation with periarticular locking plates. J Orthop Trauma 2011;25(suppl 1):S29–S34.
6. Henderson CE, Kuhl LL, Fitzpatrick DC, et al. Locking plates for distal femur fractures: is there a problem with fracture healing? J Orthop Trauma 2011;25(suppl 1):S8–S14.
7. Kammerlander C, Riedmuller P, Gosch M, et al. Functional outcome and mortality in geriatric distal femoral fractures. Injury 2012;43(7):1096–1101.
8. Leung KS, Shen WY, Mui LT, et al. Interlocking intramedullary nailing for supracondylar and intercondylar fractures of the distal part of the femur. J Bone Joint Surg Am 1991;73A:332–340.
9. Lujan TJ, Henderson CE, Madey SM, et al. Locked plating of distal femur fractures leads to inconsistent and asymmetric callus formation. J Orthop Trauma 2010;24(3):156–162.
10. Markmiller M, Konrad G, Sudkamp N. Femur-LISS and distal femoral nail for fixation of distal femoral fractures: are there differences in outcome and complications? Clin Orthop Relat Res 2004;426:252–257.
11. Nork SE, Segina DN, Aflatoon K, et al. The association between supracondylar-intercondylar distal femoral fractures and coronal plane fractures. J Bone Joint Surg Am 2005;87A:564–569.
12. Otto RJ, Moed BR, Bledsoe JG. Biomechanical comparison of polyaxial-type locking plates and a fixed-angle locking plate for internal fixation of distal femur fractures. J Orthop Trauma 2009;23:645–652.
13. Rademakers MV, Kerkhoffs GMMJ, Sierevelt IN, et al. Intra articular fractures of the distal femur: a long-term follow-up study of surgically treated patients. J Orthop Trauma 2004;18:213–219.
14. Ricci WM, Streuble PN, Morshed S, et al. Risk factors for failure of locked plate fixation of distal femur fractures: an analysis of 335 cases. J Orthop Trauma 2014;28(2):83–89.
15. Schatzker J. Fractures of the distal femur revisited. Clin Orthop Relat Res 1998;347:43–56.
16. Starr AJ, Jones AL, Reinert CM. The "Swashbuckler": a modified anterior approach for fractures of the distal femur. J Orthop Trauma 1999;13:138–140.
17. Vallier HA, Hennessey TA, Sontich JK, et al. Failure of LCP condylar plate fixation in the distal part of the femur: a report of six cases. J Bone Joint Surg Am 2006;88A:846–853.
18. Wilkens KJ, Curtiss S, Lee MA. Polyaxial locking plate fixation in distal femur fractures: A biomechanical comparison. J Orthop Trauma 2008;22:624–628.
19. Zlowodzki M, Bhandari M, Marek DJ, et al. Operative treatment of acute distal femur fractures: systematic review of 2 comparative studies and 45 case series (1989 to 2005). J Orthop Trauma 2006;20:366–371.

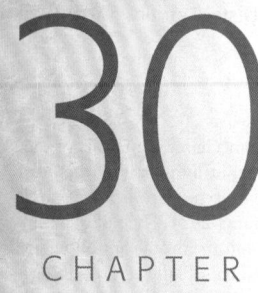

# Pediatric Tibial Fractures

Craig P. Eberson

## DEFINITION

- Fractures of the tibia are common in children.
- Severity ranges from nondisplaced "toddler's" fracture to high-energy open injury.
- Open growth plates at the ends of the tibia preclude standard adult treatment options such as solid interlocked nails.
- Many cases can be managed nonoperatively, but orthopaedists need to maintain familiarity with operative techniques.

## ANATOMY

- Relevant anatomy includes muscle compartments (anterior, posterior, superficial, and deep posterior), cross-sectional shape, and growth plates (**FIG 1**).
- Neurovascular structures are at risk from direct trauma or compartment syndrome.
- Understanding the anatomy of the growth plates is crucial when planning fixation techniques.

## PATHOGENESIS

- The most common injury scenarios are either low-energy injuries, such as those sustained during sports (twisting injury), or high-energy ones, such as seen in car versus pedestrian accidents (direct blow, comminuted fracture).
- Many injuries fall somewhere along the spectrum.
- High-energy injuries often are seen with concomitant injuries, such as ipsilateral femoral injuries (the so-called floating knee), compartment syndromes, and intra-articular injuries of the proximal or distal tibia.[11]
- Occasionally, the fracture may be pathologic through an underlying bone lesion (eg, nonossifying fibroma, aneurysmal bone cyst, osteomyelitis, osteosarcoma).
- As in all fractures in young children, child abuse must be suspected if the history is unclear or multiple fractures are present.

## NATURAL HISTORY

- Because of the significant remodeling potential in young children, most patients heal without sequelae.
- Morbidity from associated injuries, however, may be significant (ie, compartment syndrome), so a thorough evaluation is of paramount importance.
- General guidelines are available to define acceptable healing alignment (Table 1).

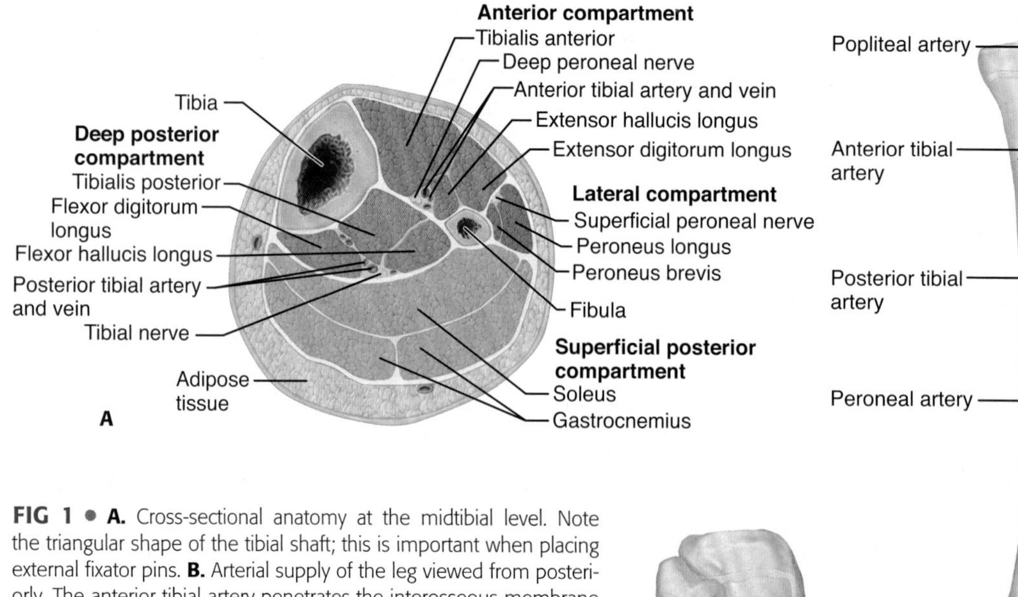


**FIG 1** • **A.** Cross-sectional anatomy at the midtibial level. Note the triangular shape of the tibial shaft; this is important when placing external fixator pins. **B.** Arterial supply of the leg viewed from posteriorly. The anterior tibial artery penetrates the interosseous membrane proximally and is tethered there, putting it at risk for injury in proximal fractures. **C.** Proximal tibial physis viewed laterally. It is important to appreciate the continuity of the tubercle and proximal tibial growth plates. Injury to the tubercle growth plate will result in a recurvatum deformity.

**Table 1 Acceptable Deformity for Fractures of the Tibia**

| | Acceptable Deformity by Patient Age | |
|---|---|---|
| **Parameter** | **Under 8 Years** | **8 Years or Older** |
| Valgus | 5 degrees | 5 degrees |
| Varus | 10 degrees | 10 degrees |
| Apex anterior/posterior | | |
| Angulation | 10 degrees | 5 degrees |
| Shortening | 10 mm | 5 mm |
| Malrotation | 5 degrees | 5 degrees |

Adapted from Heinrich SD. Fractures of the shaft of the tibia and fibula. In: Beaty JH, Kasser JR, eds. Rockwood and Wilkins' Fractures in Children, ed 5. Philadelphia: Lippincott Williams & Wilkins, 2001:1077–1119; Wilkins KE. Principles of fracture remodelling in children. Injury 2005;36(suppl 1):A3–A11.

## PATIENT HISTORY AND PHYSICAL FINDINGS

- The history should include mechanism of injury, antecedent pain, neurologic symptoms, and other areas of pain (eg, femur, abdominal pain, headache).
- A high-energy injury should also prompt a full trauma workup using standard Advanced Trauma Life Support protocols.
- The physical examination should focus on assessing initial displacement and skin condition (ie, open injury) as well as swelling of the compartments.
- The limb should be splinted, in the case of gross deformity, before obtaining films using a material that permits high-quality radiographs.
- A thorough neurovascular examination is needed to assess for vascular injury or compartment syndrome.[1]
  - Pulses should be palpated or obtained with Doppler assistance.
  - Sensation in the deep and superficial peroneal nerve and tibial nerve distributions should be assessed as well as motor function (toe flexors–extensors).
  - Pain with passive motion of the toes may represent an evolving compartment syndrome. More specifically, increasing pain, or pain out of proportion to the injury, is often the first early warning sign and should be taken seriously. Splitting or removal of casting material should be performed if any question exists. In young children, anxiety and fearfulness may be the presenting feature.
- Compartment pressure measurements should be obtained in cases of concern (**FIG 1A**).
  - Compartment syndrome is signaled by tense swelling of the compartment, pain with gentle squeezing of the compartment, pain with passive extension–flexion of toes, and paresthesias in involved nerve distributions. Loss of pulse is a late finding.
    - Patients with any of these signs should be considered at risk.
- A low threshold should be present for measuring compartment pressures and performing fasciotomy as needed.
- Vigilance is required to prevent permanent sequelae due to missed compartment syndrome.

## IMAGING AND OTHER DIAGNOSTIC STUDIES

- Standard anteroposterior (AP) and lateral radiographic views should be obtained.
- For complex fractures, dedicated knee and ankle films can be helpful to evaluate for extension into the physeal or articular regions.
- Computed tomography can be helpful to assess these regions if radiographs do not provide sufficient clarity.
- Contralateral full-length films are helpful for determining length in comminuted fractures.

## DIFFERENTIAL DIAGNOSIS

- Isolated tibial fracture
- Floating knee
- Pathologic fracture
- Intra-articular or intraphyseal injury
- Compartment syndrome
- Child abuse

## NONOPERATIVE MANAGEMENT

- Most tibial fractures can be managed with closed reduction and cast immobilization in an above-the-knee cast.
- The cast should be molded to the anatomy of the tibia.
  - A supracondylar "squeeze" mold above the knee and 15 to 20 degrees of knee flexion can prevent cast slippage.
  - To truly avoid weight bearing, however, the cast must be flexed at least 70 to 80 degrees (if appropriate for a specific fracture).
- In cases of acute fracture, the cast can be univalved or bivalved to allow for swelling. It can then be overwrapped before initiating weight bearing.
- Weekly radiographs are obtained for the first 3 weeks, with the cast being wedged or changed as needed for loss of alignment.
- Weight bearing is dictated by patient comfort.
- The cast is changed to a short-leg or patellar-bearing cast after 4 to 6 weeks, and immobilization is continued until healing is complete.
- Surgical management is required for inability to maintain satisfactory alignment (see Table 1).

## SURGICAL MANAGEMENT

- Indications for surgical treatment of tibial fractures in children include open injuries, compartment syndrome, multiple injuries, and fractures for which closed treatment fails.
- Treatment in mature adolescents is the same as for adults with reamed, locked intramedullary nails.
- Younger children's open physes require techniques that avoid the proximal and distal tibia, such as external fixation, plate fixation, and elastic intramedullary nailing.
- Traditionally, external fixation was used primarily for fractures with significant comminution or soft tissue injury, where intramedullary fixation was considered impractical. However, recent work challenges this paradigm for surgeons experienced with elastic nailing.[12]
  - Rapid stabilization of the multiply injured child is often accomplished using external fixation as well.[4,7,9,13]
- Plate fixation is a helpful technique for fractures not amenable to elastic nail fixation.
  - It is particularly helpful in patients who present with late loss of reduction and require an open approach to remove callus and align the fracture.

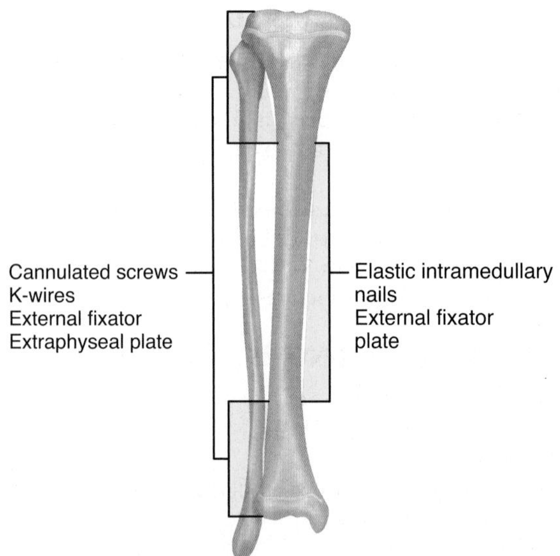


**FIG 2** • Suggested fixation techniques for the pediatric tibia.

- It is used at our institution primarily for distal-third fractures.
- After successful use in the treatment of pediatric femur fractures, the elastic intramedullary nail technique has also been successfully applied to the tibia.[3,6,14]

## Preoperative Planning

- Full-length radiographs of the tibia and fibula should be obtained.
  - Views of the contralateral side can be helpful to determine proper length in comminuted fractures.
  - A clinical examination of the well side can guide the surgeon in determining rotational alignment.
- The choice of fixation is determined by fracture location, comminution, and soft tissue envelope (**FIG 2**).

## Positioning

- The patient is positioned supine on the operating table (**FIG 3**).
- The fluoroscopy machine can be brought in from the opposite side of the table so that it is out of the surgeon's way.
- A small bump placed under the ipsilateral hip is helpful to counter external rotation of the femur so that the patella is pointed directly up.

## Approach

- The approach for treatment of tibial fractures depends on the technique used.
- Elastic nails and external fixation pins are placed through stab incisions.
- Open reduction and internal fixation approaches are the same as described for adult injuries elsewhere in this text.

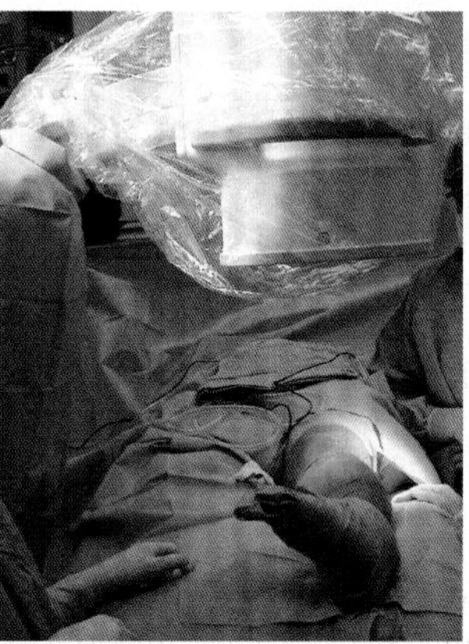

**FIG 3** • Positioning for operative treatment of tibia fractures. The hip is elevated on a towel roll so that the patella points directly anteriorly. The fluoroscopic unit is brought in from the opposite side of the table to avoid interference with the surgeon.

TECHNIQUES

# External Fixation

- In the supine position, traction is used to roughly align the fracture.
- Pins are placed using fluoroscopic guidance to avoid the physis.
  - Particular care is required when placing the most proximal pin.
  - The tibial tubercle physis is not easily seen on the AP radiograph.
  - A lateral view is required to avoid injury to this structure and a late procurvatum deformity.
- An array of pin sizes should be available.
  - Full-sized adolescents may require 5-mm pins as in adults, but smaller children require smaller pins to avoid an overly stiff construct.
  - Four-millimeter pins should be used for younger children (ie, younger than 10 years old), and I have found an adult wrist external fixator with 2.5-mm pins useful for treatment of toddlers with open injuries requiring fixation such as lawnmower injuries.
- Multiple pins are placed on each side of the fracture, one close (within several centimeters of the fracture line) and one far (at least 2 to 3 cm away from the physis).
- Children's bone is often quite hard. Despite using "self-drilling" pins, I prefer to predrill the anterior cortex before placing the pin.
  - Ring sequestra may develop from the heat generated in hard bone if pins are drilled directly in some children.
- The roughly triangular shape of the tibia should be noted (see **FIG 1A**).
  - The pins should be started on the tip of the anterior tibia or just medial and aimed slightly medially.
  - Laterally aimed pins may be unicortical, as the lateral cortex of the tibia is vertically oriented.
- The fracture is then manually reduced, using the pins for traction if necessary, and the frame is connected (**TECH FIG 1A**).
- In cases of soft tissue injury requiring the ankle to be immobilized, extending the frame to the first or fifth metatarsal can allow easier wound management (**TECH FIG 1B**).
- The pin sites are covered with iodine-soaked gauze.
  - I have caregivers begin cleaning the pin sites with half-strength hydrogen peroxide once or twice daily after the 1-week follow-up visit.
- A posterior splint is applied to immobilize the ankle and allow soft tissue healing. It is removed after 2 to 3 weeks to begin ankle range of motion.

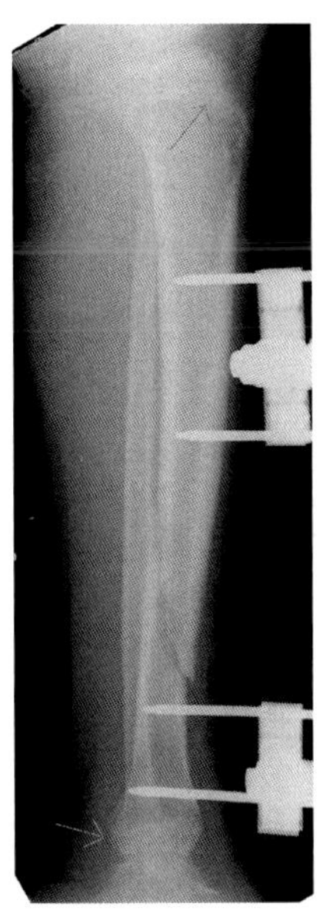

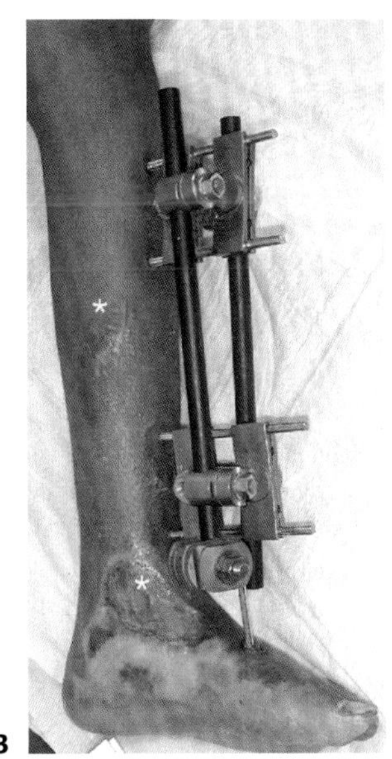

**TECH FIG 1** • **A.** External fixation in a patient with a compartment syndrome. *Arrows* mark the proximal and distal growth plates. The proximal pins start fairly distally to avoid the tubercle physis. **B.** In this patient, an external fixator was used for a grade 2 open fracture treated with delayed closure. The patient also had a degloving injury requiring a flap and skin graft over the medial ankle. The frame was extended to the first metatarsal to immobilize the foot during healing. Although somewhat bulky, the "double stack" configuration of the frame allows for easy dynamization.

## Plate Fixation

- Treatment is essentially the same as for adult injuries, but several points bear emphasis.
- It is helpful to make the incision slightly laterally over the anterior compartment so it will not lie directly over a medially placed plate (**TECH FIG 2A**).
- The fracture is reduced using standard techniques. Care should be taken to avoid unnecessary stripping of the fracture.
- I prefer to make an incision over the fracture large enough to reduce the fragments but not the entire length of the plate.
  - The plate can be slid under the skin, over the periosteum, and the screws placed through stab incisions, as for percutaneous plating in adults (**TECH FIG 2B**).
- For larger children, many adult fracture systems include precontoured 3.5-mm plates for the distal tibia.
  - For smaller children, a small fragment plate may be contoured to fit appropriately.
  - It is important to avoid injury to the perichondral ring at the distal extent of the plate.
- If the plate is applied on the medial side of the tibia, as it often is for fractures with valgus angulation, it will usually need to be removed after healing due to prominence.
- If applied laterally, I usually make a longer incision because percutaneously placed screws will traverse the anterior compartment and potentially injure the neurovascular bundle. I prefer open placement in this case.
- The wound is closed using standard techniques. A posterior splint is applied to protect the soft tissues.

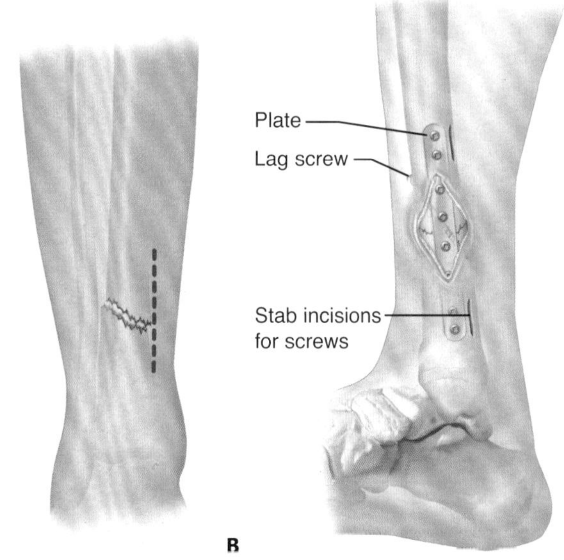


**TECH FIG 2** • **A.** Incision for open reduction and internal fixation is made laterally over the anterior compartment, and the skin can then be mobilized to gain access to the fracture site. It is important not to incise the skin directly over the proposed location of the plate. **B.** Medial view of internally fixed tibia. A lag screw compresses the fragment, and the plate stops short of the physis. The skin incision is centered over the fracture to allow an accurate reduction, but the proximal and distal screws can be placed percutaneously through a medially applied plate. It is helpful to make one stab incision for every two holes, centered between them.

## Elastic Intramedullary Nail Fixation

- The surgeon begins by selecting the proper nail size. Usually, nails should be 0.4 times the diameter of the tibial isthmus.
- The nails are contoured so that there is a C shape with its apex at the fracture site. This will cause cortical contact at the apex, yielding three-point fixation (proximal, cortical at fracture level, and distal).
- By contouring rods of equal diameter symmetrically, the elasticity of the nails resists deformation of the fracture, as opposed to reamed nailing, where the fracture is statically supported by the strength of the nail.

### Preparation for Nail Insertion

- The nails are inserted in the tibial metaphysis.
  - The proper starting point is at least 1 cm distal to the proximal tibial physis and 2 cm posterior to the tibial tubercle physis (**TECH FIG 3A,B**).
- The relevant landmarks should be identified fluoroscopically and marked on the skin (physis, tubercle, starting points) before proceeding (**TECH FIG 3B**).
- The incision should be 1 to 1.5 cm long, with its most distal extent roughly 1 cm proximal to the physis.
  - This will allow an oblique passage of the nail at the correct proximal to distal angle.
- A small hemostat is used to carefully spread through the tissue down to bone, and a drill sleeve and drill are placed on the bone. The drill should be 1 to 1.5 mm larger than the diameter of the nail.
- After checking the position of the drill tip with fluoroscopy (**TECH FIG 3C**), a starting hole is drilled along the proposed path of the nail (**TECH FIG 3D**).
  - Care is taken not to drill across the tibia out the opposite cortex.
- Alternatively, an awl can be used by hand to create this opening in the cortex.

### Nail Pattern and Placement

- Multiple nail patterns have been described,[6] but the standard is one medial and one lateral nail (**TECH FIG 4A,B**).
- Alternately, if soft tissue compromise precludes the use of an entry site, the first nail is bent into a C shape, with the second bent into an S shape. The apex of the more distal curve in the nail should be at the fracture site.
- The first nail is contoured into a C shape. It should be placed on the tibia and a fluoroscopic image obtained (**TECH FIG 4C,D**).
  - A gentle bend is placed in the nail, centered at the fracture.
- The nail is placed up to the fracture site under fluoroscopic guidance. Initially, it is helpful to direct the bend posteriorly, as in the passage of a guidewire for a standard reamed nail, but it is important to rotate the bend into the proper plane to prevent a recurvatum deformity (**TECH FIG 4E,F**).
- The second nail is placed in the same fashion.

### Fracture Reduction and Fixation

- The fracture is then manually reduced.
  - It is rarely necessary to open the fracture to obtain a reduction, as the fracture can be easily manipulated.

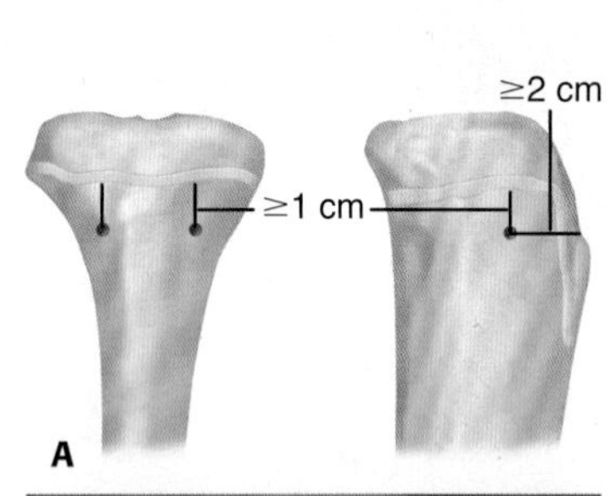


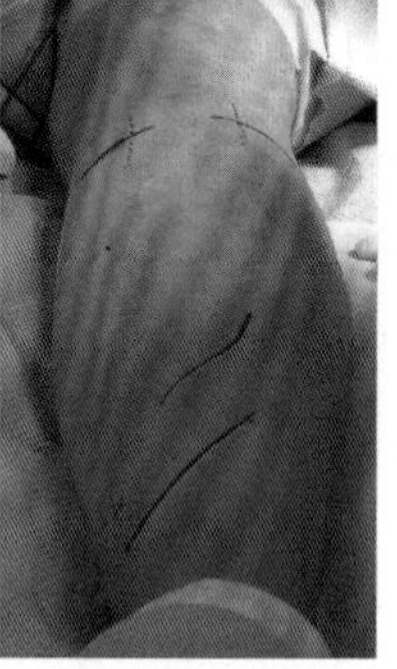


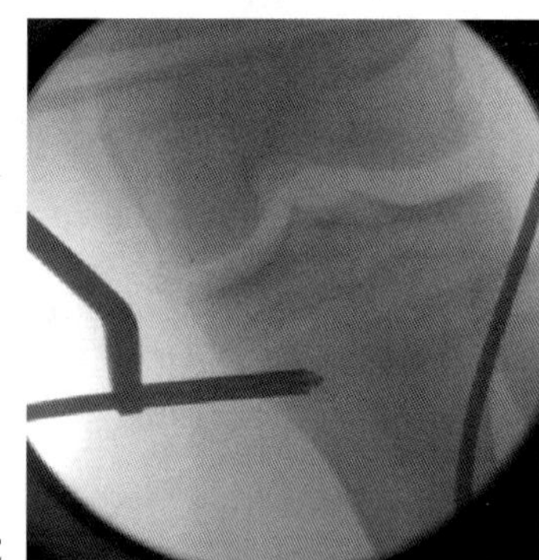


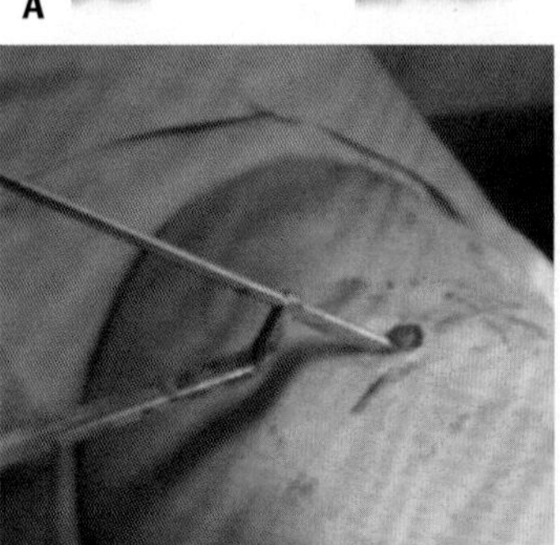


**TECH FIG 3** • **A.** The proper starting point for nail insertion lies at least 1 cm distal to the proximal tibial growth plate and 2 cm posterior to the tubercle physis. **B.** Patient undergoing elastic intramedullary nailing of the tibia. Marked on the skin are the proximal growth plate and proposed entry sites as well as the fracture. The incision is made proximal to the line of the physis, and an oblique angle matching the final path of the nail is dissected with a hemostat down to the bone. **C.** After confirming the entry site radiographically, a drill is used through a guide to open the cortex 1 to 2 mm larger than the nail diameter. **D.** The drill starts perpendicular to the bone and is advanced distally. Care is taken not to drill into a previously placed nail or through the far cortex.

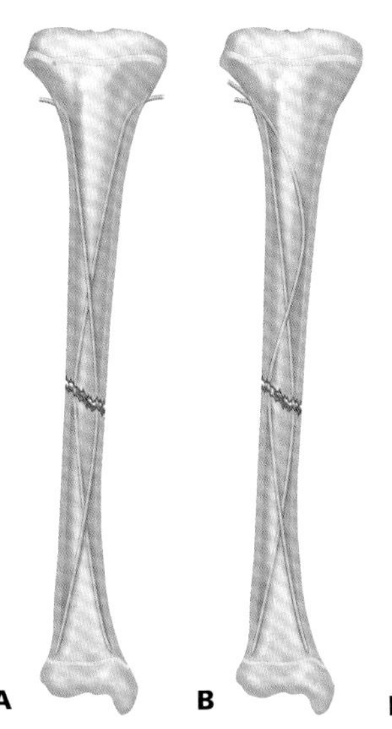


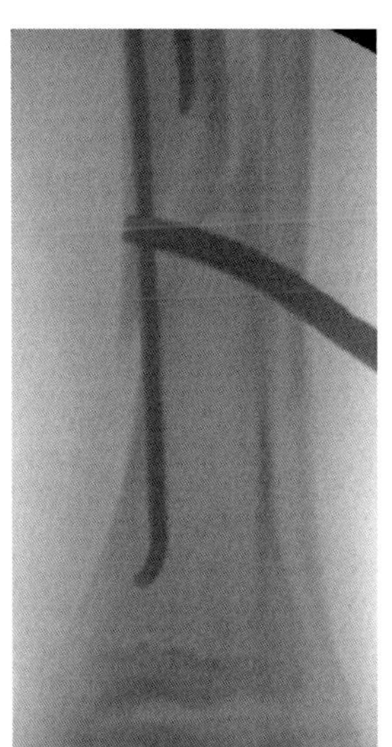


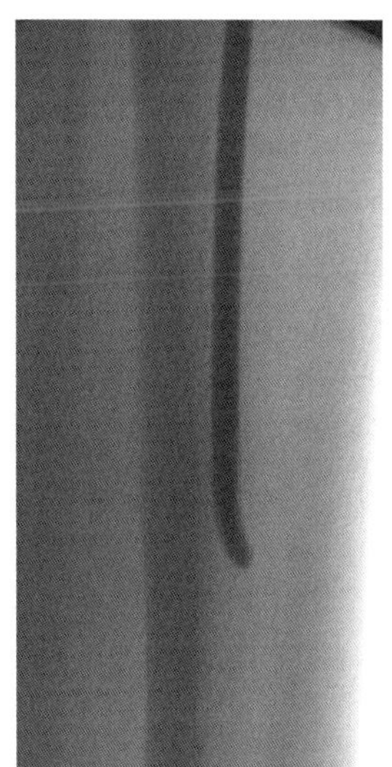


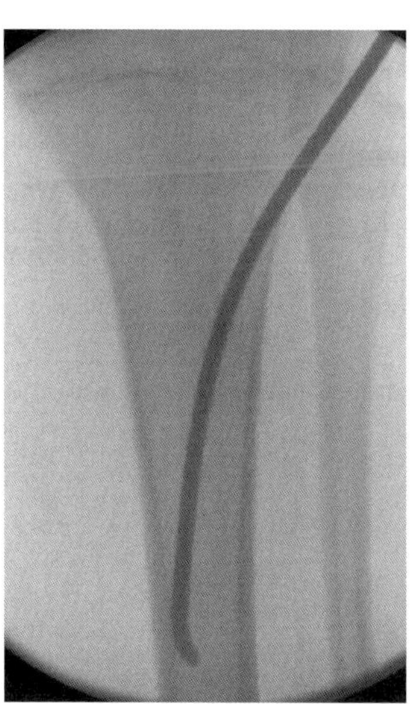


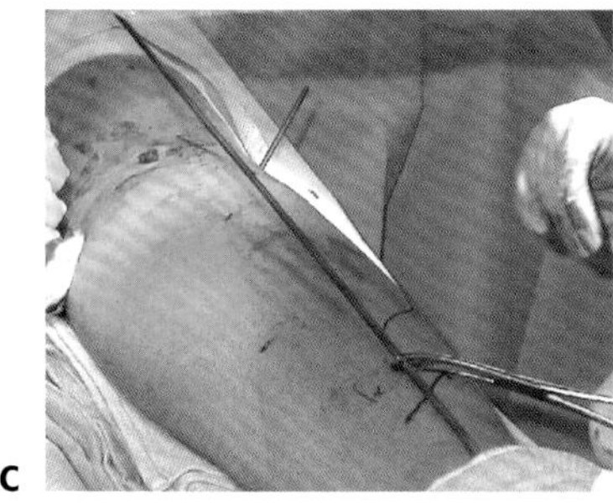


**TECH FIG 4** • **A,B.** Potential patterns of nail insertion. The standard pattern (**A**) entails one medial and one lateral nail. Alternately, both nails are inserted from the same side to avoid compromised skin (**B**). In the tibia, the former technique is far easier. **C.** The nail is placed on the skin, with the tip at the proposed final location, as confirmed radiographically. **D.** The nail is marked at the fracture site and bent to place the apex at that location. **E.** When starting a nail, it is helpful to rotate the nail so that the tip points anteriorly, bouncing off the posterior cortex. **F.** The nail is then turned so that the bend in the nail lies in the coronal plane.

  - The bent tip of the nail can be used to assist in reduction as well.
- To pass the nails across the fracture, it is helpful to consider the initial deformity of the fracture.
  - For example, if the fracture tends to lie in valgus, it may be helpful to pass the medial nail first to apply a varus force. The second nail is then directed across the fracture site.
  - Care should be taken to stop the nails short of the distal physis and to avoid distraction at the fracture site.
- When passing the nails, it is often helpful to pass them both to the level of the fracture and sequentially crossing the fracture site.
  - In oblique fractures, the first nail will deform the fracture and make passing the second nail difficult if the first nail is passed all the way down initially.
  - In simple fractures, the order of passage is less important.

## Cutting the Nails and Wound Closure

- The nails are then cut, pulling them away from the bone without exceeding the elastic modulus of the nail, so they lie against the bone after they are cut, with about 2 cm of the nail extending out of the bone to facilitate later.
  - Alternately, the nails can be withdrawn a few centimeters, cut short, and then impacted back down the tibia, again leaving 2 cm of exposed nail beyond the entry site.
  - This step is important because if the nails are left too long or are bent out away from the bone, they can cause symptoms from nail prominence before fracture healing. This is especially true medially, where the rod is subcutaneous (**TECH FIG 5**).
- The incisions are closed with subcuticular suture, and a posterior splint is applied to allow tissue healing.

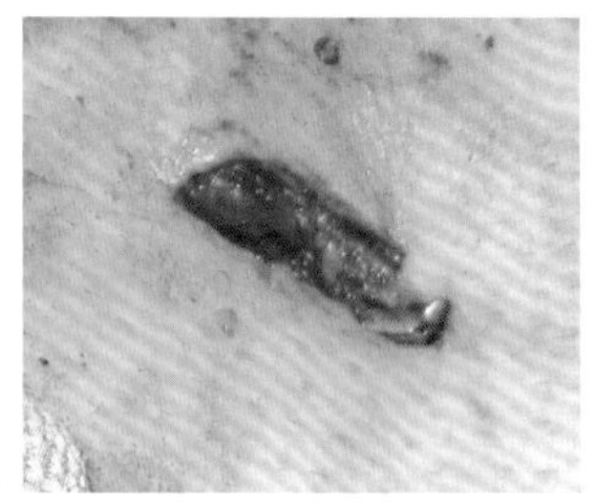


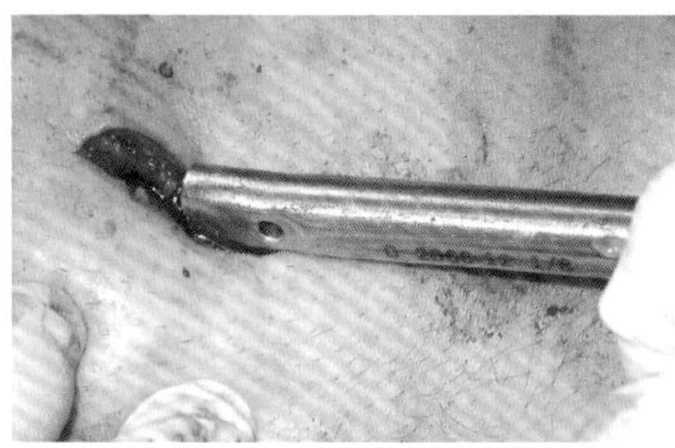


**TECH FIG 5** • Instead of cutting the nail under the skin, it can be withdrawn, cut at skin level (**A**), and tamped in to prevent irritation (**B**).

## PEARLS AND PITFALLS

| | |
|---|---|
| **Compartment syndrome** | ■ A high index of suspicion is required.<br>■ The surgeon must maintain vigilance throughout the postoperative period for late development.<br>■ Increasing pain and anxiety are the first signs of pediatric compartment syndrome. |
| **External fixation** | ■ Rigid frames may lead to delayed union.<br>■ Care should be taken to use appropriately sized pins and to dynamize early.<br>■ Fluoroscopic guidance is used to avoid growth plates. |
| **Plate fixation** | ■ Incisions should be carefully chosen to avoid compromised skin.<br>■ Low-profile plates may help avoid irritation from the plate before fracture healing. |
| **Elastic intramedullary** | ■ Fractures that are very distal or proximal, or highly comminuted, should be treated by other techniques.<br>■ Proper nail contouring and size selection are important to maintain stability of the fracture.<br>  ■ The nails should be the same diameter to provide balanced fixation (**FIG 4A**).<br>  ■ Nails should be passed carefully to avoid the "creeping vine" effect.<br>  ■ If the nails spiral around each other, the elastic recoil, and thus the stability of the technique, will be lost (**FIG 4B**).<br>■ Care should be taken to avoid physeal injury.<br>■ Nails should be cut short to avoid irritation. |

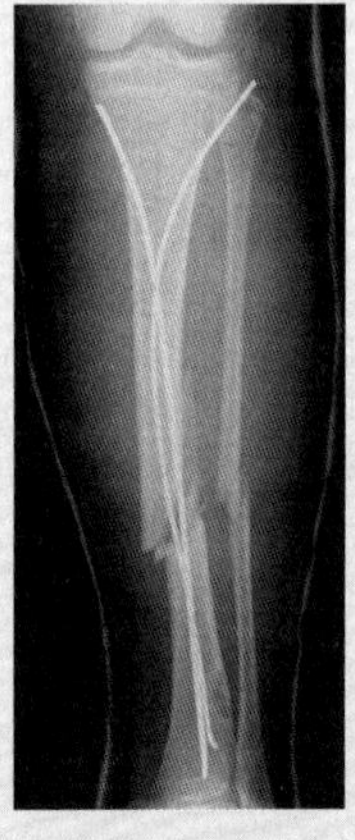
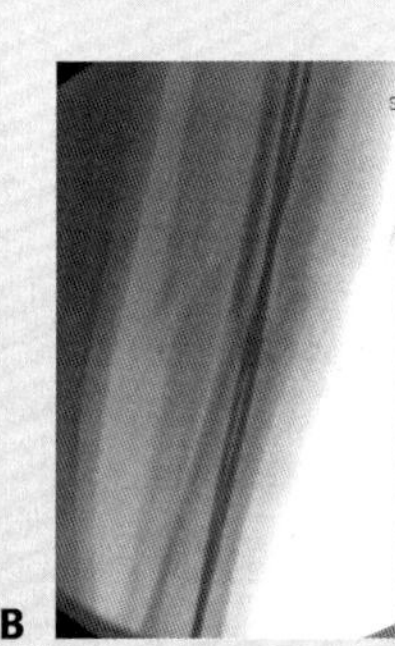

**FIG 4** • Potential pitfalls in nail placement. **A.** The nails are of differing diameter, inducing a valgus moment that needs to be controlled in a cast. Note the incidental nonossifying fibroma. **B.** "Spiraling nails." The elasticity afforded by three-point fixation is lost, making the construct less stable.

## POSTOPERATIVE CARE

- For patients treated with external fixation, a splint is used for 7 to 10 days to allow the tissues to recover.
  - For stable fractures, progressive weight bearing is initiated in reliable patients.
  - Unstable or comminuted fractures require waiting until visible callus is present before weight bearing.
  - Depending on fracture stability, dynamization of the fixator is initiated early, after sufficient callus is seen. The frame is removed in the office or the operating room after healing is noted radiographically.
  - Most patients benefit from short-term support with a bivalved cast after removal.
- Patients treated with plate fixation begin a progressive weight-bearing program, with immobilization discontinued after sufficient radiographic healing is present, usually by 6 weeks.
- Patients treated with elastic intramedullary fixation are usually splinted for 7 to 10 days, followed by progressive weight bearing. The plan is modified based on fracture stability, soft tissue injury, and patient reliability.
  - Patients with substantial (over 50%) cortical contact may begin weight bearing as tolerated after soft tissue healing has occurred.
- In general, prolonged stiffness is unusual in pediatric patients.
  - It is better to overimmobilize in questionable cases to avoid malalignment and regain motion later with aggressive physiotherapy.
- Removal of symptomatic hardware (ie, nails or plate) should be delayed until fracture healing and remodeling are complete.
  - I prefer to remove elastic nails electively in all patients 6 to 12 months after injury, as the nails will become completely intramedullary with significant continued growth, thus making late removal extremely difficult.
  - Ideally, plate removal is delayed for a year, after remodeling is complete.

## OUTCOMES

- Most tibial fractures in children will heal uneventfully, although healing difficulties can occur, especially in older patients.[5,10]
- Slongo[15] noted that most complications seen in his series were a result of improperly applied technique, particularly residual distraction at the fracture site, leading to a "pseudarthrosis model" even in children.
- Bar-On and associates[2] noted increased callus formation and shorter time to union in the elastic intramedullary nailing group versus external fixation (7 weeks compared with 10) in a femur model.

- Myers and coworkers[12] reported a significant complication rate in high-energy tibial fractures treated with external fixation, including delayed union, malunion, leg length discrepancies, and pin tract infections.
- Kubiak and colleagues[8] reported 2 delayed unions, 2 malunions, and 3 nonunions in a series of 15 patients managed with external fixation, although these appear to have occurred in open injuries.
  - They reported higher functional scores in their patients treated with elastic intramedullary nailing compared to external fixation.
- Operative techniques usually require additional procedures for removal of pins or prominent nails or plates.
- Obviously, operative complications do not occur in nonoperatively treated patients. Knowledge of proper indications is crucial to maximize outcomes.

## COMPLICATIONS

- Malunion
- Delayed union
- Leg length discrepancy
- Compartment syndrome
- Symptomatic hardware
- Infection

## REFERENCES


1. Bae DS, Kadiyala RK, Waters PM. Acute compartment syndrome in children: contemporary diagnosis, treatment, and outcome. J Pediatr Orthop 2001;21:680–688.
2. Bar-On E, Sagiv S, Porat S. External fixation or flexible intramedullary nailing for femoral shaft fractures in children. A prospective, randomised study. J Bone Joint Surg Br 1997;79(6):975–978.
3. DeLong WG Jr, Born CT, Marcelli E, et al. Ender nail fixation in long bone fractures: experience in a level I trauma center. J Trauma 1989;29:571–576.
4. Furlan D, Pogorelić Z, Biočić M, et al. Elastic stable intramedullary nailing for pediatric long bone fractures: experience with 175 fractures. Scand J Surg 2011;100(3):208–215.
5. Gicquel P, Giacomelli M, Basic B, et al. Problems of operative and non-operative and healing in tibial fractures. Injury 2005;36(suppl 1):A44–A50.
6. Goodwin RC, Gaynor T, Mahar A, et al. Intramedullary flexible nail fixation of unstable tibial diaphyseal fractures. J Pediatr Orthop 2005;25:570–576.
7. Hunter JB. The principles of elastic stable intramedullary nailing in children. Injury 2005;36(suppl 1):A21–A24.
8. Kubiak EN, Egol KA, Scher D, et al. Operative treatment of tibial fractures in children: are elastic stable intramedullary nails an improvement over external fixation? J Bone Joint Surg Am 2005;87(8):1761–1768.
9. Lascombes P, Huber H, Fay R, et al. Flexible intramedullary nailing in children: nail to medullary canal diameters optimal ratio. J Pediatr Orthop 2013;33(4):403–408.
10. Lascombes P, Nespola A, Poircuitte JM, et al. Early complications with flexible intramedullary nailing in childhood fracture: 100 cases managed with precurved tip and shaft nails. Orthop Traumatol Surg Res 2012;98(4):369–375.
11. Moulton SL. Early management of the child with multiple injuries. Clin Orthop Relat Res 2000;(376):6–14.
12. Myers SH, Speigel D, Flynn JM. External fixation of high-energy tibia fractures. J Pediatr Orthop 2007;27:537–539.
13. Norman D, Peskin B, Ehrenraich A, et al. The use of external fixators in the immobilization of pediatric fractures. Arch Orthop Trauma Surg 2002;122:379–382.
14. O'Brien T, Weisman DS, Ronchetti P, et al. Flexible titanium nailing for the treatment of unstable pediatric tibial fracture. J Pediatr Orthop 2004;24:601–609.
15. Slongo T. Complications and failures of the ESIN technique. Injury 2005;36:A78–A85.

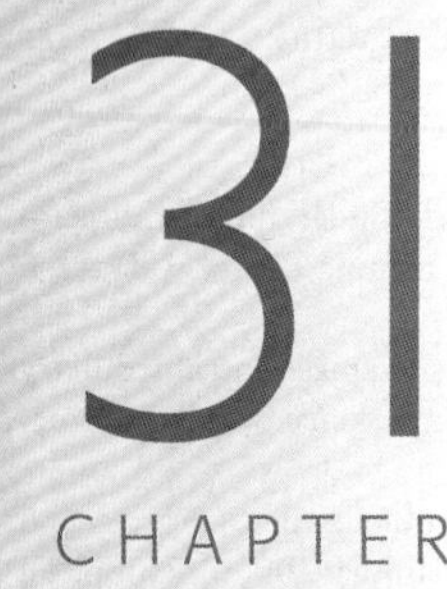

# External Fixation of the Mature Tibia

J. Tracy Watson

## DEFINITION

- Indications for external fixation of the tibial shaft in trauma applications include the treatment of open fractures with extensive soft tissue devitalization and contamination. Other indications include the stabilization of closed fractures with high-grade soft tissue injury or compartment syndrome. External fixation is favored when the fracture configuration extends into the metaphyseal/diaphyseal junction or the joint itself, making other treatment options problematic.
  - For patients with multiple long bone fractures, external fixation has been used as a method for temporary, if not definitive, stabilization.[3]
  - With the introduction of circular and hybrid techniques, indications have been expanded to include the definitive treatment of complex periarticular injuries, which include high-energy tibial plateau and distal tibial pilon fractures.[4]
  - Hexapod fixators can be used to perform gradual reductions of the tibial shaft or periarticular injuries in cases of severe soft tissue injury where soft tissue coverage procedures are contraindicated and in cases of delayed presentation where acute distraction and reduction would compromise neurovascular elements[12] (**FIG 1F**).
- Contemporary external fixation systems in current clinical use can be categorized according to the type of bone anchorage used.
  - Fixation is achieved either using large threaded pins, which are screwed into the bone, or by drilling small-diameter transfixion wires through the bone. The pins or wires are then connected to one another through the use of longitudinal bars or circular rings.
  - The distinction is thus between monolateral external fixation (longitudinal connecting pins to bars) and circular external fixation (wires and/or pins connecting to rings).
- Acute trauma applications primarily use monolateral frame configurations and are the focus of techniques described here.
  - The first type of monolateral frame is modular with individual components: separate bars, attachable pin–bar clamps, bar-to-bar clamps, and Schanz pins (**FIG 1A,B**). These "simple monolateral" frames allow for a wide range of flexibility with "build-up" or "build-down" capabilities.

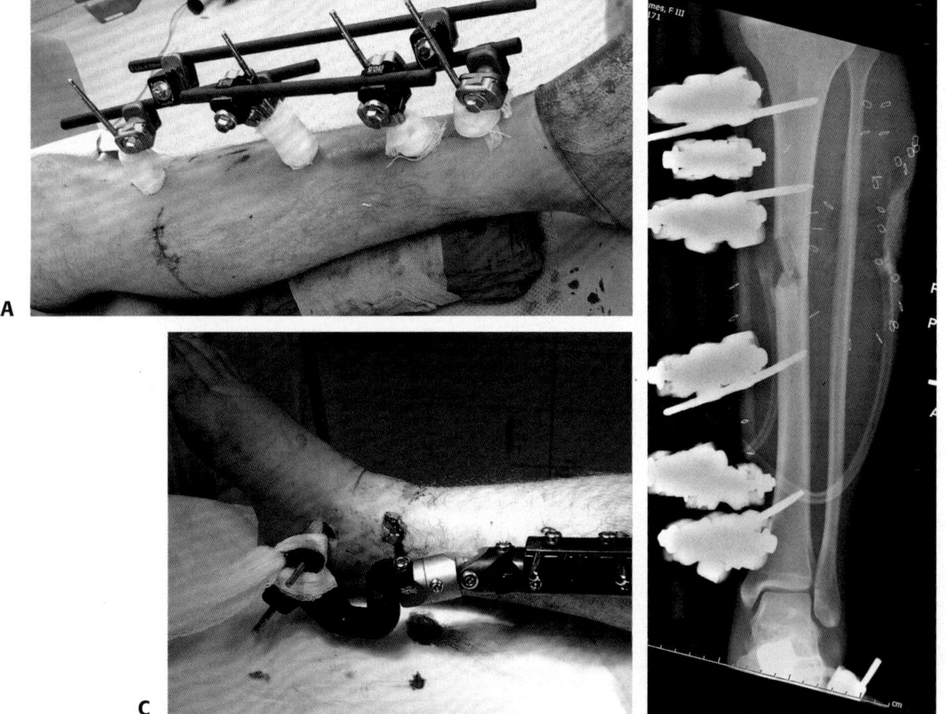

**FIG 1** • **A.** Simple monolateral four-pin frame with a double-stack connecting bar to increase frame stability. **B.** X-ray demonstrating ability to connect the fixation pins to each limb segment in a variety of ways to achieve a congruent reduction. **C.** Large monotube fixator spanning the ankle for a severe pilon fracture. This was applied to temporize the soft tissues before definitive open stabilization of the injury. *(continued)*

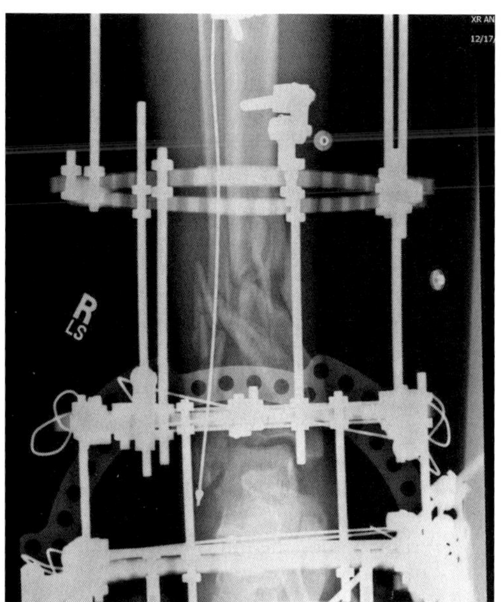

D

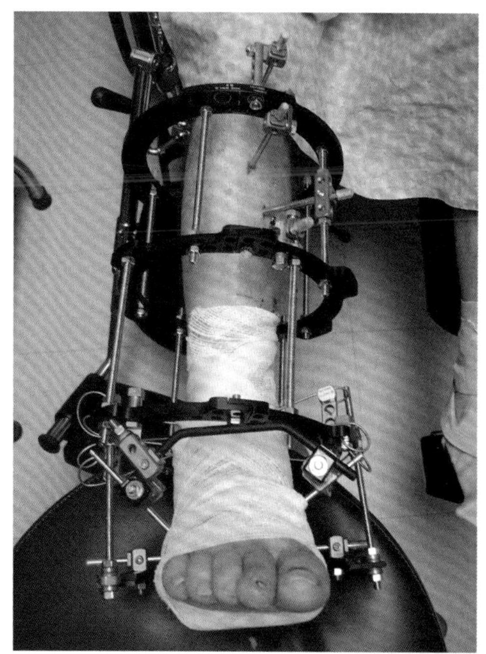

E

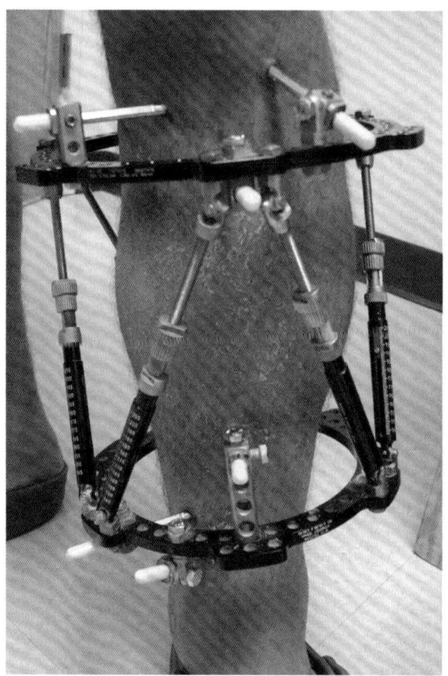

F

**FIG 1** • *(continued)* **D,E.** Small tensioned wire circular fixator used for definitive management of a distal tibial periarticular fracture with proximal shaft extension. The versatility of these frames allows for spanning into the foot to maintain a plantigrade position. **F.** A hexapod frame attached to the bone with large Schanz pins. This frame allows for gradual correction of fracture displacement over time by adjusting the six distractors.

- The second type of monolateral frame is a more constrained type of fixator that comes preassembled with a multipin clamp at each end of a long rigid tubular body. The telescoping tube allows for axial compression or distraction of this so-called monotube-type fixator (**FIG 1C**).
- For diaphyseal injuries, the most common type of fixator application is the monolateral frame using large pins for skeletal stabilization.
  - Simple monolateral fixators have the distinct advantage of allowing individual pins to be placed at different angles and varying obliquities while still connecting to the bar. This is helpful when altering the pin position to avoid areas of soft tissue compromise (ie, open wounds or severe contusion).[9]
  - The advantage of the monotube-type fixator is its simplicity. Pin placement is predetermined by the multipin clamps. Loosening the universal articulations between the body and the clamps allows these frames to be easily manipulated to reduce a fracture.
- Many high-energy fractures involve the metaphyseal regions, and transfixion techniques using small tensioned wires are ideally suited to this region. They have better mechanical stability and longevity than traditional half-pin techniques.
  - Small tensioned wire circular frames or hybrid frames (frames using a combination of large half-pins and transfixion wires) can be useful in patients with severe tibial metaphyseal injuries that occur in concert with other conditions such as soft tissue compromise or compartment syndrome or in patients with multiple injuries (**FIG 1D,E**).

- Hexapod fixators are ring fixators consisting of six distractors and 12 ball joints which allow for 6 degrees of freedom of bone fragment displacement. By adjusting the simple distractors, gradual three-dimensional corrections or acute reductions are possible without the need for complicated frame mechanisms (**FIG 1F**).

## ANATOMY

- The bulk of the tibia is easily accessible in that most of the diaphyseal portions are subcutaneous.
  - The hard cortical bone found in this location is ideally suited to the placement of large Schanz pins, which achieves excellent mechanical fixation.
  - The cross-sectional anatomy of the diaphysis and the lateral location of the muscular compartments allow placement of half-pins in a wide range of subcutaneous locations. This facilitates pin placement "out of plane" or divergent to each other, which helps achieve excellent frame stability (**FIG 2**).
- The proximal and distal periarticular metaphyseal regions of the tibia are also subcutaneous except for their lateral surfaces. The bone in these locations is primarily cancellous, with thin cortical walls.
  - The mechanical stability achieved with half-pins depends on cortical purchase and therefore may not be adequate for fixation in this cortex-deficient region.
  - Excellent stability is afforded in these areas by using small-diameter tensioned transfixion wires in conjunction with circular external fixators. Metaphyseal transfixion wires can be combined with diaphyseal half-pins can be combined to produce frames for periarticular fracture fixation for complex pilon and plateau fractures.

## PATHOGENESIS

- Open tibial diaphyseal fractures are primarily candidates for closed intramedullary nailing, but there are occasions when external fixation is indicated.
  - External fixation is favored when there is significant contamination and severe soft tissue injury or when the fracture configuration extends into the metaphyseal–diaphyseal junction or the joint itself, making intramedullary nailing problematic.

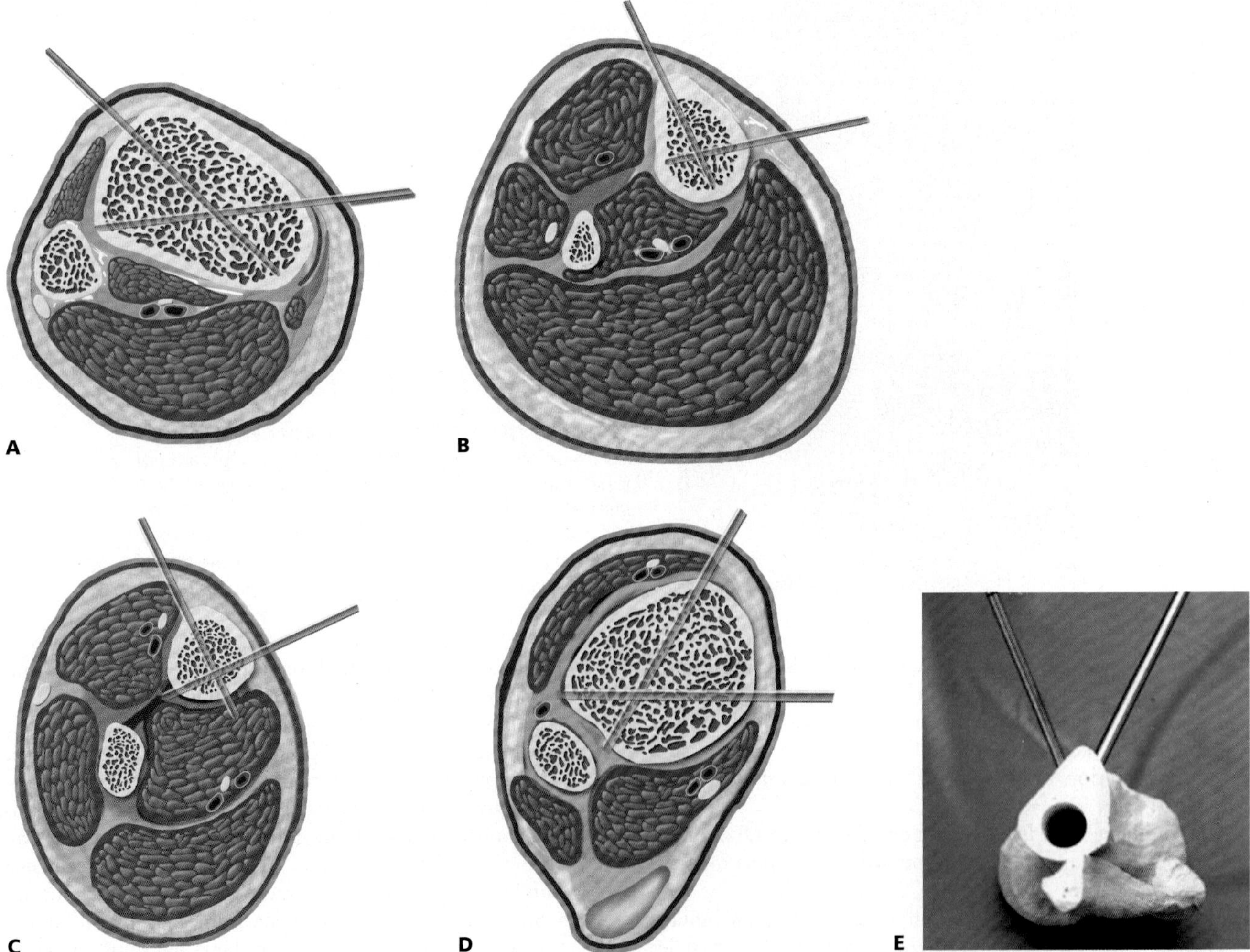

**FIG 2 • A–D.** Cross-sectional anatomy of the tibia at all levels. The proximal cross-section demonstrates the ability to achieve at least 120 degrees of pin divergence in this region with progressively smaller diversion angles as the pins are placed distally. It is important to avoid tethering of any musculotendinous structures. To accomplish this, pins are placed primarily along the subcutaneous border of the tibia. **E.** Model showing similar pin placement avoiding the anterolateral and posterior muscular compartments. Posterior cortex pin protrusion is minimal to avoid damaging any posterior neurovascular structures.

- The choice of external fixator type depends on the location and complexity of the fracture as well as the type of wound present when dealing with open injuries.
  - The less stable the fracture pattern (ie, the more comminution), the more complex a frame needs to be applied to control motion at the bone ends.
  - If possible, weight bearing should be a consideration.
  - If periarticular extension or involvement is present, the ability to bridge the joint with the frame provides satisfactory stability for both hard and soft tissues.
  - It is important that the frame be constructed and applied to allow for multiple débridements and subsequent soft tissue reconstruction. This demands that the pins are placed away from the zone of injury to avoid potential pin site contamination with the operative field.
- Fractures treated with external fixation heal with external bridging callus. External bridging callus is largely under the control of mechanical and other humoral factors and is highly dependent on the integrity of the surrounding soft tissue envelope. This type of fracture healing has the ability to bridge large gaps and is very tolerant of movement.
  - Micromotion with the external fixator construct has been found to accentuate fracture union. It results in the development of a large callus with formation of cartilage due to the greater inflammatory response caused by increased micromovement of the fragments.
  - There appears to be a threshold at which the degree of micromotion becomes inhibitory to this overall remodeling process, however, so hypertrophic nonunion can result from an unstable external frame.
- Temporary spanning fixation for complex articular injuries is used routinely. The ability to achieve an initial ligamentotaxis reduction substantially decreases the amount of injury-related swelling and edema by reducing large fracture gaps.
  - It is important to achieve an early ligamentotaxis reduction: A delay of more than a few days will result in an inability to disimpact and adequately reduce displaced metaphyseal fragments with distraction alone.
  - Once the soft tissues have recovered, definitive open reconstruction can be accomplished with relative ease as the operative tactic can be directed to the area of articular involvement.[13]
- Application of these techniques in a polytrauma patient is valuable when rapid stabilization is necessary for a patient in extremis. Simple monolateral or monotube fixators can be placed rapidly across long bone injuries, providing adequate stabilization to facilitate the management and resuscitation of the polytrauma patient (**FIG 3**).

## NATURAL HISTORY

- The stability of all monolateral fixators is based on the concept of a simple "four-pin frame."
  - Pin number, pin separation, and pin proximity to the fracture site, as well as bone bar distance and the diameter of the pins and connecting bars, all influence the final mechanical stability of the external fixator frame.[1]
- Large pin monolateral fixators rely on stiff pins for frame stability. On loading, these pins act as cantilevers and produce eccentric loading characteristics. Shear forces are regarded as inhibitory to fracture healing and bone formation, and this may be accentuated with pins placed in all the same orientation.

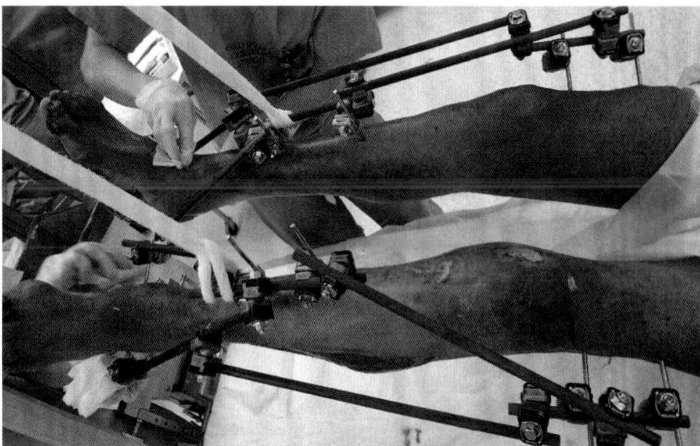

**FIG 3** • Polytrauma patient with bilateral temporary spanning fixators. External fixation on the *right side* spans bicondylar tibial plateau fracture with an ipsilateral pilon fracture. The left knee is bridged to stabilize a tibial plateau fracture and a severe bimalleolar ankle fracture. The left leg injury is complicated by a compartment syndrome with open fasciotomy wounds.

- After stable frame application, the soft tissue injury can be addressed. Once the soft tissues have healed, conversion to definitive internal fixation can be safely accomplished. In some cases, the external device is the definitive treatment. Dynamic weight bearing is initiated at an early stage once the fracture is deemed stable.
  - In fractures that are highly comminuted, weight bearing is delayed until visible callus is achieved and sufficient stability has been maintained. As healing progresses, active dynamization of the frame may be required to achieve solid union.
- Dynamization converts a static fixator, which seeks to neutralize all forces including axial motion, and allows the passage of forces across the fracture site. As the elasticity of the callus decreases, bone stiffness and strength increase and larger loads can be supported.[7] Thus, axial dynamization helps to restore cortical contact and to produce a stable fracture pattern with inherent mechanical support.[2] This is accomplished by making adjustments in the pin–bar clamps with simple monolateral fixators or in releasing the body on a monotube-type fixator.
- Bony healing is not complete until remodeling of the fracture has been achieved. At this stage, the visible fracture lines in the callus decrease and subsequently disappear. The fixator can be removed at this point.

## PATIENT HISTORY AND PHYSICAL FINDINGS

- History should focus on the mechanism of injury.
  - Determining whether the injury was high energy versus low energy gives the surgeon an idea of the extent of the soft tissue zone of injury and will help determine the possible location of fixation pins.
- Determining the location of the accident is helpful in cases of open fracture (ie, open field with soil contamination vs. slip and fall on ice and snow).
  - These parameters give the surgeon an idea as to the extent of intraoperative débridement that might be required to cleanse the wound and the necessary antibiotic coverage for the injury.

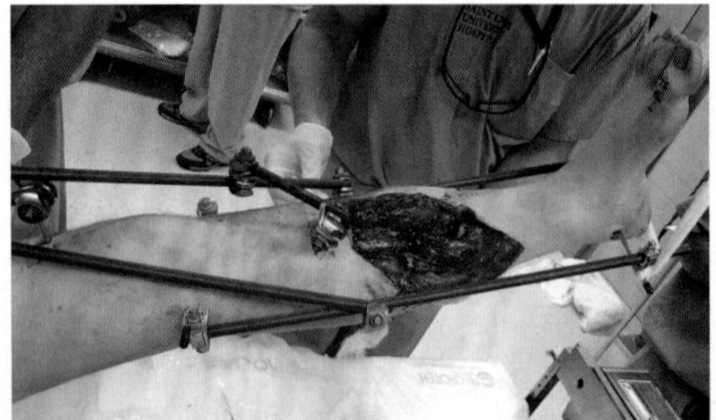

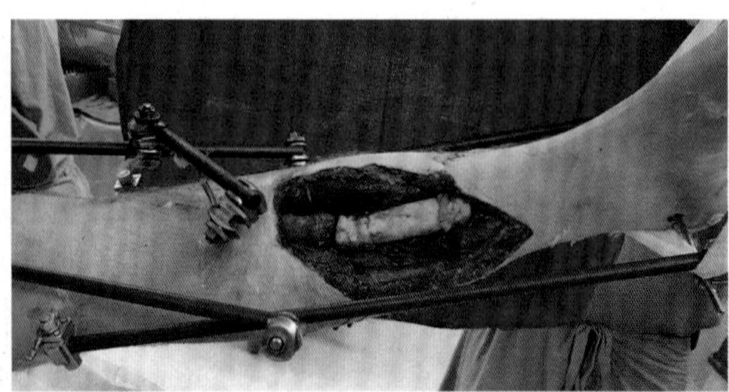

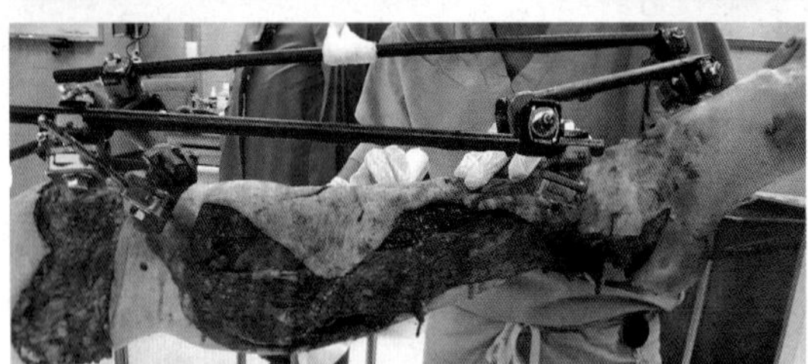

**FIG 4** • **A.** Extensive open grade 3b injury with bone and soft tissue loss dictates judicious pin placement to avoid placing pins directly into the open wound. **B.** The ability to place fixation pins out of the zone of injury allows multiple débridements to be performed with disturbing the original fixation montage. An intercalary antibiotic spacer was inserted in the skeletal defect to augment the overall frame stability. **C.** The extensive lacerations in this grade 3b injury determined the variable pin placement of this monolateral frame spanning the large zone of injury and helped facilitate multiple débridement procedures for this complex tibial shaft fracture. The frame was spanned across the ankle to control the hindfoot due to a partial heel pad avulsion.

- The neurovascular status should be documented, specifically the presence or absence of the anterior and posterior tibial pulses at the ankle.
  - A weak or absent pulse may be an indication of vascular injury and may dictate further evaluation with ankle–brachial indices, compartment pressure evaluation, or a formal arteriogram.
  - Evaluation of compartment pressures is often indicated in open fractures and closed high-energy fractures with severe soft tissue contusion.
- Evaluation of soft tissues and grading of the open fracture with regard to the size, orientation, and location of the open wounds aid in decision making about pin placement and the configuration of the fixator to allow access to open wounds (**FIG 4**).

## IMAGING AND OTHER DIAGNOSTIC STUDIES

- Imaging of the tibia should include at least two orthogonal views, anteroposterior and lateral.
  - Radiographs of the knee and ankle are necessary to evaluate any articular fracture involvement or associated knee or ankle subluxation or dislocation.
  - Identifying any occult fracture lines aids in the preoperative planning of potential pin placement.
  - Many patients with high-energy tibial fractures have associated foot injuries, and views of the foot and ankle are necessary to identify this injury pattern.
- Traction radiographs of articular injuries of the tibia are useful to identify the nature and orientation of metaphyseal fragments as well as degree of articular impaction. This aids in determining whether a joint-spanning fixator is necessary.
- Distraction computed tomography (CT) scans should be obtained *after* the knee- or ankle-spanning fixator has been applied. These studies indicate the effectiveness of the ligamentotaxis reduction. This allows the surgeon to determine the preoperative plan for definitive fixation once the soft tissues have recovered[14] (**FIG 5**).

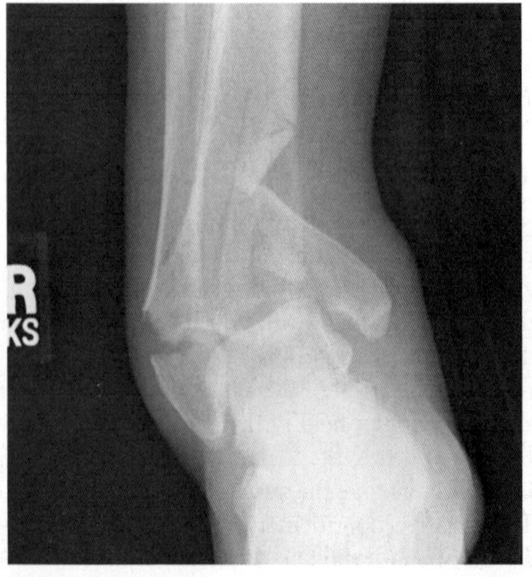

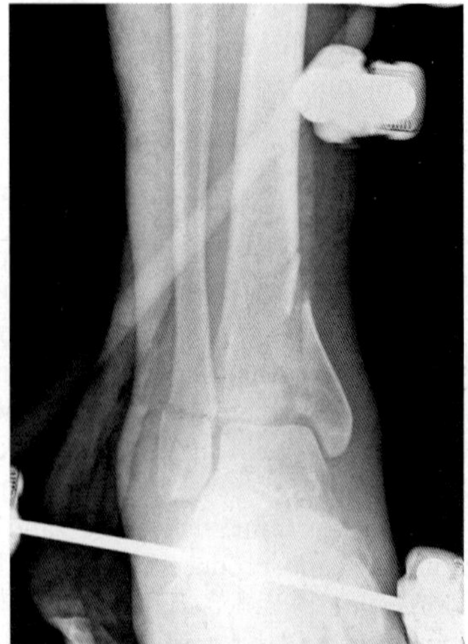

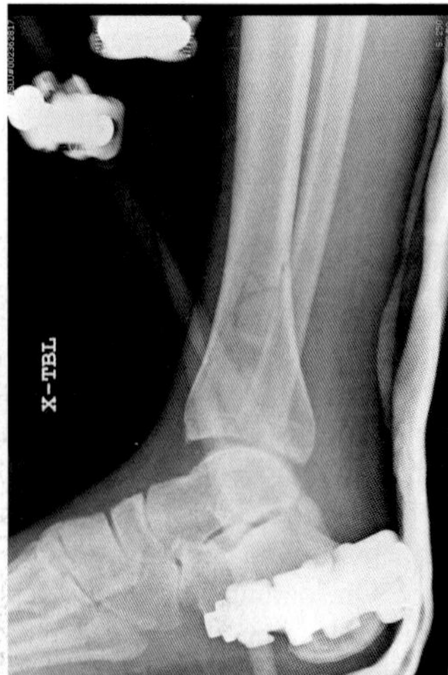


**FIG 5** • **A–C.** Injury and post external fixation films demonstrating an ankle-spanning frame stabilizing a complex pilon fracture. *(continued)*

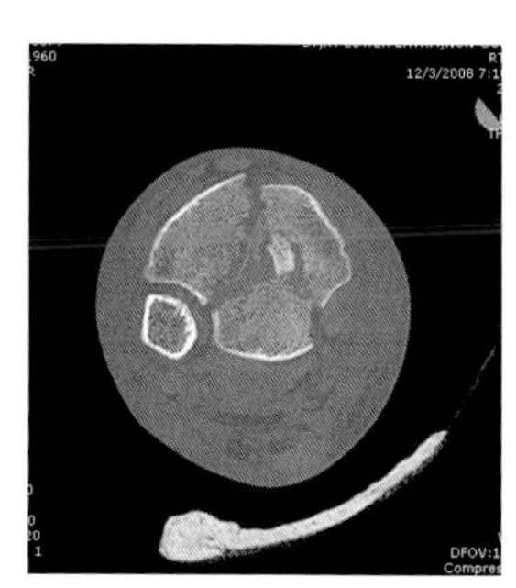

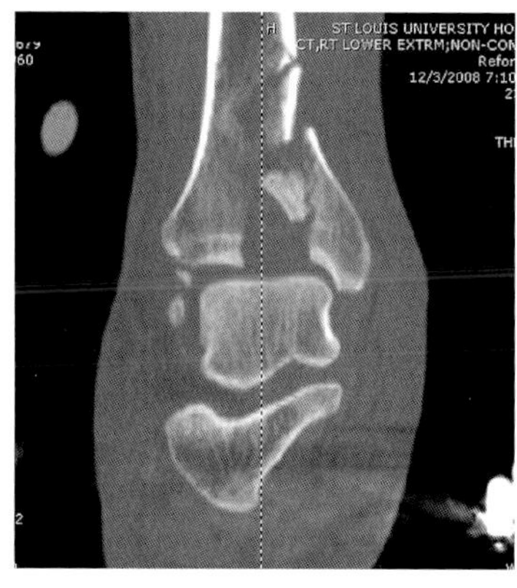

**FIG 5** • *(continued)* **D,E.** CT scan obtained post distraction in the frame provides valuable information to help determine the preoperative plan for delayed definitive reconstruction once the soft tissues have recovered.

## SURGICAL MANAGEMENT

- The surgical decisions relate to the configuration of the external device to be applied. These generally will fall into two categories of treatment options.
- The first category is a temporary device intended to allow the soft tissues to recover or the patient's overall condition to improve until definitive fixation of the injury can be safely carried out.
  - Temporary frames include knee- or ankle-spanning fixators used in cases of periarticular injuries requiring ligamentotaxis reduction and relative stabilization and simple frames spanning a tibial shaft fracture in the case of a polytrauma patient who needs emergent stabilization of injuries. These frames are later converted to intramedullary nails once the patient can undergo additional surgery.[6]
  - They are simplistic and not intended for long-term treatment times.
- Definitive treatment fixators are primarily applied to diaphyseal injuries with severe soft tissue compromise (open and closed).
  - These devices are maintained throughout the entire treatment period to allow access to soft tissues and facilitate secondary procedures such as rotational or free flap coverage as well as delayed bone grafting.
  - These frames are more involved and are intended to remain in place for the entire treatment period (ie, hexapod fixators).

### Preoperative Planning

- Evaluation of injury radiographs should identify any distal or proximal articular extension into the knee or ankle joint.
- Location of the primary fracture is noted in terms of proximal or distal locations to help decide on a particular fixator construct and to help determine if a joint-spanning fixator is required.

### Positioning

- The patient's entire lower extremity is elevated using bumps or a beanbag patient positioner under the ipsilateral hip (**FIG 6**). This elevates the tibia off the operating table.

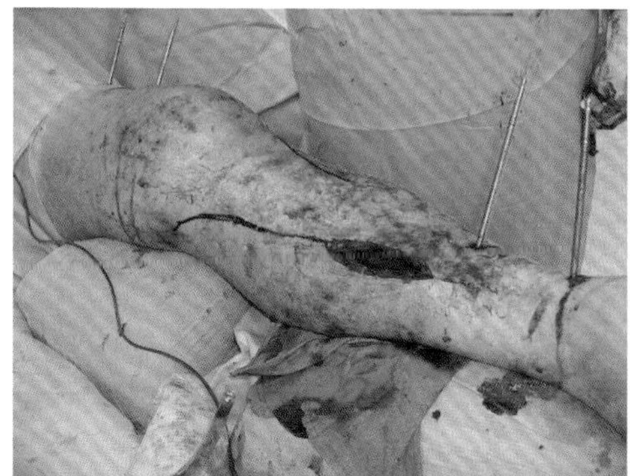

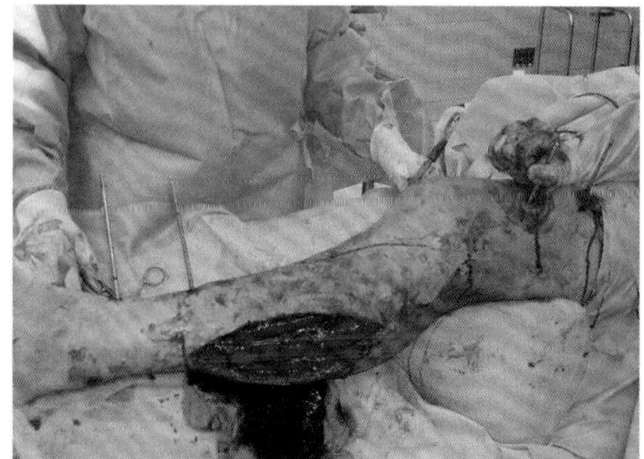

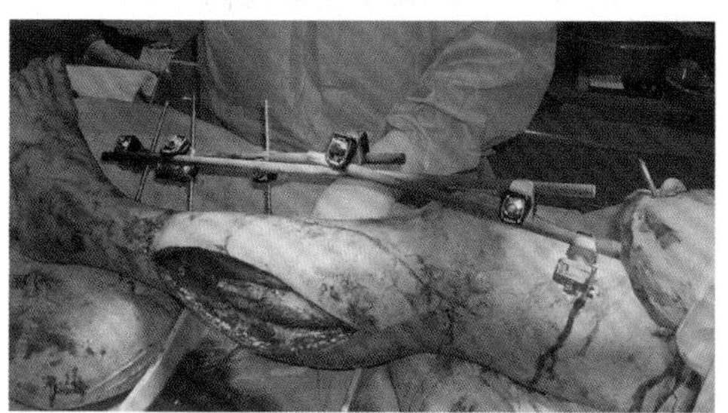

**FIG 6** • **A–C.** A knee-spanning frame is applied for a complex plateau fracture with associated compartment syndrome. The injured limb is elevated using sterile bumps or a beanbag patient positioner placed under the ipsilateral hip. This allows the injured leg to be visualized via fluoroscopy without interference from the opposite "down" leg. A sterile bump is also used to support the ankle, allowing 360-degree access to the injured tibial plateau region and providing clearance for any fixator configuration or secondary procedure necessary.

- The foot can be supported with a sterile bump, thus suspending the limb and allowing full 360-degree access and visualization of the limb.
  - Elevating the limb positions the nonoperative leg below the operative limb, which aids in placing out-of-plane pins as well as circular frame components.
- The image intensifier is positioned opposite the operative leg. This aids in fluoroscopic visualization of the femur and knee, which is important when applying a knee-spanning fixator for a severe tibial plateau fracture.
- The location of any proposed periarticular incisions should be carefully marked on the skin to ensure that eventual pin placement does not encroach into this region[8] (see **FIG 6**).

## Approach

- The integrity of the pin–bone interface is a critical factor in determining the longevity of an applied external fixation pin.
- Pin insertion technique is important in achieving an infection-free, stable pin–bone interface and thus maintaining frame stability.



## Pin Insertion Technique

- The correct insertion technique involves incising the skin directly at the side of pin insertion.
- After a generous incision is made, dissection is carried directly down to bone and the periosteum is incised where anatomically feasible (**TECH FIG 1A**).
- A small Penfield-type elevator is used to gently reflect the periosteum off the bone at the site of insertion (**TECH FIG 1B**). Extraneous soft tissue tethering and necrosis is avoided by minimizing soft tissue at the site of insertion.
- A trocar and drill sleeve are advanced directly to bone, minimizing the amount of soft tissue entrapment that might be encountered during predrilling (**TECH FIG 1C,D**). A sleeve should also be used if a self-drilling pin is selected.
- After predrilling, an appropriate-size depth of pin is advanced by hand to achieve bicortical purchase. Any offending soft tissue tethering should be released with a small scalpel (**TECH FIG 1E,F**).
- Fluoroscopy is used to ensure that transcortical pin placement is avoided (**TECH FIG 1G**).

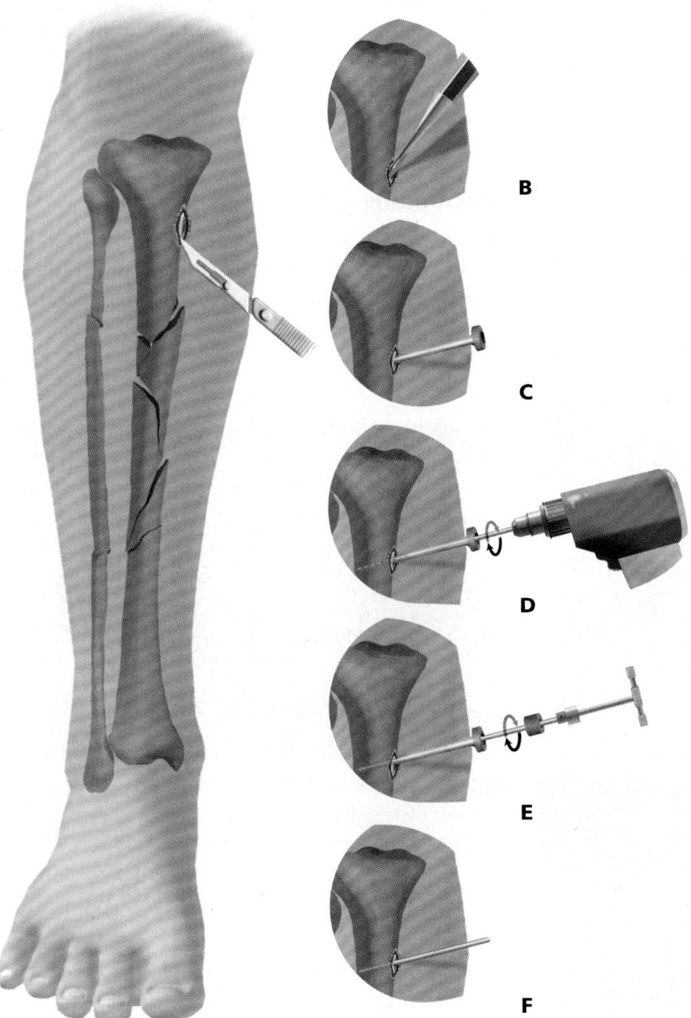


**TECH FIG 1** • Proper pin insertion technique. **A.** A generous incision is made over the location of the pin site. **B.** A small elevator is used to elevate all soft tissues, including the periosteum, off the bone to help avoid the tethering of excessive soft tissues during predrilling and pin insertion. **C.** A trocar is advanced to bone to protect the soft tissues. **D.** The pin site is predrilled through the trocar to avoid incarcerating and tethering soft tissues. **E,F.** A T-handle insertion chuck is used to hand-torque the pin into position, achieving purchase in both the near and far cortices. *(continued)*

TECHNIQUES

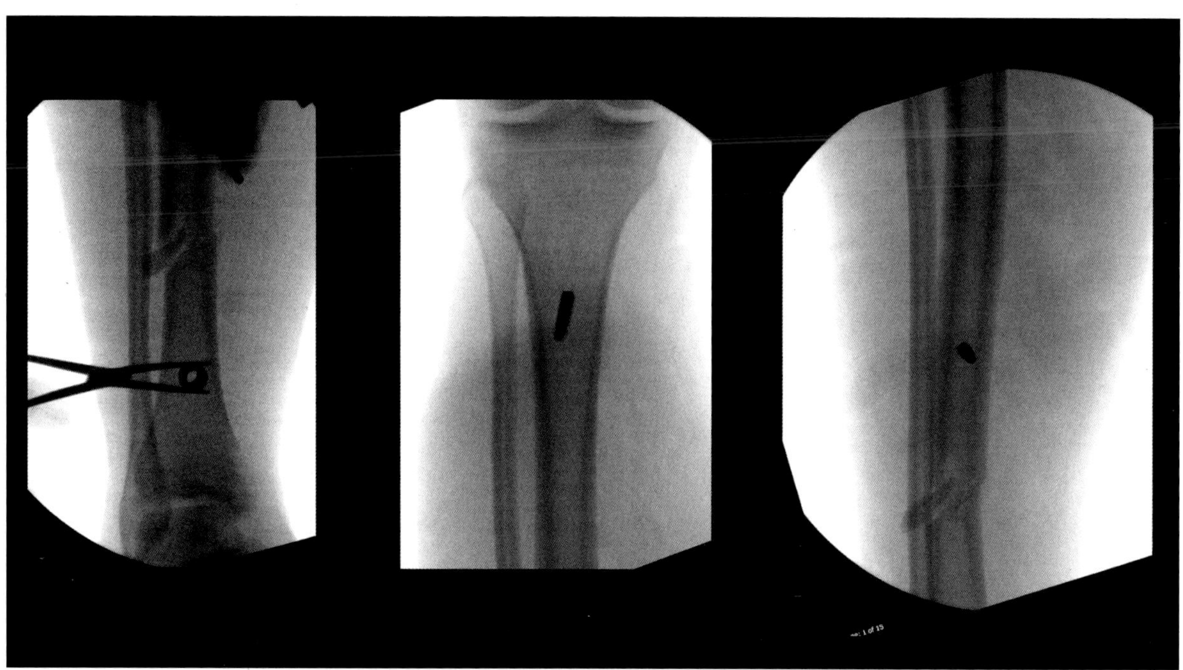

TECH FIG 1 • *(continued)* **G**. It is important to place the trocar over the center of the medullary canal and confirm its location to ensure that the pin captures the near cortex, medullary canal, and far cortex. This confirms that a transcortical pin is avoided, as these pins can be stress risers and may lead to pin-related fracture or pin infection due to the drilling and placement in only hard, dense cortical bone.

## Monolateral Four-Pin Frame Application for Tibial Shaft Fracture

- Contemporary simple monolateral fixators have clamps that allow independent adjustments at each pin–bar interface, allowing wide variability in pin placement, which helps to avoid areas of soft tissue compromise.
  - Because of this feature, simple four-pin placement may be random on either side of the fracture.

### Option 1

- The initial two pins are first inserted as far away from the fracture line as possible in the proximal fracture segment and as distal as possible in the distal fracture segment (**TECH FIG 2A**).
- A solitary connecting rod is attached close to the bone to increase the rigidity of the system.
- Longitudinal traction is applied and a gross reduction is achieved (**TECH FIG 2B–F**).
- The intermediate pins can then be inserted using the pin fixation clamps attached to the rod to act as templates with drill sleeves as guides.
- These pins should not encroach on the open wound or severely contused skin in the immediate zone of injury.
- After placement of these two additional pins, the reduction can be achieved with minimal difficulty by additional manipulation of the fracture.
- Once satisfactory reduction has been accomplished, the clamps are tightened and reduction is confirmed via fluoroscopy.

### Option 2

- Alternatively, all the fixation pins can be inserted independent of each other, with two pins proximally and two pins distally (**TECH FIG 3**).
- The two proximal pins are connected to a solitary bar and the distal two pins are connected to a solitary bar.
- Both proximal and distal bars are then used as reduction tools to manipulate the fracture into alignment.
- Once reduction has been achieved, an additional bar-to-bar construct between the two fixed-pin couples is connected.
- Reduction is confirmed under fluoroscopy.

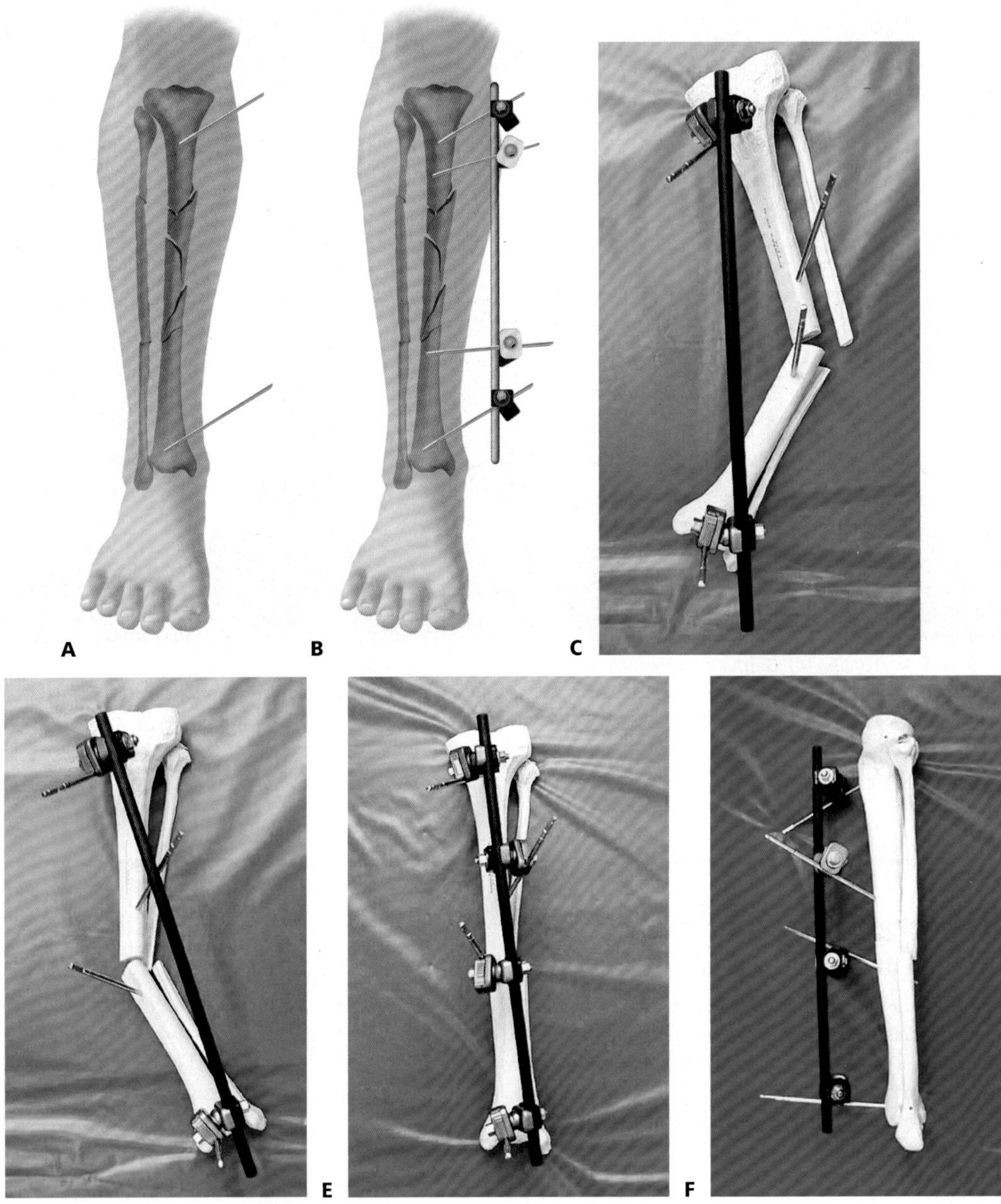

**TECH FIG 2** • Placement of a simple four-pin monolateral fixator. **A.** Two pins are placed on either side of the fracture as far from the fracture as possible. A connecting bar is then attached to the two pins (**B**) and a gradual reduction is performed (**C–F**). Two pins are then placed as close to the fracture as possible on either side, after longitudinal traction has accomplished a reduction. The inner pins are then attached, and the reduction is fine-tuned.

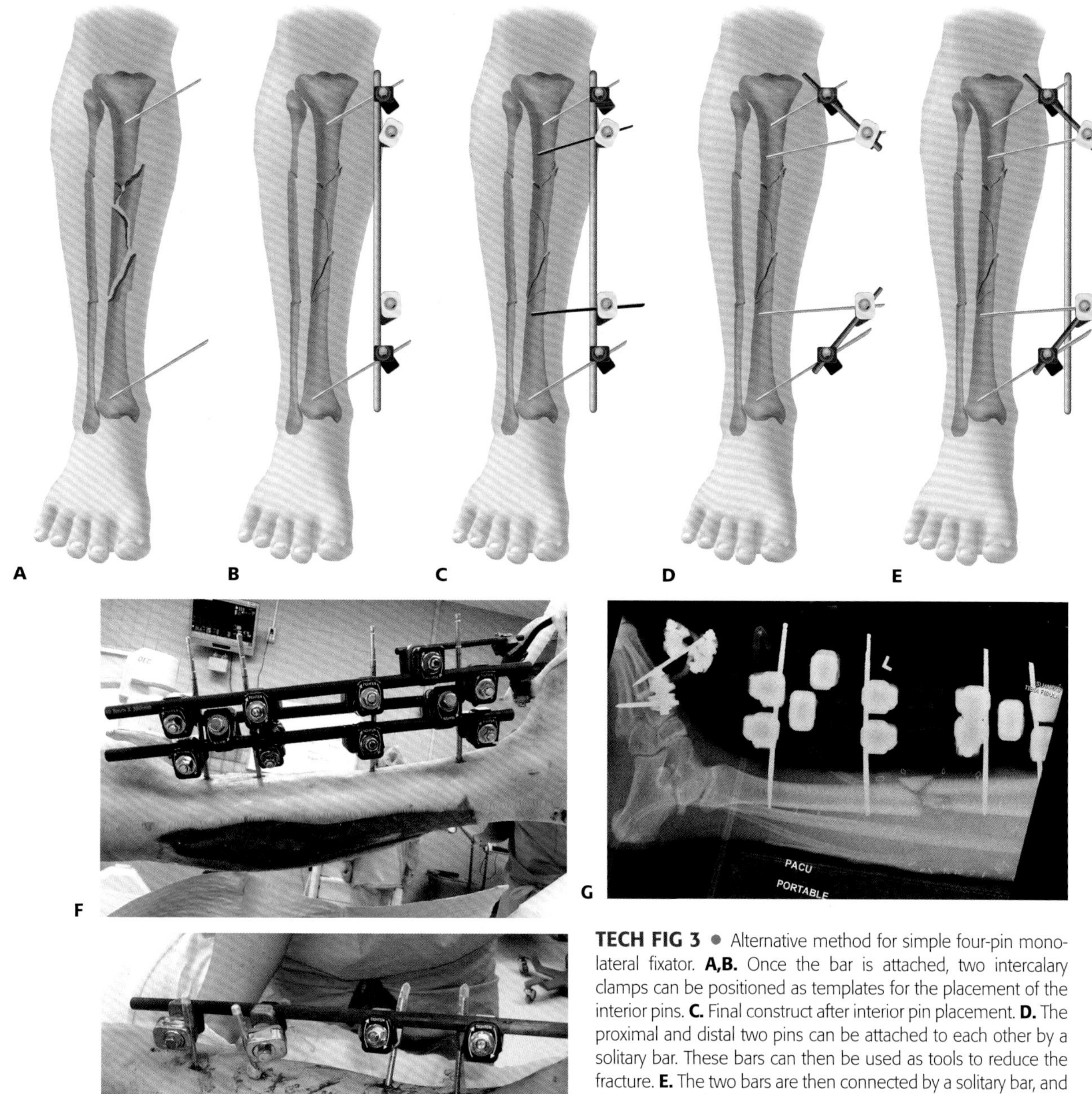


**TECH FIG 3** • Alternative method for simple four-pin monolateral fixator. **A,B.** Once the bar is attached, two intercalary clamps can be positioned as templates for the placement of the interior pins. **C.** Final construct after interior pin placement. **D.** The proximal and distal two pins can be attached to each other by a solitary bar. These bars can then be used as tools to reduce the fracture. **E.** The two bars are then connected by a solitary bar, and the fracture reduction is maintained. **F,G.** Closed fracture with associated compartment syndrome is reduced and stabilized using a four-pin fixator with a double stack bar for stability, and the foot is spanned to maintain a plantigrade foot. **H.** Similar tibial fracture reduced with four pins and a single bar. Note pins out of plane to each other to facilitate ease of pin insertion.

## Monotube Four-Pin Frame Application for Tibial Shaft Fracture

- Use of the large monotube fixators facilitates rapid placement of these devices, with the fixed-pin couple acting as pin templates (**TECH FIG 4**).
- Two pins are placed through the fixator pin couple proximal to the fracture. They are inserted parallel to each other at fixed distances set by the pin clamp itself. These are usually oriented along the direct medial or anteromedial face of the tibial shaft.
  - Once the pins are inserted, the pin clamp is tightened to secure them in place.

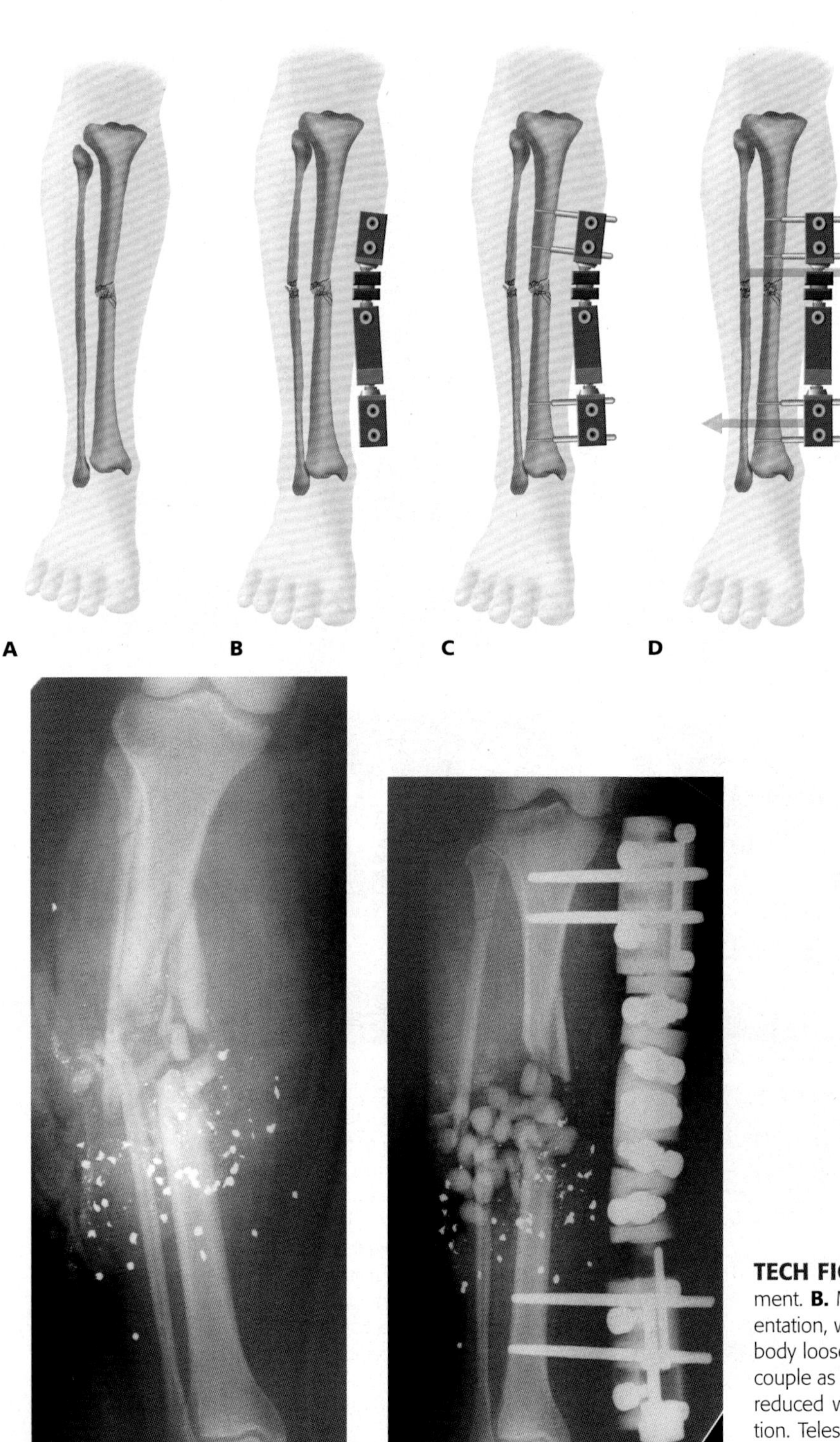


**TECH FIG 4** • **A.** Tibial shaft fracture with displacement. **B.** Monotube fixator adjusted to length and orientation, with all ball joints and the telescoping central body loosened. **C.** Proximal two pins applied using pin couple as template. **D.** Distal pins inserted and fracture reduced with all ball joints locked to maintain reduction. Telescoping body is also locked to maintain axial alignment. **E,F.** Injury and reduction radiographs using a large-body monotube fixator for an open comminuted tibial shaft fracture.

- The monotube body is then attached to the proximal pin couple and longitudinal traction applied to achieve a "gross" reduction. The fixator body and distal multipin clamp are oriented along the shaft of the tibia.
  - The proximal and distal ball joints should be freely movable with the telescoping body extended.
- Two pins are placed through the pin couple distal to the fracture and tightened.
  - Care must be taken to allow adequate length of the monotube frame before final reduction and tightening of the body.[11]

- Using the proximal and distal pin clamps as reduction aids, the fracture is manually reduced. The proximal and distal ball joints are then tightened, accomplishing a reduction.
- At this point, the telescoping body can be extended or compressed to dial in the axial alignment. When length is achieved, the body component is tightened to maintain axial length.
- Monotube bodies have a very large diameter, which limits the amount of shearing, torsional, and bending movements of the fixation construct.
  - Axial compression is achieved by releasing the telescoping mechanism.
- Dynamic weight bearing is initiated at an early stage once the fracture is deemed stable.
  - In fractures that are highly comminuted, weight bearing is delayed until visible callus is achieved and sufficient stability has been maintained.
- The telescopic body allows dynamic movement in an axial direction, which is a stimulus for early periosteal healing.

## Knee-Spanning Fixator of Tibial Plateau Fracture

- Two Schanz pins are placed along the anterolateral thigh. These pins are placed in the midshaft region of the femur (**TECH FIG 5**).
- Two Schanz pins are then inserted into the midshaft and distal tibia.
- Apply the tibial pins far enough away from the distal extension of the proximal tibia such that any future incisions required to perform definitive open reduction and internal fixation of the plateau fracture would not impinge on the pins.
- A solitary bar can then be used to span all pins.
  - Longitudinal traction is applied and reduction confirmed under fluoroscopy.
  - Slight flexion of the knee is maintained and all connections are tightened to maintain the ligamentotaxis reduction.
- Alternatively, the proximal two femur pins can be connected using a single bar and the two tibial pins with a second bar. These two bars can then be manipulated to achieve a reduction of the plateau, and a third bar connecting the proximal femoral and distal tibial bars is then attached and tightened to maintain the reduction.
- A large monotube fixator can also be used in this fashion to span the knee and maintain a temporary reduction.

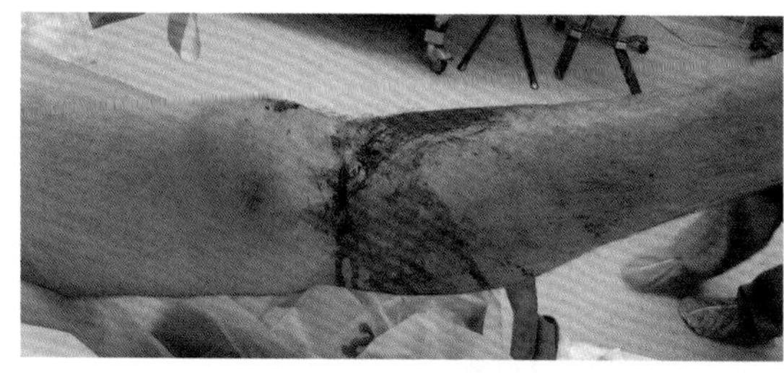

A

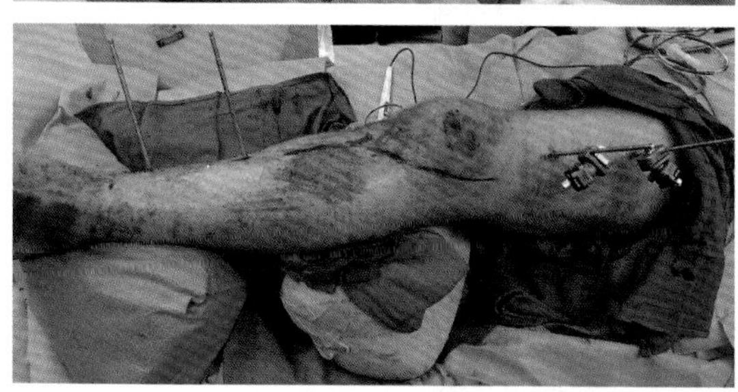

C

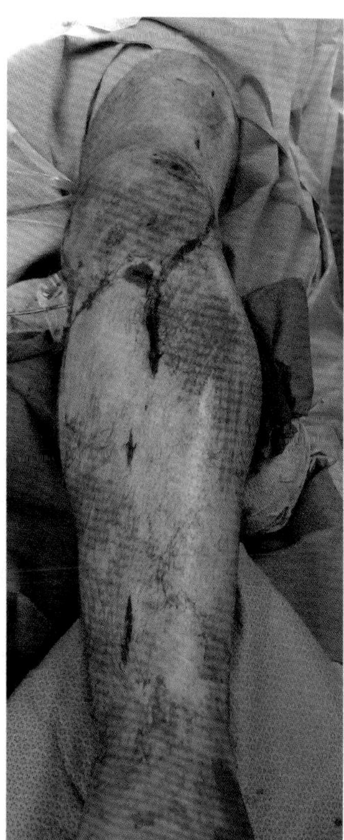

B

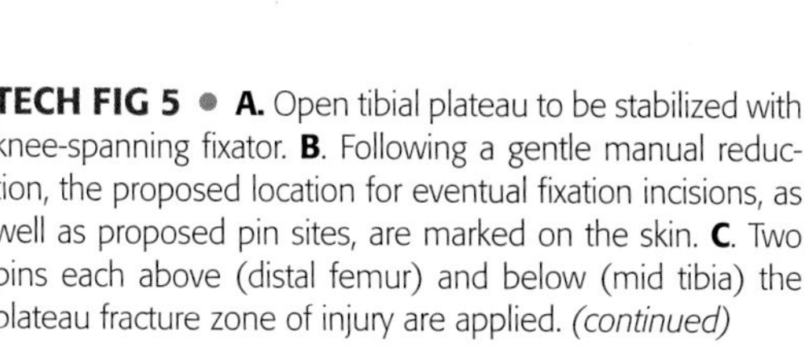

**TECH FIG 5** • **A.** Open tibial plateau to be stabilized with knee-spanning fixator. **B**. Following a gentle manual reduction, the proposed location for eventual fixation incisions, as well as proposed pin sites, are marked on the skin. **C**. Two pins each above (distal femur) and below (mid tibia) the plateau fracture zone of injury are applied. *(continued)*

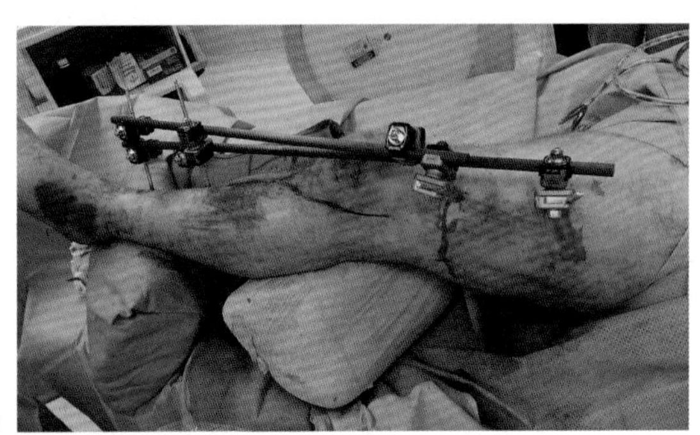

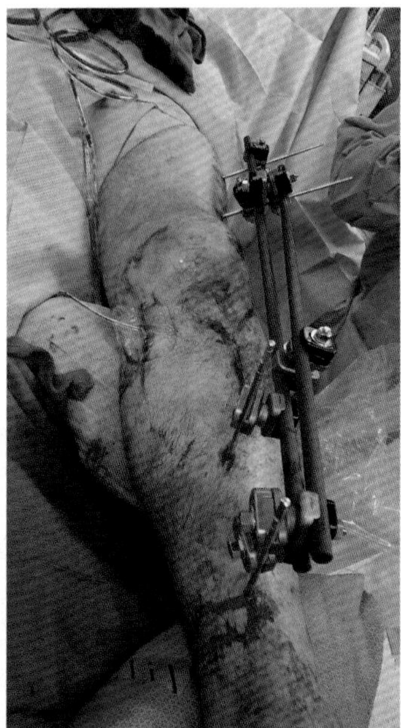

**TECH FIG 5** • *(continued)* **D,E.** One single bar connects the proximal two pins to the distal two pins. The fracture is then reduced and the clamps tightened. A second bar was added for stability, bridging the fracture.

## Ankle-Spanning Fixator for Tibial Pilon Fracture

- Two Schanz pins are placed into the midshaft tibial region (**TECH FIG 6**).
  - Avoid any compromised soft tissues and possible fracture extension if spanning the ankle for a severe pilon fracture with shaft extension.
- A centrally threaded transfixion pin is then placed through the calcaneal tuberosity from medial to lateral, avoiding the posterior tibial artery.
  - The appropriate location for this pin is 1.5 cm anterior to the posterior aspect of the heel and 1.5 cm proximal to the plantar aspect of the heel.
  - This location is confirmed via fluoroscopy.
- A solitary bar is connected to the tibial pins.

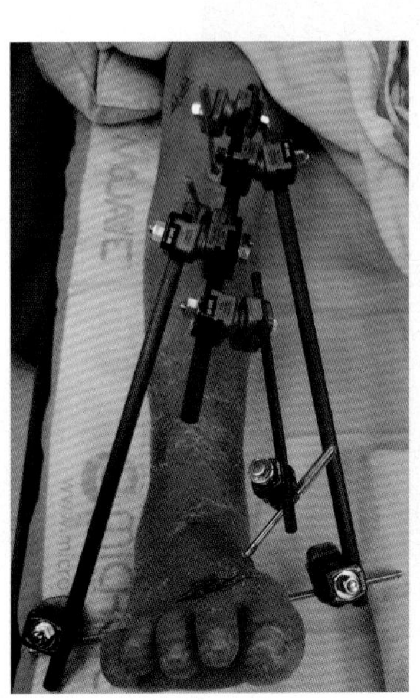

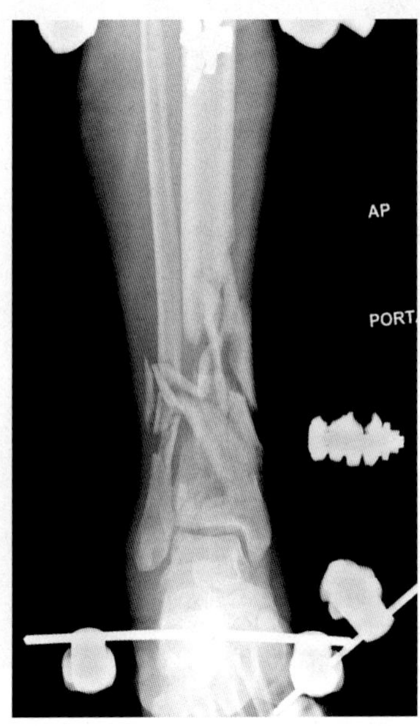


**TECH FIG 6** • Ankle-spanning fixators bridging a severe pilon fracture. **A,B.** Two pins are placed into the proximal tibia, out of the distal fracture zone of injury. A calcaneal transfixion pin is placed through the calcaneal tuberosity and subsequent medial-lateral triangulation connecting bars are attached. Longitudinal traction is applied, and all bars are tightened to maintain reduction. A forefoot pin is placed into the first metatarsal to maintain the foot in a neutral position and avoid equinus contracture. *(continued)*

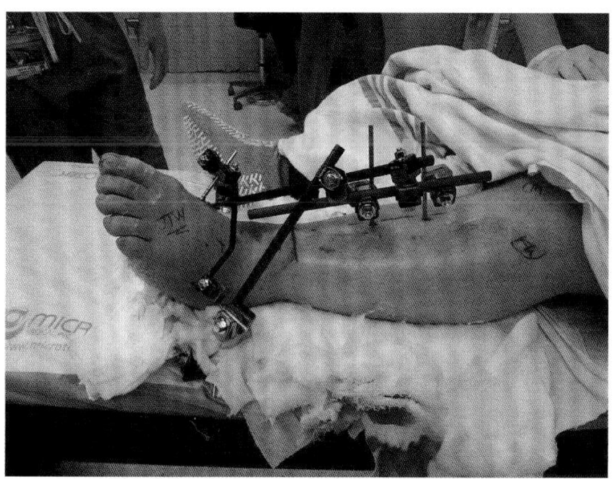

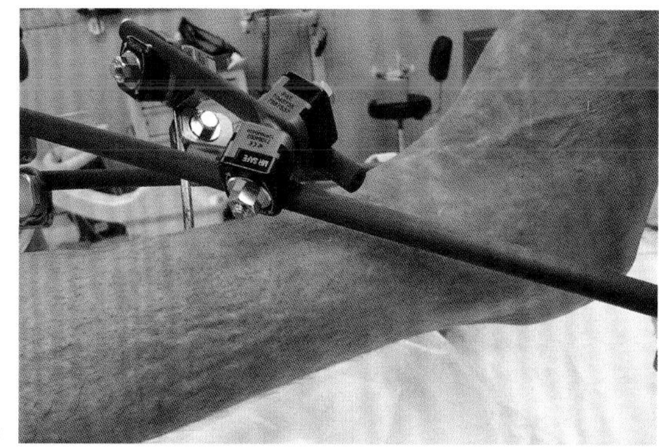

**TECH FIG 6** • *(continued)* **C.** Similar pin configuration with a triangular frame. First and fifth metatarsal pins with a forefoot bar were applied to maintain a neutral foot position. **D.** Skin demonstrates wrinkles and at this time is amenable to formal open reconstructive procedures.

- Medial and lateral bars are then connected to each side of the heel pin, making a triangular configuration.
  - Longitudinal traction is carried out to obtain length, and care is taken to achieve appropriate anteroposterior reduction.
- To maintain a plantigrade foot and to maintain alignment, a pin is placed into the base of the first or second metatarsal.[15]
  - This forefoot pin is then connected to the main frame with a connecting bar and the foot is held in neutral dorsiflexion.

## Two-Pin Fixator: Temporary Stabilization for Tibial Shaft, Pilon, or Plateau Fractures

- This is a temporary frame designed for rapid distraction and gross reduction used for all types of tibial pathology.
- A proximal centrally threaded transfixion pin is applied one fingerbreadth proximal to the tip of the proximal fibula. It is inserted from lateral to medial (**TECH FIG 7A,B**).
  - Alternatively, this pin can be placed into the distal femur at the level of the midpatella along the midlateral condyle of the femur.
- A second transfixion pin is placed through the calcaneal tuberosity, similar to the ankle-spanning frame described earlier.
- Two long connecting bars are then attached to the pins on each side of the leg.
  - Longitudinal traction is applied and a gross reduction is achieved.
- In some circumstances, a third pin is placed into the tibial shaft and attached to one of the longitudinal bars by a third connecting bar (**TECH FIG 7C,D**). This is done to add stability to this very simple frame (**TECH FIG 7E–G**).

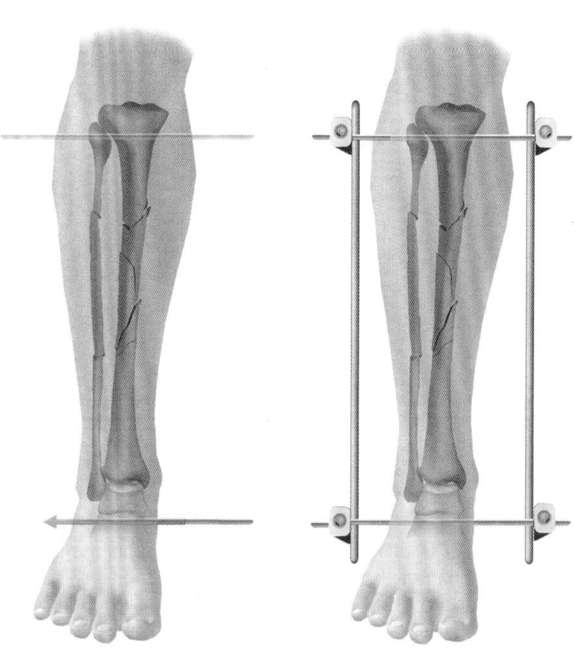

**TECH FIG 7** • **A,B.** Application of spanning two-pin fixator "traveling traction" with attachment of medial and lateral bars. This is used as a very temporary frame to stabilize a variety of conditions. *(continued)*

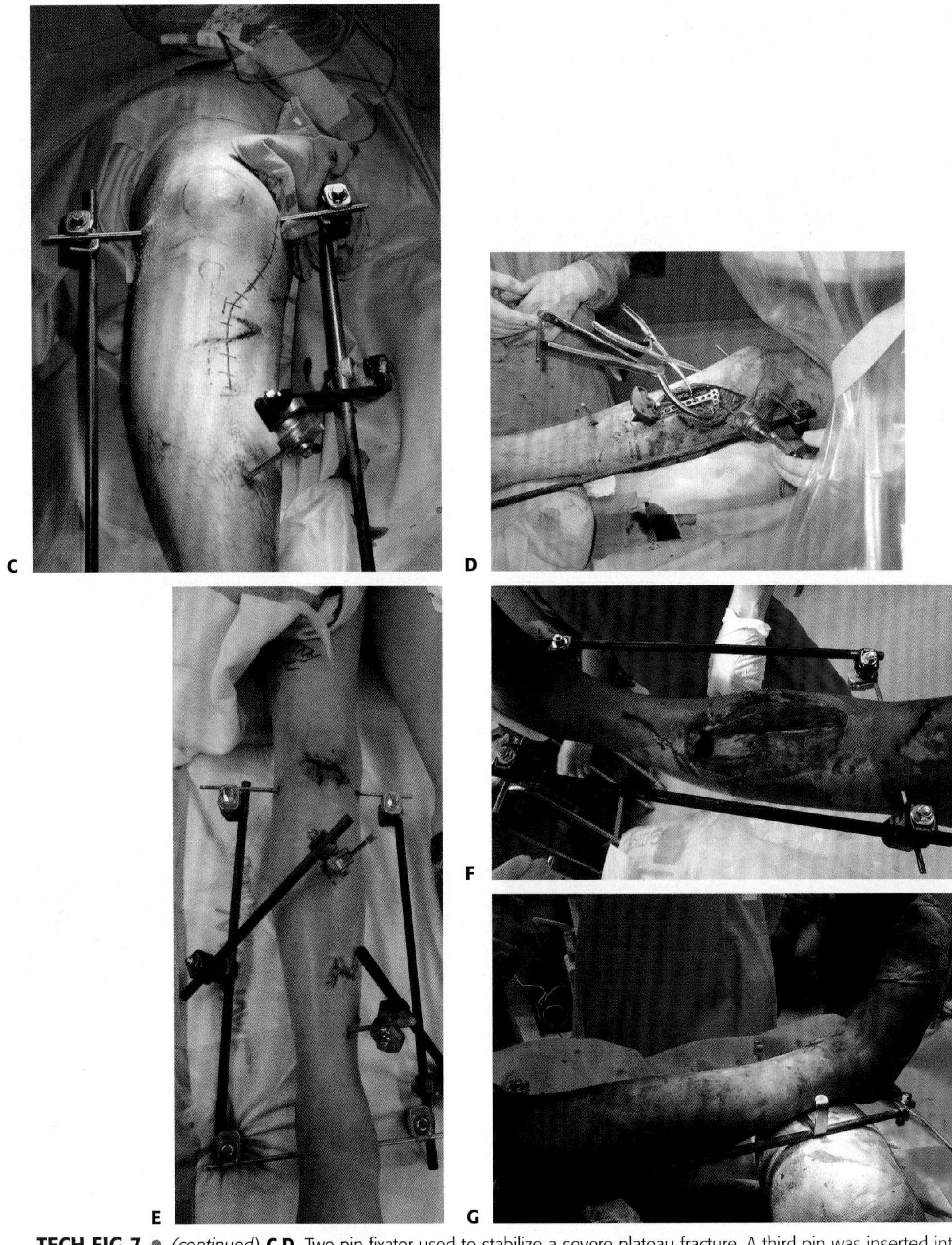

**TECH FIG 7** • *(continued)* **C,D.** Two-pin fixator used to stabilize a severe plateau fracture. A third pin was inserted into the distal third of the tibia to provide additional stability. The frame is prepped directly into the operative field at the time of secondary surgery to definitively stabilize the fracture using a medial buttress plate. **E.** Modified two-pin fixator with an additional half-pin placed above and below the fracture for added stability prior to intramedullary nailing of the shaft injury. **F.** Spanning two-pin frame providing initial stabilization to a severe open tibia with soft tissue and bone loss. This temporizes the injury and allows for additional staging procedures. **G**. Simple two-pin frame previously applied, now used as a reduction aid at the time of definitive intramedullary nailing.

## PEARLS AND PITFALLS

| | |
|---|---|
| **Pin placement location** | ▪ Areas of soft tissue compromise, open wounds, and occult fracture lines as identified on CT scans should be avoided. This prevents any associated pin tract infection from involving the fracture site. The frame must be constructed and applied to allow for multiple débridements, subsequent soft tissue reconstruction, and definitive secondary internal fixation conversions. Thus, the pins must be placed away from the zone of injury to avoid potential pin site contamination with the operative field. (Mark proposed incisions on skin prior to pin placement.) |
| **Pin insertion technique** | ▪ Adequate skin release is provided to avoid tethering or bunching of soft tissues around pins. Pins are overwrapped with small gauze wrap to provide a stable pin–skin interface and to avoid excessive pin–skin motion and development of tissue necrosis and infection. |
| **Temporary frames require adjunctive splinting of knee, leg, ankle, and foot.** | ▪ Temporary spanning frames are *not* excessively rigid and require additional splinting to maintain the foot in neutral and to avoid the development of equinus contractures. Alternatively, span frame into foot using metatarsal pins to maintain a plantigrade foot. |

## POSTOPERATIVE CARE

- A compressive dressing should be applied to the pin sites immediately after surgery to stabilize the pin–skin interface and thus minimize pin–skin motion, which can lead to the development of necrotic debris.
- Compressive dressings can be removed within 10 days to 2 weeks once the pin sites are healed.
- If appropriate pin insertion technique is used, the pin sites will completely heal around each individual pin. Once healed, only showering, without any other pin cleaning procedures, is necessary.[10]
  - Removal of a serous crust around the pins using dilute hydrogen peroxide and saline may occasionally be necessary.
- Ointments should not be used for pin care. They tend to inhibit the normal skin flora and alter the normal skin bacteria and may lead to superinfection or pin site colonization.
- If pin drainage does develop, pin care should be provided three times per day.
  - This may also involve rewrapping and compressing the offending pin site in an effort to minimize the abnormal pin–skin motion.
- Following a standardized protocol that involves precleaning the external fixator frame, followed by alcohol wash, sequential povidone-iodine preparation, paint, and spray with air drying followed by draping the extremity and fixator directly into the operative field, additional surgery can be safely performed without an increased rate of postoperative wound infection.
- Definitive treatment with an external fixator demands close scrutiny of the radiographs to ensure that the fracture has completely healed before frame removal. Various techniques have been described, including CT scans, ultrasound, and bone densitometry, to determine the adequacy of fracture healing.
  - In general, the patient should be fully weight bearing with minimal pain at the fracture site. The frame should be fully dynamized such that the load is being borne by the patient's limb rather than by the external fixator.

## OUTCOMES

- Staged management of high-energy tibial plateau and tibial pilon fractures using spanning external fixation to allow the recovery of soft tissues has reduced the overall rates of soft tissue complications. With secondary plating procedures after soft tissue recovery, infection rates have been reported to be less than 5% for complex plateau fractures and less than 7% for complex pilon fractures.
- No severe complications related to the temporary external fixator alone have been reported.
- Immediate external fixation followed by early, closed, interlocking nailing has been demonstrated to be a safe and effective treatment for open tibial fractures if early (<21 days after injury) conversion to intramedullary nailing is performed.
- Early soft tissue coverage and closure is the primary determinant of delayed infection, highlighting the need for effective soft tissue management and early closure of open injuries.
- Definitive treatment of open tibial fractures with external fixation has a higher rate of malunion compared with intramedullary nailing. No difference in union rates is noted. Slightly higher rates of infection are noted in the external fixation group.
  - The severity of the soft tissue injury rather than the choice of implant appears to be the predominant factor influencing outcome. External fixation is preferentially used in patients with the most severe soft tissue injuries or wound contamination.

## COMPLICATIONS

- Wire and pin site complications include pin site inflammation, chronic infection, loosening, or metal fatigue failure.
  - Minor pin tract inflammation requires more frequent pin care consisting of daily cleansing with mild soap or half-strength peroxide and saline solution.
  - Occasionally, an inflamed pin site with purulent discharge will require antibiotics and continued daily pin care.
- Severe pin tract infection consists of serous or seropurulent drainage in concert with redness, inflammation, and radiographs showing osteolysis of both the near and far cortices.
  - Once osteolysis occurs with bicortical involvement, the offending pin should be removed immediately, with débridement of the pin tract.[5]
- Late deformity after removal of the apparatus usually presents as a gradual deviation of the limb. This often occurs if the patient and surgeon become "frame weary," which results in frame removal before healing is complete.
  - One should always err on the conservative side and leave the frame on for an extended time to ensure that the fracture has healed.

- When late deformity occurs, it usually has an unsatisfactory outcome unless collapse is detected early and the frame is reapplied.
  - If untreated, the resulting malunion requires secondary osteotomy procedures.
  - Early detection of delayed union often requires adjunctive bone grafting for previously open shaft fractures.

## REFERENCES


1. Behrens F, Johnson W. Unilateral external fixation: methods to increase and reduce frame stiffness. Clin Orthop Relat Res 1989;(241): 48–56.
2. Chao EY, Aro HT, Lewallen DG, et al. The effect of rigidity on fracture healing in external fixation. Clin Orthop Relat Res 1989;(241): 24–35.
3. Della Rocca GJ, Crist BD. External fixation versus conversion to intramedullary nailing for definitive management of closed fractures of the femoral and tibial shaft. J Am Acad Orthop Surg 2006;14(10) (suppl):S131–S135.
4. Egol KA, Tejwani NC, Capla EL, et al. Staged management of high-energy proximal tibia fractures (OTA type 41): the results of a prospective, standardized protocol. J Orthop Trauma 2005;19:448–455.
5. Green SA. Complications of External Skeletal Fixation: Causes, Prevention, and Treatment. Springfield, IL: Charles C Thomas, 1981.
6. Haidukewych GJ. Temporary external fixation for the management of complex intra- and periarticular fractures of the lower extremity. J Orthop Trauma 2002;16:678–685.
7. Kenwright J, Richardson JB, Cunningham JL, et al. Axial movement and tibial fractures: a controlled randomised trial of treatment. J Bone Joint Surg Br 1991;73B:654–659.
8. Laible C, Earl-Royal E, Davidovitch R, et al. Infection after spanning external fixation for high-energy tibial plateau fractures: is pin site-plate overlap a problem? J Orthop Trauma 2012;26(2):92–97.
9. Lenarz C, Bledsoe G, Watson JT. Circular external fixation frames with divergent half pins: a pilot biomechanical study. Clin Orthop Relat Res 2008;466(12): 2933–2939.
10. Lethaby A, Temple J, Santy J. Pin site care for preventing infections associated with external bone fixators and pins. Cochrane Database Syst Rev 2008;(4):CD004551.
11. Marsh JL, Bonar S, Nepola JV, et al. Use of an articulated external fixator for fractures of the tibial plafond. J Bone Joint Surg Am 1995;83A:733–736.
12. Nho SJ, Helfet DL, Rozbruch SR. Temporary intentional leg shortening and deformation to facilitate wound closure using the Ilizarov/Taylor spatial frame. J Orthop Trauma 2006;20(6):419–424.
13. Sirkin M, Sanders R, DiPasquale T, et al. A staged protocol for soft tissue management in the treatment of complex pilon fractures. J Orthop Trauma 1999;13:78–84.
14. Watson JT, Moed BR, Karges DE, et al. Pilon fractures: treatment protocol based on severity of soft tissue injury. Clin Orthop Relat Res 2000;375:78–90.
15. Ziran BH, Morrison T, Little J, et al. A new ankle spanning fixator construct for distal tibia fractures: optimizing visualization, minimizing pin problems, and protecting the heel. J Orthop Trauma 2013;27(2):e45–e49.

# Intramedullary Nailing of the Mature Tibia

32

CHAPTER

Mark A. Lee, Jonathan G. Eastman, and Brett Crist

## DEFINITION

- Intramedullary nailing techniques are typically used for closed and open displaced diaphyseal tibial fractures.
- The indications for intramedullary nailing can be extended to proximal and distal metaphyseal tibia fractures, including those associated with simple articular involvement.
- Both traditional peripatellar and semiextended approaches are used to attain the entry site for nailing all levels of tibial fractures.

## ANATOMY

- The triangular-shaped proximal tibia is narrowest medially, and the proximal medial cortex tibia is obliquely oriented to the frontal plane. The medullary canal of the tibia exits at the margin of the lateral articular facet. As a result of this complex proximal anatomy, there is less sagittal plane space for an intramedullary nail within the tibia metaphysis with a medial or central insertion path. With a medial start site, the anteromedial metaphyseal cortex can deflect the nail and create a valgus deformation. Due to these factors, a tendency toward a more lateral start site is favored.
- The patellar tendon inserts on the tibial tubercle and extends the proximal fracture segment in proximal fracture patterns. This displacement is accentuated with further flexion of the knee, which typically is required to attain the proper starting point for intramedullary nailing (**FIG 1A**).
- Gerdy tubercle—the origin of the anterior compartment muscles and insertion site of the iliotibial band—is palpable along the proximal lateral tibia. In addition to the deforming forces of the patellar tendon, the anterior compartment muscles and the iliotibial band contribute to the shortening and valgus deformity typically seen with more proximal fractures.
- The anterior tibial crest corresponds to the vertical lateral surface of the tibia. When it is palpable, it is an excellent reference for the anatomic axis and nail path (**FIG 1B**).
- The anteromedial tibial surface is subcutaneous and often is the site of traumatic open wounds.
- The anterior neurovascular bundle and tibialis anterior tendon are at risk with anterior to posterior distal interlocking screw paths; internal rotation of the nail may decrease the risk of iatrogenic nerve injury[3] (**FIG 1C**).
- The Hoffa fat pad and intermeniscal ligament are commonly injured during all tibial intramedullary nail insertion techniques, especially during lateral parapatellar and patellar tendon-splitting approaches.[27,34]

## PATHOGENESIS

- Tibial shaft fractures may occur from high-energy mechanisms of injury, as when a pedestrian is struck by a motor vehicle. Many fractures, however, result from low-energy mechanisms such as simple falls in elderly patients or those with poor bone quality or sports-related injuries (common in soccer players) in younger patients.[6]
- In this low-energy fracture group, elderly patients are more likely to have comminuted and open fractures due to simple falls.

## NATURAL HISTORY

- The long-term outcome of tibial malunion is not clearly defined in the trauma literature.
  - A weak association is seen between a tibial shaft fracture malunion and ipsilateral knee and ankle arthritis.[12,19,32]
- Knee pain is reported in up to 58% of cases after intramedullary nailing. This pain typically is anterior, associated with activity, and exacerbated by kneeling activities.[6,11]
  - Knee pain improves in about 50% of patients after hardware removal.[6]
  - Attempts to detect a correlation between start sites and knee pain have been inconclusive, and comparative evaluations between traditional start sites and semiextended start sites (ie, suprapatellar) are underway.

## PATIENT HISTORY AND PHYSICAL FINDINGS

- Understanding the mechanism of injury and the environment in which the injury occurred is important for evaluating a patient's risk for associated injuries and compartment syndrome. In open fractures, it can help determine the choice of prophylactic antibiotic therapy.
- All patients who sustain tibial shaft fractures from high-energy mechanisms should undergo standard advanced trauma and life support (ATLS) protocol to have a thorough examination for life- and other limb-threatening injuries. Seventy-five percent of patients with open tibia fractures have associated injuries.[1]
- To evaluate a patient's risk for potential complications, other medical conditions should be investigated, including a history of diabetes mellitus, renal disease, inflammatory arthropathies, tobacco use (which increases healing time by up to 40%), and peripheral vascular disease.[4]
- It also is important to find out about the patient's normal activities and employment requirements to give them a reasonable expectation for when they will be able to resume those activities.
- Pain at the fracture site, swelling, and deformity are common findings in patients with tibial shaft fractures.
- A thorough examination of the skin is important to avoid missing open fracture wounds.
- Evaluation of the soft tissue envelope for abrasions, contusions, and fracture blisters can help determine whether

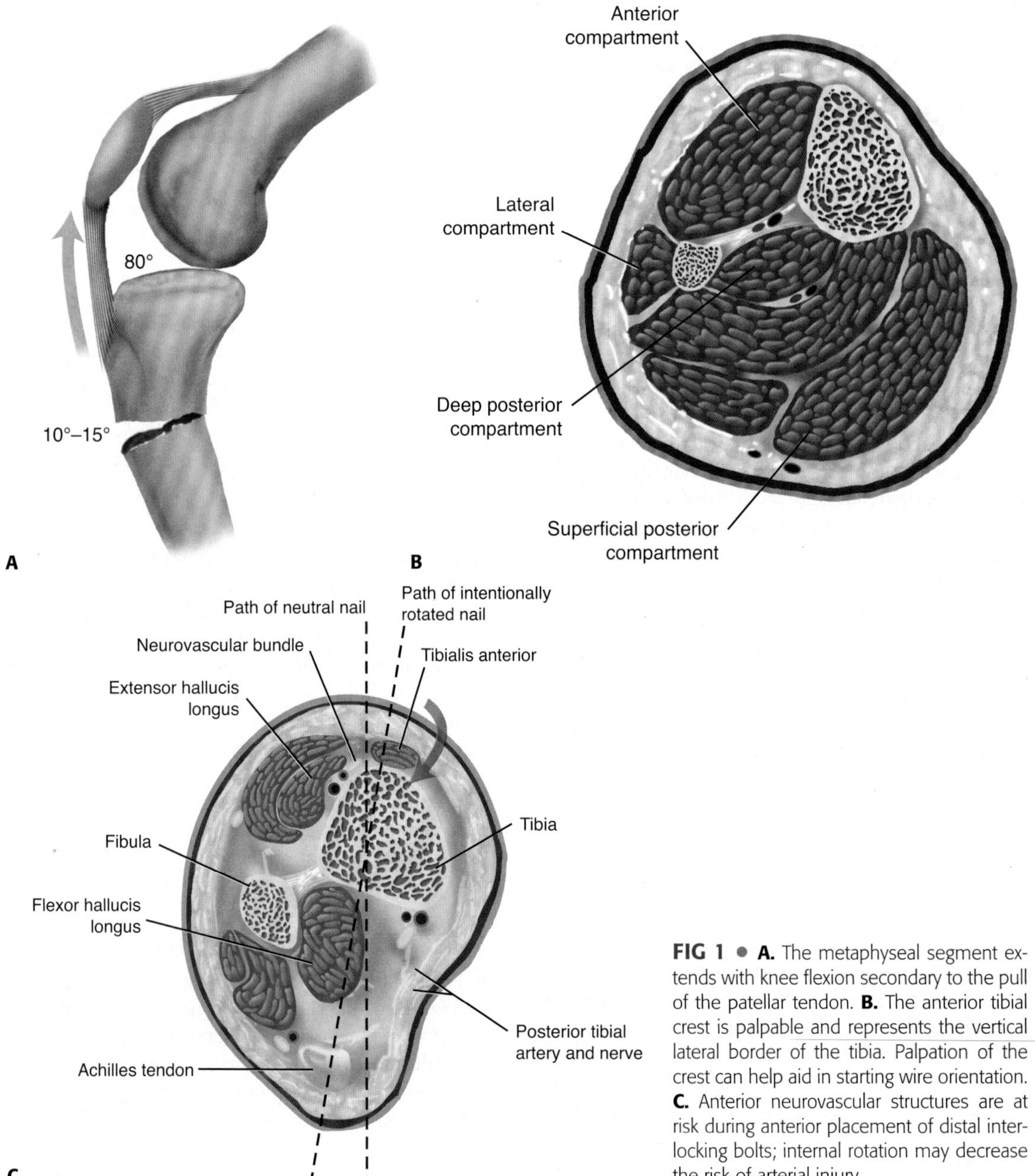


**FIG 1** • **A.** The metaphyseal segment extends with knee flexion secondary to the pull of the patellar tendon. **B.** The anterior tibial crest is palpable and represents the vertical lateral border of the tibia. Palpation of the crest can help aid in starting wire orientation. **C.** Anterior neurovascular structures are at risk during anterior placement of distal interlocking bolts; internal rotation may decrease the risk of arterial injury.

definitive treatment can be done primarily or if a staged or delayed approach is required.

- A detailed neurovascular examination is critical to avoid the devastating complications associated with compartment syndrome, which can occur in both closed and open fractures (see Chap. 38).

## IMAGING AND OTHER DIAGNOSTIC STUDIES

- Full-length anteroposterior (AP) and lateral plain radiographs are necessary to adequately evaluate the tibia and fibula. Complete orthogonal views of the tibia and fibula help evaluate for concurrent fractures or dislocation and any preexisting deformity or implants.
  - Orthogonal radiographic views of the knee and ankle are required to rule out articular involvement.
- Axial computed tomography (CT) scan can be used for proximal and distal fractures to rule out intra-articular fracture extension.
  - Nondisplaced fracture lines are common.
  - Gunshot wounds may merit CT evaluation to rule out intra-articular bullet fragments and intra-articular fracture extension.
- Magnetic resonance imaging (MRI) is not useful for most diaphyseal or metadiaphyseal fractures.
- Ankle–brachial index (systolic pressure in injured leg below injury divided by systolic pressure of the brachium) after fracture reduction should be used to rule out vascular injuries in severely displaced fractures or fractures with severe soft tissue injury. Values of less than 0.9 may be indicative of vascular injury, requiring further investigation.[18]

- Compartment pressure evaluation with a commercially available handheld single-stick monitor or with a side-ported catheter connected to a pressure monitor (using the arterial line setup) is indicated in patients who have severe or increasing swelling and are not able to comply with physical examination and questioning.
  - Observe for early signs of compartment syndrome in all patients with tibial diaphyseal fractures.
  - Open fracture does not preclude development of compartment syndrome.
  - Measure the pressure difference between the diastolic pressure and the intracompartmental pressure—a differential value of less than 30 mm Hg is considered an indication for a four-compartment fasciotomy.[17]

## NONOPERATIVE MANAGEMENT

- Nonoperative management is indicated in ambulatory patients for closed and open fractures that do not require flap coverage and that do not present with excessive initial shortening or unacceptable angulation when a cast is applied (**FIG 2**).
- An intact fibula with an axially unstable fracture pattern (ie, short oblique, butterfly fragment, or comminuted) is at risk for shortening and varus deformities and is a relative contraindication to nonoperative management.
- A higher rate of malunion and nonunion with nonoperative management is seen in higher energy fractures.[2,9]
- Joint stiffness, especially hindfoot, is common with all forms of prolonged immobilization.[7,22]
- Initial treatment includes ~2 weeks of a long-leg splint, then a long-leg cast for 2 to 4 weeks.
  - When the initial swelling has subsided, the patient is graduated to a patellar tendon or functional brace. Weight bearing is allowed and encouraged.
  - Radiographs are evaluated at 1- to 2-week intervals over the first month of treatment to confirm maintenance of acceptable alignment.

## SURGICAL MANAGEMENT

### Classification and Relative Indications

- Tibia fractures usually are classified according to the AO Foundation and Orthopaedic Trauma Association (AO/OTA) classification (Table 1).
- Several relatively well-accepted indications and contraindications have been established for the intramedullary nailing of tibia fractures (Table 2).
- A thorough evaluation of the patient's soft tissue envelope will determine when the patient can proceed with definitive fixation.
- Complete orthogonal radiographs of the entire tibia and fibula are important to determine whether the patient's intramedullary canal is large enough to accommodate an intramedullary nail (approximately 8 mm) and identify any preexisting deformity that may preclude nail placement. Most modern cannulated nail designs start near 8 mm in diameter. Complete radiographs also identify any proximal or distal articular involvement.
  - Preoperative measurement of the intramedullary canal and the length of the tibia will help determine which size nail can be used.
    - The lateral radiograph is the most accurate to use for measuring the appropriate nail length.
    - Measuring the narrowest diameter of the diaphysis on the AP and lateral views will determine the appropriate nail diameter and whether intramedullary reaming will be necessary.

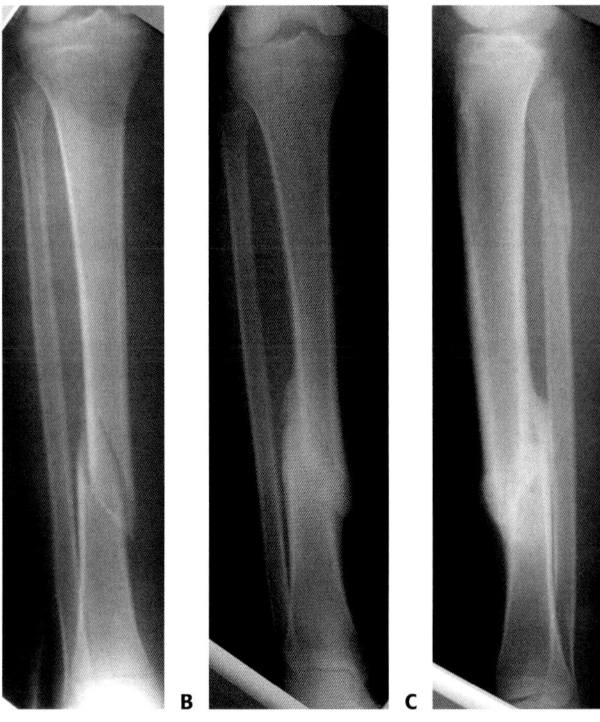


**FIG 2** • **A–C.** An oblique diaphyseal tibial shaft fracture treated nonoperatively to union. (Courtesy of Paul Tornetta III, MD.)

**Table 1 The AO/OTA Classification of Diaphyseal Tibial Fractures**

| Classification | Description | Illustration | Classification | Description | Illustration |
|---|---|---|---|---|---|
| 42-A | Simple | | 42-B3 | Fragmented wedge | 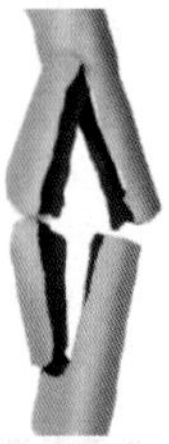 |
| 42-A1 | Spiral | 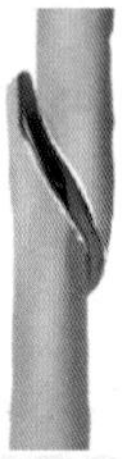 | | | |
| | | | 42-C | Complex | |
| 42-A2 | Oblique (≥30 degrees) | 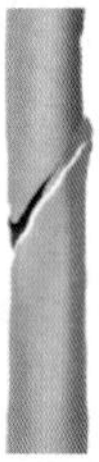 | 42-C1 | Spiral | 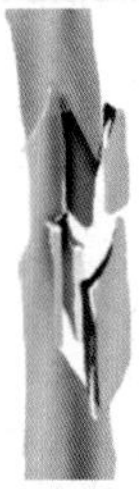 |
| 42-A3 | Transverse (<30 degrees) | 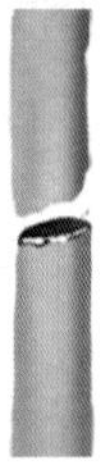 | 42-C2 | Segmented | 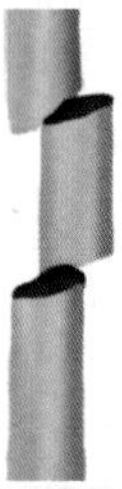 |
| 42-B | Wedge | | | | |
| 42-B1 | Spiral wedge | 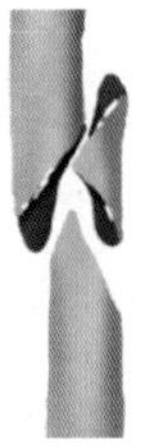 | 42-C3 | Irregular | 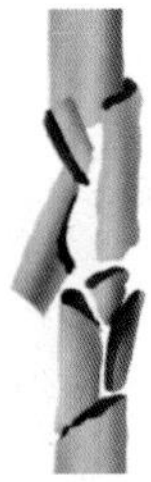 |
| 42-B2 | Bending wedge | 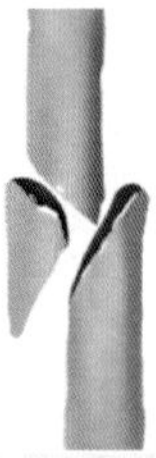 | | | |

**Table 2 Relative Indications and Contraindications for Intramedullary Nailing of Tibial Fractures**

| Relative indications |
|---|
| • High-energy mechanism<br>• Moderate to severe soft tissue injury precluding cast or brace<br>• Angular deformity ≥5 to 10 degrees<br>• Rotational deformity ≥5 to 10 degrees<br>• Shortening >1 cm<br>• Displacement >50%<br>• An ipsilateral fibula fracture at the same level<br>• An intact fibula<br>• Compartment syndrome<br>• Ipsilateral femoral fracture<br>• Inability to maintain reduction<br>• Older age, inability to manage with cast or brace |
| **Contraindications** |
| • Intramedullary canal diameter <6 mm<br>• Gross contamination of intramedullary canal<br>• Severe soft tissue injury where limb salvage is uncertain<br>• Preexisting deformity precluding nail insertion<br>• Ipsilateral total knee arthroplasty or knee arthrodesis<br>• Significant articular involvement<br>• Previous cruciate ligament reconstruction |

Baumgartner M, Tornetta P, eds. Orthopaedic Knowledge Update: Trauma 3. Rosemont, IL: American Academy of Orthopaedic Surgeons, 2005; Schmidt A, Finkemeier CG, Tornetta P. Treatment of closed tibia fractures. In: Tornetta P, ed. Instructional Course Lectures: Trauma. Rosemont, IL: American Academy of Orthopaedic Surgeons, 2006:215–229.

- Orthogonal radiographs of the uninjured tibia can be used as templates for determining the appropriate length, alignment, and rotation in comminuted fractures or open fractures with bone loss.

## Positioning

- Supine positioning is standard.
- A fracture table can be used with boot traction, calcaneal traction, or an arthroscopy leg holder that supports the leg and provides mechanical traction when no assistants are available. However, knee hyperflexion is difficult, and the guidewire insertion angle is suboptimal for proximal fractures[16] (**FIG 3A**).
- The patient is placed on the radiolucent table in one of the following positions:
  - Supine with the leg free (**FIG 3B**)
    - Mechanical traction is helpful to achieve reduction when the leg is draped free (**FIG 3C,D**).
    - The proximal posterior Schanz pin (**FIG 3E**) is inserted medial to lateral and parallel to the tibial plateau.
    - The distal Schanz pin (**FIG 3F**) is inserted parallel to the plafond and inferior to the projected end of the nail.
  - Supine with the leg flexed over a bolster or radiolucent triangle (**FIG 3G**)
    - Maximizing knee flexion makes it easier to attain a start site and to obtain an optimal insertion vector, which approaches a parallel path with the anterior tibial border.

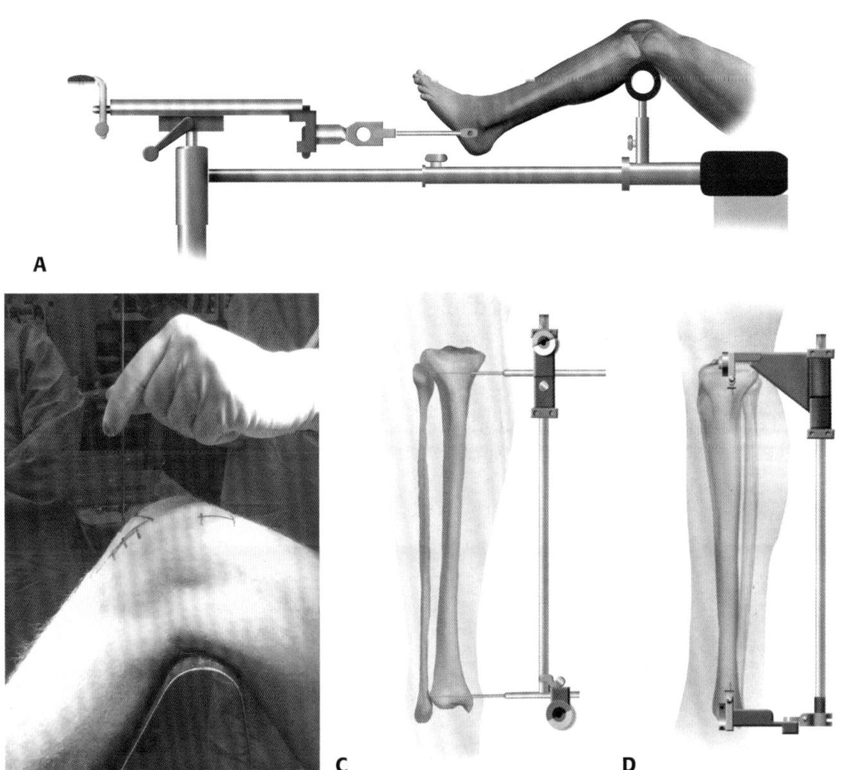


**FIG 3** • **A.** The fractured leg is positioned in calcaneal skeletal traction on the fracture table. This provides excellent mechanical traction but limits limb mobility, especially knee flexion. **B.** The knee is flexed over a positioning triangle in preparation for the surgical approach. **C,D.** The tibial fracture is distracted and reduced using a mechanical distraction device with proximal and distal half-pins. *(continued)*

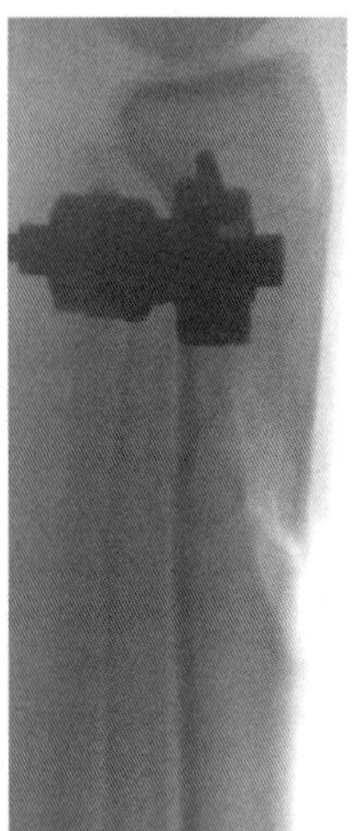
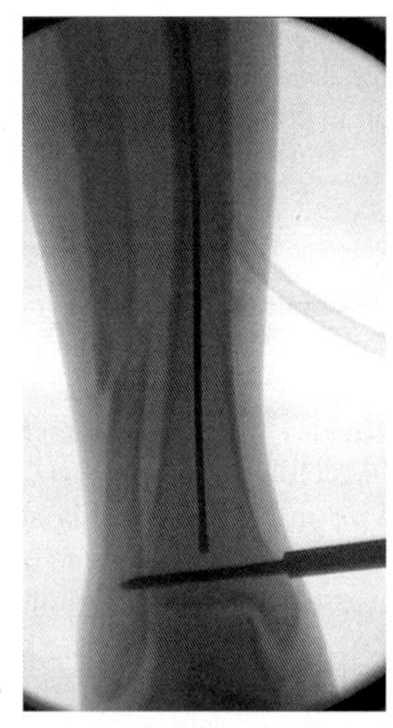
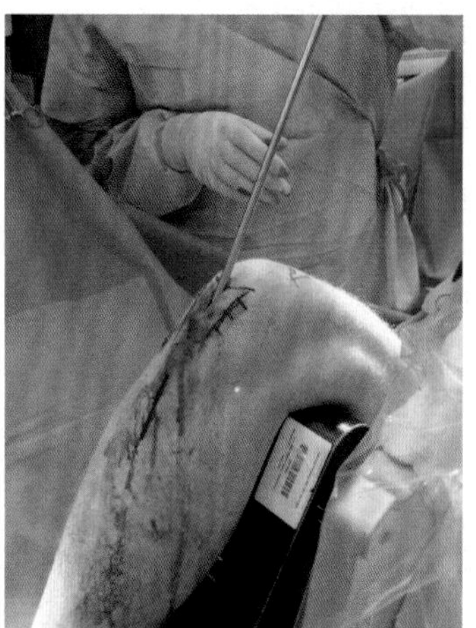
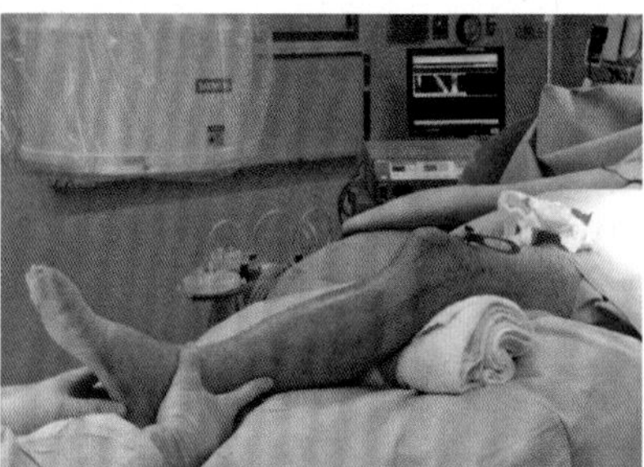

**FIG 3** • *(continued)* **E.** A posteriorly positioned half-pin can be placed behind the projected nail path. **F.** A distal half-pin placed just over and parallel to the plafond can be helpful for aligning the distal fragment and lies inferior to the projected end of the nail. **G.** The knee is maximally flexed over the triangle to allow for the proper starting wire insertion angle. **H.** Typical setup for semiextended nailing with a small bolster for limited knee flexion and easy access to the limb for reduction and imaging.

- Semiextended position
  - For proximal fractures, extending the knee to 20 to 30 degrees of flexion counters the pull of the patellar tendon and helps reduce the flexion deformity that is typical for these fractures.[26] Either a radiolucent triangle or bolster can be used (**FIG 3H**).

## Approach

- Use fluoroscopy to determine which approach will allow the starting point to be placed just medial to the lateral tibial spine on the AP view and at the anterior articular margin on the lateral view.[27] A guidewire can be used to assess the relationship between the anatomic axis of the tibia and the appropriate start site (**FIG 4**). Externally rotated views are common and can be misleading in selecting the ideal start point.[33]
- For diaphyseal and distal metaphyseal fractures, any of the following approaches are appropriate. As mentioned earlier, the patient's anatomy and fracture deformity can be used to determine which approach allows for appropriate starting point placement.
  - Medial parapatellar
  - Transpatellar tendon (This approach may be avoided by some surgeons due to previous retrospective series that showed an increased likelihood of knee pain with this approach.[11,21] However, other retrospective series and more recent prospective trials have found no association between knee pain and the surgical approach used.)[5,29–31]
  - Lateral parapatellar
- Fractures at the transition between metaphysis and diaphysis
  - The lateral parapatellar approach allows for guidewire and nail placement in the more lateral position, which is beneficial in countering the valgus deformity associated with these fractures. It also allows intramedullary nailing in the familiar hyperflexed knee position.
    - The semiextended position assists for reduction of the flexion deformity associated with these fractures.
    - The limited or formal medial parapatellar may be used if the surgeon is unfamiliar with the suprapatellar approach and special instrumentation is not available.
    - If the suprapatellar approach is being performed, a superomedial or superior midline is used and special instrumentation is required.
    - All of the surgical approaches are performed with the knee in the semiextended position.

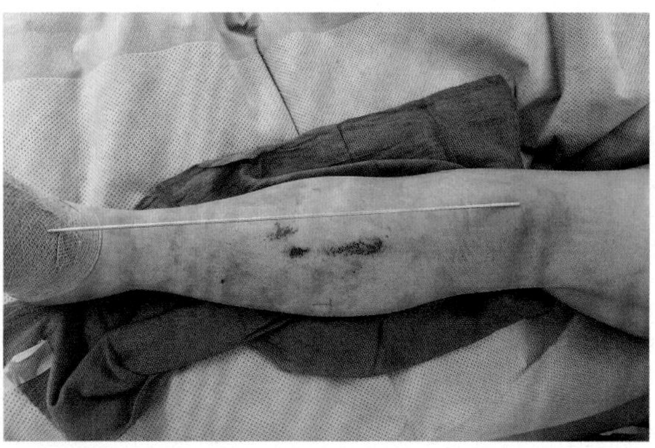
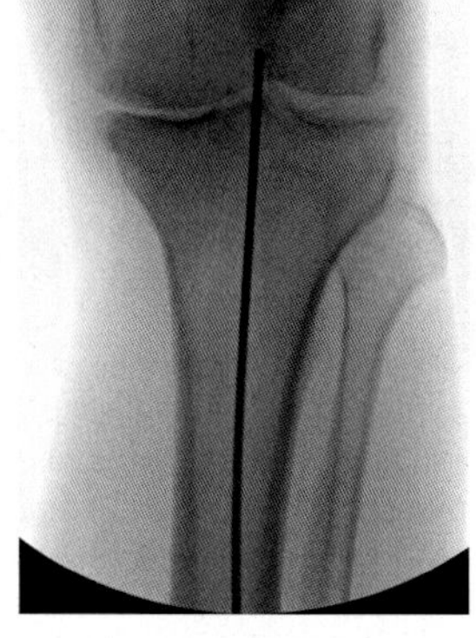

**FIG 4** • Clinical and fluoroscopic examples demonstrating usage of a guidewire to determine tibial anatomic axis and appropriate start site. **A.** Guidewire placed along tibial crest. **B.** Correlating fluoroscopic AP view showing guidewire at the medial aspect of the lateral tibial spine.

## Surgical Approach

### Medial Parapatellar Tendon Approach

- Palpate and mark the medial border of the patellar tendon (**TECH FIG 1**, line *A*).
- Incise the skin at the medial border of the patellar tendon.
- Full-thickness skin flaps are developed.
- Dissection is carried down to the retinaculum.
- The retinaculum is then split, and the patellar tendon is retracted laterally.
- Do not incise the capsule.

### Transpatellar Tendon Approach

- Palpate and mark the medial and lateral border of the patellar tendon, the inferior border of the patella, and the tibial tubercle (**TECH FIG 1**, line *B*).
- Incise the skin starting at the inferior margin of the patella and continue distally in the middle of the patellar tendon.
- Full-thickness skin flaps are developed.
- Incise the paratenon in the midline, and elevate medial and lateral flaps to identify the margins of the patellar tendon.
- Make a single full-thickness incision in the midline of the patellar tendon. Do not incise the capsule and avoid injuring the menisci at the inferior margin of the incision.

### Lateral Parapatellar Tendon Approach

- Palpate and mark the lateral border of the patellar tendon (**TECH FIG 1**, line *C*).
- Incise the skin at the lateral border of the patellar tendon.
- Full-thickness skin flaps are developed.
- Dissection is carried down to the retinaculum.
- The retinaculum is then split, and the patellar tendon is retracted medially.
- Do not incise the capsule.

### Semiextended Position[26]

#### *Medial Parapatellar Approach*

- Either a standard midline or limited medial skin incision can be used (**TECH FIG 2**).
- Full-thickness skin flaps are developed.
- The distal portion of the quadriceps tendon is incised, leaving a 2-mm cuff of tendon medially for later repair.
- A formal medial arthrotomy is done extending around the patella, leaving a 2-mm cuff of capsule and retinaculum for later repair, and continuing along the medial border of the patellar tendon.

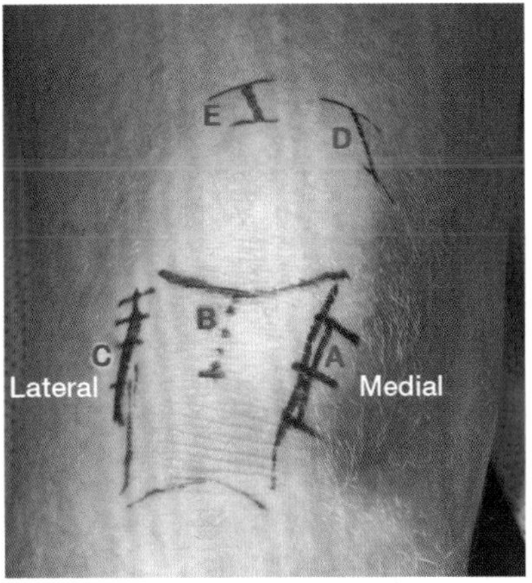


**TECH FIG 1** • Options for surgical incisions in relation to the patella and patellar tendon. Medial parapatellar tendon incision (*A*). Transpatellar tendon incision (*B*). Lateral parapatellar tendon (*C*). Superomedial tendon incision (*D*). Suprapatellar incision (*E*).

#### *Suprapatellar Approach*[28]

- The suprapatellar approach requires special nail insertion instrumentation as well as cannulas for guide pin placement and reaming.
- The skin incision is made at the superomedial edge of the patella (**TECH FIG 3**).
  - Full-thickness skin flaps are developed.
  - Make a superomedial arthrotomy large enough to place the special instrumentation.
- An alternative skin incision can be made extending from the midline of the superior pole of the patella proximally (see **TECH FIG 1**, line *E*).
  - Full-thickness skin flaps are developed.
  - Incise the quadriceps tendon in the midline, extending proximally from the superior pole of the patella, and make an arthrotomy.
  - Mobilize the patella and free up any adhesions in the patellofemoral joint.

### Extra-articular Extended[14]

- Semiextended nailing is performed with the goal of remaining outside knee synovium/joint.
  - Medial or lateral parapatellar approach is selected based on patellar laxity.
  - A curvilinear incision begins at the medial border of the proximal third of the patellar tendon and extends proximally

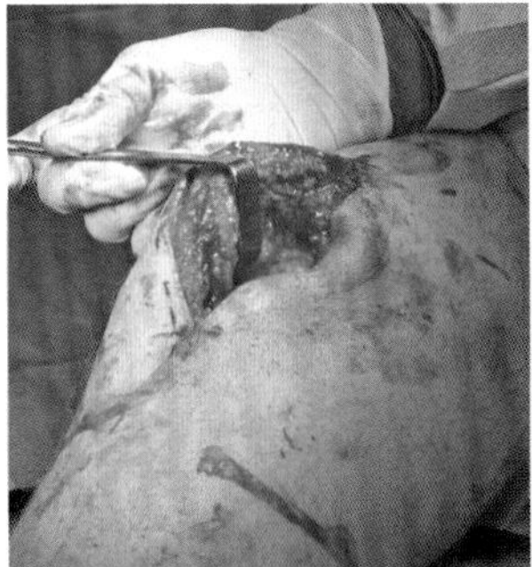
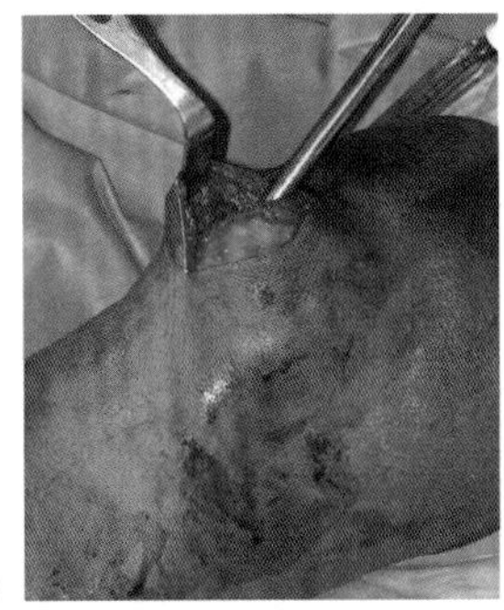

**TECH FIG 2** • **A.** A formal full medial parapatellar approach allows for easy patellar subluxation and start site localization but requires significant dissection. **B.** The alternative is a limited medial approach. (**B:** Courtesy of Paul Tornetta III, MD.)

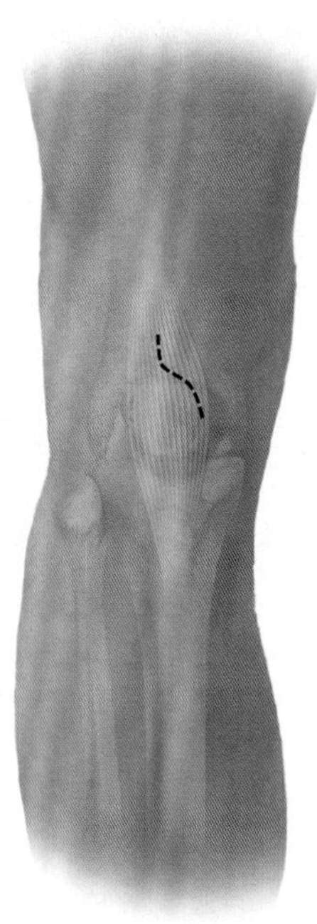

**TECH FIG 3** • A partial medial parapatellar arthrotomy that is carried into the intermedius allows enough subluxation of the patella to perform semiextended nailing. (Courtesy of Paul Tornetta III, MD.)

to the medial border of the patella and then to the level of the proximal pole.

- Dissect synovium from retinaculum; divide retinaculum sharply.

## Standard Intramedullary Nailing

### *Initial Guidewire Placement*

- Drape the leg free, including the proximal thigh. Draping the leg more distally can limit knee flexion due to bunching of the drapes.
- Flex the knee over a bolster or radiolucent triangle.
  - A padded thigh tourniquet can be applied and inflated during the surgical approach, but it must not be inflated during reaming because of the risk of thermal injury to the intramedullary canal. For this reason, a thigh tourniquet is usually omitted.
- The starting guidewire is placed on the skin and radiographically aligned with the anatomic axis and in line with the lateral tibial spine on a true AP fluoroscopic image. The skin can be marked along the guidewire path to allow visualization of the anatomic axis without fluoroscopy (**TECH FIG 4A**).
- The appropriate surgical approach is performed.
- The knee is maximally flexed, and the guidewire is aligned with the anatomic axis of the tibia.
  - Typically, achieving an appropriate insertion vector will require the wire to be pushed against the patella or the peripatellar tissues.
- The anterior tibial crest is palpated for frontal plane wire alignment.
- Lateral plane fluoroscopy is necessary to place the wire at the proximal and superior aspect of the "flat spot" and near parallel with the anterior tibial cortical line (**TECH FIG 4B**).
- The guidewire is directed 8 to 10 cm into the metaphysis.
  - Guidewire position is verified in the AP and lateral planes.
  - The frontal plane wire position should be in line with the anatomic axis and proximally should be just medial to the lateral tibial spine. Lateral alignment should be nearly parallel with the anterior tibial cortex, and all efforts should be made to avoid a posteriorly directed vector (**TECH FIG 4C**).

### *Creating and Reaming the Starting Hole*

- The opening reamer (matching the proximal nail diameter) is introduced via a tissue sleeve and inserted while carefully maintaining knee hyperflexion and biplanar alignment.
- If the knee is allowed to extend or posterior pressure is not maintained on the tissue sleeve, the starting hole will become enlarged anteriorly, and the proximal anterior cortex will be violated.
  - Imprecise reaming technique leads to anteriorization of the nail and violation of the proximal anterior cortex (**TECH FIG 5**).
- Place a 15-degree bend 2 cm from the distal extent of the ball-tipped guidewire to allow for directional control during wire advancement.
  - Alternatively, a straight ball-tipped guidewire can be used with an intramedullary reduction instrument (ie, a cannulated finger device), which can precisely direct the wire and simplify passage across the fracture.
- A ball-tipped guidewire is introduced into the proximal segment, and the knee is slightly extended for fracture reduction and instrumentation.

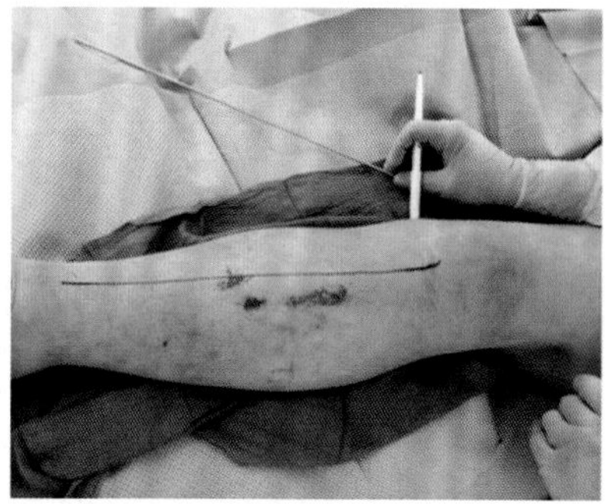
A

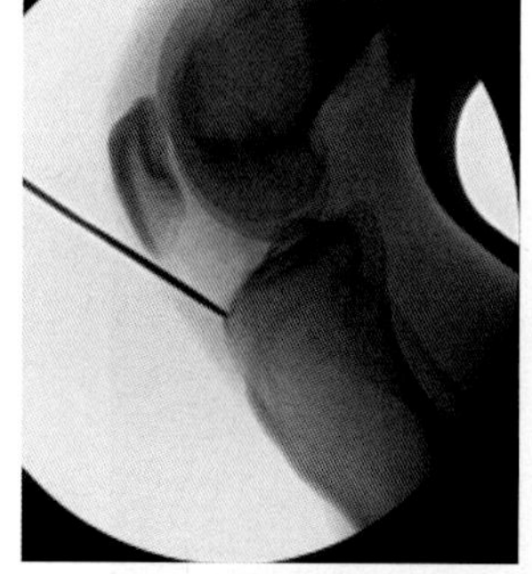
B

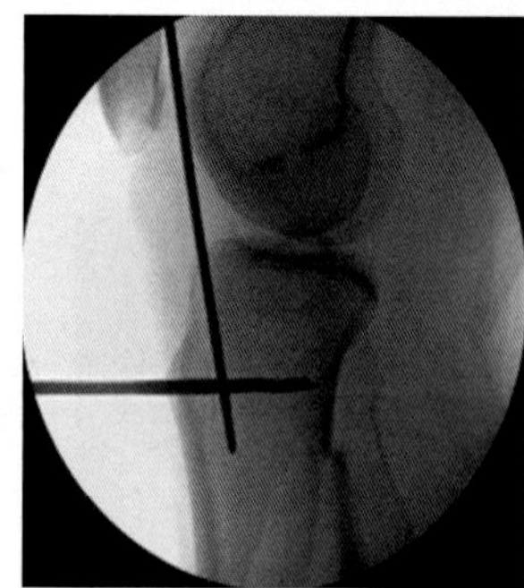
C

**TECH FIG 4** • **A.** Marking the skin along the crest can assist in aligning the guidewire with the path of the intramedullary canal and lessen the need for fluoroscopic guidance. **B.** Ideal proximal extra-articular start site as seen on lateral fluoroscopic image; this is near the articular margin. **C.** An ideal insertion vector approaches a parallel path with anterior cortex and minimizes the likelihood of fragment extension with seating of the nail.

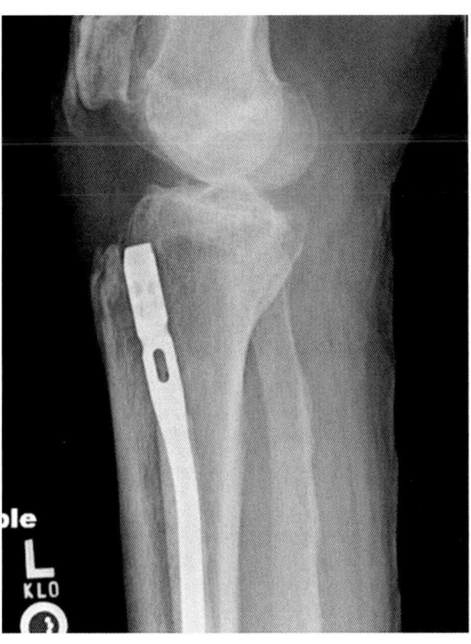

**TECH FIG 5** • If flexion is not maintained during reaming, or reaming is started before entrance into the starting hole, the anterior tibial cortex will be violated by the reamer, and an anterior nail path will be produced.

## *Fracture Reduction*

### Simple Middle Diaphyseal Fractures (Transverse or Short Oblique)

- Manual traction with gross manipulation will reduce simple transverse mid-diaphyseal fractures.
- Medially based external fixation or distraction with a large universal distractor is helpful for reduction when no assistants are available, in large patients, or when used for provisional fixation.
- Muscular paralysis is often helpful.
- Placement of percutaneous pointed reduction forceps can be helpful in oblique and short oblique patterns to achieve anatomic or near-anatomic reduction.
  - Use fluoroscopy to mark the level and orientation of the fracture on the skin to facilitate the reduction clamp orientation and ideal placement of skin incisions.
  - Introduce a small or large pointed clamp under and through skin stab wounds; care must be taken to maintain clamp points against bone (**TECH FIG 6A–C**).
  - Typically, the spike on the distal fragment is posterolateral.

### Highly Comminuted Middle Diaphyseal Fractures

- Have comparison radiographic images of the uninjured extremity available to be used as a template for length and rotational reduction landmarks.

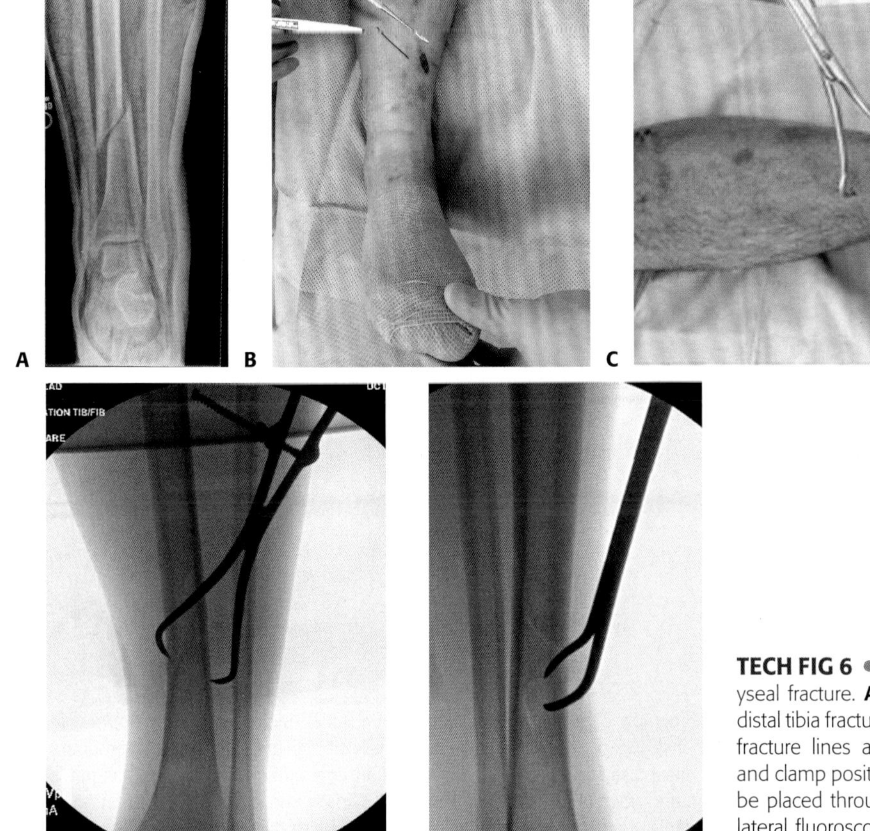

**TECH FIG 6** • Reduction of a simple middle diaphyseal fracture. **A.** AP radiograph of an oblique spiral distal tibia fracture. **B.** Use fluoroscopy to demonstrate fracture lines and localize clamp incision locations and clamp positions. **C.** Pointed reduction clamps can be placed through small stab incisions. **D,E.** AP and lateral fluoroscopic image demonstrating fracture reduction with percutaneous clamp application.

- Mechanical traction with medially based half-pin fixation is very helpful.
  - A large external fixator or large universal distractor is equally effective.
  - The proximal Schanz is placed posteriorly and parallel to the tibial plateau (**TECH FIG 7A**).
  - The distal Schanz pin is placed just above and parallel to the plafond (**TECH FIG 7B**).
- The intramedullary reduction tool available in most nail or reamer sets can be used to manipulate the proximal fragment in order to advance the tool across the fracture, which achieves fracture reduction and guidewire placement.

### Open Middle Diaphyseal Fractures

- Large segmental and butterfly fragments that are completely devitalized and void of soft tissue attachments should be removed and cleaned of contamination.
- These pieces can be reintroduced into the fracture site and used to perform anatomic open reduction following passage of the intramedullary rod and interlocking. These pieces should be removed after fixation is completed because they represent a large amount of nonviable material in a high-risk wound.
- Occasionally, an osteotome is required to free near-circumferential fragments (**TECH FIG 8A–C**).
- If reduction is difficult, a small fragment unicortical plate can be used to maintain the reduction during reaming and nail placement. Once interlocking is completed, the plate should be removed (**TECH FIG 8D**).

### *Passing the Guidewire*

- Once optimal AP and lateral plane reduction is achieved, the wire is advanced past the level of the fracture. Verify that the wire is within the canal on both the AP and lateral views to avoid advancing too far and damaging extramedullary structures.
- In metadiaphyseal fractures, the wire must be centered in the metaphyseal segment.
  - In proximal and distal fractures, blocking screws or half-pins may be required to ensure centralized positioning of the guidewire (**TECH FIG 9A**).

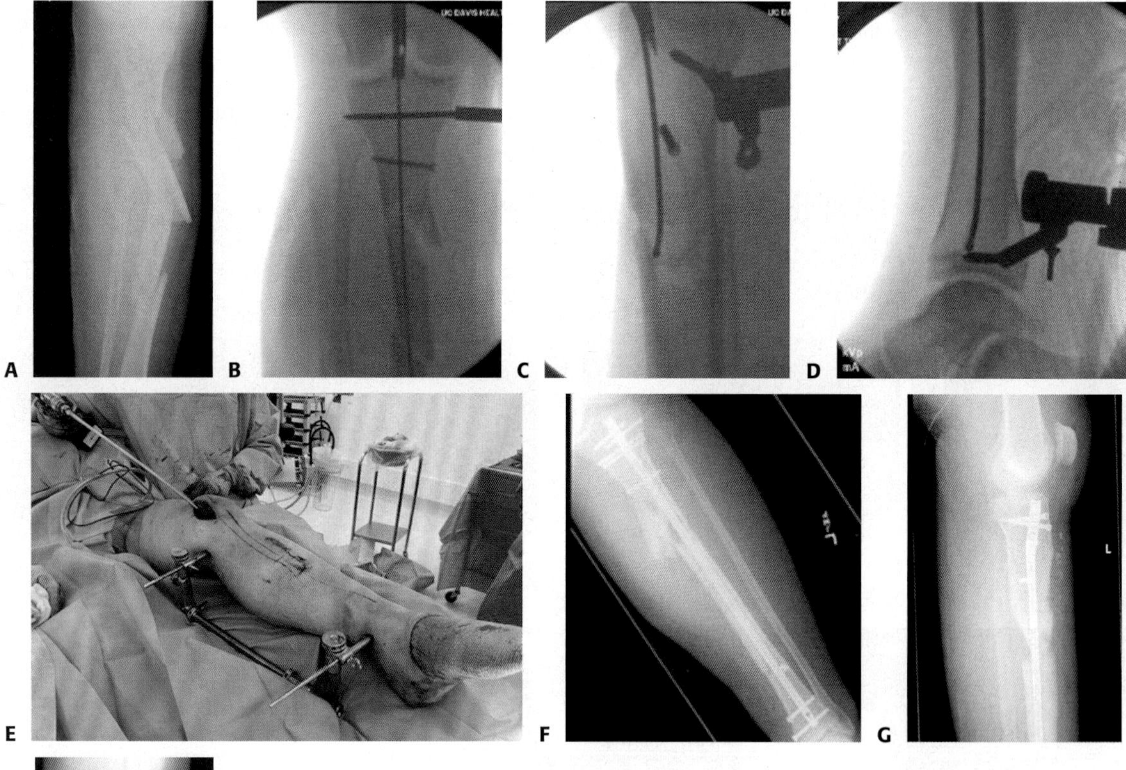

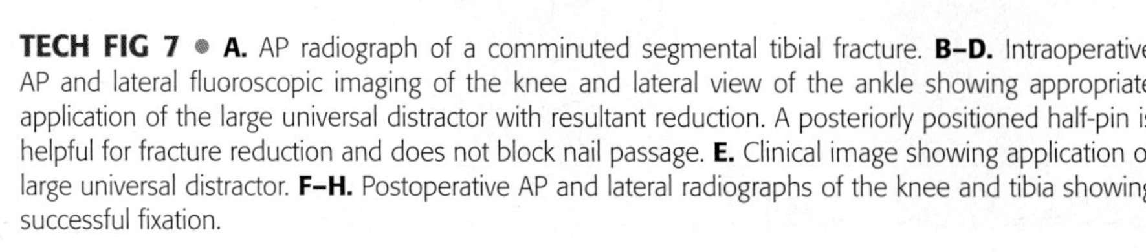

**TECH FIG 7** • **A.** AP radiograph of a comminuted segmental tibial fracture. **B–D.** Intraoperative AP and lateral fluoroscopic imaging of the knee and lateral view of the ankle showing appropriate application of the large universal distractor with resultant reduction. A posteriorly positioned half-pin is helpful for fracture reduction and does not block nail passage. **E.** Clinical image showing application of large universal distractor. **F–H.** Postoperative AP and lateral radiographs of the knee and tibia showing successful fixation.

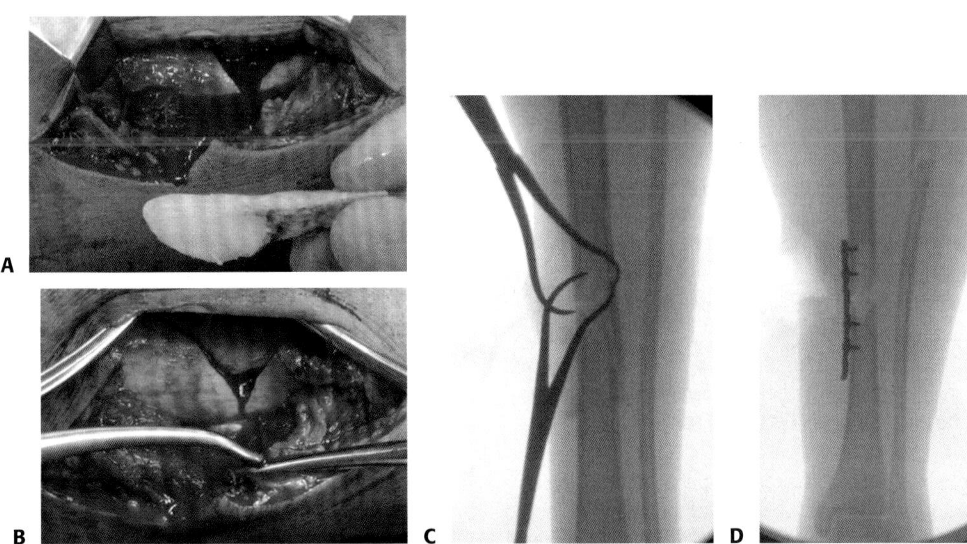

**TECH FIG 8** • Reduction of an open middle diaphyseal fracture. **A.** A large segment of stripped cortical bone has been removed and cleaned on the back table. **B.** The cortical fragment has been placed into the fracture site and clamped in reduced position to reduce the fracture anatomically. **C.** Intraoperative fluoroscopic image of the fracture with the fracture fragment clamped in reduced position; note that this fragment will be removed after reaming and nail passage. **D.** Unicortical plates are useful for maintaining reduction during nail passage.

- Once centralized, the ball-tipped wire must be impacted into the subchondral bone of the tibial plafond at the level of the physeal scar. This decreases the risk of inadvertently removing the guidewire during reaming.
- Nail length measurement is performed using supplied length gauges and should be verified with lateral fluoroscopic measurement (**TECH FIG 9B**). The lateral view is used because it is more accurate in determining the level of the articular surface and avoiding nail prominence.
    - Alternatively, inserting a guidewire of the same length to the nail entry site and then measuring the length differential between wires also provides an accurate measurement. However, this introduces the significant cost of a second guidewire.
- Device manufacturers supply nails in variable increments. When a length measurement falls in between lengths, choose the shorter length. A threaded end cap (usually 5, 10, and 15 mm) can be used if it is desired to bring the nail to top of the canal opening.
- Leaving the nail countersunk below the bone surface does not compromise stability in middle and distal fractures but may complicate future nail extraction.

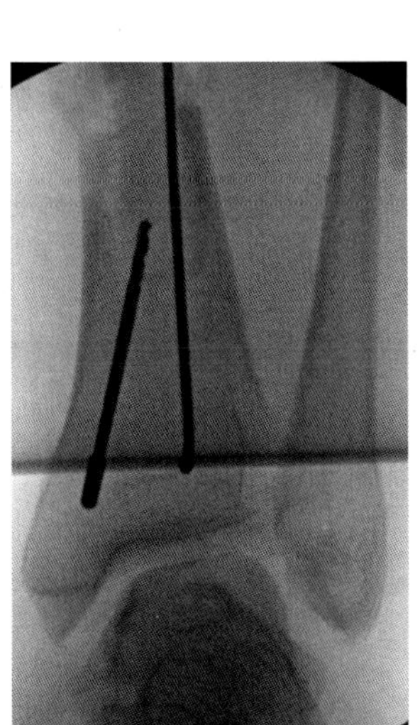

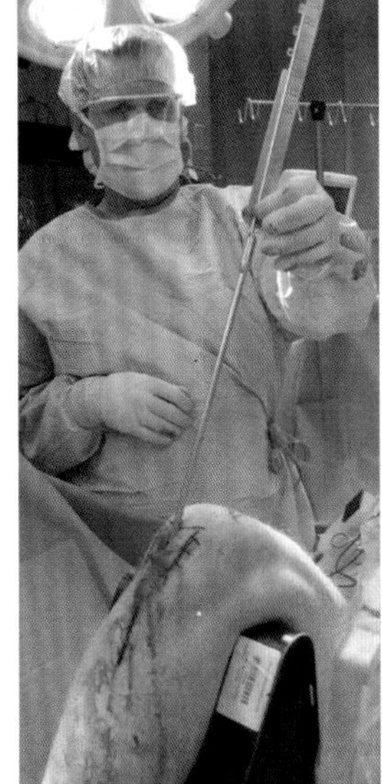

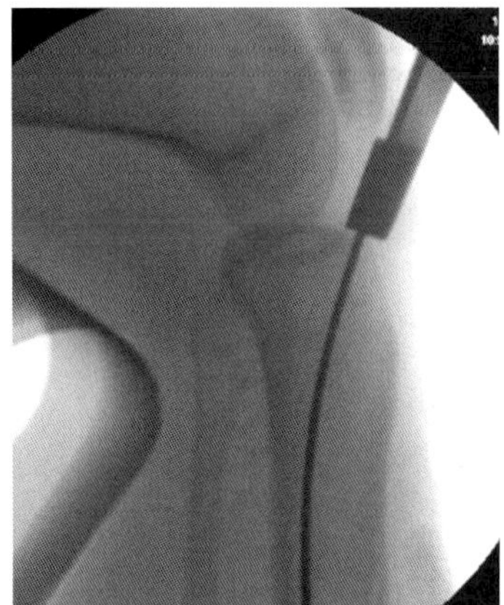

**TECH FIG 9** • **A.** A drill bit is used to ensure the guidewire is placed centrally in the distal segment of this distal metadiaphyseal fracture. **B,C.** The nail length guide is pushed to the opening of the tibia and verified with lateral fluoroscopic imaging.

## Reaming the Canal

- Before reaming, estimate the narrowest canal diameter using both AP and lateral plain radiographs. Alternatively, intramedullary reamer sets typically have a radiolucent ruler that allows for intraoperative fluoroscopic verification, which should be done on both the AP and lateral views. The canal typically is reamed at least 1 mm over the isthmic diameter to minimize the risk of nail incarceration.
- Reaming should begin with an end-cutting reamer—the 8.5- or 9-mm size in most systems.
- Reamer heads should be evaluated before insertion and should be sharp and free of defects.
- Insert the reamer head into the proximal metaphysis with the knee in maximal flexion before applying power to avoid distorting the entrance hole (**TECH FIG 10A**).
- Reamers are advanced at a slow pace under full power.
  - If the reamer shafts are not solid, but are wound, be sure to avoid using reverse when drilling because that would cause the reamers to unwind if resistance is encountered within the intramedullary canal.
- Care must be taken not to inadvertently extract the guidewire when the reamers are removed.
  - Multiple techniques are used. First, manual downward pressure can be applied to the wire with specialized instruments, medicine cups, or cleaning cannulas (**TECH FIG 10B**).
  - Once the reamer has cleared the opening, it can be clamped and held in position (**TECH FIG 10C**).
- For the minimally reamed technique, a single end-cutting reamer (usually 9 mm) is passed down the canal to ensure the smallest diameter nail can pass through the narrowest segment of the intramedullary canal.
- In an effort to minimize thermal damage to the endosteal cortex, reaming should be discontinued within 0.5 to 1 mm of hearing the reamer head catching ("chatter") on the endosteal cortex.
  - Care also should be used when there are butterfly or oblique fracture fragments. Continued reaming after encountering chatter may result in iatrogenic comminution and loss of reduction.

## Unreamed Technique

- Standard preparation technique is used for the starting hole, and the fracture is reduced.
- Precise evaluation of the lateral isthmic diameter is repeated, and a small-diameter nail is selected, typically in the 7- to 9-mm range.
- A good guideline is to use a nail 1 to 1.5 mm smaller than the narrowest measure of the isthmus on the lateral radiograph.
- If lateral plane imaging is suggestive of canal diameter very close to nail size, a single pass with an end-cutting reamer usually is performed to decrease the possibility of nail incarceration.
- The nail is inserted and impacted in standard fashion. If significant resistance is encountered when the nail reaches the isthmus, the nail is removed to avoid incarceration or iatrogenic fracture propagation. A reamer 0.5 to 1.0 mm larger than the nail is passed down the canal, and nail passage is attempted again.

## Nail Insertion

- Once the nail insertion handle is attached, pass a drill through the proximal screw insertion attachment and screw insertion cannulas before inserting the nail to ensure accurate alignment of the attachment jig.
- Maintain nail rotation during insertion by aligning the center of the insertion handle with the tibial crest. Consider internal rotation of the nail if distal AP interlocking bolts are deemed necessary to minimize damage to distal neurovascular structures.
  - Maintain knee hyperflexion during nail insertion to minimize the risk of posterior cortical abutment and iatrogenic fracture.
- Impact the nail to the final depth using lateral plane fluoroscopy.

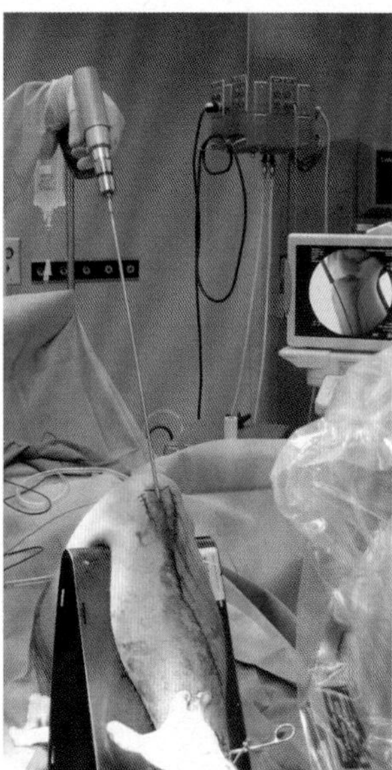
A

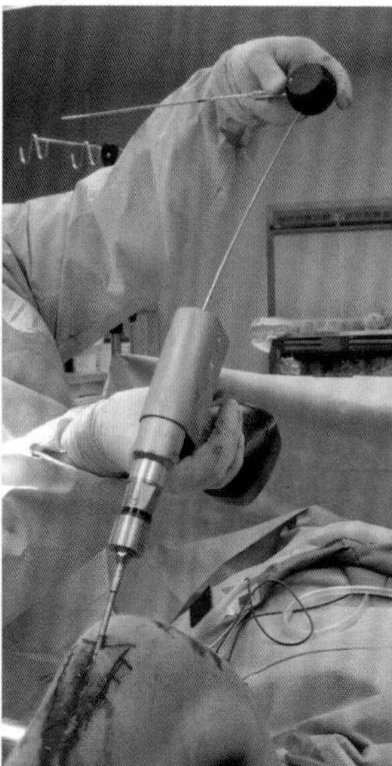
B

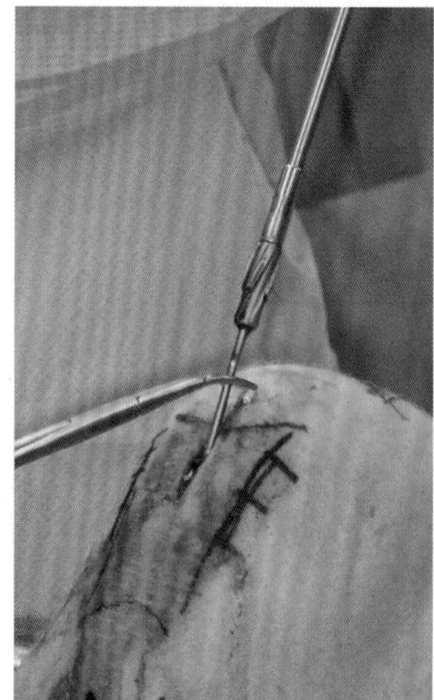
C

**TECH FIG 10** • **A.** Maintenance of maximal knee flexion protects the entrance hole from being inadvertently enlarged by the reamer. **B.** If the guidewire is rotating during reaming, it must be held down as the reamer is pulled back to avoid inadvertent removal of the guidewire. **C.** A clamp can be used to grasp the guidewire when the reamer head clears the soft tissues.

### *Interlocking Bolt Insertion*

- In simple transverse fractures, place distal interlocks first to allow for backslapping for interfragmentary compression and gap minimization.
- Usually, distal interlock bolts are placed medial to lateral.
- Position the leg in slight extension and stable neutral rotation.
- Rotate the C-arm to lateral imaging position and pull the tube back away from the medial side of the leg to allow for drill placement.
- Rotate the leg and C-arm individually and sequentially to create a perfect circle image; optimize this view before drilling attempts (**TECH FIG 11A**).
- After localizing the interlocking hole using a clamp and fluoroscopy, make an incision large enough to place the locking bolt. Use blunt clamp dissection until the cortex is reached.
- Use a sharp drill point and place the center of the point in the center of the circle.
  - Hold the drill obliquely to the nail axis to simplify repositioning (**TECH FIG 11B**).
- Once the central location is achieved; align hand and drill with imaging axis.
  - Fluoroscopes with laser alignment guides can be helpful to assist with alignment by centering the laser on the skin incision and then placing the laser in the center of the back of the drill when preparing to drill the hole (**TECH FIG 11C**).
  - Drill to the midsagittal point in the tibia. Then, disengage the drill from the drill bit and check the fluoroscopic image.
    - If the drill is accurately positioned in the center of the hole, advance the drill bit with power through the far cortex; avoid broaching the far cortex by impacting with a mallet to avoid iatrogenic fracture.
    - Drill the second interlock hole using the same technique but maintaining a parallel axis with the first successful drill passage.
- Replace the drill with the appropriate depth gauge and check an AP image before screw length selection.
- Once interlock lengths and position are verified, "backslapping" can occur to optimize compression.
  - Using the slotted mallet attachment on the insertion handle, superiorly directed mallet blows can be used while pressure is applied to the foot in order to compress the fracture site. Fluoroscopy should be used to monitor the amount of compression and the nail position proximally. If backslapping is planned, the nail should be slightly overinserted to avoid nail prominence after compression is performed.
- Place proximal interlocks through drill guides.
  - Because the tibia is a triangle, oblique views may be used to more accurately judge screw length for transverse locking bolt measurement.
  - If oblique locking bolts are chosen proximally, oblique fluoroscopic views should be used prior to insertion handle removal to avoid placing long screws that are particularly symptomatic on the medial side of the knee and to avoid injury to the peroneal nerve posterolaterally.

## Lateral Parapatellar Tendon Approach

- After completing the lateral parapatellar approach described, the standard patient positioning is used.
- The lateral parapatellar approach allows the guide pin to be more easily placed just medial to the lateral tibial spine on the AP view and along the lateral cortex to correct the valgus angulation.
  - If a true AP view is not obtained and the leg is externally rotated, the starting point will be more medial than desired.[4]
- It is important to get enough knee flexion over the radiolucent triangle or bolster to allow for the guide pin to be placed as proximal as possible and parallel along the anterior tibial cortex to help correct the typical flexion deformity.[20]

## Semiextended Technique

- The benefit of the semiextended technique is that the leg position helps neutralize the associated flexion deformity.[26]
- The patient is placed in the semiextended position as described earlier.
- The open medial parapatellar approach can be used (see **TECH FIG 2**).
  - Using the previously described surgical approach, the patella is subluxated to allow for guide pin placement, reaming, and nail placement, with the knee remaining in the semiextended position.
  - No special instruments are required.
- Suprapatellar approach[28]
  - Either the superomedial or direct superior approach is used.
  - Special instrumentation is required; which instrumentation is needed depends on the specific system used.

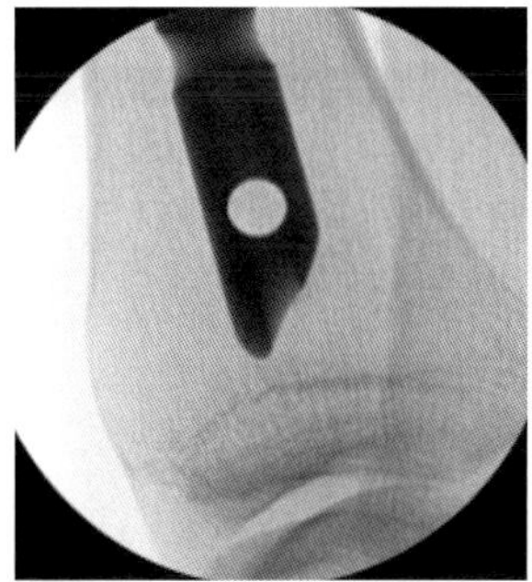
A

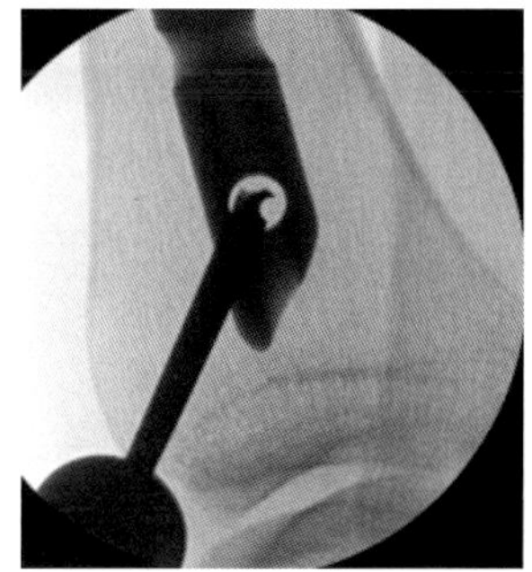
B

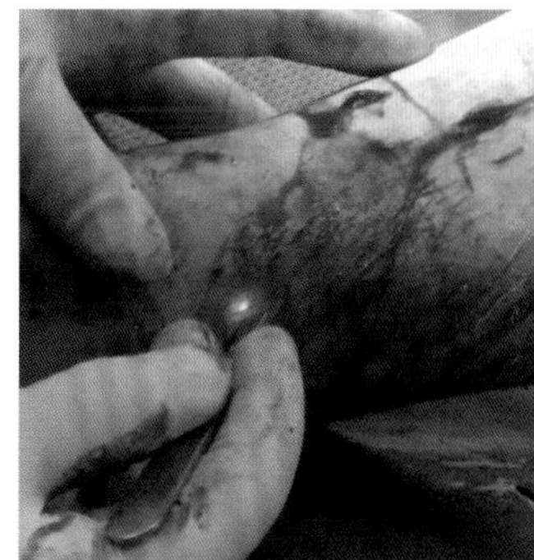
C

**TECH FIG 11** • **A.** A perfectly rotated lateral fluoroscopic image will appear as a perfect circle and should be achieved before drilling is attempted. **B.** The drill point must be aligned in the center of the perfect circle before drilling. **C.** The laser alignment guide can be helpful for localizing the skin incision.

- The patella is subluxated using an elongated cannula (**TECH FIG 12A**).
- The cannula is advanced to the standard starting point using fluoroscopy.
- The guide pin is placed in the standard position (**TECH FIG 12B**).
- The typical steps—using the opening drill, placing the guidewire, and reaming—are all completed through the elongated cannula.
- Standard intramedullary reamers can be used but reamer extensions are helpful, especially in taller patients.
- Fracture reduction and passing of the guidewire are performed before reaming.
- A special elongated nail insertion handle is required for nail insertion (**TECH FIG 12C**).
- Proximal locking bolt insertion is done using the aiming arm.
- Distal locking bolts are placed using the standard freehand technique, as previously described.

## Adjunct Reduction and Fixation Techniques

### *Blocking/Pöller Screws*

- Screws can be placed across the intramedullary canal to create a "false" cortex outside of the isthmus that narrows the potential space for the nail. This aids in both fracture reduction as the nail is being placed and maintenance of the reduction once the nail is seated.[13,24]
- Locking bolts found in the nailing set or screws made from the same metal as the nail should be used.
- Blocking screws can either be placed prior to initial nail insertion or, if the nail is inserted and residual deformity exists, the nail can be removed and blocking screws can be inserted.
  - Coronal and sagittal plane correction can be performed by placing a screw at the concavity of the deformity.
    - To correct valgus, the screw is placed laterally (**TECH FIG 13A**). To correct lateral plane extension, the screw is placed posteriorly (**TECH FIG 13B**).
  - The appropriately sized drill bit is placed with fluoroscopic assistance.
  - The appropriately sized screw replaces the drill bit.
  - The guidewire is then inserted and seated distally.
  - Intramedullary reaming is necessary to ensure the nail follows the newly created path.
    - When a screw that blocks the way is encountered, simply push the reamer head past the screw without reaming. This avoids dulling the reamer head and potentially displacing the blocking screw.
    - Once passed the screw, resume reaming.
    - After reaming is complete, insert the intramedullary nail.
    - If the displacement has not been corrected, it will be necessary to remove the nail, and additional screws may be added. Reaming and reinsertion of the guidewire are required before reinserting the nail.
  - Interlocking bolts through the nail are placed in the standard fashion (**TECH FIG 13B,C**).

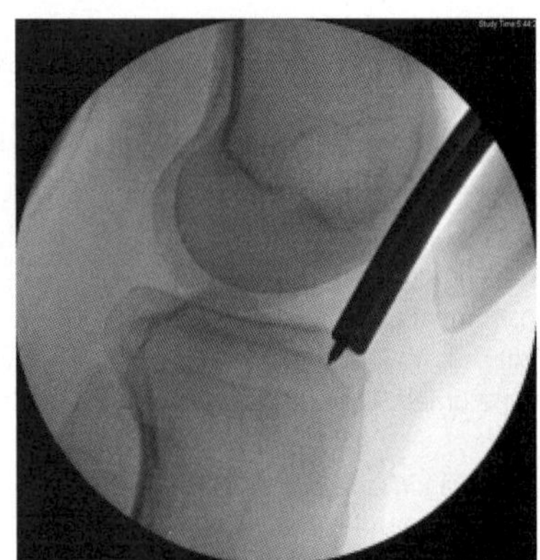

A

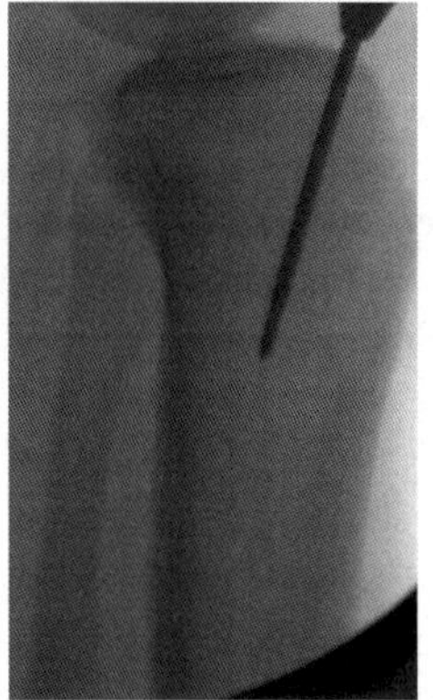

B

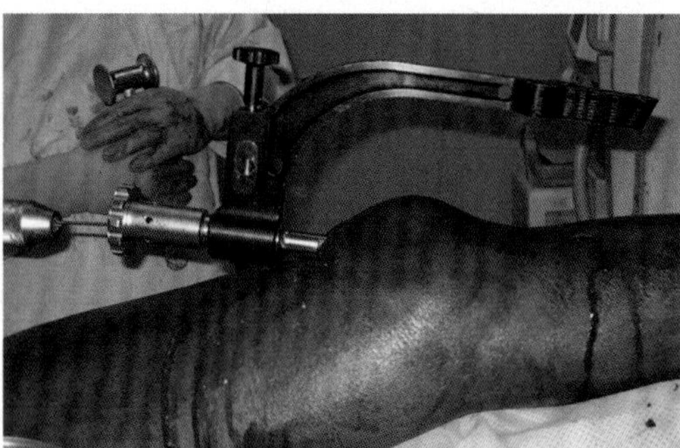

C

**TECH FIG 12** • **A.** Suprapatellar approach: A specially designed cannula is used to subluxate the patella and pass through the patellofemoral joint and is positioned at the appropriate starting point. **B.** The guide pin is advanced appropriately and the cannula is used for the opening reamer, guidewire placement, and intramedullary reaming—but not nail insertion. Long reamer extensions are helpful for intramedullary reaming. **C.** A specialized, long insertion handle is required for suprapatellar techniques to reach the tibial start site.

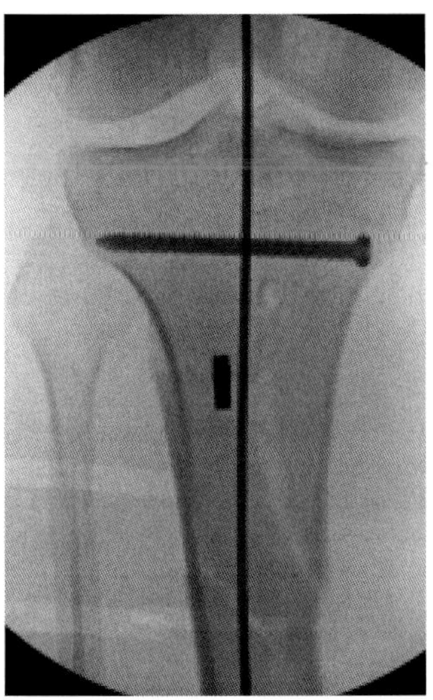

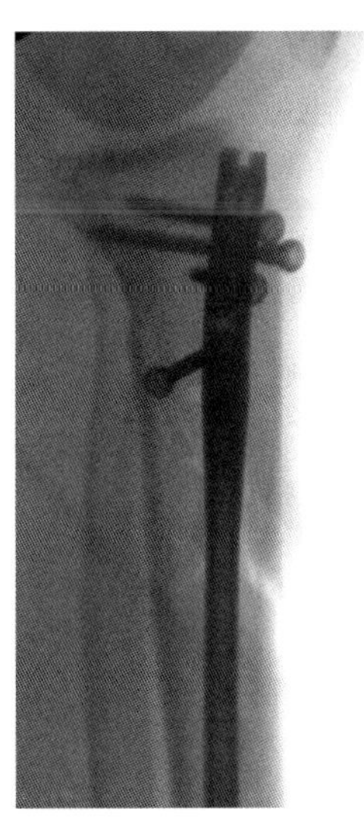

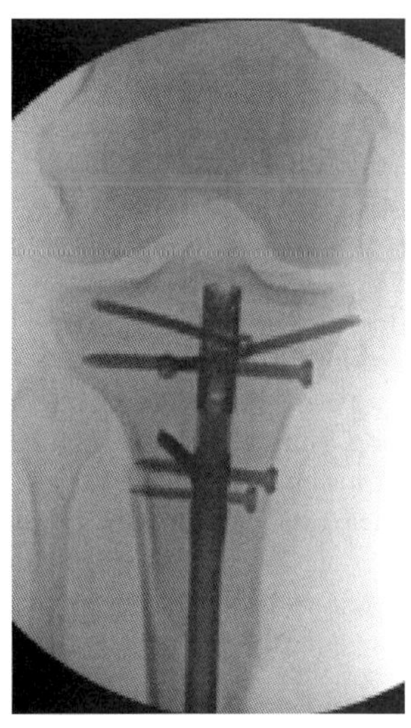

**TECH FIG 13** • **A.** A blocking screw positioned just lateral to the ideal nail path to prevent valgus deformation. **B.** A posterior blocking screw limits proximal fragment extension by limiting the effective anterior to posterior canal diameter. **B,C.** Lateral and AP fluoroscopic imaging showing oblique and medial to lateral interlocking bolts placed through the nail.

## PEARLS AND PITFALLS

| | |
|---|---|
| **Starting point** | ▪ The starting point should be at the anterior articular margin and just medial to the lateral tibial spine. Starting too medial and distal for proximal metaphyseal fractures results in a valgus and flexed malunion. |
| **Centering the guidewire** | ▪ Center the guidewire distally on the AP and lateral views. If not centered, the nail will follow the path of the reamer and guidewire, which will malreduce the fracture. |
| **Measuring nail length** | ▪ Measure on the lateral view. Measuring on the AP view will potentially lead to a nail that is too long, with articular prominence causing knee pain or articular surface damage. |
| **Femoral distractor or external fixator for reduction** | ▪ Half-pins can be placed outside of the path of the nail. The best positions are posterior in the proximal tibia and distally very close to the subchondral bone of the tibial plafond. Placement of the proximal pin too anteriorly and the distal pin too proximally may impede reaming and nail insertion. |
| **Unicortical plates for reduction** | ▪ Metadiaphyseal plates contribute to stability and maintenance of reduction and removal can lead to loss of reduction after nail passage. Diaphyseal reduction plates, however, should be removed to prevent rigid fixation of the fracture gap. |
| **Blocking screws/Pöller screws** | ▪ Use interlocking bolts from nail instrumentation rather than small fragment screws to avoid screw breakage during nail passage.<br>▪ Do not remove screws because they provide stability and help maintain reduction.<br>▪ Use caution when using a drill bit because it is prone to breakage during nail insertion and removal after nail passage may destabilize the construct. |
| **Posterior malleolus** | ▪ Critically evaluate the posterior malleolus in distal diaphyseal and metaphyseal fractures pre-, intra-, and postoperatively.<br>▪ If a posterior malleolar fracture or articular involvement is missed, ankle subluxation or displacement of the articular surface can occur with weight bearing. |

## POSTOPERATIVE CARE

- Weight bearing as tolerated, unless there is articular involvement
- Posterior splint or cam walker
- Early range of motion
- Suture removal at 2 to 3 weeks postoperatively
- Strengthening after at 6-week clinic visit
  - Consider a quadriceps-specific program.
- After the 6-week visit, return clinic visits are made at 6- to 8-week intervals until the bone is clinically and radiographically healed.

## OUTCOMES

- Long-term follow-up of patients treated nonoperatively reveals persistent functional deficits and dysfunction, including stiffness, pain, and loss of muscle power.[7,15,22,23]

- Anterior knee pain is common (50% to 60%), and patients should be informed of this preoperatively.[5,11]
  - This knee pain is more common in young patients. It typically is mild and may be exacerbated by kneeling, squatting, or running.
  - Its occurrence is not dependent on surgical approach.
  - Nail removal leads to pain resolution in about one-half of patients and decreased pain in another one-fourth.[6]
- At late follow-up after tibial nailing, patients' function is comparable to population norms, but objective and subjective evaluation shows persistent sequelae, including knee pain, persistent swelling, muscle weakness, and arthritis—many of which are not insignificant.
- Malunion has an unclear association with development of arthritis.
  - Some authors have associated even mild deformity with increased risk of osteoarthritis.[12,32]

## COMPLICATIONS[4,25]

### Infection

- Closed fractures: about 1%
- Open fractures
  - Type I: 5%
  - Type II: 10%
  - Type III: over 15%
- Condition of the soft tissues is key for risk of infection and for outcome.

### Nonunion

- Closed fractures: 3%
- Open fractures: about 15% and may be higher, depending on the soft tissue injury
- Risk factors
  - Unreamed smaller diameter nails with smaller locking bolts are associated with delayed or nonunion and an increased risk of locking bolt breakage.
  - Closed fractures carry a risk of severe soft tissue injury, that is, internal degloving.
  - Open fractures may be accompanied by severe soft tissue injury.
    - Delayed bone grafting may be warranted for treatment of bone loss.
    - The use of recombinant human bone morphogenetic protein 2 (RhBMP-2) is U.S. Food and Drug Administration (FDA) approved in open tibia fractures.[8] It decreases the nonunion rate by 29% and decreases secondary interventions. BMP-2 combined with allograft for delayed bone grafting procedures in tibia fractures with cortical defects have shown a similar rate of healing to autograft with the benefit of decreased donor site morbidity.[10]
  - Compartment syndrome
  - Fracture pattern—transverse
  - Host factors
    - Tobacco use
    - Medications: bisphosphonates, nonsteroidal anti-inflammatory drugs
    - Diabetes mellitus
    - Vascular disease
    - Malnutrition—albumin level lower than 34 g/L and a lymphocyte count below 1500/mm$^3$
  - Infection

### Malunion

- Occurs in up to 37% of all tibial nailing procedures
  - Malunion is seen in as many as 84% of patients with proximal metaphyseal tibia fractures.
  - These can be avoided with proper surgical techniques.

## REFERENCES

1. Baumgartner M, Tornetta P, eds. Orthopaedic Knowledge Update: Trauma 3. Rosemont, IL: American Academy of Orthopaedic Surgeons, 2005.
2. Bone LB, Sucato D, Stegemann PM, et al. Displaced isolated fractures of the tibial shaft treated with either a cast or intramedullary nailing. An outcome analysis of matched pairs of patients. J Bone Joint Surg Am 1997;79(9):1336–1341.
3. Bono CM, Sirkin M, Sabatino CT, et al. Neurovascular and tendinous damage with placement of anteroposterior distal locking bolts in the tibia. J Orthop Trauma 2003;17:677–682.
4. Cannada LK, Anglen JO, Archdeacon MT, et al. Avoiding complications in the care of fractures of the tibia. J Bone Joint Surg Am 2008;90(8):1760–1768.
5. Court-Brown CM, Gustilo T, Shaw AD. Knee pain after intramedullary tibial nailing: its incidence, etiology, and outcome. J Orthop Trauma 1997;11:103–105.
6. Court-Brown CM, McBirnie J. The epidemiology of tibial fractures. J Bone Joint Surg Br 1995;77(3):417–421.
7. Digby JM, Holloway GM, Webb JK. A study of function after tibial cast bracing. Injury 1983;14:432–439.
8. Govender S, Csimma C, Genant HK, et al. Recombinant human bone morphogenetic protein-2 for treatment of open tibial fractures: a prospective, controlled, randomized study of four hundred and fifty patients. J Bone Joint Surg Am 2002;84-A:2123–2134.
9. Hooper GJ, Keddell RG, Penny ID. Conservative management or closed nailing for tibial shaft fractures. A randomised prospective trial. J Bone Joint Surg Br 1991;73(1):83–85.
10. Jones AL, Bucholz RW, Bosse MJ, et al. Recombinant human BMP-2 and allograft compared with autogenous bone graft for reconstruction of diaphyseal tibial fractures with cortical defects: a randomized, controlled trial. J Bone Joint Surg Am 2006;88(7):1431–1441.
11. Keating JF, Orfaly R, O'Brien PJ. Knee pain after tibial nailing. J Orthop Trauma 1997;11:10–13.
12. Kettelkamp DB, Hillberry BM, Murrish DE, et al. Degenerative arthritis of the knee secondary to fracture malunion. Clin Orthop Relat Res 1988;(234):159–169.
13. Krettek C, Miclau T, Schandelmaier P, et al. The mechanical effect of blocking screws ("Poller screws") in stabilizing tibia fractures with short proximal or distal fragments after insertion of small-diameter intramedullary nails. J Orthop Trauma 1999;13:550–553.
14. Kubiak EN, Widmer BJ, Horwitz DS. Extra-articular technique for semiextended tibial nailing. J Orthop Trauma 2010;24(11):704–708.
15. Kyro A, Lamppu M, Bostman O. Intramedullary nailing of tibial shaft fractures. Ann Chir Gynaecol 1995;84:51–61.
16. McKee MD, Schemitsch EH, Waddell JP, et al. A prospective, randomized clinical trial comparing tibial nailing using fracture table traction versus manual traction. J Orthop Trauma 1999;13:463–469.
17. McQueen MM, Christie J, Court-Brown CM. Acute compartment syndrome in tibial diaphyseal fractures. J Bone Joint Surg Br 1996;78(1):95–98.
18. Mills WJ, Barei DP, McNair P. The value of the ankle-brachial index for diagnosing arterial injury after knee dislocation: a prospective study. J Trauma 2004;56:1261–1265.
19. Milner S, Greenwood D. Degenerative changes at the knee and ankle related to malunion of tibial fractures. J Bone Joint Surg Br 1997;79(4):698.
20. Nork SE, Barei DP, Schildhauer TA, et al. Intramedullary nailing of proximal quarter tibial fractures. J Orthop Trauma 2006;20:523–528.

21. Orfaly R, Keating JE, O'Brien PJ. Knee pain after tibial nailing: does the entry point matter? J Bone Joint Surg Br 1995;77(6):976–977.
22. Pun WK, Chow SP, Fang D, et al. A study of function and residual joint stiffness after functional bracing of tibial shaft fractures. Clin Orthop Relat Res 1991;(267):157–163.
23. Puno RM, Teynor JT, Nagano J, et al. Critical analysis of results of treatment of 201 tibial shaft fractures. Clin Orthop Relat Res 1986;(212):113–121.
24. Ricci WM, O'Boyle M, Borrelli J, et al. Fractures of the proximal third of the tibial shaft treated with intramedullary nails and blocking screws. J Orthop Trauma 2001;15:264–270.
25. Schmidt A, Finkemeier CG, Tornetta P. Treatment of closed tibia fractures. In: Tornetta P, ed. Instructional Course Lectures: Trauma. Rosemont, IL: American Academy of Orthopaedic Surgeons, 2006:215–229.
26. Tornetta P III, Collins E. Semiextended position of intramedullary nailing of the proximal tibia. Clin Orthop Relat Res 1996;(328):185–189.
27. Tornetta P III, Riina J, Geller J, et al. Intraarticular anatomic risks of tibial nailing. J Orthop Trauma 1999;13:247–251.
28. Tornetta P III, Steen B, Ryan S. Tibial metaphyseal fractures: nailing in extension. Presented at Orthopaedic Trauma Association Annual Meeting, Denver, October 16–18, 2008.
29. Väistö O, Toivanen J, Kannus P, et al. Anterior knee pain after intramedullary nailing of fractures of the tibial shaft: an eight-year follow-up of a prospective, randomized study comparing two different nail-insertion techniques. J Trauma 2008;64:1511–1516.
30. Väistö O, Toivanen J, Kannus P, et al. Anterior knee pain and thigh muscle strength after intramedullary nailing of a tibial shaft fracture: an 8-year follow-up of 28 consecutive cases. J Orthop Trauma 2007:21:165–171.
31. Väistö O, Toivanen J, Paakkala T, et al. Anterior knee pain after intramedullary nailing of a tibial shaft fracture: an ultrasound study of the patellar tendons of 36 patients. J Orthop Trauma 2005;19:311–316.
32. van der Schoot DK, Den Outer AJ, Bode PJ, et al. Degenerative changes at the knee and ankle related to malunion of tibial fractures. 15-year follow-up of 88 patients. J Bone Joint Surg Br 1996;78:722–725.
33. Walker RM, Zdero R, McKee MD, et al. Ideal tibial intramedullary nail insertion point varies with tibial rotation. J Orthop Trauma 2011;25:726–730.
34. Weninger P, Schultz A, Traxler H, et al. Anatomical assessment of the Hoffa fat pad during insertion of a tibial intramedullary nail—comparison of three surgical approaches. J Trauma 2009;66: 1140–1145.

# Intramedullary Nailing of Metaphyseal Proximal and Distal Fractures of the Mature Tibia

Robert Ostrum and Michael Quackenbush

## DEFINITION

- A fracture of the proximal or distal tibial metaphysis can occur from a variety of high- and low-energy trauma.
- Fractures may be confined to the metaphysis or extend into the articular surface.
- Simple fractures suggest lower energy injuries, whereas comminution signifies a greater amount of energy and a higher velocity mechanism.

## ANATOMY

- Proximal metaphyseal fractures of the tibia are those that occur proximal to the isthmus of the tibia (**FIG 1A**).
- Distal metaphyseal fractures of the tibia are those that occur distal to the isthmus of the tibia (**FIG 1B**).

## PATHOGENESIS

- Common causes of tibial fractures include high-energy collisions (pedestrian vs. car bumper) such as an automobile or motorcycle crash.
- Lower energy injuries, such as certain sports injuries or falls, can also cause fractures of both the proximal or distal tibial metaphysis.

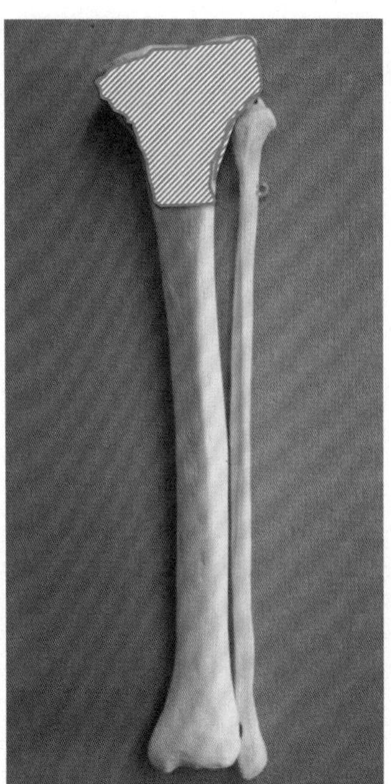
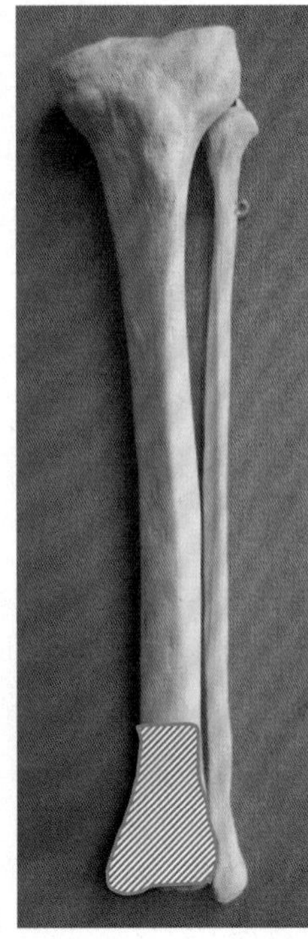

**FIG 1** • **A.** AP view of synthetic tibia model. *Shading* of the proximal tibial metaphysis is shown. **B.** AP view of synthetic tibia model. *Shading* of the distal tibial metaphysis is shown.

## NATURAL HISTORY

- Fractures of the tibia can occur in all age groups and from a variety of mechanisms.
- Goals of treatment should include restoration of length, rotation, and alignment of the tibia with a return to previous level of activity and function.
- Recognition and treatment of associated injuries including those to nerves, blood vessels, or compartment syndrome should be an integral part of the assessment and treatment to prevent complications.

## PATIENT HISTORY AND PHYSICAL FINDINGS

- Patients will often present with a recent history of trauma.
- Tibial fractures may present with a variety of findings:
  - Pain in the affected extremity with an inability to bear weight
  - Leg length inequality
  - Visual deformity including tenting of the skin
  - Contusions/abrasions
  - Nerve injury
  - Open fractures
  - Compartment syndrome
  - Sensory deficits in the foot (less common)

## IMAGING AND OTHER DIAGNOSTIC STUDIES

- Diagnosis of a proximal or distal tibia (**FIG 2A,B**) fracture can usually be made with standard orthogonal anteroposterior (AP) and lateral x-rays.
  - Dedicated knee and ankle x-rays are necessary to decrease the chance of missing a fracture at the articular surface.
- Fractures that extend proximally or distally into the articular surface may require a computed tomography (CT) scan to evaluate joint involvement and/or displacement to aid in preoperative planning (**FIG 3A,B**).

## DIFFERENTIAL DIAGNOSIS

- Trauma
  - Fractures of the knee
  - Fractures of the ankle
- Soft tissue injury
  - Ankle injury
  - Knee injury
- Compartment syndrome
- Peripheral vascular injury
- Pathologic process (tumor/malignancy)
- Infection

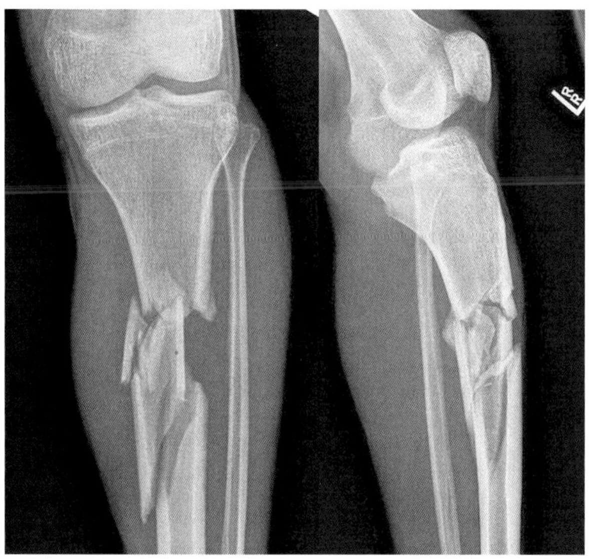

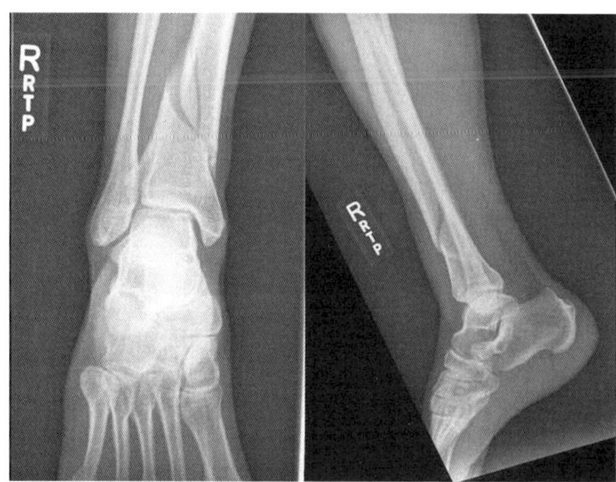

**FIG 2 • A.** AP and lateral x-ray of a proximal tibia fracture. **B.** AP and lateral x-ray of a distal tibia fracture.

## NONOPERATIVE MANAGEMENT

- Nonoperative management is normally reserved for lower energy injuries with minimal or no displacement.
- Patients with low functional demands (ie, paraplegic) or significant medical comorbidities can be successfully treated without surgical intervention.
- Nonoperative management of the proximal or distal tibia often involves a long-leg splint with conversion to a long-leg cast once swelling has resolved.
  - Distal fractures may be converted to a short-leg cast or brace once there is radiographic evidence of healing.
- Non–weight bearing for the first 6 weeks with progression to full weight bearing, with or without a brace, once there is physical evidence of healing (decrease in pain) and/or radiographic evidence of healing (callus formation)

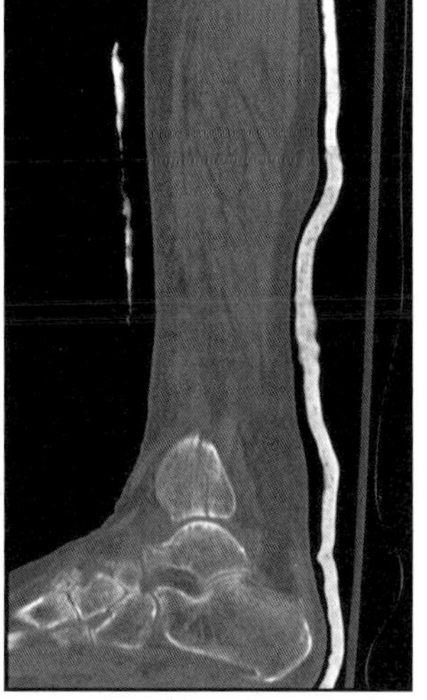

**FIG 3 • A.** CT of distal tibia with axial cut demonstrating intra-articular extension of distal tibia fracture. **B.** CT of distal tibia with sagittal cut demonstrating intra-articular extension of distal tibia fracture.

## SURGICAL MANAGEMENT

### Proximal Tibia Fractures

- The proximal tibia presents a challenge for intramedullary (IM) nailing due to deforming forces from the patella and the eccentric starting point for the IM nail.
- Flexion of the knee past 60 degrees to allow access to the tibial nail starting point causes the quadriceps, patella, and patellar tendon to extend the proximal fracture fragment leading to an extreme procurvatum deformity.
  - In addition, starting the IM nail at the "usual" starting point, just medial to the lateral tibial spine, in the coronal plane will produce a valgus deformity. Techniques to prevent these deformities include the following:
    - Judicious use of blocking screws
    - Suprapatellar IM nailing
    - Semiextended IM nailing
    - Clamps, plates for reduction prior to IM nailing

### Preoperative Planning

- A review of all images will help to plan the surgical approach.
- Fractures that extend into the proximal plateau or across the distal plafond may require closed or open reduction and fixation prior to IM nailing.
  - Cancellous screws (6.5 mm) placed posteriorly in the tibial plateau will be out of the way of the tibial nail and its entry site.
  - Depending on the fixation required, small fragment screws and/or plates should be readily available for distal fractures.
- Obtaining and maintaining the reduction may require additional equipment. Planning ahead of time will avoid unnecessary delays in the operating room.
  - Some examples of other items you may wish to have available include (**FIG 4A,B**) the following:
    - Clamps, "spike" pushers, K-wires
    - Small fragment set (for provisional plate fixation)
    - Large fragment (6.5, 7.3 mm) cannulated cancellous screws
    - External fixator/universal distractor
    - Skeletal traction tray (calcaneal traction)

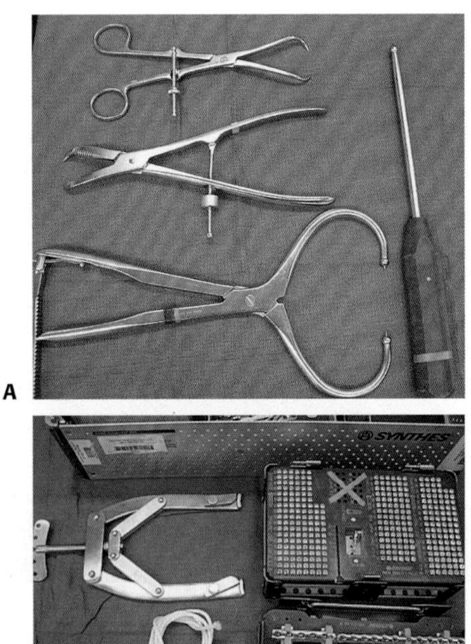

**FIG 4** • **A,B.** Preoperative planning may include additional equipment. This may include small fragment plates and screws (Synthes, Paoli, PA), specific clamps, or traction sets.

## Positioning

- Patients are positioned in the supine position on a radiolucent table. A bolster may be placed under the ipsilateral hip.
- Radiolucent triangles may be used to assist with hyperflexion of the knee for standard nailing (**FIG 5**), whereas smaller bumps may be placed under the knee for semiextended approaches (**FIG 6**).

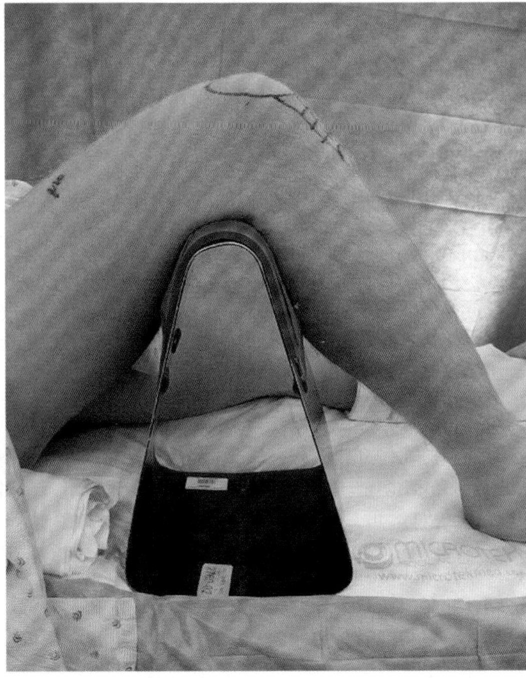

**FIG 5** • Standard tibial nailing requires hyperflexion of the knee. Radiolucent triangles may help with positioning.

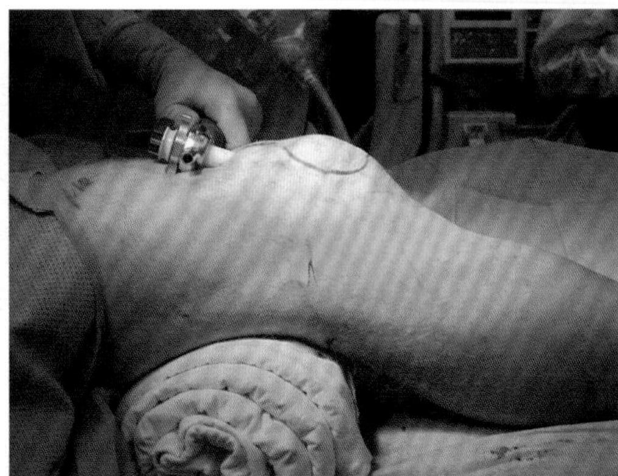

**FIG 6** • Patient positioning for semiextended or suprapatellar nailing. Notice a small bump under the knee to provide 30 to 40 degrees of knee flexion. Suprapatellar nailing requires specific instruments seen here.

## Approach

- Standard nailing uses an incision between the inferior pole of the patella and the tibial tubercle (**FIG 7**).
- Incision is carried down through skin and subcutaneous tissue and should be carried distally to the proximal tibia.
- The patellar tendon is identified and an incision can be made medial to the patellar tendon or through the tendon.
  - Guidewire placement and correct starting point are extremely important, especially with proximal fractures.
  - Avoid an incision too medial which could make it difficult to achieve the correct starting point.
- Semiextended nailing uses a suprapatellar portal.
  - The incision is made from the superior pole of the patella proximally in line with the quadriceps tendon (**FIG 8**). A deeper incision is then made through the quadriceps tendon.
  - If the knee joint is too tight to enter through this portal, the skin incision can be carried distally and a medial parapatellar arthrotomy can be made to help elevate the patella out of way and provide access to the correct starting point.
  - The semiextended approaches require specific instrumentation (**FIG 9**) and soft tissue guides to help protect the cartilage in the patellofemoral joint and to avoid unnecessary damage to the joint surface.

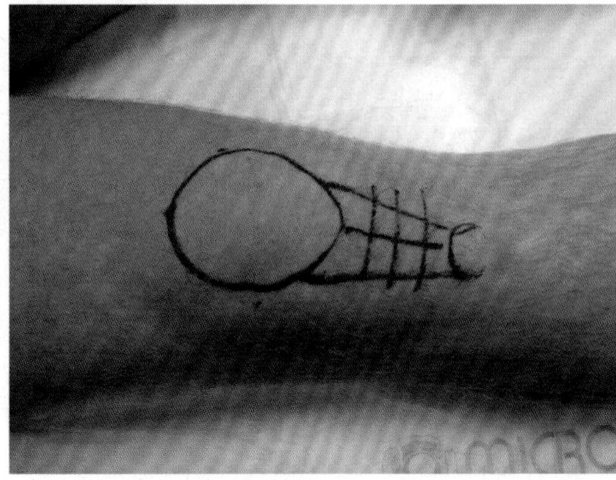

**FIG 7** • Skin incision for standard tibial nailing from inferior pole of the patella to the tibial tubercle.

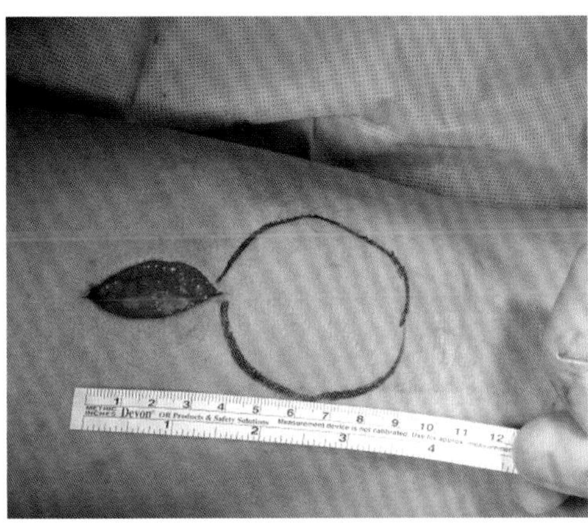

**FIG 8** • Skin incision used for a suprapatellar tibial nail is from the superior pole of the patella proximal approximately 3 cm centered over the quadriceps tendon.

- Guide pin placement and starting point are dependent on whether the tibia fracture is proximal or distal.
  - For distal fractures, a starting point just medial to the lateral tibial eminence on the frontal plane and along the proximal anterior portion of the tibia anterior to the cruciate insertion is appropriate.

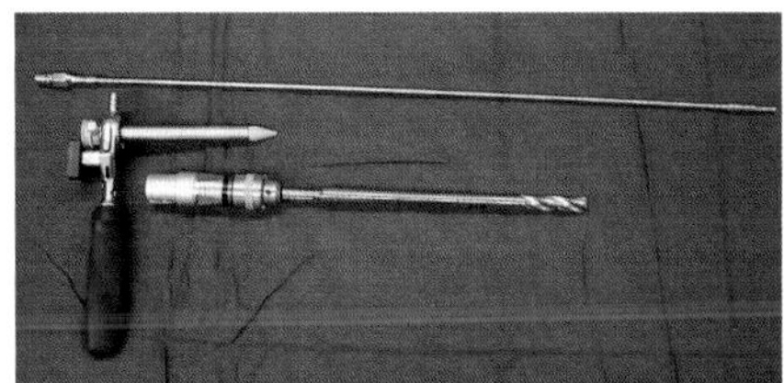

**FIG 9** • Suprapatellar nailing requires specific instrumentation. Specifically, it requires longer cannulas to protect the cartilage of the patellofemoral joint, a longer opening reamer, and longer reamer rods.

  - The wire should be aiming down the center of the canal in the AP plane and traversing parallel to the anterior cortex on the lateral view.
- For proximal fractures, the starting guide pin should be slightly more lateral, in line with the lateral tibial eminence, and parallel to the lateral cortex of the proximal tibia.
- On the lateral view, a more anterior starting point that is extra-articular but on the flat surface of the proximal tibia, avoiding the meniscus attachments, with the guidewire directed parallel to the anterior cortex of the tibia is optimal.

TECHNIQUES

## Proximal Tibia Fractures

- The starting point for IM nailing of fractures of the proximal tibia must be modified from the "classic" entry portal.
- The IM nail for proximal fractures is inserted at the "flat" anterior part of the tibial plateau and more lateral, at the lateral tibial spine, in line with the lateral cortex of the proximal tibia.
- On the sagittal view, the IM nail should be traversing parallel to the anterior cortex to avoid deformity (**TECH FIG 1A**).
- If, despite proper proximal tibial insertion site technique, deformity still occurs, then the next best intraoperative solution is the application of blocking screws.
  - These are usually the locking screws from the IM tibial nail set and are placed to prevent the IM nail from going posteriorly and causing the procurvatum deformity.
  - In the sagittal plane, the blocking screws are placed posterior to the IM nail to force it off of the posterior cortex and parallel to the anterior cortex (**TECH FIG 1B**).
  - If the deformity is present with the IM guidewire in place after fracture reduction, then the blocking screw can be placed to "block" the guidewire to a more anterior position prior to reaming.
  - Sometimes, the guidewire is so far posterior that the blocking screw has to be placed anterior to the wire that lies on the posterior proximal tibial cortex. In this case, the blocking screw is inserted in its proper position and then the guidewire is pulled back and reinserted anterior to the blocking screw prior to reaming.
  - The reamer must either hit the blocking screw or be forcibly pushed past it for the screw to work.
- Similarly, a lateral blocking screw can be added to redirect the nail centered in the proximal fragment on the coronal view (**TECH FIG 1C,D**). This strategy is most commonly employed when the proximal tibia is nailed with the knee flexed greater than 60 degrees over a triangle and a too medial starting point has been employed.

## Additional Strategies

- Two other strategies for proper insertion site and trajectory is to perform the IM nailing with the knee in less flexion to prevent the extremes of proximal deformity.
- The semiextended position allows for a small paramedian arthrotomy, with the knee in only slight flexion, and subluxation of the patella allows for a straight trajectory in the proximal fragment and a more anterior line of insertion.
- The second option is suprapatellar IM nailing. This has gained popularity lately but requires special extra-long insertion instruments and caution so as not to cause damage to the patellofemoral cartilage.
  - The best insertion angle is between 20 and 50 degrees of knee flexion but up to 22% articular damage has been reported. A small insertion site is created just above the superior pole of the patella and a cannula is inserted in the patellofemoral groove.
  - A guide pin is then placed just proximal on the "flat portion" of the proximal tibia just superior to the anterior slope.
  - This pin is directed in a direction that centers the pin in both planes using the more proximal and lateral starting points previously described.
  - All reaming is done through the cannula to prevent articular damage.
  - Bolsters are used under the knee and, with the knee in only slight flexion, the fracture stays reduced during the IM nailing procedure (**TECH FIG 2A–D**).

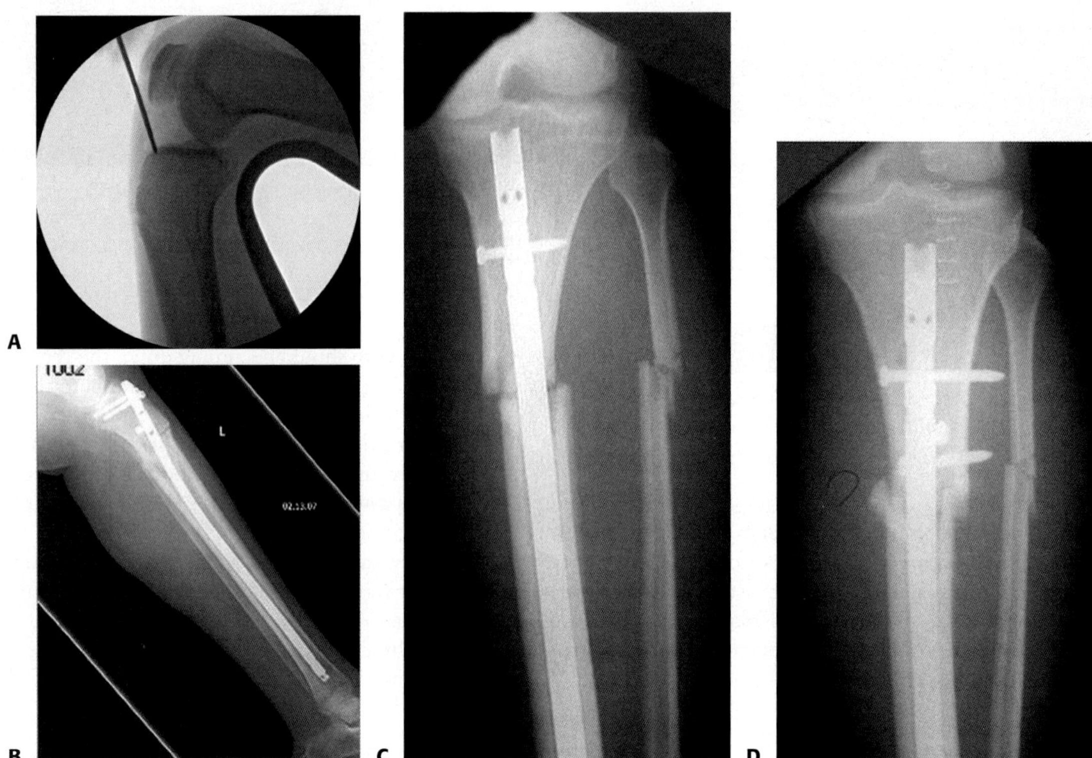

**TECH FIG 1 • A.** Guidewire positioning for proximal tibia fractures at the flat anterior part of the tibial plateau and more lateral, at the lateral tibial spine, in line with the lateral cortex of the proximal tibia. On the sagittal view, the IM nail should be traversing parallel to the anterior cortex to avoid deformity. **B.** A blocking screw in the proximal tibia will help guide the nail into the right position and aid in reduction of this common deformity. **C.** An AP radiograph demonstrating common valgus deformity with a medial starting point. **D.** Correction of the deformity can be seen with a laterally placed blocking screw in the proximal fragment. The nail will "bounce" off of the nail and center itself in the proximal deformity.

- Finally, direct reduction of the fracture through small incisions can be performed prior to IM nailing.
  - A ball spike "pusher" can be used with a small anterior incision to push the proximal fragment down and inhibit the flexion deformity (**TECH FIG 2E**).
  - Percutaneous clamps (**TECH FIG 2F**) through very small incisions, without stripping of soft tissues, that are placed to reduce the fracture allow for the surgeon to ream and place the IM nail with the fracture reduced.

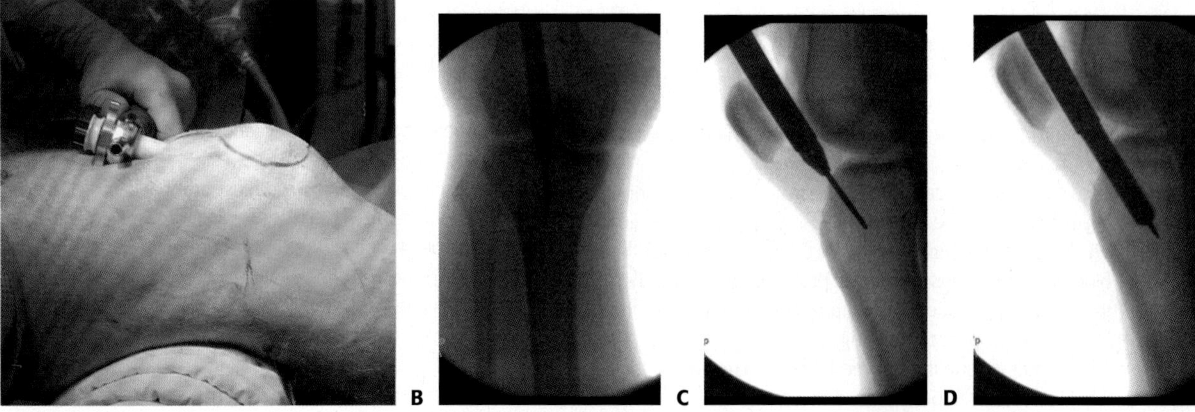

**TECH FIG 2 • A–D.** An image depicting the suprapatellar approach. A small incision is made through the quadriceps tendon. Notice the cannula protecting the cartilage and the insertion of the guidewire followed by the opening reamer. *(continued)*

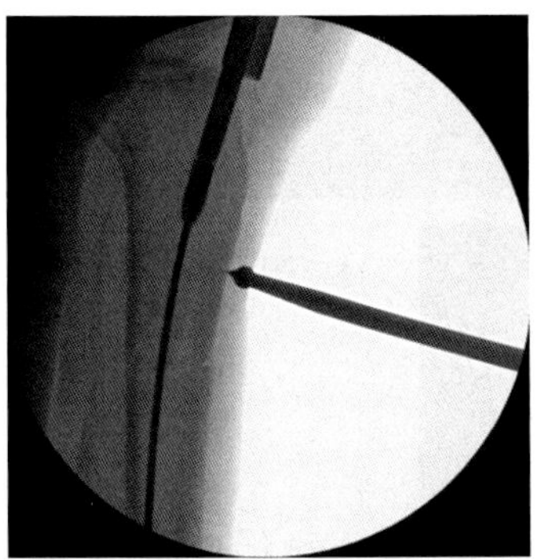

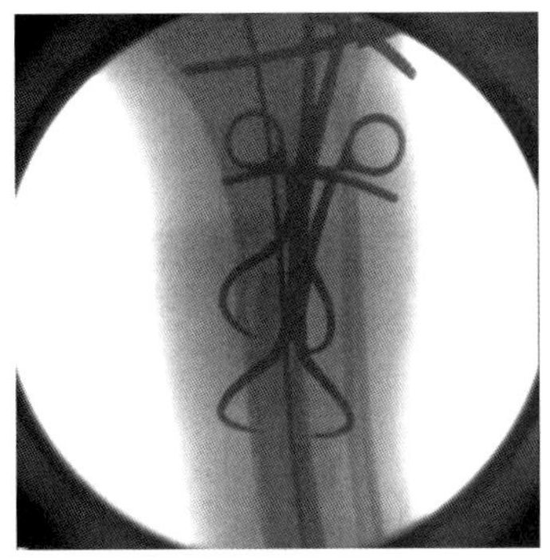

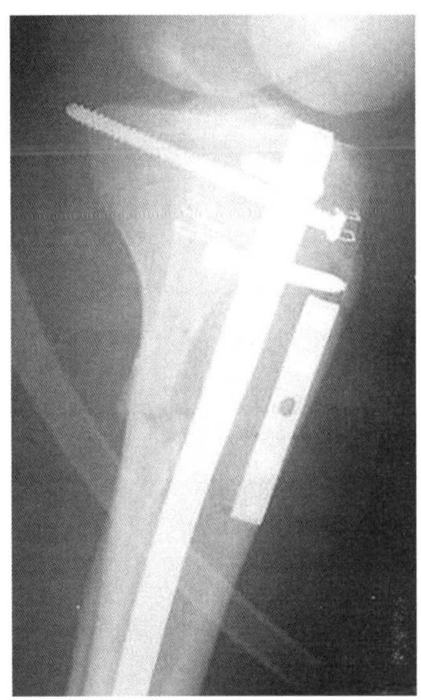

E F G

**TECH FIG 2** • *(continued)* **E.** A ball spike centered over the proximal fragment with a posteriorly directed force can hold the reduction during reaming. **F.** Percutaneous clamps can be used to hold the reduction while the guidewire, reamers, and nail are passed. This requires minimal soft tissue stripping. **G.** A one-third tubular plate was used to hold the reduction of this proximal tibia fracture. A five-hole plate with two screws on either side of the fracture is usually sufficient. Remember to place the plate anterior so that it is out of your way. Once the nail is locked, you may remove the plate or leave it in as depicted here.

- A small fragment plate, usually a one-third tubular plate, can be placed safely through a small incision (**TECH FIG 2G**) to reduce the fracture precisely prior to IM nailing.
  - An anterolateral incision centered over the proximal fracture and under the muscle mass allows for the placement of a five-hole plate with two screws on either side of the fracture line. The screws can be directed into the anterior cortex or placed unicortical to allow the subsequent passage of the IM nail. These plates can be left in place after IM nailing if adequate soft tissue coverage is present.

## Distal Fractures

- Similarly to proximal fractures, reduction is the key to IM nailing of distal tibia fractures.
- A closed reduction can be performed but is often difficult with spiral fractures that have an intact fibula or those with a proximal fibula fracture.
- Often, a small, pointed reduction clamp can be placed percutaneously, with minimal soft tissue stripping, and then the ball-tipped guide rod can be placed in a center–center position down to the epiphyseal scar.
- To correct varus or lateral translation, a blocking screw can be inserted just medial to the guidewire in the distal fragment (**TECH FIG 3A**).
  - This is done using the same drill bit and screws from the IM nailing set and should be close enough to the guide rod that the reamers and IM nail will bounce off of it.
- The other option is fixation of the fibula fracture, especially in distal one-third tibia and associated fibula fractures. There are pros and cons to this approach.
  - For the pros, the surgeon can get rotation and length correct and make the IM nail procedure much easier.
  - The cons relate to the fact that a malreduction of a comminuted fibula can lead to deformity and malunion of the tibia.
- Further, if tibial metaphyseal comminution is present, fixation of the fibula may not allow this area to compress and consolidate and later exchange procedures require an osteotomy of the fibula to allow for tibial compression and subsequent union.
- Adjunctive plating of the distal tibia with subsequent IM nailing is to be avoided as the skin of the distal leg has a limited blood supply as does the tibia; incisions with plate and subsequent IM nail insertion could lead to disastrous skin and bone healing issues.
- For distal fractures, two interlocking screws should be inserted through the IM nail into the distal fragment, preferably with screws at 90 degrees or oblique to each other as these out-of-plane screws allow for early motion and lessen the chance of screw loosening and loss of distal fixation.

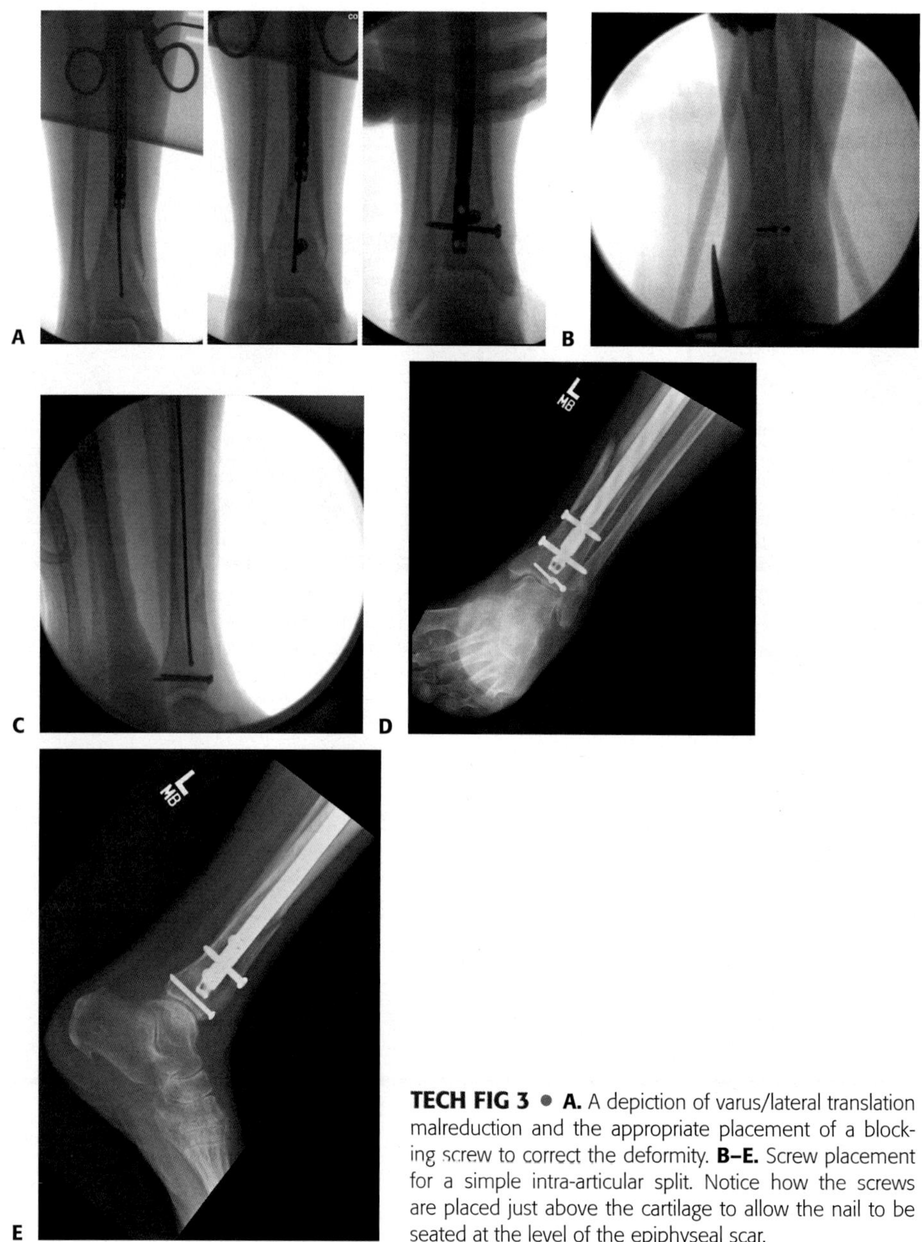


**TECH FIG 3** • **A.** A depiction of varus/lateral translation malreduction and the appropriate placement of a blocking screw to correct the deformity. **B–E.** Screw placement for a simple intra-articular split. Notice how the screws are placed just above the cartilage to allow the nail to be seated at the level of the epiphyseal scar.

## Intra-articular Splits

- Proximal and distal intra-articular splits associated with a metaphyseal fracture can be treated by percutaneous clamp and screw fixation.
- For proximal fractures, these are most commonly sagittal splits, and a cannulated or solid 6.5-mm screw with a washer can be placed across the split from lateral to medial as long as the screw is at the midportion of the plateau or posterior to this line.
  - Because the IM nail enters anteriorly, the percutaneously placed screw will not interfere with IM nail passage.
- For distal fractures, the plane of the fracture needs to be identified. If the fracture is not completely visible or understood on plain x-rays, then a CT scan is performed to elucidate the fracture configuration and morphology.
  - Once the fracture is identified, a percutaneous clamp and a partially threaded cancellous screw or fully threaded screw can be inserted perpendicular to the fracture line at the level of the epiphyseal scar.
  - This distal screw insertion site allows for the IM nail placement as far distal as possible up to this screw (**TECH FIG 3B–E**).

## PEARLS AND PITFALLS

| | |
|---|---|
| Proximal tibia fractures behave differently than diaphyseal fractures. | ■ Correct starting point is essential to eliminating valgus and flexion deformity. Slightly more lateral and proximal than the conventional starting point. |
| The starting point makes all the difference. | ■ "High on the tibia, at the edge of the articular surface of the knee, just medial to the lateral tibial spine."[2] |
| Reduce and hold the reduction prior to reaming and inserting the nail. | ■ The nail will not reduce the fracture if it is in the proximal or distal metaphysis due to a canal–nail size mismatch. Reduce and hold the reduction, then ream and insert the IM nail. Percutaneous clamps with minimal soft tissue stripping can hold proximal and distal fractures reduced during reaming and nailing. |
| Nailing of proximal fractures with the knee in extension may be technically easier. | ■ With semiextended position, there is less pull on the proximal fragment through the patellar tendon and less deformity. Suprapatellar nailing requires specialized equipment and there is the possibility of cartilage damage. |
| Proximal plate fixation can be extremely helpful. | ■ You can use any variety of plates, just be sure that it is out of the way of your nail. Can be left in, but be cautious of making an incision through the zone of injury. |
| Beware of the intra-articular extension. | ■ Any questions about the extent of the fracture should be further investigated with a CT scan. If there is intra-articular involvement, address that first then continue with the IM nail. |
| Blocking screws can help direct the nail and alleviate malreductions that come with bone/implant mismatch. | ■ They are minimally invasive and you can use the same screws as your interlocking screws. Placed in the right position, they can help redirect your nail and guide it in the right direction. |

## POSTOPERATIVE CARE

- After surgery, immobilization of the limb can be achieved by placement of a splint or boot for soft tissue protection along with elastic bandage compression, ice, and elevation.
  - The splint is typically removed prior to discharge once the patient's pain allows range of motion (ROM). This may help avoid an acquired equinus contracture.
- Antibiotics are generally discontinued after 24 hours but may continue until all wounds are closed in the presence of an open fracture or with fasciotomies performed secondary to compartment syndrome.
- Although full weight bearing is generally protected until there is radiographic evidence of healing (10 to 12 weeks), aggressive ROM including heel cord stretching and mobilization are essential to provide optimal outcomes.
  - Partial weight bearing can be started at 6 weeks, depending on the progression of healing and the inherent stability of the fracture–nail construct.
- A course of deep venous thrombosis (DVT) prophylaxis is recommended for at least 2 weeks, with longer duration for patients who may have multiple injuries or who are otherwise slow to mobilize.
  - Low-molecular-weight heparin is often used in multiply injured patients or those who are high risk, whereas low-dose aspirin may be sufficient for the ambulatory patient.
- Follow-up is generally at 2 weeks for suture removal, 6 weeks for radiographic follow-up and to assess ROM, and 3 months for advancement to weight bearing as tolerated.
- Follow-up beyond that may be every 6 to 12 weeks thereafter, depending on healing and return to function.

## OUTCOMES

- Closed tibial fractures should be expected to heal by 24 weeks.
- There is little information about the long-term, patient-reported outcomes of tibial shaft fractures.
- Factors such as smoking, comminution, quality of reduction, and whether or not the fracture is open can influence the patient's ability to heal a tibia fracture.
- Those fractures associated with intra-articular extension may have decreased joint motion despite aggressive postoperative therapy.
- Tibial IM nailing, whether using a medial patellar tendon incision or a midline tendon split, has been shown to cause knee pain in as high as 50% of patients with hardware removal alleviating pain in half of the patients.

## COMPLICATIONS

- Similar to other orthopaedic surgery
  - Infection
  - DVT
  - Malunion
  - Nonunion
  - Hardware irritation/pain (knee pain)
- Malunion can be avoided with proper starting point and ensuring that you have appropriate reduction prior to IM nailing.
  - In some instances, leaving intraoperative adjunctive fixation (ie, plate, blocking screws) indefinitely may provide additional stability and aid in healing and prevention of late deformity.
- Nonunions are not uncommon in tibia fractures and increase if the fracture is comminuted or is an open fracture with extensive soft tissue stripping.
  - Recent studies have suggested avoiding reoperations until at least 6 months after surgery in absence of infection or catastrophic failure[1] as these fractures may simply require longer to achieve union.
- Hypertrophic nonunions are usually a result of a canal–nail mismatch and instability.
  - These are most readily treated with a dynamic exchange nailing often with a fibular osteotomy to allow for

compression at the nonunion site. The nonunion in these cases does not need to be débrided.
- IM cultures should be done in all nonunions, open or closed, to rule out infection as a cause of the nonunion.

- Atrophic or oligotrophic nonunions may need an increase in stability as well but most require the addition of bone graft.
  - Options include autograft, allograft, or a combination of these adjuvants to obtain union.

## REFERENCES

1. Bhandari M, Guyatt G, Tornetta P III, et al. Randomized trial of reamed and unreamed intramedullary nailing of tibial shaft fractures. J Bone Joint Surg Am 2008;90:2567–2578.
2. Schmidt AH, Templeman DC, Tornetta P, et al. Anatomic assessment of the proper insertion site for a tibial intramedullary nail. J Orthop Trauma 2003;17:75–76.

# Tibial Tuberosity Fractures

Eric W. Edmonds

34

CHAPTER

## DEFINITION

- Tibial tuberosity fractures are rare fractures that predominately occur in adolescents with the onset of proximal tibial physeal closure.
- These apophyseal fractures occur almost exclusively in boys, but there are a few cases reported in girls.
- Most commonly, the injury occurs at the initiation of a jump.
- The association with prior tibial tuberosity traction apophysitis (Osgood-Schlatter syndrome) is possible but not always present.

## ANATOMY

- The tibial tubercle exists in an anterolateral location on the proximal tibia just distal to the physis and develops in four recognized stages[5] that are important to understanding potential pathology.[14]
  - Stage 1: The tubercle is completely a cartilage anlage without a secondary center of ossification.
  - Stage 2: known as the *apophyseal stage*, occurs between ages 8 and 12 years in girls and 9 and 14 years in boys. The secondary center of ossification is present but not contiguous with the epiphyseal ossification of the proximal tibia.
  - Stage 3: known as the *epiphyseal stage*, occurs when the apophyseal ossification connects with the epiphyseal bone; commonly occurring between ages 10 and 15 years for girls and 11 and 17 years for boys
  - Stage 4: is identified by complete fusion of the tubercle and closure of the apophyseal cartilage
- Closure of the proximal tibial physis and the tubercle apophysis occurs in a predictable pattern.[14] The proximal tibial physis closes in a posteromedial to anterolateral direction toward the tubercle apophysis, which is simultaneously closing in a proximal to distal direction.
- The patellar ligament (tendon) inserts into the apophysis with a large periosteal insertion distally.
- It is important to remember the native anterolateral position of the tubercle and therefore the fracture fragment when preoperatively planning the approach for intra-articular visualization.
- The anterior tibial recurrent artery is at risk to rupture with a displaced fracture. Bleeding from its proximal branches as it retracts into the anterolateral compartment could cause a compartment syndrome.

## PATHOGENESIS

- The injury occurs with a forceful quadriceps contraction while the foot is fixed. There is a significant eccentric force of the quadriceps mechanism that overcomes the strength of the apophysis and the surrounding periosteum.[10] A second possible mechanism of injury is sudden passive knee flexion while the quadriceps is contracted.
- It has been hypothesized that individuals with this fracture may have quadriceps strength that is greater than their peers.[8] Thus, the conditions for the fracture are present during jumping and in strong individuals.
- Many children may have preexisting Osgood-Schlatter syndrome.[1,12,13]
- The injury usually occurs at a time when the tuberosity is undergoing normal closure,[14] and the pattern of normal skeletal maturity results in specific fracture patterns.
- There have also been reports of associated injuries such as quadriceps tendon injury, cruciate ligament tears, and meniscal injury.[3,6,7,9]

## PATIENT HISTORY AND PHYSICAL FINDINGS

- Patients usually present acutely with significant pain and an inability to bear weight on the affected leg after sustaining an injury during physical activity. They are usually tender, with significant swelling over the anterior proximal tibia. An effusion may be present, and active straight-leg raise against gravity is often not possible.
  - Children with minimally displaced fractures may extend the knee but with obvious discomfort (likely due to intact retinaculum and surrounding periosteum).
- Neurovascular examination should always be performed, as there is distinct risk of injury with tibia tubercle fractures.
- There should also be an evaluation for the presence of leg compartment syndrome.
- Osgood-Schlatter syndrome has a more insidious onset and usually will not have an effusion or result in extensor lag, even though it may be significantly tender over the tubercle.

## RADIOGRAPHIC FINDINGS

- Good anteroposterior (AP) and lateral radiographs are often able to make the diagnosis, but they may be limited in the assessing the extent of injury.[14]
- The displacement is most obvious on the lateral radiograph.
  - Lateral radiographs with about 15 degrees internal rotation can place the tubercle on profile and assist with the assessment of nondisplaced or minimally displaced fractures. Contralateral images can be helpful for comparison and may help confirm the diagnosis.
- Ogden et al[13] described three types of tubercle fractures using only the lateral x-ray:
  - Type I: fractures through the apophysis only
  - Type II: fractures that exit between the epiphysis and apophysis

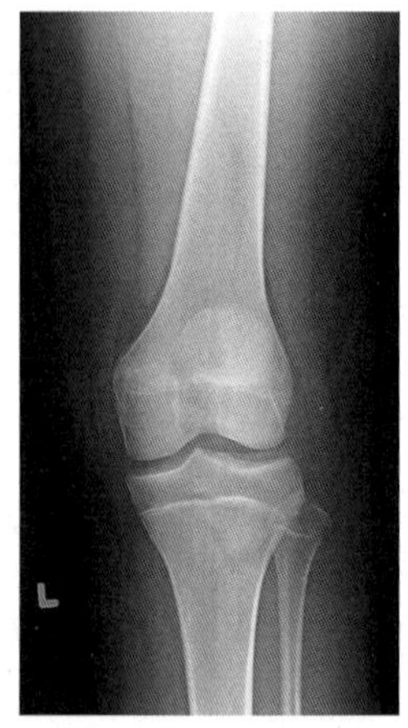


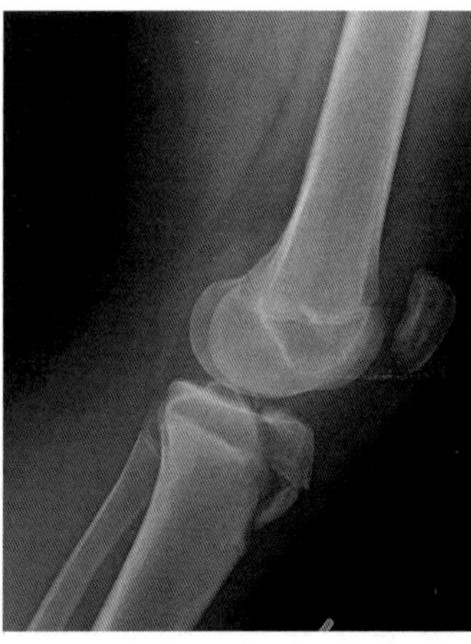

**FIG 1** • AP (**A**) and lateral (**B**) radiographs of a 16-year-old boy who sustained a tibial tuberosity fracture. The fracture is a type III or type C, which enters the knee joint.

- Type III: fractures that propagate into the anterior knee joint under the anterior meniscus attachments (**FIG 1**)
- A multiplanar imaging classification scheme has also been described that takes the skeletal development and risk for associated injuries into consideration.[14]
  - Type A (isolated tubercle, child) is isolated to the ossified tip (seen on x-ray) of the largely cartilaginous tubercle—seen predominately between stages 1 and 2 of development.
  - Type B (physeal) involves both the epiphysis and tubercle that fracture as a single unit off the metaphysis without intra-articular involvement—seen predominately during stage 2 of development.
  - Type C (intra-articular) extends into the intra-articular surface of the proximal tibia—predominately occurring during stage 3 of development.
  - Type D (isolated tubercle, teen) involves only the distal aspect of the tubercle because there has been closure of all the remaining apophysis—predominately occurring between stages 3 and 4 of development.
- Type A fractures risk apophyseal closure and possible recurvatum, whereas type D fractures carry minimal risk.
- Type B and C fractures should have computed tomography (CT) or magnetic resonance imaging (MRI) assessment to fully evaluate the extent of injury for preoperative planning.
  - Type B fractures carry the greatest risk for associated pathology including neurovascular injury and compartment syndrome.

## NONOPERATIVE MANAGEMENT

- Open reduction and internal fixation is indicated for all patients except those with completely nondisplaced fractures, especially type D fractures.
- A long-leg cast is the nonoperative management for children with nondisplaced fractures that can perform a straight-leg raise.
  - Immobilization is 6 to 8 weeks.
- Close radiographic follow-up is needed for the first 2 weeks to ensure the fracture does not become displaced.
- The disadvantage of casting even the nondisplaced fractures is the subsequent risk of stiffness that may not arise with percutaneous screw fixation (that may allow earlier mobilization).

## SURGICAL MANAGEMENT

- For fractures with displacement, open reduction and fixation with screws is recommended, whereas nondisplaced fractures can be treated with percutaneous screw fixation.

### Positioning

- Patients are positioned supine with the operative leg and knee prepared free.
- The table should allow good anterior and posterior views to be obtained with fluoroscopy.
  - Use of a radiolucent table is imperative, but even partially radiolucent tables can be used if the patient's knee is positioned on the table to confirm adequate exposure for the fluoroscopy (this assessment should be made prior to surgery).
- A thigh tourniquet can be used to keep the field dry, improving visualization of the fracture fragments and the joint reduction. However, the tourniquet can entrap the quadriceps muscle proximally, thereby limiting excursion and making the fragment reduction more challenging.
- A bump can be placed under the operative knee to keep it slightly bent during the procedure. This improves visualization by keeping the skin incision on traction and allowing any hematoma or fluid to flow away from the central aspect of the incision.

### Approach

- A midline anterior incision is appropriate in most if not all tibial tubercle fractures.
- The proximal extent is the midpatella, and the distal aspect is a few centimeters distal to the tibial tubercle fracture bed for a full, unimpeded view of the fracture and its reduction. It can be shortened on the proximal aspect if it does not involve the joint.
  - Commonly, there is a significant amount of hematoma formation and torn periosteum; thus, the incision length allows the surgeon to define the appropriate anatomy and prepare the fragment for reduction.
- Because the tubercle and the fracture are on the lateral aspect of the proximal tibia, a lateral parapatellar approach will give better visualization of the fracture and intra-articular reduction.
  - The lateral approach also limits any damage to the infrapatellar branch of the saphenous nerve.

## Dissection and Fasciotomy

- The large hematoma should be evacuated.
- Identify the long periosteal flap on the distal aspect of the elevated fracture that is commonly present, and extract it from its intercalary position if it is trapped within the fracture.
- A prophylactic anterior compartment fasciotomy is performed, if it is not already been done by the fracture itself.
- The distal, medial, and lateral extent of the fracture should be surgically defined with sharp dissection.
- For type C fractures (exiting in the knee joint), the surgeon must visualize the articular surface either through the fracture (to identify concomitant injuries such as the meniscus) or via the lateral parapatellar approach to assist reduction.

## Open Reduction

- Next, the fracture is reduced, and this is often aided by leg extension to take tension off the quadriceps muscle.
  - For type C fractures, the articular surface should be reduced first, followed by the distal aspect of the fracture.
- Tentative fixation is used, and the reduction is confirmed with both direct visualization and fluoroscopy.
- If the fracture is not reduced anatomically, it is due to soft tissue interposition or meniscal interposition (**TECH FIG 1**).

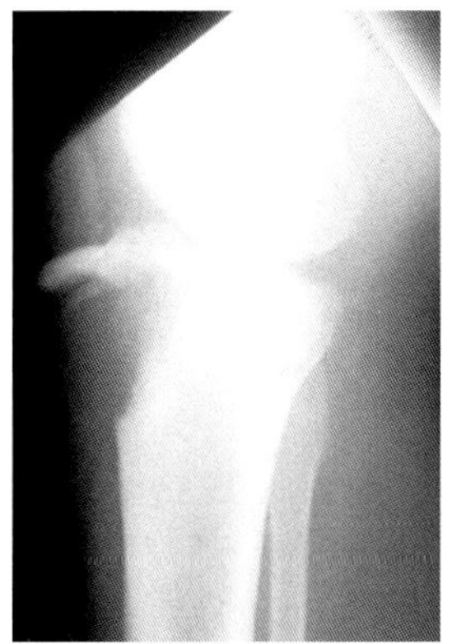
A

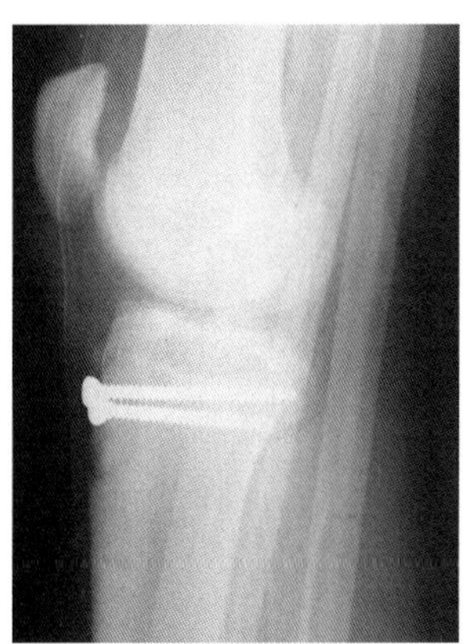
B

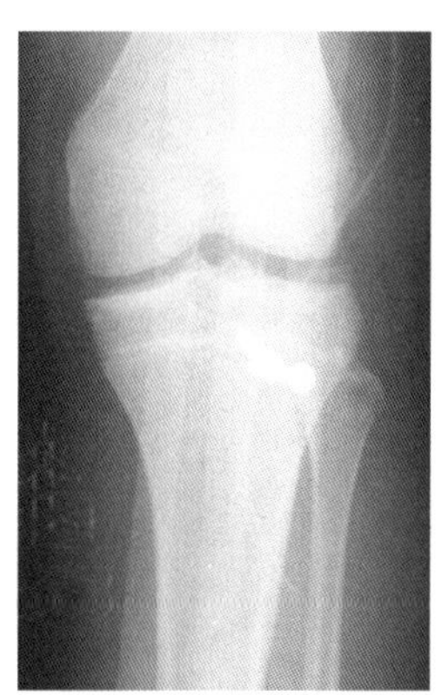
C

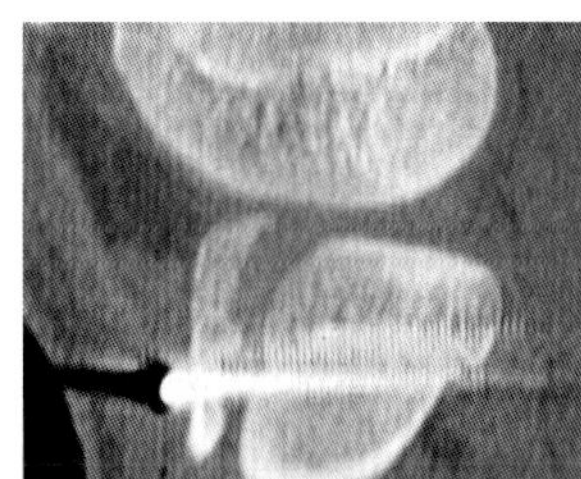
D

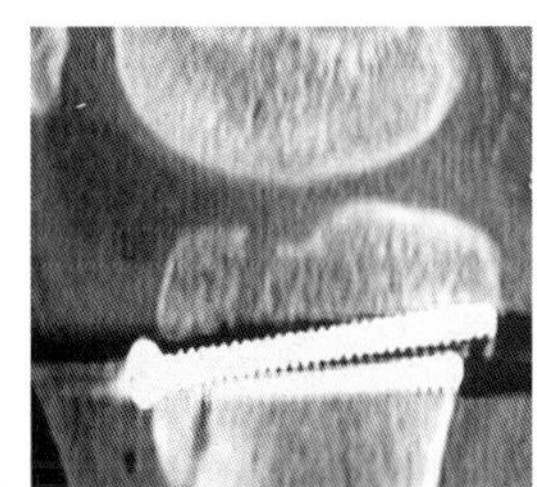
E

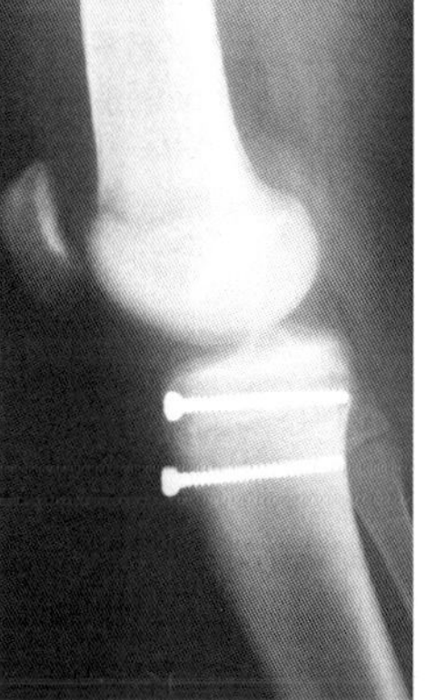
F

**TECH FIG 1** • **A.** A 15-year-old boy with a displaced tibial tuberosity fracture that enters the joint surface. **B.** Initial postoperative lateral radiograph after open reduction and internal fixation. Despite initial fluoroscopic views indicating an adequate reduction, the radiographs indicate a poor reduction. **C.** AP postoperative radiograph indicating a possible poor reduction. **D,E.** CT scans indicate the joint surface is poorly reduced. **F.** A repeat open reduction and internal fixation was performed. The lateral meniscus was impeding the prior reduction and it was removed from the fracture site. This allowed a successful reduction, as shown by the lateral radiograph.

## Fixation

- Once the fracture is reduced in an acceptable position, screw fixation is recommended. Solid screws or cannulated screws can be used.
- Provisional Kirschner wire (K-wire) fixation is best to hold the reduction before screw fixation because it is difficult to use clamps without a more extensive posterior dissection.
  - Standard K-wires can be used if solid screws are planned, and the surgeon should be cognizant to the K-wire placement so as not to interfere with later ideal screw placement. Conversely, guide pins may be used if a cannulated screw system is being used and placement should be at the ideal location.
- The screws are placed from anterior to posterior parallel to the joint surface and without crossing the proximal tibial physis, if desired (**TECH FIG 2**). Bicortical purchase is not necessary, and it is important to prevent vascular injury posterior to the knee joint in this region.
- Cancellous screws in compression are ideal for this location, and cortical screws can be used to achieve fixation distally in larger fragments.
- If there is a large bone fragment, two or three 4.5-mm screws are ideal and may lead to less screw head irritation.
  - A washer can be used for these smaller screws to resist loss of near cortical fixation.
  - Alternatively, 6.5- or 7.3-mm screws can be used, although screw head irritation may occur. Washers should not be used with these screws.
- The surgeon should avoid placing the screws directly under the incision.
- For type A fractures that involve the very young, screw fixation will guarantee developed recurvatum; therefore, smooth K-wire fixation should be used. These should also be placed parallel to the joint and avoid crossing the proximal physis as well. They can be left out of the skin and pulled after 4 weeks, during a cast change.

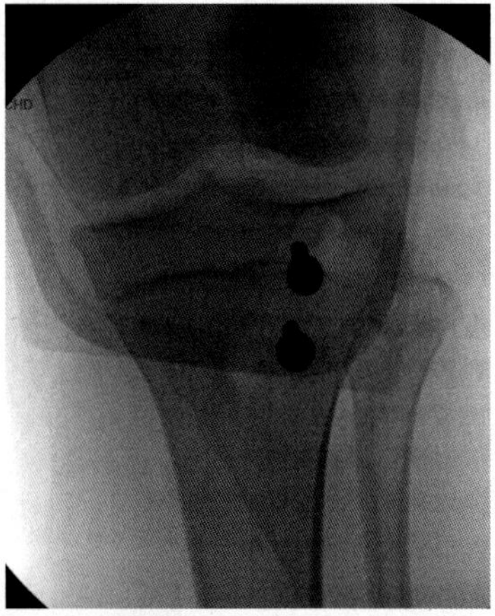

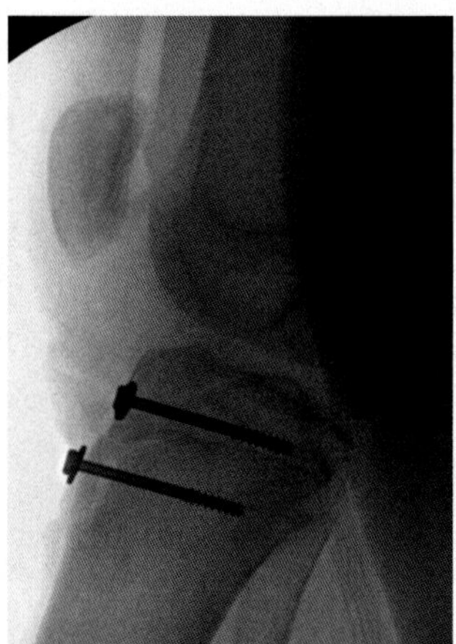

**TECH FIG 2** • Same patient as **FIG 1**, demonstrating anatomic reduction of both fragments with 4.5-mm cannulated screws and washers placed parallel to the joint surface. **A.** The AP radiograph shows the screws are lateral to the midline as the fracture is more lateral, and the screws are not directly under the incision, in an attempt to avoid painful screw heads. **B.** Lateral radiograph demonstrating fixation of both the epiphyseal fragment and the tubercle fragment.

## PEARLS AND PITFALLS

| | |
|---|---|
| **Radiographic interpretation** | ▪ Close radiographic evaluation can help the surgeon to recognize the minimally displaced fracture and the possibility of another extensor mechanism injury, such as a sleeve fracture.<br>▪ Advanced imaging can identify intra-articular extension and entrapment of meniscal tissue. |
| **Reduction techniques** | ▪ The impediments to reduction—the periosteum and meniscus (see **TECH FIG 1**)—should be removed, being sure that the tourniquet is not limiting quadriceps excursion.<br>▪ A lateral parapatellar approach is more direct to the site of injury.<br>▪ The surgeon should make sure that the joint surface is reduced in type B and C or type III fractures. Moreover, preoperative advanced imaging is important for planning purposes. |
| **Associated pathology and complications** | ▪ The surgeon should be aware of associated injuries (eg, meniscus, anterior cruciate) and look for them.<br>▪ A prophylactic anterior compartment fasciotomy should be performed.<br>▪ Smaller screw heads (4.5 mm) may lead to less complaints of screw head pain and reduce the risk of return to surgery for implant removal. |

## POSTOPERATIVE MANAGEMENT

- Postoperatively, a cylinder cast or long-leg cast can be used. A cylinder allows motion at the ankle but may have more skin issues because of that motion. For type A fractures being treated with pins, a long-leg cast that includes the foot must be used to protect the protruding pins.
- Postoperative immobilization after fixation should be done for 4 weeks. This can be followed by progression into a knee range-of-motion brace to limit activities but promote gentle range of motion if radiographs at that visit demonstrate adequate healing. With less than the ideal bone callus and healing at that 4-week visit, a knee immobilizer can be used for an additional 4 weeks, followed by range of motion and physical therapy, if needed.

## OUTCOMES

- Most of the published series have a small number of patients due to the uncommon nature of this fracture.
- All studies have been consistent in their conclusion that the fractures heal with success and patients return to normal function. Growth abnormality has not been reported in types C or D[4,9,12,13]; however, recurvatum due to premature apophyseal closure can occur in types A and B fractures.[14]

## COMPLICATIONS

- Reported complications are few for the treatment of tibial tuberosity fractures, with screw prominence and irritation being the most common.[16]
- Compartment syndrome has been reported, particularly in type B fractures.[11,14,15] A prophylactic anterior compartment fasciotomy and close observation and recognition may decrease the possibility of this complication.
- As mentioned in the Outcomes section, growth disturbance, such as a recurvatum from tibial tubercle arrest, is not of too much concern, as this fracture predominately occurs in adolescents near the end of growth.
- Loss of motion or quadriceps muscle weakness is extremely rare but may occur with a malunion or malreduction.[2]

## ACKNOWLEDGMENT

- Thank you to Ernest L. Sink, MD, who prepared this chapter for the first edition of this text.

## REFERENCES

1. Bang J, Broeng L. Spontaneous avulsion of the tibial tuberosity following Osgood-Schlatter disease [in Danish]. Ugeskr Laeger 1995;157:3061–3062.
2. Bolesta MJ, Fitch RD. Tibial tubercle avulsions. J Pediatr Orthop 1986;6:186–192.
3. Choi NH, Kim NM. Tibial tuberosity avulsion fracture combined with meniscal tear. Arthroscopy 1999;15:766–769.
4. Christie MJ, Dvonch VM. Tibial tuberosity avulsion fracture in adolescents. J Pediatr Orthop 1981;1:391–394.
5. Ehrenborg G. The Osgood-Schlatter lesion. A clinical study of 170 cases. Acta Chir Scand 1962;124:89–105.
6. Falster O, Hasselbach H. Avulsion fracture of the tibial tuberosity with combined ligament and meniscal tear. Am J Sports Med 1992;20: 82–83.
7. Lipscomb AB, Gilbert PP, Johnson RK, et al. Fracture of the tibial tuberosity with associated ligamentous and meniscal tears. A case report. J Bone Joint Surg Am 1984;66(5):790–792.
8. Maffulli N, Grewal R. Avulsion of the tibial tuberosity: muscles too strong for a growth plate. Clin J Sport Med 1997;7:129–132.
9. McKoy BE, Stanitski CL. Acute tibial tubercle avulsion fractures. Orthop Clin North Am 2003;34:397–403.
10. Mubarak SJ, Kim JR, Edmonds EW, et al. Classification of proximal tibia fractures. J Child Orthop 2009;3(3):191–197.
11. Neuschwander DC, Heinrich SD, Cenac WA. Tibial tuberosity fracture associated with a compartment syndrome. Orthopedics 1992;15:1109–1111.
12. Nimityongskul P, Montague WL, Anderson LD. Avulsion fracture of the tibial tuberosity in late adolescence. J Trauma 1988;28: 505–509.
13. Ogden JA, Tross RB, Murphy MJ. Fractures of the tibial tuberosity in adolescents. J Bone Joint Surg Am 1980;62(2):205–215.
14. Pandya NK, Edmonds EW, Roocroft JH, et al. Tibial tubercle fractures: complications, classification, and the need for intra-articular assessment. J Pediatr Orthop 2012;32(8):749–759.
15. Pape JM, Goulet JA, Hensinger RN. Compartment syndrome complicating tibial tubercle avulsion. Clin Orthop Relat Res 1993;(295): 201–204.
16. Wiss DA, Schilz JL, Zionts L. Type III fractures of the tibial tubercle in adolescents. J Orthop Trauma 1991;5:475–479.

# Pediatric Ankle Fractures

Scott J. Mubarak and Andrew T. Pennock

## DEFINITION

- Ankle fractures account for about 5% of all pediatric fractures and are second only to distal radius fractures as the most prevalent physeal fracture comprising approximately 15% of these injuries.[1]
- As in most pediatric trauma, nonoperative management is the mainstay of treatment; however, surgical indications can be specific to the pediatric population.
  - Much like adults, surgical treatment is indicated when there is any significant articular incongruity or angular deformity.
- Classification of pediatric ankle fractures can be a practical tool for both the treatment and prognosis of these fractures.
  - The most common classification scheme for pediatric ankle fractures is the Salter-Harris method for physeal fractures.
  - The Lauge-Hansen classification used in adults can be modified for pediatric ankle fractures and aids in conceptualizing the reduction technique by reversing the fracture pattern. Also, previous studies have shown that pronation-type injuries have a higher rate of premature physeal closure than supination–external rotation (SER) type injuries.[7]
  - This classification is useful as most orthopaedic surgeons are familiar with it.
  - Additional classification systems include the fibular-based Danis-Weber system as well as a more comprehensive classification suggested by Dias and Tachdjian[2] that uses the Lauge-Hansen[4] guidelines correlated with the Salter-Harris classification.
- Transitional fractures of the ankle occur near skeletal maturity and are due to the asymmetric closure of the distal tibial physis.
  - Triplane fracture is described as a complex Salter-Harris type IV fracture that consists of sagittal, transverse, and coronal components with an epiphyseal and metaphyseal fragment.
  - Tillaux fractures occur most often in adolescents within 1 year of distal tibial physeal closure. They involve an external rotational force that avulses the anterolateral aspect of the tibial epiphysis, which is attached to the anterior inferior tibiofibular ligament, which is stronger than the residual open physis.

## ANATOMY

- The ligaments of the ankle attach to the epiphyses provide stability to the ankle mortise. These ligaments contribute to the pathomechanics of transitional fractures (triplane and Tillaux fractures) because they are often more stout than the growth plate, leading children to sustain physeal fractures more readily than ankle sprains.
  - The anteroinferior tibiofibular ligament attaches to the anterolateral border of the tibial epiphysis, and with an external rotation force on the foot, it has the ability to avulse the anterolateral fragment of the tibial epiphysis; the strength imbalance between the ligament and weaker physis can create the transitional Tillaux and triplane fractures.
- The anatomy of the distal tibial physis is relevant to understanding certain ankle fractures and their management and prognosis.
  - The secondary ossific nucleus of the distal epiphysis appears between 6 and 24 months, with the apophysis of the medial malleolus often extending from an elongation from this ossific nucleus or from a separate ossification center, the os subtibiale, which ossifies between 7 and 8 years of age.
  - The distal tibial physis is primarily transverse; however, there is an anteromedial undulation that consistently appears within the first 2 years of life that has been described by Kump (termed *Kump bump*). This centromedial location is where physiologic physeal closure begins (**FIG 1**).
  - Physeal closure of the distal tibia occurs around 15 years of age in girls and 17 years of age in boys.
  - Closure progresses from the centromedial location of Kump bump medially, then laterally from this location, over about 18 months.
- The anatomy of the physis also influences ankle fractures in children.
  - The perichondral ring of LaCroix is a transitional area between the articular cartilage and the periosteum of the diaphysis. Made of perichondrium, it retains the potential for producing cartilage and bone.
  - Functionally, the perichondral ring provides stability to the physis and may play a role in certain fractures and growth plate injuries in children.
  - Adjacent periosteum which rigidly attaches to the perichondral ring can become interposed in the fracture site and obstruct anatomic reduction.

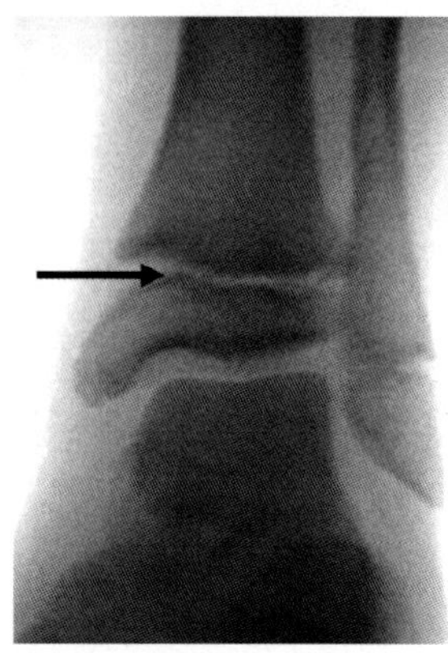

**FIG 1** • Kump bump. The *arrow* demonstrates the centromedial-located Kump bump, which is where physeal closure begins. We believe that damage to this structure may induce premature physeal closure.

## PATHOGENESIS

- The Lauge-Hansen classification system was developed in 1950 to understand the injury mechanism by reproducing fracture patterns in adult cadavers.[4]
- This classification is a two-part classification, with the initial portion describing the position of the foot at the time of injury (eg, supination, pronation) and the following portion describing the direction of the deforming force, either rotational (internal or external) or translational (abduction or adduction).
- This system grades the severity of ankle injuries as I to IV in rotational patterns and I to II in translational patterns.
- A recent series of 114 classifiable ankle fractures (Salter II) using the Lauge-Hansen system, SER composed 66%; abduction, 30%; pronation–external rotation, 3%; and axial crush injuries, 1%.[7]
- The activity that resulted in ankle fractures varied in our series, with most occurring during falls and sports.[1,7]
- SER fractures did not seem to have any specific activity that was more likely to produce premature physeal closure; however, abduction injuries occurring with soccer or skateboarding were much more likely to develop premature physeal closure when compared to other activities.
- Specific anatomy and growth plate closure patterns create certain fractures in adolescence.
  - For example, the same external rotation mechanism can produce a Tillaux or a triplane fracture, depending on the age and degree of physeal closure of the child.
  - The lateral portion of the distal tibial physis closes last. This is often an area of weakness in the skeletally maturing child, allowing an anterolateral fragment to be avulsed from the epiphysis, creating Tillaux fractures or the intra-articular fragment in the triplane fracture.

## NATURAL HISTORY

- Premature physeal closure of the distal tibia has been historically described as a rare sequela in physeal fractures, with an incidence as low as 2% to 5%.[1]
- Our recent data demonstrate an overall 38% incidence of physeal arrest in Salter-Harris I type and II fractures but maybe as high as 55% for displaced fractures. Both the mechanism of injury and and treatment modality have been shown to influence the rate of premature closure.[7,8]
  - SER injuries have a better prognosis for premature physeal closure, with a 38% overall incidence, as compared to abduction-type injuries, with a 52% overall incidence.
  - This difference in prognosis between SER and abduction injuries may be explained by the shearing force of Kump bump that may occur in abduction injuries, as opposed to less traumatic rotational force to this anatomic structure that occurs with SER injuries.
- These data have prognostic relevance in pediatric ankle fractures, as an earlier series demonstrated a 3.5-fold increase in the premature physeal closure rate if a gap of 3 mm or more was present on the postreduction imaging of Salter-Harris types I and II fractures.
  - Our experience suggests that periosteum interposed in the physis leads to residual fracture gapping and may contribute to premature physeal closure.
- The orthopaedic surgeon should discuss the potential for premature physeal closure with the family at the initial visit, particularly with an abduction type of injury.

## PATIENT HISTORY AND PHYSICAL FINDINGS

- As in adult trauma, the initial evaluation of a child's ankle injury consists of eliciting the mechanism and timing of injury.
- Basic examination should consist of evaluating the skin and soft tissues, finding areas of maximal tenderness to palpation, and obtaining an accurate sensory, motor, and vascular examination.
- Particular issues that must be considered in the diagnosis of ankle fractures in children include osteomyelitis and child abuse.
  - Osteomyelitis has a prevalence of 1 per 5000 children. It generally occurs in the vascular loops of the metaphyseal regions of bone in children and can occur because of hematogenous spread or as a result of trauma, which can further complicate diagnosis.
  - A thorough history of the proximity of pain onset relative to the inciting trauma will help differentiate trauma from infection.
  - Metaphyseal fractures of the distal tibia in children can be concerning for child abuse, as the mechanism can be attributed to forceful pulling or twisting of the extremity, fracturing the cancellous bone through the metaphysis. Additional concerns are bilateral extremity fractures and fractures at different stages of healing.
- Visualization of the skin is critical in the evaluation for potential open injuries. The quality of skin can also affect the timing of surgical fixation and give insight into the energy and location of injury.
- Palpation of the ankle can assist in locating the injury and may allow diagnosis of occult physeal fractures or ligamentous injuries not seen on radiographs.
- Establishing preoperative deficits is critical in the pre- and postoperative management of ankle fractures and may aid in establishing the need to release the extensor retinaculum compartment.
- Preoperative deficits can be due to nerve contusion or laceration, in addition to tendon disruption or mechanical block. This can affect the surgical approach.
- Vascular status is the key to the ultimate viability of the extremity. If deficits are found, the fracture should be immediately reduced. If a deficit is still present after reduction, a vascular study may be considered versus immediate operative exploration to evaluate for transient spasm or vascular injury.

## IMAGING AND OTHER DIAGNOSTIC STUDIES

- If there is any suspicion of an ankle injury, a complete radiographic ankle series should be performed consisting of an anteroposterior (AP), a lateral, and a mortise view (**FIG 2A–C**).
  - The mortise view is critical and is taken from anterior to posterior with the foot internally rotated 20 degrees to view the talus with a symmetric clear space seen medially and laterally.
  - The importance of the mortise view is seen in Tillaux fractures, where the anterolateral fragment is often obscured by the overlap of the posterior fibula on the AP view and is not well visualized on the lateral view.
- We do not advocate stress radiographs in children; however, we will use an external rotation stress view intraoperatively to evaluate for syndesmosis injury if suspected in children near skeletal maturity.
- Accessory ossicles can be commonly visualized on plain radiographs and may be confused with ankle fractures.
  - These include the os subtibiale medially (up to 20% of population), the os trigonum posteriorly (about 10% of population), and the os fibulare laterally (about 1% of population).

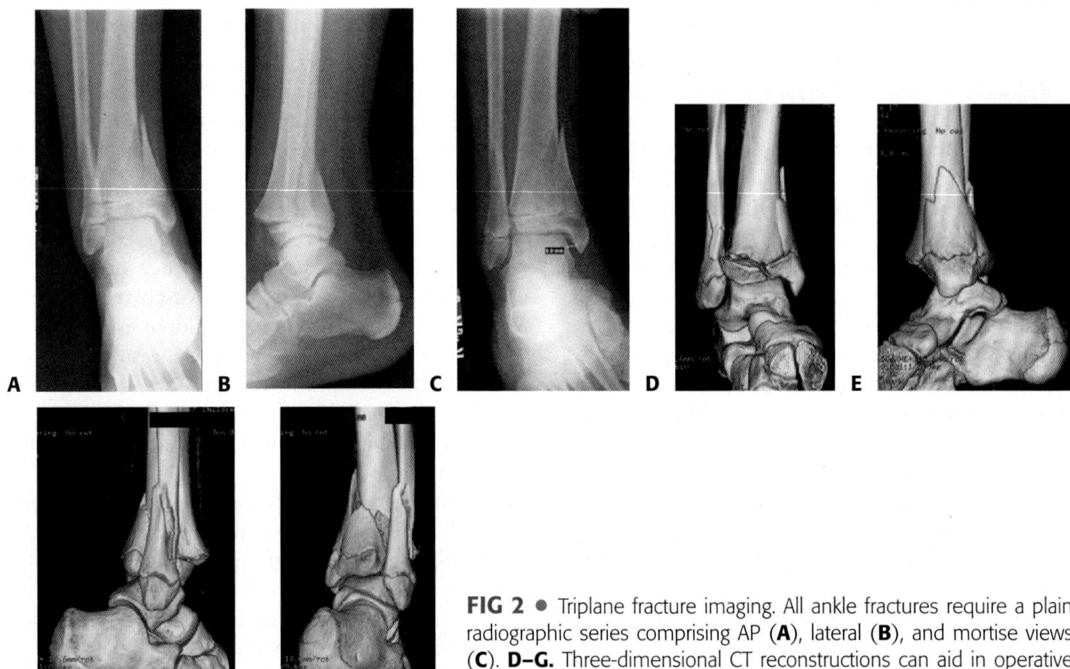

**FIG 2** • Triplane fracture imaging. All ankle fractures require a plain radiographic series comprising AP (**A**), lateral (**B**), and mortise views (**C**). **D–G.** Three-dimensional CT reconstructions can aid in operative planning, especially for the difficult to visualize intra-articular fractures.

- Contralateral comparison films may be helpful to differentiate accessory ossicles from a fracture.
- Computed tomography (CT) is required to fully understand many ankle fractures, and we often advocate three-dimensional postreduction CT scans (**FIG 2D–G**).
  - We advocate CT scans for intra-articular fractures that show residual displacement on plain radiographs after attempted closed reduction.
- At time of injury for Salter-Harris types I and II fractures and triplane fractures of the distal tibia, in addition to the standard radiographs, it can be helpful to obtain an AP view of the left hand to establish bone age and contralateral radiographs for a baseline physeal comparison.

## DIFFERENTIAL DIAGNOSIS

- Ankle sprain
- Accessory ossicle
- Osteochondral lesion (osteochondritis dissecans)
- Contusion
- Osteomyelitis

## NONOPERATIVE MANAGEMENT

- Our clinical pathway for surgery advocates that all closed ankle fractures have an attempt of closed reduction under conscious sedation in the emergency department.
- Reductions generally take place in our emergency department with the use of ketamine for conscious sedation and the aid of a portable image intensifier.
- Reduction maneuvers should reverse the established mechanism of injury derived from patient history and fracture pattern, such as the Quigley maneuver for the abduction–external rotation type of fractures.
- Patients are placed in fiberglass casts that are initially univalved with plastic spacers inserted in the cast to accommodate for swelling (**FIG 3**).
- In children with a high-energy mechanism or with any neurovascular change that has not improved after reduction, admission for serial neurovascular checks to monitor for compartment syndrome is recommended.
- For Salter-Harris types I and II and triplane fractures, if a near-anatomic reduction is obtained with 2 mm or less of residual displacement, we will proceed to a long-leg cast and non–weight bearing for 4 weeks with periodic radiographs, with the frequency depending on the stability of the fracture pattern.
- To assess residual displacement in both the physis and articular surface, CT scan provides more accurate anatomic

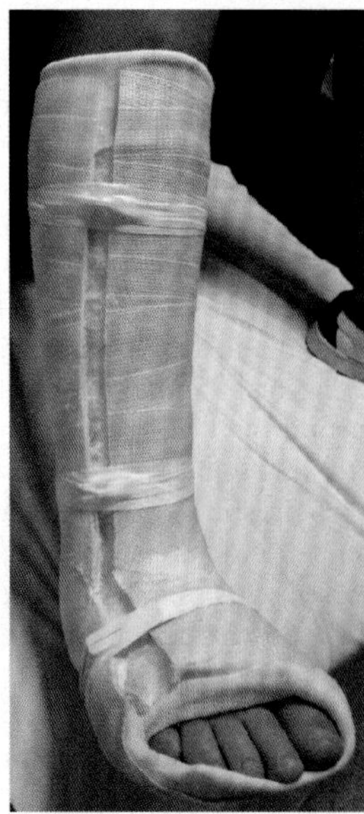

**FIG 3** • Postreduction casting. Short-leg fiberglass cast after reduction of distal tibial physeal fracture is univalved, spacers are later placed, and the cast is overwrapped with waterproof tape.

assessment, and we routinely perform plain radiographs and CT scans after reduction.
- For children with any residual intra-articular irregularity or significant angular deformity, we will proceed with open reduction and internal fixation.

## SURGICAL MANAGEMENT

### Preoperative Planning

- A repeat attempt at closed reduction may be made in the operating room under general anesthesia with or without muscle relaxation to see if the fracture would be amenable to closed reduction and casting or closed reduction and percutaneous pinning.
- CT scanning with three-dimensional reconstructions allows the surgeon to better understand ankle fracture pathoanatomy. We feel these studies are essential in the preoperative planning of many complex ankle fractures, especially triplane fractures.
  - CT scans enable understanding of the complex configuration of these fractures and ultimately allows the planning for lag screw placement in relation to the fracture planes.
  - As mentioned previously, CT scans are also important in assessment of the need for open reduction of the fracture due to gapping of the growth plate or intra-articular displacement.
- For the most part, in children with open growth plates, transphyseal fixation should involve only smooth Kirschner wires; screws may be used and should be positioned parallel to the physis.

### Positioning

- Almost all ankle fractures can be addressed in the supine position.
  - If lateral ankle exposure is necessary, a bump can be placed underneath the operative hip to improve lateral visualization.
- The image intensifier is positioned with the screen at the foot of the table angled toward the surgeon on the operative side, whereas the C-arm should come in directly from the opposite side of the operative ankle.
- The operative leg can be elevated with blankets or a foam pad to allow a pull-through lateral view unobstructed by the contralateral extremity.
- Nonsterile tourniquets are applied as proximal as possible before sterile draping.

### Approach

- The anterior approach involves an incision of 5 to 10 cm over the distal tibia.
  - The superficial peroneal nerve lies over the ankle retinaculum at this level and should be avoided.
  - The superior extensor retinaculum is incised at the interval between the extensor digitorum longus and the extensor hallucis longus.
  - Care is taken not to injure the neurovascular bundle consisting of the deep peroneal nerve and anterior tibial artery, which lies in this interval.
- The posteromedial approach to the ankle consists of an incision of 5 to 10 cm roughly midway between the medial malleolus on the medial border of the Achilles tendon.
  - The deep fascial layers are incised longitudinally to expose the flexor tendons posterior to the ankle. At this level, the flexor hallucis longus is the only muscle that still has muscle fibers.
  - Dissection is carried out along the lateral border of the flexor hallucis longus, and the ankle is exposed as the flexor hallucis longus is retracted medially.
  - Care must be taken because the neurovascular bundle is just medial to the flexor hallucis longus; the tibial nerve is relatively large in young children compared to the tendon of the flexor digitorum longus.
- The lateral approach involves an incision over the posterior margin of the fibula toward the distal end centered about the fracture site.
  - The short saphenous vein and the sural nerve run just posterior and inferior to the distal portion of the lateral malleolus.
- The medial approach can be centered more anterior or posterior depending on the location of the medial malleolar fracture and the need to visualize the posterior tibia or the intra-articular structures.
  - The incisions for these approaches should be centered over the malleolus longitudinally but should not be over the most prominent portion of the malleolus to prevent irritation.
  - Anterior to the medial malleolus run the long saphenous vein and the saphenous nerve, which should be preserved.

TECHNIQUES

## Salter-Harris Types I and II Distal Tibia Fractures

### Exposure and Reduction

- A standard anterior approach for SER fractures is used as described earlier.
- For a medially gapped, Salter-Harris type II abduction injury, a medial approach is used (**TECH FIG 1**).
  - The approach can be made slightly more medial or lateral, depending on the location of the fracture.
- The fracture and growth plate should be identified and defined.
  - The growth plate and perichondral ring should be identified and protected.
    - The physis has an identifiable white cartilaginous appearance.
  - Two Hohmann-type retractors can be placed around the distal tibia to allow for exposure.
- Once exposure is obtained, the interposed periosteum can be removed by using a Freer elevator to carefully sweep this periosteum out of the physis.
  - Care should be taken to preserve the periosteum, as it provides blood flow to aid in fracture healing and can be intimately associated with the perichondral ring.
    - The periosteum, however, may be carefully incised to ease its removal from the fracture site and to obtain an anatomic reduction.
- At this point, under direct visualization, the reduction is achieved and manually held in place.
  - Once the periosteum is atraumatically removed from the fracture site, the reduction is relatively easy and the fracture is typically stable.

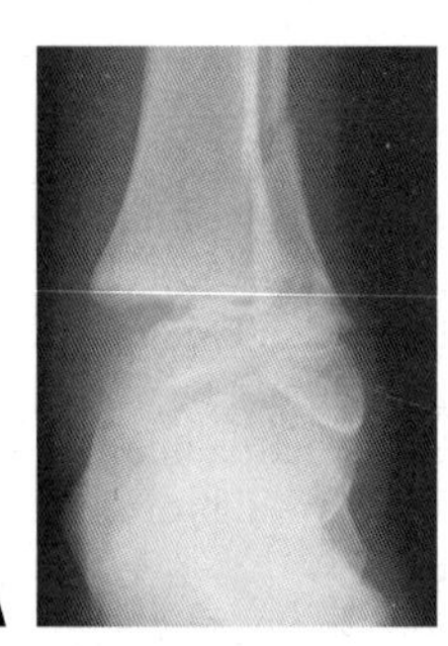
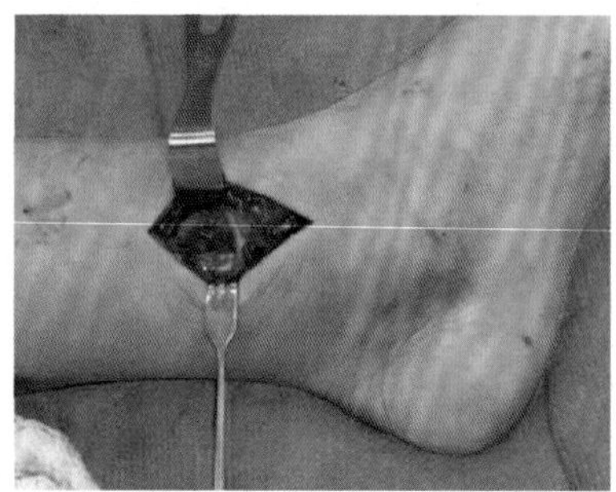
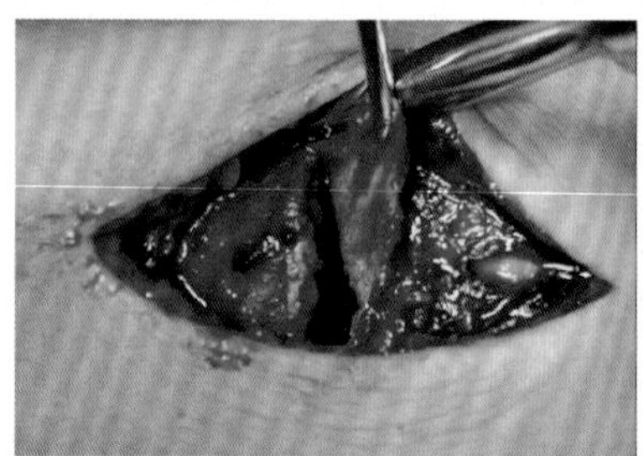

**TECH FIG 1** • Surgical approach to a medially gapped fracture. **A.** This AP radiograph demonstrates a medially gapped Salter-Harris type II abduction-type fracture. **B.** A medial approach is used to obtain open reduction of this fracture. **C.** This operative photograph highlights the periosteum interposed in the physeal fracture, which was extracted to obtain anatomic reduction and prevent medial gapping.

## Stabilization

- Many Salter-Harris type II fractures can be successfully stabilized with two 0.062-inch smooth Kirschner wires.
  - The wires are placed from distal to proximal, from the anteromedial malleolus, and from the anterolateral corner of the tibial epiphysis (**TECH FIG 2**).
  - The entry point of the percutaneous pins must be placed distally enough through the skin to enter the bone at the appropriate starting point.
  - On insertion, the Kirschner wires can be directly visualized through the open incision at their appropriate entry point into bone.
- Occasionally, there may be large metaphyseal fragments that may be more appropriately stabilized with one or two lagged cancellous bone screws.
  - These screws should be placed proximal to the physis and perpendicular to the fracture site.
- Cannulated screws can also be used, based on the surgeon's preference.

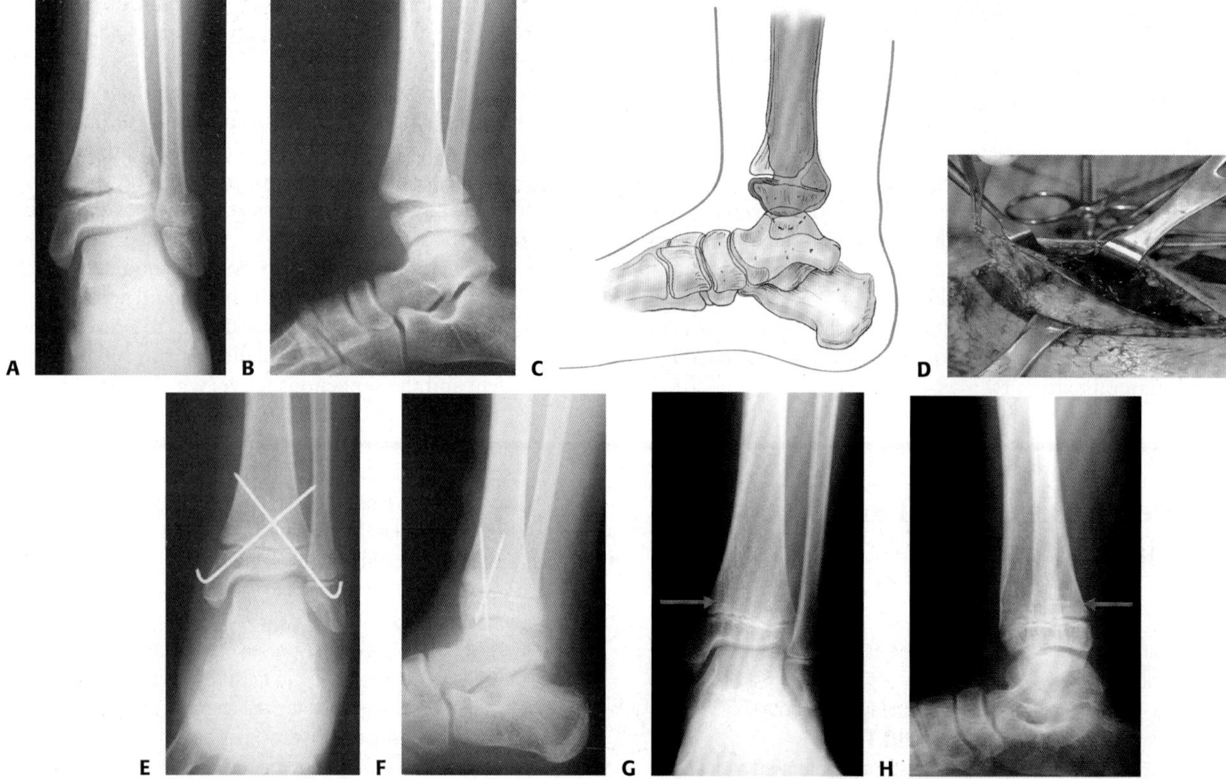

**TECH FIG 2** • Treatment of Salter-Harris type II SER type of fracture with interposed periosteum. **A,B.** Radiographs demonstrate a Salter-Harris type II SER type of fracture gapped anteriorly and medially. **C.** Periosteum (shown in *red*) is often interposed anteriorly in SER-type Salter-Harris type II fractures, which prevents closed reduction. **D.** This periosteum must be carefully extracted from the physeal fracture to obtain anatomic reduction and decrease the chance of premature physeal closure. **E,F.** Open reduction was obtained after failed closed reduction due to interposed periosteum in the physeal fracture. Then, the fracture was stabilized with two crossed Kirschner wires placed percutaneously. **G,H.** At 1 year postoperatively, the distal tibial physis appears open. The *red arrows* mark the Harris growth line, which is parallel with the physis, demonstrating symmetric growth after injury. This further supports that the tibial physis is open.

## Tillaux Fractures: Salter-Harris Type III Fractures

- An anterolateral approach to the ankle is used.
- This fracture can be fixed by a distal to proximal and anterior to posterior compressive interfragmentary cancellous screw (**TECH FIG 3**).
- Again, cannulated screw fixation may be used if the surgeon prefers it to the use of noncannulated screws.
- Crossing the physis is not contraindicated in this fracture pattern because by definition, the medial physis is closed and complete physeal closure is imminent.

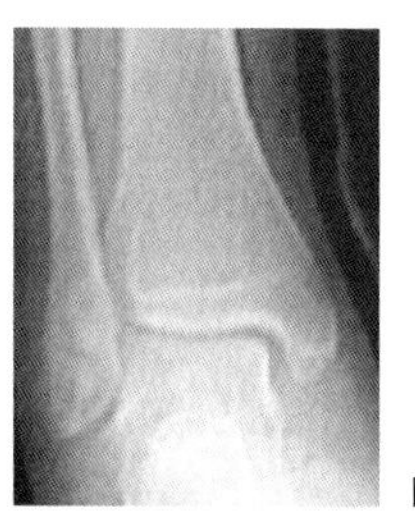
A

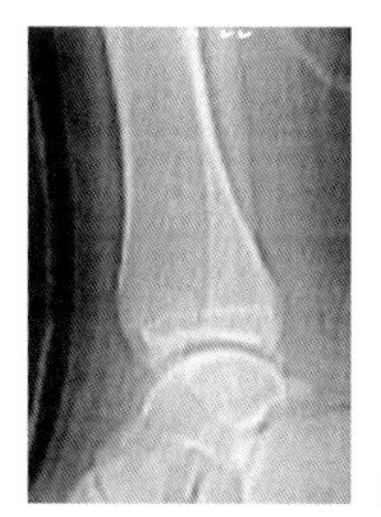
B

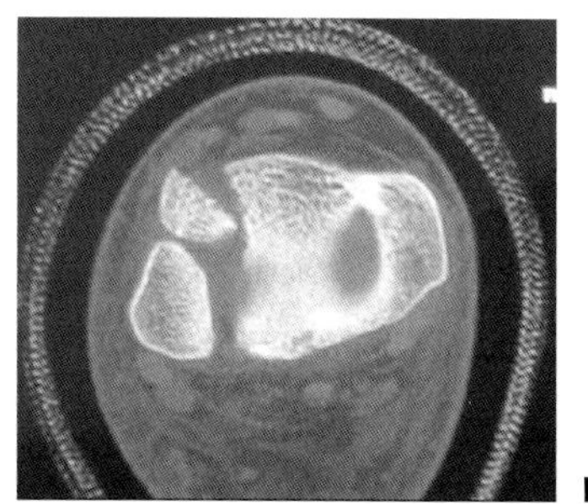
C

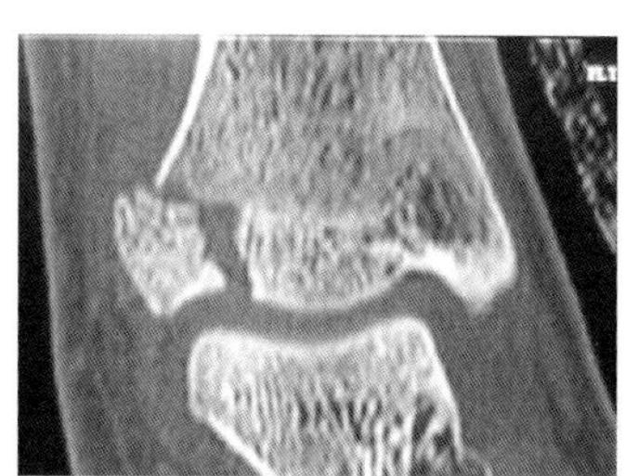
D

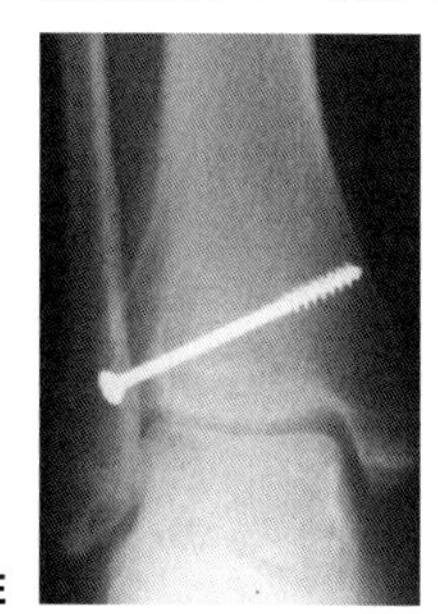
E

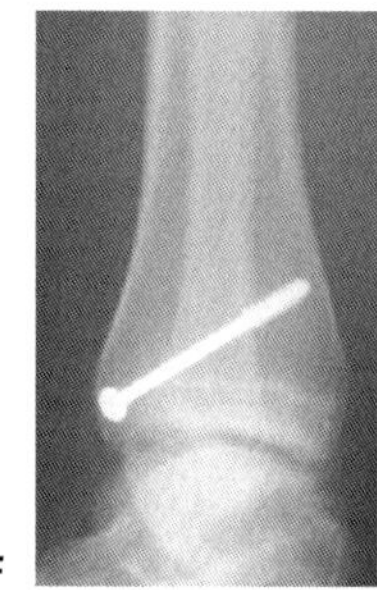
F

**TECH FIG 3** • Tillaux fracture treatment. **A,B.** Tillaux fractures are often not seen clearly on plain radiographic views, and it is important to obtain a mortise view to see the fracture fragment that is obstructed by the fibula in standard AP views. **C,D.** CT scans often aid in fracture characterization and operative planning. **E,F.** These fractures are fixed with compressive interfragmentary cancellous screws across the fracture site, without concern for transphyseal fixation as these patients are always close to skeletal maturity.

## Medial Malleolar Fractures: Salter-Harris Types III and IV Fractures

- If there is only a small metaphyseal fragment, these fractures may be fixed with 4.0-mm cancellous bone screws or Kirschner wires completely within the epiphysis and parallel to the physis and joint (**TECH FIG 4**).
  - These fractures can be treated percutaneously if anatomic reduction can be attained by closed treatment; however, a small incision can easily allow direct visualization of the reduction and the joint surface.
- If a larger metaphyseal fragment is present, another metaphyseal screw can be placed parallel to the physis in addition to the epiphyseal screw.
- If the patient is skeletally immature and the fracture is not amenable to intraepiphyseal fixation, Kirschner wires may be placed across the fracture site and physis and removed at a later date.
  - This method can also be used if there is a small avulsion fragment off the medial malleolus.
- If the patient is near skeletal maturity, these fractures can be treated as in adults with two partially threaded cannulated or noncannulated screws placed perpendicular to the fracture site.
  - Alternatively, in this population near maturity, compression across the fracture and apophysis can be obtained with two Kirschner wires compressed by means of a tension band wire loop.
- In certain cases, it has been advocated to excise and discard the metaphyseal fragment to allow improved visualization of the physis and prevent bony bridging in this area. However, we do not advocate this form of treatment.
  - We do not advocate this approach, as the goal is to ultimately restore anatomic alignment.
  - If it is necessary to remove this bony fragment, we will subsequently replace it after anatomic alignment is restored and the physis is atraumatically cleared of any mechanical blockages.

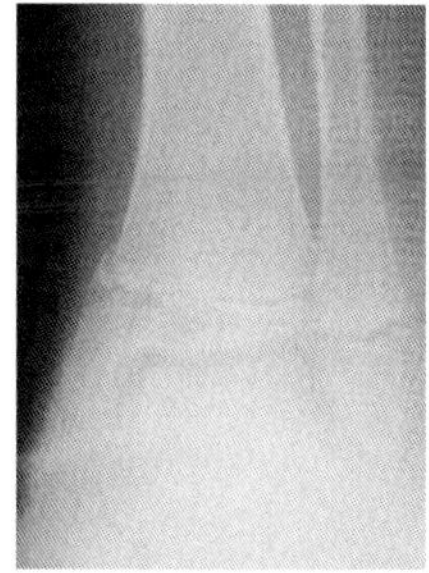
A

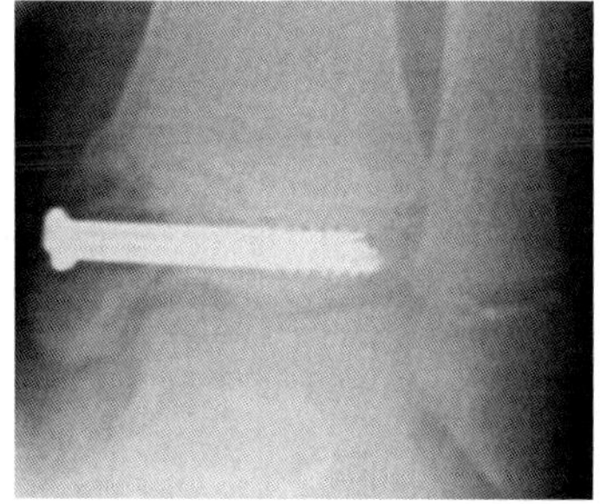
B

**TECH FIG 4** • **A,B.** Medial malleolar fracture fixation with an epiphyseal screw. If there is only a small metaphyseal fragment, medial malleolar fractures can be fixed with compressive screws placed within the epiphysis, parallel to the physis. Cannulated screws can be used to help ensure the physis is not compromised.

## Triplane Fractures: Salter-Harris Type IV Fractures

- Triplane fractures are complex transitional fractures that involve the distal tibial physis at the time of its asymmetric closure during the early teenage years.
- Because of their complexity, we advocate CT scans with three-dimensional reconstructions for preoperative planning (see **FIG 2**).
- The surgical approach depends on the complexity of the fracture, as these fractures can be two-, three-, or four-part fractures (**TECH FIG 5A–C**).
- Growth plate disturbance is rare, given the proximity to skeletal maturity in these patients.
- Anatomic alignment of the articular surface is essential.
- Two-part and sometimes three-part fractures can be anatomically reduced and fixed through an isolated anterolateral approach.
- Generally, lag screws need to be placed at the level of both the epiphysis and metaphysis, and it may be beneficial to employ a two-incision approach to obtain reduction and better access to fracture fixation (**TECH FIG 5D**).
  - The anterior incision is used to obtain lag fixation of the metaphyseal fragment, often in the coronal plane, and to visualize the joint surface.
  - The medial incision allows insertion of the epiphyseal screw.
  - Both incisions will allow direct visualization of the fracture reduction.
- If the fibula is significantly fractured and shortened, it is important to either anatomically reduce the fibula with or without fixation to obtain an appropriate template for the anatomic length of the ankle mortise.

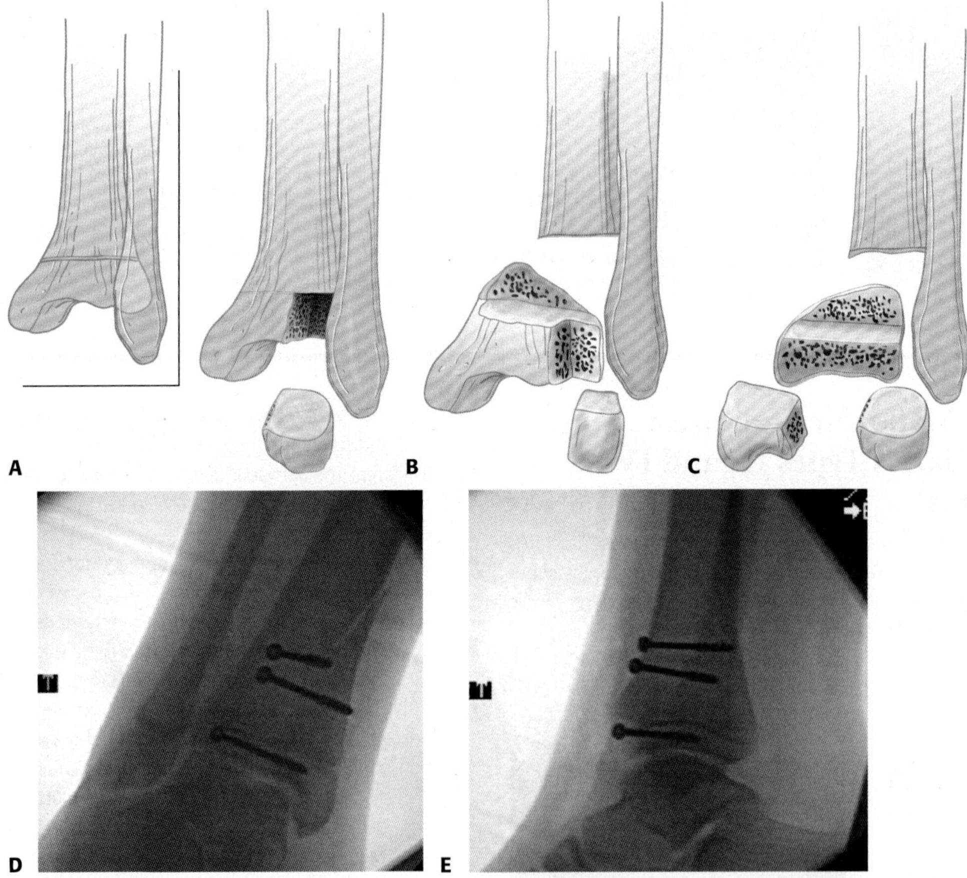

**TECH FIG 5** • Triplane fractures can be two-part (**A**), three-part (**B**), or four-part (**C**) fractures, but all involve an intra-articular epiphyseal component in addition to a metaphyseal component, making them Salter-Harris type IV fractures. **D,E.** In complex triplane fractures, screws often need to be placed both at the level of the epiphysis and the metaphysis, as dictated by the specific fracture pattern.

## Fibular Fracture Fixation

- Distal fibula fractures in patients who are skeletally immature may be treated with a large-diameter smooth Kirschner wire as an intramedullary device from a distal entry point at the tip of the lateral malleolus in a retrograde fashion.
  - The starting point should be at the distal tip of the lateral malleolus.
- Distal fibula fractures in skeletally immature patients may also be cross-pinned if the fracture pattern allows.
- For patients close to skeletal maturity, interfragmentary fixation can be used with or without a one-third tubular plate similar to a skeletally mature patient.

### Metaphyseal Distal Tibial Fractures

- Mercer Rang has given metaphyseal distal tibial fractures in children the eponym, Gillespie fractures.
- Often, these fractures need to be reduced in some equinus to allow for anatomic alignment and prevent recurvatum.
- Generally, metaphyseal distal tibial fractures that have failed closed management can be treated with cross-pinning using smooth Kirschner wires.
- Some metaphyseal fractures may be amenable to flexible intramedullary nailing in an anterograde fashion if they are not too distal.

## Alternative Techniques

- External fixation may be a useful tool in grossly contaminated fractures or fractures with significant soft tissue compromise, such as a lawnmower injury.
  - The goals of the external fixator are to maintain length and to minimize soft tissue necrosis from bony fragments.
  - External fixators can be used as temporizing devices or definitive treatment.
  - There are no pediatric-specific rules for external fixator application other than to avoid physeal damage by crossing the growth plate.
  - Large, medium, or even small external fixator sets may need to be available depending on the size of the child.
- Syndesmosis injuries generally occur in the pediatric population only at or near the time of skeletal maturity; thus, these injuries can generally be treated like adult injuries.

## PEARLS AND PITFALLS

| | |
|---|---|
| **Use of CT scans** | ▪ We advocate obtaining postreduction CT scans to evaluate joint space congruity and physeal gap if persistent displacement exists after closed reduction; plain radiographs may underestimate actual fracture displacement and comminution. |
| **Superior extensor retinaculum syndrome** | ▪ Patients presenting with severe ankle pain and swelling, hypoesthesia or anesthesia in the first dorsal web space, weakness of the extensor hallucis longus and extensor digitorum communis, and pain on passive flexion of the great toe (**FIG 4**) should be evaluated for superior extensor retinaculum syndrome. Pressure measurements should be obtained and release of the superior extensor retinaculum performed to prevent ischemic change. Untreated, the natural history of this syndrome involves a residual sensory deficit in the first dorsal web space and contracture of the extensor hallucis longus and extensor digitorum brevis.[3] |
| **Premature physeal closure** | ▪ To attempt to mitigate this complication, we have developed an algorithm:<br>  ▪ Nondisplaced fractures (<2 mm) are casted.<br>  ▪ Displaced fractures undergo closed reduction under general anesthesia or conscious sedation, then casting for 3–6 weeks.<br>▪ In addition to prereduction and postreduction ankle radiographs, we often obtain contralateral ankle radiographs and left hand bone age films and, if there are any questions about fracture displacement, a postreduction CT scan.<br>▪ Additionally, we follow-up with patients with growth plate fractures at regular intervals until skeletal maturity. |
| **Abduction injuries versus SER-type injuries** | ▪ Abduction-type injuries carry a worse prognosis compared to SER type injuries with higher rates of premature physeal closure regardless of treatment (open reduction versus closed treatment). These issues should be discussed with the family preoperatively. |
| **Postoperative follow-up** | ▪ For follow-up after physeal injuries, we often obtain baseline radiographs of the contralateral ankle and an AP view of the left hand for establishing bone age. After initial fracture management follow-up is maintained at 6-month intervals and should include bilateral ankle radiographs.<br>▪ Alignment of both the child's ankles should be assessed while weight bearing, as malalignment can be a sequela of premature physeal closure. If closure is noted, early physeal assessment with CT scans is necessary to prevent ankle deformity and leg length discrepancy. |

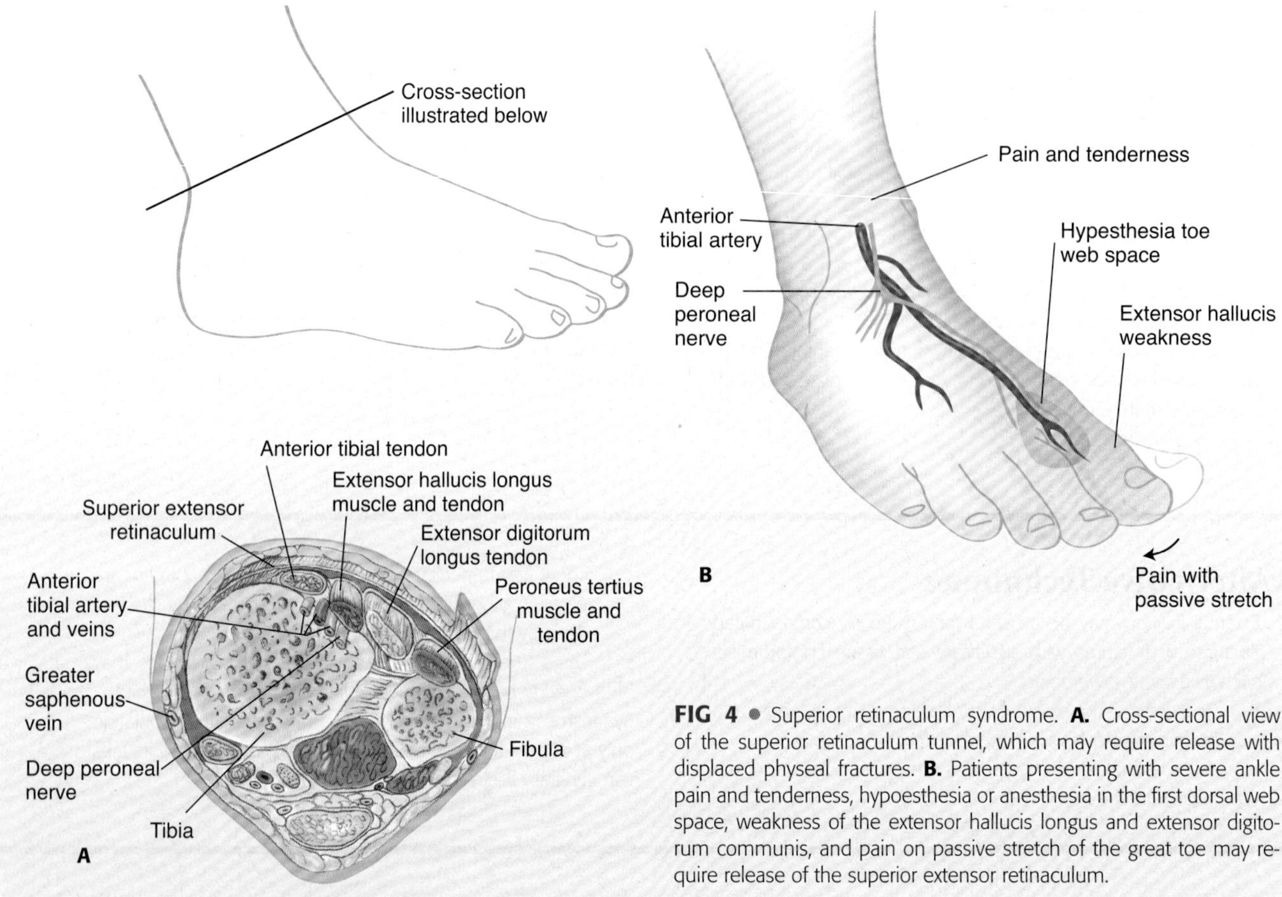


**FIG 4** • Superior retinaculum syndrome. **A.** Cross-sectional view of the superior retinaculum tunnel, which may require release with displaced physeal fractures. **B.** Patients presenting with severe ankle pain and tenderness, hypoesthesia or anesthesia in the first dorsal web space, weakness of the extensor hallucis longus and extensor digitorum communis, and pain on passive stretch of the great toe may require release of the superior extensor retinaculum.

## POSTOPERATIVE CARE

- Treatment after surgical fixation generally consists of immobilization with a short-leg cast applied in the operating room, and the patient is kept non–weight bearing for 4 weeks.
  - We univalve our fiberglass casts and place plastic spacers taped in with waterproof tape to accommodate leg swelling, with the patient returning in 1 week for removal of spacers and cast overwrap and tightening with fiberglass (see **FIG 3**).
- Four weeks postoperatively, the cast is changed to a weight-bearing cast, and the child is allowed to be weight bearing as tolerated for 2 or 3 more weeks with a cast shoe.
- With percutaneous pin fixation, we use 0.062-inch Kirschner wires left through the skin, which are removed at the 4-week cast change.
- Physical therapy is rarely needed for range of motion in the preadolescent population, as daily activity with walking often suffices to restore function. Occasionally, adolescents may benefit from physical therapy for range of motion and proprioceptive conditioning.
- We advocate follow-up for at least 1 year, at 3, 6, and 12 months, then every 6 months until skeletal maturity for children with physeal injuries to monitor for premature physeal closure.
  - At these follow-up visits, plain radiographs should include images of the affected ankle as well as AP and lateral views of the contralateral ankle.

## OUTCOMES

- As in most children's fractures, children with ankle fractures generally fare well.
- Data on long-term follow-up are sparse. However, data for intra-articular triplane fractures have shown the importance of anatomic alignment with less than 2 mm of displacement.
  - Ertl and coworkers[3] demonstrated with a follow-up of 18 to 36 months that "residual displacement of two millimeters or more after reduction was associated with a less than optimum result unless the epiphyseal fracture was outside the primary weight-bearing area of the ankle."
  - Rapariz and colleagues,[6] with a mean follow-up of 5 years, found that "prognosis is surprisingly good" and that "only when adequate reduction (<2 mm displacement) has not been achieved can degenerative changes be seen at long-term follow-up (>5 years)."
  - Rapariz and colleagues found good functional results ubiquitously, but as in the study by Ertl and associates, the follow-up was short.
  - Both these studies stressed the need to obtain CT scans to define and characterize the fracture and the degree of displacement as well as advocating a trial of closed reduction to obtain adequate reduction.

## COMPLICATIONS

- Premature physeal closure, as mentioned earlier, can lead to limb length discrepancies and malalignment, which in younger children with continued growth potential can be symptomatic and may need to be addressed surgically.[1,7]

- Reflex sympathetic dystrophy or complex regional pain syndrome can develop after these ankle injuries.
  - It is characterized by pain out of proportion that persists beyond a typical recovery time frame and may also entail swelling, skin color changes, and limited range of motion.
  - Treatment can include medications, therapy, psychological counseling, and sympathetic nerve blocks; in extreme cases, sympathectomy or implantation of a dorsal column stimulator has been proposed.
- Arthrofibrosis is a normal sequela from joint injury or prolonged immobilization. Generally, in the pediatric population, interventions such as physical therapy or manipulation under anesthesia are not necessary.
- Superior extensor retinaculum syndrome, as described earlier, can lead to residual numbness in the great toe web space and persistent pain and weakness in the toe extensors.[5]
- Acute compartment syndrome that is untreated can lead to permanent neuromuscular damage, including weakness or altered sensibilities.
- Malunion of fractures can occur with operative or nonoperative treatment or can be a secondary consequence of premature physeal closure.
- Osteochondral injury in ankle fractures can ultimately lead to symptomatic posttraumatic osteoarthritis, and studies have demonstrated that anatomic reduction is important to prevent this complication.
  - If significant chondral injury does occur in the young patient population, drilling for focal posttraumatic osteochondritis dissecans lesions can be successful. In extreme cases with osteochondral damage, osteochondral autografting or allografting can be attempted.
- Complications with casts are inherent when they are used to treat fractures.
  - These complications include cast ulceration from poorly fitted or padded casts. Casts applied too tightly or not appropriately split can lead to acute compartment syndrome. Removal of casts can lead to cast saw burns, which can permanently scar children's skin.

## REFERENCES


1. Barmada A, Gaynor T, Mubarak SJ. Premature physeal closure following distal tibia physeal fractures. J Pediatr 2003;23:733–739.
2. Dias LS, Tachdjian MO. Physeal injuries of the ankle in children: classification. Clin Orthop Relat Res 1978;(136):230–233.
3. Ertl JP, Barrack RL, Alexander AH, et al. Triplane fracture of the distal tibial epiphysis long-term follow-up. J Bone Joint Surg Am 1988;70(7):967–976.
4. Lauge-Hansen N. Fractures of the ankle. II. Combined experimental-surgical and experimental-roentgenologic investigations. Arch Surg 1950;60:957–985.
5. Mubarak SJ. Extensor retinaculum syndrome of the ankle after injury to the distal tibial physis. J Bone Joint Surg Br 2002;84(1):11–14.
6. Rapariz JM, Ocete G, González-Herranz P, et al. Distal tibial triplane fractures: long-term follow-up. J Pediatr Orthop 1996;16:113–118.
7. Rohmiller MT, Gaynor TP, Pawelek J, et al. Salter-Harris I and II fractures of the distal tibia: does mechanism of injury relate to premature physeal closure? J Pediatr Orthop 2006;26:322–328.
8. Russo F, Moor MA, Mubarak SJ, et al. Salter-Harris II fractures of the distal tibia: does surgical management reduce the risk of premature physeal closure? J Pediatr Orthop 2013;33:524–529.

# Open Reduction and Internal Fixation of the Mature Ankle

Sanjit R. Konda and Kenneth A. Egol

## DEFINITION

- The ankle is a modified hinge joint, which relies on a congruently reduced mortise to provide optimal function.
- Maintenance of normal tibiotalar contact is essential if one is to maintain function.
- Surgical treatment of displaced, unstable ankle fractures centers on anatomic restoration of the bony and ligamentous relationships that make up the ankle mortise.[12]
- This chapter will focus on the treatment of a specific pattern of injury to the ankle, specifically, the bimalleolar fracture pattern.

## ANATOMY

- The anatomy of the distal tibia and ankle joint must be taken into account when considering ankle fractures. As the tibial shaft flares in the supramalleolar region, the dense cortical bone changes to metaphyseal cancellous bone (**FIG 1A**).
- The shape of the tibial articular surface is concave, with distal extension of the anterior and posterior lips.
  - This surface has been called the *tibial plafond*, which is French for ceiling.
- The talar dome is wedge-shaped and sits within the mortise. It is wider anteriorly than posteriorly.
- The medial end of the tibia is the medial malleolus.
  - The medial malleolus is composed of the anterior and posterior colliculi, separated by the intercollicular groove (**FIG 1B**).
  - The anterior colliculus is the narrower and most distal portion of the medial malleolus and serves as the origin of the superficial deltoid ligaments.
  - The intercollicular groove and the posterior colliculus, which is broader than the anterior colliculus, provide the origin of the deep deltoid ligaments.
  - The insertions of the deltoid ligaments (medial tubercle of the talus, navicular tuberosity, and sustentaculum tali) can also be considered as part of the medial malleolar osteoligamentous complex.
- The lateral malleolus is the distal end of the fibula. It extends about 1 cm distally and posteriorly compared to the medial malleolus.
- The syndesmotic ligament complex unites the distal fibula with the distal tibia. The following ligaments make up the syndesmotic complex: the anteroinferior tibiofibular ligament, the posteroinferior tibiofibular ligament, the inferior transverse ligament, and the interosseous ligament (**FIG 1C**).

## PATHOGENESIS

- The majority of bimalleolar ankle fractures are secondary to rotation of the body about a supinated or pronated foot.[8] They are best defined by the classification of Lauge-Hansen[6] (**FIG 2**).
- The supination–external rotation pattern of ankle fracture is divided into four stages.
  - The stage I injury is tearing of the anteroinferior tibiofibular ligaments.
  - As the external rotation force continues laterally, a spiral fracture of the fibula occurs. On lateral radiograph, the fracture line will pass from the anteroinferior cortex to the posterosuperior cortex.
  - The third stage occurs when the posteroinferior tibiofibular ligaments avulse or fracture off the posterior malleolus.
  - The final stage results in a medial malleolar osteoligamentous complex injury with either a deep deltoid ligament tear or a fracture of the medial malleolus.
- The pronation–external rotation variant also has four stages. Because of the pronated position of the foot at injury, however, the medial structures are injured in the early stages.
  - The fibula fracture pattern seen with this mechanism is usually suprasyndesmotic, and the fracture pattern is an anterosuperior to posteroinferior fracture line as seen on the lateral radiograph.
- The supination–adduction pattern is heralded by a low transverse fibular fracture and a vertical shearing pattern medially. This pattern is also associated with tibial plafond impaction.
- Finally, the pronation–abduction pattern is identified by the avulsion of the medial malleolus and a transverse or laterally comminuted fibular fracture above the syndesmosis secondary to a direct bending moment.

## PATIENT HISTORY AND PHYSICAL FINDINGS

- Most patients who present with ankle pain following trauma will describe a twisting type of injury. Less frequently, they will report a direct blow to the ankle.
- Proper medical history should include the patient's current comorbid medical conditions, such as peripheral vascular disease, diabetes, or peripheral neuropathy.
- Physical examination should center on inspection, palpation, and neurovascular examination.
  - It is important to note any gross deformity, which may signify dislocation. If dislocation is present, the ankle should be reduced and splinted as soon as possible to prevent skin tenting (and subsequent skin necrosis) and neurovascular compromise.
- Inspection for any open wound about the ankle is critical as well. Open fractures imply a surgical urgency. Swelling, ecchymosis, and tenderness about the malleoli should be recorded.
- For patients with a supination–external rotation pattern isolated fibula fracture who present with an intact mortise, the gravity stress examination can be revealing. More than

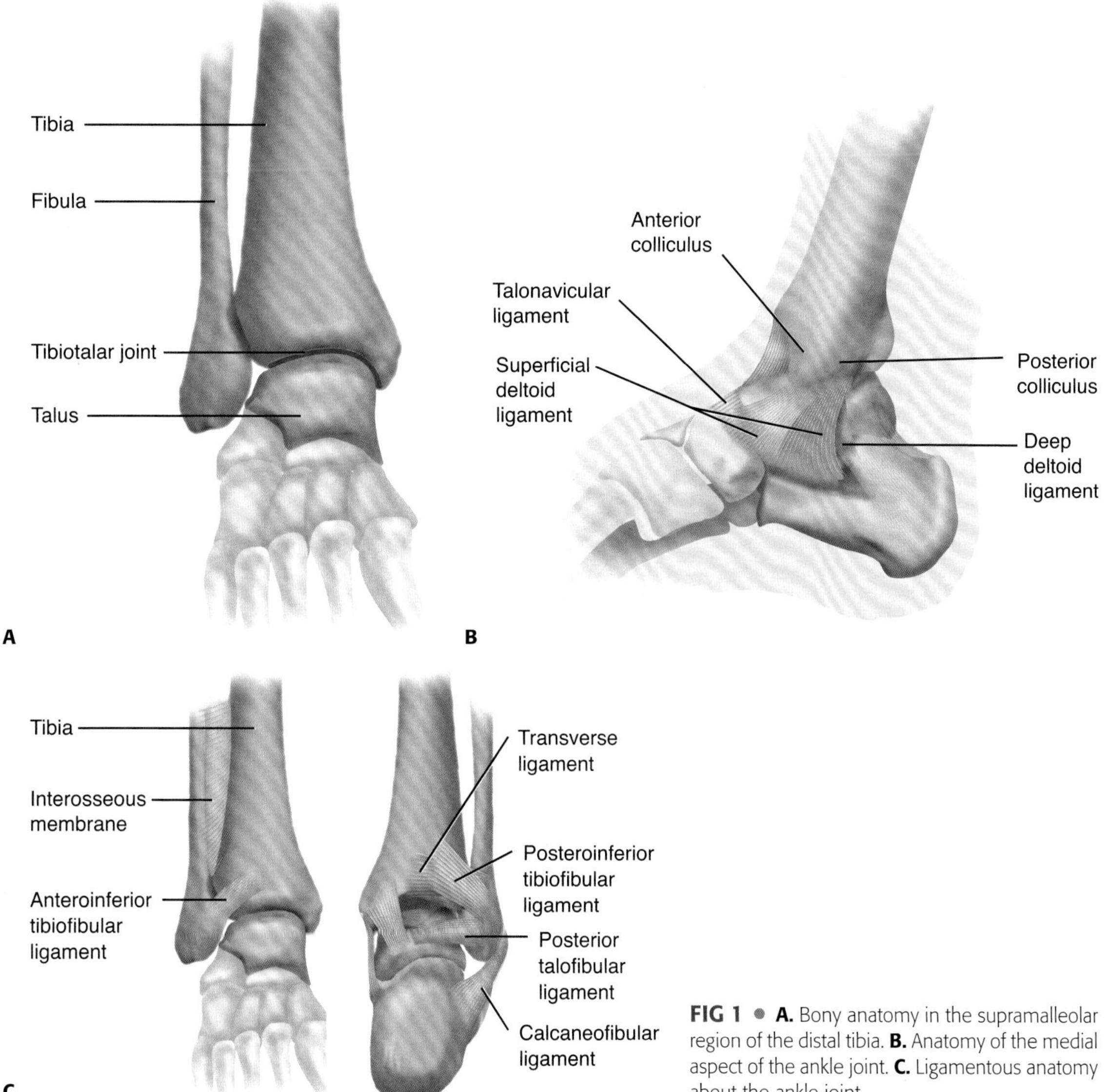


**FIG 1** • **A.** Bony anatomy in the supramalleolar region of the distal tibia. **B.** Anatomy of the medial aspect of the ankle joint. **C.** Ligamentous anatomy about the ankle joint.

5 mm of medial clear space widening in association with a lateral malleolus fracture signifies an unstable pattern.[7,9]

- Pain at the ankle along the syndesmosis during a squeeze test implies injury to the syndesmosis.
- The proximal fibula, knee, and tibia should also be examined. Palpation of pulses, detection of capillary refill, and a careful neurosensory examination must be documented prior to manipulation.

## IMAGING AND OTHER DIAGNOSTIC STUDIES

- Radiographic examination includes the ankle trauma series: anteroposterior (AP), lateral, and mortise view (**FIG 3A–C**).
- In patients with isolated lateral malleolar fractures with clinical signs of medial injury, or if there is any question of ankle stability in a supination–external rotation fracture pattern, a manual external rotation stress radiograph should be obtained to assess for instability.[2,7]
  - The tibia is held internally rotated 15 degrees with the ankle in dorsiflexion to produce a gentle external rotation moment at the ankle under fluoroscopy (**FIG 3D**).[11]
  - More than 5 mm of medial clear space widening in association with a lateral malleolus fracture signifies an unstable pattern (**FIG 3E**).[2]
- If clinically warranted, full-length tibia–fibula radiographs should be obtained.
- Restoration of medial ankle stability depends on the size and location of the medial malleolar fragment.
  - The size of the medial fragment is key to stability.
  - Anterior collicular fractures only have the superficial deltoid attached. In about 25% of supination–external rotation type 4 injuries, there will be an associated deep deltoid rupture.[10] Thus, fixation of this fragment will not enhance stability.
  - The lateral radiograph is the key. If the fragment is greater than 2.8 cm wide (supracollicular fracture), the deep deltoid will be attached and stability is restored after fixation. If the fragment is less than 1.7 cm wide (anterior collicular or intercollicular fracture), then stability is not restored with fixation. For fractures in between, an intraoperative external rotation stress examination should be performed following malleolar fixation.[16]

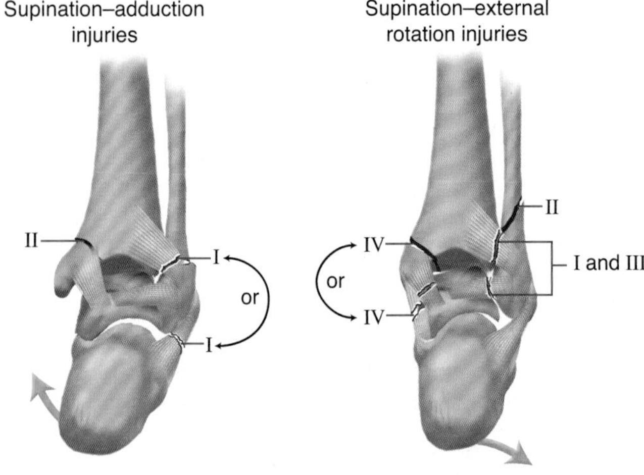


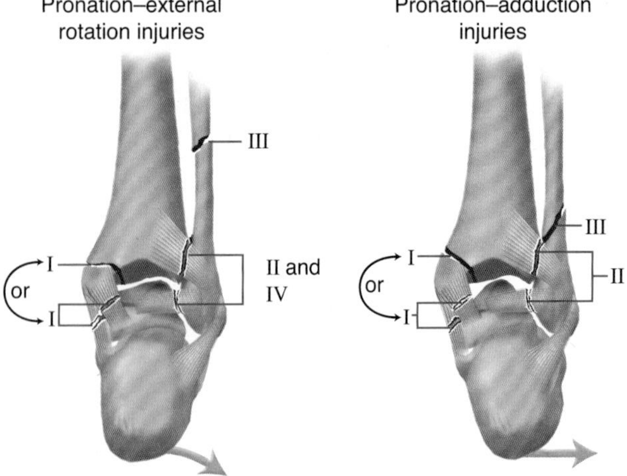


**FIG 2** • The Lauge-Hansen classification of ankle fractures.

- Computed tomography (CT) scanning may be helpful in assessing posterior malleolar fragment size in rotational ankle fractures.
- Magnetic resonance imaging (MRI) may have some use if there is an isolated lateral malleolus fracture with signs of medial injury and an equivocal stress examination.

## DIFFERENTIAL DIAGNOSIS

- Ankle sprain
- Lateral malleolus fracture
- Medial malleolus fracture
- Maisonneuve fracture
- Bimalleolar ankle fracture
- Trimalleolar ankle fracture
- Lateral process talus fracture
- Anterior process calcaneus fracture
- Subtalar dislocation

## NONOPERATIVE MANAGEMENT

- Ankle fractures in which the ankle mortise remains stable can be treated nonoperatively.
  - Isolated lateral malleolus fractures without evidence of medial-sided injury are considered supination external rotation type 2 injuries and can be treated with functional bracing and weight bearing as tolerated.
  - Unstable patterns, such as supination–external rotation type 4, either ligamentous or a true bimalleolar or trimalleolar ankle fracture, can also be treated nonoperatively in patients who are poor surgical candidates (eg, insulin-dependent diabetics), who have severe soft tissue problems, or who do not wish to undergo surgical stabilization.
- If nonoperative treatment is chosen, it is crucial to ensure anatomic mortise reduction throughout treatment until healing.
- Unstable injuries should be treated in a well-molded short-leg cast and checked on a weekly basis to ensure continued mortise reduction.

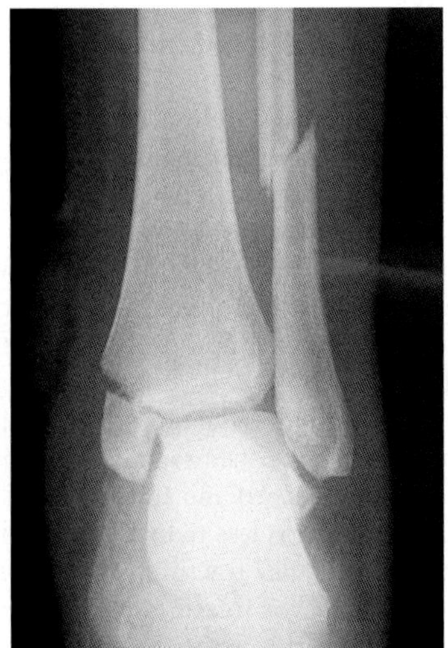


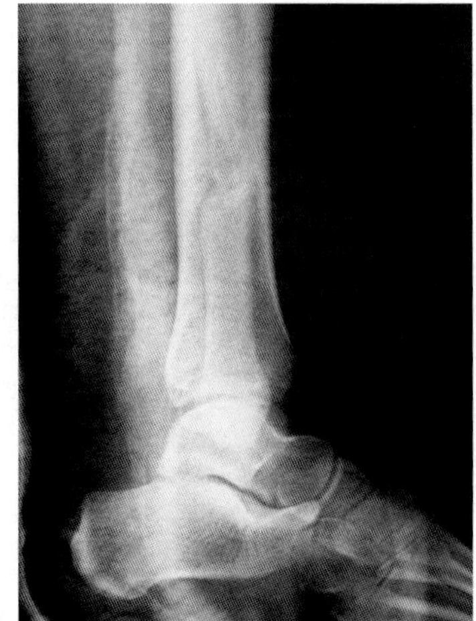


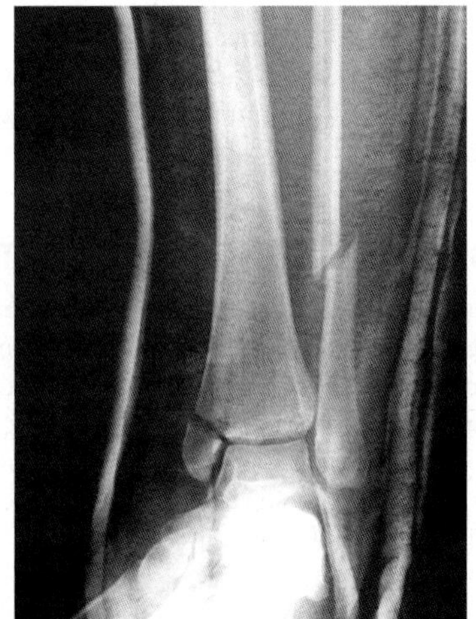


**FIG 3** • Radiographic evaluation with an ankle trauma series: AP (**A**), lateral (**B**), and mortise (**C**) views. *(continued)*

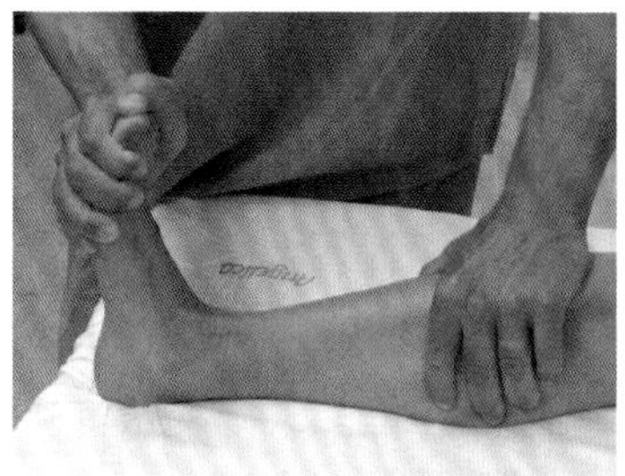
D

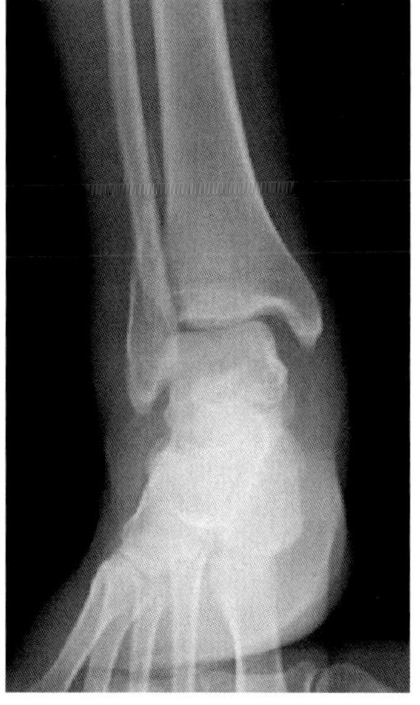
E

FIG 3 • *(continued)* Clinical (**D**) and radiographic (**E**) demonstration of a physician-assisted external rotation stress examination of the ankle.

## SURGICAL MANAGEMENT

- Any fracture of the ankle in which there is residual talar tilt or talar subluxation such that the ankle mortise is not anatomically reduced is an indication for surgical stabilization.

### Preoperative Planning

- Surgical anatomy should be reviewed prior to entering the operating room, including the bony and ligamentous structures.
  - The neurovascular anatomy about the ankle should be reviewed, including the course of the saphenous vein medially and the superficial peroneal nerve laterally.
- Equipment to be used includes a small fragment plate and screw set, large pelvic reduction clamps, small-diameter Kirschner wires, and 3.5- to 4.0-mm cannulated screw sets. If the nature of the fracture is still in question, radiographic stress examination may be performed under anesthesia.

### Positioning

- The patient is positioned supine with a small bump under the ipsilateral hip to ease access to the fibula.
- A pneumatic tourniquet can be applied to the affected thigh if desired for use during the surgical procedure. The affected limb is prepared and draped free (**FIG 4**).
- The bump may be removed after lateral fixation for easier access to the medial side.
- If a posterior approach is chosen, the patient may be placed in the prone position to allow access to the posterior tibia via the posterolateral approach.

### Approach

- The fibula is approached via a direct lateral incision.
- The medial malleolus is approached via a gently curved anteromedial incision.
- Direct access to the posterior malleolus can be obtained through a posterolateral approach to the fibula.

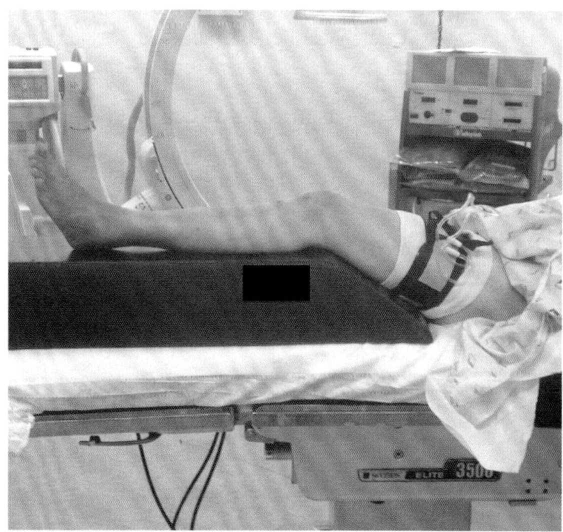

FIG 4 • Supine positioning of the injured ankle. A thigh tourniquet is applied, a rolled sheet bump is placed under the hip to internally rotate the leg so the patella is pointed directly anterior, and the ankle is elevated on an inclined bump (foam bump or sheets) to allow for lateral fluoroscopic images without moving the ankle.

## Direct Lateral Approach to the Fibula

### Exposure

- The incision is kept just off the posterior border of the fibula but may be adjusted slightly based on soft tissue considerations (**TECH FIG 1A**).
  - Deeper tissues are incised in line with the skin incision (**TECH FIG 1B**).
  - Care must be taken proximally in the wound to avoid injury to the superficial peroneal nerve, which crosses the field about 7 cm proximal to the distal tip of the fibula (**TECH FIG 1C**).
- Next, the peroneal fascia is divided, and the peroneal tendons and musculature are retracted posteriorly.
  - With gentle elevation of the periosteum about the fracture site, the fibula should be exposed.
  - Care should be taken to avoid excessive stripping of fracture fragments as well as iatrogenic disruption of the syndesmotic ligaments as they insert anteriorly on the fibula.

### Lateral Plating

- Following exposure of the fracture, the first step involves cleaning the fracture site (**TECH FIG 2A**) followed by fracture reduction.
- Usually, reduction is afforded by a small "lion jaw" clamp or pointed reduction forceps.
  - If reduction is difficult, manual traction with pronation and internal rotation will afford fracture alignment in supination–external rotation patterns.
  - Care should be taken to avoid placing clamps over fracture spikes to prevent inadvertent comminution (**TECH FIG 2B**).
- If the clamps make it difficult to place a lag screw, provisional Kirschner wires may be placed across the fracture and the clamps removed (**TECH FIG 2C**).
- At this point, if a lateral plate is chosen, the lag screw is placed in the anterior to posterior direction, perpendicular to the fracture.
  - If a posterior plate (antiglide) is chosen, the lag screw is placed through the plate in a posterior to anterior direction.
  - In either case, the near cortex is overdrilled with a 3.5-mm drill bit followed by drilling of the far cortex with a 2.5-mm drill bit (**TECH FIG 2D**).
- The length of the screw is measured and a self-tapping 3.5-mm screw is placed across the fracture in the screw track.
- Next, a one-third tubular plate is placed directly lateral on the fibula (neutralization) (**TECH FIG 2E**).
- The proximal screw holes are filled with bicortical 3.5-mm screws after drilling with the 2.5-mm drill bit.
- Distally, unicortical cancellous screws are placed, with care not to penetrate the distal tibia–fibula joint. In osteoporotic bone, locking screws can be used distally (one-third tubular locking plate used in this example) (**TECH FIG 2F,G**).
- The wound is closed (**TECH FIG 2H**).

### Obtaining Fibular Length

- In cases in which the fibula is significantly shortened (high-energy, late presentation of fracture in which callus is present), adjunctive techniques may be necessary to achieve anatomic fibular length.
  - A small bone distractor can be placed proximally to the plate in the proximal segment and through the plate in the distal segment with appropriate distraction applied to achieve fibular length (**TECH FIG 3A**).
  - Alternatively, a laterally placed fibular plate can be secured to the distal segment with a screw and a push–pull screw (3.5-mm cortical screw) can be placed proximal to the plate in the proximal segment. A laminar spreader can then be used to push the proximal end of the plate distally, which will then distract the fracture site to the appropriate fibular length (**TECH FIG 3B**).

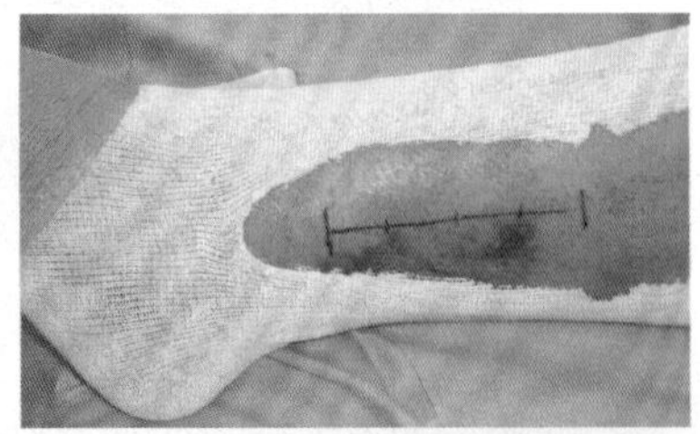

A

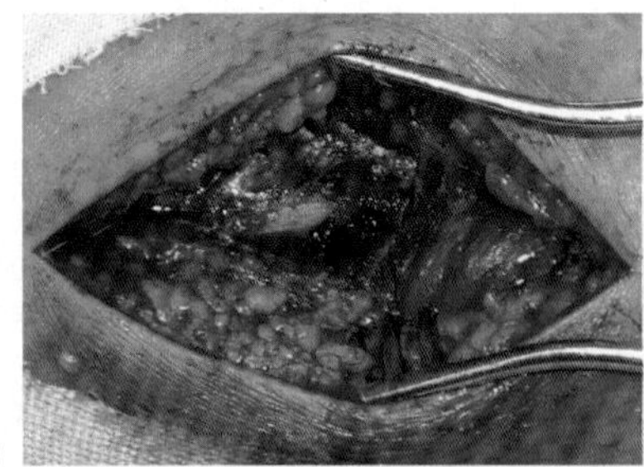

B

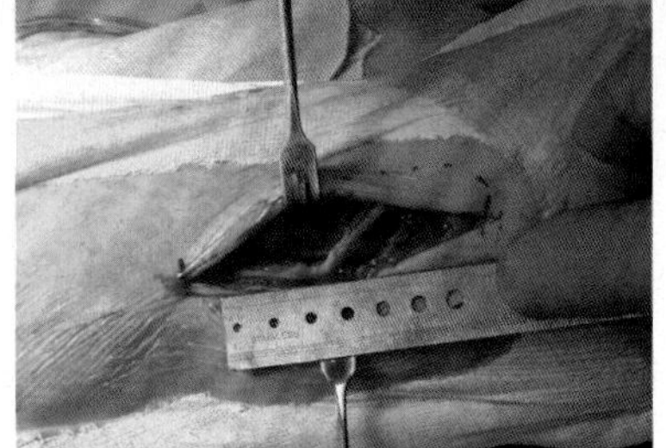

C

**TECH FIG 1** • Surgical approach to the fibula, directly lateral. **A.** Skin incision marked out just along the posterior border of the fibula, centered about the level of the fracture. **B.** Incision through the peroneal (lateral compartment) fascia, exposing the fracture site. **C.** Identification of the superficial peroneal nerve as it crosses proximally in the wound.

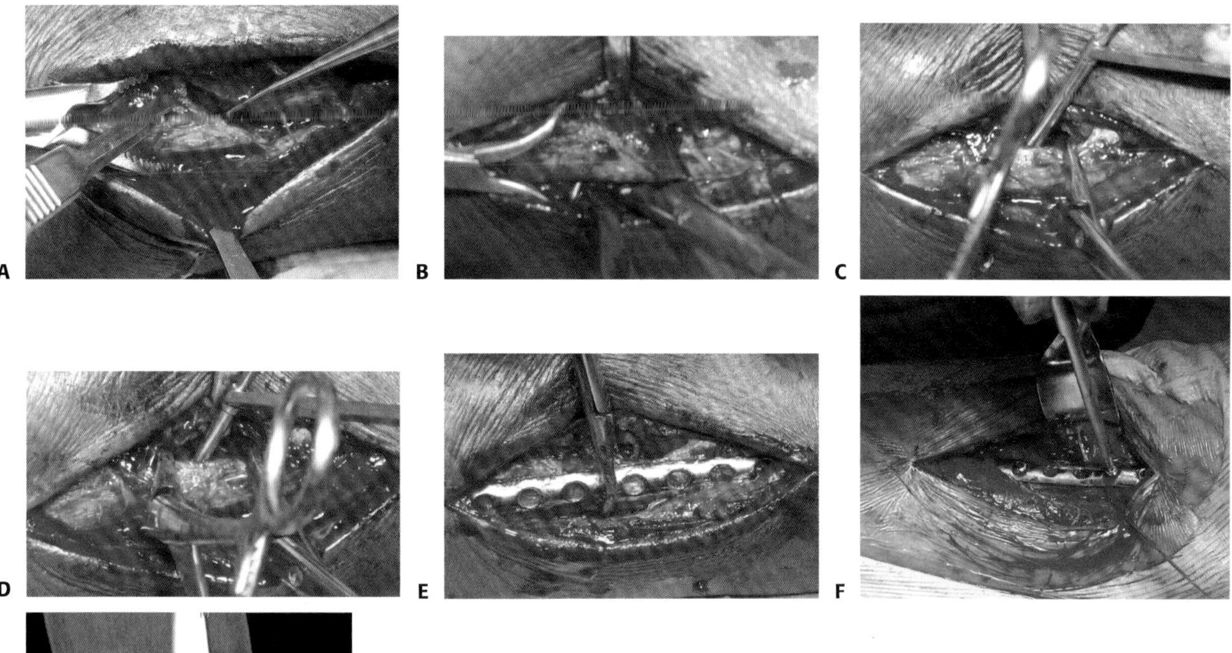

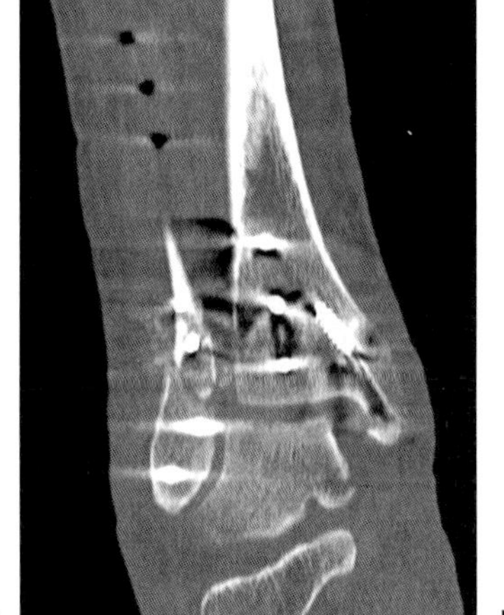

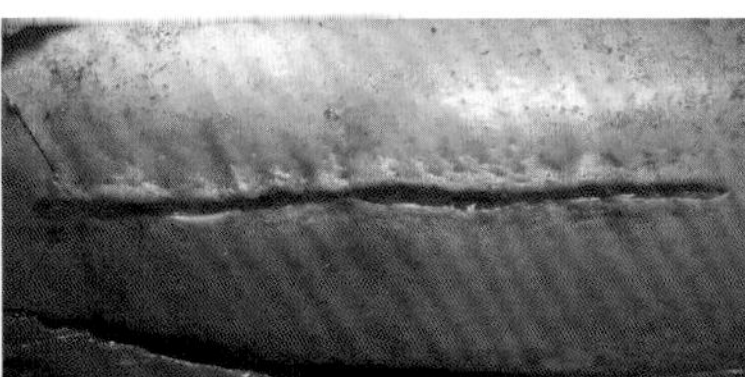

**TECH FIG 2** • **A.** Cleaning the fracture site with a small curette. **B.** An example of clamp placement across the fibular fracture site. Care is taken not to comminute the fracture spike. **C.** Lag screw placement, overdrilled with a 3.5-mm drill bit proximally. **D.** This is followed by drilling of the far cortex with a 2.5-mm drill. **E.** A neutralization plate is applied to the lateral surface of the fibula. **F.** Distal locking screws are placed through a locking one-third tubular plate in the case of osteoporotic bone. **G.** Example of distal screw penetration to be avoided. **H.** Wound closure.

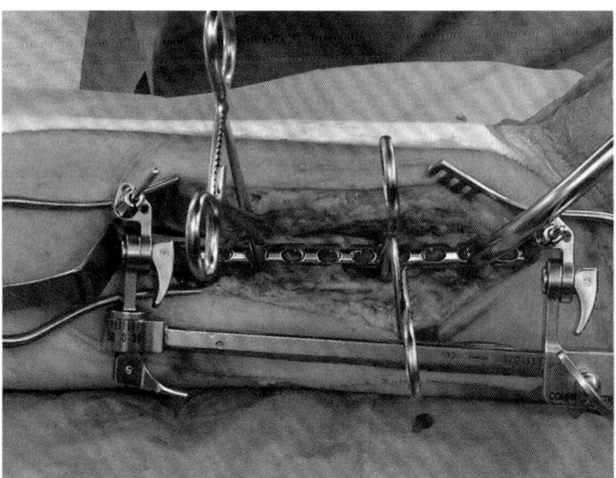

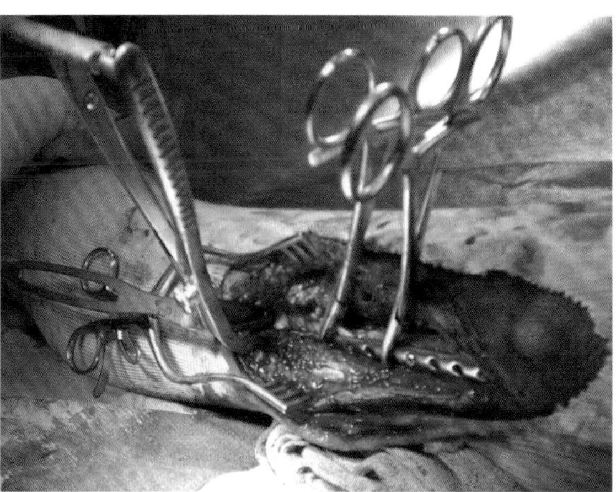

**TECH FIG 3** • **A.** Small bone distractor applied to a severely shortened fibula fracture that presented 4 weeks after the initial injury. Bone forceps are used to align the plate on the fibular shaft. **B.** Laminar spreader used to push the fibular plate (which is secured to the distal fragment only) distally causing distraction at the fracture site.

## Anteromedial Approach to the Medial Malleolus

### Exposure

- The medial malleolus is approached via a gently curved anteromedial incision (**TECH FIG 4A**).
  - An incision is made parallel to the saphenous vein that is either concave anteriorly or concave posteriorly to allow visualization of the anteromedial joint.
- After dissection of the skin, the subcutaneous tissues should be carefully dissected to prevent injury to the saphenous vein and nerve (**TECH FIG 4B**).
- With the dissection carried down sharply to the bone, the periosteum is elevated for 1 mm proximally and distally.
- The fracture should be booked open to allow visual inspection of the talar dome for chondral injury.
- The joint and medial gutter should be irrigated through the fracture for any loose hematoma or debris that may impede reduction (**TECH FIG 4C**).

### Operative Stabilization

- Following exposure, the medial malleolar fragment (usually one large piece) can be reduced with the aid of a dental tool or small, pointed reduction clamp (**TECH FIG 5A**).
- The fragment can be provisionally stabilized with small-diameter (1.25 mm) Kirschner wires placed in parallel. Alternatively, two 2.5-mm drill bits can be used to drill paths for two parallel screws, leaving the drill bits in place to gain rotational control of the malleolar fragment (**TECH FIG 5B**).
- After radiographic documentation of the reduction and wire placement, cannulated screws of appropriate length may be placed over the wires after drilling of the out cortices with a cannulated drill. Alternatively, noncannulated screws may be used independent of the provisional stabilization.
- Usually, a 4.0-mm partially threaded cancellous screw can be placed. If the fragment is small, however, 3.5- or 3.0-mm cannulated screws are now available.
  - More recent studies have advocated for the use of two bicortical 3.5-mm screws placed in lag mode.[14]
- Two screws are recommended for rotational control. If the fragment is too small, however, one screw may suffice owing to the inherent stability of the undulating fracture line.
- Countersinking the screw heads medially may help to alleviate painful prominent hardware.
- Comminuted fractures that are not amenable to screw fixation may benefit from a small buttress plate or a "suture tension band" technique using the deltoid ligament for fixation.
  - The suture or wire tension band is anchored about a more proximal screw placed parallel to the articular surface.

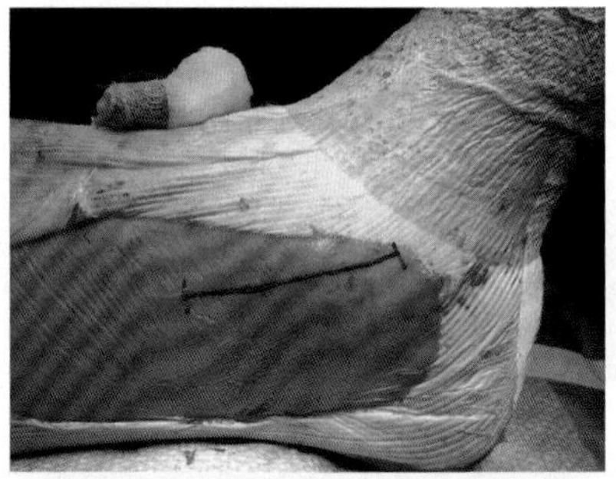
A

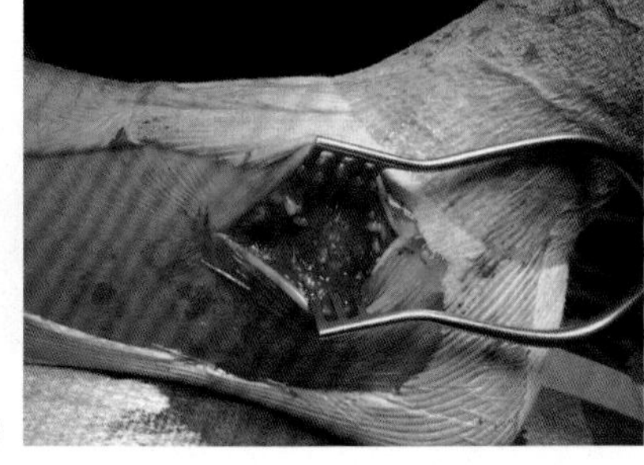
B

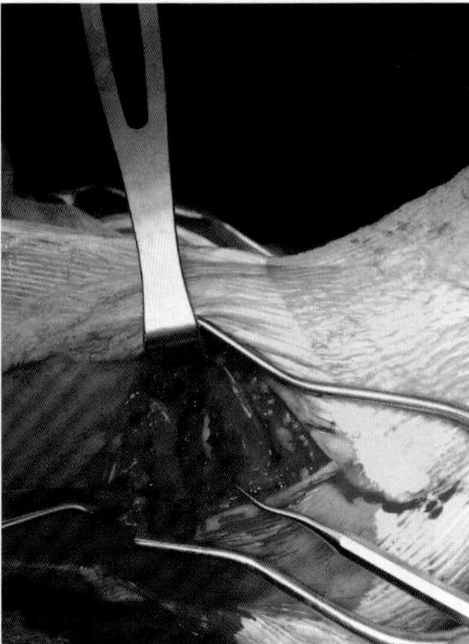
C

**TECH FIG 4** • **A.** For a medial-side injury, the skin incision is curved about the medial malleolus. **B.** Careful dissection is performed to avoid injury to the saphenous vein and nerve, which usually cross some aspect of the incision. The nerve and vein are retracted anteriorly or posteriorly. **C.** Fracture site is exposed and cleaned of hematoma and the talar dome is inspected for signs of chondral injury.

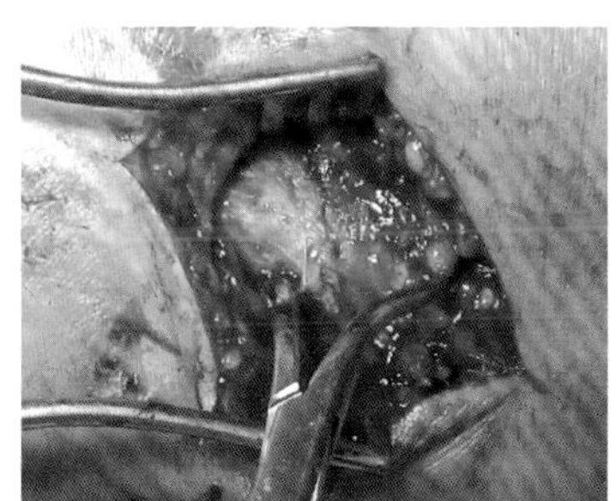

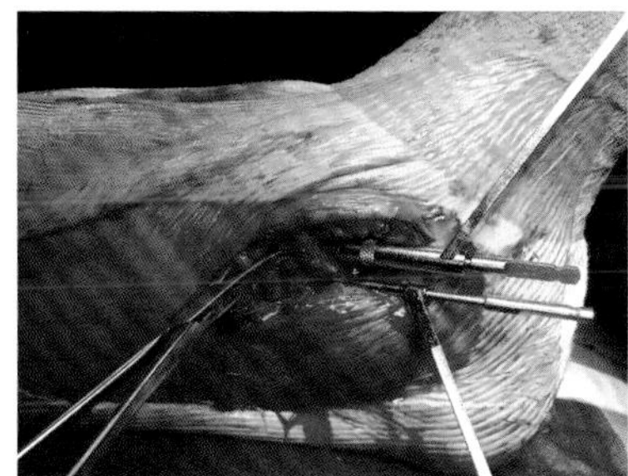

**TECH FIG 5** • **A.** Reduction is achieved with a pointed reduction clamp. **B.** Two 2.5-mm drills are placed across the fracture site in parallel fashion and left in place to maintain rotational control. One drill is left in place as the first partially threaded screw is placed.

## Posterolateral Approach to the Tibia

- Direct access to the posterior malleolus fracture (**TECH FIG 6A**) can be obtained through the posterolateral approach to the fibula (**TECH FIG 6B**).
  - The interval between the Achilles and the peroneal muscle is developed (**TECH FIG 6C**).
  - The flexor hallucis longus is taken off the fibula down to the interosseous membrane and then the rest of the deep posterior compartment is taken off the posterior tibia (**TECH FIG 6D**).

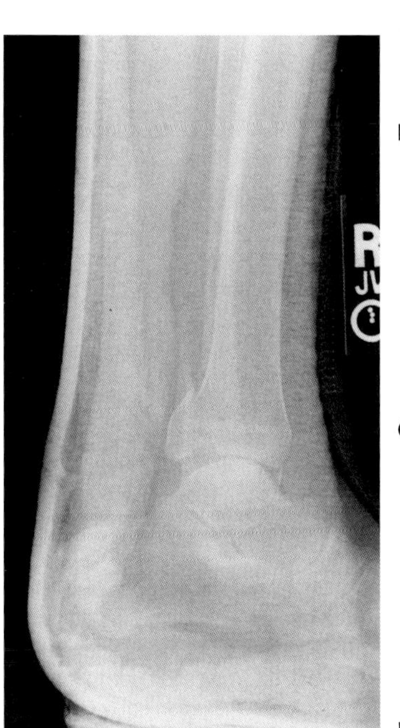

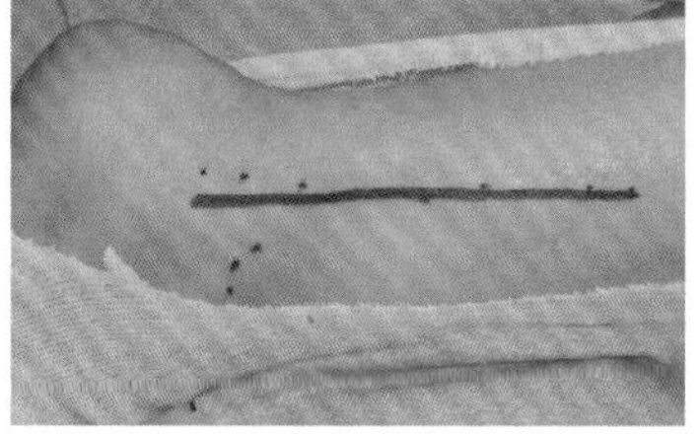

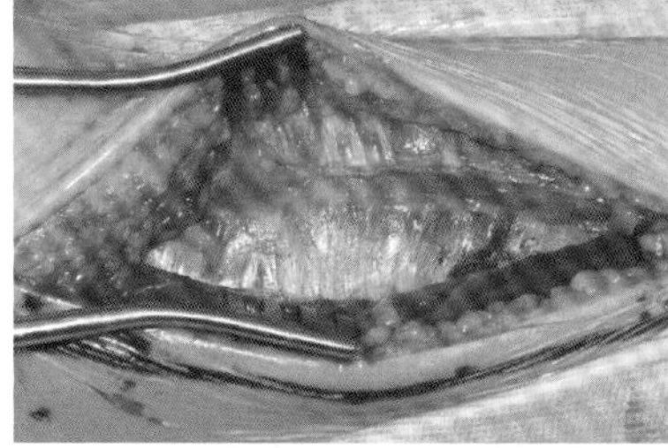

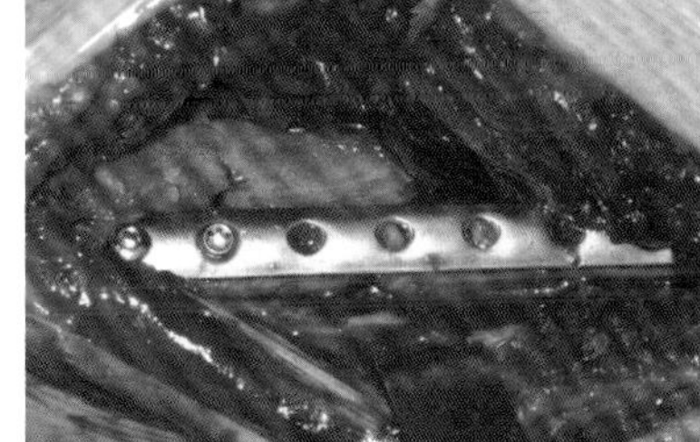

**TECH FIG 6** • Direct posterior plating is well suited for fractures involving large portions of the posterior malleolus. **A.** Postreduction lateral radiograph showing a posterior malleolus fracture involving more than one-third of the articular surface. **B.** Patient in prone position, incision between Achilles and posterior fibula border. **C.** Access is via the interval between the flexor hallucis longus and the peroneal muscle belly. **D.** Posterior malleolar fragment following fibular plating.

## Posterior Malleolus Fixation

- If an adequate reduction can be achieved via closed, indirect reduction, the fracture can be stabilized with cannulated lag screws placed in the anterior to posterior direction.
- If an open approach is used for reduction, screws placed posterior to anterior may be placed across the fracture site.
- If the fracture fragment is of sufficient size, an antiglide plate (one-third tubular) may be placed with undercontouring of the plate to provide a satisfactory buttress effect (**TECH FIG 7**).

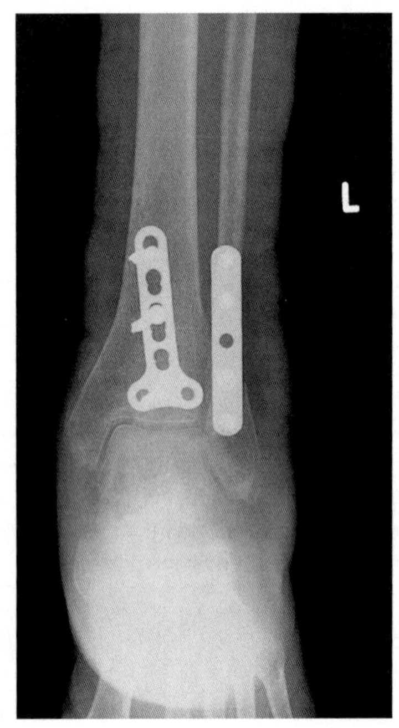


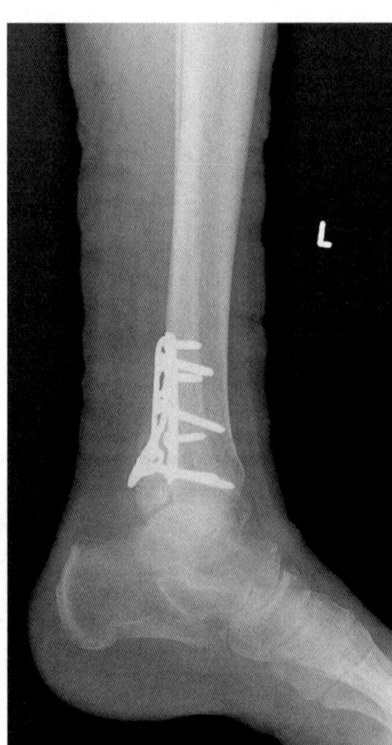


**TECH FIG 7** • Postoperative AP (**A**) and lateral (**B**) radiographs demonstrating posterior plating of the tibia to buttress the posterior malleolar fracture fragment.

## Posterior Plating of the Fibula

- In this case, the surgical approach is similar to the lateral plating technique.
- When application of a posterior or antiglide plate is chosen, placement of a lag screw or screws in the distal fracture segment is optional.
- My preferred method is to apply the plate along the flat posterior surface of the bone, using it as a reduction aid with a bone reduction clamp (**TECH FIG 8A**).
- The authors prefer to place a posterior-to-anterior–directed lag screw through the plate.
  - Because of the biomechanical properties of this plate construct, this lag screw is optional.
- Next, at least two or three bicortical screws are placed in the plate proximal to the fracture. Bicortical screws placed posterior to anterior distal to the fracture are optional.
- In osteoporotic bone, to achieve increased fixation, the authors prefer a posterior plate with bicortical posterior to anterior screws placed both proximal and distal to the fracture (**TECH FIG 8B**).

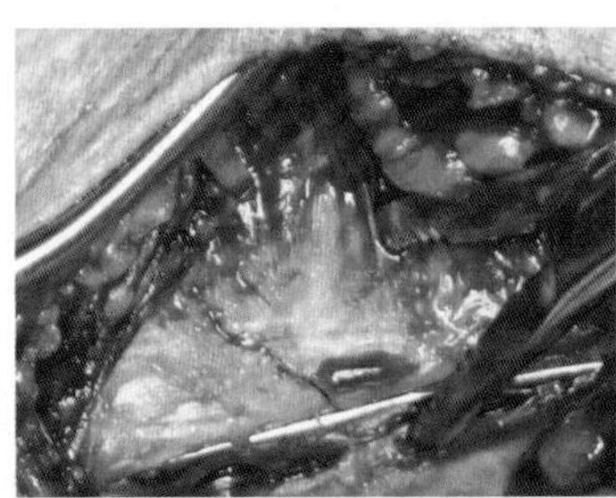

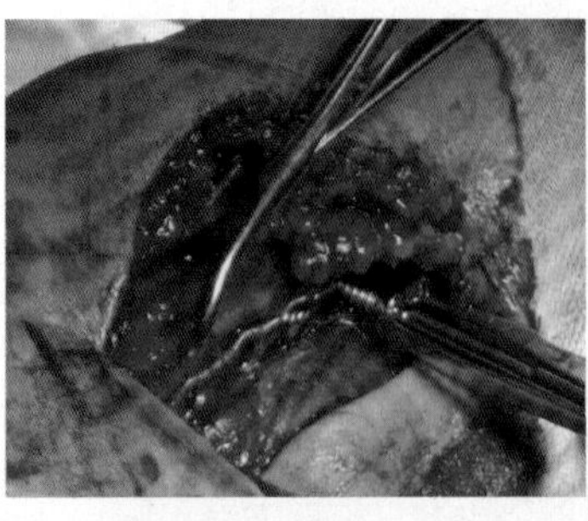

**TECH FIG 8** • An alternative for plate placement is along the posterior border of the fibula. **A.** In this construct, the implant is an antiglide plate. **B.** The lag screw can be placed from posterior to anterior with bicortical purchase achieved in each screw.

## Syndesmosis Fixation

- After stabilization of the medial and lateral sides of the ankle, syndesmotic integrity should be assessed.
  - The Cotton test involves providing a lateral force on the fibula with a bone hook or bone clamp (**TECH FIG 9A**).
  - The stress external rotation test can also be used to assess for syndesmotic integrity.
  - Lateral displacement that allows more than a few millimeters of tibiofibular widening is considered pathologic and an indication for syndesmotic fixation.

- The lateral radiograph should be scrutinized to assess the relationship of the fibula to the articular surface of the ankle joint. In general, on a true lateral view of the ankle, the tip of the fibula should be anterior to the posterior border of the diaphyseal tibia and comparisons to the contralateral ankle can be assessed.
- With a bolster behind the ankle, a large tenaculum clamp is placed across the tibiofibular joint, with one tine on the distal tibia and the other on the fibula (**TECH FIG 9B**).
- Reduction is confirmed on the AP, mortise, and lateral radiographic views.
- Although dorsiflexion of the talus has been recommended in the past to prevent overtightening of the syndesmosis, more recent studies have shown that it is virtually impossible to overtighten an anatomically reduced mortise.
- Direct reduction of the syndesmosis with visualization of the anterior distal fibula seated within the tibial incisura should be performed if there is concern for malreduction.
  - The incidence of syndesmosis malreduction is as high as 40% and is associated with worse functional outcomes.[1,15]
- Fixation choices range from one or two screws, with three or four cortices drilled and 3.5- or 4.5-mm screw diameters used. Although the size and number of screws remain controversial, some parameters are agreed on.
  - The screw should be placed 1.5 to 2 cm proximal and parallel to the joint.
  - The screw should not be placed in lag mode.
  - If a lateral plate is used, the screw is placed through one of the distal holes.
  - If a posterior plate is used, the syndesmosis screw will likely be placed outside the plate on the lateral cortex.

A 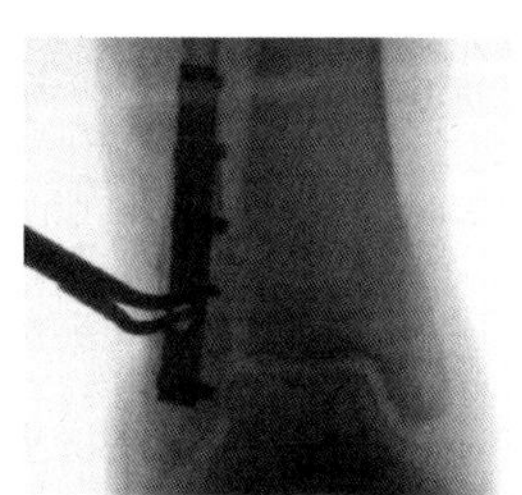

B 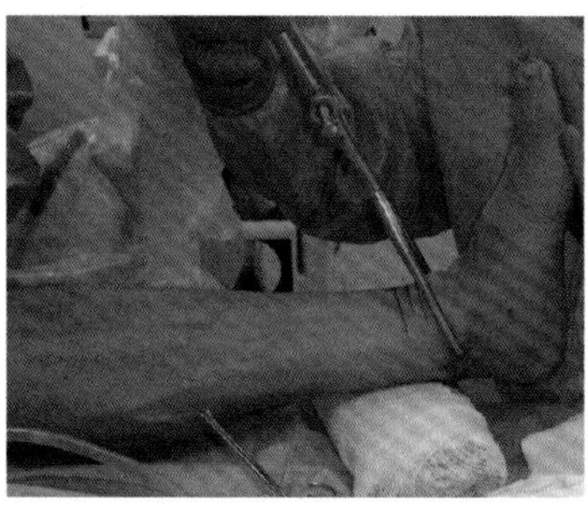

**TECH FIG 9** • **A.** The Cotton test is performed following fibular fixation by pulling laterally with a hook or clamp to assess the integrity of the syndesmosis. **B.** Reduction and stabilization of the syndesmosis is achieved with a clamp placed across the distal tibiofibular joint and a bump placed under the leg.

## PEARLS AND PITFALLS

| | |
|---|---|
| **Damage or entrapment of superficial peroneal nerve** | ■ Care must be taken to expose and mobilize the nerve proximally if in the surgical field (**FIG 5A**). This will help minimize the chance of damage during surgery and closure. |
| **Failure to obtain fibular length** | ■ This will lead to persistent medial widening.<br>■ A plate is used to push the distal fragment with a laminar spreader. The distal tibiofibular anatomic relationship is assessed and the contralateral ankle is used for comparison. |
| **Presence of osteoporotic bone** | ■ Supplementary Kirschner wires<br>■ Multiple syndesmosis screws<br>■ Posteriorly placed fibula plate with bicortical screws proximal and distal to fracture<br>■ Locked plate |
| **Intra-articular hardware penetration** | ■ Careful intraoperative radiographic assessment is important.<br>■ Distal screws in the lateral fibular plate must be unicortical.<br>■ AP radiograph is best to evaluate medial malleolus fixation. |
| **Malreduction of the syndesmosis** | ■ Bolster is placed under ankle, not foot. This will cause anterior displacement (**FIG 5B**).<br>■ A good lateral radiograph is obtained to assess reduction.<br>■ It is impossible to overtighten an anatomically reduced syndesmosis. |
| **Peroneal tendinitis and painful hardware** | ■ Laterally placed fibular hardware is associated with a higher incidence of painful hardware.<br>■ Posteriorly placed fibular fixation is associated with a higher incidence of peroneal tendinitis. |

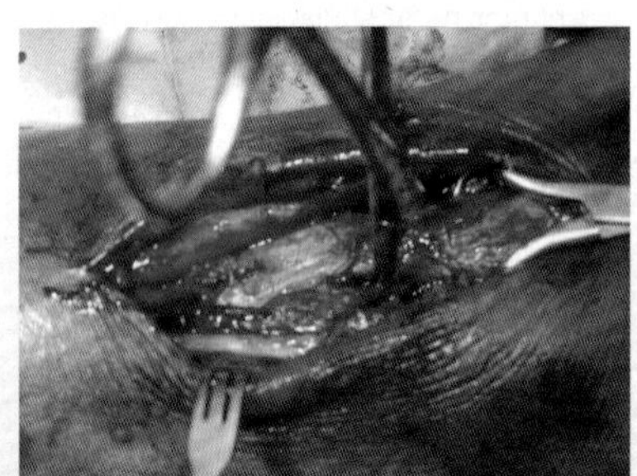

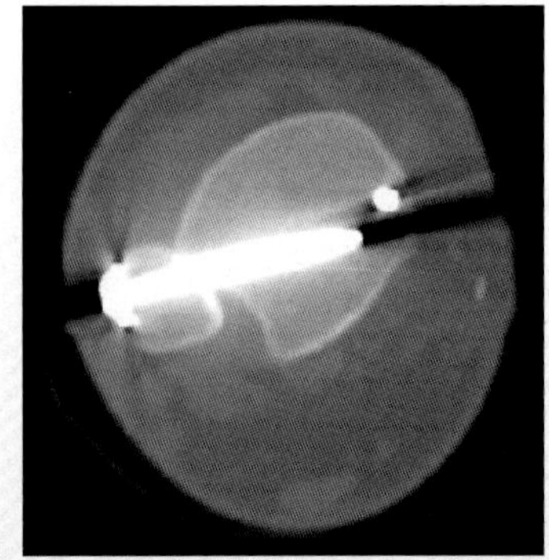

**FIG 5** • **A.** Identification and protection of the superficial peroneal nerve within the anterior flap. **B.** CT scan showing malreduction of the syndesmosis.

## POSTOPERATIVE CARE

- All ankles should be splinted in the neutral position and elevated for at least 24 hours postoperatively.
- We remove the splint at 10 or 14 days and remove the sutures.
- Patients are then placed into a removable functional brace that allows them to begin early active-assisted and passive range of ankle motion.[3]
- Patients are also allowed to begin isometric strengthening exercises.
- All patients are kept non–weight bearing for at least 6 weeks.
- At 6 weeks, patients are progressed to weight bearing as tolerated based on radiographic criteria.
  - Weight bearing can be delayed for slow healing and presence of a syndesmotic screw. In general, we do not alter the weight-bearing status because of syndesmotic injury or routinely remove the syndesmosis screw, but we advise patients of the possibility of screw breakage following weight bearing.
- Patients are restricted from operating an automobile for 9 weeks following right-sided ankle fracture.[4]

## OUTCOMES

- One year after ankle fracture surgery, patients generally do well, with most experiencing little or mild pain and few restrictions in functional activities. They have significant improvement in function compared with 6 months after surgery.
  - Younger age, male sex, absence of diabetes, and a lower American Society of Anesthesia class are predictive of functional recovery at 1 year following ankle fracture surgery.[5]
  - It is important to counsel patients and their families on the expected outcome after injury with regard to functional recovery.
- Looking specifically at elderly patients (older than 60 years), functional outcomes steadily improved over 1 year of follow-up, albeit at a slower rate than in the younger patients.[5]
  - Our results suggest that operative fixation of unstable ankle fractures in the elderly can provide a reasonable functional result at the 1-year follow-up.

## COMPLICATIONS

- Minor complications include epidermolysis (**FIG 6A**), superficial infection, and peroneal tendinitis with painful hardware.[13]
- Major problems include nonunion (**FIG 6B**), hardware failure, deep infection, and compartment syndrome.[13]

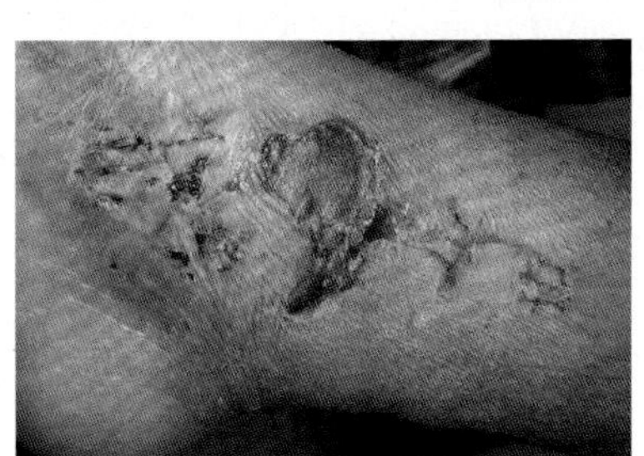

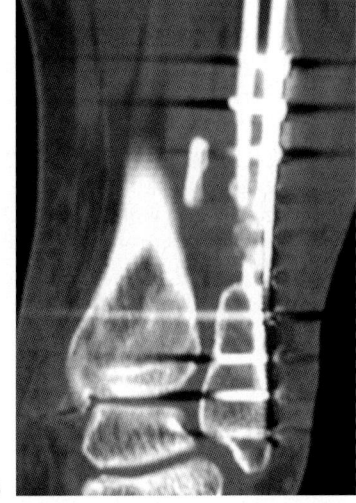

**FIG 6** • **A.** Skin necrosis and slough following surgical intervention. **B.** CT scan demonstrating fibular nonunion at 6 months following open reduction and internal fixation of a pronation–abduction injury.

## REFERENCES

1. Davidovitch RI, Weil Y, Karia R, et al. Intraoperative syndesmotic reduction: three-dimensional versus standard fluoroscopic imaging. J Bone Joint Surg Am 2013;95:1838–1843.
2. Egol KA, Amirtharajah M, Tejwani NC, et al. Ankle stress test for predicting the need for surgical fixation of isolated fibular fractures. J Bone Joint Surg Am 2004;86A:2393–2398.
3. Egol KA, Dolan R, Koval KJ. Functional outcome of surgery for fractures of the ankle: a prospective, randomised comparison of management in a cast or a functional brace. J Bone Joint Surg Br 2000;82(2):246–249.
4. Egol KA, Sheikhazadeh A, Mogatederi S, et al. Lower-extremity function for driving an automobile after operative treatment of ankle fracture. J Bone Joint Surg Am 2003;85-A(7):1185–1189.
5. Egol KA, Tejwani NC, Walsh MG, et al. Predictors of short-term functional outcome following ankle fracture surgery. J Bone Joint Surg Am 2006;88(5):974–979.
6. Lauge-Hansen N. Fractures of the ankle. II. Combined experimental-surgical and experimental-roentgenologic investigations. Arch Surg 1950;60:957–985.
7. McConnell T, Creevy W, Tornetta P III. Stress examination of supination external rotation-type fibular fractures. J Bone Joint Surg Am 2004;86-A(10):2171–2178.
8. Michelson JD. Fractures about the ankle. J Bone Joint Surg Am 1995;77A:142–152.
9. Pakarinen H, Flinkkilä T, Ohtonen P, et al. Intraoperative assessment of the stability of the distal tibiofibular joint in supination-external rotation injuries of the ankle: sensitivity, specificity, and reliability of two clinical tests. J Bone Joint Surg Am 2011;93:2057–2061.
10. Pankovich AM, Shivaram MS. Anatomical basis of variability in injuries of the medial malleolus and the deltoid ligament. II. Clinical studies. Acta Orthop Scand 1979;50:225–236.
11. Park SS, Kubiak EN, Egol KA, et al. Stress radiographs after ankle fracture: the effect of ankle position and deltoid ligament status on medial clear space measurements. J Orthop Trauma 2006;20:11–18.
12. Pettrone FA, Gail M, et al. Quantitative criteria for prediction of the results after displaced fracture of the ankle. J Bone Joint Surg Am 1983;65(5):667–677.
13. Phillips WA, Schwartz HS, Keller CS, et al. A prospective, randomized study of the management of severe ankle fractures. J Bone Joint Surg Am 1985;67A:67–78.
14. Ricci WM, Tornetta P, Borrelli J Jr. Lag screw fixation of medial malleolar fractures: a biomechanical, radiographic, and clinical comparison of unicortical partially threaded lag screws and bicortical fully threaded lag screws. J Orthop Trauma 2012;26:602–606.
15. Sagi HC, Shah AR, Sanders RW. The functional consequence of syndesmotic joint malreduction at a minimum 2-year follow-up. J Orthop Trauma 2012;26:439–443.
16. Tornetta P III. Competence of the deltoid ligament in bimalleolar ankle fractures after medial malleolar fixation. J Bone Joint Surg Am 2000;82(6):843–848.

# Open Reduction and Internal Fixation of Lisfranc Injury

Michael P. Clare and Roy W. Sanders

## DEFINITION

- A Lisfranc injury refers to bony or ligamentous compromise of the tarsometatarsal and intercuneiform joint complex and includes a spectrum of injuries ranging from a stable, partial sprain to a grossly displaced and unstable fracture or fracture-dislocation of the midfoot.

## ANATOMY

- The bony elements of the medial three tarsometatarsal joints (medial, middle, and lateral cuneiforms and first, second, and third metatarsal bases) feature a unique trapezoidal shape in cross-section, creating a concave arrangement plantarly resembling a Roman arch (**FIG 1A**).
- The second metatarsal is recessed between the medial and lateral cuneiforms in the axial plane and is positioned at the apex of the Roman arch in the coronal plane. It thus functions as the keystone of the entire midfoot complex (**FIG 1B**).
- The tarsometatarsal joints are stabilized by dorsal and plantar tarsometatarsal ligaments.
  - Dorsal and plantar intermetatarsal ligaments provide further stability between the second through fifth metatarsal bases.
  - There are no intermetatarsal ligaments between the first and second metatarsals, which may predispose the area to injury.
  - The Lisfranc ligament courses from the plantar portion of the medial cuneiform to the base of the second metatarsal (**FIG 1C**).
- The unique bony arrangement of the medial midfoot imparts inherent bony stability to the medial and middle columns of the foot, which in combination with the stout plantar ligaments prevents plantar displacement of the metatarsal bases and facilitates the weight-bearing function of the first ray (**FIG 2**).
- The medial three tarsometatarsal joints and the adjacent intercuneiform and naviculocuneiform articulations (medial and middle columns) have limited inherent motion, making these joints nonessential to normal foot function and therefore relatively expendable.
  - The medial column refers to the first tarsometatarsal and navicular–medial cuneiform articulations; the middle column includes the second and third tarsometatarsal joints and articulations between the navicular and middle and lateral cuneiforms, respectively.
- The fourth and fifth tarsometatarsal (lateral column) joints have distinctly more inherent motion and are critical in accommodation of the foot to uneven surfaces.
  - These joints are considered essential joints to normal foot function and therefore nonexpendable.

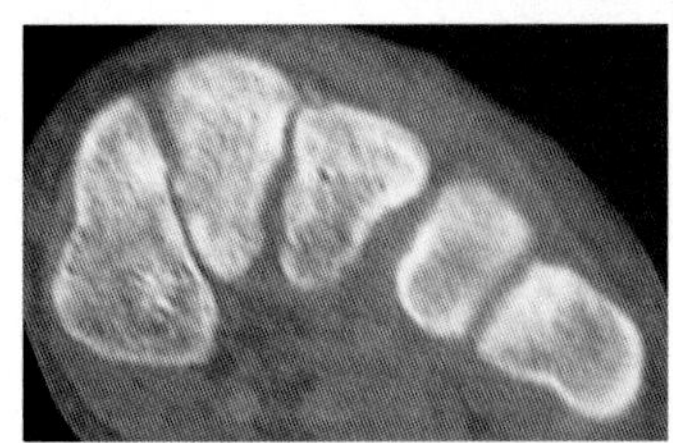

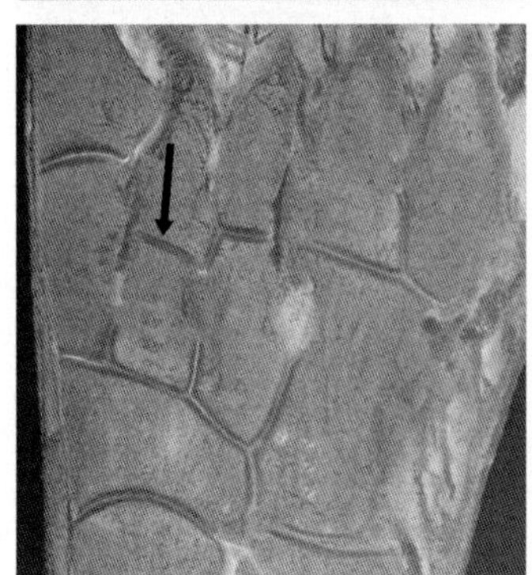

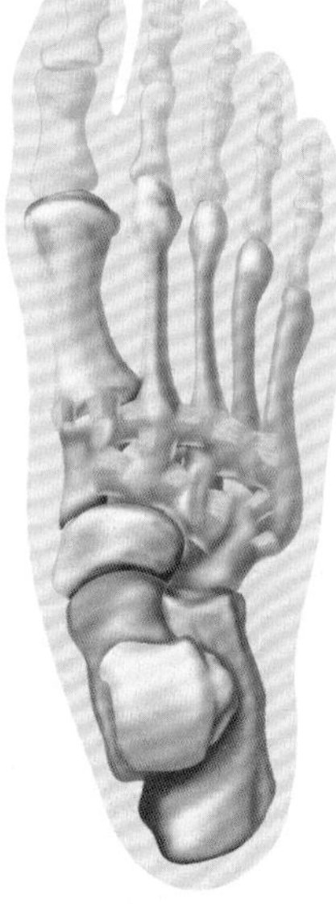

**FIG 1** • **A.** Axial CT image depicting the Roman arch configuration of the tarsometatarsal joints. **B.** Anatomic specimen demonstrating the keystone of the Roman arch: The second metatarsal base is recessed between the medial and lateral cuneiforms (*black arrow*). **C.** Ligamentous connections of the tarsometatarsal region.

## PATHOGENESIS

- Lisfranc injuries are generally the result of a high-energy injury, such as a fall from a height or a high-speed motor vehicle accident, but depending on the position of the foot, they may also result from a lower energy injury, such as a slip and ground-level fall.
- These injuries result from a combination of axial load and dorsiflexion, plantarflexion, abduction, or adduction (or variable combinations thereof) of the midfoot.

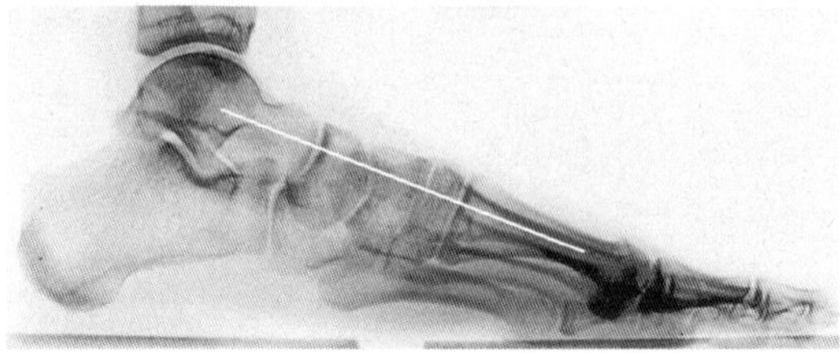

**FIG 2** • Normal weight-bearing lateral radiograph demonstrating normal alignment of the medial column and the weight-bearing first ray (*white line*).

- The pathoanatomy is individually specific and highly variable and may consist of a pure ligamentous injury, a pure bony injury (fracture), or a combination.
- Although the injury classically includes the first, second, and third tarsometatarsal joints, there may be involvement of all five tarsometatarsal articulations, extension into the intercuneiform joints, or even fracture lines into the navicular or cuboid proximally or metatarsal shafts or necks distally.
- In pure ligamentous patterns, the stability of the injury depends on the status of the plantar tarsometatarsal ligaments. Disruption of these stout structures makes the injury unstable.
- Partial injuries (sprains) occur as a result of lower energy and are more common with axial load and plantarflexion, such as in competitive sports.
  - In this instance, by definition, the plantar tarsometatarsal ligaments remain intact, making the injury stable.

## NATURAL HISTORY

- Stable injuries (partial sprains, extra-articular fractures) often require prolonged recovery time. When accurately diagnosed, however, patients with these injuries can generally expect full recovery and return to activity with minimal long-term implications.[7]
- Unstable injuries that are misdiagnosed or inadequately treated generally go on to a poor result with persistent pain, activity limitations, and progressive posttraumatic arthritis in the involved joints,[2,3] necessitating arthrodesis as salvage.[4,9]
- A high index of suspicion must therefore be maintained; historically, up to 20% of unstable Lisfranc injuries are misdiagnosed on plain radiographs.[3]

## PATIENT HISTORY AND PHYSICAL FINDINGS

- The physician should obtain a history of trauma and details of the exact injury mechanism (position of foot, direction of force, extent of energy involved).
- The physician should observe any initial swelling and inability to bear weight.
- A thorough examination of the involved foot and ankle also includes assessment of associated injuries and any other areas of swelling or tenderness to palpation.
- The physician should observe the skin and soft tissue envelope. Diffuse swelling of the midfoot or plantar ecchymosis at the midfoot suggests a Lisfranc injury.
- The physician should palpate the midfoot joints; pain at the midfoot with palpation suggests a Lisfranc injury.
- The physician should test midfoot stability with passive flexion of the metatarsal heads and passive abduction and adduction through the forefoot. Pain at the tarsometatarsal joint region with passive forefoot range of motion suggests a Lisfranc injury.

## IMAGING AND OTHER DIAGNOSTIC STUDIES

- Initial radiographic evaluation consists of non–weight-bearing anteroposterior (AP), oblique, and lateral views of the foot, which, depending on the extent of intra-articular displacement, may provide sufficient diagnostic information (**FIG 3A–C**).
- Fluoroscopic stress views may be helpful in more subtle injuries; however, these studies are painful and generally require anesthesia.
- We therefore prefer weight-bearing radiographs of the foot for more subtle injuries (**FIG 3D–H**); comparison weight-bearing radiographs of the contralateral foot may also be obtained where necessary.
  - The weight-bearing AP view of the foot will demonstrate intra-articular displacement through the first and second tarsometatarsal joints (so-called Lisfranc joint), intercuneiform joint, and naviculocuneiform joint; fractures through the first and second metatarsal bases, medial and middle cuneiforms, and proximal extension into the navicular; and the extent of columnar shortening or asymmetry.
    - The medial border of the second metatarsal should align with the medial border of the middle cuneiform (**FIG 3D**).
  - The oblique view will reveal intra-articular displacement through the third, fourth, and fifth tarsometatarsal joints and fractures of the third, fourth, and fifth metatarsal bases, lateral cuneiform, and cuboid.
    - The medial borders of the third and fourth metatarsals should align with the medial borders of the lateral cuneiform and cuboid, respectively (**FIG 3E**).
  - The lateral view may reveal dorsal–plantar displacement of fractures or dislocations as well as any flattening of the medial longitudinal arch, thereby reflecting the status of the weight-bearing medial column and first ray (**FIG 3F**).
- Computed tomography (CT) scanning may also be beneficial in the instance of a subtle Lisfranc injury, particularly in a polytrauma patient or a patient with multiple extremity injuries that preclude weight-bearing radiographs, and in delineating proximal fracture line extension into the navicular, cuboid, or cuneiforms (**FIG 4**).

## DIFFERENTIAL DIAGNOSIS

- Partial Lisfranc injury (sprain)
- Isolated metatarsal fracture
- Navicular–cuneiform fracture
- Anterior process of calcaneus fracture
- Lateral ankle sprain

## NONOPERATIVE MANAGEMENT

- Nonoperative treatment is indicated for partial Lisfranc injuries (sprains), which by definition are stable and therefore nondisplaced on weight-bearing radiographs.
- Nonoperative treatment is also indicated for nondisplaced or minimally displaced extra-articular metatarsal base fractures with no intra-articular involvement (displacement) on weight-bearing radiographs.
- Because of the often subtle nature of Lisfranc injuries and the negative consequences of misdiagnosis, if the findings are inconclusive, weight-bearing radiographs may be repeated 2 to 3 weeks after the injury.
- Nonoperative management consists of immobilization in a venous compression stocking and prefabricated fracture boot.

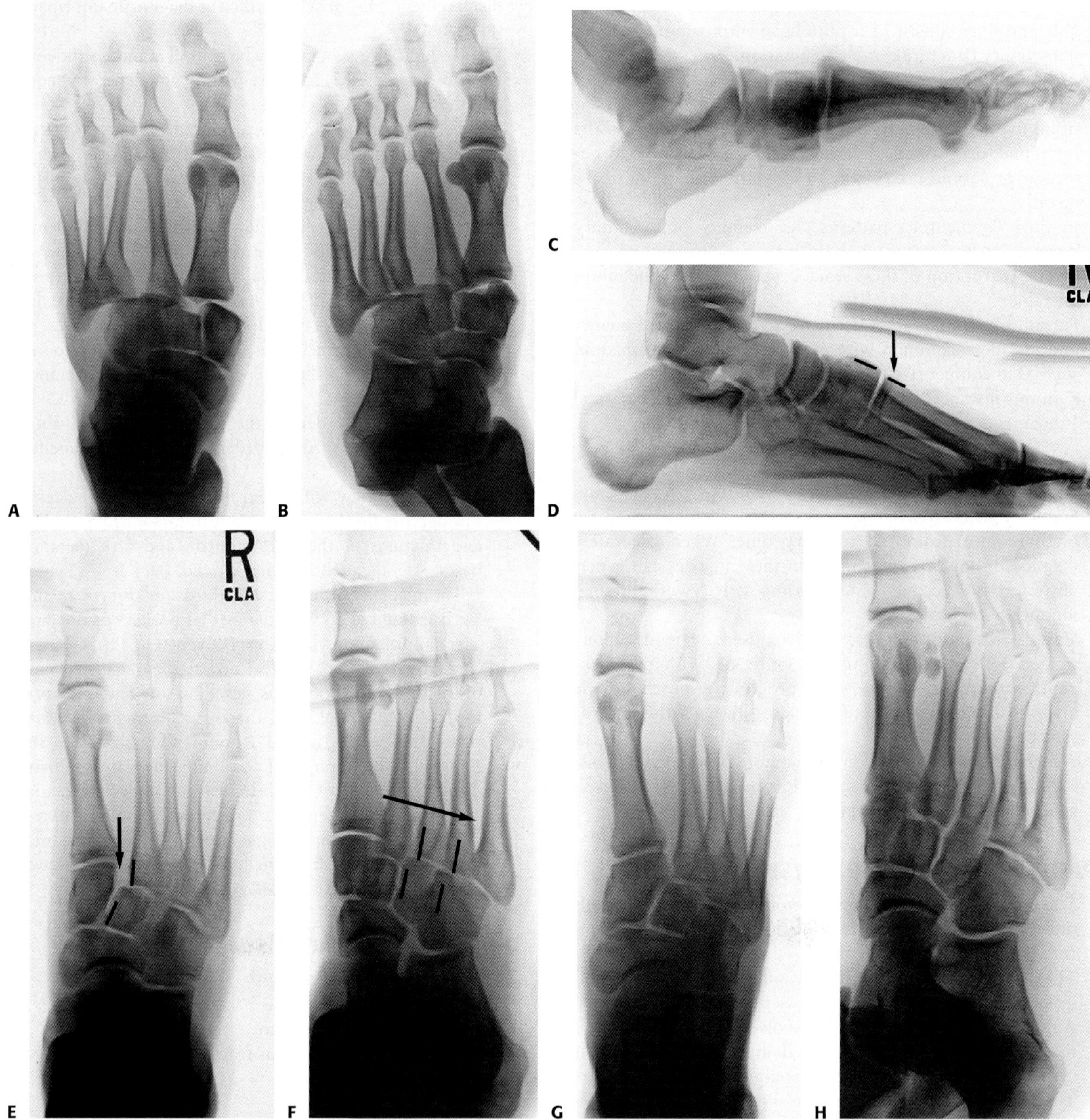


**FIG 3** • Non–weight-bearing AP (**A**), oblique (**B**), and lateral (**C**) radiographs of grossly unstable, purely ligamentous, Lisfranc dislocation involving all five tarsometatarsal articulations. Marked lateral subluxation through all five tarsometatarsal joints is evident on the AP and oblique views, and significant dorsal displacement is evident on the lateral view. Weight-bearing lateral (**D**), AP (**E**), and oblique (**F**), and non–weight-bearing (**G**) and oblique (**H**) radiographs of more subtle Lisfranc injury. Lateral and plantar subluxation (*black arrows*) is evident on the weight-bearing radiographs, and displacement of normal radiographic landmarks (*black lines*) confirms injury.

- The patient is allowed to bear weight to tolerance, and early progression to range of motion is encouraged.
- The patient continues in the fracture boot for 5 to 6 weeks, at which point maintenance of alignment or radiographic union is confirmed on repeat weight-bearing radiographs.
- The patient is then allowed to wear regular shoes, and activities are advanced as tolerated thereafter.
- Full recovery and return to sports or other rigorous activity may require up to 3 to 4 months.

## SURGICAL MANAGEMENT

- Surgical management is indicated for unstable (displaced) injuries of the midfoot, including pure ligamentous, bony, or variable combinations.

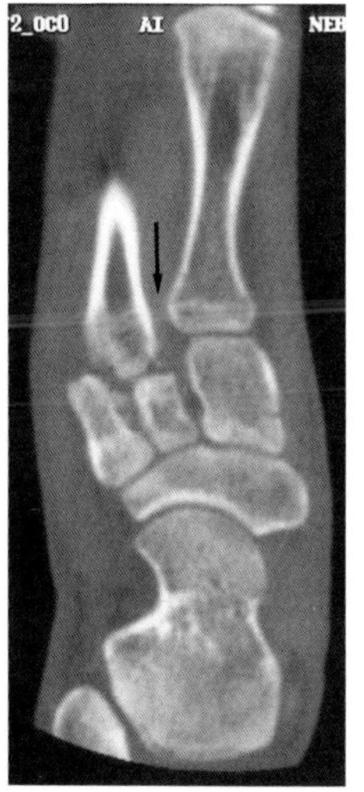
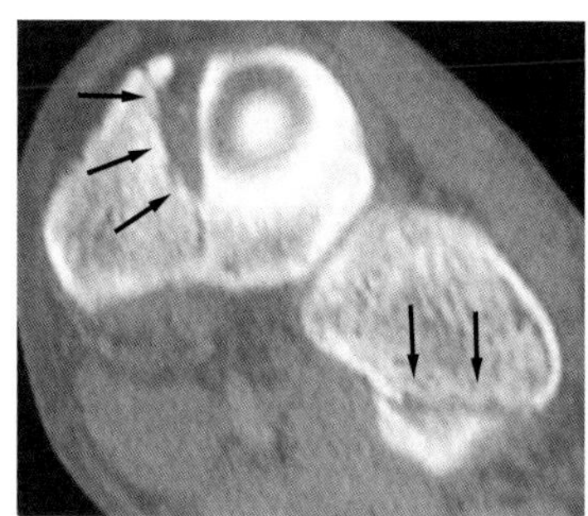

**FIG 4** • CT scan showing displacement through second tarsometatarsal and intercuneiform articulations (**A**) and intra-articular fractures of navicular and cuboid (**B**, *black arrows*) in a different patient.

- Recent studies suggest that pure ligamentous Lisfranc injuries are best managed with open reduction and primary arthrodesis of the medial and middle columns.[6]
- Any dislocation producing tension on the overlying skin and soft tissue envelope should be immediately reduced and immobilized (**FIG 5**).
- Definitive surgery is generally delayed 10 to 14 days to allow adequate resolution of soft tissue swelling.

## Preoperative Planning

- The injury and weight-bearing radiographs and CT images are reviewed and the injury is classified,[8] which allows planning for the anticipated pathoanatomy of the injury.
- Pure ligamentous injuries require rigid screw fixation for the medial and middle column joints and Kirschner wire fixation for the lateral column joints; bony injury patterns, particularly those with more comminution, may require minifragment bridge plate fixation.[1,5]

## Positioning

- The patient is placed supine with a bolster beneath the ipsilateral hip. Protective padding is placed around the contralateral limb, primarily to protect the peroneal nerve, and the contralateral limb is secured to the table.
- A sterile bolster is placed beneath the operative limb at the knee to facilitate access to the midfoot and intraoperative fluoroscopy.

## Approach

- We prefer the dual-incision approach (**FIG 6**).
  - The medial incision courses directly over the extensor hallucis longus (EHL) tendon and is centered over the first tarsometatarsal joint. It affords access to the first and second tarsometatarsal joints.
  - The lateral incision is centered over the lateral border of the third tarsometatarsal joint. If extended, it also provides exposure to the fourth and fifth tarsometatarsal joints where necessary.
- A third, more proximal and lateral incision may be required to stabilize the cuboid where necessary.
- Because of the limited soft tissue envelope overlying the midfoot, the importance of meticulous soft tissue handling and maintaining full-thickness soft tissue flaps cannot be overemphasized.

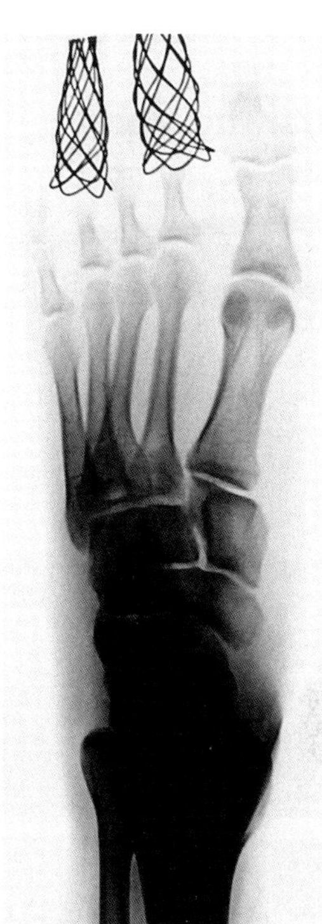

**FIG 5** • Closed reduction of Lisfranc dislocation; displaced fragments were tenting skin.

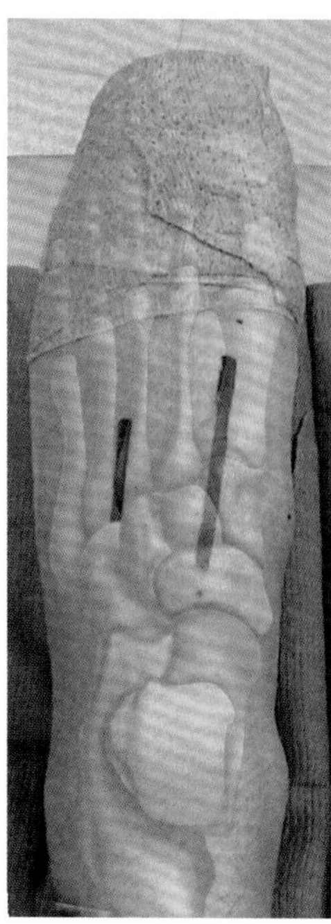

**FIG 6** • Planned incisions for dual-incision approach.

## Medial Incision

- The medial incision is made directly over the EHL tendon and is centered over the first tarsometatarsal joint.
  - The tendon sheath is incised dorsally, and the EHL is retracted laterally (**TECH FIG 1A**).
- The floor of the tendon sheath is then incised and subperiosteal dissection commences medially, extending to the medial margin of the first tarsometatarsal joint and producing a full-thickness flap.
- Subperiosteal dissection then extends laterally to the lateral margin of the second tarsometatarsal joint, again producing a full-thickness flap, while preserving the adjacent neurovascular bundle within the soft tissue flap (**TECH FIG 1B**).
- The status is noted of each of the tarsometatarsal and intercuneiform joint capsules dorsally and therefore the extent of instability of each joint (**TECH FIG 1C,D**).
- We prefer using the medial (EHL) incision for access to the second tarsometatarsal and intercuneiform joints, even if the first tarsometatarsal joint is not involved, because the neurovascular bundle remains protected within the full-thickness flap.

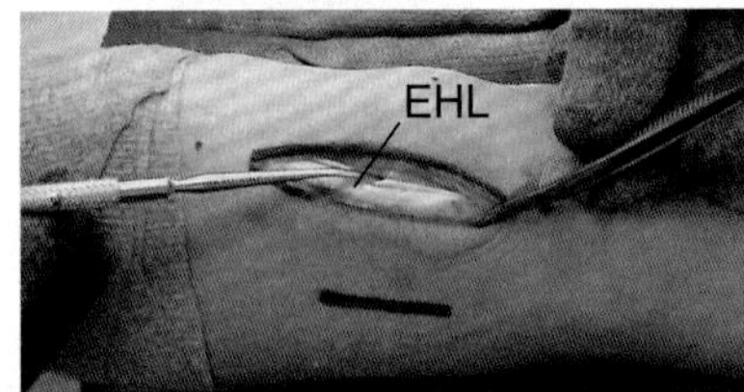


A

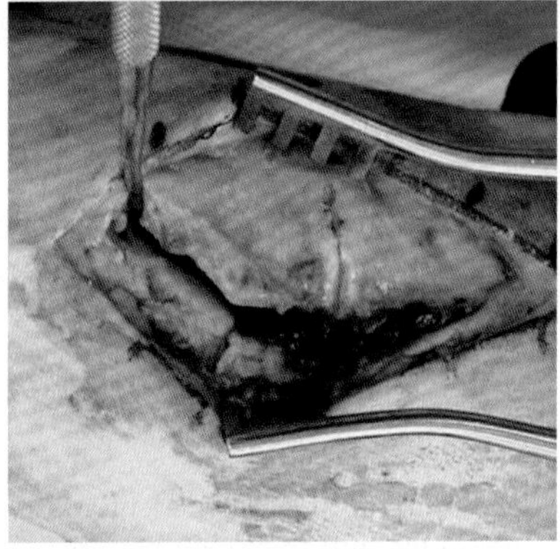

D

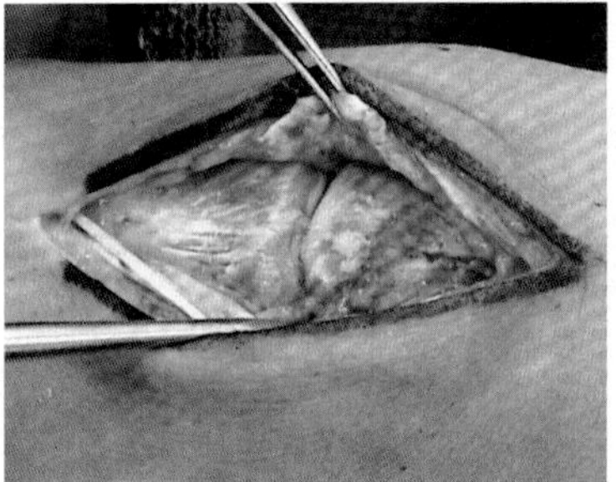

B

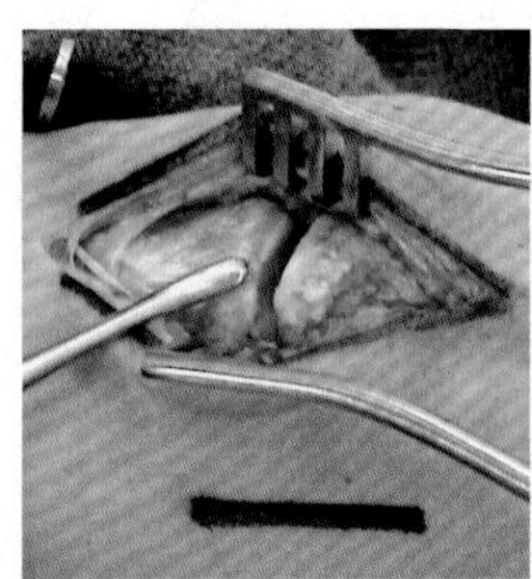

C

**TECH FIG 1** • **A,B.** Medial incision. **A.** Deep dissection continues medial to EHL tendon. **B.** Full-thickness subperiosteal flaps provide access to first and second tarsometatarsal and medial-middle intercuneiform joints. **C,D.** Gross instability through first tarsometatarsal joint (**C**) and second tarsometatarsal and intercuneiform joints (**D**) in a different patient.

## Lateral Incision

- A Freer elevator is placed beneath the full-thickness flap to the level of the third tarsometatarsal joint, and the lateral incision is made overlying the lateral border.
- Dissection extends through the overlying extensor retinaculum, exposing the extensor digitorum communis tendon and medial margin of the extensor digitorum brevis muscle, both of which are retracted laterally (**TECH FIG 2**).
  - Care is taken not to violate the adjacent neurovascular bundle, which is maintained within its soft tissue envelope.
- The underlying third tarsometatarsal joint capsule is identified and a full-thickness subperiosteal flap is developed extending medially toward the lateral portion of the second tarsometatarsal joint and laterally toward the fourth and fifth tarsometatarsal joints where necessary.
- Again, the status is noted of each of the tarsometatarsal and intercuneiform joint capsules dorsally and therefore the extent of instability of each joint.

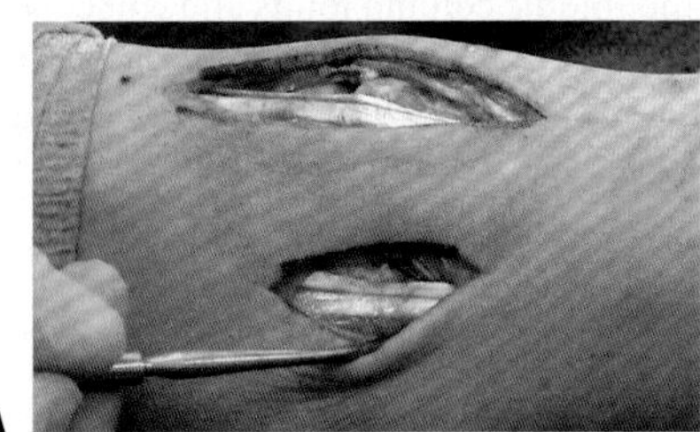

A

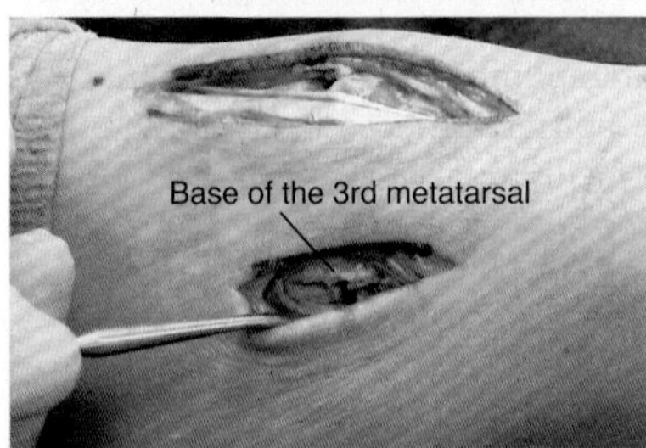


B

**TECH FIG 2** • Lateral incision. Deep dissection continues medial to extensor digitorum communis tendon and extensor digitorum brevis muscle (**A**) and exposes the third tarsometatarsal and the lateral portion of the second tarsometatarsal (not visualized here) joints (**B**).

## Articular Surface Assessment and Decision Making

- The fracture lines and articular surface of the involved joints are then débrided of residual hematoma and assessed for chondral damage.
- If more than 50% of the articular surface of the medial and middle column joints is involved, primary arthrodesis should be considered, although this is controversial.
- Arthrodesis of the fourth and fifth tarsometatarsal joints should be avoided if possible.
- If primary arthrodesis is elected, the involved joints are meticulously débrided of residual articular cartilage, preserving the underlying subchondral plate.
  - The joints are irrigated and the subchondral plate is perforated with a 2.0-mm drill bit to stimulate vascular ingrowth.
  - Supplemental allograft mixed with highly concentrated platelet aspirate is then placed within the involved joint spaces.

## Provisional Reduction and Definitive Stabilization

### First Tarsometatarsal Joint

- The provisional reduction begins medially at the first tarsometatarsal joint if injured. Although the exact reduction maneuver may vary depending on the injury pattern, the first metatarsal is typically supinated (externally rotated) relative to the medial cuneiform.
- Correction of this rotational deformity is crucial in restoring the medial column and the weight-bearing function of the first ray. The reduction of the remaining midfoot joints depends on an anatomic reduction of the first tarsometatarsal joint.
- The provisional reduction is held with a 2.0-mm Kirschner wire and confirmed under fluoroscopy (**TECH FIG 3A**).
- Definitive stabilization is then obtained at the first tarsometatarsal joint with 3.5-mm solid cortical position screws (**TECH FIG 3B–D**).
  - The first screw is placed from distal to proximal, starting at the dorsal crest and distal to the metaphyseal–diaphyseal junction, and is angled toward the plantar–proximal cortex of the medial cuneiform; this screw is generally 45 to 50 mm long.
  - A second screw is placed from proximal to distal starting at the edge of the naviculocuneiform joint and similarly angled to exit at the plantar cortex distal to the metaphyseal–diaphyseal junction. This screw typically measures 40 to 45 mm.
  - In a primary arthrodesis, these screws are placed in lag fashion.
  - For larger patients, 4.0-mm cortical screws may be used for further stability.

A 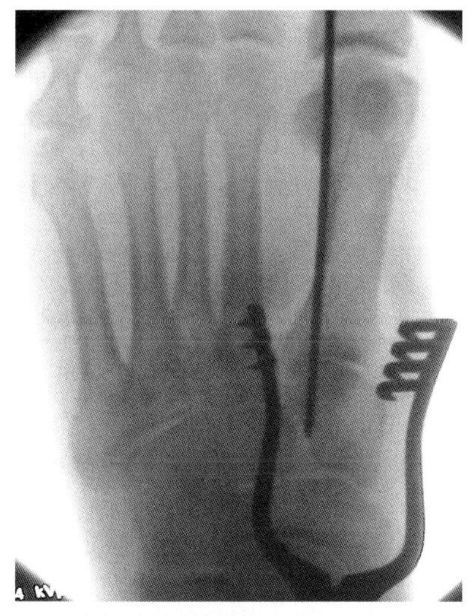

B 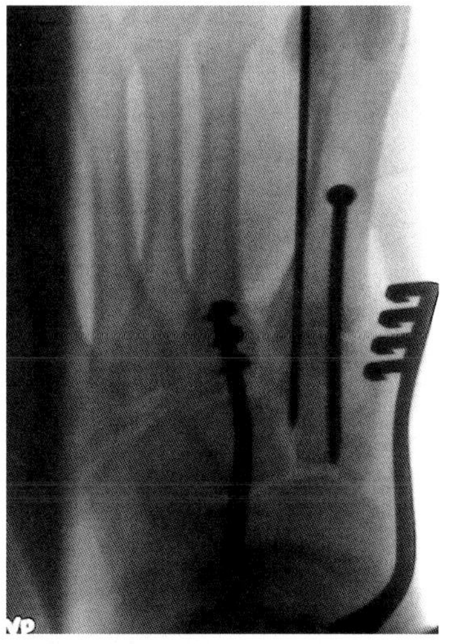

C 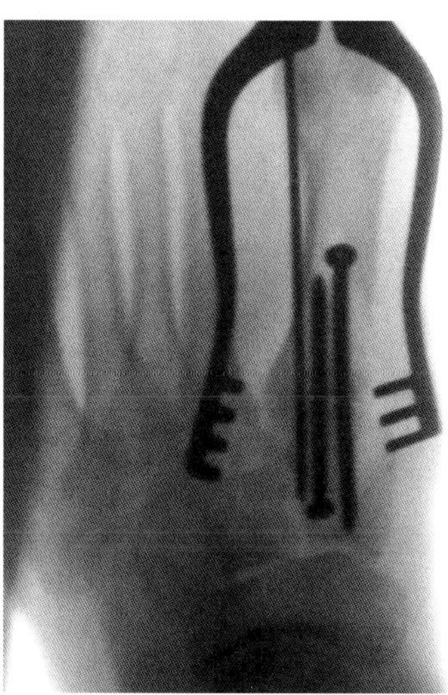

D 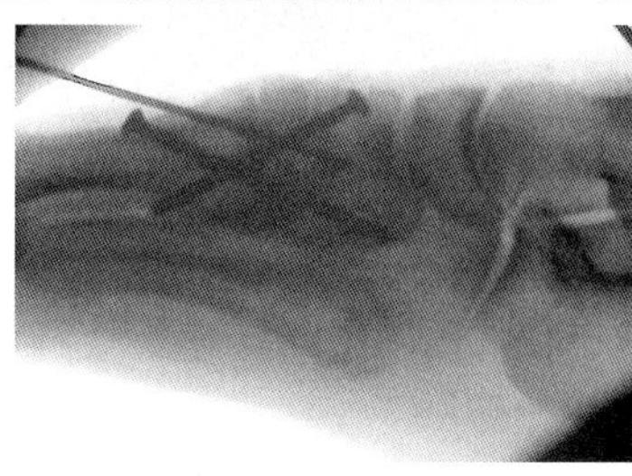

**TECH FIG 3** • Reduction and stabilization of first tarsometatarsal joint. **A.** Provisional reduction. **B.** Distal to proximal screw. **C.** Proximal to distal screw. **D.** Long bicortical trajectory of screws for enhanced stability.

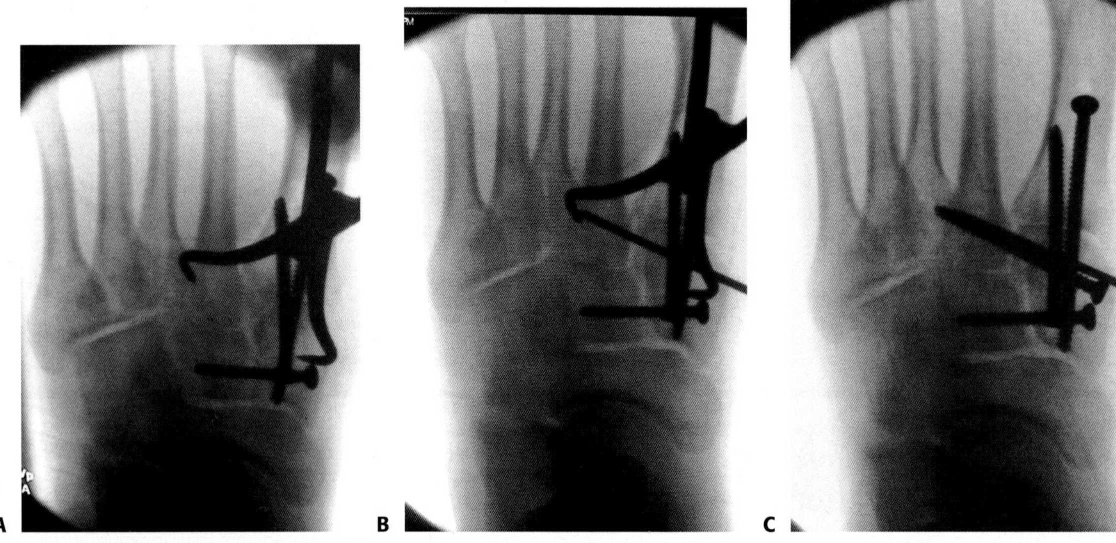

**TECH FIG 4** • Reduction and stabilization of Lisfranc joint. **A.** Pointed reduction forceps. **B.** Supplemental Kirschner wire. **C.** Screw fixation. Trajectory of screw mirrors the normal path of ligamentous structures. Intercuneiform joint was previously reduced and stabilized as initial step.

## Lisfranc Joint

- A pointed reduction forceps is then placed from the medial cuneiform to the lateral border of the second metatarsal to anatomically reduce the so-called Lisfranc joint; care is taken to ensure accurate dorsal–plantar alignment of the second tarsometatarsal joint.
- The reduction is confirmed under fluoroscopy, and a 2.0-mm Kirschner wire that mirrors the intended path of the screw is placed to provide further rotational control (**TECH FIG 4A,B**).
- There is typically a distinct cortical "shelf" on the medial cuneiform that provides an excellent buttress for screw purchase.
  - A 3.5-mm cortical screw is placed through a stab incision overlying this cortical shelf medially, angling toward the proximal metaphysis of the second metatarsal; for a primary arthrodesis, this screw is placed in lag fashion (**TECH FIG 4C**).

## Other Joints

- If the intercuneiform joint is involved, it is first reduced and stabilized before stabilizing the Lisfranc joint (**TECH FIG 5A**). Alternatively, this joint may also be reduced and stabilized before stabilizing the first tarsometatarsal joint.
  - A 3.5-mm cortical screw is again used, coursing parallel to the plane of the naviculocuneiform joint. It is placed in lag fashion for a primary arthrodesis.
  - Care is taken not to violate the articulation between the middle and lateral cuneiform.
- The second tarsometatarsal joint is then provisionally reduced and provisionally stabilized with a 1.6-mm Kirschner wire.
  - Definitive fixation is obtained with a countersunk 2.7-mm cortical screw from distal to proximal; it is placed in lag fashion for a primary arthrodesis (**TECH FIG 5B**).

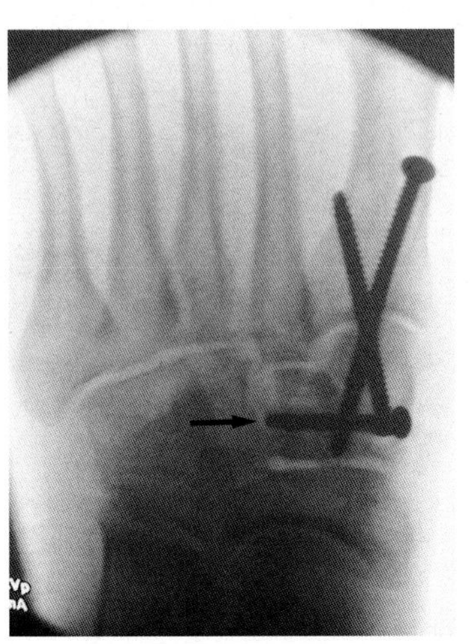

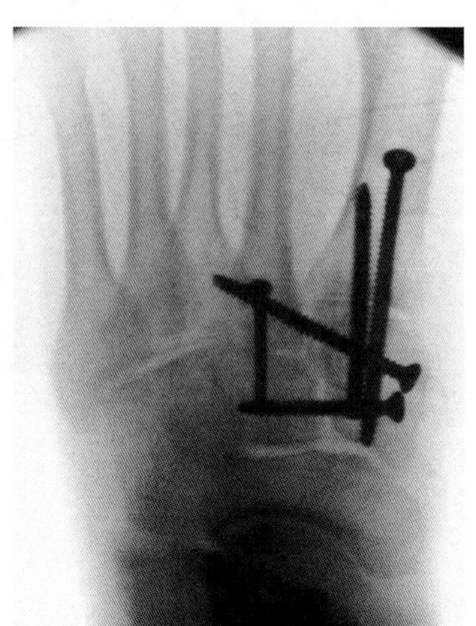

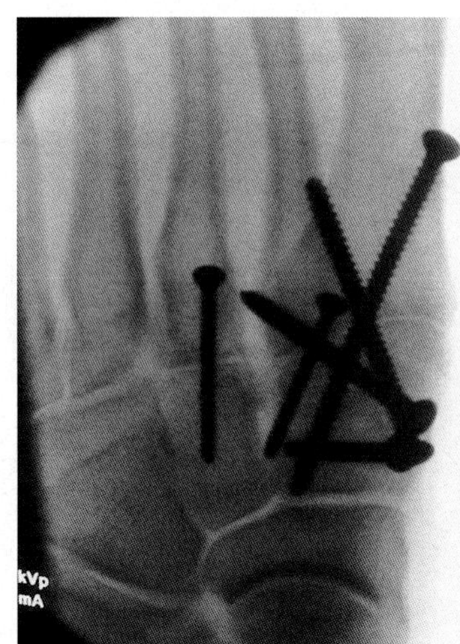

**TECH FIG 5** • **A.** Reduction and stabilization of intercuneiform joint. **B.** Reduction and stabilization of second tarsometatarsal joint. **C.** Reduction and stabilization of third tarsometatarsal joint. *(continued)*

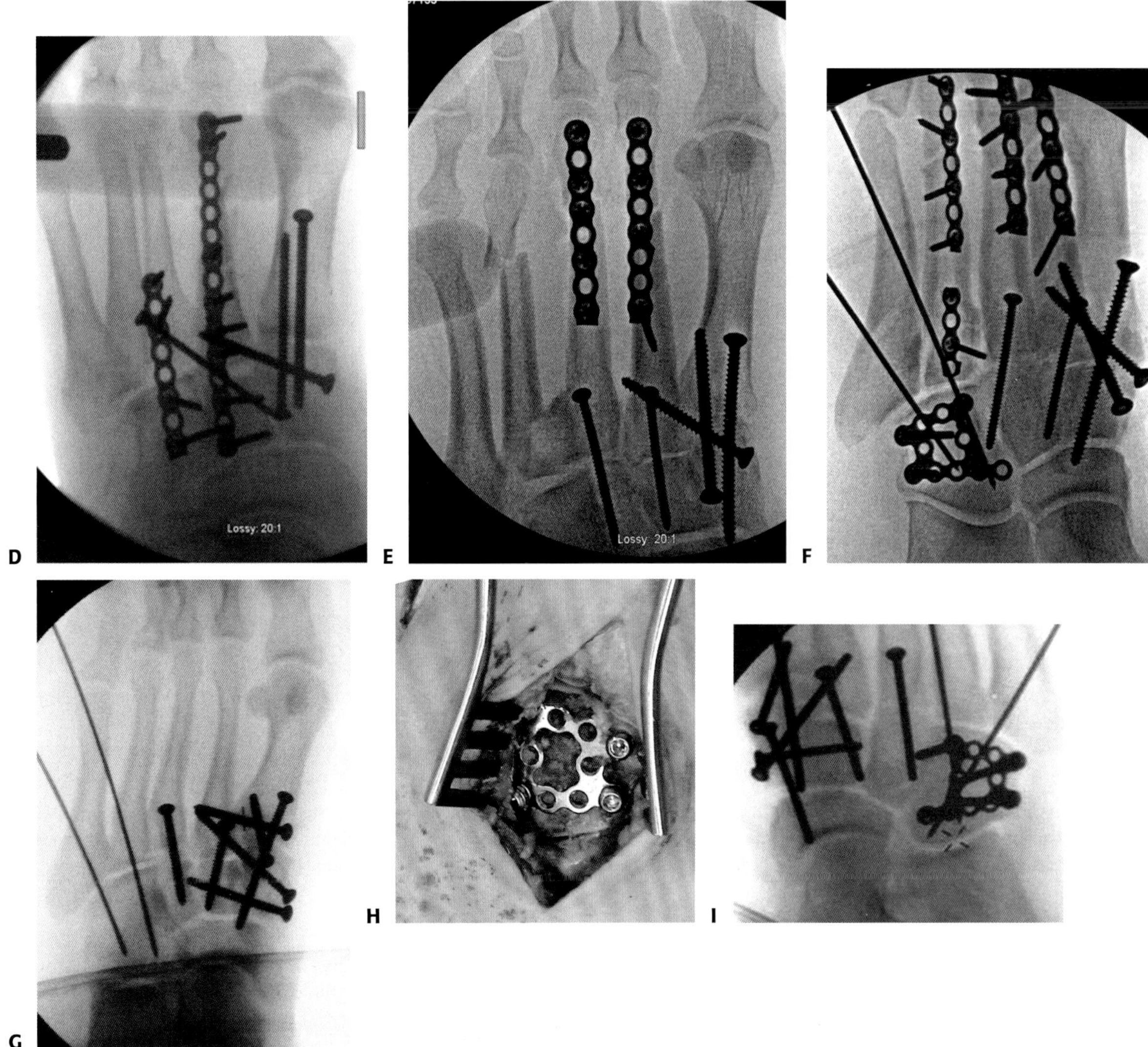


**TECH FIG 5** • *(continued)* **D.** Comminuted second metatarsal and second and third tarsometatarsal joints. **E,F.** Second and third metatarsals and segmental fourth metatarsal in a different patient. **G.** Kirschner wire fixation of fourth and fifth tarsometatarsal joints. **H.** Reduction and stabilization of cuboid through separate proximal–lateral incision. **I.** Fluoroscopic image.

- The third tarsometatarsal joint is reduced and stabilized in identical fashion (**TECH FIG 5C**).
- For a metatarsal base fracture or fracture-dislocation pattern precluding transarticular fixation, bridge plate fixation may be required.
  - We prefer a low-profile (2.0 or 2.4 mm) reconstruction plate and 2.4-mm cortical screws (**TECH FIG 5D–F**).
- The fourth and fifth tarsometatarsal joints are then reduced and definitively stabilized with 1.6-mm Kirschner wires.
  - Because the intermetatarsal ligaments between the third, fourth, and fifth metatarsals are often preserved, these joints may anatomically reduce indirectly, thereby allowing percutaneous stabilization.
  - The Kirschner wires are contoured and buried beneath the skin layer through separate stab incisions, which facilitates removal at 6 weeks postoperatively, either in the office under local anesthesia or in the operating room under sedation (**TECH FIG 5G**).
- For a cuboid fracture, the cuboid is reduced and definitively stabilized to ensure restoration of lateral column length before stabilizing the fourth and fifth tarsometatarsal joints; by definition, this is then an open reduction (**TECH FIG 5H**).
- Final fluoroscopic images are obtained, confirming articular reduction and implant placement (**TECH FIG 5I**).

TECHNIQUES

## Closure

- The wounds are irrigated, and closure commences with the medial incision. The floor of the EHL tendon sheath (and subperiosteal flaps) is closed with deep no. 0 absorbable suture, thereby sealing the intra-articular surfaces of the first and second tarsometatarsal joints and intercuneiform joints.
- The EHL tendon sheath is closed in similar fashion, thereby sealing the tendon (**TECH FIG 6A**).
- The remainder of the incision is closed in layered fashion with subcutaneous 2-0 absorbable suture and 3-0 monofilament suture for the skin layer using the modified Allgöwer-Donati technique (**TECH FIG 6B**).
- The tourniquet is deflated and sterile dressings are placed, followed by a bulky Jones dressing and Weber splint.

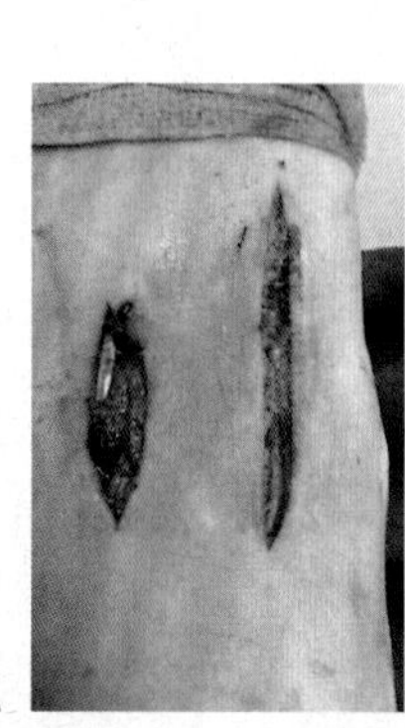
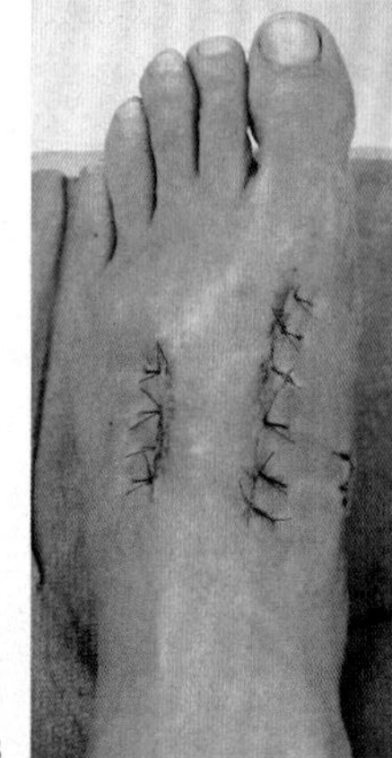

A B

**TECH FIG 6** • Wound closure. **A.** Deep layered closure sealing intra-articular contents and EHL tendon. **B.** Skin closure with modified Allgöwer-Donati technique.

## PEARLS AND PITFALLS

| | |
|---|---|
| **Misdiagnosis of proximal joint injuries (medial, middle, or lateral cuneiform; intercuneiform joint; cuboid fracture)** | ▪ Because of the highly variable injury patterns, a high index of suspicion must be maintained. Injury radiographs must be closely scrutinized preoperatively for proximal joint involvement. If radiographs are inconclusive, CT evaluation is warranted. During surgery, the status is noted of each of the intercuneiform joint capsules dorsally and therefore the extent of instability of each joint. |
| **Correcting plantar displacement or malalignment of the first and second tarsometatarsal joints** | ▪ Strict attention is paid to dorsal–plantar alignment of the first and second metatarsals and their respective cuneiforms because plantar displacement or malalignment greater than 2 mm may affect the weight-bearing metatarsal cascade, potentially resulting in a transfer (metatarsalgia) lesion. |
| **Correcting supination malrotation of first tarsometatarsal joint** | ▪ There is typically a distinct dorsal crest on both the first metatarsal and medial cuneiform. They should be precisely aligned to ensure an accurate reduction. |
| **Definitive fixation of first tarsometatarsal joint** | ▪ Because of the hard cortical bone at the diaphysis of the first metatarsal, the screw head of the distal to proximal screw is specifically countersunk to avoid compromise of the dorsal cortex and loss of fixation. |
| **Definitive fixation of Lisfranc joint** | ▪ With fixation of the Lisfranc joint, the screw must angle slightly dorsally (relative to the plantar foot) to accommodate the normal "Roman arch" configuration in the coronal plane. |

## POSTOPERATIVE CARE

- The patient is converted to a venous compression stocking and prefabricated fracture boot, and early progression to motion is initiated.
  - The Kirschner wires traversing the lateral column joints are removed 6 weeks postoperatively.
- Weight bearing is not permitted until 10 to 12 weeks postoperatively, at which point weight-bearing radiographs are obtained to confirm maintenance of reduction.
  - The patient is gradually allowed to resume regular shoes, and activity is advanced as tolerated thereafter.
- In a primary arthrodesis, the limb is immobilized in serial short-leg non–weight-bearing casts for 10 to 12 weeks after surgery, at which point radiographic union is confirmed on weight-bearing radiographs.
  - The patient is then converted to a venous compression stocking and prefabricated fracture boot, and weight bearing is advanced as described previously.
- We do not routinely remove hardware unless symptomatic or specifically requested by the patient, in which case the implants may be removed at 1 year after surgery.

## OUTCOMES

- Outcomes after open reduction and internal fixation of Lisfranc injuries are generally good overall, as patients have relatively few activity limitations. An accurate diagnosis and anatomic reduction are crucial to ensuring satisfactory results.[5]
- Outcomes for pure ligamentous patterns are less predictable after open reduction and internal fixation; these patients tend to have higher rates of posttraumatic arthritis.[5] Primary arthrodesis appears to be especially beneficial in this situation: One recent study reported a greater than 90% return to preinjury level after primary arthrodesis.[6]
- Late arthrodesis as salvage for posttraumatic arthritis provides predictable pain relief and functional improvement.[4,9]

## COMPLICATIONS

- Delayed wound healing, wound dehiscence, deep infection
- Malunion or nonunion
- Late displacement (premature implant removal)
- Neurovascular compromise
- Chronic pain

## REFERENCES


1. Arntz CT, Veith RG, Hansen ST. Fractures and fracture-dislocations of the tarsometatarsal joint. J Bone Joint Surg Am 1988;70A:154–162.
2. Curtis M, Myerson M, Szura B. Tarsometatarsal injuries in the athlete. Am J Sports Med 1994;21:497–502.
3. Goossens M, DeStoop N. Lisfranc's fracture-dislocations: etiology, radiology, and results of treatment. Clin Orthop Relat Res 1983;176: 154–162.
4. Komenda GA, Myerson MS, Biddinger KR. Results of arthrodesis of the tarsometatarsal joints after traumatic injury. J Bone Joint Surg Am 1996;78A:1665–1676.
5. Kuo RS, Tejwani NC, DiGiovanni CW, et al. Outcome after open reduction and internal fixation of Lisfranc joint injuries. J Bone Joint Surg Am 2000;82:1609–1618.
6. Ly TV, Coetzee JC. Treatment of primarily ligamentous Lisfranc joint injuries: primary arthrodesis compared with open reduction and internal fixation: a prospective, randomized study. J Bone Joint Surg Am 2006;88A:514–520.
7. Meyer SA, Callaghan JJ, Albright JP, et al. Midfoot sprains in collegiate football players. Am J Sports Med 1994;22:392–401.
8. Myerson MS, Fisher TR, Burgess RA, et al. Fracture-dislocations of the tarsometatarsal joints: end results correlated with pathology and treatment. Foot Ankle 1986;6:225–242.
9. Sangeorzan BJ, Veith RG, Hansen ST. Salvage of Lisfanc's tarsometatarsal joints by arthrodesis. Foot Ankle 1990;4:193–200.

# Fasciotomy of the Leg for Acute Compartment Syndrome

George Partal, Andrew Furey, and Robert V. O'Toole

## DEFINITION

- Compartment syndrome remains one of the most devastating orthopaedic conditions if not treated appropriately. The potential clinical sequelae and medicolegal implications of possible missed compartment syndrome make it one of the most important entities in all of orthopaedic surgery.[5]
- Compartment syndrome is a condition, with numerous causes, in which the pressure within the osteofascial compartment rises to a level that exceeds intramuscular arteriolar pressure, resulting in decreased blood flow to the capillaries, decreased oxygen diffusion to the tissue, and, ultimately, cell death. This is the rare orthopaedic emergency for which evidence indicates that delay in treatment results in worse outcomes.[10,13,29–31,34]
- The clinical sequelae of missed compartment syndrome can be life- and limb-threatening. Myonecrosis can lead to acute renal failure and multiorgan failure if not appropriately managed.[24]
- Any situation that leads to increased pressure within the compartment can result in compartment syndrome.
  - The impermeable fascia prevents fluid from leaking out of the compartment and also prevents an increase in volume that could reduce pressure within the compartment.
- The incidence of compartment syndrome is 7.3 per 100,000 male patients and 0.7 per 100,000 female patients.
- This chapter describes acute compartment syndrome (ACS), in contrast to exertional compartment syndrome.
  - Exertional compartment syndrome is a transient chronic condition brought on by exercise. Unlike ACS, exertional compartment syndrome is not an emergency, and its treatment is beyond the scope of this chapter.

## ANATOMY

- The lower leg has four compartments: anterior, lateral, superficial posterior, and deep posterior (**FIG 1**; Table 1).
- The anterior compartment is bound anteriorly by fascia, laterally by the anterior intermuscular septum, and posteriorly by the interosseous membrane between the fibula and tibia.
  - The four muscles in this compartment are the tibialis anterior, extensor digitorum longus, extensor hallucis longus, and peroneus tertius.
  - The neurovascular bundle includes the deep peroneal nerve and the anterior tibial artery.
  - The deep peroneal nerve provides sensation to the first dorsal web space of the foot and motor function to all the muscles in the anterior compartment.
  - The anterior tibial artery travels in this compartment just anterior to the tibiofibular interosseous membrane and continues in the foot as the dorsalis pedis artery.
- The lateral compartment is bordered anteriorly by the fascia, posteriorly by the posterior intermuscular septum, and medially by the fibula.
  - The lateral compartment has only two muscles: the peroneus longus and the peroneus brevis.
  - The major nerve supply to the lateral compartment is the superficial peroneal nerve, which supplies the two muscles

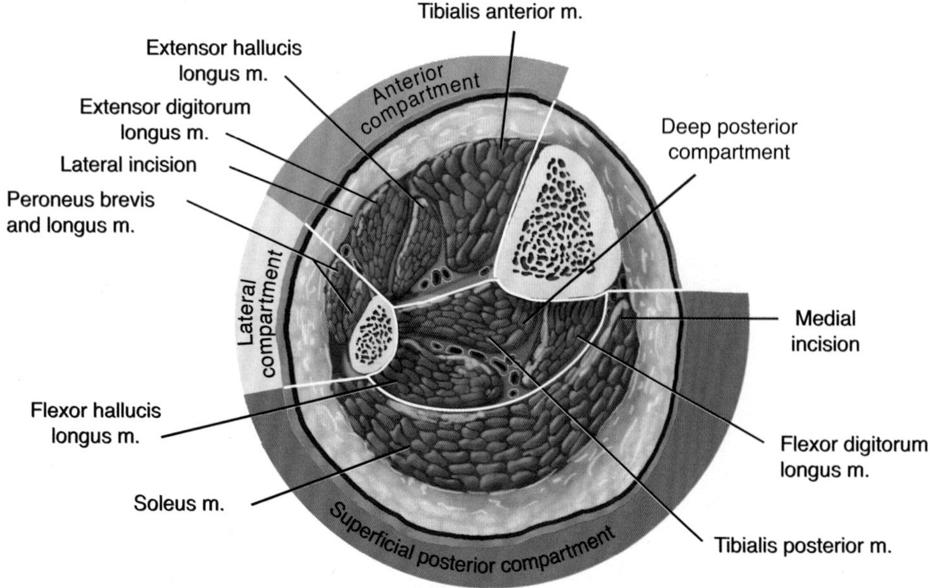


**FIG 1** • Cross-section of the lower leg at midtibial level.

**Table 1 Compartments of the Lower Leg**

| Compartment | Muscles | Major Arteries | Nerves |
|---|---|---|---|
| Anterior | Tibialis anterior<br>Extensor hallucis longus<br>Extensor digitorum longus<br>Peroneus tertius | Anterior tibial | Deep peroneal |
| Lateral | Peroneus brevis<br>Peroneus longus | None | Superficial peroneal<br>Deep peroneal (proximal in leg) |
| Deep posterior | Posterior tibialis<br>Flexor hallucis longus<br>Flexor digitorum longus | Posterior tibial<br>Peroneal | Tibial |
| Superficial posterior | Gastrocnemius<br>Soleus | None | None |

of the compartment. The nerve supplies sensation to the dorsum of the foot, except the first dorsal web space.
  - Because the deep peroneal nerve courses proximally around the fibular head, both the deep and superficial peroneal nerves travel proximally within this compartment.
  - No main vessels are present in this compartment, and the muscles receive their blood supply from the peroneal and anterior tibial arteries.
- The deep posterior compartment contains the flexor digitorum longus, tibialis posterior, and flexor hallucis longus muscles. Popliteus is thought to lie within this compartment proximally.
  - Although it is not considered a separate compartment, the tibialis posterior muscle can have its own fascial covering.
  - The deep posterior compartment contains the main neurovascular bundle of the posterior compartment, which consists of the tibial nerve, posterior tibial artery and vein, and peroneal artery and vein.
- The superficial posterior compartment contains the gastrocnemius, soleus, and plantaris muscles, which are supplied by branches of the tibial nerve, posterior tibial artery, and peroneal arteries.
  - No major artery travels in this compartment.

## PATHOGENESIS

- Although the exact pathophysiology is not completely understood, the syndrome is thought to be the result of either a decrease in the space available for the tissues within the fixed compartment or an increase in the size of the tissues within the compartment.
  - Either case can result in an increase in pressure above a critical value.
- Increased fluid content and swelling of damaged muscles can be caused by the following:
  - Bleeding into the compartment (from fractures, large vessel injury, or bleeding disorders)
    - Fractures are the most common cause of compartment syndrome. It is estimated that 9.1% of tibial plateau fractures develop compartment syndrome.[7]
    - Blunt trauma is the second most common cause, accounting for 23% of cases.[19]
  - Increased capillary permeability (eg, burns, ischemia, exercise, snake bite, drug injection, intravenous fluids)
- Decreased compartment size can be caused by the following:
  - Burns
  - Tight circumferential wrapping, dressings, casts
  - Localized external pressure, such as lying on the limb for an extended period of time or from pressure on the "well leg" in the lithotomy position on the fracture table
- Elevated pressure prevents perfusion of the tissue from the capillaries and results in anoxia and necrosis.
  - The impermeable fascia prevents fluid from escaping, causing a rise in compartment pressure, such that it exceeds the pressure within the veins, resulting in collapse of the veins or an increase in venous pressure.[22]
  - The final event is cellular anoxia and necrosis.[24]
  - During necrosis, an increase in intracellular calcium concentration occurs, coupled with a subsequent shift of water into the tissue, causing the tissue to swell further, adding to the pressure.[12] This "capillary leakage" adds to the increased pressure in the compartment, thus creating a vicious cycle. Lindsay et al[17] reported that prolonged ischemia of the muscle results in adenosine triphosphate breakdown and that the amount of energy depletion during ischemia determines the extent of the ischemic damage.
- The effects on muscle and nerve function are time-dependent.
  - Prolonged delay results in greater loss of function.
  - Red muscle fibers (eg, anterior compartment of the leg), which rely predominantly on aerobic metabolism, are far more vulnerable to ischemia than "white" muscle fibers (eg, gastrocnemius muscle), which rely on anaerobic metabolism.[14]
  - After sustained elevation of compartment pressures for more than 6 to 8 hours, nerve conduction is blocked.[10] In animal studies,[13,30] irreversible muscle damage occurred after 8 to 12 hours.
- The exact pressure at which change within the compartment occurs has been the subject of debate and has evolved over time.
  - Initially, the pressure of 30 mm Hg was reported to be the maximum pressure above which irreversible muscle damage occurred.[40]
  - Currently, clinicians have recognized the importance of the patient's blood pressure when considering the compartment pressure and use an absolute difference between diastolic blood pressure and compartment pressure of less than 30 mm Hg as an indicator of ACS.[18]

- Animal studies have highlighted the importance of the systemic pressures relative to the compartment pressure.
  - Whiteman and Heckman[40] found that irreversible ischemic changes occurred when the compartment pressure was elevated within 30 mm Hg of the mean arterial pressure and within 20 mm Hg of the diastolic pressure.
  - Research[4] on limb ischemia at the University of Pennsylvania led to similar conclusions. Bernot et al[4] coined the term *delta P*, referring to the difference between the mean arterial pressure minus the compartment pressure, with a lower number reflecting less blood flow. The authors[4] found that cellular anoxia and death occur with pressure within 20 mm Hg of the mean arterial pressure; however, at pressures within 40 mm Hg, oxygen tension was reduced, but anoxia was not indicated and aerobic metabolism persisted.
  - McQueen et al[18] used the cutoff of compartment pressure within 30 mm Hg of the diastolic blood pressure as a fasciotomy threshold. No adverse clinical outcomes occurred as a result of not releasing compartments with pressures that were more than 30 mm Hg from the diastolic blood pressure, and this has come to be the value currently used most often as a threshold for compartment syndrome.

## NATURAL HISTORY

- The outcome of compartment syndrome depends on location, trauma to the tissue, and time to intervention.
  - Six hours of ischemia currently is the accepted upper limit of viability. Rorabeck and Macnab[31] reported almost complete recovery of the limb function when fasciotomies were performed within 6 hours of the onset of symptoms.
  - Muscle undergoes irreversible change after 8 hours of ischemia, whereas nerves can incur irreversible damage in 6 hours.[10]
- Compartment syndrome can have broad effects on multiple systems.
  - As muscle necrosis occurs, myoglobin, potassium, and other metabolites are released into circulation.
  - As a result, several metabolic conditions can arise, including myoglobinuria, hypothermia, metabolic acidosis, and hyperkalemia. In turn, these biochemical phenomena can cause renal failure, cardiac arrhythmias, and, potentially, death.

## PATIENT HISTORY AND PHYSICAL FINDINGS

- Diagnosis of compartment syndrome is a clinical challenge, and significant variation among clinicians likely exists.[25] Studies of diagnosis in patients are limited by lack of a reliable gold standard other than "fasciotomy was performed," which is what typically is used in the literature.
- Compartment syndrome is, for the most part, still a clinical diagnosis. However, the use of physical examination findings to diagnose compartment syndrome has not been well validated.[38]
- The key to successful handling of compartment syndrome is early diagnosis and treatment. Therefore, the orthopaedic surgeon must be familiar with the risk factors and signs and symptoms of the diagnosis, obtain a detailed documented history, and perform a thorough physical examination.

### Risk Factors for Compartment Syndrome

- The patient's history is critical. Certain aspects of the patient's history render the syndrome more likely.
- Risk factors for compartment syndrome include age younger than 35 years, male gender, and mechanism of sport injury.[19,26,43]
- The most common cause of ACS is fracture, and the second most common cause is soft tissue injury.
- Tibial fractures are associated with a high rate of compartment syndrome, with rates for shaft fractures ranging from 1% to 11%.[25,38] Proximal tibial fractures are at particular risk, especially high-energy tibial plateau fractures, with rates of approximately 15% to 28%[3,9,33] and fracture-dislocations reported to be as high as 53%.[20,36] Ballistic proximal fibular fractures[20] also have been shown to be at particular risk for developing compartment syndrome.
  - It should be noted that open fractures can still develop ACS, and some authors have found no difference in incidence of ACS with open compared with closed fractures.[18,19]
  - The existence of any of the following characteristics should heighten the surgeon's suspicion: high-energy injury mechanism, a patient receiving anticoagulation medication, or a patient with a tight circumferential dressing.

### Physical Examination of Acute Compartment Syndrome

- Little rigorous data exist regarding the validation of clinical examination findings. The most widely cited review of the literature on this topic includes only four patients with compartment syndrome.[38]
- The classic "Ps" taught in medical schools (pain out of proportion, pain with passive range of motion, paresthesias, pulselessness, pallor, paralysis, and pressure on palpation) for diagnosing compartment syndrome are not equally useful, and little validation work has been conducted.[38]
- Pain out of proportion to the injury is a classic symptom of the diagnosis. Patient injury severity and perception and expression of pain vary substantially, rendering this judgment difficult in clinical practice. The amount of pain medicine needed by the patient is a useful predictor of compartment syndrome in a pediatric setting.[2]
- Patients in whom pain might be difficult to ascertain include those with head injuries; those using ethanol or drugs; those who are intubated or sedated; those who have major distracting injuries, such as long bone fracture; those receiving large amounts of pain medicine; and those with any other factor that might alter the patient's ability to accurately sense and communicate pain levels.
  - Pain perception can also be altered by anesthesia, and some work suggests that patients receiving epidural anesthesia are four times more likely to develop compartment syndrome than those receiving other forms of pain control.[23]
  - This type of anesthesia results in a sympathetic nerve blockade, thereby increasing the blood flow, compounding the local tissue pressures and extremity swelling.
- Similarly, local anesthesia combined with narcotics has been shown to increase the risk of compartment syndrome.[8,23]
  - Pulselessness typically is not helpful because the presence of a pulse does not rule out compartment syndrome. Most patients with ACS have normal pulses.
  - Pallor typically is not helpful either. Pallor also reflects loss of arterial flow and rarely is present during physical examination.

- Pain with passive range of motion of the muscles of the compartment is another classic sign of compartment syndrome.[12] For tibial fractures, for example, motion of the toes does not typically cause substantial pain.
- Zones of paresthesia can be a useful, but confusing, symptom of compartment syndrome.
  - It has been shown, however, that nerve function is altered after only 2 hours of ischemia; therefore, paresthesia represents a potential early symptom.[11]
- Light touch is a better indicator because it indicates change in the ability of the nerves to detect a threshold force, as opposed to two-point discrimination. Two-point discrimination is a test of nerve density, which might not change until later in the process.
  - With increased pressure in a compartment, the sensory nerves are affected first and then the motor nerves (eg, in the anterior compartment, the deep peroneal nerve is affected quickly and patients report loss of sensation between the first two toes).
  - Considering that small fiber nerves are affected first, light touch will be affected before pressure and proprioception.
- Decreased motor function of muscles in the compartment is another classic sign. However, it can be caused by ischemia, guarding, pain, or a combination of these factors, particularly in patients with distracting extremity injuries, such as tibial shaft fracture.
  - Muscle force should be documented in all compartments when ruling out compartment syndrome. Documenting that the patient "wiggles toes" is not adequate because that indicates only that either the flexors or extensors are firing. "NVI" is not useful either because it does not state the exact muscle groups that were tested.
- Palpation of tight compartments has been thought to be an important indicator of compartment syndrome. The deep posterior compartment cannot be directly palpated because of its location deep to the superficial posterior compartment. Recent data have questioned clinicians' ability to evaluate pressure based on palpation alone.[35]
- Serial examinations are critical. All complaints should be thoroughly investigated, and all findings should be carefully documented in the chart such that subsequent examiners can refer to the record as a tool for diagnosis.

## IMAGING AND OTHER DIAGNOSTIC STUDIES

- The diagnosis of compartment syndrome typically is made clinically. Intracompartmental pressure measurements are the most common data used to aid in diagnosis, particularly in patients with limited physical examinations.
- Once a patient is diagnosed with compartment syndrome, fasciotomies should be performed emergently. Any workup that could substantially delay this process should be undertaken with great caution.

### Intracompartmental Pressure Measurements

- If the patient cannot provide clinical clues because he or she is sedated or for other reasons, or if the diagnosis is in question, compartment pressures can be measured.
- The exact pressure that defines compartment syndrome is still debated, although a pressure measurement should be obtained with reference to the diastolic blood pressure.[18]
  - Some authors have argued that using single pressure measurements alone might result in high rates of false-positive diagnoses using the standard delta P of 30 mm Hg threshold.[27,41] Therefore, in our opinion, compartment pressure checks should not be performed on patients in whom there is no clinical concern for ACS.
  - The technique of measuring compartment pressures must be mastered by the surgeon.
  - Inexperience with the technique can lead to inaccurate data and potentially missed compartment syndrome.
  - When measuring the pressure, the surgeon must be familiar with the local anatomy and able to accurately measure all the compartments.
  - Location of the measurement is important.
  - Whitesides and Heckman[40] reported that the highest pressures were within 5 cm of the fracture site; pressures decreased as the measurements were obtained distally and proximally to the fracture.

### Measurement of the Compartment Pressure

- Several techniques to measure compartment pressure have been described, including the Whiteside infusion technique, the Stic technique, the Wick catheter technique, and the slit catheter technique. The two most commonly used instruments are the Whiteside side port needle and the slit catheter device.
- Numerous digital pressure monitors are commercially available and frequently used. The Stryker pressure monitor is in common clinical use (**FIG 2**).
- Inserting an arterial line (16- to 18-gauge needle) is easy to do in the operating room, but the pressure measured with a simple needle is thought to be 5 to 19 mm Hg higher than the pressure measured with a side port or wick catheter.[21]
- Pressure values should be recorded for all four compartments. Typically, each compartment is checked twice. If a fracture is present, the value will be highest within 5 cm of the fracture.[40] The contralateral limb can be checked as a control. Normal resting internal compartment pressure is approximately 8 mm Hg in adults and 13 to 16 mm Hg in children.
- Delta P (diastolic blood pressure minus intracompartmental pressure) is measured.
  - A delta P of less than 30 mm Hg generally is accepted as an indication for fasciotomy based on the work conducted by McQueen et al[19] that showed that all patients with a delta P greater than 10 mm Hg in whom fasciotomy was not performed had normal function at follow-up. Clinicians should interpret this study with caution considering it used continuous pressure measurement values averaged over 12 hours (not one-time pressure measurements, as are obtained in common clinical practice) and considering only three patients in that study had compartment syndrome.
  - Although some animal data indicate that lower thresholds might be safe and although some concern might exist that this threshold leads to a high false-positive rate,[27,41] clinicians should be reassured that delta P of 30 mm Hg seems to be highly sensitive to avoid missing any compartment syndromes.
  - Unless the patient will be in the operating room for a prolonged time period, preoperative values of diastolic

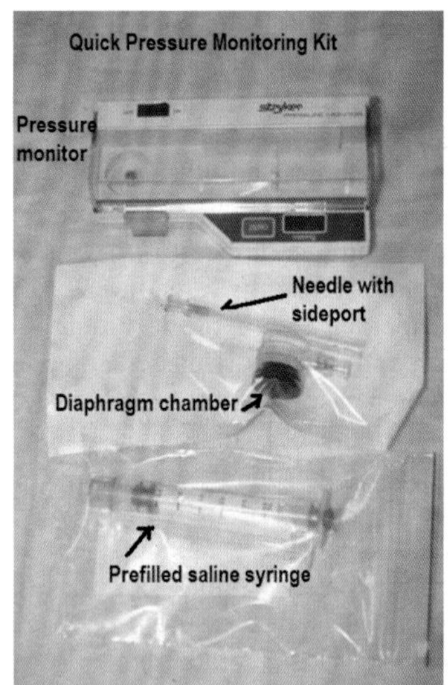


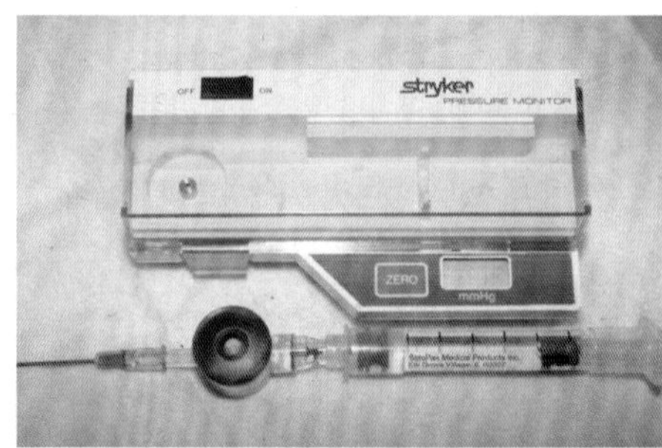


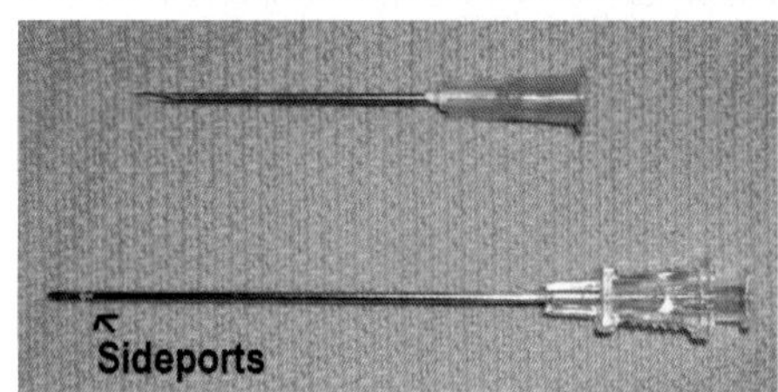


**FIG 2** • Stryker intracompartmental pressure monitor. **A.** Quick pressure monitoring kit containing the intracompartmental pressure monitor, a prefilled saline syringe, a diaphragm chamber (transducer), and a needle. **B.** The assembled pressure monitor. To assemble the monitor kit, the needle is attached to the tapered end of the tapered chamber stem (transducer). The blue cap from the prefilled syringe is removed and the syringe is screwed into the remaining end of the transducer, which is a Luer-lock connection. The cover of the monitor is opened. The transducer is placed inside the well (black surface down). The snap cover is closed. Next, the clear end cap is pulled off the syringe end, and the monitor is ready to use. To prime the monitor, the needle is held 45 degrees up from the horizontal and the syringe plunger is pushed slowly to purge air from the syringe. The monitor is then turned on. The assembled monitor is tilted at the approximate intended angle of insertion of the needle into the skin. The zero button is pressed to set the display at zero. The needle is then inserted into the appropriate location in the compartment. **C.** The intracompartmental pressure monitor needle has side ports to prevent soft tissue from collapsing around the needle opening. This is different from a regular needle that has only one opening at the end.

pressure should typically be used because diastolic blood pressure decreases 20 points, on average, with anesthesia.[15]

- McQueen et al[19] have advocated routine continuous pressure monitoring in the anterior compartment of tibial fractures. It is their center's technique for continuous monitoring that has been extrapolated to determine our current threshold of 30 mm Hg delta P even though the measurement technique used does not currently include continuous measurement. Continuous monitoring of routine tibial shaft fractures has not gained clinical popularity in North America as of yet, likely because of logistical difficulties in setting up the monitoring and some clinicians' concerns regarding the false positives associated with monitoring.[27,41]
- Near-infrared spectroscopy is a noninvasive and continuous method that determines tissue oxygenation by comparing the light emitted when comparing the concentration of venous blood oxyhemoglobin and deoxyhemoglobin. It might ultimately be a tool to monitor patients with evolving compartment syndrome, making it useful in the setting of critically ill patients.[1,28] This technology has not been validated and is not currently in routine clinical use.
  - Laboratory studies should include a complete metabolic profile, a complete blood count with differential, creatine phosphokinase (CPK), urine myoglobin, serum myoglobin, urinalysis (which might be positive for blood but negative for red blood cells, indicating myoglobin in the urine caused by rhabdomyolysis), and a coagulation profile (prothrombin time, partial thromboplastin time, international normalized ratio).
- Obtaining a complete laboratory panel should not delay operative treatment in a diagnosed case of compartment syndrome.
- Elevated CPK or creatine kinase in an intubated trauma patient might be a sign of compartment syndrome. Typical CPK values are 1000 to 5000 μg/L or higher in cases of ACS. One recent study proposed a CPK value of 4000 μg/L as indicative of ACS.[39] Myoglobinemia can also be observed in some cases.

## DIFFERENTIAL DIAGNOSIS

- Compartment syndrome is diagnosed in a patient with either of the following:
  - Suspicious clinical findings as discussed earlier
  - Pressure in a compartment within 30 mm Hg of the diastolic blood pressure
- Other diagnoses to consider
  - Normal pain response secondary to fracture or other trauma
  - Low pain tolerance secondary to preoperative substance abuse
  - Muscle rupture
  - Deep venous thrombosis and thrombophlebitis
  - Cellulitis
  - Coelenterate and jellyfish envenomations

- Necrotizing fasciitis
- Peripheral vascular injury
- Peripheral nerve injury
- Rhabdomyolysis
- Of special note, recent studies have shown that in the case of envenomations, compartment syndrome is multifactorial and fasciotomy might not prevent myonecrosis, which can be caused by the direct toxic effect of the venom and the inflammatory response.
  - In these cases, antivenom should be administered; this has been shown to decrease limb hypoperfusion.

## NONOPERATIVE MANAGEMENT

- All patients suspected of having ACS should undergo emergent fasciotomies performed in the operating room or at the bedside.
- Nonoperative treatment of ACS is almost never appropriate unless operative treatment would risk the patient's life. ACS is a life- and limb-threatening injury; the successful treatment of which is based on limiting the time until fasciotomy is performed.
- Considering that ischemic injury is the basis for compartment syndrome, additional oxygen should be administered to the patient diagnosed with compartment syndrome because it will slightly increase the blood partial pressure of oxygen.
  - The surgeon must ensure that the patient is normotensive because hypotension reduces perfusion pressure and leads to further tissue injury.
- Any circumferential bandages or casts should be removed from patients at risk for development of compartment syndrome.
  - Compartment pressure falls by 30% when a cast is split on one side and by 65% when a cast is spread after splitting. Splitting the padding reduces the pressure by an additional 10% and complete removal of the cast by another 15%. A total of 85% to 90% reduction in pressure can be achieved by removing the cast.[42]
- Elevating the limb above the heart decreases mean arterial pressure in the limb without changing the intracompartmental pressure. Thus, the affected extremity should not be elevated.
  - As shown by Wiger et al,[42] after an elevation of 35 cm, the mean perfusion pressure decreased by 23 mm Hg but the intracompartmental pressure stayed the same.
- Intravenous fluids should be administered to decrease the chance of kidney damage from myoglobin.
  - The "crush syndrome" is a sequela of muscle necrosis (ie, high CPK level, above 20,000 IU) that manifests as nonoliguric renal failure, myoglobinuria, oliguria, shock, acidosis, hyperkalemia, and cardiac arrhythmia.
  - Treatment is supportive, with ventilatory support, hydration, correction of acidosis, and dialysis.
  - It is important in this situation to decrease the metabolic load by preventing ongoing tissue necrosis and performing débridement of all dead tissue.
- The use of narcotics should be closely recorded and monitored for any patient suspected of having compartment syndrome.
  - The use of local, spinal, or epidural anesthesia for postoperative pain control generally is discouraged in patients at high risk for compartment syndrome because it limits the ability of the clinician to perform serial examinations.

### Late Presentation of Acute Compartment Syndrome

- Nonoperative treatment of missed compartment syndrome is reserved for patients presenting very late after missed compartment syndrome who already have irreversible muscle necrosis.
  - One school of thought is that these patients should not be treated operatively because doing so would increase the chance of infection and lead to amputation.
  - It often is difficult to know when compartment syndrome has occurred, however, so in situations in which it is unclear, it is probably wise to release the compartments.
  - One school of thought is that if compartment syndrome has run its course, fasciotomies should not be performed unless the pressure in the compartment is within 30 mm Hg of diastolic pressure, but this recommendation is controversial and without support in the literature.

## SURGICAL MANAGEMENT

- All patients with ACS should be treated with emergent fasciotomies of the affected compartments because compartment syndrome is limb-threatening and potentially life-threatening if allowed to progress to myonecrosis and renal failure.
- Time to diagnosis and surgical treatment of compartment syndrome is critical; nerve damage after 6 hours of ischemia might be irreversible.
- Patients with compartment syndrome should be given the highest priority, and the condition should be treated as an operative emergency.
- Fasciotomy of the involved compartment is the standard of care for ACS.
  - In a trauma setting, typically all four compartments of the leg are released, regardless of evidence of involvement of the other compartments.
- Fasciotomies ideally should be performed in the operating room.
  - If the patient is too ill to be transported to the operating room or if no operating room is available, fasciotomies can be performed at the bedside in as sterile an environment as possible.
- The only common contraindication to fasciotomy in the face of compartment syndrome is delayed presentation, in which a patient with missed compartment syndrome presents late, after irreversible injury has set in (see Nonoperative Management section).
- Fasciotomies are also often performed in a prophylactic manner for any patient with an ischemic limb for more than 6 hours to prevent reperfusion injury.

### Preoperative Planning

- Once compartment syndrome is diagnosed, every effort should be directed at getting the patient to the operating room as quickly as possible for fasciotomies.
  - All further workup should be deferred until fasciotomies are complete, except workup that is needed for a potential life-threatening injury.
  - Little preoperative planning is required for this component of the patient's treatment.

- Radiographs should be reviewed to rule out fractures and dislocations; however, additional radiographs can be obtained in the operating room after fasciotomies have been completed.
- Only essential preoperative workup should be conducted before the patient is taken to the operating room. The case should not be delayed for additional, nonessential radiographic workup.

## Positioning

- The patient usually is positioned supine on the operating room table to facilitate fasciotomies. A small bump can be placed under the hip on the affected side.
- The leg is prepared in a sterile fashion, and a thigh tourniquet is applied but not inflated.

## Approach

- Two separate techniques have been used for decompression of the lower leg compartments.
  - The two-incision technique is the most commonly used method, but a one-incision technique involving a lateral (perifibular) approach also exists.
  - The two-incision technique is more straightforward and requires less experience to ensure a complete compartment release and is therefore typically advocated. Draw both planned incisions on the skin before making them to avoid a narrow skin bridge.
  - Some have argued that the one-incision technique can be useful in cases of defined anterior tibial artery injuries to help prevent loss of anterior skin.



## Double-Incision Technique

### Anterolateral Incision

- The anterolateral incision decompresses the anterior and lateral compartments.
  - The anterolateral incision is made halfway between the fibula and the crest of the tibia and lies just above the intermuscular septum dividing the anterior and lateral compartments (**TECH FIG 1A**).
- Fasciotomies have also been accomplished through small incisions. However, we prefer using generous incisions to allow for full decompression of the compartments.
  - We recommend incisions that typically are at least 15 to 20 cm both medially and laterally.
- A small transverse incision is made to identify the intermuscular septum, after which scissors are used to split the fascia of the anterior and lateral compartments.
  - Care must be taken to avoid injuring the superficial peroneal nerve by making separate incisions in each compartment and not cutting the intermuscular septum (**TECH FIG 1B–F**).

### Posteromedial Incision

- The posteromedial approach decompresses the superficial and deep posterior compartments.
  - The incision lies approximately 2 cm posterior to the posterior tibial margin (**TECH FIG 2A**).
  - Care is taken to avoid injury to the saphenous vein and nerve, which are retracted anteriorly.
- Each fascia of the deep and superficial posterior compartments is incised longitudinally in line with the incision (**TECH FIG 2B–E**).
- The deep posterior compartment is initially released distally, and then the scissors are oriented proximally through and under the soleus bridge. If the posterior tibia is visualized, the deep posterior compartment has been released.
- Some surgeons release the soleus attachment to the tibia more than halfway. Also, the fascia over the posterior tibial muscle should be released.
- One useful tip is to keep the tips of the scissors away from major neurovascular structures.

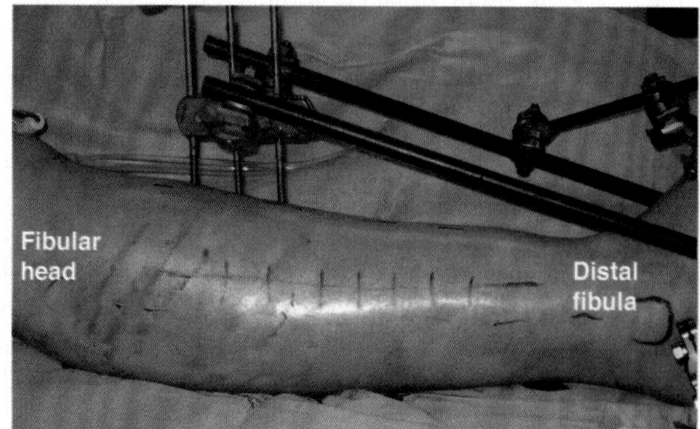


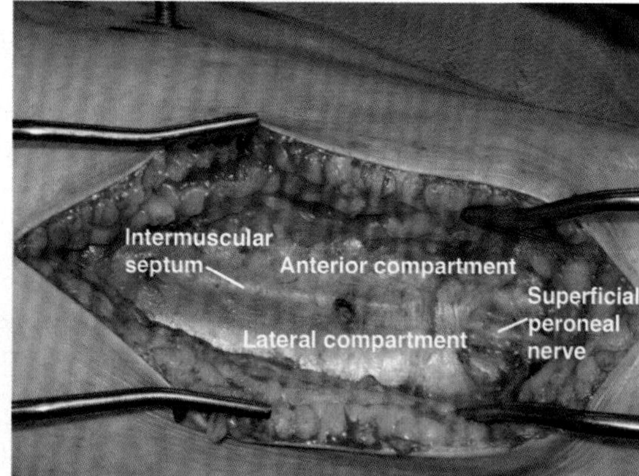


**TECH FIG 1** • Lateral incision of the two-incision technique. **A.** The anterolateral incision is made halfway between the fibula and the tibial crest overlying the intermuscular septum dividing the anterior and lateral compartments. **B.** Close-up picture of the fasciotomy site after skin incision before the fascia is open, showing the intermuscular septum between the lateral and anterior compartments and the course of the superficial peroneal nerve. *(continued)*

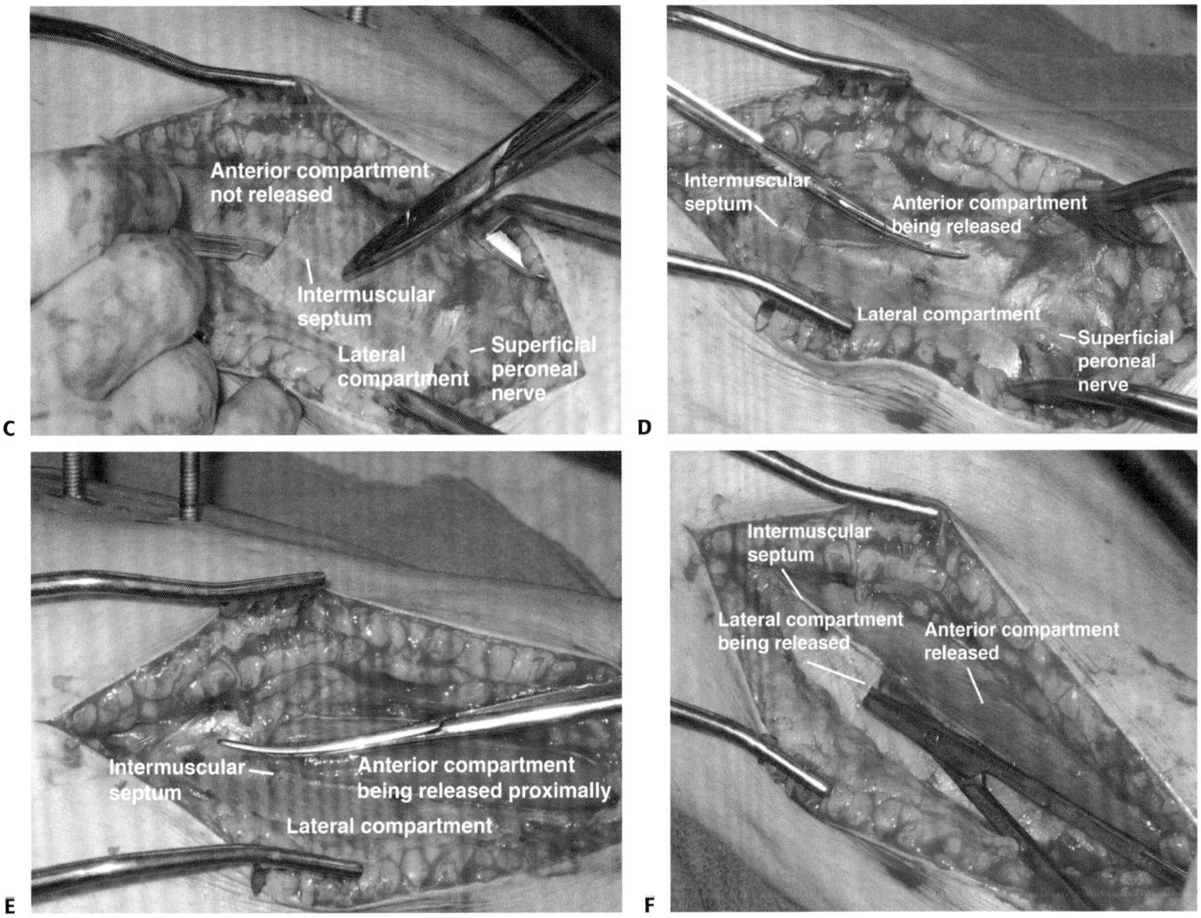

**TECH FIG 1** • *(continued)* **C.** With a knife, a small transverse incision is made over the intermuscular septum. Care is taken to avoid injury to the superficial peroneal nerve. **D.** The surgeon inserts the tips of the scissors into the small rent in the fascia, and keeping the tips of the scissors up and away from the superficial peroneal nerve, the surgeon incises the fascia over the anterior compartment distally. **E.** The scissors are turned with the tips proximally, and the fascia of the anterior compartment is released proximally. **F.** The tips of the scissors are then inserted into the rent created in the fascia of the lateral compartment. Keeping the tips of the scissors up and away from the superficial peroneal nerve, the surgeon releases the fascia over the lateral compartment proximally and distally.

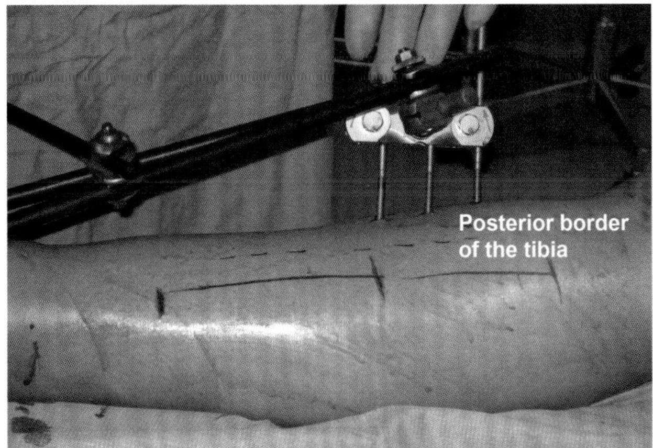


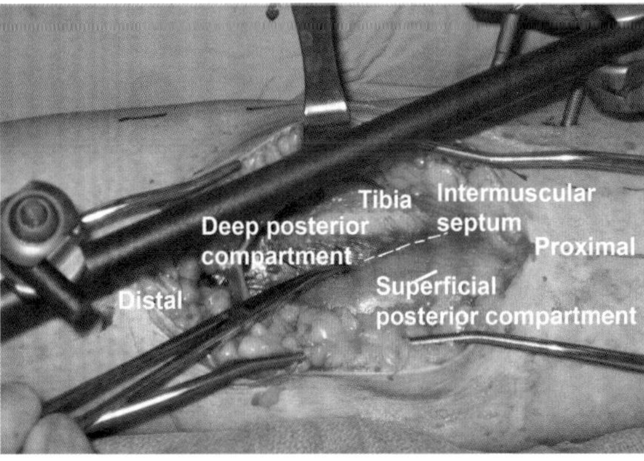


**TECH FIG 2** • Medial incision of the two-incision technique. **A.** The medial incision lies approximately 2 cm posterior to the posterior tibial margin. **B.** Care is taken to avoid injury to the saphenous vein. The picture shows the posterior border of the tibia exposed along with the deep and superficial posterior compartments. The tips of the dissecting scissors lie on the deep posterior compartment. *(continued)*

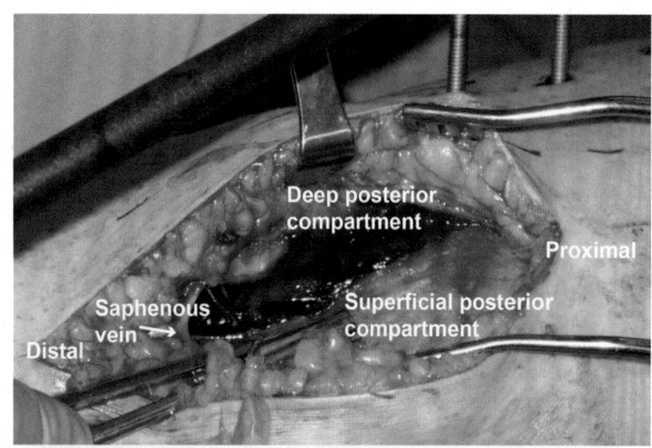


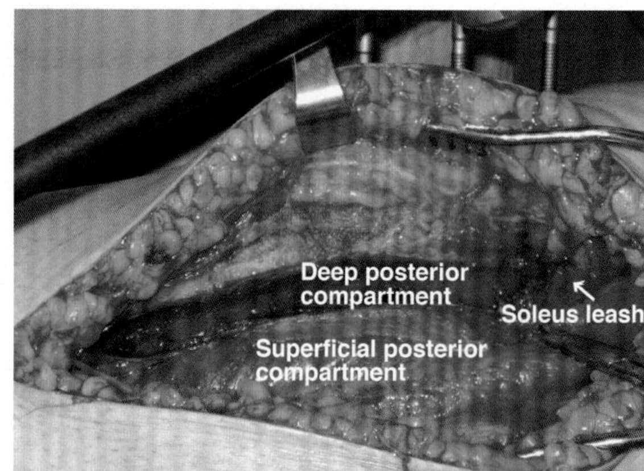


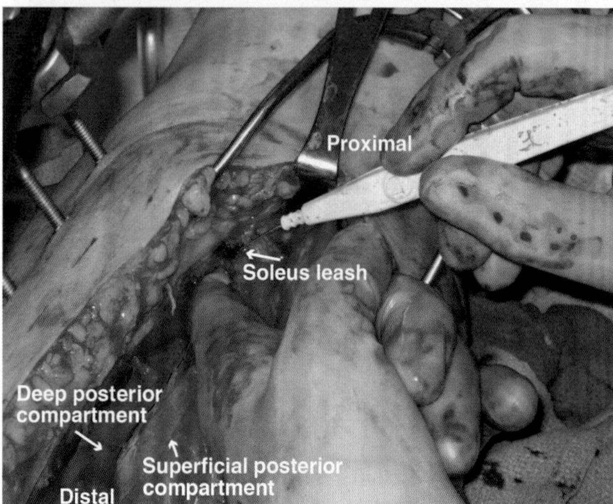


**TECH FIG 2** • *(continued)* **C.** A small transverse incision is made to identify the intermuscular septum between the deep and superficial posterior compartments. Dissecting scissors are used to release the fascia over the deep posterior compartment proximally and distally. Proximally, the fascia is released under the soleus bridge. Scissors are shown under the fascia of the superficial posterior compartment. **D.** The deep and superficial compartments are released. The superficial posterior compartment looks healthy, whereas the deep posterior compartment is dusky. The tips of the clamp lie under the soleus bridge, which also needs to be released from its origin on the tibia. **E.** The surgeon releases the soleus bridge using electrocautery, taking care to protect the deep structures.

## One-Incision Technique

- The one-incision technique often requires more careful dissection around major neurovascular structures and can prove to be more challenging. For this reason, it is less often used. Bible et al[6] showed no difference in infection or nonunion rates between a one- and two-incision fasciotomy technique.
- A straight lateral incision is created that originates just posterior and parallel to the fibula at the level of the fibular head (protecting the peroneal nerve) to a point above the tip of the lateral malleolus (**TECH FIG 3A**).
- Posterior to the fibula, access is gained to the deep and superficial posterior compartments (**TECH FIG 3B**).
  - The fascia between the soleus and flexor hallucis longus is identified distally and released proximally to the level of the soleus origin (**TECH FIG 3C**).[16]
- Anterior to the fibula, the anterior and lateral compartments are decompressed, taking care to avoid injury to the superficial peroneal nerve.

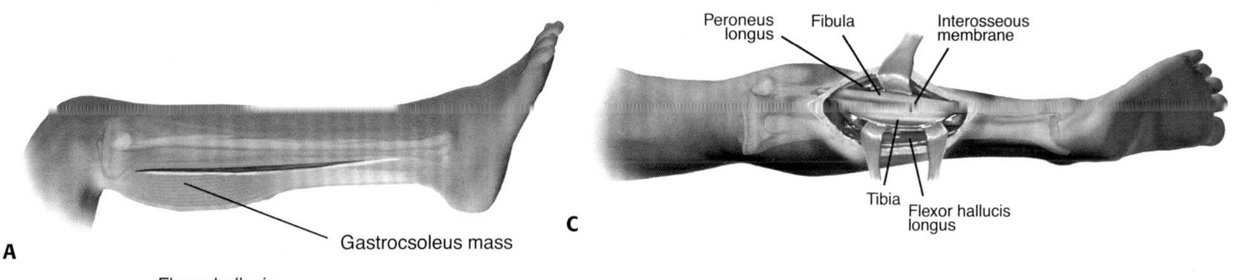


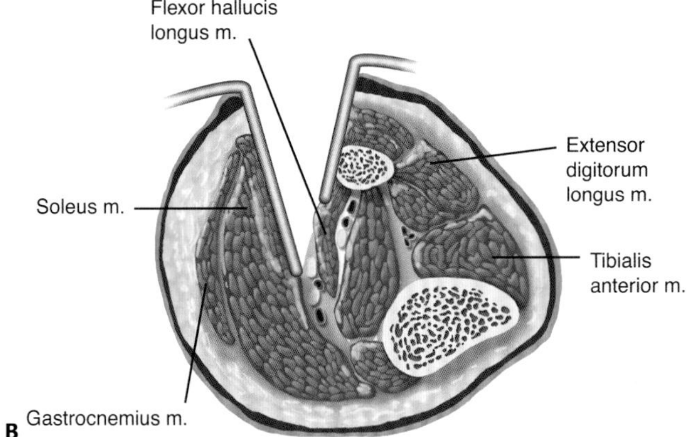


**TECH FIG 3** • One-incision technique. **A.** Schematic shows the incision laterally, just posterior and parallel to the fibula. Again, care is taken to avoid injury to the superficial peroneal nerve. **B.** Cross-section of the midtibia shows dissection posterior to the fibula, allowing access to the deep and superficial posterior compartments. Here, the fascia between the soleus and flexor hallucis longus is identified distally and released proximally to the level of the soleus origin. **C.** Schematic showing access to the posterior tibia and thus release of the deep posterior compartment. Dissection anterior to the fibula allows identification of the intermuscular septum between the lateral and anterior compartments. The fascia overlying these two compartments is released proximally and distally with the tips of dissecting scissors, taking care to avoid injury to the superficial peroneal nerve.

## Muscle Débridement

- Regardless of the choice of fasciotomy performed, devitalized muscle undergoes débridement as necessary.
  - Muscle viability is ascertained by the presence of healthy color and the ability to contract when pinched gently or touched with the electrocautery.
  - Necrotic muscle serves no function and must eventually be removed because it will form a culture medium for infection after fasciotomy.
- Extensive débridement typically is not undertaken until the second look at 36 to 72 hours, when muscle viability is more readily determined.
- When fasciotomies are performed in the setting of fractures, the fractures are stabilized with either internal or external fixation, which eliminates the need for constrictive casts and allows access for clinical examination, repeat pressure measurements, and wound care.
  - Fixation of fractures can trigger compartment syndrome through traction and reaming.

## Closure of Fasciotomies

- Fasciotomies typically are not closed acutely because the skin itself can constrict muscle.
- Most often, fasciotomy wounds are either packed with moist dressings (**TECH FIG 4A**) or covered with a sterile vacuum sponge and kept under suction until the next débridement procedure (**TECH FIG 4B**).
- After a lower leg fasciotomy, a useful technique has been the shoelace closure, which involves using a vessel loop and skin staples to gradually close large areas of gaping skin.
  - This allows gradual approximation of the skin edges over the course of several days, thus potentially obviating the need for a skin graft (**TECH FIG 4C**).
- It is our opinion that if two surgical wounds are present, the surgeon should attempt to close the medial wound secondarily before the lateral wound.
  - The lateral side of the leg has better soft tissue coverage and consequently is easier to skin graft over if one of the wounds cannot be closed.
- Sometimes, small relaxing incisions around the fasciotomy wound can decrease the tension, enhancing the chance of healing (**TECH FIG 4D**).

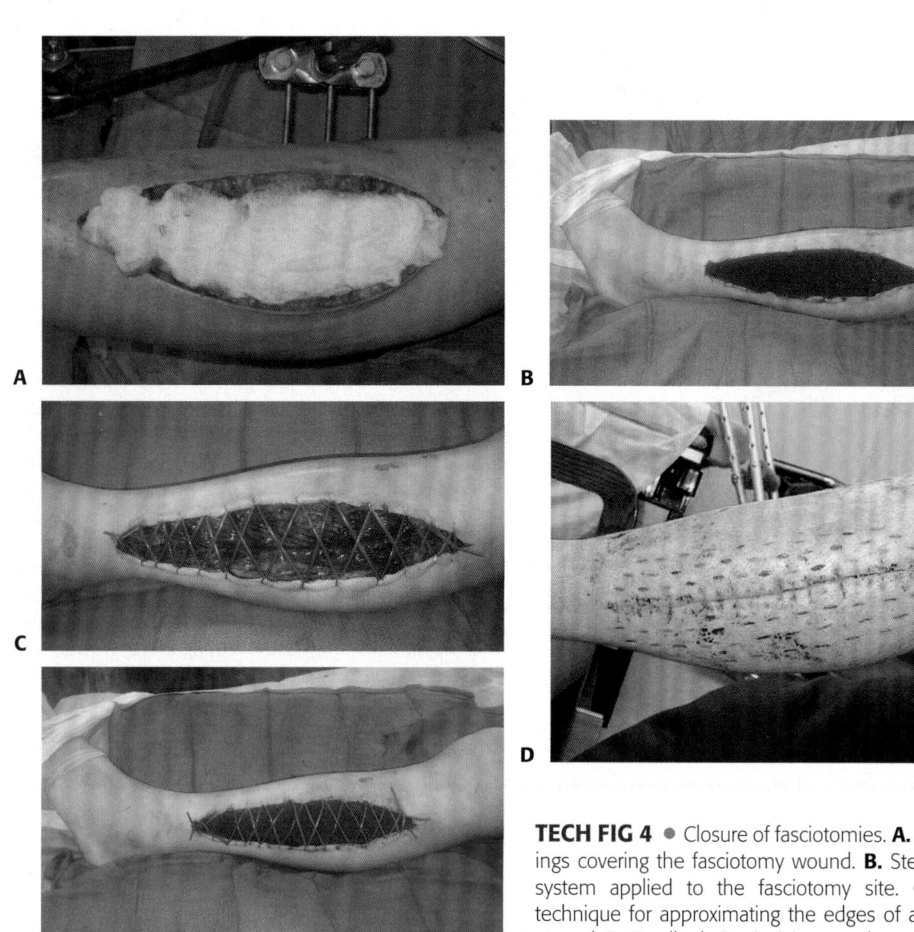

**TECH FIG 4** • Closure of fasciotomies. **A.** Moist dressings covering the fasciotomy wound. **B.** Sterile vacuum system applied to the fasciotomy site. **C.** Bootlace technique for approximating the edges of a fasciotomy wound. **D.** Small relaxing incisions made around the fasciotomy site to release tension and allow easier closure. **E.** Bootlace technique combined with sterile vacuum system.

## PEARLS AND PITFALLS

| | |
|---|---|
| **Medicolegal pitfalls** | ▪ When in doubt, the surgeon should measure and document pressure in all compartments of the involved extremity. The surgeon should clearly document in the patient's chart that the patient does not have compartment syndrome at this time if the clinical examination findings and pressures are negative.<br>▪ In 1993, the average litigation award was $280,000 for eight cases of missed compartment syndrome (in all eight cases, no compartment pressures had been measured).[37]<br>▪ The surgeon should consider the possibility of equipment error.<br>▪ Needles can be misplaced in tendons, fascia, or the wrong compartment. All pressure readings must be interpreted within the context of the clinical presentation.<br>▪ The surgeon should fully release all four compartments along with the soleal leash and posterior tibial fascia.<br>▪ No tight postoperative dressings should be used.<br>▪ Skin can cause increased pressure, so the surgeon should not close acutely. |

## POSTOPERATIVE CARE

- Once decompressed, the extremity should be covered in a bulky dressing, splinted with the foot in neutral position, and elevated above the level of the heart to promote venous drainage and reduce interstitial fluid.
  - The foot should be splinted in neutral position to prevent equinus contracture.
- The patient must be closely monitored for the systemic effects of compartment syndrome. See the discussion in the Nonoperative Management section regarding administration of supplemental oxygen, intravenous hydration, mannitol, and hyperbaric oxygen.
  - Intravenous hydration is important to help prevent rhabdomyolysis.

- The timing of skin closure varies depending on the cause and severity of compartment syndrome.
  - Most fasciotomies can be closed in 5 to 7 days.
  - If the skin is not easily closed secondarily, a split-thickness skin graft is needed to prevent excessive granulation and to lessen exposure of muscle and tendon. A flap might be needed if nerves, vessels, or bone is exposed.
  - If delayed primary closure is planned, a small relaxing incision can be made.
- Hyperbaric oxygen has been used because it reduces tissue edema through oxygen-induced vasoconstriction while maintaining and increasing oxygen perfusion.
  - However, its opponents argue that hyperbaric oxygen leads to reperfusion injury after compartment syndrome.
- Other agents that have been found to affect recovery from compartment syndrome include allopurinol and oxypurinol, superoxide dismutase, deferoxamine, and pentafraction of hydroxyethyl starch. These agents are antioxidants that scavenge for damaging free radicals.

## OUTCOMES

- Outcomes generally are poor if compartment syndrome is diagnosed and treated in a delayed fashion. Results are better with earlier treatment.
- In a study by Sheridan and Matsen,[34] 50% of patients underwent decompression within 12 hours and 50% underwent decompression after 12 hours. Sixty-eight percent of the patients who underwent decompression within 12 hours had normal leg function, whereas only 8% of the delayed group had normal function.
- If untreated, Volkmann ischemic contractures develop, leading to claw toes, weak dorsiflexors, sensory loss, chronic pain, and, eventually, amputation.
- ACS results in hospital stays that are increased threefold and hospital charges that are more than doubled. It is important in this day and age to avoid unnecessary fasciotomies.[32]

## COMPLICATIONS

- Most patients (77%) complain of altered sensation within the margins of the wound.[18]
- Forty percent report dry, scaly skin; 33% pruritus; 30% discolored skin; 25% swollen extremity; 26% tethered scars; 13% recurrent ulcerations; 13% muscle herniation; 10% pain related to the wound; and 7% tethered tendons.
- Severe prolonged tissue ischemia resulting in necrosis of the muscles leads to fibrosis of the muscles and contracture that can continue over a period of several weeks.
  - This is known as *Volkmann ischemic contracture*.
- The late sequelae of compartment syndrome are weak dorsiflexors, claw toes, sensory loss, chronic pain, and, eventually, amputation.
- Delayed fasciotomy beyond 12 hours is associated with a reported infection rate of 46% and an amputation rate of 21%.[34]
  - The complication rate associated with delayed fasciotomies is also much higher (54%) than that associated with early fasciotomies (4.5%). Therefore, the current recommendation is that if the compartment syndrome has existed for more than 24 to 48 hours and the compartment pressures are not within 30 mm Hg of diastolic pressure, supportive treatment for acute renal failure should be considered, the skin should not be violated, and plans should be made for later reconstruction.

## REFERENCES


1. Arbabi S, Brundage SI, Gentilello LM. Near-infrared spectroscopy: a potential method for continuous, transcutaneous monitoring for compartment syndrome in critically injured patients. J Trauma 1999;47: 829–833.
2. Bae DS, Kadiyala RK, Waters PM. Acute compartment syndrome in children: contemporary diagnosis, treatment, and outcome. J Pediatr Orthop 2001;21:680–688.
3. Barei DP, Nork SE, Mills WJ, et al. Complications associated with internal fixation of high-energy bicondylar tibial plateau fractures utilizing a two-incision technique. J Orthop Trauma 2004;18:649–657.
4. Bernot M, Gupta R, Dobrasz J, et al. The effect of antecedent ischemia on the tolerance of skeletal muscle to increased interstitial pressure. J Orthop Trauma 1996;10:555–559.
5. Bhattacharyya T, Vrahas MS. The medical-legal aspects of compartment syndrome. J Bone Joint Surg Am 2004;86:864–868.
6. Bible JE, McClure DJ, Mir HR. Analysis of single-incision versus dual-incision fasciotomy for tibial fractures with acute compartment syndrome. J Orthop Trauma 2013;27:607–611.
7. Blick SS, Brumback RJ, Poka A, et al. Compartment syndrome in open tibial fractures. J Bone Joint Surg Am 1986;68:1348–1353.
8. Dunwoody JM, Reichert CC, Brown KL. Compartment syndrome associated with bupivacaine and fentanyl epidural analgesia in pediatric orthopaedics. J Pediatr Orthop 1997;17:285–288.
9. Egol KA, Tejwani NC, Capla EL, et al. Staged management of high-energy proximal tibia fractures (OTA types 41): the results of a prospective, standardized protocol. J Orthop Trauma 2005;19:448–455.
10. Hargens AR, Romine JS, Sipe JC, et al. Peripheral nerve-conduction block by high muscle-compartment pressure. J Bone Joint Surg Am 1979;61:192–200.
11. Hargens AR, Schmidt DA, Evans KL, et al. Quantitation of skeletal-muscle necrosis in a model compartment syndrome. J Bone Joint Surg Am 1981;63:631–636.
12. Heppenstall RB, McCombs PR, DeLaurentis DA. Vascular injuries and compartment syndromes. In: Bucholz RW, Heckman JD, eds. Rockwood and Green's Fractures in Adults, vol 1, ed 5. Philadelphia: Lippincott Williams & Wilkins, 2001:331–352.
13. Heppenstall RB, Scott R, Sapega A, et al. A comparative study of the tolerance of skeletal muscle to ischemia: tourniquet application compared with acute compartment syndrome. J Bone Joint Surg Am 1986;68:820–828.
14. Jennische E. Ischemia-induced injury in glycogen-depleted skeletal muscle: selective vulnerability of the FG-fibres. Acta Physiol Scand 1985;125:727–734.
15. Kakar S, Firoozabadi R, McKean J, et al. Diastolic blood pressure in patients with tibia fractures under anesthesia: implications for the diagnosis of compartment syndrome. J Orthop Trauma 2007;21:99–103.
16. Kelly RP, Whitesides TE Jr. Transfibular route for fasciotomy of the leg. J Bone Joint Surg Am 1967;49:1022–1023.
17. Lindsay TF, Liauw S, Romaschin AD, et al. The effect of ischemia/reperfusion on adenine nucleotide metabolism and xanthine oxidase production in skeletal muscle. J Vasc Surg 1990;12:8–15.
18. McQueen MM, Christie J, Court-Brown CM. Acute compartment syndrome in tibial diaphyseal fractures. J Bone Joint Surg Br 1996;78:95–98.
19. McQueen MM, Gaston P, Court-Brown CM. Acute compartment syndrome: who is at risk? J Bone Joint Surg Br 2000;82:200–203.
20. Meskey T, Hardcastle J, O'Toole RV. Are certain fractures at increased risk for compartment syndrome after civilian ballistic injury? J Trauma 2011;71:1385–1389.
21. Moed BR, Thorderson PK. Measurement of intracompartmental pressure: a comparison of the slit catheter, side-ported needle, and simple needle. J Bone Joint Surg Am 1993;75:231–235.
22. Morrow BC, Mawhinney IN, Elliott JR. Tibial compartment syndrome complicating closed femoral nailing: diagnosis delayed by an epidural analgesic technique: case report. J Trauma 1994;37:867–868.

23. Mubarak SJ, Wilton NC. Compartment syndrome and epidural analgesia. J Pediatr Orthop 1997;17:282–284.
24. Olson SA, Glasgow RR. Acute compartment syndrome in lower extremity musculoskeletal trauma. J Am Acad Orthop Surg 2005;13:436–444.
25. O'Toole RV, Whitney A, Merchant N, et al. Variation in diagnosis of compartment syndrome by surgeons treating tibial shaft fractures. J Trauma 2009;67:735–741.
26. Park S, Ahn J, Gee AO, et al. Compartment syndrome in tibial fractures. J Orthop Trauma 2009;23:514–518.
27. Prayson MJ, Chen JL, Hampers D, et al. Baseline compartment pressure measurements in isolated lower extremity fractures without clinical compartment syndrome. J Trauma 2006;60:1037–1040.
28. Reisman WM, Shuler MS, Kinsey TL, et al. Relationship between near infrared spectroscopy and intra-compartmental pressures. J Emerg Med 2013:44:292–298.
29. Rorabeck CH. The treatment of compartment syndromes of the leg. J Bone Joint Surg Br 1984;66:93–97.
30. Rorabeck CH, Clarke KM. The pathophysiology of anterior tibial compartment syndrome: an experimental investigation. J Trauma 1978;18:299–304.
31. Rorabeck CH, Macnab L. Anterior tibial-compartment syndrome complicating fractures of the shaft of the tibia. J Bone Joint Surg Am 1976;58:549–550.
32. Schmidt AH. The impact of compartment syndrome on hospital length of stay and charges among adult patients admitted with a fracture of the tibia. J Orthop Trauma 2011;25:355–357.
33. Shah SN, Karunaker MA. Early wound complication after operative treatment of high energy tibial plateau fractures through two incisions. Bull NYU Hosp Jt Dis 2007;65:115–119.
34. Sheridan GW, Matsen FA III. Fasciotomy in the treatment of the acute compartment syndrome. J Bone Joint Surg Am 1976;58:112–115.
35. Shuler FD, Dietz MJ. Physicians' ability to manually detect isolated elevations in leg intracompartmental pressure. J Bone Joint Surg Am 2010;92:361–367.
36. Stark E, Stucken C, Trainer G, et al. Compartment syndrome in Schatzker type VI plateau fractures and medial condylar fracture-dislocations treated with temporary external fixation. J Orthop Trauma 2009;23:502–506.
37. Templeman D, Varecka T, Schmidt R. Economic costs of missed compartment syndromes. Presented at the Annual Meeting of the American Academy of Orthopaedic Surgeons, San Francisco, 1993.
38. Ulmer T. The clinical diagnosis of compartment syndrome of the lower leg: are clinical findings predictive of the disorder? J Orthop Trauma 2002;16:572–577.
39. Valdez C, Schroeder E, Amdur R, et al. Serum creatine kinase levels are associated with extremity compartment syndrome. J Trauma Acute Care Surg 2013;74:441–445.
40. Whitesides TE, Heckman MM. Acute compartment syndrome: update on diagnosis and treatment. J Am Acad Orthop Surg 1996;4:209–218.
41. Whitney A, O'Toole RV, Hui E, et al. Do one-time intracompartmental pressure measurements have a high false positive rate in diagnosing compartment syndrome? J Trauma 2014;76(2):479–483.
42. Wiger P, Blomqvist G, Styf J. Wound closure by dermatotraction after fasciotomy for acute compartment syndrome. Scand J Plast Reconstr Surg Hand Surg 2000;34:315–320.
43. Wind TC, Saunders SM, Barfield WR, et al. Compartment syndrome after low-energy tibia fractures sustained during athletic competition. J Orthop Trauma 2012;26:33–36.

# Elbow Arthroscopy for Panner Disease and Osteochondritis Dissecans

Theodore J. Ganley, Christine M. Goodbody, J. Todd R. Lawrence, and R. Jay Lee

## DEFINITION

### Panner Disease

- Panner disease is a condition in which there is compromised subchondral bone, potentially due to repetitive microtrauma and diminished blood supply to the developing ossific nucleus within the distal humerus chondral epiphysis in preadolescents.[9]
- Those affected are typically 6 to 10 years old, and symptoms usually respond to a reduction of the offending repetitive microtrauma.[9]

### Osteochondritis Dissecans of the Capitellum

- This term is used to describe the condition of compromised subchondral bone in the capitellum of adolescents, which can lead to secondary articular surface separation.[8]
- Osteochondritis dissecans (OCD) of the capitellum is most commonly seen in children ages 10 to 17 years old, particularly those who engage in overhead throwing sports and activities in which the elbow serves as a load-bearing joint.

## ANATOMY

- The three articulations in the elbow are the ulnohumeral joint, the radiocapitellar joint, and the proximal radioulnar joint.
- The ulnohumeral joint is a hinge joint that allows for flexion and extension of the elbow, whereas the radiocapitellar and radioulnar joints are trochoid joints that allow for axial rotation and pivoting of the elbow.
- The capitellum articulates with the rim of the radial head throughout flexion–extension and pronation–supination.
- Secondary ossification centers are involved in the formation of the distal humerus, proximal radius, and ulna. The ossification center of the capitellum appears at 18 months and completely fuses by age 14 years.
- Descending extraosseous branches of the brachial artery supply the capitellum. Chondral vessels supply the osseous nucleus, which in turn supplies the chondroepiphysis.

## PATHOGENESIS

- It is theorized that both Panner disease and OCD of the capitellum arise from repetitive submaximal stresses, which in summation result in abnormal valgus forces exerted across the radiocapitellar joint.[3,4,11,13]
- The result of this abnormal stress on the radiocapitellar joint may depend on the age of the patient, with those exposed to the stress at a younger age (6 to 10 years) developing Panner disease and those exposed to the stress at a later age (10 to 17 years) developing OCD of the capitellum.
- The development of the lesions also depends on the limited blood supply of the capitellum, which allows for limited repair potential.

## NATURAL HISTORY

- With activity restriction, reossification and resolution of symptoms typically occur in Panner disease.[7]
- The natural history of OCD is articular surface separation for patients who do not restrict their activities. Even with activity modification and brief periods of immobilization, elbow OCD lesions will progress in most patients treated nonoperatively.
- In OCD of the capitellum, radiographs will initially show irregularity and fragmentation of the capitellum. Erosion, lysis, and sclerosis may be observed in later stages.

## PATIENT HISTORY AND PHYSICAL FINDINGS

- Early stages
  - Patients have full motion but complain of vague aching lateral elbow discomfort during throwing and load-bearing activities as well as swelling at the lateral elbow. They typically have full range of motion.
  - Synovitis: occasional mild palpable effusion
- Later stages: Patients complain of mechanical symptoms, including locking and catching, and limited flexion and extension.
  - Examination may reveal palpable synovial thickening, elbow effusion, decreased range of motion, and tenderness over the radiocapitellar joint.

## IMAGING AND OTHER DIAGNOSTIC STUDIES

- Anteroposterior (AP) and lateral radiographs of the elbow are needed to evaluate both conditions. In Panner disease, the size of the ossific nucleus and the degree of radiolucency can be determined from the radiographs. In OCD lesions, fragmentation, erosion, subchondral lysis, or cystic changes may be seen on radiographs (**FIG 1A**).
- Magnetic resonance imaging (MRI) findings in OCD may reveal bone edema, synovitis, and loose bodies as well as subchondral and cartilage separation (**FIG 1B**).

## DIFFERENTIAL DIAGNOSIS

- Familial OCD
- Hemophilia and variants
- Multiple epiphyseal dysplasia

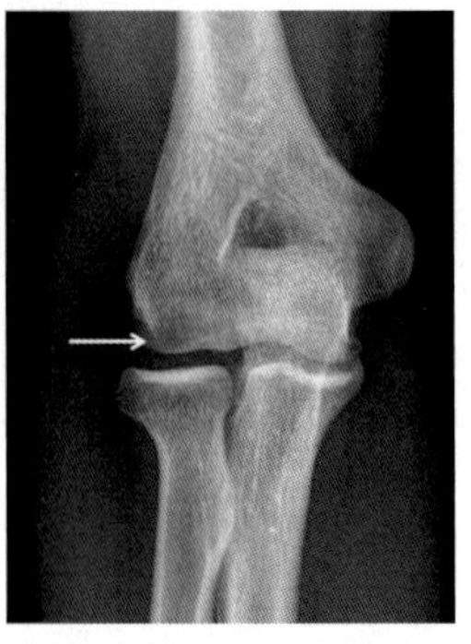

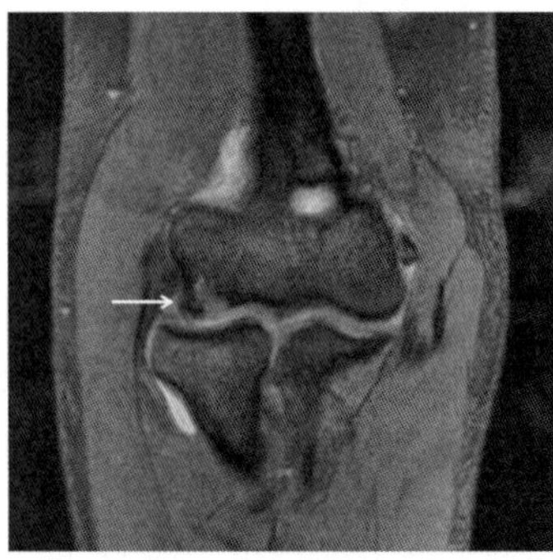

**FIG 1** • **A.** AP radiograph of the elbow showing an area of subchondral lysis in the capitellum, representing a large osteochondral lesion (*arrow*). **B.** MRI image showing the same OCD lesion of the capitellum with subchondral separation (*arrow*).

- Autoimmune vasculitis
- Steroid-induced avascular necrosis

## NONOPERATIVE MANAGEMENT

- Treatment for Panner disease consists of the following:
  - Sling for 4 to 6 weeks
  - Range-of-motion exercises
  - Cessation of all offending activity
  - Follow-up radiographs through resorption and reconstitution phases at 3-month intervals prior to resumption of sport-specific exercises.
- Nonoperative treatment of OCD is reserved for cases in which the cartilage is intact. It consists of the following:
  - Immobilization in a posterior splint or sling for 6 weeks
  - Removal of the splint or sling for a few minutes several times per day to perform range-of-motion exercises
  - Rest until symptoms resolve
  - Follow-up radiographs through resorption and reconstitution phases prior to resumption of sport-specific exercises

## SURGICAL MANAGEMENT

- Surgical management is largely dependent on the character of the lytic lesion (stable vs. unstable, intact vs. partially or completely detached articular cartilage) and the presence or absence of symptoms.
- Surgery is generally reserved for unstable lesions with partially or completely detached articular cartilage.
- Persistent pain and swelling despite intact cartilage may warrant arthroscopic evaluation with a search for loose bodies as well as consideration of lesion drilling to stimulate subchondral bone healing.

### Preoperative Planning

- All imaging studies obtained before surgery should be reviewed. An MRI may be helpful to determine the extent of the lesion and the location and size of chondral or small osteochondral loose bodies in the joint.
- A thorough physical examination should be performed under anesthesia to note range of motion and appropriate or pathologic degrees of laxity.

### Positioning

- The patient is adequately padded and placed in the lateral decubitus position.
- The involved elbow is placed over a padded bump that places the elbow in 90 degrees of flexion.
- The extremity is then prepared and draped, allowing unhindered flexion and extension of the elbow and internal and external rotation of the shoulder (**FIG 2A**).
- The landmarks over the elbow are marked (**FIG 2B**).

### Approach

- Arthroscopy-assisted miniarthrotomy (Children's Hospital of Philadelphia approach) is used for large to massive loose bodies and osteochondral defects.
- After the patient is positioned, prepared, and draped and the anatomic landmarks are identified, a 3- to 5-cm incision is carried over the capitellum (**FIG 2C**).
- The incision is carried down to the fascia, and the plane between the anconeus and the extensor carpi ulnaris is identified and entered.
- Alternatively, if during the course of arthroscopy a larger incision is required, then the superior and inferior arthroscopy

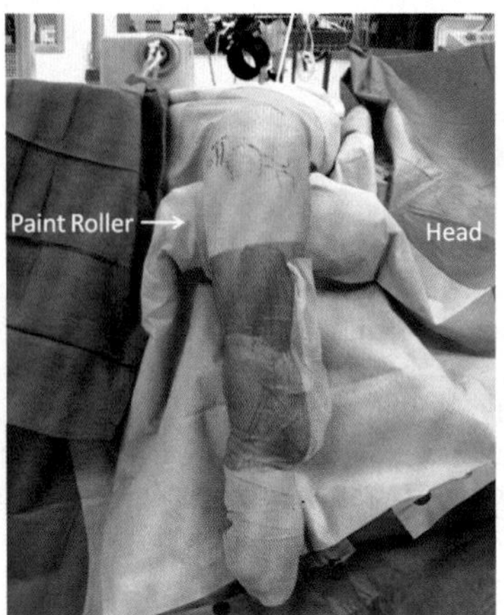


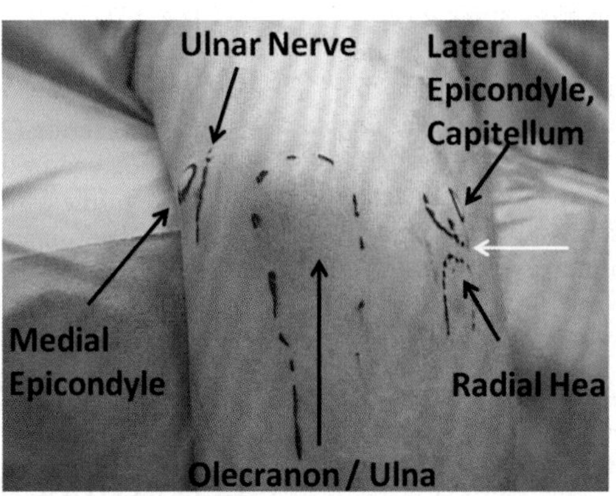


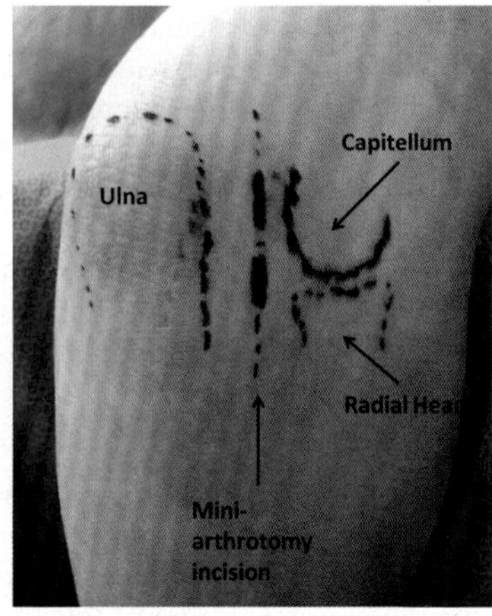


**FIG 2** • **A.** The patient is positioned in the lateral decubitus position with the elbow in 90 degrees of flexion over a paint roller. **B.** The landmarks, including the path of the ulnar nerve located posterior to the medial epicondyle, as well as the radiocapitellar interval (*white arrow*), and the olecranon are identified with a marking pen. **C.** Both the incision for the arthroscopy-assisted miniarthrotomy approach (*dashed line*) and the incision for arthroscopy portals only (*solid portion of line*) are marked out of the skin.

portals can be incorporated into an incision of 1.5 cm. Again, the deep dissection can be in the plane of the anconeus–extensor carpi ulnaris interval.

- For both miniarthrotomy and connecting the superior and inferior arthroscopy portals, care is taken to avoid the annular ligament during the deep dissection. Then, the joint capsule is incised to allow adequate visualization of the lesion.
- A 30-degree arthroscope is then inserted and used to view the joint surface. The arthroscope is placed on the outer border of the radiocapitellar joint and angled to allow a complete view of the capitellum and radiocapitellar interval.

TECHNIQUES

## Arthroscopic Treatment

- The patient is positioned, prepared, and draped in a lateral decubitus position as previously described.
- After the landmarks in the elbow are drawn with a marking pen and the tourniquet is inflated, 15 mL of sterile saline is injected into the joint, depending on the size of the patient.
- A smaller set of instruments (2.9 mm) is used.
- The arthroscopic portals are identified using the palpable landmarks (**TECH FIG 1A**).
    - In the soft spot between the lateral epicondyle or capitellum and radial head laterally and olecranon medially, a position equidistant from the lateral epicondyle or capitellum or radial head is marked.
    - Just inferior to this position is the location of the inferior lateral coaxial portal, and just superior to this position is the location of the superior lateral coaxial portal.
- The inferior lateral coaxial portal is created first. A no. 15 scalpel is brought through the skin and subcutaneous tissues. A hemostat is used to enter the capsule bluntly. If there is the potential for creating a miniarthrotomy, the skin incision should be oriented so that it would easily connect with the superior portal.
- The arthroscope is inserted, and a careful and thorough inspection of the elbow is performed, examining the chondral surfaces of the radial head and capitellum, An 18-gauge needle may be placed into the olecranon fossa under direct visualization to act as an outflow (**TECH FIG 1B,C**).
- A portal 1 cm superior to the initial portal is made under direct visualization for insertion of graspers and shavers. A spinal needle is used to confirm the location and trajectory, and again, a no. 15 blade is used as before to incise the skin.
- Definitive management depends on the intraoperative findings.
    - For stable and intact lesions, we prefer drilling of the lesion to stimulate healing.
    - For unstable lesions that are partially detached or "hinged" with appropriate subchondral bone, we prefer screw fixation.
    - For completely detached lesions that are contained defects, we prefer marrow stimulation.
    - For completely detached lesions that are uncontained, we prefer osteochondral autograft transfer through an arthroscopic-assisted miniarthrotomy. The osteochondral transplant procedure is described elsewhere in this textbook (check Index).

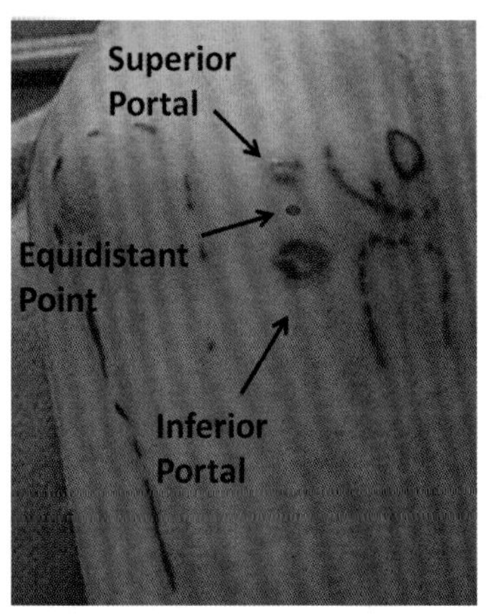


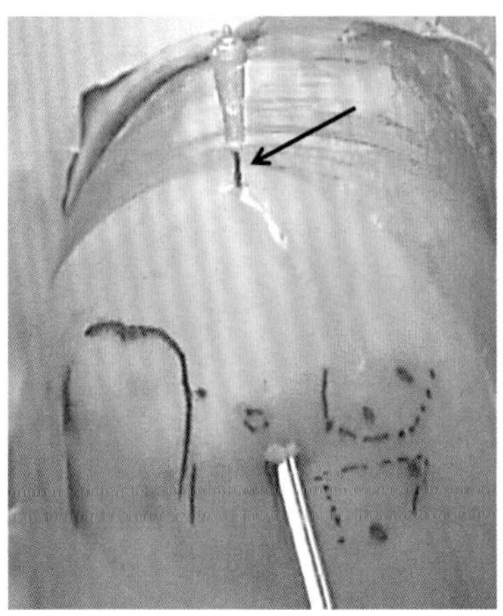


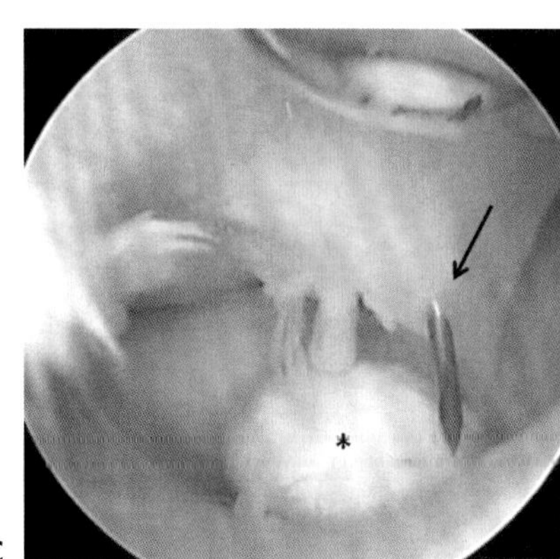


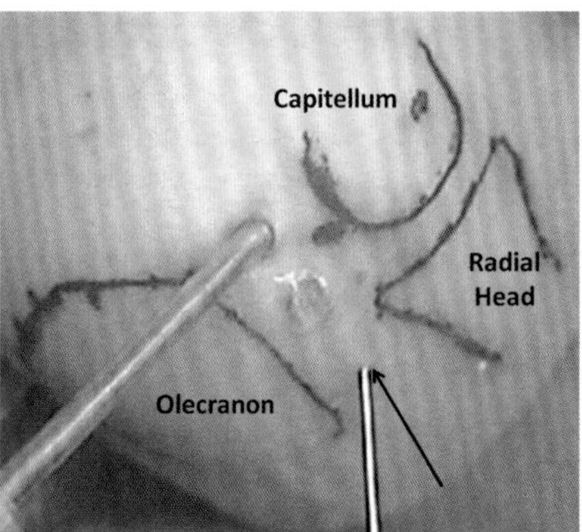


**TECH FIG 1** • **A.** The arthroscopic portals are identified, just superior and inferior to an equidi stant point. **B,C.** The arthroscope is placed through the inferior lateral portal, and an 18-gauge needle placed into the olecranon fossa can be used as both an outflow portal (*arrow* in **B**) and as an instrument to secure loose bodies (*asterisk* in **C**) to prevent them from migrating (*arrow* in **C**). **D.** Drilling is performed through the inferior percutaneous approach with a 0.62-mm Kirschner wire (*arrow*). At times, it is helpful to place the wire percutaneously and flex the elbow to ensure that it is always placed perpendicular to the surface of the capitellum. Care is taken to use a posterior starting point to avoid the posterior interosseous nerve.

### Cartilage Stable and Intact

- Drilling of the lesion is performed to stimulate healing.
- A 0.62 or 0.45-mm Kirschner wire is used to drill into the subchondral bone. Drilling is performed as perpendicular to the capitellum as possible, in a distal to proximal direction. The Kirschner wire may be placed through the inferior portal or via an inferior percutaneous approach distal and posterior to the inferior portal.
  - For the inferior percutaneous approach, the entry point is between the radial head-neck junction and olecranon. The wire is biased toward the olecranon and away from radius to avoid the posterior interosseous nerve (**TECH FIG 1D**).
- After satisfactory bleeding is obtained, final inspection of the area is performed and the arthroscope is removed, and the wounds are closed using no. 4-0 Monocryl subcuticular sutures, followed by Steri-Strips.
- A sterile dressing and a posterior splint are applied.

### Cartilage Unstable and Partially Detached or "Hinged" with Appropriate Subchondral Bone

- Débridement and fixation of the lesion is performed to both stimulate healing and provide stability for healing.
- After thorough inspection of the joint, the lesion is explored.
- For lesions with appropriate viable subchondral bone, the lesion can be secured with compression screws arthroscopically.
- For lesions with underlying granulation tissue or nonviable bone, this can be débrided to a healthy subchondral base for healing.
  - If a bony defect is present after débridement, bone grafting and fixation via arthrotomy may be necessary.
- For lesions with fractured cartilage, without healthy subchondral bone, the fractured hinged piece is removed, and salvage procedures such as marrow stimulation and osteochondral transplant are performed.

### Cartilage Completely Detached from a Contained Lesion

- Curettage and drilling of the lesion is performed to stimulate formation of fibrocartilage.
- After thorough inspection of the joint is performed, any loose bodies found within the joint are removed.
- The defect is identified, and curettage of the defect is performed to remove all granulation tissue and to ensure that a stable rim of cartilage exists circumferentially (**TECH FIG 2A,B**).
- The underlying sclerotic bone is exposed.
- Drilling of the lesion is performed using a 0.62 or 0.45-mm Kirschner wire. Drilling is performed as perpendicular to the capitellum as possible, in a distal to proximal direction. The previously described inferior percutaneous approach is performed (see **TECH FIG 1D**).
- Final inspection of the area is performed and the arthroscope is removed, and the wounds are closed using no. 4-0 Monocryl subcuticular sutures, followed by Steri-Strips.
- A sterile dressing and a posterior splint are applied.

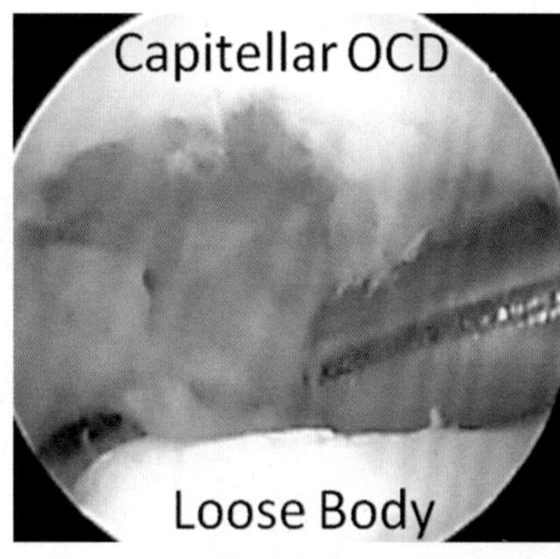


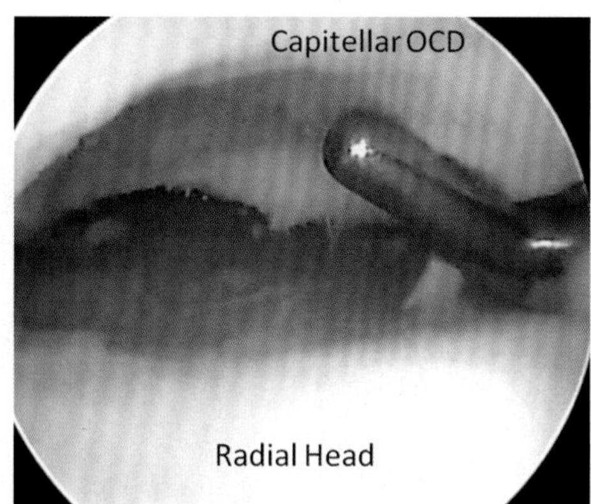


**TECH FIG 2 • A,B.** A capitellar OCD débrided back to a stable base.

## Arthroscopic-Assisted Miniarthrotomy

- The patient is positioned, prepared, and draped as previously described.
- The miniarthrotomy approach is carried through the plane of the anconeus and extensor carpi ulnaris. The capsule is incised to access the lesion (**TECH FIG 3A**).[9]
- A 30-degree arthroscope is inserted through the arthrotomy site to view and assess the entire lesion (**TECH FIG 3B**).
- The arthroscope can be used to assess the portions of the capitellum not clearly visualized through the arthrotomy site, much like a dental mirror (**TECH FIG 3C**).
- Once the entire lesion is visualized and assessed, removal of any loose bodies is performed, with débridement and drilling of the lesion with Kirschner wires as described in the arthroscopic technique.
  - For massive or uncontained lesions, osteochondral transplant can be performed (**TECH FIG 3D**).
- Final inspection of the area is performed and the arthroscope is removed.
- The capsule is repaired. A layer-by-layer closure is then performed.
- A sterile dressing and a posterior splint are applied.

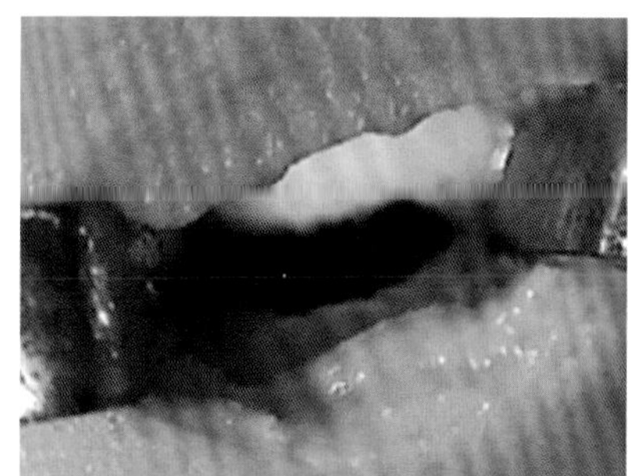

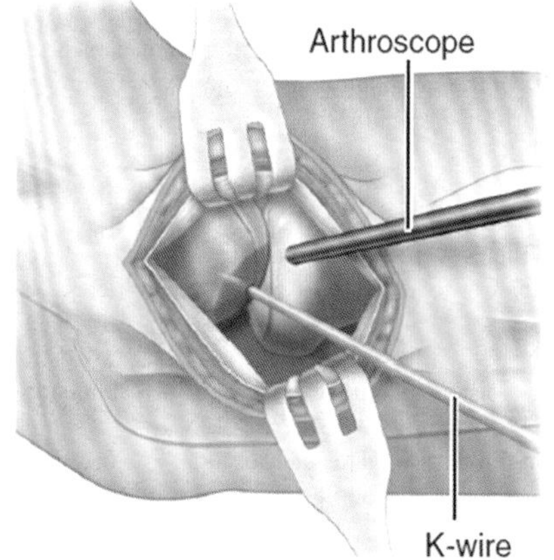


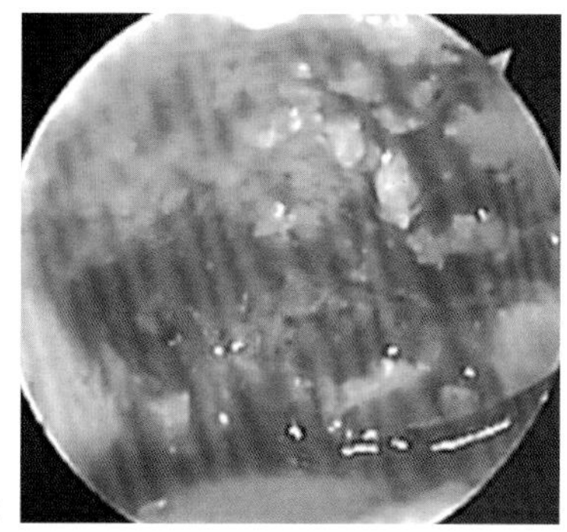

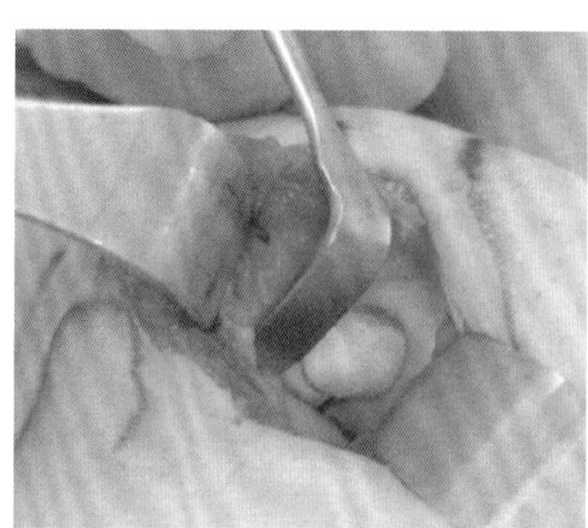

**TECH FIG 3 • A.** For massive lesions and loose bodies, a miniarthrotomy can be performed through the plane of the anconeus and extensor carpi ulnaris. **B.** A 30-degree arthroscope is inserted, and the lesion is identified. When a miniarthrotomy is performed, the arthroscope can be used like a dental mirror to enhance visualization and minimize the need for extensive open dissection. **C.** The arthroscopic view of the prepared lesional bed. **D.** Image of the elbow demonstrating an uncontained lesion treated with multiple osteochondral grafts.

## PEARLS AND PITFALLS

| | |
|---|---|
| **Surgical technique** | ■ When performing the miniarthrotomy, posterior dissection of the capitellum is avoided to prevent devascularization. |
| **Drilling of the lesion** | ■ When drilling the lesion, the Kirschner wires should be maintained perpendicular to the capitellum. They may be inserted through the inferior portal with the elbow flexed or through a portal placed distal to the radiocapitellar joint. Care should be taken to place this adjacent ulna and not the radial head to avoid injury to the posterior interosseous nerve. |
| **Arthroscopic technique** | ■ The bony landmarks and the location of the ulnar nerve are drawn carefully before the procedure to avoid inadvertent neurovascular injury. Draping the hand free also allows for more flexibility in the procedure. |

## POSTOPERATIVE CARE

- For stable and intact lesions where drilling is performed, strengthening and range of motion are the early goals of therapy. A gradual return to activity and axial loading is permitted, as healing is seen radiographically.
- For unstable and detached lesions where fixation is performed and for full-thickness defects where marrow stimulation is performed, a sling is used and early-assisted motion is instituted. Patients are sent to physical therapy to ensure appropriate elbow range of motion and core strengthening, although impact loading of the elbow is avoided. After 6 weeks, a gradual return to activity of daily living is instituted; however, axial loading, impact loading, and throwing are prohibited for up to 6 months.

## OUTCOMES

- Panner disease
  - Full recovery is expected in 12 to 18 months, but long-term noncompliance can result in lesion progression.
- OCD of the capitellum
  - The arthroscopic-assisted miniarthrotomy procedure described has demonstrated promising midterm results. Twenty-five patients, 10 with arthroscopic débridement and drilling alone and 12 requiring miniarthrotomies for bone grafting or loose body removal, were shown at 48 months postoperatively to have gained an average of 17 degrees of extension and 10 degrees of flexion compared to their preoperative range of motion.[6] Average elbow function rating using the Single Assessment Numerical Evaluation score (0% to 100%) was 87%. Eighteen out of 21 patients returned to sport at their preinjury level.
  - Ruch and coworkers[10] reported on 12 patients treated for OCD of the capitellum by arthroscopic débridement; 11 of them were highly satisfied. The average age was 14.5 years and the average follow-up was 3.2 years. Clinical presentation showed a contracture improvement from 23 degrees to 10 degrees.

- Byrd and Jones[2] reported on 10 baseball players treated for OCD of the capitellum by arthroscopic débridement; 4 of them were able to resume playing competitively. The average age was 14.5 years, and the average follow-up was 3.9 years. However, in this study, the outcomes were poorly correlated with the lesion grade.
- Baumgarten and associates[1] reported on 14 young athletes (gymnastics or throwing sports) whose OCD of the capitellum was treated by arthroscopic débridement. Three were forced to give up their sport. The average age was 13.8 years, and the average follow-up was 4 years. In this review, contracture was noted to improve by 14 degrees.
- Shimada et al[12] reported on 26 patients with advanced OCD of the capitellum treated by cylindrical costal osteochondral autograft, with an average follow-up of 36 months. All patients had rapid functional recovery and returned to sport. Extension improved by 7 degrees and flexion by 13 degrees postoperatively. Five patients required minor additional procedures such as screw removal, loose body removal, and articulate cartilage shaving, but all remaining patients showed full recovery within 1 year.
- Iwasaki et al[5] described 19 male athletes who underwent autologous osteochondral transfer for capitellar OCD. Mean total arc of elbow motion improved by an average of 16 degrees. All patients except one had a good or excellent clinical result, and all but two returned to their prior level of sport.

## COMPLICATIONS

- Angular deformity
- Avascular necrosis of the capitellum
- Detachment and capitellum overgrowth
- Early arthritis

## REFERENCES


1. Baumgarten TE, Andrews JR, Satterwhite YE. The arthroscopic classification and treatment of osteochondritis dissecans of the capitellum. Am J Sports Med 1998;26:520–523.
2. Byrd JW, Jones KS. Arthroscopic surgery for isolated capitellar osteochondritis dissecans in adolescent baseball players: minimum three-year follow-up. Am J Sports Med 2002;30:474–478.
3. Douglas G, Rang M. The role of trauma in the pathogenesis of the osteochondroses. Clin Orthop Relat Res 1981;(158):28–32.
4. Duthie RB, Houghton GR. Constitutional aspects of the osteochondroses. Clin Orthop Relat Res 1981;(158):19–27.
5. Iwasaki N, Kato H, Ishikawa J, et al. Autologous osteochondral mosaicplasty for osteochondritis dissecans of the elbow in teenage athletes: surgical technique. J Bone Joint Surg Am 2010;92(suppl 1, pt 2): 208–216.
6. Jones KJ, Wiesel BB, Sankar WN, et al. Arthroscopic management of osteochondritis dissecans of the capitellum: mid-term results in adolescent athletes. J Pediatr Orthop 2010;30(1):8–13.
7. Kobayashi K, Burton KJ, Rodner C, et al. Lateral compression injuries in the pediatric elbow: Panner's disease and osteochondritis dissecans of the capitellum. J Am Acad Orthop Surg 2004;12:246–254.
8. Krijnen MR, Lim L, Willems WJ. Arthroscopic treatment of osteochondritis dissecans of the capitellum: report of 5 female athletes. Arthroscopy 2003;19:210–214.
9. Pill SG, Ganley TJ, Flynn JM, et al. Osteochondritis dissecans of the capitellum: arthroscopic-assisted treatment of large, full-thickness defects in young patients. Arthroscopy 2003;19:222–225.
10. Ruch DS, Cory JW, Poehling GG. The arthroscopic management of osteochondritis dissecans of the adolescent elbow. Arthroscopy 1998;14:797–803.
11. Ruch DS, Poehling GG. Arthroscopic treatment of Panner's disease. Clin Sports Med 1991;10:629–636.
12. Shimada K, Tanaka H, Matsumoto T, et al. Cylindrical costal osteochondral autograft for reconstruction of large defects of the capitellum due to osteochondritis dissecans. J Bone Joint Surg Am 2012;94:992–1002.
13. Singer KM, Roy SP. Osteochondrosis of the humeral capitellum. Am J Sports Med 1984;12:351–360.

# Arthroscopic Treatment of Elbow Loss of Motion

Laith M. Al-Shihabi, Chris Mellano, Robert W. Wysocki, and Anthony A. Romeo

## DEFINITION

- Loss of motion is a common sequela of elbow trauma or the natural progression of nontraumatic conditions of the elbow, significantly impairing function of the upper extremity and hindering performance of activities of daily living (ADLs).
  - A functional arc of 100 degrees (30 to 130 degrees) in flexion and extension, along with 100 degrees in pronation and supination (50 degrees each), is required for most ADLs.[19]
  - Neighboring joints offer little compensatory function, making elbow stiffness poorly tolerated.
- Stiffness may be due to intrinsic (intra-articular) or extrinsic (extra-articular) causes (Table 1) or a combination of both.[6,14]
- Posttraumatic stiffness is most common, but osteoarthritis, inflammatory conditions, systemic injuries (head trauma), and neurologic disorders may also cause elbow joint contractures.
- Loss of extension is most common, although loss of flexion is more poorly tolerated due to an inability to reach the face for eating or grooming.[18]
- The key to treatment is identifying and correcting the functional and occupational impairment; decisions should not be based solely on the absolute loss of motion of the elbow.[11]
- Arthroscopic treatment of elbow stiffness is intended to restore motion, function, and relieve pain when present.[23]

**Table 1 Classification of Elbow Stiffness Based on Location of Structure in Relation to the Elbow Joint**

| Type | Location | Description |
|---|---|---|
| Intrinsic | Within the elbow joint | Articular incongruity after fracture, degenerative changes and loss of cartilage, intra-articular adhesions, loose bodies, synovitis, infection |
| Extrinsic | Tissues immediately adjacent | Soft tissue and capsular contracture, muscle fibrosis (brachialis especially), collateral ligament stiffness, to the elbow joint heterotopic ossification, skin contractures |
| Peripheral | Factors anatomically separate from the elbow | Stroke, neurologic problems, peripheral nerve disorder, head injury, cerebral palsy |

From Jupiter JB, O'Driscoll SW, Cohen MS. The assessment and management of the stiff elbow. AAOS Instr Course Lect 2003;52:93–111.

- Arthroscopic treatments may range from capsular release alone to osteocapsular arthroplasty, including the removal of loose bodies, osteophytes, and capsulectomy.[22]

## ANATOMY

- The elbow is anatomically predisposed to stiffness by virtue of the close relationship of the capsule to the surrounding ligaments and muscles, along with the presence of three joints within a synovial-lined joint cavity—(a hinge ginglymus) ulnohumeral articulation and rotatory (trochoid) radiocapitellar and radioulnar joints.[11]
- The anterior elbow capsule attaches proximally above the coronoid fossa and distally extends to the coronoid medially and annular ligament laterally. The posterior capsule starts proximally just above the olecranon fossa and inserts at the articular margin of the sigmoid notch and annular ligament (**FIG 1**).
- The anterior capsule is taut in extension and lax in flexion, with strength derived from the cruciate orientation of its fibers.
- The greatest capsular capacity is at 80 degrees flexion.[9,24] The normal capacity of 25 mL can be reduced to as little as 6 mL in a contracted state.[9,24]
- The joint capsule is innervated by branches from all the major nerves crossing the joint along with the musculocutaneous nerve.[16]
- The cubital tunnel, which houses the ulnar nerve at the elbow, becomes compressed in flexion (due to stretching of the retinaculum between the olecranon and medial epicondyle) and loosens in extension.
- Flexion contractures may adversely compress the ulnar nerve, leading to ulnar neuropathy (**FIG 2**).

## PATHOGENESIS

- O'Driscoll[23] describes four stages of posttraumatic elbow stiffness:
  - Bleeding: minutes to hours
  - Edema: hours to days. Both bleeding and edema cause swelling within the joint and surrounding tissues, and the capsule become biomechanically less compliant. Early elbow range of motion through an entire range during stages 1 and 2 can help prevent stiffness.
  - Granulation tissue: days to weeks. Splints can be used to regain range of motion.
  - Fibrosis: Maturation of the granulation tissue further decreases compliance. More aggressive splinting is necessary, along with possible surgical management.

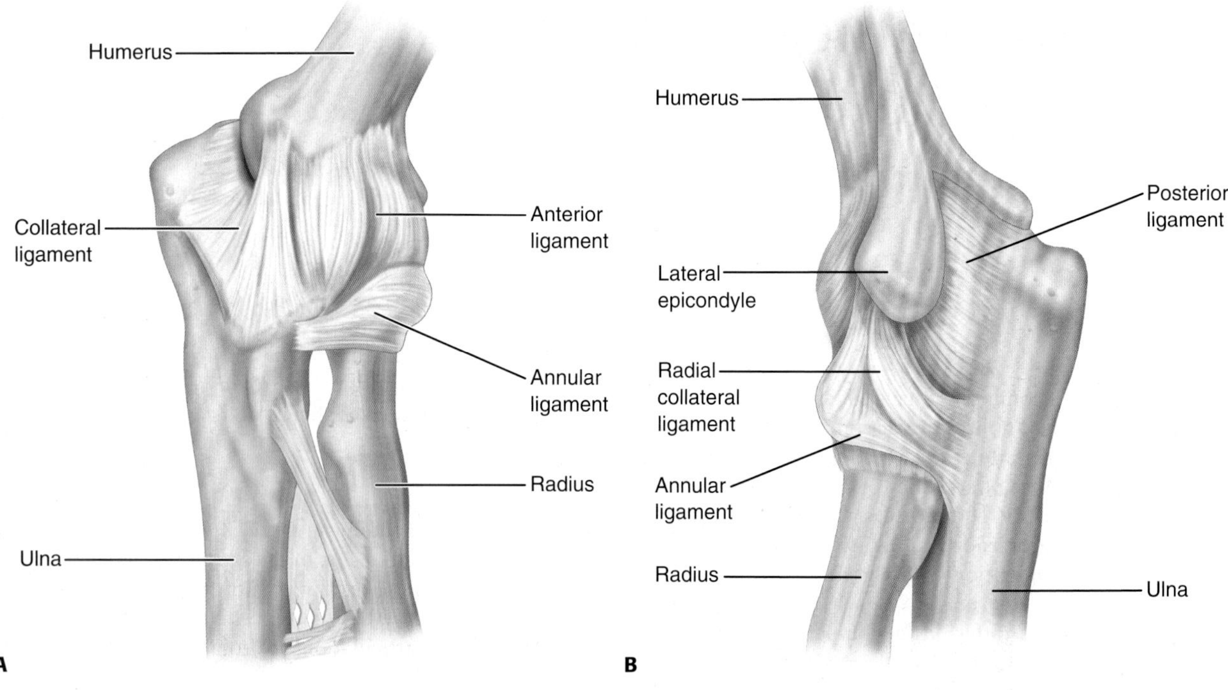


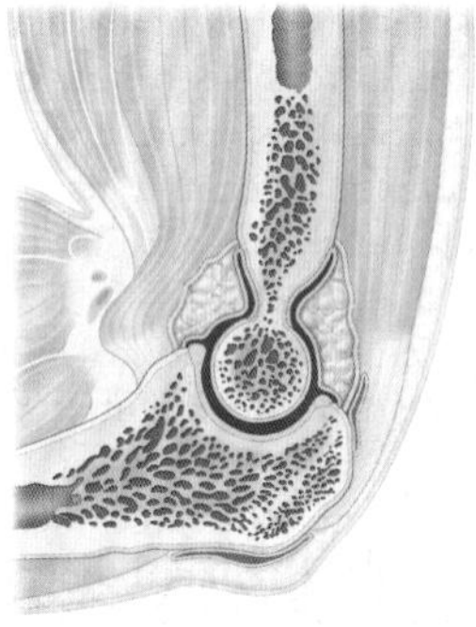


**FIG 1** • Anatomic drawing of elbow capsular structures. The anterior (**A**) and posterior capsular areas (**B**) are highlighted. The anterior capsule distally extends to the coronoid medially and annular ligament laterally. **C.** Lateral diagram of the elbow shows the capsular size and fat pad.

- The posttraumatic joint capsule is sensitive to contracture, secondary to an increase in disorganized collagen fiber deposition at the cellular level, resulting in thickening that translates into loss of flexibility and joint volume.[9,16,23]
- The reasons for altered capsular properties are multifactorial and not completely known.
  - Myofibroblasts, cells that enhance collagen production and tissue contraction, increase in number in the posttraumatic anterior capsule.[10]
  - Collagen formation, cross-linking, and hypertrophy increase while water and proteoglycan content decrease in the contracted elbow tissue.[1]
  - Increased matrix metalloproteinase activity and collagen disorganization have also been described in the contracted capsular tissue.[10]
  - Growth factors and other cellular mechanisms may be involved. This is highly variable among individuals.[17]
- Heterotopic ossification may also occur in conjunction with capsular thickening and act as a bony block to motion. Patients most at risk are those with combined head and elbow trauma, burn patients, and those who have undergone surgical approaches to the elbow, all of which are believed to incite a complex inflammatory chain that leads to elbow contracture and heterotopic ossification.[7]

## NATURAL HISTORY

- The onset and progression of elbow stiffness is closely related to its inciting causes (see Table 1); most contractures have mixed elements.[14]
  - Posttraumatic contracture is most common and is associated with a failure to regain motion after a direct traumatic injury to the elbow joint rather than progressive elbow motion loss. A posttraumatic contracture will typically remain stable over the long-term unless intra-articular degenerative changes ensue that would worsen motion further.
  - Contractures associated with degenerative or inflammatory arthritis may slowly progress with time due to capsular contraction and impingement on osteophytes or hypertrophic synovium. Such cases will often have episodic flares of swelling and stiffness in combination with steady baseline progression.
- Morrey[17] has also characterized elbow stiffness as static or dynamic based on tissue involvement (Table 2).

## PATIENT HISTORY AND PHYSICAL FINDINGS

- It is critical to determine the degree of functional impairment and duration of symptoms for each patient. Management decisions should be based on subjective

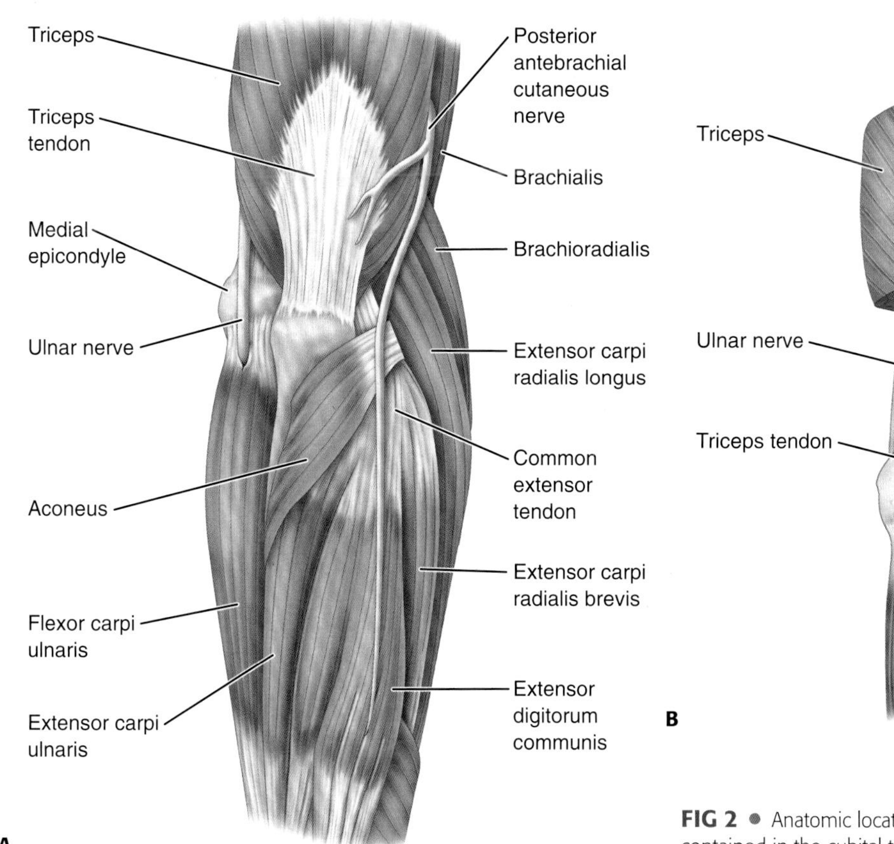


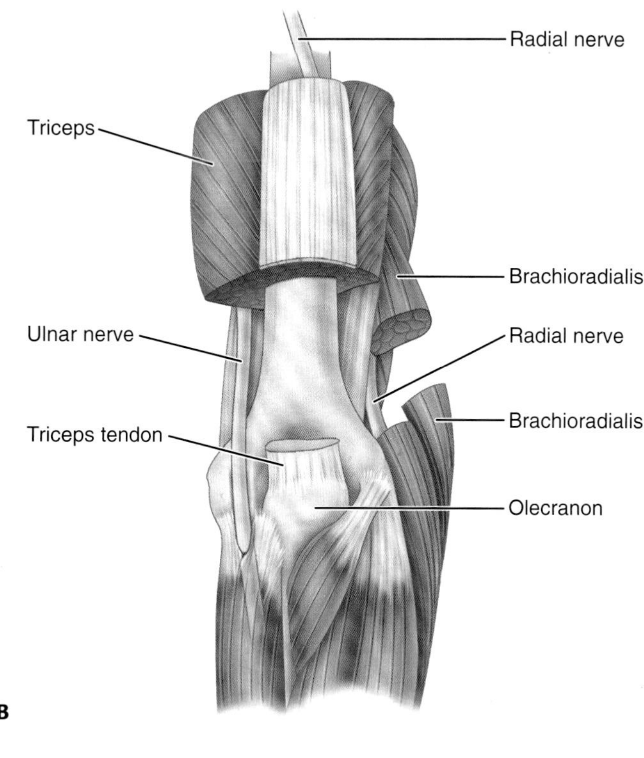


**FIG 2** • Anatomic location of the ulnar nerve at the elbow (**A**), which is contained in the cubital tunnel (**B**).

impairment and demands, not necessarily the amount of motion loss.[11]

- Associated disorders should be identified, as peripheral or central neurologic pathology may influence management decisions.
- Hand dominance, the patient's occupation, and the extent of prior therapy should be noted.
- The function of the entire ipsilateral and contralateral upper extremities should be tested.
- Physical examination
  - The cranial nerves and cervical spine should be examined to assess for neurologic pathology.
  - Shoulder motion and strength is assessed.
  - Careful assessment of the ulnar nerve
    - The physical examination is critical, as the patients will often not even recognize the presence of ulnar neuropathy in the setting of their adjacent elbow pathology. The elbow flexion and ulnar nerve compression test is the most sensitive for detection of ulnar nerve entrapment at the elbow.[21]
    - Two-point discrimination: Although less than 6 mm is considered normal, careful comparison to the ipsilateral median nerve and contralateral ulnar nerve is necessary to detect subtle signs of nerve damage.
    - Froment sign and intrinsic hand muscle function: Weakness of the adductor pollicis or interossei may also signify ulnar neuropathy.
    - The cubital tunnel is palpated to assess for tenderness or a positive Tinel sign.
  - Elbow range of motion: Flexion and extension are tested with the shoulder flexed to 90 degrees, whereas pronation and supination are evaluated with the elbow held in flexion at the side of the body.
    - Measure the flat surface of the forearm just proximal to the wrist in comparison to the axis of the humerus. Measurements in supination can be erroneous if tested through the palm because patients can often compensate with significant intercarpal supination.

**Table 2 Characterization of Elbow Stiffness by Tissue Involvement**

| Classification | Relative Occurrence | Location | Description |
|---|---|---|---|
| Static | Most common | Tissues in and around the elbow joint | Capsule, ligaments, heterotopic ossification, articular and cartilaginous components |
| Dynamic | Less common | Involves muscles around the joint | Poor muscle tone, nerve injuries, and poor excursion of the muscles that cross the elbow joint |

From Morrey BF. The stiff elbow with articular involvement. In: Jupiter JB, ed. The Stiff Elbow. Rosemont, IL: American Academy of Orthopaedic Surgeons, 2006:21–30.

- Measurements can also be erroneous in obese patients who cannot fully adduct the arm to the side, as they will appear to have a deficit in supination if the measurement is compared to the trunk axis and not the abducted humerus, which stresses the importance of using the humerus and not the trunk as the reference point.
- Elbow instability: The surgeon should check the ligamentous restraints to varus and valgus stress, as concomitant elbow instability and stiffness may occur after elbow dislocation or subluxation.
  - Ligaments are assessed with varus and valgus stress at 0 and 30 degrees of flexion as allowed by the patient's range of motion.

## IMAGING AND OTHER DIAGNOSTIC STUDIES

- Plain radiographs (anteroposterior [AP] and lateral) are usually adequate.
  - The AP provides joint line and subchondral bone visualization.
  - If an elbow is contracted more than 45 degrees, the AP view of the joint line is usually distorted.[17]
- The lateral view may show osteophytes on the olecranon or coronoid processes or within their respective fossae (**FIG 3A,B**).
- Radiographs can be used to follow the maturation process of heterotopic ossification, which usually signifies multiple extrinsic causes of elbow contracture that preclude arthroscopic treatment (**FIG 3C**).
- Computed tomography (CT) is useful to better characterize impinging osteophytes, loose bodies, and intra-articular non- or malunions. These studies are often more for preoperative planning than for diagnostic purposes
- Magnetic resonance imaging (MRI) has a limited role in the management of elbow stiffness but is the favored imaging study for staging and diagnosis of osteochondritis dissecans lesions and ulnar collateral ligament insufficiency, both of which not uncommonly will be accompanied by loss of motion. Fortunately, the age and history in these patients are quite specific, which helps narrow the differential diagnosis.

## DIFFERENTIAL DIAGNOSIS

- Elbow fracture-dislocation
- Osteoarthritis/posttraumatic arthritis
- Inflammatory arthropathy
- Osteochondritis dissecans
- Ulnar collateral ligament insufficiency with posteromedial impingement
- Heterotopic ossification
- Closed head injury
- Burns
- Dysplastic radial head (congenital)
- Neuromuscular disease
- Stroke

## NONOPERATIVE MANAGEMENT

- Nonoperative management should be considered up to 6 months after contracture onset.[14]
- Response is better if there is a soft "spongy" end point during range of motion[14,23]; bony blocks to motion such as heterotopic ossification or osteophytes are unlikely to respond to stretching protocols.
- The goal is to gain motion gradually without causing additional trauma to the capsule and, subsequently, development of additional capsular contracture (more pain, inflammation, and swelling leads to more contracture).
- Edema control is critical, and therapy should focus on this, not exercises that induce inflammation around the elbow.
- Static-progressive splinting is indicated as a first-line treatment for capsular contracture and should be used three times daily in between therapy sessions.[11,18] Dynamic splints yield results comparable to static progressive but are often less well tolerated as they provide a constant tension over time rather than allowing stress relaxation of soft tissues.[16,20] Care should be taken not to be overly aggressive in stretching as this may incite an inflammatory process leading to further capsular contracture. Regardless of whether static or dynamic splinting is chosen, this type of splinting can be beneficial for up to 1 year in treating posttraumatic elbow stiffness.[16]

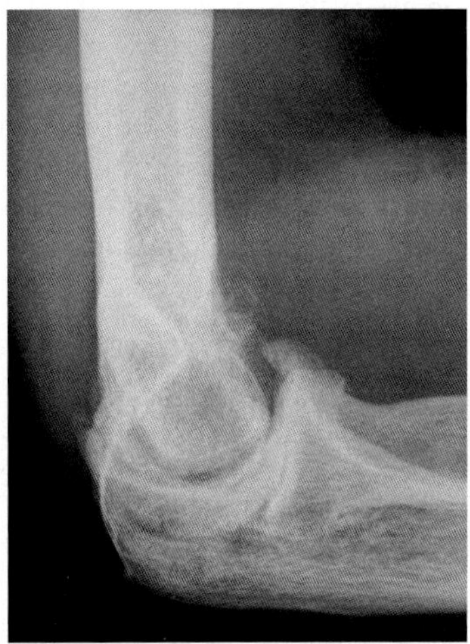


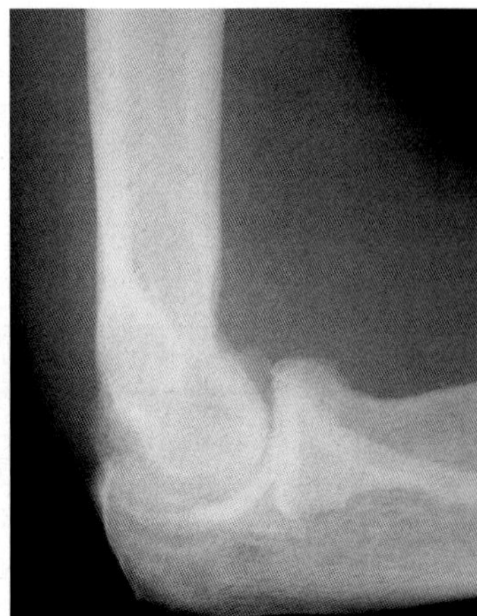


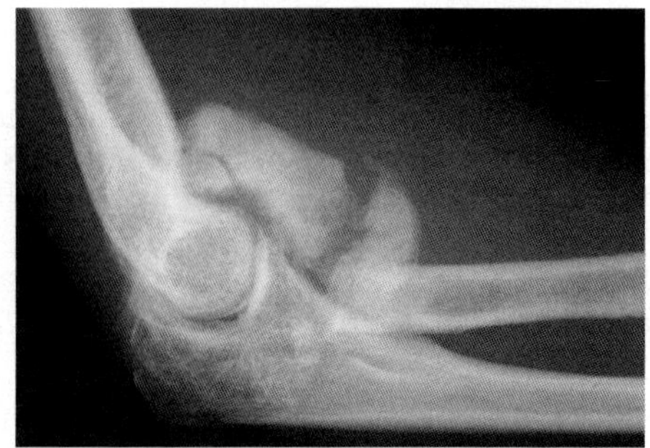


**FIG 3** • **A.** Preoperative lateral radiograph of an elbow before arthroscopic resection of osteophytes at the olecranon and coronoid, with associated anterior capsular contracture. Heterotopic ossification is absent. **B.** Postoperative radiograph after resection of osteophytes. **C.** Lateral radiograph of an elbow with heterotopic ossification. Arthroscopic resection is not recommended in this type of patient.

- Nonoperative improvements in range of motion vary widely. A systematic review by Müller[20] found an average improvement of 40 degrees with static-progressive splinting, but results of 10 to 50 degrees or more have been reported.[14,17,23]

## SURGICAL MANAGEMENT

- The key is to identify the functional disability of the patient—pain, loss of motion, or both—and what would be most beneficial to correct.
- The indications include a loss of function precluding the patient from performing ADLs and occupational or vocational activities.
- Arthroscopic treatment of elbow stiffness should be undertaken only if the offending structures can be treated from an arthroscopic approach. Capsular contractures and intra-articular osteophytes are ideally suited for arthroscopic treatment, whereas articular malunion, heterotopic ossification, or skin and muscle contractures are not amenable to arthroscopic release.
- Appropriate counseling with the patient should cover realistic expectations of range of motion and functional recovery. Will patients be able to get their hand to their mouth, comb their hair, or reach behind their back, or are more extensive demands required?
- There are several contraindications to arthroscopic release:
  - Prior surgery that has altered the neurovascular anatomy, especially of the radial nerve from previous surgery in the area of the radial head
  - Joint deformity that would compromise arthroscopic viewing, such as with severe posttraumatic malunion or inflammatory arthritis
  - Arthroscopy is also less favored for pathology best treated through an open approach such as heterotopic ossification or a fracture malunion that requires osteotomy.[3,26,27]

### Preoperative Planning

- An examination under anesthesia helps to distinguish static versus dynamic elbow stiffness and should confirm the preoperative clinical diagnosis.
- A thorough understanding of the pathoanatomy will allow the surgeon to plan the surgical order of events to maximize surgical efficiency and optimize patient safety.
  - In the presence of osteophytes or loose bodies, a CT scan with two-dimensional coronal and sagittal reconstructions as well as three-dimensional surface renderings may be helpful to provide a "road map" for the osteocapsular arthroplasty.
  - If the posterior compartment medial and lateral gutters require extensive work, it may be technically easier to perform this first before significant soft tissue swelling evolves. Visualization of the anterior compartment in the presence of soft tissue swelling can be better accommodated by the use of arthroscopic retractors.
- If the preoperative examination documented ulnar nerve irritation or neuropathy or if the patient has a subluxating ulnar nerve,[3] it should be exposed and an in situ release across the elbow joint be performed.
  - We recommend that the ulnar nerve be released before arthroscopy for ease of soft tissue dissection before fluid distention.
  - In patients with elbow flexion of less than 100 degrees, the nerve should be prophylactically released to prevent compression once flexion is restored postsurgically.[17]
  - Exploration and identification of the nerve prior to arthroscopy is also mandatory for patients who have undergone a prior ulnar nerve transposition. Open release may be preferable for these patients.
  - Following release, the nerve must be protected during placement of the anteromedial portal to prevent iatrogenic injury.

### Positioning

- Either the lateral decubitus or prone position can be used, with the operative extremity supported by either an arm cradle or rolled sheets (**FIG 4A,B**).
- A well-padded sterile tourniquet is used to optimize viewing by limiting intra-articular bleeding.
- The remainder of the arthroscopic setup has been described elsewhere.
- The surgeon should clearly mark the course of the ulnar nerve, portal sites, and bony landmarks with surgical marker (**FIG 4C**).

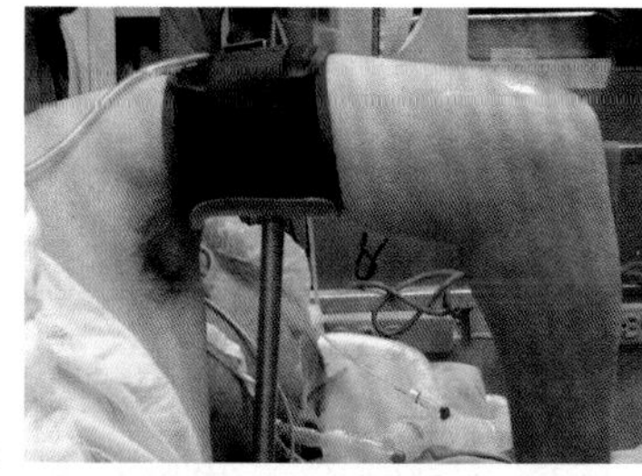
A

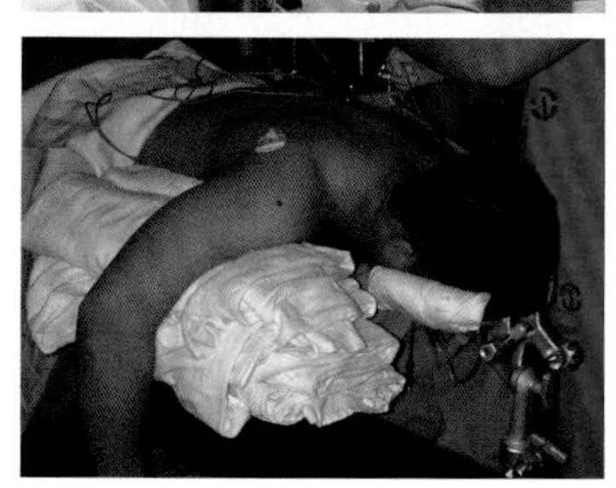
B

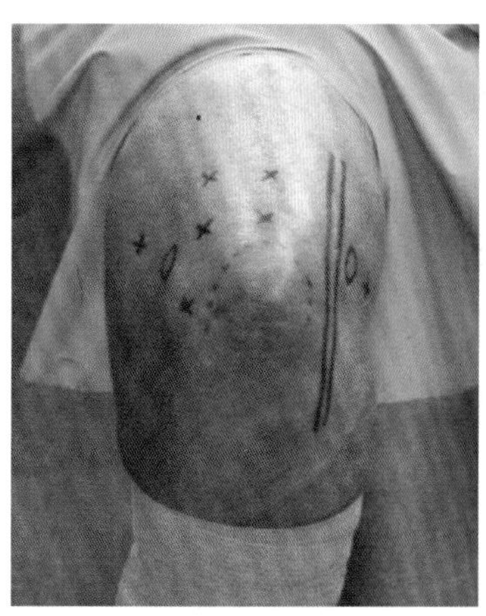
C

**FIG 4** • **A,B.** Setup of patient for elbow arthroscopy in lateral (**A**) and prone (**B**) positioning. **C.** Landmarks of the elbow drawn for operative incisions and to identify at-risk structures, including the ulnar nerve, in the prone position.

## Approach

- Arthroscopic elbow osteocapsular arthroplasty should proceed in a stepwise fashion.
  - Establish a view—get into the joint and confirm your anatomic orientation.
  - Create a working space—synovectomy and removal of debris
  - Bone removal—retractor is used to hold soft tissue away from burr or shaver blade.
  - Capsulectomy—using a large shaver can optimize fluid outflow and act as a periosteal elevator to strip soft tissue off bone before resection.
- Capsular contraction and loss of volume complicates arthroscopic visualization of the stiff elbow but can be greatly facilitated through the use of arthroscopic retractors placed through proximal medial and proximal lateral portals 1 to 2 cm above the standard medial and lateral portals.[22,23]
- Avoiding nerve injury during the approach and during capsular treatment is critical.
- If required, the ulnar nerve is decompressed and protected prior to arthroscopy in order to avoid soft tissue distortion due to fluid extravasation (**FIG 5**).

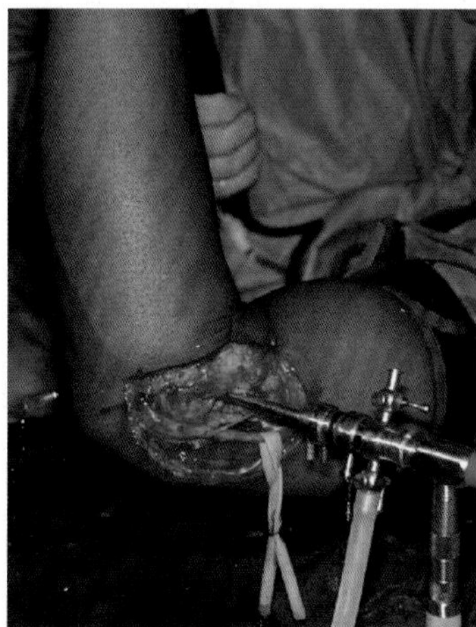

**FIG 5** • If the ulnar nerve is thought to be involved, it may be released before starting the arthroscopy to facilitate dissection without the soft tissue changes that occur after fluid extravasation from the elbow joint. The ulnar nerve is marked with a vessel loop.



## Ulnar Nerve Release and Transposition

- Subcutaneous transposition or in situ decompression of the ulnar nerve can be performed; these techniques are described elsewhere within this text.
- The ulnar nerve is exposed before performing the arthroscopic release to allow gentle fluid extravasation from the soft tissue posteromedially.[23]
  - Gentle retraction on the nerve with a Penrose drain can help protect it while performing arthroscopic releases in this area, especially posteromedial osteophytes.

## Portal Establishment in the Contracted Elbow

- The joint is distended with saline through the "soft spot" portal (up to 40 mL, as allowed by contracture).
- Portals are established.
  - The proximal anteromedial portal is established first (2 cm proximal to the medial epicondyle and 1 cm anterior to the intermuscular septum). A 4.5-mm, 30-degree scope is used for visualization (**TECH FIG 1A,B**).[2]
  - The proximal anterolateral portal (1.5 to 2 cm proximal to lateral epicondyle) is useful as a retractor portal to improve distention and visualization. The portal is established with either a blunt-tipped Wissinger rod as an inside-out technique or a spinal needle under direct visualization using an outside-in technique. (**TECH FIG 1C**).
- Blunt elevation with the Wissinger rod, a freer elevator, or specially designed retractors will help create a working space by lifting the capsule away from the joint and anterior humerus.

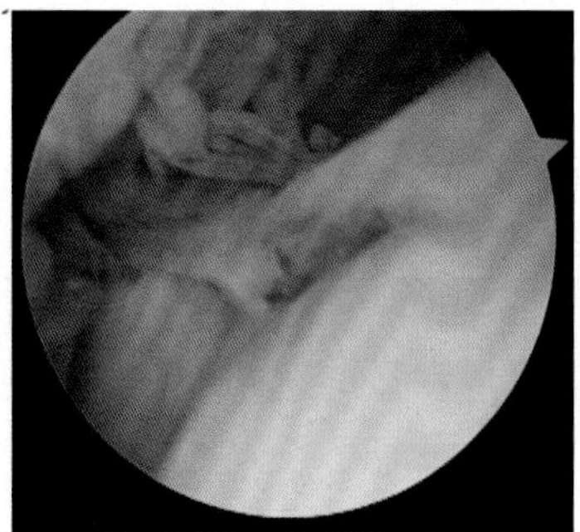

A

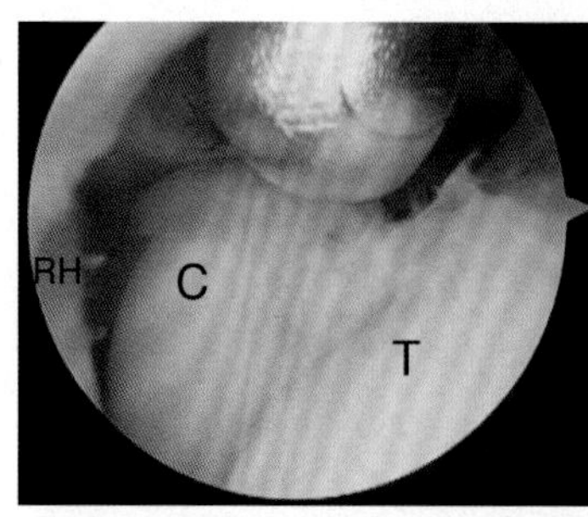


B

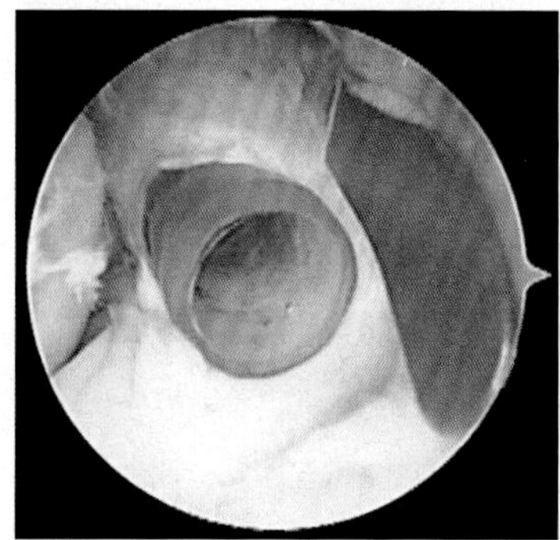

C

**TECH FIG 1** • **A.** Arthroscopic view of a right elbow joint after first obtaining scope entry into the proximal anteromedial portal, looking laterally. There is synovitis in the joint. **B.** After the synovitis is gently débrided with an arthroscopic shaver, the bony overgrowth of the coronoid and radial fossa is revealed. There is a lack of concavity in the trochlea and capitellum area. **C.** Arthroscopic view of elbow joint viewed from the medial portal, showing the increased visualization of the elbow joint that is obtained with the use of intra-articular retractors. *C*, capitellum; *RH*, radial head; *T*, trochlea.

- Avoid excessive inflow and high-pump pressures (>35 mm Hg), which will lead to increased fluid extravasation and extra-articular soft tissue distention that will impair visualization.
- A 4.5-mm shaver (oscillate function) débrides intra-articular synovitis or loose flaps of articular cartilage.
- A small radiofrequency device can also be used to ablate scar tissue within the joint. Inflow should be increased during the use of thermal energy to prevent cartilage injury.
- Impinging osteophytes of the coronoid tip and coronoid or trochlear fossae can be resected with a burr or shaver, if necessary.
  - Direct the burr away from the capsule to prevent accidental injury to the anterior neurovascular structures.
- The capsule is débrided superficially to define it as a structure and clear any synovitis; however, it is not removed until all intra-articular débridement, both bony and soft tissue, has already been carried out so as to limit fluid extravasation.

## Anterior Capsular Release

- Capsulotomy of the anterior capsule is performed with an arthroscopic basket cutter or radiofrequency ablation, from lateral to medial, along the nonarticular distal humerus.
  - The radial nerve rests on the anterior capsule at the level of the radial head. To prevent injury to it, the capsulotomy should be performed as close to the humerus as possible.
  - The posterior interosseous nerve (PIN) is adjacent to the anterolateral capsule at the level of the radial neck.[26]
  - The capsulotomy can be continued to the level of the collateral ligaments on each side, but the ligaments are not incised.
- The brachialis muscle can be visualized and the plane between the capsule and brachialis developed from the lateral working portal (**TECH FIG 2A**).
  - The brachialis protects the median nerve, so the surgeon should avoid penetrating this muscle. The fibers of the brachialis serve as the marker that the capsule has been released to an appropriate depth.
- The arthroscope is then moved to the anterolateral portal and the same steps of capsular release performed to ensure adequate medial release (**TECH FIG 2B**).
- Check passive extension after excision of posterior osteophytes and anterior capsulotomy alone, and if sufficient extension is restored, then complete capsulectomy can be avoided.
- A wide capsulotomy fully from medial to lateral off the humerus is often sufficient for the anterior release without endangering the neurovascular structures that are more at risk with a complete capsulectomy.

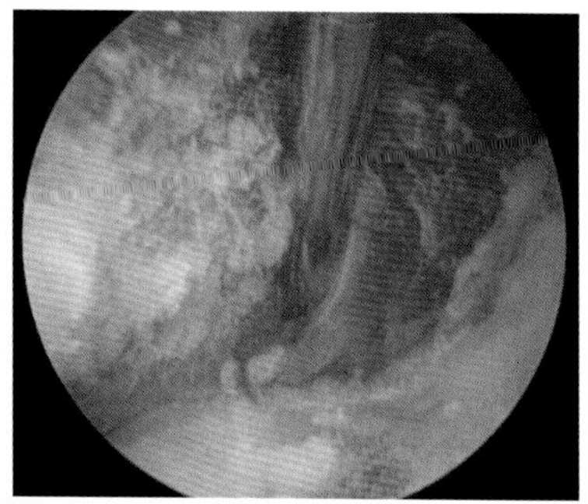
A

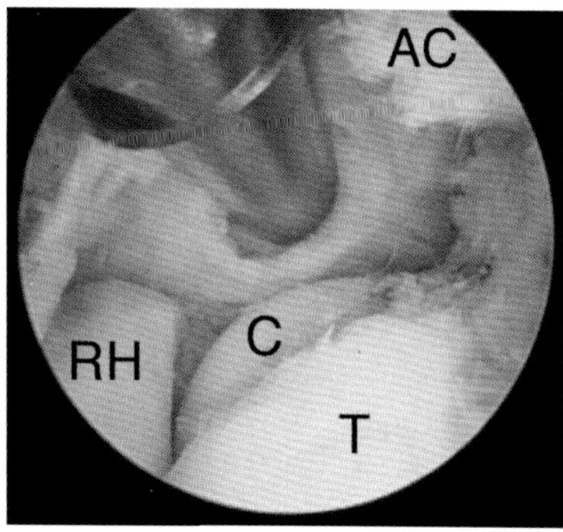

B

**TECH FIG 2** • **A.** Arthroscopic view of the elbow joint after capsulectomy and deepening of the coronoid and radial fossae. The dissection is carried down to the fibers of the brachialis muscle but does not violate the brachialis (retracted structure). **B.** View from the lateral portal shows the partially completed release. Bony work and resection are completed before capsulectomy. The concavity of the coronoid and trochlear fossae areas is restored, but anterior capsulectomy is not yet completed. *AC*, anterior capsule; *C*, capitellum; *RH*, radial head; *T*, trochlea.

## Posterior Capsular Release

- Portals are established:
  - The posterocentral viewing portal (3 to 4 cm proximal to the olecranon tip, through the triceps) is established first; it must be placed sufficiently proximal to clear the olecranon tip and enter the olecranon fossa.
  - A proximal posterolateral working portal (2 cm proximal to the olecranon tip and lateral to the triceps) is also established using an outside-in technique.
- A shaver is used to débride the posterior fat pad and open the posterior working space, avoiding shaving medial to the midline and certainly in and along the medial gutter until full visualization is obtained.
- The capsule is elevated from the distal humerus using blunt dissection or an elevator.
- Visualization and débridement of the posterior radiocapitellar joint can be facilitated using a midlateral (soft spot) working portal.
  - Viewing through the posterolateral portal, the midlateral portal is made under direct visualization using a spinal needle placed through the soft spot toward the posterior radiocapitellar joint.
  - An arthroscopic shaver is in used in this portal to débride the posterior capsule and arthrofibrosis. Suction is avoided in and along the medial gutter.
- Loose bodies and impinging osteophytes are removed before capsular resection to optimize visualization.

- Osteophytes are resected from the olecranon fossa, posterior capitellum, and olecranon tip using an arthroscopic burr or shaver.
- When necessary, osteophytes involving the medial gutter should be removed with care. Using a burr or serrated shaver may inadvertently draw the ulnar nerve into harm's way. For this reason, it is recommended to use a shaver blade instead.
- Up to 14 mm of the olecranon tip can be resected without injury to the triceps tendon.[12]
- A small open arthrotomy may be required at times for removal of larger loose bodies.

- The posterior capsule is released with a basket cutter or arthroscopic elevator on the medial and lateral sides; care should be taken to avoid capsular release medial to the olecranon fossa to avoid injury to the ulnar nerve.
- The posteromedial capsule (posterior band of the medial collateral ligament) should be resected in the setting of significant flexion loss. Release of this tissue does not risk medial-sided elbow instability.[25]
  - Care should be taken to protect the ulnar nerve, as this tissue represents the floor of the cubital tunnel. If a posteromedial release is planned, a limited open ulnar nerve decompression or full transposition should be performed prior to arthroscopy.
  - Release is performed along the olecranon, rather than the humerus, as this portion of the capsule is furthest from the ulnar nerve.
  - Use of radiofrequency ablation or suction medially should also be avoided to protect the nerve.
- An open arthrotomy through the ulnar nerve incision carries minimal morbidity and can be very useful to access the posteromedial capsule for release and the olecranon tip for excision in cases where the arthroscopic visualization is limited.
- Final inspection from both portals is done to ensure adequate release (**TECH FIG 3**).

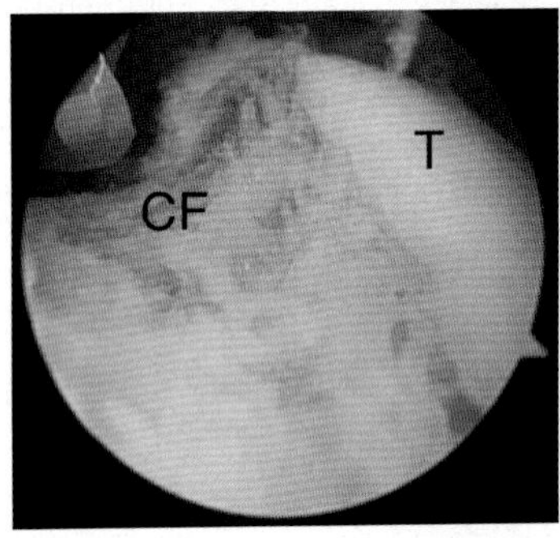


A

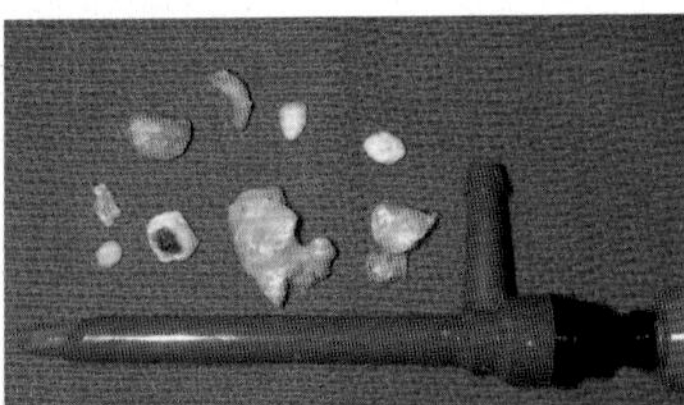

B

**TECH FIG 3** • **A.** View from the lateral portal after medial release showing completed capsulectomy and bony débridement in the coronoid fossa area. **B.** Loose bodies are removed during this procedure via a 5-mm smooth cannula. *CF*, coronoid fossa; *T*, trochlea.

## Wound Closure and Intraoperative Splinting

- A drain is placed through the proximal anterolateral portal because accumulation of fluid and postoperative bleeding will compromise range of motion.
- Our postoperative dressing is a soft bulky dressing with Webril, Kerlix, and Ace bandages from wrist to shoulder. Material is cut out from the antecubital fossa in order to facilitate flexion (**TECH FIG 4**). Continuous passive motion (CPM) can be initiated on postoperative day 0 at the surgeon's discretion.
  - Alternatively, an anterior plaster slab is placed to keep the elbow near full extension and alternating resting flexion and extension splints are used.
- Indwelling catheters, a long-acting regional block, or cryotherapy may be used to facilitate CPM (from full flexion to extension).

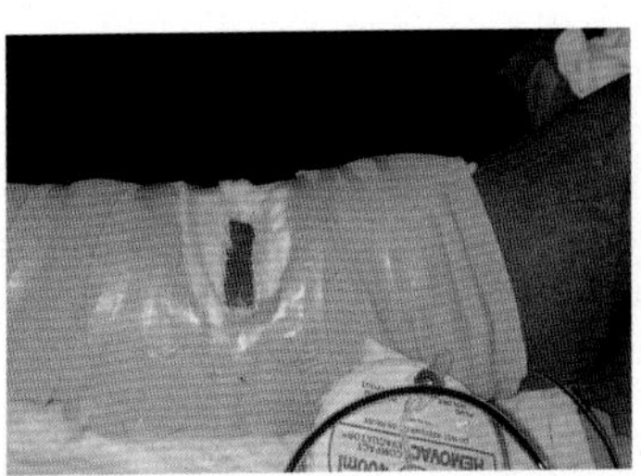

A

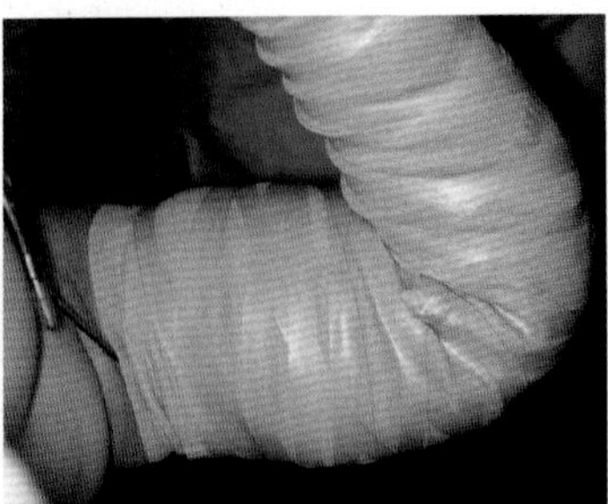

B

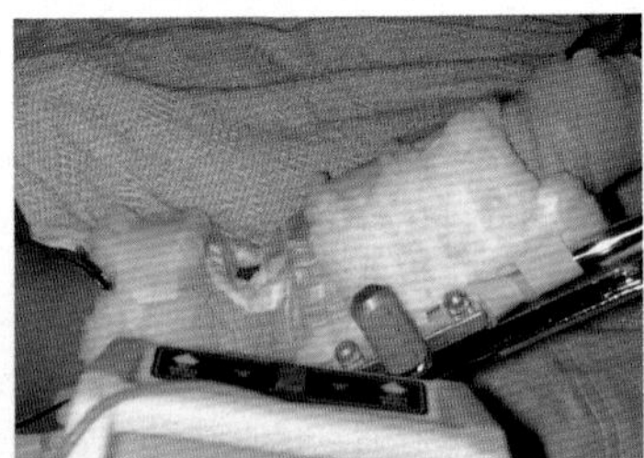

C

**TECH FIG 4** • **A.** Postoperative dressing is applied to the patient after capsular release in the operating room with a drain. **B.** Flexion obtained after removing splint material from the antecubital fossa. **C.** Immediate continuous passive motion is instituted.

## PEARLS AND PITFALLS

| | |
|---|---|
| **Managing the ulnar nerve** | ■ Prophylactic release before arthroscopy if flexion contracture is significant or if examination consistent with neuropathy or neuritis. |
| **Optimizing visualization** | ■ Use arthroscopic retractors to aid visualization in anterior and posterior compartments. |
| **Avoiding neurovascular injury** | ■ The surgeon should avoid motorized burrs. No suction should be used on the shaver in at-risk areas. Use of arthroscopic retractors is recommended. |
| **Anterior osteocapsular release** | ■ Using a basket and retractor, develop the plane between capsule and brachialis until the defined fat stripe over the midportion of radiocapitellar joint, which represents the radial nerve. Watch for PIN adjacent to anterolateral capsule distally. |
| **Posterior osteocapsular release** | ■ Consider performing first if working in medial and lateral gutters. Retract the ulnar nerve and use a shaver blade to avoid iatrogenic nerve injury. |

## POSTOPERATIVE CARE

- CPM can be continued at home up to 4 weeks and should be used in full range of motion (0 to 145 degrees) with a bolster behind the elbow.[26]
- Daily physiotherapy is instituted immediately postoperatively, with home static- (preferred) or dynamic-progressive splinting.
- The surgeon should consider prophylaxis of heterotopic ossification with indomethacin. Single-dose external beam irradiation is only considered in the most severe cases of heterotopic ossification, in which case, the release is typically performed open.

## OUTCOMES

- Patients usually regain about 50% of lost motion.[11,23]
- About 80% of patients obtain a functional arc of motion greater than 100 degrees.[11]
- A systematic review by Kodde et al[15] found a mean gain in arc of motion of 40 degrees (from 84 to 124 degrees) with arthroscopic elbow release, although gains of up to 80 degrees have been reported.[26]
- Ball et al[3] reported high patient satisfaction and recovery of function after surgery, with all patients in the series stating they wound undergo surgery again.
- In high-level athletes undergoing arthroscopic release for loss of terminal extension (<35 degrees), the average loss of flexion improved from 27 degrees to 6 degrees, and 23 of 26 athletes returned to the previous level of performance.[4]
- It is difficult to compare arthroscopic versus open capsular releases as arthroscopic surgery is typically performed for less severe disease, whereas open release is preferred for more complex cases.[15]

## COMPLICATIONS

- The overall complication rate for arthroscopic release is low (5% vs. 23% for open surgery).[15]
- Blona et al[5] reported no permanent neurologic injuries in a series of over 500 elbow arthroscopic releases for stiffness. In less experienced hands, a neurologic injury is more likely and the learning curve should be appreciated.
- Persistent stiffness requiring a second surgical release is the most common complication.[15]
- Ulnar nerve
  - Although the overall rate of ulnar nerve injury with elbow arthroscopy is low (1%), the preoperative diagnosis of elbow contracture and performance of a capsulectomy are both risk factors for transient ulnar nerve palsy.[13]
  - In the medial aspect of joint, the surgeon should use retractors to move the capsule medially and avoid resection along the humerus, or identify and protect the ulnar nerve through a small open incision prior to any work in the posteromedial gutter.
- Ulnar neuritis
  - If present preoperatively, or there will be a significant increase in flexion after surgery, the ulnar nerve should be released.
  - Postoperatively, it may be transient; there is a much lower incidence if it is transposed during the initial surgery.
- Radial or PIN
  - The overall rate of radial or PIN nerve palsy with elbow arthroscopy is 1%.[13]
  - Iatrogenic injury can be avoided by refraining from use of suction when working near the capsule anterior to the midline of the radiocapitellar articulation.
  - Retractors of soft tissue are used to improve visualization and distention.
- Median or anterior interosseous nerve
  - Iatrogenic injury is avoided by not penetrating the brachialis muscle.
  - The surgeon should place portals carefully, avoiding moving more anterior than necessary.
- Excessive bony resection leading to iatrogenic fracture or inadvertently aggressive resection of soft tissues surrounding the radial head leading to violation of the collateral ligament and elbow instability
  - When working in the anterolateral joint, avoid débriding further posterior than the equator of the radiocapitellar joint, as this corresponds to the superior margin of the lateral collateral ligament.[8]

## REFERENCES


1. Akai M, Shirasaki Y, Tateishi T. Viscoelastic properties of stiff joints: a new approach in analyzing joint contracture. Biomed Mater Eng 1993;3:67–73.
2. An K, Morrey BF. Biomechanics of the elbow. In: Morrey BF, ed. The Elbow and Its Disorders. Philadelphia: WB Saunders, 2000: 43–74.
3. Ball CM, Meunier M, Galatz LM, et al. Arthroscopic treatment of post-traumatic elbow contracture. J Should Elbow Surg 2002;11:624–629.

4. Blonna D, Lee G, O'Driscoll SW. Arthroscopic restoration of terminal elbow extension in high-level athletes. Am J Sports Med 2010;38:2509.
5. Blonna D, Wolf JM, Fitzsimmons J, et al. Prevention of nerve injury during arthroscopic capsulectomy of the elbow utilizing a safety-driven strategy. J Bone and Joint Surg Am 2013;95:1373–1381.
6. Bruno RJ, Lee ML, Strauch FJ, et al. Posttraumatic elbow stiffness: evaluation and management. J Am Acad Orthop Surg 2002;10:106–116.
7. Cohen MS. Heterotopic ossification of the elbow. In: Jupiter JB, ed. The Stiff Elbow. Rosemont, IL: American Academy of Orthopaedic Surgeons, 2006:31–40.
8. Cohen MS, Romeo AA, Hennigan SP, et al. Lateral epicondylitis: anatomic relationships of the extensor tendon origins and implications for arthroscopic treatment. J Should Elbow Surg 2008;17:954–960.
9. Gallay S, Richards R, O'Driscoll SW. Intraarticular capacity and compliance of stiff and normal elbows. Arthroscopy 1993;9:9–13.
10. Hildebrand K, Zhang M, van Snellenberg W, et al. Myofibroblast numbers are elevated in human elbow capsules after trauma. Clin Orthop Relat Res 2004;419:189–197.
11. Jupiter JB, O'Driscoll SW, Cohen MS. The assessment and management of the stiff elbow. AAOS Instr Course Lect 2003;52:93–111.
12. Keener JD, Chafik D, Kim HM, et al. Insertional anatomy of the triceps brachii tendon. J Should Elbow Surg 2010;19:399–405.
13. Kelley ED, Morrey BF, O'Driscoll SW. Complications of elbow arthroscopy. J Bone Joint Surg Am 2001;83:25–34.
14. King GJ, Faber KJ. Posttraumatic elbow stiffness. Orthop Clin North Am 2000;31:129–143.
15. Kodde IF, van Rijn J, van den Bekerom MP, et al. Surgical treatment of post-traumatic elbow stiffness: systemic review. J Should Elbow Surg 2013;22:574–580.
16. Lindenhovius AL, Doornberg JB, Brower KM, et al. A prospective randomized control trial of dynamic versus static progressive elbow splinting for posttraumatic elbow stiffness. J Bone Joint Surg Am 2012;94:694–700.
17. Morrey BF. Anatomy of the elbow joint. In: Morrey BF, ed. The Elbow and Its Disorders. Philadelphia: WB Saunders, 2000:13–42.
18. Morrey BF. The stiff elbow with articular involvement. In: Jupiter JB, ed. The Stiff Elbow. Rosemont, IL: American Academy of Orthopaedic Surgeons, 2006:21–30.
19. Morrey BF, Askey LJ, Chao EY. A biomechanical study of normal functional elbow motion. J Bone Joint Surg Am 1981;63:872–877.
20. Müller AM, Sadoghi P, Lucas R, et al. Effectiveness of bracing in the treatment of nonosseous restriction of elbow mobility: a systematic review. J Should Elbow Surg 2013;22:1146–1152.
21. Novak CB, Lee GW, Mackinnon SE, et al. Provocative testing for cubital tunnel syndrome. J Hand Surg 1994;19:817–820.
22. O'Driscoll SW. Arthroscopic osteocapsular arthroplasty. In: Yamaguchi K, King G, McKee M, et al, eds. Advanced Reconstruction Elbow, 1 ed. Rosemont, IL: American Academy of Orthopaedic Surgeons, 2007:59–68.
23. O'Driscoll SW. Clinical assessment and open and arthroscopic treatment of the stiff elbow. In: Jupiter JB, ed. The Stiff Elbow. Rosemont, IL: American Academy of Orthopaedic Surgeons, 2006:9–19.
24. O'Driscoll SW, Morrey BF, An K. Intra-articular pressure and capacity of the elbow. Arthroscopy 1990;6:100–103.
25. Ruch DS, Shen J, Chioros GD, et al. Release of the medial collateral ligament to improve flexion in post-traumatic elbow stiffness. J Bone Joint Surg Br 2008;90:614–618.
26. Savoie FH III, Field LD. Arthrofibrosis and complications in arthroscopy of the elbow. Clin Sports Med 2001;20(1):123–129.
27. Tucker SA, Savoie FH, O'Brien MJ. Arthroscopic management of the post-traumatic stiff elbow. J Should Elbow Surg 2011;20:S83–S89.

41

CHAPTER

# Acute Patellar and Chronic Patellar Instability

Eric J. Wall, Jay C. Albright, and Sarah R. Steward

## DEFINITION

- Patellar instability in children and adolescents usually involves an episode of complete dislocation of the patella from the trochlear groove. Occasionally, there can be episodes of patellar subluxation without gross dislocation.
- There are two main types of patellar dislocation:
  - Acute traumatic patellar dislocation in athletic, nonlax individuals
  - Atraumatic dislocations or subluxation secondary to ligamentous laxity
- Children between the ages of 10 and 17 years have the highest risk for traumatic and atraumatic patellar dislocation.[12] The incidence of primary patellar dislocation in this age group is reported at 29 per 100,000 annually and is more common in females.[9]
- Acute traumatic patellar dislocation is frequently (28% to 39%) associated with articular surface fractures of the patella or of the lateral femoral condyle.[3,22]
- Most traumatic patellar dislocations tear the medial patellofemoral ligament (MPFL), which is the primary restraint to patellar dislocation. This may lead to persistent apprehension or recurrent instability of the patellofemoral joint.
- Nonoperative treatment is indicated for patellar dislocation associated with ligamentous laxity and for first-time traumatic patellar dislocation that is not associated with a repairable articular surface injury.
- Care must be taken to avoid realignment surgery for patients with patellofemoral pain and no clear evidence of instability.

## ANATOMY

- The medial restraints of the patellofemoral joint are made up predominantly of the medial retinaculum and the MPFL. Forty percent to 60% of the resistance to lateral translation is supplied by the MPFL.[19] The MPFL provides 50% to 80% of the restraining force to lateral patellar displacement.[13]
- Traumatic dislocation of the patella occurs almost exclusively in the lateral direction and often results in a tear of the MPFL at its femur insertion, patellar origin, or in its midsubstance (**FIG 1A**). The MPFL can tear in multiple sites during a single dislocation.
- The MPFL is a flat band adjacent to the medial retinaculum that is about 15 mm wide. It extends from the superomedial aspect of the patella, about 10 to 15 mm distal to the superior pole, to the medial epicondylar area, just above and posterior to the origin of the medial collateral ligament, and distal to the adductor tubercle[25] (**FIG 1B**).
- During limited-incision surgical approaches, anatomic landmarks are not reliably identified due to small incisions. Fluoroscopy and isometry is needed to confirm the proper site of MPFL reattachment location (see **TECH FIG 1A,B**).
- Although there is some controversy, most believe that the native MPFL arises from the femur just distal to the growth plate near the medial epicondyle in a skeletally immature patient.[12,16,20,32]
- The common finding of a lateral femoral condyle bone bruise at the sulcus terminalis suggests that dislocation usually occurs at 70 to 80 degrees of flexion.[29]

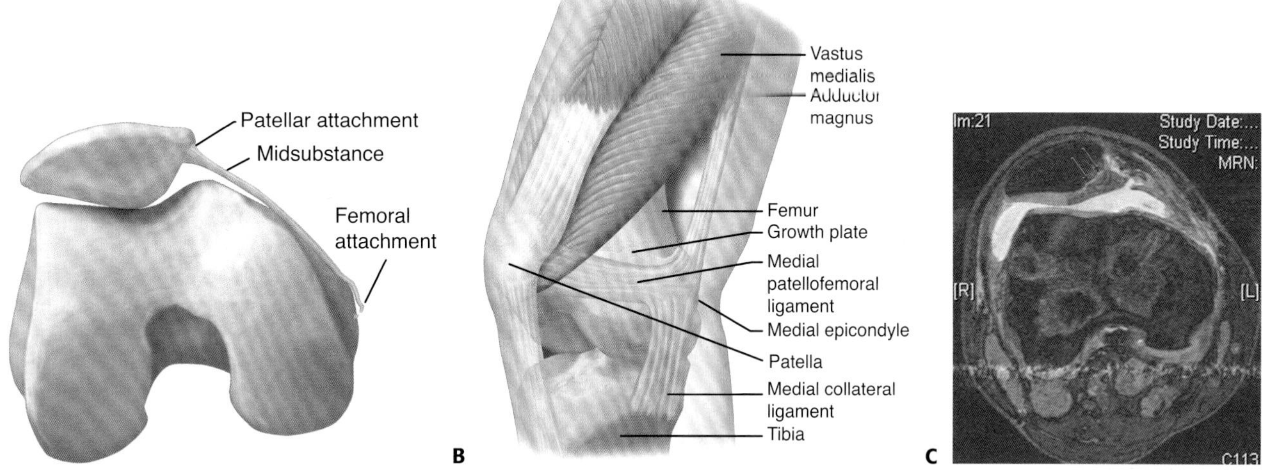


**FIG 1** ● **A.** The MPFL can tear at its patellar origin, its femoral origin, or in its midsubstance. **B.** The MPFL tethers the medial patella to the medial condyle of the femur. It arises from the superior two-thirds of the medial border of the patella and inserts between the adductor tubercle and medial epicondyle. Its insertion is just distal to the growth plate. **C.** The entire medial cartilaginous facet of the patella has separated from the underlying bone after a primary traumatic patellar dislocation. *(continued)*

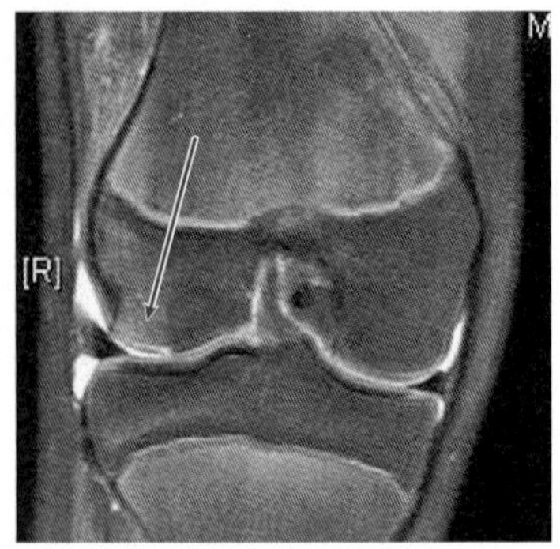


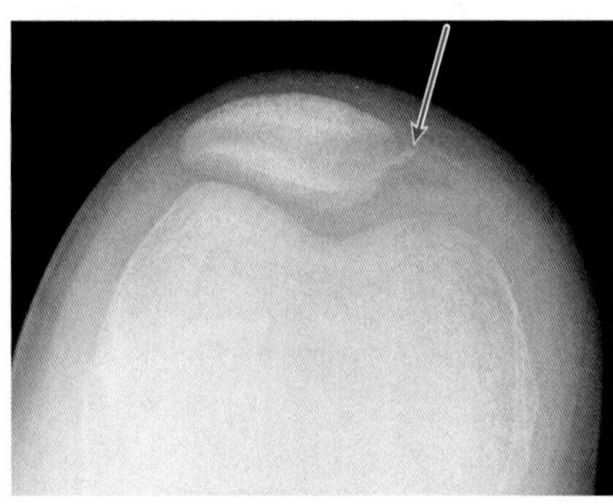

**FIG 1** • *(continued)* **D.** After patellar dislocation, this patient has an osteochondral fracture of the lateral femoral condyle (*arrow*). **E.** Insignificant avulsion fracture off medial patella (*arrow*), which is pathognomonic for patellar dislocation.

- Traumatic dislocation can cause a serious fracture of the medial patellar facet (**FIG 1C**) or the lateral femoral condyle (**FIG 1D**) and can be cartilaginous or osteocartilaginous.
- Stanitski and Paletta[33] found a 71% incidence of osteochondral injury at arthroscopy after patellar dislocation, most of which was radiographically occult.
- More frequently, there is a less serious nonarticular avulsion fracture of the MPFL off the medial patella. There can be an immediate or delayed appearance of an ossific lesion, which rarely needs removal or reattachment, at the avulsion site off the medial patella (**FIG 1E**).

## PATHOGENESIS

- Noncontact patellar dislocation during sports usually involves lower extremity internal rotation combined with knee valgus on a planted foot (a mechanism very similar to anterior cruciate ligament injury).
- Less commonly, patellar dislocation is caused by a direct blow on a valgus bent knee that pushes the kneecap laterally.
- The bony anatomy of the patellofemoral joint may be abnormal with a deficient lateral femoral slope of the trochlear groove, a shallow trochlear groove, patella alta, patellar tilt, or a lateralized and/or hypoplastic tibial tubercle. These factors can increase the risk of dislocation by decreasing the force needed to laterally translate or dislocate the patella.[7]
- The lateral retinaculum may also be tight, characterized by less than 12 mm of medial translation.[15]
- The alignment of the lower extremities must also be considered. The quadriceps angle may be greater than average, increasing the lateral translational force.
- So-called miserable malalignment syndrome may exist, including excessive femoral anteversion with or without increased external tibial torsion.[14,15]
- Multiple anatomic factors are theorized to increase the risk of patellar dislocation, such as family history, increased Q angle, femoral intorsion, tibial extorsion, knee valgus, trochlear groove dysplasia, and foot pronation. Only patella alta is a proven risk factor.[2] MPFL reconstruction results are not diminished by patella alta or tibial tuberosity–trochlear groove (TT-TG) distances of up to 25 mm.[21]

## NATURAL HISTORY

- Patients with an atraumatic presentation of instability or dislocation of the patellofemoral joint have a higher likelihood of repeat instability episodes, despite aggressive physical therapy and bracing.[14,15]
- A recent study on adolescents with traumatic first-time patellar dislocation reports a 70% recurrence rate.[28]
- Young age was also associated with recurrence, as was a positive family history.[9]
- At 6 months after patellar dislocation, only 69% of patients had returned to sports.[2]
- At 2 to 5 years of follow-up after patellar dislocation, Fithian and coworkers[9] showed no radiographic or scintigraphic evidence of degenerative joint disease.
- At 6 to 26 years of follow-up after nonoperative treatment for patellar dislocation, 22% of knees showed arthritic changes, compared to 11% of each patient's opposite uninjured knee.[17]
- At least 30% to 50% of patients with patellar dislocation will have knee pain more than 2 years after injury, and 69% of athletes will decrease their sports activity.[11]
- Young age and skeletal immaturity, especially in females, is associated with worse prognosis.[23]
- Patellar dislocation, especially recurrent patellar dislocation, is associated with patellofemoral arthritis in adulthood.[34]

## PATIENT HISTORY AND PHYSICAL FINDINGS

- Patients with an acute traumatic patellar dislocation often present to the emergency room with a history of a noncontact or contact injury to their knee. Many do not recognize the injury as a patellar dislocation.
- An effusion is usually present after traumatic dislocation but is rarely present after atraumatic dislocations.
- Like an anterior cruciate ligament injury, it is common to hear or feel a "pop" at the time of injury. If the patella completely dislocates, the athlete may be found to have a deformity of the knee and may be unable to actively extend the knee.
- Most episodes of patellar dislocation spontaneously reduce in the field.
  - If the patella is still dislocated, the emergency physician usually performs a reduction by slowly extending the knee from its flexed position.
  - Patellar dislocation that spontaneously reduces in the field may mimic the history and presentation of an anterior cruciate ligament tear.
- A thorough examination will include the following:
  - Examination for effusion
  - Patellar glide (Patellar stability) test: With the knee flexed 25 to 30 degrees, the patella is gently translated laterally and compared to the opposite knee, which show less

translation. An intact MPFL will usually have a solid end point near the limit of lateral translation. Unfortunately, the patellar stability examination is often unreliable in the awake patient due to extreme apprehension to lateral translation. In this case, an examination under anesthesia can help confirm the diagnosis when the history and magnetic resonance imaging (MRI) are unclear.

- Patella apprehension sign: With the knee flexed over a bolster at 25 degrees, the patella is translated laterally. If the patient exhibits apprehension, the test is positive. This is the best test for patellar instability.
- J sign: Observe and palpate the patella for lateral subluxation during active range of motion. A positive sign occurs when the patella pulls laterally as the knee reaches full extension, tracing the path of an upside-down "J." This can identify proximal alignment issues.
- Femoral rotation: Average rotation is external rotation greater than or equal to internal motion.
- Tibial alignment: Average axis is 10 to 15 degrees of external tibial torsion.
- Patients with obvious genu valgum should have a standing alignment film with their patellas pointing forward. A plumb line drawn between the femoral head center and the center of ankle tibial plafond that passes lateral to the notch may be an indication for a guided growth hemiepiphysiodesis.
- Assess for generalized hypermobility using the Beighton hypermobility score, which ranges from 0 to 9. One point accrues for each elbow that hyperextends greater than 10 degrees, each little finger that shows greater than 90 degrees extension across the metacarpophalangeal (MCP) joint, each thumb that can touch the volar forearm, each knee that hyperextends greater than 10 degrees, and one point if the patient can bend forward and touch their palms flat on the floor.
  - Beighton scores of four or greater may indicate generalized hypermobility.

## IMAGING AND OTHER DIAGNOSTIC STUDIES

- Knee radiographs should include the anteroposterior (AP), lateral, and sunrise (or Merchant) views.
- The sunrise or Merchant view requires a patient to flex the knee 30 to 45 degrees, which may be impossible owing to pain at the initial time of presentation in the emergency department. The sunrise view can usually be obtained at the first follow-up visit.
- Each radiograph is evaluated for fracture or loose fragment necessitating more emergent surgical indications.
- Plain radiographs can miss 40% of arthroscopically documented chondral or osteochondral lesions. Many reparable osteochondral injuries show only a sliver of bone on one view in the plain radiographic series, which can be easily overlooked (**FIG 2A**).
- Because of the high rate of occult articular or osteoarticular injury, we recommend an MRI scan on patients who present with a large traumatic effusion after patellar dislocation.
  - The site of MPFL ligament disruption can often be identified on MRI. MRI is reported to be 85% sensitive and 70% accurate[30] (**FIG 2B**). The MPFL is torn or stretched at multiple sites after a patellar dislocation episode in 27% to 46% of cases.[8,16]
  - MRI after acute traumatic patellar dislocation shows a signature bone contusion pattern (**FIG 2C**). There was a 100% occurrence of anterior third of the lateral femoral condyle bone bruises and 96% occurrence of medial patellar bone bruises in one study.[27] This bone bruise pattern is distinct from that associated with anterior cruciate ligament tears.

## DIFFERENTIAL DIAGNOSIS

- Anterior cruciate, medial collateral, lateral collateral, or posterior cruciate ligament tear
- Meniscal tear
- Knee contusion
- Osteochondral injury
- Sinding-Larsen-Johansson disease
- Patellofemoral pain syndrome

## NONOPERATIVE MANAGEMENT

- Some 17% to 70% of adolescent patients will suffer a recurrent patellar dislocation after nonoperative management of their first patellar dislocation.[9,28]

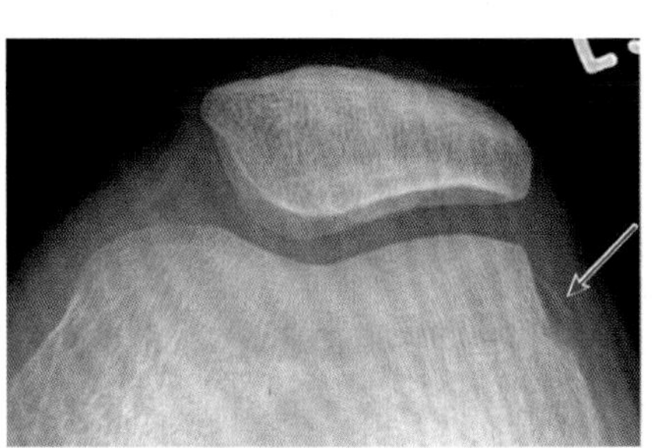

A

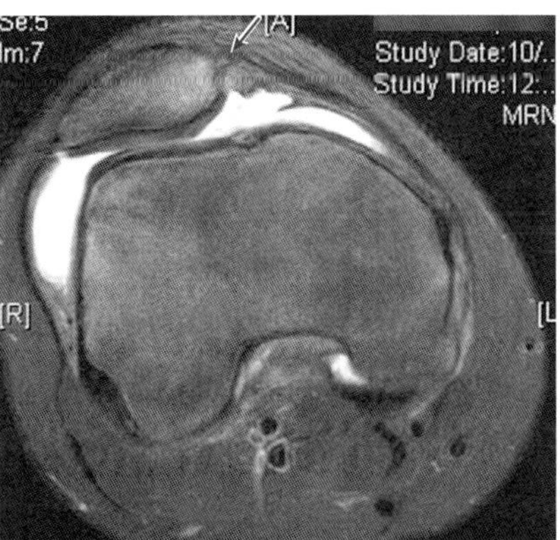


B

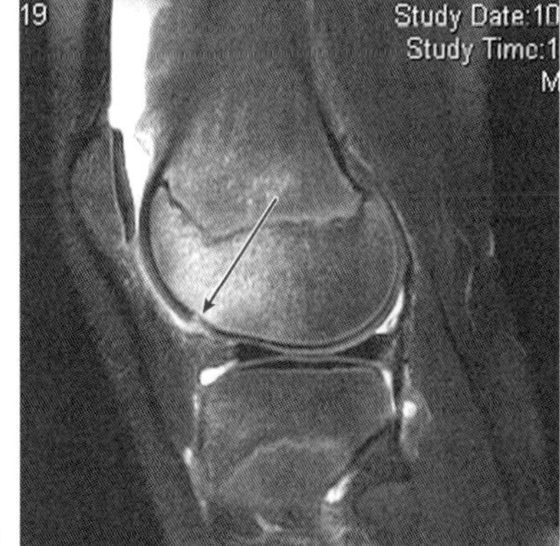


C

**FIG 2** • **A.** Osteochondral fragment. Postpatellar dislocation radiographic sunrise view shows a subtle sliver of bone (*arrow*), which on arthroscopy proved to be a large osteochondral fracture from the lateral condyle that was repaired with screw fixation. **B.** MPFL tear off from the patella. MRI shows disruption of MPFL off its origin from the patella (*arrow*), with increased signal on medial patella. **C.** Lateral femoral condyle bone bruise on MRI scan after a patellar dislocation. There is a subtle break in the articular cartilage (*arrow*). The location of the bruise provides evidence that the patella usually dislocates with the knee in 70 to 80 degrees of flexion.

- Nonoperative treatment is appropriate initial treatment for first time dislocators or subluxators who do not have a chondral facture, especially those who have generalized ligamentous laxity or an atraumatic type of presentation.
- Controversy exists as to the best treatment of first-time dislocators who are ligamentously tight, with or without a traumatic (but usually forceful) event.
- Some advocate early surgical intervention to repair the MPFL and medial retinaculum, even without fractures or loose body; however, pediatric and adult controlled studies show no advantage of surgical treatment (predominantly medial reef procedures +/− lateral release) over nonsurgical treatment.[23,24,28]
- A recent randomized controlled trial of predominantly adults found that MPFL reconstruction gave significantly better outcome than nonoperative treatment.[4]
- Nonoperative regimen for an acute traumatic dislocation includes the following:
  - Rest, ice, compression, and elevation for acute pain and swelling
  - Anti-inflammatory medications and oral narcotics in the initial phase, if needed
  - Initial knee immobilization for pain followed by early ROM, physical therapy and a patellar stabilizing sleeve starting at about 1–2 weeks after injury.
    - In one study, the risk of redislocation is reported as three times higher in patients treated with immediate mobilization versus immobilization with cast or brace.[18]
  - Weight bearing as tolerated with crutches
  - Early physical therapy with modalities and exercise used to control effusion, restore normal range of motion, and initiate quadriceps activation.
  - A patellar protection program of hip, core, quadriceps, and hamstrings strengthening to provide dynamic stability once symptoms have resolved.
  - Bracing, with a lateral patellar restraint type of brace, for return to activity
- Treatment options for recurrent subluxation should include the following:
  - Bracing with a lateral patellar restraint type of brace
  - Physical therapy: a patellar protection program emphasizing strengthening of the hip flexors, abductors (which are routinely weak in this patient population), and quadriceps in particular.
  - The clinician should emphasize to the patient that therapy requires participation at home as well as at therapy sessions.

## SURGICAL MANAGEMENT

- MPFL reconstruction is revolutionizing the functional outcomes and redislocation rates after patellar stabilization surgery in both adults and children[4,5,21,35] as compared to the previously mentioned studies showing no benefit to soft tissue repair surgery after first-time dislocation.
- Operative treatment is indicated for first-time patellar dislocation that fails to reduce concentrically or that involves osteochondral damage necessitating repair or removal of a loose body.
- Osteochondral or pure chondral lesions larger than 1 cm in diameter should be repaired if surgically possible. Fixation devices should be countersunk 2 to 4 mm beneath the thick cartilage surface.
- The MPFL can be repaired at the time of surgery for osteochondral lesions in acute dislocations, but the recurrence rate is higher with MPFL repair versus MPFL reconstruction. MPFL reconstruction should not be performed at the time of chondral or osteochondral repair if the fixation devices will need an arthrotomy for future removal. The reconstruction can be staged with implant removal surgery.
- Operative intervention should not be considered in chronic subluxators unless they prove that instability remains problematic despite a good effort in therapy and bracing over 6 to 12 months.
  - Recurrent traumatic patellar dislocation, especially after the patient has complied with a rigorous physical therapy program after the first patellar dislocation, is an indication for surgical stabilization.
- The surgeon should be wary of operative treatment for patients with pain without instability.
- MPFL reconstruction is not indicated for malalignment, patellofemoral pain, or arthrosis.
- Lateral release is rarely necessary with repair or reconstruction of the MPFL.
- Tibial tubercle realignment procedures should be avoided in skeletally immature patients with open growth plates because of the risk of creating iatrogenic genu recurvatum from growth arrest.
- Patella alta, trochlear dysplasia, and TT-TG axial distance seem to have an insignificant bearing on outcomes after MPFL reconstruction for traumatic patellar instability in children and adolescents, so these are not contraindications to isolated MPFL surgery.[21]

### Preoperative Planning

- All imaging studies are reviewed for concurrent pathology. MRI scans best determine the size and location of osteochondral fractures and their potential for repair versus removal.
- Before positioning, an examination of the knee under anesthesia should be performed.
  - Test overall knee stability: Lachman, pivot shift, varus–valgus stress test, and AP drawer
  - Test lateral patellar tracking and medial and lateral patellar stability at 45 degrees of knee flexion. Results should be compared with those from the opposite knee.
  - Translation of the patella over 50% of the width of the patella laterally indicates an incompetency of the MPFL (**FIG 3**).
- Small metallic or bioabsorbable screws or pins should be available for osteochondral fracture repair.

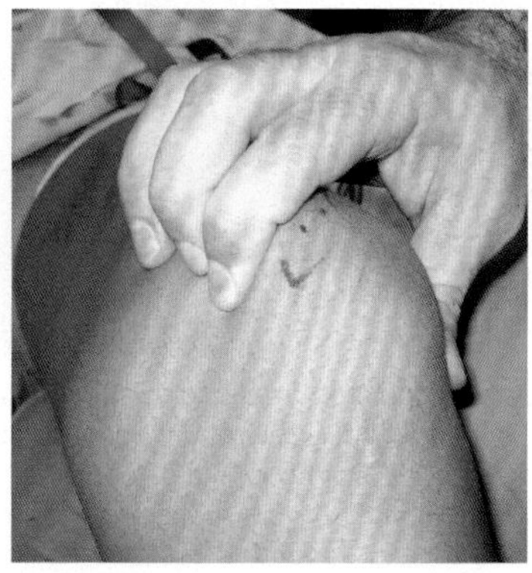

**FIG 3** • Complete dislocation of the patella at the time of surgery.

## Positioning

- The patient is positioned supine on a table that will allow knee imaging.
- The operative leg is free with a nonsterile tourniquet on the proximal thigh.
- A lateral post is used to apply a valgus moment and thus improve visualization of the medial compartment.
- The table can be kept flat with a 1 L bag of intravenous (IV) fluid taped on the end of the table to allow blocking the knee at about 45-degree flexion during patellar tunnel drilling and during final tensioning (**FIG 4**). Alternatively, the foot of the table is flexed about 30 to 45 degrees.
- The opposite leg can be positioned per the surgeon's preference.

## Approach

- Some surgeons perform diagnostic arthroscopy in all cases, but this procedure may be eliminated if a preoperative high-resolution MRI shows no articular damage of the patella of the lateral femoral condyle. Arthroscopy is indicated when there has been a new traumatic dislocation after the MRI was obtained.
- A lateral release is rarely necessary in combination with an MPFL reconstruction and may increase lateral instability.
- If an arthroscopic lateral release is being perfomed as part of the modified Insall procedure, a 4 to 5 cm limited medial parapatellar approach may be used, centering on the widest portion of the patella (**FIG 5**). Subcutaneous flaps can be elevated to allow great mobility of the prepatellar skin to limit the size of the incision.
- Alternatively, for the modified Insall procedure, and open subcutaneous lateral release can be performed through a 1-cm incision, along with the medial plication–imbrication, or both may be done through a midline incision.
- If needed, the hamstring semitendinosus graft is harvested through a standard proximal medial tibial approach with a tendon stripper.

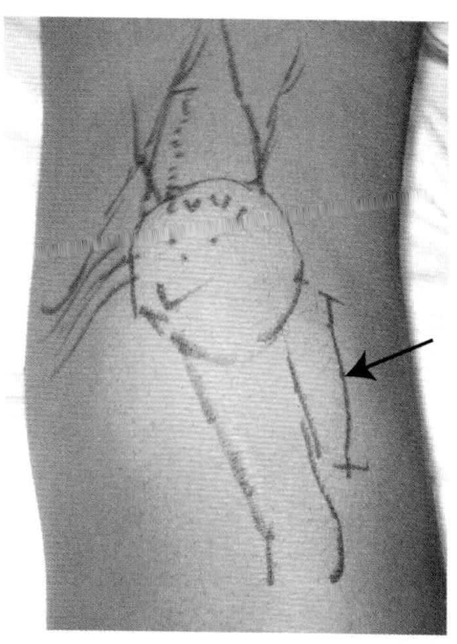

**FIG 5** ● For the modified Insall procedure, first an arthroscopic examination and limited lateral release (*arrow*) are performed. The surgical incision is centered over the medial aspect of the widest portion of the patella.

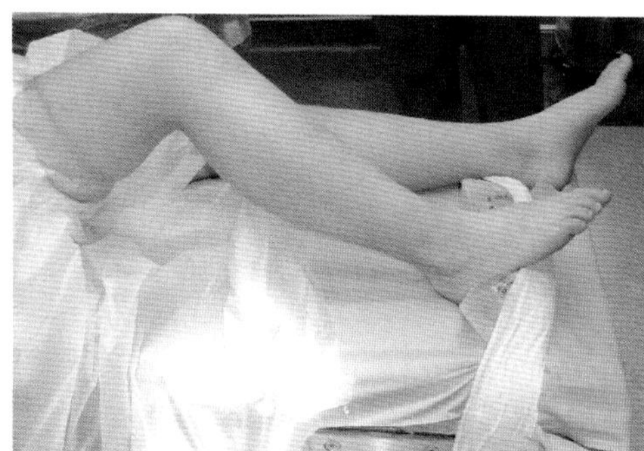

**FIG 4** ● Operating room position. Patients are positioned supine on a radiolucent operating room table. A bump is placed under the ipsilateral hip to help balance the knee in flexed position so it does not flop medial or lateral. An IV fluid bag is taped to the table to act as a block to hold the knee in about 45 degrees flexion during tensioning of the reconstruction.

# Medial Patellofemoral Ligament Reconstruction (Hamstring Autograft)

## Exposure and Tunnel Creation

- The semitendinosis or gracilis tendon (single tendon) is harvested using standard technique with a tendon stripper and trimmed if necessary to fit through a 3.5- to 4-mm diameter sizing device.
- A 3-cm medial patellar longitudinal skin incision is carried down sharply to the anteromedial border of the patella.
- All medial patellar soft tissue except the joint synovium is sharply elevated of the medial patella, and a tissue plane is developed in the extrasynovial fatty plane under the medial retinaculum, using Metzenbaum or curved tenotomy scissors.
  - This extrasynovial soft tissue tunnel is expanded down toward the medial epicondyle of the femur between layers 2 and 3. A pocket should easily be identified, and the insertion of the native MPFL can be palpated with a finger medially.
  - It is not necessary to enter the joint space.
- The extra-articular portion of the medial patella face is drilled with a 3.5-mm drill bit about 3 mm posterior to the thick anterior cortex and just superior to the equator of the patella. A 3.5-mm socket is drilled about 10 mm deep transversely from medial to lateral.
- A 3.5-mm tunnel is then drilled through the anterior cortex that meets up with the deep end of the 10-mm transverse socket, leaving a 10 mm bone bridge in the anterior cortex.
- No. 0 and no. 1 curettes are used to expand the tunnel up to about 3.5 to 4 mm, especially at the narrow isthmus where the medial and anterior sockets connect. A folded 22-gauge steel wire is placed from medial to lateral through the tunnel and is left as a marker.

## Pin Placement

- A finger is placed back under the medial retinaculum and down to the medial reflection (medial gutter) of the native MPFL, near the medial epicondyle, to estimate placement of a short Beath pin. The pin is positioned over the skin, and fluoroscopy verifies

TECHNIQUES

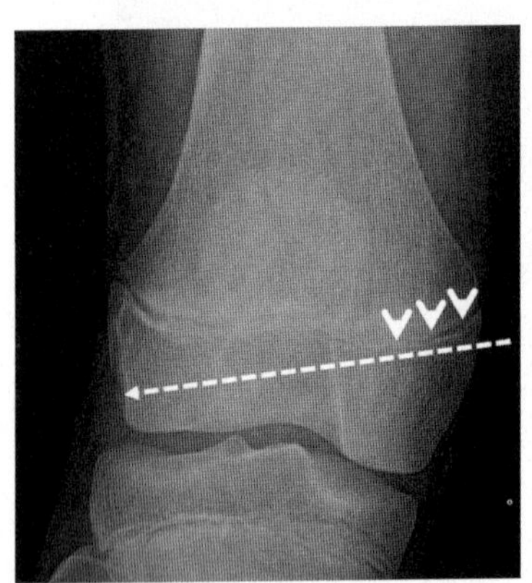
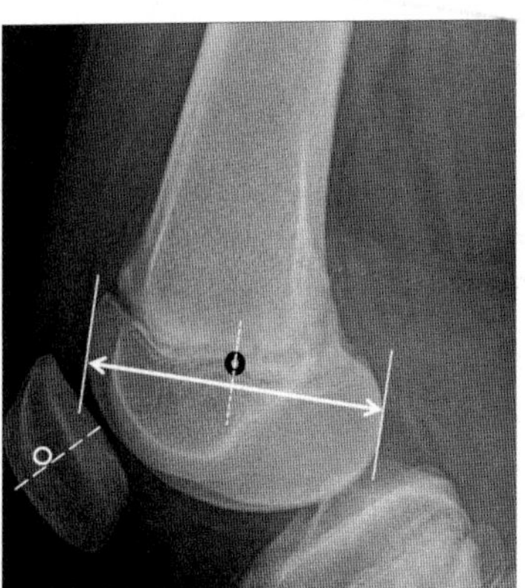

**TECH FIG 1** ● **A.** On the AP fluoroscopy view, the femoral guide pin is placed just distal to the medial femoral growth plate. Because the edge of the growth plate is cupped proximally (*arrowheads*), the pin trajectory is distal and lateral. **B.** On the lateral view, the knee is rotated so to obtain a perfect lateral with the posterior condyles superimposed. The femoral pin position (*black circle*) appears to overlie the growth plate due to the cupping. The pin entry point is halfway between the anterior and posterior condyles, which is slightly anterior to the adult Schöttle point. The patellar tunnel is placed just proximal to the equator of the patella.

that the pin is about 4 mm distal to the medial femoral growth plate before the tip is drilled or tapped a few millimeters into the medial femoral condyle.

- Because of proximal cupping of the medial distal femur growth plate, the Beath pin should be angled slightly distal across the epiphysis (**TECH FIG 1A**).
- Placement distal to the growth plate will avoid relative migration of the reconstructed MPFL up the femoral shaft with growth.

- A cross-table lateral fluoroscopic view is taken with the femoral condyles lined up perfectly. Because of proximal cupping of the edges of the distal femur condyle, the pin tip will project over the growth plate on the lateral view.[21] The pin is usually placed about halfway between the anterior and posterior border of the femoral condyle projections that are perfectly aligned on the lateral view (**TECH FIG 1B**).
  - This is slightly anterior to "Schöttle point," as described for adult MPFL surgery.[31]
- If the pin is driven all the way across the condyle and out the skin, it will bind on the on the IT band and make isometery and motion testing difficult. A 1-cm incision is made over the pin, stabbing down to the condyle to make a soft tissue tunnel down to the bone.

## Isometric Testing

- Isometry should be pretested before drilling the femoral tunnel. An umbilical tape is looped around the femoral guide pin and then passed under the medial patella retinaculum using a tonsil clamp placed through the anteromedial patellar incision. With the 22-gauge steel wire, the umbilical tape is pulled through the patellar tunnel.
- The ends of the umbilical tape are then clamped together with the knee at about 45 degrees. With a finger palpating the tension in the umbilical tape, the knee is flexed to 120 degrees and then extended to full hyperextension.
  - If the tape is too tight with hyperextension, the patella will pull medially. The guidewire should be moved slightly anterior, which is the most common correction.
  - If the tape is too tight in flexion, the pin should be moved slightly posterior.
  - About one-third of the time, the pin position needs to be readjusted to optimize isometry.

## Graft Placement and Completion

- Once isometry is acceptable, the thinnest end of the semitendinosus graft is pulled through the patellar tunnel and folded back on itself so it is a doubled graft. Then the two free ends of the tendon are sewn together with a no. 2 nonabsorbable suture using locking Krackow technique so that about 25 mm of tendon will pull into the femoral socket (**TECH FIG 2A**).
- The doubled tendon end is sized (usually to 5 to 6 mm in diameter). The femoral socket is drilled to the tendon diameter and about two times the anticipated depth, so as not to "bottom out" in the socket during tensioning.

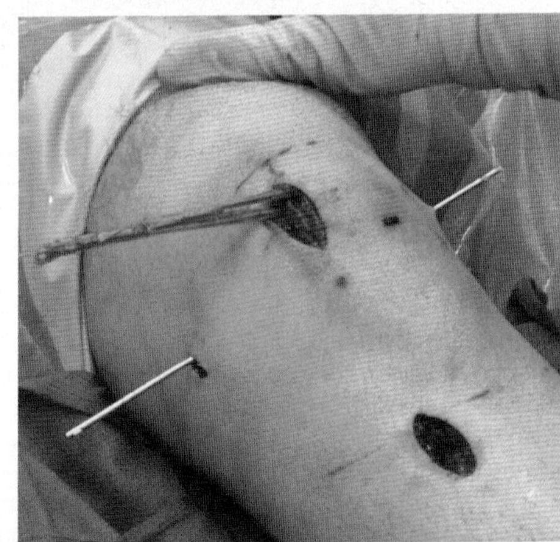

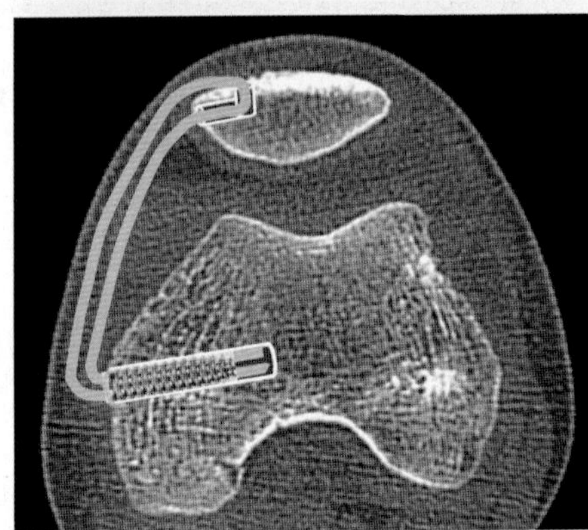

**TECH FIG 2** ● **A.** The hamstring graft is looped through the patellar tunnel, folded back on itself, and then the two free ends are sewn together. The doubled tendon ends are sized, and the femoral guide pin is reamed to the same diameter. The tendon is routed under the soft tissue and out the femoral incision and then drawn back into the femoral socket with the guide pin, which is pulled out laterally. **B.** Axial view showing the hamstring graft in its final position being looped through the patellar tunnel and the doubled ends fixed into the femoral socket with an interference screw.

- The tendon graft is then drawn under the medial retinaculum and brought out through the medial soft tissue tunnel surrounding the guide pin. The suture is placed in the guide pin eyelet. The interference screw's guidewire is placed in the socket before pulling the Beath pin across the distal femur and out the lateral side to sink the graft in the femoral socket.
- Light tension is placed on the tendon at 45 to 60 degrees of flexion, and the knee is fully flexed and extended to allow the graft to seek its level of zero tension.
- The graft is then fixed with a biocomposite interference screw (same diameter as the tunnel and usually 25 mm long) placed over the previously placed screw guide pin (**TECH FIG 2B**).
  - Ultimately, the graft should have no tension placed on it but instead should act as a leash that prevents patellar dislocation.
- Standard closure is performed, and a knee immobilizer is placed.

## Medial Patellofemoral Ligament Reconstruction (Quadriceps Turndown Graft)

- The incision in the quadriceps mechanism and retinaculum is kept as extrasynovial as possible, especially directly medial to the patella and distally.
- The retinaculum is dissected from the subcutaneous tissue superficially back to the medial intermuscular septum (**TECH FIG 3A**).
- It is then dissected from the synovium deep back to the intermuscular septum.
- A puncture hole is made in the retinaculum immediately anterior to the intermuscular septum, superficial to the medial epicondylar insertion of the natural ligament, and immediately distal to the VMO.
- The distance from the widest portion of the patella to the planned puncture site is measured.
- The medial 6 to 8 mm of full-thickness quadriceps tendon is taken typically as a 50- to 60-mm long graft remaining attached to the superior pole of the patella (**TECH FIG 3B**).
- The graft is subperiosteally reflected distally about 10 to 12 mm from the superior pole of the patella (more distally laterally than medially to allow it to fold over on itself during fixation and tensioning).
- A nonabsorbable suture is placed in the free end of the graft, with a whipstitch or other graft stitch performed with two ends.
- The graft is then passed deep to the retinaculum through the puncture hole to the superficial side of the retinaculum (**TECH FIG 3C**).
- The tension is then set via the medial retinaculum suture plication as described earlier before setting the tension of the graft.
- At 45 degrees of knee flexion, the graft is then tensioned to allow no more than 25% lateral translation of the patella. (**TECH FIG 3D**).
- The graft is secured into position with no. 1 or 2 nonabsorbable suture placed through the medial intermuscular septum periosteum of the medial epicondyle and the graft and retinaculum at the puncture hole in the retinaculum.
- It is further secured by 0 absorbable sutures in the graft and retinaculum, catching the graft superficial and deep to the retinaculum as the free end of the graft is directed back toward the patella.
- The suture in the free end of the graft is also used to secure it into position.
- Once the graft is secured and imbrication is complete, the knee is flexed to 90 degrees to ensure that no overtightening of the quadriceps mechanism has occurred and that the sutures stay in place.
- Tracking of the patella is also checked as described earlier.[26]

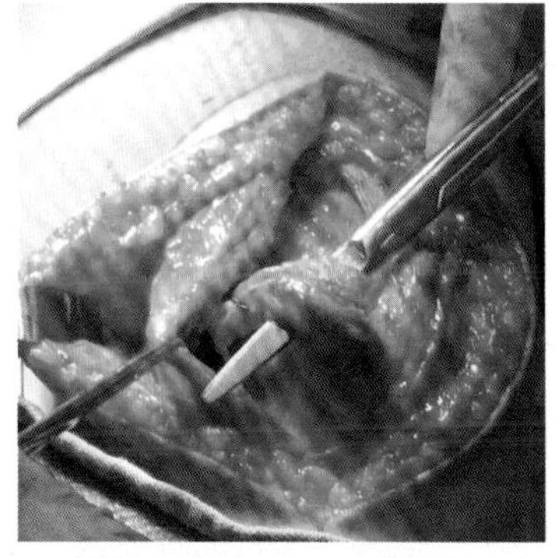
A

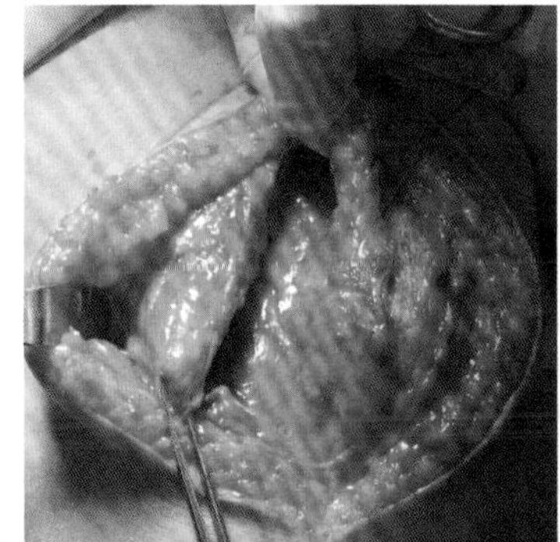
B

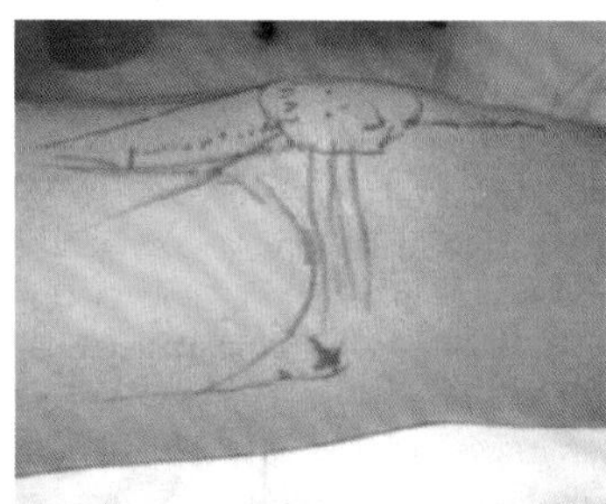
C

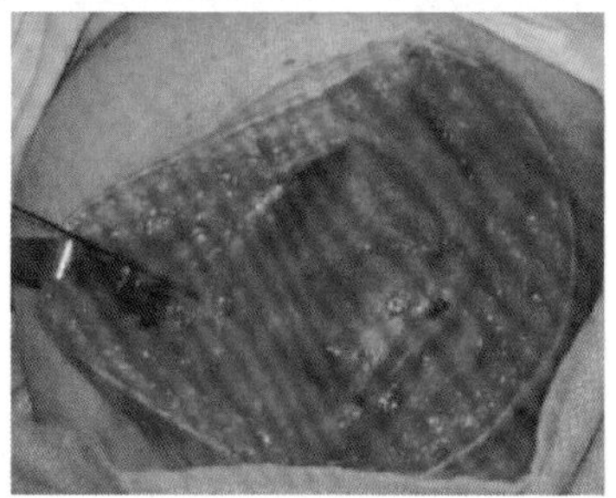
D

**TECH FIG 3** • **A.** The surgeon dissects deep to the medial retinaculum, posterior to the medial epicondyle and the medial intermuscular septum. **B.** If the MPFL is to be reconstructed, the surgeon measures the length of graft needed. A full-thickness quadriceps tendon graft 6 to 8 mm wide is obtained, with attachment to the patella maintained at its widest portion. **C.** The medial retinaculum is punctured at the point marked by placement anterior to the intermuscular septum, distal to the VMO, and superficial to the medial epicondyle. **D.** The graft is tensioned and secured to the medial retinaculum–intermuscular septum, also at 45 degrees.

## Medial Retinaculum Plication (Modified Insall)

- After dissection of the subcutaneous tissues, a medial parapatellar incision is made, leaving about 2 mm of tendon with the vastus medialis obliquus (VMO) (**TECH FIG 4A**).
- This incision in the tendon and the retinaculum is made from about 3 to 4 cm above the superior pole of the patella distally to 3 to 4 cm distal to the inferior pole of the patella medial to the tendon, leaving enough retinaculum with the tendon to suture to.
- The entire depth of the tendon and retinaculum is incised.
- The knee is then held in 45 degrees of flexion, and the patella is held in position in the center of the trochlea (**TECH FIG 4B**).
- Three nonabsorbable no. 1 or no. 2 sutures are placed, but not tied, in a horizontal mattress fashion.
- These are typically placed 25% to 40% across the width of the patella from medial to lateral, imbricating the edge of the tendon of the VMO and the retinaculum distally and laterally.
- With the three sutures held tight, the knee is placed through a range of motion, from full extension to 90 degrees of flexion, to check that enough imbrication has been performed.
- The sutures are then tied and a 0 absorbable suture is used above and below the imbrication to reinforce the tension set by these sutures.
- A running 0 absorbable suture then can be sutured over the imbrication to help reinforce the imbrication as well as lower its profile.
- The wound is irrigated and closed in layers.
- Absorbable 3-0 or 4-0 monofilament should be used in the skin.[10,11]

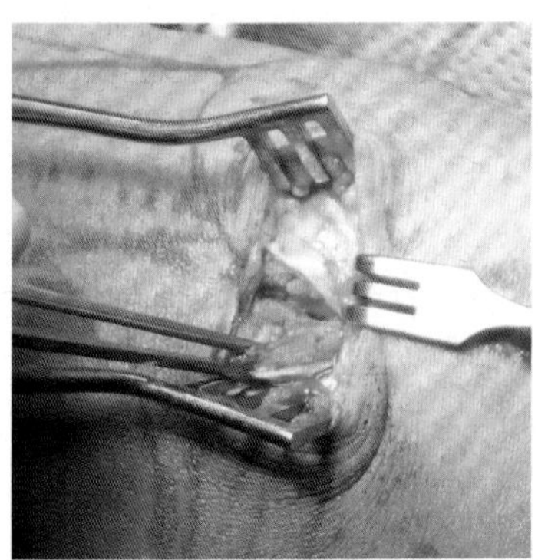

A

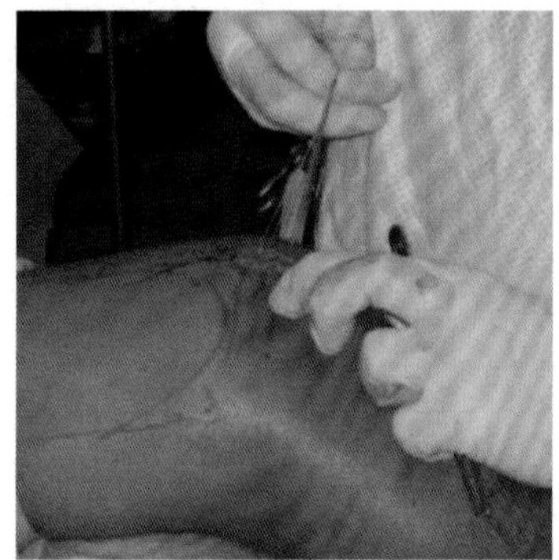

B

**TECH FIG 4** • **A.** Medial parapatellar incision is made with 2 to 3 mm of quadriceps tendon left attached to the VMO. **B.** The knee is placed at 45 degrees of flexion, with the patella centered in the femoral groove; set the tension of the medial side by imbricating the medial retinaculum.

## Galeazzi Procedure (Semitendinosus Tenodesis)

- The semitendinosus tendon (posterior and distal to the gracilis) is harvested with an open tendon stripper, and the distal tendon is left attached to the proximal tibia.
- The free end of the tendon is secured with a Krackow type of locking stitch of no. 2 nonabsorbable suture.
- Through a midline incision, the patella is exposed to allow an oblique 4- to 5-mm drill hole placed from proximal lateral to distal medial in the coronal plane of the patella.
- A lateral release is performed about 1 cm lateral to the patella, extending from the proximal tibia to 1 cm above the proximal patella.
- The free end of the semitendinosus is passed retrograde up through the oblique tunnel, and the free end is folded back across the anterior surface of the patella periosteum and sutured to the anterior patella or sewn back to itself if its length permits (**TECH FIG 5**).
- The graft should be tensioned and fixed with the knee at 45 to 60 degrees flexion.
- A knee immobilizer is placed, and the patient may bear weight as tolerated. Early motion is encouraged.
  - The Galeazzi procedure was reported to have an 82% redislocation rate and a poor functional outcome on the Kujala and International Knee Documentation Committee (IKDC) scales.[10]

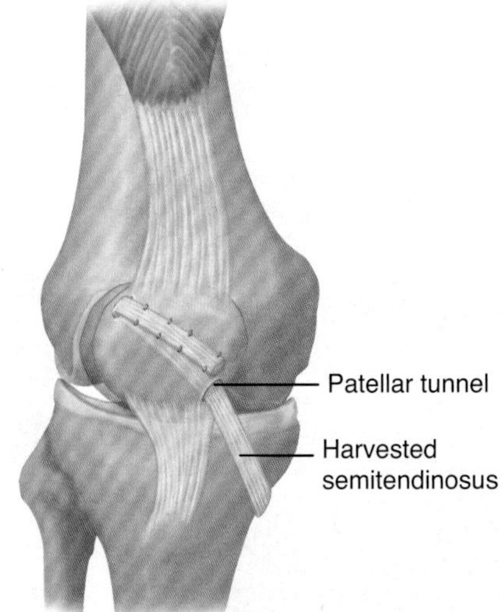


**TECH FIG 5** • Galeazzi procedure. Semitendinosus is harvested and left attached distally. The free end of the graft is fixed into the oblique patellar tunnel.

TECHNIQUES

## Roux-Goldthwaite Patellar Tendon Hemitransfer

- A midline incision about 5 to 6 cm long is taken down to the patellar tendon and the proximal tibia.
- A lateral release is performed from about 1 to 2 cm above the proximal pole of the patella, distal to the tibial tubercle.
- The patella tendon is split in its midline, and the distal end of the lateral half is released from the proximal tibia insertion without damaging the cartilaginous tibial tubercle.
- The free end of the lateral tendon is passed posterior to the medial tendon and brought out and sewn into the soft tissue of the medial proximal tibia, preferably into the insertion of the sartorius muscle (**TECH FIG 6**).
- The hemitransfer is tensioned in 45 to 60 degrees of flexion, with equal tension on both halves of the tendon.
- The knee is immobilized for 4 to 6 weeks.

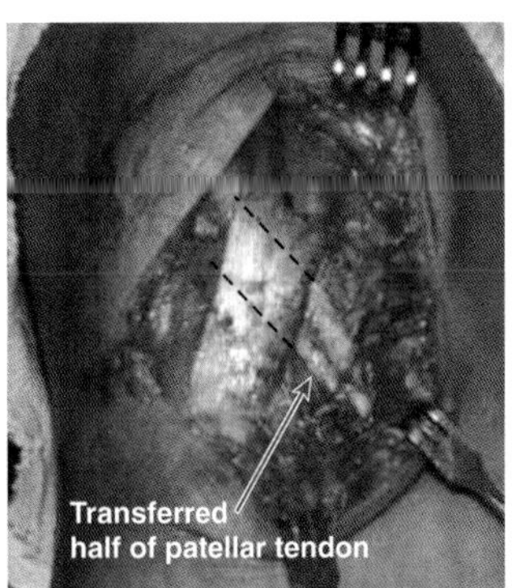


**TECH FIG 6** • Roux-Goldthwaite procedure in which the lateral half of the patella tendon is transferred into the soft tissue of the medial proximal tibia.

## PEARLS AND PITFALLS

| | |
|---|---|
| **Indications** | ■ Carefully select patients with proven instability.<br>■ Patients with patellofemoral pain and no instability signs are not good candidates for patellar stabilization.<br>■ MPFL reconstruction has excellent results in adolescents with recurrent traumatic patellar dislocation. |
| **Tension setting** | ■ The surgeon should make sure that the patella translates close to 25% of its width laterally after graft fixation. It should not be rigidly trapped in the trochlear groove.<br>■ This is best done by setting the tension with the knee flexed about 45 degrees.<br>■ Before closure, the knee is taken through the range of motion from 0 to greater than or equal to 120 degrees to ensure good alignment and to make sure that the graft is not under too much tension.<br>■ When placing the interference screw in the femoral tunnel avoid pushing the graft deeper into the tunnel which will cause over-tensioning. Twist the screw in rather than push the screw in. |
| **Quadriceps graft management** | ■ Care must be taken not to detach the quadriceps graft from the patella completely.<br>■ Dissecting more distally on the lateral aspect of the patellar attachment allows for the graft to lay down on itself.<br>■ The puncture site is positioned distal to the most inferior aspect of the VMO and immediately anterior to the intermuscular septum.<br>■ When passing the graft through the puncture hole in the retinaculum, a snap or Kocher clamp is used to hold the stitch in the free end. It is pulled through in line with the graft (the surgeon should push anterior to posterior, not pull posterior to anterior). |
| **Fixation problems (quadriceps)** | ■ The quadriceps graft is sutured at the patellar attachment as it folds over itself. |
| **MPFL reconstruction (hamstring)** | ■ The isometry of the femoral guidewire should be checked to avoid patellar maltracking before drilling the medial epicondyle tunnel.<br>■ The tendon is passed through the patellar tunnel with a Hewson suture passer or a folded 22-gauge steel wire. |
| **Galeazzi procedure** | ■ The hamstring tendon is passed retrograde through the patellar tunnel using a Hewson suture passer or a guide pin with an eyelet.<br>■ The transferred hamstring tendon is tensioned with the knee flexed 30–60 degrees. |
| **Roux-Goldthwaite procedure** | ■ The surgeon should avoid overtensioning the transferred lateral half of the patellar tendon to keep adequate tension on the untransferred half. |

## POSTOPERATIVE CARE

- MPFL reconstruction patients are placed in a hinged postoperative knee brace locked in full extension or a knee immobilizer.
- Weight bearing is as tolerated but is protected with crutches until the patient regains quadriceps control resisted straight-leg raise (hamstring graft) or is comfortable to walk with the knee fully extended in a knee brace (quadriceps graft).
- Physical therapy for range of motion (passive and active assisted) should be started in the first few days to combat arthrofibrosis.
- During the initial phase of therapy, patellar mobilization, quadriceps activation, straight-leg raises, pain modalities, and edema control are important.

- Range of motion is unrestricted with the hamstring graft technique.
  - With the quadriceps turndown graft, knee motion is restricted to 0 to 90 degrees for the first 3 to 4 weeks postoperatively. At 4 weeks, full range of motion is allowed with progressive quadriceps strengthening, edema control, and pain control, and gait training is initiated.
- Brace use in community settings is continued until adequate quadriceps strength has returned (about 6 weeks).
- From 6 to 12 weeks, there is continued progression of quadriceps strengthening and the addition of plyometrics.
- Functional return to activities starts at 3 to 6 months postoperatively.
- Galeazzi procedure patients have similar rehabilitation due to solid fixation if the tendon is sewn to itself.
- Roux-Goldthwaite procedure patients are kept toe-touch weight bearing for 6 weeks postoperatively, owing to the less secure fixation of the transferred tendon into medial proximal tibia soft tissue.

## OUTCOMES

- Child and adolescent patellar dislocation, particularly recurrent traumatic dislocation, can often be improved or cured with reconstructive surgery of the MPFL.[21] This is in sharp contrast to the poor functional results of medial imbrication/reef procedures, VMO transfer, and lateral release procedures, all of which usually result in redislocation at a rate equal to nonoperative treatment in adult and pediatric studies.[23,28]
- Andrish[1] suggested that failed MPFL reconstructions associated with trochlear or patellar dysplasia often necessitate a trochleoplasty, tibial tubercle transfer, or both.
- Examination of the results of MPFL repairs (not reconstructions), many with suture anchoring into the patella, showed an unacceptably high rate of redislocation.
- Paradoxically, lateral release has been shown to increase the tendency for lateral patellar dislocation rather than to relieve lateral tension and let the patella centralize.[6]
- The time-honored Galeazzi procedure has recently been shown to have an 82% redislocation rate and poor overall outcome measured on the IKDC and Kujala scores.[10]

## COMPLICATIONS

- Failure of fixation is typically seen at the time of surgery if knee is tested from 0 to 90 degrees (quadriceps MPFL).
- Late fixation failure is uncommon but can happen if flexion beyond 90 degrees is started too soon postoperatively (quadriceps MPFL).
- Arthrofibrosis should be treated aggressively with manipulation under anesthesia if greater than 90 degrees of flexion is not obtained by 6 weeks.
- Injury to the cutaneous nerves is common, and patients should be warned of this risk. It can be minimized with well-placed small incisions.
- Recurrence is seen in less than 10% of patients after MPFL reconstruction.
- Continued pain may occur, especially if not enough or too aggressive of a lateral release was performed, leading to either increased pressure on the patella or medial pressure and instability.
- Patellofemoral pain is often unchanged from the preoperative condition. Apprehension sensation is often improved.
  - Patients with severe patellofemoral arthrosis and patellofemoral pain syndrome may not benefit from these procedures.
  - Skeletally mature patients with patellofemoral arthrosis may benefit from a procedure that moves the tibial tubercle more anterior (Fulkerson osteotomy).
- Overtightening of medial soft tissue can result in medial dislocation. This is especially possible if a medial repair is tensioned in full extension or is combined with an extensive lateral release.
- Care must be taken to avoid patellar articular cartilage penetration when drilling patella holes, especially with the Galeazzi procedure.
- With the Roux-Goldthwaite procedure, there are reports of patellar tendon rupture of the untransferred tendon.

## REFERENCES


1. Andrish JT. Surgical reconstruction of the medial patellofemoral ligament. Tech Knee Surg 2006;5:121–127.
2. Atkin DM, Fithian DC, Marangi KS, et al. Characteristics of patients with primary acute lateral patellar dislocation and their recovery within the first 6 months of injury. Am J Sports Med 2000;28(4):472–479.
3. Beran MC, Samora WP, Klingele KE. Weight-bearing osteochondral lesions of the lateral femoral condyle following patellar dislocation in adolescent athletes. Orthopedics 2012;35(7):e1033–e1037.
4. Bitar AC, Demange MK, D'Elia CO, et al. Traumatic patellar dislocation: nonoperative treatment compared with MPFL reconstruction using patellar tendon. Am J Sports Med 2012;40(1):114–122.
5. Camanho GL, Viegas Ade C, Bitar AC, et al. Conservative versus surgical treatment for repair of the medial patellofemoral ligament in acute dislocations of the patella. Arthroscopy 2009;25(6):620–625.
6. Christoforakis J, Bull AM, Strachan RK, et al. Effects of lateral retinacular release on the lateral stability of the patella. Knee Surg Sports Traumatol Arthrosc 2006;14(3):273–277.
7. Dejour H, Walch G, Nove-Josserand L, et al. Factors of patellar instability: an anatomic radiographic study. Knee Surg Sports Traumatol Arthrosc 1994;2(1):19–26.
8. Felus J, Kowalczyk B. Age-related differences in medial patellofemoral ligament injury patterns in traumatic patellar dislocation: case series of 50 surgically treated children and adolescents. Am J Sports Med 2012;40(10):2357–2364.
9. Fithian DC, Paxton EW, Cohen AB. Indications in the treatment of patellar instability. J Knee Surg 2004;17(1):47–56.
10. Grannatt K, Heyworth BE, Ogunwole O, et al. Galeazzi semitendinosus tenodesis for patellofemoral instability in skeletally immature patients. J Pediatr Orthop 2012;32(6):621–625.
11. Hawkins RJ, Bell RH, Anisette G. Acute patellar dislocations. The natural history. Am J Sports Med 1986;14(2):117–120.
12. Hennrikus W, Pylawka T. Patellofemoral instability in skeletally immature athletes. J Bone Joint Surg Am 2013;95(2):176–183.
13. Hinton RY, Sharma KM. Acute and recurrent patellar instability in the young athlete. Orthop Clin North Am 2003;34(3):385–396.
14. Insall J, ed. Disorders of the patella. In: Surgery of the Knee. New York: Churchill Livingstone, 1984:191–260.
15. Insall J, Bullough PG, Burstein AH. Proximal "tube" realignment of the patella for chondromalacia patellae. Clin Orthop Relat Res 1979;(144):63–69.
16. Kepler CK, Bogner EA, Hammoud S, et al. Zone of injury of the medial patellofemoral ligament after acute patellar dislocation in children and adolescents. Am J Sports Med 2011;39(7):1444–1449.
17. Mäenpää H, Lehto MU. Patellar dislocation. The long-term results of nonoperative management in 100 patients. Am J Sports Med 1997;25(2):213–217.
18. Mäenpää H, Lehto MU. Patellofemoral osteoarthritis after patellar dislocation. Clin Orthop Relat Res 1997;(339):156–162.

19. Mountney J, Senavongse W, Amis AA, et al. Tensile strength of the medial patellofemoral ligament before and after repair or reconstruction. J Bone Joint Surg Br 2005;87(1):36–40.
20. Nelitz M, Dornacher D, Dreyhaupt J, et al. The relation of the distal femoral physis and the medial patellofemoral ligament. Knee Surg Sports Traumatol Arthrosc 2011;19(12):2067–2071.
21. Nelitz M, Dreyhaupt J, Reichel H, et al. Anatomic reconstruction of the medial patellofemoral ligament in children and adolescents with open growth plates: surgical technique and clinical outcome. Am J Sports Med 2013;41(1):58–63.
22. Nietosvaara Y, Aalto K, Kallio PE. Acute patellar dislocation in children: incidence and associated osteochondral fractures. J Pediatr Orthop 1994;14(4):513–515.
23. Nikku R, Nietosvaara Y, Aalto K, et al. Operative treatment of primary patellar dislocation does not improve medium-term outcome: a 7-year follow-up report and risk analysis of 127 randomized patients. Acta Orthop 2005;76(5):699–704.
24. Nikku R, Nietosvaara Y, Kallio P, et al. Operative versus closed treatment of primary dislocation of the patella. Similar 2-year results in 125 randomized patients. Acta Orthop Scand 1997;68(5):419–423.
25. Nomura E, Horiuchi Y, Inoue M. Correlation of MR imaging findings and open exploration of medial patellofemoral ligament injuries in acute patellar dislocations. Knee 2002;9(2):139–143.
26. Noyes FR, Albright JC. Reconstruction of the medial patellofemoral ligament with autologous quadriceps tendon. Arthroscopy 2006; 22(8):904.
27. Paakkala A, Sillanpää P, Huhtala H, et al. Bone bruise in acute traumatic patellar dislocation: volumetric magnetic resonance imaging analysis with follow-up mean of 12 months. Skeletal Radiol 2010;39(7): 675–682.
28. Palmu S, Kallio PE, Donell ST, et al. Acute patellar dislocation in children and adolescents: a randomized clinical trial. J Bone Joint Surg Am 2008;90(3):463–470.
29. Sallay PI, Poggi J, Speer KP, et al. Acute dislocation of the patella. A correlative pathoanatomic study. Am J Sports Med 1996;24(1):52–60.
30. Sanders TG, Morrison WB, Singleton BA, et al. Medial patellofemoral ligament injury following acute transient dislocation of the patella: MR findings with surgical correlation in 14 patients. J Comput Assist Tomogr 2001;25(6):957–962.
31. Schöttle PB, Schmeling A, Rosenstiel N, et al. Radiographic landmarks for femoral tunnel placement in medial patellofemoral ligament reconstruction. Am J Sports Med 2007;35(5):801–804.
32. Sillanpää PJ, Mattila VM, Maenpää H, et al. Treatment with and without initial stabilizing surgery for primary traumatic patellar dislocation: a prospective randomized study. J Bone Joint Surg Am 2009;91(2):263–273.
33. Stanitski CL, Paletta GA Jr. Articular cartilage injury with acute patellar dislocation in adolescents. Arthroscopic and radiographic correlation. Am J Sports Med 1998;26(1):52–55.
34. Vollnberg B, Koehlitz T, Jung T, et al. Prevalence of cartilage lesions and early osteoarthritis in patients with patellar dislocation. Eur Radiol 2012;22:2347–2356.
35. Zhao J, Huangfu X, He Y. The role of medial retinaculum plication versus medial patellofemoral ligament reconstruction in combined procedures for recurrent patellar instability in adults. Am J Sports Med 2012;40:1355–1364.

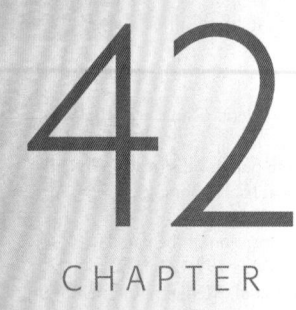

# Tibial Tubercle Transfer

John P. Fulkerson

## DEFINITION

- Tibial tubercle transfer is a versatile surgical alternative in the treatment of difficult and resistant patellofemoral disorders ranging from patellofemoral instability to patellofemoral arthritis.
- Patients with combined instability and arthritis often benefit from tibial tubercle transfer.
- Tibial tubercle transfer may be best regarded as "compensatory." In other words, if a multiplicity of structure and alignment factors leads to patellar instability or arthritis, carefully planned repositioning of the tibial tubercle can compensate for other deficiencies, providing permanent relief of pain and instability.

## ANATOMY

- The patella articulates within the femoral trochlea in such a way that the distal aspect of the patella enters the trochlea from a slightly lateralized position upon initiation of knee flexion. Normally, the patella enters the trochlea promptly within the first 10 degrees of flexion, first making contact with the distal aspect of the patella.
- As the knee flexes further, load is transferred more proximally on the patella such that in full flexion, contact is on the proximal aspect of the patella. The intervening flexion transfers load more gradually along the patella, moving proximally with each degree of flexion load.[11]
- As the patella enters the trochlea with further knee flexion, the trochlea becomes deeper, so that containment of the patella is improved. Therefore, in most people, the point of greatest instability is early flexion of the knee, when the trochlea is at its shallowest and containment of the patella is most limited.
- The position of the tibial tuberosity relative to the femoral trochlea further complicates the process of patella entry into the trochlea.[4]
  - This relationship has been referred to as the *tibial tuberosity to trochlear groove (TT–TG) index*, measured in millimeters using superimposed tomographic images of the position of the central trochlea and the tibial tubercle (**FIG 1**).
- The patella is contained within a soft tissue investing layer of tendon and retinacular structure.
  - The lateral retinaculum extends to the iliotibial band but also proximally to the lateral femur and to the tibia (the patellofemoral and patellotibial components, respectively, of the lateral retinaculum).
  - On the medial side is the medial retinaculum including the medial patellofemoral ligament (MPFL) and the medial quadriceps tendon–femoral ligament (MQTFL), which extends from the proximal half of the peripatellar extensor mechanism to the adductor tubercle region.[1] This medial retinaculum is complex and is predominantly a blend of restraint fibers from the adductor tubercle region into the extensor expansion, not so much into the patella itself.
  - The patellar tendon is located distally, with the quadriceps tendon proximally connecting the patella to the quadriceps muscle. The quadriceps tendon is a massive tendon,

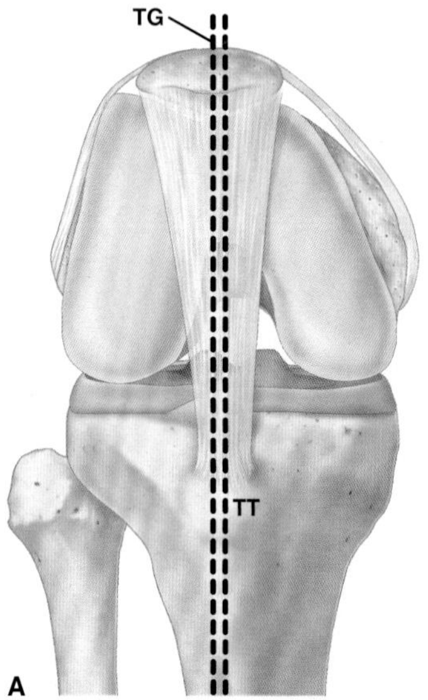


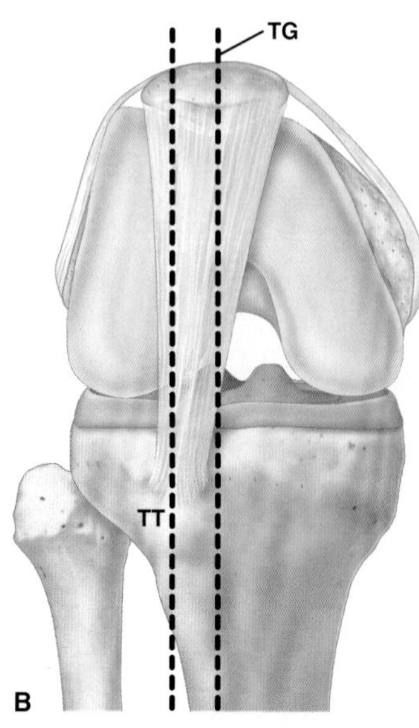


**FIG 1** • The relation of the tibial tubercle (*TT*) to the central trochlear groove (*TG*)—the TT–TG relationship—pertains to patellar instability. **A.** Normal TT–TG relationship, in which the tibial tubercle and trochlear groove are lined up. **B.** Lateralized tibial tubercle.

including a major vastus lateralis tendon component on the proximal lateral aspect of the patella.

- The superolateral corner of the patella is supported dynamically by the vastus lateralis obliquus, which interdigitates with the lateral intermuscular septum.[14]

## PATHOGENESIS

- The pathogenesis of problems around the patellofemoral joint relates to dysplasia of anterior knee anatomy, malalignment, and trauma.
- Most patients with significant dysplasia have a congenital underlying imbalance of the extensor mechanism and/or lower extremity, which leads to improper morphologic development.
- A chronically lateralized extensor mechanism is likely to cause abnormally high lateral pressure on the femoral trochlea, thereby leading to developmental flattening of the lateral trochlea and also flattening of the lateral patella (**FIG 2**).

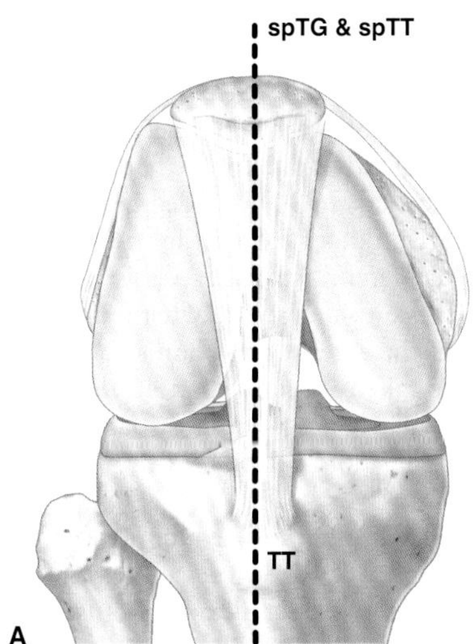


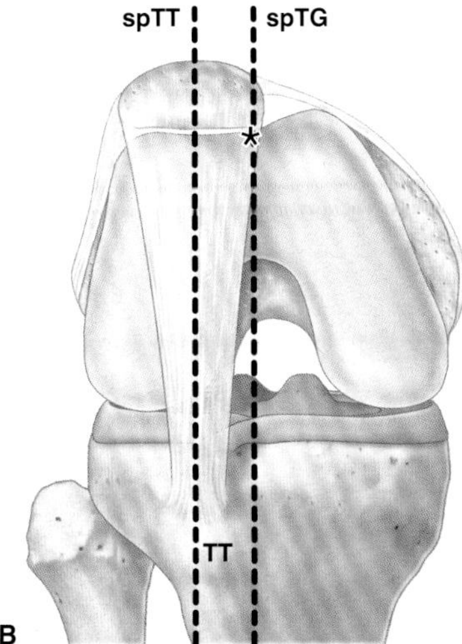


**FIG 2** • **A.** Normal trochlear groove. **B.** With prolonged lateral patella tracking, the lateral trochlea becomes flattened, further aggravating lateral patellar instability and stretching the medial patella support structure (including the MPFL). *asterisk*, center of trochlea; *spTG*, sagittal plane of trochlear groove; *spTT*, sagittal plane of tibial tubercle; *TT*, tibial tubercle.

Although it is not always the case, this pattern of development most likely explains the poor development of the lateral trochlea, trochlea dysplasia, and persistent instability in patients with abnormal extensor mechanism alignment. Such patients stretch the medial patella support structure over time, leading to subluxation and tilt of the patella in many cases.

  - This stretching can lead to chronic instability, chronic overload of the lateral patellofemoral joint, dislocation (which often causes *medial* patella articular damage as the dislocated patella reenters the lateral trochlea forcefully after a dislocation), breakdown of the lateral patellofemoral joint, and pain related to overload of the joint and peripatellar retinacula.[13]

- Some patients have anterior knee pain as the result of blunt trauma causing subchondral bone or retinacular injury, usually with the knee flexed.
- An impact to the flexed knee and resulting trauma to the patellofemoral joint usually leads to proximal patella injury. This is important because anteriorization of the tibial tubercle shifts contact on the patella proximally and can, therefore, exacerbate a lesion on the proximal patella related to blunt injury.
- Because lateral tracking of the patella is not a factor in the injury of most patients who have had blunt trauma, the problem usually is not one of abnormal extensor mechanism alignment requiring correction.

## NATURAL HISTORY

- The natural history of patellofemoral pain, instability, or arthrosis often relates to the imbalance noted earlier. With chronic lateral tracking of the patella in the trochlea, overload occurs with increased point loading on the patella and trochlea, particularly the patella.
- Eventually, this can lead to breakdown of articular cartilage and what Ficat[7] has called *excessive lateral pressure syndrome* (**FIG 3**).
  - Schutzer et al[21] demonstrated a high incidence of patellofemoral tilt and subluxation in patients with patellofemoral pain, compared with controls.
- With dislocation of the patella, the MPFL is torn and, even after healing, elongated. This further exacerbates any tendency toward lateral displacement of the patella out of the trochlea.
- With blunt trauma, pain is related to impact and subchondral bone injury, generally on the proximal patella. This pain, then, originates from injured subchondral bone because there are no nerves in cartilage.

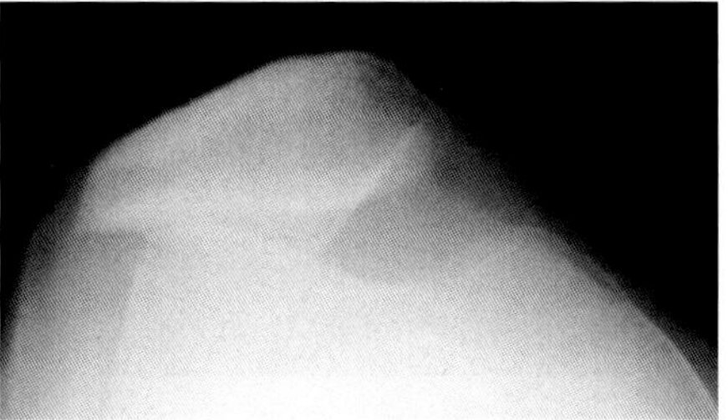

**FIG 3** • Excessive lateral pressure leads to lateral patellar chondropathy and breakdown. (Courtesy of David Dejour.)

## PATIENT HISTORY AND PHYSICAL FINDINGS

- In the patient who may be a candidate for tibial tubercle transfer, it is important to establish that this definitive surgery truly is indicated because of a structural alignment imbalance or articular overload condition leading to instability or pain.
  - The physical examination should emphasize a very critical look at patella tracking within the femoral trochlea, the condition of the medial retinacular structure, evidence of focal articular breakdown of the patellofemoral joint, evidence of retinacular or soft tissue pain, and a search for other possible causes of pain such as medial or lateral compartment disease or referred pain from the hip or back.
- Careful palpation of the retinacular structure around the patella will indicate whether there is soft tissue or retinacular overload contributing to pain.[18]
  - In some cases, simple release of the painful retinacular structure may be all that is needed.
- When examining the medial retinaculum including MPFL and MQTFL, holding the patella laterally in extension is recommended, then slowly flexing the knee to see whether the medial supports deliver the patella into the central trochlea by 20 to 30 degrees of knee flexion. A distinct pressure, pushing the examining finger back as the patella enters the trochlea, should be encountered using this technique.
  - If the patella remains lateralized with the examining finger holding it lateral as the knee is flexed to 20 to 30 degrees of flexion, the medial retinacular supports are incompetent.[10]
- Similarly, in a patient who has had previous extensor mechanism surgery, the examiner should hold the patella medially in extension and flex the knee abruptly to 30 to 40 degrees of flexion (**FIG 4**).
  - If the patella enters the trochlea very suddenly and reproduces the patient's symptom, he or she actually may have a *medial instability* problem (ie, medial subluxation) that requires repair or reconstruction of the lateral support structure or even lateralization of the tibial tubercle if it previously was overmedialized.

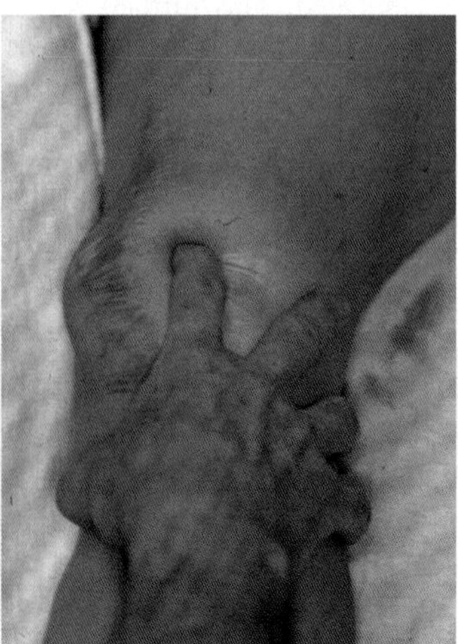

**FIG 4** • Test for medial patellar subluxation. The patella is held medial and the knee is flexed abruptly. If patella relocation reproduces the patient's symptom, pathologic medial subluxation probably is present.

- The patella is held in the central trochlea, and the knee is flexed with compression of the patella to see if this elicits crepitus or pain. The degree of flexion at which this crepitus or pain occurs is important in localizing the location of the lesion, bearing in mind that the articulation surface of the patella moves proximally as the knee is flexed. This compression of the patella in the trochlea should be repeated as the patient extends the knee actively against resistance of the other examining hand from full flexion up to full extension, taking note of where pain or crepitus occurs with active extension against resistance.
- Every patient should be examined prone so that the hip can be rotated internally and externally to see if there is a source of pain within the hip. With the patient prone, the pelvis is flat, and, therefore, flexion of the knee may be completed to compare with the contralateral side to establish whether the quadriceps and extensor mechanism are overly tight. The patient should be taught at this time how to stretch the extensor mechanism.
- Nonoperative treatment should be exhausted before considering surgical intervention.

## IMAGING AND OTHER DIAGNOSTIC STUDIES

- In diagnosis of the anterior knee, a standardized office posteroanterior radiograph with the knee flexed 45 degrees and standardized axial radiograph of the patellofemoral joint with the knee flexed exactly to 30 or 45 degrees is very important.[15]
  - By 45 degrees of knee flexion, the patella normally is centralized in the femoral trochlea. This is a good screening test in the office to determine whether there is significant imbalance of the extensor mechanism.
  - Radiographs taken in more than 45 degrees knee flexion are not particularly useful in most patients.
  - Our practice has not found 30-60-90–degree radiographs useful.
  - Many patients present for evaluation with axial radiographs taken only at 90 degrees of flexion. This probably is easier for radiology technicians because they can simply hang the patient's legs over the side of an examining table and take the axial radiograph in this fashion. It is very important to standardize flexion to 30 or 45 degrees, using a support frame as needed.
- The other important office radiograph is the true lateral view[16] (**FIG 5**), which is taken with the knee at 30 degrees of

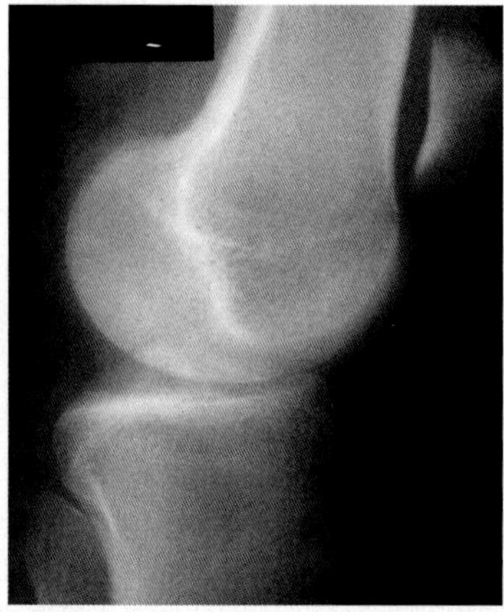

**FIG 5** • The true lateral radiograph defines the osseous structure of the trochlea most accurately.

flexion and standing. The posterior femoral condyle should be overlapped.

- This view is technically demanding, but most radiology technicians with reasonable experience can palpate the posterior condyles and, with one or sometimes two tries, obtain a good lateral view with overlap (or near-complete overlap) of the posterior condyles.
- This study shows the femoral trochlea completely so that the central sulcus can be identified as well as both medial and lateral aspects of the trochlea from proximal to distal.

- Other imaging studies include computed tomography (CT), magnetic resonance imaging (MRI), and radionuclide scan. Relatively few patients require these studies.
  - If CT is done, it is best performed at 0, 15, 30, and 45 degrees of knee flexion, obtaining midpatellar transverse images to see how the patella enters the trochlea. This should be done with reproduction of normal standing alignment on the tomographic table.
  - MRI is less useful in many patients but can be helpful in evaluating articular cartilage and soft tissue structure as well as gaining insight into subchondral bone reaction. Additionally, the caregiver may be able to measure the relationship between the tibial tubercle and the trochlear groove by scrolling between these locations on the axial images and using the ruler from toolbar. It is important to acknowledge here, though, that such TT–TG measurements are approximations and not absolute indicators for whether or not to do a tibial tubercle transfer.
  - Radionuclide scanning is not often used but can be extremely helpful in determining subchondral bone reaction to overload.[5] It may be most applicable in patients with trauma to the anterior knee, unexplained anterior knee pain, or chronic patella overload and in cases involving workers' compensation litigation where objective findings beyond the normal studies needed to determine appropriate treatment are particularly important.
  - In some cases, a single-photon emission computed tomographic (SPECT) scan also can be helpful in accurately locating a source of subchondral bone overload. SPECT may play a role, selectively, in patients who require a patella unloading or resurfacing procedure.

## NONOPERATIVE MANAGEMENT

- Before tibial tubercle transfer is considered, all patients must exhaust nonoperative management, including complete lower extremity core stability therapy, patellofemoral taping and bracing (I prefer the Tru-Pull brace that I helped design [DJ ORTHO, Vista, CA]), and modification of activity.
- Viscosupplementation may be helpful in some patients with patellofemoral arthritis but has not been very helpful in most patellofemoral arthrosis patients.

## SURGICAL MANAGEMENT

- In patients with more severe extensor mechanism imbalance, instability, pain, and eventual articular cartilage breakdown are fairly common. When specific factors such as disruption of the medial retinacular (MQTFL, MPFL) structures cause instability, reconstruction of the deficient structure should be considered first.
  - In many patients with patellar instability, restoration of medial support, either by imbrication (open or arthroscopic) or reconstruction of the MPFL and release of tight lateral retinaculum, may be the procedure of choice when dysplasia and trochlea structure are normal or near normal. In general, this is the first line of surgical treatment after failed nonoperative measures in a patient with patellar instability related to deficiency of medial support structure.
- In patients with more severe dysplasia, a high TT–TG index (see **FIG 1B**), and degenerative change in the patella or trochlea, tibial tubercle transfer offers an opportunity to improve balance permanently and provide long-term relief of instability.
- Tibial tubercle transfer in the treatment of patellar instability is best used when the TT–TG index is high (>20 is a rough guideline), the Q angle is high (usually >20 degrees), or the lateral trochlea is dysplastic, such that soft tissue reconstruction alone will either be less likely to succeed or require excessive tension resulting in overload of the medial patellofemoral joint.[20]
  - Anteriorization alone is best reserved for patients with painful distal patella articular degeneration alone without abnormal lateral tracking of the patella.
  - MPFL reconstruction alone is insufficient in the face of more serious tracking dysfunction because of the need to "pull" the patella in a posteromedial direction to gain stability and achieve central tracking, thereby adding load to the patella that eventually might lead to patellofemoral joint degeneration. One must recognize the inherent benefit of tibial tubercle transfer in patients with more severe patella lateral tracking
  - Tibial tubercle transfer also provides immediate fixation and stability, making early range of motion (ROM) possible, further reducing the risk of stiffness, tightness, and chronic pain in the anterior knee following reconstructive surgery for instability.
- In the treatment of patellofemoral arthritis, tibial tubercle anteromedialization or anteriorization plays an important role in joint preservation.
  - Many patients have patellofemoral arthritis as a result of excessive lateral pressure, as originally described by Ficat.[7] This excessive lateral pressure eventually causes erosion of the lateral patellofemoral joint, sometimes to bone, because of the constant lateralization of the patella related to lateral subluxation and high lateral pressure on the lateral patella facet. Lateral release has been used to reduce this pressure and is helpful in the early stages when patella tilt is prominent.
  - Tibial tubercle transfer is a powerful procedure for unloading and rebalancing the extensor mechanism, placing the patella into the center trochlea, and maintaining it there through an ROM.
- By adding some anteriorization to a medial tibial tubercle transfer (ie, anteromedial tibial tubercle transfer), the distal articular surface of the patella may be unloaded.[19] This is important because many patients with patellofemoral chondrosis or arthrosis have distal patella articular breakdown or pain. Anteriorization of the tibial tubercle unloads the distal articular surface of the patella permanently, and the

medialization component of this procedure rebalances the patella in the central trochlea, unloading the lateral facet.

- Most patients with chronic lateralization of the extensor mechanism develop lateral facet breakdown and distal patella degeneration over time because of the abnormal shear stress and lateral overload. Anteromedial tibial tubercle transfer compensates for this and is, therefore, the procedure of choice for treating articular degeneration and pain emanating from the distal or lateral patella articular surface.[6]
- Anterolateral tibial tubercle transfer[9] may be best regarded as a salvage procedure in patients who have had previous overmedialization of the tibial tubercle. It has been helpful in relieving pain related to chronic medial patellofemoral arthritis resulting from a previous Hauser procedure in which the tibial tubercle was moved posteriorly, medially, and distally to stabilize the extensor mechanism at an earlier time.
- Distalization of the tibial tubercle is only necessary in more extreme cases of patella alta, generally when distalization is necessary to maintain stability. Distalization, in my experience, however, carries considerable risk of pain and/or patella overload, so I have not found it useful except in fairly extreme cases in which it is needed to create a stable patellofemoral joint beyond what can be achieved with medial reconstruction, lateral release/elongation, and medial or anteromedial tibial tubercle transfer.



# Medial Tibial Tubercle Transfer

## Incision and Dissection

- Medial tibial tubercle transfer is best approached through a midline incision from the midpatella to a region approximately 5 to 7 cm distal to the tibial tubercle.[3]
- The medial and lateral borders of the patellar tendon are identified, the anterior tibialis muscle is reflected posteriorly and retracted, the skin edges are retracted, and a cut is made deep to the tibial tubercle.

## Osteotomy

- A flat incision is made posterior to the tibial tubercle, tapered anteriorly at its distal extent such that only about 1 mm of bone is left at the distal tip of the osteotomy and the proximal cut is made about 2 mm above the patellar tendon insertion.
    - This cut should be made perpendicular to the anterior surface of the tibia such that a flat ledge is left to add additional stability to the transferred tibial tubercle. This proximal cut must be made in such a way that the tibial tubercle may be freely moved medially, that is, the medial side of the proximal cut is more proximal than the lateral side of the proximal cut, open medially.
    - The thickness of the cut deep to the tibial tubercle will vary depending on the individual patient's need for medialization.
        - In patients with a severe dysplasia requiring more than 1 cm of medialization, a deeper cut will be required.
        - In patients requiring 1 cm of medialization, a proximal tibial tubercle anteroposterior thickness of 1 to 1.5 cm is ample in most cases.
    - Care must be taken to taper this osteotomy anteriorly at the distal extent of the cut to allow for easy greenstick fracturing of the tip of the osteotomy to move the tubercle medially.

## Completion of the Transfer

- After the osteotomy has been completed with an oscillating saw, the proximal cut usually is made with a 1- to 2-inch osteotome.
- The osteotomized fragment is elevated and then displaced medially. If there is an overhang of bone medially, it can be removed with the saw or a rongeur.
- The fragment is then stabilized securely with two cortical lag screws (**TECH FIG 1**), carefully measuring the depth of the drill hole, overdrilling the proximal fragment, and lagging the fragment down using the posterior cortex to hold the cortical screw.
    - Care must be taken not to allow the cortical screw tip to protrude any more than necessary beyond the posterior cortex.
    - The surgeon releases the lateral retinaculum either arthroscopically or by open surgery to achieve the needed balance of the extensor mechanism upon tibial tubercle transfer.
    - Some thickening and even mild infrapatellar contracture may be observed in patients who have had longstanding and more severe imbalance of the extensor mechanism. This also should be released at the time of surgery.
    - Tracking of the patella within the central trochlea should be confirmed arthroscopically or openly after the tibial tubercle transfer.

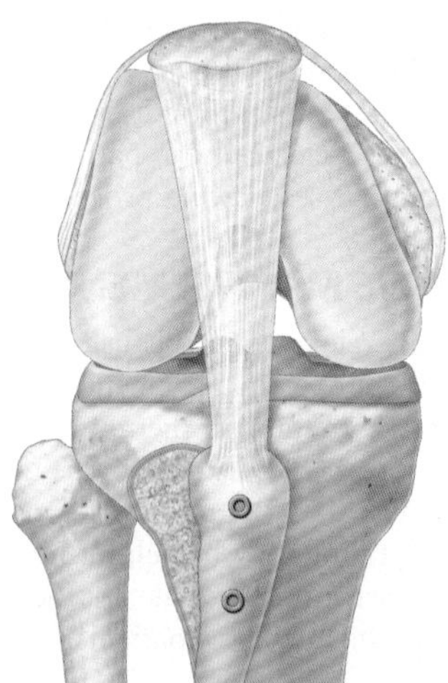

**TECH FIG 1** • Correction of abnormal TT–TG relationship by medialization of tibial tubercle.

## Anteromedial Tibial Tubercle Transfer

### Incision and Dissection

- To unload both the distal and lateral aspects of the patella, an oblique osteotomy must be created deep to the tibial tubercle and the tibial tubercle transferred in both anterior and medial directions.[8,12]
- To perform anteromedial tibial tubercle transfer, a longitudinal incision close to midline extending from a region about halfway between the patella and the tibial tubercle to about 7 cm distal to the tibial tubercle usually is sufficient.
- After isolating the patellar tendon, the anterior tibialis muscle is released and reflected posteriorly.
- Because an oblique osteotomy will be made from medial to lateral, a large retractor must be placed to retract the anterior tibialis muscle laterally to view the saw making the osteotomy cut as it exits on the posterolateral aspect of the tibia. The entire lateral side of the tibia must be under direct view[11] (**TECH FIG 2**).

### Osteotomy

- At this point, it usually is best to use a guide, such as the Tracker guide (Mitek, Norwood, MA) or Arthrex AMZ guide (Naples, FL), to ensure an accurate osteotomy cut. With experience, some surgeons can make this cut without a guide, but only a surgeon who is doing this type of surgery on a regular basis will feel comfortable without guide control.
- An external fixator block also may be used to create an appropriate orientation for the osteotomy (**TECH FIG 3A**). A drill bit is left at the top and bottom of the osteotomy.
- The osteotomy usually extends from the level of the tibial tubercle to a level of about 7 to 9 cm distally on the tibia and again must exit at the level of the anterior cortex of the tibia to avoid a cortical notch distally.
  - Making a deep cut (notch) distally increases the risk of tibia fracture; this should be avoided.
- After the guide is placed at the desired angle to create an oblique osteotomy from medial to lateral, a cut is made from the region immediately adjacent to the patellar tendon insertion medially and angled posterolaterally so that the saw blade will exit on the lateral cortex (**TECH FIG 3B**) under direct visualization at all times.
  - This strategy avoids injury to the anterior tibial artery and deep peroneal nerve, which are around the posterolateral corner of the tibia posteriorly.
  - The cut should start distally first where it is most visible, and as the oblique cut proceeds proximally, it will become more posterior.
- Once the proximal extent of the cut has reached the level of the mid to posterior portion of the lateral tibia cortex, it should be stopped at the lateral side. An osteotome or saw then is used to make a back cut from the corner of the proximal lateral corner of the osteotomy up to a point proximal to the patellar tendon laterally.
  - This allows for release of the lateral cortex when the osteotomy has been completed, and the osteotomized fragment will be displaced anteromedially.
- The third cut for anteromedial tibial tubercle transfer is directly proximal to the patellar tendon insertion on the tibia, about 2 mm above the patellar tendon insertion.
  - This cut usually is made with a 1/4- or 1/2-inch osteotome under direct vision using an Army-Navy retractor to hold the patellar tendon anteriorly.
  - It is best made from medial to lateral and connects the proximal extent of the medial osteotomy cut to the oblique back cut on the lateral side so that the osteotomy is now free to displace anteromedially.
  - It is moved anteromedially by greenstick fracturing the anterior cortex distally, which should be no more than 1 to 2 mm thick at its distal extent.
  - The osteotomized fragment is moved about 1 cm but may be moved slightly more, as needed, to achieve more anteriorization or medialization.
  - The obliquity of this osteotomy will be determined by how much anteriorization and how much medialization the surgeon wants (**TECH FIG 3C,D**).
    - When there is a greater need for realignment of the extensor mechanism, the cut should be made flatter so that more medialization can be achieved.
    - When it is more urgent to unload a damaged or painful distal patella, the cut should be made more oblique (steeper), allowing more anteriorization.
    - Thus, this osteotomy is customized for each patient, depending on the specific need.

### Completion of the Transfer

- The osteotomized fragment is fixed securely with two cortical lag screws.
  - These screws must be carefully positioned to ensure that they remain within the cortex and that they have good cortical bone purchase on both sides.

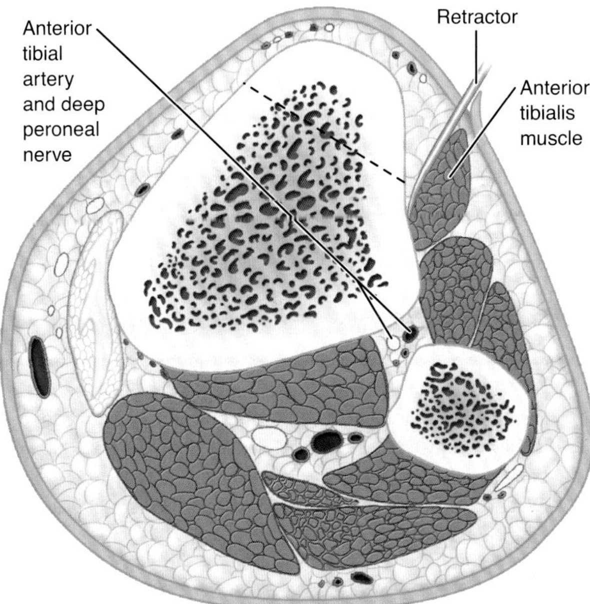


**TECH FIG 2** • Retraction of the tibialis anterior gives a full view of the entire lateral proximal tibia.

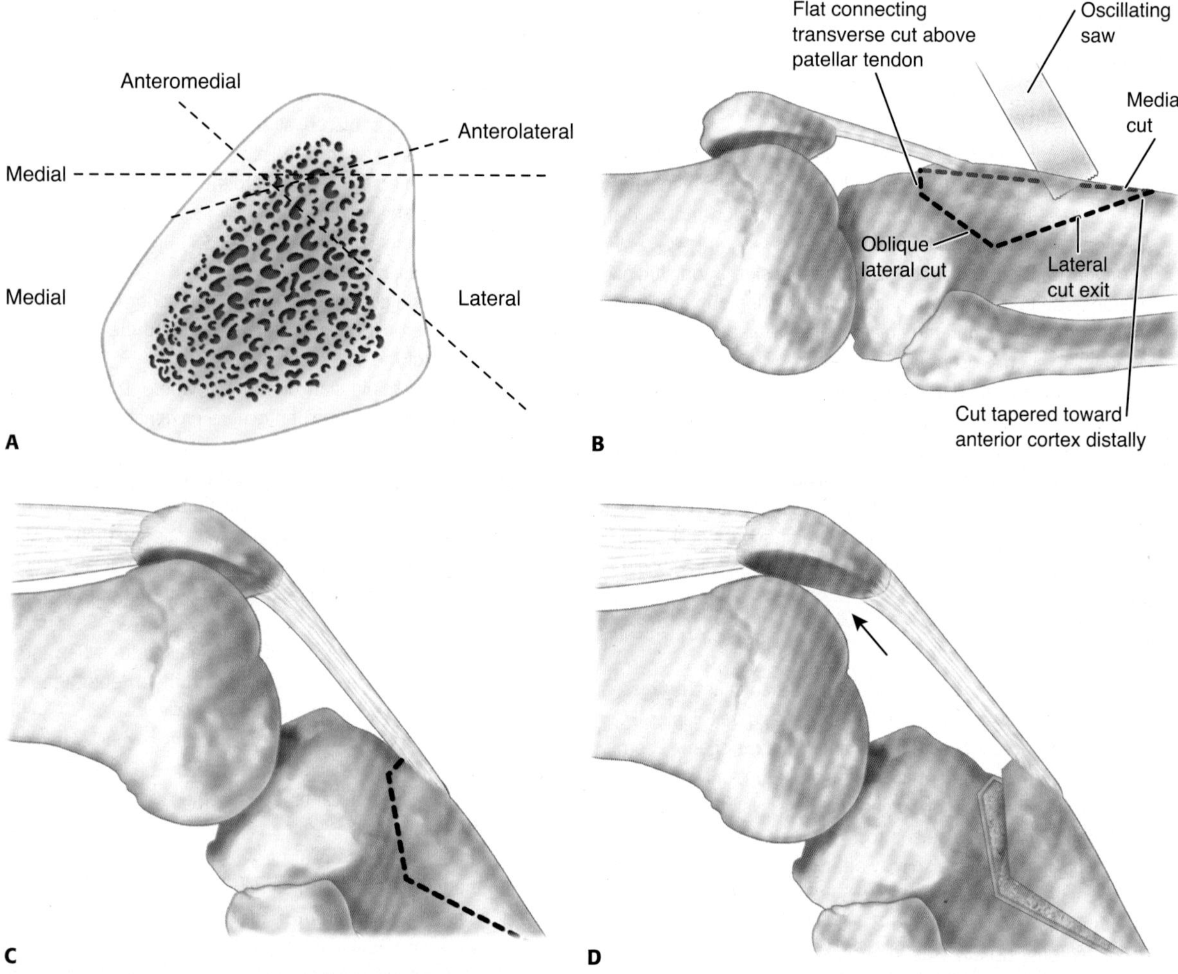


**TECH FIG 3 • A.** Displacement of the tibial tubercle transfer showing planes for cuts. **B.** For anteromedial tibial tubercle transfer, the cut proceeds obliquely from medial to lateral, tapering toward the anterior crest distally. After transferring the tibial tubercle along the osteotomy (**C**), both anteriorization and medialization of the tibial tubercle are achieved (**D**).

- If the most proximal cut has been made carefully, there will be a ledge of bone on which the osteotomized fragment will rest, which will add stability to the osteotomy beyond what the screws offer.
- Lateral release or lengthening is accomplished as needed to free the patella. In patients with any retropatellar tendon contracture, this tendon also is released to free up the extensor mechanism. One great advantage of this procedure is the release and distraction of the fat pad and retropatellar scar.
- After tibial tubercle transfer, hemostasis must be meticulous, and then the subcutaneous tissue and skin are closed. We prefer skin sutures or skin clips rather than subcuticular sutures to ensure skin integrity over the osteotomy.

## Anterolateral Tibial Tubercle Transfer

- In the very small number of patients who have had previous overmedialization of the tibial tubercle, an osteotomy cut deep to the previously transferred tibial tubercle may be made in a slightly oblique lateral-to-medial direction and the tibial tubercle transferred anterolaterally.
- Fixation and rehabilitation are similar to anteromedial tibial tubercle transfer.

## PEARLS AND PITFALLS

**Avoiding complications**

- Patients should stay on crutches for at least 6 weeks because fracture is a risk with weight bearing that is too aggressive.
- Smoking should be stopped before surgery and not resumed for at least 2 months because of its adverse effect on bone healing.
- Surgery should be accurate and fixation secure.
- Patients should start ROM very soon after surgery to avoid stiffness.
- All patients should receive some form of postoperative anticoagulation and should have prophylactic antibiotics at the time of surgery.
- Hemostasis should be meticulous, and proper drainage of hematoma is implemented as needed.

## POSTOPERATIVE CARE

- Following tibial tubercle transfer, immediate ROM is important.
  - If stability is secure, patients are started immediately on ROM exercises.
  - These may start with a single cycle of flexion a day if proximal reconstruction has been done and there is concern about stretching out a proximal repair.
  - In such cases, a short period of immobilization in extension may be appropriate for soft tissue healing, but a single cycle of knee flexion daily after the first 10 to 12 days is important to ensure full ROM later and maximal ROM ultimately.
- Patients are kept on crutches for 6 to 8 weeks and resume weight bearing as tolerated after 6 weeks.
- During the initial 6 weeks, we recommend toe-touch or light weight bearing on the affected side.
- We recommend anticoagulation with aspirin for at least 4 to 6 weeks for most patients.
- Most of our patients go home from same-day surgery and are seen in 1 to 3 days as needed and then for suture removal and radiographs at 10 to 12 days.
- Steri-Strips are applied and kept in place for 4 to 6 weeks to minimize wound spread.

## COMPLICATIONS

- The primary concerns following tibial tubercle transfer are fracture of the tibia,[22] stiffness, thrombophlebitis, nonunion, infection, and hematoma.
- These complications usually can be avoided with proper care.
- Gross obesity increases the risk of complications.

## OUTCOMES

- Buuck and Fulkerson[2] reviewed the results of anteromedial tibial tubercle transfer in patients 4 to 12 years following the procedure and demonstrated that good results are maintained over time.
- Our follow-up studies have consistently revealed a satisfactory outcome in 85% to 90% of patients. Pidoriano et al[17] demonstrated that results are closely related to the location of articular lesions. Patients with lateral and distal patellar lesions are more likely to experience relief than patients with proximal (dashboard) or medial (s/p dislocation) lesions.

## REFERENCES

1. Amis AA, Firer P, Mountney J, et al. Anatomy and biomechanics of the medial patellofemoral ligament. Knee 2003;10:215–220.
2. Buuck DA, Fulkerson JP. Anteromedialization of the tibial tubercle: a 4- to 12- year follow-up. Oper Tech Sports Med 2000;8:131–137.
3. Cox JS. Evaluation of the Roux-Elmslie-Trillat procedure for knee extensor realignment. Am J Sports Med 1982;10:303–310.
4. Dejour H, Walch G, Nove-Josserand L, et al. Factors of patellar instability: an anatomic radiographic study. Knee Surg Sports Traumatol Arthrosc 1994;2:19–26.
5. Dye SF, Chew MH. The use of scintigraphy to detect increased osseous metabolic activity about the knee. J Bone Joint Surg Am 1993;75A:1388–1406.
6. Farr J, Schepsis A, Cole B, et al. Anteromedialization: review and technique. J Knee Surg 2007;20(2):120–128.
7. Ficat P. The syndrome of lateral hyperpressure of the patella [in French]. Acta Orthopaedica Belgica 1978;44(1):65–76.
8. Fulkerson JP. Anteromedialization of the tibial tuberosity for patellofemoral malalignment. Clin Orthop Rel Res 1983;177:176–181.
9. Fulkerson JP. Anterolateralization of the tibial tubercle. Tech Orthop 1997;12:165–169.
10. Fulkerson JP. A clinical test for medial patella tracking. Tech Orthop 1997;12:144.
11. Fulkerson JP. Disorders of the Patellofemoral Joint. Philadelphia: Lippincott Williams & Wilkins, 2005.
12. Fulkerson JP, Becker GJ, Meaney JA, et al. Anteromedial tibial tubercle transfer without bone graft. Am J Sports Med 1990;18:490–497.
13. Fulkerson JP, Tennant R, Jaivin JS, et al. Histologic evidence of retinacular nerve injury associated with patellofemoral malalignment. Clin Orthop Rel Res 1985;197:196–205.
14. Hallisey MJ, Doherty N, Bennett WF, et al. Anatomy of the junction of the vastus lateralis tendon and the patella. J Bone Joint Surg Am 1987;69A:545–549.
15. Merchant AC, Mercer RL, Jacobsen RH, et al. Radiographic analysis of patellofemoral congruence. J Bone Joint Surg Am 1974;56A:1391–1396.
16. Murray TF, Dupont JY, Fulkerson JP. Axial and lateral radiographs in evaluating patellofemoral malalignment. Am J Sports Med 1999;27:580–584.
17. Pidoriano AJ, Weinstein RN, Buuck DA, et al. Correlation of patellar articular lesions and results from anteromedial tibial tubercle transfer. Am J Sports Med 1997;25:533–537.
18. Post WR. Clinical evaluation of patients with patellofemoral disorders [current concepts]. Arthroscopy 1999;15:841–851.
19. Saleh KJ, Arendt EA, Eldridge J, et al. Operative treatment of patellofemoral arthritis. J Bone Joint Surg Am 2005;87A:659–671.
20. Schepsis AA, DeSimone AA, Leach RE. Anterior tibial tubercle transposition for patellofemoral arthrosis: a long-term study. Am J Knee Surg 1994;7:13–20.
21. Schutzer SF, Ramsby GR, Fulkerson JP. Computed tomographic classification of patellofemoral pain patients. Orthop Clin North Am 1986;17:235–248.
22. Stetson WB, Friedman MJ, Fulkerson JP, et al. Fracture of the proximal tibia with immediate weightbearing after a Fulkerson osteotomy. Am J Sports Med 1997;25:570–574.

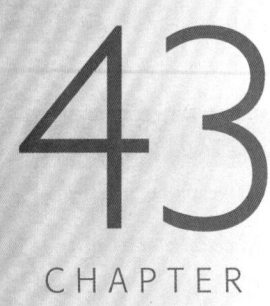

# Knee Lateral Release

Andrea M. Spiker, Carl H. Wierks, and Andrew J. Cosgarea

## DEFINITION

- Patellofemoral pain is a common symptom in active adolescents and adults.
- The diagnosis of patellofemoral pain is nonspecific. It may be caused by trauma, instability, overuse, or anatomic abnormalities such as bipartite patella, maltracking, or malalignment. It may also be caused by a tight lateral retinaculum causing excessive compression of the patella on the lateral femoral trochlea.
- The patella acts to enhance the extensor mechanism of the knee as it glides through its normal course within the femoral trochlea. Static bone and soft tissue stabilizers as well as dynamic muscular stabilizers maintain the patella within the femoral sulcus.[18]
- The lateral retinaculum and patellofemoral ligament make up the lateral static soft tissue stabilizers of the patella. If these structures are abnormally tight, the patella can be excessively compressed against the femur with knee flexion, causing pain.[18]
- This scenario of exaggerated patellar compression on the lateral femoral trochlea has been described as *excessive lateral pressure syndrome* (ELPS),[10] *patellar compression syndrome*,[18] and *patellofemoral stress syndrome*.[25]
- This chapter describes lateral retinacular release of the knee, which is the surgical treatment for patients with ELPS who exhibit patellofemoral pain, a tight lateral retinaculum, and lateral patellar tilt. This surgical intervention is indicated for patients with ELPS only after nonoperative treatment has failed.
- Lateral retinacular release has also been used to treat other patellofemoral disorders with varying success, including chondromalacia patellae, patella malalignment, and instability.[2,4,8,15,20–22,29] In this chapter, we will focus our discussion on ELPS, the most widely accepted indication for knee lateral retinacular release.

## ANATOMY

- The patella is a sesamoid bone that acts as a fulcrum in knee extension, providing a smooth surface over which the extensor mechanism can function while protecting the anterior knee.[7]
- The patella also acts to centralize the converging forces of the four quadriceps muscles.
- The thickest articular cartilage in the body is located in the patellofemoral joint.
- Forces across the patellofemoral joint are approximately three times the body weight during ascending and descending stairs and can reach up to 20 times the body weight during activities such as jumping.[1]
- As the knee flexes from full extension, the patella is drawn into the trochlear groove at approximately 20 degrees.
- In extension, the medial patellofemoral ligament is the primary restraint to excessive lateral translation. As the knee flexes beyond 20 degrees, the lateral trochlear ridge becomes the primary restraint.
- A tight lateral retinaculum and patellofemoral ligament may be responsible for excessively constricting the patella and causing symptoms of knee pain in patients with ELPS.

## PATHOGENESIS

- An abnormally tight lateral retinaculum can tether the patella against the lateral femoral trochlear during knee flexion, at which point patients may describe a sensation of pressure, grating, or symptoms of pain. With chronic excessive pressure, degeneration of articular cartilage in the lateral patellofemoral joint can occur.
- Some conditions, such as a weak vastus medialis obliquus normal alignment (abnormal Q angle, lateralized tibial tuberosity, valgus deformity, internal tibial torsion, and femoral anteversion), predispose to lateral patellar tracking.
- Direct trauma (eg, dashboard injury or patellar dislocation) can also result in degeneration of the lateral patellofemoral articular cartilage.

## NATURAL HISTORY

- No long-term natural history studies of ELPS have been reported to date.
- It is well accepted, however, that disruption of articular cartilage results in progressive degenerative changes.

## PATIENT HISTORY AND PHYSICAL FINDINGS

- Patients typically report insidious onset of anterior knee pain that is activity related, although some may have a history of traumatic injury.
- Pain is typically exacerbated by prolonged sitting, stair-climbing, or an increase in activity.
- Symptoms and clinical findings of instability have no role in ELPS.
- A thorough physical examination should include the following:
  - Examination for effusion. Effusion may indicate traumatic or degenerative disruption of the articular surface.
  - Observation of patellar tracking. A positive J sign, indicating patellar maltracking, occurs if the patella sits laterally in extension, then suddenly glides medially as it engages in the trochlear with flexion.
  - Patellar tilt test. The examiner attempts to lift the lateral border of the patella. If the lateral facet cannot be elevated to neutral, the lateral retinaculum is abnormally tight.

- Patellar glide test. Patellar lateral glide of up to two to three quadrants is normal. Excessive lateral translation indicates incompetence of the medial retinaculum and the medial patellofemoral ligament. Comparison should be made to the contralateral leg.
- Patellar apprehension test. As with the patellar glide test, examiner pushes the patella laterally. If the patient is apprehensive, it suggests that he or she is sensing patellar instability.
- Examination of the quadriceps. Quadriceps tightness has been associated with patellofemoral pain. Quadriceps weakness, especially involving the vastus medialis, indicates a predisposition to instability.
- Patellar grind test. With the knee in full extension, the examiner pushes directly down onto the patella, compressing it against the femoral sulcus. Pain may indicate patellofemoral arthritis but can also occur with normal articular surfaces.
- Inspection for elevated Q angle. The Q angle is measured with the patient in a supine position as the angle formed by a line from the anterior superior iliac spine to the center of patella and a line from the center of the patella to the tibial tubercle. An angle of more than 15 to 20 degrees is abnormal and can predispose to lateral patellar subluxation.

## IMAGING AND OTHER DIAGNOSTIC STUDIES

- Radiographs of the knee should include anteroposterior, tunnel, axial (sunrise), and 30-degree lateral views. If arthritis is suspected, a posteroanterior flexed 45-degree view should be obtained.
- Lateral subluxation can be measured on the axial radiograph. If a line drawn from the patellar apex to the center of the trochlear sulcus is lateral to a line bisecting the trochlear sulcus angle, then the patella is subluxed laterally (**FIG 1A**). A computed tomography scan is the best way to evaluate patellar tilt radiographically. Using an axial image, a line is drawn along the posterior femoral condyles. This line is then compared to a line drawn along the lateral patellar facet. If these lines converge laterally, then the patella is determined to have excessive lateral tilt (**FIG 1B**).
- A computed tomography scan can also be used to measure the tibial tubercle–trochlear groove (TT–TG) distance.
- Magnetic resonance imaging may be beneficial in evaluating the integrity of articular cartilage and may also reveal concomitant meniscal and ligamentous pathology (**FIG 1C**).

## DIFFERENTIAL DIAGNOSIS

- Patellofemoral pain (without ELPS)
- Patellar instability
- Lateral meniscal tear
- Patellar fracture
- Iliotibial band syndrome
- Prepatellar bursitis
- Neuroma
- Osteochondritis dissecans of the patella or trochlea
- Bipartite patella
- Patellofemoral arthritis
- Medial patellar plicae[6]

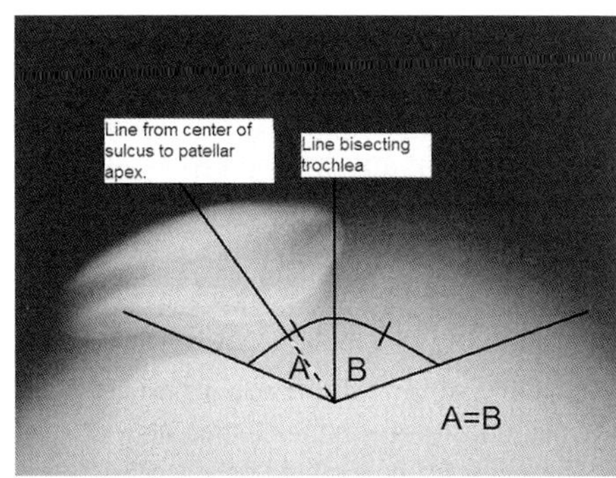


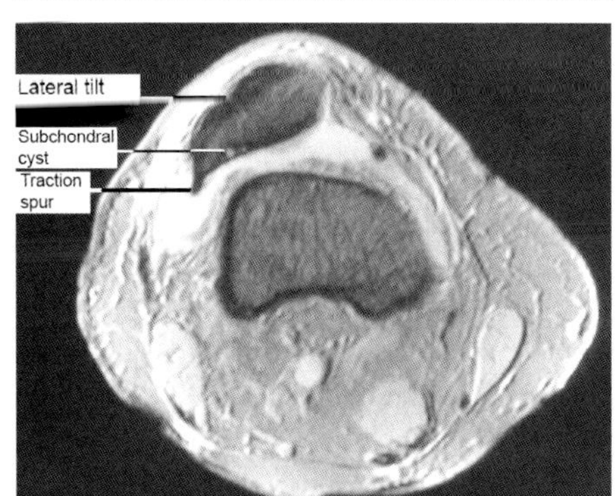


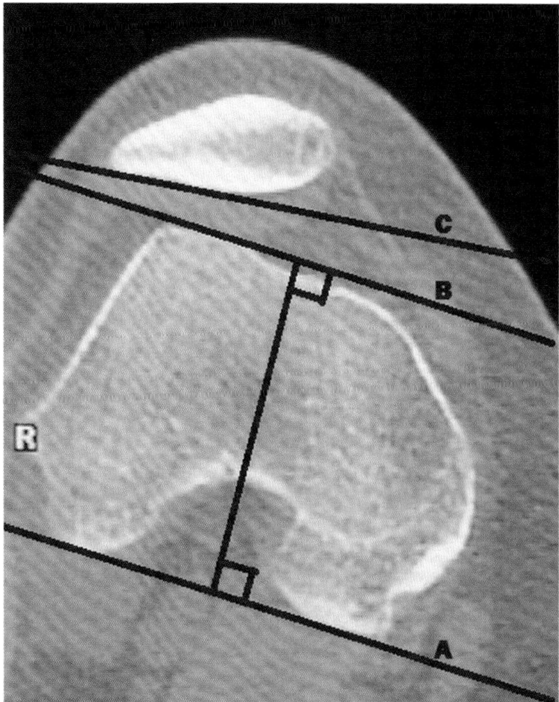


**FIG 1** • **A.** Axial radiograph of a right knee showing lateral subluxation of the patella, as the line from the patellar apex to the trochlear sulcus is lateral to the line bisecting the trochlear sulcus angle. **B.** Axial computed tomography image of the right knee showing measurement of patellar tilt. A line (**A**) is drawn across the posterior femoral condyles, and a parallel line (**B**) is drawn and placed at the lateral trochlear ridge. A third line (**C**) is drawn along the lateral patellar facet. Radiographic confirmation of an excessively tight lateral retinaculum is demonstrated if lines **B** and **C** converge laterally. **C.** An axial magnetic resonance imaging of the right knee of a patient with ELPS, illustrating changes associated with chondral damage.

## NONOPERATIVE MANAGEMENT

- The mainstay of treatment is nonoperative, with the great majority of patients seeing improvement in patellofemoral knee pain after quadriceps stretching, strengthening, and physical therapy.[12,16]
- Oral analgesics can be beneficial for a limited period of time.
- Corticosteroid injection or viscosupplementation may be helpful in patients with concomitant chondral degeneration or arthritis.

## SURGICAL MANAGEMENT

- The indication for lateral retinacular release is failure of an adequate trial of rehabilitation in a patient with symptomatic patellofemoral pain, excessive lateral retinacular tightness, and lateral tilt.[11] Before consideration for surgery, physical therapy should be attempted and deemed unsuccessful.[27]
- Isolated lateral release is usually not a successful treatment strategy for lateral patellar instability and, in some cases, can result in iatrogenic medial patellar instability. In patients undergoing a tibial tuberosity osteotomy, the addition of lateral retinacular release may improve overall results.[9] Successful lateral retinacular release can be performed using arthroscopic or open techniques.

### Preoperative Planning

- Knee range of motion, retinacular tightness, and ligamentous laxity should be examined while the patient is under anesthesia.
- Particular attention should be paid to patellar tracking as the knee is taken through a range of motion and whether the patella is dislocatable.
- The symptomatic knee should be compared to the contralateral side.

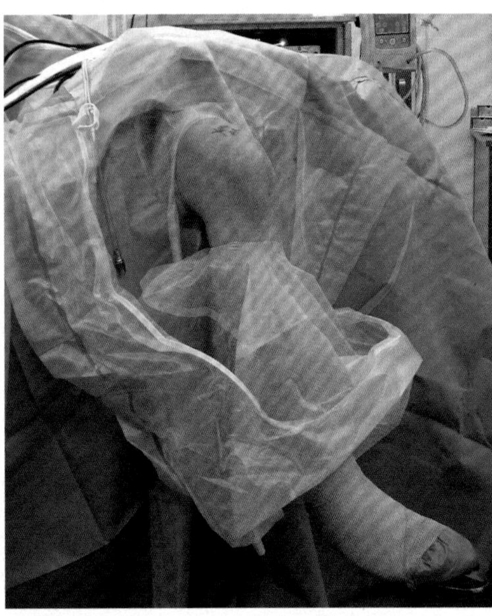

**FIG 2** • Patient positioning for standard knee arthroscopy using a leg holder.

### Positioning

- The patient is placed in the supine position with the operative leg supported according to the surgeon's preference for standard knee arthroscopy (**FIG 2**).
- A nonsterile tourniquet is placed around the thigh.

### Approach

- For arthroscopic lateral release, a superolateral inflow portal is established just proximal to the superior pole of the patella and lateral to the vastus lateralis obliquus. Standard inferomedial and inferolateral arthroscopy portals are used.

TECHNIQUES

## Arthroscopic Lateral Release

- Diagnostic arthroscopy is performed with the 30-degree arthroscope placed in the anterolateral portal.
- The entire knee is examined to rule out concomitant intra-articular pathology.
- The posteromedial and posterolateral compartments are visualized by passing the arthroscope through the intercondylar notch.
- Meniscal tears, articular cartilage lesions, and loose bodies are identified and addressed surgically when indicated.
- Patellofemoral tracking is visualized as the knee is taken through its full range of motion.
- Once the diagnostic arthroscopy is completed, an Esmarch bandage can be used to exsanguinate the leg if the surgeon chooses to use a tourniquet.
- The camera is placed in the inferomedial portal, and a hooked coagulation device is placed in the inferolateral portal. Other techniques have been described using the holmium:YAG laser or hook knife.[5]
- Under direct arthroscopic visualization, the release is started just distal to the inflow cannula (**TECH FIG 1A**).
- First, the synovium is cut, exposing the underlying retinaculum.
- The retinaculum, which has a distinct firm feel, is then cut using multiple passes with the electrocautery device (**TECH FIG 1B**).
- The release should extend distally to the level of the inferolateral portal.
- Great care should be taken to avoid cutting the vastus lateralis muscle or tendon (**TECH FIG 1C**).
- If the superior lateral geniculate vessels are seen (**TECH FIG 1D**), they should be aggressively coagulated. The ability to coagulate these vessels immediately upon encountering them is one advantage of using electrocautery devices for this step.
- Patellar tilt is assessed after release. The surgeon should be able to tilt the patella approximately 30 degrees laterally with the knee fully extended.
- Excessive lateral release, which may result in medial patellar instability, must be avoided.
- If a tourniquet was used, it is gradually deflated after completion of the release to evaluate for excessive bleeding under direct visualization.
- The portal sites are closed, and a sterile compression dressing along with a cryotherapy device are applied.

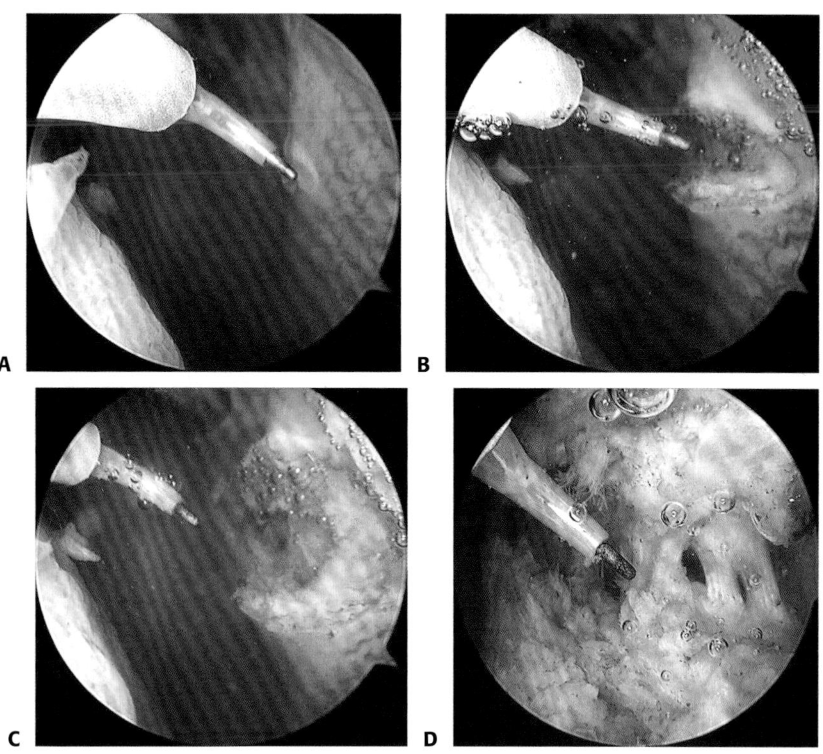

**TECH FIG 1** ● **A.** The proximal starting point for the lateral retinacular release is just distal to the superolateral inflow cannula. **B.** The synovium is cut first, revealing the retinaculum. **C.** The retinaculum is cut using multiple passes of the electrocautery. **D.** Here, the superior lateral geniculate artery can be seen.

## Open Lateral Retinacular Release

- A skin incision approximately 3 cm long is made just lateral to the patella.
- The retinaculum is incised in line with the skin incision, approximately 2 cm lateral to the lateral patellar margin.
- The superior lateral geniculate artery should be identified and cauterized.
- The proximal and distal extent of the incision is adequate when the patella can be laterally elevated to an adequate angle from the epicondylar axis.[26]
- Excessive release should be avoided in order to decrease the risk of iatrogenic medial instability, which has led some surgeons recommending performing a lateral retinacular lengthening.

## Lateral Retinacular Lengthening

- After making the longitudinal skin incision lateral to the patella, the lateral retinaculum is incised superficially in line with the skin incision, approximately 1 cm lateral to the lateral patellar border (**TECH FIG 2A**). The deep fibers of the retinaculum in close contact with the joint capsule are not cut.
- A flap of retinaculum is then created by dissecting laterally in this plane approximately 2 cm.
- An incision is then made through the deep fibers of the retinaculum and the superficial capsule, leaving a thin layer of capsule intact (**TECH FIG 2B**).
- The deep incision is continued proximally and distally until the patella can be everted adequately.
- The superior lateral geniculate artery should be identified and coagulated.
- The free edge of the medial capsule with deep retinacular fibers and the free edge of the superficial lateral retinaculum are sutured together with the knee flexed (**TECH FIG 2C**).

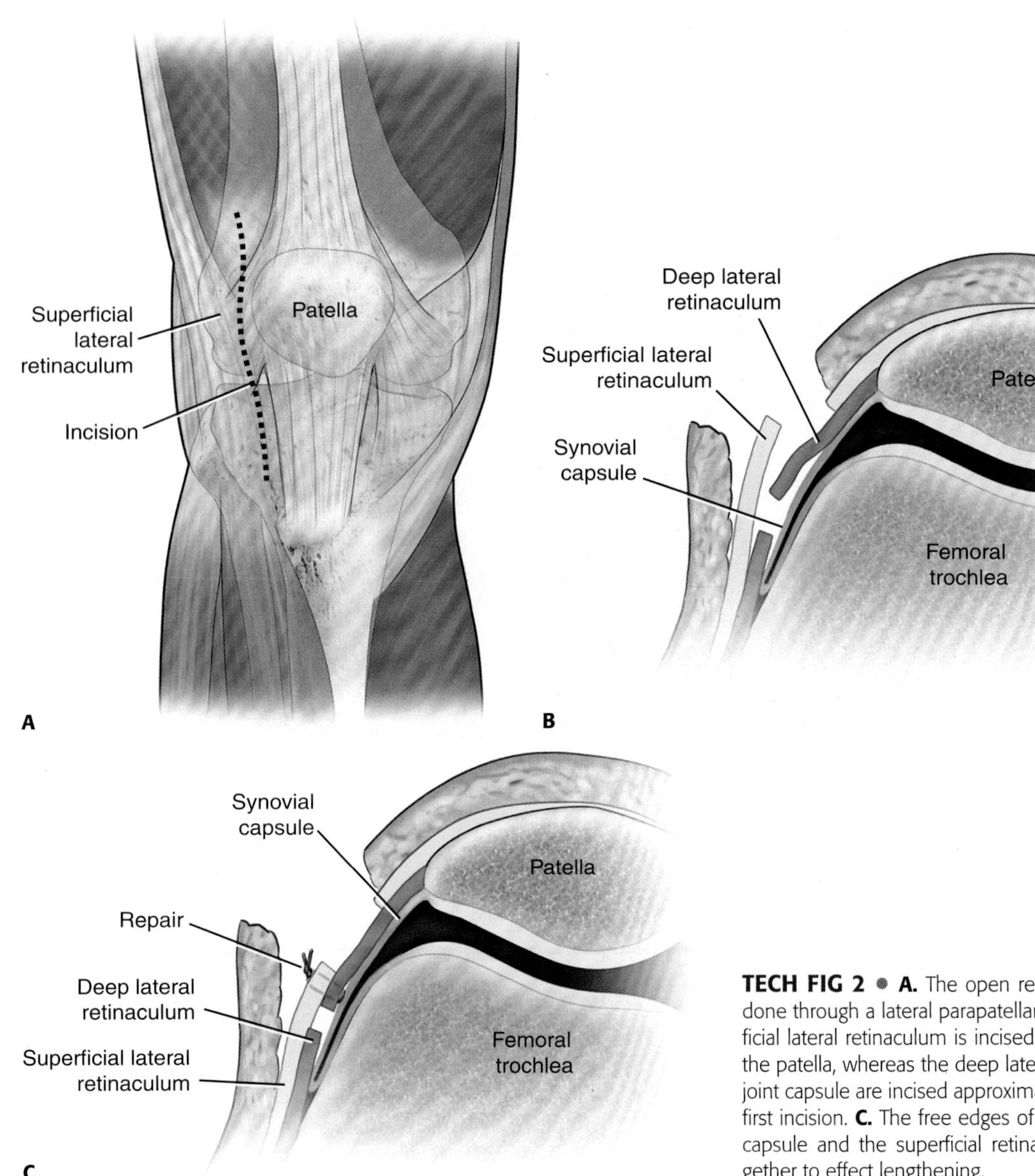


**TECH FIG 2 • A.** The open retinacular lengthening is done through a lateral parapatellar incision. **B.** The superficial lateral retinaculum is incised longitudinally lateral to the patella, whereas the deep lateral retinaculum and the joint capsule are incised approximately 2 cm lateral to the first incision. **C.** The free edges of the deep retinaculum/capsule and the superficial retinaculum are sutured together to effect lengthening.

## PEARLS AND PITFALLS

| | |
|---|---|
| **Indications** | ■ The indication for isolated lateral release is retropatellar pain from the lateral patellofemoral joint secondary to soft tissue tightness but only after nonoperative management has failed. Lateral retinacular release should not be performed as an isolated procedure if patellar instability is the primary problem.[11,30] |
| **Instability** | ■ It is important to not transect the vastus lateralis obliquus muscle and tendon during release because doing so can predispose to medial instability. |
| **Hemostasis** | ■ The superior lateral geniculate artery is at risk during lateral release (see **TECH FIG 1D**). If a tourniquet is used in an arthroscopic release, deflating it before closure can help identify excessive bleeding. Use of a cryotherapy device and a compression dressing will also decrease the risk of hemarthrosis. Use of a drain may be considered on a case-by-case basis in any of the arthroscopic or open approaches. |
| **Landmarks guiding length of release** | ■ The superolateral inflow cannula is an excellent guide for the most proximal starting point of release. The release should extend distally to the inferolateral portal. |

## POSTOPERATIVE CARE

- A compression dressing and a cryotherapy device are used to decrease the risk of hemarthrosis.
- Patients are allowed to progress to weight bearing as tolerated and discard crutches when they are ambulating safely.
- Patients are initially seen 1 week after surgery to assess knee motion and quadriceps function and to remove sutures.
- Time spent strengthening the quadriceps and hamstrings has been shown to directly correlate with results.[23]

## OUTCOMES

- Arthroscopic and open techniques have similar success rates.[7,18,20,24,27]
- Success rates range from 70% to 93%.[19,20,24,27]
- Arthroscopic release may result in less postoperative incisional pain and better cosmesis than open techniques.
- One study found that lateral lengthening had better clinical outcomes, less medial instability, and less quadriceps atrophy at 2 years than open lateral release.[26]
- One prospective, randomized study[24] found that 93% of patients returned to presymptomatic activity level and, although 40% of patients had quadriceps strength deficits, in almost all cases, the strength was within 10% of that of the normal leg.
- The success rates of lateral release are lower when it is performed for instability alone.[3,8,16]

## COMPLICATIONS

- There is no significant difference in postoperative complications (hemarthrosis, infection, need for reoperation) when comparing open versus arthroscopic techniques,[19] and hemarthrosis is the most common complication followed by infection.[13,17]
- Medial instability from overaggressive release can be especially difficult to diagnose.
- Patients may report a sensation of lateral instability if the patella sits in a medially subluxed position during early flexion and then snaps laterally during continued flexion.
- If a patient with medial instability is initially misdiagnosed with lateral instability, surgical treatment with a medial stabilization procedure could result in exacerbating the problem.[28]
- An open lateral closure procedure can be used to treat medial patellar instability that results after lateral retinacular release.[14]
- Other potential complications include quadriceps tendon weakness or rupture, patella baja, thermal injury/subcutaneous burns, arthrofibrosis,[17] paradoxical increased lateral patellar instability, anterior knee pain, reflex sympathetic dystrophy,[14] synovial herniation, or recurrence of ELPS.[26]

## REFERENCES


1. Aglietti P, Menchetti PPM. Biomechanics of the patellofemoral joint. In: Scuderi GR, ed. The Patella. New York: Springer-Verlag, 1995: 25–48.
2. Aglietti P, Pisaneschi A, Buzzi R, et al. Arthroscopic lateral release for patellar pain or instability. Arthroscopy 1989;5:176–183.
3. Betz RR, Magill JT III, Lonergan RP. The percutaneous lateral retinacular release. Am J Sports Med 1987;15:477–482.
4. Bigos SJ, McBride GG. The isolated lateral retinacular release in the treatment of patellofemoral disorders. Clin Orthop Relat Res 1984;186:75–80.
5. Calpur OU, Ozcan M, Gurbuz H, et al. Full arthroscopic lateral retinacular release with hook knife and quadriceps pressure-pull test: long-term follow-up. Knee Surg Sports Traumatol Arthrosc 2005;13: 222–230.
6. Calpur OU, Tan L, Gurbuz H, et al. Arthroscopic mediopatellar plicaectomy and lateral retinacular release in mechanical patellofemoral disorders. Knee Surg Sports Traumatol Arthrosc 2002;10:177–183.
7. Ceder LC, Larson RL. Z-plasty lateral retinacular release for the treatment of patellar compression syndrome. Clin Orthop Relat Res 1979;144:110–113.
8. Christensen F, Soballe K, Snerum L. Treatment of chondromalacia patellae by lateral retinacular release of the patella. Clin Orthop Relat Res 1988;(234):145–147.
9. Christodoulou NA, Tsaknis RN, Sdrenias CV, et al. Improvement of proximal tibial osteotomy results by lateral retinacular release. Clin Orthop Relat Res 2005;441:340–345.
10. Ficat P. The syndrome of lateral hyperpressure of the patella [in French]. Acta Orthop Belg 1978;44:65–76.
11. Fithian DC, Paxton EW, Post WR, et al. Lateral retinacular release: a survey of the International Patellofemoral Study Group. Arthroscopy 2004;20:463–468.
12. Fu FH, Maday MG. Arthroscopic lateral release and the lateral patellar compression syndrome. Orthop Clin North Am 1992;23:601–612.
13. Fulkerson JP. Diagnosis and treatment of patients with patellofemoral pain. Am J Sports Med 2002;30:447–456.
14. Heyworth BE, Carroll KM, Dawson CK, et al. Open lateral retinacular closure surgery for treatment of anterolateral knee pain and disability after arthroscopic lateral retinacular release. Am J Sports Med 2012;40:376–382.
15. Jackson RW, Kunkel SS, Taylor GJ. Lateral retinacular release for patellofemoral pain in the older patient. Arthroscopy 1991;7:283–286.
16. Kolowich PA, Paulos LE, Rosenberg TD, et al. Lateral release of the patella: indications and contraindications. Am J Sports Med 1990; 18:359–365.
17. Kunkle KL, Malek MM. Complications and pitfalls in lateral retinacular release. In: Malek MM, ed. Knee Surgery: Complications, Pitfalls and Salvage. New York: Springer-Verlag, 2001:161–170.
18. Larson RL, Cabaud HE, Slocum DB, et al. The patellar compression syndrome: surgical treatment by lateral retinacular release. Clin Orthop Relat Res 1978;(134):158–167.
19. Lattermann C, Drake GN, Spellman J, et al. Lateral retinacular release for anterior knee pain: a systematic review of the literature. J Knee Surg 2006;19:278–284.
20. McGinty JB, McCarthy JC. Endoscopic lateral retinacular release: a preliminary report. Clin Orthop Relat Res 1981;(158):120–125.
21. Merchant AC, Mercer RL. Lateral release of the patella. A preliminary report. Clin Orthop Relat Res 1974;(103):40–45.
22. Metcalf RW. An arthroscopic method for lateral release of subluxating or dislocating patella. Clin Orthop Relat Res 1982;(167):9–18.
23. Micheli LJ, Stanitski CL. Lateral patellar retinacular release. Am J Sports Med 1981;9:330–336.
24. O'Neill DB. Open lateral retinacular lengthening compared with arthroscopic release. A prospective, randomized outcome study. J Bone Joint Surg Am 1997;79:1759–1769.
25. O'Neill DB, Micheli LJ, Warner JP. Patellofemoral stress. A prospective analysis of exercise treatment in adolescents and adults. Am J Sports Med 1992;20:151–156.
26. Pagenstert G, Wolf N, Bachmann M, et al. Open lateral patellar retinacular lengthening versus open retinacular release in lateral patellar hypercompression syndrome: a prospective double-blinded comparative study on complications and outcome. Arthroscopy 2012;28: 788–797.
27. Panni AS, Tartarone M, Patricola A, et al. Long-term results of lateral retinacular release. Arthroscopy 2005;21:526–531.
28. Post WR. Anterior knee pain: diagnosis and treatment. J Am Acad Orthop Surg 2005;13:534–543.
29. Schonholtz GJ, Zahn MG, Magee CM. Lateral retinacular release of the patella. Arthroscopy 1987;3:269–272.
30. Shea KP, Fulkerson JP. Preoperative computed tomography scanning and arthroscopy in predicting outcome after lateral retinacular release. Arthroscopy 1992;8:327–334.

# Arthroscopy-Assisted Management or Open Reduction and Internal Fixation of Tibial Spine Fractures

Itai Gans and Theodore J. Ganley

## DEFINITION

- Tibial spine fractures are bony avulsions of the anterior cruciate ligament (ACL) from its attachment on the anteromedial portion of the intercondylar tibial eminence.[26] Some authors consider them to be equivalent to the midsubstance ACL injuries seen in the adult population.
- This injury most commonly occurs in the younger age group, particularly children aged 8 to 14 years with open growth plates, but can also occur in adults.
- Tibial spine fractures have an incidence of 3 per 100,000 children each year.[21]
- Meyers and McKeever[16] classified tibial spine fractures into three types based on the degree of displacement. This classification was later modified by Zaricznyj[27] to include a fourth type, signifying a comminuted fracture fragment (**FIG 1**):
  - Type I: nondisplaced fracture with minimal anterior margin elevation
  - Type II: posterior hinged fracture with partial displacement of the anterior margin (one-third to one-half of the tibial spine lifting from the epiphyseal bed)
  - Type III: completely displaced fracture fragment
    - Type IIIA: no rotational malalignment
    - Type IIIB: Fracture fragment has rotated such that the cartilaginous surface of the fracture fragment faces the raw bone of the epiphyseal bone bed.
  - Type IV: completely displaced and comminuted fracture fragment(s)

## ANATOMY

- The tibial eminence is found lying in the intercondylar area of the tibia (**FIG 2**).
- It is anatomically divided into four distinct regions: a medial and lateral triangular elevation (or medial and lateral tibial spines) and an anterior and posterior recess.
  - The ligamentous ends of the medial and lateral menisci insert into the intercondylar eminence.
  - The medial elevation provides the attachment for the fibers of the ACL with the anterior attachment of the medial meniscus just anterior to the ACL insertion and the anterior attachment of the lateral meniscus just posterior to the ACL insertion.
    - The intermeniscal ligament is vulnerable to entrapment within fractures of the tibial spine where it traverses between the medial and lateral menisci, just anterior to the tibial spine, thereby blocking reduction[8] (**FIG 3**).
  - There are no structures that attach to the lateral portion of the eminence.
  - The tibial eminence also serves as an insertion for the posterior cruciate ligament (PCL); the fibers of the PCL typically arise from the posterior portion of the intercondylar eminence.[16]
- In the younger child, the majority of the anterior portion of the tibial eminence is cartilaginous.[16]

## PATHOGENESIS

- Avulsions of the tibial spine are usually traumatic in nature. This injury is more common in children, particularly those with incomplete ossification and open growth plates.
- The usual mechanism of injury is a hyperextension injury, with or without a forced valgus or external rotational force about the knee.[17] These fractures may also occur following a direct blow to the distal femur when the knee is flexed.

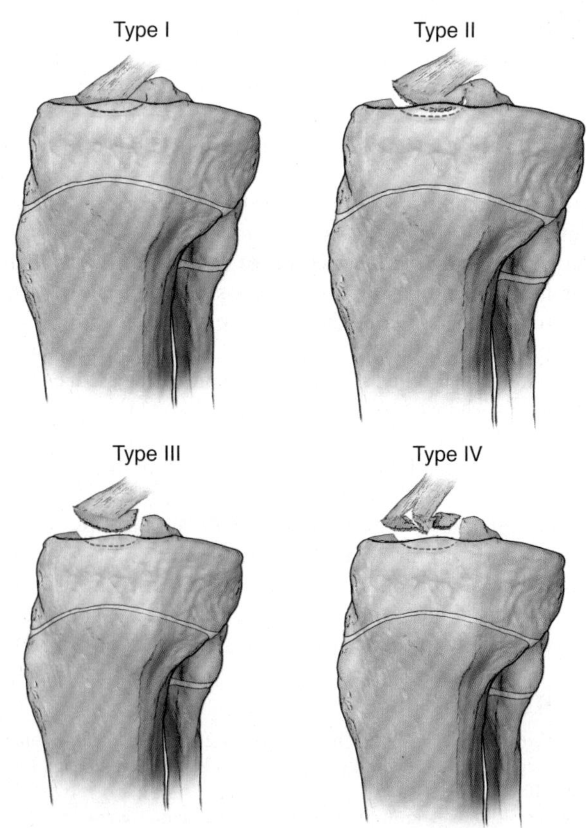


**FIG 1** • Meyers and McKeever classification with Zaricznyj modification. Type I has minimally displaced fragments. Type II has displacement through the anterior portion of the fracture with an intact posterior hinge. Type III has complete displacement of the fracture fragments. Type IV has complete displacement and comminution of the fracture fragments.

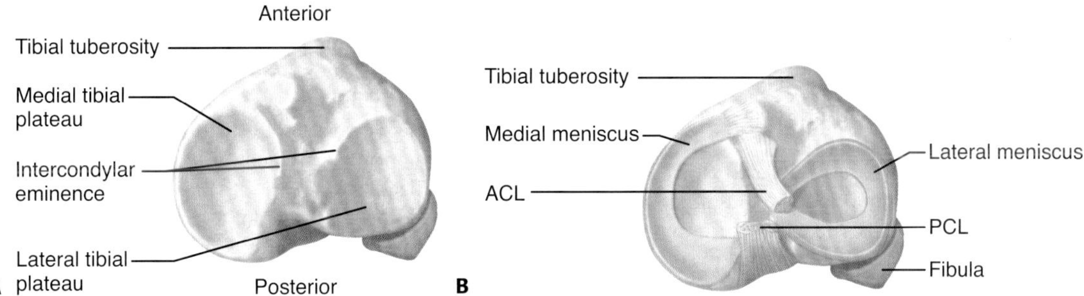


**FIG 2** • Axial view of the tibial plateau. **A.** The intercondylar eminence lies between the medial and lateral condyles. **B.** The medial portion serves as the attachment of the ACL.

- The injury occurs because of a tensile load placed on the ACL. The ligamentous ACL is much stronger in resisting tensile forces than the immature, incompletely ossified and primarily cartilaginous, osteochondral surface; this often results in failure and avulsion of the osteochondral attachment of the ACL.
- Before bone failure, in situ stretch injury of the ACL may occur[18] and may result in clinical laxity despite adequate reduction of the fracture fragment.[10,22]
- Different loading mechanisms are likewise implicated in the development of the injury. Experimental models have shown that rapid loading rates result in midsubstance ACL tears, whereas gradual loading results in tibial spine avulsion fractures.[18,26]
- The inherent anatomy of the knee has likewise been implicated. Kocher and colleagues[11] compared 25 skeletally immature knees with tibial spine fractures against 25 age-matched skeletally immature knees with midsubstance ACL tears and found a narrower notch width (intercondylar notch) in individuals who had sustained the midsubstance ACL tears.

## PATIENT HISTORY AND PHYSICAL FINDINGS

- Fractures of the tibial spine are usually precipitated by an acute traumatic event. The clinical presentation usually coincides with the severity of injury.
- Usually, a patient with a tibial spine injury will have a history of trauma or sports-related injury; the most common mechanism is historically a fall from a bicycle. With increasing numbers of children playing in competitive athletics, sports-related tibial spine fractures have been reported with increasing frequency. High-velocity trauma may also cause tibial spine injuries.
- The patient will usually present with a painful swollen knee. Swelling is secondary to hemarthrosis from the intra-articular knee injury.
- Gentle palpation and examination of the knee are undertaken. Most patients have some degree of swelling due to hemarthrosis secondary to the intra-articular fracture. Other superficial injuries are related to the degree and nature of the traumatic event.
- Knee joint laxity is often present, and patients typically have an inability to bear weight on the affected extremity.
  - It is important to note that patients will typically only have positive anterior drawer tests or Lachman tests with complete fractures (ie, type III and type IV) of the tibial spine. However, due to stretch of the ACL complex during injury, subclinical laxity may be noticed in incomplete fractures.
  - A positive anterior drawer test indicates knee joint laxity. However, this is not as sensitive as the Lachman test in assessing for ACL deficiency.
  - A positive result on the Lachman test indicates deficiency of the ACL complex. The test has greater sensitivity and specificity for ACL tears.
  - In the presence of a deficient ACL complex, during the pivot shift test (usually done intraoperatively when the patient is anesthetized), the femur falls posteriorly in relation to the tibia as the leg is raised and rotated internally. The valgus force applied to the leg along with slight flexion of the knee results in the pivot shift phenomenon. The intact iliotibial band reduces the femur when the knee is brought into 20 to 30 degrees of flexion.
- The knee should also be carefully examined for any concomitant injury including meniscal and collateral ligament injury.

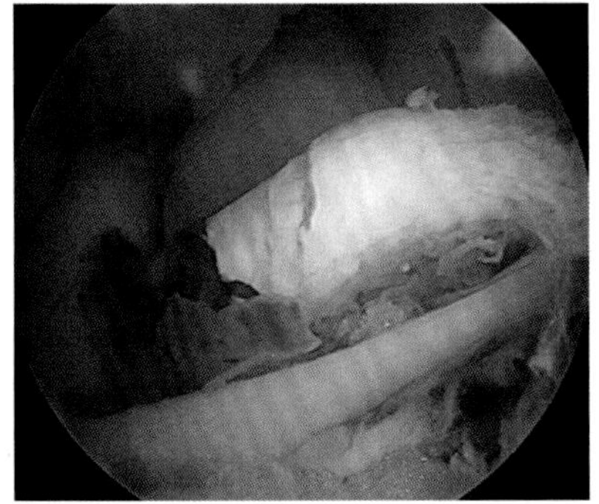

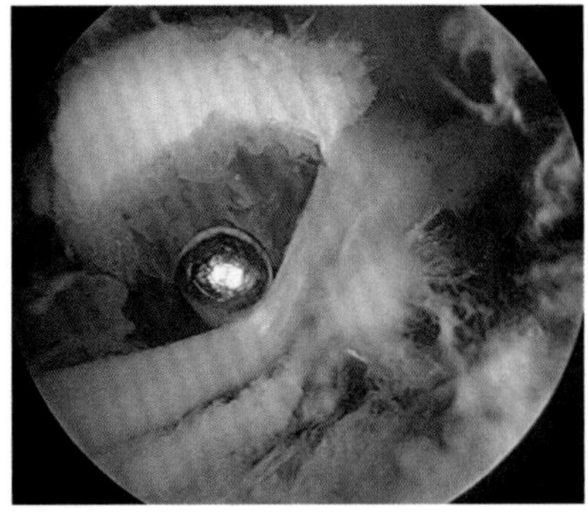

**FIG 3** • Arthroscopic view of the knee. **A.** A completely displaced tibial spine fracture with interposition of the intermeniscal ligament blocks reduction of the fracture. **B.** Probe helps remove the entrapped intermeniscal ligament to allow proper reduction of the tibial spine fracture fragment.

## IMAGING AND OTHER DIAGNOSTIC STUDIES

- Good imaging is crucial in the assessment and management of tibial spine fractures as appropriate classification of the fracture pattern dictates treatment (see section on Nonoperative Management).
- Standard anteroposterior (AP) and lateral views of the knee are usually adequate in making the diagnosis. These views help to define and identify the extent of bony injury.
  - A precise lateral radiograph is necessary as this is the best view to accurately assess fracture classification and fracture fragment position.
  - In lesions that are predominantly cartilaginous, radiographs may sometimes detect a small piece or a fleck of avulsed bone, which may be indicative of the avulsed osteochondral fragment, and underestimate the true size of the fracture fragment (**FIG 4**).
- Magnetic resonance imaging (MRI) is a good imaging modality for suspected tibial spine injuries, especially in the immature knee, where the tibial spine is predominantly cartilaginous and radiation exposure is of concern. MRI can help differentiate between a midsubstance ACL injury and a true avulsion fracture of the tibial spine and allow for classification of the fracture pattern. MRI can also allow assessment for fracture displacement and help to detect concomitant injuries around the knee joint.[9]
- Computed tomography is helpful in the older age group and in cases of severe trauma, where the fracture configuration may be severely comminuted and there is no suspicion of concomitant meniscal or collateral ligament injury.

## DIFFERENTIAL DIAGNOSIS

- ACL tear
- Osteochondral lesion or osteochondral fracture
- Tibial plateau fracture
- Other ligamentous or meniscal injuries about the knee

## NONOPERATIVE MANAGEMENT

- Nonoperative management is reserved for nondisplaced type I fractures and reducible type II fractures.
- Type II fractures may be reduced by first aspirating the hematoma and injecting a local anesthetic agent into the joint space.
  - The knee is extended in an attempt to reduce the fracture fragment. The mechanism of reduction is through direct pressure exerted by the lateral femoral condyle.
    - This maneuver may be effective for lesions that are large enough to include part of the tibial plateau.
    - In small lesions, or in lesions where the intermeniscal ligament is interposed between fracture fragments, the maneuver may not afford adequate reduction.
- The reduction is assessed with radiographs, and the knee is immobilized.
- A hinged knee brace or long-leg cast is placed to immobilize the leg and maintain reduction.
  - There has been controversy about the optimal position for cast placement.
  - Previous authors have recommended varying knee positions, ranging from 0 to 40 degrees of flexion.[3,5,17] The arguments in favor of flexing the knee relate to the relative relaxation of the ACL in flexion.[15]
  - Immobilization in hyperextension is *not* recommended due to patient discomfort and the risk of putting the popliteal artery under tension, potentially causing the development of a compartment syndrome.
  - The authors recommend immobilization in a hinged knee brace in full extension for 4 to 6 weeks.
- The reduction should be checked radiographically after 1 week and at 2 weeks. Any loss of reduction warrants an operative reduction of the fracture.

## SURGICAL MANAGEMENT

- The general indications for surgical management of tibial spine fractures include the following:
  - Type II tibial spine fractures with inadequate closed reduction
  - Completely displaced tibial spine fractures (type III and type IV)
    - Historically, type III and type IV tibial spine fractures were sometimes treated with nonoperative management. However, a recent systematic review has shown very high rates of nonunion in type III and type IV tibial spine fractures treated without surgical fixation, and as such, we recommend surgical management for all completely displaced tibial spine fractures.[7]

### Preoperative Planning

- Careful preoperative evaluation and preparation are always imperative to the success of treatment.
- All imaging studies obtained before surgery should be reviewed.
  - If the avulsed fragment has a relatively large osseous component, plain radiographs will usually suffice in determining treatment.

A B

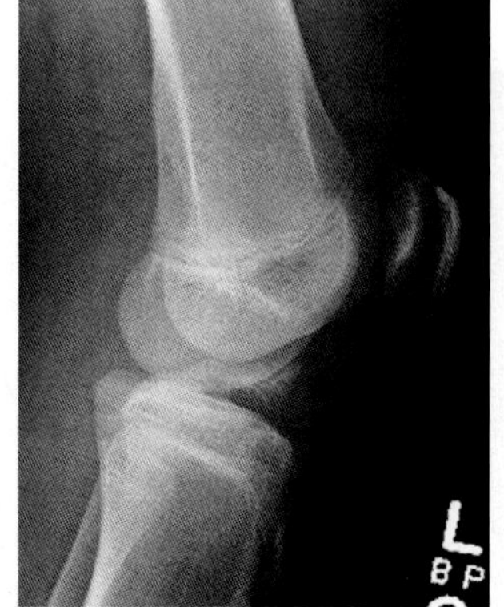

**FIG 4** • AP (**A**) and lateral (**B**) radiographs of the knee showing a displaced tibial spine fracture (type III).

- In lesions that are primarily cartilaginous, MRI may be required to determine the extent of the lesion. Any other lesion noted on imaging studies should likewise be addressed.
- A thorough physical examination should be performed under anesthesia.
- The choice of surgical treatment (open vs. arthroscopic reduction) as well as the choice of fixation device largely depends on the preference and experience of the surgeon and the character of the lesion. Most surgeons now favor arthroscopic treatment.[7]
  - Larger lesions with an adequate osseous component, for example, may allow for screw fixation, whereas a lesion that is primarily cartilaginous or an osseous lesion with a lot of comminution may be better treated with suture or anchor fixation.
  - Inevitably, the final decision as to which fixation device is best is made intraoperatively.
  - The surgeon should be prepared to offer fixation techniques that will provide stable anatomic fixation by arthroscopy or open methods.

## Positioning

- For arthroscopic procedures, the position largely depends on the surgeon's preference. A variety of positions can be used.
  - The leg can be placed on the operating table with the knee joint spanning the break in the table. This allows the knee to flex 90 degrees when the lower end of the table is dropped down, allowing the knee to hang off the table. This position can be done with or without a leg holder.
  - The leg can be placed supine on the operating table, with the hip flexed and the knee flexed 90 degrees. The knee is allowed to angle off the table as needed. A bump positioned under the knee may be helpful to achieve appropriate knee flexion for hardware placement (**FIG 5**).

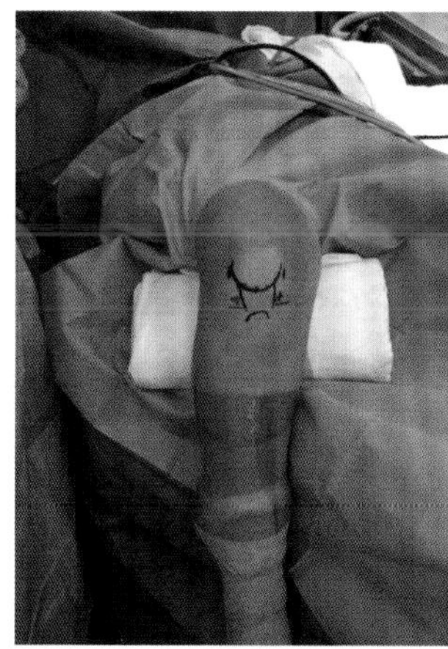

**FIG 5** ● Position of the knee in the leg holder.

- For open reduction techniques, the patient is placed supine on the operating table, a tourniquet is placed on the thigh, and the knee is draped in a standard fashion. The leg is exsanguinated.

## Approach

- The standard arthroscopic portals used for ACL reconstruction can be used. We recommend use of standard anteromedial and anterolateral portals as well as medial and lateral mid-parapatellar portals (**FIG 6**).
- For open reduction and internal fixation (ORIF), the knee is approached through a limited parapatellar approach.

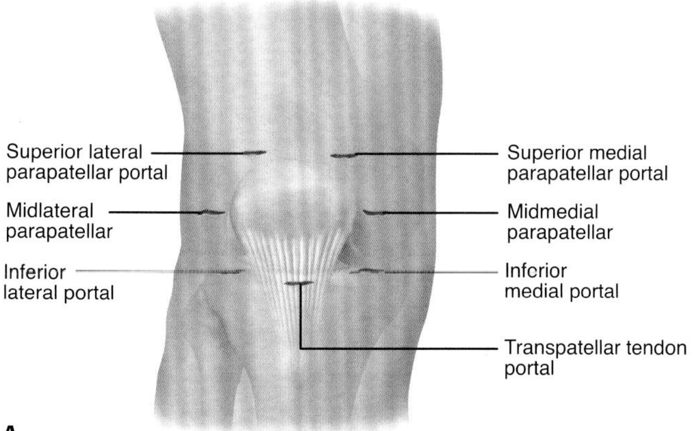


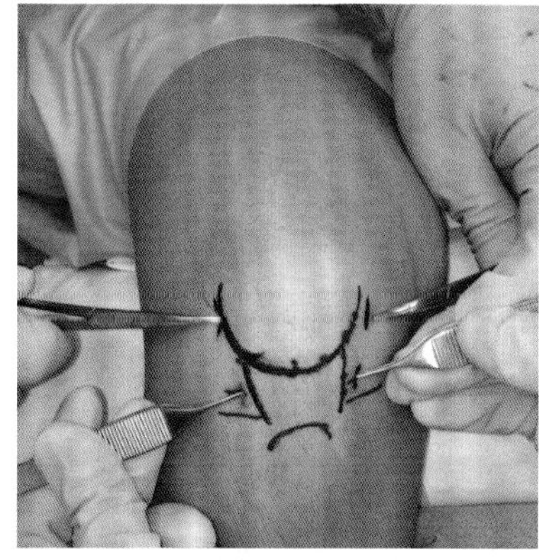


**FIG 6** ● **A.** The standard portals used for ACL reconstruction are the same ones commonly used for arthroscopic treatment of tibial spine fractures. **B.** We recommend use of standard anteromedial and anterolateral portals (marked by forceps) and medial and lateral mid-parapatellar portals (marked by hemostats).

## Fracture Reduction

- Once adequate visualization and exposure of the knee joint are achieved (either arthroscopically or open), the fracture fragments as well as any concomitant injuries are identified.
- Ninety degrees of flexion with slight posterior drawer stress is usually the best position to hold the leg for evaluation and treatment of the tibial spine fracture.
- Each fracture, however, has its own characteristics. The surgeon should evaluate various degrees of flexion and extension from approximately 70 to 110 degrees as well as rotation and posterior drawer stressing to find the best position for fracture reduction.
- Once reduction is achieved, the leg is held in the appropriate position by the assistant to allow for fixation by the surgeon.

## Arthroscopy-Assisted Tibial Spine Repair

### Arthroscopic Fixation

- An anterolateral portal is made for visualization, a superomedial portal is used as an outflow tract, and an anteromedial portal is made for instrumentation.
- The hemarthrosis is evacuated to allow for direct inspection and evaluation of the knee joint. This may require 1 to 2 minutes of irrigation and débridement in order to achieve adequate visualization.
- Identify any concomitant injuries.
- The base of the fracture fragment is débrided using shavers and curettes, and the fracture hematoma is carefully removed.
- Attempt to reduce the fracture fragments as described earlier in the section "Fracture Reduction" (**TECH FIG 1**).
- If any interposing structure is found preventing reduction, it should be carefully retracted and sutured or repaired if necessary.
- Mid-parapatellar portals are recommended, as they will allow easy use of accessory probes and instruments.

### Screw Fixation

- Once anatomic reduction of the fracture has been achieved, a 0.045-inch Kirschner wire is passed through the fracture fragment through the mid-parapatellar portal in the desired location of the final screw (**TECH FIG 2A,B**).
  - The position of the Kirschner wire is checked under fluoroscopy to ensure proper placement and to avoid traversing the growth plate.
- A second Kirschner wire may be introduced, depending on the stability of the fracture reduction and whether fixation will be achieved with metal or resorbable screw to maintain the fragments in place and prevent rotation during screw placement.

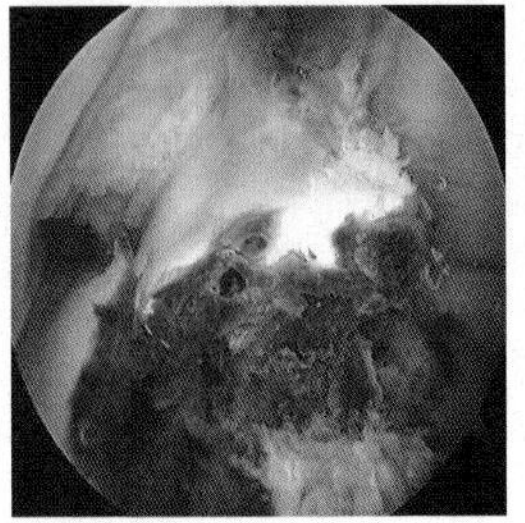
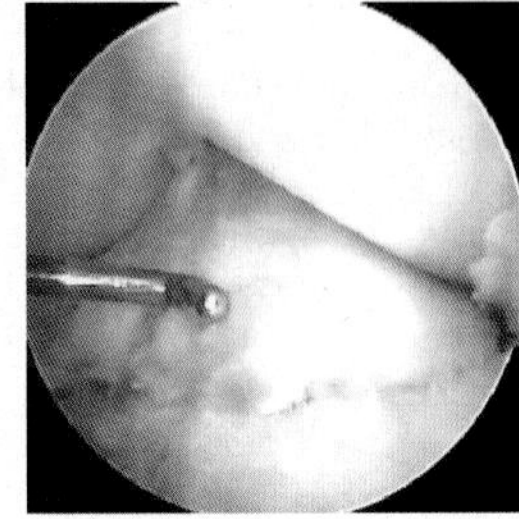

**TECH FIG 1** ● **A.** Arthroscopic image taken of a type III tibial spine fracture. **B.** Arthroscopic image showing anatomic reduction of the fracture fragments.

- A screw of appropriate size and length is chosen.
  - Metal or resorbable screws can be used for fixation (**TECH FIG 2C**).
  - With metal screws, a 3.5- or 4.0-mm cannulated, self-drilling self-tapping screw is used. The screw size is largely dependent on whether the fracture fragments will accommodate the screw.
  - With resorbable screws (noncannulated), a cannulated drill and cannulated tap may be used over the Kirschner wire. With a second Kirschner wire holding fixation, the original Kirschner wire is removed, allowing placement of the noncannulated reabsorbable screw in the position of the removed Kirschner wire.
  - One or two screws may be placed, depending on the size of the fragment.
- With reduction maintained, the screw is gradually advanced under fluoroscopic guidance, making sure that the growth plate is not traversed.
- Once adequate fixation has been obtained, the Kirschner wires are removed.
- The knee is gently flexed and extended while the stability of the reduction is checked under direct arthroscopic visualization.
- AP and lateral radiographs of the knee are taken to document appropriate positioning of the screw and to document adequate reduction before closure (**TECH FIG 2D,E**).
- Once satisfactory reduction is documented, the instruments are removed, and the arthroscopic portals are closed.
- The knee is placed in a hinged knee brace locked in full extension.

### Suture Fixation

- Two 1-0 polydioxanone (PDS) sutures are passed through the base of the ACL proximal to its insertion on the tibial spine (**TECH FIG 3**). This is most easily achieved through the mid-parapatellar portal.
- An incision is made 1 to 2 cm medial to the tibial tubercle to allow for placement of an ACL tibial guide.
- Two parallel 2-mm transphyseal tunnels are made.
- A suture passer is passed through each tunnel and the suture ends are retrieved.
- The tibial spine is reduced in its own bed and the suture ends are tied over a bone bridge in the anteromedial portion of the tibia.
  - If desired, provisional fixation using a resorbable compression screw (discussed earlier) can be used with suture fixation for secondary support. The provisional fixation with a resorbable compression screw prevents the fracture fragments from displacing during suture fixation.[6]
- Once adequate reduction has been achieved, gentle flexion and extension of the knee is performed under direct arthroscopic visualization to check for stability of reduction.

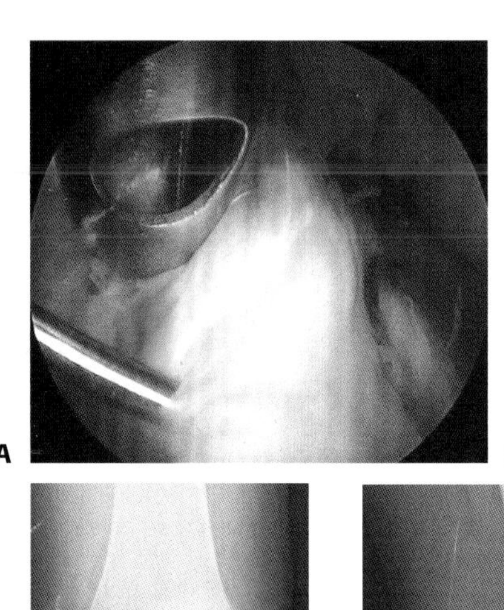
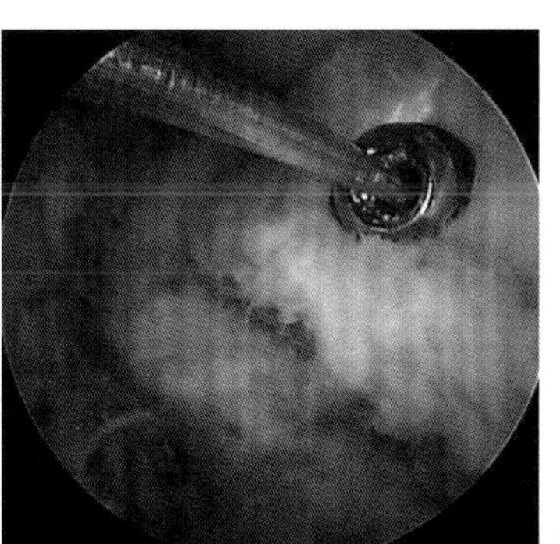
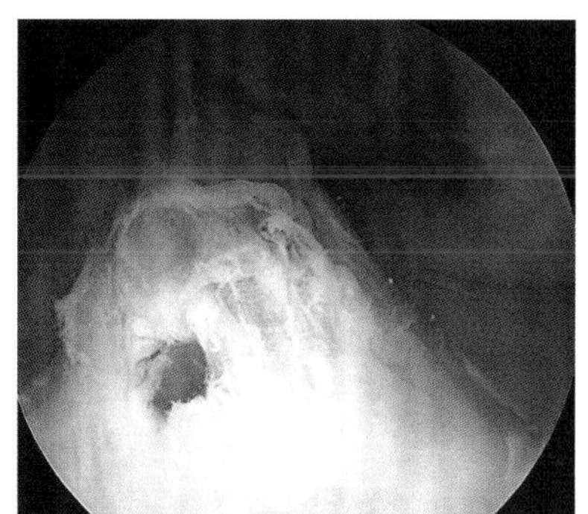
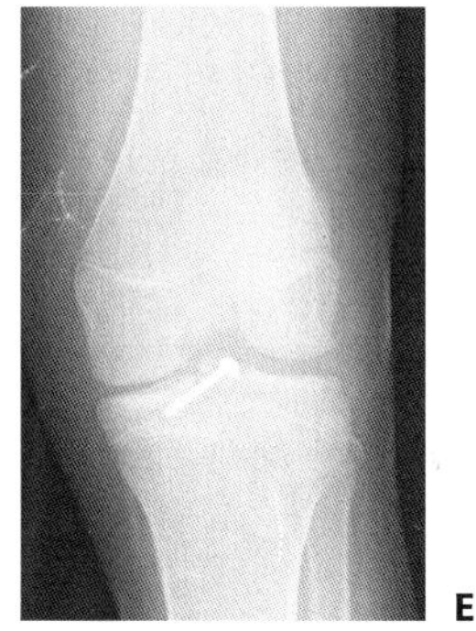
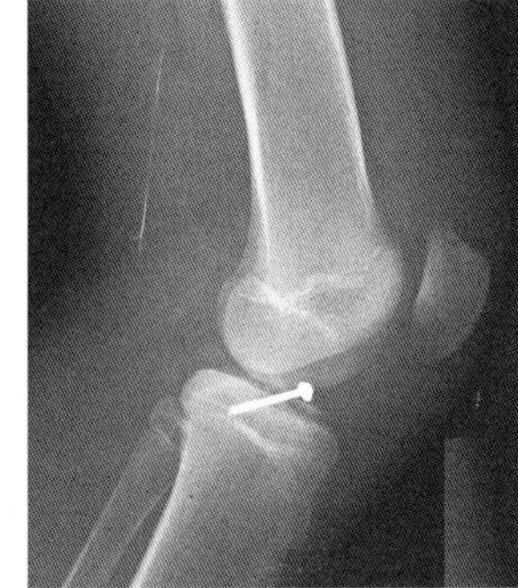

**TECH FIG 2** • Arthroscopic screw fixation. **A.** The fracture fragment is maintained using Kirschner wire(s). **B.** A cannulated metal screw is inserted under fluoroscopic guidance. **C.** A resorbable screw in position. As resorbable screw are not typically cannulated, placement requires removal of the Kirschner wire. A second Kirschner wire maintains reduction while the resorbable screw is inserted. **D,E.** AP and lateral radiographs, respectively, showing the tibial spine fracture fixed with a single cannulated screw with washer. Care should be taken to avoid crossing the physis with the screw.

- When satisfactory reduction of the fracture is obtained and documented, the instruments are removed and the arthroscopic portals are closed.
- The knee is placed in a hinged knee brace locked in full extension.

## Suture Anchor (Shoulder Anchor) Fixation

- Two 1-0 PDS sutures are passed through the base of the ACL proximal to its insertion on the tibial spine as in the suture fixation method described earlier. A technique similar to basic shoulder labral repair is then performed.
- The limbs of suture are luggage tagged around the base of the ACL (**TECH FIG 4A**), and then passed through the suture anchors.
- The tibial spine fracture is reduced and the anchors are then secured anterior to the tibial eminence, angled slightly anterior to posterior (**TECH FIG 4B,C**).
  - If desired, provisional fixation using a resorbable compression screw (discussed earlier) can be used with secondary suture anchor fixation. The provisional fixation with a resorbable compression screw prevents the fracture fragments from displacing during anchor fixation. This method is most recommended for use in type IV (comminuted) fractures.[6]
- After adequate reduction had been achieved, gentle flexion and extension of the knee is performed under direct arthroscopic visualization to check for stability of reduction.
- Once satisfactory reduction of the fracture is obtained and documented, the instruments are removed and the arthroscopic portals are closed.
- The knee is placed in a hinged knee brace locked in full extension.

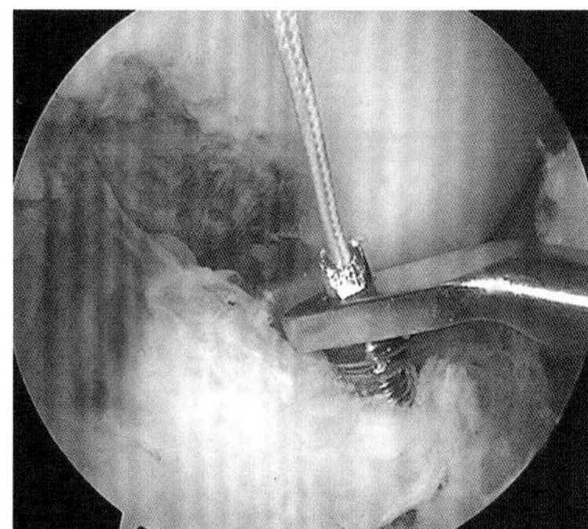
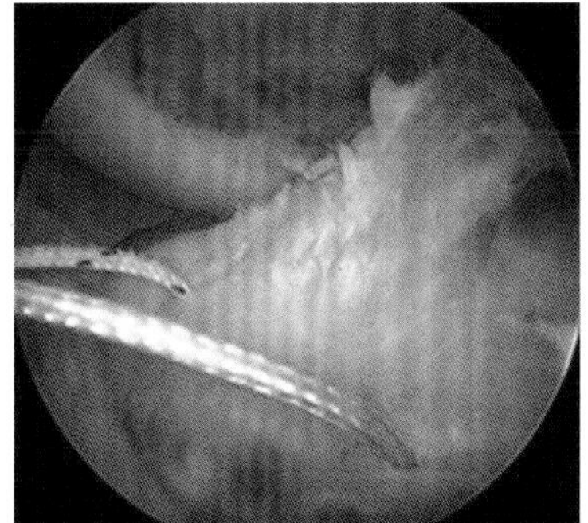
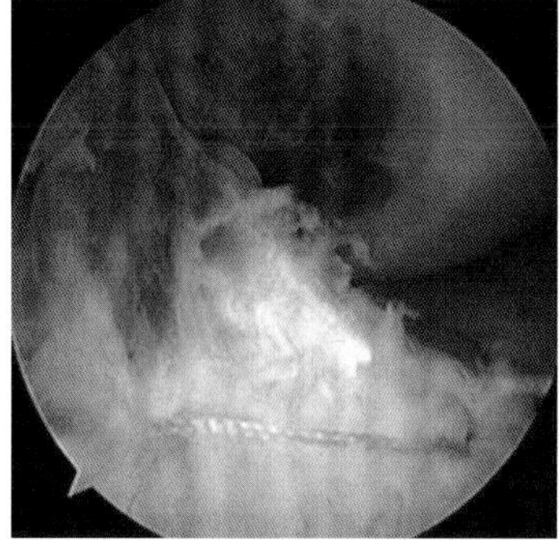

**TECH FIG 3** • Arthroscopic suture fixation. **A,B.** Two 1-0 PDS sutures are passed through the base of the ACL. A suture passer is used to grab the suture ends through a transphyseal tunnel and the suture ends are tied in the anteromedial border of the tibia. **C.** Final suture fixation of a tibial spine fracture.

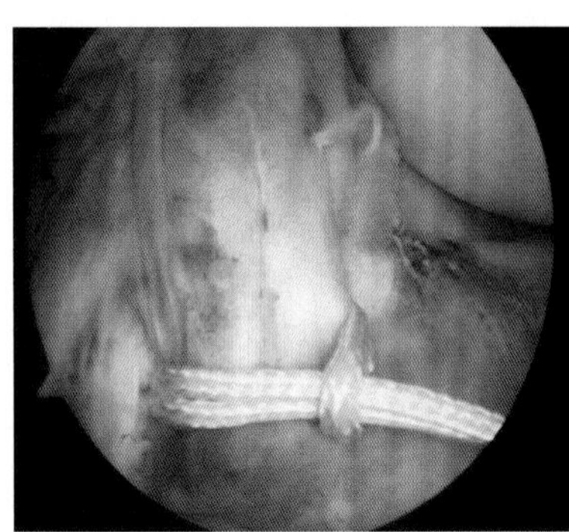

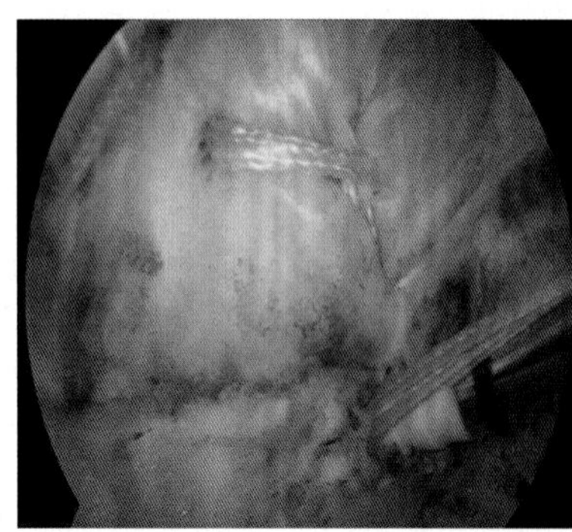

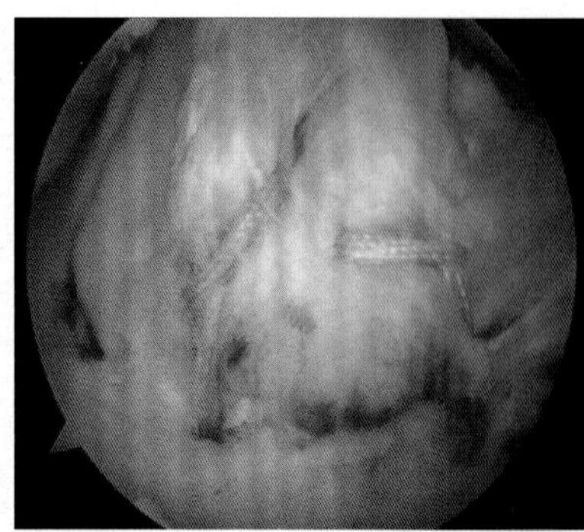

**TECH FIG 4** • Arthroscopic suture anchor fixation. **A.** Two limbs of 1-0 PDS suture are passed through the base of the ACL at its insertion onto the tibial eminence and luggage tag the sutures. **B.** The limbs of suture are passed through suture anchors and secured anterior to the tibial eminence, angled slightly anterior to posterior. **C.** Final suture anchor fixation of a tibial spine fracture.

## Open Reduction and Internal Fixation

### Exposure

- The procedure begins with a standard medial parapatellar approach. The skin incision may be parapatellar or midline.
- The medial parapatellar incision is started at the inferior pole of the patella and follows the medial border of the patellar tendon down to the level of the tibial tubercle. The incision can be extended as needed (**TECH FIG 5**).
- When performing the medial parapatellar skin incision, care should be taken to avoid inadvertent transection of the infrapatellar branch of the saphenous nerve; if a branch is cut, it should be buried in fat to decrease the risk of developing a neuroma.
- The skin incision is carried down to the fascia. The skin and subcutaneous tissues are retracted and reflected.
- Dissection is carried through the medial border of the patellar retinaculum, making sure to retain at least a 2- to 3-mm cuff of soft tissue to allow for adequate closure and then down along the medial border of the patellar tendon.
- The patella and patellar tendon are retracted laterally to allow for direct visualization of the ACL and tibial spine fracture.

### Fracture Fixation

- Once fracture reduction is achieved, fixation materials are used to hold the fragment in place, including sutures, screws, Kirschner wires, and suture anchors—similar to those described in the arthroscopic techniques earlier.
- Once fixation of the fracture has been achieved, stability is tested by gentle flexion and extension of the knee.
- Any concomitant injuries about the knee joint may be addressed.
- Copious washing of the knee joint is done before closure to clear the knee joint of any remaining debris.
- Meticulous hemostasis and layer-by-layer closure are performed.
- The knee is placed in a hinged knee brace locked in extension.

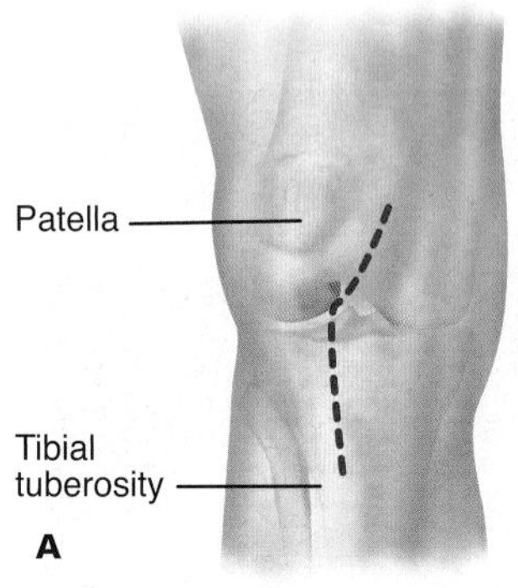


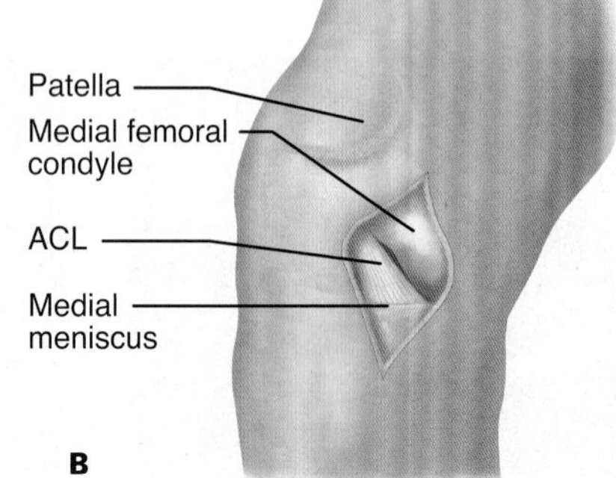


**TECH FIG 5** • **A.** The medial parapatellar approach to the knee can be done through a straight midline incision. **B.** The parapatellar incision is carried through to the knee joint and the patella is reflected laterally.

## PEARLS AND PITFALLS

| | |
|---|---|
| **Diagnosis** | ■ As treatment is based on appropriate classification of the fracture pattern, it is important to have an adequate lateral radiograph in order to avoid missing diagnosis of tibial spine fractures and to avoid misclassification. The mechanism of injury is typically the same as that for ACL tears. Although more commonly seen in pediatric patients than in adults, tibial spine fractures are not specific to either group. |
| **Indications** | ■ A careful assessment of the injury is done before treatment; any concomitant injuries such as meniscal tears or injuries to the collateral ligaments should be carefully evaluated and incorporated into the surgical plan. |
| **Surgical preparation** | ■ Even with proper preoperative planning, the surgeon should be prepared to use a variety of fixation devices and techniques. This is often dictated by the size and character of the fracture fragment. A large fragment may accommodate more than one screw; a smaller fragment, however, may be better treated with suture fixation or suture anchor fixation. |
| **Fracture reduction** | ■ Difficult reduction is often secondary to soft tissue interposition. The fracture bed should be cleared and any interposing soft tissue should be retracted or removed as deemed necessary. Often, the intermeniscal ligament or the anterior horn of the medial meniscus become entrapped; performing an anterior drawer maneuver may allow the entrapped fragment to be liberated. The fragment may then be reduced onto the fracture bed and fixed accordingly. |
| **Fracture fixation** | ■ The fracture fragment should be assessed and carefully fixed. Multiple attempts at obtaining purchase with the use of fixation devices should be avoided, as this may cause comminution of the fragment.<br>■ In skeletally immature individuals, care must be taken to avoid crossing the physis, particularly with the use of screw fixation. Fluoroscopic guidance should be used when radiopaque implants are used and the physis identified and avoided during fixation.<br>■ Midpatellar portals allow for easy placement of screws, sutures, and suture anchors. |
| **Mobilization** | ■ Early treatment, secure fixation, and early postoperative mobilization can help avoid complications such as postoperative stiffness, arthrofibrosis, and loss of knee extension.[19] Mobilization is allowed depending on the stability of fixation. If prolonged immobilization is needed, immobilizing in extension is preferred, as flexion contractures are more difficult to treat than stiffness. |

## POSTOPERATIVE CARE

- Postoperatively, the knee is immobilized in full extension if adequate fixation is achieved. If adequate fixation is not obtained, the knee may be placed in 5 to 10 degrees of flexion; hyperextension should always be avoided. The authors prefer immobilization in a hinged knee brace locked in extension.
- Radiographs are taken to document adequate reduction of the fracture fragment.
- Early range of motion may be started at 1 to 2 weeks postoperatively when the swelling has subsided and if good fixation of the fracture fragment is obtained. Early mobilization reduces the risk of development of arthrofibrosis and loss of range of motion.[19]
- In more severe cases, where stability may be in question, range-of-motion exercises are generally instituted once adequate healing of the fracture can be ascertained radiographically; this is usually 4 to 6 weeks after surgery.

## OUTCOMES

- Residual laxity of the knee is commonly seen, even with anatomic reduction of the fracture, and is due to the inherent stretch of the ACL before the tibial spine fails. In most cases, the residual laxity is subclinical. As long as reduction is maintained, excellent functional outcomes have been reported, despite the residual laxity with both closed management and operative treatment of tibial spine fractures.[2,14,24,25]
- Good to excellent outcomes have been reported with ORIF as well as arthroscopic reduction with suture fixation,[1,4,14] arthroscopic reduction with screw fixation,[10,20] and arthroscopic reduction with suture anchor fixation.[12,13,23]
- Gans, et al[7] performed a systematic review using meta-analytic technique on observational studies to look at the optimal method of reduction and fixation of tibial spine fractures in pediatric patients based on outcomes and complications. They found that nonoperative treatment of completely displaced (type III and type IV) fractures resulted in higher rates of nonunion. There were no observable differences in outcome with open versus closed operative technique or screw versus suture fixation.

## COMPLICATIONS

- Nonunion
- Malunion
- Arthrofibrosis
- Residual laxity—although usually subclinical
- Implant-related complications and retained metal hardware in the case of metal screw fixation
- Growth disturbance
- Loss of motion

## REFERENCES

1. Ahn JH, Yoo JC. Clinical outcome of arthroscopic reduction and suture for displaced acute and chronic tibial spine fractures. Knee Surg Sports Traumatol Arthrosc 2005;13:116–121.
2. Baxter MP, Wiley JJ. Fractures of the tibial spine in children. An evaluation of knee stability. J Bone Joint Surg Br 1988;70(2):228–230.
3. Beaty JH, Kumar A. Fractures about the knee in children. J Bone Joint Surg Am 1994;76:1870–1880.
4. Binnet MS, Gürkan I, Yilmaz C, et al. Arthroscopic fixation of intercondylar eminence fractures using a 4-portal technique. Arthroscopy 2001;17:450–460.

5. Fyfe IS, Jackson JP. Tibial intercondylar fractures in children: a review of the classification and the treatment of malunion. Injury 1981;13:165–169.
6. Gans I, Babatunde OM, Ganley TJ. Hybrid fixation of tibial eminence fractures in skeletally immature patients. Arthrosc Tech 2013;2(3):e237–e242.
7. Gans I, Baldwin KD, Ganley TJ. Treatment and management outcomes of tibial eminence fractures in pediatric patients: a systematic review. Am J Sports Med 2013;4:1743–1750.
8. Hunter RE, Willis JA. Arthroscopic fixation of avulsion fractures of the tibial eminence: technique and outcome. Arthroscopy 2004;20:113–121.
9. Ishibashi Y, Tsuda E, Sasaki T, et al. Magnetic resonance imaging aids in detecting concomitant injuries in patients with tibial spine fractures. Clin Orthop Relat Res 2005;(434):207–212.
10. Kocher MS, Foreman ES, Micheli LJ. Laxity and functional outcome after arthroscopic reduction and internal fixation of displaced tibial spine fractures in children. Arthroscopy 2003;19:1085–1090.
11. Kocher MS, Mandiga R, Klingele K, et al. Anterior cruciate ligament injury versus tibial spine fracture in the skeletally immature knee: a comparison of skeletal maturation and notch width index. J Pediatr Orthop 2004;24:185–188.
12. Louis ML, Guillaume JM, Launay F, et al. Surgical management of type II tibial intercondylar eminence fractures in children. J Pediatr Orthop B 2008;17(5):231–235.
13. Lu XW, Hu XP, Jin C, et al. Reduction and fixation of the avulsion fracture of the tibial eminence using mini-open technique. Knee Surg Sports Traumatol Arthrosc 2010;18(11):1476–1480.
14. Mah JY, Adili A, Otsuka NY, et al. Follow-up study of arthroscopic reduction and fixation of type III tibial-eminence fractures. J Pediatr Orthop 1998;18:475–477.
15. McLennan JG. Lessons learned after second-look arthroscopy in type III fractures of the tibial spine. J Pediatr Orthop 1995;15:59–62.
16. Meyers MH, McKeever FM. Fracture of the intercondylar eminence of the tibia. J Bone Joint Surg Am 1959;41(2):209–222.
17. Meyers MH, McKeever FM. Fracture of the intercondylar eminence of the tibia. J Bone Joint Surg Am 1970;52(8):1677–1684.
18. Noyes FR, DeLucas JL, Torvik PJ. Biomechanics of anterior cruciate ligament failure: an analysis of strain-rate sensitivity and mechanisms of failure in primates. J Bone Joint Surg Am 1974;56:236–253.
19. Patel NM, Park MJ, Sampson NR, et al. Tibial eminence fractures in children: earlier posttreatment mobilization results in improved outcomes. J Pediatr Orthop 2012;32(2):139–144.
20. Reynders P, Reynders K, Broos P. Pediatric and adolescent tibial eminence fractures: arthroscopic cannulated screw fixation. J Trauma 2002;53:49–54.
21. Skak SV, Jensen TT, Poulsen TD, et al. Epidemiology of knee injuries in children. Acta Orthop Scand 1987;58:78–81.
22. Tudisco C, Giovarruscio R, Febo A, et al. Intercondylar eminence avulsion fracture in children: long-term follow-up of 14 cases at the end of skeletal growth. J Pediatr Orthop B 2010;19(5):403–408.
23. Vega JR, Irribarra LA, Baar AK, et al. Arthroscopic fixation of displaced tibial eminence fractures: a new growth plate-sparing method. Arthroscopy 2008;24(11):1239–1243.
24. Wiley JJ, Baxter MP. Tibial spine fractures in children. Clin Orthop Relat Res 1990;(255):54–60.
25. Willis RB, Blokker C, Stoll TM, et al. Long-term follow-up of anterior tibial eminence fractures. J Pediatr Orthop 1993;13:361–364.
26. Woo SL, Hollis JM, Adams DJ, et al. Tensile properties of the human femur-anterior cruciate ligament–tibia complex: the effects of specimen age and orientation. Am J Sports Med 1991;19:217–225.
27. Zaricznyj B. Avulsion fracture of the tibial eminence treated by open reduction and pinning. J Bone Joint Surg Am 1997;59(8):1111–1114.

# Anterior Cruciate Ligament Reconstruction in the Skeletally Immature Patient

45
CHAPTER

J. Todd R. Lawrence, R. Jay Lee, and Mininder S. Kocher

## DEFINITION

- Skeletally immature patients have open growth plates, or physes, and thus have growth potential remaining.
- Intrasubstance anterior cruciate ligament (ACL) injuries were once considered rare in this population, with tibial eminence avulsion fractures considered the pediatric ACL injury equivalent.[14] However, intrasubstance ACL injuries in children and adolescents are being seen with increasing frequency and result in an "ACL-deficient knee" as in adult patients.
- ACL deficiency in the skeletally immature patient usually results in an unstable knee at risk for further injury and accelerated degeneration.
- Conventional surgical reconstruction techniques risk potential iatrogenic growth disturbance due to physeal violation, and thus special consideration must be given to this patient population.[10]
- The physiologic age of the patient reflects the amount of remaining growth potential and knee size and thus heavily influences the treatment options.

## ANATOMY

- The ACL originates from a semicircular area on the posterior portion of the medial aspect of the lateral femoral condyle and courses obliquely to the anteromedial aspect of the tibial plateau at the anterior tibial eminence (or spine).
- The primary role of the ACL is to resist anterior translocation and rotation of the tibia on the femur.
- The ligament is composed of two anatomically and biomechanically distinct bundles: the anteromedial and the posterolateral bundles.
  - The anteromedial bundle is more anterior and vertical in orientation. It largely resists anterior translation and tightens in the last 30 degrees of extension.
  - The posterolateral bundle is more posterior and oblique in orientation. It is more isometric and plays a greater role in rotational control.
- Not all skeletally immature patients are the same. Some have a tremendous amount of growth remaining, whereas others are essentially done growing.
- Most of the longitudinal growth of the lower extremities comes from the distal femur and the proximal tibia. The tibial physis can be as close as 15 to 20 mm to the tibial spine. The femoral physis comes within millimeters of the femoral attachment of the ACL at the most posterior aspect of its insertion (**FIG 1**).

## PATHOGENESIS

- The etiology of ACL injury in skeletally immature patients is similar to that in the adult population. It is usually due to a noncontact injury involving a cutting, pivoting, or rapid deceleration maneuver.
- Patients often report hearing a "pop" followed by swelling of the knee. ACL injury has been reported in up to 65% of pediatric patients with acute traumatic hemarthrosis.[17]
- The "shift" that occurs with the ACL-deficient knee at the time of injury causes an impaction injury on the posterior aspect of the tibial plateau against the distal femur at the sulcus terminalis as the tibia translates anteriorly on the femur. Characteristic bone bruises in this location on magnetic resonance imaging (MRI) are pathognomonic for ACL injury (**FIG 2**).
- Ligamentous, meniscal, and chondral injuries are commonly associated with ACL injury.
  - The medial collateral ligament is commonly injured with the ACL.
  - The posterolateral corner is less often injured with the ACL but is a common cause of failure of ACL reconstruction if it is not addressed as well.
  - Tears of the lateral meniscus are associated with acute tears of the ACL.

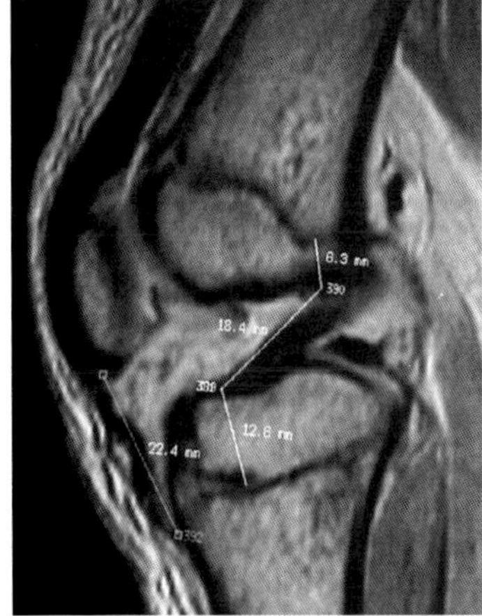


**FIG 1** • Sagittal MRI demonstrating the relationship of the ACL to the distal femoral and proximal tibial physes. (From Kocher MS, Garg S, Micheli LJ. Physeal sparing reconstruction of the anterior cruciate ligament in skeletally immature prepubescent children and adolescents. Surgical technique. J Bone Joint Surg Am 2006;88[suppl, 1 pt 2]:283–293.)

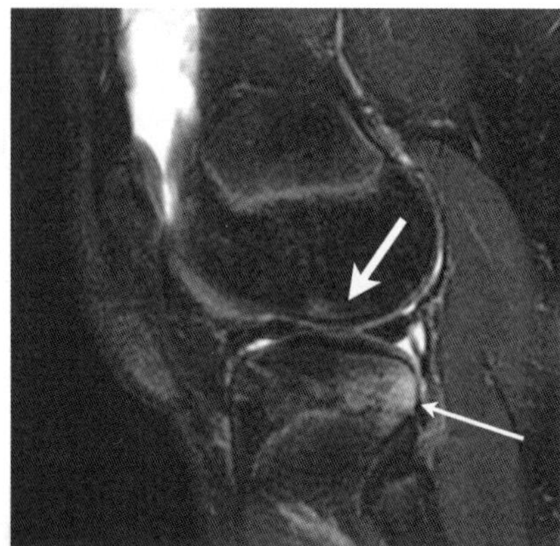

**FIG 2** ● Sagittal MRI through the lateral aspect of the knee demonstrating characteristic bone bruise pattern for an acute ACL injury (*thin arrow*). Note increased signal on the posterior aspect of the lateral tibial plateau and the distal aspect of the femur at the sulcus terminalis (*thick arrow*).

- The posterior horn of the medial meniscus is a secondary restraint to anterior translation of the tibia. In the chronically ACL-deficient knee, the posterior horn of the medial meniscus assumes a greater role in preventing anterior translation and is thus at increased risk of injury.

## NATURAL HISTORY

- *Partial tears* may be successfully managed nonoperatively in some patients.[9]
- *Complete tears* in skeletally immature patients generally have a poor prognosis, with instability leading to further meniscal and chondral injury.[1,12]
- Over half of patients show evidence of early degenerative changes 4 to 5 years after their injury with nonoperative management.[12]
- Patients who have a greater amount of instability, as measured objectively with KT-1000 arthrometry, or pursue higher level cutting and jumping sports, are at greater risk for recurrent injury.[3]
- ACL reconstruction can reduce the risk of ongoing mechanical meniscal and chondral injury associated with instability. However, how this influences the risk of developing degenerative joint disease is not clear at this time.

## PATIENT HISTORY AND PHYSICAL FINDINGS

- Adolescents are notoriously bad historians, but every attempt should be made to garner an appreciation for the mechanism of injury, a history of acute or recurrent effusions, and a sense of instability with activities or mechanical symptoms.
- Physiologic age should be established informally in the office using the Tanner staging system.[18] This can be confirmed in the operating room after the induction of anesthesia. Skeletal age can be determined via hand and wrist radiographs per the method of Greulich and Pyle.[4]
- A complete examination of the knee should be performed. Particular attention should be given to evaluating the knee for associated pathology.
- Overall, lower extremity alignment, angular deformity, and any leg length discrepancy should be noted.
- Patellar ballottement and fluid wave test should be done to evaluate for the presence of an effusion.
- Range of motion (ROM) is important to assess because regaining full ROM before ACL reconstruction may be critical to prevent postoperative arthrofibrosis. Loss of extension should alert the clinician to the possibility of a displaced bucket-handle tear or preoperative arthrofibrosis. Loss of flexion may be due to pain secondary to a tense effusion.
- Tenderness to palpation should be assessed and localized specifically as it can greatly direct the diagnosis of related injuries.
  - Tenderness to palpation along the joint line, particularly the posterior aspect of the joint line, should alert the clinician to the possibility of a meniscal tear. Pain or palpable popping with provocative maneuvers, such as McMurray, Apley compression, or duck walk, will help to confirm this finding.
  - Pain along the course of or at the femoral or tibial insertion points for the collateral ligaments should alert the clinician to the possibility of a collateral ligament tear.
  - Pain at the physis should prompt an investigation for a physeal injury, although in our experience, this is not commonly associated with complete ACL injuries.
  - Tenderness along the medial retinaculum or the course of the medial patellofemoral ligament can indicate an acute patellar dislocation that reduced spontaneously.
- Ligamentous evaluation should include the anterior and posterior cruciate ligaments, the medial and lateral collateral ligaments, and the posterolateral corner.
  - Skeletally immature athletes have a greater degree of physiologic laxity than adult athletes and as such a comparison should always be made to the uninjured knee.
  - Evaluation of the ACL is best done with the Lachman test in the cooperative patient. In the patient who voluntarily or involuntarily guards against traditional Lachman testing, the prone Lachman or the anterior drawer tests may encourage relaxation and give a more reliable examination.
  - Pivot shift testing may be performed in the office but is usually not well tolerated by pediatric patients. It should be performed in the operating room as part of the preoperative evaluation of every patient.
  - The posterior cruciate ligament should be evaluated using the posterior drawer test. The relative starting point should always be assessed first and compared to the contralateral side. The use of posterior drawer stress radiographs is unclear at this time. Injuries of grade II and above should alert the clinician to the possibility of an associated posterolateral corner injury.
  - Medial and lateral collateral ligament injuries are assessed through stress opening with valgus and varus stress at 0 and 30 degrees of knee flexion. In the pediatric patient, opening with varus and valgus stress can be due to physeal injuries, and the clinician should always be vigilant for this.
  - Evaluation of the posterolateral corner is best done with the dial test. The posterolateral drawer and the external rotation recurvatum tests are also useful for evaluating posterolateral corner injuries.
- Evaluation for patellar instability with apprehension testing should be performed.
- Evaluation of quadriceps bulk and strength is important for postoperative recovery.

## IMAGING AND OTHER DIAGNOSTIC STUDIES

- All pediatric patients with a complaint of knee pain should receive an initial plain radiographic evaluation including anteroposterior (AP), lateral, and patellar views. With a traumatic injury, both oblique views should be obtained. If there is a concern for an osteochondritis dissecans lesion in the differential, a notch view should also be obtained. In scrutinizing the radiographs, special attention should be given to evaluate for physeal injuries as well as other injuries on the differential diagnosis.
- AP and frog-leg lateral plain radiographs of the hip should be considered in the evaluation of all pediatric patients with complaints of knee pain.
- Overall varus and valgus malalignment or leg length discrepancies, if present clinically, should be evaluated with full-length, hip-to-ankle radiographs.
- MRI is the diagnostic imaging test of choice for further evaluation of ACL tears in the skeletally immature patient. Recent high-field strength magnets with quality imaging has shown high sensitivity and specificity for diagnosing ACL injuries in this population[15] despite earlier reports noting decreased diagnostic value compared with the adult population.[6] Findings on MRI signifying an ACL tear include a discontinuity in the fibers on the ACL and a characteristic bone bruise pattern on the distal femur and the posterior tibial plateau of the lateral hemijoint.
  - MRI in the pediatric population has a high false-positive rate for meniscal tears. This is likely due to the increased vascularity of the meniscus, which is often interpreted as intrasubstance degeneration or a tear of the meniscus.[6]

## DIFFERENTIAL DIAGNOSIS

- Tibial eminence (spine) fracture
- Other intra-articular or physeal fracture
- Patellar dislocation
- Meniscal tear
- Posterior cruciate ligament tear
- Medial or lateral collateral tear
- Posterolateral corner injury
- Physiologic laxity
- Hip etiology

## NONOPERATIVE MANAGEMENT

- Partial or incomplete tears can be successfully managed nonoperatively in some patients if clinical and functional stability is present. The following criteria have been shown to be associated with successful nonoperative treatment of partial tears[9]:
  - Tears of less than 50% of the ligament
  - Relative preservation of the posterolateral bundle
  - Age younger than 14 years
  - Normal or near-normal Lachman or pivot shift test
- Up to a third of patients may require subsequent reconstruction and should be made aware of that risk at the onset of treatment.
- Successful treatment based on the earlier criteria includes the following:
  - A hinged knee brace is worn for 12 weeks.
  - Touchdown weight bearing is maintained for 6 to 8 weeks.
  - Passive terminal extension is restricted for the first 6 weeks.
  - Open-chain activities and active terminal extension is restricted for 12 weeks.
  - Physical therapy emphasizes hamstring muscle strengthening.
  - Return to sports and active play is permitted at 3 to 6 months if strength and functional testing are symmetric with good form on all activities. A functional knee brace is recommended for 2 years for cutting and pivoting activities.
- Nonoperative management of complete tears in skeletally immature patients generally has a poor prognosis.
- For prepubescent patients with a complete ACL tear but without a concurrent chondral injury requiring stabilization or meniscal injury requiring repair, we still discuss nonoperative treatment with activity modification, functional bracing, and continued rehabilitation.
- In our experience, compliance with activity modification and brace use and effectiveness limits the success of this treatment.
- Delay in surgical stabilization can lead to further meniscal and chondral injury due to recurrent instability.
- Although results of nonoperative management are generally poor, the risk of further intra-articular injury by waiting until skeletal maturity to undergo reconstruction must be weighed against the risk of growth disturbance with early reconstruction.
- Some patients are able to cope with their ACL insufficiency or modify their activities, allowing for further growth and aging such that the reconstruction may be performed when little or no growth remains, minimizing risk for growth disturbance.
- For prepubescent patients with ongoing instability, early reconstruction with a physeal-avoiding procedure is indicated.
- For adolescent patients with growth remaining who have a complete ACL tear, we do not advocate initial nonoperative treatment because the risk of functional instability resulting in injury to the meniscal and articular cartilage is high and there are anatomic reconstruction options that have a minimal risk of growth disturbance.

## SURGICAL MANAGEMENT

- Conventional adult ACL reconstruction techniques risk potential iatrogenic growth disturbance due to physeal violation, and cases of growth disturbance have been reported in animal models and clinical series.[10]
- The following principles should always be followed with any reconstructive strategy:
  - No hard fixation, such as with an interference screw, should cross the physis because it has a high risk of inducing a growth disturbance.
  - No bone, such as that associated with a bone–patellar tendon–bone graft, should cross the physis because it also has a high risk of inducing a growth disturbance.
- The following principles should be taken into consideration and approached with great caution when deciding on a reconstructive strategy:
  - Drill holes across the physis should be as small and as central in the physis as possible.
  - Oblique drill holes across the physis affect a larger portion of the physis than do perpendicular drill holes of the same diameter. This is especially important when considering placement of the femoral tunnel.
  - A tensioned soft tissue graft in a bone tunnel across the physis can also induce a growth disturbance.
  - Excessive dissection around the posterolateral aspect of the femoral physis or performance of an aggressive

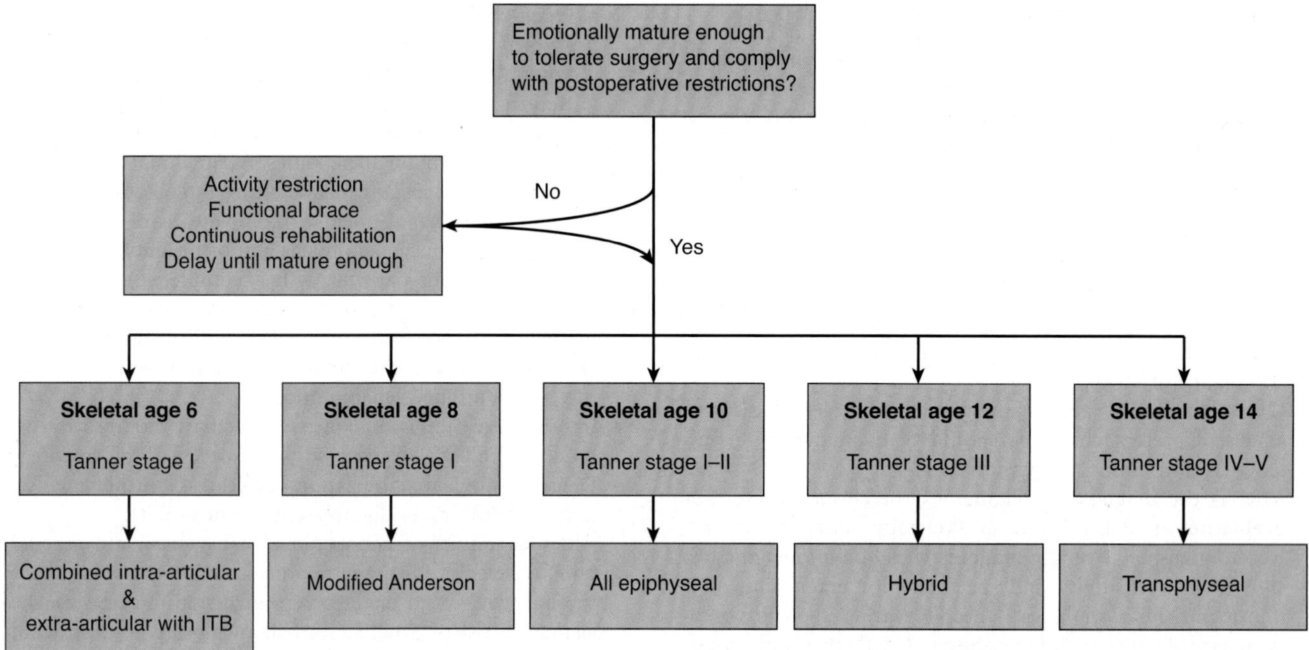


**FIG 3** • Algorithm for management of complete ACL injuries in skeletally immature patients.

notchplasty should be avoided to prevent injury to the perichondral ring and subsequent deformity.

- The approach to ACL reconstruction in the skeletally immature patient should be based on physiologic age and growth remaining. Knee size can also be considered in the feasibility of various techniques (**FIG 3**).
- A variety of reconstructive techniques have been used, including physeal-sparing, partial transphyseal, and transphyseal methods using various grafts.
- In prepubescent patients with large amounts of growth potential remaining, and smaller knees, a physeal-sparing, combined intra-articular and extra-articular reconstruction using autogenous iliotibial band should be considered.
  - Recognizing that the combined intra-articular and extra-articular reconstruction using autogenous iliotibial band described here is nonanatomic, we still counsel patients and families that revision reconstruction may be needed if recurrent instability develops, but this procedure may temporize for further growth such that the patient may then undergo a more conventional reconstruction with drill holes.
  - However, we have found that few revision reconstructions are necessary with the combined intra-articular and extra-articular reconstruction and that long-term function is similar to other reconstructions.
- In prepubescent patients with large amounts of growth potential remaining, and larger knees, an all-epiphyseal reconstruction using autogenous hamstrings may be considered.
- In adolescent patients with significant growth remaining, transphyseal ACL reconstruction with autogenous hamstring tendons with fixation away from the physes can be considered.
- In adolescent patients approaching skeletal maturity, we perform conventional adult ACL reconstruction with interference screw fixation using either autogenous central-third patellar tendon or autogenous hamstrings.
- A variety of other physeal-sparing or physeal-respecting hybrid reconstructions have been described and may be used in cases where patients are in between the previously noted categories (**FIG 4**). One common reconstruction technique is the epiphyseal femoral tunnel combined with the transphyseal tibial tunnel to avoid creating such an oblique femoral tunnel in a younger adolescent with significant growth remaining.
- In skeletally immature patients, as in adult patients, ACL reconstruction should be performed with caution in the acute inflammatory phase after the injury to minimize the risk of arthrofibrosis.
- Rehabilitation is performed to regain ROM, decrease swelling, and resolve the reflex inhibition of the quadriceps prior to proceeding with reconstruction.
- Skeletally immature patients must be emotionally mature enough to actively participate in the extensive rehabilitation and adhere to the restrictions required after ACL reconstruction.

## Preoperative Planning

- All imaging studies, including plain radiographs and MRI, should be reviewed and associated injuries identified.
- In general, associated injuries, such as meniscal, articular cartilage, or other multiple ligament injuries, should be addressed at the time of ACL reconstruction. However, reconstruction may be staged in some cases, such as nonoperative treatment of a medial collateral ligament injury before ACL reconstruction.
- Consideration should be given to using pediatric anesthesia services, given the age of the patient.
- Tanner staging should be confirmed at the time of surgery after the induction of general anesthesia.
- A complete ligamentous knee examination, including Lachman, pivot shift, varus and valgus stress, posterior drawer, and dial tests, should be performed and the findings compared to the contralateral side to confirm the diagnosis.

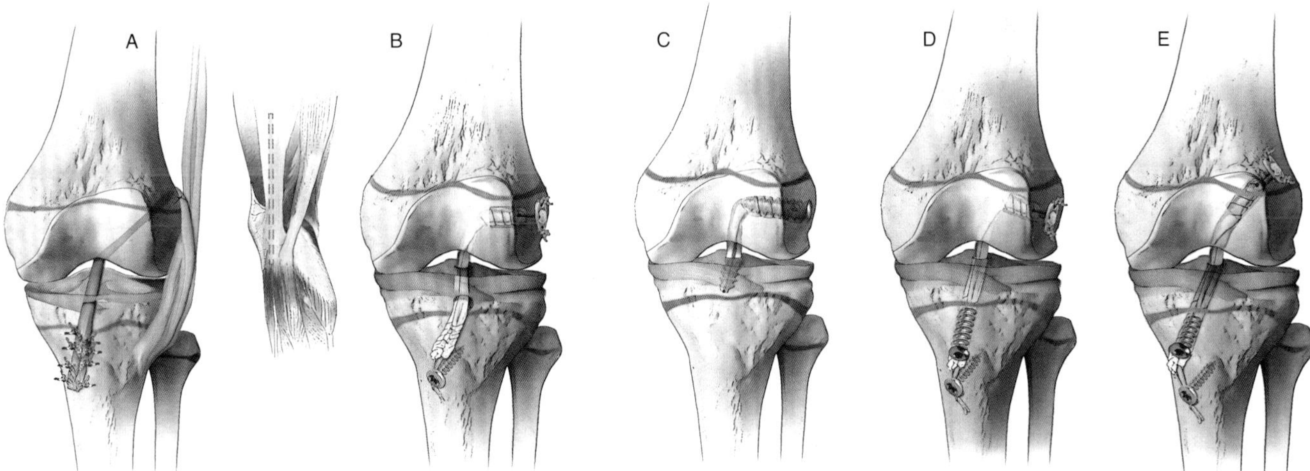


**FIG 4** ● Examples of repairs in male patients aged 6 to 14 years old. **A.** Skeletal age 6: combined intra-articular and extra-articular with iliotibial band. **B.** Skeletal age 8: modified Anderson. **C.** Skeletal age 10: all-epiphyseal. **D.** Skeletal age 12: hybrid. **E.** Skeletal age 14: transphyseal.

## Positioning

- For the procedures described here, positioning and setup are very similar.
- The procedure is performed under general anesthesia and can usually be done on an outpatient basis. Young children may benefit from overnight observation.
- Regional anesthesia can assist with pain relief but is not required. Local anesthesia with sedation may not be reliable in this population and has the potential for a paradoxical effect of sedation.
- The patient is placed supine on the operating room table and moved close to the operative side of the table such that the operative leg easily drapes over the edge of the table.
- A tourniquet is placed high about the upper thigh. It is routinely used during the combined intra-articular and extra-articular reconstruction using autogenous iliotibial band but is not routinely used during the all-epiphyseal and transphyseal technique.
- A side post is placed two fingerbreadths above the flexed knee as it drapes over the side of the bed. It is used in the "up" position for the diagnostic arthroscopy and dropped to the "down" position to provide a ledge for supporting the knee during the ACL reconstruction.

## Approach

- The approach depends on the technique employed and the choice of graft.
- Autograft is preferred because of a potential of decreased risk of retear compared with allograft,[5,13] but soft tissue allograft could be considered based on patient preference. Allograft would negate the need for hamstring harvest.

TECHNIQUES

# Physeal-Sparing, Combined Intra-articular and Extra-articular Reconstruction with Autogenous Iliotibial Band in Prepubescent Patients with Smaller Knees

## Harvest of Iliotibial Band Graft

- An incision of about 6 cm is made obliquely from the lateral joint line to the superior border of the iliotibial band.
- Proximally, the iliotibial band is separated from subcutaneous tissue using a periosteal elevator under the skin of the lateral thigh.
- The anterior and posterior borders of the iliotibial band are incised and the incisions carried proximally under the skin using curved meniscotomes (**TECH FIG 1A**).
- The iliotibial band is detached proximally under the skin using a curved meniscotome or an open tendon stripper. Alternatively, a counterincision can be made at the upper thigh to release the tendon.
- Dissection is performed distally to separate the iliotibial band from the joint capsule and from the lateral patellar retinaculum (**TECH FIG 1B**).
- The iliotibial band is left attached distally at the tubercle of Gerdy (**TECH FIG 1C**).
- The free proximal end of the iliotibial band is tubularized with a no. 5 Ethibond whipstitch and wrapped in a moist sponge until needed later.

## Arthroscopy

- Diagnostic arthroscopy of the knee is performed through standard anterolateral viewing and anteromedial working portals.
- Management of meniscal injury or chondral injury is performed if present.
- The ACL remnant is excised with the use of biting instruments and the shaver.
- The over-the-top position on the femur and the over-the-front position under the intermeniscal ligament are identified and cleared of excess tissue to allow passage of the graft.
- Minimal notchplasty is performed to avoid iatrogenic injury to the perichondral ring of the distal femoral physis, which is very close to the over-the-top position.[2]

## Graft Passage

- The free end of the iliotibial band graft is brought through the over-the-top position using a full-length clamp (**TECH FIG 2A**)

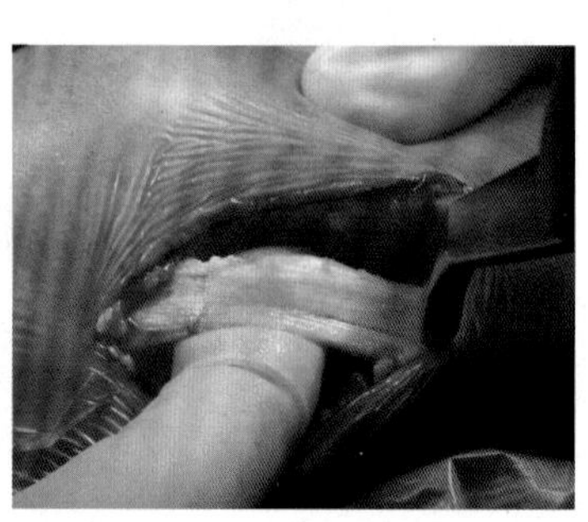
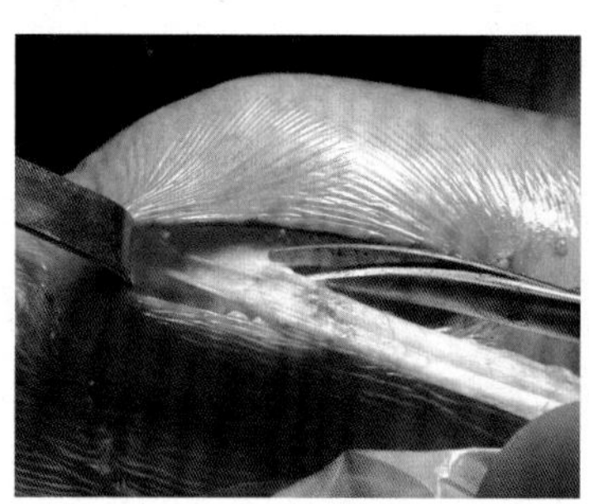
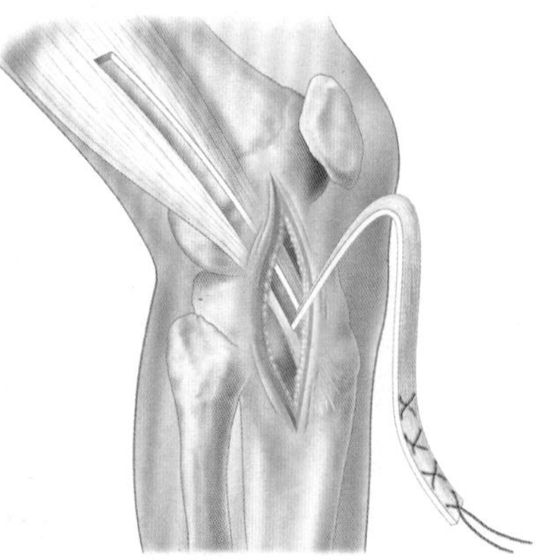

**TECH FIG 1** • Harvest of iliotibial band graft for physeal-sparing ACL reconstruction. The anterior and posterior aspects of the iliotibial band are identified through a laterally based incision at the knee. **A.** A meniscotome or an open tendon stripper is then used to harvest the proximal aspect of the graft. **B.** The graft is then freed distally. **C.** The free proximal aspect of the graft is tubularized and left attached distally to the tubercle of Gerdy. (**A,B:** From Kocher MS, Weiss JM. ACL reconstruction in the skeletally immature patient. In: Tolo VT, Scaggs DL, eds. Master Techniques in Orthopaedic Surgery: Pediatrics. Philadelphia: Lippincott Williams & Wilkins, 2008:277–287.)

or a two-incision rear-entry guide (**TECH FIG 2B**) and out the anteromedial portal (**TECH FIG 2C,D**).

- A second incision of about 4.5 cm is made over the proximal medial tibia in the region of the pes anserinus insertion.
- Dissection is carried through the subcutaneous tissue to the periosteum.
- A curved clamp is placed from this incision into the joint under the intermeniscal ligament (**TECH FIG 2E**).
- A small groove is made in the anteromedial proximal tibial epiphysis under the intermeniscal ligament using a curved rat-tail rasp to bring the tibial graft placement more posterior.

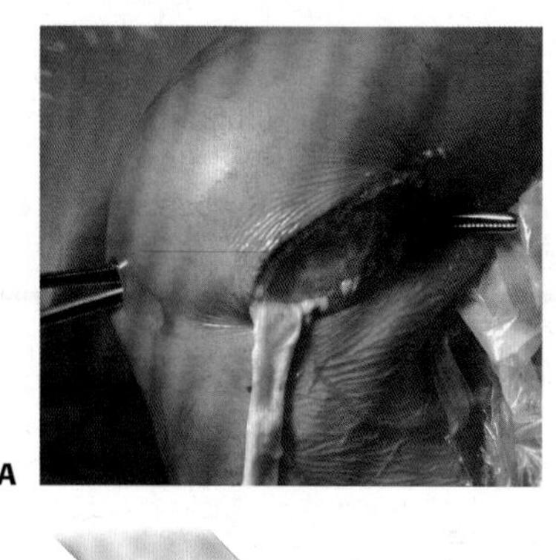
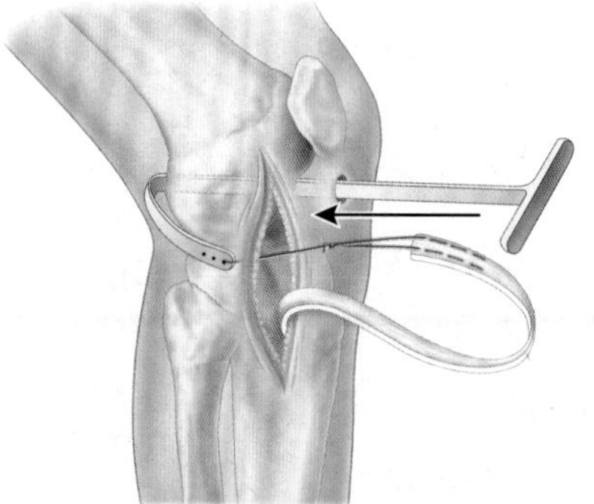
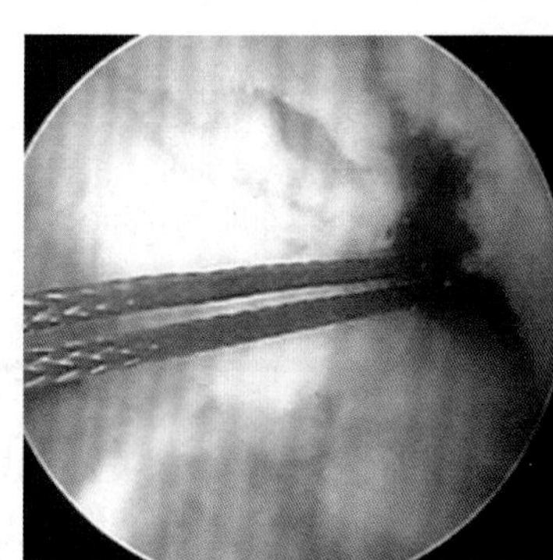
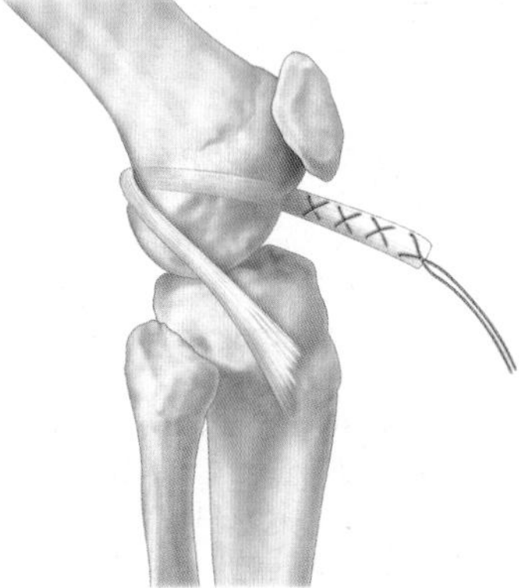
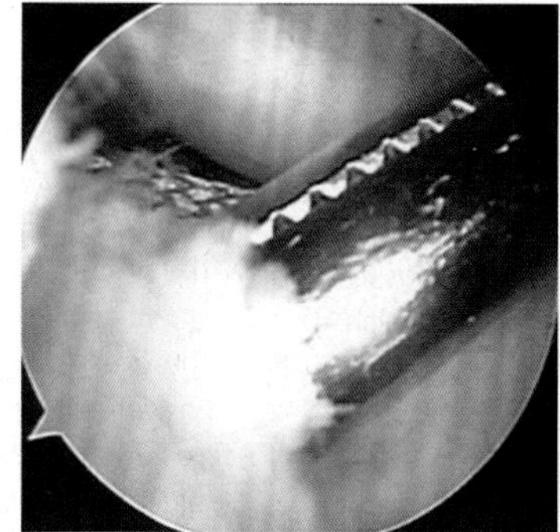
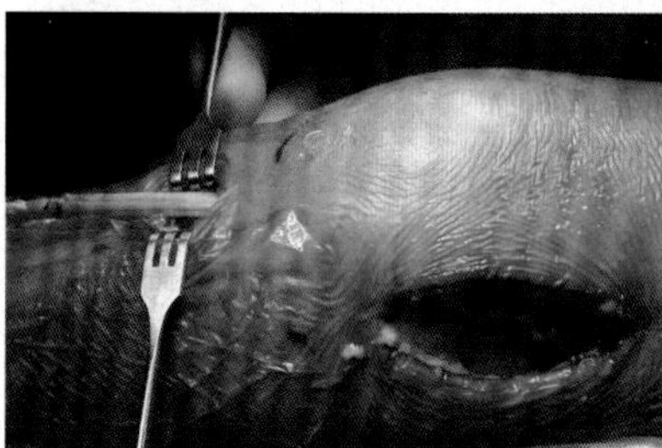

**TECH FIG 2** • Graft passage for physeal-sparing ACL reconstruction. **A.** The graft is brought through the knee in the over-the-top position using a full-length clamp introduced through the anteromedial portal and out the lateral incision. **B.** Alternatively, a two-incision rear-entry guide can be used. **C,D.** The lead sutures are used to bring the graft through the notch and out the anteromedial portal. **E.** After a rasp is used to create a groove in the anterior tibia under the intermeniscal ligament, a curved clamp is placed under the intermeniscal ligament (**F**) and the graft is brought to the anterior aspect of the knee. (**A,C,E,F:** From Kocher MS, Weiss JM. ACL reconstruction in the skeletally immature patient. In: Tolo VT, Scaggs DL, eds. Master Techniques in Orthopaedic Surgery: Pediatrics. Philadelphia: Lippincott Williams & Wilkins, 2008:277–287.)

- The free end of the graft is then brought through the joint, under the intermeniscal ligament in the anteromedial epiphyseal groove, and out the medial tibial incision (**TECH FIG 2F**).

## Graft Fixation

- Through the lateral incision, the iliotibial band graft is sutured near the over-the-top position to the intermuscular septum and the periosteum of the posterior lateral femoral condyle with the knee flexed 90 degrees, tension on the graft, and the foot externally rotated 30 degrees (**TECH FIG 3A**).
- Fluoroscopic imaging is used to assess the location of the proximal tibial physis.
- A longitudinal incision is made in the periosteum distal to the proximal tibial physis.
- The edges are gently elevated and a trough is made in the proximal tibial medial metaphyseal cortex.
- The knee is flexed 20 degrees and tension applied to the graft.
- The graft is sutured to the periosteum at the roughened margins with mattress sutures (**TECH FIG 3B**).
- The knee is checked for stability to Lachman testing and ROM.

## Wound Closure

- The wounds are copiously irrigated.
- The tourniquet is deflated and meticulous hemostasis is achieved.
- The wounds are then closed in layers in a standard fashion.

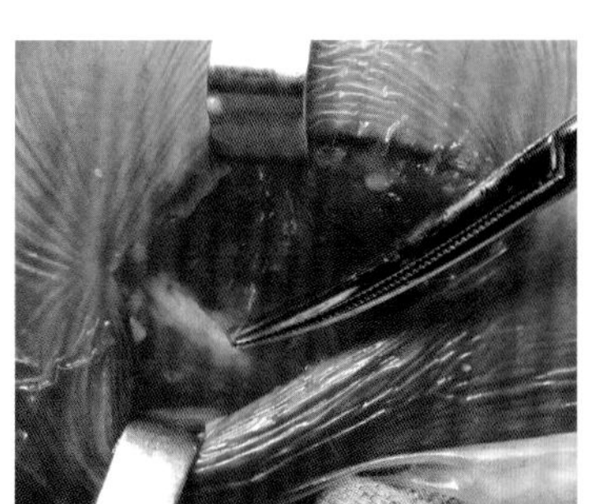
A

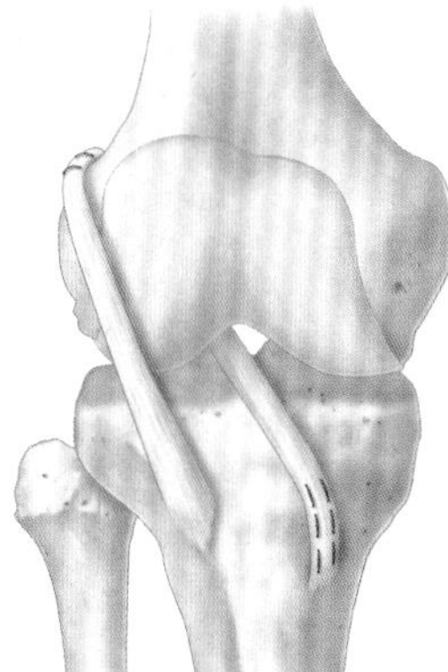
B

**TECH FIG 3** • Graft fixation for physeal-sparing ACL reconstruction. **A.** With the knee flexed 90 degrees, tension on the graft, and the foot externally rotated 30 degrees, the graft is secured to the intermuscular septum and the periosteum of the posterior lateral femoral condyle near the over-the-top position. **B.** With the knee flexed to 20 degrees, the tensioned graft is secured to the periosteum at the roughened margins of a trough in the proximal tibia. Fluoroscopic imaging is used to ensure that the proximal tibial physis is not disturbed. (**A:** From Kocher MS, Weiss JM. ACL reconstruction in the skeletally immature patient. In: Tolo VT, Scaggs DL, eds. Master Techniques in Orthopaedic Surgery: Pediatrics. Philadelphia: Lippincott Williams & Wilkins, 2008:277–287.)

# Physeal-Sparing Reconstruction with Autogenous Hamstring with All-Epiphyseal Fixation in Prepubescent Patients with Larger Knees

- This all-epiphyseal reconstruction[11] restores the native ACL attachments and keeps the graft and fixation entirely in the epiphysis.
- Intraoperative fluoroscopy or CT scanning is used to confirm the precise localization of the all-epiphyseal femoral and tibial tunnels.
- This technique uses an all-soft tissue graft with epiphyseal fixation. We describe fixation with an epiphyseal RetroScrew (Arthrex, Inc., Naples, FL) on the tibia side and an epiphyseal interference screw on the femoral side, but other suspensory fixation methods are also possible especially when using all-inside ACL reconstruction techniques.

## Harvest and Preparation of Autogenous Hamstrings Tendon Graft

- Hamstrings are routinely harvested at the start of the case if the diagnosis is not in question. However, if the diagnosis is in doubt, arthroscopy can be performed first to confirm ACL tear.
- The leg is placed in a slightly externally rotated position with the knee slightly bent.
- A 4-cm incision is made over the palpable pes anserinus tendons on the medial side of the proximal tibia.
- Dissection is carried through skin to expose the sartorius fascia.
  - The underlying gracilis (superior) and semitendinosus (inferior) tendons are identified by palpation.
- A longitudinal incision is made in the flat sartorius fascia. The cordlike gracilis and semitendinosus tendons are identified on its deep surface.
- The tendons are dissected free distally and their free ends whipstitched with no. 2 high tensile strength suture or no. 5 Ethibond suture.
- They are dissected proximally using sharp and blunt dissection. Fibrous bands to the medial head of the gastrocnemius should be sought and must be completely released before proceeding with tendon stripping.
- A closed tendon stripper is used to dissect the tendons free proximally. Firm, steady longitudinal retraction is placed on the tendons individually as the tendon stripper is gently and slowly advanced proximally collinear to the vector of pull of the tendon.
  - Alternatively, the tendons can be left attached distally and an open tendon stripper is used to release the tendons proximally.
- The tendons are taken to the back table and excess muscle is removed by scraping with the side of a no. 15 blade or a Freer.
- The ends are whipstitched with no. 2 high tensile strength suture or no. 5 Ethibond suture.

- The tendons are folded over a no. 5 Ethibond suture and the end 2 cm of folded-over graft is whipstitched with no. 2 high tensile strength suture or no. 5 Ethibond suture.
- The graft diameter is sized and the graft is placed under tension with wet gauze around it.

## Arthroscopy

- Arthroscopy of the knee is then performed through standard anterolateral viewing and anteromedial working portals.
- Management of meniscal injury or chondral injury is performed if present.
- The ACL remnant is excised with the use of biting instruments and the shaver to reveal the anatomic footprint on the tibia and the femur.
- Minimal notchplasty is performed to avoid iatrogenic injury to the perichondral ring of the distal femoral physis, which is very close to the over-the-top position.[2]

## Femoral Tunnel Preparation

- An outside-in femoral guide is set at 95 degrees and placed through the medial portal into the center of the femoral ACL footprint.
- A 1.5- to 2-cm incision is made over the lateral femur (**TECH FIG 4A**), anterior and distal to the lateral epicondyle. Blunt dissection is performed down to bone.
- A guidewire is then passed through the femoral guide, distal to the femoral physis, to the center of the femoral ACL footprint. The guidewire is left in while the femoral guide is removed (**TECH FIG 4B**).
  - The guidewire, when properly placed, is usually running slightly distal to proximal upon insertion into the knee and usually has about a 45-degree angle relative to the floor when the knee is in extension and with the patella straight-up.

## Tibial Tunnel Preparation

- Preoperatively, the distance from the tibial ACL footprint to the physis is measured. Based on the expected slight obliquity of the tunnel, at least 20 mm of epiphyseal bone is needed for this technique.
- A RetroDrill targeting guide (Arthrex), with a cutting blade appropriate for the graft size, is inserted over the center of the tibial ACL footprint.
- The guide pin for the RetroDrill is advanced through the targeting guide, capturing the cutting blade. It is then drilled back about 17 to 18 mm or about 2 to 3 mm less than the distance from the tibial ACL footprint to the physis measured preoperatively.
- The guide pin, with the engaged cutting blade seated at the most distal aspect of the tibial tunnel, is left in place, whereas the RetroDrill targeting guide is removed (see **TECH FIG 4B**).

## Epiphyseal Tunnel Position Confirmation

- Imaging is used to confirm the position of the guidewires and their distance from the physis.
- The undulating nature of the distal femoral physis makes accurate assessment of pin placement on plain imaging challenging.

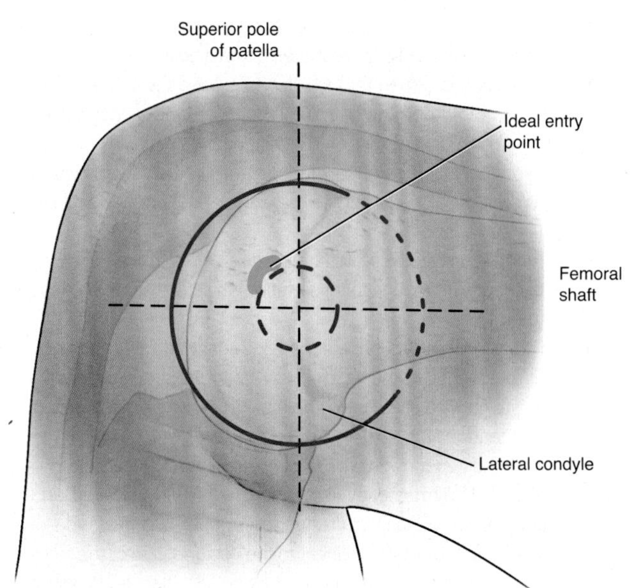


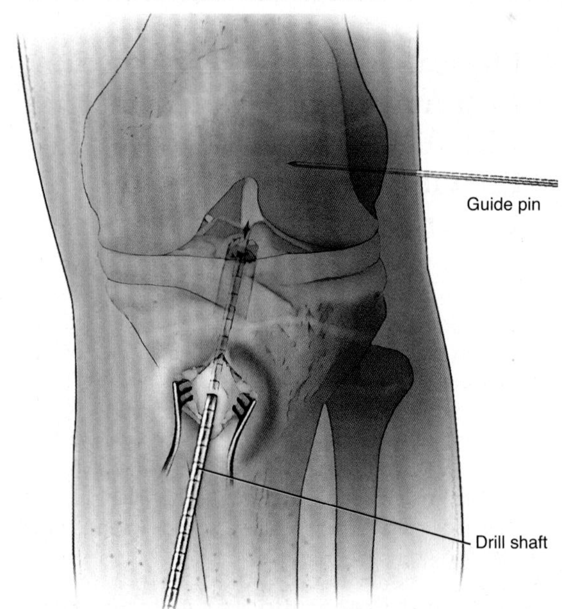


**TECH FIG 4 • A.** For the femoral epiphyseal tunnel, we draw a "bull's-eye" to approximate our desired entry point using the palpable landmarks. First, a semicircle is drawn for the lateral femoral condyle. Then a line is drawn parallel to the femoral shaft (*solid line*). A second line, perpendicular to the first, is drawn starting at the level of the superior pole of the patella. The intersection of these two lines represents a safe starting point. Proximal to the line off of the superior pole of the patella lies the physis and perichondral ring. Posterior to the line along the femoral shaft lies neurovascular structures and a greater risk for violating the cartilaginous surfaces. Any deviation from the ideal starting point should be anterior and distal. **B.** With the femoral guide pin seated in the femoral epiphysis, and the engaged cutting blade and its guide pin seated at the most distal aspect of the tibial tunnel, imaging is used to confirm their positions.

- A low-dose, limited-cut CT scan may be performed with an O-arm (Medtronic, Inc., Minneapolis, MN) to provide accurate three-dimensional assessment of pin placement relative to the physis (**TECH FIG 5**).
- Alternatively, AP and lateral fluoroscopy can also be used, but again, the undulating nature of the femoral physis can make interpretation challenging.
- The position of the femoral guide pin and the depth of the tibial RetroDrill are adjusted accordingly.

## Completion of Femoral and Tibial Tunnel Preparation

- The femoral tunnel is drilled outside-in over the femoral guidewire using standard cannulated reamers. Frequent pauses in drilling are appropriate to decrease the zone of thermal necrosis.
- The femoral tunnel is then examined arthroscopically to ensure that the femoral physis has not been violated.
- The RetroDrill targeting guide is replaced, and the cutting blade is then advanced back into the joint, disengaged, and removed. A FiberStick suture (Arthrex) is passed through the tibial tunnel and out the femoral tunnel before the RetroDrill targeting guide is removed.
- The intra-articular tunnel openings are smoothed with the back of a curette.

## Graft Passage and Fixation

- The FiberStick suture is used to pass the lead suture of the graft and a separate Nitinol wire (Arthrex) for the RetroScrew from the femoral tunnel out the tibial tunnel (**TECH FIG 6A**).
- The Nitinol wire is retrieved from the femoral socket and shuttled out the anteromedial portal to place it on the anterior portion of the tibial socket (**TECH FIG 6B**).
- The graft is advanced through the femoral socket and seated firmly into the tibial socket.
- The RetroScrew screwdriver is inserted through the tibial tunnel over the Nitinol wire, past the graft seated in the tibial socket and just into the joint.
- The Nitinol wire is removed and replaced with another FiberStick suture which is brought out the anteromedial portal. A RetroScrew is placed on the FiberStick and mulberry knot is tied behind it (**TECH FIG 6C**).
- The RetroScrew is advanced into the joint, flipped onto the screwdriver, and screwed into place while tension is held on the graft and it is firmly seated in the tibial tunnel.
- Each limb of the graft is tensioned, the knee cycled 20 times and brought into full extension.
- In full extension with a slight posterior drawer, the graft is tensioned and an interference screw is placed to secure the graft into the femoral tunnel (**TECH FIG 6D**).

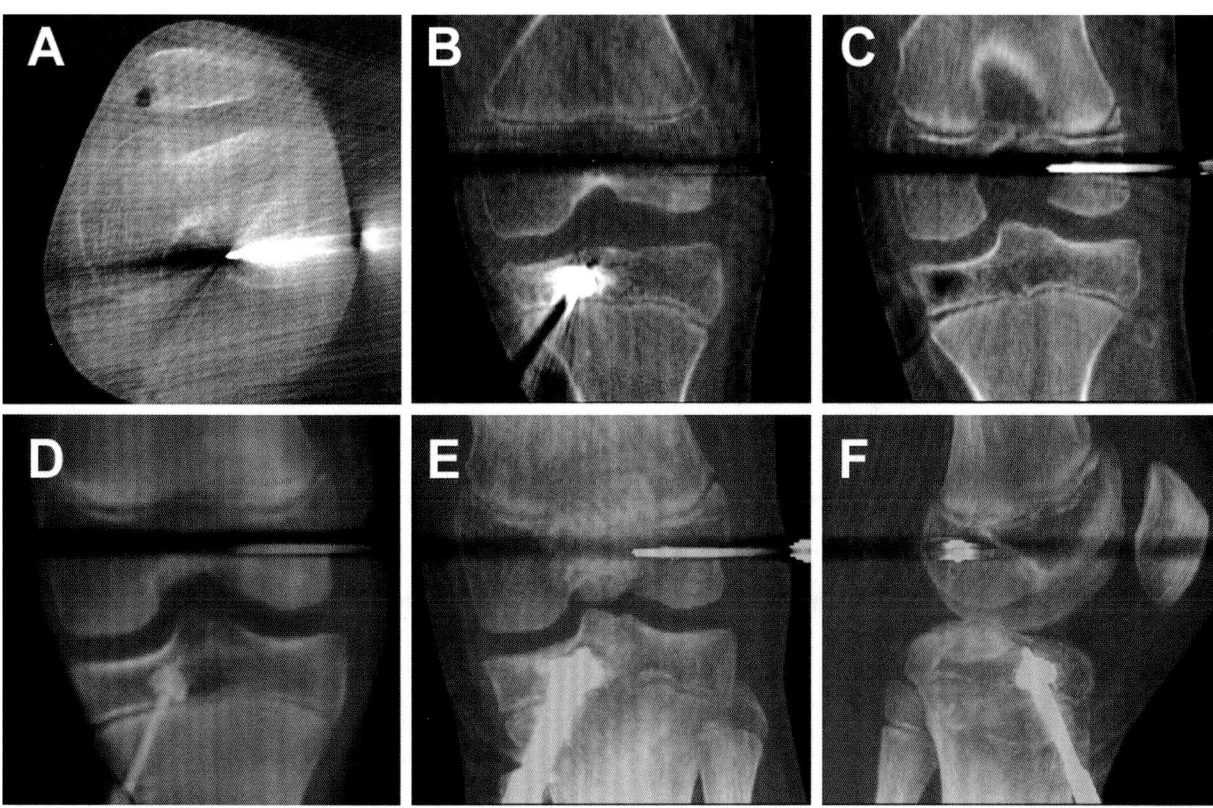


**TECH FIG 5** ● Intraoperative images from a limited-cut CT scan with the femoral guide pin in the epiphysis and the engaged cutting blade and its guide pin seated at the most distal aspect of the tibia tunnel.

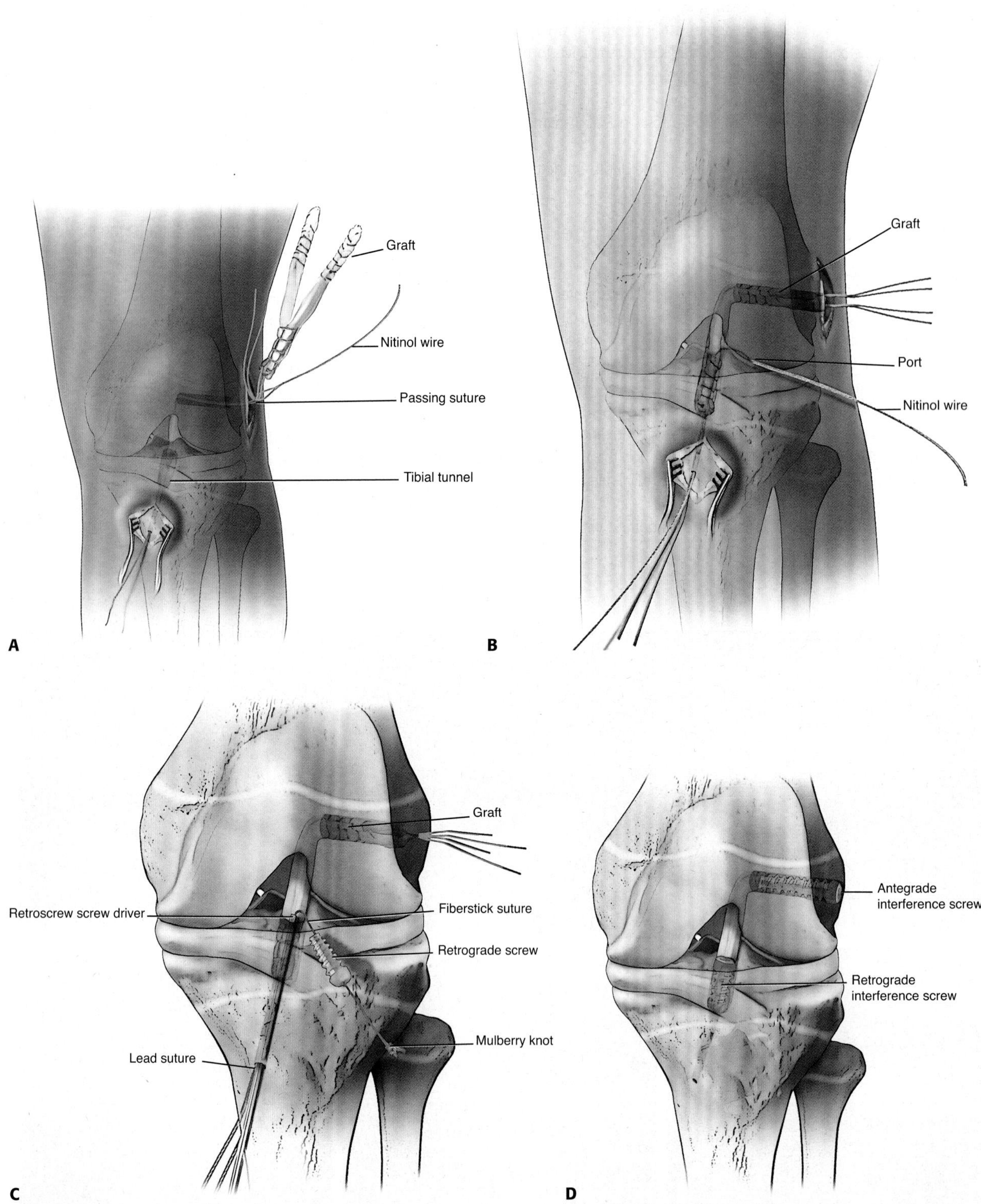


**TECH FIG 6** • **A.** The FiberStick suture is used to pass the lead suture of the graft and a separate Nitinol wire in from the femoral socket. **B.** The Nitinol wire is retrieved from the femoral socket and shuttled out the anteromedial portal. **C.** The RetroScrew is placed on a second FiberStick suture placed up the retroscrewdriver and mulberry knot tied behind it. **D.** The final construct with the femoral interference screw having been placed.

## Transphyseal Reconstruction with Autogenous Hamstring with Metaphyseal Fixation in Adolescent Patients with Growth Remaining

- The transphyseal reconstruction is similar to the anatomic single-bundle ACL reconstruction technique.
- The basic principles of graft harvest, notch preparation, tunnel placement, and tunnel creation are the same.
- This technique uses an all–soft tissue graft with metaphyseal fixation. We describe fixation with a cortical button on the femoral side and an all-metaphyseal interference screw on the tibial side, but other all-metaphyseal options exist.
- Most prior studies noting the relative safety of the transphyseal procedure with respect to growth disturbance have used more vertical and central femoral tunnels than the more anatomic independent and anteromedial portal femoral tunnel techniques now routinely used to place grafts closer the center of the anatomic footprint of the ACL. Because of concerns with creating oblique and eccentric tunnels in patients with more growth remaining, many surgeons favor creating an epiphyseal femoral tunnel and paring it with a transphyseal tibial tunnel in younger adolescents (see **FIG 4D**).

### Harvest and Preparation of Autogenous Hamstrings Tendon Graft

- Hamstrings harvest and preparation is performed the same way as in all-epiphyseal reconstruction except the tendons are folded over the loop of a cortical button fixation device instead of a no. 5 Ethibond suture. We prefer self-cinching devices, as they maximize the amount of graft in the tunnel.

### Arthroscopy

- Arthroscopy of the knee is performed the same way as in the other reconstructions.

### Femoral Tunnel Preparation

- A femoral tunnel is drilled independently of the tibial tunnel using an anteromedial portal technique or an outside-in retrodrilling technique. We describe here the outside-in retrodrilling technique because it can be used to place the femoral tunnel either in a transphyseal or an epiphyseal location.
- For both techniques, the center of the femoral footprint should be marked and visualized via the medial portal.
- An outside-in femoral targeting guide is placed at the center of the femoral footprint and a guidewire inserted from outside-in.
- A 7-mm stepped drill sleeve is then placed over guidewire and malleted securely into place. The guide contains a 7-mm offset preventing reaming out the lateral femoral cortex. The guidewire is removed.
- A appropriately sized FlipCutter (Arthrex) is drilled into the center of the femoral footprint. The drill bit is then deployed and drilled back 25 to 30 mm or until it engages the stepped drill sleeve 7 mm from the lateral femoral cortex.
- The FlipCutter is removed and a Nitinol guidewire placed through the stepped drill sleeve. The stepped drill sleeve is then removed.
- The edge of the femoral tunnel is smoothed by slight impaction with the back of a curette.

### Tibial Tunnel Preparation

- A tibial tunnel guide (set at 60 to 65 degrees) is used through the anteromedial portal. The tunnel should be about 50 mm to allow for placement of a short interference screw distal to the physis.
- The hamstrings harvest incision is used and a guidewire is drilled into the center of the ACL tibial footprint.
- The guidewire entry point on the tibia should be kept medial to avoid injury to the tibial tubercle apophysis.
- The guidewire is reamed with the appropriate-diameter reamer based on the size of the graft. Frequent pauses in drilling are appropriate to decrease the chance of thermal necrosis.
- Excess soft tissue around the tibial tunnel is excised to avoid the formation of a cyclops lesion, which may limit postoperative ROM.
- The posterior rim of the tunnel is smoothed with a rasp or impacted with the smooth side of a curette to prevent graft abrasion over a sharp tunnel edge.
- The looped Nitinol wire is brought out the tibial tunnel to the anterior tibia.

### Graft Passage and Fixation

- The passing sutures on the cortical button device are placed in the loop of the Nitinol wire and pulled through the tibial tunnel, through the femoral tunnel, and out the lateral thigh (**TECH FIG 7A**).
- The cortical button is passed just to the femoral cortex and flipped (**TECH FIG 7B**). Then, the graft is cinched up to the button until fully seated in the femoral tunnel.
- Alternatively, the cortical button is passed through the lateral femoral cortex until the graft is fully seated in the femoral tunnel. Then, the cortical button is cinched down to the lateral femoral cortex.
- Fixation of the self-cinching mechanism can be reinforced by a couple of overhand knots tied over the button.
- Tension is applied to each limb of the graft to ensure that there is even tension in all strands and no graft slippage.
- The knee is then extended to ensure that there is no graft impingement and cycled about 10 to 20 times with tension applied to the graft.
- The knee is flexed to 20 to 30 degrees, tension is applied to the graft, and a posterior drawer force placed on the tibia.
- On the tibial side, the graft is fixed either with a soft tissue interference screw if there is adequate tunnel distance (at least 30 mm) below the physis to ensure metaphyseal placement of the screw (**TECH FIG 7C**) or with a post and spiked washer (**TECH FIG 7D**).
- Fluoroscopy can be used to ensure that the fixation is away from the physis if there is any question.

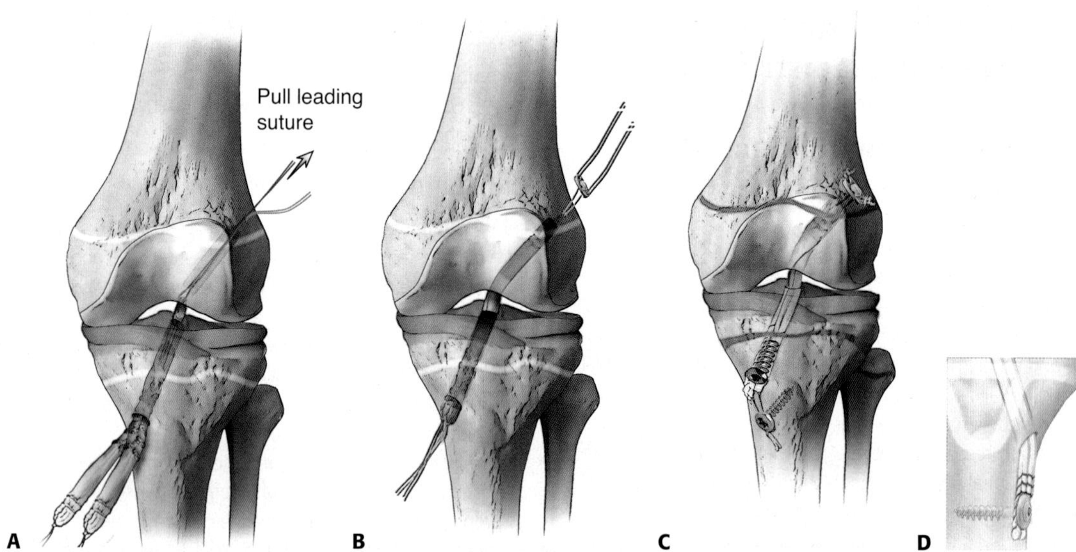


**TECH FIG 7** • Graft passage and fixation for transphyseal reconstruction with metaphyseal fixation. **A.** The Nitinol wire is used to pass the cortical button device and graft through the tibial tunnel and into the femoral tunnel. **B.** The cortical button is flipped and seats perpendicular to the cortex. **C.** Tibial fixation is with an interference screw if enough graft and tunnel length is present inferior to the proximal tibial physis. **D.** Alternatively, a post and spiked washer may be used.

## PEARLS AND PITFALLS

| | |
|---|---|
| **History and physical examination** | ▪ Because of normal physiologic laxity in adolescents, physical examination findings should always be compared to the opposite side. |
| **Diagnostic imaging** | ▪ MRI in skeletally immature knees is less sensitive and specific for evaluating meniscal injuries and so a careful evaluation at the time of arthroscopy should be performed. |
| **Graft preparation** | ▪ With the physeal-sparing approach, the surgeon should avoid having too short of a graft to adequately secure to the tibia by harvesting a long enough strip of iliotibial band fascia.<br>▪ With autograft hamstring harvest, care should be taken to clear all bands attached to the hamstring tendons before performing tendon stripping.<br>▪ Grafts should be handled carefully and secured while waiting for insertion. |
| **Arthroscopy** | ▪ The surgeon should avoid excess dissection around the posterolateral aspect of the femoral condyle and aggressive posterior notchplasty to avoid potential injury to the perichondral ring and subsequent deformity. |
| **Tunnel preparation** | ▪ Large and oblique tunnels should be avoided, as the likelihood of arrest is increased with greater violation of epiphyseal plate cross-sectional area. |
| **Graft fixation** | ▪ The surgeon should avoid fixation that crosses the physis, particularly across the lateral distal femoral epiphyseal plate, which seems to have the greatest risk of producing a growth disturbance.[8,10]<br>▪ For tibial fixation while performing the physeal-sparing technique, the surgeon should stay medial to avoid damage to the vulnerable tibial tubercle physis. |
| **Postoperative care** | ▪ The patient's emotional maturity and ability to comply with postoperative rehabilitation protocols should be factored into the clinician's recommendations. Slower rehabilitation protocols should be used for some patients. |

## POSTOPERATIVE CARE

- Rehabilitation after ACL reconstruction in skeletally immature patients is essential to ensure a good outcome, allow return to sports, and avoid reinjury.
- Rehabilitation in prepubescent children can be challenging. A therapist who is used to working with children and can make therapy interesting and fun is very helpful.
- Compliance with therapy and restrictions should be carefully monitored.
- Weight bearing is limited to touchdown weight bearing for 6 weeks for physeal-sparing, combined intra-articular and extra-articular reconstruction with autogenous iliotibial band; 4 weeks for the all-epiphyseal with autogenous hamstrings; and 2 weeks for the transphyseal technique in adolescents with growth remaining.

- A protective brace is used for 6 weeks postoperatively.
- ROM is limited from 0 to 90 degrees for the first 2 weeks, followed by progressive full ROM.
- A continuous passive motion (CPM) machine from 0 to 90 degrees and cryotherapy are used for 2 weeks postoperatively.
- Progressive supervised rehabilitation consists of ROM exercises, patellar mobilization, electrical stimulation, pool therapy (if available), proprioception exercises, and closed-chain strengthening during the first 3 months postoperatively. A running program that progresses through straight-line jogging, plyometric exercises, and finally sport-specific exercises follows.
- Return to full activity, including cutting sports, is usually allowed at a minimum of 9 months for transphyseal and 1 year for all-epiphyseal reconstructions and then only if the patient has achieved full ROM, has 90% to 95% strength compared to the uninjured leg, and can perform a series of functional tests including single-leg hop to 90% to 95% of the uninjured leg with good form.
- A functional knee brace is routinely used during cutting and pivoting activities for the first 2 years after return to sports.

## OUTCOMES

- Performed properly, physeal-sparing reconstruction in preadolescent skeletally immature patients appears to provide an excellent functional outcome, with a low revision rate and a minimal risk of growth disturbance.
- The largest study of outcomes after physeal-sparing, combined intra-articular and extra-articular ACL reconstruction noted a 4.5% revision rate for graft failure at 4.7 and 8.3 years postoperatively.[7,16]
- No cases of significant angular deformity measured radiographically or leg length discrepancy measured clinically were noted in this series.

## COMPLICATIONS

- Growth disturbance
  - Leg length discrepancy
  - Distal femoral valgus
  - Tibial recurvatum with an arrest of the tibial tubercle apophysis
- Arthrofibrosis, particularly loss of extension
- Graft failure
- Recurrent instability despite an intact graft, requiring revision to more anatomic reconstruction at skeletal maturity
- Tunnel widening
- Infection
- Deep venous thrombosis

## REFERENCES


1. Aichroth PM, Patel DV, Zorrilla P. The natural history and treatment of rupture of the anterior cruciate ligament in children and adolescents. A prospective review. J Bone Joint Surg Br 2002;84(1):38–41.
2. Behr CT, Potter HG, Paletta GA Jr. The relationship of the femoral origin of the anterior cruciate ligament and the distal femoral physeal plate in the skeletally immature knee. An anatomic study. Am J Sports Med 2001;29:781–787.
3. Daniel DM, Stone ML, Dobson BE, et al. Fate of the ACL-injured patient. A prospective outcome study. Am J Sports Med 1994;22: 632–644.
4. Greulich WW, Pyle SI. Radiographic Atlas of Skeletal Development of the Hand and Wrist. Stanford, CA: Stanford University Press, 1959.
5. Kaeding CC, Aros B, Pedroza A, et al. Allograft versus autograft anterior cruciate ligament reconstruction: predictors of failure from a MOON prospective longitudinal cohort. Sports Health 2011;3:73–81.
6. Kocher MS, DiCanzio J, Zurakowski D, et al. Diagnostic performance of clinical examination and selective magnetic resonance imaging in the evaluation of intraarticular knee disorders in children and adolescents. Am J Sports Med 2001;29:292–296.
7. Kocher MS, Garg S, Micheli LJ. Physeal sparing reconstruction of the anterior cruciate ligament in skeletally immature prepubescent children and adolescents. J Bone Joint Surg Am 2005;87(11):2371–2379.
8. Kocher MS, Hovis WD, Curtin MJ, et al. Anterior cruciate ligament reconstruction in skeletally immature knees: an anatomical study. Am J Orthop 2005;34:285–290.
9. Kocher MS, Micheli LJ, Zurakowski D, et al. Partial tears of the anterior cruciate ligament in children and adolescents. Am J Sports Med 2002;30:697–703.
10. Kocher MS, Saxon HS, Hovis WD, et al. Management and complications of anterior cruciate ligament injuries in skeletally immature patients: survey of the Herodicus Society and the ACL Study Group. J Pediatr Orthop 2002;22:452–457.
11. Lawrence JT, Bowers AL, Belding J, et al. All-epiphyseal anterior cruciate ligament reconstruction in skeletally immature patients. Clin Orthop Relat Res 2010;468:1971–1977.
12. Mizuta H, Kubota K, Shiraishi M, et al. The conservative treatment of complete tears of the anterior cruciate ligament in skeletally immature patients. J Bone Joint Surg Br 1995;77(6):890–894.
13. Pallis M, Svoboda SJ, Cameron KL, et al. Survival comparison of allograft and autograft anterior cruciate ligament reconstruction at the United States Military Academy. Am J Sports Med 2012;40:1242–1246.
14. Rang M. Children's Fractures. Philadelphia: JB Lippincott, 1983.
15. Schub DL, Altahawi F, F Meisel A, et al. Accuracy of 3-Tesla magnetic resonance imaging for the diagnosis of intra-articular knee injuries in children and teenagers. J Pediatr Orthop 2012;32:765–769.
16. Spindler KP, Kuhn JE, Freedman KB, et al. Anterior cruciate ligament reconstruction autograft choice: bone-tendon-bone versus hamstring: does it really matter? A systematic review. Am J Sports Med 2004;32:1986–1995.
17. Stanitski CL, Harvell JC, Fu F. Observations on acute knee hemarthrosis in children and adolescents. J Pediatr Orthop 1993;13:506–510.
18. Tanner JM, Whitehouse RH. Clinical longitudinal standards for height, weight, height velocity, weight velocity, and stages of puberty. Arch Dis Child 1976;51:170–179.

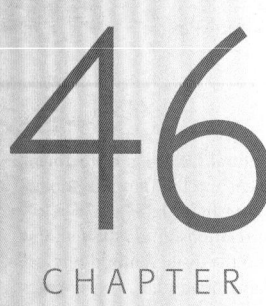


# Posterior Cruciate Ligament Surgery

Amanda L. Weller, Craig S. Mauro, and Christopher D. Harner

## DEFINITION

- The posterior cruciate ligament (PCL) serves as the primary restraint to posterior translation of the tibia relative to the femur.
- PCL injuries are uncommon, may be partial or complete, and rarely occur in isolation.
- Our understanding of the PCL with respect to its natural history, surgical indications and technique, and postoperative rehabilitation is improving rapidly.

## ANATOMY

- The PCL has a broad femoral origin in a semicircular pattern on the medial femoral condyle.
  - It inserts on the posterior aspect of the tibia, in a depression between the medial and lateral tibial plateaus, 1.0 to 1.5 cm below the joint line.
  - Its cross-section area is 11 mm$^2$ on average, which is variable along its course; the average length is 32 to 38 mm.[24]
- Anatomic studies have delineated separate characteristics of the anterolateral (AL) and posteromedial (PM) bundles within the PCL.
  - The AL bundle origin is more anterior on the intercondylar surface of the medial femoral condyle, and the insertion is more lateral on the tibia, relative to the PM bundle.
  - The larger AL bundle has increased tension in flexion, whereas the PM bundle becomes more taut in extension.
- The meniscofemoral ligaments, which arise from the posterior horn of the lateral meniscus and insert on the posterolateral aspect of the medial femoral condyle, also contribute to the overall strength of the PCL.

## PATHOGENESIS

- Acutely, there usually is a history of a direct blow to the anterior lower leg. Common mechanisms include high-energy trauma and athletic injuries.
  - In motor vehicle trauma, the "dashboard injury" occurs when the proximal tibia strikes the dashboard, causing a posteriorly directed force to the proximal tibia.
  - Athletic injuries usually involve a direct blow to the anterior tibia or a fall onto a flexed knee with the foot in plantar flexion.
- Hyperextension injuries, which often are combined with varus or valgus forces, often result in combined ligamentous injuries.

## NATURAL HISTORY

- There is little conclusive clinical information regarding the natural history of patients with PCL tears treated nonoperatively.
  - Some studies suggest that patients with isolated grade I to II PCL injuries usually have good subjective results, but few achieve good functional results.[17,21,23]
    - More recent literature suggests that although PCL deficient knees may have increased laxity, patients with grade 1 to 2 laxity still have good functional results and return to activity.[22,20]
- A high incidence of degeneration, primarily involving the medial femoral condyle and patellofemoral joint, has been noted in patients treated nonoperatively. This finding is especially prevalent in those patients with grade III injuries or combined ligamentous injuries.
- Consequently, pain rather than instability may be the patient's primary symptom following a PCL injury treated nonoperatively.
  - Biomechanical studies have shown that asymptomatic PCL deficient knees do function with altered kinematics compared to PCL intact knees.[5,6]

## PATIENT HISTORY AND PHYSICAL FINDINGS

- The initial history should focus on the mechanism of injury, its severity, and associated injuries.
- With acute injuries, the patient often does not report feeling a "pop" or "tear," as often is described with anterior cruciate ligament (ACL) injuries.
- The history also should focus on assessing the chronicity of the injury and the instability and pain experienced by the patient.
- A complete knee examination, including inspection, palpation, range-of-motion (ROM) testing, neurovascular examination, and special tests, should be performed.
  - Posterior drawer test: The most accurate clinical test for PCL injury.
  - Posterior sag (Godfrey) test: A positive result is an abnormal posterior sag of the tibia relative to the femur from the force of gravity. This result suggests PCL insufficiency if it is abnormal compared to the contralateral side.
  - Quadriceps active test: useful in patients with combined instability. A posteriorly subluxed tibia that reduces anteriorly is a positive result.
  - Reverse pivot shift test: A palpable reduction of the tibia occurring at 20 to 30 degrees indicates a positive result. The contralateral knee must be examined because a positive test may be a normal finding in some patients.
  - Dial test: A positive test is indicated by asymmetry in external rotation. Asymmetry of more than 10 degrees at 30 degrees rotation indicates an isolated posterolateral corner (PLC) injury, whereas asymmetry at 30 and 90 degrees suggests a combined PCL and PLC injury.

- Posterolateral external rotation test: Increased external rotation of the tibia is a positive result. Increased posterior translation and external rotation at 90 degrees indicate a PLC or PCL injury, whereas subluxation at 30 degrees is consistent with an isolated PLC injury.
- It is important to assess the neurovascular status of the injured limb, especially if there is a history of a knee dislocation.

## IMAGING AND OTHER DIAGNOSTIC STUDIES

- Radiographs of the knee should be performed following an acute injury to assess for a fracture. An avulsion of the tibial insertion of the PCL may be identified on a lateral radiograph (**FIG 1A**).
  - In the chronic setting, radiographs may identify posterior tibial subluxation (**FIG 1B**) or medial and patellofemoral compartmental arthrosis.
  - Stress radiographs may be used to confirm and quantify dynamic posterior tibial subluxation.[12]
  - Long cassette films should be obtained if coronal malalignment is suspected.
- MRI is important to confirm a PCL injury, determine its location and completeness, and assess for concomitant injury, including meniscal and PLC pathology.

## DIFFERENTIAL DIAGNOSIS

- Combined ligament injury
- PLC injury
- ACL tear
- Tibial plateau fracture
- Articular cartilage injury
- Medial or lateral collateral ligament tear
- Meniscal tear
- Patellar or quadriceps tendon rupture
- Patellofemoral dislocation

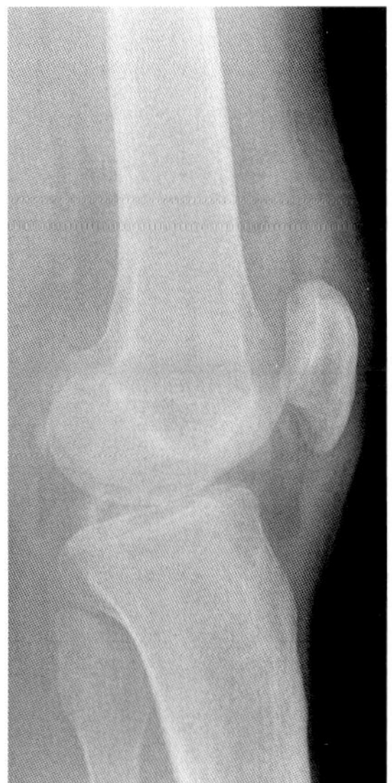
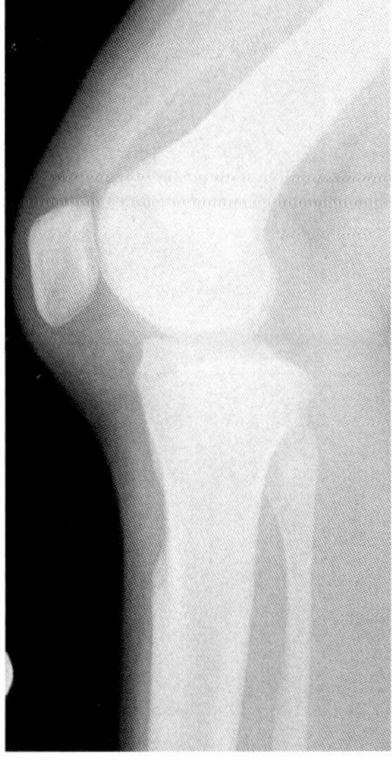

**FIG 1** • **A.** Avulsion fracture of the tibial insertion of the PCL. **B.** Posterior subluxation of the tibia in a case of chronic PCL deficiency.

## NONOPERATIVE MANAGEMENT

- Most experts advocate nonoperative management of isolated, partial PCL injuries (grades I and II).[15]
  - In these cases, we recommend immobilization in full extension with protected weight bearing for 2 weeks. The goal is to protect the healing PCL/PLC.
- ROM exercises are advanced as tolerated, and strengthening is focused on the quadriceps muscles.
  - Closed-chain exercises (foot on the ground) are recommended.
  - Applying an axial load across the knee causes anterior translation of the tibia because of the sagittal slope.[4] This important biomechanical principle allows early ROM exercises and protects PCL/PLC healing.
- The patient usually can return to athletic activities after isolated grade I and II PCL injuries in 4 to 6 weeks. It is important to protect the knee from injury during this time to prevent progression to a grade III injury.
  - Functional bracing is of little benefit after return to sports activities.
- Isolated grade III injuries are more controversial, and nonoperative management may be appropriate in certain patients.
  - We recommend immobilization in full extension for 4 weeks to prevent posterior tibial subluxation. Weight bearing is protected for the first 2 weeks, then slowly advanced.
  - Quadriceps strengthening such as quadriceps sets and straight-leg raises is encouraged; hamstring loading is prohibited until later in the rehabilitation course.
  - During the bracing period, the patient can participate in closed-chain mini-squat exercises which do not stress the PCL or interfere with healing.
  - After 1 month, ROM, full weight bearing, and progression to functional activities are instituted.
  - Return to sports usually is delayed for 2 to 4 months in patients with grade III injuries.

## SURGICAL MANAGEMENT

- Surgical indications include those patients with displaced bony avulsions, acute grade III injuries with concomitant ligamentous injuries, and chronic grade II to III injuries with symptoms of instability or pain.
  - With any PCL injury, it is imperative to assess the PLC to rule out injury because surgery is indicated for combined injuries.
- In higher level athletes, surgical treatment may be considered for acute isolated grade III PCL injuries.
- The timing of PCL reconstruction depends on the severity of the injury and the associated, concomitant ligamentous injuries.
  - Displaced bony avulsions and knees with multiligamentous injuries should be addressed within the first 3 weeks to provide the best opportunity for anatomic repair.[6]
- A number of graft options are available for PCL reconstruction.
  - Autologous tissue options include bone–patellar tendon–bone, hamstring tendons, and quadriceps tendons.
  - Allograft options include tibialis anterior tendon, Achilles tendon, bone–patellar tendon–bone, and quadriceps tendon.
  - Advantages of allograft tissue include decreased surgical time and no harvest site morbidity. Disadvantages include the possibility of disease transmission. The operating surgeon should discuss these issues with the patient preoperatively.
- Currently, allograft tibialis anterior tendon is our graft of choice for single- and double-bundle PCL reconstructions (**FIG 2**).

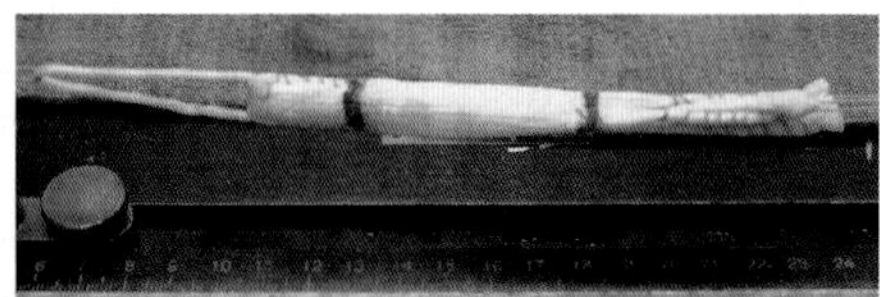

**FIG 2** • Double-stranded tibialis anterior allograft sutured through an Endoloop.

## Preoperative Planning

- In the office setting, the surgeon should have a variety of options available and explain that the final surgical plan will depend on the examination under anesthesia (EUA) and the diagnostic arthroscopy.
- In the preoperative holding area, sciatic and femoral nerve block catheters may be placed by the anesthesiology staff.
  - No anesthetic is introduced, however, until neurologic assessment has been completed.
- After anesthesia induction in the operating room, an EUA is performed on both the nonoperative and the operative knees.
  - A detailed examination is performed to determine the direction and degree of laxity.
  - Data from the contralateral knee may be particularly helpful with combined injuries.
- Fluoroscopy may be used after the EUA to assess posterior tibial displacement.

## Positioning

- The patient is positioned supine on the operating room table.
- We do not use a tourniquet.
- Depending on the anticipated length of the planned procedure, a Foley catheter may be used.
- A padded bump is taped to the operating room table to hold the knee flexed to 90 degrees. A side post is placed on the operative side just distal to the greater trochanter to support the proximal leg with the knee in flexion (**FIG 3A**). Padded cushions are placed under the nonoperative leg.
- For the inlay technique, a gel pad bump is placed under the contralateral hip to facilitate later exposure to the posteromedial knee of the operative extremity in the figure-4 position.
- After prepping and draping the operative site, a hole is cut in the stockinette for access to the dorsalis pedis pulse throughout the case (**FIG 3B**).

## Approach

- Several techniques have been described for PCL reconstruction. We have developed the following treatment algorithm:
  - For acute injuries, we employ the single-bundle technique.
  - If some component of the native PCL remains, we spare this tissue and use the augmentation technique.
    - This technique can be time-consuming and difficult, but preservation of PCL tissue may provide enhanced posterior stability of the knee and may promote graft healing.
  - We most commonly perform the double-bundle technique in the chronic setting, when any remaining structures are significantly incompetent.
  - Some authors advocate the tibial inlay technique for all settings. We typically do not use this technique but have included a description of an open double-bundle technique here as part of a comprehensive overview. All arthroscopic tibial inlay techniques also have recently been described.[8,13] A description of the arthroscopic inlay technique is also included.
  - In cases of displaced tibial avulsion, we use the technique described in the Techniques box.

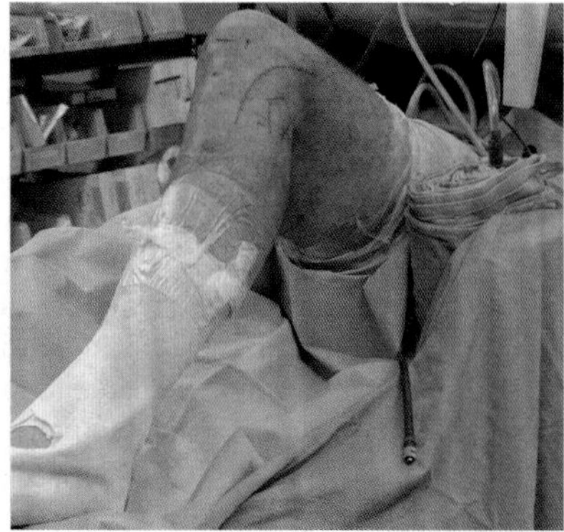

A B

**FIG 3** • **A.** Operative field setup, demonstrating the bump holding the knee flexed to 90 degrees and a side post supporting the proximal leg with the knee in flexion. **B.** Stockinette with hole cut out to palpate the dorsalis pedis pulse.

## Single-Bundle Technique

### Diagnostic Arthroscopy

- A bump is placed between the post and the leg to stabilize the knee in a flexed position while the foot rests on the prepositioned sandbag.
    - The knee is flexed to 90 degrees, and the vertical arthroscopy portals are delineated.
- The anterolateral portal is placed just lateral to the lateral border of the patellar tendon and adjacent to the inferior pole of the patella.
- The anteromedial portal is positioned 1 cm medial to the medial border of the superior aspect of the patellar tendon.
- Diagnostic arthroscopy is conducted to determine the extent of injury and evaluate for other cartilage or meniscal derangements.
    - The notch is examined for any remaining intact PCL fibers. If augmentation is to be performed, care should be taken to preserve these fibers (see Single-Bundle Augmentation Technique).
    - Using an arthroscopic electrocautery device and shaver, overlying synovium and ruptured PCL fibers are débrided, and the superior interval between the ACL and PCL is defined.
- An accessory posteromedial portal is created just proximal to the joint line and posterior to the medial collateral ligament (MCL).
    - A 70-degree arthroscope is placed between the PCL remnants and the medial femoral condyle to assess the posterior horn of the medial meniscus and to localize the posteromedial portal with a spinal needle (**TECH FIG 1**).
    - A switching stick can be placed into the posteromedial portal to facilitate exchange of the arthroscope. The 30-degree arthroscope is used when viewing via the posteromedial portal.
    - A transseptal portal also may be created for better visualization of and access to the tibial PCL insertion.[1,2,14]

### Preparation and Exposure of the Tibia

- Correct preparation and exposure of the tibia is essential for drilling the tunnel safely in the appropriate position.

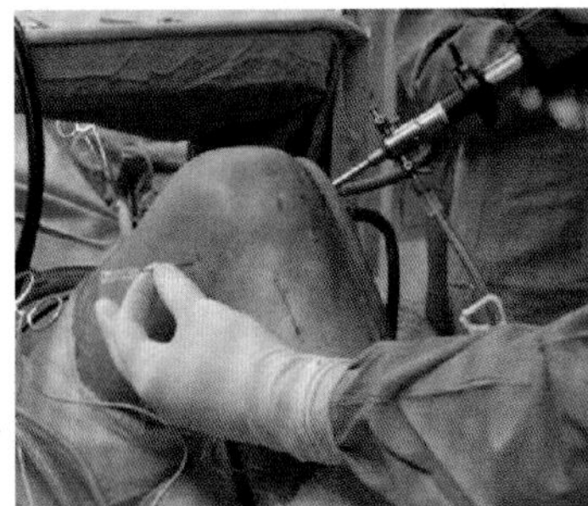

**TECH FIG 1** • The posteromedial portal is established under direct visualization using a spinal needle.

- First, the 70-degree arthroscope is placed into the anterolateral portal, and a commercially available PCL curette is introduced through the anteromedial portal.
    - A lateral fluoroscopic image can be obtained to confirm its position.
- The 30-degree arthroscope is then introduced through the posteromedial portal. The soft tissue on the posterior aspect of the tibia is carefully elevated centrally and slightly laterally.
- A shaver can be placed through the anterolateral portal to débride some of the surrounding synovium.
- The 70-degree arthroscope is returned to the anterolateral portal and the shaver placed in the posteromedial portal to complete the exposure.

### Creating the Tibial Tunnel

- A commercially available PCL tibial drill guide set to 55 degrees is advanced through the anteromedial portal and placed just distal and lateral to the PCL insertion site, 1.5 cm distal to the articular edge of the posterior plateau along the sloped face of the posterior tibial fossa (**TECH FIG 2A**).
    - The position is checked fluoroscopically using a lateral view and arthroscopically via the posteromedial portal.
- An incision and dissection through periosteum to bone is made on the anteromedial aspect of the tibia in line with the guide.
- The PCL guide is set, and its position is confirmed with fluoroscopy and arthroscopy (**TECH FIG 2B**).
- A guidewire is drilled to but not through the posterior cortex.
    - Fluoroscopy is used to confirm the path of the guidewire (**TECH FIG 2C,D**).
- With the 30-degree arthroscope in the posteromedial portal, the PCL curette is introduced through the anteromedial portal and is used to protect the posterior knee structures as the guidewire is carefully advanced through the posterior cortex under arthroscopic visualization.
    - A parallel pin guide can be used to make small pin placement corrections if necessary.
- A cannulated compaction reamer is used to drill the tibial tunnel.
    - The tibial cortex is cautiously perforated by hand reaming under arthroscopic visualization.
    - The tunnel is irrigated, and increasing serial dilators are used under arthroscopic visualization up to the graft size.

### Creating the Femoral Tunnel

- An angled awl, via the anterolateral portal, is used to create a starting hole at the 1 o'clock (right knee) or 11 o'clock (left knee) position.
    - The anteroposterior position depends on the size of the graft, but the hole should be positioned so the tunnel edge is located at the junction with the articular cartilage (**TECH FIG 3**).
    - A guidewire is impacted into the starting hole via the anterolateral portal.
    - An appropriately sized cannulated acorn reamer is carefully passed over the guidewire, taking into consideration the close proximity of the patellar articular surface.

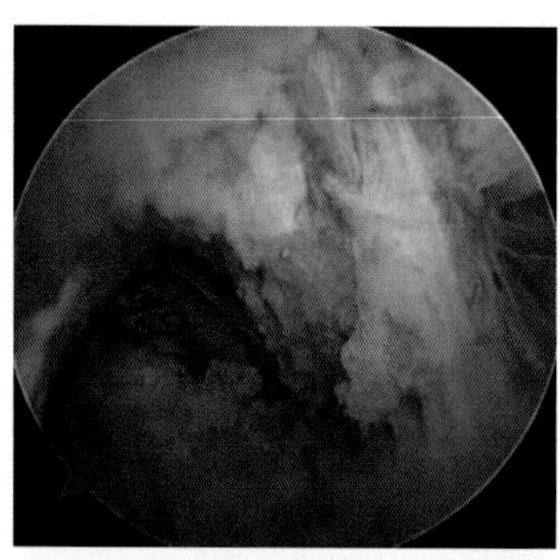

A

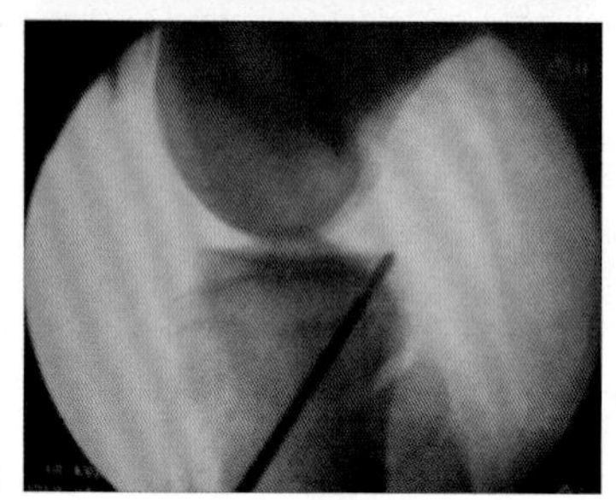

D

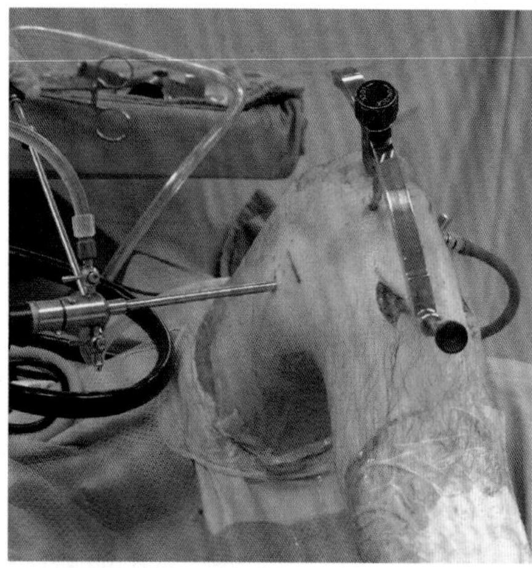

B

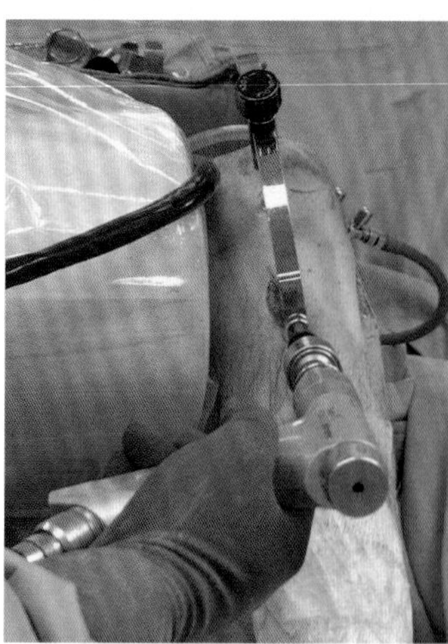

C

**TECH FIG 2** • **A.** PCL drill guide positioned to facilitate guide pin exit at the PCL insertion. **B.** Once the PCL drill guide is set, it is confirmed arthroscopically and fluoroscopically. **C.** The tibial guidewire is drilled under fluoroscopic guidance. **D.** The tibial guidewire position is confirmed with fluoroscopy.

- The tunnel is drilled to a depth of approximately 30 mm, taking care to avoid penetrating the outer cortex of the medial femoral condyle.
  - Increasing serial dilators are passed to match the size of the graft.
- A smaller EndoButton drill (Smith & Nephew, Andover, MA) is used to perforate the outer cortex of the medial femoral condyle, and a guidewire is inserted through the anterolateral portal into the femoral tunnel.
- An incision is made parallel to Langer lines over the anteromedial aspect of the distal medial femoral condyle, at the estimated exit of the guidewire from the bone.
  - The vastus medialis obliquus fascia and muscle is split in line with their fibers, and the muscle and periosteum are elevated off the anteromedial distal femur.
  - The drill hole is exposed and guidewire is removed.

## Graft Passage

- Passage of the graft may require enlarging the anterolateral portal.
- The 30-degree arthroscope is placed in the posteromedial portal, and a long 18-gauge bent wire loop is passed with the loop bent upward from anterior and distal to posterior and proximal through the tibial tunnel.
  - A tonsil is introduced through the anterolateral portal and through the notch to retrieve the bent wire loop (**TECH FIG 4**).
  - Leading sutures from the free ends (tibial side) of the graft are placed through the wire loop.
  - The wire and sutures are pulled back through the tibial tunnel in an anterograde fashion.
- A small scooped malleable retractor is introduced through the anterolateral portal and placed just posterior to the femoral tunnel to retract the fat pad and provide an unobstructed path for a Beath pin.
  - A Beath pin is then passed through the anterolateral portal and through the femoral tunnel.
  - The lead suture limbs from the Endoloop (Ethicon, Inc., Somerville, NJ) side of the graft are threaded through the eye of the Beath pin.
  - The pin, with the suture limbs, is pulled proximally.
- Traction on the suture limbs pulls the graft into the femoral tunnel to the marked line, whereas traction of the tibial suture limbs pulls the graft into the tibial tunnel.
  - The position of the graft is confirmed arthroscopically.

**TECH FIG 3** • The femoral tunnel is positioned so the tunnel edge is located at the junction with the articular cartilage.

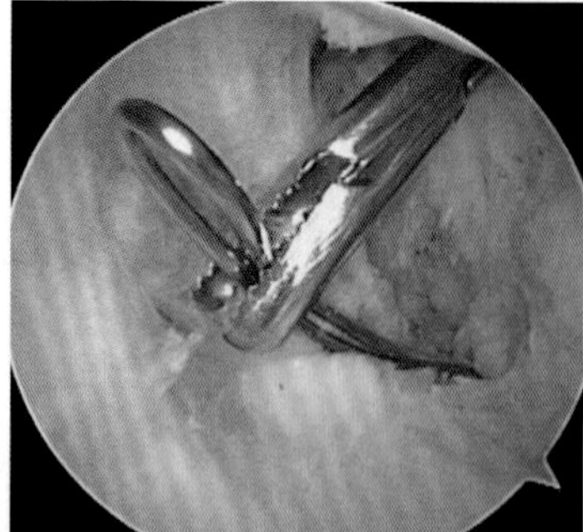

**TECH FIG 4** • A long 18-gauge bent wire loop, used to pass the sutures through the tibial tunnel in an anterograde fashion, is retrieved through the anterolateral portal.

## Graft Fixation

- Graft fixation is achieved by placing the Endoloop along the medial femur with a tonsil to estimate its most proximal extent.
- A 3.2-mm drill bit is used to make a unicortical hole at the most proximal extent of the Endoloop.
  - After the hole is measured and tapped, a 6.5-mm cancellous screw and washer are placed through the Endoloop into the femur.
  - The screw is tightened as the graft is pulled tight distally.
- The fixation is palpated to ensure the Endoloop limbs are tight distal to the screw and washer.
- An anterior tibial force is applied to reduce the tibia before and during final tibial fixation.
  - A cortical 4.5-mm screw and washer are placed from anteromedial to posterolateral within the proximal tibia.
  - The graft is fixed at 90 degrees flexion.
  - Before the screw advances to the second cortex, the suture limbs from the tibial side of the graft are tied with tension over the post. The screw is then tightened.
- The arthroscope is inserted to confirm adequate position, tension, and fixation of the graft.

## Wound Closure

- The incisions are irrigated, and the fascia in the anterolateral femoral incision is closed with size 0 Vicryl suture.
- The subcutaneous layer is approximated with interrupted, inverted 3-0 chromic suture, and the skin is closed with a running 4-0 absorbable suture.
- The portals are closed with 3-0 nylon suture.
- The dorsalis pedis and posterior tibialis pulses are assessed by palpation and a Doppler ultrasound examination if necessary.
- The incisions are covered with Adaptic gauze and sterile gauze, then wrapped in cast padding and bias wrap.

# Single-Bundle Augmentation

- For single-bundle augmentation, much of the technique is identical to the single-bundle technique already described.
  - Often, the AL bundle is ruptured and the PM bundle remains intact. Consequently, for the purposes of this chapter, AL bundle augmentation will be described.
- The diagnostic arthroscopy is performed.
- If any fibers of the AL bundle are found to be intact, special care is taken to preserve these intact fibers while the overlying synovium and ruptured PCL fibers are débrided (**TECH FIG 5A**).
- When preparing the posterior aspect of the tibia, preservation of the PCL origin is essential.
- Tibial tunnel preparation is performed similarly to the single-bundle technique.
  - The exit point for the guide pin along the sloped face of the posterior tibial fossa is just distal and lateral to the intact PCL insertion site (**TECH FIG 5B**).
- When preparing the medial femoral condyle for tunnel drilling, care again is taken to preserve the intact PCL bundle.
  - The starting hole is placed at the 1 o'clock (right knee) or 11 o'clock (left knee) position.
  - The hole should be positioned in the anteroposterior plane so the tunnel edge is located at the junction with the articular cartilage.
  - This location depends on the size of the graft and the distance from the intact PM bundle.
- The graft is passed around the intact bundle, which is the final augmentation consideration.
- Fixation and closure are then performed.

A
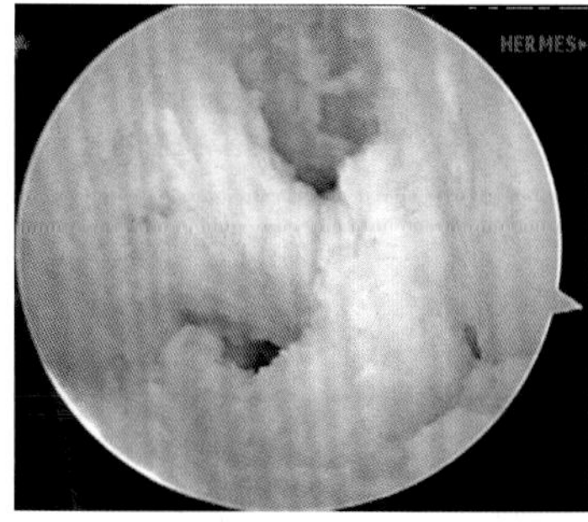


B
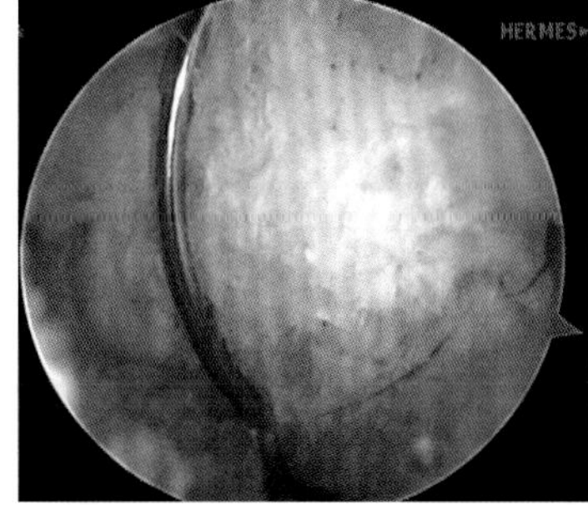


**TECH FIG 5** • **A.** An intact AL bundle is preserved and the overlying synovium and ruptured PCL fibers are débrided. **B.** The exit point for the tibial tunnel along the sloped face of the posterior tibial fossa is just distal and lateral to the intact PCL insertion, as demonstrated by a long 18-gauge bent wire loop.

# Double-Bundle Reconstruction

- For double-bundle PCL reconstruction, the initial aspects of the technique are identical to those of single-bundle reconstruction, including portal placement, arthroscopy, and preparation for drilling.

## Tibial Tunnel Creation

- Throughout this process, care must be taken to avoid tunnel convergence and ensure an adequate bony bridge between the two tibial tunnels.

- First, the guide pin for the AL tunnel is positioned using the same technique as with single-bundle reconstruction.
  - It exits the tibia just distal and lateral to the PCL insertion site, 1.5 cm distal to the articular edge of the posterior plateau.
- The PCL guide is reintroduced into the joint.
- The same steps and precautions are repeated for placement of the PM tibial guidewire.
  - The PM tibial guidewire enters the tibia on the anteromedial aspect of the tibia, slightly more proximal and medial than the AL guidewire.
  - Conversely, the PM guidewire can be introduced through the anterolateral tibia, crossing the AL guidewire on the coronal view, but remaining proximal to the AL guidewire throughout its course on the sagittal view. It exits the tibia in the footprint more medial and slightly proximal to the AL tibial guidewire (**TECH FIG 6A**).
  - It is important to ensure adequate separation between the two guide pins to accommodate both tunnels with a bony bridge separation.
- Once the guidewire positions are satisfactory, a cannulated compaction reamer is used to first drill the AL tibial tunnel.
  - The drill is advanced under fluoroscopic guidance.
  - The posterior tibial cortex is cautiously perforated by hand reaming under arthroscopic visualization.
  - The tunnel is irrigated, and increasing serial dilators are used under arthroscopic visualization.
- The steps are repeated for drilling the PM tibial tunnel with a 7-mm cannulated compaction reamer (**TECH FIG 6B**).

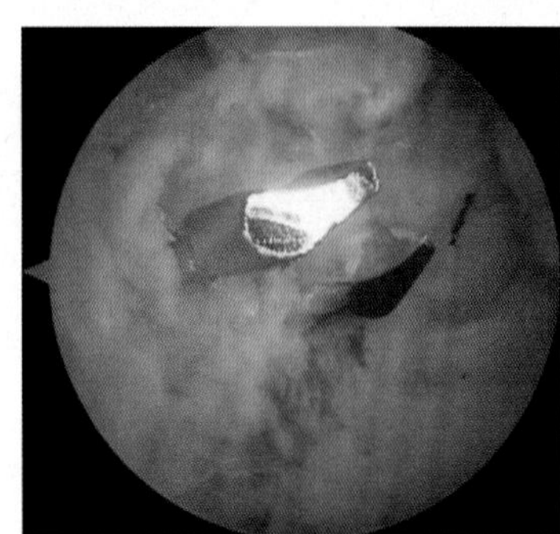

A

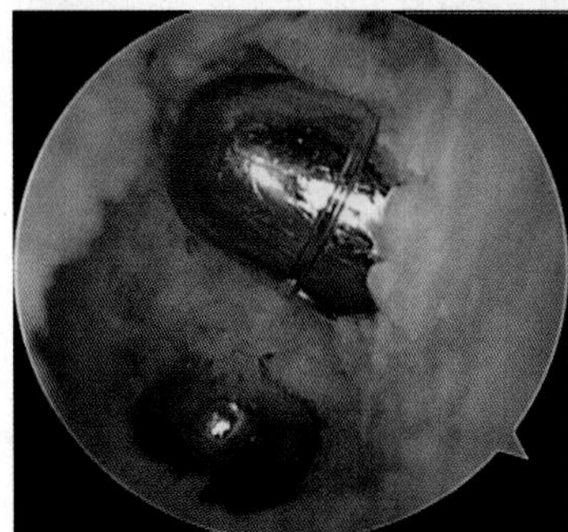

B

**TECH FIG 6** • **A.** Both the AL and PM guidewires are positioned in the proximal posterior tibia. The PM guidewire, and subsequently the tunnel, exits the tibia in the footprint more medial and slightly proximal to the AL tibial guidewire. **B.** Dilators demonstrate the position of the AL and PM tunnels in the proximal posterior tibia.

## Femoral Tunnel Creation

- An angled awl is used to create the starting holes.
- For the AL bundle, the starting hole is placed at the 1 o'clock (right knee) or 11 o'clock (left knee) position.
  - The hole should be positioned in the anteroposterior plane so the tunnel edge is located at the junction with the articular cartilage.
  - The guidewire is passed via the anterolateral portal and impacted into the starting hole.
  - The appropriately sized cannulated acorn reamer is passed over the guidewire.
  - The reamer should be passed carefully, given the close proximity of the patellar articular surface.
  - The tunnel is drilled to a depth of about 30 mm, with care taken to avoid penetration of the outer cortex of the medial femoral condyle.
  - Increasing serial dilators are passed to match the size of the graft.
  - A smaller EndoButton drill is used to perforate the outer cortex of the medial femoral condyle.
- This inside-out femoral tunnel preparation technique is then repeated for the PM tunnel.
  - The angled awl is used to create the starting hole at the 3 o'clock (right knee) or 9 o'clock (left knee) position.
  - The PM tunnel is placed parallel or slightly posterior to the AL tunnel.
  - The guide pin is then placed via the anterolateral portal and impacted into the starting hole.
  - A 7-mm acorn reamer is passed over the guidewire and drilled to a depth of approximately 30 mm (**TECH FIG 7**).
  - The medial femoral condylar cortex is perforated with the EndoButton drill.

## Graft Placement and Fixation

- The AL graft is passed first, using the same technique as with single-bundle reconstruction.
- This process is then repeated for the PM graft (**TECH FIG 8**).
  - It is helpful to keep tension on the AL graft suture ends when passing the PM graft to ensure that the AL graft does not get pulled into the joint.
- Graft fixation is performed first on the femoral side.
  - The AL bundle is secured as previously described.
  - This process is repeated for the PM bundle, ensuring that adequate separation exists between the two screws and washers to prevent overlap.

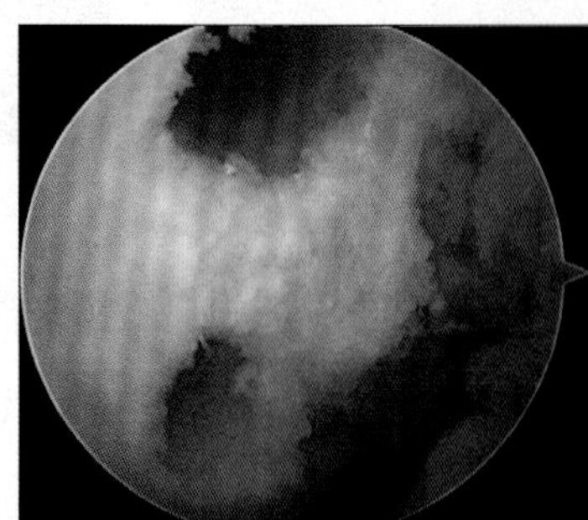

**TECH FIG 7** • The femoral tunnels, with the AL tunnel at the 11 o'clock position and the PM tunnel at the 9 o'clock position.

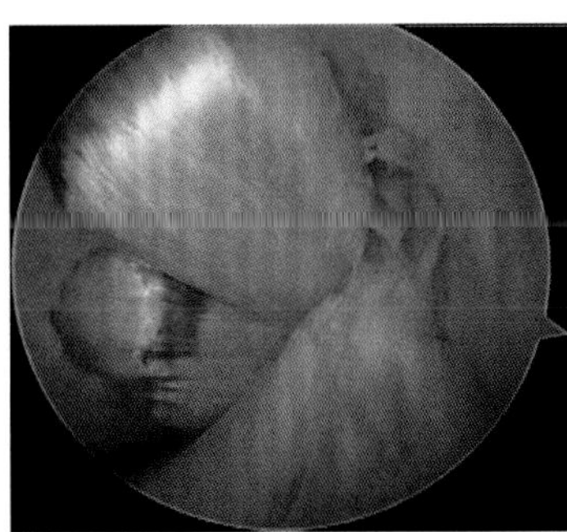

**TECH FIG 8** • The double-bundle reconstruction with the grafts in place.

- An anterior tibial force is applied to reduce the tibia before and during final tibial fixation.
  - Two 4.5-mm cortical screws and washers are placed from anteromedial to posterolateral within the proximal tibia, just distal to the respective tunnels.
  - As with the single-bundle technique, before the screw advances to the second cortex, the suture limbs from the tibial side of the graft are tied with tension over the post, and then the screw is tightened.
  - The AL graft is secured first at 90 degrees flexion, and the PM bundle then is secured at 15 degrees of flexion.
  - The arthroscope is inserted to confirm adequate position, tension, and fixation of the grafts.



## Tibial Inlay, Open

- For the double-bundle tibial inlay PCL reconstruction, the initial aspects of the technique are similar to those for single-bundle reconstruction, including portal placement, arthroscopy, and débridement.
- A whole, nonirradiated, frozen patellar tendon allograft is prepared with two bundles attached to a common tibial bone block and distinct femoral bone blocks.
  - The tibial bone block is fashioned from the tibial side of the graft and should measure 20 mm long, 13 mm wide, and 12 mm thick.
    - A single 4.5-mm gliding hole is placed in the center of the block for later fixation.
  - The tendon bundles stemming from the tibial bone block should measure 11 mm (AL bundle) and 9 mm (PM bundle).
  - The femoral bone plugs from the patellar side of the graft are shaped to 20 mm in length and 11 mm (AL bundle) and 9 mm (PM bundle) in diameter.
    - The femoral bone plugs are each drilled with two separate 2.0-mm holes, through which FiberWire (Arthrex, Inc. Naples, FL) passing sutures are placed (**TECH FIG 9A**).
- The leg is brought into a figure-4 position, with the knee flexed to 90 degrees and the bump repositioned under the lateral ankle.
  - A 6-cm incision is made over the posterior border of the tibia from the crease of the popliteal fossa and curving distally along the posteromedial border of the tibia (**TECH FIG 9B**).
- The dissection is continued through the subcutaneous fat to the sartorius fascia and the fascia overlying the medial head of the gastrocnemius.
  - The fascia is incised along the palpable posteromedial tibial border.
  - The semimembranosus and pes anserinus tendons are retracted anteriorly and proximally.
  - The medial head of the gastrocnemius is elevated from the tibial cortex and retracted posteriorly.
  - The medial border of the gastrocnemius is followed distally along the posterior tibia, and the proximal border of the popliteus muscle is identified. The popliteus muscle is elevated subperiosteally off the posteromedial surface of the tibia and mobilized laterally and distally (**TECH FIG 9C**).
- Attention is then turned to drilling an 11-mm AL and a 9-mm PM femoral tunnel, performed as described for the double-bundle technique.
- The leg is returned to the figure-4 position, and the tibial trough is prepared by creating a vertical arthrotomy between the palpable prominences of the medial and lateral tibial plateaus at the native PCL tibial insertion.
- The remaining PCL is identified and débrided, and a ¼-inch curved osteotome is used to create a trough measuring 13 mm wide, 12 mm deep, and 20 mm long (**TECH FIG 9D**).
  - A 3.2-mm transtibial drill hole is placed in the trough that corresponds to the 4.5-mm gliding hole in the tibial bone block.
- The graft is passed through the joint via an enlarged anteromedial portal into the tibial trough.
  - A 4.5-mm fully threaded cortical screw is used to lag the bone block into the trough.
  - Fluoroscopy is used to verify the position of the graft.
- A 4-cm incision is made along the posterior border of the vastus medialis at the center of the medial femoral condyle, and the femoral tunnels are identified.
  - The AL and PM bundle grafts are then passed through their respective femoral tunnels using a suture passer.
  - Several cycles of flexion and extension are performed to pretension the graft.
- The bundles are secured with metal interference screws placed outside-to-in (**TECH FIG 9E,F**).
  - The AL graft is secured first at 90 degrees flexion, and the PM bundle then is secured at 15 degrees of flexion.
  - A gentle anterior drawer is applied during screw insertion to recreate the natural tibial step-off.
  - Any remaining bone plug protruding from the femoral tunnels is removed with a rongeur, and sutures are tied together over the tunnel bone bridge or additional fixation can be achieved by tying the sutures over a post.

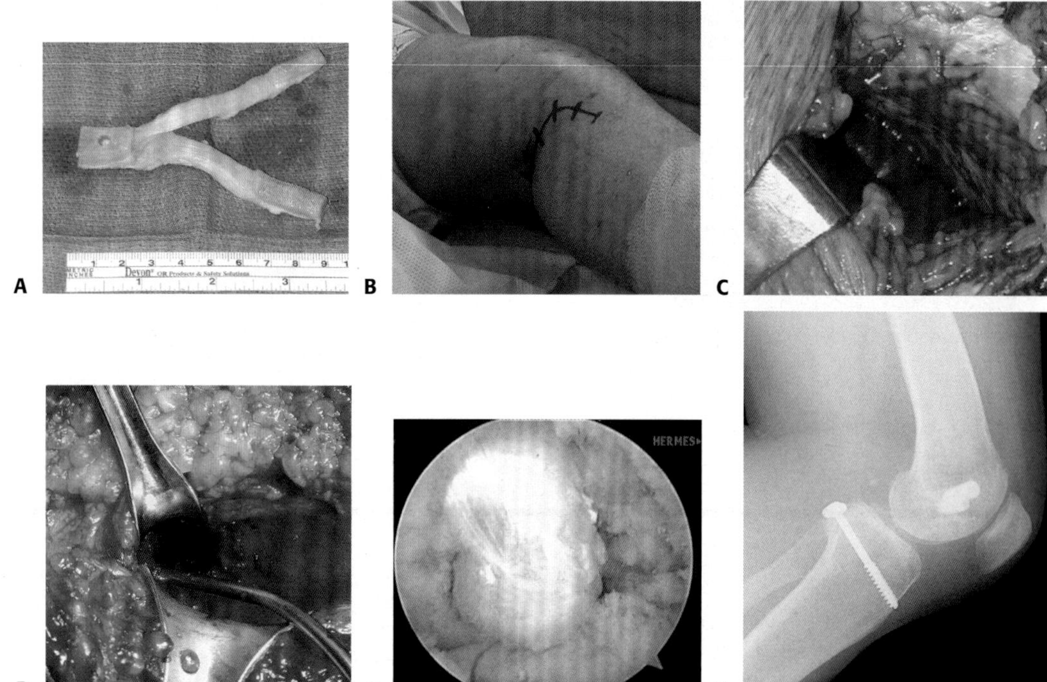

**TECH FIG 9** • **A.** The tibial inlay graft. **B.** The approach for the tibial inlay begins with a 6-cm incision over the posterior border of the tibia from the crease of the popliteal fossa, which curves distally along the posteromedial border of the tibia. **C.** The posterior aspect of the tibia after the popliteus muscle has been elevated subperiosteally off the posteromedial surface of the tibia and mobilized laterally and distally. **D.** The posterior aspect of the tibia after the inlay trough has been created. **E.** The double-bundle tibial inlay graft after being positioned in the tunnels. **F.** Lateral radiograph demonstrating the tibial inlay fixation with a 4.5-mm fully threaded cortical screw on the tibial side and interference screws on the femoral side.

## Tibial Inlay, Arthroscopic

- Although we do not typically use this technique, it has been well described by Salata and Sekiya.[18]
- As with other types of PCL reconstruction, this technique begins with an EUA and a diagnostic arthroscopy of the knee.
  - Most of the procedure is done between 45 and 90 degrees of flexion.
- The anterolateral arthroscopy portal is made as previously described; however, the anteromedial portal is made closer to the patellar tendon for better access to the posteromedial joint. A posteromedial portal 1 cm proximal to the posteromedial joint line is also used.
  - After portal placement, the PCL remnant is débrided to expose the femoral and tibial footprints.
- The tibial socket is created using a PCL guide (Arthrex, Inc.).
  - The target for the guidewire is 7 mm distal to the proximal tibial footprint.
  - The guidewire is overreamed with a 3.5-mm cannulated drill using direct vision and fluoroscopy to avoid plunging. The wire and drill are then removed.
  - A FlipCutter (Arthrex, Inc.) is then pushed through the tunnel until it is visualized inside the knee and then is "flipped" into an inverted L configuration to drill a 13-mm diameter tibial socket to a depth of 10 to 12 mm. Once this has been drilled, the FlipCutter is withdrawn.
- A fresh frozen whole Achilles tendon allograft with a minimum tendon length of 7 cm is preferred.
  - A no. 10 blade is used to divide the graft into two bundles along its natural raphe stopping 1 cm from the calcaneal bone plug; the larger portion is used from the AL bundle (8 to 11 mm) and the small for the PM bundle (6 to 9 mm). Each end is whipstitched with a no. 2 braided nonabsorbable suture.
  - The calcaneal bone plug is made into a single cylindrical 12-mm plug using a coring reamer (for a 13-mm socket).
  - A central tunnel is created in the plug with a 3.5-mm cannulated drill system; the 1 cm of tendon adjacent to the bone plug left in continuity is then whipstitched with a no. 2 braided nonabsorbable suture and the ends are passed through the bone plug tunnel from cortical to cancellous and used to guide the bone plug into the tibial socket and can be tied over a post.
  - Alternatively, these sutures can be passed through a PCL tightrope construct (Arthrex, Inc.) using buttons on the tibial bone plug and for tibial fixation.
- The femoral tunnels can then be created as previously described for the double-bundle arthroscopic reconstruction and open tibial inlay technique.
- The anteromedial portal again is typically extended for graft passage.

- A right angle clamp or arthroscopic probe can be used to seat the tibial bone plug into the socket and position is confirmed with fluoroscopy.
- The tibial bone plug is press-fit into the socket and further fixation is achieved on the tibial side by tying the sutures over a post (**TECH FIG 10 A,B**).

- The femoral limbs can be passed into their respective tunnels using an 18-gauge looped wire.
  - The graft is cycled prior to femoral fixation.
  - The graft is tensioned as previously described in the double-bundle technique and can be secured with interference screws and/or tied over a post or with suspensory fixation (**TECH FIG 10C**).

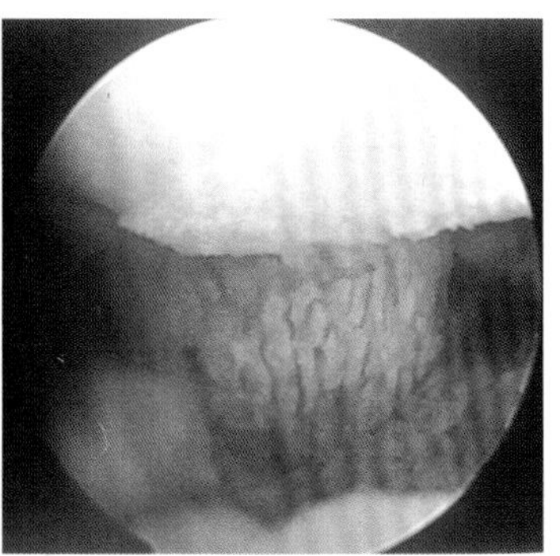
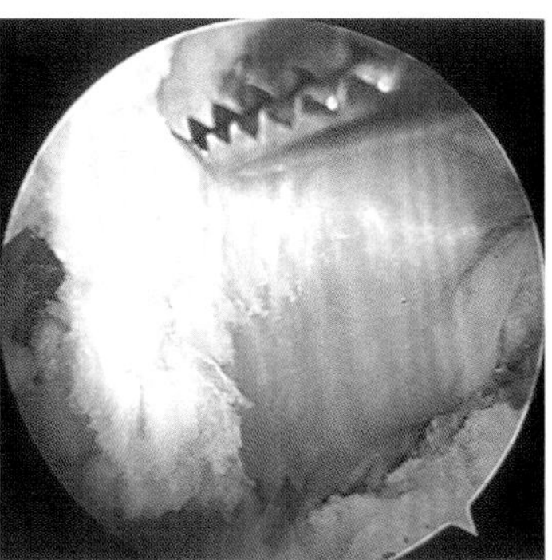
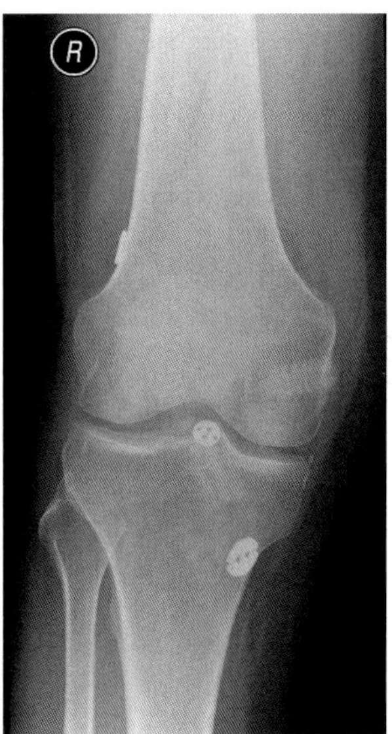


**TECH FIG 10** • **A.** Graft bone plug seating into the tibial socket. **B.** Graft bone plug set completely into the tibial socket. **C.** Postoperative radiograph after arthroscopic tibial inlay PCL reconstruction using single-bundle suspensory fixation.

## Tibial Avulsion

- The PCL tibial avulsion is approached similarly to tibial inlay reconstruction.
- The patient is positioned supine, as in the tibial inlay technique, to facilitate arthroscopic examination.
- The skin incision and the dissection are performed as described for the tibial inlay technique.
- A vertical arthrotomy is made, and the avulsed fragment of the tibia with the attached PCL is identified.
- The bone fragment and PCL are reduced and secured with a 4.0-mm cortical or a 6.5-mm cancellous screw and spiked washer, depending on the size of the fragment.
- The reduction is confirmed with fluoroscopy or a radiograph (**TECH FIG 11**).

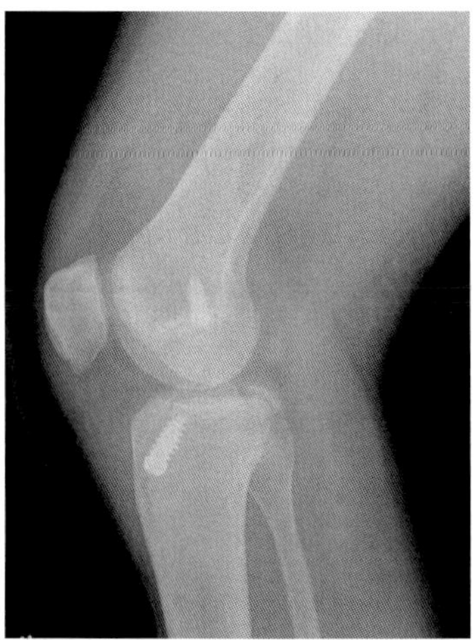
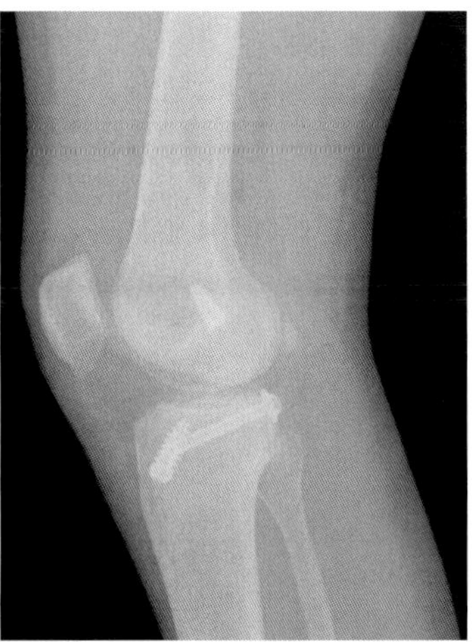
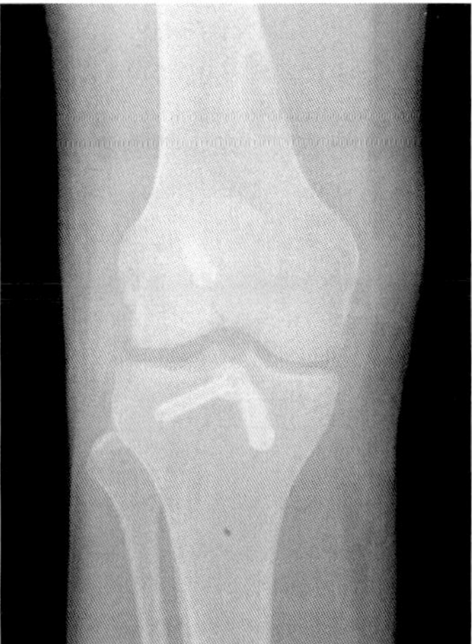

**TECH FIG 11** • **A.** PCL tibial avulsion in a patient with a previous ACL reconstruction. **B,C.** Lateral and PA radiographs after fixation of the tibial avulsion.

## PEARLS AND PITFALLS

| | |
|---|---|
| **Indications** | ■ Assess for concomitant PLC injury on the EUA and following PCL reconstruction because deficiency of these structures may lead to PCL graft failure.<br>■ Employ the appropriate technique based on the chronicity of the injury and remaining native PCL. |
| **Arthroscopy** | ■ Exposure of the posterior tibia may be tedious but is essential for appropriate, safe tunnel placement.<br>■ When working in the posterior knee joint, be certain the shaver or electrocautery device always faces anteriorly, away from the popliteal vessels.<br>■ Fluid extravasation and lower extremity compartments must be monitored throughout the procedure. |
| **Tunnel placement** | ■ A parallel pin guide can be used to make small corrections in tunnel placement.<br>■ Perforate the posterior tibial cortex by hand with the guide pins or reamers in a controlled fashion under direct arthroscopic visualization to avoid neurovascular injury.<br>■ If the patella causes resistance to the acorn reamer when drilling the femoral tunnels, use a smaller reamer to make a starting hole, then hand-dilate the tunnel to the appropriate size with larger reamers. |
| **Graft management** | ■ An arthroscopic switching rod, placed via the posteromedial portal between the graft and the posterior tibial cortex, can facilitate graft passage by decreasing friction.<br>■ Avoid penetrating soft tissue with the Beath pin while passing through the anterolateral portal to prevent the graft from getting caught in the soft tissue. |
| **Fixation** | ■ An anterior tibial force should be applied during fixation to prevent posterior subluxation. |
| **Rehabilitation** | ■ Closed-chain exercises that apply an axial load across the knee protect the PCL reconstruction owing to the sagittal slope of the tibial plateau. |

## POSTOPERATIVE CARE

- A hinged knee brace is applied and locked in extension. The patient is awakened and taken to the recovery room, where pain and neurovascular status are reevaluated.
- Patients may be kept overnight for pain management and to monitor their neurovascular status.
- Patients are given instructions for exercises (quadriceps sets, straight-leg raises, calf pumps, and mini-squats) and crutch use.
- All dressing changes are performed while an anterior tibial force is applied.
- Patients are instructed to maintain touchdown weight bearing for 1 week.
- Partial weight bearing is initiated after the first postoperative visit.
- The brace is unlocked after 4 to 6 weeks and usually is discontinued after 8 weeks.
- Symmetric full hyperextension is achieved, and passive prone knee flexion, quadriceps sets, and patellar mobilization exercises are performed with the assistance of a physical therapist for the first month.
- Mini-squats are performed from 0 to 60 degrees after the first week and from 0 to 90 degrees after the third week.
- Once full, pain-free ROM is achieved, strengthening is addressed.
- The goals for achievement of flexion are 90 degrees at 4 weeks and 120 degrees at 8 weeks.

## OUTCOMES

- Choice of graft (autograft vs. allograft) has not been shown to affect overall outcome.[3,15]
- Acute single-bundle reconstructions have been demonstrated to have significantly better outcomes than chronic reconstructions.[19]
- The clinical outcomes after single-bundle and tibial inlay reconstructions have produced a satisfactory return of function and improvement in symptoms.[3,7,9,16,19]
- Neither transtibial or tibial inlay has been shown to be superior with regard to overall outcome.[11,15]
- No studies have specifically addressed the long-term clinical outcomes of double-bundle reconstructions and PCL augmentation reconstructions.
  - No clear clinical advantage has been shown regarding double-bundle reconstruction versus single-bundle reconstruction.[10]
  - Single-bundle PCL reconstruction has not been shown to prevent degenerative osteoarthritis despite improvements in knee function.[7,9]
  - Despite reconstruction, knee kinematics may not return to normal.[24]

## COMPLICATIONS

- Failure to carefully position the extremity with adequate padding may result in neurapraxia.
- Loss of motion (usually decreased flexion) can result from errors in graft positioning or excessive tensioning during graft fixation. Inadequate rehabilitation also may lead to loss of motion.
- Residual laxity also can occur as a result of graft positioning or failure to address concomitant ligamentous injury.
- Injury to the popliteal vessels is rare but may be a very serious complication. Care must be taken to prevent overpenetration of the posterior tibial cortex.
- The thigh and calf should be routinely palpated to ensure no compartment syndrome develops from fluid extravasation into the soft tissues.

## REFERENCES

1. Ahn JH, Ha CW. Posterior trans-septal portal for arthroscopic surgery of the knee joint. Arthroscopy 2000;16:774–779.
2. Ahn JH, Yoo JC, Wang JH. Posterior cruciate ligament reconstruction: double-loop hamstring tendon autograft versus Achilles tendon allograft: clinical results of a minimum 2-year follow-up. Arthroscopy 2005;21:965–969.

3. Cooper DE, Stewart D. Posterior cruciate ligament reconstruction using single-bundle patella tendon graft with tibial inlay fixation: 2- to 10-year follow-up. Am J Sports Med 2004;32:346–360.
4. Giffin JR, Vogrin TM, Zantop T, et al. Effects of increasing tibial slope on the biomechanics of the knee. Am J Sports Med 2004;32:376–382.
5. Goyal K, Tashman S, Wang JH, et al. In vivo analysis of the isolated posterior cruciate ligament-deficient knee during functional activities. Am J Sports Med 2012;40:777–785.
6. Harner CD, Waltrip RL, Bennett CH, et al. Surgical management of knee dislocations. J Bone Joint Surg Am 2004;86A:262–273.
7. Hermans S, Corten K, Bellemans J. Long-term results of isolated anterolateral bundle reconstructions of the posterior cruciate ligament: a 6- to 12-year follow-up study. Am J Sports Med 2009;37:1499–1507.
8. Kim SJ, Park IS. Arthroscopic reconstruction of the posterior cruciate ligament using tibial-inlay and double-bundle technique. Arthroscopy 2005;21:1271.
9. Kim YM, Lee CA, Matava MJ. Clinical results of arthroscopic single-bundle transtibial posterior cruciate ligament reconstruction: a systemic review. Am J Sports Med 2011;39:425–434.
10. Kohen RB, Sekiya JK. Single-bundle versus double-bundle posterior cruciate ligament reconstruction. Arthroscopy 2009;25(12):1470–1477.
11. MacGillivray JD, Stein BE, Park M, et al. Comparison of tibial inlay versus transtibial techniques for isolated posterior cruciate ligament reconstruction: minimum 2-year follow-up. Arthroscopy 2006;22:320–328.
12. Margheritini F, Mancini L, Mauro CS, et al. Stress radiography for quantifying posterior cruciate ligament deficiency. Arthroscopy 2003;19:706–711.
13. Mariani PP, Margheritini F. Full arthroscopic inlay reconstruction of posterior cruciate ligament. Knee Surg Sports Traumatol Arthrosc 2006;14:1038–1044.
14. Mauro CS, Margheritini F, Mariani PP. The arthroscopic transeptal approach for pathology of the posterior joint space. Tech Knee Surg 2005;4:120–125.
15. Montgomery SR, Johnson JS, McAllister DR, et al. Surgical management of PCL injuries: indications, techniques, and outcomes. Curr Rev Musculoskelet Med 2013;6:115–123.
16. Panchal HB, Sekiya JK. Open tibial inlay versus arthroscopic transtibial posterior cruciate ligament reconstructions. Arthroscopy 2011;27(9):1289–1295.
17. Parolie JM, Bergfeld JA. Long-term results of nonoperative treatment of isolated posterior cruciate ligament injuries in the athlete. Am J Sports Med 1986;14:35–38.
18. Salata MJ, Sekiya JK. Arthroscopic posterior cruciate ligament tibial inlay reconstruction: a surgical technique that may influence rehabilitation. Sports Health 2011;3(1):52–58.
19. Sekiya JK, West RV, Ong BC, et al. Clinical outcomes after isolated arthroscopic single-bundle posterior cruciate ligament reconstruction. Arthroscopy 2005;21:1042–1050.
20. Shelbourne KD, Clark M, Gray T. Minimum 10-year follow up of patients after an acute, isolated posterior cruciate ligament injury treated nonoperatively. Am J Sports Med 2013;41:1526–1533.
21. Shelbourne KD, Davis TJ, Patel DV. The natural history of acute, isolated, nonoperatively treated posterior cruciate ligament injuries. A prospective study. Am J Sports Med 1999;27:276–283.
22. Shelbourne KD, Muthukaruppan Y. Subjective results of nonoperatively treated, acute, isolated posterior cruciate ligament injuries. Arthroscopy 2005;21(4):457–461.
23. Toritsuka Y, Horibe S, Hiro-Oka A, et al. Conservative treatment for rugby football players with an acute isolated posterior cruciate ligament injury. Knee Surg Sports Traumatol Arthrosc 2004;12:110–114.
24. Voos JE, Mauro CS, Wente T, et al. Posterior cruciate ligament: anatomy, biomechanics, and outcomes. Am J Sports Med 2012;40(1):222–231.

# Arthroscopic Drilling and Fixation of Osteochondritis Dissecans

**Theodore J. Ganley, Kevin G. Shea, and Nathan L. Grimm**

## DEFINITION

- Osteochondritis dissecans (OCD) is described as a focal, idiopathic alteration of subchondral bone with risk for instability and disruption of adjacent articular cartilage that may result in premature osteoarthritis.[25]

## ANATOMY

- The most common location for OCD lesions to occur is in the knee; more specifically, on the lateral aspect of the medial femoral condyle.
- The morphology of the OCD in this anatomic position varies and can appear as an initial softening of the subchondral bone and overlying articular cartilage, which can progress to early articular cartilage separation and later osteochondral separation (**FIG 1**).

## PATHOGENESIS

- Although the exact pathogenesis of OCD remains unclear, several hypotheses about the etiology of OCD have been proposed—ischemia, trauma, accessory centers of ossification, and genetic factors.
- Ischemia
  - In 1870, Sir James Paget had described what was later thought to be OCD as "quiet necrosis."[24] Green and Banks[14] also theorized that OCD was due to ischemia of subchondral bone leading to the development of OCD.
  - Later studies on the epiphyseal artery construct, however, would conclude that this hypothesis is less likely to explain the etiology.
- Microtrauma
  - Fairbank's[12] early work described trauma as an etiology for OCD. Smillie[27] strongly supported Fairbank's "tibial spine" theory for the etiology of OCD. Although this may offer an explanation for the classic location on the lateral aspect of the medial femoral condyle, it does not account for other locations of OCD in the knee.
  - A theory of repetitive microtrauma is appealing given that multiple studies have shown up to 60% of patients with OCD report being involved in sporting activities.[3,15,21]

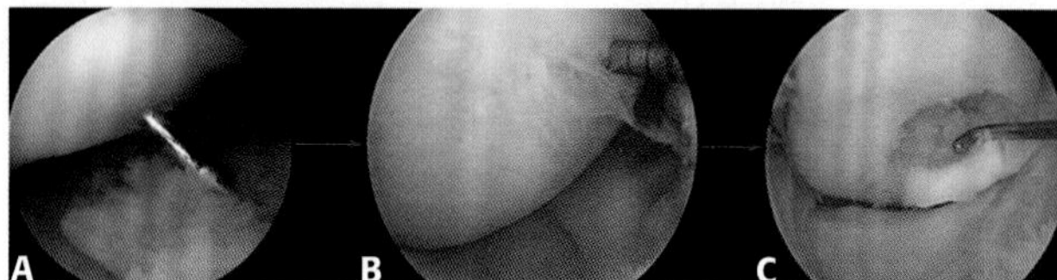


**FIG 1** • Showing three common morphologies of OCD lesions of the knee. **A.** Ballotable, intact cartilage lesion. **B.** Fissured "locked door" lesion. **C.** Hinged trap door lesion.

  - Reports of acute traumatic events that lead to delayed development of lesions that resemble OCD have been reported in the knee and elbow.[9,13,28]
- Accessory centers of ossification
  - The one hypothesis that may unite all previous evidence is that of epiphyseal endochondral ossification described by Ribbing.[26]
  - These "accessory centers of ossification" were described by Ribbing[26] and shown to occur in the classic location of the medial femoral condyle.
- Genetic
  - Although a solitary lesion is the most common finding of OCD, cases of joint bilaterality, multiple lesions in a single joint, and reports of OCD in twin studies have provided support for a hypothesis of genetic predisposition.

## NATURAL HISTORY

- Hughes et al[16] documented the natural history of skeletally immature OCD of the knee through serial magnetic resonance imaging (MRIs) over a 5-year period, which they correlated with arthroscopy and clinical outcomes.
- In this small series, they demonstrated that all lesions with intact cartilage will likely heal with conservative treatment; however, if the lesion shows evidence of cartilage breakdown or subchondral bone fragmentation, it loses its mechanical support and may progress to further breakdown resulting in extrusion into the joint.[16]

## PATIENT HISTORY AND PHYSICAL FINDINGS

- The presentation of OCD of the knee is variable, and the symptomatology is in large part due to the stage of the lesion when the particular symptoms present.
- A stable lesion which remains in situ may present as nonspecific knee pain that is poorly localized by the patient, externally rotated gait, and a possible effusion.[29]
- A lesion that has progressed to instability may become a "trap door"–type lesion with mobility or a loose body. Both lesion types may present with mechanical symptoms that may be described as a "catching" or "locking" sensation.
- In 1967, Wilson[29] describes a clinical examination finding which he suggests is diagnostic of OCD of the knee: "[With the patient] in the supine position, the knee on the affected side is flexed through about 90° and the tibia is medially rotated. The knee is then gradually extended and at a point of about 30° short of full extension the [patient] will complain of pain over the anterior part of the medial femoral condyle. Lateral rotation of the tibia relieves this pain immediately."
- However, Wilson sign has been shown to be unreliable and nonspecific.[8]

## IMAGING AND OTHER DIAGNOSTIC STUDIES

- Imaging protocols have received close attention in the literature as a result of the varied success of nonoperative treatment. The goals of imaging are to characterize the lesion, determine the prognosis of nonoperative management, and monitor the healing of the lesion.
- Radiographs are useful for making the diagnosis of OCD and should be the first imaging modality of choice, as they usually characterize and localize the lesion and rule out other bony pathology of the knee region. In a significant number of cases, however, OCD lesions may not be readily apparent on plain radiographs.
  - Imaging workup begins with plain radiographs, including anteroposterior (AP), tunnel, and lateral views (**FIG 2A–C**).
  - A Merchant view should be included to best reveal any OCD lesions of the patella or trochlea.
- MRI is most useful for determining the size of the lesion and the status of the cartilage and subchondral bone in addition to further characterizing the OCD lesions (**FIG 2D–F**).
  - The extent of bony edema, the presence of a high-signal zone beneath the fragment, and the presence of other loose bodies are also important findings on MRI. Arthroscopy continues to be the gold or reference standard for diagnosing stability.[4]
- Scintigraphy and computed tomography (CT)
  - Although CT can better differentiate bone contour and congruency, this are rarely ordered especially in juvenile cases of OCD.
  - Similarly, technetium bone scans have been employed to provide information about the biologic capacity of an OCD lesion to heal. However, with the advent of MRI and its ability to be used without exposure to radiation yet still provide quality images of OCD lesions, scintigraphy is less commonly used.
  - Use of ionizing radiation in OCD lesions should be carefully considered, as other imaging options may provide excellent diagnostic and prognostic information with none or minimal exposure to radiation.

## DIFFERENTIAL DIAGNOSIS

- Irregular ossification
- Acute osteochondral fractures
- Meniscal injuries

## NONOPERATIVE MANAGEMENT

- An initial course of nonoperative management is the treatment of choice for skeletally immature children with small intact lesions with the goal of nonoperative intervention to promote healing in the subchondral bone and potentially prevent chondral collapse, subsequent fracture, and crater formation.
- Controversy exists regarding the ideal nonoperative management for these patients. Clinicians who adhere to treating the subchondral bone as the primary source of pathology favor a period of immobilization. Those whose focus is on

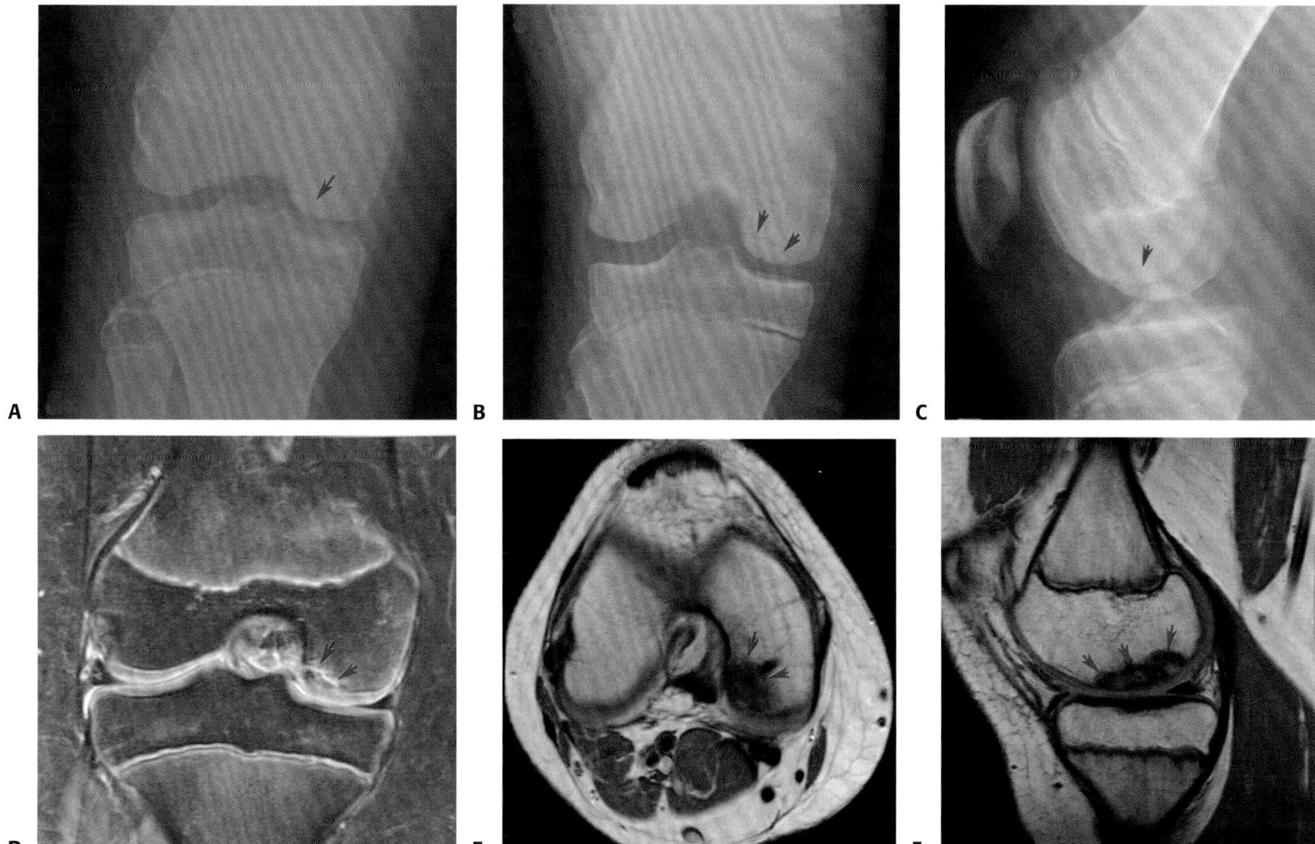


**FIG 2** • Three-view series of OCD lesion: AP (**A**), tunnel view (**B**), and lateral view (**C**). MRI sequence of OCD: coronal (**D**), axial (**E**), and sagittal slice (**F**). *Red arrows* point to OCD lesion.

**Table 1 Three-Phase Approach to Nonoperative Management of Skeletally Immature Osteochondritis Dissecans**

| | |
|---|---|
| **Phase I** (wk 1–6) | Knee immobilization in a hinged brace. The patient may walk with the hinged brace locked in extension. The brace may be unlocked to work on range of motion for 5 minutes five times per day. |
| **Phase II** (wk 6–12) | If the patient is pain-free and radiographs show signs of healing after 6 weeks, he or she is allowed to begin weight bearing without immobilization and to begin a physical therapy protocol to improve knee range of motion and quadriceps and hamstring strength. |
| **Phase III*** (wk 8–12) | Running, jumping, and cutting sports are permitted under close observation. High-impact activities and activities that might involve shear stress to the knee should be restricted until the child has been pain-free for several months and the radiographs show a healed lesion. |

* This phase begins typically 3 months after treatment and is instituted if the patient continues to remain pain-free and shows radiographic evidence of healing.

the articular cartilage as a source of pathology tend to favor mobilization.

- The options for immobilization include casting, bracing, and standard knee immobilizers.
- We recommend a three-phase approach to the nonoperative management of OCD lesions (Table 1).

## SURGICAL MANAGEMENT

- The goals of operative treatment are to promote healing of the native articular cartilage and subchondral bone when possible, to maintain joint congruity, to rigidly fix unstable fragments, and to replace osteochondral defects with cells that can replace and grow cartilage.
- It is widely accepted that operative treatment should be considered for patients with unstable or detached lesions and in patients whose lesions have not resolved with an appropriate period of nonoperative management, especially in those approaching skeletal maturity.
- Operative treatment is recommended if one or more of the following conditions are met:
  - Persistently symptomatic juvenile lesions
  - Presence of symptomatic loose bodies
  - Predicted physeal closure within 1 year
  - Evidence of fragment detachment/instability
- Optimal surgical treatment provides a stable construct of subchondral bone, calcified tidemark, and cartilage repair with viability and biomechanical properties equivalent to or similar to native hyaline cartilage.

### Preoperative Planning

- Careful preoperative evaluation and preparation are always imperative to the success of treatment.
- All imaging studies obtained before surgery should be reviewed. If the displaced fragment has a relatively large osseous component, then plain radiographs will usually demonstrate the lesion.
  - Radiographs do not demonstrate the actual size of the cartilaginous component. To demonstrate the cartilaginous component, MRI may be required to determine the extent of the lesion. Any other lesion noted on imaging studies should likewise be addressed.
- A thorough physical examination should be performed under anesthesia.

### Positioning

- For arthroscopic procedures, the position largely depends on the surgeon's preference. A variety of positions can be used:
  - The leg can be placed in a leg holder on the operating table with the knee joint past the end of the operating table, thus allowing the knee to flex 90 degrees and the lower leg to hang freely.
  - The leg can be placed supine on the operating table, with the hip flexed and the knee flexed 90 degrees. The knee can be flexed, and the lower leg can, in this case, hang freely over the side of the operating table.
  - The leg can be placed supine on the operating table, with the hip flexed and the knee flexed 90 degrees, using a thigh post and foot post to hold the leg in this position. The lower leg in this case may remain on the flat table and does not need to hang off the end of the table.

### Approach

- Standard arthroscopic parapatellar portals are initially used (**FIG 3A**).
  - Key: Accessory portals may be created higher or lower to the standard parapatellar portals if the lesion is excessively large or in an atypical location.
- Transarticular drilling can be used for intact lesions, but it is particularly valuable when the lesion is detached, partially detached, or unstable (**FIG 3B**).
- Retroarticular drilling is reserved for cases with intact lesions (**FIG 3C**).

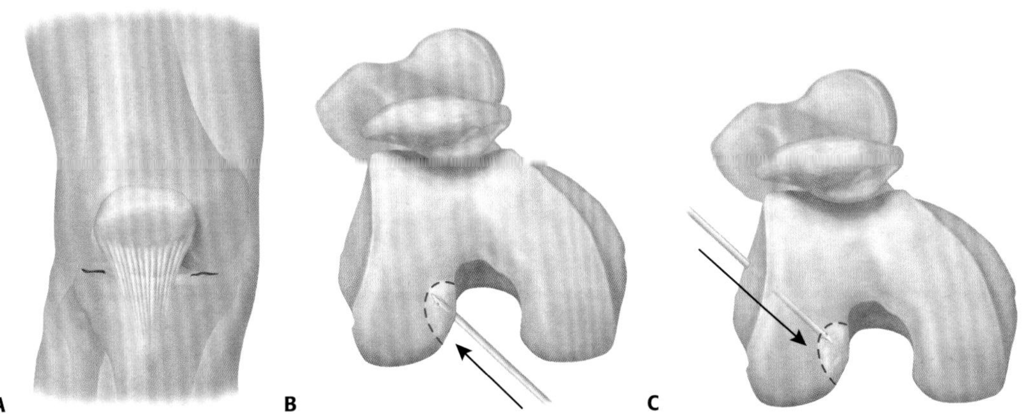

**FIG 3** • Standard arthroscopic portals are used for arthroscopic drilling techniques. **A.** Accessory portals can be used for visualizing or treating lesions of the patellotrochlear interval. **B.** Transarticular drilling of OCD lesion. **C.** Retroarticular drilling of OCD lesion.



## Transarticular Drilling of Osteochondritis Dissecans Lesion

- This procedure can be completed with or without exsanguinating the knee and applying a tourniquet depending on surgeon preference.
- An anterolateral portal and anteromedial portals are made for visualization and instrumentation.
- A complete arthroscopic inspection of the knee is performed. Any other pathologies in the knee are recorded and treated accordingly.
- The lesion is identified (**TECH FIG 1A**).
- A 0.45- or 0.62-inch Kirschner wire is positioned perpendicular to the lesion (**TECH FIG 1B**). The portal used depends on the location of the lesion.
  - The key is to keep the Kirschner wire as perpendicular as possible. Additional portals as well as varying the degree of knee flexion and extension may be used as needed to achieve adequate position.
- The drilling is performed under arthroscopic visualization. Having the radiographs and MRI images in the operating theatre can be used as visual aids to confirm the location and orientation of drilling of the lesion.
- Appropriate depth of penetration is confirmed by the efflux of blood or fat from the drilled holes (**TECH FIG 1C,D**).
- The drilling should be performed through the calcified tidemark in immature patients, taking care not to penetrate the physis.

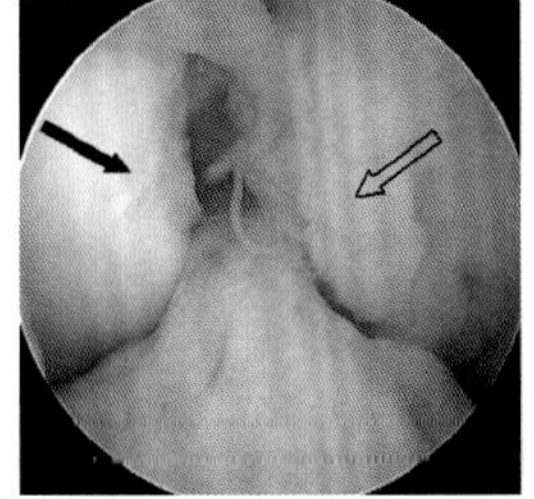

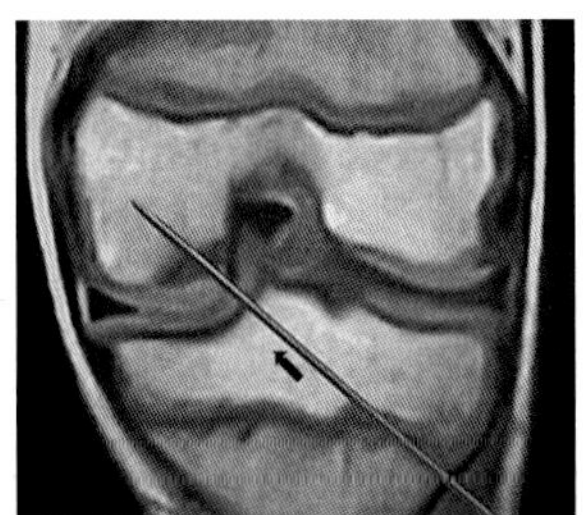

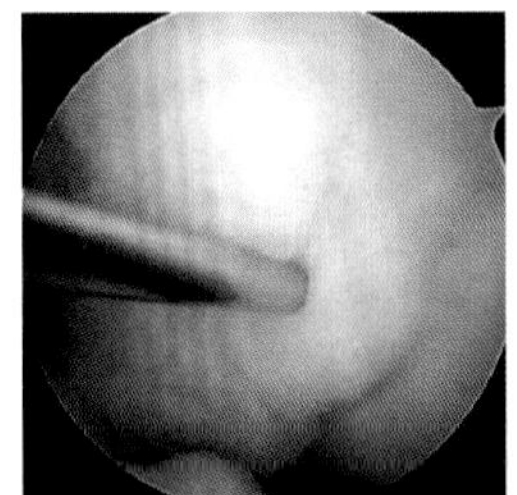

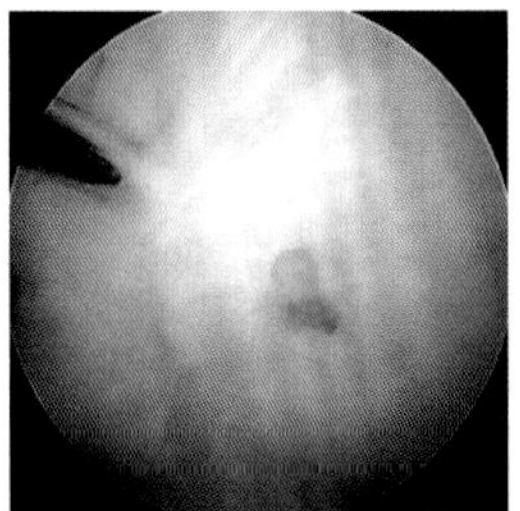

**TECH FIG 1** • **A.** The knee is inspected and the lesion is identified. The *solid arrow* shows the intact cartilage side and the *open arrow* shows the OCD side. **B.** A Kirschner wire is shown superimposed over a T1-weighted MRI. The *arrow* shows the direction of drilling. The smooth 0.62-inch Kirschner wire should be kept as perpendicular to the lesion as possible to prevent undermining the defect. **C,D.** The appearance of fat or blood demonstrates that subchondral bone has been penetrated.

## Retroarticular Drilling of Osteochondritis Dissecans Lesion

- This procedure can be completed with or without exsanguinating the knee and applying a tourniquet depending on surgeon preference.
- Anterolateral and anteromedial portals are made for visualization and instrumentation.
- A complete arthroscopic inspection of the knee is performed. Any other pathologies in the knee are recorded and treated accordingly.
- Once complete inspection has been performed, a 0.62-inch Kirschner wire is directed toward the lesion in a proximal to distal direction with fluoroscopic guidance and a guide to help maintain an appropriate angle.
  - The starting point of the Kirschner wire is immediately distal to the physis to avoid any damage.

- The Kirschner wire is slowly advanced through the subchondral bone, taking care not to penetrate the articular cartilage.
- The Kirschner wire is kept as perpendicular to the lesion as possible.
- The position and depth of the Kirschner wires are confirmed using fluoroscopy.
- Kirschner wires are inserted through the lesion several millimeters apart as needed. A small drill guide that allows parallel pin placement may assist with repeat drilling.
- Final inspection of the knee is performed, and the Kirschner wires and instrumentation are removed.
- Closure of the knee is performed, and sterile dressing is applied before placing the knee in a knee immobilizer.

## Fixation of Unstable Osteochondritis Dissecans Lesion

### Metallic or Bioabsorbable Screws

- The entire lesion is assessed, and the bed is prepared. A débridement is performed until all granulation tissue and sclerotic bone beneath the flap is removed, and subchondral bone is reached.
- In deep lesions, autograft or allograft cancellous bone grafting may be required to ensure that the hinged portion of the lesion is not recessed relative to the remaining unaffected cartilage within the knee.
- The lesion is reduced into its bed and fixed with a variety of implants, such as cannulated screws or variable pitch screws. The fixation devices may be made of metal or bioabsorbable materials. The implant used depends on the surgeon's preference.
- We prefer to use small metal double-ended threaded compression screws for hinged lesions in which there is appropriate subchondral support that allows for adequate screw thread to engage the subchondral progeny bone of the lesion. In some cases, the subchondral progeny bone may not be of adequate thickness to allow this type of fixation (**TECH FIG 2**).
- Once the lesion is secured, drilling of the surrounding parent and progeny bone may be performed to augment healing.

### Matchstick Technique

- Anterolateral and anteromedial portals are made for visualization and instrumentation.
- A complete arthroscopic inspection of the knee is performed. Any other pathologies in the knee are recorded and treated accordingly.
- A 2.5-cm longitudinal incision is made approximately 1 cm medial to the tibial tubercle, which will be the site of bone stick harvest.
- Using a microsaw, bone sticks are created and harvested from the tibia (**TECH FIG 3A,B**).
- Using a large diameter cannula no. 1, the perforation of the focus is oriented and performed with a Steinmann pin that has a diameter similar to the internal diameter of cannula no. 2. Cannula no. 2 contains the bone stick and is introduced into cannula no. 1 (**TECH FIG 3C,D**).
- The trocar is introduced into cannula no. 2 to introduce the bone stick into the center of the OCD lesion.
  - This step is repeated with as many bone sticks as need to obtain a secure rigid fixation of the OCD lesion.

### Autologous Osteochondral Grafting

- Anterolateral and anteromedial portals are made for visualization and instrumentation.
- A complete arthroscopic inspection of the knee is performed, taking care to assess the position and size of the lesion, which is used to estimate the number of needed osteochondral plugs to harvest.
- The bed of the lesion is inspected, and a débridement is performed to remove any granulation tissue and sclerotic bone.
  - The estimation of osteochondral plug length is based on preoperative MRI findings.
- The number of osteochondral plugs are then harvested from non–weight-bearing aspects of the medial and/or lateral trochlea (**TECH FIG 4**).

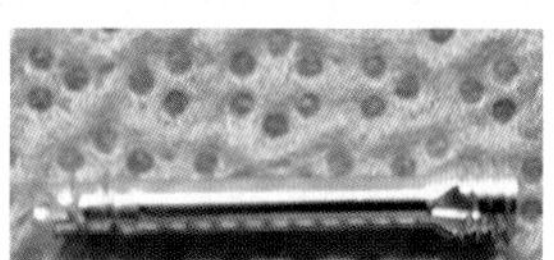

**TECH FIG 2** • Small metallic variable pitch compression screws are the authors' preferred choice for fixation used for hinged lesions—although many options are available.

A

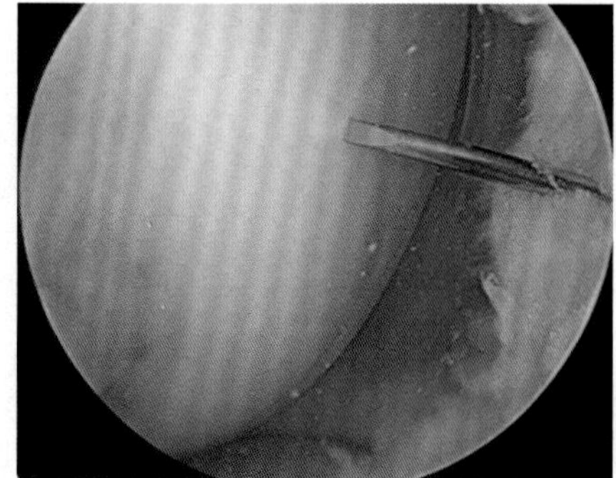

B

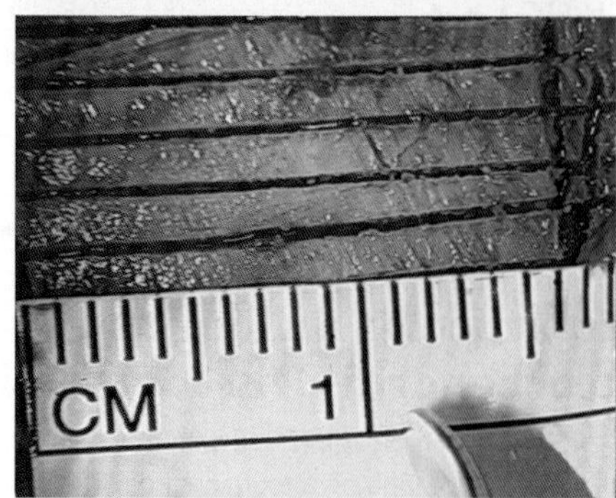


**TECH FIG 3** • Showing preparation of skeletally immature OCD lesion for autologous cortical bone stick tunnels (**A**), measuring of bone sticks being harvested from the tibia (**B**), *(continued)*

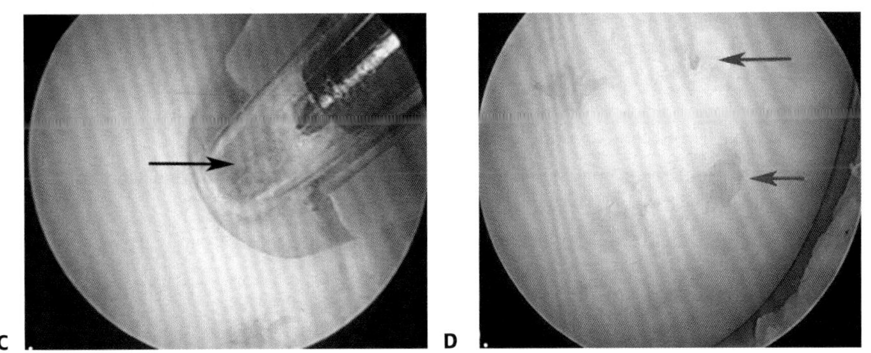


**TECH FIG 3** • *(continued)* tamping of 1- × 16-mm bone sticks (*black arrow*) into lesion (**C**), and showing cortical bone sticks (*red arrows*) in place with cartilaginous congruency (**D**).

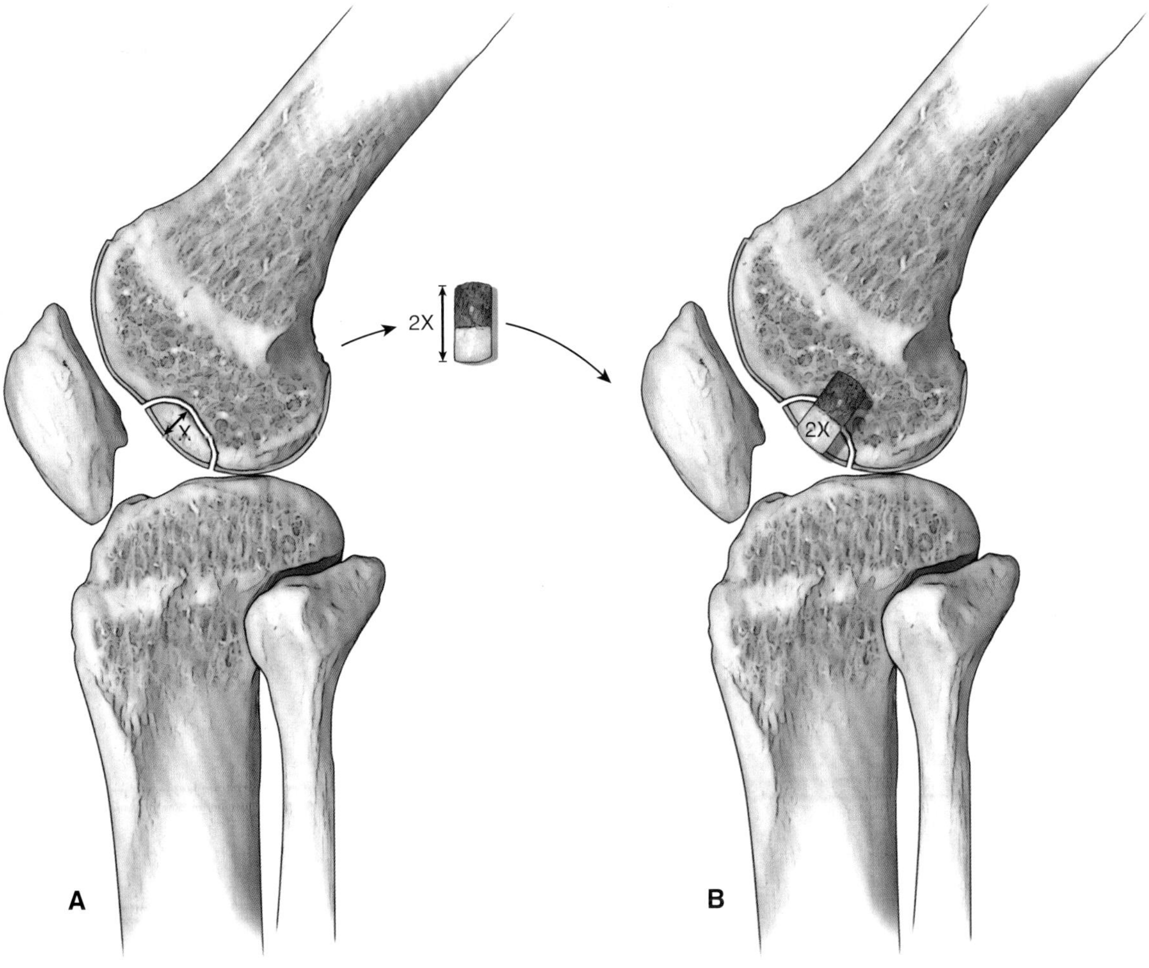

**TECH FIG 4** • **A.** Depth of lesion at midpoint (X). **B.** Length of bone plug and drill hole, which should be twice that of X.

- Using a 4.5-mm mosaicplasty drill and delivery guide, the bone plugs are inserted into the center of the lesion—or various locations depending on the number of plugs used.
  - Care must be taken to ensure that the osteochondral plug is not proud and there is clear cartilage congruence compared to the adjacent cartilage.
- The joint is inspected before final closure.
- The arthroscopic instrumentation is removed, and the arthroscopic portals are closed.
- The knee is placed in a hinged knee brace.

## PEARLS AND PITFALLS

| | |
|---|---|
| **Surgical technique** | ■ Careful review of all prior imaging modalities and a complete clinical evaluation is performed before surgery. |
| **Transarticular drilling** | ■ The Kirschner wires should be kept as perpendicular to the lesion as possible to prevent undermining the lesion. This technique is indicated for intact OCD lesions. |
| **Matchstick technique** | ■ Care should be taken when establishing the harvest site on the medial aspect of the tibia to avoid and not compromise the insertion of the pes anserinus. |
| **Autologous osteochondral grafting technique** | ■ To assure rigid fixation the graft should be passed into the normal underlying subchondral bone as far it had been passed through the lesion and the interface. |

## POSTOPERATIVE CARE

- Our postoperative rehabilitative protocol is outlined in Table 2.

## OUTCOMES

- Nonsurgical treatment is often regarded as the treatment of choice for small stable lesions in skeletally immature patients. Typically, a period of 3 to 6 months of nonoperative treatment is instituted, with numerous authors reporting a success rate of 50% to 94%.[1,2,6,7]
- Skeletally immature patients with wide open physes and no signs of instability on MRI are more likely to respond to nonoperative measures.
- Drilling
  - Both retroarticular drilling and transarticular drilling appear to have very favorable short-term clinical outcomes. Transarticular drilling has been reported as successful in 91% to 100% of patients.[2,7,19] Retroarticular drilling has similar success rates and been reported as 75% to 96% of cases.[1,11,17]
  - Edmonds et al[11] in the largest OCD case series reviewed 59 knees in 53 children with retroarticular drilling after 6 months conservative management reported complete radiographic healing in only 75% of cases but found complete resolution of pain and full return to activities in all patients after treatment. However, 13% of patients did require a repeat surgery.
  - Boughanem et al[6] retrospectively reviewed 34 knees in 31 children treated with arthroscopic retroarticular drilling and noted that 95% of patients had radiologic improvement.
  - Kocher et al[19] reviewed 30 knees in 23 patients treated with arthroscopic transarticular drilling after 6 months of conservative therapy. All patients who failed to respond to nonoperative measures were noted to have healed after drilling.
- Screw fixation
  - Kouzelis et al[20] reported successful fixation of unstable lesions in patients aged 14 to 26 years old using variable pitch screw fixation. In this small series of 10 patients, with a mean follow-up of 27 months, radiologic union was observed in 9/10 patients and return to previous level of activity was also seen in 9/10 patients.
  - In contrast to the variable pitch screw, Cugat et al[10] report on a small series of 14 patients (15 knees), with OCD lesions using cannulated screws as a means of fixation. In this series, there was a mean follow-up of 43 months, and Cugat et al[10] reported good to excellent results in 93% of this series with minimal complications.
- Matchstick technique
  - Navarro et al[23] describe this technique in a series of 11 patients aged 11 to 20 years old with OCD, with a mean follow-up of 48 months. With satisfactory results in 90% of cases, Navarro et al[23] state the advantages of this technique include obviation of large incisions or arthrotomy, solid fixation, and no need for hardware removal.
- Autologous osteochondral grafting
  - Miniaci and Tytherleigh-Strong[22] report on a series of 20 patients (age range of 12 to 27 years) with OCD of the knee who underwent autogenous osteochondral grafting (mosaicplasty) technique. Similar to other reports using fixation with mosaicplasty,[5,18] the series of Miniaci and Tytherleight-Strong[22] series showed excellent 1 year outcomes.

**Table 2 Rehabilitation Protocol following Fixation of Unstable Skeletally Immature Osteochondritis Dissecans**

| | |
|---|---|
| **Phase I** (wk 1–6) | 1. Use of hinged brace for 6 wk, locked in extension for walking<br>2. Home physical therapy: unlock or remove brace to perform ROM, straight-leg raises<br>3. WBAT with brace locked in extension |
| **Phase II**[*] (wk 6–12) | 1. Brace removed<br>2. WBAT without brace: activities of daily living, no running or jumping<br>3. Physical therapy ROM, straight-leg raises, modalities |
| **Phase III**[††] (wk 8–12) | 1. Weight-bearing exercises, sport-specific exercises<br>2. Gradual return to spot |

[*] Follow-up x-ray performed prior to phase III. If healed, phase III is initiated. If unhealed, phase II is repeated.
[††] ROM, range of motion; WBAT, weight-bearing as tolerated.

## COMPLICATIONS

- Primary complications include the potential failure to heal, especially in older adolescents treated nonsurgically.
- The prognosis for OCD lesions is worse in those patients who have reached skeletal maturity.

- Patients who have been treated nonsurgically and have not shown progressive healing and those patients with large lesions that are approaching skeletal maturity are therefore treated surgically to promote healing.

## REFERENCES


1. Adachi N, Deie M, Nakamae A, et al. Functional and radiographic outcome of stable juvenile osteochondritis dissecans of the knee treated with retroarticular drilling without bone grafting. Arthroscopy 2009;25(2):145–152.
2. Aglietti P, Buzzi R, Bassi PB, et al. Arthroscopic drilling in juvenile osteochondritis dissecans of the medial femoral condyle. Arthroscopy 1994;10(3):286–291.
3. Aichroth P. Osteochondritis dissecans of the knee. A clinical survey. J Bone Joint Surg Br 1971;53(3):440–447.
4. American Academy Orthopaedic Surgeons. The Diagnosis and Treatment of Osteochondritis Dissecans: Guideline and Evidence Report. Rosemont, IL: American Academy of Orthopaedic Surgeons, 2010. http://www.aaos.org/research/guidelines/guide.asp. Accessed June 11, 2014.
5. Berlet GC, Mascia A, Miniaci A. Treatment of unstable osteochondritis dissecans lesions of the knee using autogenous osteochondral grafts (mosaicplasty). Arthroscopy 1999;15(3):312–316.
6. Boughanem J, Riaz R, Patel RM, et al. Functional and radiographic outcomes of juvenile osteochondritis dissecans of the knee treated with extra-articular retrograde drilling. Am J Sports Med 2011;39(10):2212–2217.
7. Bradley J, Dandy DJ. Results of drilling osteochondritis dissecans before skeletal maturity. J Bone Joint Surg 1989;71(4):642–644.
8. Conrad JM, Stanitski CL. Osteochondritis dissecans: Wilson's sign revisited. Am J Sports Med 2003;31(5):777–778.
9. Conway FM. Osteochondritis dissecans: description of the stages of the condition and its probable traumatic etiology. Am J Surg 1937;38(3):691–699.
10. Cugat R, Garcia M, Cusco X, et al. Osteochondritis dissecans: a historical review and its treatment with cannulated screws. Arthroscopy 1993;9(6):675–684.
11. Edmonds EW, Albright J, Bastrom T, et al. Outcomes of extra articular, intra-epiphyseal drilling for osteochondritis dissecans of the knee. J Pediatr Orthop 2010;30(8):870–878.
12. Fairbanks H. Osteo-chondritis dissecans. Br Journal Surg 1933;21(81): 67–82.
13. Green JP. Osteochondritis dissecans of the knee. J Bone Joint Surg Br 1966;48(1):82–91.
14. Green WT, Banks HH. Osteochondritis dissecans in children. J Bone Joint Surg Am 1953;35-A(1):26–47.
15. Hefti F, Beguiristain J, Krauspe R, et al. Osteochondritis dissecans: a multicenter study of the European Pediatric Orthopedic Society. J Pediatr Orthop B 1999;8(4):231–245.
16. Hughes JA, Cook JV, Churchill MA, et al. Juvenile osteochondritis dissecans: a 5-year review of the natural history using clinical and MRI evaluation. Pediatr Radiol 2003;33(6):410–417.
17. Kawasaki K, Uchio Y, Adachi N, et al. Drilling from the intercondylar area for treatment of osteochondritis dissecans of the knee joint. Knee 2003;10(3):257–263.
18. Kobayashi T, Fujikawa K, Oohashi M. Surgical fixation of massive osteochondritis dissecans lesion using cylindrical osteochondral plugs. Arthroscopy 2004;20(9):981–986.
19. Kocher MS, Micheli LJ, Yaniv M, et al. Functional and radiographic outcome of juvenile osteochondritis dissecans of the knee treated with transarticular arthroscopic drilling. Am J Sports Med 2001;29(5): 562–566.
20. Kouzelis A, Plessas S, Papadopoulos AX, et al. Herbert screw fixation and reverse guided drillings, for treatment of types III and IV osteochondritis dissecans. Knee Surg Sports Traumatol Arthrosc 2006;14(1):70–75.
21. Lindén B. The incidence of osteochondritis dissecans in the condyles of the femur. Acta Orthop Scand 1976;47(6):664–667.
22. Miniaci A, Tytherleigh-Strong G. Fixation of unstable osteochondritis dissecans lesions of the knee using arthroscopic autogenous osteochondral grafting (mosaicplasty). Arthroscopy 2007;23(8):845–851.
23. Navarro R, Cohen M, Filho MC, et al. The arthroscopic treatment of osteochondritis dissecans of the knee with autologous bone sticks. Arthroscopy 2002;18(8):840–844.
24. Paget J. On the production of some of the loose bodies in joints. St Bartholomew's Hosp Rep 1870;6:1–4.
25. Research in osteochondritis dissecans of the knee Web site. http://kneeocd.org. Accessed January 23, 2014.
26. Ribbing S. The hereditary multiple epiphyseal disturbance and its consequences for the aetiogenesis of local malacias—particularly the osteochondrosis dissecans. Acta Orthop Scand 1955;24(4):286–299.
27. Smillie IS. Treatment of osteochondritis dissecans. J Bone Joint Surg Br 1957;39-B(2):248–260.
28. Uozumi H, Sugita T, Aizawa T, et al. Histologic findings and possible causes of osteochondritis dissecans of the knee. Am J Sports Med 2009;37(10):2003–2008.
29. Wilson JN. A diagnostic sign in osteochondritis dissecans of the knee. J Bone Joint Surg Am 1967;49(3):477–480.

CHAPTER 48

# Meniscoplasty for Discoid Lateral Meniscus

Jay C. Albright

## DEFINITION

- A discoid meniscus is abnormal in both thickness and amount of covering or interposition of the compartment or plateau.
- Over 99% of cases occur on the lateral side of the knee, with an overall incidence of 1% to 15% of the general population.
- Ten percent of children found to have a discoid meniscus will have it bilaterally.

## ANATOMY

- Three types of discoid meniscus are described: complete (covering entire compartment), incomplete (on partial compartment covering), and Wrisberg (complete or incomplete compartment covering with no peripheral attachments).[5]
- Wrisberg type is by definition unstable, allowing displacement, popping, and locking as well.

## PATHOGENESIS

- It arises either congenitally or through abnormal development. No cases have been found in autopsies of fetal deaths or stillborns.

## NATURAL HISTORY

- Discoid menisci have frequently been found at autopsy in elderly, reportedly asymptomatic people.
- Frequently, it is an incidental finding.
- Symptoms typically present in the late first or early second decade of life but may occur at any age.[6]
- Symptoms are pain with or without loss of motion.

## PATIENT HISTORY AND PHYSICAL FINDINGS

- The common presentation is a young child (younger than 10 years) with a catch or popping of the lateral side of the knee with motion, with or without pain.
- Some patients describe true mechanical locking symptoms.
- The patient may present with painful or painless loss of motion.
- The clinical examination may show a hypermobile lateral meniscus with palpable, audible, and frequently visual meniscal instability.
- Effusion is a common finding. Objective signs of swelling with or without activity indicate irritation of the joint and possible tearing.
- Loss of extension and joint line tenderness are also common.[4]
- A discoid meniscus with a tear or instability will click or pop and may be uncomfortable. The results of the McMurray test will help with diagnosis.
  - Positive: pain and a pop or click
  - Negative: no pain and no pop or click
  - Equivocal: pop or click or pain without the other
- Significant mobility of the lateral meniscus, although not uncommon, normally may indicate a discoid meniscus.
- In children, varus instability may be due to accommodation of the large discoid lateral meniscus. Collateral ligament test results are important.
  - Normal: symmetric to the opposite side
  - Mild: 1 to 3 mm of increased laxity from the opposite side

## IMAGING AND OTHER DIAGNOSTIC STUDIES

- Radiographs may show flattening or sloping of the lateral femoral condyle, with widening of the lateral compartment compared to the medial compartment (**FIG 1A**).
- Magnetic resonance imaging (MRI) will show the discoid meniscus the best (**FIG 1B**).
  - A discoid meniscus will be thicker and wider than a normal meniscus.
  - Frequently, signal change is present in the center of the discoid meniscus; this could represent a tear or degenerative tissue.[1]
  - There should be no more than three consecutive 3-mm cuts of the body of a meniscus on the sagittal view before

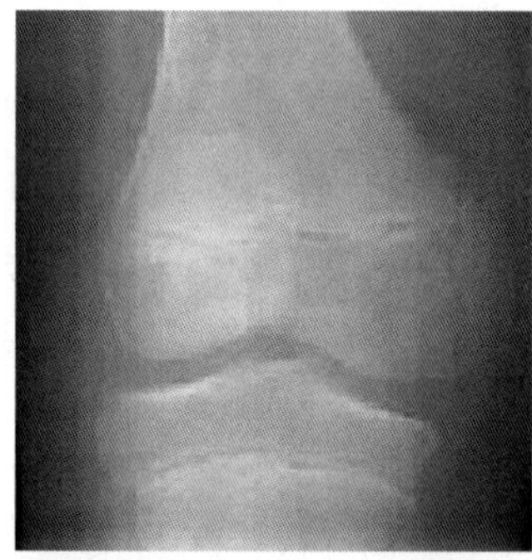

A

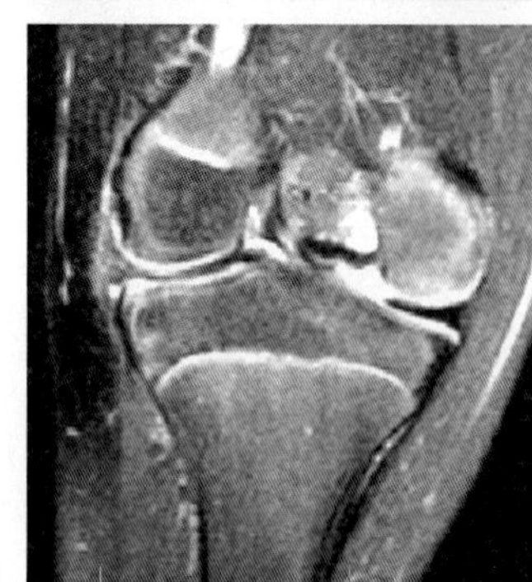

B

**FIG 1** • **A.** Radiographs may show no significant changes, although there may be a widened lateral joint on weight-bearing views, and relative flattening of the lateral femoral condyle may be present. **B.** MRI shows the discoid meniscus clearly with a thickened, wide meniscus that also has abnormal signal intensity throughout the lateral meniscus.

it is separated into an anterior and posterior horn. Coronal cuts may also show a wide, thickened meniscus (more than 12 to 15 mm).

## DIFFERENTIAL DIAGNOSIS

- Meniscal cyst
- Tear in a normal meniscus
- Anterior cruciate ligament tear
- Hypermobile lateral meniscus
- Osteochondritis dissecans
- Patellofemoral instability or dislocation

## NONOPERATIVE MANAGEMENT

- If there is no loss of motion or locking, a period of nonoperative management is the first line of defense.
- Nonoperative treatment consists of activity modifications, anti-inflammatory medications, and swelling control (ice, elevation, and compression).
- Patients with intermittent symptoms only that can be controlled with mild doses of nonsteroidal anti-inflammatories are candidates for nonoperative management.

## SURGICAL MANAGEMENT

- If locking, loss of motion, or persistent pain and disability exists despite nonoperative management, surgical intervention is indicated.[3]

### Preoperative Planning

- The surgeon should review imaging studies to evaluate the likelihood of a tear or the presence of other pathology.
- The knee examination is repeated under anesthesia, including ligamentous testing, range of motion, and the McMurray test to evaluate whether significant lateral meniscal instability is present.
- May indicate higher likelihood of the Wrisberg type of discoid meniscus

### Positioning

- The patient is positioned supine.
- A tourniquet is placed on the proximal thigh of the operative leg over padding.
- A leg holder is placed over the tourniquet.
- The opposite leg is padded and is placed in slight flexion at the hip.
- The foot of the bed is flexed 90 degrees, allowing both legs to flex 90 degrees over the edge of the table.

### Approach

- Three standard arthroscopic portals are established with a no. 11 blade through stab incisions: inferolateral parapatellar portal for scope visualization, inferomedial parapatellar portal for instruments, and lateral suprapatellar pouch portal for outflow.
- An accessory anterolateral portal may be established for another working portal.
- If the remnant of the discoid meniscus is unstable or torn, requiring fixation or stabilization, a posterolateral approach should be made for inside-out suture fixation.
- A lateral incision is made from the joint line distally by 2 cm, longitudinally in line with the posterior aspect of the fibular head.
- The interval between the biceps femoris and the iliotibial band is entered, as is the space deep to the lateral head of the gastrocnemius.
- A posterior knee retractor is placed in this interval as far medially as possible to protect the neurovascular bundle.

TECHNIQUES

## Arthroscopic Saucerization of a Discoid Lateral Meniscus

- After systematic arthroscopic evaluation of the knee is performed, the lateral compartment is opened in the figure-4 position.
- The type of discoid meniscus is determined using a probe sequentially over and under the posterior horn of the meniscus, pulling forward to evaluate displacement.
- Displacement of more than 40% to 50% anteriorly is unstable and requires stabilization with suture fixation.
- Determining peripheral instability may be difficult until the meniscoplasty is at least partly completed.
- Starting in the notch, the free edge of the discoid meniscus is identified (**TECH FIG 1A–C**).
- At this point, an arthroscopic basket or a meniscal knife can be used to incise and remove the meniscus coronally from the notch toward the body of the meniscus.
- The surgeon should stop about 15 mm from the lateral edge of the meniscus to leave ample residual rim.
- A combination of arthroscopic baskets (angled, straight, upbiters, backbiters, and 90-degree side biters) and shaver is employed to piecemeal the posterior and anterior aspects of the discoid meniscus (**TECH FIG 1D–G**).
  - A meniscal rim of about 15 mm is maintained.
- Attempts to thin the remainder of the thickened remnant should be done with care but can be performed with an aggressive shaver, baskets, or both.[2]

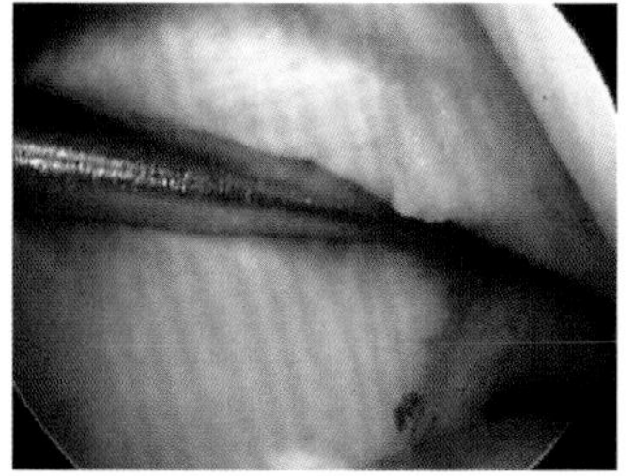


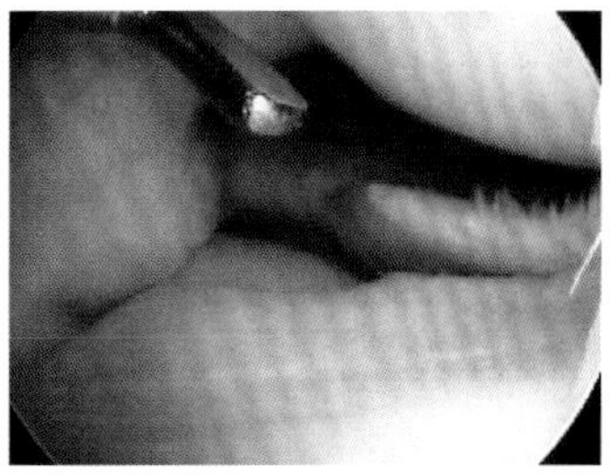


**TECH FIG 1** • Complete discoid lateral meniscus, visualization, and probing of anterior cruciate ligament (**A**) and complete discoid with a tear visualized through the notch (**B**). *(continued)*

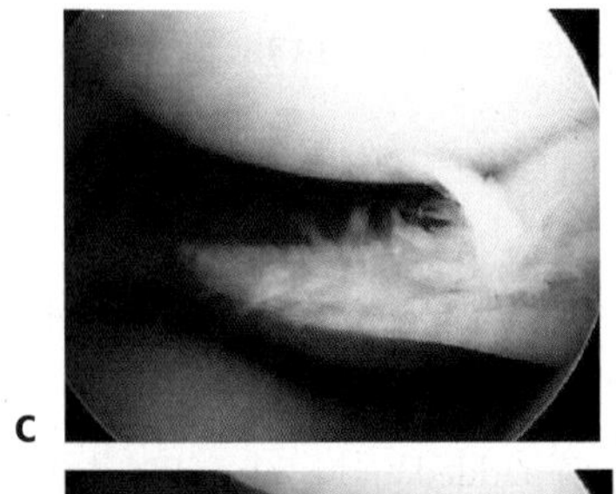
C

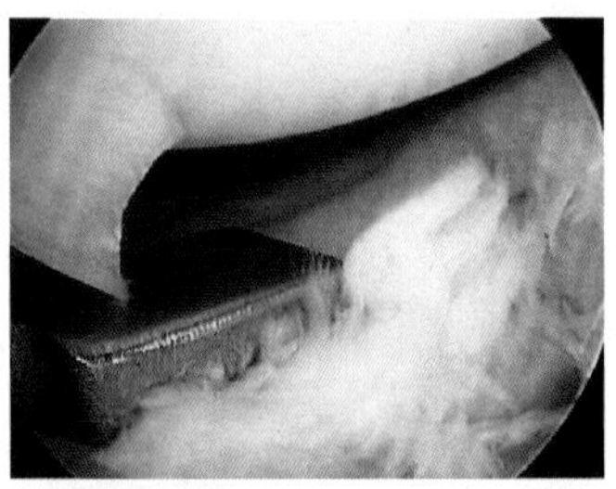
D

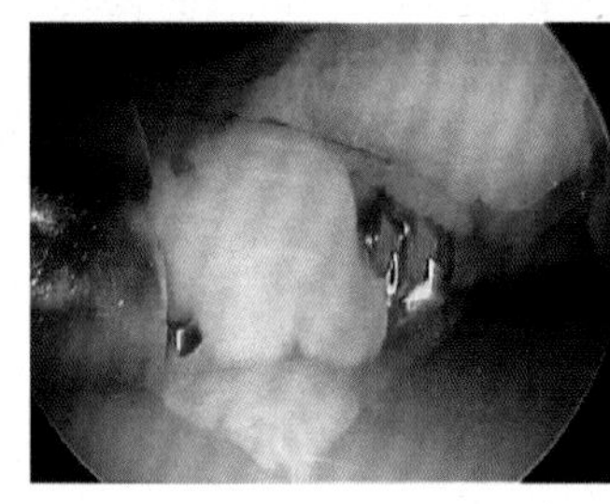
E

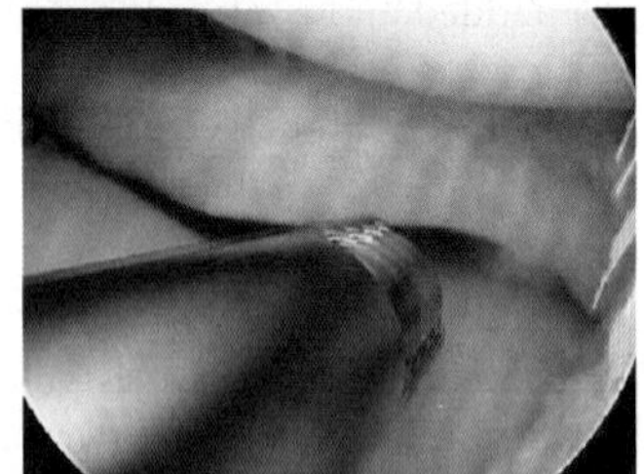
F

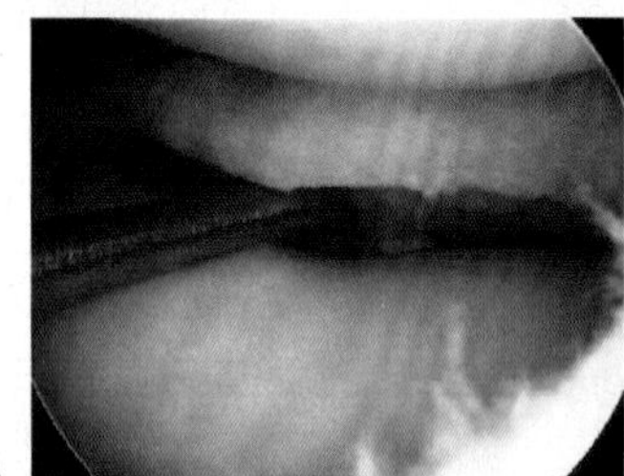
G

**TECH FIG 1** • *(continued)* **C.** Evaluation of the depth of the tear. **D.** Initiation of saucerization through access point of the notch. **E.** Use of a shaver to remove loose pieces as well as shape the meniscus. **F.** Final appearance after saucerization. **G.** When the meniscus is unstable, suture techniques may be necessary for stabilization, as demonstrated with repeat probing after one all-inside device was needed to stabilize this meniscus.

## Alternative Technique for Meniscoplasty

- The accessory anterolateral portal is made under direct visualization to ensure that there is no inadvertent damage of the peripheral meniscus.
- The free edge of the discoid meniscus is grabbed with an arthroscopic locking grasper through the medial portal.
- A meniscal knife is carefully placed through the accessory lateral portal, ideally with a protective cannula or a sheath.
- Under tension, the discoid meniscus is incised from the anterior notch, leaving about 15 mm of anterior rim, directed toward the junction of the anterior horn and body.
- The surgeon should keep in mind the normal curved architecture of the meniscus.
- At this point, the surgeon may need to regrasp the free edge of the discoid meniscus closer to the leading edge of the incised meniscus.
- The knife is then turned to cut along the body of the meniscus.
- The surgeon amputates and removes the flap of the cut discoid, leaving the posterior portion of the discoid left to finish.
- The surgeon piecemeals the remaining excess posterior aspect of the discoid with arthroscopic biters and shaver.
- The remnant is smoothed or thinned with a shaver, biters, or both.

## PEARLS AND PITFALLS

| | |
|---|---|
| **Indications** | ■ Locking, loss of motion, or persistent pain |
| **Portal placement** | ■ Accessory portals are potentially dangerous; they should be placed under direct arthroscopic vision and control.<br>■ A spinal needle is used to identify the level of portal before making the incision. |
| **Meniscal handling** | ■ The abnormal meniscus is typically difficult to handle arthroscopically owing to its thickness. All the tools at the surgeon's disposal (biters, shaver, meniscal knives) should be used to shape the meniscus. |
| **Failure to recognize instability** | ■ Snapping or pain may be due to a tear of the discoid or an unstable variant.<br>■ It may be difficult to identify some unstable menisci on initial evaluation.<br>■ After saucerization is underway or completed, probing and stability testing are repeated to ensure that an unstable variant or tear is not missed. |
| **Failure of stabilization** | ■ Stabilization of a congenitally unstable meniscus may fail even with meticulous technique.<br>■ All inside techniques are less successful when used for the lateral meniscus, especially with larger tears.<br>■ Inside-out technique should be used when an unstable or Wrisberg variant is encountered.<br>■ The surgeon should rasp, irritate, or freshen the vascular portion of the meniscus and the synovial lining of the lateral compartment before fixation. |
| **Leaving the right amount** | ■ The surgeon should aim to leave about 8 mm of meniscus behind. |

## POSTOPERATIVE CARE

- Weight bearing depends on whether a meniscal repair or stabilization was performed. Immediate weight bearing as tolerated with crutches may be instituted if the discoid meniscus was saucerized only.
- If a stabilization or repair was needed, touchdown weight bearing with crutches, or wheelchair non–weight bearing for young children, is maintained for 4 to 6 weeks.
- Immediate motion (at least 0 to 90 degrees) should be initiated in all children, with full range of motion for saucerization without repair.
- An Ace bandage is used for edema control as needed.
- Bracing is typically not needed. For repairs or stabilizations to limit meniscal stress, a range-of-motion brace (0 to 90 degrees) may be used.
- Physical therapy is useful for obtaining range of motion as well as initiation of quadriceps activation and strengthening.

## COMPLICATIONS

- Infection
- Arthrofibrosis
- Iatrogenic damage
- Subtotal or total meniscectomy
- Nerve or peroneal damage
- Failure of stabilization or repair
- Additional surgery

## REFERENCES


1. Araki Y, Ashikaga R, Fujii K, et al. MR imaging of meniscal tears with discoid lateral meniscus. Eur J Radiol 1998;27:153–160.
2. Dimakopoulos P, Patel D. Partial excision of discoid meniscus. Arthroscopic operation of 10 patients. Acta Orthop Scand 1990;61: 40–41.
3. Good CR, Green DW, Griffith MH, et al. Arthroscopic treatment of symptomatic discoid meniscus in children: classification, technique, and results. Arthroscopy 2007;23:157–163.
4. Habata T, Uematsu K, Kasanami R, et al. Long-term clinical and radiographic follow-up of total resection for discoid lateral meniscus. Arthroscopy 2006;22:1339–1343.
5. Klingele KE, Kocher MS, Hresko MT, et al. Discoid lateral meniscus: prevalence of peripheral rim instability. J Pediatr Orthop 2004;24: 79–82.
6. Rao PS, Rao SK, Paul R. Clinical, radiologic, and arthroscopic assessment of discoid lateral meniscus. Arthroscopy 2001;17:275–277.

# Osteochondritis Dissecans and Large Osteochondral Defects of the Knee

Kevin G. Shea, John Polousky, and Noah Archibald-Seiffer

## DEFINITION

- Osteochondritis dissecans (OCD) is a focal idiopathic alteration of subchondral bone with risk for instability and disruption of adjacent articular cartilage that may result in premature osteoarthritis.
- OCD and other traumatic injuries can lead to large osteochondral defects of the knee.

## ANATOMY

- Many of these injuries will include the medial or lateral femoral condyle, in both OCD and acute cartilage injury.

## PATHOGENESIS

- The etiology of OCD is not known, although many theories have been suggested, including trauma, vascular anomaly/injury, overuse or repetitive stress injury, genetic predisposition, etc.
- Acute traumatic injuries can cause displacement of preexisting OCD lesions or the development of acutely displaced cartilage fragment on otherwise normal bone and cartilage structures.

## NATURAL HISTORY

- The natural history of OCD runs a variable course.
- Many patients, especially those who are skeletally immature, with significant growth remaining, have good potential for healing with appropriate activity modification, and in select cases, subchondral bone drilling.
- Patients close to or beyond skeletal maturity have a worse prognosis for healing with activity modifications.
- The older patients may not respond to less invasive surgeries such as subchondral bone drilling.
- Patients with acute, traumatic cartilage injury with displaced fragments may be candidates for surgery.
- Cases in which the cartilage damage is so severe that the fragment is unsalvageable, osteochondral defects may be addressed with a variety of cartilage restoration procedures.
  - This chapter focuses on the use osteochondral allografts to address these large, irreparable defects.

## PATIENT HISTORY AND PHYSICAL FINDINGS

- Review of previous imaging studies (typically radiographs and/or magnetic resonance imaging [MRI]), operative reports, and arthroscopic imaging is critical in the evaluation of these patients. In many of these patients, previous surgery and arthroscopic imaging have been performed. Reviewing these studies can provide useful information about the location, depth, and perimeter of the lesion (**FIG 1**).
- The presence of a "kissing lesion" on the opposite articular surface is important, as its presence may alter or preclude certain allograft approaches. Significant osteoarthritis, especially if more diffuse, rather than focal, may be a contraindication to osteochondral allograft use.
- Patient factors: Individual patient factors, including patient preferences, alignment of the lower extremities, social resources, work/job demands, and medical comorbidities must be considered when evaluating these patients. Some research has also shown factors such as age older than 30 years and a history of two or more previous surgeries on the joint are associated with poorer outcomes.[14]
- In patients with more advanced osteochondral pathology, the history frequently includes episodes of pain, mechanical symptoms, giving way, and swelling. Both traumatic injuries and patients with OCD may present after months or years of milder symptoms.
  - These patients may describe the feeling of a loose body within the joint that can occasionally be palpated on the anterior aspect of the knee.
  - Notable findings include effusion, joint line tenderness, and, in some cases, a mobile free body may be palpated.

## IMAGING AND OTHER DIAGNOSTIC STUDIES

- The most valuable tools for evaluating osteochondral lesions are high-quality imaging studies, the most basic of which is the weight bearing, plain radiograph of the knee. The authors prefer standing anteroposterior, tunnel, lateral, and Merchant views.
- A wealth of information can be gleaned from properly performed radiographs, including the approximate dimensions and location of the lesion and the precedence of diffuse osteoarthritis. Long-standing radiographs are valuable in assessing limb length discrepancy and malalignment.

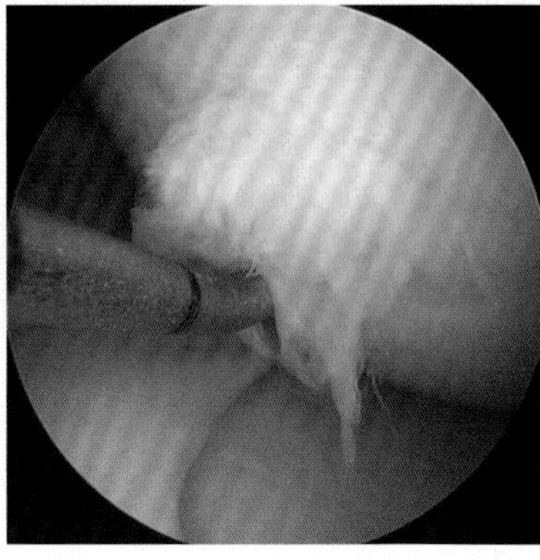

**FIG 1** • Arthroscopic view of failed microfracture, subsequent allograft.

- MRI provides a more detailed look at the condition of the lesion and surrounding cartilage. The MRI may also reveal kissing lesions, in which there is chondral injury on opposing articular surfaces. Careful inspection for malalignment, kissing lesions, or signs of more diffuse cartilage injury is essential, as these factors may change the surgical management of the patient.[14] The lesions are less common in younger patients but may increase in frequency in older patients or those with a prolonged history of symptoms.

## DIFFERENTIAL DIAGNOSIS

- OCD
- Acute osteochondral fracture
- Osteochondral defect

## NONOPERATIVE MANAGEMENT

- Nonoperative management may consist of activity modifications, maintenance of ideal body weight, and low-impact conditioning programs.
- Significant mechanical symptoms may not be addressed with this approach.

## SURGICAL MANAGEMENT

- With regard to stable OCD lesions, many procedures are designed to promote healing, including subchondral drilling, both antegrade[11,15,24] and retrograde.[26,28] For unstable lesions, drilling in combination with internal fixation, bone grafting, and other procedures may promote healing. Excision of loose fragments may provide reasonable short-term results, but long-term outcomes are generally poor.[17,18] Although less invasive procedures may improve mechanical symptoms, they may not address the long-term impact of the cartilage or bone defect in a weight-bearing region of the joint.
- For patients in whom native cartilage and bone cannot be successfully repaired, or those that have failed previous attempts at repair of native tissue, osteochondral allograft is one option to be considered. Other options to be considered for cartilage loss are outlined in the following text, although some of them may have limitations especially in larger lesions and those with deep subchondral bone loss.
- For patients that have focal, full-thickness cartilage defects, several techniques can be used to restore the joint cartilage surface. These techniques include the following:
  - Marrow stimulation (microfracture)
  - Osteochondral autograft transfer (OAT)
  - Cell-based therapies, including autologous cartilage amplification and implantation
  - Osteochondral allograft implantation

### Marrow Stimulation

- Marrow stimulation, although relatively simple to perform, has several limitations.
- Clot formation secondary to marrow stimulation produces disorganized fibrocartilage characterized by a high concentration of type I collagen rather than type II collagen, which comprises hyaline cartilage.
- Fibrocartilage lacks the mechanical integrity and ultrastructural organization of hyaline cartilage and often deteriorates after a few years.[9]
- In addition to poor wear properties, the fibrocartilage formed after marrow stimulation may not restore congruity of the articular surface in cases of OCD, where loss of the subchondral bone and débridement of fibrous tissue results in a deep crater with significant bone loss.
- Restoring this subchondral bone loss can present many challenges to the surgeon, both with microfracture, and other cartilage restoration procedures.[21]

### Osteochondral Autograft

- OAT may have some advantages for treating OCD, as it can directly address the loss/abnormalities of subchondral bone.
- The depth of the osteochondral autograft donor plug can be adjusted to fill the entire defect with viable bone and articular cartilage, which has the capacity to integrate with the adjacent tissue.
- There are limitations to the OAT procedure.
  - Large defects cannot be filled due to donor site morbidity, and there may be problems with articular cartilage incongruence.
  - The technique precludes filling the entire defect when multiple grafts are used and fibrocartilage forms around the periphery of the grafts.
- Wang[27] and Horas et al[10] reported poor results when osteochondral autografting was used to treat lesions[24] larger than 6 cm.
- This approach may be reasonable for smaller OCD lesions. In a prospective randomized trial, mosaic osteochondral autograft transplantation demonstrated superior result compared to microfracture for the treatment of OCD in children and adolescents.[9]
  - At an average follow-up of 4.2 years, 63% of the microfracture group had good or excellent outcomes, but this group had some deterioration in outcome over 1 to 4 years.
  - For the mosaic osteochondral autograft transplantation group, 83% had good or excellent outcomes.
  - There were 41% failures in the microfracture group compared with none in the mosaic osteochondral autograft transplantation group at the final follow-up.
  - Consequently, in lesions that are small, mosaic osteochondral autograft transplantation is a reasonable procedure that produces outcomes that are superior to microfracture.
  - As mentioned, one challenge with mosaic osteochondral autograft transplantation is donor site morbidity as well as the differences in cartilage thickness in donor and recipient sites.

### Autologous Cartilage Implantation

- The use of autologous cartilage implantation (ACI) has been reported for treatment of OCD.[23]
- The subchondral bone abnormalities may present special challenges to ACI techniques.
- Due to the loss and/or abnormalities of the subchondral bone base, special ACI approaches have been developed.
  - Collagen-covered ACI (ACI-C) has been described in a case series, showing positive clinical results at 4 years, but most cases that underwent biopsy revealed fibrocartilage.[12]
  - Another multicenter case series using ACI for OCD demonstrated significant improvements, but more than a third of patients required secondary surgical débridement.[6]

- In cases in which the subchondral bone is minimally involved, standard ACI may be considered.
- In cases with more significant loss of subchondral bone, staged procedures to supplement regional bone loss may be an option.[14]

## Fresh Osteochondral Allograft

- For larger cartilaginous or osteocartilaginous defects, marrow stimulation, osteochondral autografts, and ACI have limitations.
- Restoring both bone and cartilage loss is especially challenging in larger lesions. Fresh osteochondral allografts address both the cartilage and bone deficits. In addition, osteochondral allografts produce enough graft material to resurface larger lesions.[4]
  - Osteochondral allograft transplantation has a long history, dating back to 1957, when Smillie proposed its use for OCD.[27] Several centers in North America developed osteochondral allograft transplantation programs in the 1970s.[29]
- The rationale for fresh osteochondral allograft transplantation is to replace diseased, unsalvageable bone, and cartilage defects in the context of an otherwise healthy joint.
  - The living chondrocytes from the transplant become a viable part of the recipient's cartilage matrix, and the transplanted bone is incorporated by the host bone.[3]
  - The osseous component of the graft incorporates in the host bone through creeping substitution, in a manner similar to that seen with bone grafting for bone defects or allograft tumor reconstruction.
- Chondrocytes and cartilage matrix in allograft transplantation generates minimal host immunologic response. The lack host tissue response to the allograft means immune suppression medications are not necessary.
  - Unlike solid organ transplantations, human leukocyte antigen (HLA)/immune marker matching has not been required. In both rat and rabbit models,[13] transplantation of chondrocytes in an intact matrix produced no host cellular immune response. In contrast, when either chondrocytes without matrix or cartilage shavings were transplanted, a host cell-mediated immune response was generated. Furthermore, transplantation of intact cartilage produced no immune response, even in a previously sensitized host.
  - More recently, Williams and colleagues[29] demonstrated no evidence of immune rejection in 26 retrieval specimens, which had failed at a mean survival of 42 months following implantation. These grafts failed for a variety of reasons, but there was no evidence that a host immune response was a contributing factor.
  - Recent studies have used MRI to evaluate host immune response, and in some cases, evidence of humoral immune responses have been suggested. Further research in this area will be helpful to evaluate immune response in grafts.
  - Histologic studies on failed grafts have not identified significant signs of graft rejection, and chondrocytes remain viable for years after implantation.[29]
- Providing viable tissue for treating large cartilage defect includes the transfer of living cartilage cells between the donor and recipient. The need for both thorough testing of donor tissue to ensure recipient safety and rapid turnaround to preserve living tissue must be considered during the harvest and implantation process.
- There is a long history of bone, ligament, and cartilage transplantation, and disease transmission is thought to be exceedingly rare. Unfortunately, a standard reporting system for these events does not exist.
  - A preoperative discussion with the patients, which outlines these risks, is an important part of the informed consent process and patient-centered care.
  - Most tissue banks are members of the American Association of Tissue Banks (AATB), which publishes standards for tissue procurement. These standards include extensive medical history review of donors, serologic testing, bacterial cultures, storage requirements, and expiration periods. The standards for live, fresh osteochondral transfer are critical to ensure that these processes do not significantly alter the viability of the cartilage/chondrocyte tissues. For any practitioner involved with these procedures, a thorough review of the tissue bank accreditation and processes is important.
  - Many steps are taken to ensure graft safety, which include the following:
    - Review of the donor medical record
    - Review of serologies and cultures
  - These processes may require 10 to 14 days. During this interval, chondrocyte preservation is critical. Different preservation solutions include physiologic saline solutions or more complex media that may include amino acids, glucose, and inorganic salts.
- The more complex solutions may increase both quality and duration of chondrocyte viability.[27]
  - Williams et al[30] demonstrated chondrocyte viability to remain unchanged for up to 14 days when preserved in culture medium. These solutions may work optimally for 10 to 14 days, but after this time, chondrocyte viability starts to decrease, with changes in cellular contents, and extracellular matrix.
  - Current AATB requirements include harvest within 24 hours of donor demise and grafts stored at 4° C within culture medium. For these reasons, earlier transplantation within 14 to 28 days may be ideal, after donor testing is completed.
  - Other studies have evaluated the relationship between time of harvest and chondrocyte viability,[1] and early implantation is correlated with higher cell viability, especially at the articular surface of the grafts.[19]
  - Frozen grafts have significantly lower cellular viability compared with fresh, non-frozen grafts.[20]
- The dowel and shell techniques are commonly used in the setting of unsalvageable OCD.[7]
  - Both techniques begin with a medial or lateral parapatellar arthrotomy, and appropriate retractor use precludes the need for patellar dislocation in most cases (**FIG 2**).
  - Unlike posttraumatic chondral defects, which often have associated ligamentous instability and mechanical axis malalignment, OCD is generally a focal defect in an otherwise healthy knee in a younger patient.
  - If associated pathology is present, such as varus or valgus malalignment, or ACL deficiency, many authors agree that these should be addressed in conjunction with osteochondral allografting procedures.[7,24]

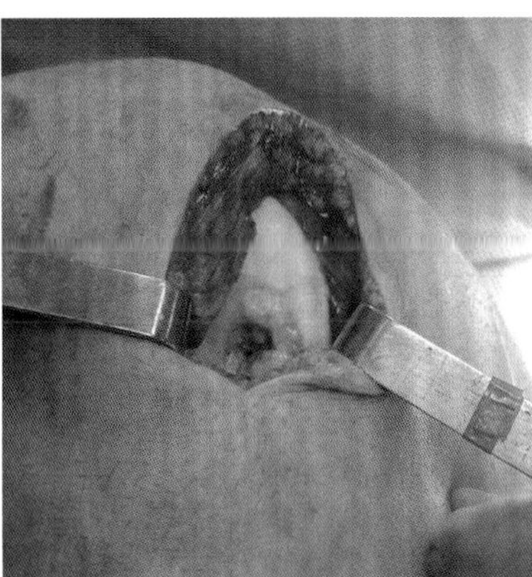

**FIG 2** • Medial parapatellar arthrotomy with retractors.

- As the surgeon gains experiences, more complicated osteochondral techniques may be employed. The techniques are used to address larger lesions or those with irregular contours.
- There are several approaches to larger lesions, including "snowman" and "shell" techniques. Using multiple grafts, the snowman technique can increase the area covered by the dowel graft technique.
  - The dowel technique is simply repeated adjacent to the first graft. The second graft is placed in such a manner that it interdigitates with the first graft.
- Most OCD lesions lend themselves to the single-graft dowel technique, which is relatively straightforward, and we encourage surgeons to perform this both with sawbone skill sessions and cadaver labs, prior to clinical use. Participation with an experienced surgeon for the first several cases may also be advantageous.
- Several companies provide instrumentation for these dowel procedures to allow a size-matched press-fit technique. Steps in the process are well outlined in these instrumentation sets.

## Preoperative Planning

- Patient-centered decision making is a critical part of the planning process. A thorough discussion of the risk, benefit, and alternatives are important. Risks associated with allograft tissue, including disease transmission, need to be reviewed with the patients.
- If the patient is interested in proceeding with an allograft, the first step is to confirm an anatomic match between the donor and recipient anatomy, based on donor and recipient radiographs and/or MRI. Although these measurements may not ensure exact matching, the assessment should show minimal deviations of a few millimeters or less in the frontal and coronal planes. After confirmation of anatomic match is completed, surgery scheduling may proceed.
- Evaluation of the lower extremity alignment is an important step, as significant deformities may require surgery to address alignment. Preoperative clinical evaluations, and if indicated, appropriate alignment images may be helpful in surgical planning. Examination under anesthesia may include the evaluation of ligamentous laxity.

## Positioning

- The patient may be placed in a traditional arthroscopic position, if knee arthroscopy is part of the planned surgery.
- Another option is to position the patient supine, without using an arthroscopic knee holder.
- The lower extremity portion of the operating table is left at full extension rather than using a bend at the knee, which is commonly used in some arthroscopic procedures.
- An adjustable foot rest and thigh post can be used to hold the knee on the table at around 90 degrees of flexion and adjusted for more or less flexion, depending on the location of the lesion on the femoral condyle.
- This position allows for the knee to be held at the appropriate degree of flexion throughout the procedure, to optimize surgical exposure, and allow the surgical assistant to have two free hands to assist with the procedure (**FIG 3**).

## Approach

- In most cases, smaller miniarthrotomies over the medial or lateral condyle are adequate, and patellar dislocation is usually not necessary for exposure.
- The use of Z retractors can improve tissue retraction, allow for excellent exposure, and prepare the recipient bed for the allograft.
- Caution is advised with all retractors to avoid inadvertent injury to other cartilaginous areas about the condyles, tibial plateau, and the patella.
- The use of regular physiologic saline application to the exposed cartilaginous surfaces is also advised.
- Tourniquet use is at the discretion of the surgeon, although in our experience, tourniquets are not routinely used for osteochondral allograft cases.

A

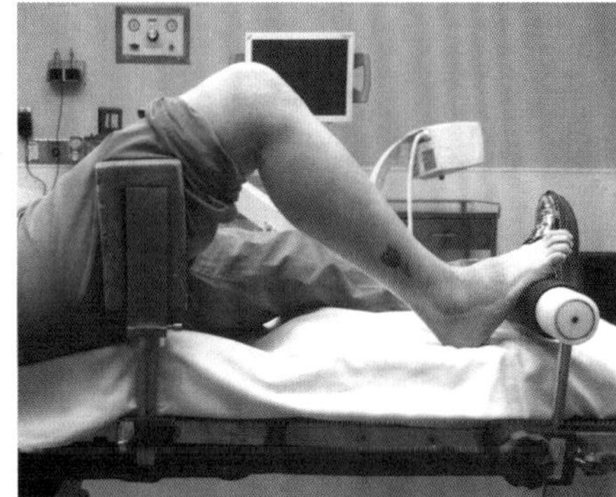

B

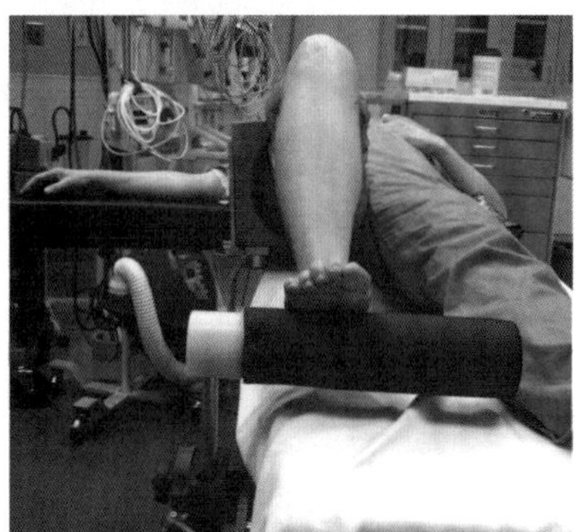

**FIG 3** • Lateral leg holder.

## Dowel Technique

### Recipient Site Reaming

- The technique includes the use of "hole saws" to harvest the graft from the donor and reamers to prepare the recipient bed. Size matching of these instruments is critical to ensure appropriate fit and stability of the allograft.
- The selection of the proper diameter is first determined with a set of sizers. These sizers are placed over the defect to ensure the hole saw will remove the entire defect, leaving a peripheral zone of mostly normal cartilage and bone (**TECH FIG 1A**).
- Once the size is determined, a guide pin is placed through the center of the sizer with the sizer in even contact with the articular surface; this ensures that the trajectory of the reamer is perpendicular to the articular surface.
  - It is critical that this step place the pin as normal as possible to the cartilage surface to ensure both donor and recipient bed have well-matched chondral surface contour.
  - The guide pin is left in place, and the edge of the area to be prepared is scored to prevent peeling of the surrounding cartilage during reaming (**TECH FIG 1B**).
- The corresponding recipient site reamer is selected, and the site is reamed over the guide pin until healthy, bleeding subchondral bone is encountered, generally 7 to 15 mm from the chondral surface (**TECH FIG 1C**).
- We prefer to drill no deeper than necessary to identify viable bone throughout the base of the lesion (**TECH FIG 1D**).
- The vascularity of the recipient bed is best assessed if the tourniquet is not used during the case, and for this reason, we prefer not to use tourniquets during these procedures.
- The visible edge of this reamer has metal-etched markers to look for the depth of penetration circumferentially around the recipient bed. In many cases, the recipient bed depth of penetration is nearly equivalent circumferentially, but in some cases, differences of 1 to 2 mm may occur.
- These differences will be addressed during the preparation of the donor graft.

### Preparation of the Donor Graft

- Following reaming of the recipient site, the 12 o'clock position is marked on the articular surface. Depth measurements are taken and recorded at the 12, 3, 6, and 9 o'clock positions. A written record and diagram of these measurements will be helpful later in the case.
- The donor condyle is now positioned precisely in the drilling jig. This step of the procedure is critical to ensure contour match of the recipient bed and donor graft.
  - Prior to surgery, it is advisable that the surgeon become familiar with the constraints of using this jig and each of the adjustable components for precisely and securing holding the condyle.

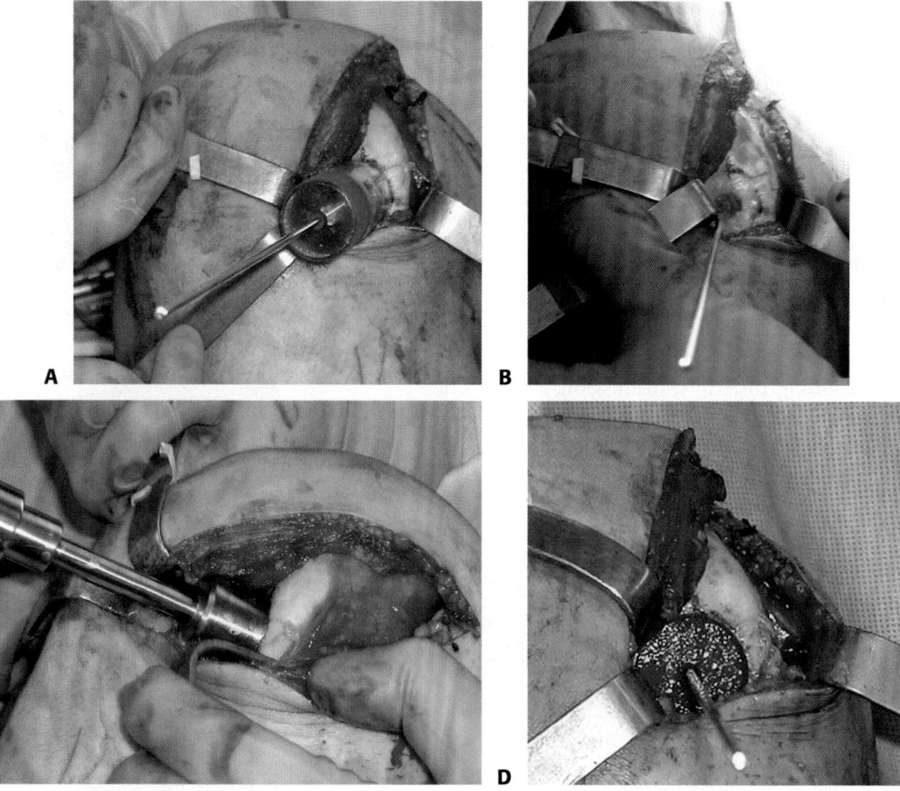

**TECH FIG 1** • **A.** Use of sizing dowel for osteochondral implantation. **B.** Use of guide pin for drilling. **C.** Use of appropriate-sized reamer for drilling donor bed. **D.** View of recipient bed, confirm complete vascularization of the bone.

- The surgeon can compare the size, arc, and width of the harvest site by placing the donor condyle next to the recipient condyle and also using the sizing dowels to ensure the location of harvest is appropriate.
- At least four points of fixation to the graft are ideal to ensure that the graft does not move during the drilling (**TECH FIG 2A**).

- After securing the donor condyle to the jig, the orientation of the hollow saw for drilling is performed. This step is also critical to ensure graft recipient contour match (**TECH FIG 2B**).
- A guide pin can be placed through the sizer to assist with maintaining a perpendicular trajectory with the reamer. Again, the cartilage of the donor is scored, the 12 o'clock position is marked, and the appropriately sized dowel reamer is used to ream the graft.
- The graft is then reamed to a depth well beyond the depth of the recipient site so that it may be trimmed. The graft is then removed from the donor condyle with a sagittal saw, taking care to preserve the appropriate depth (**TECH FIG 2C**).
- Several authors recommend that the osteochondral allograft be limited in depth to approximately 10 mm. This may be related to the clinical observations in tumor allograft surgery that creeping substitution occurs over a limited distance. Levy et al[14] recommends that for recipient depth more than 10 mm, supplemental recipient autograft be used to elevate the depth of the recipient bed to about 10 mm.
- While releasing the graft from the donor condyle, the surgeon should be prepared for the dowel graft to be ejected from the donor condyle, possibly sending the graft to the floor, which significantly complicates this procedure.
- When the dowel is free, the corresponding depths from the 12, 3, 6, and 9 o'clock positions are marked, and the sagittal saw and cutting guide are used to achieve the proper depth (**TECH FIG 2D**).
- Pulsatile irrigation is used to remove marrow elements from the donor bone.

## Graft Placement

- The graft is placed and trimmed if proud.
- Care must be taken to remove the graft for trimming. Forcibly prying the graft out can damage both the recipient site and graft. The blunt end of the guide pin can be placed into the guide pinhole to gently toggle the graft from the recipient site (**TECH FIG 3A**).
- Generally, the graft is very secure with a press-fit. If further fixation is desired, small, absorbable pins may be used.
- Recent studies have suggested that high-impact forces on osteochondral allografts may have an impact on chondrocyte viability.[2] For these reasons, we recommend firm, intermittent pressure, and impact forces as low as possible, rather than significant impacts, to help seat the graft[22] (**TECH FIG 3B**).

A 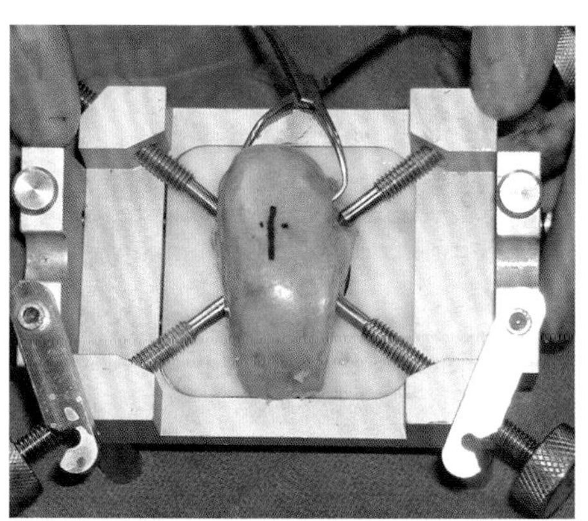

B 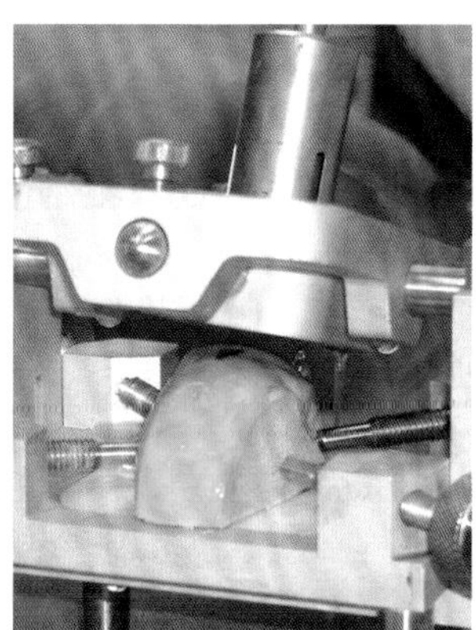

C 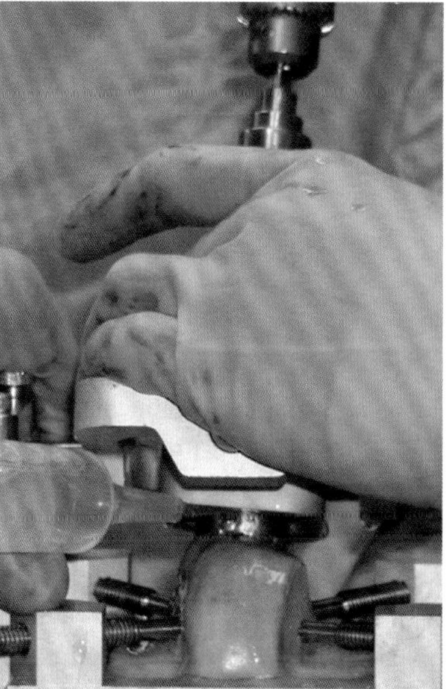

D 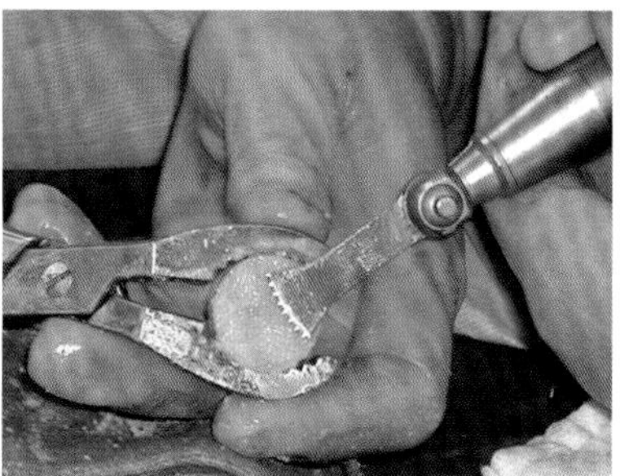

**TECH FIG 2** • **A.** Initial securing of the donor condyle in jig. **B.** Orientation of drill guide. **C.** Drilling the osteochondral allograft for removal from condyle. **D.** Trimming the osteochondral allograft to match the donor bed depth in all four quadrants.

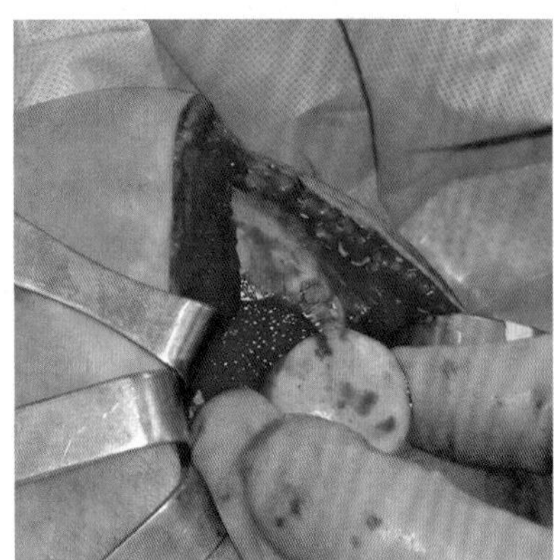
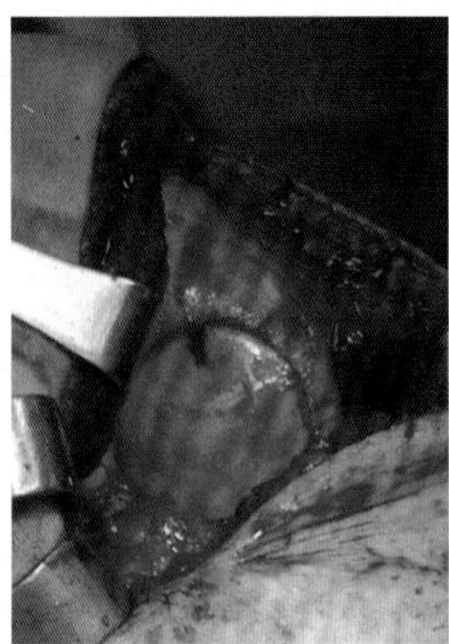

**TECH FIG 3** • **A.** Graft position prior to implantation. Note the 12 o'clock position on the graft to maintain orientation. **B.** Final position of osteochondral implant.

## PEARLS AND PITFALLS

| | |
|---|---|
| MRI sequences may underestimate size of cartilage defect. | ▪ Preoperative evaluation of images is essential for planning. |
| Contours of the graft and recipient do not match. | ▪ Cut the allograft dowel from the same area of the condyle as the recipient site. |
| Graft edges are proud on one side but recessed on another. | ▪ Make sure that both the reaming of the recipient site and allograft dowel are performed at an angle perpendicular to the surrounding articular surface. This can be aided by placing a guide pin in the graft to guide the dowel saw. |
| Graft is uncontained and feels loose after implantation. | ▪ Supplement "press-fit" fixation with small absorbable pins. |
| Mechanical axis malalignment causes overload of the compartment receiving the graft, leading to a higher failure rate. | ▪ Perform a realignment osteotomy as a staged procedure or in conjunction with the osteochondral allograft. |

## POSTOPERATIVE CARE

- Postoperative care consists of immediate range of motion to allow for optimal environment for cartilage healing.
- Deep venous thrombosis (DVT) pharmacologic prophylaxis is not given routinely in younger patients, unless risk factors for DVT exist. The use of DVT prophylaxis continues to evolve, and in some cases, prophylaxis may be advantageous, even in younger patients.
- We encourage early motion in the first 24 hours, and start formal PT-supervised physical therapy sessions at 48 to 72 hours when possible.
- Weight bearing is generally protected for 6 to 12 weeks with resumption of full activity at 4 to 6 months.[7]
- We encourage our patients to develop an exercise fitness lifestyle that emphasizes lower impact exercises, including swimming, cycling, and elliptical training. Although running is not prohibited, we do encourage them to incorporate other lower impact fitness activities.
- We also emphasize optimal body mass index, as this may also have an impact on long-term outcome.

## OUTCOMES

- Good results have been reported using fresh osteochondral allografts for the reconstruction of posttraumatic cartilage defects about the knee.[16,25]
- Emmerson et al[7] reported on the long-term results of fresh osteochondral allografting in a group of patients with the specific diagnosis of OCD.
  - The study group included 66 knees in 64 patients, with a mean age of 28.8 years.
  - The mean follow-up was 7.7 years (range 2 to 22 years).
  - The authors reported 72% good or excellent results with a 15% reoperation rate.
  - Factors associated with reoperation were older age and larger lesions.
  - The 5-year survivorship was 91%.
- Garret[8] reported his experience with osteochondral allografts for OCD of the lateral femoral condyle.
  - Defects up to 3 cm showed good results at 2 to 9 years follow-up for 16/17 patients.
  - One large lesion (3 × 4.5 cm) failed early in this series.

- Levy et al[14] reported a relatively long-term follow-up (91% of 129 grafts) of osteochondral allografts at 10 years.
  - Thirty-one knees (24%) failed at a mean of 7.2 years. Survivorship was 82% at 10 years, 74% at 15 years, and 66% at 20 years.
  - Age older than 30 years at time of surgery and having two or more previous surgeries for the operated knee were associated with allograft failure.

## COMPLICATIONS

- In a systematic review, Chahal et al[5] reported on the complications associated with osteochondral allograft transplantation.
- Overall, the short-term complication rate was low at 2.3% (14 of 595 knees reported across 19 eligible studies).
- These postoperative complications included removal of hardware (n = 3), repeat arthroscopy (n = 3), superficial infection (n = 2), deep infection (n = 2), DVT (n = 1), hyperemic reaction (n = 1), and early loosening of the graft (n = 1).
- The most frequent long-term complication rate was failure, which was reported variably as graft fragmentation or conversion to total knee arthroplasty.
- The overall failure rate was approximately 18%, based on the individual authors' definitions.
- The failure rate of bipolar grafts (opposing femoral and tibial grafts) was 65%.

## REFERENCES


1. Allen RT, Robertson CM, Pennock AT, et al. Analysis of stored osteochondral allografts at the time of surgical implantation. Am J Sports Med 2005;33(10):1479–1484.
2. Borazjani BH, Chen AC, Bae WC, et al. Effect of impact on chondrocyte viability during insertion of human osteochondral grafts. J Bone Joint Surg Am 2006;88(9):1934–1943.
3. Bugbee WD. Fresh osteochondral allografts. J Knee Surg 2002;15(3): 191–195.
4. Bugbee W, Cavallo M, Giannini S. Osteochondral allograft transplantation in the knee. J Knee Surg 2012;25(2):109–116.
5. Chahal J, Gross AE, Gross C, et al. Outcomes of osteochondral allograft transplantation in the knee. Arthroscopy 2013;29(3):575–588.
6. Cole BJ, DeBerardino T, Brewster R, et al. Outcomes of autologous chondrocyte implantation in study of the treatment of articular repair (STAR) patients with osteochondritis dissecans. Am J Sports Med 2012;40(9):2015–2022.
7. Emmerson BC, Gortz S, Jamali AA, et al. Fresh osteochondral allografting in the treatment of osteochondritis dissecans of the femoral condyle. Am J Sports Med 2007;35(6):907–914.
8. Garrett JC. Fresh osteochondral allografts for treatment of articular defects in osteochondritis dissecans of the lateral femoral condyle in adults. Clin Orthop Relat Res 1994;(303):33–37.
9. Gudas R, Simonaityte R, Cekanauskas E, et al. A prospective, randomized clinical study of osteochondral autologous transplantation versus microfracture for the treatment of osteochondritis dissecans in the knee joint in children. J Pediatr Orthop 2009;29(7):741–748.
10. Horas U, Pelinkovic D, Herr G, et al. Autologous chondrocyte implantation and osteochondral cylinder transplantation in cartilage repair of the knee joint. A prospective, comparative trial. J Bone Joint Surg Am 2003;85-A(2):185–192.
11. Kocher MS, Tucker R, Ganley TJ, et al. Management of osteochondritis dissecans of the knee: current concepts review. Am J Sports Med 2006;34(7):1181–1191.
12. Krishnan SP, Skinner JA, Carrington RW, et al. Collagen-covered autologous chondrocyte implantation for osteochondritis dissecans of the knee: two- to seven-year results. J Bone Joint Surg Br 2006;88(2): 203–205.
13. Langer F, Gross AE. Immunogenicity of allograft articular cartilage. J Bone Joint Surg Am 1974;56(2):297–304.
14. Levy YD, Gortz S, Pulido PA, et al. Do fresh osteochondral allografts successfully treat femoral condyle lesions? Clin Orthop Relat Res 2013;471(1):231–237.
15. Louisia S, Beaufils P, Katabi M, et al. Transchondral drilling for osteochondritis dissecans of the medial condyle of the knee. Knee Surg Sports Traumatol Arthrosc 2003;11(1):33–39.
16. Maury AC, Safir O, Heras FL, et al. Twenty-five-year chondrocyte viability in fresh osteochondral allograft. A case report. J Bone Joint Surg Am 2007;89(1):159–165.
17. Michael JW, Wurth A, Eysel P, et al. Long-term results after operative treatment of osteochondritis dissecans of the knee joint-30 year results. Int Orthop 2008;32(2):217–221.
18. Murray JR, Chitnavis J, Dixon P, et al. Osteochondritis dissecans of the knee; long-term clinical outcome following arthroscopic debridement. Knee 2007;14(2):94–98.
19. Pallante AL, Chen AC, Ball ST, et al. The in vivo performance of osteochondral allografts in the goat is diminished with extended storage and decreased cartilage cellularity. Am J Sports Med 2012;40(8):1814–1823.
20. Pallante-Kichura AL, Chen AC, Temple-Wong MM, et al. In vivo efficacy of fresh versus frozen osteochondral allografts in the goat at 6 months is associated with PRG4 secretion. J Orthop Res 2013;31(6):880–886.
21. Pascual-Garrido C, McNickle AG, Cole BJ. Surgical treatment options for osteochondritis dissecans of the knee. Sports Health 2009;1(4):326–334.
22. Patil S, Butcher W, D'Lima DD, et al. Effect of osteochondral graft insertion forces on chondrocyte viability. Am J Sports Med 2008;36(9):1726–1732.
23. Peterson L, Minas T, Brittberg M, et al. Treatment of osteochondritis dissecans of the knee with autologous chondrocyte transplantation: results at two to ten years. J Bone Joint Surg Am 2003;85-A(suppl 2):17–24.
24. Pruthi S, Parnell SE, Thapa MM. Pseudointercondylar notch sign: manifestation of osteochondritis dissecans of the trochlea. Pediatr Radiol 2009;39(2):180–183.
25. Shasha N, Krywulak S, Backstein D, et al. Long-term follow-up of fresh tibial osteochondral allografts for failed tibial plateau fractures. J Bone Joint Surg Am 2003;85-A(suppl 2):33–39.
26. Tis JE, Edmonds EW, Bastrom T, et al. Short-term results of arthroscopic treatment of osteochondritis dissecans in skeletally immature patients. J Pediatr Orthop 2010;32(3):226–231.
27. Wang CJ. Treatment of focal articular cartilage lesions of the knee with autogenous osteochondral grafts. A 2- to 4-year follow-up study. Arch Orthop Trauma Surg 2002;122(3):169–172.
28. Watanabe A, Wada Y, Obata T, et al. Time course evaluation of reparative cartilage with MR imaging after autologous chondrocyte implantation. Cell Transplant 2005;14(9):695–700.
29. Williams SK, Amiel D, Ball ST, et al. Analysis of cartilage tissue on a cellular level in fresh osteochondral allograft retrievals. Am J Sports Med 2007;35(12):2022–2032.
30. Williams SK, Amiel D, Ball ST, et al. Prolonged storage effects on the articular cartilage of fresh human osteochondral allografts. J Bone Joint Surg Am 2003;85-A(11):2111–2120.

# Chronic Exertional Compartment Syndrome

Jonathan A. Godin, Jocelyn R. Wittstein, L. Scott Levin, and Claude T. Moorman III

## DEFINITION

- Compartment syndrome can be either acute or chronic.
- Acute compartment syndrome is usually due to trauma to, or reperfusion of, the extremity. Chronic exertional compartment syndrome (CECS) is often associated with the repetitive loading or microtrauma of endurance activities.
- Both acute and chronic compartment syndromes are due to increased interstitial pressure within a compartment, resulting in decreased perfusion and ischemia of soft tissues.
  - In contrast to the reversible nature of CECS, acute compartment syndromes progress rapidly and require urgent fasciotomy to avoid irreversible soft tissue necrosis in the affected compartment.
- Wilson first described the concept of CECS in 1912, but Mavor[16] was the first to successfully treat a patient with anterior compartment syndrome of the leg using a fasciotomy.
- Clinical manifestations of compartment syndrome include exercise-induced pain relieved by rest, swelling, numbness, and weakness of the extremity.[8,23]
- The reported incidence ranges between 14% and 33% among individuals with lower leg pain.[3,21,30]
- CECS is often bilateral and is equally prevalent among males and females.
- Diabetic patients may be at increased risk of developing CECS.[6]
- Case reports of CECS of the forearm, thigh, and gluteal regions exist but are rare.[10,12,13,25]
  - The leg is the most common site, with the anterior and lateral compartments most frequently affected. Although this chapter focuses on CECS of the leg, the clinical features, diagnostic strategy, and treatment methods are similar for all locations.

## ANATOMY

- The leg contains four compartments: anterior, lateral, superficial posterior, and deep posterior (**FIG 1**).
- The anterior compartment contains the anterior tibial artery, the deep peroneal nerve, and four muscles (tibialis anterior, extensor digitorum longus, extensor hallucis longus, and peroneus tertius). Its borders are the tibia, fibula, interosseous membrane, anterior intermuscular septum, and deep fascia of the leg.

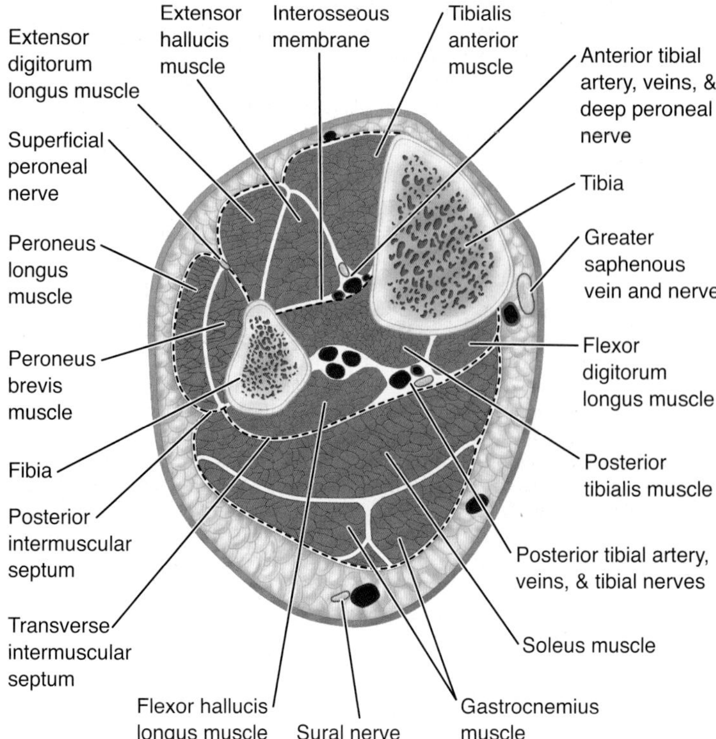


**FIG 1** • Cross-sectional anatomy of the leg.

- The lateral compartment contains the superficial peroneal nerve and two muscles (peroneus longus and peroneus brevis). Its borders are the anterior intermuscular septum, the fibula, the posterior intermuscular septum, and the deep fascia.
  - The common peroneal nerve branches into the superficial and deep peroneal nerves within the substance of the peroneus longus after passing along the neck of the fibula.
  - The superficial peroneal nerve continues within the lateral compartment, whereas the deep peroneal nerve wraps around the fibula deep to the extensor digitorum longus until reaching the anterior surface of the interosseous membrane.
  - The lateral compartment does not contain a large artery; the peroneal muscles receive their blood supply via several branches of the peroneal artery.
- The superficial posterior compartment contains the sural nerve and three muscles (gastrocnemius, soleus, and plantaris) and is surrounded by the deep fascia of the leg.
- The deep posterior compartment contains the posterior tibial and peroneal arteries, tibial nerve, and four muscles (flexor digitorum longus, flexor hallucis longus, popliteus, and tibialis posterior). It is bordered anteriorly by the tibia, fibula, and interosseous membrane and posteriorly by the deep transverse fascia.
- A fifth compartment that encloses the tibialis posterior muscle has been described,[4] but its existence is controversial. It has been suggested that the presence of an extensive fibular origin of the flexor digitorum longus muscle may create a subcompartment within the deep posterior compartment that may develop elevated pressures.[11]

## PATHOGENESIS

- The etiology of CECS is not entirely understood. It is thought to be due to an abnormal increase in intramuscular pressure during exercise resulting in impaired local perfusion, tissue ischemia, and pain.
  - One study demonstrated a 20% increase in muscle volume during exercise.[15]
  - Contributing factors may include exertion-induced swelling of the muscle fibers, increased perfusion volume, and increased interstitial fluid volume within a constrictive compartment.
  - The elevated intramuscular pressure decreases arteriolar blood flow and diminishes venous return.
  - This, in turn, results in tissue ischemia and accumulation of metabolites.
  - Elevated lactate levels and water content have been documented in muscle biopsies from compartments with elevated pressures following exercise.[21]
- Muscle hypertrophy and increased perfusion volume with exertion do not explain the elevated resting pressure seen in patients with CECS, however. The mechanical damage theory hypothesizes that heavy exertion results in myofibril damage, release of protein-bound ions, increased osmotic pressure in the interstitial space, and, therefore, decreased arteriolar flow in the compartment.
- Additionally, in some cases, focal fascial defects may be a contributing factor.
  - Anterolateral fascial hernias are present in 39% to 46% of patients with CECS, as compared to less than 5% of asymptomatic individuals.[9,31]

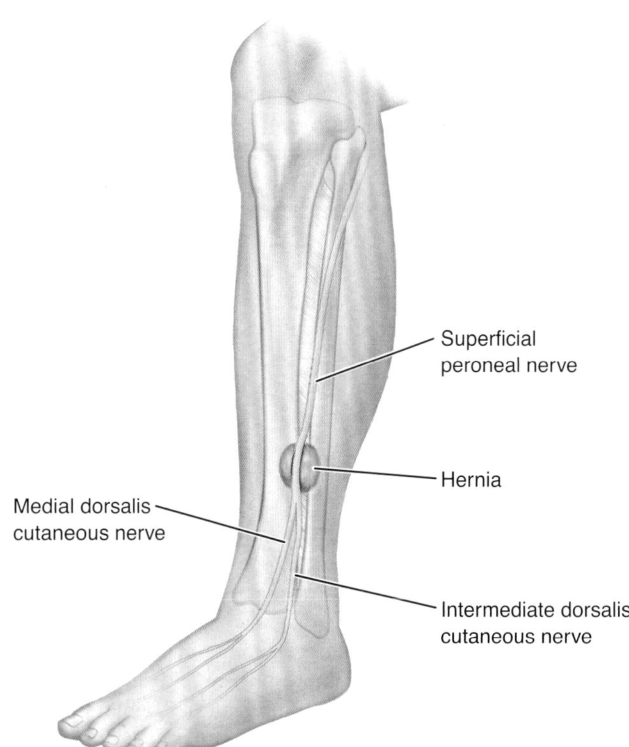


**FIG 2** • The superficial peroneal nerve can become entrapped at a fascial defect.

  - These defects typically are located near the anterior intermuscular septum between the anterior and lateral compartments, and they can entrap the superficial peroneal nerve exiting the junction of the middle and distal thirds of the leg (**FIG 2**).
- Evidence suggests that patients with CECS have a lower capillary density in relation to muscle fiber size compared to controls. This decreased capillarity leads to decreased structural capacity for muscle blood flow.[7]
- None of the existing theories explain all of the available data on the etiology of CECS. Most likely, the pathogenesis of the elevated intracompartmental pressures seen in CECS is multifactorial.

## NATURAL HISTORY

- CECS of the leg is a common injury in people involved in running and endurance sport activities, such as young athletes and military personnel.
- Pain, as well as occasional numbness and weakness, develops at a predictable interval after initiation of a repetitive, endurance-type activity and resolves with rest.
- The symptoms are long-standing and recurrent because patients tend to self-limit before subsequently attempting to resume activities.

## PATIENT HISTORY AND PHYSICAL FINDINGS

- The following symptoms may be present upon exertion and resolve with rest:
  - A sensation of cramping, burning, aching, or tightness in the region of the affected compartment(s)

- Numbness or weakness in the extremity
    - A transient foot drop may develop if the deep peroneal nerve is affected.
    - A temporary loss of eversion strength may occur if the superficial peroneal nerve is affected.
- Physical examination of the resting lower extremity often is unremarkable.
- Examination following exercise may reveal the following:
  - Tightness or tenderness to palpation of the involved compartments
  - If a fascial defect is present, a focal area of tenderness and swelling may develop as the underlying muscle bulges through the defect.
    - A positive Tinel sign over the defect if the superficial peroneal nerve is compressed
  - Numbness and/or motor weakness may be present in the superficial peroneal, deep peroneal, or tibial nerve distributions.
- When the history and physical examination findings are consistent with CECS, the diagnosis should be confirmed with pre- and postexercise compartment pressure measurements.
  - Most clinicians follow the diagnostic criteria of Pedowitz et al,[20] in which a resting pressure greater than or equal to 15 mm Hg or a 1-minute postexercise measurement greater than or equal to 30 mm Hg or a 5-minute postexercise measurement greater than or equal to 20 mm Hg is considered abnormal and diagnostic of CECS.
  - The exercise performed at the time of testing must be intense enough to reproduce the patient's symptoms; otherwise, the postexercise pressure measurements may result in a false-negative result.
  - Several methods for measuring compartment pressures have been described in the literature.
    - These include the slit catheter, wick catheter, needle manometry, digital pressure monitor, microcapillary infusion, and solid-state transducer intracompartmental catheter methods.[1,2,17,18,25,31]
    - The Stryker Intra-Compartmental Pressure Monitor (Kalamazoo, MI) is a handheld digital monitor that can be used to check multiple compartments. It can be used either with a side port needle or an indwelling slit catheter to obtain serial measurements in a single compartment.
    - A new handheld digital device recently developed by Synthes (Paoli, PA) also allows placement of indwelling catheters and may be useful for obtaining serial measurements.
- Near-infrared spectroscopy has been used to determine tissue oxygen saturation.[32] This may be a noninvasive, painless alternative to intracompartmental pressures in the diagnosis of CECS but is not currently standardized or readily available.
- The vibration test consists of placing a vibrating tuning fork over bone at the area of suspected stress; an elicitation of pain is consistent with a stress fracture.
- Pain when performing resisted ankle dorsiflexion and inversion is consistent with tibialis posterior tendinitis or posteromedial periostitis.

## IMAGING AND OTHER DIAGNOSTIC STUDIES

- When pressure measurements are not consistent with CECS, further diagnostic studies may be necessary to explore the differential diagnosis.
- Plain radiographs may demonstrate a periosteal reaction in patients with tibial stress fractures or posteromedial tibial periostitis.
- Bone scan will show increased uptake, and MRI may show edema or a black line at the site of a stress fracture.
- Ultrasound may play a role in diagnosis by identifying anterior compartment thickness.[22]
- Tingling, numbness, or a positive Tinel sign at a specific location may warrant an electromyogram (EMG) and nerve conduction velocity (NCV) studies to evaluate for peripheral nerve entrapment.
- Pain and coolness with paradoxical claudication may warrant an angiogram to evaluate for popliteal artery entrapment.

## DIFFERENTIAL DIAGNOSIS

- Tibial stress fractures
- Posteromedial tibial periostitis
- Tenosynovitis of posterior tibialis or ankle dorsiflexors
- Peripheral nerve entrapment
- Radiculopathy secondary to lumbar pathology
- Complex regional pain syndrome
- Peripheral vascular disease
- Popliteal artery entrapment syndrome
- Deep venous thrombosis

## NONOPERATIVE MANAGEMENT

- Nonoperative management usually requires activity limitation or cessation.
  - Adjuncts to activity modification include anti-inflammatory medications, stretching, and foot orthotics.
- Symptoms usually return with resumption of prior activity level. Surgery, therefore, is indicated in patients who cannot tolerate activity restriction.

## SURGICAL MANAGEMENT

- Surgical treatment involves fasciotomy of the affected compartments, sometimes with partial fasciectomy.
- Patients who are unable to maintain their desired activity level owing to symptoms of CECS are appropriate operative candidates.

### Preoperative Planning

- It is critical to identify which compartments are affected.
  - All symptomatic compartments should be addressed at the time of surgery. It is common for a failed index procedure to be due to a failure to release all affected compartments.
- The appropriate approach should be selected based on the compartments that need to be released.

### Positioning

- The patient is placed in the supine position for each technique.

### Approach

- A single- or dual-incision technique can be used to release the lateral and anterior compartments.

- The perifibular approach can be used to access all four compartments.
- A posteromedial approach offers easier access to the superficial and deep posterior compartments.
- Endoscopically assisted fasciotomies allow access to the entire length of the compartment, allow visualization of fascial hernias, and may minimize surgical complications such as postsurgical fibrosis and injury to the superficial peroneal nerve.
  - The safety and effectiveness of endoscopically assisted compartment release have been demonstrated.[14,34]
  - A technique using balloon dissectors and carbon dioxide insufflation is described in the Techniques section.[34,35]



## Single-Incision Lateral Approach for Anterior and Lateral Compartment Fasciotomy

- The patient is placed in the supine position on the operating table.
- A 5-cm vertical incision is made halfway between the fibular shaft and the tibial crest at the midportion of the leg. The incision should lie over the anterolateral intermuscular septum (**TECH FIG 1A**).
  - If a focal fascial defect is present, the incision should be adjusted so that the defect can be incorporated.
- A small transverse incision is made through the fascia, and the septum and superficial peroneal nerve, which lie near the septum in the lateral compartment and exit the fascia near the distal aspect of the incision, are identified (**TECH FIG 1B**).
- Longitudinal releases of the anterior and lateral compartments are performed using long Metzenbaum scissors in a proximal and distal direction from the transverse incision in the fascia that crosses over the anterolateral intermuscular septum (**TECH FIG 1C**).
- A partial fasciectomy may be performed, particularly in cases of recurrence following a prior fasciotomy.
- The fascia is left open.
- The subcutaneous tissue is approximated using 2-0 absorbable suture material.
- The skin is closed with a running subcuticular 4-0 nonabsorbable suture material and Steri-Strips.

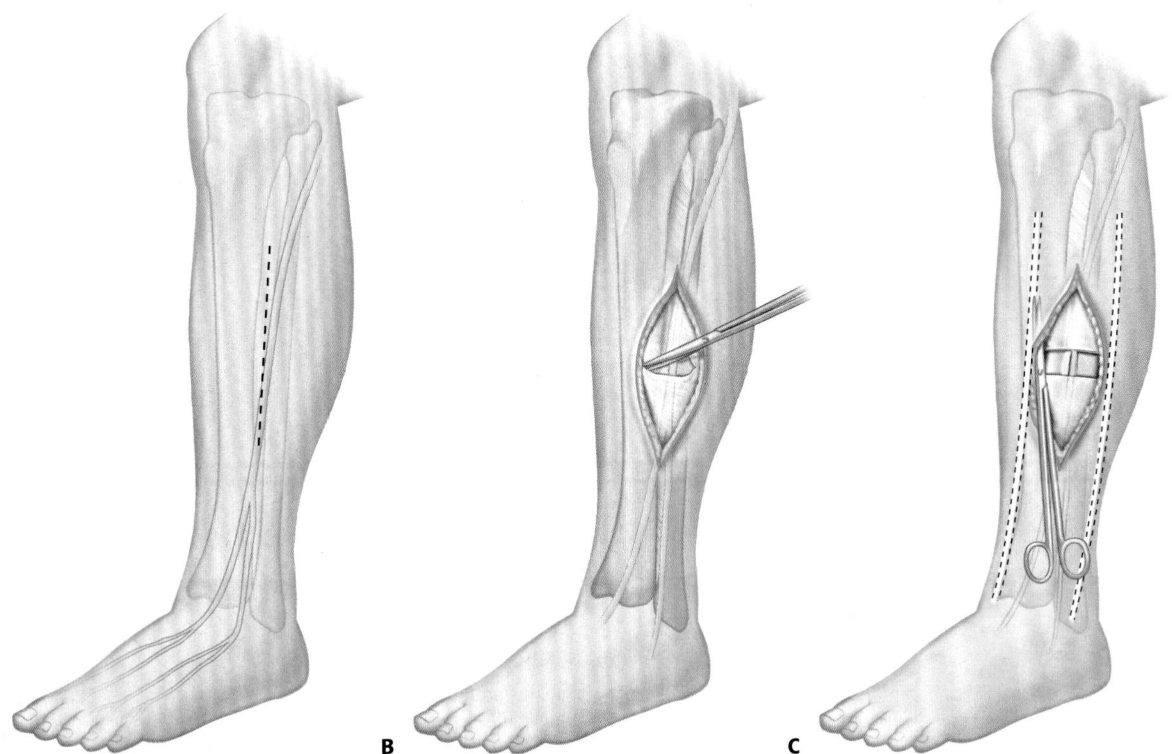


**TECH FIG 1** • Single-incision lateral approach. **A.** A 5-cm vertical incision is made halfway between the fibular shaft and the tibial crest over the anterolateral intermuscular septum. **B.** A small transverse incision is made just through the fascia, and the superficial peroneal nerve is identified. **C.** Longitudinal releases of the anterior and lateral compartments are performed using long Metzenbaum scissors.

## Dual-Incision Lateral Approach for Anterior and Lateral Compartment Fasciotomy

- The patient is placed in a supine position.
- The leg is divided into thirds, and two 3-cm incisions are placed at the junctions of the thirds over the anterolateral intermuscular septum (**TECH FIG 2A,B**).
- The superficial peroneal nerve is identified as it exits the fascia near the distal incision (**TECH FIG 2C**).
- Fasciotomies of the anterior and lateral compartments are performed on each side of the intermuscular septum (**TECH FIG 2D**).
- The incisions in the fascia are connected using Metzenbaum scissors to divide the fascia from the proximal incision toward the knee (**TECH FIG 2E**), then from the proximal incision toward the distal incision, and finally from the distal incision toward the ankle (**TECH FIG 2F**).
  - Distally, the fasciotomy should extend to 4 to 6 cm proximal to the ankle.
  - At the distal aspect of the anterior compartment, the release should be directed toward the midline to minimize risk of injuring cutaneous sensory nerves in the lateral aspect of the compartment.
  - The distal aspect of the lateral compartment fasciotomy should be directed laterally.
- The subcutaneous tissue is closed with 2-0 absorbable suture material.
- The skin is closed with running subcuticular 4-0 sutures and Steri-Strips.

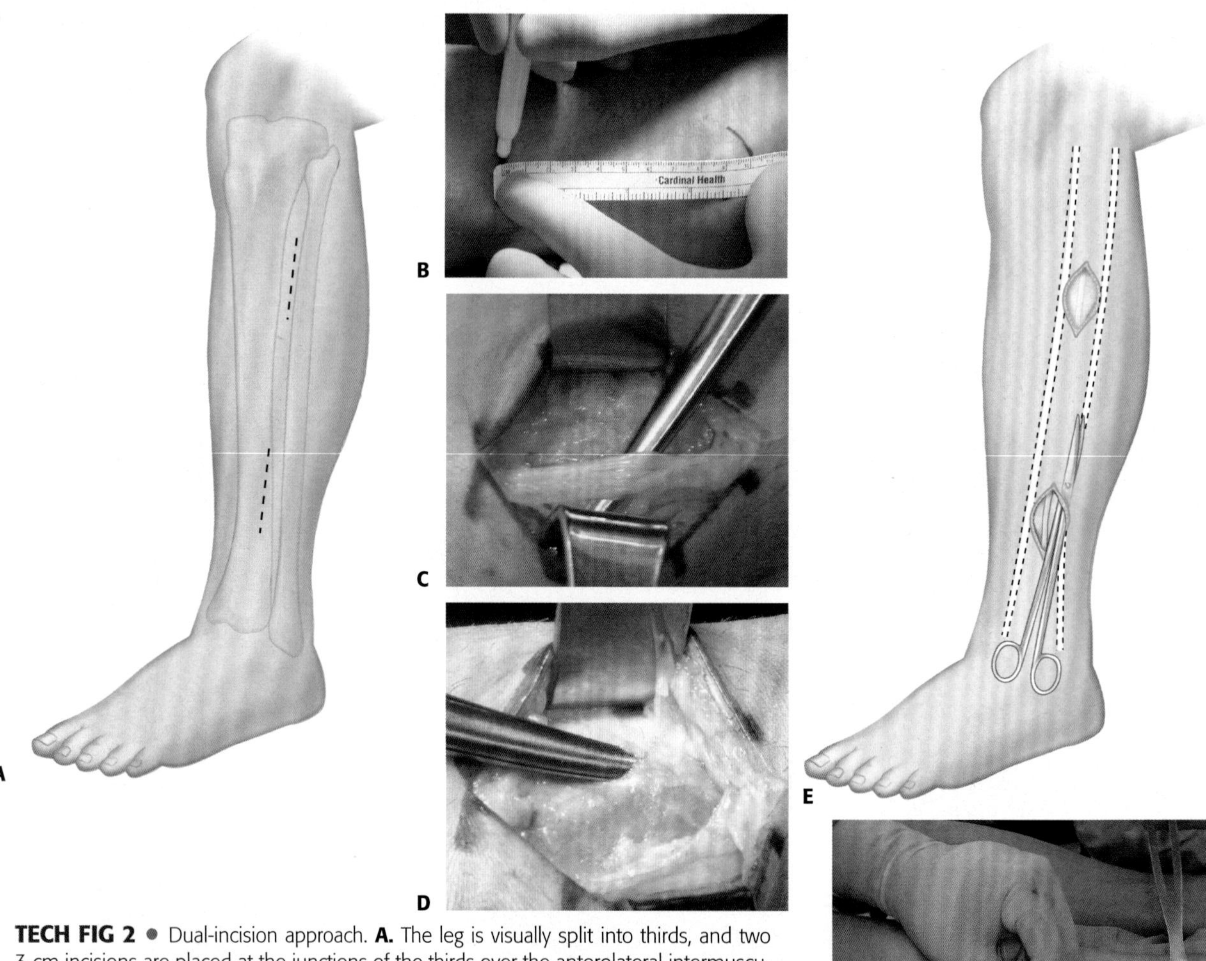


**TECH FIG 2** • Dual-incision approach. **A.** The leg is visually split into thirds, and two 3-cm incisions are placed at the junctions of the thirds over the anterolateral intermuscular septum. **B.** The superficial peroneal nerve is located 10 to 12 cm proximal to the tip of the lateral malleolus. The inferior incision is centered over this area. **C.** Dissection of the superficial peroneal nerve. **D.** A fascial defect often is present in this area, and compartment releases should be centered over these areas if possible. **E.** The incisions in the fascia are connected using Metzenbaum scissors to divide the fascia. **F.** Long scissors are used and are opened only slightly at the tips. (**B–D,F:** Courtesy of Mark D. Miller, MD.)

## Perifibular Approach for Four-Compartment Fasciotomy

- The patient is placed in the supine position.
- A 10-cm incision is made directly over the midportion of the fibula (**TECH FIG 3A**).
- The skin is retracted anteriorly and the fascia of the anterior and lateral compartments is released longitudinally in a proximal and distal direction (**TECH FIG 3B**).
- The skin is retracted posteriorly.
- The fascia overlying the lateral head of the gastrocnemius is released.
  - The fascia over the superficial posterior compartment is incised for a distance of about 15 cm.
- The anterior and lateral compartments are retracted anteriorly and the superficial posterior compartment is retracted posteriorly. The soleal bridge must be released from the fibula (**TECH FIG 3C**).
- The fascia over the flexor hallucis longus is identified and incised.
- The gastrocsoleus is retracted posteriorly and the flexor hallucis longus laterally to expose the posterior tibial artery, tibial nerve, and peroneal artery overlying the tibialis posterior.
- The fascia is incised around the tibialis posterior and the interval between the muscle and the origins of the flexor hallucis longus is widened if constrictive.
- The subcutaneous tissue is approximated with 2-0 absorbable suture.
- The skin is closed with running subcuticular nonabsorbable 4-0 suture.

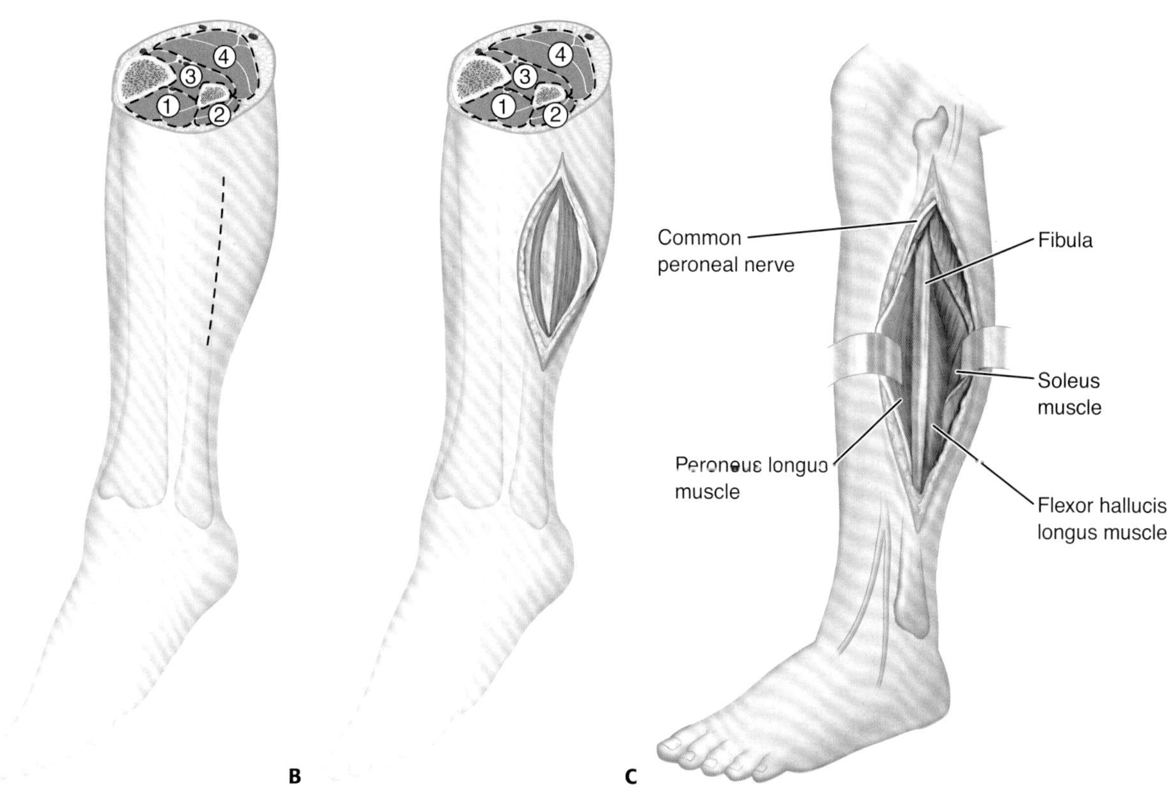


**TECH FIG 3** • Perifibular approach. **A.** A 10-cm incision is made directly over the midportion of the fibula. **B.** The skin is retracted anteriorly, and the fascia of the anterior and lateral compartments is released longitudinally. **C.** The anterior and lateral compartments are retracted anteriorly and the superficial posterior compartment posteriorly, and the soleal bridge is released from the fibula.

## Posteromedial Incision for Fasciotomy of the Posterior Compartments

- A vertical incision 8 to 10 cm in length is made over the midportion of the leg approximately 1 cm posterior to the posteromedial edge of the tibia (**TECH FIG 4A**).
- The saphenous vein and nerve are identified in the subcutaneous tissue and retracted anteriorly.
- The fascia over the superficial posterior compartment is incised for a distance of about 15 cm (**TECH FIG 4B,C**).
- To fully access the deep posterior compartment, the origin of the soleus from the proximal tibia and fibula must be detached (**TECH FIG 4D**).
- The deep fascia can then be sharply divided with Metzenbaum scissors (**TECH FIG 4E–G**).
  - The fasciotomy should extend distally to 8 to 10 cm above the ankle.
- The opening between the origins of the flexor hallucis longus and the tibialis posterior is enlarged if constrictive.
- The subcutaneous tissue is closed with 2-0 absorbable suture.
- The skin is closed with running subcuticular nonabsorbable 4-0 suture.

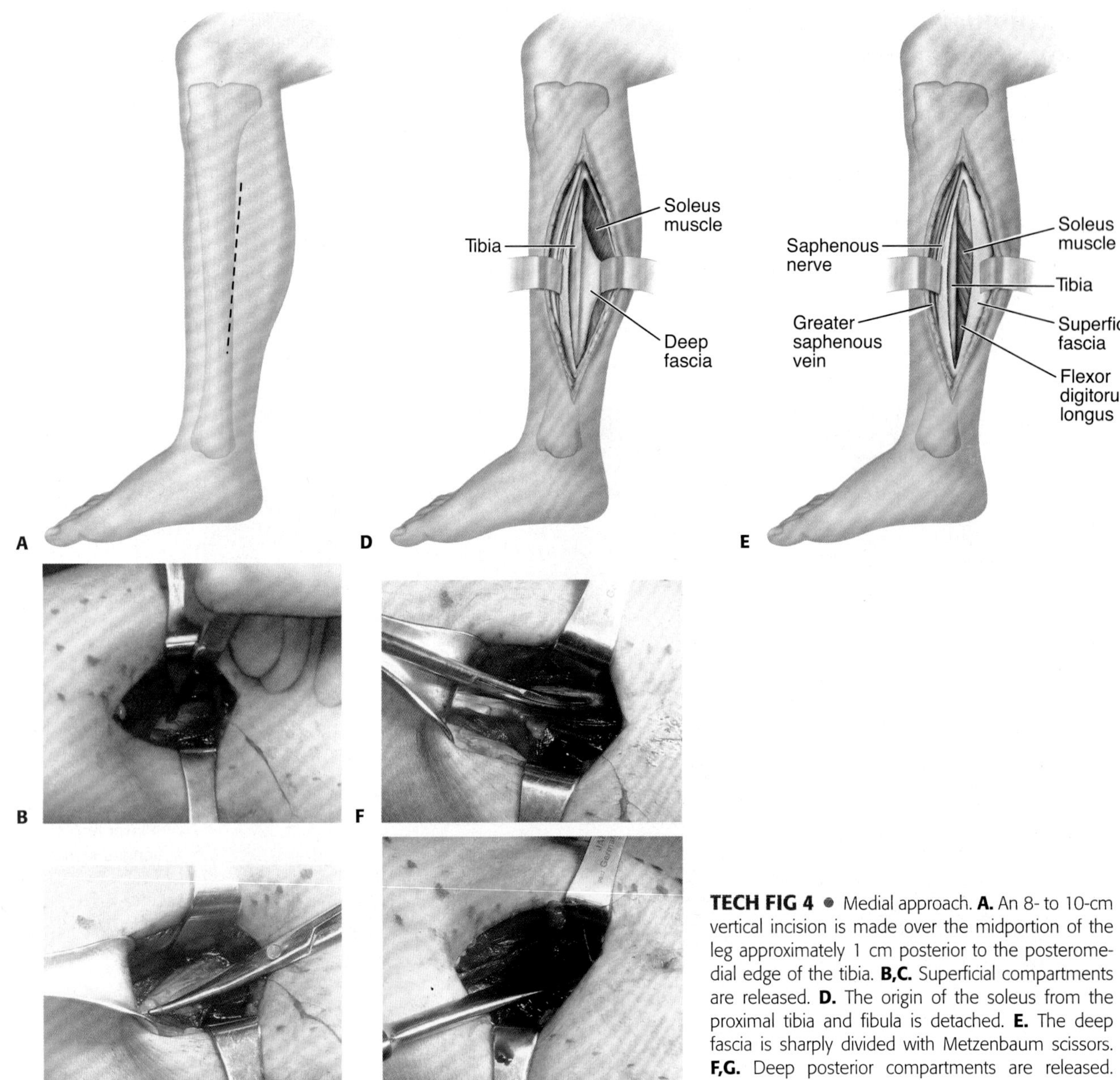


**TECH FIG 4** ● Medial approach. **A.** An 8- to 10-cm vertical incision is made over the midportion of the leg approximately 1 cm posterior to the posteromedial edge of the tibia. **B,C.** Superficial compartments are released. **D.** The origin of the soleus from the proximal tibia and fibula is detached. **E.** The deep fascia is sharply divided with Metzenbaum scissors. **F,G.** Deep posterior compartments are released. (**B,C,F,G:** Courtesy of Mark D. Miller, MD.)

## Endoscopically Assisted Compartment Release

- The patient is placed in a supine position.
- Balloon dissectors can be used to create an optical cavity at the fascial cleft, which is the potential space between the superficial fascia (the deepest layer of the skin and subcutaneous tissue) and the deep fascia (the fascia overlying a muscle compartment).
  - To insert the balloon dissector, a 2-cm transverse incision is made either at the anterolateral aspect of the knee between the fibular head and Gerdy's tubercle or at the posteromedial aspect of the knee at the level of the tibial crest (**TECH FIG 5A**).
  - Dissection is carried down through the subcutaneous fat and superficial fascia until the deep fascia overlying the muscle is visualized (**TECH FIG 5B**).
  - The balloon dissector with a sheath around it is inserted between the superficial and deep fascial layers under direct observation and manual palpation to the level of the ankle (**TECH FIG 5C**).
  - The sheath is removed and the balloon is inflated to create a cavity within the fascial cleft (**TECH FIG 5D**).
  - The balloon is then deflated and removed.

- The optical cavity is maintained using towel clips (**TECH FIG 5E**).
  - Alternatively, the optical cavity between the superficial and deep fascial layers can be maintained with 15 mm Hg of carbon dioxide insufflation to allow adequate visualization of the fascia to be released and to allow adequate space to perform soft tissue dissection with the endoscopic equipment.
- A one-way cone-shaped cannula is inserted in the skin at the site of balloon insertion.

- Next, the fascia overlying the anterior compartment is released with endoscopic scissors down to the level of the ankle under direct vision (**TECH FIG 5F**).
  - The intermuscular septum between the anterior and lateral compartments, as well as the superficial peroneal nerve, can be visualized (**TECH FIG 5G**).
- If a lateral compartment release is indicated, perform a second fasciotomy posterior to the intermuscular septum.
- If posterior compartment releases are indicated, make a 2-cm transverse incision proximally along the medial aspect of the leg just posterior to the edge of the tibia.
  - The balloon dissector and sheath are inserted into the fascial cleft overlying the superficial and deep posterior compartments to the level of the ankle.
  - As described earlier, the balloon is inflated, deflated, and removed. Towel clips are used to maintain the cavity.
  - The fascia of the deep posterior compartment is released directly off the posteromedial border of the tibia, anterior to the intermuscular septum, from proximal to distal under direct visualization with endoscopic scissors.

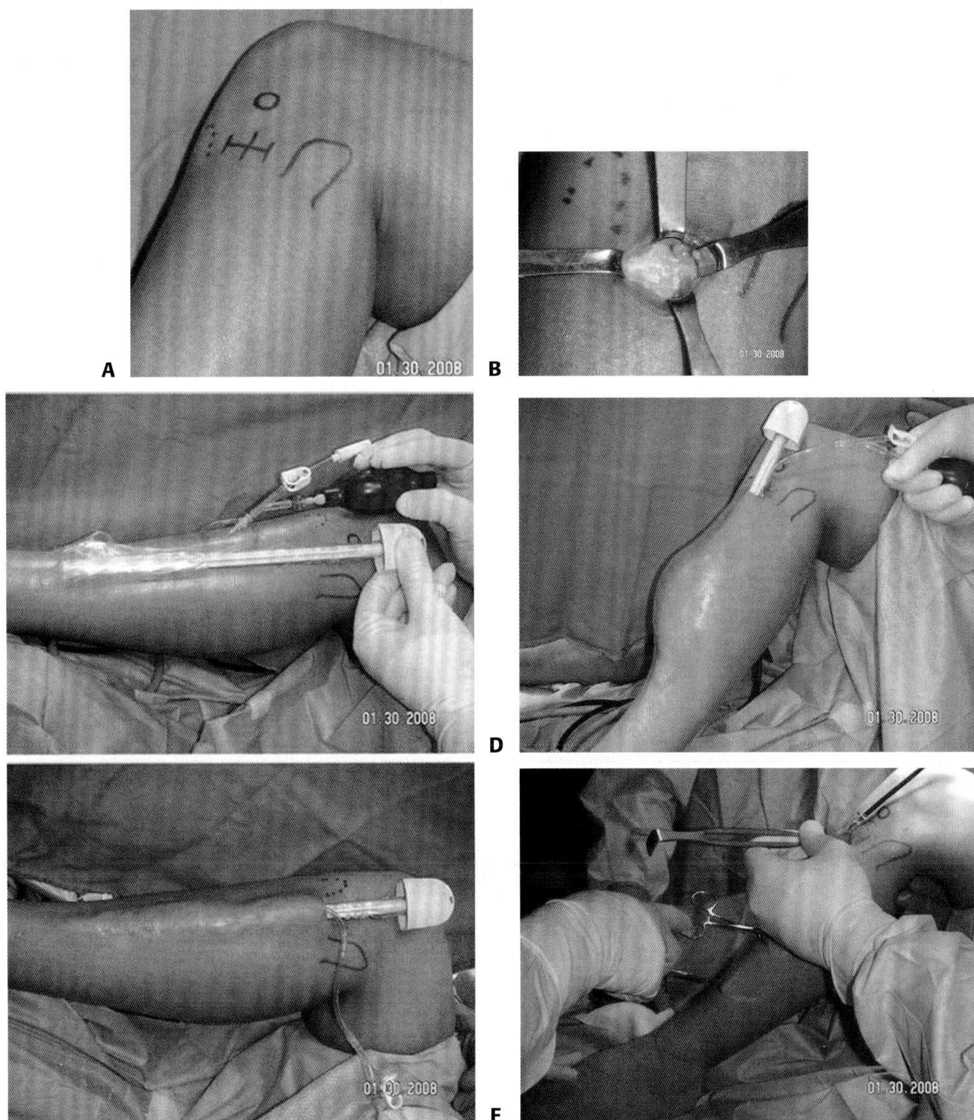

**TECH FIG 5** ● Sequential demonstration of balloon placement in the lower extremity. **A.** A transverse incision at the anterolateral aspect of the knee between the fibular head and Gerdy's tubercle is used. **B.** Dissection is carried out to the level of the deep fascia. **C.** Entry of balloon to the level of the ankle under direct visualization. **D.** The balloon is inflated. **E.** Towel clips are used to maintain the visual cavity. *(continued)*

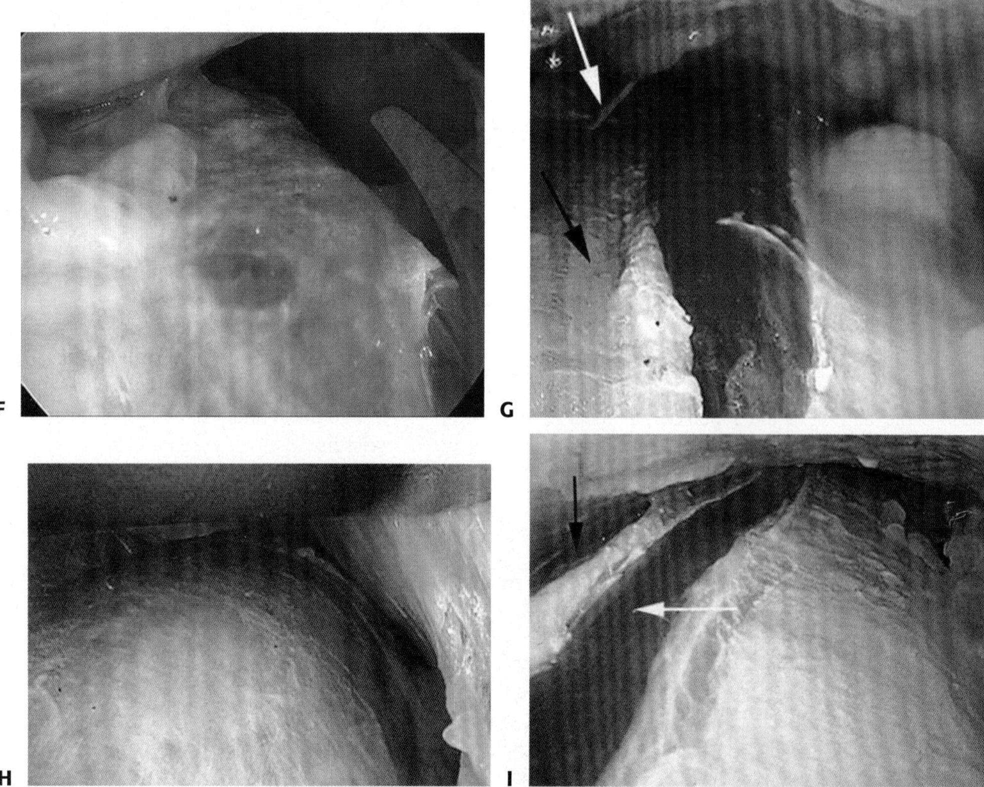


**TECH FIG 5** • *(continued)* **F.** The anterior compartment fascia is visualized and released with endoscopic scissors. **G.** Anterior compartment release in a left leg. The *black arrow* denotes the intermuscular septum between the anterior and lateral compartments. The *white arrow* points to the superficial peroneal nerve exiting the fascia of the lateral compartment distally. **H.** Endoscopic visualization of the posterior fascia of a left leg. **I.** The *black arrow* points to the deep posterior release directly off the tibia. The *white arrow* denotes the superficial compartment release.

- The fascia of the superficial posterior compartment posterior to the intermuscular septum is released in the same fashion (**TECH FIG 5H,I**).
- If necessary, a distal instrument portal with a pneumatic lock can be placed, but the fasciotomies usually are carried out proximal to distal through the initial portal.
- After the release, the cannula is removed and the cavity is deflated.
- The wound is closed in a two-layer fashion with 2-0 Vicryl for the deep layer and a running subcuticular stitch for the skin over a medium Hemovac drain.

## PEARLS AND PITFALLS

| | |
|---|---|
| **Superficial peroneal nerve injury** | ■ Identify the nerve as it exits the fascia at the junction of the distal and middle thirds of the leg; direct the anterior fasciotomy medially and the lateral fasciotomy posteriorly at the distal extent. |
| **Saphenous vein and nerve injury** | ■ Identify the structures in the subcutaneous tissue at the medial aspect of the leg. Avoid excessive traction on the saphenous nerve, which results in a traction paresthesia. |
| **Incomplete fascial release** | ■ Muscle herniates at the bottom of the "V" of the fasciotomy, resulting in pain. Extend lateral and anterior fasciotomies to 4–6 cm above the ankle and posterior fasciotomies to 8–10 cm above the ankle. |

## POSTOPERATIVE CARE

- Active range of motion at the ankle and knee should begin immediately.
- Crutches can be used as needed in the initial postoperative period, but patients are encouraged to bear weight as tolerated and perform light activities.
- Elevation of the legs while at rest may help to decrease pain and swelling.
- Full activity usually can be resumed 4 to 6 weeks after surgery.

## OUTCOMES

- Various techniques of compartment release have reports of success rates ranging from 78% to 100%.[5,9,19,20,24,26,28,30,33,34]
  - These techniques include open fasciotomies, one- or two-incision minimally invasive subcutaneous fasciotomies, and fasciotomies with partial fasciectomies.
- Adequate long-term follow-up is lacking in the literature.
  - Slimmon et al[29] reported on long-term follow-up of patients treated with fasciotomy with partial fasciectomy and noted a good or excellent outcome in 60% at a mean follow-up of 51 months. Thirteen of 62 had reduced activity levels due to recurrence of symptoms or development of a different lower extremity compartment syndrome.
- Fasciotomy appears to be less effective in alleviating pain in the deep posterior compartment than in other compartments.
  - Some authors have postulated that failure of the fasciotomy may be due to an incomplete fasciotomy or not identifying and releasing the fascia around the tibialis posterior.[4,24,26]

## COMPLICATIONS

- Recurrence rates of 3% to 17% have been reported after fasciotomy.[5,24,26,28]
  - Recurrence may be due to a number of factors, including inadequate fascial releases, failure to decompress a compartment that was believed to be asymptomatic, nerve compression by an unrecognized fascial hernia, and the development of prolific scar tissue.[27]
- Other reported complications of fasciotomies with some degree of subcutaneous or blind dissection include arterial injury, hematoma or seroma formation, superficial wound infections, peripheral cutaneous nerve injuries, and deep venous thromboses.[5,9,29,34]
  - The superficial peroneal nerve is particularly vulnerable as it exits the fascia over the lateral aspect of the leg at the junction of the middle and distal thirds.

## REFERENCES


1. Awbrey BJ, Sienkiewicz PS, Mankin HJ. Chronic exercise-induced compartment pressure elevation measured with a miniaturized fluid-pressure monitor. A laboratory and clinical study. Am J Sports Med 1988;16:610–615.
2. Brace RA, Guyton AC, Taylor AE. Reevaluation of the needle method for measuring interstitial fluid pressure. Am J Physiol 1976;229: 603–607.
3. Clanton TO, Solcher BW. Chronic leg pain in the athlete. Clin Sports Med 1994;4:743–759.
4. Davey JR, Rorabeck CH, Fowler PJ. The tibialis posterior muscle compartment. An unrecognized cause of exertional compartment syndrome. Am J Sports Med 1984;12:391–397.
5. Detmer DE, Sharpe K, Sufit RL, et al. Chronic compartment syndrome: diagnosis, management, and outcomes. Am J Sports Med 1985;13: 162–170.
6. Edmundsson D, Toolanen G. Chronic exertional compartment syndrome in diabetes mellitus. Diabet Med 2011;28:81–85.
7. Edmundsson D, Toolanen G, Thornell L, et al. Evidence for low muscle capillary supply as a pathogenic factor in chronic compartment syndrome. Scand J Med Sci Sports 2010;6:805–813.
8. French EB, Price WH. Anterior tibial pain. Br Med J 1962;2:1290–1296.
9. Fronek J, Mubarak SJ, Hargens AR, et al. Management of chronic exertional compartment syndrome of the lower extremity. Clin Orthop Relat Res 1987;220:217–227.
10. Hallock GG. An endoscopic technique for decompressive fasciotomy. Ann Plast Surg 1999;43:668–670.
11. Hislop M, Tierney P, Murray P, et al. Chronic exertional compartment syndrome: the controversial "fifth" compartment of the leg. Am J Sports Med 2003;31:770–776.
12. Kuklo TR, Tis JE, Moores LK, et al. Fatal rhabdomyolysis with bilateral gluteal, thigh, and leg compartment syndrome after the Army Physical Fitness Test. A case report. Am J Sports Med 2000;28:112–116.
13. Kutz JE, Singer R, Linday M. Chronic exertional compartment syndrome of the forearm: a case report. J Hand Surg Am 1985;10: 302–304.
14. Leversedge FJ, Casey PJ, Seiler JG, et al. Endoscopically assisted fasciotomy: description of technique and in vitro assessment of lower-leg compartment decompression. Am J Sports Med 2002;30:272–278.
15. Lundvall J, Mellander S, Westling H, et al. Fluid transfer between blood and tissues during exercise. Acta Physiol Scand 1972;2:258–269.
16. Mavor GE. The anterior tibial syndrome. J Bone Joint Surg Br 1956; 38B:513–517.
17. McDermott AG, Marble AE, Yabsley RH, et al. Monitoring dynamic anterior compartment pressures during exercise: a new technique using the STIC catheter. Am J Sports Med 1982;10:83–89.
18. Murabak SJ, Hargens AR, Owen CA, et al. The wick catheter technique for measurement of intramuscular pressure: a new research and clinical tool. J Bone Joint Surg Am 1976;58A:1016–1020.
19. Packer JD, Day MS, Nguyen JT, et al. Functional outcomes and patient satisfaction after fasciotomy for chronic exertional compartment syndrome. Am J Sports Med 2013;2:430–436.
20. Pedowitz RA, Hargens AR, Mubarak SJ, et al. Modified criteria for the objective diagnosis of chronic compartment syndrome of the leg. Am J Sports Med 1990;18:35–40.
21. Qvarfordt P, Christenson JT, Eklof B, et al. Intramuscular pressure, muscle blood flow, and skeletal muscle metabolism in chronic anterior tibial compartment syndrome. Clin Orthop Relat Res 1983;179:284–290.
22. Rajasekaran S, Beavis C, Aly AR, et al. The utility of ultrasound in detecting anterior compartment thickness changes in chronic exertional compartment syndrome: a pilot study. Clin J Sports Med 2013;4: 305–311.
23. Reneman RS. The anterior and the lateral compartment syndrome of the leg due to intensive use of muscles. Clin Orthop Rel Res 1975; 113:69–80.
24. Rorabeck CH, Bourne RB, Fowler PJ. The surgical treatment of exertional compartment syndrome in athletes. J Bone Joint Surg Am 1983;65A:1245–1251.
25. Rorabeck CH, Castle GS, Hardie R, et al. Compartment pressure measurements: an experimental investigation using the slit catheter. J Trauma 1981;21:446–449.
26. Rorabeck CH, Fowler PJ, Nott L. The results of fasciotomy in the management of chronic exertional compartment syndrome. Am J Sports Med 1988;16:224–227.
27. Schepsis AA, Fitzgerald M, Nicoletta R. Revision surgery for exertional compartment syndrome of the lower leg. Am J Sports Med 2005;33:1040–1047.
28. Schepsis AA, Martini D, Corbett M. Surgical management of exertional compartment syndrome of the lower leg: long-term follow up. Am J Sports Med 1993;21:811–817.
29. Slimmon D, Bennell K, Brunker P, et al. Long-term outcome of fasciotomy with partial fasciectomy for chronic exertional compartment syndrome of the lower leg. Am J Sports Med 2002;30:581–588.

30. Styf JR, Korner LM. Chronic exertional compartment syndrome of the leg: results of treatment by fasciotomy. J Bone Joint Surg Am 1986;68A:1338–1347.
31. Styf JR, Korner LM. Microcapillary infusion technique for measurement of intramuscular pressure during exercise. Clin Orthop Rel Res 1986;207:253–262.
32. Van den Brand JGH, Verleisdonk EJMM, van der Werken C. Near infrared spectroscopy in the diagnosis of chronic exertional compartment syndrome. Am J Sports Med 2004;32:452–456.
33. Waterman B, Laughlin M, Kilcoyne K, et al. Surgical treatment of chronic exertional compartment syndrome of the leg: failure rates and postoperative disability in an active patient population. J Bone Joint Surg Am 2013;95:592–596.
34. Wittstein J, Moorman CT, Levin LS. Endoscopic compartment release for chronic exertional compartment syndrome. Am J Sports Med 2010;8:1661–1666.
35. Zobrist R, Aponte R, Levin LS. Endoscopic access to the extremities: the principle of fascial clefts. J Orthop Trauma 2002;16:264–271.

# Femoral Rotational Osteotomy (Proximal and Distal)



Robert M. Kay

## DEFINITIONS

- Femoral anteversion is the angle in the transverse (rotational) plane between the neck of the femur and the distal femur, as defined by the intercondylar axis.
- The term *femoral torsion* may be used in lieu of *femoral anteversion* and is favored by those who believe that the torsion often occurs in the femoral shaft rather than the neck.[6,23]
- Because the femoral neck is typically directed anteriorly, the vast majority of people have femoral anteversion. Femoral retroversion is rare and is present when the neck is directed posteriorly.

## ANATOMY

- Femoral anteversion is measured as the angle of the femoral neck relative to the distal femoral transcondylar axis. The transcondylar axis is measured along the posterior distal femoral condyles (**FIG 1**).

## PATHOGENESIS

- Femoral anteversion varies throughout growth and development, both prior to and after birth.
- Femoral anteversion predominates in all age ranges and peaks at birth at a mean of 30 to 50 degrees, decreases to approximately 20 degrees by age 10 years, and 15 degrees by age 15 years.[2,7]
- During normal development, forces between the hip and anterior iliofemoral ligaments with the hip extended appear to lead to the decrease in femoral anteversion.
- The natural remodeling process may be impaired in a variety of circumstances leading to persistent increased femoral anteversion in conditions including developmental dysplasia of the hip (DDH), cerebral palsy (CP), and Legg-Calvé-Perthes.[7,12,20,24,25]

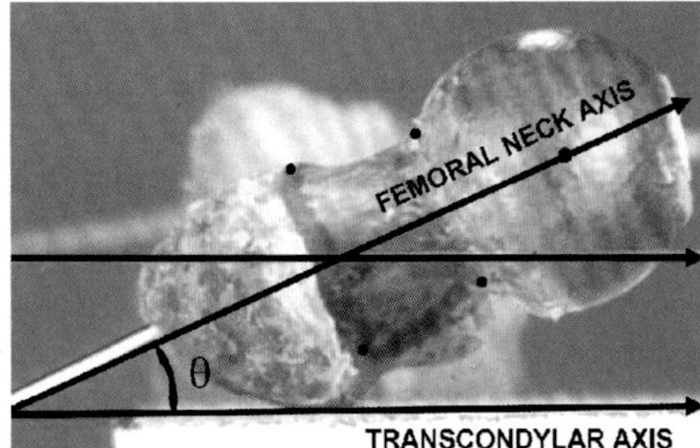


**FIG 1** • Femoral anteversion is the angle in the transverse plane by which the neck of the femur is directed (forward) relative to the transcondylar or coronal plane.

- Femoral anteversion can have a genetic component and has a predilection to occur in certain families.

## NATURAL HISTORY

### Physiologic Anteversion

- As noted, femoral anteversion decreases from 30 to 50 degrees at birth to approximately 20 degrees by age 10 years and 15 degrees by age 15 years.[2,7]
- Despite these mean values, variability is significant, and femoral anteversion is a common cause of persistent intoeing gait in children.[7,10]
- In typically developing children, persistent femoral anteversion is rarely of functional consequence because they have normal balance, strength, and coordination.
- Occasionally, the combination of persistent femoral anteversion and external tibial torsion (so-called "malignant malalignment") may be seen in a child. If this combination results in significant patellofemoral pain and/or patellar instability, osteotomy may be indicated.[5,16]
- There is conflicting evidence linking abnormally increased or decreased femoral anteversion with osteoarthritis of the hip and knee.[13,26,27]

### Cerebral Palsy

- CP affects approximately 1 in 500 children in the United States and is associated with motor and cognitive delays.
- CP has long been known to be associated with increased femoral anteversion throughout childhood, thought to be due to developmental delays, contractures and abnormal forces across the hip.[3,4,9,15,20]
- More recent work has shown that the strongest correlation with femoral anteversion in children with CP is the Gross Motor Functional Classification System (GMFCS) level.[20] For children functioning at GMFCS I, anteversion is near normal, and anteversion increases in a stepwise fashion in GMFCS II and III children, being significantly persistently elevated in GMFCS III, IV, and V children.
- Femoral anteversion (with resultant internal hip rotation during gait) is a common cause of intoeing in ambulatory children with CP and contributes to lever arm dysfunction and crouch gait in these children.[15,18,19]
- In children with severe nonambulatory CP (GMFCS IV and V), increased anteversion and coxa valga are features of the hip at risk for subluxation or dislocation.[20]
- Increased anteversion is a component of malignant malalignment syndrome, which has been implicated as a source of patellofemoral pain and instability.

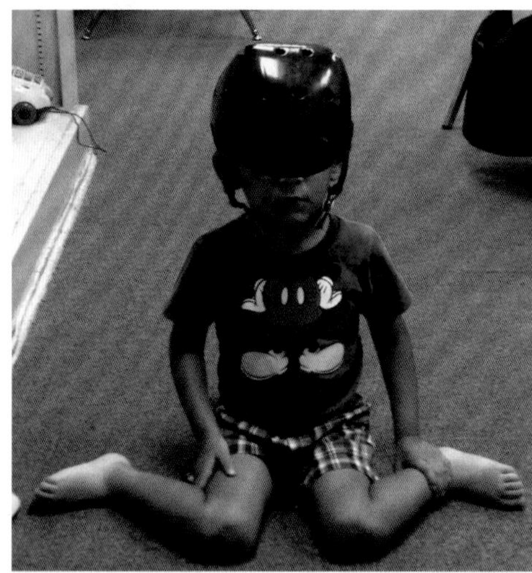

**FIG 2** • Classic "W-sitting" in a child with increased femoral anteversion. (Courtesy of Children's Orthopaedic Center, Los Angeles.)

## PATIENT HISTORY AND PHYSICAL FINDINGS

- Parents often note that children with anteversion often sit in a "W" position and may have difficulty sitting cross-legged (**FIG 2**).
- Intoeing is common in children with persistent femoral anteversion, including typically developing and special needs children.[7,10]
- Intoeing in typically developing children typically does not result in functional limitations, although it frequently results in significant functional deficits (including tripping and falls) in special needs children, such as those with CP.[9,19]
- Internal hip rotation during gait results in internal knee progression angle throughout the gait cycle.
- In most children with internal hip rotation during gait, the foot progression angle is also internal.
- Foot progression angle may be neutral (or external) if femoral anteversion and internal hip rotation are combined with ipsilateral external tibial torsion and/or significant pes valgus deformity. (The combination of femoral anteversion and external tibial torsion is known as *malignant malalignment*.)
- The rotational profile of the entire limb is checked with the child in the prone position.
- In the presence of increased femoral anteversion, hip internal rotation markedly exceeds external rotation.
- The amount of femoral anteversion can be assessed by the trochanteric prominence angle test (TPAT). The anteversion is the amount of hip internal rotation (from vertical) when the greater trochanter is palpated most laterally.[3,22]

## IMAGING AND OTHER DIAGNOSTIC STUDIES

- A number of imaging techniques have been described to estimate femoral anteversion, including plain radiography, fluoroscopy, computed tomography (CT), ultrasonography, and magnetic resonance imaging (MRI).[1,11] None of these tests is routinely necessary in the assessment of children with femoral anteversion.

## DIFFERENTIAL DIAGNOSIS

- Increased anteversion is most commonly encountered in the following situations:
  - Isolated "idiopathic" femoral anteversion
  - Malignant malalignment syndrome
  - CP
  - DDH
- In addition to femoral anteversion, other common causes of intoeing include the following:
  - Tibial torsion
  - Foot deformity (including pes varus and/or metatarsus adductus)
  - Internal pelvic rotation (in some neuromuscular diseases)[18]

## NONOPERATIVE MANAGEMENT

- There is no nonoperative intervention which changes the rotational profile of the long bones.
- Nonoperative treatment of intoeing is geared toward trying to get the child to position the affected hip(s) in more external rotation during gait. Such interventions may include mechanical devices such as twister cables or derotation straps or use of a home program to teach the child to actively externally rotate the hip(s).

## SURGICAL MANAGEMENT

### Indications

- The most common indication is persistent femoral anteversion associated with intoeing interfering with function in children with CP. The anteversion and intoeing typically impact function by causing tripping and/or lever arm dysfunction.
- Isolated idiopathic femoral anteversion rarely requires surgical correction. The rare exceptions are children at, or nearing, adolescence with severe anteversion accompanied by marked internal foot and knee progression angles resulting in functional limitations.
- Malignant malalignment (the combination of femoral anteversion and external tibial torsion) results in anterior knee pain and/or patellar instability recalcitrant to nonoperative measures.

### Preoperative Planning

#### *Location of the Osteotomy*

- The first decision which should be made in planning femoral rotational osteotomy is whether to perform the osteotomy proximally or distally.
  - Benefits of a distal femoral osteotomy fixed with Kirschner wires (K-wires) include (1) smaller incision, (2) less soft tissue dissection, and (3) no need for reoperation for retained hardware (as the K-wires are removed in the office 1 month postoperatively).[14,15]
  - Benefits of a proximal femoral osteotomy (typically fixed with a blade plate) include (1) rigid internal fixation and (2) the ability to correct coxa valga and hip subluxation by including a varus component when planning and performing the osteotomy.[14,15]

- Given the relative merits of the two techniques, distal femoral osteotomies are preferred for pure rotational correction in children before adolescence.
- Proximal femoral osteotomies are typically preferred for children with coxa valga (often with associated hip subluxation, as in CP, DDH and/or Legg-Calvé-Perthes disease) and in children nearing adolescence (in order to avoid casting).
- Even when a distal femoral osteotomy is being considered, an anteroposterior (AP) pelvis x-ray should be performed preoperatively to make sure that there is no significant hip uncovering requiring a proximal femoral osteotomy.

### Amount of Correction

- Preoperatively, the surgeon determines the amount of intraoperative rotational correction to be performed based on both physical examination measurements and the assessment of gait.
- It is imperative that other deformities impacting transverse plane kinematic (rotational) data are thoroughly assessed.[8,14,15] These include pelvic asymmetry and rotation, tibial torsion, and any foot deformities.
  - Remember that pes valgus contributes to outtoeing, and pes varus contributes to intoeing.
- Physical examination (as described earlier) allows quantification of osseous deformity in these children. Radiographic imaging to assess rotation is not typically necessary.
- Gait should be assessed thoroughly, preferably with a computerized gait study, in order to quantify the contributors to transverse plane alignment, including pelvic rotation, hip rotation, tibial torsion, and foot deformity. Although gait analysis is most commonly thought of for children with CP (or other neuromuscular maladies), it is also helpful to quantify gait deviations in typically developing children with significant torsional malalignment who are being considered for surgical intervention.
- The amount of rotation performed at surgery is based on the static and dynamic measures. Typically, the distal fragment should be rotated 1.5 to 2.0 times the amount of abnormal internal hip rotation on gait preoperatively.[15,17] (For example, if there is 20 degrees of internal hip rotation preoperatively, the femur should be rotated 30 to 40 degrees intraoperatively.) Less derotation results in undercorrection.
- If a proximal femoral osteotomy is planned (based on patient age and/or radiographic findings of coxa valga and/or hip subluxation), plain pelvis radiographs facilitate the planning regarding any varus correction to be incorporated into the osteotomy.

### Hardware Choice

#### Proximal Femoral Osteotomy

- Proximal femoral osteotomies are typically fixed with blade plates. A plate should be chosen with a long enough blade to ensure stable fixation while stopping short of the proximal femoral physis (**FIG 3**).
- For small children, a rough guide for AO (Synthes, Paoli, PA) blade plate size follows:
  - Less than or equal to 18 kg: AO "infant" blade plate
  - Eighteen to 24 kg: AO "toddler" blade plate
  - Greater than or equal to 25 kg: AO "child" blade plate

#### Distal Femoral Osteotomy

- Three or four 2.4-mm (3/32 inches) K-wires are typically used for fixation.

## Positioning

- Proximal and distal femoral osteotomies are both easily accomplished with the patient supine on a radiolucent operating table. Supine positioning also facilitates the performance of numerous other concomitant procedures, particularly in children with CP or other neuromuscular diseases.
- Some other authors advocate the prone position for proximal femoral osteotomies and cite the ability to perform the same intraoperative assessment of the torsional profile as the preoperative assessment.[21]
  - Prone positioning precludes pelvic osteotomy and hip flexor lengthening.

## Approach

### Proximal Femoral Osteotomy

- A standard lateral approach is used.
- The proximal end of the incision is at the level of the vastus ridge (origin of the vastus lateralis).

### Distal Femoral Osteotomy

- A direct lateral, subvastus approach is used.
- The distal tip of the incision is at the level of the physis. With experience, in thin children, the surgery can be accomplished through a 4- to 5-cm incision, although larger incisions (typically 7 to 10 cm) are typical until ample experience is gained.

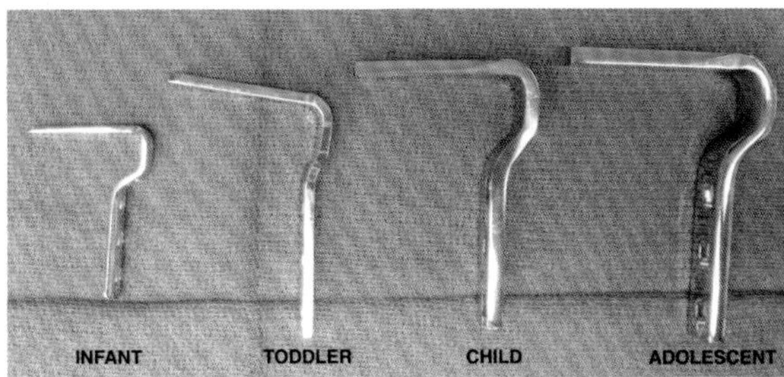


**FIG 3** • Infant, toddler, child, and adolescent size blade plates show relative sizes. Small fragment (3.5-mm cortical) are used with the infant and toddler plates, and large fragment (4.5-mm cortical) with the child and adolescent plates. (Courtesy of Children's Orthopaedic Center, Los Angeles.)

## Proximal Femoral Derotational Osteotomy with Blade Plate: Supine Technique

### Positioning, Incision, and Exposure

- The patient is positioned supine on the radiolucent table with a small "bump" placed under the sacrum.
- The image intensifier is set up on the contralateral side of the patient with the image monitor at the foot of the bed. (The image intensifier is switched to the other side of the bed subsequently for bilateral procedures.)
- Because most cases require bilateral surgery, both lower extremities are typically prepped and draped free. The prep is typically up to the level of the 12th rib, particularly if open hip reduction and/or pelvic osteotomy may be needed.
- The proximal end of the incision is at the level of the vastus lateralis ridge.
- Typically, when gaining experience with the procedure, the incision is 3 to 5 cm longer than the selected blade plate. In thin children, as experience is gained, the incision length is typically only slightly (~1 to 2 cm) longer than the blade plate (**TECH FIG 1A**).
- Electrocautery is used extensively in the dissection to minimize bleeding in these often small children, with correspondingly low blood volumes.
- The tensor fascia lata is identified (**TECH FIG 1B**) and then split in line with the skin incision, thus exposing the vastus lateralis (**TECH FIG 1C**). Exposure of the vastus lateralis may be facilitated by removal of the trochanteric bursa.
- The vastus lateralis is elevated transversely off the vastus ridge and extended in an "L" fashion in order to facilitate exposure and later closure (**TECH FIG 1D**).
- Staying just anterior to the insertion of the gluteus maximus and the linea aspera with the dissection makes the dissection much easier as the periosteum easily peels off the femur.
- Circumferential subperiosteal dissection is needed at the osteotomy site in order to allow appropriate rotational correction. This is usually best accomplished using a set of curved (Crego-type) elevators (**TECH FIG 1E**).

### Preparation for Osteotomy and Fixation

- A guide pin is inserted with the aid of the image intensifier. The guide pin insertion point is typically approximately 1 cm distal to the greater trochanteric apophysis and should be located in the mid-coronal plane of the femur (**TECH FIG 2A**).
- Prior to pin insertion, the hip is internally rotated until the greater trochanter is most lateral, indicating that the femoral neck is parallel to the ground. With the hip in this position, if the guidewire is inserted parallel to the floor, it should be parallel to the axis of the femoral neck in the transverse plane.

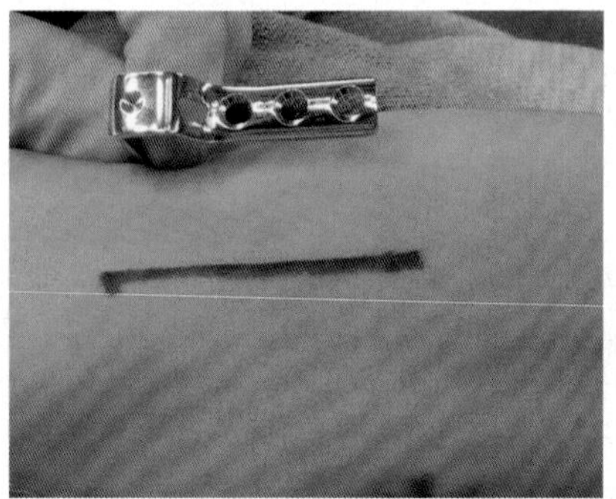
A

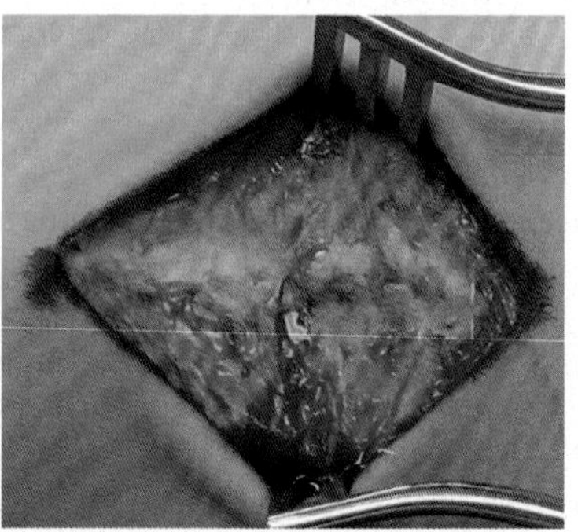
B

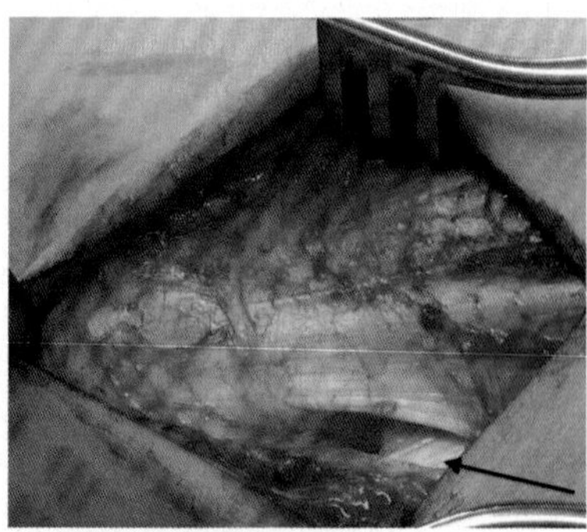
C

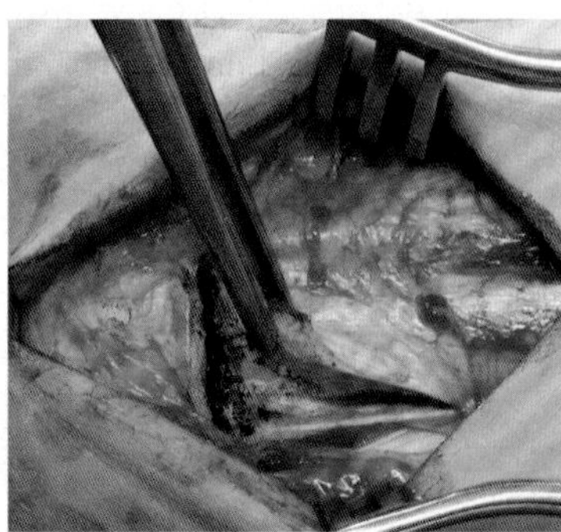
D

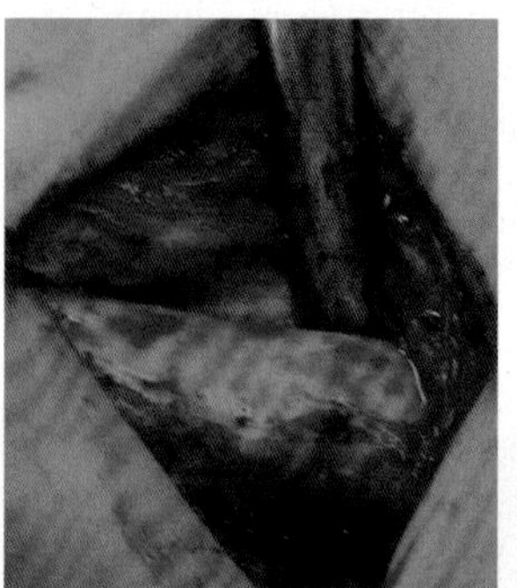
E

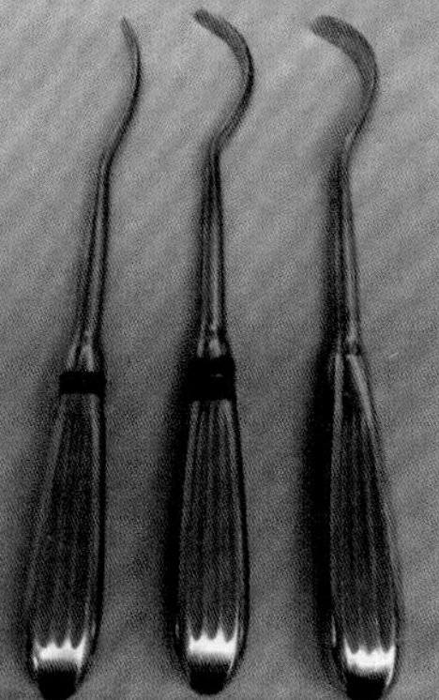
F

**TECH FIG 1** • Exposure of the proximal femur through a standard lateral approach. **A.** The incision starts proximally at the vastus ridge and extends in line with the femur distal enough to accommodate the appropriate size plate. **B.** The tensor fascia lata (TFL) is exposed (and subsequently incised) in line with the skin incision. **C.** After the TFL is split, the vastus lateralis is visualized. Sometimes, adequate visualization of the vastus lateralis is facilitated by removal of the trochanteric bursa. The *arrow* points to the gluteus maximus inserting into the femur. **D.** Detaching the vastus lateralis from the trochanteric ridge in L-shaped cut. **E.** Exposure of the lateral surface of proximal femur, with the vastus lateralis reflected anteriorly. The pickups are holding the periosteum, and the cut is just anterior to the linea aspera and gluteus maximus insertion to facilitate subperiosteal dissection. **F.** A typical set of Crego elevators used for subperiosteal dissection. (Courtesy of Children's Orthopaedic Center, Los Angeles.)

- The angle of the guidewire and chisel in the coronal plane is based on whether or not a varus component is needed for the osteotomy.
- Although using fluoroscopy in the AP view, the guidewire should be inserted in the direction desired for the ultimate position of the blade plate chisel while maintaining the wire parallel to the ground to allow appropriate position in the femoral neck on the lateral view (**TECH FIG 2B**).
- Because it is often difficult to read the depth directly off the blade plate chisel, it is easiest to insert the guidewire to the depth the seating chisel will be inserted. The depth of the wire in the femur should be equal to the length of the blade of the blade plate to be used. This is most easily accomplished by placing a second K-wire adjacent to the guidewire and advancing it to the lateral femoral cortex. The difference in the lateral prominence of the second wire relative to the first is the depth of the guidewire in the femur, which measures 38 mm in this picture (**TECH FIG 2C**).
- The chisel chosen must be the one which matches the size of the blade plate (ie, infant, toddler, child, adolescent, or adult).

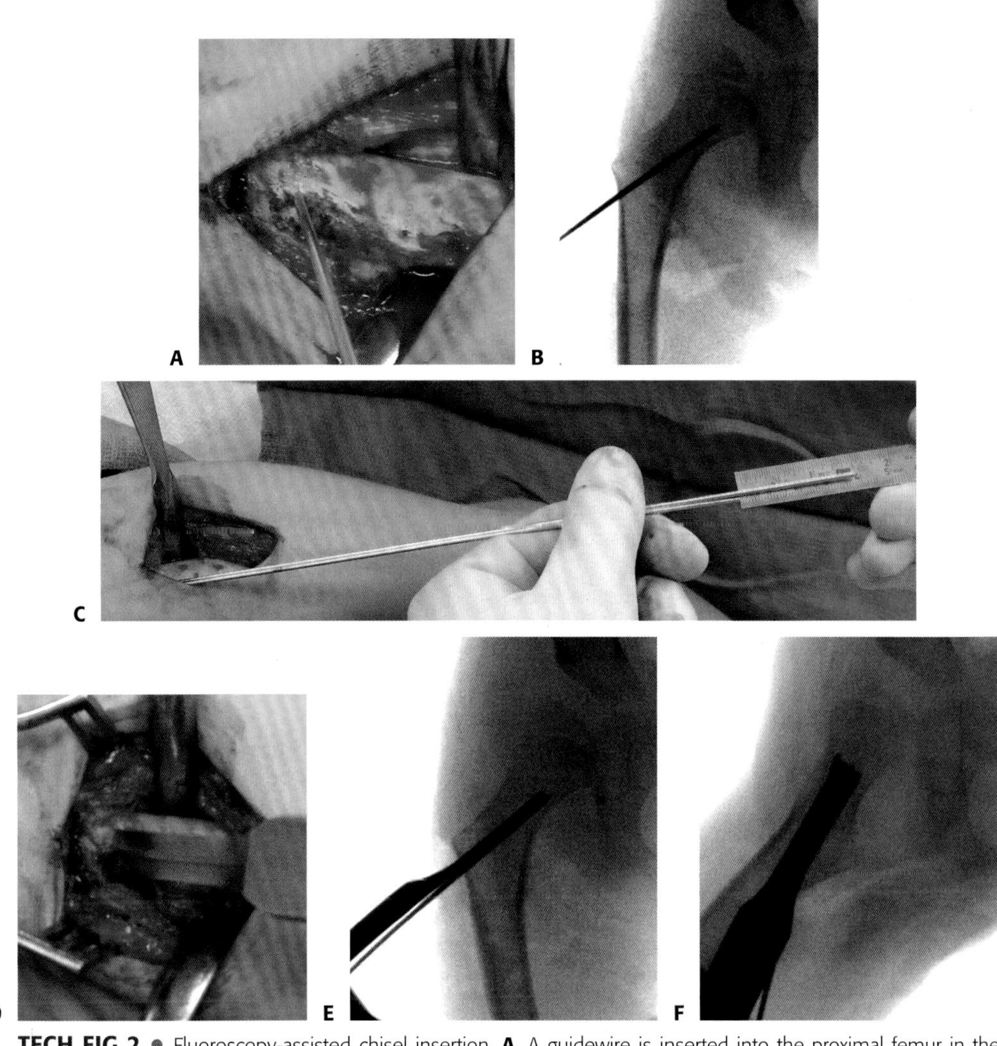

**TECH FIG 2** • Fluoroscopy-assisted chisel insertion. **A.** A guidewire is inserted into the proximal femur in the mid-coronal plane, typically starting ~1 cm distal to the vastus ridge. The hip is internally rotated until the greater trochanter is directly lateral prior to wire insertion and the wire inserted parallel to the floor. **B.** Position of the guide pin on the AP view. This pin position is more vertical than for isolated rotation, unless the plate has an angle matching the pin–shaft (and chisel–shaft) angles. **C.** The guide pin should be inserted to the depth to which the chisel will be inserted. The depth is confirmed by manually placing a second pin adjacent to the first pin and placing it against the lateral femoral cortex. The difference between the prominence of the second wire relative to the first is the depth of the guidewire in the femur, which measures 38 mm in this picture. **D.** Insertion of the seating chisel parallel to the guide pin. The chisel should be backed out several millimeters from the fully inserted position prior to osteotomy in children with strong bone, although it was rarely necessary in small children being treated with infant or toddler blade plates. **E.** Fluoroscopic imaging showing the chisel inserted parallel, and just cephalad to, the guide pin on the AP view. **F.** Position of the seating chisel in the center of the neck on the frog lateral view. Because a cannulated system was not used, the chisel does not need to be completely parallel to the pin on this view. *(continued)*

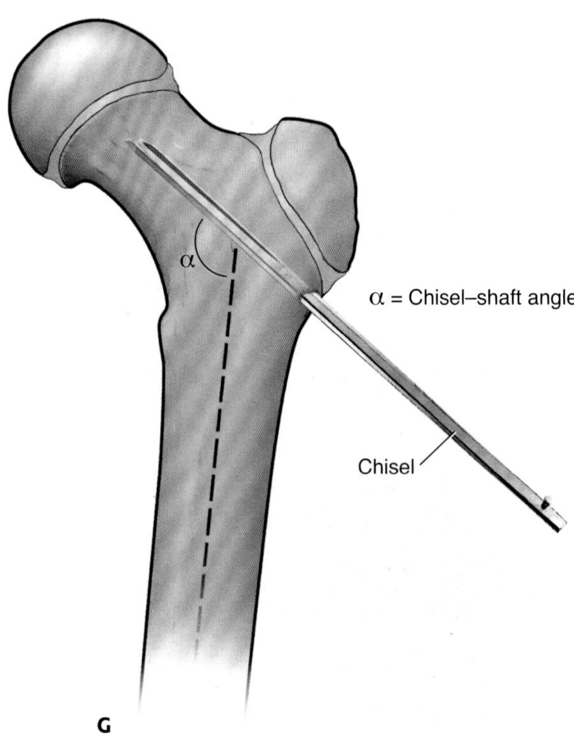


**TECH FIG 2** • *(continued)* **G.** The chisel–shaft angle is the angle between the chisel and the shaft of the femur. For a pure rotational osteotomy, the chisel–shaft angle should equal the angle of the plate to be inserted. For varus osteotomies, the chisel–shaft angle exceeds the angle of the plate to be inserted, and for valgus osteotomies, the chisel–shaft angle is less than that of the plate. (**A–F:** Courtesy of Children's Orthopaedic Center, Los Angeles.)

It is important to remember that the chisel used for child and adolescent plates is the same.

- The seating chisel is inserted immediately cephalad to the guidewire (**TECH FIG 2D**). Several AP and lateral fluoroscopic images are obtained during chisel insertion to make sure that the position is optimal on AP and frog lateral views.
  - Care must be taken to insert the chisel such that the face of the chisel is perpendicular to the shaft of the femur in the sagittal plane (in order to avoid flexion or extension at the osteotomy site).
  - The chisel is inserted to the tip of the guidewire and checked for position in AP and lateral planes (**TECH FIG 2E,F**). This is an easier way to insert the chisel to the correct depth than if one attempts to read the depth off the underside of the chisel when it is in the femur.
  - For a pure rotational osteotomy, the blade plate should be placed in a direction so that the "chisel–shaft angle" (the angle between the chisel and the shaft of the femur) equals the angle of the blade plate to be used (**TECH FIG 2G**).
    - Although many authors advocate using a 90-degree blade plate for proximal femoral rotational osteotomies, a plate with a larger angle (≥100 degrees) typically allows the surgeon to insert the blade deeper into the femoral neck, enhancing fixation, and facilitating early weight bearing.
  - For an osteotomy which requires a varus component, the chisel should be inserted at an angle which will result in the necessary varus correction. (For example, if 20 degrees of varus is desired, the chisel–shaft angle should exceed the angle of the blade plate by 20 degrees. In other words, if a 90-degree blade plate were going to be used, the guidewire and blade plate chisel should be inserted at an angle resulting in a 110-degree chisel–shaft angle.)
- If a cannulated system is used, the guidewire must be inserted in precisely the desired position for the chisel and blade plate. As a result, this may add time to the surgery as the guide pin location must be exact.
  - In ambulatory children with healthy bone, the seating chisel should be intermittently backed during insertion to facilitate chisel removal prior to blade plate insertion. The chisel should be backed out from its deepest insertion point prior to the osteotomy for the same reason.

## Osteotomy

- The level of the transverse osteotomy is marked with electrocautery perpendicular to the femoral shaft. The distance from the chisel insertion site is based on which side plate will be used: 1 cm for infant plates; 1.2 cm for toddler plates; and 1.5 cm for child, adolescent, and adult plates (**TECH FIG 3A**).
- If a femoral shortening will be performed (typically indicated when performing bilateral varus derotational osteotomies [VDROs] in children with CP), then a second osteotomy site should be marked distal and parallel to the first osteotomy site. Typically, when shortening is performed, it should be 1.5 to 2.0 cm.
- Two smooth derotation pins (1.6- or 2.0-mm K-wires) are placed in an anterior to posterior direction parallel to each other in the transverse plane, one just distal to the blade plate chisel and the second distal to the most distal transverse osteotomy (**TECH FIG 3B**).
- A transverse osteotomy is made using an oscillating saw at the osteotomy site marked 1 to 1.5 cm distal to the chisel based on plate size (as mentioned earlier) (**TECH FIG 3C**).
  - A large Crego elevator is used to protect the anterior and medial structures, and a medium or large Chandler elevator protects the posterior structures.
  - For children with strong bone, frequent irrigation is used to minimize the risk of thermal necrosis of the bone at the

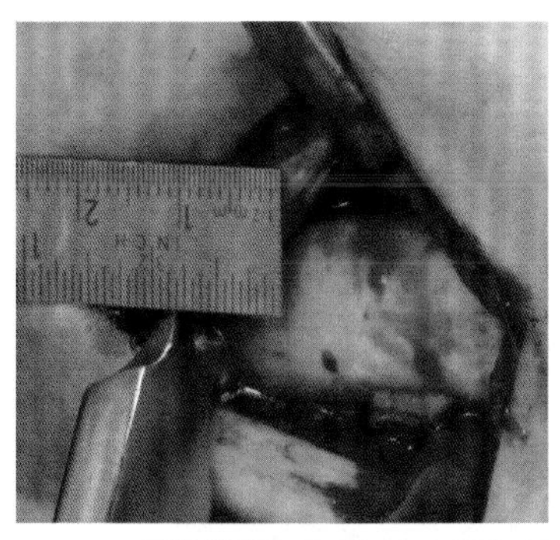
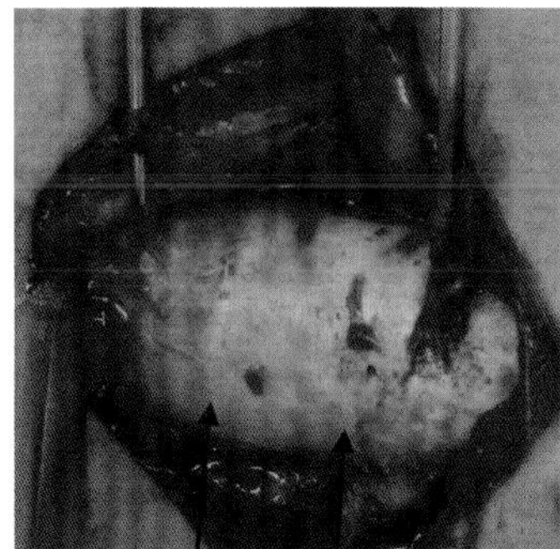
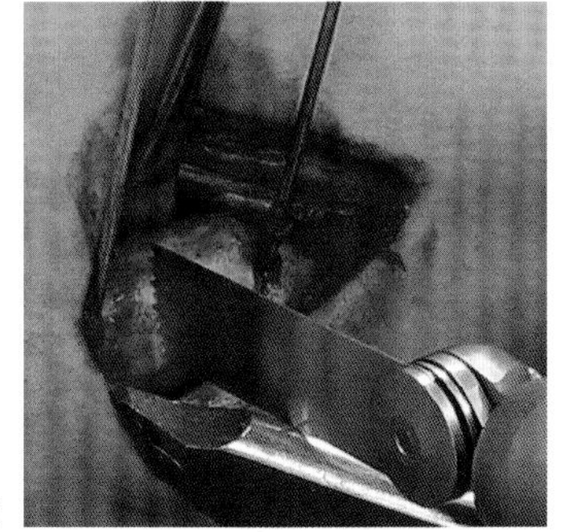
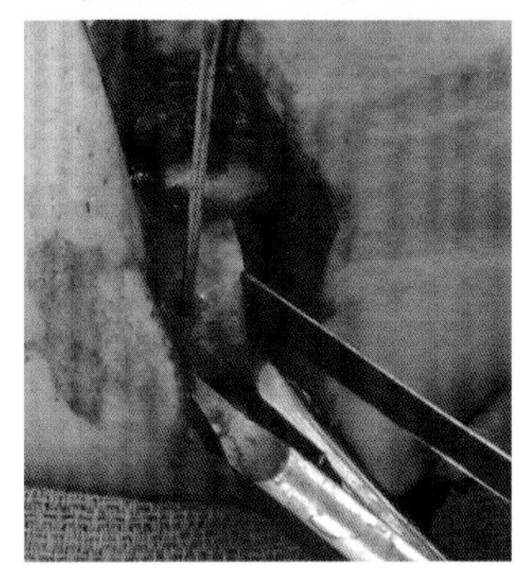

**TECH FIG 3** • Identification of osteotomy site(s) and completion of osteotomy(ies). **A.** The site for the osteotomy is localized with the use of a ruler. The distance of the osteotomy from the chisel insertion site is 1.0 cm for infant blade plates, 1.2 cm for toddler plates, and 1.5 cm for child and adolescent plates. **B.** Two parallel AP guide pins proximal and distal to the transverse osteotomy line(s) are used to judge the magnitude of derotation. In this case, there are two transverse osteotomies to be made to allow femoral shortening in this child with CP and hip subluxation. The location for the osteotomies are denoted with *arrows*. **C.** Transverse osteotomy (perpendicular to the long axis of the femur). *This is the only osteotomy needed if the osteotomy is being done for derotation only.* **D.** When varus is a necessary component of the osteotomy (as in most children with CP and other neuromuscular disorders), this cut starts halfway across the femur and should be perfectly parallel to the chisel in all planes if a 90-degree plate is being used. This medial closing wedge osteotomy is *not* needed if pure derotation is performed without varus. (Courtesy of Children's Orthopaedic Center, Los Angeles.)

osteotomy site. The periosteum is elevated circumferentially at this level to allow placement of protective retractors during the osteotomy.

- For pure rotational osteotomies, the transverse osteotomy cut is the only one needed.
- For VDROs, two or three osteotomy cuts are needed:
  - The transverse osteotomy is described earlier.
  - In children in whom a femoral shortening is being performed (particularly in children with spastic CP), a second transverse osteotomy cut is made parallel to the first cut.
  - In all cases of varus osteotomy, a medial closing wedge osteotomy of the proximal fragment is performed; this osteotomy does not start at the lateral cortex but rather approximately 50% of the distal from lateral to medial. If a 90-degree plate is to be used, this osteotomy should be parallel to the blade plate chisel in all planes (**TECH FIG 3D**).
    - If a plate other than a 90-degree blade plate is to be used, then the osteotomy needs to be adjusted accordingly. For an 80-degree plate, the osteotomy should angle 10 degree *toward* the chisel. For plates with angles greater than 90 degrees, the osteotomy should angle *away* from the plate (10 degrees away for 100-degree plates, 20 degrees away for 110-degree plates, 30 degrees for 120-degree plates, etc.).

## Derotation and Fixation

- The blade plate chisel is removed and replaced by the previously chosen blade plate (**TECH FIG 4A**).
- The position of the proximal femur is controlled (typically with anteriorly and posteriorly placed Hohmann retractors) prior to chisel removal.
- The blade plate can often be inserted at least part-way into the path created by the blade plate chisel with gentle manual pressure. A mallet can be used to gently tap the plate into the femur along the same path. Forceful striking with the mallet should be avoided in order to minimize the risk of creating a new path and penetrating the cortex medially, anteriorly, and/or posteriorly.
- The plate is impacted into final position with the impactor and mallet (**TECH FIG 4B**).

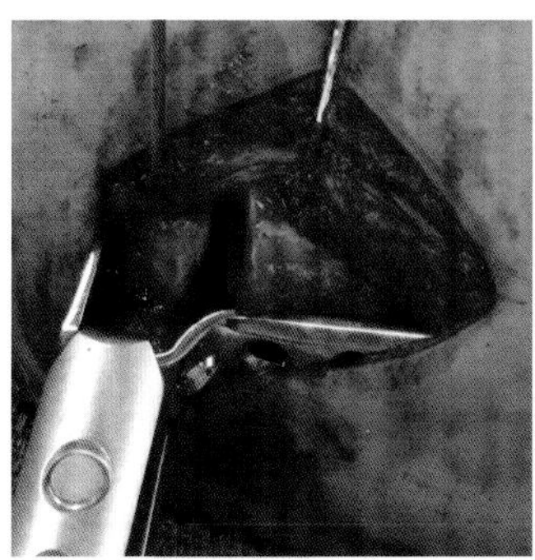
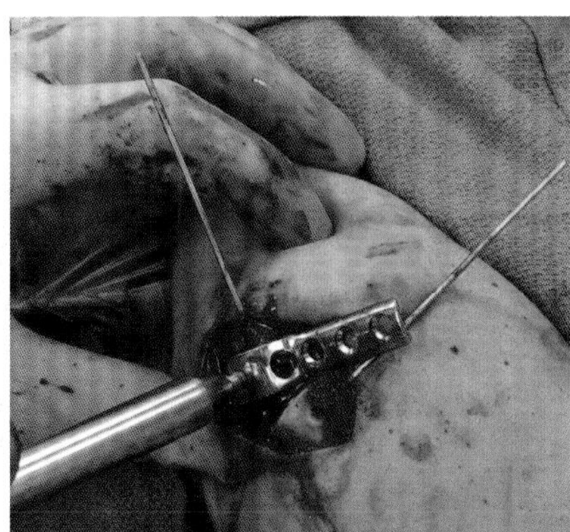

**TECH FIG 4** • Blade plate insertion and osteotomy fixation. **A.** After chisel removal, the blade plate is inserted in the same path. Whenever possible, inserting the plate as far as possible with gentle manual pressure ensures correct insertion angle and alignment. The mallet is then used to gently tap the inserter and advance the plate deeper into place. **B.** After the insertion handle is removed, an impactor is used to complete seating of the blade plate. It is common that the proximal fragment is quite flexed (analogous to proximal femur fractures) following these osteotomies; this will be important to remember in the next step. *(continued)*

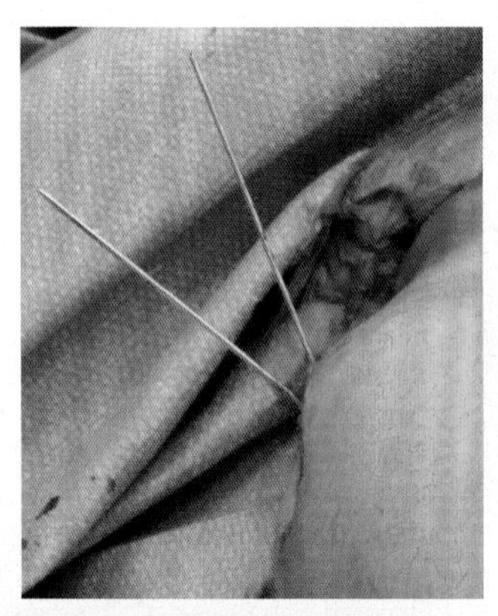

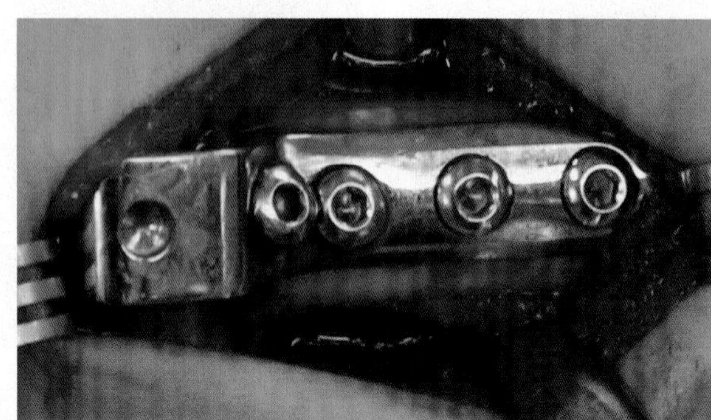

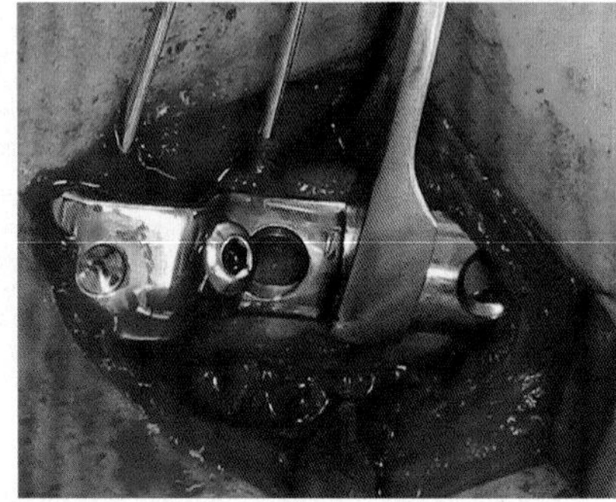

**TECH FIG 4** • *(continued)* **C.** The osteotomy is reduced (with appropriate derotation), stabilized with a Verbrugge bone-holding clamp, and the amount of rotation can be assessed by measuring the angle between the two pins with a sterile goniometer. Of note, reduction is often facilitated by flexing the hip to 90 degrees prior to reduction. **D.** The blade plate is held against the femur with a Verbrugge clamp. **E.** Fixation following cortical screw insertion. (Courtesy of Children's Orthopaedic Center, Los Angeles.)

- The distal femoral fragment is approximated to the plate with a bone-holding clamp such as a Verbrugge clamp. Reduction of the osteotomy is facilitated by flexing the hip to approximately 90 degrees.
- Prior to application of the Verbrugge clamp, the distal femoral fragment is externally rotated until the angle between the previously parallel guidewires matches the amount of derotation desired (**TECH FIG 4C**). A sterile goniometer is used to confirm the amount of correction.
- Screws are used to fix the plate to the distal femoral fragment (3.5-mm cortical screws for infant and toddler blade plates and 4.5-mm screws for the child, adolescent, and adult plates). At least one of the screws in the distal fragment is inserted in compression to hasten bone healing (except for infant plates, which cannot be compressed) (**TECH FIG 4D, E**).
  - After fixation with one or two distal screws, the arc of hip rotation is evaluated. External rotation should typically exceed internal rotation at this time.

## Wound Closure

- The vastus lateralis is approximated to the vastus ridge and repaired with two figure-8 sutures of size 0 absorbable suture, such as Vicryl (Ethicon, West Somerville, NJ). A running size 0 absorbable suture is used to close the posterior aspect of the vastus lateralis (**TECH FIG 5**).
- The fascia lata is closed with a running size 0 absorbable suture.
- The subcutaneous tissue is closed with simple, interrupted, inverted 2-0 absorbable sutures and a running 3-0 absorbable monofilament, such as Monocryl (Ethicon, West Somerville, NJ), is used to close the subcuticular layer.

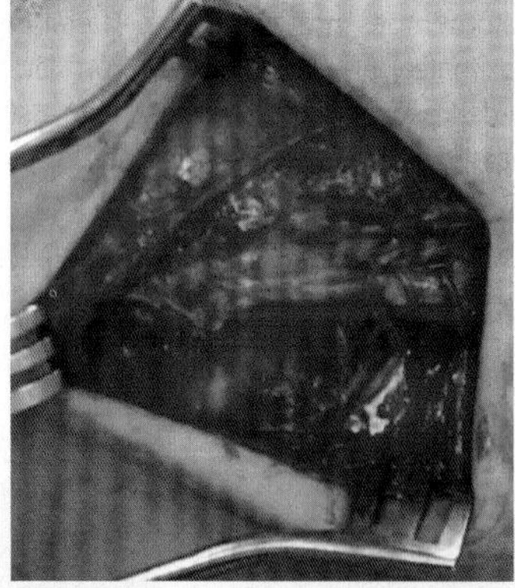

**TECH FIG 5** • Repair of vastus lateralis to its origin to cover the blade plate. (Courtesy of Children's Orthopaedic Center, Los Angeles.)

## Proximal Femoral Derotational Osteotomy with 90-Degree AO Blade Plate: Prone Technique[27]

- The patient is positioned prone on appropriate (low) bolsters to support the chest and iliac crests, keeping pressure off the abdomen and the genitalia.[27]
- The table mattress padding under the thigh segments can be built up to keep the hips relatively extended.
- The approach and dissection are identical to those described for the supine technique; only the orientation must be remembered with the anterior vastus lateralis now falling away from the operative field (**TECH FIG 6A**).
- The torsional profile in the prone position can be verified and compared with the contralateral side (**TECH FIG 6B,C**).
- Postoperative care is as described earlier for the supine technique.

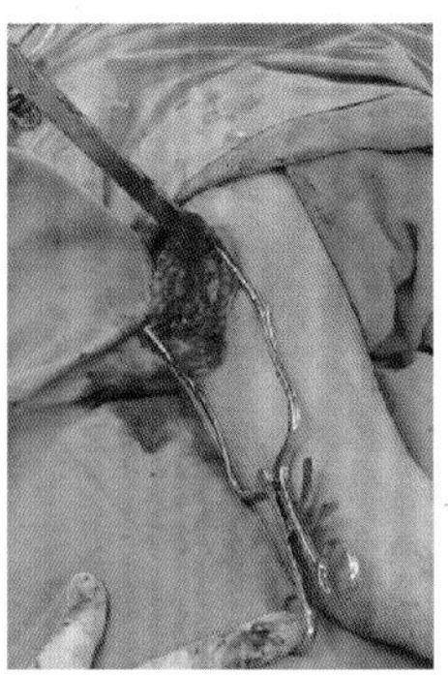
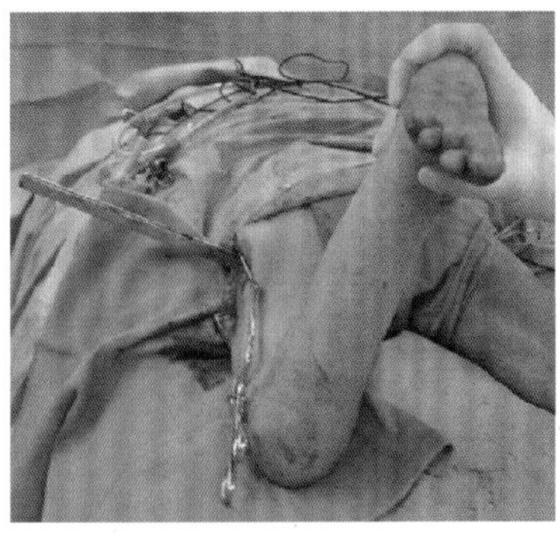
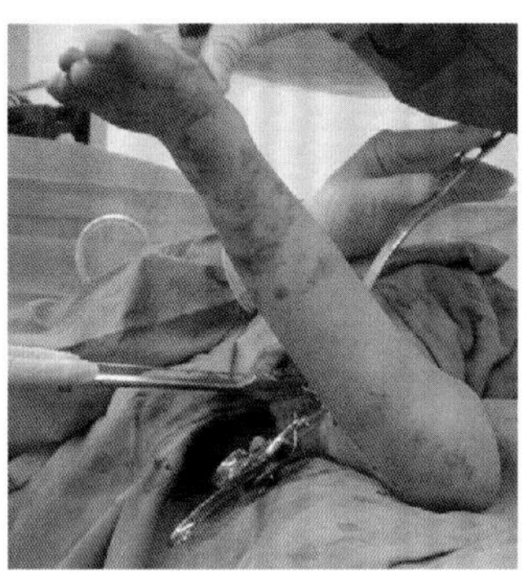

**TECH FIG 6** • Proximal femoral derotation osteotomy using the prone technique. **A.** Orientation of the exposure in the prone position. **B,C.** Intraoperative ability to estimate the torsional profile.

## Distal Femoral Derotational Osteotomy with K-Wire Fixation

### Positioning, Incision, and Exposure

- The patient is positioned supine on a radiolucent table. The leg is prepped up to the inguinal crease, unless other more proximal surgery (such as adductor lengthening or pelvic osteotomy) is needed.
- The image intensifier is set up on the contralateral side of the patient with the image monitor at the foot of the bed. (The image intensifier is switched to the other side of the bed subsequently for bilateral procedures.)
- A Freer elevator is used to localize the distal femoral physis. In the absence of patella alta, the physis is located at the junction of the middle and distal thirds of the patella (**TECH FIG 7A**).
- A longitudinal incision is made over the lateral distal femur, with the distal tip at the level of the physis. When first learning this procedure, the incision will typically be 7 to 10 cm, but as experience is gained, a 4- to 5-cm incision may be used in a thin child (**TECH FIG 7B**).
- The iliotibial (IT) band is incised in line with the skin incision, and a subvastus approach is made to the distal femur (**TECH FIG 7C,D**). The vastus lateralis is elevated off the intermuscular septum, and bleeders are coagulated as they are identified.

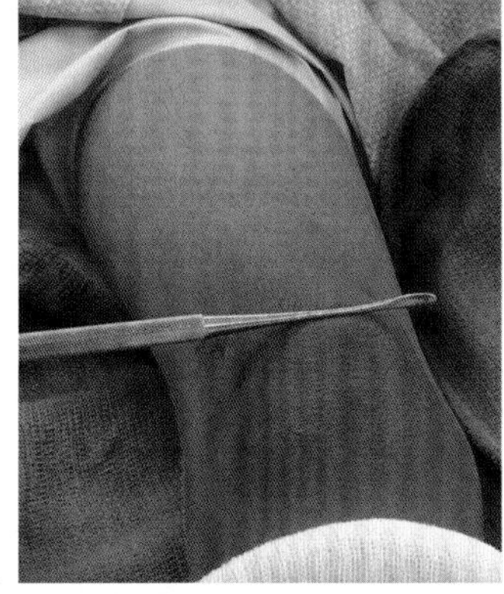
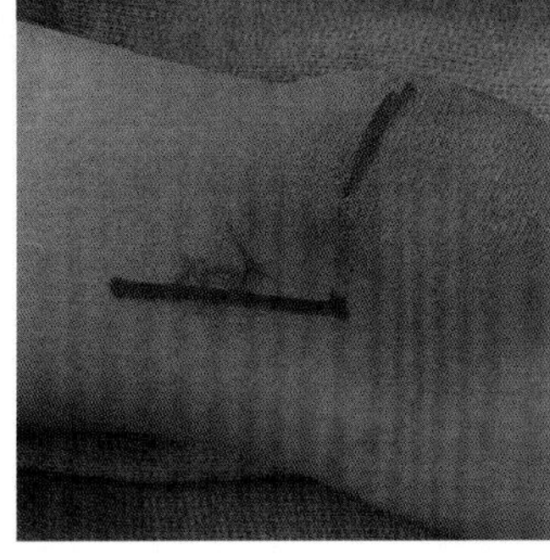

**TECH FIG 7** • Exposure of the distal femur through a lateral approach. **A.** Localization of the physis is performed using fluoroscopic guidance. The physis is typically at the junction of the middle and distal thirds of the patella. **B.** The distal end of the incision is at the level of the physis. When first using this technique, a 7- to10-cm incision is needed, although after much experience is gained, the incision may be 4 to 5 cm. *(continued)*

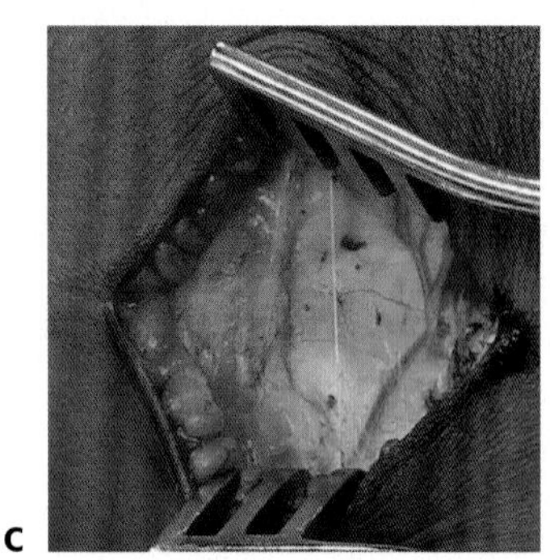

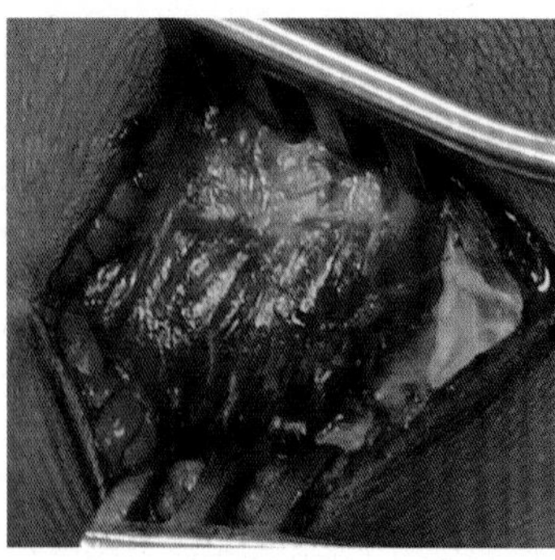

**TECH FIG 7** • *(continued)* **C.** Exposure of the IT band (ITB) prior to splitting the ITB. **D.** The appearance of the vastus lateralis after the ITB is split. A subvastus approach is made, elevating the vastus lateralis off the intermuscular septum. (Courtesy of Children's Orthopaedic Center, Los Angeles.)

## Preparation for Osteotomy and Fixation

- The osteotomy site (in the metaphysis, typically 3 to 4 cm proximal to the physis) is identified using fluoroscopic guidance (**TECH FIG 8A**). The periosteum is split in a "T" fashion, with a longitudinal cut distal to proximal and then with anterior and posterior cuts to complete the T distally, just distal to the level of the osteotomy, and at least 2 cm proximal to the physis (**TECH FIG 8B**).
- Subperiosteal dissection is performed with Crego elevators anteriorly and posteriorly. Posteriorly, a large Chandler elevator is used to complete the dissection because this Chandler elevator is used to protect the soft tissues posteriorly during the osteotomy (**TECH FIG 8C**).
- Derotation pins (1.6 or 2.0 mm) are placed parallel to each other in the transverse (rotation) plane and parallel to the physis in the coronal plane. One pin is proximal and the other is distal to the osteotomy site (**TECH FIG 8D,E**).

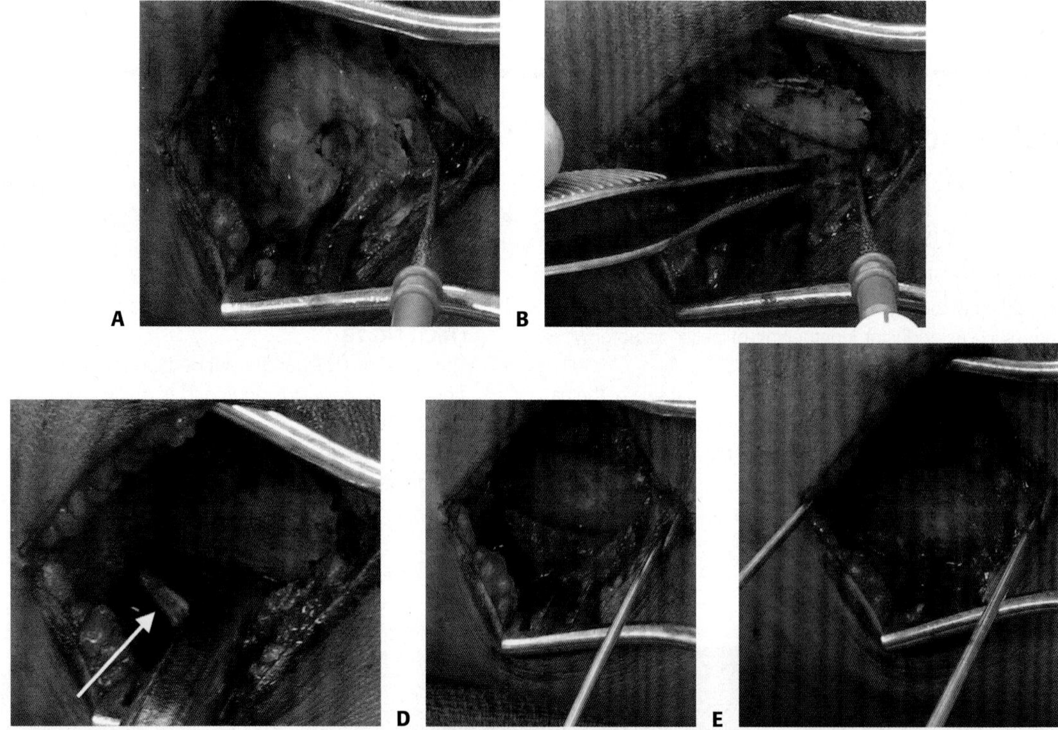

**TECH FIG 8** • **A.** Before the periosteum is incised, fluoroscopy is used to confirm that the electrocautery tip is in the correct location. **B.** The periosteum has been split longitudinally and is now being "T'ed" posteriorly. The forceps are seen holding the periosteum. **C.** Chandler elevator in place subperiosteally. The *arrow* points to the periosteum. **D.** A guidewire is inserted parallel to the physis, just distal to where the periosteum was T-ed earlier. This guidewire must be parallel to the physis because it will serve as a visual guide during the osteotomy. This wire should not penetrate through the medial metaphysis in order to minimize the risk of soft tissue binding when rotating the distal fragment prior to fixation. **E.** After placement of the second wire. These wires need to be parallel in the transverse (rotational) plane but not in the coronal plane. The distal wire (as mentioned earlier) must be parallel to the physis to guide the osteotomy. (Courtesy of Children's Orthopaedic Center, Los Angeles.)

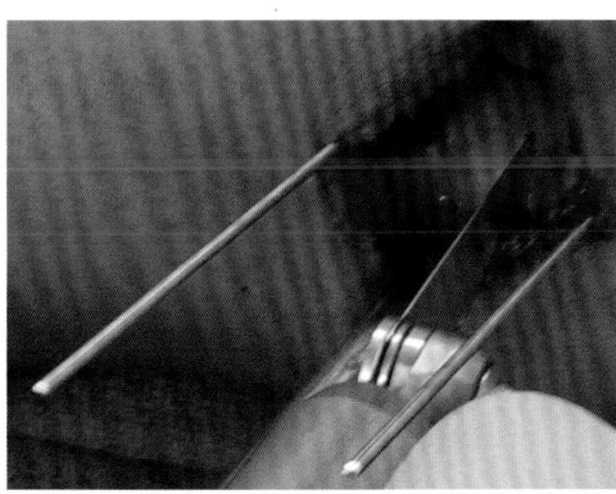

**TECH FIG 9** • A metaphyseal osteotomy is made with an oscillating saw, parallel to the distal pin (and to the physis). The distal pin is used as a guide to direct the osteotomy. (Courtesy of Children's Orthopaedic Center, Los Angeles.)

## Osteotomy

- A large Chandler elevator is placed behind the femur and a Hohmann retractor anteriorly at the level of the osteotomy.
- A metaphyseal osteotomy is performed with an oscillating, making sure to cut the femur parallel to the distal guidewire (which is parallel to the physis) (**TECH FIG 9**).
- A ½- or ¾-inch osteotome may be needed to complete the osteotomy.

## Derotation and Fixation

- A "lobster claw" clamp is placed on the proximal fragment, just proximal to the osteotomy. During insertion, care is taken to maintain subperiosteal position of the clamp (**TECH FIG 10A**).
- The knee is flexed to 90 degrees, the leg is grabbed at the ankle, and the distal fragment is rotated externally until the angle between the guidewires matches the desired amount of rotational correction planned (**TECH FIG 10B**).
- Three or four 2.4-mm smooth K-wires (1 to 2 from medial and 1 to 2 from lateral) are inserted retrograde using fluoroscopic guidance. The starting points are in the metaphysis just proximal to the physis (**TECH FIG 10C**). The pins should be advanced until the cortex is encountered on the other side of the bone. Prior to penetrating the cortex, a fluoroscopic image is obtained to make sure the wire looks like it has reached the other (medial or lateral) cortex, thus indicating that the wire will exit the femur near the mid-coronal plane. Once this is confirmed, the cortex can be penetrated with the wire. (If the wire hits the cortex and fluoroscopic imaging demonstrates that the tip of the wire is near the middle of femoral canal, then this indicates that the wire is directed too anteriorly or

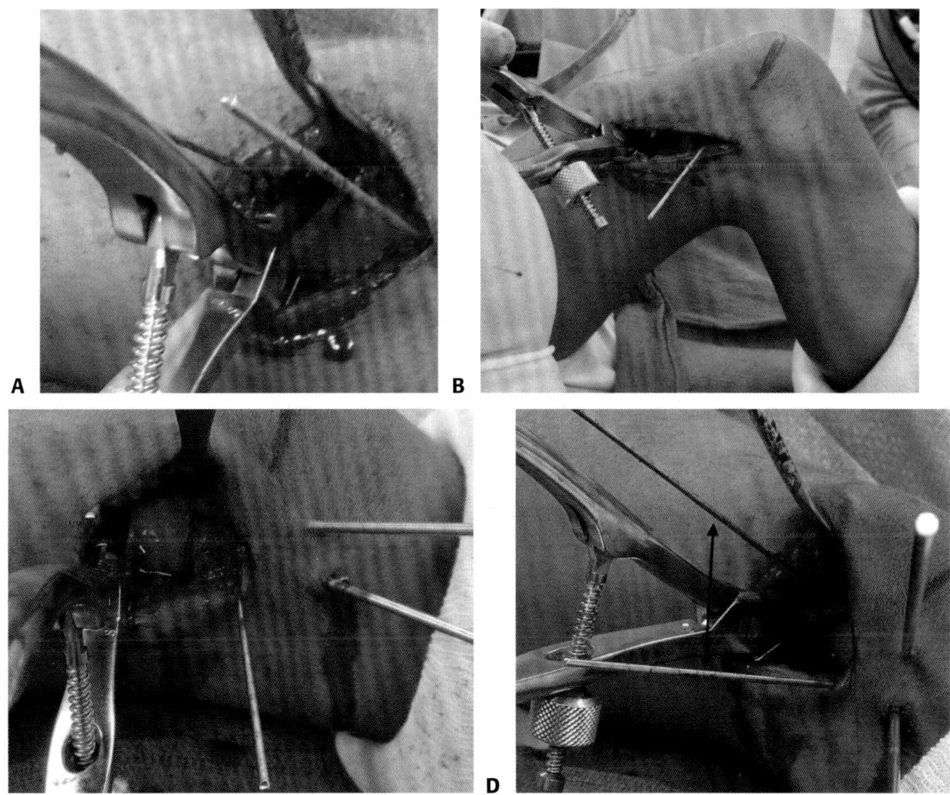


**TECH FIG 10** • **A.** A lobster claw clamp is placed on the proximal fragment to control the proximal fragment while the distal fragment is rotated. The clamp is placed subperiosteally. **B.** The distal fragment is externally rotated with the knee flexed to approximately 90 degrees, one hand controlling the proximal fragment with the clamp and the other hand at the ankle to derotate the distal fragment. The knee must be flexed sufficiently to control the distal fragment and facilitate derotation. Control of the distal fragment is hard derotation is difficult to achieve. **C.** After rotation and fixation with 2.4-mm K-wires, the osteotomy has some step-off laterally (which is common) due to the amount of derotation and intact periosteum anteriorly, posteriorly, and medially. **D.** The amount of rotation (depicted by the *arrows*) can be measured between the derotation pins. (Courtesy of Children's Orthopaedic Center, Los Angeles.)

posteriorly and should be redirected prior to penetrating the cortex.)

- The angle between the derotation pins is used to measure the amount of derotation (**TECH FIG 10D**).
- The pins are bent and cut superficial to the skin to allow for removal in the office.

## Wound Closure

- The IT band is closed with a running size 0 absorbable suture.
- The subcutaneous layer is closed with simple, interrupted size 2-0 absorbable sutures.
- A running 3-0 absorbable monofilament suture is used to close the subcuticular layer.

## PEARLS AND PITFALLS

### Supine and Prone Techniques

| | |
|---|---|
| **Preoperative determination of level of rotation** | ▪ AP pelvis x-ray must be obtained. If coxa valga and/or hip subluxation are present, then proximal femoral osteotomy is needed. In the absence of these, either proximal or distal osteotomy may be performed. |
| **Preoperative determination of the amount of rotation needed** | ▪ Thorough assessment of the rotational profile and dynamic gait parameters are requisite to determine the amount of derotation needed.<br>▪ The amount of rotation necessary is typically 1.5–2 times the amount of excessive internal hip rotation during gait. |
| **Location of the osteotomy (relative to the blade plate)** | ▪ Length distal to the chisel insertion site is based on the plate to be inserted:<br>▪ Infant plate: 1.0 cm distal<br>▪ Toddler plate: 1.2 cm distal<br>▪ Larger plates: 1.5 cm distal |
| **Chisel–shaft angle (the angle measured between the blade plate chisel and the femoral shaft)** | ▪ For purely rotational osteotomies, the chisel–shaft angle should be equal to the angle of the blade plate to be inserted (**FIG 4**).<br>▪ For osteotomies with a varus component, the chisel–shaft angle should exceed the angle of the blade plate by the amount of varus correction desired. |

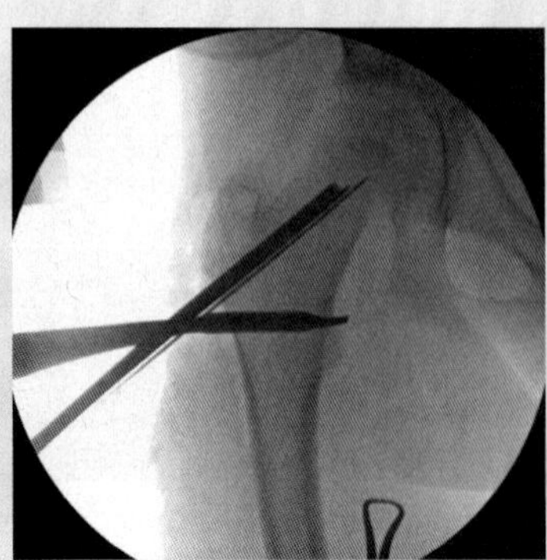

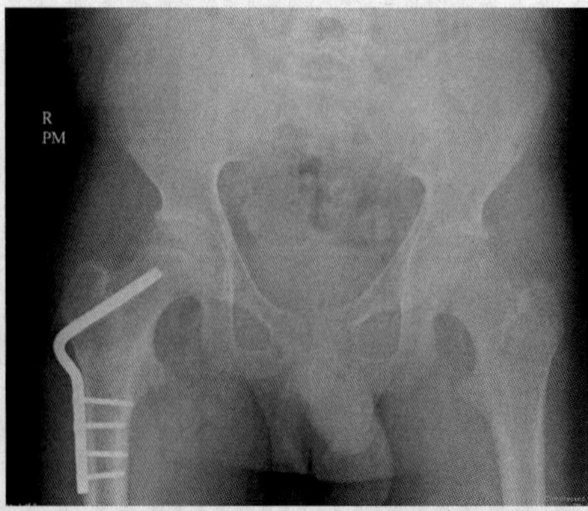


**FIG 4** ● Matching the chisel–shaft angle to the angle of the blade plate for a pure rotational osteotomy. **A.** Adult blade plate chisel inserted such that the chisel–shaft angle is 120 degrees. Use of a plate with an angle of at least 100 degrees allows a long blade to be placed in the femoral neck, thus affording excellent fixation. **B.** Healed osteotomy with 120-degree angle blade plate in place. (Courtesy of Children's Orthopaedic Center, Los Angeles.)

| | |
|---|---|
| **Angle of "varus" osteotomy cut if varus component of osteotomy needed (for all patients undergoing VDRO)** | ■ The varus cut should be oriented differently relative to the chisel depending on the angle of the blade plate being used:<br>■ 90-degree plate: Cut is parallel to the chisel in all planes.<br>■ 80-degree plate: Cut angles 10 degrees toward chisel.<br>■ Greater than 90-degree plate: cut angles α-90-degree away from chisel (eg, 10 degrees away from the chisel for a 100-degree plate; 20 degrees away for a 110-degree plate, 30 degrees away for a 120-degree plate, etc.) |
| **Intraoperative determination of amount of rotation achieved** | ■ Derotation pins are placed parallel to one another proximal and distal to the osteotomy site prior to the osteotomy.<br>■ The angle between the pins is measured with a goniometer after the derotation to measure the amount of correction. |
| **Distal Femoral Derotational Osteotomy with K-wire Fixation** | |
| **Preoperative determination of level of rotation** | ■ AP pelvis x-ray must be obtained. If the hips are well located without significant coxa valga, distal femoral osteotomy may be used. |
| **Preoperative determination of the amount of rotation needed** | ■ Thorough assessment of the rotational profile and dynamic gait parameters are requisite to determine the amount of derotation needed.<br>■ The amount of rotation necessary is 1.5–2 times the amount of excessive internal hip rotation during gait. |
| **Localization of the distal femoral physis** | ■ The physis is located at the junction of the middle and distal thirds of the patella in the absence of patella alta. |
| **Derotation technique** | ■ A lobster claw clamp is placed above the osteotomy site, the knee flexed to 90 degrees, the ankle grabbed with the other hand, and the distal fragment externally rotated. |
| **Intraoperative determination of amount of rotation achieved** | ■ Two parallel derotation pins are placed, one proximal and the other distal to the osteotomy site prior to the osteotomy.<br>■ The angle between the pins is measured with a goniometer after the derotation to measure the amount of correction. |
| **Fixation** | ■ Three to four smooth 2.4-mm K-wires are used.<br>■ The pins are bent and cut superficially to the skin to allow removal in the office 4 weeks postoperative. |

## POSTOPERATIVE CARE

### All Children

- At surgery, the child is placed in a non–weight-bearing long-leg cast.
- At 4 weeks postoperative, the cast is changed, all pins are removed in the office, and the child is placed into a long-leg walking cast.
- At 8 weeks postoperative, assuming sufficient healing, the long-leg cast is removed, and the child may weight bear fully. Physical therapy is begun and focuses on gait, strengthening, and range of motion.

### Typically Developing Children

- For typically developing children with idiopathic anteversion (either in isolation or combined with tibial torsion), fixation is typically quite secure and external immobilization is not requisite. However, an ipsilateral knee immobilizer is often used to put the leg at rest and decrease the child's activity.
- For unilateral procedures, non–weight bearing or touch-down weight bearing with crutches is started immediately. For bilateral procedures, walking is not feasible initially, and bed to chair transfers are taught on postoperative day 1.
- Assuming standard healing, 50% weight bearing is allowed 4 weeks postoperatively, and weight bearing as tolerated is allowed 6 to 8 weeks postoperatively.

### Special Needs Children (eg, Children with CP)

- For children with CP (and other special needs children), proximal femoral osteotomies are almost always performed in combination with other lower extremity soft tissue and/or osseous procedures.
- Postoperative immobilization in children with CP who are younger than approximately 10 years old is typically with an A-frame cast (even if VDRO is performed in combination with open hip reduction and/or pelvic osteotomy). Casting is for 4 weeks, unless open hip reduction was performed (which requires 6 weeks of casting). Spica casting is almost never needed and is typically reserved for those with extremely poor bone quality in whom fixation is poor.
- For older children, a knee immobilizer and hip abduction pillow are typically used nearly full time for 4 weeks.
- At 4 weeks postoperative, bone healing is typically sufficient in these children to allow for weight bearing as tolerated (6 weeks for pelvic osteotomies and/or hip open reduction) (**FIG 5**).
- Physical therapy focusing on range of motion, gait, and strengthening begins 4 to 6 weeks postoperative.

## OUTCOMES

- Supine and prone techniques
  - Correction of gait is typically very successful.
  - Ambulatory patients can expect improved transverse plane alignment with improved foot and knee progression angles.

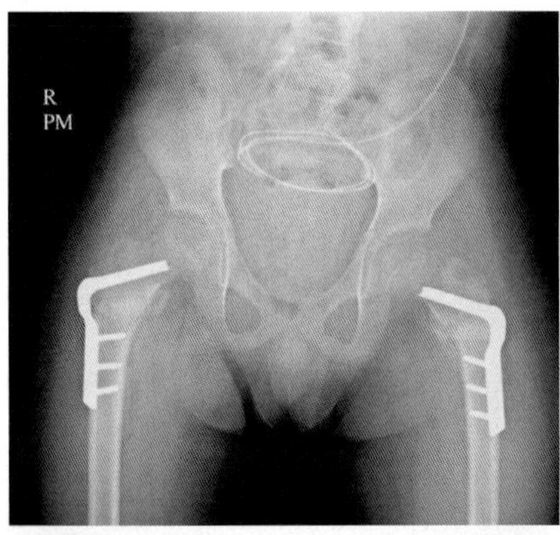


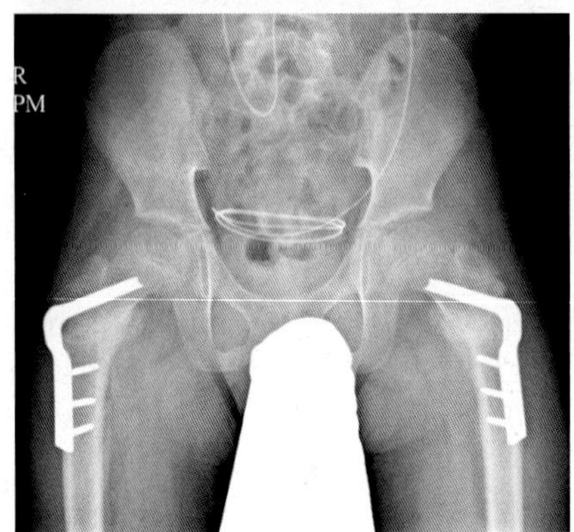


**FIG 5** • Typical healing following bilateral proximal femoral VDROs in a 9-year-old male with CP who functions at GMFCS level III. **A.** At 6 weeks postoperatively. **B.** At 3 months postoperatively. (Courtesy of Children's Orthopaedic Center, Los Angeles.)

- In CP and similar conditions, recurrence rates are higher, although correction is most typically maintained over time if the correction recommended earlier is obtained at surgery.
- K-wire technique
  - Little is known about the long-term outcomes of femoral derotational osteotomies, as these are seldom done in isolation.
  - If adequate correction is achieved, ambulatory patients can expect to experience noticeable benefits in the appearance of their gait. Whether there are measurable functional improvements is less clear.
  - In conditions such as CP, the primary pathology in the brain cannot be addressed. Consequently, the abnormal forces that created the increased anteversion in the first place may contribute to its recurrence in the growing child.
  - There is no clear indication for routine removal of hardware following proximal femoral osteotomy. K-wires are removed in the office 1 month postoperatively, following distal femoral osteotomy.

## COMPLICATIONS

- Supine and prone techniques
  - Undercorrection (common if derotation at surgery is 1:1 instead of 1.5:1 or 2:1)
  - Overcorrection (rare)
  - Recurrence (more common in children with CP)
  - Unsuccessful correction of transverse plane gait deviations if preoperative assessment does not elucidate transverse plane malalignment in the remainder of the lower extremity (ie, pelvis, tibia, and/or foot).
- K-wire technique
  - Loss of fixation (rare with K-wire fixation)
  - Undercorrection—common if 1:1 correction is used (instead of 1.5:1 or 2:1)
  - Overcorrection (rare)
  - Recurrence (more common in children with CP)
  - Knee stiffness—typically resolves by 2 months following cast removal
  - Unsuccessful correction of transverse plane gait deviations if preoperative assessment does not elucidate transverse plane malalignment in the remainder of the lower extremity (ie, pelvis, tibia, and/or foot) (**FIG 6**).

## ACKNOWLEDGMENT

- With thanks to Unni Narayanan, MD, for his contributions as the author of the Proximal Femoral Rotational Osteotomy chapter in the previous edition of this book.

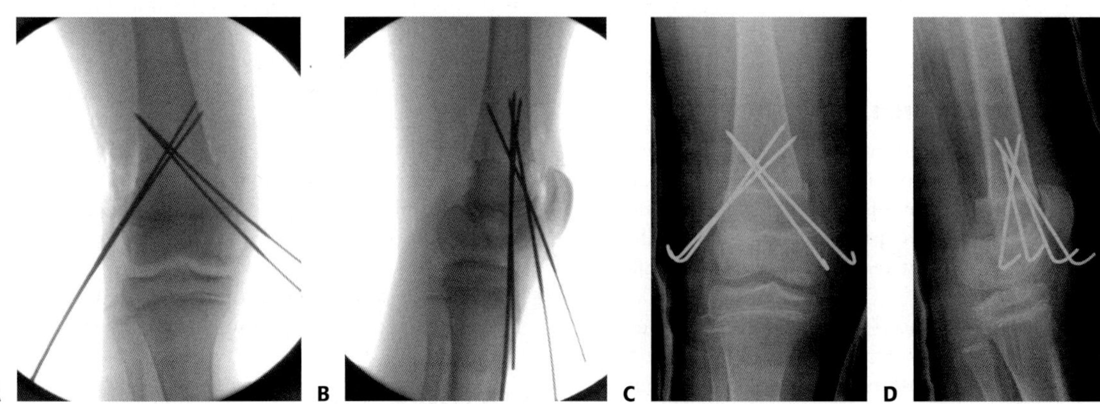

**FIG 6** • Typical healing following bilateral distal femoral rotational osteotomy in a 10-year-old female with CP who functions at GMFCS level I. **A,B.** Intraoperative AP and lateral x-rays. Because the femur is not cylindrical, there will be step-off(s) anteriorly and/or posteriorly at the time of surgery when distal femoral osteotomies are performed. The step-off(s) will resolve with time as the femur remodels. **C,D.** AP and lateral x-rays 1 month postoperative (on the date of pin removal) showing good alignment and appropriate heeling. *(continued)*

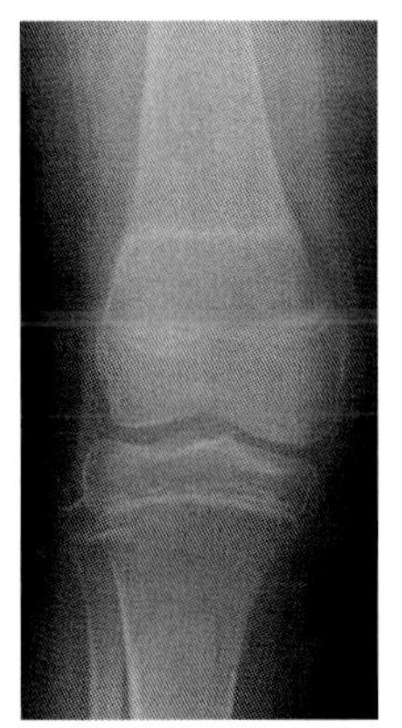


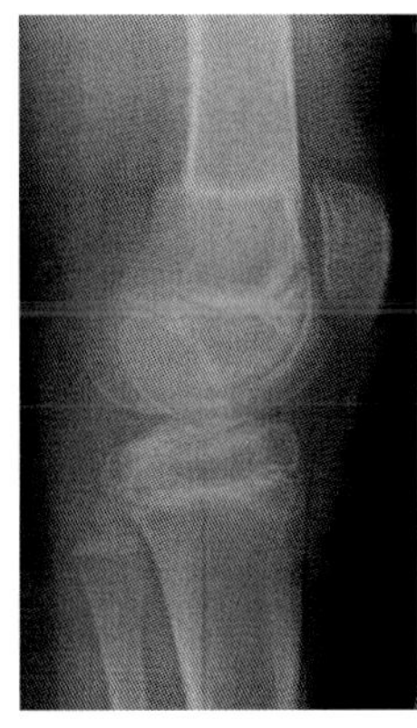


**FIG 6** • *(continued)* **E,F.** X-rays 2 months postoperative (on the day of cast removal) show good healing and alignment. (Courtesy of Children's Orthopaedic Center, Los Angeles.)

## REFERENCES


1. Botser IB, Ozoude GC, Martin DE, et al. Femoral anteversion in the hip: comparison of measurement by computed tomography, magnetic resonance imaging, and physical examination. Arthroscopy 2012;28(5):619–627.
2. Crane L. Femoral torsion and its relation to toeing-in and toeing-out. J Bone Joint Surg Am 1959;41-A(3):421–428.
3. Davids JR, Benfanti P, Blackhurst DW, et al. Assessment of femoral anteversion in children with cerebral palsy: accuracy of the trochanteric prominence angle test. J Pediatr Orthop 2002;22(2):173–178.
4. Davids JR, Marshall AD, Blocker ER, et al. Femoral anteversion in children with cerebral palsy. Assessment with two and three-dimensional computed tomography scans. J Bone Joint Surg Am 2003;85-A(3):481–488.
5. Delgado ED, Schoenecker PL, Rich MM, et al. Treatment of severe torsional malalignment syndrome. J Pediatr Orthop 1996;16(4):484–488.
6. Dunlap K, Shands AR Jr, Hollister LC Jr, et al. A new method for determination of torsion of the femur. J Bone Joint Surg Am 1953;35-A(2):289–311.
7. Fabry G, MacEwen GD, Shands AR Jr. Torsion of the femur. A follow-up study in normal and abnormal conditions. J Bone Joint Surg Am 1973;55(8):1726–1738.
8. Gage JR. Gait Analysis in Cerebral Palsy. Oxford: MacKeith Press, 1991.
9. Gage JR, Novacheck TF. An update on the treatment of gait problems in cerebral palsy. J Pediatr Orthop B 2001;10(4):265–274.
10. Gelberman RH, Cohen MS, Desai SS, et al. Femoral anteversion. A clinical assessment of idiopathic intoeing gait in children. J Bone Joint Surg Br 1987;69(1):75–79.
11. Høiseth A, Reikeras O, Fønstelien E. Evaluation of three methods for measurement of femoral neck anteversion. Femoral neck anteversion, definition, measuring methods and errors. Acta Radiol 1989;30(1):69–73.
12. Howell FR, Newman RJ, Wang HL, et al. The three-dimensional anatomy of the proximal femur in Perthes' disease. J Bone Joint Surg Br 1989;71(3):408–412.
13. Hubbard DD, Staheli LT, Chew DE, et al. Medial femoral torsion and osteoarthritis. J Pediatr Orthop 1988;8(5):540–542.
14. Kay RM. Lower extremity surgery in children with cerebral palsy. In: Tolo VT, Skaggs DL, eds. Master Techniques in Orthopaedic Surgery: Pediatrics. Philadelphia: Lippincott Williams & Wilkins, 2008:83–119.
15. Kay RM, Rethlefsen SA, Hale JM, et al. Comparison of proximal and distal rotational femoral osteotomy in children with cerebral palsy. J Pediatr Orthop 2003;23(2):150–154.
16. Moussa M. Rotational malalignment and femoral torsion in osteoarthritic knees with patellofemoral joint involvement. A CT scan study. Clin Orthop Relat Res 1994;(304):176–183.
17. Pirpiris M, Trivett A, Baker R, et al. Femoral derotation osteotomy in spastic diplegia. Proximal or distal? J Bone Joint Surg Br 2003;85(2):265–272.
18. Rethlefsen SA, Healy BS, Wren TA, et al. Causes of intoeing gait in children with cerebral palsy. J Bone Joint Surg Am 2006;88(10):2175–2180.
19. Rethlefsen SA, Kay RM. Transverse plane gait problems in children with cerebral palsy. J Pediatr Orthop 2013;33(4):422–430.
20. Robin J, Graham HK, Selber P, et al. Proximal femoral geometry in cerebral palsy: a population-based cross-sectional study. J Bone Joint Surg Br 2008;90(10):1372–1379.
21. Root L, Siegal T. Osteotomy of the hip in children: posterior approach. J Bone Joint Surg Am 1982;62(4):571–575.
22. Ruwe PA, Gage JR, Ozonoff MB, et al. Clinical determination of femoral anteversion. A comparison with established techniques. J Bone Joint Surg Am 1992;74(6):820–830.
23. Ryder CT, Crane L. Measuring femoral anteversion; the problem and a method. J Bone Joint Surg Am 1953;35-A(2):321–328.
24. Somerville EW. Persistent foetal alignment of the hip. J Bone Joint Surg Br 1957;39-B(1):106–113.
25. Staheli LT, Duncan WR, Schaefer E. Growth alterations in the hemiplegic child. A study of femoral anteversion, neck-shaft angle, hip rotation, C.E. angle, limb length and circumference in 50 hemiplegic children. Clin Orthop Relat Res 1968;60:205–212.
26. Tönnis D, Heinecke A. Acetabular and femoral anteversion: relationship with osteoarthritis of the hip. J Bone Joint Surg Am 1999;81(12):1747–1770.
27. Wedge JH, Munkacsi I, Loback D. Anteversion of the femur and idiopathic osteoarthrosis of the hip. J Bone Joint Surg Am 1989;71(7):1040–1043.

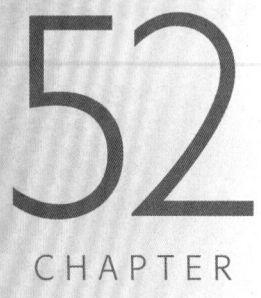

CHAPTER

# Proximal Femoral Varus Osteotomy Using a 90-Degree Blade Plate

Tom F. Novacheck

## DEFINITION

- Proximal femoral varus osteotomy can be useful for many conditions:
  - Coxa valga deformity
  - Hip subluxation (nearly all etiologies)
  - Containment for Perthes disease
  - Degenerative arthrosis
- Correction in other planes can be accomplished simultaneously (derotation and extension–flexion). Proximal femoral varus osteotomy can be accomplished at any age, as satisfactory implants are available for all bone sizes.
- In some situations (eg, neuromuscular disease), it may be necessary to address the etiology of the proximal femoral deformity and hip disease simultaneously.

## ANATOMY

- The normal femoral neck–shaft angle is 135 degrees (range 120 to 150 degrees).
- The true neck–shaft angle cannot be directly assessed from an anteroposterior (AP) pelvis radiograph unless femoral anteversion is compensated for by internally rotating the femur to eliminate it.
- The tip of the greater trochanter is at the level of the center of the femoral head.
- The neck–shaft angle at birth is typically 150 degrees, decreasing to 135 degrees by skeletal maturity.
- Normal anteversion at birth is 45 degrees, decreasing to 10 degrees in boys and 15 degrees in girls by 8 years of age.

## PATHOGENESIS

- The development of normal femoral anatomy and resolution of fetal bone alignment requires the attainment of gross motor activities at a typical age and is dependent on normal musculoskeletal forces. Both of these can be affected by neuromuscular conditions such as cerebral palsy or myelomeningocele.
- Patients with Perthes disease may have a subluxated or uncovered femoral head even with proximal femoral anatomy that is normal except for the avascular femoral head segment. Even so, with good neuromuscular function, varusizing the femur can be well tolerated and can improve the containment of the diseased femoral head.
- Contributing factors to the hip joint pathology may include musculotendinous contractures, ligamentous laxity, and coexistent acetabular dysplasia. If present, these may also require direct treatment. Adductor lengthening, psoas lengthening, open reduction of the hip with capsulorrhaphy, and acetabuloplasty may need to be considered.
- Proximal femoral deformity can have an adverse effect on hip joint development and exacerbates or contributes to muscle imbalance about the hip.[1]

## NATURAL HISTORY

- In neuromuscular conditions, if femoral head uncoverage exceeds 50% based on the Reimer migration index, then further subluxation and dislocation are likely.[4]
- Femoral head uncoverage during the resorption and reossification stages of Perthes disease puts the hip at risk for a poor outcome with permanent deformity of the femoral head.[2]
- A poor outcome radiographically predisposes to early hip degeneration.[5]

## PATIENT HISTORY AND PHYSICAL FINDINGS

- There are no physical findings that are diagnostic for coxa valga.
- The typical history for neuromuscular conditions, developmental dysplasia of the hip, or Perthes disease will be present in patients who may be candidates for a proximal femoral varus osteotomy.
- In these cases, the associated musculotendinous or joint contractures may be present on physical examination and could include hip flexion contracture, hip adduction contracture, or altered transverse plane rotation.
  - In Perthes disease, restricted internal hip rotation and abduction are common.
- Femoral anteversion is tested by palpation of the greater trochanter in the prone position.
  - When the trochanter is most prominent laterally, the femoral neck is horizontal. In the absence of tibial deformity (varus or valgus), the tibial shaft is essentially perpendicular to the posterior aspect of the femoral condyles. The angular difference between the tibial shaft and a vertical line indicates the anteversion. In an otherwise normal hip, the anteversion is about 20 degrees less than the maximum internal rotation range of motion (ROM).
  - Excessive femoral anteversion is typically seen in neuromuscular conditions and in developmental dysplasia of the hip and leads to excessive internal hip rotation and a corresponding lack of external hip rotation when tested in the prone position.
- Examining the hip ROM is essential for a differential diagnosis and to evaluate associated problems such as joint contracture, muscle imbalance, and musculotendinous contracture.
  - Normal total transverse plane ROM of the hip is about 90 degrees. Normally, one-third of the available ROM is internal and two-thirds is external.
    - Restricted ROM can indicate a joint abnormality, capsular contracture, or spasticity of the internal or external rotators of the hip.

- Excessive ROM indicates relative ligamentous laxity.
- Shifted ROM (eg, excessive internal ROM) indicates excessive femoral anteversion.

- In adolescents and young adults being evaluated for early degenerative arthrosis, pain may be found at the extremes of ROM. Severe ROM restrictions could be a contraindication to consideration of realignment osteotomy in these cases.

## IMAGING AND OTHER DIAGNOSTIC STUDIES

- A plain AP pelvis radiograph with anteversion eliminated is diagnostic of coxa valga.
  - If anteversion is normal, no compensation for hip rotation is necessary.
  - If anteversion is excessive, the AP pelvis radiograph should be taken with the hip internally rotated to obtain a true AP view of the proximal femur.
    - Hip flexion and adduction deformities can be identified by asymmetries in femoral position or asymmetric pelvic position.
    - Acetabular dysplasia should be ruled out.
    - Hip subluxation or femoral head uncoverage is assessed. Signs of degenerative arthrosis are sought.
- Computed tomography (CT) scans (including three-dimensional reconstruction) are not useful or needed for primary proximal femoral deformities but can be helpful in evaluating acetabular dysplasia or potentially in revision cases.
- Magnetic resonance imaging (MRI) may be useful in evaluating associated problems, including labral tears, hip joint effusions, articular cartilage pathology, and femoral head vascularity.

## DIFFERENTIAL DIAGNOSIS

- Hip joint contracture
- Hip joint subluxation
- Femoral anteversion or retroversion
- Musculotendinous contracture
- Acetabular dysplasia

## NONOPERATIVE MANAGEMENT

- Nonoperative management may be helpful for one of the associated conditions listed earlier.
- There is no nonoperative treatment for bone deformity that is clinically significant and adversely affecting hip joint development.

## SURGICAL MANAGEMENT

### Preoperative Planning

- The AP pelvis radiograph is reviewed.
- The size of implant is chosen based on radiographic templates.
- The amount of varusization can be determined based on radiographs preoperatively or on intraoperative findings. Other associated problems (musculotendinous contracture, joint instability, and acetabular dysplasia) are addressed concurrently.
- There is no examination under anesthesia to determine the amount of varusization to accomplish. An examination under anesthesia can guide decision making regarding concurrent tendon lengthening.
- Varusization will inevitably shorten the extremity. The effect on leg length can be controlled by altering the amount of varusization and the size of the wedge of bone removed (if any) depending on preoperative leg length assessment. Varus can be accomplished using a medial closing or lateral opening osteotomy.

### Positioning

- Although some surgeons prefer to perform proximal femoral varus osteotomy with the patient supine, I prefer the prone position with the leg draped free (**FIG 1**).
- This allows ease of exposure posterior to the muscle belly of the vastus lateralis.
- The prone position also allows accurate control of femoral torsion comparable to the prone physical examination for femoral anteversion by palpation, thereby improving accuracy and consistency of surgical realignment.

### Approach

- A direct lateral approach to the proximal femur is routine. The procedure involves placing the chisel for the blade plate in the appropriate position in the femoral neck corresponding to the amount of varus to accomplish (eg, 20-degree varus correction corresponds to 70-degree chisel placement relative to the lateral femoral cortical surface: 90-degree blade plate minus 70 degrees equals 20 degrees varusization), completing the osteotomy, and placing the 90-degree blade plate as detailed in the Techniques section.

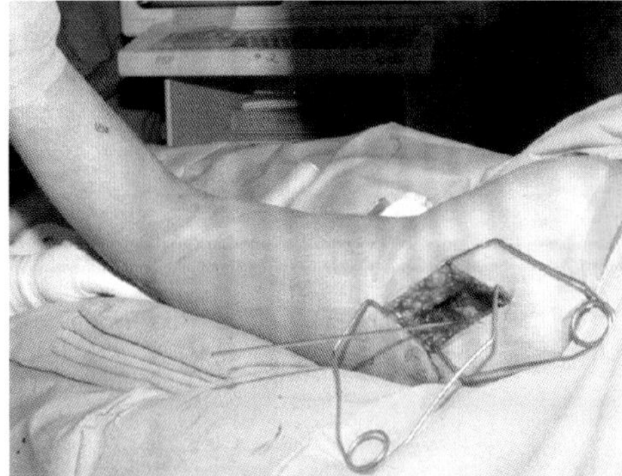

**FIG 1** • Prone positioning allows easy access to divide the vastus lateralis posteriorly and replicates the position for physical examination for femoral anteversion, allowing improved accuracy and reliability of assessment and correction of femoral torsional alignment.

## Exposure

- A longitudinal lateral incision is made over the proximal femur matching the length of the blade plate.
- The fascia lata is divided in line with the skin incision (**TECH FIG 1A**).
- The vastus lateralis is reflected from its proximal and posterior origins and elevated to expose the proximal femur subperiosteally.
- Circumferential subperiosteal elevators are placed in the intertrochanteric area to protect the soft tissues (**TECH FIG 1B**).

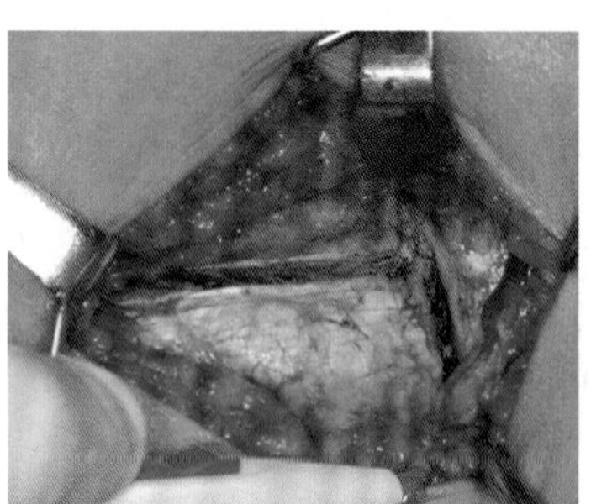

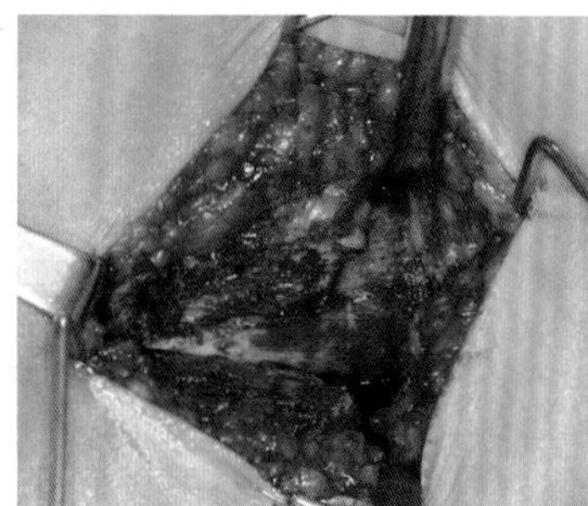

**TECH FIG 1** • **A.** The fascia of the vastus lateralis is divided transversely at the greater trochanteric apophysis and extended posteriorly to divide the periosteum in the intertrochanteric area. The vastus lateralis fascia is then divided longitudinally just anterior to the insertion of the gluteus maximus and the linea aspera (in the prone position, up is posterior). **B.** The vastus lateralis is elevated subperiosteally, and Crego retractors are placed circumferentially at the intertrochanteric level.

## Guidewire Placement

- A fluoroscope is used to guide placement of a guidewire in both the AP and lateral views.
- The entry point is just below the greater trochanteric apophysis if the patient is skeletally immature and through the greater trochanter after maturity.
  - The entry point is chosen to allow insertion of the guidewire and chisel without violating the medial calcar.
- The anterior to posterior placement is determined in the view obtained by flexing the hip and knee (with the knee over the edge of the operating table) and internally and externally rotating the hip until the fluoroscopic image shows the femoral neck and femoral shaft collinear with the guidewire placed centrally and parallel to the neck and shaft of the femur (**TECH FIG 2A**).
- The orientation of the pin on the AP view is controlled with an osteotomy triangle (**TECH FIG 2B,C**).
  - If preoperative planning indicated a 15-degree varusization goal, a 75-degree triangle would be used (see the Approach section earlier).
  - Alternatively, determination can be made based on preoperative and desired postoperative alignment; for example, the preoperative neck–shaft angle (150 degrees) minus the desired postoperative neck–shaft angle (120 degrees) equals 30 degrees of varusization. In this case, the guidewire would be placed at a 60-degree angle to the femoral shaft when using the 90-degree plate.
  - The anteversion is determined (transverse plane) by the angle between the pin (placed as described earlier) and the tibial shaft (perpendicular to the posterior aspect of the femoral condyles when the knee is flexed, provided there is no tibial varus or valgus).

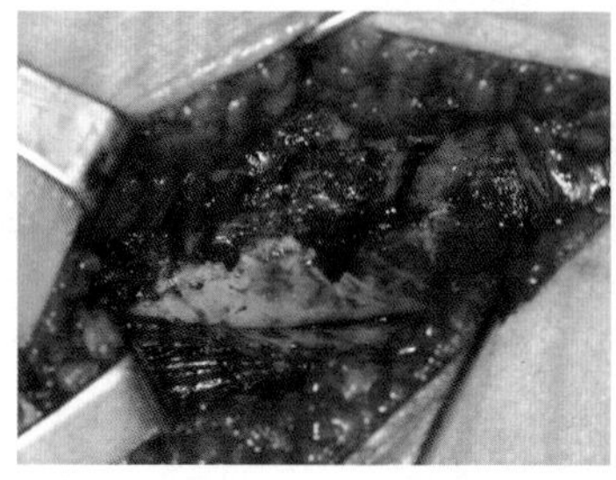

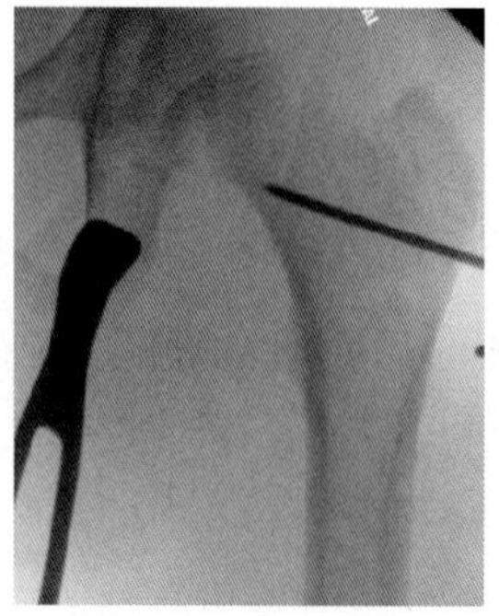

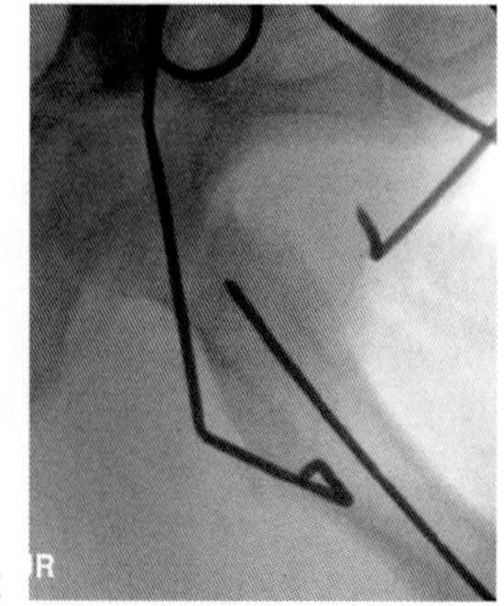

**TECH FIG 2** • **A.** A guidewire placed just below the apophysis and in line with the femoral shaft. **B.** Intraoperative C-arm view showing the guidewire at a 70-degree angle to the femoral shaft. **C.** The ideal lateral projection with femoral neck, femoral shaft, and guidewire coplanar improves accuracy and consistency.

## Placement of the Blade Plate Chisel

- The appropriate-sized chisel for the blade plate is then placed just below and exactly parallel to the pin to the desired depth (greatest depth possible depending on anatomy and available length of the blade plate; **TECH FIG 3**).
- The chisel should be dislodged 5 to 10 mm before the osteotomy to allow for ease of later removal.

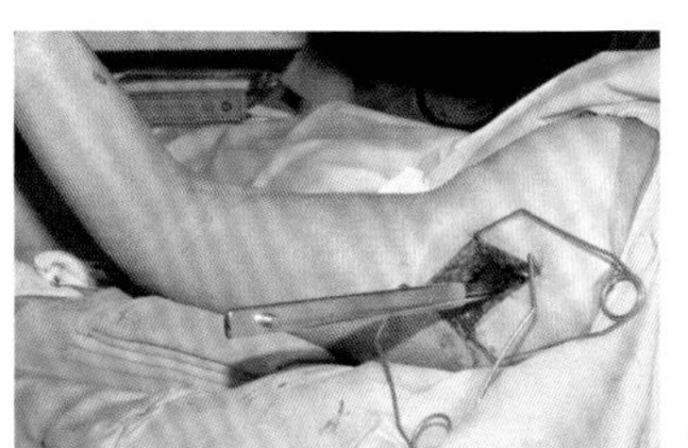
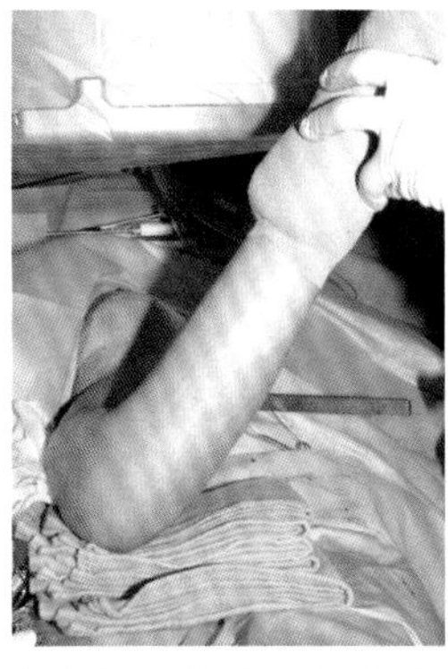
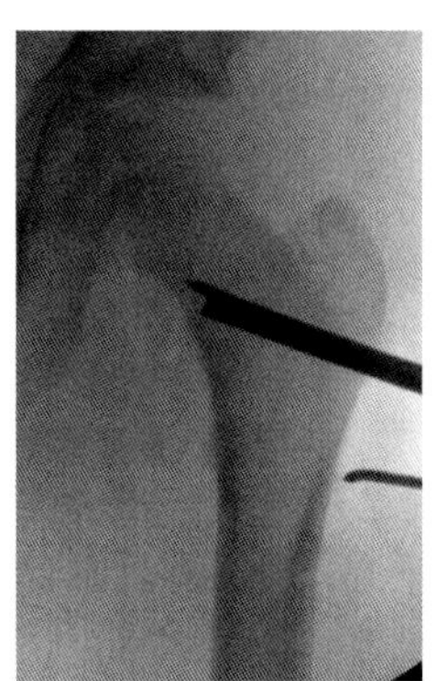
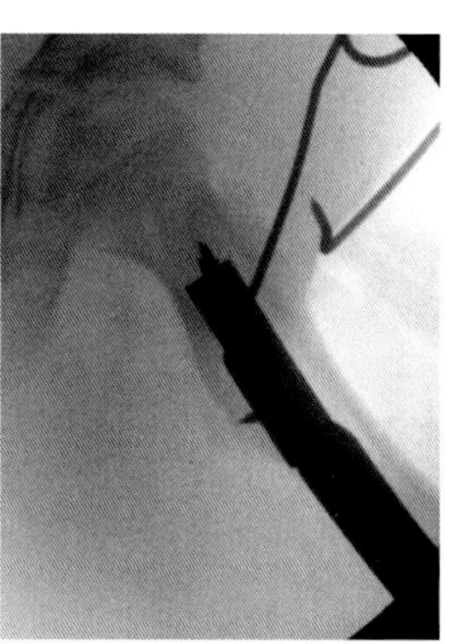

**TECH FIG 3** • **A.** The chisel is placed exactly in line with the pin. **B.** Anteversion in this case is 35 degrees. **C,D.** Chisel position confirmed in the AP and lateral projections.

## Performing the Osteotomy

- The details of the osteotomy are based on preoperative planning.
- To minimize the shortening effect of the osteotomy on leg length in a child, a single transverse osteotomy can be performed in the intertrochanteric area (**TECH FIG 4**).
  - This will result in a lateral opening osteotomy.
- Alternatively, a wedge of bone can be removed to accomplish a medial closing osteotomy.

### Wedge Osteotomy

- The first osteotomy is performed parallel to the chisel.
  - The entry point for the osteotomy saw blade is determined by the implant (distance between the blade and the subsequent angle in the plate for medialization).
- A second osteotomy is then performed perpendicular to the femoral shaft.
  - The starting level for this osteotomy varies depending on the desired amount of shortening of the extremity.
- A beginning point identical to the entry point for the first osteotomy achieves full contact of the osteotomy after fixation.
- A lateral starting level distal to the first removes a portion of the lateral femoral cortex, achieving more shortening, but is limited by the insertion of the psoas tendon on the lesser trochanter (typically should not be violated).
- An entry point proximal (within the cut of the first osteotomy) leads to less shortening but incomplete final apposition of the osteotomy surfaces.

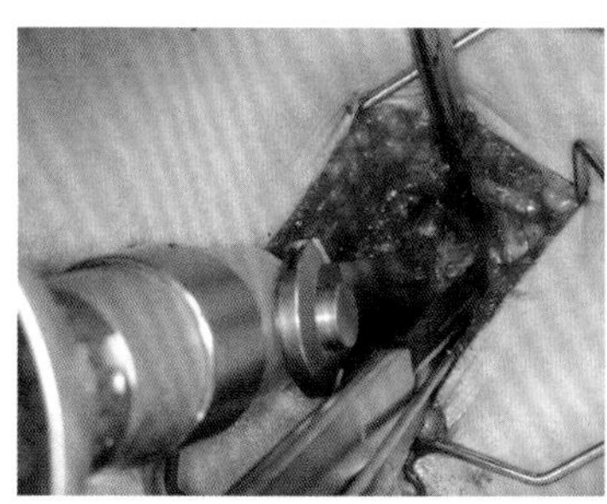
 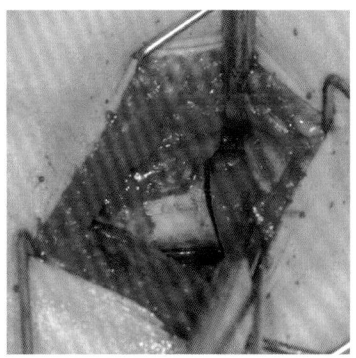

**TECH FIG 4** • **A.** An oscillating saw is used 10 to 12 mm distal and parallel to the chisel. **B.** The completed osteotomy. A second (optional) osteotomy could be performed at this point.

## Placement of the Blade Plate

- Realignment and fixation of the osteotomy are achieved by placing the blade plate.
- The chisel is removed, and the blade plate is placed in the chisel path parallel to the guidewire and impacted to its final position (**TECH FIG 5A**).
- The femoral shaft is reduced to the plate and held in position with a Verbrugge clamp (**TECH FIG 5B**).
- Final anteversion alignment is controlled at this point (**TECH FIG 5C**).
- The first two screws are typically placed in compression to optimize fixation and promote rapid healing (**TECH FIG 5D**).
- Alignment is checked after placement of the first screw both radiographically and by physical examination.
- If satisfactory, the final screws are placed. If not, alignment is adjusted accordingly.
- Final radiographs are taken in both views (**TECH FIG 5E,F**).
- The wound is closed in layers.

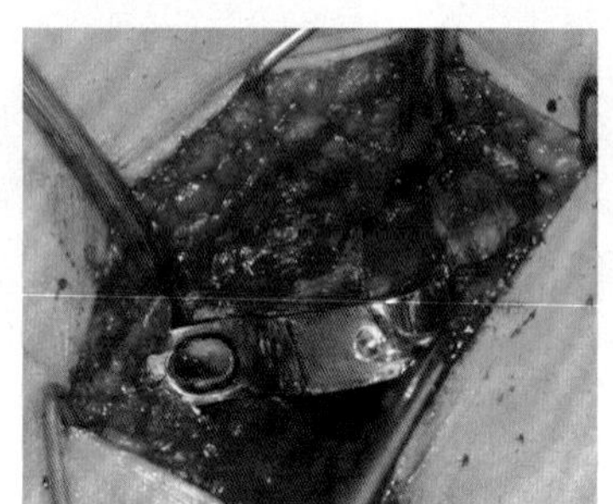
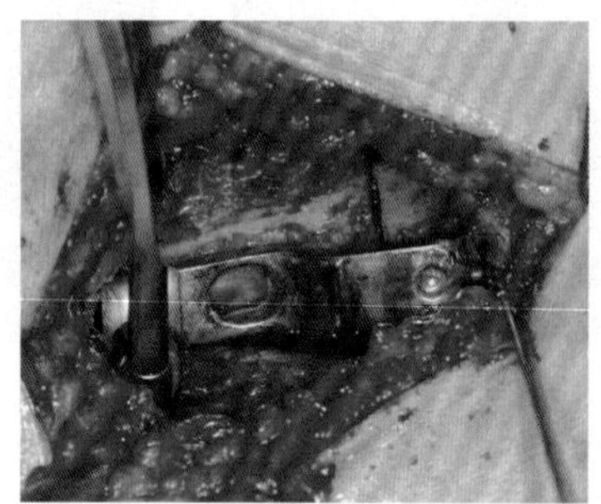
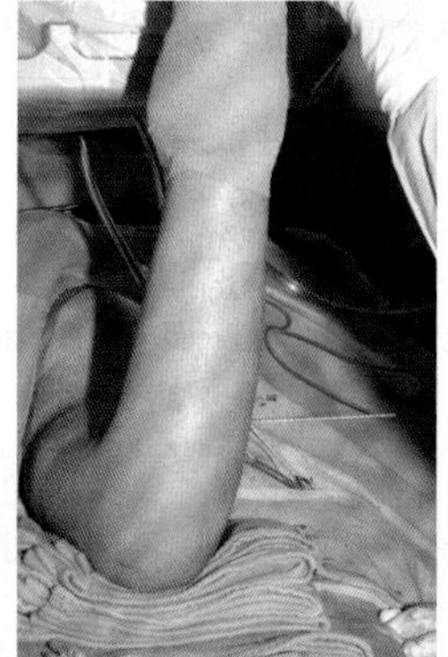
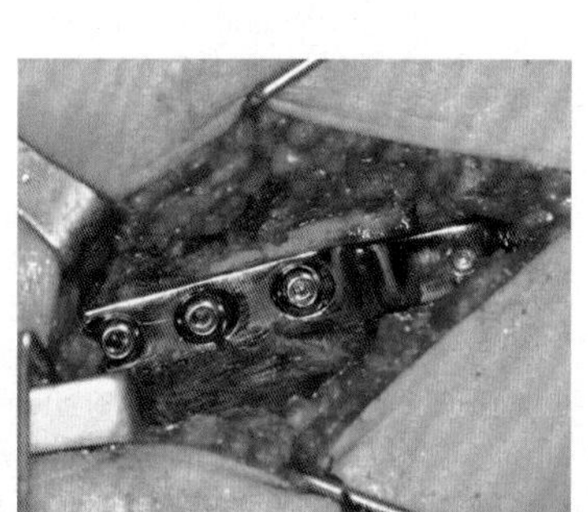
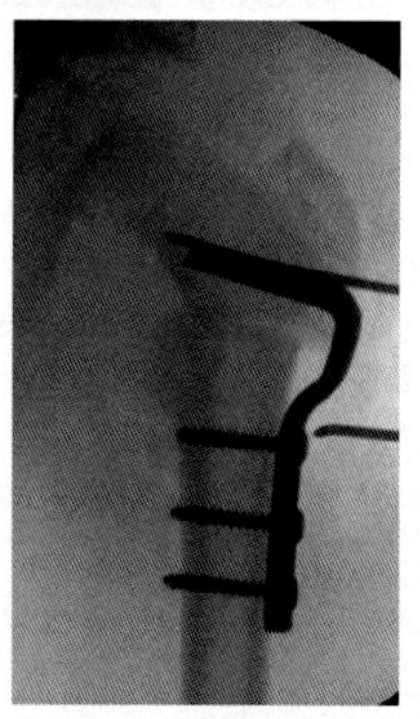
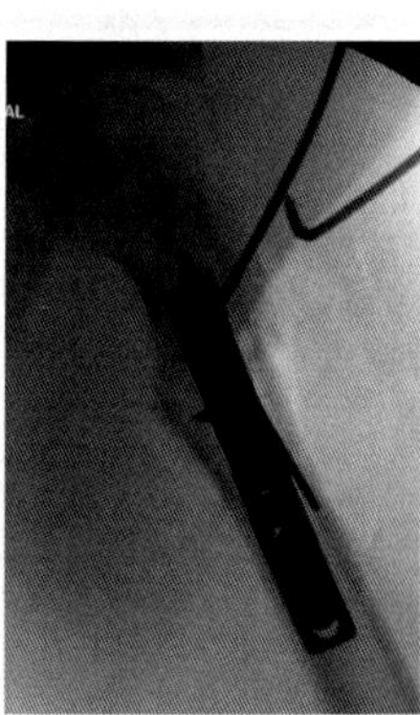

**TECH FIG 5** • **A.** The chisel has been replaced with the blade plate (guidewire is still in place). **B.** Correction of deformity by reducing the plate to the femoral shaft with a Verbrugge clamp. **C.** Anteversion is assessed before guide pin removal (corrected to 10 degrees). **D.** Fixation is complete (note well-apposed osteotomy surfaces). **E,F.** Postoperative AP and lateral views confirming implant placement, proper osteotomy alignment, and appropriate medialization of the femoral shaft to align the piriformis fossa with the intramedullary canal.

## PEARLS AND PITFALLS

| | |
|---|---|
| **Guidewire placement** | ■ Accurate placement of the guidewire is crucial to all steps of the procedure.<br>■ Care must be taken to ensure its proper placement. |
| **Indications** | ■ Adequate ROM must be available.<br>■ Hip joint pathology must not preclude repositioning of the femoral head within the acetabulum in a functional position of the leg. |
| **Accurate realignment** | ■ Prone positioning promotes accurate control, correction, or both of femoral torsion.<br>■ Final alignment depends only on the angle of pin/chisel insertion and the choice of blade plate angle (in this case, 90 degrees).<br>■ Apposition of the osteotomy surfaces themselves also depends on the orientation of the osteotomy cuts. |

## POSTOPERATIVE CARE

- Weight-bearing status and immobilization depend on patient age, condition being treated, compliance, bone size, implant size, and bone quality.
  - Weight bearing can vary from toe-touch to non–weight bearing for the first 3 to 6 weeks.
  - With poor bone quality, small bone size, small implant size, or poor compliance, a spica cast should be applied.
  - In intermediate situations, bilateral short-leg casts with a Fillauer bar can be applied along with knee immobilizers (**FIG 2**).
  - Unrestricted ROM without external immobilization may be allowed (eg, most adults).
- A ROM and strengthening program often is instituted at 3 to 4 weeks postoperatively.
- Advancement to full weight bearing can be accomplished within 6 to 8 weeks of the procedure, depending on muscle strength.

## OUTCOMES

- Patients older than 8 years of age with moderate Perthes disease (lateral pillar B or B/C border) have a better outcome with surgery.[2]

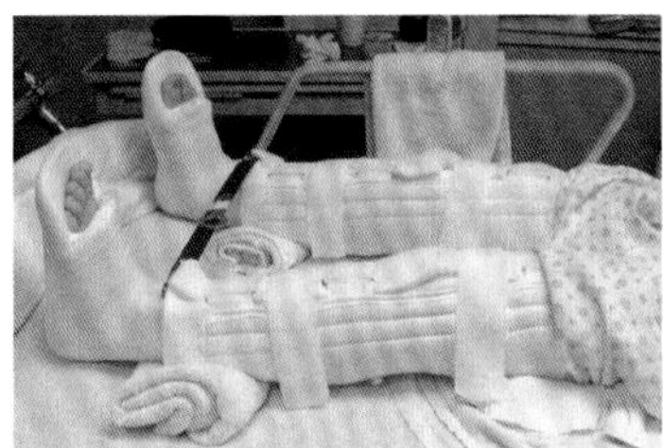

**FIG 2** ● Bilateral short-leg casts with a Fillauer bar incorporated controls rotational alignment postoperatively. Knee immobilizers improve comfort by preventing flexion–extension caused by spasms of the hip flexors and hamstrings.

- The complex spectrum of cerebral palsy hip subluxation, hip dysplasia, and dislocation can be treated successfully in most cases using a treatment algorithm that incorporates femoral varus and derotation osteotomy. Although there is a risk of recurrence and complications, McNerney and associates[3] reported excellent results with aggressive surgical management with a low rate of complications and repeat acetabuloplasty or varus osteotomy.

## COMPLICATIONS

- Excessive varusization leading to hip abductor insufficiency
- Implant failure
- Malunion
- Nonunion
- Deep venous thrombosis in adults
- Infection
- Avascular necrosis
- Implant irritation contributing to Trendelenburg gait
- Overcorrection or undercorrection

## REFERENCES


1. Gage JR. Gait and lever arm dysfunction. In: Gage JR, ed. Treatment of Gait Problems in Cerebral Palsy. London: MacKeith Press, 2004:180–204.
2. Herring JA, Kim HT, Browne R. Legg-Calve-Perthes disease. Part II: prospective multicenter study of the effect of treatment on outcome. J Bone Joint Surg 2004;86-A(10):2121–2134.
3. McNerney NP, Mubarak SJ, Wenger DR. One-stage correction of the dysplastic hip in cerebral palsy with the San Diego acetabuloplasty: results and complications in 104 hips. J Pediatr Orthop 2000;20: 93–103.
4. Reimers J. The stability of the hip in children. A radiological study of results of muscle surgery in cerebral palsy. Acta Orthop Scand Suppl 1980;184:1–100.
5. Stulberg SD, Cooperman DR, Wallensten R. The natural history of Legg-Calvé-Perthes disease. J Bone Joint Surg 1981;63(7): 1095–1108.

# Treatment of Congenital Femoral Deficiency

Dror Paley

## DEFINITION

- The term *proximal focal femoral deficiency* (PFFD) is used to describe congenital femoral deficiency and deformity of the proximal femur to be distinguished from the congenital short femur.[6] However, the more comprehensive term *congenital femoral deficiency* (CFD)[15] better describes the spectrum of deficiency, deformity, and discrepancy ranging from the congenital short femur to the most severe PFFD.
- The severity of the deformity varies widely, and this condition can be diagnosed in the prenatal period using ultrasound examination.[12]
- In most cases, CFD is not simple coxa vara. Patients with CFD lack integrity, stability, and mobility of the hip and knee, with concurrent joint malorientation, bony deformity, and soft tissue contractures. The affected limb grows at an inhibited rate depending on the severity of the underlying deficiency. The resulting limb length discrepancy (LLD) can be accurately predicted using the multiplier method.[1,2,11]

## ANATOMY

- Although existing classification systems for PFFD are descriptive, these classification systems are not helpful in determining the final femoral morphology or treatment strategies.[15]
- The Paley classification system (**FIG 1**) is based on factors that reflect the severity of pathology and reconstructability of the congenitally deficient femur. This classification is based on pathologic factors that determine surgical reconstruction strategies.[9]
- The abnormal anatomy of CFD consists of coxa vara of the proximal femur with abduction contracture of the hip (ie, tensor fascia lata [TFL], gluteus maximus, gluteus medius, and gluteus minimus muscles), proximal femoral flexion deformity with concurrent hip flexion contracture (ie, rectus femoris, TFL, iliopsoas, gluteus medius and minimus muscles), and external femoral torsion–retroversion with concurrent external soft tissue contracture (ie, piriformis muscle).
- The best way to understand the proximal femoral deformity of the more severe cases is to imagine creating the deformity de novo: start with a proximal femoral segment that ends in the subtrochanteric region. Perform all of these movements relative to the coronal plane of the pelvis in its normal anatomic position:
  - First, flex the proximal femur 90 degrees.
  - In the flexed position, abduct the proximal femur 45 degrees.
  - Connect the distal femoral diaphyseal segment to it with the distal femur rotated externally 45 degrees relative to the pelvis.
  - The resulting deformity is that seen with severe CFD (**FIG 2**).
- The proximal femur can also present a region of delayed ossification in either the subtrochanteric region or the neck region or both. Ossification of the cartilaginous proximal femur differentiates Paley type 1a CFD (ie, normal ossification) from Paley type 1b CFD (ie, delayed ossification). The latter can be subclassified as Paley type 1b subtrochanteric type, neck type, or combined subtrochanteric–neck type (see **FIG 1**).
- Once treated with realignment and in some cases insertion of bone morphogenetic protein (BMP), the unossified cartilage of the proximal femur in the type 1b will ossify changing the femur into type 1a. This area of delayed ossification is often mistaken for a pseudarthrosis (it could be referred to as a *stiff cartilaginous pseudarthrosis* to differentiate it from type 2, in which there is a true mobile, fibrous pseudarthrosis).
- A more severe form of CFD is classified as Paley type 2; this type has a true mobile pseudarthrosis between the greater trochanter and femoral head or complete absence of the femoral head (see **FIG 1**).
- The most severe proximal deficiencies are classified as Paley type 3 (diaphyseal deficiencies). In these cases, the greater trochanter is absent and the knee joint is affected to a greater (range of motion [ROM] <45 degrees) or lesser (ROM more than 45 degrees) extent. Complete absence of the femur is included in this group.
- In very rare cases, there is a distal deficiency of the femur (ie, Paley type 4). Cases of distal deficiency present with very severe knee varus but a well-developed, intact hip joint.
- Acetabular dysplasia is almost always present in patients with CFD. This deformity must be recognized and corrected to prevent subluxation or dislocation of the hip during lengthening.
- Congenital knee abnormalities also exist with CFD. Absent or hypoplastic cruciate ligaments (ie, anterior cruciate ligament [ACL], posterior cruciate ligament [PCL]); hypoplastic lateral femoral condyle resulting in genu valgum; and hypoplastic patella with lateral maltracking, subluxation, or dislocation are common. Rotatory instability of the tibiofemoral joint and knee flexion contractures (ie, biceps femoris muscle, posterior knee joint capsule, iliotibial band) are also common.

## PATHOGENESIS

- The cause of an isolated single-limb abnormality remains unknown in most cases. Unilateral CFD is usually not related to a genetic syndrome. Bilateral CFD, multiple limb deficiencies, and associated tibial hemimelia are usually related to a genetic origin.
- A patient with CFD presenting for initial evaluation does not require a genetic consultation unless multiple limb deficiencies or other congenital malformations are present.

**Type 1:** Intact Femur with Mobile Hip and Knee

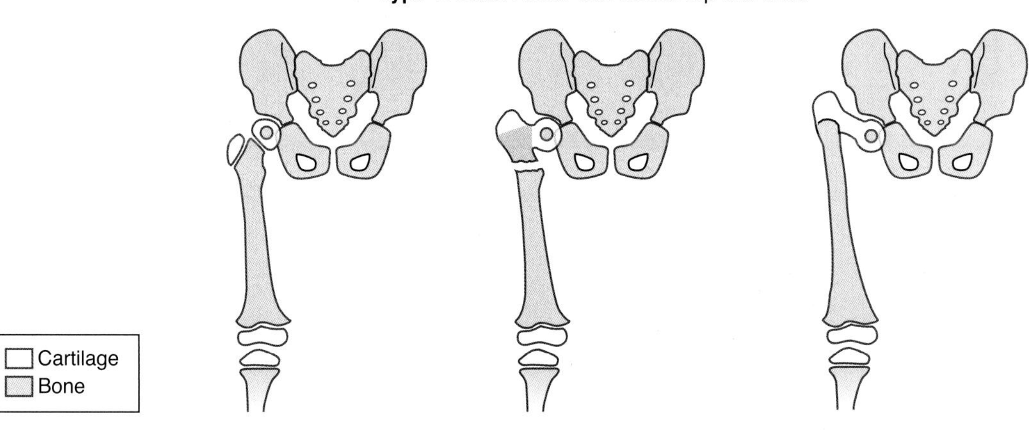


**a:** Normal ossification

**b:** Delayed ossification – Subtrochanteric type

**b:** Delayed ossification – Neck type

**Type 2:** Mobile Pseudarthrosis with Mobile Knee

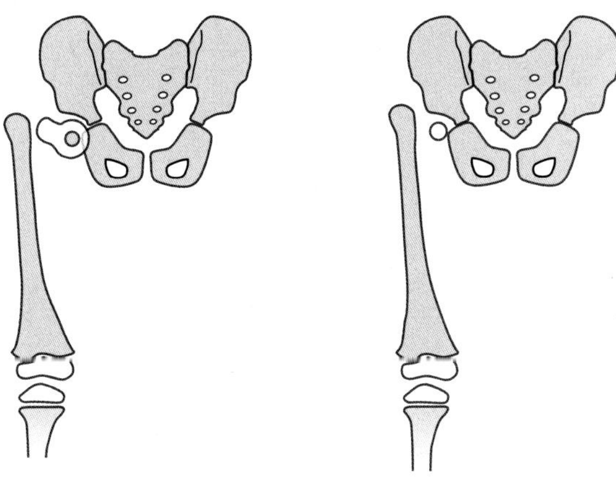

**a:** Femoral head mobile in acetabulum

**b:** Femoral head absent or stiff in acetabulum

**Type 3:** Diaphyseal Deficiency of Femur

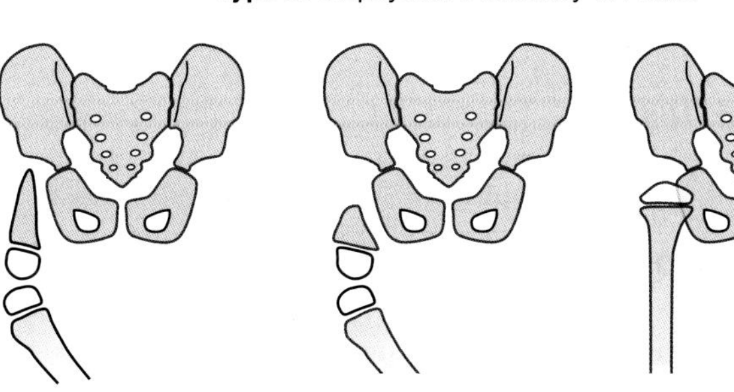

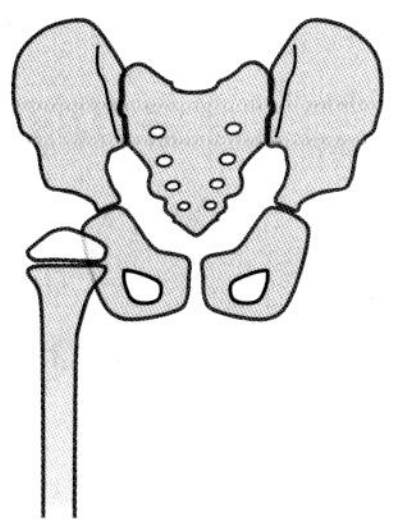

**a:** Knee motion ≥ 45 degrees

**b:** Knee motion < 45 degrees

**c:** Complete absence of femur

**Type 4:** Distal Deficiency of Femur

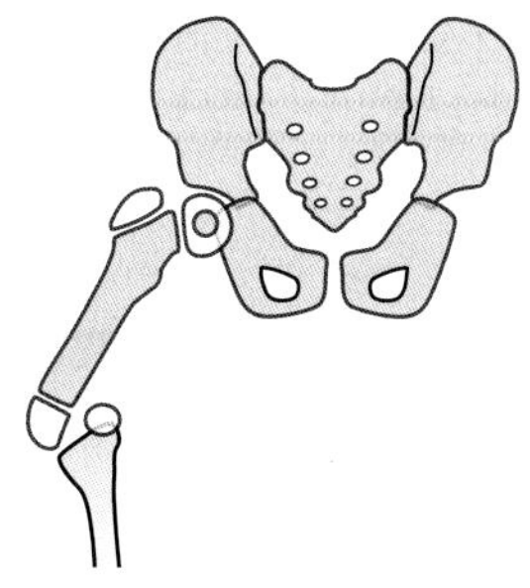

**FIG 1** ● Paley classification of CFD.

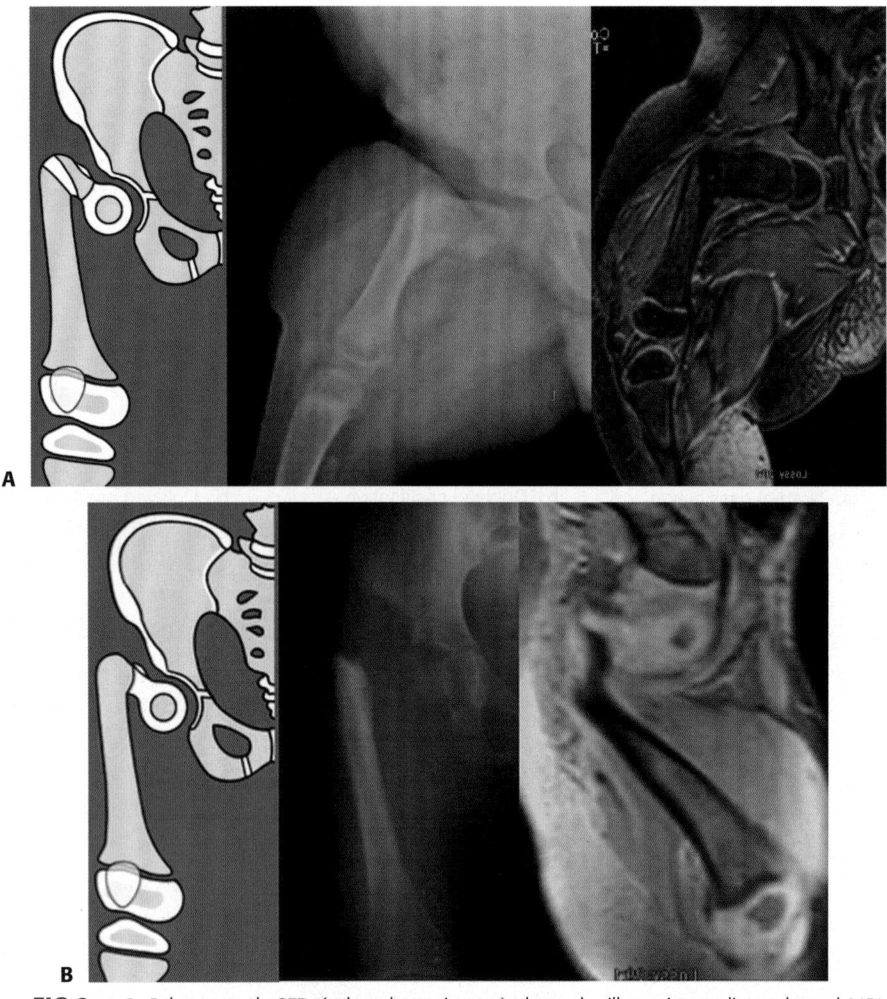

**FIG 2** • **A.** Paley type 1b CFD (subtrochanteric type) shown by illustration, radiograph, and MRI. Note the nonossified subtrochanteric cartilage **B.** Paley type 1b CFD (neck type) shown by illustration, radiograph, and MRI. Note the nonossified neck.

## NATURAL HISTORY

- The natural history of CFD is a progressive LLD in unilateral cases. The deformities and soft tissue contractures described above persist but do not progress.
- The Paley type 1b hip shows eventual ossification of the cartilaginous femoral neck or subtrochanteric region.[15] Although ossification occurs over time, the bony deformities and soft tissue contractures persist.
- Progressive LLD can be accurately predicted using the Paley multiplier method.[1,2,11] Determining the LLD at maturity and using the Paley classification system allows the surgeon to formulate an overall strategy for deformity correction and limb lengthening.
- The number and timing of surgical procedures can be presented as a general overall plan to the parents during the initial consultation.

## PATIENT HISTORY AND PHYSICAL FINDINGS

- A general history and physical examination should be performed.
  - The clinician should concentrate on family history or concurrent known congenital abnormalities, which could indicate a genetic syndrome that could require further workup and genetic consultation.
- The facies, upper extremities, and spine are also examined, looking for abnormal appearance or multiple congenital anomalies, which can indicate a genetic syndrome. In such cases, genetic consultation should be obtained.
- Hip ROM
  - Abduction–adduction and flexion ROM are examined in the supine position. Thomas test (hip extension) is performed to measure fixed flexion deformity of the hip. Hip internal rotation–external rotation is measured in the prone position, together with the thigh–foot angle to determine a rotation profile for the femur and tibia, respectively. Muscle length tests include popliteal angle (hamstring length), prone knee bend Ely test (rectus femoris muscle), and Ober test (tensor fascia lata–iliotibial band). The latter is performed with the patient in the lateral decubitus position pulling the hip into extension with the knee flexed to 90 degrees. If the leg does not drop into adduction by gravity, there is a positive Ober sign, indicating a contracture of the TFL and iliotibial band.
  - ROM is measured, and contractures are identified and quantified in degrees. A popliteal angle of more than 0 degree

and prone knee bend less than supine knee bend indicate tightness of the hamstring and rectus femoris muscles, respectively. A positive Ober sign is almost always present.
  - Contractures need to be treated in preparation for lengthening. Lengthening of the rectus femoris and hamstring muscles is recommended for positive muscle tightness. Lengthening or excision of the fascia lata and iliotibial band is always recommended prior to or at the time of femoral lengthening.
- Knee ROM
  - Flexion and extension knee ROM is measured in the supine and prone positions.
  - Greater than 10 degrees of fixed flexion deformity should be corrected during preparatory procedures. A fixed flexion deformity may be present.
- Knee stability (anteroposterior [AP])
  - The Lachman test and the anterior and posterior drawer tests are performed. The clinician looks for posterior sag and rotatory instability. The amount of instability is measured:
    - Grade I: mild with end point
    - Grade II: moderate with end point
    - Grade III: moderate or severe with no end point
  - AP knee instability is common. It is often difficult to tell if the instability is anterior, posterior, or both.
- Knee stability (rotatory)
  - The rotatory stability of the knee joint is examined by internally and externally rotating the tibia on the distal femur in flexion and extension. The presence of subluxation with rotation of the tibia on the distal femur is noted.
  - External rotatory instability is a common finding that is secondary to a contracted iliotibial band and biceps femoris tendons and can lead to rotatory subluxation of the knee and patellar dislocation.
- Patellar stability
  - The clinician should flex the knee and palpate the alignment of the patella to the notch in flexion. Tracking of the patella is assessed from 0 to 90 degrees. The clinicians should attempt to push a thumb into the intercondylar notch.
  - If the examiner's thumb is able to palpate the intercondylar notch with the patient's knee flexed, this denotes lateral subluxation or dislocation of the patella.
  - Patellar instability is common and can be an indication of lateral rotatory instability of the knee and contracture of the iliotibial band.
- The clinician should look at the overall appearance of the foot and ankle.
  - Any missing rays or positional abnormalities are noted. Ankle ROM is tested with knee flexed and extended. Inversion and eversion ROM is tested.
  - The amount of dorsiflexion, plantarflexion, inversion, and eversion is recorded. Equinovalgus deformity with missing lateral rays indicates concurrent fibular hemimelia. Subtle increase in eversion ROM indicates fibular hypoplasia or a ball-and-socket ankle joint.

## IMAGING AND OTHER DIAGNOSTIC STUDIES

- During the initial evaluation of an infant with CFD, pull down supine long AP and lateral view radiographs should be obtained that include the pelvis and both lower extremities. Both lower limbs are "pulled down" to make sure both knees are in maximum extension (**FIG 3**).

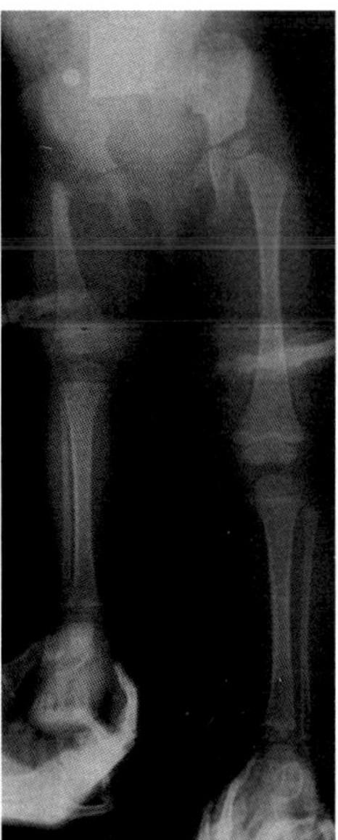

**FIG 3** • Pull down view long x-ray to assess leg length difference in infancy. Note the hands of the parent.

- The supine, long AP view radiograph should be assessed for the overall appearance of the ossific anatomy. This radiograph should allow the physician to classify the type of CFD.
  - The lengths of both femora and both tibiae should be measured. The difference between them is the LLD, not including the foot. The clinicians should measure from the lateral acetabular edge to the midpoint of the knee joint space for the femoral lengths and from the same midpoint of the knee joint space to the end of the talar ossific nucleus for the tibial lengths. The amount of current LLD can be used with the multiplier method to predict the overall LLD at maturity.[1,2,11]
  - The acetabulum should be assessed for dysplasia using the center–edge (CE) angle (even in infants) and the acetabular index (AI).
- The long lateral view radiograph of the lower extremity is assessed for underlying fixed flexion deformity of the knee.
  - The anterior cortical line of the distal femur should normally be colinear with the anterior cortical line of the proximal tibia. A flexion angle between these lines represents fixed flexion deformity of the knee. It is important that the lateral x-ray be taken with the patella forward to avoid mistaking knee valgus for flexion (the valgus of an externally rotated knee will appear to be flexed).
- Other imaging studies that are useful include magnetic resonance imaging (MRI) and arthrography of the hips. All Paley types 1b and 2 should have an MRI after age 18 months to confirm whether there is a cartilaginous connection between the femoral head and shaft (**FIG 4**).
- Arthrography under general anesthesia is also helpful to determine the presence of pseudarthrosis versus delayed ossification of the proximal femur. Although the arthrogram is obtained, the lower extremity is manipulated and the proximal femur is visualized.
  - If the proximal femur and femoral head move as a unit, this usually denotes a cartilaginous connection

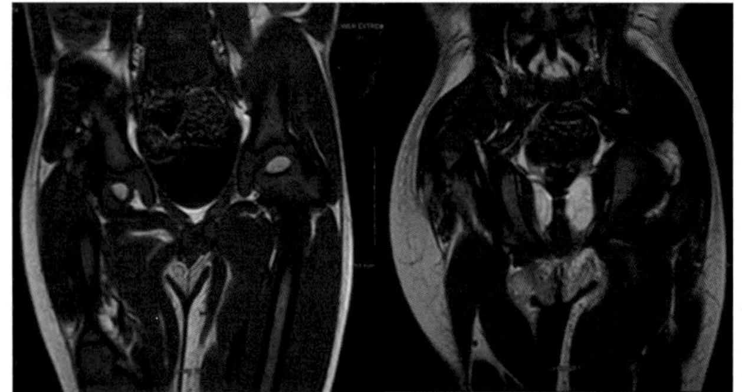

**FIG 4** • MRIs of Paley type 2 CFD. The femoral head is clearly seen (**A**), and in a separate cut, one sees the proximal femur in a different plane (**B**).

in the proximal femur, and the CFD is classified as type 1b. The arthrogram is also useful to differentiate between Paley types 2a and 2b. Both 2a and 2b might have a femoral head present; the difference is whether the femoral head is fused to the acetabulum or not. If dye can be injected into a joint space, the hip can usually be classified as type 2a. In some cases of type 2a, the dye can be seen to outline a cleft through the femoral neck.

## DIFFERENTIAL DIAGNOSIS

- If the patient has bilateral CFD, the clinician must consider the following differential diagnoses:
  - Camptomelic syndrome
  - Femoral hypoplasia with unusual facies syndrome

## NONOPERATIVE MANAGEMENT

- Shoe lifts, orthoses, and prostheses are used for the nonoperative management of LLD. All children should receive a shoe or prosthesis with a lift when they begin to cruise the furniture. A simple shoe lift of an amount equal to 1 cm less than the LLD is used in most cases in which LLD is less than 10 cm (**FIG 5**).
- It is helpful to supplement the lift with an articulated ankle–foot orthosis (AFO) for ankle support from the long lever arm of the shoe lift. If the lift is more than 10 cm, a prosthetic foot connected to an articulated AFO is preferred both to reduce weight and improve cosmesis.
- The clinician should avoid splinting the foot in equinus because it might cause an equinus contracture.
- In children younger than 6 years, a limb length radiograph should be obtained every 6 months to assess LLD and prescribe a new lift.
- After age 6 years, annual assessment and prescription is adequate.
- In more severe cases with hip and knee fixed flexion deformity, it might be necessary to extend the orthotic or prosthetic support above the knee with ischial bearing support.

## SURGICAL MANAGEMENT

- Patients with types 1a, 1b, 2a, and 2b CFD can be managed successfully with lengthening reconstruction surgery as opposed to prosthetic reconstruction surgery.
- Before undergoing lengthening reconstruction surgery, patients with certain knee and hip deformities and deficiencies should undergo preparatory procedures to prevent complications during lengthening and to reconstruct the knee and hip joints. This chapter will present the preparatory surgical procedures of the hip and knee and the external fixation method we prefer for CFD lengthening surgery.

### Type 1 Congenital Femoral Deficiency

- Type 1 CFD is the most reconstructable.
- Before lengthening, hip stability should be determined radiographically. The best indicator is the CE angle. If the CE angle is less than 20 degrees, a Dega osteotomy should be performed before lengthening. In addition, the AI should be less than 30 degrees. If the CE angle is borderline 20 degrees but the AI or inclination of the sourcil is high, it is better to err on the side of caution and perform a Dega osteotomy (**FIG 6**).
- Coxa vara should be corrected before lengthening if the neck–shaft angle is less than 120 degrees. When coxa vara and hip dysplasia are present and when the coxa vara is severe, the superhip procedure is performed. The pelvic and femoral osteotomies should be performed 12 months before the first lengthening. The superhip procedure is a

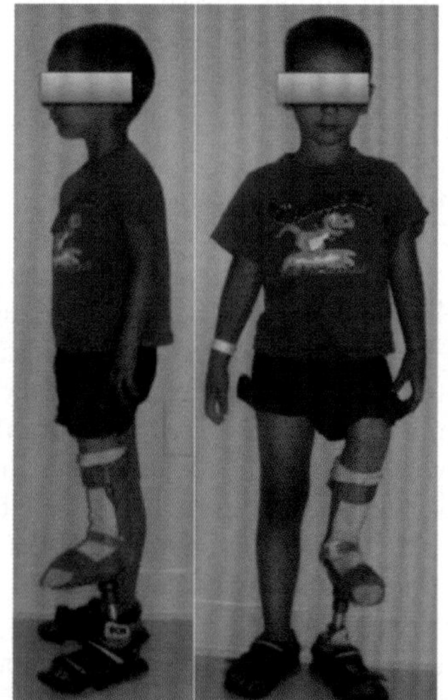

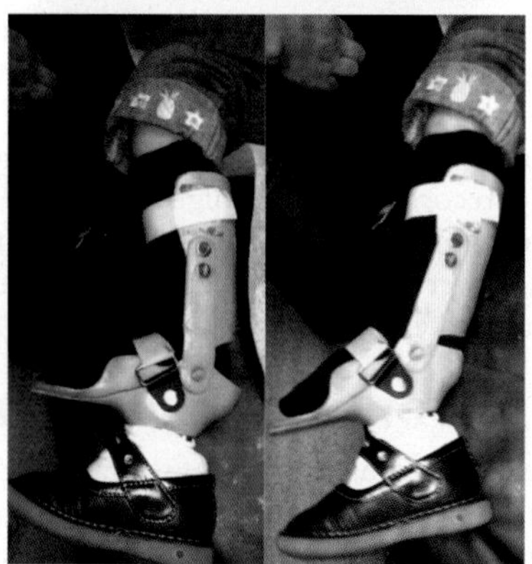

**FIG 5** • **A.** Articulated AFO prosthesis. **B.** Plantar flexion and dorsiflexion. The ankle motion aids with walking.

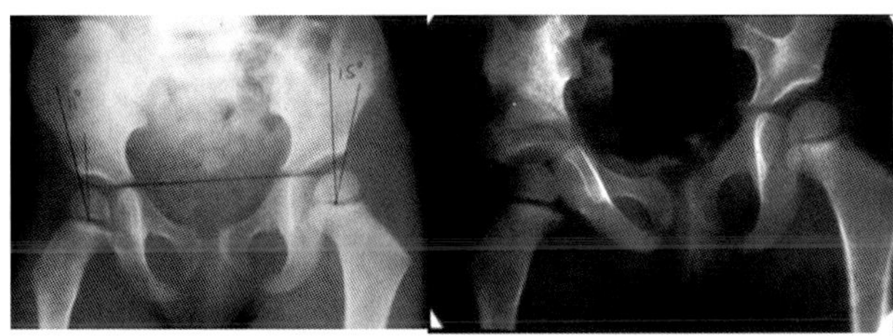

**FIG 6** • Paley type 1a CFD with dysplastic acetabulum. The CE angle is 11 degrees. The patient underwent a Dega osteotomy.

comprehensive surgery to correct the proximal femoral and hip deformities with concurrent soft tissue releases.

- At the conclusion of a successful superhip procedure, the proximal femur has been anatomically and biomechanically reconstructed and the delayed ossification of the femoral neck has ossified. The femur can now be reclassified from 1b to 1a. This ossification occurs within 3 to 12 months of the superhip procedure (often aided by the insertion of BMP). Lengthening is usually not performed in type 1b cases until they convert to type 1a. If lack of full ossification of the femoral neck or subtrochanteric region persists, despite the superhip procedure, repeat insertion of BMP is indicated. As a final measure to allow lengthening to begin in such hips at risk, the external fixation can be extended to the pelvis to protect the hip.

## Types 2 and 3 Congenital Femoral Deficiency

- The strategies that should be used to treat types 2 and 3 CFD are complex and beyond the scope of this chapter. A summary of the strategies is provided in the following text.

### *Type 2 Congenital Femoral Deficiency*

- The presence or absence of a mobile femoral head in the acetabulum determines the treatment strategy. MRI will show if the femoral head is fused to the acetabulum by a bone or cartilage bridge. If a fusion is present, it is always between the femoral head and the posterior wall of the acetabulum (ischium).
- If the femoral head is mobile, it can be connected to the remainder of the femur by a complicated procedure in which the femoral neck is reconstructed (superhip 2 procedure). If the femoral head does not move in the acetabulum, there are three options:
  - Separate it from the acetabulum creating a mobile head and proceed with a superhip 2 procedure.
  - Enucleate the femoral head from the acetabulum and perform a superhip 3 procedure.
  - Do a soft tissue release and lengthen the femur. Near skeletal maturity perform a pelvic support osteotomy.[13]
- The superhip 2 procedure converts types 2a and 2b CFD to type 1a. The proximal femur including the greater trochanter is converted into a femoral neck. An osteotomy is performed just distal to the psoas tendon insertion and the bone rotated 135 degrees. All the muscles except the quadriceps are detached from the proximal femur. The quadriceps acts as the vascular pedicle for this segment of bone. The distal diaphysis is osteotomized at a 45-degree angle and shortened to allow fixation to the new neck segment. This produces a femur with a femoral neck-shaft angle of 135 degrees. The new neck is connected to the ossific nucleus of the femoral head with threaded k-wires or a screw. All of the muscles are reattached to the femur.
- If the femoral head is not worthy of reconstruction, a superhip 3 procedure can be performed instead. This is a form of trochanteric arthroplasty. The quadriceps again serves as the vascular pedicle. All other muscles are detached. The femur is osteotomized and shortened. The hooked greater trochanter fits nicely in the acetabulum. If the acetabulum needs to be enlarged to accommodate the trochanter, the bone distal to the triradiate cartilage is burred allowing the triradiate to act as part of the dome. The anterior ischium is also burred to deepen the posterior wall, and interposition capsule is applied over the exposed bone.

### *Type 3 Congenital Femoral Deficiency*

- Type 3a can be treated like type 2b. Patients can undergo hip release, serial lengthenings, and pelvic support osteotomy or superhip 2 or 3 followed by serial lengthenings or they can be treated by prosthetic fitting options, including prosthetic reconstruction surgery (ie, Syme amputation or rotationplasty[3]).
- Prosthetic reconstruction surgery is recommended for most type 3 CFD due to the extensive deficiency present. This is especially the case for type 3b because there is a stiff knee joint (<45 degrees of motion). Although type 3a can be converted to type 2b, the treatment would consist of four or more lengthenings. Rotationplasty is recommended for most type 3a because it provides a more predictable functional result than does lengthening (**FIG 7**).

## Lengthening

- The number of lengthenings that are required for type 1 CFD is determined by the initial LLD prediction. Patients that do not require any preparatory surgery can undergo their first lengthening as early as age 2 years and preferably before age 4 years. Patients that do require preparatory surgery (eg, superhip, Dega) can undergo their first lengthening 1 year or more after the preparatory surgery. This is usually between ages 3 and 4 years. Between 5 and 8 cm can be obtained during each lengthening.
- For type 1 CFD, the femur should be lengthened by using a distal femoral osteotomy instead of a proximal femoral osteotomy.
  - Distal osteotomies allow for better regenerate bone formation because they have a broader cross-sectional diameter and because the bone is not sclerotic or dysvascular, which often is the case in the proximal femur of patients with CFD. Distal osteotomies can also be used to simultaneously correct the valgus deformity of the distal femur.
  - Proximal osteotomies are used to correct the external femoral torsion and proximal varus deformities and are usually part of the preparatory surgery and not the lengthening surgery. Proximal osteotomies are not used for lengthening because of poor regenerate bone formation. A proximal osteotomy can be used for deformity correction with a concurrent distal osteotomy for lengthening.
- Soft tissue releases are performed during lengthening to prevent subluxation and stiffness of the knee and hip. Soft tissue

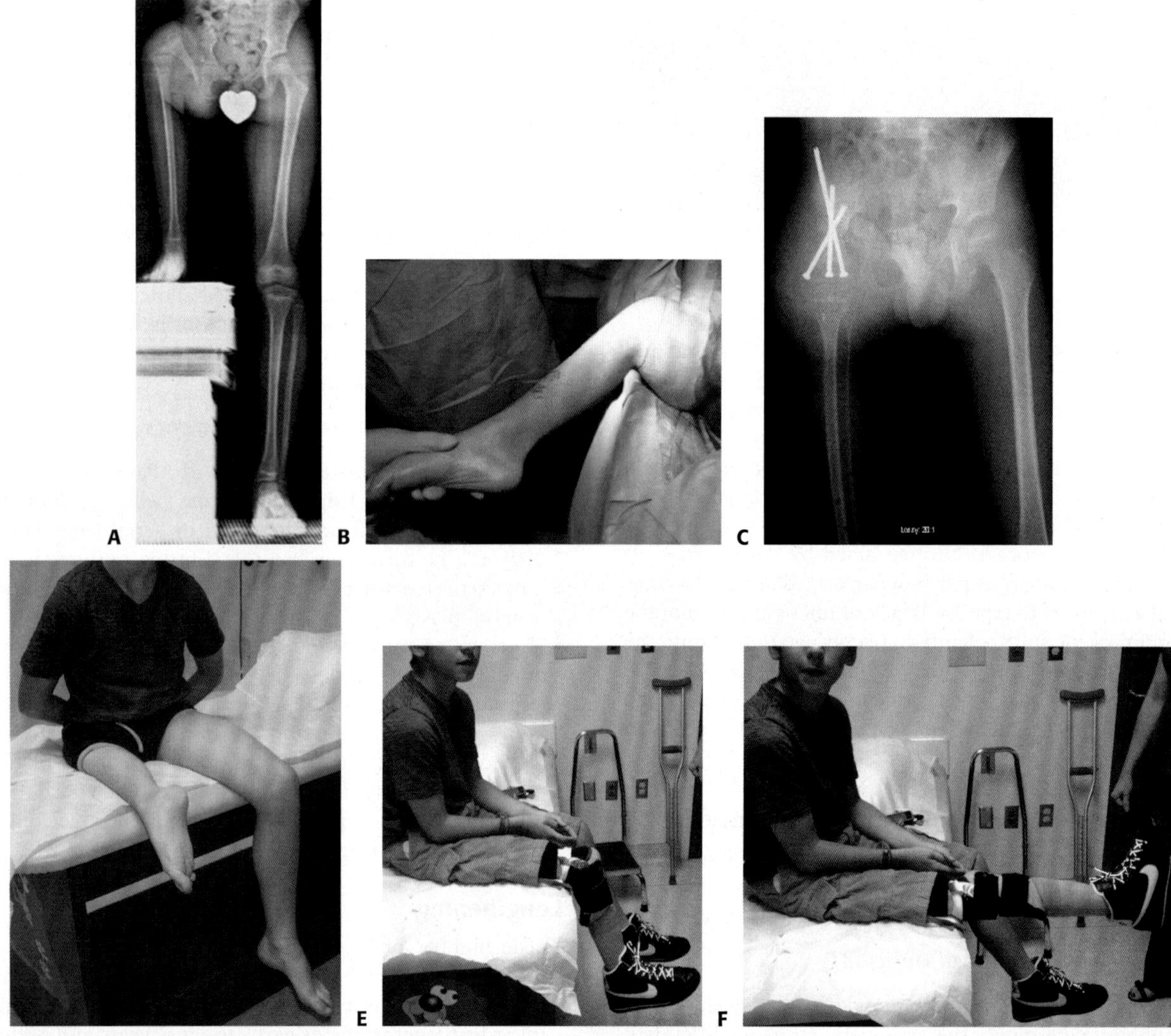

**FIG 7** • **A.** Patient with Paley type 3b CFD with severe leg length difference and knee flexion contracture. **B.** Clinical photo just prior to rotationplasty. **C.** Radiograph after Paley modified Brown rotationplasty. **D.** Photograph showing the appearance after rotationplasty. **E,F.** Side views showing knee flexed (ankle at neutral) and knee extended (ankle plantar flexed).

releases that were addressed during a previous superhip or superknee procedure do not need to be repeated.

### *Lengthening via External Fixators*

- Femoral lengthening with an external fixator can be performed with various devices.
- The essential principle of lengthening with external fixation is to stabilize the knee during lengthening while allowing for knee motion. This is accomplished by using hinges and external fixation of the tibia.
- From 1987 to 2000, the author used only the Ilizarov apparatus with fixation across the knee joint with a hinge for all CFD lengthening cases. This method has previously been described.[9] A monolateral external fixator was not used because it could not articulate across the knee joint.
- From 2000 to 2009, the author modified the Orthofix Limb Reconstruction System (LRS) rail (Orthofix, Inc., McKinney, TX) with the Sheffield Ring Fixation System arch (Orthofix) to articulate across the knee with fixation to the tibia. This method was used for all CFD cases between January 2000 and May 2009.
- From 2009 to the present, the author designed a special external fixator specifically for articulated spanning of the hip and knee joints. The Modular Rail System (Smith & Nephew, Memphis, TN) has been used in all CFD cases since June 1, 2009.

## Preoperative Planning

- Preoperative evaluation consists of obtaining radiographs and performing a physical examination as previously described.
- The radiographs are assessed as previously described, and the CFD is reclassified if progressive ossification has occurred.
- During each visit before the first surgical reconstruction, LLD is recalculated to increase accuracy so that the overall strategy can be altered as needed.[11]

## Superhip Procedure

### Positioning and Exposure

- The patient undergoing the superhip procedure is placed supine on the operating table with a bump placed under the ipsilateral sacrum to tilt the pelvis about 40 degrees. The entire lower extremity (including the groin, iliac crest, and gluteal region) is prepared to the subcostal margin (**TECH FIG 1A**).
- Landmarks: apex of iliac crest, proximal femoral bump, tibial tuberosity
- Make a straight midlateral incision from the apex of the iliac crest to just below the tibial tuberosity. Do not curve the incision.
  - This incision should pass over the bump of the proximal femur (the bump is the lateral prominence in the region where one would usually find the greater trochanter; this bump in most patients is not the trochanter but rather the bend in the femur).
- The anterior flap of skin and the subcutaneous tissues are reflected in a full-thickness fashion off the deep fascial layer until the anterior superior iliac spine (ASIS) proximally and the midpatella distally. The posterior flap is reflected to the level of the intermuscular septum (**TECH FIG 1B**).
- The fascia lata is incised longitudinally, anteriorly from proximal to distal, from the interval between the sartorius and the TFL proximally, to the lateral border of the patella distally. It is then incised longitudinally, posteriorly, from distal to proximal from just posterior to the intermuscular septum distally, to the gluteus maximus muscle proximally.
- The fascia is then cut proximally at the TFL muscle tendon junction.

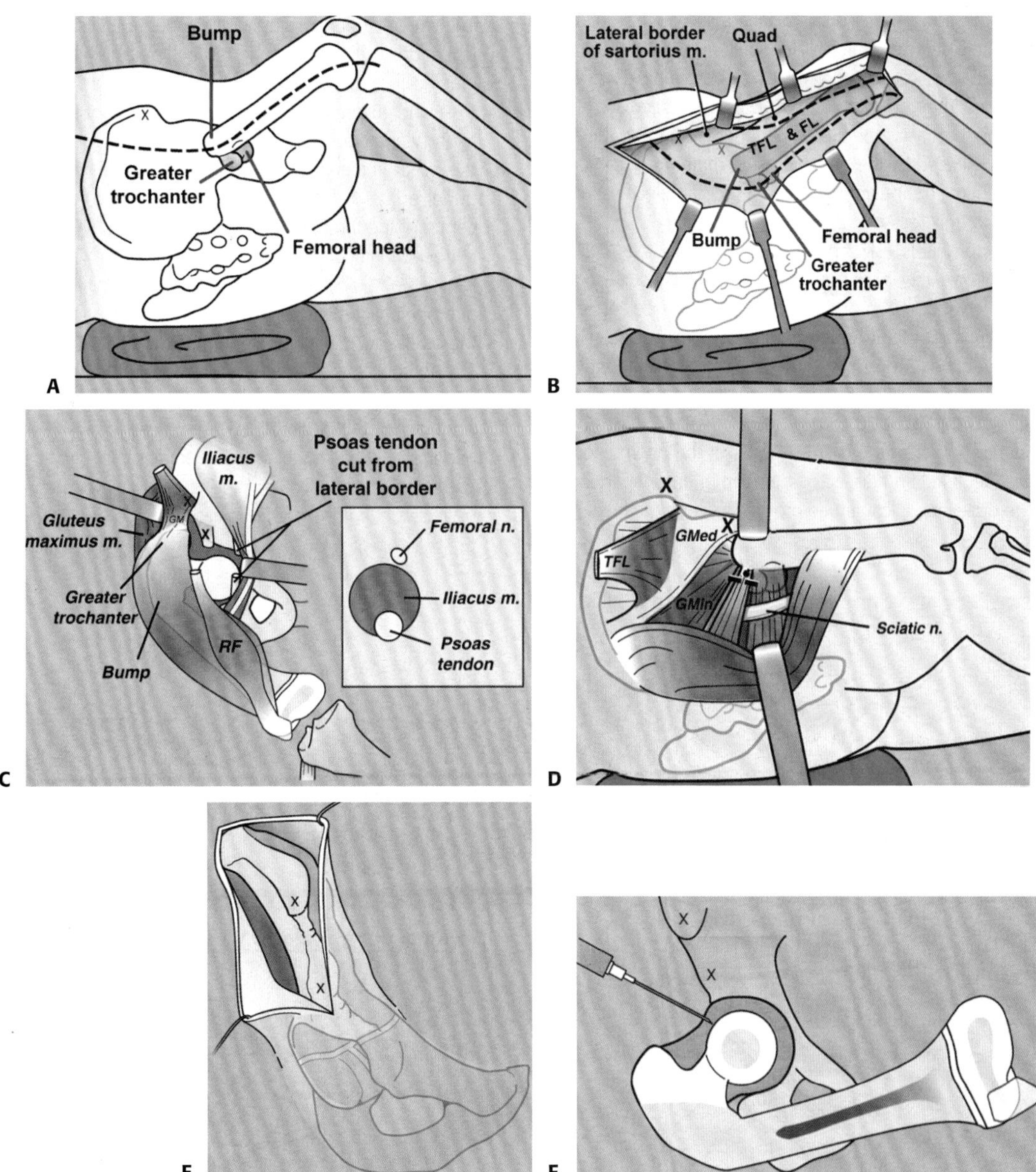


**TECH FIG 1** • **A.** Patient positioning with bump. **B**. The posterior flap is reflected to the level of the intermuscular septum **C**. The conjoint tendon of the rectus femoris is transected just distal to the AIIS. **D.** With the femur internally rotated, the piriformis tendon is released. **E.** The iliac apophysis is divided. **F**. Dye is injected to visualize the femoral head and neck.

- The gluteus maximus is separated from the TFL and reflected posteriorly.
- The conjoint tendon of the rectus femoris, before it divides into the direct and reflected heads, is transected just distal to the anterior inferior iliac spine (AIIS) (**TECH FIG 1C**).
- The iliacus muscle is lifted off the ilium, and the underlying psoas tendon is exposed and released at the level of the pelvic brim. The surgeon must realize that the femoral nerve is much closer to both the rectus femoris muscle and psoas tendon in patients with CFD. Therefore, the femoral nerve is identified, decompressed, and protected before the aforementioned releases.
- If the anterior fascia of the thigh and the fascia of the sartorius muscle are tight, they are released. The lateral femoral cutaneous nerve is identified and protected before releasing the fasciae.
- The trochanter of the femur is palpated posteriorly, and the femur is retracted using a rake anteriorly to visualize the piriformis tendon. The sciatic nerve can also be identified, decompressed, and protected. The contracted piriformis tendon is cut (**TECH FIG 1D**).
- The last contracted muscle that needs to be released are the hip abductors. They act both as abductors and flexors of the hip when the femur has the aforementioned deformity. The abductors are released by the abductor slide method. This avoids weakening them. The previously described distal release should be avoided for this reason.
- The iliac apophysis is now split from the AIIS to the ASIS to two-thirds of the way back along the iliac crest just past the apex of the crest. The hip abductor muscles are peeled off of the lateral ilium with their underlying periosteum. This is called the *abductor slide*. Similarly, the medial half of the apophysis is stripped off of the ilium with the iliacus muscle producing a flexor slide (**TECH FIG 1E**).
- The posterior border of the vastus lateralis at the intermuscular septum is identified and dissected free of the femur subperiosteally. The dissection is continued proximally along the posterior aspect of the greater trochanter to the bone cartilage junction. Distally, the quadriceps is elevated for most of the length of the congenitally short femur.
- An arthrogram of the hip is carried out using a spinal needle. The femoral head and neck are placed in a neutral orientation to the pelvis by extending and maximally adducting the hip joint (**TECH FIG 1F**).
- The femur can now be freely extended, adducted, and internally rotated such that the proximal femur is in a normal anatomic position.

## Femoral Osteotomy

- The preferred method of fixation is the 130-degree pediatric cannulated blade plate (Smith & Nephew, Memphis, TN).
- The first step is to place a guidewire from the tip of the greater trochanter to the center of the femoral head (**TECH FIG 2A**). The greater trochanter is cartilaginous and its tip is found by palpation. The center of the femoral head is determined radiographically after injection of arthrographic dye.
- A second guidewire is inserted in the center of the femoral neck to the center of the femoral head, at a 45-degree angle with the initial guidewire. The second guidewire is then visualized under a lateral fluoroscopic view to confirm its position in the center of the femoral head ossific nucleus (**TECH FIG 2B**). The correct orientation on the lateral fluoroscopic view is when one can see a "bull's eye" created by the concentric circles of the arthrographic outline of the femoral head and femoral neck with the ossific nucleus in the center (**TECH FIG 2C**).
- The appropriate-sized cannulated blade plate chisel is driven over the femoral neck guidewire to create a path for the corresponding size blade plate (**TECH FIG 2D**). The chisel should be oriented perpendicular to the straight posterior border of the greater trochanter. The chisel is removed, and the correct length cannulated blade plate is inserted over the femoral neck guidewire (**TECH FIG 2E**).

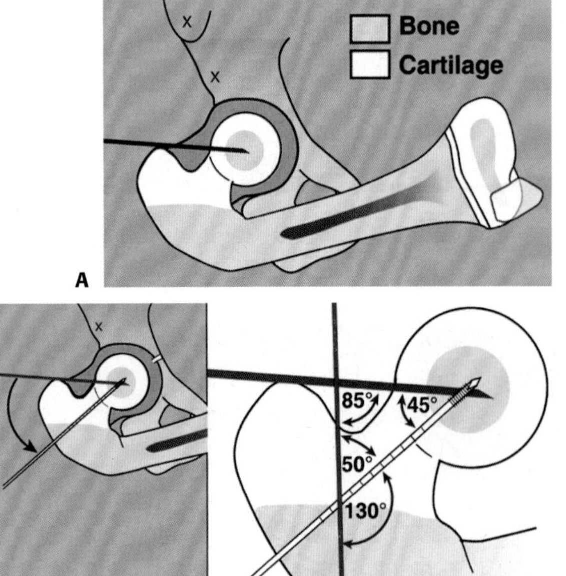


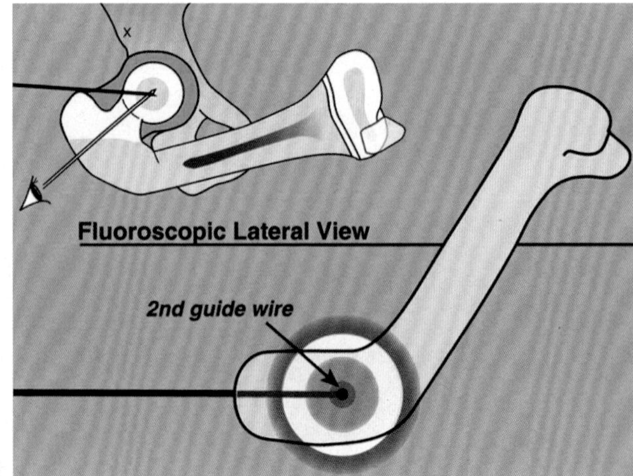


**TECH FIG 2** • **A.** A K-wire is inserted from the greater trochanter to the center of the femoral head. **B,C.** A second guidewire is inserted in the center of the femoral neck to the center of the femoral head, at a 45-degree angle with the initial guidewire (**B**), and confirmed fluoroscopically (**C**). *(continued)*

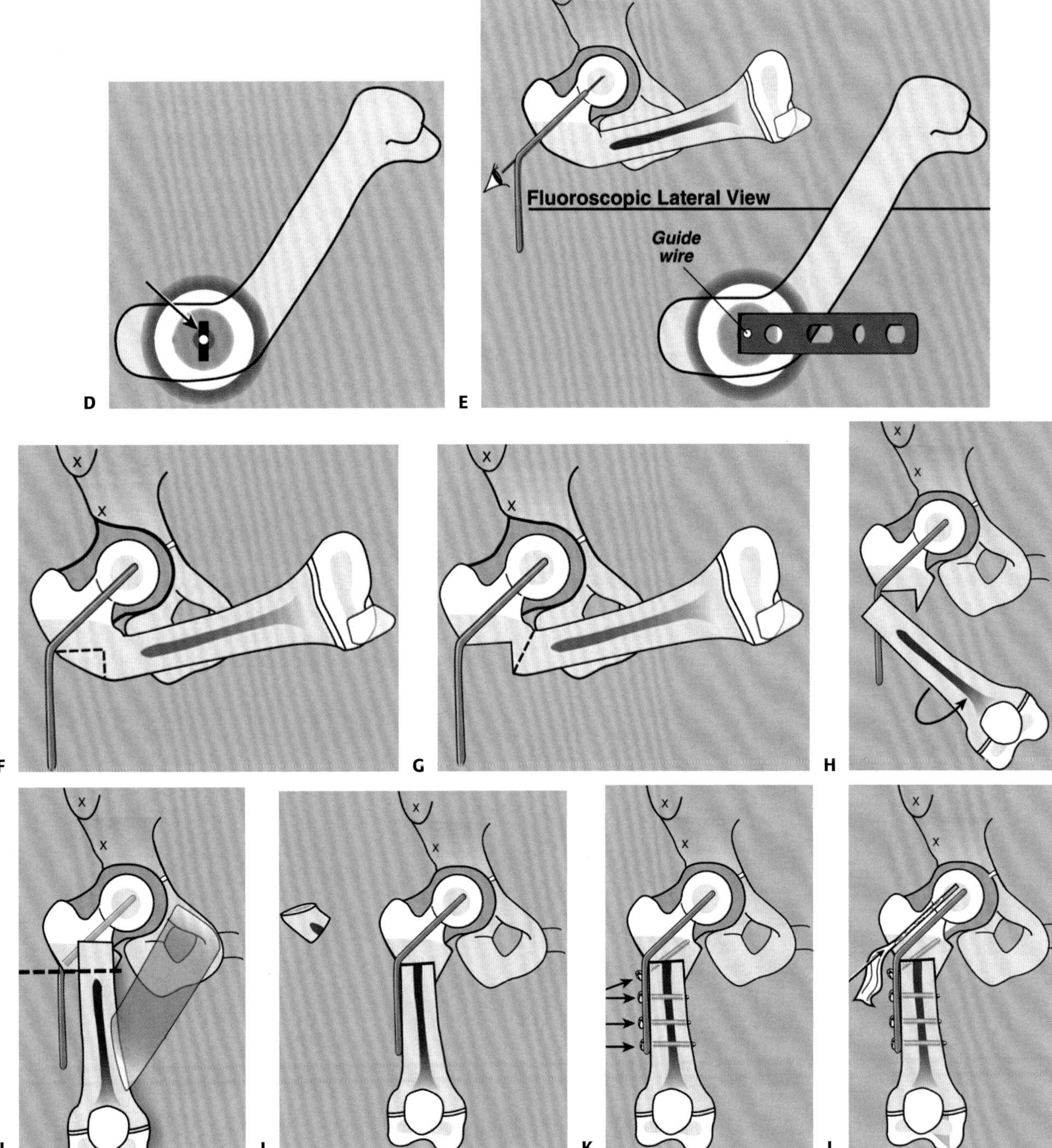


**TECH FIG 2** • *(continued)* **D.** The appropriate-sized cannulated blade plate chisel is driven over the femoral neck guidewire (*arrow*). **E.** The cannulated blade plate is inserted over the femoral neck guidewire. **F.** An osteotomy wedge is made perpendicular and parallel to the blade plate. **G.** A second osteotomy is made from the distal end of the notch across the femur. **H.** The distal femur is then extended, abducted, and internally rotated. **I.** The distal femur is approximated to the blade plate, with the osteotomy level noted (*dashed line*). The length of the distal femur is limited by the length of the adductor muscles (*pink area* at right). **J.** With the osteotomy completed, the distal femoral segment is reduced to the proximal segment. **K.** The plate is fixed with screws. **L.** The channel in the femoral neck is packed with BMP.

- Just distal to the bend in the blade plate, two wires are inserted perpendicular and parallel to the side plate. A sagittal saw is used to remove a triangular segment of bone. The first cut is parallel to the plate, and the second cut is perpendicular to the plate. The width of the second cut is equal to the diameter of the femoral diaphysis (**TECH FIG 2F**).
- A second subtrochanteric osteotomy is performed by cutting obliquely from the apex of the triangle (**TECH FIG 2G**).
- The distal femoral segment is stripped of its periosteum. The periosteum is often incised transversely to gain some length. The distal femur is then extended, abducted, and internally rotated (**TECH FIG 2H**) and aligned with the plate allowing the femoral segments to overlap (**TECH FIG 2I**). The bone ends have to overlap because of the constraints of the surrounding soft tissues. The amount of overlap determines the amount of shortening of the distal segment that is required (**TECH FIG 2J**).
- A third osteotomy is performed perpendicular to the distal femoral shaft at the level of overlap (usually 2 to 4 cm distal to the second osteotomy site). The distal femoral segment is reduced to the plate. The version of the femoral neck is adjusted by rotation, the femur with the knee flexed, and a wire inserted in the cannulation of the blade to represent the orientation of the neck. Fixation is completed with four screws (**TECH FIG 2K**). The resected bone segment is used in the Dega osteotomy at the end of the procedure.
- For type 1b subtrochanteric type, the unossified segment is resected as part of the shortening.
- For type 1b neck type, BMP (INFUSE Bone Graft, Medtronic, Inc., Memphis, TN) is inserted into the femoral neck to induce ossification of the femoral neck (**TECH FIG 2L**).

## Pelvic Osteotomy

- The next step is to perform the author's modification of the Dega osteotomy. The ilium is already exposed from the abductor slide. The outer table of the ilium is subperiosteally dissected down to the sciatic notch and toward the triradiate cartilage separating the ilium from the ischium (**TECH FIG 3A**).
- The pelvic osteotomy is curved along the lateral cortex from the AIIS to the triradiate cartilage posteriorly. At the AIIS, the osteotomy goes through both tables of the ilium. It is important to cut the apophysis and periosteum transversely at this level to allow the osteotomy to separate anteriorly. The osteotomy does not enter the sciatic notch but passes just anterior to the sciatic notch and parallel to the level of the triradiate cartilage. The apex of the osteotomy should start 2 cm above the hip joint and is inclined to the triradiate cartilage medially.
- The osteotomy is levered distally and laterally to cover the femoral head. The large opening wedge is maintained by inserting the resected femoral segment (**TECH FIG 3B**). The end point of correction is a horizontal sourcil.
- The stability of the graft is tested by attempting to pull the graft from the osteotomy site with a Kocher clamp. The graft should be fully within the lateral cortical margins of the ilium. Typically, the graft is extremely stable and no further fixation is needed.

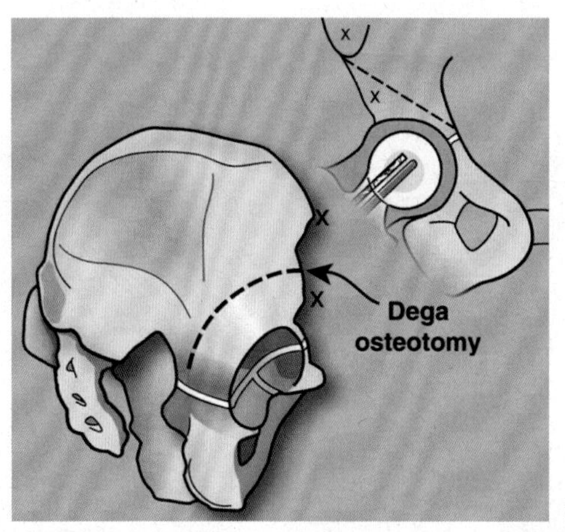


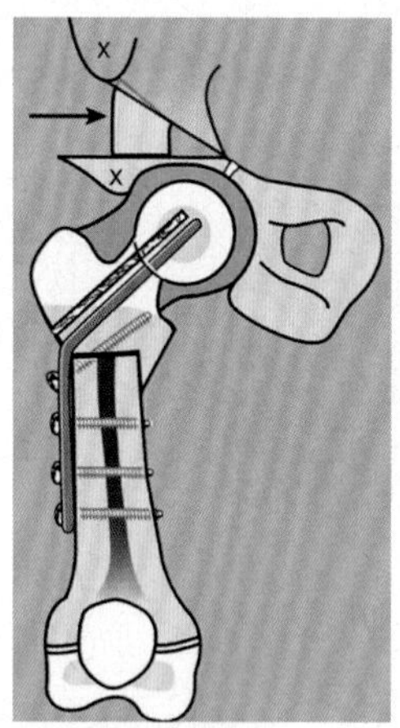


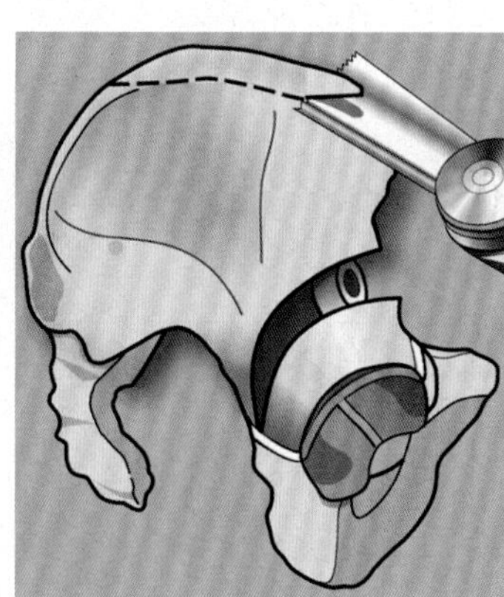


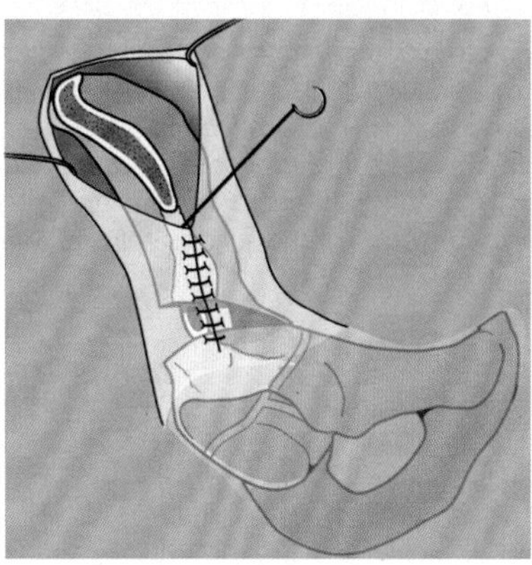


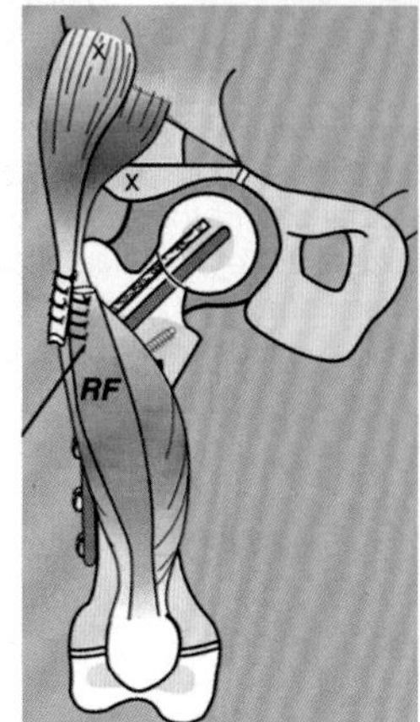


**TECH FIG 3** • **A.** A Dega osteotomy is performed (*dashed lines*). **B.** Bone graft from the femur is inserted to maintain the osteotomy site. **C.** The crest is removed to ease tight abductors. **D.** The apophysis is closed. **E.** The TFL is sutured to the rectus femoris (RF).

- Because of the correction of the abduction contracture and the opening wedge of the Dega, it is not possible to close the apophysis. The apophysis is pulled up and the level marked with a pen. The crest is then resected using a saw until the medial and lateral apophysis can be repaired without excessive tension (**TECH FIG 3C,D**). This is called the *abductor slide technique*.
- The TFL is then sutured to the rectus femoris (**TECH FIG 3E**).
- The incision is closed in layers. A suction drain is used and is left in place until the drainage stops (<10 mL per 24 hours), which can take several days. Prophylactic antibiotics are administered intravenously until the drain is removed.
- A spica cast is applied with the hip in full extension, neutral abduction, and neutral rotation. The knee is splinted in full extension. The cast is bivalve to allow for swelling. One week after surgery, the cast is made removable and gentle flexion and extension ROM of the hip and knee started.
- **TECH FIGS 4** and **5** are two case examples of superhip procedures.

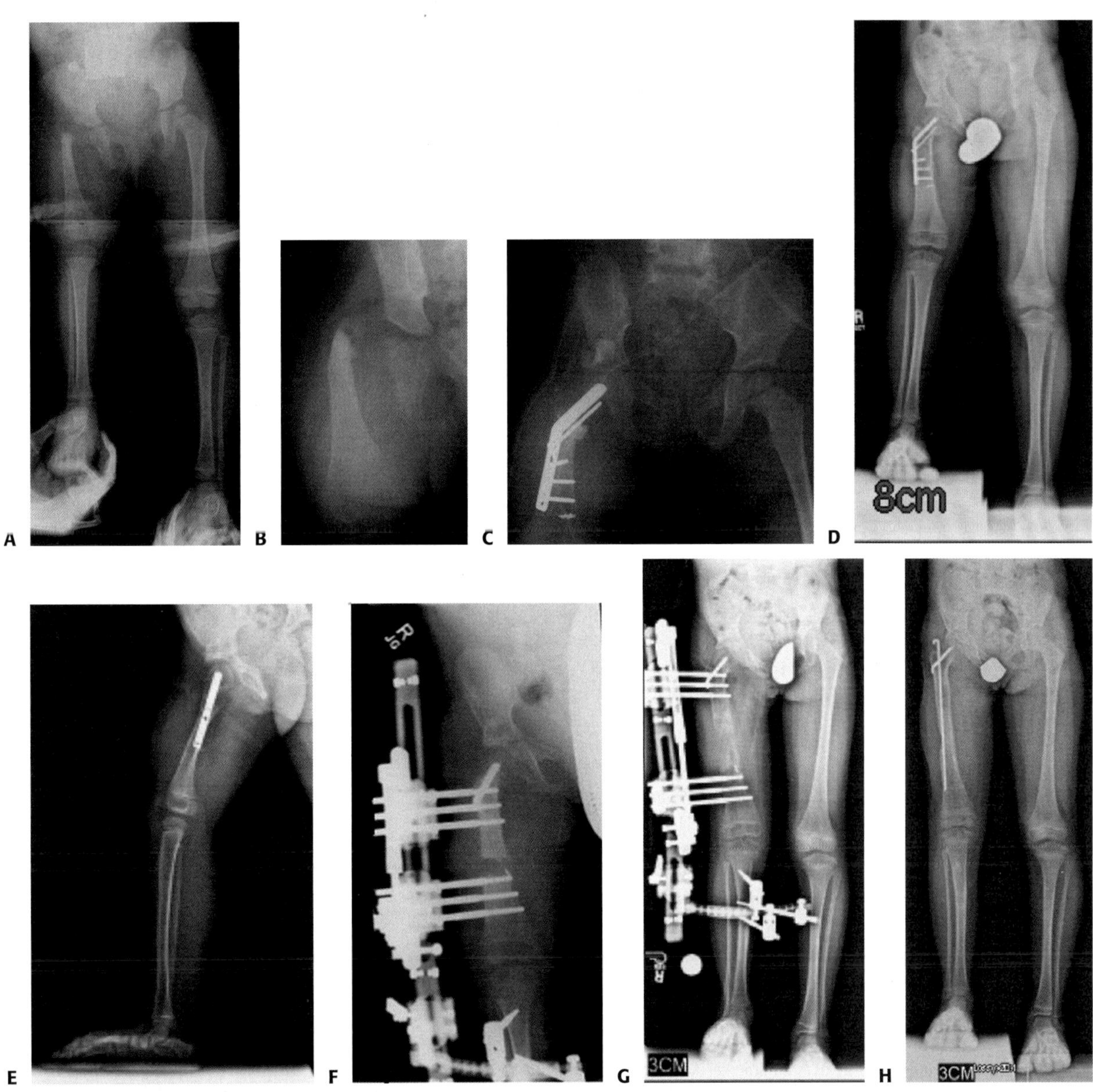


**TECH FIG 4 • A,B.** CFD Paley type 1b with delayed ossification of femoral neck. **C.** Superhip procedure at age 2 years including insertion of BMP in femoral neck. **D.** The neck is fully ossified by age 3 years. **E,F.** First lengthening is performed at age 4 years with Smith & Nephew Modular Rail System external fixator with articulation across the knee joint. **G.** Eight centimeters of lengthening is achieved. **H.** Removal of external fixator with Rush rodding of bone to prevent fracture.

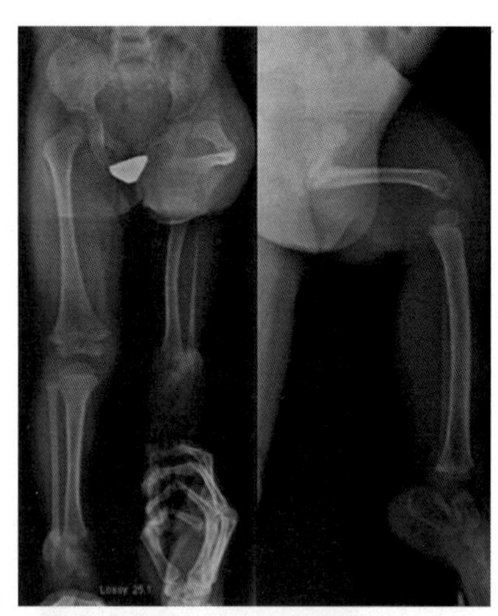
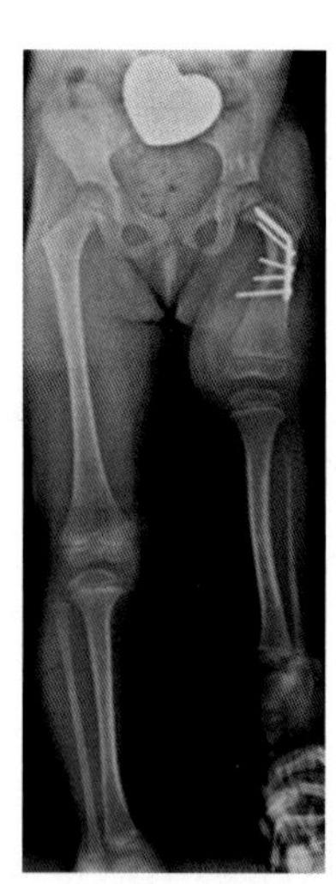
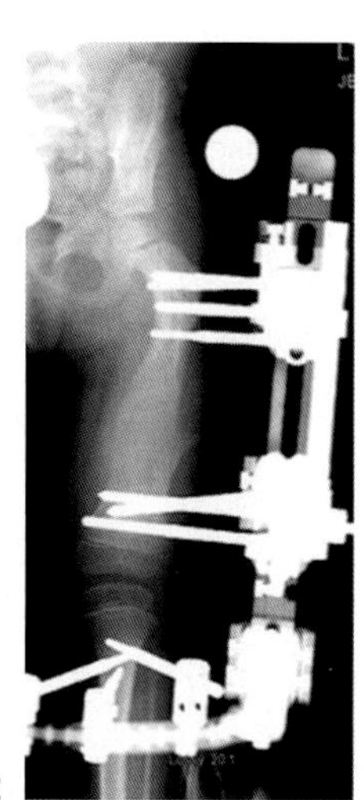
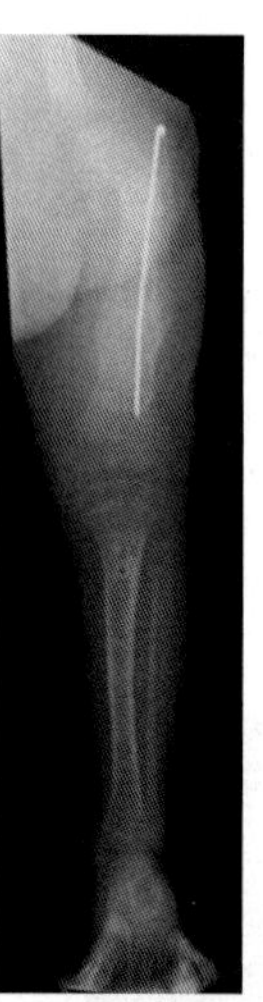
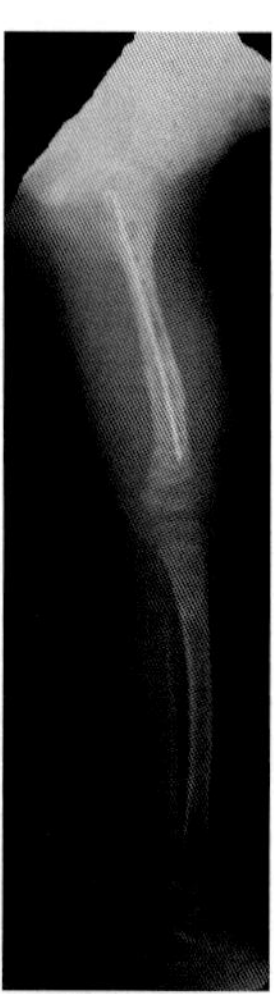

**TECH FIG 5** • **A.** Two-year-old girl with CFD Paley type 1b with delayed ossification and severe angulation of the subtrochanteric level of the femur. **B.** The deformity is fully corrected, and the femur is healed after the superhip surgery. **C.** Lengthening of the femur was performed at age 4 years. **D,E.** X-rays after lengthening of the femur 7 cm and insertion of Rush rod.

## Superknee Procedure

### Exposure

- If significant knee instability is present, a superknee procedure should be performed conjointly with the superhip procedure.[9] The superknee procedure can address ACL and PCL insufficiency, patellar subluxation or dislocation, and maltracking. Different parts of the procedure can be used depending on the knee pathology.
- If performed independently, the same midlateral straight incision is used. The anterior and posterior margins of the fascia lata are incised longitudinally. The fascia lata is transected as proximally as possible and reflected distally until its insertion onto the tibia (**TECH FIG 6A**).
- The fascia lata is split into two longitudinal strips to make two ligaments. A Krackow whipstitch[5] is used to run a nonabsorbable suture from the free end of the fascia lata toward the tubercle of Gerdy in a tubular fashion (**TECH FIG 6B**).
- A lateral release of the capsule leaving the synovium intact is performed if the patella is maltracking.
- The lateral release is extended distally to the lateral aspect of the patellar tendon. If a Grammont procedure[4] is to be performed, the incision is extended past the tibial tuberosity along the crest of the tibia so that the proximal periosteum is elevated.

### Anterior Cruciate Ligament Reconstruction

- A MacIntosh intra-articular and/or extra-articular ACL reconstruction is performed. The lateral collateral ligament (LCL) is identified. Two tunnels are made. One tunnel is placed under the LCL and does not enter the knee joint (**TECH FIG 7A**). The other tunnel is made subperiosteally, from anterior and proximal to posterior and distal, over the lateral intramuscular septum of the femur (**TECH FIG 7B**).
- A hole is made in the posterior knee joint capsule by inserting a curved clamp from the "over-the-top" position.
- The posterior limb of the fascia lata is passed under the LCL. An ACL reamer is used over a guidewire to create a bony tunnel in the proximal tibial epiphysis. The wire is inserted from the anteromedial aspect of the tibia and is directed to the center of the tibial epiphysis. The outer diameter of the actual graft is measured, and the hole in the epiphysis is reamed to this diameter.

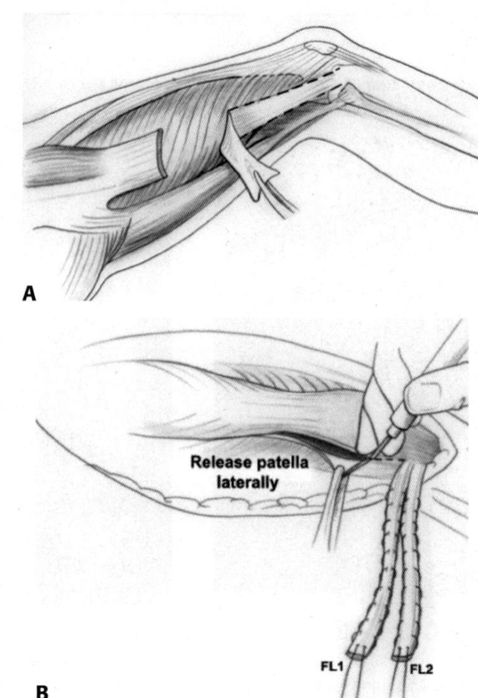


**TECH FIG 6** • **A.** The fascia lata is incised and reflect to Gerdy tubercle. **B.** The fascia lata is split into two longitudinal strips (FL1 and FL2) to make two ligaments. A Krackow whipstitch is used to run a nonabsorbable suture from the free end of the fascia lata toward the tubercle of Gerdy in a tubular fashion.

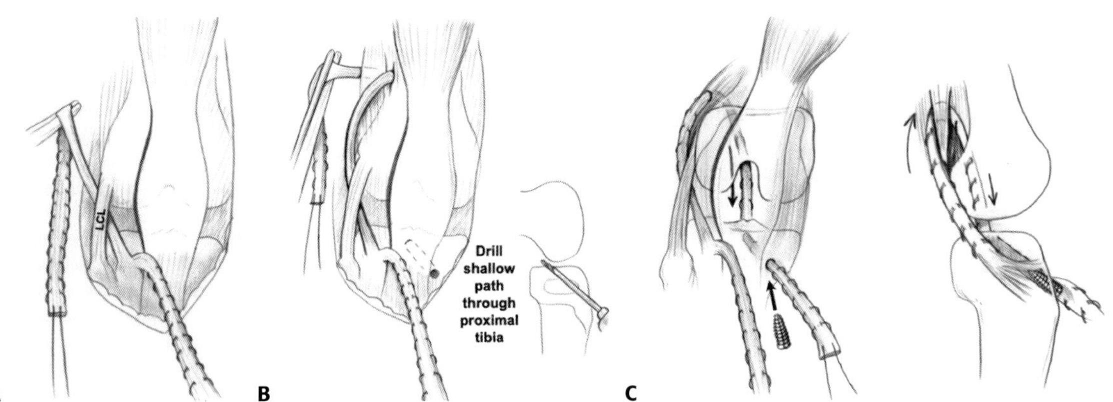


**TECH FIG 7** • One strip of the fascia lata (FL1) is tunnelled under the (**A**) and then under the intramuscular septum of the femur (**B**). **C.** FL1 is passed through the intercondylar notch, through the epiphyseal tunnel, and secured with an interference screw.

- A suture passer is passed through the tibial epiphyseal tunnel and out the posterior capsule of the knee to exit laterally anterior to the septum. The fascia lata suture is pulled through the knee and the bony tunnel using the suture passer. A bioabsorbable headless screw is used to secure the graft to the tunnel (**TECH FIG 7C**). The ACL graft is tensioned and sutured with the knee reduced and in full extension to prevent creation of a fixed flexion deformity of the knee.
- If only an extra-articular ACL repair is needed, the fascia lata is looped back after passing under the LCL and the lateral intramuscular septum. The fascia lata is sutured to itself and no tunnel is made. To prevent loosening, the graft can be reinforced and retensioned after fixation by passing a nonabsorbable suture anchor through bone at the point at which the graft loops over the intermuscular septum.

## Extra-articular Posterior Cruciate Ligament Reconstruction (Reverse MacIntosh Procedure)[9]

- The anterior skin flap is elevated off the knee and dissected and reflected medially until the entire vastus medialis muscle can be visualized.
- The anterior limb of the fascia lata is usually not tubularized. It is passed first under the patellar tendon and then through a medial retinacular tunnel (**TECH FIG 8A**). The graft is then passed through a subperiosteal tunnel around the adductor magnus tendon. Finally, it is sutured to itself with nonabsorbable suture (**TECH FIG 8B,C**).
- This extra-articular ligament is tensioned with the knee in 90 degrees of flexion to prevent an extension contracture.
- The end of the ACL is sutured to the end of the extra-articular PCL to prevent any slippage.

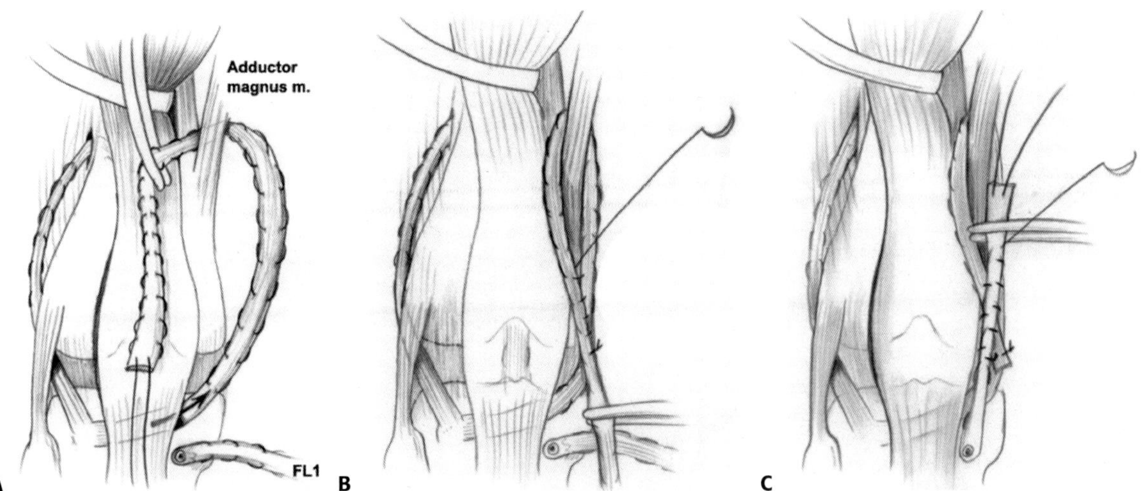


**TECH FIG 8** • The second strip of fascia lata (FL2) is tunneled under the patellar ligament, then passed through the intermuscular septum (**A**), and then sutured back onto itself (**B**). **C.** FL1 and FL2 are sutured together, and a bioabsorbable headless screw secures the graft to the tunnel.

## Intra-articular Posterior Cruciate Ligament Reconstruction

- Intra-articular PCL reconstruction is rarely needed, but if it is, the peroneal nerve is identified, decompressed, and protected.
- The lateral head of the gastrocnemius muscle is then released from the femur. The posterior aspect of the proximal tibial epiphysis is identified to the midline.
- An anterior to posterior drill hole is made through the epiphysis from Gerdy tubercle to the center of the proximal tibial epiphysis. The anterior limb of the fascia lata is passed from anterior to posterior, exiting near the midline posteriorly.
- Another drill hole that passes through the medial distal femoral epiphysis from anteromedial to posterolateral is made. The ligamentized fascia lata is pulled through the posterior capsule and into the medial femoral epiphyseal tunnel using its leading suture. It is fixed in place with a biotenodesis absorbable screw after tensioning in flexion.

### Alternative Step for Patellar Realignment: Langenskiöld Reconstruction

- A modified Langenskiöld procedure is performed when fixed patellar subluxation or dislocation is present. If there is a flexion deformity or rotatory subluxation of the tibia on the femur, the biceps tendon should be Z-lengthened and the peroneal nerve decompressed.[10]
- The lateral capsule is cut to, but not through, the synovium. The vastus lateralis muscle is elevated off the intermuscular septum.
- The retinaculum is released on both the medial and lateral aspect of the patella. This is the same incision used for the lateral release (**TECH FIG 9A**).
  - The incision is taken down to the synovial layer without violating the synovium. The synovium is then carefully dissected free of the undersurface of the quadriceps muscle proximally and from the patellar tendon distally (**TECH FIG 9B**).
  - Medially, the capsule is incised proximally in a longitudinal fashion, separating the vastus medialis muscle from the vastus intermedius muscle.
  - The distal medial capsule is cut transversely at the level of the joint line. The capsule is separated from the synovium as far as the medial gutter.
- Once the synovial layer has been separated completely from the overlying tissues, its connection to the patella is incised circumferentially (**TECH FIG 9C**). The quadriceps and patellar tendon are left attached to the patella, and the entire extensor mechanism can be shifted medially.
  - The synovium is now a free tissue layer with a patella-sized hole in the center.
  - The synovial hole is sutured longitudinally with absorbable suture (**TECH FIG 9D**). The patella is left extra-articular at this point.
- The Grammont procedure is performed by elevating the patellar tendon off of the tuberosity cartilage and the patellar tendon is shifted medially. The patellar tendon is secured with absorbable suture (**TECH FIG 9E**).
- The patella with the quadriceps muscle is now realigned medially to its new position and a marking pen is used to mark its new location on the synovium (**TECH FIG 9F**).
- The synovium is incised longitudinally with the knee in full extension (**TECH FIG 9G**). The patella is inserted into this new position and sutured circumferentially to the synovium with a continuous absorbable suture (**TECH FIG 9H,I**).
- The medial retinacular flap is now advanced over the patella and sutured to the lateral side of the patella (**TECH FIG 9J**).
- Once the modified Langenskiöld reconstruction is completed, the ACL and PCL knee ligamentous reconstruction, as previously described, is performed (**TECH FIG 9K**).

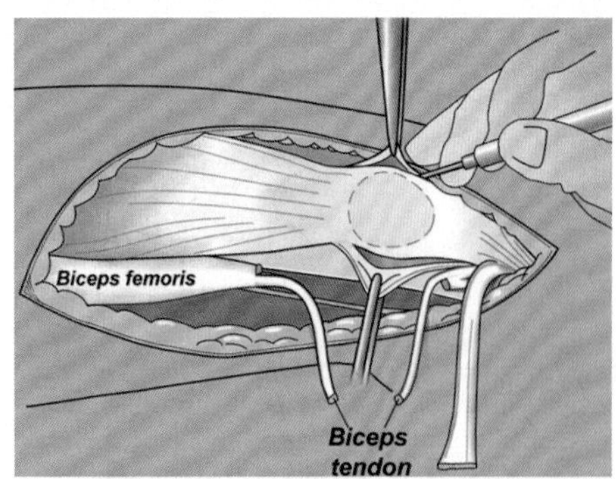


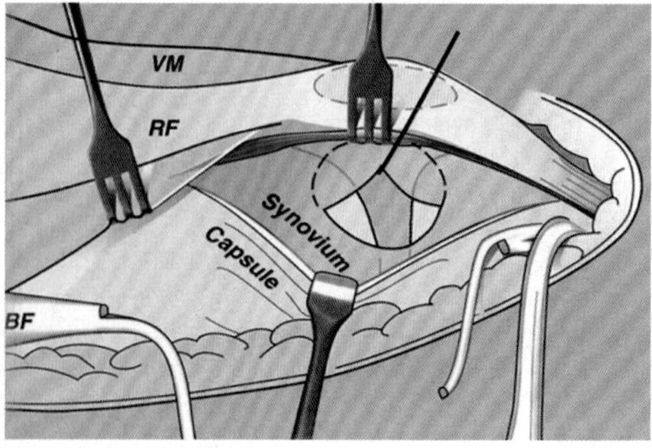


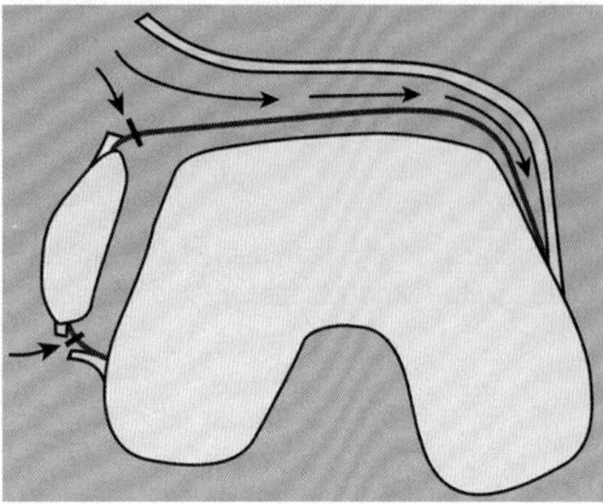


**TECH FIG 9** • **A.** The capsule is opened laterally. **B.** The capsule is released from the synovium. **C.** The synovium is released from the patella in a circumferential cut. *(continued)*

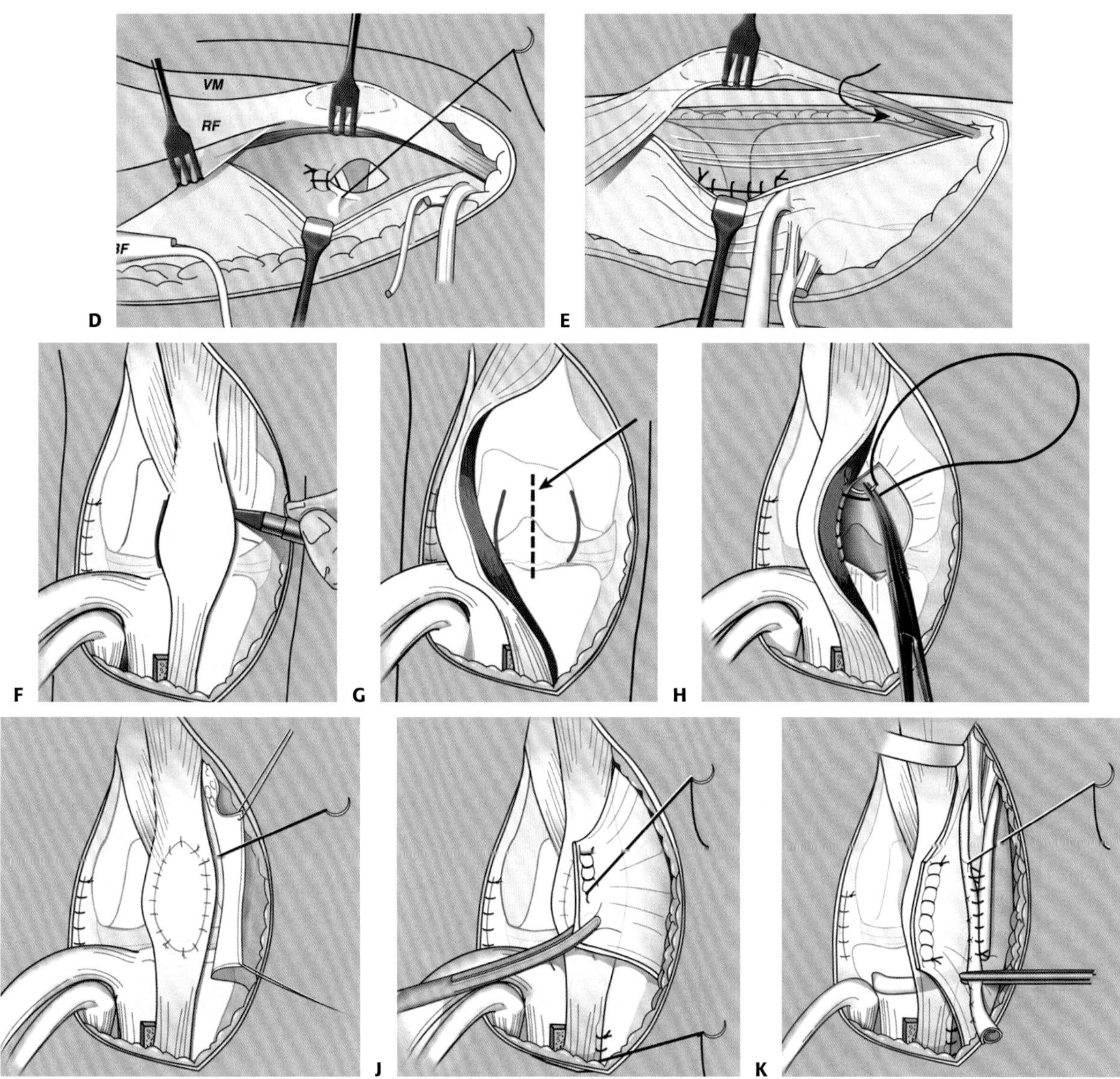


**TECH FIG 9** • *(continued)* **D.** The synovium is sutured closed. **E.** A Grammont elevation of the patellar tendon is performed. **F.** The new position for the patella is marked on the synovium. **G.** The synovium is opened between the markings. **H,I.** It is then sutured to the patella circumferentially. **J.** The medial capsule is sutured to the patella (*top*) and the patellar tendon is sutured to the tibia (*bottom*). **K.** Finally, the fascia lata graft is sutured back onto itself.

## Femoral Lengthening of Type 1 Congenital Femoral Deficiency: Orthofix Fixator Technique

### Preparatory Surgery

- If there are no indications for hip or knee surgery, the fascia lata and rectus femoris proximally and the iliotibial band and biceps tendon distally should be released at the time of the lengthening surgery.
- If these tissues were released with a previous Dega, superhip, or superknee procedure, there is no need to do any soft tissue releases.

### Placement of Femoral Fixator

- An arthrogram of the involved knee is obtained under fluoroscopy. In the lateral view, the femoral condyles are rotated until they superimpose each other. This is considered a "true lateral of the knee." (Note that this is not the patella-forward position—actually, the patella will be externally rotated approximately 10 degrees in this position.)
- The center of knee rotation is identified. The center of rotation is the intersection of the posterior cortical line and the distal femoral physeal line.

- A 2-mm Steinmann pin is inserted into the distal femoral physis at the center of rotation and parallel to the distal femoral joint line in the frontal plane (**TECH FIG 10A**).
  - A half-pin is inserted into the femur at its proximal end parallel to this hinge-axis pin.
  - To accurately place the half-pin, use the cannulated drill technique. Insert a wire into the femur and check if it is in the correct location with the image intensifier. Then over drill it with a cannulated drill. The half-pin is then inserted in a perfect position.
  - Half-pins placed in the anterior half of the femoral diaphysis can result in a fracture either during the lengthening process or after frame removal.
- The preconstructed modular rail system (MRS) (Smith & Nephew, Memphis, TN) is applied so that distally the Steinmann pin goes through the cannulated hinge bolt and proximally the half-pins goes through the proximal clamp.
- The most distal half-pin is placed one hole proximal and anterior to the knee axis reference wire.
  - At this point, the position of the hinge axis is a fixed point to the initial distal half-pin.
- The additional half-pins are placed proximal and distal. Three frontal plane half-pins should be placed in each segment (**TECH FIG 10B**).
- The osteotomy is made immediately proximal to the distal pin group. This is done through a 1-cm lateral incision, followed by multiple drill holes with an osteotome, followed by completion of the osteotomy with an osteotome.
- If concurrent distal valgus deformity is being corrected, the proximal and distal pins are placed at angles to each other and the osteotomy performed after there are two proximal and two distal pins. The rail is placed only after the deformity is corrected. The deformity is corrected acutely and the rest of the fixation is as for the underformed bone.
- The external fixation is completed with insertion of two AP pins (**TECH FIG 10C–E**).

## Placement of Tibial Fixator

- A distal rail segment is used to suspend a floating arch. The tibial fixation is attached to this arch.
- A single-hole Ilizarov cube is placed on the arch, and an AP half-pin is placed in the proximal tibia. The knee should be in full extension and reduced.
- After the first half-pin is inserted into the tibia, the hinge is tested with gentle ROM of the knee.
- If the motion is smooth, a drop leg test is performed.
  - The drop leg test consists of lifting the lower extremity off the bed and fully extending the knee. The thigh is supported and the foot dropped.
  - If the knee flexes with no catching or friction, two additional half-pins are placed in the tibia.
  - If there is friction during the drop leg test, connection to the pin needs to be adjusted (eg, fix it in flexion first). After the adjustment, the drop leg test is repeated until knee ROM is smooth, with no friction.
- The floating arch is not connected to the rail. It therefore does not impede growth of the distal femoral and proximal tibial physes.
- A knee extension bar is built using Ilizarov parts between the rail and the arch.
  - This knee extension bar can be removed to allow knee motion. It should be used all night and part time during the day to prevent knee flexion contracture.
- If hip stabilization is required, a hip hinge clamp is used. It is centered on the center of the femoral head. Three pins are placed in the pelvis and fixed with an arch (see **TECH FIG 8E**).
- At the conclusion of the procedure, Botox, 10 units per kilogram of body weight, is injected into the proximal quadriceps using multiple injection sites.
  - This is to reduce quadriceps muscle spasms and pain during knee flexion stretches.

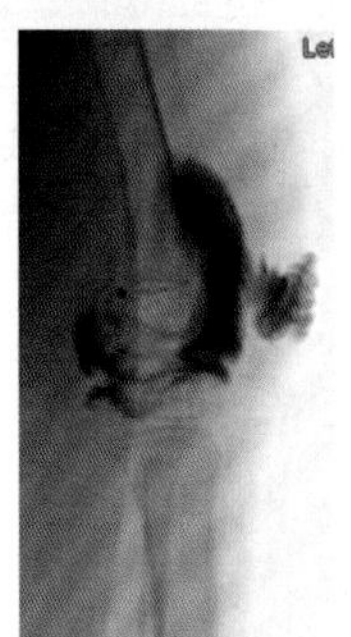
A

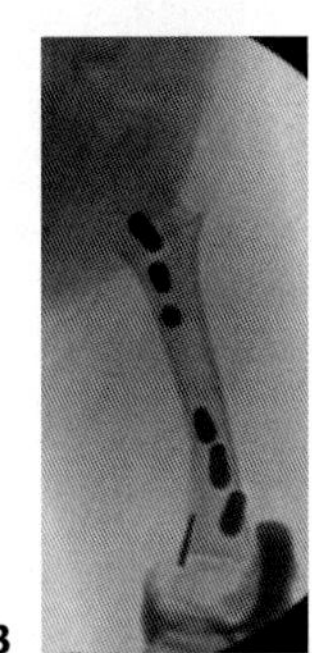
B

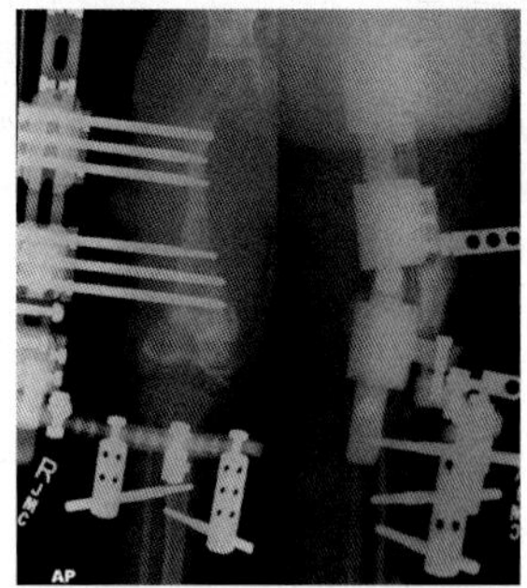

C

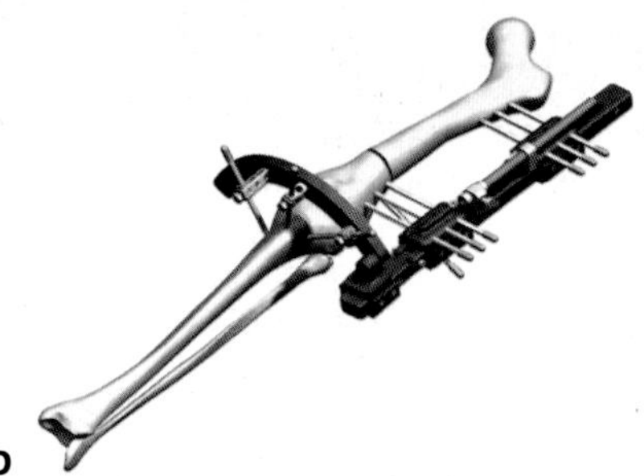
D

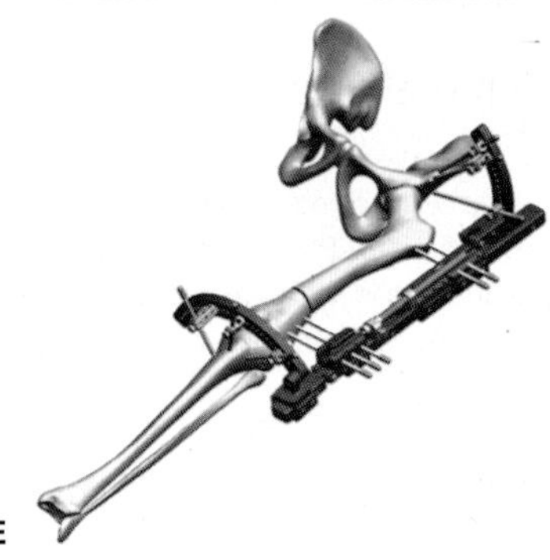
E

**TECH FIG 10** • **A.** Steinmann pin is inserted into the distal femoral physis at the center of rotation of the knee with a knee arthrogram lining up the two posterior femoral condyles. **B.** The other half pins are placed parallel to the Steinmann pin. The external fixator is used as a template. **C.** The external fixator is removed and the osteotomy performed. The fixator is then reapplied to the femur and the tibial frame and pins added. **D.** The MRS with knee hinge and articulated fixation to the tibia from the femur. **E.** The MRS with hip and knee hinge with articulated fixation to the pelvis and tibia from the femur.

## PEARLS AND PITFALLS

| | |
|---|---|
| **Superhip—initial dissection** | ■ Rectus femoris and iliopsoas tendons are located closer to the femoral nerve than expected. The surgeon should first identify the femoral nerve before performing any releases or tenotomies. |
| **Superknee—knee flexion contracture** | ■ Knee flexion contracture should be released with biceps femoris lengthening and posterior capsular release. A concurrent ligamentous reconstruction should not be performed unless absolutely necessary to reduce the incidence of a stiff knee. |
| **Femoral lengthening** | ■ Positioning the hinge-axis wire is the crucial step when applying the external fixator. Great care should be taken to ensure precise placement of the wire at the center of rotation of the knee (intersection of the posterior femoral cortical line and the distal femoral physis). This must be performed after an arthrogram of the knee is obtained, which allows exact visualization of the overlapped posterior femoral condyles in the lateral fluoroscopic view. In young children, the posterior femoral condyles are not ossified and can only be visualized using the arthrogram. |
| **External fixator removal** | ■ At the time of external fixator removal, a Rush pin (Zimmer, Inc., Warsaw, IN) should be placed prophylactically as described in the following text. Activities, to include physical therapy, should be modified for 4 weeks after removal. |
| **Femoral lengthening** | ■ If the initial distal femoral half-pin is positioned too far anterior, the initial hinge-axis pin is too far anterior. The surgeon should carefully examine the hinge-axis wire and ensure that it is at the level of the posterior femoral cortical line. |
| **Postoperative therapy and preservation of knee motion** | ■ Knee flexion should be maintained at greater than 45 degrees. If knee flexion is 40 degrees or less, lengthening should be slowed or discontinued and knee rehabilitation increased. |

## POSTOPERATIVE CARE

- Patients who have undergone the superhip or superknee procedures are placed into a one-and-a-half hip spica cast.
  - The involved limb is placed in neutral abduction, neutral rotation, and 0 degree of extension. The knee is held in full extension, and the foot is included.
  - The cast is made removable and gentle physical therapy is started. The cast is discontinued at 6 weeks, and gentle ROM of all joints is performed as well as weight bearing as tolerated.
- Patients undergoing femoral lengthening require close follow-up and intensive rehabilitation. Patients are usually discharged on postoperative day 3 or 4.
  - The lengthening begins on day 5 to 7 at a rate of 0.75 to 1.0 mm per day.
  - The patient is assessed every 2 weeks in the outpatient clinic with radiographic and clinical examinations.
    - Pin site problems, nerve function, hip and knee ROM, and knee subluxation are assessed.
    - The joint location, limb alignment, regenerate bone quality, and length gained are assessed radiographically.
  - The rate of distraction is adjusted according to regenerate bone quality and joint ROM.
  - Physical therapy is begun on postoperative day 1. During the distraction phase, physical therapy is continued daily, with formal therapy occurring 5 days per week.
  - The formal therapy consists of one or two sessions with a therapist each day, with 1 hour of land therapy and 1 hour of hydrotherapy.
  - The patient also undergoes two physical therapy sessions at home each day with the parents.
- During therapy, the patient should perform exercises that obtain knee flexion and maintain knee extension.
  - Knee flexion should be maintained at greater than 45 degrees.
  - If knee flexion is 40 degrees or less, lengthening should be discontinued or slowed and knee rehabilitation should be increased.
  - If there is no improvement, lengthening is discontinued.
- During the distraction phase, passive exercises are most important; during the consolidation phase, passive plus active exercises are important. Hip abduction and extension are two important hip exercises.
- During the consolidation phase, the formal therapy can be reduced to three sessions per week if the patient is doing well. Weight bearing is allowed as tolerated.
- The frame can be removed from the femur and tibia after the regenerate bone has healed.
  - A prophylactic Rush pin is placed in the femur at the time of external fixation removal. Application of the Rush pin prevents refracture after lengthening. Without this, O'Carrigan et al[8] noted a 34% refracture rate.
  - The frame is removed under general anesthesia, and radiographs in the AP and lateral views are obtained.
  - At this point, the pin sites are cleaned, prepared, and then isolated with Tegaderm dressings (3M Healthcare Ltd, St. Paul, MN). The entire lower extremity to include the hip, iliac crest, and gluteal region is prepared and draped.
  - A 1.8-mm Ilizarov wire is inserted into the tip of the greater trochanter and driven into the center of the proximal femur. An intraoperative lateral view radiograph after external fixation removal is used to place the starting point on the greater trochanter. The 1.8-mm wire is drilled or tapped into the femur and then overdrilled with a cannulated 3.2- or 4.8-mm drill to create the starting hole for the prophylactic Rush pin insertion, depending on whether a 3.1- (1/8 inch) or 4.6-mm (3/16 inch) Rush pin is used.
  - After the reaming is complete, the Rush pin is inserted and should reach just above the distal femoral physis. Its tip might need to be slightly bent to navigate the curves of the femur.
  - The small proximal incision is closed, and the pin sites are dressed. The pin sites are not manipulated or released to decrease the risk of concurrent infection.
  - Antibiotics are administered intravenously during the procedure, and oral antibiotics are used for 14 days postoperatively.

- If a significantly problematic pin site or pin site infection is present, it should be removed prior to frame removal to reduce the incidence of deep infection.
- Physical therapy is discontinued for 1 month to avoid fracture through the regenerate bone or a pin hole.
- Physical therapy is restarted 1 month after frame removal and Rush pin application. With the Rush pin in place, no cast or brace is needed. The patient is allowed partial weight bearing.

## OUTCOMES

- Saghieh and associates[14] studied our first 79 consecutive patients with Paley type 1 CFD. The patients underwent 99 femoral lengthenings between January 1988 and December 2000. Medical charts and radiographs were retrospectively reviewed. Fifty-nine patients (73 lengthenings) had Paley type 1a and 20 patients (26 lengthenings) had Paley type 1b CFD. Forty-six (58%) were female and 33 (42%) were male patients. The mean patient age was 12.3 years (age range, 1.5 to 62.3 years). The lengthenings were divided into three age groups: toddler (younger than 6 years), juvenile (between 6 years and skeletal maturity), and adult (skeletally mature). Because 19 patients each underwent more than 1 lengthening (18 underwent 2 lengthenings and 1 underwent 3 lengthenings), each lengthening was evaluated independently as a separate lengthening and studied for its own results and complications.
- Distraction gap, percent of femur lengthened, external fixation time index, degree of preservation of knee motion, result score, and complications were compared among the groups. The complications and ROM data were routinely recorded, and the data were obtained from a review of the charts. Radiographic measurements were obtained from preoperative lower limb alignment AP view radiographs (teleroentgenograms), compensating for magnification, and from lateral view radiographs of the femur and tibia. The CE angle and neck–shaft angle also were measured, preferably by using an AP view radiograph of the pelvis. The average follow-up from the time of removal of the external fixator was 69 months (range, 19 to 132 months).
- The average discrepancy in femoral length was 9.1 cm (range, 1.2 to 22.1 cm) preoperatively and 4.1 cm (range, 14.7 to 2.3 cm) postoperatively. The mean distraction gap was 5.8 cm (range, 2.4 to 12.0 cm). The average duration of treatment with external fixation was 5.9 months (range, 2 to 15.9 months) with an external fixation time index of 1.07 months per centimeter (range, 0.49 to 2.38 months per centimeter). The result score was excellent in 61 (61.6%) lengthenings, good in 29 (29.3%), fair in 7 (7.1%), and poor in 2 (2%).
- Excellent and good results were achieved in 91% of patients. No significant differences in most of the studied parameters, including result score, were observed among the different groups. The two younger groups experienced a higher incidence of fracture (no prophylactic rodding was used in this group). The adult group experienced a higher incidence of delayed union and joint stiffness. However, the overall complication rates were similar among the three groups. We prefer to begin lengthening at an early age so that additional needed lengthenings can be spaced in time.
- Since this first study, more than 750 patients have been treated either by the Orthofix with Sheffield hinge technique or the MRS device. This group is undergoing review.

## COMPLICATIONS

- Flexion contracture of the knee
  - A significant knee flexion contracture places the knee at risk for posterior subluxation.
  - One of the primary goals of physical therapy is to maintain knee extension and to continue to obtain knee flexion. Both the surgeon and therapist need to closely monitor the patient's ROM and must be in regular communication if difficulties arise.
  - To prevent fixed flexion deformity, a knee extension bar is used every night and part time during the day. If the patient experiences a loss of motion, therapy must be increased and the patient assessed immediately.
  - Acute pin site infections can lead to increased pain and decreased motion and should be immediately treated with oral or intravenous antibiotics.
  - If significant soft tissue tightness is present in the quadriceps muscle, the distraction rate should be decreased. However, decreasing the distraction rate should be followed closely with radiographs to prevent premature consolidation. If Botox was not used at the index procedure, the surgeon should consider injecting the quadriceps muscle with 10 units of Botox solution per kilogram of body weight. We perform the Botox injection under anesthesia or sedation for the younger patient.
- Adduction and flexion contractures of the hip
  - Hip adduction contractures place the hip joint at risk for subluxation and dislocation during the lengthening process. Hip adduction should be assessed at the time of the lengthening surgery. If a contracture is present, an adductor tenotomy should be performed.
  - Hip ROM and stretching is addressed by the therapist on a daily basis. If a contracture is a concern initially, an abduction pillow is used at night. If the patient has subluxated or dislocated the hip in a previous procedure, the external fixator should be extended above the hip with a hinge device similar to that used for the knee. Hip flexion contracture might occur when the patient is positioned in a wheelchair for prolonged periods of time.
  - The patient should not only stretch during the therapy sessions but also should be placed in a prone position on a daily basis. Iliopsoas contracture does not occur during the lengthening because the distraction site is distal to the psoas insertion.
- Nerve injury
  - Nerve injury is unusual with femoral lengthening. Complaints of pain in the foot are usually referred pain from nerve entrapment. Quantitative sensory testing is the best method to identify early nerve entrapment.[7]
  - The nerve problem can be treated by slowing the distraction or nerve decompression. The peroneal nerve should be decompressed at the neck of the fibula if symptoms continue or pressure-specified sensory device testing is positive.[10]
- Premature consolidation
  - Premature consolidation usually occurs during the first 2 cm of distraction and is rare after 4 cm of distraction. In a young child, the latency period can be reduced to 3 days.
  - Increasing pain with distraction or difficulty while turning the distracting unit are signs of possible preconsolidation. Radiographs should be obtained to assess the regenerate bone. If the fibrous interzone disappears, the turning rate

should be increased (ie, five quarter-turns per day) and additional radiographs obtained within 1 week.
- If one of the cortices has bridged with narrow bone, continued distraction at an increased rate can be performed.
- The physician must warn the parents that the patient may experience or hear an audible "pop" during distraction. This will be followed by a mild to moderate increase in pain. However, the distraction will become easier and surgery can be avoided.
- If the regenerate site is consolidated with abundant bone, the pins might bend or become deformed. This type of preconsolidation is addressed with a repeat osteotomy 1 to 2 cm proximal to the original site. The surgeon should not attempt to repeat an osteotomy at the same regenerate site because the patient will have increased bleeding and poor regenerate bone formation. If the fibrous interzone is greater than 5 mm, lengthening should be slowed (ie, two or three turns per day).

- Regenerate bone failure
  - Partial defects in the bone are not uncommon on the lateral cortex. Sequential radiographs obtained during the distraction phase must be closely followed for increasing fibrous interzone distance and poor regenerate bone formation.
  - Regenerate bone failure is prevented by slowing the distraction rate when signs of poor regenerate formation are present. During the consolidation phase, a partial defect can be treated with dynamization to increase healing of the regenerate bone.
  - If the defect persists and encompasses less than 25% of the bone diameter, a rigid intramedullary rod placed at the time of removal will allow for ossification during a prolonged time period (6 to 12 months).
  - If the regenerate bone failure is more severe, open autogenous bone grafting should be performed after first excising the interposing fibrous tissue.

## ACKNOWLEDGMENT

- The author wishes to acknowledge Dr. Shawn Standard, from the Rubin Institute in Baltimore, who co-authored the first edition of this chapter.



## REFERENCES

1. Aguilar JA, Paley D, Paley J, et al. Clinical validation of the multiplier method for predicting limb length at maturity, part I. J Pediatr Orthop 2005;25:186–191.
2. Aguilar JA, Paley D, Paley J, et al. Clinical validation of the multiplier method for predicting limb length discrepancy and outcome of epiphysiodesis, part II. J Pediatr Orthop 2005;25:192–196.
3. Brown KL. Resection, rotationplasty, and femoropelvic arthrodesis in severe congenital femoral deficiency. A report of the surgical technique and three cases. J Bone Joint Surg Am 2001;83-A(1): 78–85.
4. Grammont PM, Latune D, Lammaire IP. Treatment of subluxation and dislocation of the patella in the child: Elmslie technic with movable soft tissue pedicle (8 year review) [in German]. Orthopade 1985;14:229–238.
5. Krackow KA, Thomas SC, Jones LC. A new stitch for ligament-tendon fixation. Brief note. J Bone Joint Surg Am 1986;68(5):764–766.
6. Levinson ED, Ozonoff MB, Royen PM. Proximal femoral focal deficiency (PFFD). Radiology 1977;125:197–203.
7. Nogueira MP, Paley D, Bhave A, et al. Nerve lesions associated with limb-lengthening. J Bone Joint Surg Am 2003;85-A(8):1502–1510.
8. O'Carrigan, Paley D, Herzenberg JE. Obstacles in limb lengthening: fractures. In: Rozbruch SR, Ilizarov S, eds. Limb Lengthening and Reconstruction Surgery. New York: Informa Healthcare, 2007: 485–494.
9. Paley D. Lengthening reconstruction surgery for congenital femoral deficiency. In: Herring JA, Birch JG, eds. The Child with a Limb Deficiency. Rosemont: American Academy of Orthopaedic Surgeons, 1998:113–132.
10. Paley D. Principles of Deformity Correction, rev ed. Berlin: Springer-Verlag, 2005.
11. Paley D, Bhave A, Herzenberg JE, et al. Multiplier method for predicting limb-length discrepancy. J Bone Joint Surg Am 2000;82-A(10): 1432–1446.
12. Paley J, Gelman A, Paley D, et al. The prenatal multiplier method for prediction of limb length discrepancy. Prenat Diagn 2005;25: 435–438.
13. Rozbruch SR, Paley D, Bhave A, et al. Ilizarov hip reconstruction for the late sequelae of infantile hip infection. J Bone Joint Surg Am 2005:87(5);1007–1018.
14. Saghieh S, Paley D, Kacaoglu M, et al. Strategies and results for lengthening reconstruction surgery in congenital femoral deficiency. Paper presented at 66th Annual Meeting of the American Academy of Orthopaedic Surgeons, February 4–8, 1999, Anaheim, CA.
15. Sanpera I, Sparks LT. Proximal femoral focal deficiency: does a radiologic classification exist? J Pediatr Orthop 1994;14:34–38.

54

CHAPTER

# Surgical Repair of Irreducible Congenital Dislocation of the Knee

Matthew B. Dobbs

## DEFINITION

- Congenital dislocation of the knee (CDK) is a rare deformity that presents at birth as recurvatum.
- The incidence of CDK is estimated at 1 per 100,000 live births, which is approximately 1% of the incidence of congenital dislocation of the hip.[7]
- It may be an isolated entity or occur with associated musculoskeletal anomalies such as dislocated hips, clubfoot, and congenital vertical talus. It can also occur with myelodysplasia, Larsen syndrome, and arthrogryposis.
- It varies in severity and has been classified as simple hyperextension, subluxation, and anterior dislocation of the tibia on the femur (**FIG 1**).[3]

## ANATOMY

- The fundamental pathologic feature in CDK involves the quadriceps muscle. The amount of quadriceps muscle is small, and the muscle as well as the lateral retinaculum adheres to the femur.
- The quadriceps femoris tendon is shortened and fibrosed, which is thought to be secondary to the dislocation rather than its cause.[3]
- The patella is often laterally displaced.
- There is hypoplasia of the suprapatellar pouch.
- The hamstrings are often deficient, subluxed anteriorly, or both.
- The anterior knee articular capsule is tight.
- The menisci are usually present and normal.
- The pathology in the cruciate ligaments is variable, from absent to elongated.[5]

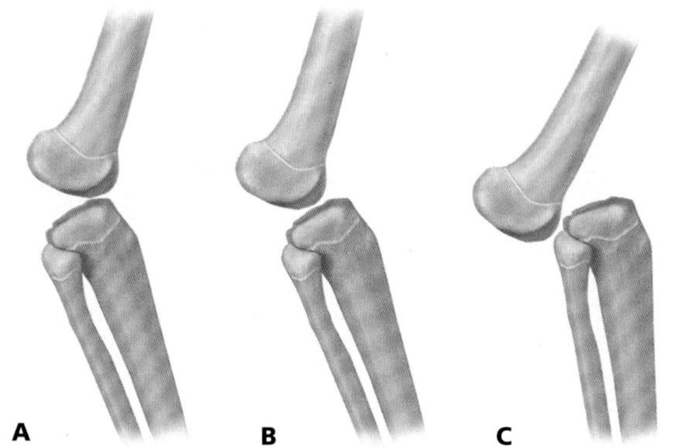


**FIG 1** • Congenital knee dislocation can vary from simple hyperextension (**A**) to subluxation (**B**) to complete anterior dislocation of the tibia on the femur (**C**).

## PATHOGENESIS

- The exact cause of CDK remains unknown.
- A genetic etiology is supported by the presence of familial occurrence in some cases as well as the association of CDK with developmental hip dysplasia, idiopathic clubfoot, and congenital vertical talus; all three of which have a known or presumed genetic basis.[1,11]
- Simple hyperextension of the knee in newborns may be caused by aberrations in intrauterine positions, such as frank breech presentation, which slowly stretches the hamstrings and posterior knee soft tissues.[7,13] Chronic knee hyperextension results in anterior subluxation of the hamstrings, allowing them to function as knee extensors.
- Severe CDK often occurs in association with disorders with muscle imbalance, such as myelodysplasia, arthrogryposis, Larsen syndrome, Ehlers-Danlos syndrome, Streeter syndrome, and oligohydramnios.[3,8,11]

## NATURAL HISTORY

- The natural history of CDK depends on the severity of the disorder on presentation. Simple hyperextension of the knee tends to resolve spontaneously or with splinting.[2,6]
- In cases of subluxation and dislocation, spontaneous resolution is not common, and most patients require surgical correction.
- Left untreated, these patients have great difficulty with ambulation owing to the inability to flex the knees. These patients often have associated neuromuscular or genetic syndromes.[3]

## PATIENT HISTORY AND PHYSICAL FINDINGS

- The physical findings of CDK are readily apparent at birth but of variable severity (**FIG 2**).

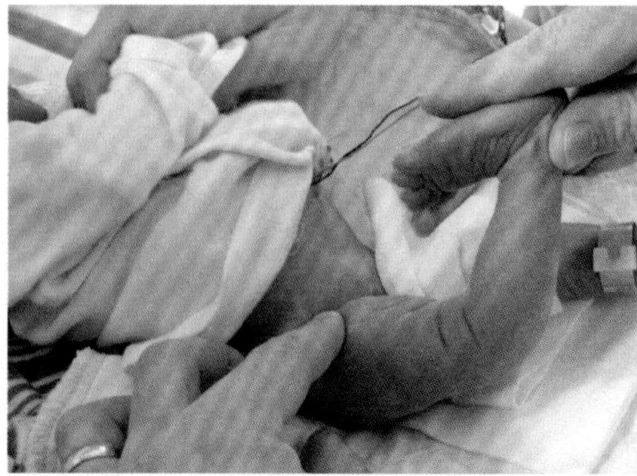

**FIG 2** • This infant has a unilateral knee dislocation. Note, the deep skin creases across the front of the knee.

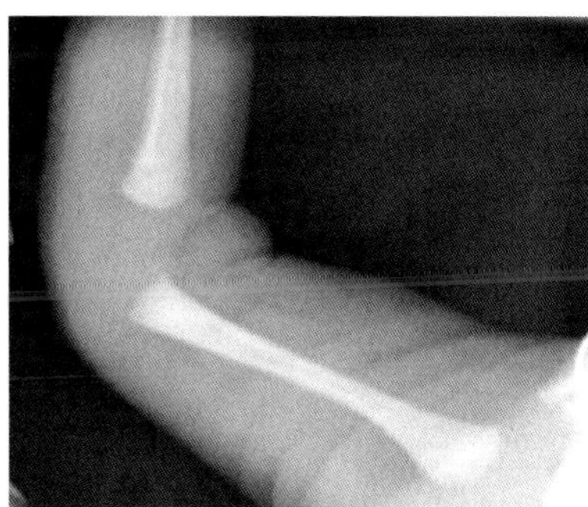

**FIG 3** ● A lateral radiograph of a newborn demonstrating complete dislocation of the tibia on the distal femur. The anterior aspect of the knee is on the right. Note, the deep skin creases anteriorly.

- The knee is hyperextended, in severe cases to such a degree that the foot rests against the baby's face.
- In cases of simple hyperextension, the knee can be passively brought into flexion.
- In the more common scenario of subluxation, passive flexion is limited but improves with splinting, casting, or both.
- In cases of dislocation, the knee cannot be easily passively flexed with simple manipulation. The patella is often laterally displaced and difficult to palpate. A deep crease may be present over the anterior aspect of the knee.
- The more severe cases are more likely to have associated musculoskeletal anomalies.

## IMAGING AND OTHER DIAGNOSTIC STUDIES

- Anteroposterior and lateral radiographs of the knee help to differentiate the mild hyperextension deformity from the more severe type of subluxation or fixed anterior dislocation of the tibia on the distal femur (**FIG 3**).
- The ossification centers of the distal femur and proximal tibia are usually present in the full-term infant.
- The patella is not yet ossified in the infant.
- Ultrasound can also be used to make the diagnosis.

## DIFFERENTIAL DIAGNOSIS

- Simple hyperextension of the knee

## NONOPERATIVE MANAGEMENT

- Nonoperative treatment should be started as soon as possible.
- Nonoperative treatment consists of serial manipulations and long-leg plaster castings.[2,4,6,10,12]
- Using the correct technique of manipulation and casting is extremely important.[4,12]
- With the patient relaxed with a bottle of milk, gentle traction is applied to the tibia to stretch the contracted quadriceps muscle. After several minutes of stretching, a long-leg plaster cast is applied from the toes to the top of the thigh. The cast is applied in one section and is carefully molded to maintain the position achieved with stretching and to avoid skin sores.
- The casts are changed on a weekly basis in the clinic. Once the tibia reaches the distal femur with traction, flexion of the knee is begun.
  - In cases of simple hyperextension, flexion of the knee can often be started quite early (**FIG 4**).
  - In cases of subluxation and complete dislocation of the knee, however, flexion of the knee often cannot be started for several weeks until the quadriceps muscle is adequately stretched.
- It is very important to obtain a lateral radiograph of the knee once knee flexion reaches 45 degrees and again if 90 degrees of flexion is reached during serial casting. It is possible to create an iatrogenic physeal separation of the distal femur or to deform the proximal tibia plastically.
  - Closed treatment should be stopped if anatomic reduction of the tibia cannot be confirmed.
- If 90 degrees of flexion is obtained and a normal restoration of the femoral–tibial articulation is demonstrated on a lateral radiograph, it is unlikely that any surgical intervention will be necessary.
- When done correctly, this casting technique is successful in correcting even severe cases of dislocation.
- For those cases where casting alone is not enough to gain full correction, smaller a la carte procedures can be done as discussed in the following text to finish the correction initiated with casting.
- This approach should greatly reduce the number of extensive surgical reconstructions.

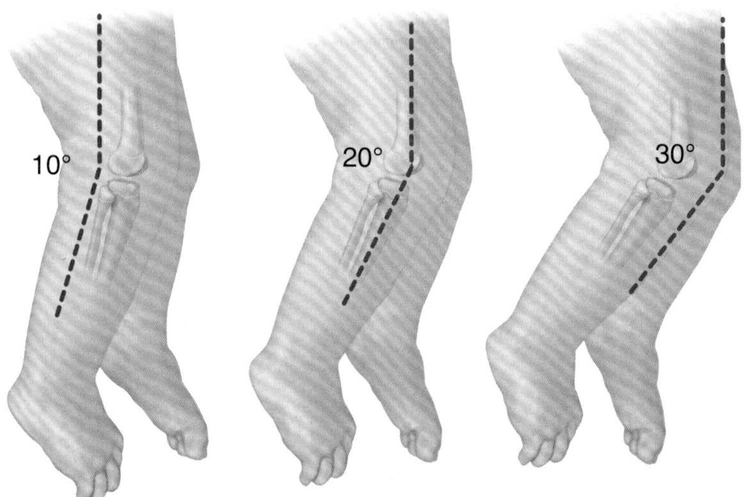


**FIG 4** ● Approximate amount of knee flexion achieved each week during serial castings.

## SURGICAL MANAGEMENT

### Preoperative Planning

- If serial casting fails to obtain a reduction of the anteriorly dislocated tibia on the end of the femur, which is verified on a lateral radiograph of the knee, surgical management should be considered.
- Timing of the surgical correction depends on the particular technique that the surgeon chooses but usually ranges from 1 month of age to 2 years.

### Positioning

- The patient is positioned supine on a radiolucent table. No tourniquet is used, as this interferes with the location of the surgical incision.
- The entire leg is prepared into the field from the hip to the tip of the toes to allow easy manipulation of the knee (**FIG 5**).

### Approach

- The approach depends on the surgeon's preference but varies from minimally invasive approaches to extensile approaches with quadriceps mechanism reconstruction.

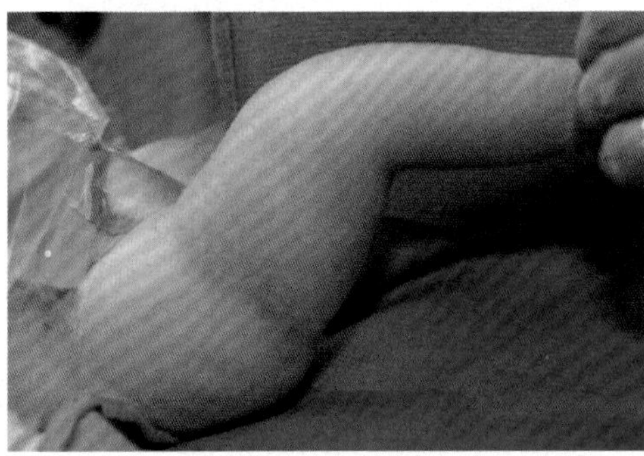

**FIG 5** • The entire leg is prepared into the field to allow easy manipulation of the knee.



## Percutaneous Quadriceps Recession

- This procedure is ideally performed at 1 to 2 months of age and is described by Roy and Crawford.[11]
- An assistant holds the affected leg and attempts to flex the knee.
- A small stab incision is made one to two patellar lengths superior to the patella in the midline of the thigh, and the fascia overlying the rectus femoris is released (**TECH FIG 1**).
- Medial and lateral stab incisions are then made at the superior border of the patella to release the medial and lateral quadriceps tendon and retinaculum.
- After the release is performed, the knee is flexed to 90 degrees.
- Sterile dressings are applied, followed by a long-leg plaster cast with the knee flexed at 90 degrees or greater.
- The cast is worn for 4 to 6 weeks.
- After cast removal, the patient is placed in a Pavlik harness to maintain knee flexion for an additional 4 to 6 weeks.

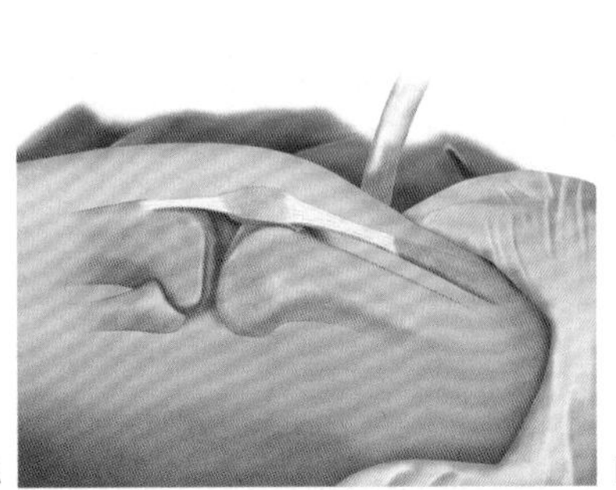



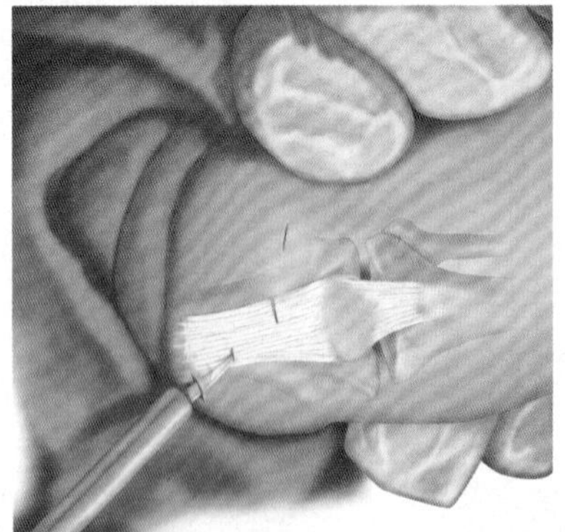



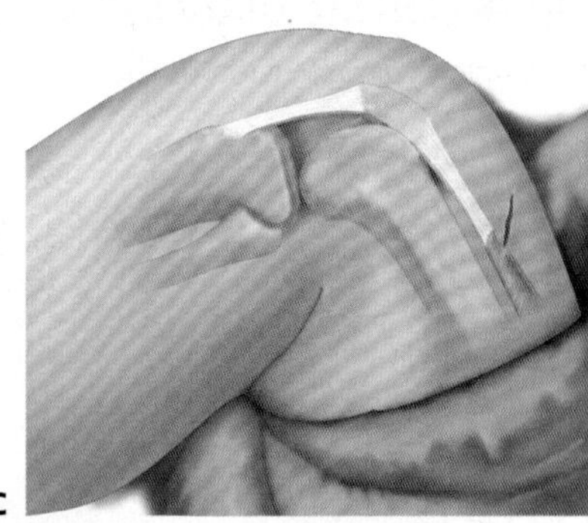



**TECH FIG 1** • Percutaneous quadriceps recession. **A.** The knee is held in maximum flexion. **B.** Medial and lateral stab incisions are made at the superior border of the patella to release the quadriceps and retinaculum. **C.** The knee is flexed to 90 degrees after release of the retinaculum is achieved.

## Mini-Open Quadriceps Tenotomy

- This approach is ideally performed between 1 and 6 months of age and has been described by Dobbs et al[4] and Shah et al[12] (TECH FIG 2).
- A 2-cm vertical midline incision is made just above the superior pole of the patella.
- Dissection is carried down to the patella and the quadriceps tendon.
- The quadriceps tendon is carefully isolated with blunt dissection using a hemostat.
- The quadriceps tendon is transected completely about 1 cm proximal to its insertion on the superior pole of the patella leaving the medial and lateral retinaculum intact.
- The knee is then gently flexed until at least 90 degrees of flexion is obtained.
- If 90 degrees of flexion cannot be obtained after the quadriceps tenotomy, the anterior knee capsule is released as well as the lateral retinaculum until 90 degrees of flexion is obtained.
- An intraoperative lateral knee radiograph is obtained to ensure anatomic reduction of the tibia on the distal femur.
- After wound closure, a sterile dressing is applied, followed by a long-leg plaster cast with the knee in 90 degrees of flexion.

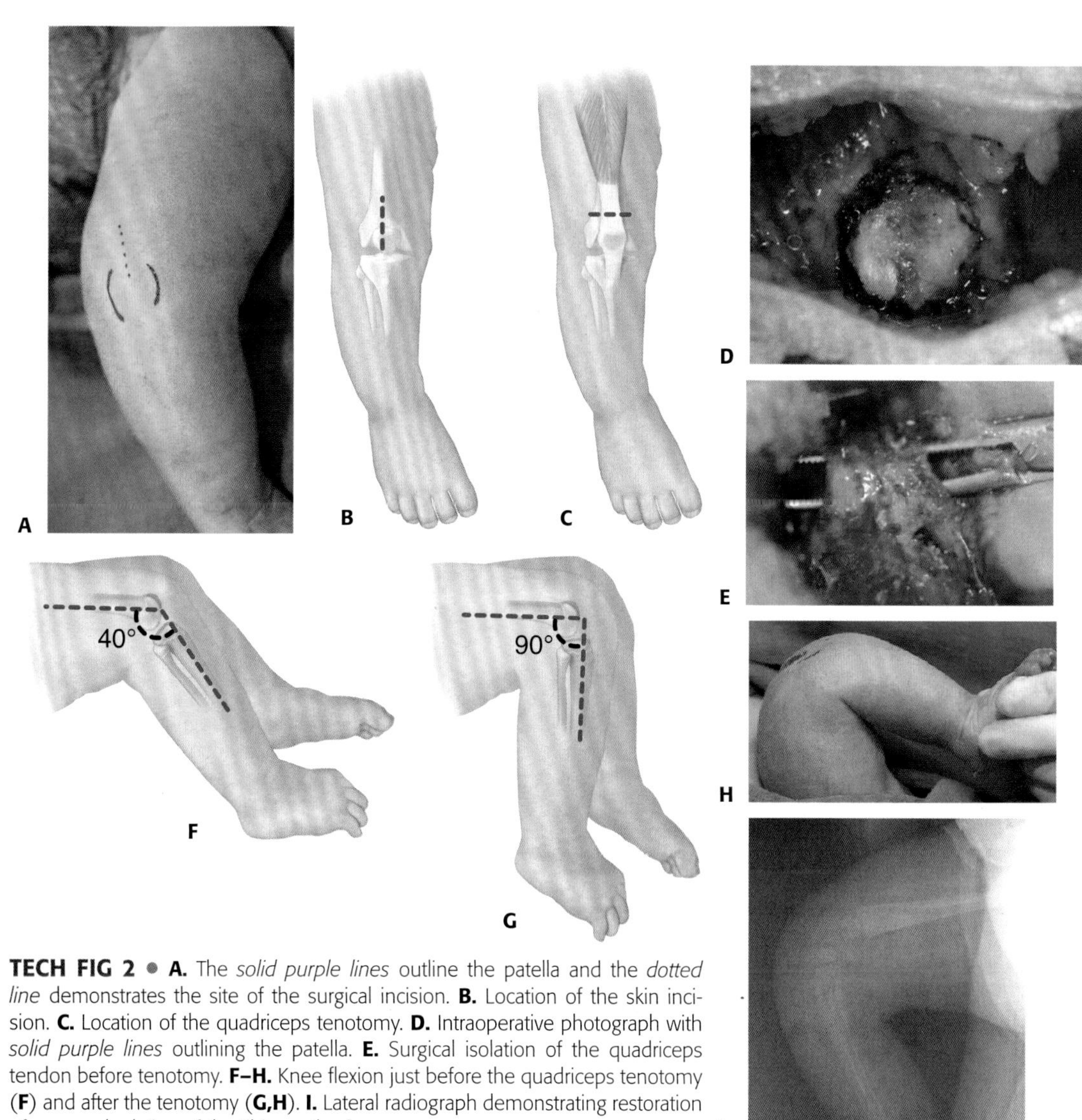


**TECH FIG 2** • **A.** The *solid purple lines* outline the patella and the *dotted line* demonstrates the site of the surgical incision. **B.** Location of the skin incision. **C.** Location of the quadriceps tenotomy. **D.** Intraoperative photograph with *solid purple lines* outlining the patella. **E.** Surgical isolation of the quadriceps tendon before tenotomy. **F–H.** Knee flexion just before the quadriceps tenotomy (**F**) and after the tenotomy (**G,H**). **I.** Lateral radiograph demonstrating restoration of a normal relation of the tibia on the femur.

## Extensile Reconstruction of Congenital Knee Dislocation

- This approach is usually performed between 6 months and 1 year of age.
- A midline longitudinal incision or serpentine incision can be used. The midline incision extends from the tibial tubercle to the middle of the thigh; the serpentine incision extends from the tibial tubercle to the proximal thigh.[3,7]
- The serpentine incision may facilitate wound closure and result in fewer wound healing problems than the straight incision.
- The patella, the quadriceps muscle and tendon, the patellar tendon, and the lateral retinaculum are all carefully exposed.
- The quadriceps muscle is striking in that it is small, fibrosed, and often adherent to the distal femur.
- In severe cases, the patella is subluxed laterally.
- The quadriceps is lengthened using a V-Y advancement (**TECH FIG 3**).
- If the tibia is in valgus and external rotation, the iliotibial band should be divided at this point.
- The anterior knee joint capsule is released transversely to the collateral ligaments.
- The quadriceps muscle and the lateral retinaculum must be dissected free from the distal femur. This usually allows the knee to be flexed to 90 degrees.
- The hamstrings and the cruciate ligaments can be left alone, as these structures do not prevent knee flexion in the vast majority of cases.
- The quadriceps tendon is repaired with the knee in 30 to 40 degrees of flexion.[1,3]
- A spica cast is used for immobilization with the knee in about 45 degrees of flexion to prevent recurrent subluxation.[7]

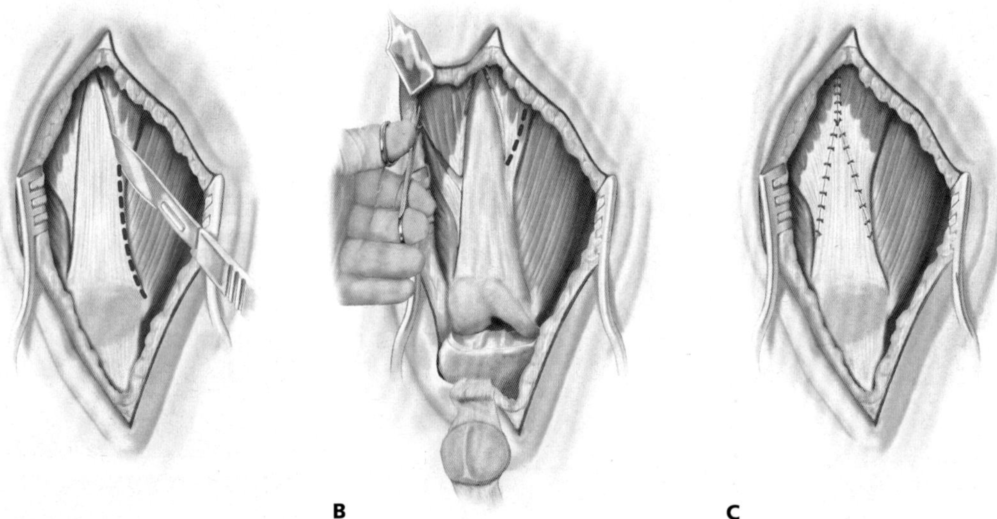


**TECH FIG 3** • V-Y quadriceps advancement. **A.** The quadriceps tendon is exposed proximal to the patella, and most of the medial and lateral fibers are detached from the tendon. The medial and lateral retinaculum is divided to the collateral ligaments. The iliotibial band is divided if the tibia is in valgus and externally rotated. **B.** The posterior borders of the lateralis and the medialis are divided sharply and the flap of muscle created is dissected free of underlying attachments to the femur. This will permit the tibia and collateral ligaments to slide posteriorly and allow sufficient mobilization of the quadriceps. **C.** With the knee flexed at about 40 degrees, the medialis and lateralis are reattached to the quadriceps tendon, creating the V-Y advancement and repair. The retinaculum is not closed.

## PEARLS AND PITFALLS

| | |
|---|---|
| **Indications** | ■ A complete history and physical examination should be performed.<br>■ Associated diagnoses must be recognized as this can alter the prognosis and treatment strategy. |
| **Nonoperative treatment** | ■ Care must be taken during manipulation and casting not to create iatrogenic fractures in the distal femur or proximal tibia.<br>■ Use of radiographs can confirm anatomic reduction of the tibia on the distal femur. |
| **Extensile surgical approach** | ■ Reapproximation of the quadriceps mechanism must be done in 30–40 degrees of flexion.[1,3] Flexing the knee less than 30 degrees often results in recurrent subluxation, and flexion greater than 40 degrees is too much to permit reconstruction of the quadriceps tendon.[3] |

| | |
|---|---|
| **Postoperative management** | ■ No matter what treatment method is used to correct the deformity, splinting and range-of-motion exercises are essential to maintain flexion and minimize loss of extension. A knee flexion contracture can be more debilitating than a lack of full flexion. |
| **Management of associated musculoskeletal problems** | ■ Associated clubfoot deformity can be treated at the same time as the CKD by incorporating the foot into the long-leg cast using the Ponseti method.<br>■ Management of associated hip dislocation should be done later as a staged procedure. |

## POSTOPERATIVE CARE

- A lateral radiograph of the knee is essential to ensure anatomic reduction of the tibia on the distal femur.
- Casting is required after each treatment method. The degree of knee flexion in the cast and the duration of casting vary with technique.
  - Percutaneous quadriceps recession
  - A long-leg plaster cast with the knee flexed at least 90 degrees is applied at the end of the procedure and worn for 4 to 6 weeks.
  - After cast removal, the patient is placed in a Pavlik harness to maintain knee flexion for an additional 4 to 6 weeks.
- Mini-open quadriceps tenotomy
  - The initial long-leg plaster cast with the knee in 90 degrees of flexion is removed at 3 weeks in the clinic.
  - Formal physical therapy is begun on an outpatient basis emphasizing both knee flexion and extension. Removable nighttime extension splints are also used for 4 to 6 weeks.
  - Parents are instructed on range-of-motion exercises as well.
  - Extensile reconstruction: spica cast with the knee in about 45 degrees of flexion
- Once casting is complete, close follow-up is mandatory to ensure maintenance of knee motion.
- Splinting is also important after each treatment method to maintain maximal flexion and minimize loss of knee extension.
- Physical therapy is also an essential part of postoperative rehabilitation and is done on an outpatient basis several times a week for up to 3 months.

## OUTCOMES

- Patients with a hyperextension deformity that requires only serial manipulation and castings do very well long term both clinically and radiographically.[2,5,9,10]
- Roy and Crawford[11] report good short-term results using the percutaneous quadriceps tenotomy, but there are no long-term data with this technique. This technique was successful only in patients without associated syndromes or neuromuscular deformities.
- Dobbs et al[4] and Shah et al[12] report good short-term results using the mini-open quadriceps tenotomy in patients with isolated CDK as well as in many children with associated genetic and neuromuscular conditions.
- Patients with severe dislocation who have undergone an extensive open procedure, but do not have any other associated musculoskeletal problem, generally do well long term if knee flexion is 80 degrees or greater.
- Children with associated neuromuscular disorders or genetic syndromes do not do as well long term.
- Children with bilateral deformities do not do as well as those with unilateral deformity.
- Early correction has a more satisfactory result than late repair.[4,7,11]

## COMPLICATIONS

- Wound healing problems have been reported with extensile approaches.
- Loss of flexion initially gained at surgery can be a late complication.
- Development of a flexion contracture can occur postoperatively and compromise long-term outcome.
- Iatrogenic fractures of the distal femur, proximal tibia, or both can occur with casting and manipulation.

## REFERENCES


1. Bell MJ, Atkins RM, Sharrard WJ. Irreducible congenital dislocation of the knee. Aetiology and management. J Bone Joint Surg Br 1987;69(3):403–406.
2. Bensahel H, Dal Monte A, Hjelmstedt A, et al. Congenital dislocation of the knee. J Pediatr Orthop 1989;9:174–177.
3. Curtis BH, Fisher RL. Heritable congenital tibiofemoral subluxation. Clinical features and surgical treatment. J Bone Joint Surg Am 1970; 52(6):1104–1114.
4. Dobbs MB, Boehm S, Grange DK, et al. Case report: congenital knee dislocation in a patient with Larsen syndrome and a novel filamin B mutation. Clin Orthop Relat Res 2008;466:1503–1509.
5. Ferris B, Aichroth P. The treatment of congenital knee dislocation. A review of nineteen knees. Clin Orthop Relat Res 1987;(216): 135–140.
6. Iwaya T, Sakaguchi R, Tsuyama N. The treatment of congenital dislocation of the knee with the Pavlik harness. Int Orthop 1983;7: 25–30.
7. Johnson E, Audell R, Oppenheim WL. Congenital dislocation of the knee. J Pediatr Orthop 1987;7:194–200.
8. Katz MP, Grogono BJ, Soper KC. The etiology and treatment of congenital dislocation of the knee. J Bone Joint Surg Br 1967;49(1): 112–120.
9. Ko JY, Shih CH, Wenger DR. Congenital dislocation of the knee. J Pediatr Orthop 1999;19:252–259.
10. Nogi J, MacEwen GD. Congenital dislocation of the knee. J Pediatr Orthop 1982;2:509–513.
11. Roy DR, Crawford AH. Percutaneous quadriceps recession: a technique for management of congenital hyperextension deformities of the knee in the neonate. J Pediatr Orthop 1989;9:717–719.
12. Shah NR, Limpaphayom N, Dobbs MB. A minimally invasive treatment protocol for the congenital dislocation of the knee. J Pediatr Orthop 2009;29:720–725.
13. Uhthoff HK, Ogata S. Early intrauterine presence of congenital dislocation of the knee. J Pediatr Orthop 1994;14:254–257.

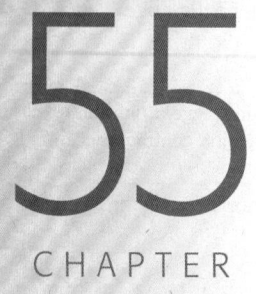

CHAPTER

# Surgical Management of Blount Disease

Richard S. Davidson

## DEFINITION

- Blount disease, also known as *idiopathic tibia vara* and *osteochondritis deformans tibiae*, is characterized by abnormal growth of the proximal tibia physis with progressive varus deformity.
- Blount disease is classified into three types based on age of clinical onset: infantile (0 to 3 years), juvenile (4 to 10 years), and adolescent (11 years and older).[9]
  - Infantile tibia vara is most prevalent in African American females and is associated with obesity, internal tibial torsion, and leg length discrepancy. Radiographs reveal a prominent medial metaphyseal beak, and the origin of the varus deformity is in the proximal tibia only. About 80% of cases are bilateral, and the potential for deformity is the greatest in this group.
  - Adolescent tibia vara is most prevalent in African American males with marked obesity, minimal internal tibial torsion, mild medial collateral ligament laxity, and mild leg length discrepancy. The site of the deformity is in the proximal tibia and sometimes in the distal femur as well. About 50% of cases are bilateral, and pain rather than deformity is more commonly the presenting complaint.

## ANATOMY[7]

- When evaluating patients with Blount disease, the normal development of the tibiofemoral angle in children must be considered.
- The normal tibiofemoral angle in newborns is approximately 15 degrees varus. It decreases with growth, so that the tibiofemoral angle approaches 0 degrees around 18 months of age.
- The tibiofemoral angle progresses to maximum valgus around 3 years of age and then decreases until adult physiologic valgus is achieved between 7 years of age and skeletal maturity.
- One standard deviation of the anatomic tibiofemoral angle throughout growth is approximately 8 degrees.

## PATHOGENESIS[7]

- Blount disease is likely due to a combination of genetic factors and a cycle of increased stress across the medial physis, which leads to decreased medial endochondral ossification, further varus deformity, and, subsequently, further medial physeal stress. The medial physeal stress is aggravated by obesity and progressive genu varum.
- Histopathologic studies of infantile and late-onset tibia vara are similar to those of patients with slipped capital femoral epiphysis. Findings include fissuring and clefts in the physis, fibrovascular and cartilaginous repair at the physeal–metaphyseal junction, foci of necrotic cartilage, and marked disorganization of the medial degenerative physeal zone.
- These findings are consistent with an arrest of the normal endochondral growth mechanism.

## NATURAL HISTORY

- A varus alignment of the lower extremity places excess stress on the medial compartment of the knee. This stress places the knee at increased risk for arthritis.
- The goal of intervention is to restore the normal anatomic orientation of the knee and ankle joints and to restore the normal mechanical axis of the leg.

## PATIENT HISTORY AND PHYSICAL FINDINGS

- The chief complaint in infantile tibia vara is usually deformity. In late-onset tibia vara, in contrast, knee pain is the primary complaint. The characteristics of the pain should be elicited.
- Patients may exhibit a limp, with or without a leg length discrepancy. Observe the patient's gaiting, noting a limp or lateral thrust.
- The mechanical axis of the lower leg is in varus. Genu recurvatum and internal tibial torsion may be present as well.
  - Inspect the sagittal profile for the presence of genu recurvatum; if present, it may be necessary to address it at the time of surgery.
- The Q angle provides a clinical estimate of the anatomic tibiofemoral angle.
- Range of motion and collateral ligament laxity also should be assessed.

## IMAGING AND OTHER DIAGNOSTIC STUDIES

- Anteroposterior (AP) long-leg radiographs (which include the hips, knees, and ankles) should be obtained (**FIG 1**). The patella (not the foot) must be pointing forward.

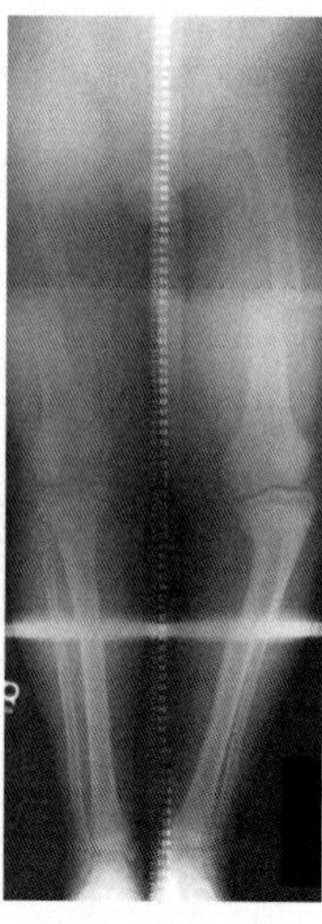

**FIG 1** • Orthoradiograph of patient with adolescent Blount disease.

- Infantile Blount disease has several characteristic radiographic findings.
  - To help differentiate infantile Blount disease from physiologic varus, the metaphyseal–diaphyseal angle is drawn. A metaphyseal–diaphyseal angle less than 10 degrees is consistent with physiologic varus, whereas an angle of more than 16 degrees is consistent with infantile Blount disease.
  - Acute angulation of the medial proximal tibia, medial beaking, fragmentation of the medial metaphysis, progressive varus, and unilateral involvement are consistent with infantile Blount disease.
    - Care must be taken that the radiographs are taken with the patella forward.
    - If tibial torsion is present, the feet must cross medially so that the patella is forward. The medial and lateral flares of the distal femurs will be equal if the patella is forward.
  - The proximal tibia is examined to determine the Langenskiöld stage.
    - Stage I: age younger than 3 years; medial and distal beaking of metaphysis with irregularity of entire metaphysis
    - Stage II: age 2.5 to 4 years; sharp anteromedial depression in ossification line of wedge-shaped medial metaphysis
    - Stage III: age 4 to 6 years; deepening of metaphyseal beak
    - Stage IV: age 5 to 10 years; enlargement of epiphysis
    - Stage V: age 9 to 11 years; cleft in epiphysis, appearance of double epiphysis
    - Stage VI: age 10 to 13 years; closure of medial proximal tibial physis
- Late-onset Blount disease is characterized by less obvious changes in the proximal tibia.
  - These changes include wedging of the medial portion of the epiphysis, a mild posteromedial articular depression, a serpiginous curved physis of variable width, and mild or no fragmentation of the proximal medial metaphysis.
- Radiographic analysis for deformity has been well described by Paley et al.[4]
  - The magnitude of the overall lower extremity malalignment can be determined by the anatomic tibiofemoral angle or the mechanical axis deviation. The *anatomic tibiofemoral angle* is the angle between the midshaft lines of the femur and the tibia. The *mechanical axis deviation* is the distance from the center of the knee to the mechanical axis line of the leg.
  - Analysis of the frontal plane deformity begins with the malalignment test.
    - The mechanical axis line is drawn from the center of the hip to the midpoint of the ankle plafond.
    - To identify whether the source of the deformity is the femur, the tibia, or both, joint orientation angles are measured.
    - The mechanical lateral distal femoral angle (mLDFA, normal value is 85 to 90 degrees) and medial proximal tibial angles (MPTA, normal value is 85 to 90 degrees) are measured to determine which is/are abnormal.
    - The joint line convergence angle is measured to determine whether the joint line is an additional source of deformity.
    - If the midpoints of the femur and tibia are over 3 mm apart, then frontal plane subluxation is a source of deformity as well.
    - Finally, the joint lines are inspected for intra-articular sources of deformity.
- The malorientation test is applied to the ankle and hip to determine whether these joints are oriented normally to the mechanical axis line.
  - Abnormal joint orientation angles indicate which joints are contributing to the deformity.
- Sagittal plane radiographs are obtained and analyzed as appropriate.
- Leg lengths are measured in order to identify a leg length discrepancy.
- The location of the deformity point, or center of rotation of angulation (CORA), is identified during preoperative planning.

## DIFFERENTIAL DIAGNOSIS

- Physiologic varus
- Pathologic causes
  - Rickets
  - Skeletal dysplasias
  - Focal fibrocartilaginous dysplasia
  - Renal osteodystrophy
  - Osteogenesis imperfecta

## NONOPERATIVE MANAGEMENT

- Nonoperative treatment with bracing may be indicated in patients with infantile Blount disease.
- Bracing should be considered for varus deformity greater than 15 degrees in children older than 2 years of age with Langenskiöld stage I or II Blount disease.[2]
- Bracing usually is not helpful in obese African American girls older than the age of 3 years.
- Nonoperative treatment with bracing is not successful in adolescent Blount disease.

## SURGICAL MANAGEMENT

- The surgical treatment of infantile Blount disease is distinct from that for adolescent Blount disease.
  - In patients with infantile Blount disease, the proximal tibial physis has several years of growth remaining. A proximal tibial osteotomy should be performed with the goal of correcting the anatomic tibiofemoral angle to within 5 degrees of neutral. In addition to the osteotomy, medial proximal tibial physeal bar resection, lateral proximal tibial hemiepiphysiodesis (guided growth plates), or tibial plateau elevation can be performed to improve the alignment of the physis and to allow for proper future growth.
    - Definitive surgery for infantile Blount disease should be done before 5 years of age because recurrence may develop if surgery is performed after this age.
  - In patients with adolescent Blount disease, treatment options are hemiepiphysiodesis and osteotomy. However, if insufficient growth remains for hemiepiphysiodesis to be effective, osteotomy is the best option for correction of the deformity. Hemiepiphysiodesis of an already short limb may leave the patient with a significant limb length inequality. If such limb length inequality will require

osteotomy for lengthening, the tibia vara should be corrected by osteotomy for angular and linear correction with external fixation.

- The objective of the osteotomy is to obtain a neutral mechanical axis with a horizontal knee joint. Many different types of osteotomies have been described for the treatment of adolescent Blount disease, including opening and closing wedge osteotomies, dome osteotomies, and oblique osteotomies.
- Following the osteotomy, fixation may be achieved with external or internal fixation. The use of cast immobilization alone has been associated with a loss of correction.
  - Internal fixation after osteotomy for Blount disease has been associated with problems. Loder et al[3] reported poor results in patients treated with internal fixation and noted many were internally fixed in malposition, likely due to difficulty in assessing intraoperative alignment. Crossed K-wires have been associated with a loss of fixation. The use of plates has been associated with stress shielding, delayed and nonunion, and hardware breakage, and requires a second surgical procedure to remove the implant.
  - External fixation allows for acute or gradual correction and for later adjustments as clinically and radiographically indicated. In addition, external fixation allows for correction of the coexistent leg length discrepancy. Price et al[5] reported the successful use of dynamic external fixation to stabilize osteotomies for tibia vara without supplemental casting. Monolateral, hybrid, or circular external fixators may be used.
- In this chapter, we describe the technique for correction of adolescent Blount's disease via osteotomy and external fixation. The external fixator used in this technique is the EBI Multi-Axial Correction System (EBI, Parsippany, NJ). This fixator allows gradual or acute correction of deformity in two planes of angulation, two planes of translation, rotation, and lengthening without the disadvantages of a ring fixator.

## Preoperative Planning[1,6]

- Standing lower extremity alignment radiographs are obtained (see **FIG 1**). The location of the CORA in the tibia in Blount disease cannot be determined by simply drawing two shaft lines because the deformity is metaphyseal or juxta-articular.
  - If the mechanical axis method of preoperative planning is used, the mechanical axis of the proximal tibia may be estimated by extending the femoral mechanical axis (if mLDFA is normal) or by drawing the MPTA of the contralateral MPTA (if normal) or the population normal value (87 degrees).
  - The distal tibia mechanical axis of the tibia is represented by a line that begins at the center of the ankle and extends parallel to the shaft. If the distal tibia has insufficient shaft length on which to base the line, the line is drawn using the contralateral lateral distal tibia angle (LDTA) or the population normal value (90 degrees).
  - The intersection of these lines is the CORA.
  - If the femur also was found to be a source of deformity during the alignment test, then CORA in the femur is identified as described by Paley et al.[4]
- The technique described in this chapter is for adolescent Blount disease with deformity located solely in the proximal tibia metaphysis not amenable to guided growth because of age or Langenskiöld classification.
- The external fixator used in this technique can be applied in three different locations with respect to the CORA: CORA-centric, CORA-perpendicular, and CORA-proximal.
  - The CORA-centric method places the fixator hinge directly over the CORA and minimizes unintended translation.
  - The CORA-perpendicular application places the fixator hinge on the bisector of the deformity, which, when placed on the convex side of the deformity, produces simultaneous lengthening during angular correction. CORA-perpendicular application is advisable only when lengthening is required.
  - The CORA-proximal application places the hinge near the CORA. This application is used when the hinge cannot be placed on the CORA or the bisector and relies on the flexibility of the hinges and translation screws to correct secondary translation.

## Positioning

- The patient is placed supine on a radiolucent table. The use of an OSI table with Jackson imaging top (Mizuho Osi, Orthopaedic Systems, Inc., Union City, CA) permits fluoroscopic images to be taken with minimal difficulty. A bump may be placed under the ipsilateral buttock.
- A tourniquet typically is not used because the thigh circumference of patients with Blount disease often is too large for a tourniquet to be used effectively and can possibly cause increased bleeding from venous tourniquet.
- The entire lower extremity is prepared and draped. The toes are left uncovered so that muscle contraction caused by inadvertent nerve irritation during pin placement is visible.

## Approach

- The procedure is divided into fibular osteotomy, external fixator application, proximal tibial osteotomy, and completion of the surgery. Prophylactic fasciotomies are performed during exposure for the fibular and tibial osteotomies.
- The lateral approach to the fibula is used for the fibular osteotomy and lateral compartment fasciotomy. Small medial and lateral incisions are made for the tibial osteotomy, and the anterior compartment is released from the lateral incision.
- The surgeon must have thorough knowledge of the cross-sectional anatomy of the lower leg and the half-pin positions for safety.

## Surgical Management of Blount Disease

### Fibula Osteotomy

- A longitudinal incision is made just lateral to the fibula at the intersection of the middle and distal thirds of the lower leg. Dissection is carried down to the deep fascia.
- A prophylactic subcutaneous lateral compartment fasciotomy is then performed. Care is taken to avoid injury to the superficial peroneal nerve and its branches.
- The peroneus longus and peroneus brevis muscles are visualized. These muscles are then retracted either anteriorly or posteriorly (depending on exposure), and the fibula is visualized. Subperiosteal exposure of the fibula is then developed using a Cobb elevator or right angle, and retractors are placed around the fibula to protect the soft tissues.
- The tibia is corrected in the direction of valgus. Because the fibula is lateral to the tibia, correction will push the fibula proximally.
- To prevent damage to the peroneal nerve at the proximal fibula, a 1-cm segment of bone is removed from the fibula. Oblique cuts in the fibula are made with the most proximal end aspect of the cut in the posterior edge of the fibula (**TECH FIG 1**). The cut is made carefully so that the saw is not inadvertently pushed past the posteromedial edge of the fibula with resultant injury to the peroneal artery.
- Wound closure is performed at this point because this is easier to do before the external fixator is applied.

### External Fixator Application

- The external fixator can be assembled before the procedure begins or just before application.
- A rotating arc is selected that will allow for correction of coexisting rotational deformity or rotation inadvertently caused by misplacement of the fixator.
- The ring size (130, 150, 180, or 220 mm) is based on the leg circumference at the level of the proximal tibia.
- The arc should match the curvature of the anterior proximal tibia with two fingerbreadths between the ring and the leg.
- The adult multiaxial correction (MAC) central component is then attached to the center of the rotating ring such that the primary arc on the MAC central component is facing anteriorly.
- The MAC female adapter is placed at the other end of the MAC central component, and the telescoping arm is attached to the female adapter.
- The primary hinge of the MAC central component is adjusted so that the fixator matches the angular deformity of the tibia.

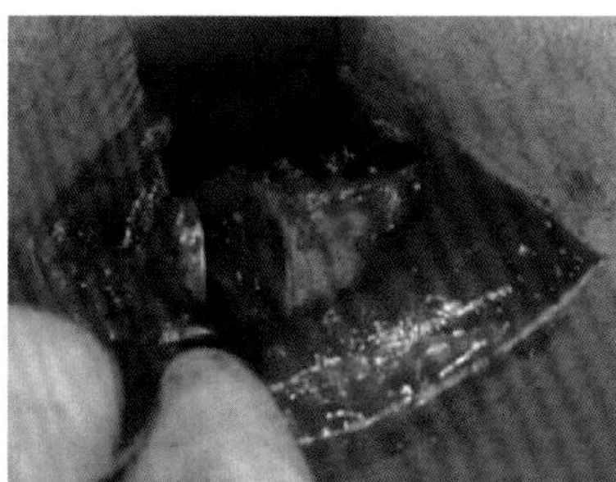

**TECH FIG 1** • An oblique 1-cm wedge is removed from the fibula.

- In the example illustrated in this section, the MAC is applied in the CORA-centric location.
- The CORA, as identified during preoperative planning, is localized under fluoroscopy, and an appropriately sized guide pin (supplied with the MAC) is placed from anterior to posterior into the CORA (**TECH FIG 2A**).
- The guidewire should be perpendicular to the tibial diaphysis (in the true deformity axis). Although placement of the guidewire exactly into the CORA can be difficult, the multiangular or translation and rotation ability of the MAC device can correct any secondary deformity due to misplacement of the MAC off the CORA.
- Sterile Webril padding (Kendall Co., Mansfield, MA) is then placed around the K-wire to serve as a two-fingerbreadth spacer (**TECH FIG 2B**).
- The centering hole of the primary hinge of the MAC fixator is placed over the K-wire so that the fixator rests on top of the spacer (**TECH FIG 2C**).
- Universal screw carriages are locked onto the rotation arc and used as guides for placement of two or three proximal screws.
- Three proximal half-pins are then placed in the safe zones of the proximal tibia.
- At least one pin is placed from anteromedial to posterolateral and one is placed from anterolateral to posteromedial.
- The pins are placed distal to the physis (which may be open).
- Care should be taken not to place the screws so close to the MAC device as to block rotation.
- Holes are predrilled bicortically with the 4.8-mm drill bit and 6.0-mm pins are placed.
- We prefer to use hydroxyapatite-coated pins to reduce the risk of loosening and, therefore, infection. Pin size typically is around 60 mm thread length and 160 to 180 mm overall length (**TECH FIG 2D**).
- The size of the bone screw depends on the size of the patient, the tibia at the level of screw insertion, and the size of the arc chosen.
- The carriages are tightened after the pins are placed. The MAC is then adjusted to the tibial deformity, ensuring that the distal bone screw block is parallel to the distal tibial diaphysis at the medial subcutaneous face of the tibia (**TECH FIG 2E**).
- Three distal half-pins are placed through the telescoping arm in the midshaft of the tibia (**TECH FIG 2F**). Pin size typically is 120 mm overall and 40 mm of thread length.
- If the MAC is aligned such that the pins placed through the telescoping arm will not go through the tibia, the CORA pin should be removed and the device rotated, angulated, or translated so that the pins are aligned. (If this is done, rotation must be corrected first before the remainder of the deformity is corrected to realign the primary hinge to the bone deformity.)
- At this point, all the pins (bone screws) have been inserted.

### Tibial Osteotomy

- Using the MAC external fixator, placing the guide pin at the CORA allows deformity correction to occur at the CORA. The osteotomy does not have to be made at the CORA. It should be performed just below the insertion of the tibial tubercle, decreasing the risk of damage to the nearby physis and joint line. Placement of the osteotomy below the tibial tubercle will also avoid pulling the patella distally during distraction.
- The tibial osteotomy may be performed using one of several different techniques. Our preference is to perform the osteotomy

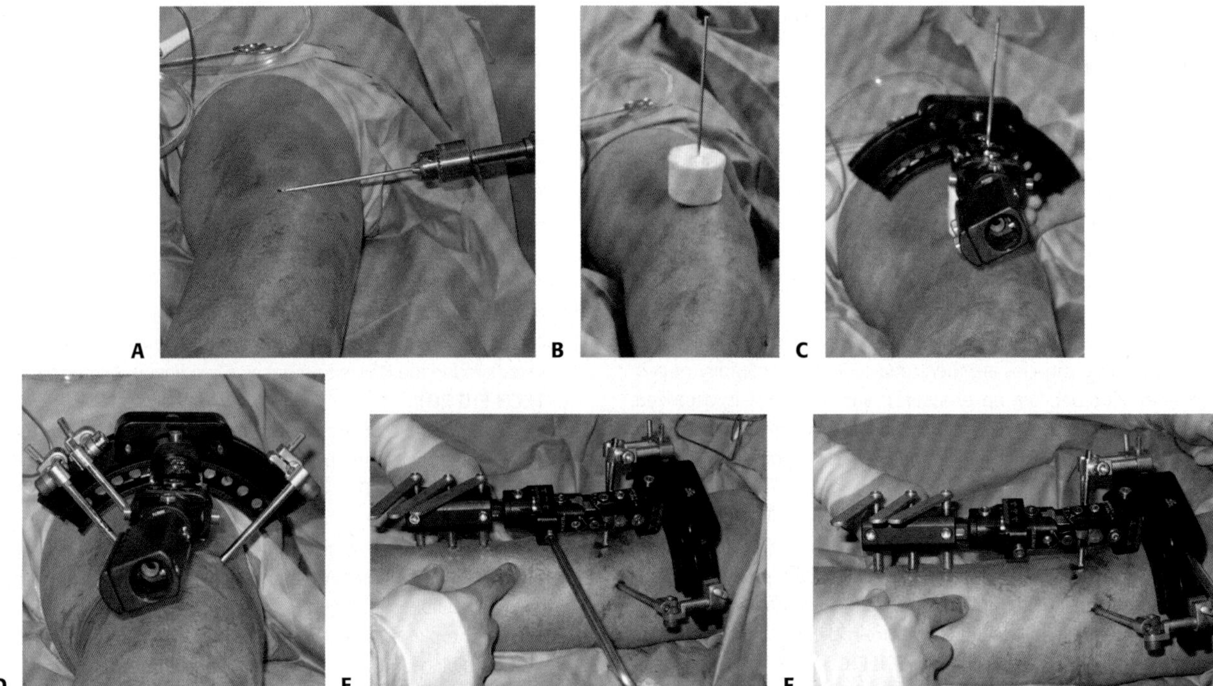

**TECH FIG 2 • A.** Fluoroscopy is used to localize the CORA (which was identified during preoperative planning). **B.** Sterile web roll padding is placed over the guidewire to serve as a spacer. **C.** The MAC external fixator is placed on top of the spacer. **D.** Two or three bone screws are placed in the proximal tibia. **E.** The length and angulation of the MAC external fixator are adjusted to match the deformity. **F.** Three bone screws are placed in the tibial shaft.

through small transverse anteromedial and anterolateral incisions with a Gigli saw passed subperiosteally.

- Fluoroscopy is used to identify the metaphyseal–diaphyseal junction where the osteotomy will be made.
- The guide pin is removed.
- Two 2-cm transverse incisions are made, one on the medial and one on the lateral aspects of the anterior tibia at the level for the osteotomy. The incision is made transversely to avoid skin injury from the Gigli saw.
- From the lateral incision, dissection is carried down to the fascia of the anterior compartment.
- A prophylactic subcutaneous release of the anterior compartment is then performed through this incision.
- A hemostat is used to expose the tibia subperiosteally at the level of the osteotomy (**TECH FIG 3A**).
- A no. 5 suture is then held taut by a right angle clamp and passed, subperiosteally, around the back of the tibia (**TECH FIG 3B**). A hemostat is placed posterior to the tibia from the opposite side, and the suture is grasped and pulled out the opposite side of the leg (**TECH FIG 3C**).
- To verify that the saw has not been placed around the anterior or posterior tibial arteries, the ends of the suture are pulled taut while palpating the pedal pulses for occlusion.
- The Gigli saw is then tied to the suture to pass the saw around the back of the tibia.
- The osteotomy is then performed with the Gigli saw.

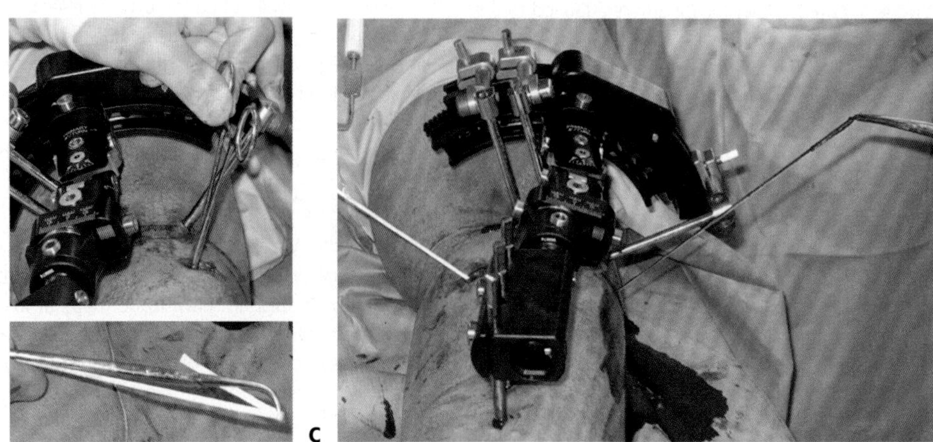

**TECH FIG 3 • A.** Subperiosteal exposure of the tibia is developed at the level of the osteotomy. **B.** Umbilical tape is held taut by a right angle clamp. **C.** The umbilical tape is pulled posterior to the tibia.

- Care is taken to avoid injury to the skin.
- Fluoroscopy is used to verify the completion of the osteotomy and alignment of the proximal and distal fragments with the external fixator.

## Completion of Surgery

- The lengthening device is then inserted onto the telescoping arm and turned such that it slides into the telescoping arm (**TECH FIG 4A**). Both screws of the lengthening device are then tightened.
- All screws of the external fixator are then given their final tightening.
- All wounds are closed, and a sterile dressing is applied (**TECH FIG 4B**).
- Acute correction typically is not performed if there is risk of stretching neurovascular tissues.
- During the first postoperative week, the patient learns to walk with crutches, 10 pounds partial weight bearing.
- On the eighth day, the patient is taught to lengthen through the compression distraction mechanism at a rate of one 90-degree turn of the Allen wrench four times a day. This will cause lengthening of 1 mm per day.
- On the 14th day, a radiograph should show that the ends of the osteotomized tibia are separated by a distance of about 7 mm (**TECH FIG 4C,D**).
- Angular correction can now begin. The patient is taught to place the Allen wrench into the primary angulation screw and turn 90 degrees in the direction for angular correction. This 90-degree turn will correct 1 degree of angular deformity and can comfortably be performed four times a day for a correction of about 4 degrees per day until the deformity is corrected (**TECH FIG 4E,F**).
- Long radiographs are then taken to assess the correction.
- Secondary deformity (flexion or extension) can be corrected through the secondary hinges, translation screws (one 360-degree turn translates 1 mm), lengthening screws, and the rotation arc (one 90-degree turn corrects 1 degree of rotation).
- Once the deformity is corrected, all screws and locks on the MAC device are secured. The device can be safely removed after passage of at least 1 month per centimeter of lengthening and a minimum of about 3 months.
- Radiographs should also demonstrate healing of at least three cortices on each of the AP and lateral views before removal of the fixator.
- Training and experience with external fixation and deformity correction is always advised.

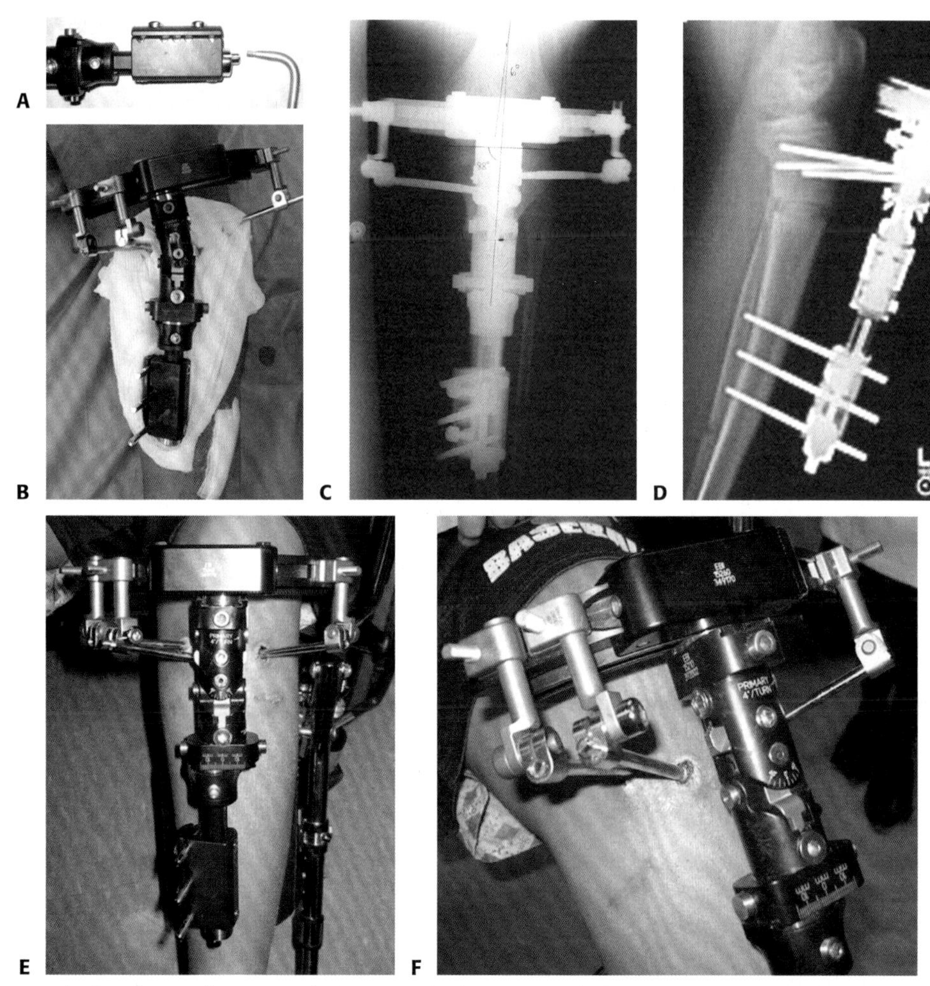


**TECH FIG 4 • A.** The lengthening device is applied. **B.** A sterile dressing is applied. **C,D.** Radiographs are taken to verify that there is distraction at the osteotomy site prior to correcting angulation. **E,F.** Correction is performed until the angulation has been rectified.

## PEARLS AND PITFALLS

| | |
|---|---|
| **Indications** | ■ A correct diagnosis of Blount disease must be made before treatment is initiated. Treatment alternatives, including hemiepiphysiodesis (if there is sufficient growth remaining), must be discussed with the patient and family. |
| **Deformity planning** | ■ Radiographs must be evaluated carefully and systematically so that the location of the CORA and coexistent deformities of the femur or sagittal plane are identified. |
| **Neurovascular injury** | ■ All half-pins must be placed into safe zones of the leg to avoid inadvertent neurovascular injury.<br>■ Careful neurovascular examinations must be performed postoperatively. |
| **Postoperative care** | ■ Patients must be followed closely during correction so that malalignment does not occur. Pin site infections must be recognized and treated appropriately. |

## POSTOPERATIVE CARE

- Patients are admitted to the hospital and monitored closely for signs and symptoms of neurovascular injury and compartment syndrome for 1 to 3 days.
- Patients initially are allowed touchdown weight bearing only. Range-of-motion exercises are begun immediately.
- Pin care is begun on postoperative day 2. Patients are instructed on the signs and symptoms of pin site infections.
- No adjustments or corrections are made to the external fixator for the first 7 days. A 7-day latency allows fracture callus to develop at the site of the osteotomy. Then, the correction phase is begun.
- The correction phase begins with lengthening the leg by 7 to 8 mm at a rate of 1 mm per day (0.25 mm four times per day) to separate the bone ends. Angulation is then corrected. The patient is evaluated clinically and radiographically to follow correction of the mechanical axis. Scanograms can then be obtained to determine leg length inequality, which can be corrected by lengthening with the fixator. The rotational deformity (internal tibial torsion) is corrected last. Placing white adhesive tape with arrows onto the device helps patients remember how to turn the screws appropriately for angular, linear, and rotational correction.
- Weight bearing is increased during the consolidation period. The consolidation period is approximately twice the correction period. Most patients treated with this technique for adolescent Blount disease will have the external fixator on for 3 to 4 months. They can walk with crutches initially and progress to full weight bearing as the osteotomy heals. They can shower within 3 days of application of the fixator.
- When radiographs show that the osteotomy and distraction gap have healed, the external fixator is removed. Removal can be done in the office or in the operating room. Considerable torque is required to remove hydroxyapatite pins and this must be done in the operating room with adequate sedation and analgesia.

## OUTCOMES

- Because adolescent Blount disease is relatively uncommon, there are few outcome studies in the literature.
- Price et al[5] reported on the treatment of 31 tibiae in 23 patients with dynamic external fixation. All osteotomies healed. There was an average correction of 20 degrees, and no postoperative loss of correction occurred.

## COMPLICATIONS

- High complication rates have been reported for proximal tibial osteotomies.
  - Steel et al[8] reported a 20% rate of neurologic complications in 46 tibial osteotomies. The neurologic complications are related to the location of the osteotomy, which must be done in the metaphysis to avoid damaging the proximal tibial epiphysis.
  - Deformity correction at this level can stretch or compress the anterior tibial artery because of its proximity to the tibia at that level. Although arterial stretch or compression is more common than laceration or edema in anterior compartment following correction, prophylactic fasciotomies of the anterior and lateral compartments are still indicated to decrease the risk of neurovascular complications.
- Other complications include delayed union and nonunion.

## ACKNOWLEDGMENT

- With thanks to Dr. Eric D. Shirley,[†] the author of this chapter in the first edition.

[†]Deceased.

## REFERENCES

1. Birch JG, Samchukov ML. Use of the Ilizarov method to correct lower limb deformities in children and adolescents. J Am Acad Orthop Surg 2004;12:144–154.
2. Laville JM, Chau E, Willeman L, et al. Blount's disease: classification and treatment. J Pediatr Orthop B 1999;8(1):19–25.
3. Loder RT, Schaffer JJ, Bardenstein MB. Late-onset tibia vara. J Pediatr Orthop 1991;11:162–167.
4. Paley D, Herzenberg JE, Tetsworth K, et al. Deformity planning for frontal and sagittal plane corrective osteotomies. Orthop Clin North Am 1994;25:425–465.
5. Price CT, Scott DS, Greenberg DA. Dynamic axial external fixation in the surgical treatment of tibia vara. J Pediatr Orthop 1995;15:236–243.
6. Salenius P, Vankka E. The development of the tibiofemoral angle in children. J Bone Joint Surg Am 1975;57(2):259–261.
7. Schoenecker PL, Meade WC, Pierron RL, et al. Blount's disease: a retrospective review and recommendations for treatment. J Pediatr Orthop 1985;5:181–186.
8. Steel HH, Sandrow RE, Sullivan PD. Complications of tibial osteotomy in children for genu varum or valgum. Evidence that neurological changes are due to ischemia. J Bone Joint Surg Am 1971;53(8):1629–1635.
9. Thompson GH, Carter JR. Late-onset tibia vara (Blount's disease), Current concepts. Clin Orthop Relat Res 1990;(255):24–35.

# Percutaneous Distal Femoral or Proximal Tibial Epiphysiodesis for Leg Length Discrepancy

56

CHAPTER

Emily R. Dodwell and Roger F. Widmann

## DEFINITION

- Epiphysiodesis involves manipulation of a physis (growth plate) to cause temporary or permanent, partial or complete growth inhibition to correct length or angular deformity in children with growth remaining.
  - In the setting of leg length discrepancy, epiphysiodesis must cause growth inhibition symmetrically across the physis such that shortening results without development of angular deformity. Epiphysiodesis can be achieved by obliteration of the growth cells through physical disruption (drill, curettage, radioablation, or similar) or tethering with various devices (screws crossing the physis or staples/small plates at the periphery of the physis) or various forms of bone grafting such as the open Phemister technique.[22]
  - Today, the two most common techniques are percutaneous drill and percutaneous screw epiphysiodesis.[7]
- Growth of the longer extremity is inhibited by prematurely arresting or tethering growth at one or more physes so that remaining growth of the shorter extremity may "catch up" thus approximating limb lengths at maturity.
- Patients with a predicted leg length discrepancy of less than 2 to 2.5 cm do not typically require surgical intervention and may be treated with observation or a shoe lift/insert.
- Epiphysiodesis is usually considered when the final limb length discrepancy of the lower extremity is predicted to be in the range of 2 to 5 cm. Patients with leg length discrepancies greater than 5 cm may be considered for other procedures, including lengthening. Some patients with large discrepancies may undergo lengthening on their short side, as well as epiphysiodesis on their long side, to minimize the number of lengthening procedures required.
- Limb equalization surgery is considered successful if residual leg length discrepancy is less than 2 cm.
- In order to optimize leg length equalization, the surgeon must understand the etiology of the leg length discrepancy and be able to predict growth based on the underlying cause of growth inequality, the child's maturity by chronologic and bone age, and the child's own height percentile and parental and sibling heights.

## ANATOMY

- The physis is made up of cartilage cells that are replicating and growing away from the physis.
  - The germinal cells are on the epiphyseal side of the physis.
  - The distal femoral physis and proximal tibial physes are undulating and slightly curved.
- The neurovascular bundle is posterior and midline at the level of the distal femoral physis.
- The common peroneal nerve at the knee runs obliquely along the lateral side of the popliteal fossa, close to the medial border of the biceps femoris muscle and the lateral head of the gastrocnemius muscle, toward the head of the fibula.
  - The nerve winds posteriorly around the neck of the proximal fibula and passes deep to the peroneus longus muscle, where it divides into the superficial and deep peroneal nerves.

## EPIDEMIOLOGY

- Approximately 25% of people have a leg length discrepancy of 1 cm or more, and the incidence of leg length discrepancy of 2 cm or greater is estimated at 1 in 1000 cases.
- Epiphysiodesis is the most frequently used operative procedure in North America for the equalization of limb lengths.

## PATHOGENESIS

- The etiology of a limb length discrepancy can be congenital/developmental; related to tumor; neuromuscular disease; skeletal dysplasia; or otherwise acquired through trauma, infection radiation, or other causes. A partial list of causes includes the following:
  - Congenital shortening: proximal focal femoral deficiency, coxa vara, congenital short femur, fibular and tibial hemimelia, hemiatrophy
  - Congenital lengthening: overgrowth syndromes such as hemihypertrophy, Beckwith-Wiedemann syndrome, Klippel-Trenaunay-Weber syndrome, and Parkes-Weber syndrome
  - Skeletal dysplasia or tumor: Multiple hereditary exostoses may result in limb shortening on the affected side, as growth cartilage cells are diverted to the cartilage tumor. Radiation for malignancies adjacent to the physis may result in growth suppression or complete destruction of physeal cartilage cells, resulting in limb length discrepancy or angular deformity.
  - Infection: Physeal destruction may result from physeal invasion from adjacent metaphyseal or epiphyseal bacterial osteomyelitis or direct physeal involvement in the case of intracapsular joint physes such as at the hip and shoulder.
  - Paralysis: Poliomyelitis and cerebral palsy as well as other nervous system afflictions in children typically result in shortening on the more affected side.
  - Trauma: direct injury to growth plate, posttraumatic bone loss or shortening, and overgrowth following femoral fracture
- Miscellaneous: slipped capital femoral epiphysis, Legg-Calvé-Perthes disease

## NATURAL HISTORY

- Depending on the underlying cause of the leg length discrepancy, a discrepancy may be static or increase or decrease with remaining growth.
  - Congenital limb length discrepancies typically maintain proportional growth over time. For instance, a tibia that is 10% shorter than the normal side at birth will be approximately 10% shorter than the normal side at maturity.
- Leg length discrepancies under 2 cm are typically well tolerated.
  - Untreated leg length discrepancy of more than 3 cm may result in pelvic obliquity, visual gait disturbance, short-legged gait, or structural/nonstructural scoliosis.
- Leg length discrepancy greater than 5.5% of the long leg has been shown to decrease the efficiency of gait, as determined from kinetic data.[23]
- No causative relationship has been proved between leg length discrepancy and knee or hip pain or arthritis. A large population study has shown an association between leg length discrepancy and knee arthritis, but there was no evidence of causation.[9]
- Although scoliosis has been associated with leg length discrepancy, there is no evidence that leg length discrepancy causes structural curvature of the spine. Assessing the spine with a block under the short leg, with the pelvis level, permits assessment of true scoliosis.
- Following drill epiphysiodesis, bony bridges form between the epiphysis and the metaphysis, preventing further physeal growth. Growth arrest has been documented within 3 months of the procedure using radiostereotactic (RSA) three-dimensional imaging.[11]
- Following screw epiphysiodesis, there is compression or tethering across the physis. Physeal closure may be slightly delayed compared to ablative techniques. Growth inhibition has been documented within 6 months of screw epiphysiodesis but has not been measured using RSA or other highly accurate techniques.

## PATIENT HISTORY AND PHYSICAL FINDINGS

- The underlying cause of a leg length discrepancy can typically be elucidated by careful history and physical examination.
- The common symptoms at presentation are limp, compensatory gait mechanics, pelvic obliquity, and nonstructural scoliosis.
- Physical findings depend on the etiologic factors.
- In hemihypertrophy (both syndromic and nonsyndromic), the affected extremity may be larger in both length and girth. In classic hemihypertrophy, upper extremity hypertrophy as well as hemifacial asymmetry may be present. Vascular overgrowth syndromes may be associated with cutaneous or deep hemangiomas, which may alter surgical approaches to attempted limb equalization.
- Clinically, leg length discrepancy is best measured by the block test, in which the shorter leg is placed on increasingly larger measured blocks until the posterior iliac crest is level. Discrepancies as small as 2 cm are accurately detected by this method, and detection of discrepancies is largely unaffected by patient size or body mass.
- True leg length is measured from the anterior superior iliac spine to the tip of the medial malleolus. It is important to place the legs in identical positions to measure true leg length, and for this reason, this measurement is less accurate than the block test.
  - If the patient has a 20-degree abduction deformity of right hip, the left hip is placed in 20 degrees of abduction to measure true length.
- Apparent leg length is measured with the patient supine with the legs parallel to each other. The landmarks are the umbilicus to the tip of medial malleolus. Pelvic obliquity and fixed deformities of the hip and knee affect the reading. This method is also significantly less accurate than block measurement.
- Range of motion is noted for all joints, primarily the hip, knee, ankle, and subtalar joints. The ankle joint range of motion is measured with the knee in extension and flexion.

## IMAGING AND OTHER DIAGNOSTIC STUDIES

- Plain radiographs have traditionally been used to document the objective measurement of leg length discrepancy.
- Full-length (hip to ankle) anteroposterior (AP) radiographs are obtained in standing position with both patellae facing directly anteriorly. The appropriate-sized block is placed beneath the shorter leg to level the pelvis. A long x-ray cassette (51-inch) is used with the x-ray beam center focused on the knee from a distance of 10 feet. A radiolucent ruler often is used to assist in calculation of limb discrepancies.
  - A lateral hip to ankle view can be included to further assess length, as contractures in the sagittal plane may result in inaccuracies on AP measurements. This view can also assess for angular deformities in the coronal plane.
  - Computed tomography (CT) scanogram has been the gold standard for low-dose accurate imaging of leg length discrepancy.
  - CT scanogram is as precise in measuring leg length discrepancy as the slit scanogram and it has the added benefit of more easily measuring leg length discrepancy in the setting of joint contractures. Slit scanogram is of historical interest only and is no longer typically used for measuring leg length discrepancy.
  - EOS[8] is a low-dose, high-resolution radiologic imaging system that captures standing simultaneous posteroanterior (PA) and lateral radiographs and full-body radiographs.[17]
  - Recently, EOS biplanar imaging systems have been shown to be equally accurate/reliable with the added benefit of imaging the patient in a standing position such that leg length and alignment can be obtained from a single low-dose image. Radiation exposure is also lower with EOS.[6]
- Skeletal age can be determined by a left hand/wrist radiograph in combination with the Greulich and Pyle method.[10]
  - Alternatively, the Hospital for Special Surgery (HSS) shorthand method can be used. This method was derived from Greulich and Pyle and uses a single radiographic criteria is used for each age, allowing for rapid bone age determination.[12]
- The leg length discrepancy at maturity can be predicted in a variety of ways:
  - The arithmetic method[18]
  - The growth remaining method[1,2]
  - The Moseley straight line method[20]
  - The Paley multiplier technique[21]
- Applications/programs that incorporate the Paley multiplication factors are readily available on smartphones/computers for clinical use. These allow calculation of length

discrepancy at maturity for both congenital and acquired deformities.

- Parental and sibling height may be useful in interpreting predicted height be the above methods.
- In leg length discrepancy secondary to physeal growth arrest, graphical or arithmetic methods are helpful in determining appropriate timing of epiphysiodesis.

## DIFFERENTIAL DIAGNOSIS

- True shortening (eg, femoral or tibial)
- Apparent shortening due to dislocated hip
- Apparent shortening from contractures
- Angular deformity causing apparent shortening
- Overgrowth syndrome with both increased length and limb girth: hemihypertrophy
- Congenital limb deficiency
  - Trauma, radiation, tumor, infection, burns, and other causes.

## NONOPERATIVE MANAGEMENT

- No treatment is required for a predicted limb length discrepancy of less than to 2.5 cm at maturity.
- A shoe lift can be used as treatment for leg length discrepancies at maturity below 2 cm.
  - Often, a lift is used in children until an appropriate skeletal age is reached to perform an equalization procedure.

## SURGICAL MANAGEMENT

- Epiphysiodesis is most commonly performed at the distal femoral physis or the proximal tibia with or without fibular physis.
- Ablation of the medial and lateral physis causes bony bridges to form between the epiphysis and metaphysis that accomplish growth inhibition in that physis (epiphysiodesis).
  - This can be accomplished by different instruments, including a curette, a drill, a burr, a reamer, or radioablation.
- Some authors recommend ablation only at the periphery, as bony bridge formation at the peripheral margins of the physis both medially and laterally has been shown to cause spontaneous closure of the central physis.
- The authors' preferred method for mechanical ablation involves ablating the majority of the physis, including the central portion.
  - Due to intact cortex at the physis (with the exception of two small drill holes), stability of the bone is maintained postoperatively and the patient may weight bear as tolerated, although traditionally, the child is protected with a brace and crutches for the first few weeks.
  - There is no clear evidence to support when a child should return to sports, although given the potential destabilizing effect of disruption the physis and theoretical concern for Salter Harris fracture, it is reasonable to delay return to sports for the first 6 weeks following mechanical ablation of the physis.
    - Transphyseal screws are another option for longitudinal growth inhibition. This technique tethers the physis causing growth inhibition.

### Preoperative Planning

- Anticipated remaining growth is determined by obtaining bone age and using one of the prediction methods mentioned earlier.
- A proximal fibular epiphysiodesis should be performed in addition to the proximal tibial epiphysiodesis if the final discrepancy between the tibia and fibula is anticipated to be more than 2 cm.
  - No method is completely accurate, with an error for each method of up to 1.5 cm.
  - The authors' preference is to use the multiplier method.
  - Charts are available for both acquired and congenital leg length discrepancies, and predicted growth can be easily calculated with a calculator or a multiplier specific software program or smartphone application.
  - Some studies suggest that growth inhibition with screw epiphysiodesis may be less than with drill/curettage, although this has not been the authors experience.[15]

### Positioning

- For both drill/curette and screw epiphysiodesis, the patient is placed supine on a radiolucent table.
  - A bump below the hip on the operative side may aid in maintaining the patella forward.
- A tourniquet is placed on the proximal thigh but is not inflated unless bleeding occurs.
  - Elevating the operative leg on a bump or wedge will help facilitate lateral fluoroscopy and passage of wires/drills/screws from both the medial and lateral starting points (**FIG 1**).
  - Fluoroscopy can be brought in from the patient's nonoperative side.

### Approach

- Drill/curette
  - Distal femoral epiphysiodesis
    - Longitudinal incisions of 5 mm medially and laterally are made in the skin at the level of the physis.
  - Proximal tibial epiphysiodesis
    - Longitudinal incisions of 5 mm medially and laterally are made in the skin at the level of the physis, with the lateral incision just anterior to the fibular head.
  - Proximal fibular epiphysiodesis
    - The same incision is used for the fibular epiphysiodesis as for the lateral physeal area of the tibia; however, in the epiphysiodesis of the fibula, the drill and curette

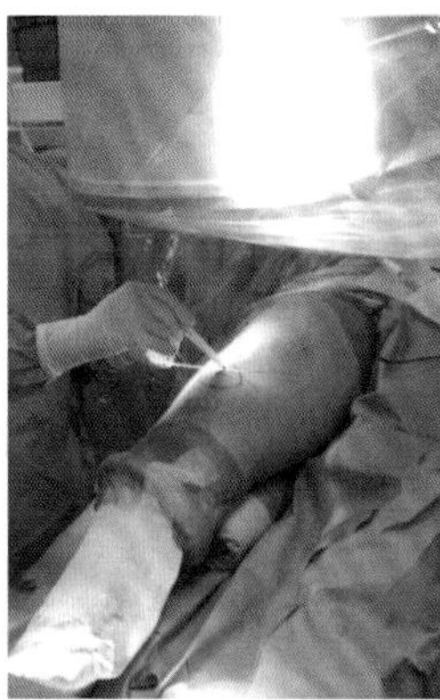

**FIG 1** • The patient is placed supine on a radiolucent table, with the operative leg elevated on a bump or wedge for ease of AP and lateral fluoroscopy, and passage of instruments from both medial and lateral starting points, across the physis.

enter at the anterior/superior aspect of the fibula and longitudinally cross the physis.

- Screw
  - Distal femoral epiphysiodesis
    - Longitudinal incisions of 8 mm are made medially and laterally proximal to the physis by approximately 4 to 6 cm.
  - Proximal tibial epiphysiodesis
    - Longitudinal incisions of 8 mm are made medially and laterally distal to the physis by approximately 4 to 6 cm.
    - The incision for the lateral screw is made just lateral to the tibial crest, and the anterior compartment muscles are retracted laterally.



## Drill/Curette Epiphysiodesis of the Distal Femoral Physis or the Proximal Tibial Physis

### Preparation of the Physis

- The level of the physis is identified both medially and laterally using fluoroscopy and a metal marker on the skin (**TECH FIG 1A**).
- A 5-mm skin incision is made with a scalpel at the level of the physeal plate both medially and laterally (**TECH FIG 1B**).
- A 4.5-mm drill is used to enter the medial cortex and is passed across the physis toward the lateral side (**TECH FIG 1C**). It is directed straight across, and then the drilling hand is raised and lowered to redirect the drill such that it passes anteriorly and posteriorly. Care is taken to avoid exiting the cortex anteriorly or posteriorly. When drilling the proximal tibial physis, care should be taken to avoid injury to the tibial tubercle apophysis (**TECH FIG 1D,E**).
- We prefer making a second incision to repeat the process from the lateral side of the physis. However, it is possible to perform

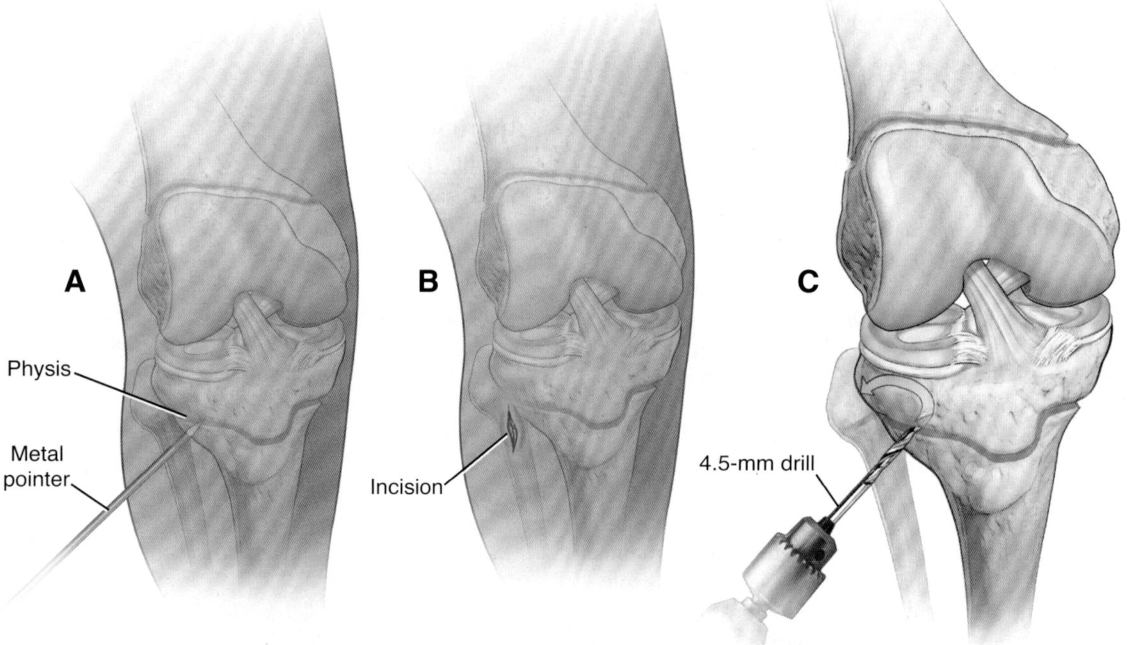


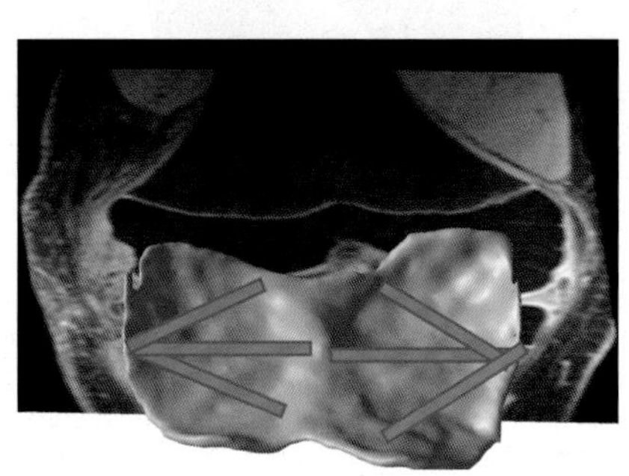


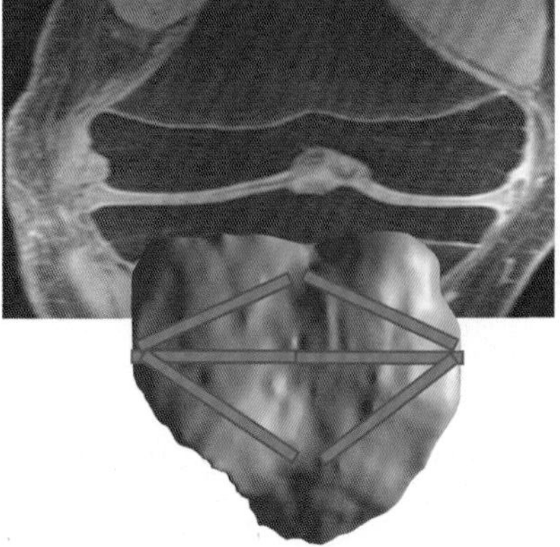


**TECH FIG 1** • **A.** A metal pointer is used to identify the level of the physis under fluoroscopy. **B.** A 5-mm longitudinal incision is made at the level of the physis. **C.** A 4.5-mm drill is used to enter the physis medially and laterally. **D,E.** Magnetic resonance imaging (MRI) physeal map of distal femoral and proximal tibial physis showing the intended path of the drills/curettes for percutaneous drill/curette epiphysiodesis.

the femoral and/or tibial epiphysiodesis from a single incision (medial or lateral).

## Physeal Plate Ablation

- A curette is advanced through the drill holes (**TECH FIG 2A–C**) and is used to scrape out physeal cells anterior, posterior, laterally, cephalad, and caudad. Care is taken to avoid breaching the cortex anteriorly, posteriorly, or proximally.
- Fluoroscopy images are saved to confirm passage of instruments across the desired region of the physis.
- Radiopaque dye can be injected into the site of the physeal disruption to confirm ablation of the physis (**TECH FIG 2D,E**).
  - The goal is to ablate at least 50% of the physis medially and laterally.
- Following epiphysiodesis, the physis is no longer easily distinguished on radiographs (**TECH FIG 2F,G**).

## Wound Closure

- The wound is closed in a layered fashion as per the surgeon's preferences.

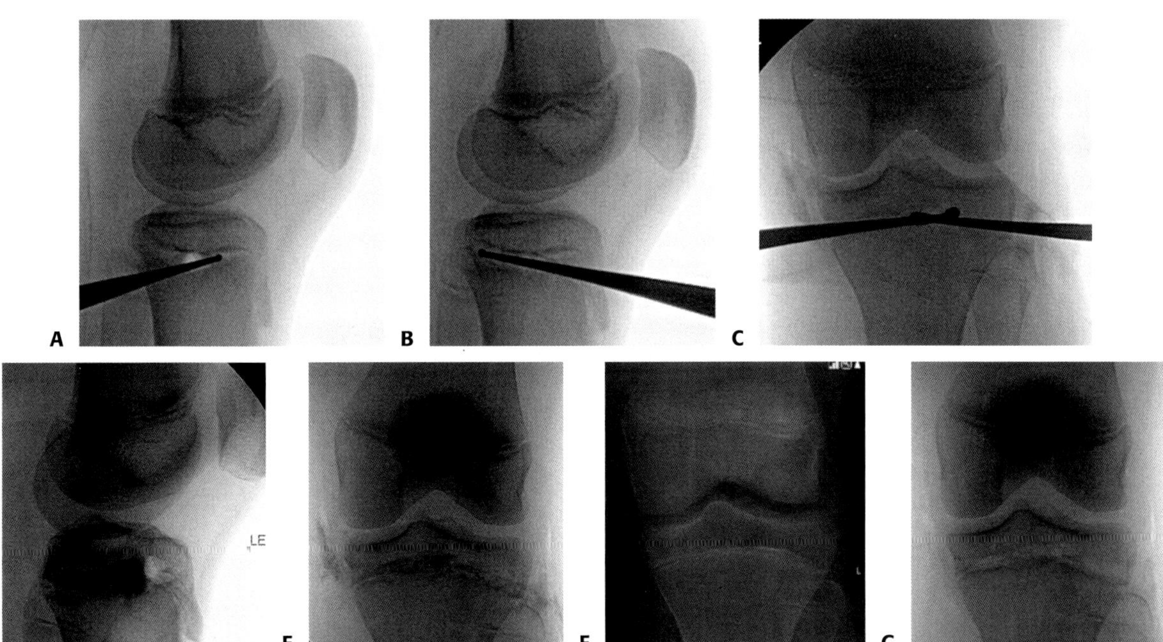


**TECH FIG 2** • Curettes are passed through the medial and lateral drill holes to the midline (**A**), centrally (**B**), anteriorly, and posteriorly (**C**). **D,E.** Following curettage, radiolucent dye can be injected into the physis to demonstrate surface area that has been mechanically disrupted. **F.** The proximal tibial physis preoperatively, prior to mechanical disruption of the physis. **G.** The proximal tibial physis post drill and curette epiphysiodesis, showing removal of the physis.

# Drill/Curette Epiphysiodesis of the Proximal Fibula

- The anterolateral incision used for epiphysiodesis of the lateral tibia can be used for epiphysiodesis of the proximal fibula.
- Directing the drill in the plane of the fibular physis puts the common peroneal nerve at risk (**TECH FIG 3A**).
  - To avoid injury to the common peroneal nerve, the fibular cortex is entered at the anterior superior aspect of the fibula, through the epiphysis (**TECH FIG 3B**).
  - The drill and curette are passed from proximal to distal across the physis.
  - The most proximal aspect of the fibula is usually at the level of the tibial physis.
- The curette is used to ablate the entire central area of the physis of the fibula to achieve epiphysiodesis (**TECH FIG 3C**).

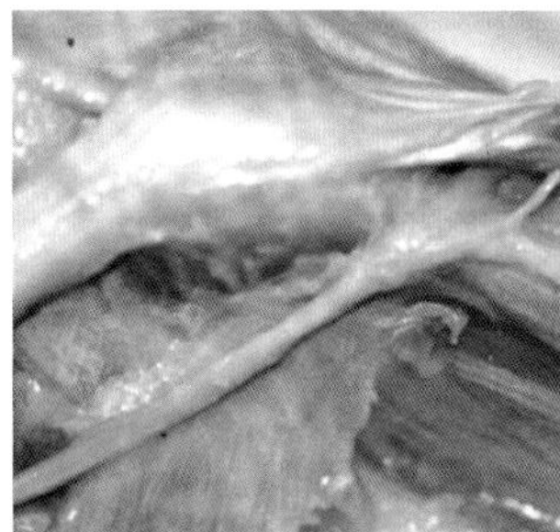


**TECH FIG 3** • **A.** Dissection of the common peroneal nerve at the level of the fibular head. *(continued)*

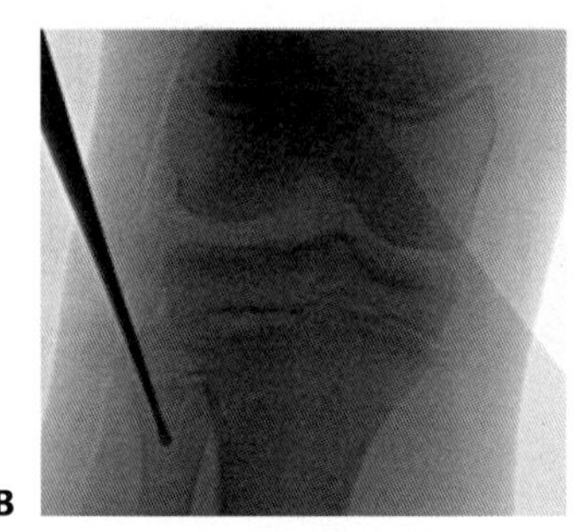
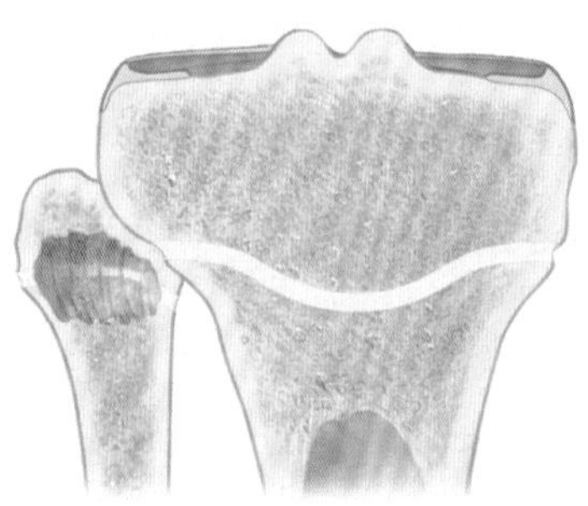

**TECH FIG 3** • *(continued)* **B.** A drill is used to enter the anterior superior aspect of the proximal fibula, followed by a curette. **C.** Disruption at the central portion of the proximal fibular physis results in bridging bone across the physis.

## Screw Epiphysiodesis

### Femoral Screw

- Fluoroscopy is used to mark the physis and the desired entry site of the guidewires both medially and laterally (**TECH FIG 4A**).
- In the distal femur, guidewires are placed in an antegrade fashion, with an 8-mm skin incision placed approximately 5 cm proximal to the physis both medially and laterally.
- The guidewire is placed such that the medial wire crosses the lateral half of the physis and the lateral guidewire crosses the physis at the medial half of the physis (**TECH FIG 4B,C**).
- The wires extend into the epiphysis and avoid entry into the joint.
- The guidewires are then over drilled with a 5-mm drill, and 7.3-mm fully threaded cannulated screws are placed across the growth plate (**TECH FIG 4D,E**).
  - Fully threaded screws are used for ease of removal.

### Tibial Screw

- For tibial screw placement, the wires are retrograde, with 8-mm incisions made medially and laterally approximately 5 cm distal to the physis, and guidewires directed with a distal starting point, aiming proximally.
- Care should be taken to avoid penetrating the subchondral bone with the screw tips.
- Due to posterior tibial slope, AP x-rays with variable degrees of flexion can help to demonstrate the joint surface and true position of the screw tips.

### Wound Closure

- The incisions are irrigated and closed in the surgeon's preferred method. Sterile dressings are applied. The patient can weight bear as tolerated with crutches and is counseled to wean off crutches and gradually increase activity as tolerated.

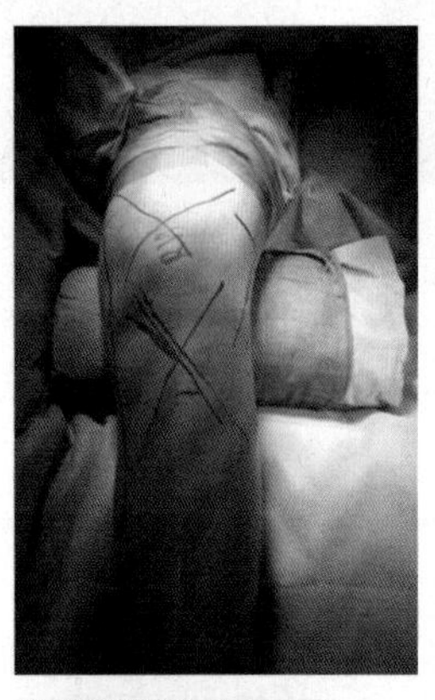
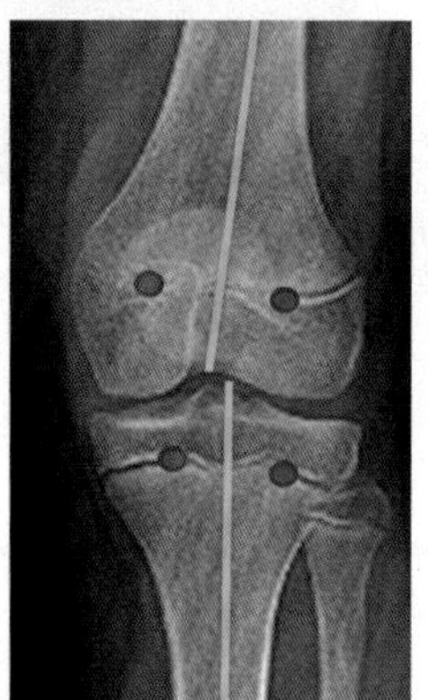
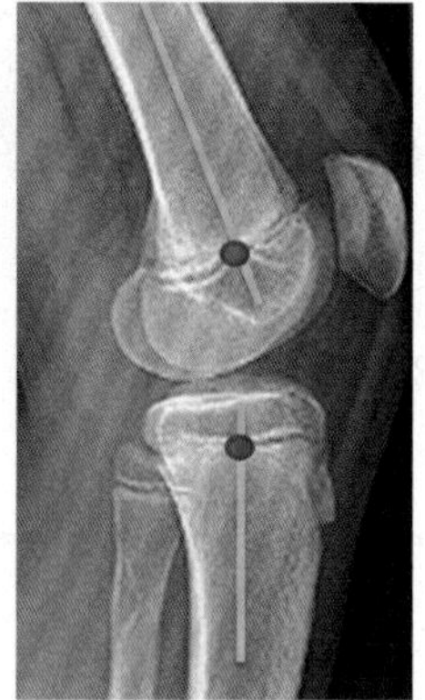
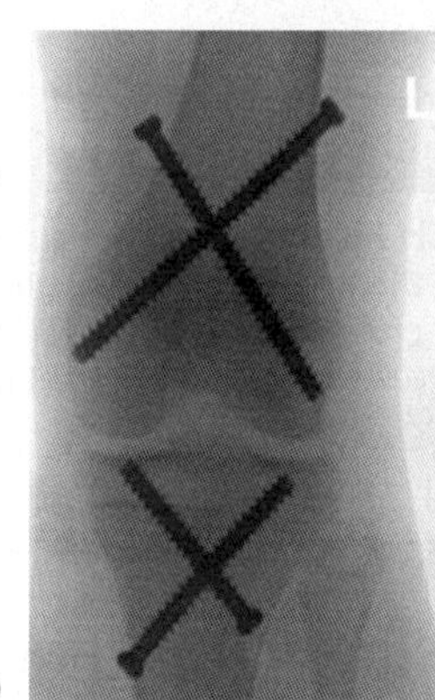
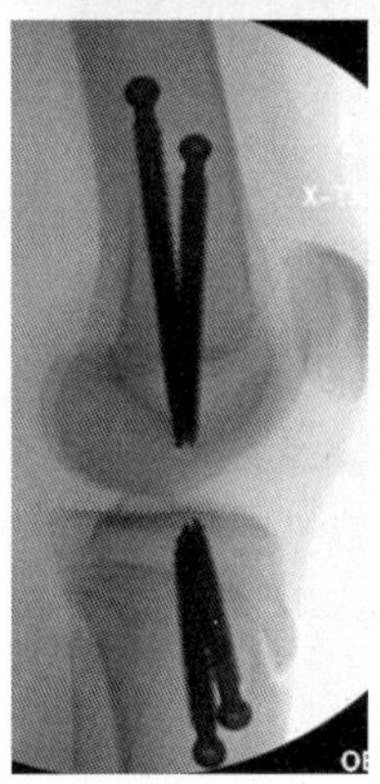

**TECH FIG 4** • **A.** Fluoroscopy is used to mark out the planned trajectory of the screws. **B.** On the AP view, the medial femoral screw should cross the physis at the middle of the lateral half of the physis and the lateral femoral screw should cross the physis at the middle of the medial half of the physis. **C.** On the lateral view, both screws should pass as close to midline as possible. *Green lines* indicate midline. *Red dots* indicate ideal crossing point for the screws. **D,E.** Two fully threaded 7.3-mm cannulated screws are shown directed antegrade in the distal femur and retrograde in the proximal tibia.

## PEARLS AND PITFALLS

| | |
|---|---|
| **Discrepancy between bone age and chronologic age** | ■ Bone age is typically used for calculations of remaining growth. |
| **Imaging** | ■ Recently, EOS biplanar imaging systems have been shown to be equally accurate/reliable with the added benefit of imaging the patient in a standing position such that leg length and alignment can be obtained from a single low-dose image. |
| **Prominent hardware** | ■ Patients should be advised that screws may be palpable. Using a fully threaded screw and removing the screw as soon as possible following complete physeal closure will facilitate ease of screw removal. |
| **Screw placement** | ■ Screws placed asymmetrically, outside of the preferred location, and those with less than 4 threads across the physis may be at higher risk for failure of epiphysiodesis or development of an angular deformity. |
| **Neuromuscular, weak and short extremity** | ■ Patients with hemiplegia, foot drop, or other neurologic conditions may have difficulty with toe-catch and/or tripping. Leaving the affected leg short by 1–1.5 cm may be beneficial in this setting. |
| **Follow-up to maturity** | ■ Some diseases tend to produce growth in a manner that is poorly predictable. If the limb lengths correct and remaining growth causes overshortening of the long side, contralateral epiphysiodesis may be required. |

## POSTOPERATIVE CARE

- Drill epiphysiodesis disrupts a large surface area of the physis. Although the cortex is intact with the exception of the medial and lateral drill holes, this procedure is considered potentially destabilizing. For this reason, patients are typically provided with a knee immobilizer, in extension. They may weight bear as tolerated. Crutches and modified weight bearing may be used as symptoms require. Patients are typically kept out of sports and high-impact activities for 4 to 6 weeks.
- Screw epiphysiodesis is not typically considered destabilizing. Patients can be discharged in a soft dressing. They may weight bear as tolerated. Crutches, a knee immobilizer, and modified weight bearing may be used as symptoms require. As this is not considered a destabilizing procedure, patients are not restricted from returning to sports and may return as tolerated.[7]
  - Clinical examination should be performed at 2 weeks postoperatively and clinical and radiographic examinations every 6 months until maturity to determine closure of the physis and assess for possible complications, including angular deformity or failure of growth arrest.
- Full-length standing plain films or EOS are the preferred radiographic modality, although CT scanogram or plain x-rays may also be used.
  - Physeal closure following mechanical ablation (drill/curette) has been reported as early as 1 month, and complete closure has been documented at 3 months by radiostereotactic analysis.[11]
- Growth inhibition may be delayed by at least 6 months in screw epiphysiodesis, and one study[23] has reported physeal closure to be delayed to approximately 1 year following screw epiphysiodesis.

## OUTCOMES

- Outcomes and complications associated with the two percutaneous techniques are summarized in Table 1.
- Both percutaneous drill epiphysiodesis and percutaneous screw epiphysiodesis[13] provide for improved cosmesis and more rapid recovery than traditional open techniques of epiphysiodesis.[3]
- In a small retrospective series, drill epiphysiodesis was compared to medial and lateral 8-plates (peripheral tether). Growth inhibition was significantly less with 8-plate epiphysiodesis, and the authors recommended against the use of medial and lateral 8 plates for equalization of leg lengths.[24]
- Medial and lateral staples used for limb length equalization has been associated with mechanical axis deviation in over 50% of cases, and authors have advised caution in using medial and lateral staples for equalization of leg lengths.

**Table 1 Outcomes and Complications Associated with the Two Percutaneous Techniques**

| Parameter | Drill | Screw |
|---|---|---|
| Time to distal femoral physeal closure | 3 mo by RSA[11] | Within 6 mo[19] |
| Time to proximal tibial physeal closure | 3 mo by RSA[11] | Within 6 mo[19] |
| Reoperation rate | 0%–17%[5,24] | 0%–18% |
| Development of angular deformity | 0%[5,14] | 0%–20% |
| Failure of growth arrest | 0%–13% | 0%–20% |
| Infection | 0%–7% | 0% |
| Hematoma | 2%–5% | 0% |
| Knee effusion | 4%–5% | Not assessed |
| Skin blisters | 9% | Not assessed |
| Peroneal nerve palsy | 5% (fibular epiphysiodesis) | Not assessed |
| Fracture | 2% | 0% |
| Joint penetration | 2% | Not assessed |
| Hardware failure | N/A | 2.3% |
| Exostosis/heterotopic bone formation | 3%[16] | Not assessed |

RSA, radiostereotactic.

## COMPLICATIONS

- Complication rates range from 2.9% to 33% for percutaneous mechanical ablation technique and 16% to 27% for percutaneous transphyseal screw techniques.[4]
- Reported complications and rates summarized from multiple published series are given in Table 1.

## REFERENCES


1. Anderson M, Green WT, Messner MB. Growth and predictions of growth in the lower extremities. J Bone Joint Surg Am 1963;45-A:1–14.
2. Anderson M, Messner M, Green WT. Distribution of lengths of the normal femur and tibia in children from one to eighteen years of age. J Bone Joint Surg Am 1964;46:1197–1202.
3. Babu LV, Evans O, Sankar A, et al. Epiphysiodesis for limb length discrepancy: a comparison of two methods. Strategies Trauma Limb Reconstr 2014;9(1):1–3. doi:10.1007/s11751-013-0180-9.
4. Campens C, Mousny M, Docquier PL. Comparison of three surgical epiphysiodesis techniques for the treatment of lower limb length discrepancy. Acta Orthop Belg 2010;76(2):226–232.
5. Craviari T, Bérard J, Willemen L, et al. Percutaneous epiphysiodesis: analysis of a series of 60 full-grown patients [in French]. Rev Chir Orthop Reparatrice Appar Mot 1998;84:172–179.
6. Escott BG, Ravi B, Weathermon AC, et al. EOS low-dose radiography: a reliable and accurate upright assessment of lower-limb lengths. J Bone Joint Surg Am 2013;95(23):e1831–e1837.
7. Ghanem I, Karam JA, Widman RF. Surgical epiphysiodesis indications and techniques: update. Curr Opin Pediatr 2011;23(1):53–59.
8. Gheno R, Nectoux E, Herbaux B, et al. Three-dimensional measurements of the lower extremity in children and adolescents using a low dose biplanar X-ray device. Eur Radiol 2012;22(4):765–771.
9. Golightly YM, Allen KD, Renner JB, et al. Relationship of limb length inequality with radiographic knee and hip osteoarthritis. Osteoarthritis Cartilage 2007;15(7):824–829.
10. Greulich WW, Pyle S. Radiographic Atlas of Skeletal Developmental of the Hand and Wrist, ed 2. Stanford: Oxford University Press, 1959.
11. Gunderson RB, Horn J, Kibsgard T, et al. Negative correlation between extent of physeal ablation after percutaneous permanent physiodesis and postoperative growth: volume computer tomography and radiostereometric analysis of 37 physes in 27 patients. Acta Orthop 2013;84(4):426–430.
12. Heyworth BE, Goldstein M, Schneider R, et al. A new validated shorthand method for determining bone age. Hospital for Special Surgery. Available at http://www.hss.edu/files/HSSBoneAgePoster.pdf. Accessed August 18, 2014.
13. Hofmann SR, Roesen-Wolff A, Hahn G, et al. Update: cytokine dysregulation in chronic nonbacterial osteomyelitis (CNO). Int J Rheumatol 2012;2012:310206.
14. Horton GA, Olney BW. Epiphysiodesis of the lower extremity: results of the percutaneous technique. J Pediatr Orthop 1996;16:180–182.
15. Ilharreborde B, Gaumetou E, Souchet P, et al. Efficacy and late complications of percutaneous epiphysiodesis with transphyseal screws. J Bone Joint Surg Br 2012;94(2):270–275.
16. Inan M, Chan G, Littleton AG, et al. Efficacy and safety of percutaneous epiphysiodesis. J Pediatr Orthop 2008;28(6):648–651.
17. Lazennec JY, Rangel A, Baudoin A, et al. The EPS imaging system for understanding a patellofemoral disorder following THR. Orthop Traumatol Surg Res 2011;97(1):98–101.
18. Menelaus M. Correction of leg length discrepancy by epiphyseal arrest. J Bone Joint Surg Br 1966;48(2):336–339.
19. Métaizeau JP, Wong-Chung J, Bertrand H, et al. Percutaneous epiphysiodesis using transphyseal screws (PETS). J Pediatr Orthop 1998;18(3):363–369.
20. Moseley C. A straight-line graph for leg-length discrepancies. J Bone Joint Surg Am 1977;59(2):174–179.
21. Paley D, Bhave A, Herzenberg JE, et al. Multiplier method for predicting limb-length discrepancy. J Bone Joint Surg Am 2000;82-A(10):1432–1446.
22. Phemister DB. Epiphysiodesis for equalizing the length of the lower extremities and for correcting other deformities of the skeleton. Mem Acad Chir 1950;76:758–763.
23. Song MH, Choi ES, Park MS, et al. Effects and complications of percutaneous epiphysiodesis using transphyseal screws in the management of leg length discrepancy: optimal operation timing and techniques to avoid complications [published online ahead of print June 26, 2014]. J Pediatr Orthop.
24. Stewart D, Cheema A, Szalay EA. Dual 8-plate technique is not as effective as ablation for epiphysiodesis about the knee. J Pediatr Orthop 2013;33(8):843–846.

# Excision of Physeal Bar

Anthony A. Stans

57 CHAPTER

## DEFINITION

- A physeal bar, or partial premature physeal arrest, is an osseous connection that forms across a physis and has the potential to affect physeal growth.[7]
- Partial physeal arrest may result in three clinically significant consequences:
  - Angular deformity
  - Limb length discrepancy
  - Bone length discrepancy in a two-bone limb segment such as the forearm or leg
- When evaluating a patient with a physeal bar, one must critically consider whether there is sufficient growth remaining to cause a clinically significant length discrepancy or angular deformity.
- One should consider the linear magnitude of anticipated growth remaining as well as the years of remaining growth.

## ANATOMY

- The normal physis acts as a physical cartilage barrier separating the trabecular bone of the epiphysis from the metaphysis (**FIG 1**).

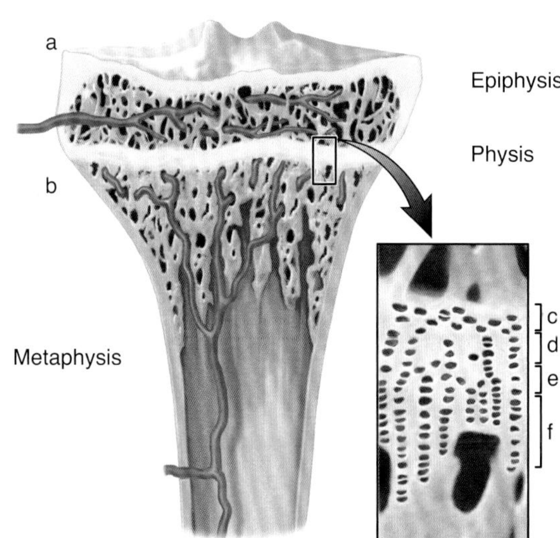


**FIG 1** • The physis acts as a physical barrier separating the trabecular bone of the epiphysis from the trabecular bone of the metaphysis. The physis also acts as a barrier to blood flow, separating the epiphyseal blood supply (*a*) from the metaphyseal blood supply (*b*). Magnification of the physis illustrates the four physeal cell layers: the resting cell zone (*c*), the proliferating cell zone (*d*), the hypertrophying cell zone (*e*), and the endochondral ossification zone (*f*). Insults that breach the physical separation between metaphyseal and epiphyseal trabecular bone that significantly compromise epiphyseal blood flow or that critically injure the resting or proliferating cell layers may result in physeal bar formation.

- Blood vessels typically do not traverse the physis, necessitating an independent blood supply for the epiphysis and metaphysis.[1]
- The physis consists of four cell layers: resting zone, proliferative zone, hypertrophic zone, and endochondral ossification zone.

## PATHOGENESIS

- Physeal bars form when the cartilage barrier is breached as the result of trauma, infection, or cell death, and trabecular bone heals in continuity between the epiphysis and the metaphysis across the physis.[9]
- Variation in physeal anatomy may predispose certain physes to physeal bar formation. For example, the distal radius physis is relatively two-dimensional and uniplanar, whereas the distal femoral physis has a more complex three-dimensional biconcave configuration.
- Distal radius physeal fractures are quite common, yet subsequent premature physeal bar formation is relatively rare. In contrast, distal femoral physeal fractures are uncommon but distal femoral physeal bar formation is much more prone to occur after injury.
- The three-dimensional configuration of the distal femoral physis contributes to the considerable energy required to fracture through the distal femoral physis, and the complex geometry increases the likelihood for violation of the physeal cartilage barrier between epiphyseal and metaphyseal bone, thereby increasing the risk of partial physeal bar formation after injury.
- Breach of the physeal cartilage barrier is most frequently caused by fracture, followed by infection.
- Less common pathogenesis for partial physeal bar formation may occur when the germinal or proliferating cells on the epiphyseal side of the physeal plate are injured by ischemia, infection, heat, laser, electricity, or other insult. As the germinal cells die and cell division in this region of the physis stops, partial physeal bar formation may occur.[6]

## NATURAL HISTORY

- In almost all situations, once a physeal bar has formed, length discrepancy, angular deformity, or both will continue to increase so long as the patient is skeletally immature and the affected physis (or its contralateral counterpart) continues to grow.

## PATIENT HISTORY AND PHYSICAL FINDINGS

- Questioning the patient quickly reveals the cause for physeal bar formation in most cases. The most common causes of physeal bar formation, fracture and infection, are typically memorable events that the patient can quickly recall.

- The examiner should ask the patient and family if they have noticed a progressive limb length discrepancy, limp, angular deformity, or bony prominence; this may confirm the presence of a physeal bar.
- Ideally, the orthopaedist is aware of the physeal injury, is anticipating possible physeal bar formation after injury, and is monitoring the patient at 6-month intervals with clinical examination and radiographs.
- The patient is examined for lower extremity limb length discrepancy using blocks of known height under the shorter limb until the pelvis is level.
- The patient is also examined for lower extremity angular deformity. The alignment at knee and ankle is assessed and compared to the contralateral limb.
- The patient is also examined for upper extremity limb length deformity. Length of the affected limb is compared to that of the contralateral limb.

## IMAGING AND OTHER DIAGNOSTIC STUDIES

- Appropriate imaging is critical for the evaluation of a potential physeal bar. Initial imaging is performed to determine whether the patient has sustained a clinically significant physeal injury and therefore should demonstrate limb length discrepancy and angular deformity.
- True scanograms use a slit beam that is perpendicular to the patient that scans the length of the limb and therefore has no magnification. The scanogram provides limb length and angular information with a single image (**FIG 2A**).
- A teleoroentgenogram, or full-length, standing, hip-to-ankle radiograph taken at a distance, does result in some magnification of the limb.
  - By placing blocks of known height beneath the shorter limb, a teleoroentgenogram can also provide information about length and angular deformity with a single radiograph.
  - A ruler or magnification markers can also be placed next to the limb to allow more accurate measurement of limb length.
- Orthoroentgenograms (separate exposures of the hip, knee, and ankle on a single film with a ruler) or computed tomography (CT) scout images can be used to determine limb length.
  - These must be supplemented by a full-length image of the limb to assess angular deformity.
- If the distal tibial physis is the injured physis in question, standing anteroposterior (AP) and lateral ankle radiographs are indicated to assess angular deformity.
- If limb length discrepancy or angular deformity is confirmed, additional imaging is indicated to determine the size and location of the physeal bar.
- Either fine-cut CT or magnetic resonance imaging (MRI) may be used, and axial, coronal, and sagittal plane images are obtained.
  - The CT or MRI images are used to create a map that illustrates the location and approximate cross-sectional area of the physeal bar (**FIG 2B,C**).
  - The relative cross-sectional area of the bar is important because physeal bars occupying greater than 50% of the cross-sectional area of the physis have a less favorable result after resection. Excision of bars greater than 50% of the physeal cross-sectional area may still be indicated in young patients, such as a 5-year-old patient with a 65% bar of the distal femoral physis.
- A skeletal age radiograph of the hand and wrist may be helpful in older patients if one is trying to determine if there is sufficient growth remaining for physeal bar resection to be indicated.

## DIFFERENTIAL DIAGNOSIS

- Physeal injury without growth abnormality
- Idiopathic limb length discrepancy
- Developmental cause for limb length discrepancy or angular deformity
- Blount disease
- Madelung deformity of the distal radius

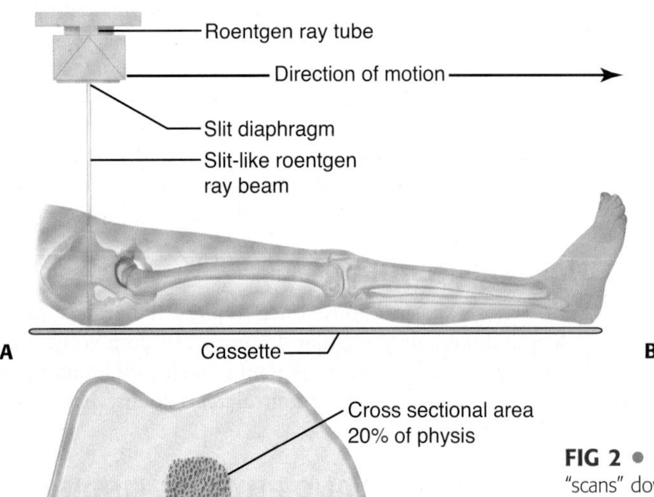


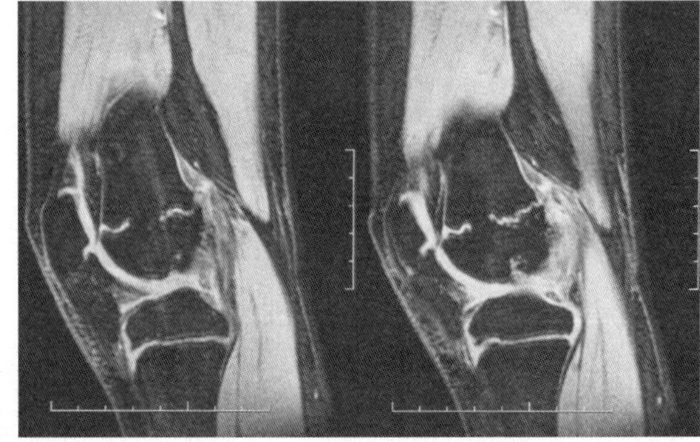


**FIG 2** • **A.** A true scanogram uses a slit beam of radiation that moves or "scans" down the length of the extremity. Because the radiation beam always remains perpendicular to the film, there is no magnification of the radiographic image, and distances can accurately be measured directly on the radiograph. The entire limb is included on the image so angular deformity can be measured as well as length. Using multiple CT or MRI images (**B**), a map of the physeal bar is created (**C**) and the relative cross-sectional area of the bar is estimated.

## NONOPERATIVE MANAGEMENT

- Anticipated lower extremity limb length discrepancy of less than 1 cm requires no treatment.
- The simplest means of correcting a lower extremity limb length discrepancy is to place a lift either inside or on the bottom of the shoe on the shorter limb.
- Anticipated lower extremity discrepancy of 1 or 2 cm is most easily treated with a shoe lift inside the shoe.
- Discrepancy greater than 2 cm treated nonoperatively is typically managed by a lift placed on the shoe sole.
- There is no effective nonoperative treatment to correct clinically significant angular deformity caused by a physeal bar.

## SURGICAL MANAGEMENT

- Lower extremity physeal arrest resection should be considered in patients with an anticipated growth remaining from the affected physis of about 2 years or 2 cm.
- Pure length discrepancy in the upper extremity caused by a physeal bar in the proximal humerus causes little functional problem, and anticipated discrepancy of up to 5 cm may be observed.
- Bone length discrepancy in a two-bone limb segment such as the forearm or leg is less well tolerated. Anticipated bone length discrepancy of greater than 1 cm at the wrist may warrant surgical treatment either by physeal bar resection or complete epiphysiodesis of both bones to prevent bone length discrepancy.
- Surgical treatment for a physeal bar may consist of physeal bar resection, complete epiphysiodesis of the involved physis, epiphysiodesis of the adjacent bone in leg or forearm, epiphysiodesis of the contralateral physis, or an approach combining more than one of these.[8] The surgical technique for physeal bar resection alone will be discussed in the following text.
- If the decision has been made to perform physeal bar excision and an angular deformity is present, one is faced with the question whether an osteotomy should be performed at the time of physeal arrest resection to correct angular deformity.
  - Our philosophy is to first perform physeal bar resection alone.
  - Physeal bar resection is a relatively minor procedure with rapid recovery and the potential to correct (at least partially) the angular deformity. Accurate prediction of angular correction after physeal bar resection is not possible, making it very difficult to know with certainty the degree of osteotomy angular correction to perform.
  - We would prefer to perform physeal bar resection alone first, then correct any residual angular deformity when physeal growth is complete.
  - At skeletal maturity, the target is no longer moving and any additional adjustment in limb length can be addressed as well.

### Preoperative Planning

- Imaging studies are reviewed, and a map of the size and location of the physeal bar is created.
- A strategy is determined to provide the safest and most direct surgical approach to the physeal bar.

### Positioning

- The patient is positioned to facilitate a direct approach to the physeal bar. For example, if a lateral approach is determined to be the most direct and safe route to a distal femoral bar, the patient is positioned with a generous bump elevating the hemipelvis and affected limb, with a tourniquet placed on the proximal thigh.
- Fluoroscopy is used to guide physeal bar resection, so the patient must be placed on a radiolucent table in a position to facilitate AP and lateral fluoroscopic images.

### Approach

- The particular approach for each patient is determined by the location of the physis affected by the physeal bar and the location of the bar within the physis.
- A direct approach to the bone surface at the level of the physis is used for peripheral bars.
- Central physeal bar resection is typically performed by approaching the physis through the metaphysis adjacent to the physeal bar.
- The general strategy for central physeal bar excision in a long bone is to access the bar through a metaphyseal bone tunnel, resect the bar, and place an interposition material that will prevent recurrent bar formation (**FIG 3**).

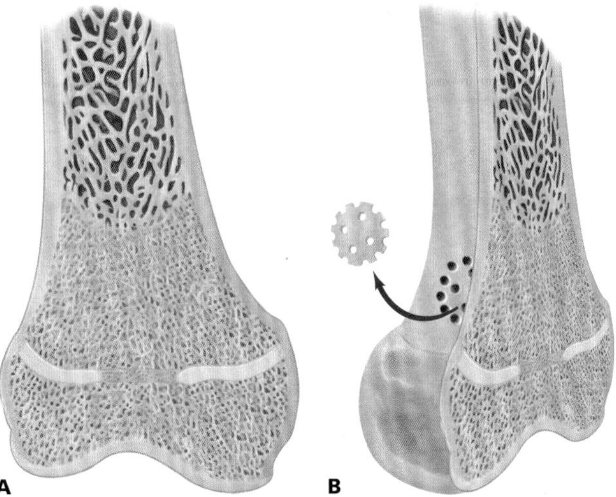


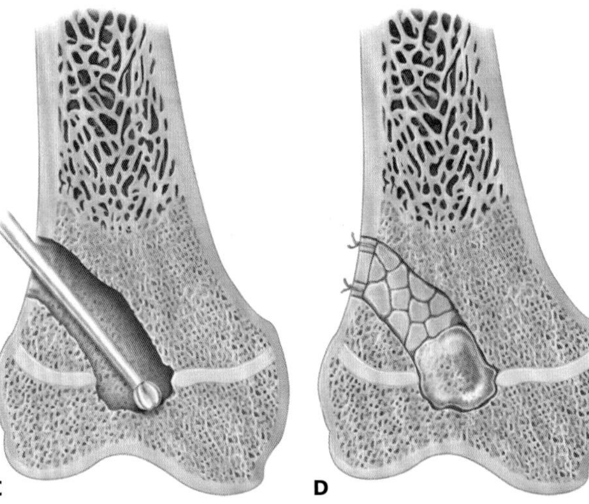


**FIG 3** • The general strategy for central physeal bar resection (**A**) is to create a cortical window (**B**) through which the surgeon can excise the bar (**C**) and then place interposition material (**D**) to prevent bar recurrence. (Adapted from Peterson HA. Partial growth plate arrest and its treatment. J Pediatr Orthop 1984;4:246–258.)

## Physeal Bar Localization

- With the patient prepared and draped, fluoroscopy is brought into the field and the location of the physis is marked on the skin surface.
- Next, using a blunt pin or straight instrument, mark on the skin the desired approach trajectory to the physeal bar.
- Draw the skin incision line on the approach trajectory (**TECH FIG 1A**).
- Exsanguinate the limb and incise the skin longitudinally where an internervous plane can be used.
- With metaphyseal bone exposed, using AP and lateral fluoroscopic imaging, consider advancing a Kirschner wire or Steinmann pin along the approach trajectory from the metaphysis into the center of the physeal bar.
  - This Kirschner wire will act as a guide to the location and depth of the physeal bar (**TECH FIG 1B**).
- Using multiple drill holes and an osteotome, create an oval cortical window in metaphyseal bone (**TECH FIG 1C**).
- Remove and save the cortical window and superficial metaphyseal bone to be used for later closure.
- As the tip of the reference Kirschner wire is approached, use a motorized burr to carefully remove bone until the center of the physeal bar is reached, as confirmed fluoroscopically.
- Within the center of the physeal bar, no physis will be seen. Under fluoroscopic guidance, use the motorized burr to carefully expand the area of resection until normal physis is encountered (**TECH FIG 1D**).
- Computer navigation has also been described as another technique used to assist with physeal bar localization and resection.[3]

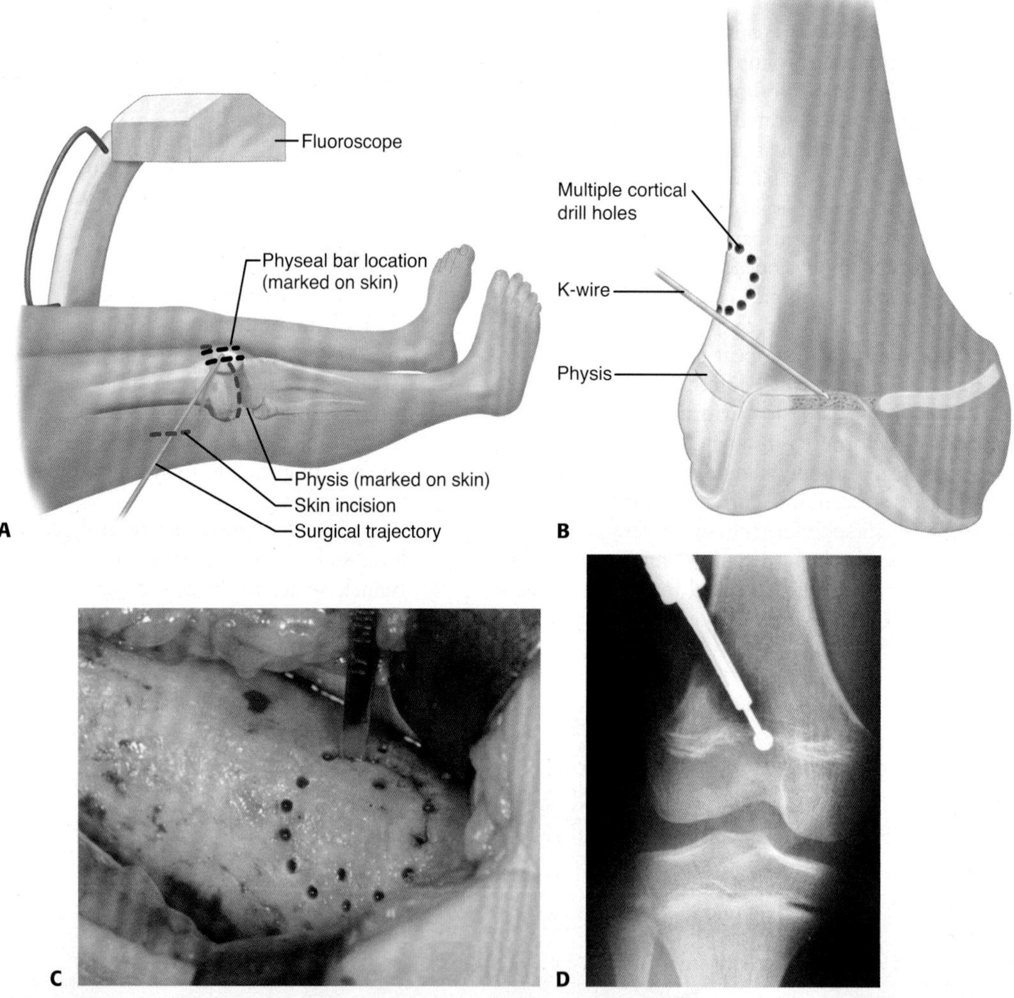


**TECH FIG 1** • **A.** Before making a skin incision, fluoroscopy is brought into the surgical field and the surgeon draws on the skin the physis location, the physeal bar location, the surgical approach trajectory, and the skin incision location that will permit the desired approach. **B.** Under fluoroscopic guidance, a Kirschner wire is advanced to the level of the physeal bar along the desired surgical approach trajectory. Multiple drill holes are then made that incorporate the Kirschner wire into the periphery of an elliptical cortical window. The Kirschner wire will act as a guide to the location and depth of the physeal bar. **C.** Multiple drill holes are connected with a narrow osteotome to create a cortical window. The window is saved and replaced during closure. (Kirschner wire guide is not shown in this photograph.) **D.** After removing metaphyseal bone with a curette, a burr is guided by fluoroscopy to expand the bar resection cavity until normal physis is visualized within the cavity. (**C,D:** From Peterson HA. Epiphyseal Growth Plate Fractures. Heidelberg: Springer, 2007. With kind permission of Spring Science and Business Media.)

## Bar Resection

- Once the physis is identified within the resection cavity, the motorized burr is used to remove bone along the leading edge of the exposed physis until normal-appearing physis is exposed throughout the entire circumference of the resection cavity.
  - The exposed normal physis should appear flat and smooth (**TECH FIG 2A**).
- A surgical headlight is helpful to visualize the physis within the resection cavity.
- If a region of the resection area cannot be seen by direct vision, use a dental mirror to visualize the physis and confirm complete physeal bar excision (**TECH FIG 2B**).
- A 70-degree arthroscope may also be used to visualize the physis.[5]
- Topical liquid thrombin may be applied to the resection cavity bone surface to reduce hematoma formation, which in theory might promote recurrent bar formation.

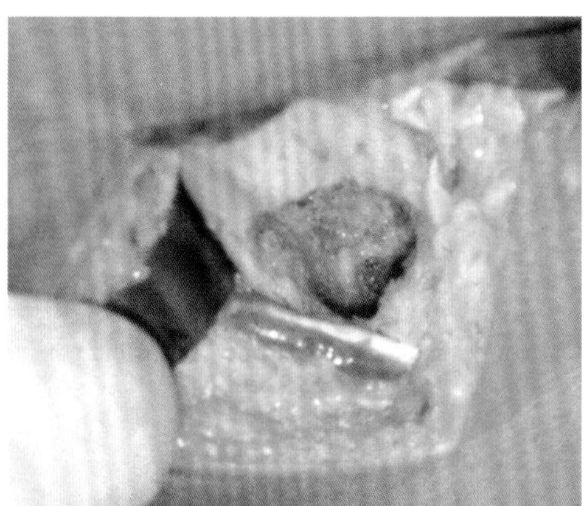
A

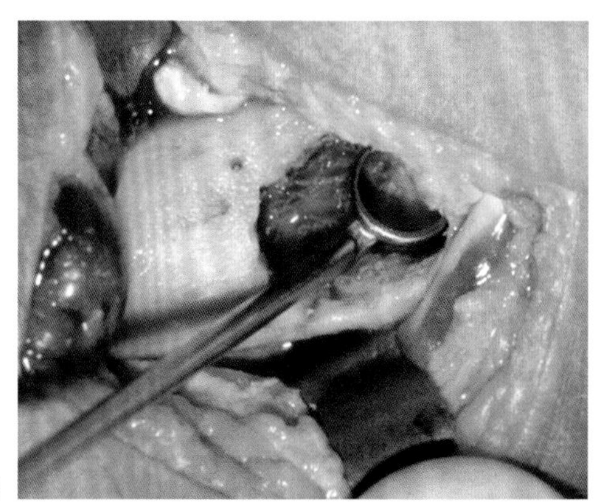
B

**TECH FIG 2 • A.** Within the resection cavity, the physis should appear smooth, flat, and healthy after bar resection. **B.** A dental mirror is used to look back at the physis in regions within the cavity where the physis cannot be directly visualized. At the conclusion of bar resection, normal physis should be visualized as a continuous cartilage line around the full circumference of the resection cavity.

## Marker Placement

- Place titanium markers in the epiphysis and metaphysis to facilitate later measurement of physeal growth (**TECH FIG 3A**).
  - Marker position in the center of the bone prevents the metaphyseal marker from becoming extraosseous with future remodeling.
  - Our preference is a titanium 0.062 Kirschner wire notched 10 mm from the tip, which can be broken off within bone (**TECH FIG 3B**).
  - Titanium markers avoid artifact on subsequent MRI or CT scans.

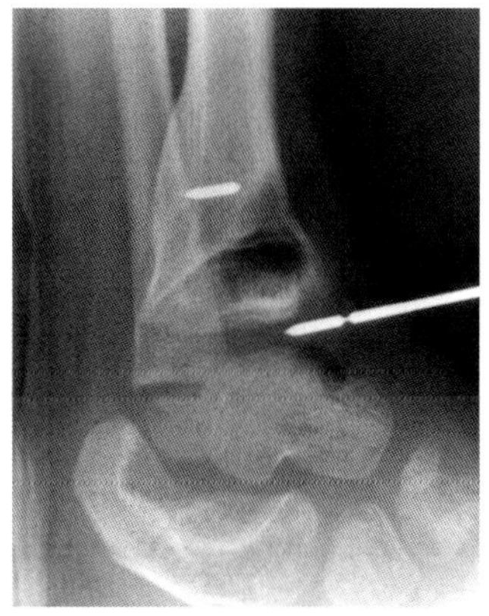
A

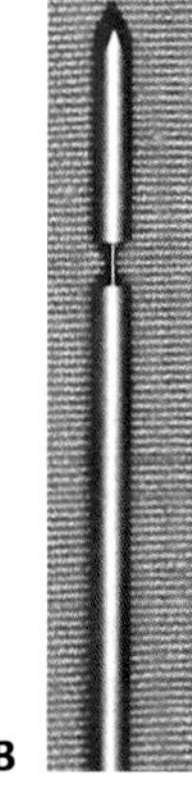
B

**TECH FIG 3 • A.** The first titanium marker has been placed centrally within the metaphysis proximal to the physis. A second marker is going to be placed within the epiphysis distal to the physis. **B.** A 0.062 titanium Kirschner wire notched 10 mm from the end makes an ideal radiographic marker that will not interfere with future MRI imaging. (From Peterson HA. Epiphyseal Growth Plate Fractures. Heidelberg: Springer, 2007. With kind permission of Spring Science and Business Media.)

## Cranioplast Interposition

- An interposition material is then placed in the physeal bar defect. Some authors have recommended fat as an interposition material, but we prefer cranioplast polymethylmethacrylate for several reasons:
  - Cranioplast has a slow polymerization rate and does not generate heat, which might be harmful to the physis.
  - Cranioplast confers immediate structural strength to the resection area, allowing full weight bearing after surgery.
  - No loosening has ever been reported after physeal bar resection.
  - Cranioplast stays securely within the resection bed and cannot "float" out of the resection bed on hematoma.
  - An additional incision to harvest fat interposition material is avoided.
- Cranioplast can be injected into the resection defect in its liquid state, or it can be allowed to polymerize to the consistency of putty, then gently digitally pressurized into the cancellous bone of the resection bed, preventing displacement.

## Fat Interposition

- If fat is chosen as the interposition material, a donor site must be chosen.
  - Rarely, in a patient with a small physeal bar, local fat may be harvested.
  - Most patients require harvesting fat from a distant site and the gluteal region is typically used.
- Our current indications for fat interposition material include the following:
  - Physeal bars caused by infection, where this is a concern for recurrent infection
  - Peripheral physeal bar resection, where cranioplast may become prominent during future growth and remodeling (**TECH FIG 4**)
- Not being adherent to tissue, fat has the potential to become displaced from the bar resection area, resulting in recurrent physeal arrest.[2]

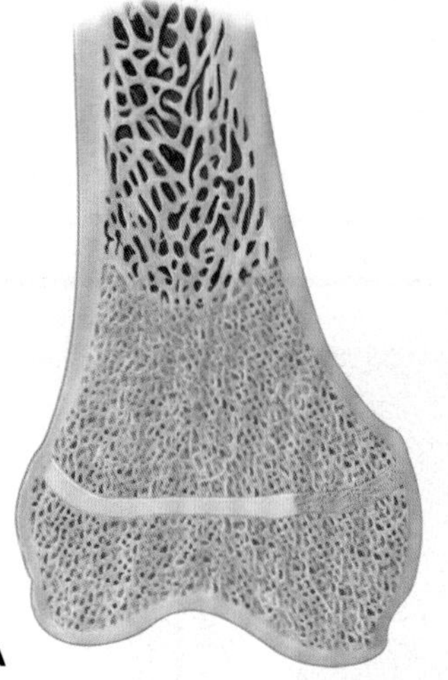


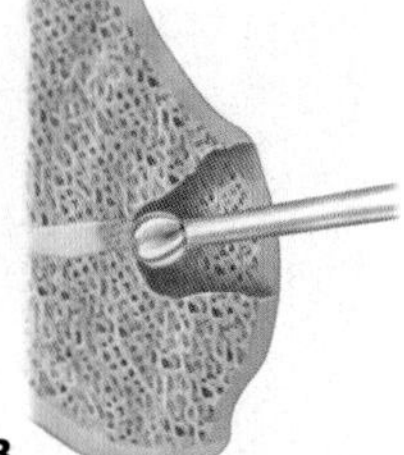


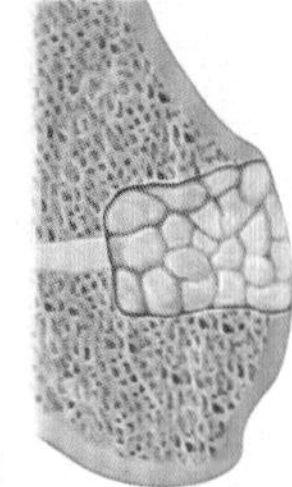


**TECH FIG 4** • Peripheral physeal bar resection (**A**) is performed by approaching the bar directly (no bone tunnel) and excising the bar with a burr (**B**). Fat works well as an interposition material for peripheral bars (**C**) because bone remodeling and growth may result in cranioplast becoming prominent with time. (Adapted from Peterson HA. Partial growth plate arrest and its treatment. J Pediatr Orthop 1984;4:246–258.)

## Closure

- After placement of the interposition material, cancellous bone saved during exposure is gently packed into the remaining bone cavity.
- The cortical window of bone is replaced and may be sutured in place if desired.
- Periosteum is closed over the cortical bone window.

## PEARLS AND PITFALLS

| | |
|---|---|
| **Detection** | ▪ Absence or angulation of a Harris growth "resumption" line at the injured physis, especially when present at the contralateral physis, may be an early sign of physeal bar formation (**FIG 4**). |

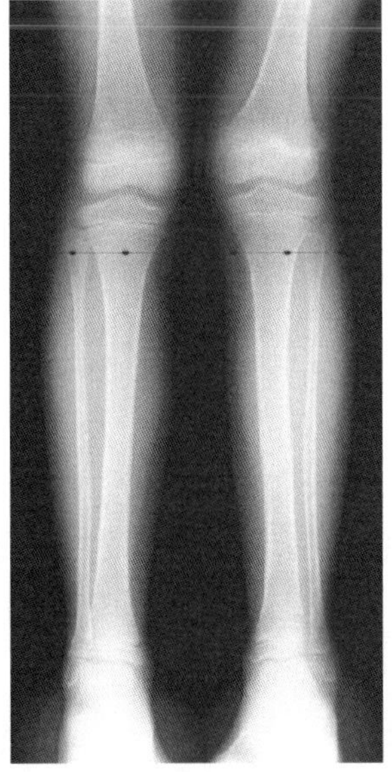
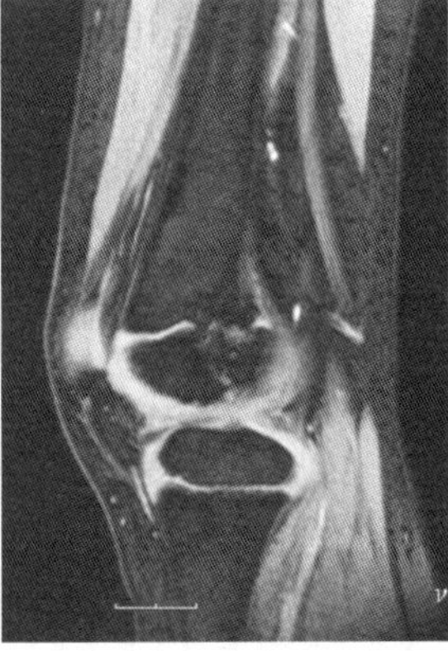

**FIG 4** ● A 7-year-old girl was referred for evaluation of limb length discrepancy 9 months after sustaining a Salter-Harris type IV fracture of the distal left femur. **A.** Scanogram demonstrates the presence of a Harris growth resumption line on the right but absent on the left and a 9-mm limb length discrepancy. **B.** MRI confirms the presence of an eccentric physeal bar.

| | |
|---|---|
| **Indications** | ▪ For older patients with limited growth remaining, the surgeon should consider epiphysiodesis to prevent angular deformity or limb or bone length discrepancy from occurring. |
| **Technique** | ▪ Placement of a reference Kirschner wire along the line of resection into the center of the physeal arrest is very helpful in providing guidance while the surgeon is working "blind" until normal physis is exposed.<br>▪ Removing initial bone with a curette and saving it to fill the resection cavity after interposition material has been placed facilitates rapid healing and return to full strength. |
| **Inadequate resection** | ▪ Insufficient physeal bar resection may lead to recurrent bar formation. The physis should appear relatively normal around the entire circumference of the resection cavity, not narrowed and irregular. |
| **Inadequate follow-up** | ▪ On average, each patient is likely to benefit from at least one additional procedure as a consequence of their physeal bar. Follow-up until skeletal maturity is essential. |

## POSTOPERATIVE CARE

- At the conclusion of the operation, local anesthetic is injected into the incision site, ketorolac (Toradol) is administered unless there is a medical contraindication, and the patient is placed in a gentle compressive dressing, which is removed on the first postoperative day.
- Patients are allowed to bear weight as tolerated with crutches as needed for comfort, and early active joint range of motion is encouraged.
- Noncontact sports are typically permitted 3 months after surgery and full-contact sports are allowed 6 months postoperatively in most patients.

## OUTCOMES

- One hundred patients treated at the Mayo Clinic with physeal bar resection in the femur or tibia were followed to skeletal maturity.[10]
  - Thirteen percent of the patients required no additional treatment; the physeal bar was definitively treated by a single physeal bar resection procedure.
  - Ninety-four patients of the patients did experience some growth after physeal arrest resection.
  - Restored physeal growth was, on average, 86% of the contralateral physeal growth rate.
  - 118 additional procedures were performed, for an average of 1.2 additional procedures per patient.
  - In all patients (except the six in whom there was no growth), any subsequent surgery was of lesser magnitude than would have been necessary had physeal bar resection not been performed.

## COMPLICATIONS

- In 100 patients treated at the Mayo Clinic with physeal bar resection and cranioplast interposition followed to skeletal maturity, 2 patients had a surgical wound infection and 2 patients had a late fracture at the cranioplast site, for a total complication rate of 4%.[10]
- Fracture through the resection cavity after using fat as an interposition material has also been reported.[4]

## REFERENCES


1. Dietz FR, Morcuende JA. Embryology and development of the musculoskeletal system. In: Morrissy RT, Weinstein SL, eds. Lovell and Winter's Pediatric Orthopaedics, ed 6. Philadelphia: Lippincott Williams & Williams, 2005:1–33.
2. Hasler CC, Foster BK. Secondary tethers after physeal bar resection: a common source of failure? Clin Orthop Relat Res 2002;(405):242–249.
3. Kang HG, Yoon SJ, Kim JR. Resection of a physeal bar under computer assisted guidance. J Bone Joint Surg Br 2010;92(10):1452–145.
4. Langenskiöld A. Surgical treatment of partial closure of the growth plate. J Pediatr Orthop 1981;1:3–11.
5. Marsh JS, Polzhofer GK. Arthroscopically assisted central physeal bar resection. J Pediatr Orthop 2006;26(2):255–259.
6. Ogden JA. Injury to the growth mechanisms of the immature skeleton. Skeletal Radiol 1981;6:237–253.
7. Peterson HA. Epiphyseal Growth Plate Fractures. Heidelberg: Springer, 2007.
8. Peterson HA. Partial growth plate arrest and its treatment. J Pediatr Orthop 1984;4:246–258.
9. Salter RB, Harris WR. Injuries involving the epiphyseal plate. J Bone Joint Surg Am 1963;45A:587–622.
10. Stans AA, Klassen RA, Shaughnessy WJ, et al. Excision of partial physeal arrest followed to skeletal maturity. Presented at AAOS Annual Meeting, Chicago, IL, 2006.

# Repair of Congenital Pseudarthrosis of the Tibia with the Williams Rod

58

CHAPTER

Perry L. Schoenecker and Margaret M. Rich

## DEFINITION

- Congenital pseudarthrosis of the tibia follows pathologic fracture of a tibia.[2,4]
- In most cases, the pseudarthrosis is preceded by increasing anterolateral bowing of the tibia.[8]
- Spontaneous healing does not occur; shortening and angulation with instability are progressive and impair ambulation.
- Surgical treatment with a solid intramedullary rod and bone graft and long-term protection with a total contact orthosis can provide lasting consolidation and minimize secondary deformity.[1,3,5,7,9]
- Inability to achieve stable union may necessitate amputation.[5,7]

## ANATOMY

- The tibia is abnormal from birth; however, this may not become apparent until weight bearing begins. The remainder of the extremity is normal.
- Most patients will have anterolateral bowing that increases to the point of pathologic fracture.
- Shortening is common and tends to increase after fracture.
- As the anterior bowing increases, the foot may assume a dorsiflexed position to maintain contact with the floor.
- Involvement of the fibula is variable and may worsen as the tibial pseudarthrosis progresses.
- Nearly all cases are unilateral.

## PATHOGENESIS

- Anterolateral bowing, when present, increases with weight bearing as the mechanical axis falls farther behind the axis of the tibia. Additionally, the calf musculature acts like a bowstring and increases tension within the tibia, leading to failure.
- Most pseudarthroses occur in the middle to distal third of the tibia.
- The pseudarthrosis comprises hamartomatous fibrous tissue, not neurofibroma.
- Fibular bowing or pseudarthrosis compounds the deformity and further compromises stability.[7,8]

## NATURAL HISTORY

- Rarely, bowing or sclerosis is present and does not progress to fracture and pseudarthrosis.
- Once established, the pseudarthrosis remains and does not resolve spontaneously. The resultant instability and shortening interferes with normal ambulation.
- Use of a total contact orthosis may slow the progression and postpone, but, not eliminate the need for surgical intervention.
- More severe deformities become symptomatic at an earlier age, occasionally presenting in infancy.

## PATIENT HISTORY AND PHYSICAL FINDINGS

- The most common presenting complaint is anterolateral bowing of the tibia (**FIG 1**).[2,4] Shortening of the involved extremity may not be apparent at presentation.
- Pain is absent unless the tibia has fractured acutely.
- Limp or dull aching may precede pathologic fracture.
- Over half of these patients have neurofibromatosis (NF) type I.[4,8]
- The skin should be closely inspected for café-au-lait spots, axillary or inguinal freckles, or neurofibromas as signs of underlying NF.
- A family history of NF may be present.
- Referral to a geneticist is recommended for confirmation of the diagnosis and genetic counseling.

## IMAGING AND OTHER DIAGNOSTIC STUDIES

- Anteroposterior (AP) and lateral plain radiographs of the affected tibia are sufficient for diagnosis (**FIG 2**).
- The radiographic appearance of the tibia is variable: it may be cystic, sclerotic, or atrophic. There may be involvement throughout the tibia.[2–4]

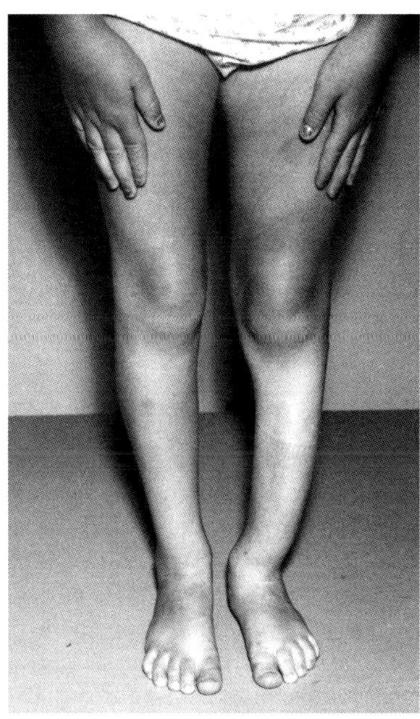

**FIG 1** • Standing AP photo of lower extremities. Anterior and lateral bowing is present in the left tibia of this 4-year-old girl. Shortening is minimal. The foot, knee, and thigh appear normal. Note multiple café-au-lait spots on the thighs and lateral side of the right leg, one of the major criteria of type I NF.

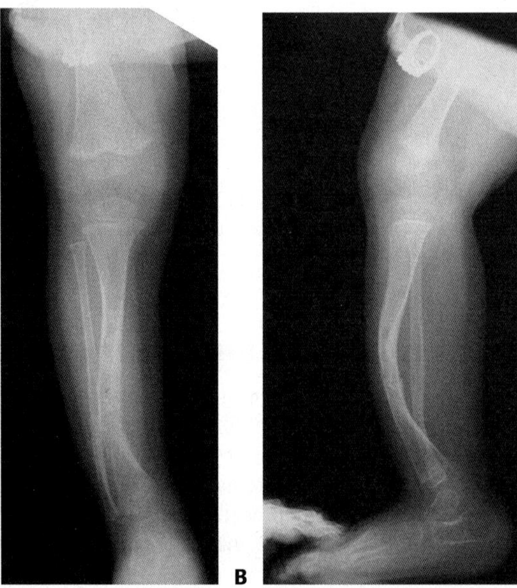


**FIG 2** • **A.** AP radiograph of the tibia at age 13 months demonstrates lateral bowing of the tibia and fibula. The medullary canal of the tibia is widened and has a cystic appearance. **B.** The accompanying lateral view shows the anterior bow with a mixed cystic and sclerotic medullary canal of the tibia. Note the relative dorsiflexed position of the foot as compensation for the anterior angulation of the distal tibia. A total contact orthosis is used to support the extremity and slow progression of the deformity.

- Mild deformities present with bowing and mild sclerosis at the apex. The medullary canal can be narrow or expanded, with a cystic appearance.
- After fracture, little callus forms and the bone tends to become more atrophic in appearance.
- Severe deformities show resorption of bone at the pseudarthrosis, increasing fibular deformity, and tapering of the bone ends (the "pulled taffy" appearance).

## DIFFERENTIAL DIAGNOSIS

- Ring constriction or amniotic band syndrome
- Fibrous dysplasia
- Osteofibrous dysplasia
- Osteomyelitis
- Fibrosarcoma of infancy
- Fibular hemimelia (total absence of the fibula)

## NONOPERATIVE MANAGEMENT

- Use of a total contact ankle–foot orthosis (AFO) or knee-ankle-foot orthosis (KAFO) provides mechanical support for the tibia, particularly in toddlers and young children.[8]
- Pathologic fracture in a very young child can be treated with cast immobilization if the bowing deformity is mild.
- Nonoperative measures are useful to postpone the age for surgical treatment, allowing the use of a larger intramedullary rod and greater volume of available autologous bone graft.

## SURGICAL MANAGEMENT

- The presence of a pseudarthrosis warrants operative treatment to stabilize the tibia and provide a sufficient biologic framework for healing.[1,3,5–9]
- The intramedullary rod is designed to provide long-term stabilization of the tibial pseudarthrosis as the child grows. The rod remains in place, anchored by press-fit in the medullary canal. The proximal tibia and the distal tibia grow away from the ends of the rod.[10]
- Younger children may require exchange with a longer rod if needed to maintain support of the tibia and stabilization of the pseudarthrosis.

### Preoperative Planning

- The dimensions of an appropriate-sized rod can be determined from the plain films. The width of the medullary canal adjacent to the pseudarthrosis dictates the diameter of rod to be used. The length of the rod is determined from the lateral film.[6]
- The anticipated length of tibia to be resected to healthy bone is also measured; it is usually 1 to 2 cm.
- In young children (younger than 8 years) and in those with a very distal pseudarthrosis, the intramedullary rod should cross the ankle and subtalar joints to provide maximum stabilization because of the short distal tibial segment. The distance from the proximal tibial physis to the bottom of the calcaneus is measured. That length minus the amount to be resected is the length of intramedullary rod to be used.
- In older children (more than 8 years), the rod can be placed within the tibia and does not need to remain across the ankle or subtalar joints. The distance from the proximal tibial physis to the distal tibial physis minus the amount of tibia to be resected is the length of rod that will be needed.
- The Williams rod is made up of two sections: The section with the female coupling remains within the tibia and the piece with the male coupling is used as an introducer or pusher rod and is not considered in the selection of rod length (**FIG 3**). The rod can be cut or trimmed intraoperatively if needed to adjust the length.[6]
- If additional angular deformity is present in the tibia, an osteotomy may be needed to allow passage of the straight rod within the medullary canal.
- If a fibular pseudarthrosis is also present, it should also be stabilized using an intramedullary Kirschner wire. If the fibula is intact, osteotomy may be needed to facilitate preparation of the tibia and introduction of the intramedullary rod.[7,8]

### Positioning

- The patient is supine for preparation and rodding of the tibia. Before this, an iliac bone graft is obtained.
  - For small children, the graft should be obtained from the posterior iliac crest. In those cases, the child is positioned in the lateral decubitus position and is prepared from the waist to the toes.
  - For larger children, a bump can be placed under the buttock to facilitate positioning for an anterior iliac crest graft. It is removed before proceeding with the tibial exposure.

### Approach

- The tibia is approached directly along the anterior subcutaneous border. The incision is centered over the pseudarthrosis and extends 3 to 4 cm above and below that level.
- The fibula is approached through a longitudinal incision, centered over the fibular pseudarthrosis, anterior to the peroneal muscles.

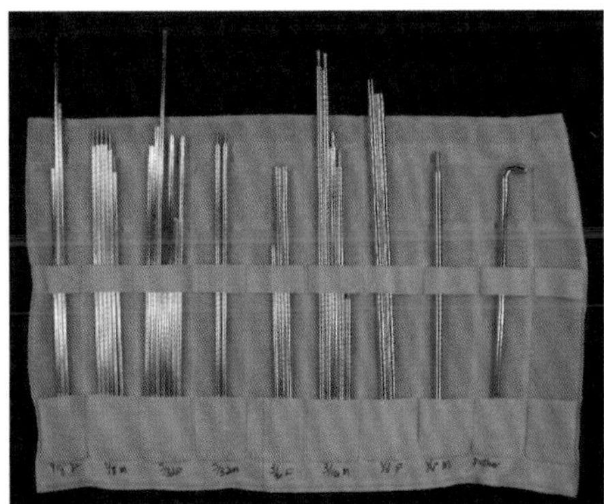

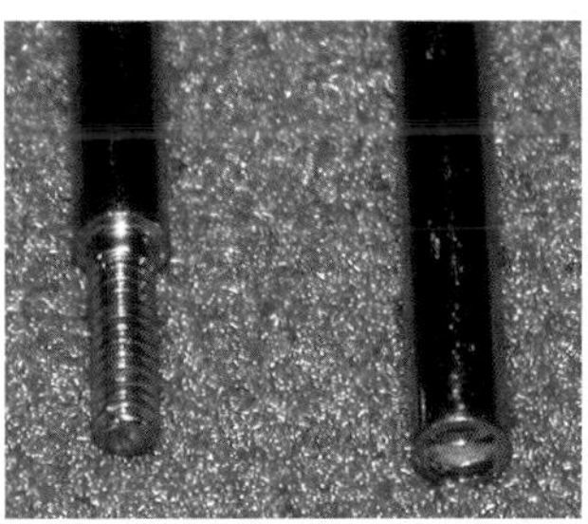

**FIG 3** • **A.** This assortment of Williams rods includes the female rod, which will remain within the tibia, and the complementary male rod used for insertion. Ideally, variable lengths and widths should be available. Selection of the appropriate-sized rod is based on the width of the medullary canal on the AP and lateral plain films. The length is estimated using the lateral film, measuring from the proximal tibial physis to the distal physis or bottom of the calcaneus, depending on the need to include the ankle and subtalar joints, and subtracting the length of the pseudarthrosis to be resected. The rod is to be coaxial with the tibia and of maximum length to minimize recurrent bowing above and below the rod as growth continues. **B.** Close-up view of the ends of the male and female sections. The male rod with the knurled end is the distal section and will be removed. The female flat, threaded end will be left in place. If the rod chosen is too long, it can be shortened using a bolt cutter and the tip of the rod removed, leaving the threaded end intact.

TECHNIQUES

## Obtaining the Iliac Crest Bone Graft

### Posterior Iliac Graft

- A 6-cm incision is made following the contour of the posterior medial corner of the iliac crest.
- The incision is carried down through the subcutaneous tissue, exposing the fascia overlying the iliac crest and abductor musculature.
- The apophyseal cartilage is exposed along the ilium and is split in half, sharply, along the course of the iliac crest. The lateral (superficial) half of the apophyseal cartilage and attached periosteum is elevated to expose the outer table of the ilium, subperiosteally.
- An osteotome is used to cut the outer table. Cortical and cancellous strips are obtained.
- The apophysis is reapproximated with interrupted sutures. A drain is used at the surgeon's discretion. The subcutaneous layer and skin are closed, and the patient is then rolled to the supine position.

### Anterior Iliac Crest Graft

- In larger children, the anterior iliac crest can be used.
- The approach is similar except that the incision is centered over the anterolateral ilium.

## Preparation of the Tibia

- A sterile thigh tourniquet is applied and inflated.
- A 6- to 8-cm longitudinal incision is made over the tibial pseudarthrosis, along the subcutaneous border.
- The tibia is exposed subperiosteally and circumferentially around the pseudarthrosis.
  - The plane for subperiosteal dissection is more readily identified proximal and distal to the pseudarthrosis rather than directly over it.
  - The fibrous tissue within the pseudarthrosis is removed to expose the bone. A combination of sharp dissection, rongeur, and curettage is used.
  - The pseudarthrosis must be excised in addition to the abnormal dense, sclerotic bone adjacent to it.
  - The medullary canal can be probed and identified with a small curette.
- A drill bit, smaller in diameter than the intramedullary rod to be inserted, is used to open and enlarge the medullary canal above and below the pseudarthrosis (**TECH FIG 1A**).
  - The C-arm image is used to ensure that the canal preparation is not eccentric.
- If secondary bowing is present, it may not be possible to remain within the central medullary canal. Osteotomy of the tibia at that level should allow passage of the drill bit, remaining central in the medullary canal.
- Distally, the drill bit is passed through the tibia, stopping at the physis.
- If the rod will be left across the ankle and subtalar joints, a similar-sized smooth Kirschner wire is used to perforate the talus and calcaneus. Care must be taken to hold the foot and ankle in a neutral position during this process.
- Preparation of the tibia is complete when the drill bit can be passed through the proximal fragment up to the physis and distally to the physis.
  - The drill bit should be centered within the tibia in both the AP and lateral images (**TECH FIG 1B**).

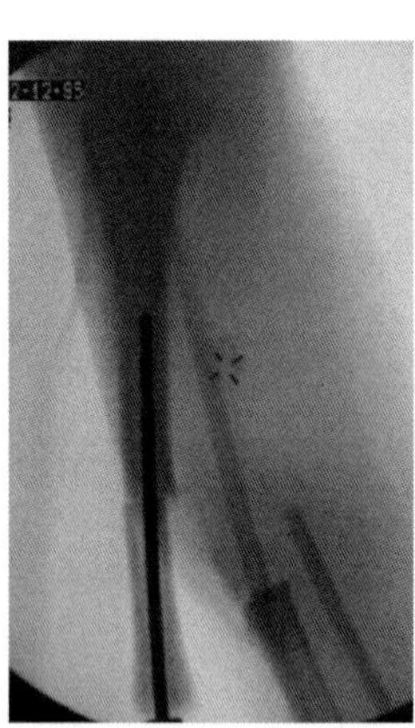

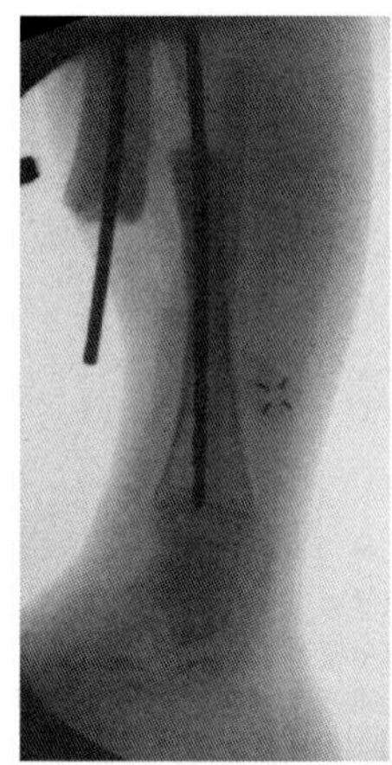

**TECH FIG 1** • Preparation of the tibia. **A.** A drill bit is used to open the medullary canal proximal and distal to the pseudarthrosis. C-arm image intensification is used to maintain central positioning within the medullary canal on the AP and lateral views. If there is severe bowing of the tibia, an osteotomy may be needed to prevent eccentric reaming, as in this patient. **B.** Lateral C-arm image of the distal tibia showing central position of the drill bit, stopping just above the distal physis. A similar-sized Kirschner wire can be used to cross the physis, talus, and calcaneus if needed prior to rod insertion.

## Preparation of the Fibula

- A fibular pseudarthrosis is approached through a lateral incision, anterior to the peroneals. The fibula is exposed subperiosteally and the fibrous tissue and adjacent pathologic bone are removed, as in the tibia.
  - Care must be taken to avoid injury to the deep motor branches of the peroneal nerve just medial to the fibula.
- Ideally, the fibula is stabilized with an intramedullary Kirschner wire. This is inserted through the distal fragment, exiting the skin at the tip of the fibula. After insertion of the tibial rod, the wire is then drilled into the proximal fibula. In some cases, this cannot be accomplished because the fibula is too atrophic.
- An intact fibula may interfere with preparation of the tibia, as it can limit mobilization of the proximal and distal fragments. It can also prevent contact of the tibial fragments. Osteotomy of the fibula will resolve the issue. It may be necessary to resect a portion to allow compression across the tibia.

## Stabilization with the Williams Rod

- The length of the rod is checked before insertion by reducing the tibia, laying the rod next to the leg, and noting the position of the rod proximally and distally.
  - The proximal point should be just below the proximal tibial physis.
  - The flat, distal end (female) should be at the distal tibial physis (if the rod is to remain within the tibia) or within the calcaneus (if the rod will stabilize the ankle and subtalar joints).
  - If the rod is too long, the pointed end can be cut on an angle to the appropriate length.
- The rod sections are assembled by twisting the two sections together. A power drill is used to insert the pusher section into the distal fragment and it is advanced antegrade, across the ankle and subtalar joints, exiting the bottom of the foot through the heel pad (**TECH FIG 2A**).
  - The foot must be kept in a neutral position both in plantarflexion and dorsiflexion as well as varus–valgus alignment.
  - A small incision may be needed to relieve the skin tension around the rod (**TECH FIG 2B**).
- The drill is detached from the proximal rod section and reattached to the distal rod, exiting the foot. The rod is drawn into the distal fragment (**TECH FIG 2C**).
- The tibia is reduced and the rod advanced retrograde across the pseudarthrosis into the proximal tibia, stopping adjacent to the tibial physis (**TECH FIG 2D,E**).
  - C-arm imaging is used to ensure concentric location of the rod within the tibia (**TECH FIG 2F,G**).
- The rod is grasped through the pseudarthrosis; with the drill on reverse, the pusher rod will disengage the female section (**TECH FIG 2H**). Spot C-arm images are used to confirm satisfactory position of the rod before the pusher is completely removed.
- Contact of the tibial fragments is confirmed visually. If the fragments are distracted, the surgeon should osteotomize or remove more fibula to ensure contact is made.
- The fibular Kirschner wire is advanced into the proximal fibula and cut flush with the tip of the fibula.
- The bone graft is placed circumferentially about the tibia (**TECH FIG 2I**). Cortical strips can be secured with loops of suture placed around the tibia. Cancellous bone is placed within and across the pseudarthrosis.
- The tourniquet is deflated and circulation assessed around the repair and in the foot.
- The periosteum usually cannot be closed over the bone graft. The wound is closed in layers over a drain.

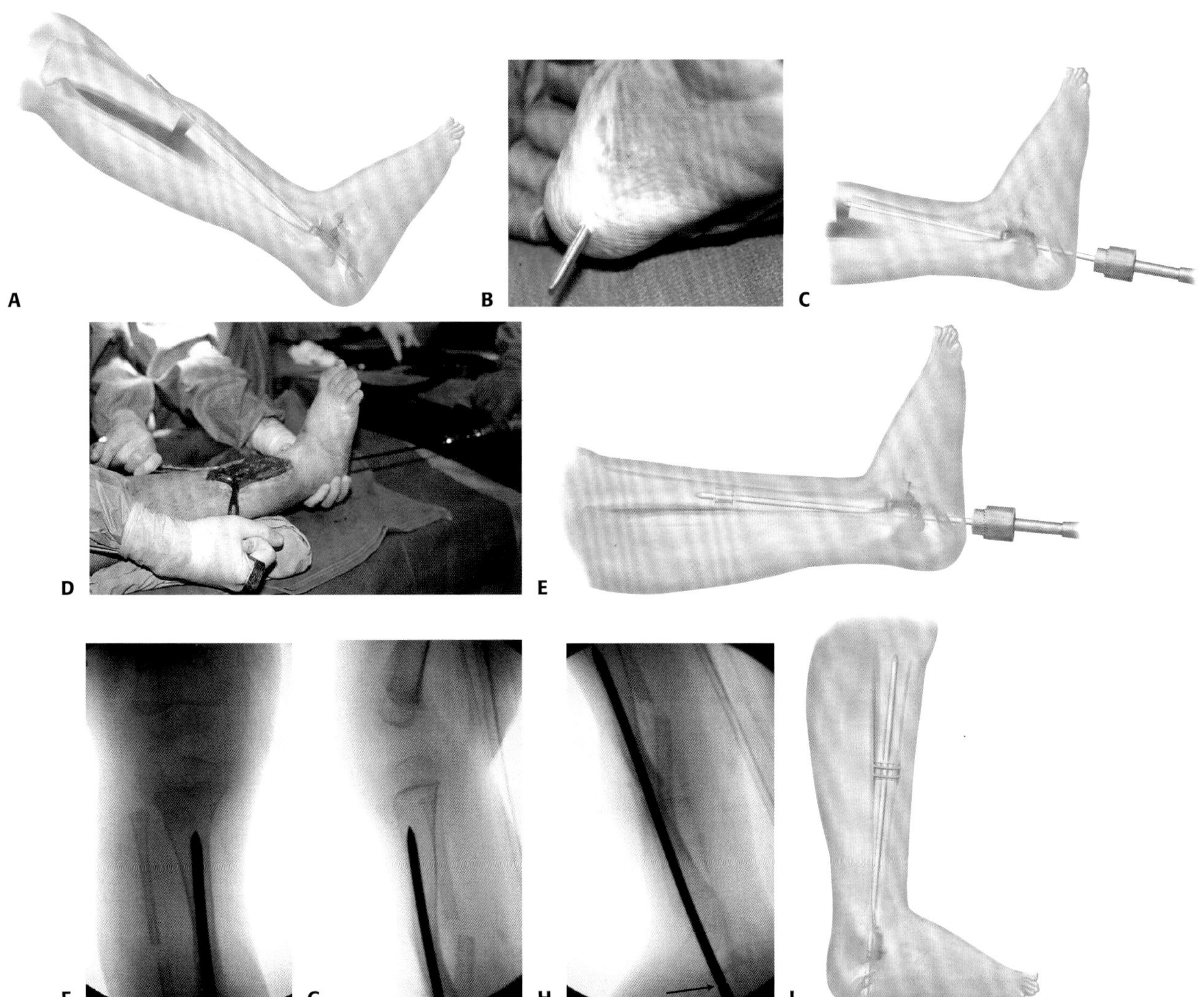

**TECH FIG 2** ● **A.** The male section of the Williams rod is inserted antegrade into the distal segment and advanced through the talus and calcaneus. The foot must be held in neutral flexion and mediolateral angulation as the rod is passed. **B.** The Williams rod is pushed through the heel pad as it exits the foot. A small incision may be needed to relieve the skin tension around the rod. **C.** The Williams rod is assembled by twisting the male and female sections together. The drill is attached to the exposed tip of the male section, and the rod is drawn into the distal fragment. Note the neutral position of the foot relative to the tibia. **D,E.** The tibial fragments are approximated, and the rod is advanced retrograde into the proximal tibia. **F.** As the rod is advanced, C-arm images are used to confirm satisfactory coaxial positioning of the rod in both planes. This AP view shows satisfactory position. The rod fills the middle of the canal. A fibular shortening osteotomy has also been completed to allow contact of the tibial fragments. This is usually necessary to avoid distraction by an intact fibula after resection of the pseudarthrosis. **G.** Lateral C-arm image of the advancing rod. The rod is slightly anterior and can be withdrawn and redirected posteriorly to achieve a satisfactory position. In the presence of more severe bowing, an osteotomy would be needed to achieve satisfactory alignment. **H.** Once the rod is in satisfactory position within the proximal tibia, the male section is partially untwisted from the female section. It may be necessary to grasp the rod through the pseudarthrosis to disengage the two sections. The lateral C-arm image reveals the position of the distal end of the rod before the sections are completely disengaged. The separation of the sections is shown at the *arrow*. The proximal–distal position of the rod can easily be adjusted if needed. Once contact of the tibial fragments is also confirmed by direct vision and C-arm, the male end is detached and removed. **I.** The corticocancellous strips are placed circumferentially about the pseudarthrosis. If preferred bone morphogenetic protein (BMP)-soaked sponges are wrapped around the tibia and bone graft. No attempt is made to achieve periosteal coverage.

## PEARLS AND PITFALLS

| | |
|---|---|
| **Patient selection** | ■ This procedure should be considered only for patients with an established pseudarthrosis. Infants and young children with anterolateral bowing (prepseudarthrosis) should be observed and treated with a total contact orthosis. |
| **Alignment and centering of the rod** | ■ Residual anterior angulation increases the potential for recurrent bowing and refracture. Placement of the rod in a colinear fashion within the tibia—that is, a straight rod within a straight tibia—optimizes protection of the tibia from deformity and fracture (**FIG 4A**). As the tibia grows away from the ends of the rod, bowing may increase through this unprotected segment. |
| **Foot position** | ■ If the ankle and subtalar joints are transfixed by the rod, it is important to maintain neutral alignment and a plantigrade foot (**FIG 4B**). Because of the anterior bow, the foot tends to assume a dorsiflexed position; the lateral bow promotes a valgus deformity at the ankle. A calcaneus foot position potentiates posterior muscle weakness of the leg. Angular deformity may require treatment by hemiepiphysiodesis or guided growth. |
| **Distraction** | ■ An intact or overly long fibula may distract the tibia and compromise consolidation. Osteotomy with shortening as needed to permit contact of the tibial fragments resolves the issue. |
| **Rod selection** | ■ Ideally, the rod spans enough of the tibia to provide long-term mechanical support and protection of the pseudarthrosis. As growth occurs, more of the tibia is exposed to stresses that promote recurrence of bowing. Selection of the longest and greatest diameter rod is best. Preoperative measurements from plain films provide a reliable guide for the length and width needed. An assortment of rod sizes are available (Zimmer) and may need to be modified—that is, cut to an appropriate length—before surgery. |
| **Orthotic management** | ■ Use of a total contact orthosis is essential throughout growth to reduce stress through the pseudarthrosis and maintain consolidation. A solid AFO is used if the rod transfixes the ankle and subtalar joints. A KAFO is used in young children (younger than 5 years). |

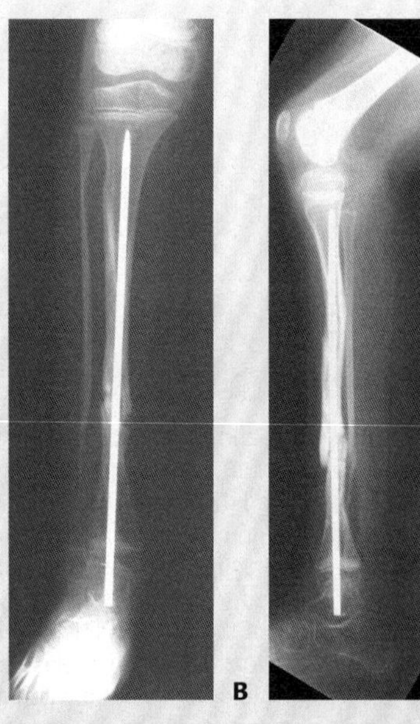


**FIG 4** • **A.** AP view of tibia after rodding in this 5.5-year-old girl shows ideal rod placement centrally within the tibia. The proximal tip of the rod is just below the physis, the fragments are in contact, and the distal rod is central within the tibia and also fills the medullary canal. The ankle is in neutral varus–valgus alignment. The fibula is very atrophic and could not be stabilized even with a small-diameter Kirschner wire. **B.** Lateral view of the same patient. The rod crosses the ankle, which is held in neutral flexion. The rod controls a maximum length of the tibia and centers the proximal tibia over the plafond.

## POSTOPERATIVE CARE

- Cast immobilization is used postoperatively until consolidation of the pseudarthrosis occurs, usually at least 12 weeks. A one-and-a-half spica cast is used for infants and young children (younger than 6 years) to minimize stress across the pseudarthrosis. A long-leg, non–weight-bearing cast is used in older children.
- A total contact orthosis is used long term to protect the area of consolidation and reduce mechanical stresses on the lower leg that promote anterior bowing. Initially, a nonarticulated KAFO is used in young children and in those with the rod across the ankle and subtalar joints. This is changed to an articulated AFO when the rod is positioned within the tibia, no longer transfixing the ankle.
- Once the ankle is no longer transfixed, an ankle rehabilitation program is implemented that includes range of motion and calf strengthening.
- Periodic follow-up is necessary throughout growth to monitor the quality of healing and maintenance of good rod position (**FIG 5**).
- Ambulation and activities are unrestricted as long as the orthosis is used. Once skeletal maturity is reached, the orthotic use is recommended for sports and high-stress activities.

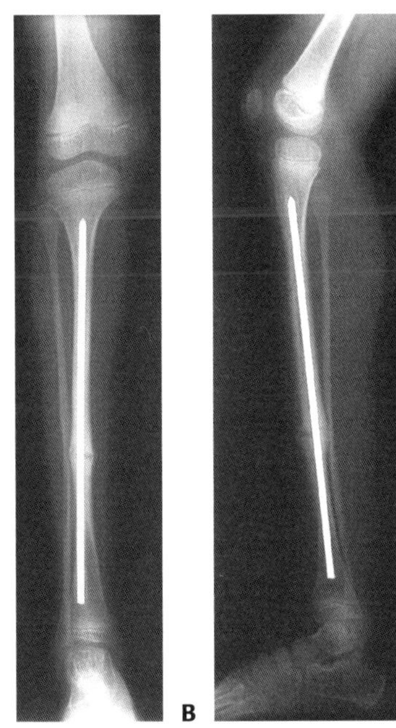


**FIG 5** • Follow-up AP (**A**) and lateral (**B**) views of another child 2 years after Williams rod placement and bone graft. The rod now lies within the tibia. The proximal and distal tibial physes have grown away from the ends of the rod. Bowing has not recurred, and the consolidation is stable. An articulated total contact AFO is used as additional support and protection. Refracture is common but manageable with cast immobilization if deformity is minimal. Supplemental bone graft can be used if healing is delayed. In the presence of recurrent deformity, revision surgery using a larger diameter, longer rod, bone graft, and osteotomy, if needed, is recommended.

## OUTCOMES

- Patients resume independent ambulation with long-term orthotic protection.
- Consolidation reliably occurs in 90% of cases with this technique.[1,3,5,7–9]
- Two long-term studies assessed the quality of maintenance of healing, with variable results. Both studies emphasized the importance of paying attention to details regarding the technique of rod insertion, continued orthotic use, and long-term follow-up care.[7,8]
- Anterior bowing may recur and lead to refracture. If the rod is in good position, healing can be obtained by simple cast immobilization. If healing is delayed, the addition of bone graft will generally lead to union.[1]
- Valgus angulation may also occur and may need to be managed by guided growth or hemiepiphysiodesis.[8]
- Limb length inequality is variable. It is more common with patients with severe deformity, those requiring greater length of pseudarthrosis resection, and those with recurrent fracture.
- Although most patients realized long-term satisfactory healing and function, some patients ultimately chose amputation after multiple recurrent fractures resulting in loss of function or limb length inequality.[7,8]

## COMPLICATIONS

- Complications include those routinely associated with musculoskeletal procedures, such as swelling, wound healing, and pain, with similar incidence.
- The most likely intraoperative complication is neurovascular injury, particularly to the deep motor branches of the peroneal nerve. These are at risk during fibular osteotomy.
- None of the studies have reported occurrence of a compartment syndrome, although this could be produced by overzealous use of bone graft, which may compress the tibial vessels. Fasciotomy is usually incidental with the surgical approach to the tibia.
- Refracture with progressive shortening and loss of stability may compromise function sufficiently to warrant amputation.
- Satisfying the primary goal of a healed pseudarthrosis is easier to accomplish than maintaining union, which serves to emphasize the recalcitrant nature of this pathologic process.

## REFERENCES

1. Anderson DJ, Schoenecker PL, Sheridan JJ, et al. Use of an intramedullary rod for the treatment of congenital pseudarthrosis of the tibia. J Bone Joint Surg Am 1992;74(2):161–168.
2. Boyd HB. Pathology and natural history of congenital pseudarthrosis of the tibia. Clin Orthop Relat Res 1982;(166):5–13.
3. Charnley J. Congenital pseudarthrosis of the tibia treated by the intramedullary nail. J Bone Joint Surg Am 1956;38 A(2):283–290.
4. Crawford AH. Anterolateral bowing. Presented at Pediatric Orthopedic Society of North America One-Day Course, Orlando, FL, May 16, 1999.
5. Dobbs MB, Rich MM, Gordon JE, et al. Use of an intramedullary rod for treatment of congenital pseudarthrosis of the tibia. A long-term follow-up study. J Bone Joint Surg Am 2004;86-A(11):1186–1197.
6. Dobbs MB, Rich MM, Gordon JE, et al. Use of an intramedullary rod for the treatment of congenital pseudarthrosis of the tibia. Surgical technique. J Bone Joint Surg Am 2005;87(suppl 1, pt 1):33–40.
7. Johnson CE. Congenital pseudarthrosis of the tibia: results of technical variations in the Charnley-Williams procedure. J Bone Joint Surg Am 2002;84-A(10):1799–1810.
8. Schoenecker PL, Rich MM. Bowing of the tibia: congenital pseudarthrosis of the tibia. In: Morrissy RT, Weinstein SL, eds. Lovell and Winter's Pediatric Orthopedics, ed 6. Philadelphia: Lippincott Williams & Wilkins, 2005:1189–1197.
9. Umber JS, Moss SW, Coleman SS. Surgical treatment of congenital pseudarthrosis of the tibia. Clin Orthop Relat Res 1982;(166): 28–33.
10. Williams PF. Fragmentation and rodding in osteogenesis imperfecta. J Bone Joint Surg Br 1965;47:23–31.

# Limb Lengthening Using the Ilizarov Method or a Monoplanar Fixator

Roger F. Widmann, Emily R. Dodwell, Purushottam A. Gholve, and Arkady Blyakher

## DEFINITION

- Limb lengthening is a surgical procedure performed to lengthen a bone.
- In the Ilizarov method, lengthening is accomplished by gradual bone distraction through a low-energy, atraumatic corticotomy site. The bone fragments are controlled via stable bone fixation using half-pins and tensioned wires through bone that are rigidly fixed to an external ring fixator or arch.[11]
- When a monoplanar fixator is used, lengthening is accomplished by distraction of the atraumatic corticotomy of the bone.[9,19] The bone fragments are controlled via stable bone fixation using half-pins that are rigidly fixed to a single rail or plane external fixator.

## ANATOMY

- Using the Ilizarov method, one can lengthen bones of both the upper and lower extremities, including bones of the hand and foot and the surrounding soft tissue.
- The most commonly lengthened bones in the lower extremity include the tibia and fibula, the femur, and the metatarsals. In the upper extremity, the most commonly lengthened bones are the humerus, the radius and ulna, and the metacarpal bones.
- Consideration is given to lengthening of the surrounding soft tissues, which include the muscle tendon unit, neurovascular bundle, and skin.[11]
- During bone lengthening, the tension in the surrounding soft tissue may predispose the lengthened segment to deformity.[13,20] Frequently encountered deformities include the following:
  - Femur: varus and procurvatum
  - Tibia: valgus and procurvatum
  - Humerus: varus and procurvatum
  - Radius and ulna: has a tendency to collapse in the interosseous space, which may cause synostosis
  - Metatarsal and metacarpal: apex dorsal angulation
- During large lengthenings, care is necessary to prevent subluxation or dislocation of the adjacent joint.[20]
- Femoral lengthening, especially in the setting of congenital short femur, may result in hip or knee subluxation or dislocation secondary to associated deficient acetabular coverage at the hip and the high frequency of deficient cruciate ligaments at the knee.
- Tibial lengthening may cause knee or ankle subluxation and progressive equinus deformity of the foot.
- Metatarsal and metacarpal lengthening can cause metatarso- or metacarpophalangeal subluxation.
- All of these issues are considered during any lengthening procedure.

## PATHOGENESIS

- The term *distraction osteogenesis* implies synthesis of new bone by slow, gradual (no more than 1 mm per 24 hours) controlled distraction of the bone fragments under conditions of rigid fixation.[11]
- The new bone is formed mostly by intramembranous ossification and, to a lesser extent, through endochondral ossification.[9,11]
- To provide maximum construct stability and to minimize soft tissue trauma, it is important to maintain the two fragments well apposed to each other following the corticotomy.
- Distraction is a good tool for influencing reparative regeneration of both the bone and the soft tissue ("stretching tension," as described by Ilizarov). However, the new regenerate ossifies and remodels slowly.
- Gradually removing distraction and applying mild compression increases the rate of remodeling. Therefore, the regenerate becomes more rigid against bending loads.
- Functional load is a strong stimulus for the improvement of blood flow and allows organic remodeling of the regenerated osseous part. The extent of load depends on the stability of fragments and the amount of regenerate.

## NATURAL HISTORY

- The natural history of the limb length discrepancy (LLD) depends on the condition causing the LLD.[22] A partial list of causes are as follows:
  - Congenital shortening: proximal focal femoral deficiency, coxa vara, congenital short femur, fibula and tibia hemimelia, hemiatrophy
  - Congenital lengthening: overgrowth syndromes such as hemihypertrophy, Beckwith-Weidemann syndrome, Klippel-Trenaunay-Weber syndrome, and Parke-Weber syndrome
  - Skeletal dysplasia or tumor: Multiple hereditary exostoses may result in limb shortening on the affected side as growth cartilage cells are diverted to the cartilage tumor.[19] Radiation for malignancies adjacent to the physis may result in growth suppression or complete destruction of physeal cartilage cells, resulting in LLD or angular deformity.
  - Infection: Physeal destruction may result from physeal invasion from adjacent metaphyseal or epiphyseal bacterial osteomyelitis or direct physeal involvement in the case of intracapsular joint physes such as at the hip and shoulder.
  - Paralysis: Poliomyelitis and cerebral palsy as well as other nervous system afflictions in children typically result in shortening on the more affected side.
  - Trauma: direct injury to growth plate, posttraumatic bone loss or shortening, and overgrowth following femoral fracture

- Miscellaneous: slipped capital femoral epiphysis, Legg-Calvé-Perthes disease
- Upper extremity discrepancy or shortening usually does not cause major functional problems but may result in significant cosmetic deformities.
- Predicted lower extremity discrepancy of 2 to 5 cm may be dealt with by long-leg epiphysiodesis in children or by leg lengthening using the Ilizarov technique. LLD greater than 5 cm usually is amenable to leg lengthening.[22]
- Untreated LLD of more than 3 cm may result in pelvic obliquity, visual gait disturbance, short-legged gait, or structural/nonstructural scoliosis.[22]
  - LLD greater than 5.5% of the long leg has been shown to decrease the efficiency of gait, as determined from kinetic data.

## PATIENT HISTORY AND PHYSICAL FINDINGS

- The underlying cause of a leg length discrepancy can typically be elucidated by careful history and physical examination.
- The common symptoms at presentation are limp, compensatory gait mechanics, pelvic obliquity, and nonstructural scoliosis.
- Physical findings depend on the etiologic factors.[22]
- In hemihypertrophy (both syndromic and nonsyndromic), the affected extremity may be larger in both length and girth. In classic hemihypertrophy, upper extremity hypertrophy as well as hemifacial asymmetry may be present. Vascular overgrowth syndromes may be associated with cutaneous or deep hemangiomas, which may alter surgical approaches to attempted limb equalization.
- Clinically, LLD is best measured by the block test, in which the shorter leg is placed on increasingly larger measured blocks until the posterior iliac crest is level. Discrepancies as small as 2 cm are accurately detected by this method, and detection of discrepancies is largely unaffected by patient size or body mass.[25] Direct measurement of leg length from anterior superior iliac spine to the tip of medial or lateral malleolus is significantly less accurate.
- True leg length is measured from the anterior superior iliac spine to the tip of the medial malleolus. It is important to place the legs in identical positions to measure true leg length.
  - If the patient has a 20-degree abduction deformity of right hip, the left hip is placed in 20 degrees of abduction to measure true length.[22]
- Apparent leg length is measured with the patient supine with the legs parallel to each other. The landmarks are the umbilicus to the tip of medial malleolus. Pelvic obliquity and fixed deformities of the hip and knee affect the reading. This method is also significantly less accurate than block measurement.
- Range of motion is noted for all joints, primarily the hip, knee, ankle, and subtalar joints. The ankle joint range of motion is measured with the knee in extension and flexion.[22]

## IMAGING AND OTHER DIAGNOSTIC STUDIES

- Plain radiographs have traditionally been used to document the objective measurement of LLD (**FIG 1**).
- Full-length (hip to ankle) anteroposterior (AP) radiographs are obtained in standing position with both patellae facing directly anteriorly. The appropriate-sized block is placed beneath the shorter leg to level the pelvis. A long x-ray cassette

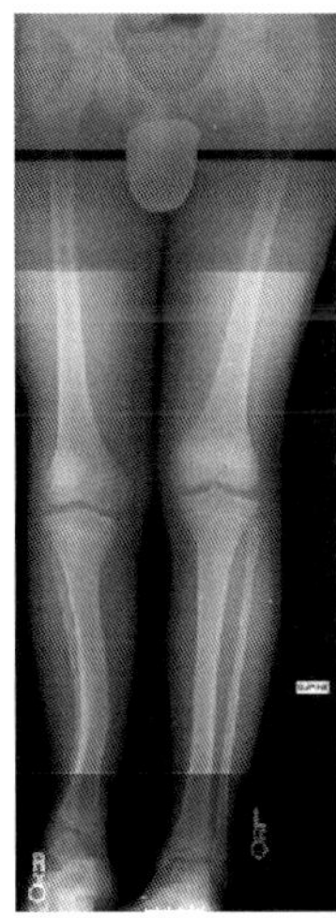


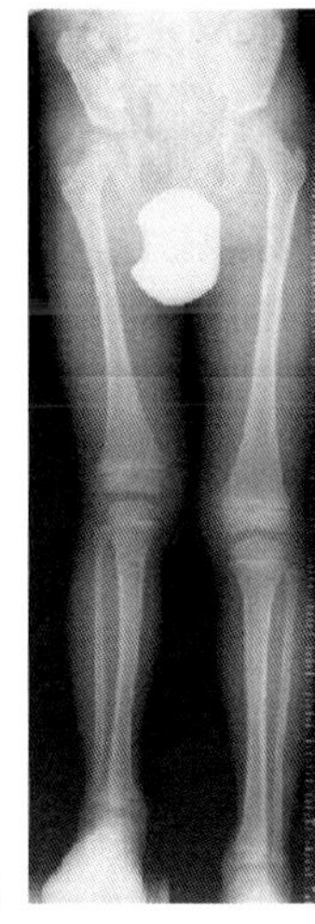


**FIG 1** • **A.** Supine radiograph of a 10-year-old boy with a posteromedial bow of the tibia and a 4.5-cm leg length discrepancy. **B.** AP standing radiograph of a 6-year-old boy with a congenital short femur and a 4-cm LLD.

(51 inches) is used with the x-ray beam center focused on the knee from a distance of 10 feet. A radiolucent ruler often is used to assist in calculation of limb discrepancies.
  - A lateral hip to ankle view can be included to further assess length, as contractures in the sagittal plane may result in inaccuracies on AP measurements. This view can also assess for angular deformities in the coronal plane.
  - Computed tomography (CT) scanogram has been the gold standard for low-dose, accurate imaging of leg length discrepancy.
  - CT scanogram is as precise in measuring LLD as the slit scanogram and it has the added benefit of more easily measuring LLD in the setting of joint contractures. Slit scanogram is of historical interest only and is no longer typically used for measuring LLD.
  - EOS[7] is a low-dose, high-resolution radiologic imaging system, which captures both simultaneous posteroanterior (PA) and lateral radiographs and full body radiographs.[12,26]
  - Recently, EOS biplanar imaging systems have been shown to be equally accurate/reliable with the added benefit of imaging the patient in a standing position such that leg length and alignment can be obtained from a single low-dose image. Radiation exposure is also lower with EOS.[6]
- Skeletal age can be determined by a left hand/wrist radiograph in combination with the Greulich and Pyle method.[8]
  - The Hospital for Special Surgery (HSS) shorthand method. This method was derived from Greulich and Pyle and uses a single radiographic criteria used for each age, allowing for rapid bone age determination.[10]
  - The LLD at maturity can be predicted in a variety of ways:
    - The arithmetic method[15]
    - The growth remaining method[1]
    - The Moseley straight-line method[17]
    - The Paley multiplier technique[21]
  - Applications/programs that incorporate the Paley multiplication factors are readily available on phones/computers for clinical use. These allow calculation of length discrepancy at maturity for both congenital and acquired deformities.
- Parental and sibling height may be useful in interpreting predicted height in the previously mentioned methods.

- In LLD secondary to physeal growth arrest, graphical or arithmetic methods are helpful in determining appropriate timing of epiphysiodesis.

## DIFFERENTIAL DIAGNOSIS

- True shortening (eg, femoral or tibial)
- Apparent shortening due to dislocated hip
- Apparent shortening from contractures
- Angular deformity causing apparent shortening
- Overgrowth syndrome with both increased length and limb girth: hemihypertrophy
- Congenital limb deficiency (beware knee joint instability)

## NONOPERATIVE MANAGEMENT

- No treatment is required for a predicted LLD less than 2 to 2.5 cm at maturity.
- A shoe lift can be used as treatment for leg length discrepancies at maturity less than 2 cm.
  - Often, a lift is used in children until an appropriate skeletal age is reached to perform an equalization procedure.
- A prosthesis may be necessary if deformities are so severe that adequate length or ambulatory ability cannot be achieved by operative methods.

## SURGICAL MANAGEMENT

### Preoperative Planning

#### *Ilizarov Method*

- Accurate radiographic measurement of current discrepancy and calculation of projected LLD at maturity
- Determination of which bony segment is affected
- Assessment of compensatory mechanics used for walking: equinus gait, circumduction, vaulting, or combination
- Assessment of contractures: for example, extra- or intra-articular, bony
- Assessment of associated deformities: for example, angulation, translation, and rotation
  - Long-leg standing radiographs in both planes help determine malalignment.
- Stability or laxity of joints (hip, knee, ankle) is determined clinically and radiographically.
- Skin condition: for example, open defect, scar tissue
- Planning for corticotomy level, for lengthening as well as for correction of associated deformity with appropriate room for wire or half-pin fixation
- Determine optimum frame configuration, with or without inclusion of the adjacent joint.
- Details on ring size, half-pin, or K-wire placement
- Single-stage lengthening of 10% to 15% of bone length is associated with fewer complications.
- Technical considerations
  - The Ilizarov frame may be constructed before surgery. The design of the frame and the number of rings and arches depend on the amount of lengthening planned.
  - Separate threaded connecting rods are used between each ring block and the next. A rod spanning two or more rings allows less flexibility if adjustments are needed.
  - Adequate skin clearance of at least 2 to 3 cm must be maintained circumferentially under the ring. Small rings are more rigid than large rings, but smaller rings may hinder skin care and may cause soft tissue compression if there is postoperative swelling.
  - A template or an actual ring can be used to select the appropriate ring size (**FIG 2**).
  - Due to the changing diameter of each limb segment, different ring sizes may be required for a single limb segment (eg, the diameter of the proximal arch for the femur typically is larger than the distal ring).

#### *Monoplanar Fixation*

- True measures of current discrepancy and calculation of projected LLD
- Compensation mechanisms used during walking: equinus gait, circumduction, vaulting
- Assessment of contractures: extra- or intra-articular
- Associated deformity: angulation, translation, and rotation
- Stability or laxity of joints: for example, hip, knee, ankle
- Skin condition: for example, open defect, scar tissue
- Long-leg films showing hip, knee, and ankle for lower extremity and similar long films for the upper extremity
- Planning for corticotomy level, osteotomy level if needed for correction of associated deformity, and planning for points of fixation
- Choose appropriate size for arch, rods, rail, half-pin, and/or K-wires.
- Choose the appropriate size of the fixator (pediatric or adult).

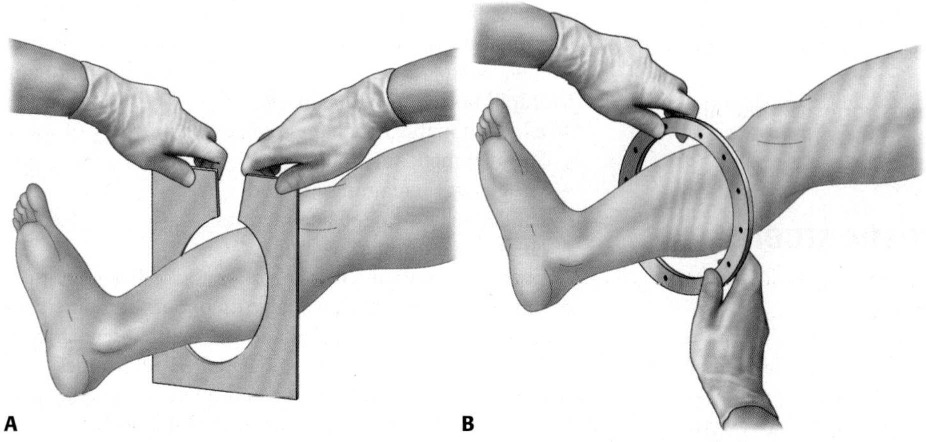


**FIG 2** • Either a template (**A**) or an actual ring (**B**) may be used to measure the ring size.

## Positioning

- Lower extremity: supine position on any radiolucent table (eg, Jackson table)
- Upper extremity: supine position with arm over a radiolucent table
- Intraoperative fluoroscopy (for both the AP and lateral images)
- For the Ilizarov method
  - Place rolled sheets (as bumps) beneath the ipsilateral buttock and proximal tibia, leaving the femur free (**FIG 3A**). Similarly, for the tibia, a rolled sheet is placed beneath distal femur and ankle to create space for the tibial frame (**FIG 3B**).
  - Place a sandbag beneath the ipsilateral shoulder/scapula and rolled sheets (as bump) beneath the humerus and radius ulna to create a space for the frame.
- For monoplanar fixator use, place rolled sheet (as bumps) beneath the femur and tibia to create working space for application of the frame.

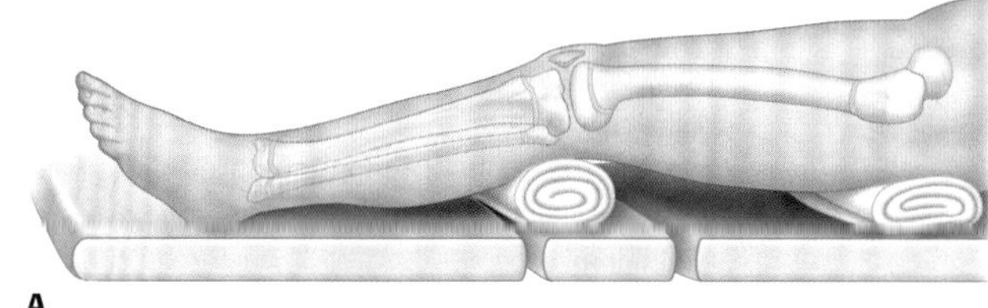

A

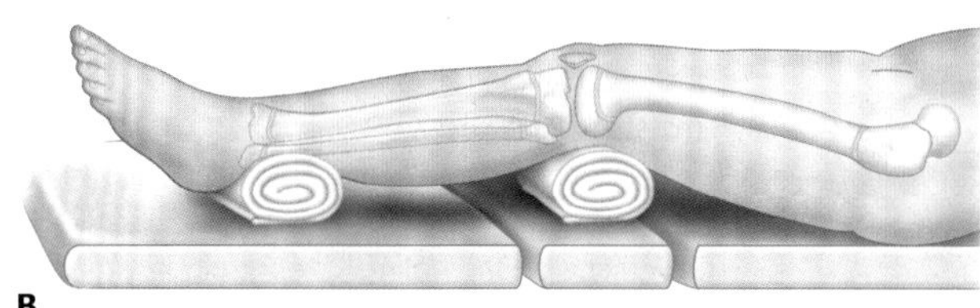

B

**FIG 3** • **A.** Patient positioned over the radiolucent table with a bump under the ipsilateral buttock and proximal tibia, leaving the femur relatively free. **B.** Patient positioned over the radiolucent table with a bump under the distal femur and ipsilateral ankle, leaving the tibia relatively free.

TECHNIQUES

# Tibial Lengthening Using the Ilizarov Method

## Wire Insertion

- The wire insertion site is determined by local anatomy and the use of cross-sectional anatomic atlases to protect and avoid damage to blood vessels, nerves, and tendons.
- In small children, 1.5-mm fixation wires are used; in adolescents and adults, 1.8-mm fixation wires are used. The wires usually are tensioned to 100 kg in children and to 130 kg in adults.
- The wire is introduced from the side nearest the neurovascular bundle. This helps prevent inadvertent injury to the neurovascular structures.
- Initially, the wire is gently pushed through the soft tissue until it hits bone cortex. The center of the bone is located, and the wire is drilled through the cortex. It is important not to bend the wire while drilling.
- The wire is prevented from bending by a short lever arm on the wire that holds the wire with a wet sponge or by use of a protective soft tissue sleeve (**TECH FIG 1**).
- After piercing the far cortex, the lowest possible drill speed is used to further insert the wire. After exiting the far skin, the wire is inserted further by tapping with a mallet.
- The wire is fixed to the ring without bending the wire. Bent wires will move the bony fragments on tensioning.
- Any tension or puckering of the skin at wire insertion or exit is corrected by releasing the surrounding skin or fascia with the help of a no. 15 blade on a scalpel.

## Half-Pin Insertion

- Hydroxyapatite-coated half-pins are recommended because they achieve better fixation and are associated with lower rates of infection and loosening.[3]
- The size of the half-pin should not exceed one-third the diameter of the bone segment being fixed.
- Freehand technique
  - Identify the optimal site for pin insertion.
  - Incise the skin over the insertion site, and then dissect down to the bone using a hemostat.

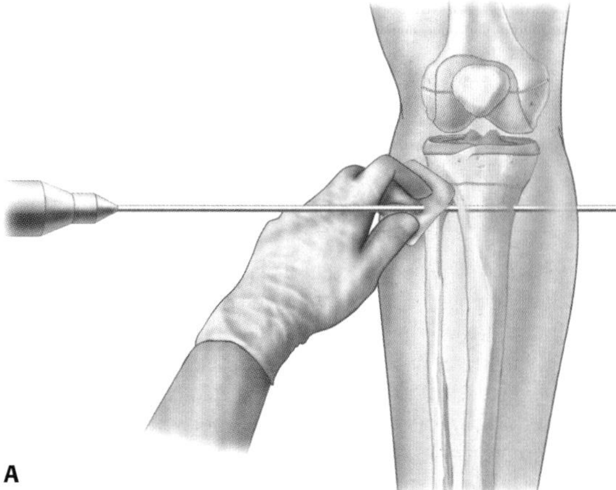

A

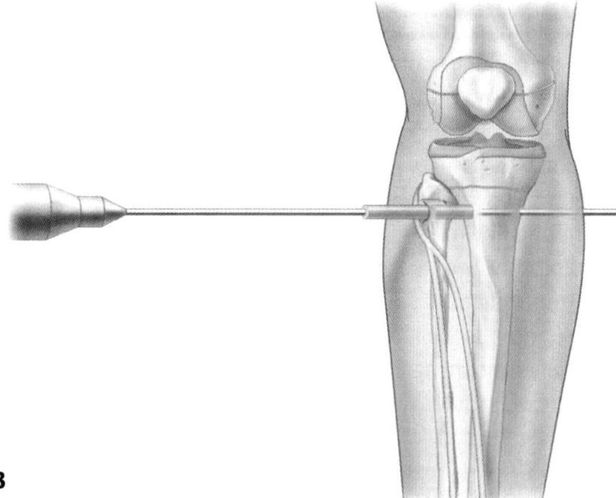

B

**TECH FIG 1** • Bending of wire during insertion is prevented by holding the wire with a wet sponge (**A**) or with a protective soft tissue sleeve (**B**).

- Now, drill the bone (both cortices) through a protective drill sleeve.
- The half-pin is introduced in the drilled track. The pin traverses only 1 to 2 mm through the far cortex, confirmed with fluoroscopy.
- The half-pin is attached to the ring or arch, which is positioned perpendicular to the bone segment.
- If the half-pin insertion is not perpendicular to the bone, a post and half-pin fixation bolt are used.

- Ring guide technique
  - First, the ring or arch is fixed perpendicular to the bone with a wire.
  - Depending on the optimal site for pin insertion, the half-pin fixation bolt or Rancho cube is attached to the ring.
  - Now, the sleeve is introduced through the half-pin fixation bolt or cube, and the skin site is marked.
  - The skin is incised and dissected to the bone using a hemostat.
  - The sleeve is advanced further to contact the bone.
  - The drill is introduced through the sleeve, and the bone is drilled (both cortices).
  - The half-pin is introduced in the drilled track. The pin traverses 1 to 2 mm through the far cortex, and this is confirmed fluoroscopically.
  - The half-pin fixation bolt or the cube is tightened over the pin.

## Fibular Osteotomy and Anterior Compartment Fasciotomy

- The osteotomy is done at the junction of the proximal and middle thirds of the fibula. Avoid osteotomies of both the tibia and fibula at same level.
- The fibula is approached laterally through the plane between the peroneus longus and the lateral intermuscular septum. The periosteum is incised with a sharp knife and is elevated circumferentially with a periosteal elevator.
- A Hohmann or Bennett retractor then is placed around the exposed fibula to protect the surrounding soft tissue.
- The fibula is osteotomized, either with an oscillating saw or using an osteotome, after placing several drill holes through both cortices. Irrigation fluid is used to prevent thermal necrosis while using the saw or drill.
- An oblique osteotomy is used to have larger contact area between the two fragments and is typically made from anterosuperior to inferoposterior.
- The skin and subcutaneous tissues are closed without closing the underlying fascia.
- Now, the skin is incised over the tibial corticotomy site. The corticotomy site usually is the proximal metaphysis.
- Prophylactic fasciotomy of the anterior compartment may be performed by releasing the anterior compartment fascia distally and proximally with a Metzenbaum scissor.
- We recommend fasciotomy before the frame is mounted because more space is available to work. However, it can be done later after mounting the frame.
- A temporary suture is placed over the proximal tibial incision, deferring the corticotomy until later in the procedure.

## Ilizarov Frame Application

- For simple lengthening (without deformity), three rings (or two rings and one arch) are used.
- Introduce a transverse proximal tibial wire perpendicular to the shaft and below the growth plate in children (**TECH FIG 2**, #1).
- To avoid penetrating the joint capsule, the transverse wire should be no closer than 14 mm to the subchondral bone of the proximal tibia.
- Attach the proximal ring (previously constructed frame) to this wire, and tension the wire with a wire tensioner. Adequate ring clearance from the soft tissues must be verified circumferentially.
- Another transverse wire is introduced in the distal metaphysis of the tibia proximal to the distal growth plate and fixed to the distal ring (**TECH FIG 2**, #2).
- The biomechanical and anatomic axis of the tibia is the same in the absence of deformity.
- The lengthening rods are placed parallel to the biomechanical axis. Radiographically, the rods should be parallel to the posterior cortex on the lateral view and parallel to the longitudinal axis of the tibia on the AP view.
- Next, a wire is placed proximally, passing from lateral to medial. This wire enters the fibular head (just distal to the proximal

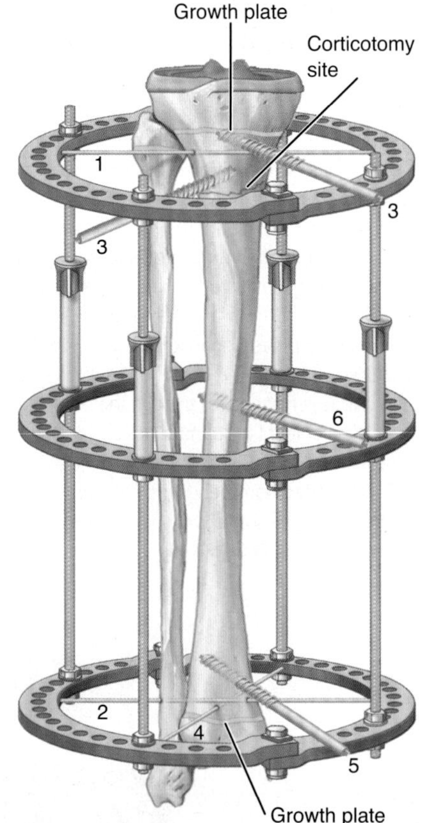


**TECH FIG 2** • The sequence and placement of K-wires or half-pins in tibial lengthening. *1*, Proximal transverse tibial wire perpendicular to the shaft and below the growth plate in children. This wire is placed anterior to the fibular head. *2*, Transverse wire in the distal metaphysis of the tibia proximal to the distal growth plate. *3*, Two half-pins are inserted proximally, one above and one below the proximal ring at an approximate angle of 90 degrees to one another. *4*, Distal wire through the fibula and tibia above the growth plate at level of syndesmosis. *5*, Distal tibial half-pin is introduced in the anteromedial direction. *6*, One or two half-pins are introduced, just above and below the middle ring.

fibular growth plate), traversing the tibia and exiting through the anteromedial tibial cortex.
  - Care is necessary to prevent damage to the peroneal nerve, which is in close proximity to the fibular neck.
- The wire is then fixed and tensioned to the proximal ring.
- Now, two half-pins are placed in the most proximal ring. In this configuration, there should ideally be 90 degrees of angulation between the two pins (**TECH FIG 2**, #3).
  - Usually, a half-pin fixation bolt is required with one half-pin and a one hole cube for the other half-pin, so that the pins are placed at slightly different levels.
  - It is important not to damage the tibial tubercle and proximal tibial physis while placing the half-pins or wires.
- Next, a wire is placed distally through the fibula and tibia just above the growth plate at the level of the syndesmosis (**TECH FIG 2**, #4). This wire is attached and tensioned to the distal ring.
- Place the fibula–tibia wire more than 12.2 mm from the distal tibia subchondral surface to avoid capsular penetration and the risk of joint sepsis.
- A half-pin is introduced just proximal to the distal ring in an anteromedial direction. It is then fixed to the distal ring (**TECH FIG 2**, #5).
- One or two half-pins are similarly introduced just above and below the middle ring and are securely fixed to the middle ring (**TECH FIG 2**, #6).
- The connecting rods between the proximal and middle rings are then disconnected, and attention is directed to the corticotomy site.
- Extraperiosteal dissection is performed at the proximal tibial metaphyseal osteotomy site.
- The periosteum is not elevated circumferentially in order to preserve the blood supply.

## Corticotomy

- Multiple drill holes are made in both tibial cortices from anterior to posterior. If necessary, additional drill holes can be made at the same level from another point over the anteromedial cortex (**TECH FIG 3A**).

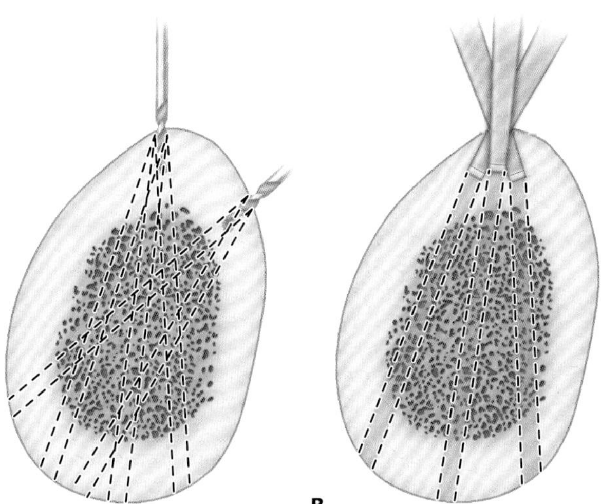


**TECH FIG 3 • A.** Multiple drill holes are made in the anterior/anteromedial tibial cortex. **B.** A 5-mm osteotome is advanced through the bone at the level of drill holes in a regulated manner. Lateral fluoroscopic imaging is helpful to judge depth.

- A 5-mm osteotome is advanced through the bone at the level of the drill holes (**TECH FIG 3B**).
- First, the anteromedial cortex is osteotomized, followed by the anterolateral cortex. Each time the osteotome passes through the far cortex, it is twisted with a wrench to cause a controlled fracture in the cortex.
- Finally, a wider osteotome is seated in the posterior cortex and twisted with a 14-mm wrench to break the posterior cortex.
- The corticotomy is confirmed by externally rotating the distal block. Internal rotation is avoided because it places tension on the common peroneal nerve. The fragments are rotated back to the normal reduced position.
- The rods between the proximal and distal blocks are reconnected as they were before the corticotomy, and the osteotomy is reduced.
- The use of square nuts or clickers on the connecting rods allows future distraction.

## Wound Closure

- The skin is closed without closing the underlying fascia.
- Check that all the nuts and bolts are tight.
- Put a dressing (eg, Xeroform [Covidien, Mansfield, MA], sponges) around the wires and half-pins. Pressure dressing is applied over the fibular and tibial corticotomy sites. Place the dressing material between the frame and the surgical wound.
- The foot is placed in a plantigrade position, and a footplate is attached. When planning a large lengthening, the foot may be included in the frame to prevent progressive equinus deformity of the ankle.
- Similar consideration is given to including the knee in the frame for large lengthening or in the setting of cruciate ligament laxity.

## Taylor Spatial Frame

- The Taylor spatial frame (TSF; Smith & Nephew, Andover, MA) has Web-based spatial software, which helps to calculate correction of deformity or lengthening of the bone.
- Deformities can be corrected using chronic deformity correction, the rings first method, or the residual deformity method.
- In the TSF, the proximal and distal blocks may or may not be connected preoperatively.
- The number and site of wire/half-pin fixation, the number of rings, and the basic construct of the frame are similar to those described earlier.
- The details of fibular osteotomy and anterior compartment fasciotomy are the same.
- Mount the frame and secure with wires and half-pins.
- The proximal and distal blocks are connected with six connecting struts. The details of the strut lengths are recorded, after which the struts are disconnected and corticotomy is completed as discussed earlier.
- The corticotomy is reduced, and the struts are reconnected the way they were before the corticotomy (**TECH FIG 4**).
- The deformity, frame, and mounting parameters are entered in the software program, which prescribes a lengthening/corrective program.
- The rate of distraction is determined based on local bone and soft tissue status. Typically, it is 1 mm per day in healthy bone and soft tissue.

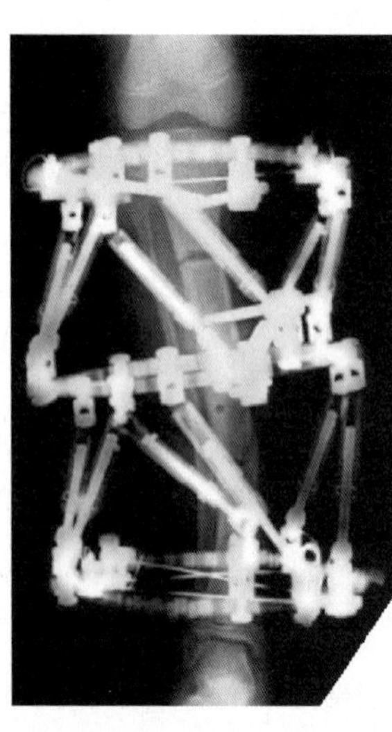

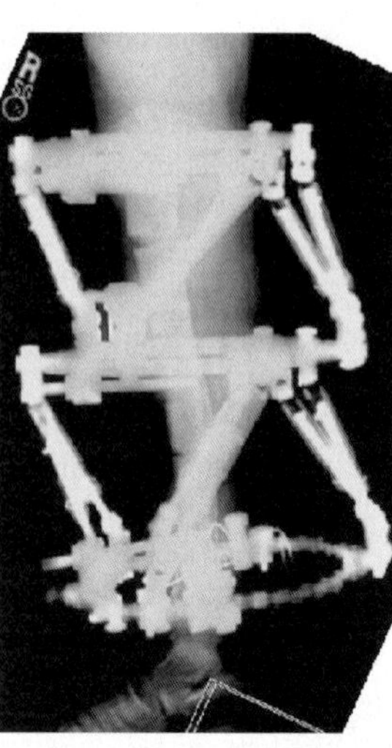

**TECH FIG 4** • A two-level osteotomy was performed on the patient shown in **FIG 1A** with the goal of distal deformity correction and proximal tibia lengthening with application of a TSF.

## Femoral Lengthening Using the Ilizarov Method

- The usual frame construct for simple femoral lengthening (without deformity) is composed of two rings and one arch.
- Initially, a transverse wire is placed in the distal femur, parallel to the knee joint line and proximal to the growth plate in children (**TECH FIG 5A**, wire 1). The direction of the wire is from lateral to medial.
- The previously constructed frame is mounted, and the distal ring is attached to this wire. The wire is then tensioned. All the rings, including the arch, should have at least one or two fingerbreadths clearance from the anterior and posterior surface of the thigh.
- The mechanical and anatomic axes of the femur are not identical as in the tibia. The mechanical axis is drawn from the center of the femoral head to the center of the knee joint, whereas the anatomic axis is the central axis of the femoral shaft. The anatomic axis forms a 7-degree angle with the mechanical axis.
- A transverse half-pin is introduced in the lateral proximal femur perpendicular to the mechanical axis, using the ring guide technique (**TECH FIG 5A**, pin 2). The pin is placed centrally in the lateral cortex and is fixed to the proximal arch.
- The frame rods are placed parallel to the mechanical axis. Radiographically, the rods are parallel to the posterior cortex on the lateral view and parallel to the mechanical axis (marker from center of femoral head to the center of knee joint) on the AP view.
- Next, two half-pins are placed in the distal femur proximal to the growth plate. The direction of these half-pins is from posterolateral to anteromedial and from posteromedial to anterolateral (**TECH FIG 5A**, pin 3).
- While introducing half-pins, it is necessary to flex the knee to avoid placement across the tendon and muscle (ie, biceps

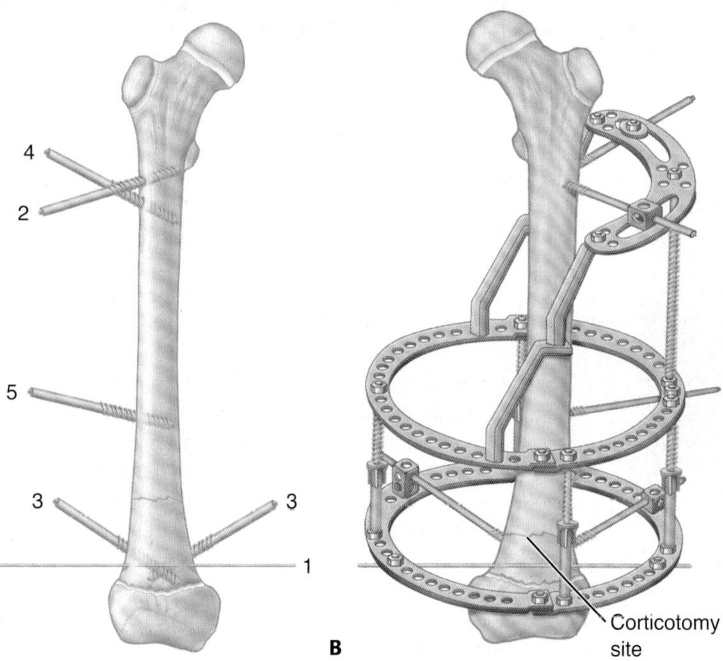


**TECH FIG 5** • **A.** The sequence and placement of K-wires or half-pins in femur lengthening. *1*, Transverse wire in the distal femur, which is parallel to the knee joint line and proximal to the growth plate in children. *2*, A transverse half-pin in the lateral proximal femur perpendicular to the mechanical axis. *3*, Two half-pins in the distal femur directed from posterolateral to anteromedial and from posteromedial to anterolateral cortex. *4*, One or two additional half-pins in the proximal femur. *5*, One or two half-pins adjacent to the middle ring. **B.** A completed femoral frame with rings, connecting rods, wire/half-pins, and distal metaphyseal corticotomy.

femoris, semitendinosus, semimembranosus). Care is necessary to prevent any damage to the common peroneal nerve, which is in close relationship with the biceps femoris.

- One or two half-pins are introduced in the proximal femur (**TECH FIG 5A**, pin 4). The half-pins are fixed to the proximal arch using different size Rancho cubes to avoid pin placement at the same level.
- Next, one or two half-pins are placed adjacent to the middle ring (**TECH FIG 5A**, pin 5).
- The rods between the middle and distal rings are disconnected for corticotomy of the distal femoral metaphysis.
- A skin incision is made over the anterolateral distal femur close to the distal metaphysis. The deep tissue is incised, and the vastus lateralis is elevated by blunt dissection to expose the lateral femoral cortex without disturbing the underlying periosteum. The osteotomy is performed approximately 1 cm proximal to the most proximal wire or half-pin attached to the distal ring.
- The cortex is drilled at the same level, with multiple drill holes at varying angles. A 5-mm osteotome is advanced through the anterior, lateral, medial, and posterior cortices.
- Each time the osteotome is fully seated through the far cortex, it is twisted with a wrench to cause an atraumatic fracture in the cortex. The corticotomy is confirmed by externally rotating the distal ring.
- The fragments are rotated back to the normal reduced position. This will decrease bleeding from the cut bony surfaces.
- The rods are reconnected as before the corticotomy. Square nuts or clickers are used with these connecting rods to allow for controlled distraction.
- The corticotomy site is closed. A check is done to tighten all nuts and bolts (**TECH FIG 5B**).
- During large lengthening and in presence of knee ligament laxity, one should consider extending the frame across the knee joint.

## Taylor Spatial Frame

- When using the TSF for femoral lengthening, the proximal and distal blocks may or may not be connected preoperatively.
- The number and site of wire/half-pin fixation, number of rings, and basic construct of the frame are similar to those described with the Ilizarov technique.
- Mount the frame and secure with wires and half-pins.
- The proximal and distal blocks are connected with six connecting struts. The details of the strut lengths are noted. Then, the struts are disconnected and corticotomy is completed as discussed earlier.
- The corticotomy is reduced, and the struts are reconnected at the same lengths as before corticotomy (**TECH FIG 6**). This results in anatomic reduction at the osteotomy site.
- The deformity, frame, and mounting parameters are entered in the software program, which prescribes a lengthening/deformity correction program. Lengthening proceeds at 1 mm per day under normal circumstances.

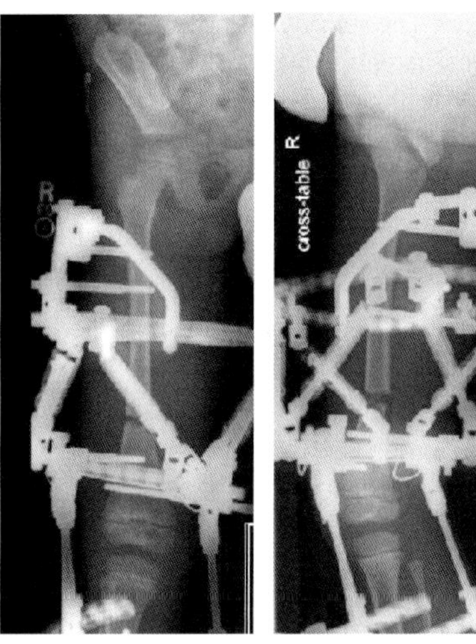


**TECH FIG 6** • A distal femur osteotomy was performed on the patient shown in **FIG 1B** after application of a femur frame with extension across the knee to include the tibia. The femur and tibia frames were connected with hinges to prevent knee subluxation during lengthening.

# Monoplanar Fixator Assembly

## Technical Considerations

- Monolateral fixators stabilize bone fragments using percutaneous half-pins to transfix the bone with external fixation of the half-pin to the clamp, rail, rod, or arch.
- Some monoplanar systems use arches or rings to achieve multiplanar fixation.
- Advantages of monoplanar fixators[22]:
  - Greater patient comfort during femur and humerus lengthening
  - Less bulky frame
  - Simple construct
- Disadvantages of monoplanar fixators[11,22]:
  - Less rigid
  - Less flexible: for example, the MAC frame (EBI, Parsippany, NJ) has a universal hinge that allows correction of angular deformity and a translation device that allows correction of translation in two directions.
  - Not recommended for large lengthening (more than 5 cm)
- The monolateral frame is constructed preoperatively. The design of the frame, including the number of clamps and arches, depends on the planned lengthening.
- Rail size depends on the planned lengthening.
- Techniques to increase frame stability include the following:
  - Increase number of half-pins
  - Increase diameter of the half-pins (pin diameter should not exceed a third of the bone diameter)
  - Greatest possible angle between half-pins (maximum, 90-degree angle)
  - Reduce distance between the bone and the external frame.
  - Increase the distance between half-pins.
  - Fixation as close to the corticotomy as possible

## Femoral Lengthening

- For simple lengthening (without deformity), three-point fixation is required in each segment.
- Use guidewire technique to place the first half-pin in the distal femur. A guidewire is introduced parallel to the knee joint line and proximal to the growth plate in children.
  - Because the femur has a natural anterior bow, the guidewire is placed slightly anterior (not central) in the lateral femoral cortex (**TECH FIG 7A**, #1).
- The bone is drilled over the guidewire with a 4.8- or 3.2-mm cannulated drill bit (depending on the size of half-pin to be used). Then, a self-tapping, hydroxyapatite-coated half-pin is introduced in the drilled track (**TECH FIG 7B**, #1).
- Attach this half-pin to the clamp, which is connected to the rail (monolateral fixator).
- At least one fingerbreadth of distance is maintained between the external frame and the lateral surface of the proximal thigh.
- A second half-pin is introduced in the proximal femur perpendicular to the biomechanical axis and fixed to the proximal clamp (**TECH FIG 7B**, #2).
- This half-pin is also placed slightly anterior (not central) in the lateral femoral cortex (**TECH FIG 7A**, #2).
- With intraoperative fluoroscopy, check the AP and lateral relationships of the frame with the femur. The frame should be located parallel to the biomechanical axis on the AP view (**TECH FIG 7B**, #3). On the lateral view, all the holes of the proximal and distal clamp should overlie the bone.
- Introduce two or more half-pins through the empty holes of the proximal clamp (**TECH FIG 7B**, #4).
- During femoral lengthening, soft tissue tension predisposes the femur to develop procurvatum deformity.
- Procurvatum deformity can be prevented by making simple adjustments during frame application. After the proximal half-pins have been placed, the rail is disengaged from the proximal clamp. The distal clamp is then angulated by 10 degrees anteriorly (**TECH FIG 7C**).
- The additional two half-pins are then placed in the distal clamp. This pin placement creates a mild recurvatum deformity (10 degrees), which compensates for the predicted procurvatum deformity.
- At this point, the frame is removed in preparation for corticotomy. The distance between the clamp and the skin is marked on the half-pins.
- Gloves are changed, and the skin at the level of the corticotomy is prepped again.
- The femoral corticotomy is completed following the same principles discussed earlier.
- After completion of the corticotomy, the frame is reapplied, maintaining the same distance between the clamps and the skin.
- Fluoroscopy is used to confirm the slight recurvatum deformity. This recurvatum deformity compensates for the procurvatum tendency during lengthening of femur.

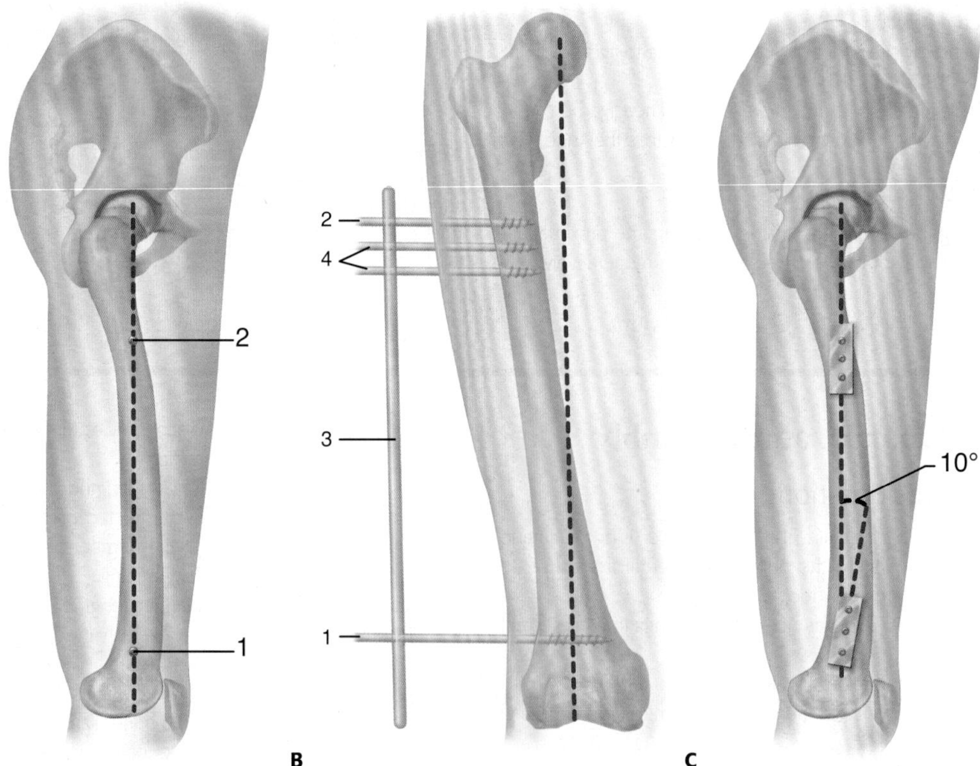


**TECH FIG 7** ● **A.** Lateral view of the femur. The guidewire and half-pin are placed just slightly anterior (not central) in the lateral femoral cortex. **B.** The sequence and placement of half-pins in femur lengthening. *1*, A half-pin is placed in the distal femur parallel to the knee joint line and proximal to the growth plate in children. *2*, The second half-pin is introduced in the proximal femur perpendicular to the biomechanical axis. *3*, The frame/rail is placed parallel to the biomechanical axis in AP view. *4*, One or two half-pins are introduced through the empty holes of the proximal clamp. **C.** The proximal part of the distal clamp is approximately angulated by 10 to 15 degrees anteriorly.

- The skin is closed after repair of the tensor fascia.
- The distraction device is connected to the clamps, and final tightening is performed.
- Half-pins are dressed with Xeroform gauze and sponges.

## Tibial Lengthening

- For simple lengthenings (without deformity), two- or three-point fixation is required in each bony segment.
- The tibial frame usually includes a proximal clamp or arch with two or three half-pins and a distal fixation clamp with two or three half-pins.
- Fibular osteotomy is performed first (as discussed previously).
- A distal tibia–fibula transfixation screw is required to prevent distal tibia–fibula subluxation.
- The skin is incised over the tibial corticotomy site, which usually is the proximal metaphysis.
- Prophylactic fasciotomy of the anterior compartment is performed under direct vision before frame application.
- Now, a temporary suture is placed at the corticotomy skin incision, and corticotomy is performed after pin fixation is complete.
- Two half-pins are introduced in the proximal tibial metaphysis perpendicular to the shaft and distal to the growth plate (**TECH FIG 8**, #1). The half-pins are placed in the anteromedial and anterolateral cortex, with care to avoid the tibial tuberosity.
- The half-pin configuration should aim for pin spread of 90 degrees. The half-pins are introduced at different levels. The first half-pin is placed freehand. The arch is placed parallel to the proximal tibial joint line, and the second half-pin is placed through the clamp.
- The anterior aspect of the arch should be at least a fingerbreadth from the anterior cortex.
- In the absence of deformity, the mechanical and anatomic axis of the tibia are the same. The mounted frame should be parallel to the biomechanical axis in both the AP and lateral views (**TECH FIG 8**, #2).
- A half-pin is then introduced in the distal tibia through the clamp (**TECH FIG 8**, #3). Once again, parallel alignment of the frame with the mechanical axis is confirmed.
- Two additional half-pins are placed distally through the distal clamp (**TECH FIG 8**, #4).
- The distance of the clamps from the skin is marked on the half-pins. The frame is then removed in preparation for the corticotomy.
- Gloves are changed, and the skin at the level of the proximal tibial metaphysis is prepared again.
- The tibial corticotomy is completed following the same principle discussed earlier (**TECH FIG 8**, #5).
- The frame is reapplied, maintaining the same distance between the clamps and the skin as measured before the corticotomy.
- A properly executed procedure will not have any residual displacement at the corticotomy site.
- The skin is closed, leaving the underlying fascia open.
- The distraction device is connected to the clamps, and final tightening is performed.
- Half-pins are dressed with Xeroform and sponges. A pressure dressing is applied over the corticotomy site.
- The foot is placed in a plantigrade position.

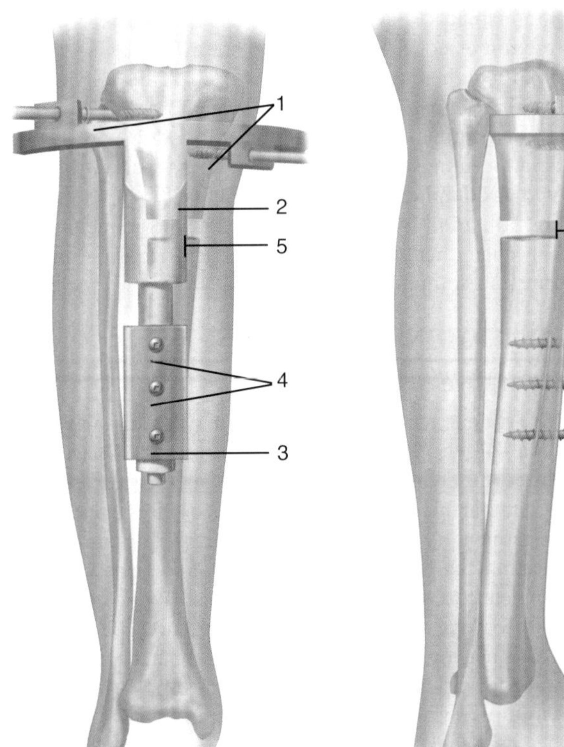

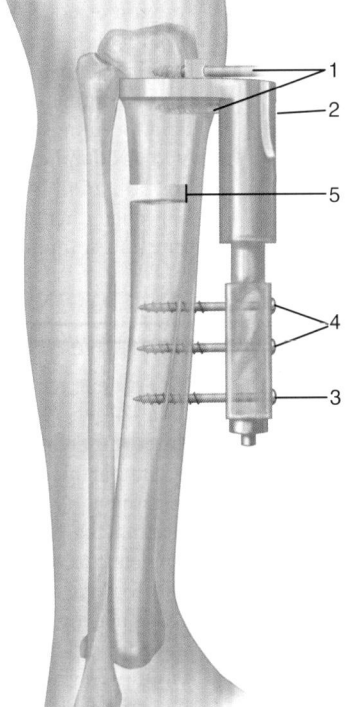

**TECH FIG 8** • The sequence and placement of half-pins in tibial lengthening: AP (**A**) and lateral views (**B**). *1*, two half-pins in the proximal tibia; *2*, the frame is parallel to the biomechanical axis; *3*, the half-pin is inserted in the distal tibia through the distal clamp; *4*, two half-pins are placed distally through the distal clamp; *5*, corticotomy site.

## PEARLS AND PITFALLS

| | |
|---|---|
| **Intraoperative** | ■ Incomplete osteotomy will not allow distraction. Identify this intraoperatively and complete the corticotomy. Confirm complete osteotomy with fluoroscopy by externally rotating the distal fragment.<br>■ Avoid neurovascular injury by placing half-pins and wires through the safe zones.[19] Use cross-sectional atlas in operating room.<br>■ Skeletal muscle relaxants may mask intraoperative nerve injury, and paralyzing agents are avoided.[19] |
| **Distraction period** | ■ Prevent joint contracture by reducing or stopping distraction temporarily, increasing physical therapy, and using static or dynamic splinting of the joint.<br>■ To prevent subluxation and dislocation of an adjacent joint during limb lengthening:<br>■ Correct hip instability before performing femur lengthening.<br>■ Extend the frame across the knee joint in the setting of cruciate ligament laxity.<br>■ Maintain full knee extension using nighttime static splinting. |

## POSTOPERATIVE CARE

- Distraction is started after a latency period of 7 to 10 days (depending on the age of the patient, the level of the corticotomy, and the local blood supply).[11,19]
- The rate of distraction is 1 mm per day, distributed as 0.25 mm four times a day.[11,19]
- Pin care is done with half-strength hydrogen peroxide and normal saline.
- Showering is allowed 1 week after the surgery, with antibacterial soap.
- Full weight bearing is encouraged as tolerated.
- Physical therapy to maintain range of motion and prevent contractures:
  - Minimum: three times a week and a home program is performed four times a day
- During active lengthening, the patient is seen once per week.
- Routine perioperative intravenous antibiotic prophylaxis is used.

## OUTCOMES

### Ilizarov Technique

- In 1995, Stanitski et al[23] reported the results of 36 femoral lengthenings in 30 consecutive patients using the Ilizarov technique. The etiology of femoral shortening was congenital in 21 femurs and acquired in 15. The average lengthening was 8.3 cm (range, 3.5 to 12 cm), with a treatment time of 6.4 months (range, 2.5 to 12 months). Complications included premature consolidation in four patients, malunion of more than 10 degrees in two patients, and residual limb length inequality (<2 cm) in two patients. Two patients developed knee subluxation. There were no reports of osteomyelitis, ring sequestra, neurologic or vascular compromise, compartment syndrome, hypertension, or hip or knee dislocations in their series. Psychological problems necessitated cessation of lengthening in two patients.
  - These results show a significant improvement over previous reports of earlier techniques of femoral lengthening in terms of greater lengthening, simultaneous deformity correction, and fewer major complications.
- Stanitski et al[24] reported tibial lengthening for 62 tibiae in 52 patients using the Ilizarov technique. The average lengthening was 7.5 cm (range, 3.5 to 12 cm). Twenty-eight (22%) patients required unplanned procedures, which included osteotomy for malunion or deformation of the regenerate and Achilles tendon for persistent equinus contracture. The complication rate decreased after the initial learning curve.
  - Aston et al[2] reported on 27 patients that underwent lengthenings for congenital short femur using the Ilizarov technique. Over 50% experienced regenerate deformation or fracture after lengthening regardless of the location of the corticotomy. This complication was resolved using placement of a Rush nail.
  - Moraal et al[16] reported pre- and postoperative quality of life in children that underwent lengthening procedures. There was a small decrease in quality-of-life scores immediately following surgery, but the long-term quality-of-life scores were similar to those for normal controls. Patients with residual length discrepancy of greater than 2 cm had lower quality of life at long-term follow-up.[16]

### Monoplanar Fixator

- Coleman and Noonan[5] reported results of distraction osteogenesis in 114 femurs and 147 tibias treated with monoplanar external fixator for a variety of different conditions. Mean femoral lengthening was 11 cm or 48% of the original femur length. The femora that gained more length (expressed as percentage of original length) had poor healing indices.
  - Interestingly, LLD was more difficult to correct with distraction osteogenesis than short stature. In tibia, the mean tibial lengthening was 9 cm or 41% of the original tibial length. The mean healing index was 32 days per centimeter of lengthening. The complication rate was 1.33 per tibia. Seemingly, obstacles or problems were also considered as complications in their study.
  - Overall, good results were obtained. They concluded that larger lengthenings are possible, but the cost is increased time and complications.

## COMPLICATIONS

### Intraoperative

- Compartment syndrome is rare but may occur early following the surgery. Pain with passive stretch and paresthesias are important clinical signs of compartment syndrome. Measure compartment pressures and decompress the affected compartment as needed. Prophylactic anterior compartment release may be performed at the time of corticotomy.[19,20]
- Incomplete corticotomy: Confirm complete corticotomy by externally rotating the distal fragment under fluoroscopic imaging.
  - Avoid neurovascular injury by placing half-pins through safe zones.[4] Use a cross-sectional atlas.
  - Avoid paralyzing anesthetic agents during surgery because they may mask nerve injury.[20]

### Distraction Period

- Pin tract infection initially is treated with a short course of oral antibiotics (7 to 10 days) and appropriate pin tract care. If infection persists, consider intravenous antibiotics or removal of the wire or half-pin with curettage of the infected site.

- Premature consolidation may be due to incomplete osteotomy, slow distraction rate, or incorrect direction of distraction.
- Neurologic symptoms may arise in the form of altered sensation or weakness of the muscle. The wire or half-pin is removed if direct contact or irritation of the nerve is suspected. Stretching of the nerve with rapid distraction may result in nerve injury, and it may be necessary to decrease the rate of distraction or even stop distraction temporarily.[20,27]
- Decompression of the peroneal nerve is an option, and many surgeons perform this routinely for lengthenings and correction of valgus deformity.[18]
- Unplanned deformity may develop during bone lengthening. Appropriate frame modifications may be required to correct the deformity.[13,20]
- Joint contractures may occur during lengthening. Treatment includes increasing the number of physical therapy sessions and use of dynamic splinting, especially to prevent equinus contracture.
- Iatrogenic deformity may develop during lengthening. Frame modifications may be required to correct the deformity and maintain a neutral mechanical axis.
- Compartment syndrome is rare (the anterior compartment is always released intraoperatively) but may occur following surgery. Paresthesia, pain with passive stretch, and pain out of proportion to the surgical procedure are clinical indicators of compartment syndrome. Compartment pressures should be measured, and compartments should be released as needed.[5]

### Consolidation Period

- Pin tract infection (as described earlier)
- Delayed consolidation of regenerate may respond to electrical or ultrasound bone stimulator. The frame can be dynamized or the regenerate can be compressed by 0.5 cm.
  - Although evidence is not conclusive regarding bone stimulators, this may be considered in the setting of delayed consolidation.[14]
  - Vitamin D deficiency has been implicated in delayed bone healing. Checking vitamin D levels and supplementing when deficient may improve bone regeneration.[5]

### After Frame Removal

- The regenerate bone may deform after premature frame removal (eg, poor regenerate, fewer than three continuous cortices). This can be prevented by frame dynamization prior to frame removal and protected weight bearing.
  - Assess the regenerate bone clinically and radiographically at the time of frame removal. Consider use of a cast or brace and protected weight bearing in the setting of questionable bone regenerate.
- Stress fracture can occur either at the site of half-pins, especially when the half-pin size exceeds one-third the diameter of the cortex, or through the regenerate bone. Fracture is treated with reapplication of the frame, casting, intramedullary rod fixation, or plate application.

## REFERENCES


1. Anderson M, Green WT, Messner MB. Growth and predictions of growth in the lower extremities. J Bone Joint Surg Am 1963;45-A:1–14.
2. Aston WJ, Calder PR, Baker D, et al. Lengthening of the congenital short femur using the Ilizarov technique: a single-surgeon series. J Bone Joint Surg Br 2009;91(7):962–967.
3. Caja VL, Piza G, Navarro A. Hydroxyapatite coating of external fixation pins to decrease axial deformity during tibial lengthening for short stature. J Bone Joint Surg Am 2003;85-A(8):1527–1531.
4. Catagni MA. Atlas for the Insertion of Transosseous Wires and Half Pins. Ilizarov Method, ed 6. Milan, Italy: Medi Surgical Video, 2002.
5. Coleman SS, Noonan TD. Anderson's method of tibial-lengthening by percutaneous osteotomy and gradual distraction. J Bone Joint Surg Am 1967;49(2):263–279.
6. Escott BG, Ravi B, Weathermon AC, et al. EOS low-dose radiography: a reliable and accurate upright assessment of lower-limb lengths. J Bone Joint Surg Am 2013;95(23):e1831–e1837.
7. Gheno R, Nectoux E, Herbaux B, et al. Three-dimensional measurements of the lower extremity in children and adolescents using a low-dose biplanar X-ray device. Eur Radiol 2012;22(4):765–771.
8. Greulich W, Pyle S. Radiographic Atlas of Skeletal Development of the Hand and Wrist, ed 2. Redwood City, CA: Stanford University Press, 1959.
9. Hamdy RC, Silvestri A, Rivard CH, et al. Histologic evaluation of bone regeneration in cases of limb lengthening by Ilizarov's technique. An experimental study in the dog [in French]. Ann Chir 1997;51:875–883.
10. Heyworth BE, Goldstein M, Schneider R, et al. A new validated shorthand method for determining bone age. Hospital for Special Surgery. Available at: http://www.hss.edu/files/HSSBoneAgePoster.pdf. Accessed August 18, 2014.
11. Ilizarov GA. Clinical application of the tension-stress effect for limb lengthening. Clin Orthop Relat Res 1990;(250):8–26.
12. Lazennec JY, Rangel A, Baudoin A, et al. The EOS imaging system for understanding a patellofemoral disorder following THR. Orthop Traumatol Surg Res 2011;97(1):98–101.
13. Leyes M, Noonan K, Forriol F, et al. Statistical analysis of axial deformity during distraction osteogenesis of the tibia. J Pediatr Orthop 1998;18:190–197.
14. Luna Gonzalez F, Lopez Arévalo R, Meschian Coretti S, et al. Pulsed electromagnetic stimulation of regenerate bone in lengthening procedures. Acta Orthop Belg 2005;71(5):571–576.
15. Menelaus MB. Correction of leg length discrepancy by epiphyseal arrest. J Bone Joint Surg Br 1966;48:336–339.
16. Moraal JM, Elzinga-Plomp A, Jongmans MJ, et al. Long-term psychosocial functioning after Ilizarov limb lengthening during childhood. Acta Orthop 2009;80(6):704–710.
17. Moseley CF. A straight line graph for leg length discrepancies. J Bone Joint Surg Am 1977;59(2):174–179.
18. Nogueira MP, Paley D. Prophylactic and therapeutic peroneal nerve decompression for deformity correction and lengthening. Oper Tech Orthop 2011;21(2):180–183.
19. Paley D. Current techniques of limb lengthening. J Pediatr Orthop 1988;8:73–92.
20. Paley D. Problems, obstacles, and complications of limb lengthening by the Ilizarov technique. Clin Orthop Relat Res 1990;(250):81–104.
21. Paley D, Bhave A, Herzenberg J, et al. Multiplier method for predicting limb-length discrepancies. J Bone Joint Surg Am 2000;82-A(10):1432–1446.
22. Stanitski DF. Limb-length inequality: assessment and treatment options. J Am Acad Orthop Surg 1999;7:143–153.
23. Stanitski DF, Bullard M, Armstrong P, et al. Results of femoral lengthening using the Ilizarov technique. J Pediatr Orthop 1995;15:224–231.
24. Stanitski DF, Shahcheraghi H, Nicker DA, et al. Results of tibial lengthening with the Ilizarov technique. J Pediatr Orthop 1996;16:168–172.
25. Terry MA, Winell JJ, Green DW, et al. Measurement variance in limb length discrepancy: clinical and radiographic assessment of interobserver and intraobserver variability. J Pediatr Orthop 2005;25(2):197–201.
26. Thometz J. EOS scanner provides higher level of imaging with less radiation. Children's Hospital of Wisconsin. Available at: http://www.chw.org/display/PPF/DocID/46705/router.asp. Accessed August 18, 2014.
27. Young NL, Davis RJ, Bell DF, et al. Electromyographic and nerve conduction changes after tibial lengthening by the Ilizarov method. J Pediatr Orthop 1993;13(4):473–477.

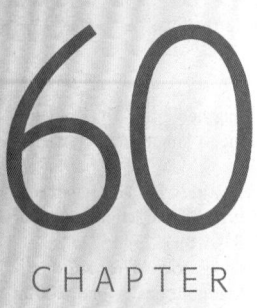

# Guided Growth to Correct Limb Deformity

Ryan D. Muchow and Kenneth J. Noonan

## DEFINITION

- The anatomic axis is the mid-diaphyseal line of a bone. The anatomic angle of the lower extremity consists of the angle between the anatomic axis of the femur and tibia (normal = 5 to 9 degrees valgus).
- The mechanical axis represents the weight-bearing alignment of a bone or an extremity in either the coronal or sagittal plane. It is a straight line connecting the proximal and distal extent of the bone regardless of its anatomic alignment. For example, the normal mechanical axis of the lower extremity in the coronal plane is a straight line from the center of the femoral head to center of the distal tibia and passes through the middle of the knee (**FIG 1**).[14]
  - The mechanical axis is used to assess coronal and sagittal plane deformity and guide surgical correction to restore a normal weight-bearing alignment. Sagittal plane deformity can also be manipulated to improve the amount of extension at the knee or dorsiflexion at the ankle.
- Symmetric physiologic varus is expected between birth and 18 to 24 months, which transitions to a physiologic valgus deformity that is maximal at 3 to 4 years and should correct by 6 to 8 years of age.[18]

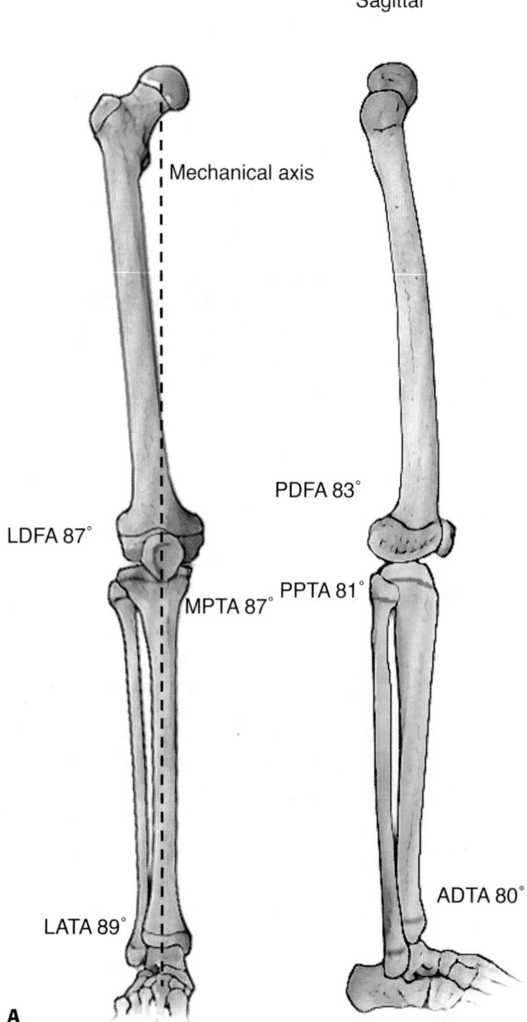


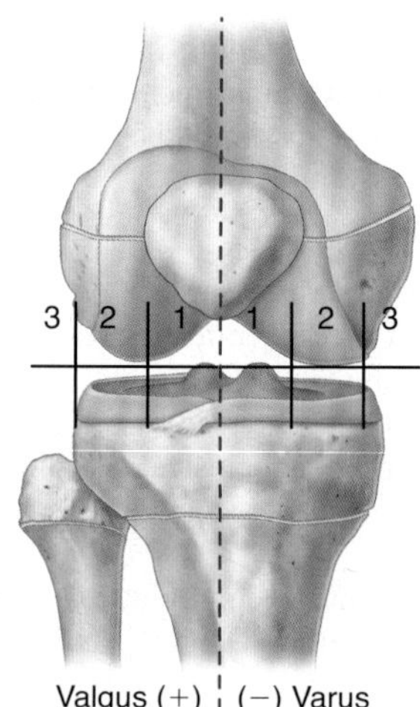


**FIG 1** • **A.** The mechanical axis is a straight line drawn on a full-length, standing AP, or lateral radiograph of the lower extremity connecting the center of the femoral head to the center of the distal tibia. The normal angles for LDFA, MPTA, and LDTA will assist in identifying the location of deformity in the coronal plane, and PDFA, PPTA, and ADTA likewise will locate deformity in the sagittal plane. **B.** Dividing the knee into zones, the mechanical axis should pass through the central one-third of the joint. Deviation into zone 2 or 3 indicates deformity which may require surgical intervention.

- The physis is located at the junction of the epiphysis and metaphysis of long bones and is responsible for longitudinal growth. Consisting of chondrocytes in an extracellular matrix, the cells are oriented longitudinally in four distinct zones: the resting zone, the proliferative zone, the zone of hypertrophy, and the zone of provisional calcification.
  - The zone of Ranvier is located at the periphery of the physis and contributes to circumferential growth of the physis.
  - The perichondrial ring of LaCroix is an extension of the diaphyseal bone and periosteum and stabilizes the physis to the periosteum of the bone enhancing the shear strength of the growth plate.[1]
- The Heuter-Volkmann principle states that compression of the growth plate results in slowing the rate of bone growth. Delpech law is related in that tension across the growth plate increases the rate of bone growth.
- Guided growth or growth modulation techniques use the Heuter-Volkmann principle to affect the rate of growth at one part of the physis relative to another to gain correction of deformity in the coronal or sagittal plane. Common lower limb deformities that are treated with guided growth include pathologic:
  - Genu varum and genu valgum[19]
  - Knee flexion contracture[8,16]
  - Ankle valgus[20]
  - Ankle plantarflexion contracture
  - Hip varus and valgus[23]

## ANATOMY

- Mechanical and anatomic axis of lower extremity (see **FIG 1A**)[15]
  - Hip
    - Neck–shaft angle (NSA) = 130 degrees
  - Knee
    - Lateral distal femoral angle (LDFA) = 87 degrees
    - Medial proximal tibia angle (MPTA) = 87 degrees
    - Posterior distal femoral angle (PDFA) = 83 degrees
    - Posterior proximal tibia angle (PPTA) = 81 degrees
  - Ankle
    - Lateral distal tibia angle (LDTA) = 89 degrees
    - Anterior distal tibia angle (ADTA) = 80 degrees
- Center of rotation of angulation (CORA) is the location of deformity in a long bone. If a single point of deformity exists, the point of intersection between the proximal mechanical axis and the distal mechanical axis is the CORA and it should correspond to anatomic deformity. If a constructed CORA does not correspond with obvious anatomic deformity, another deformity must exist. Therefore, deformity correction should occur at the CORA to restore the mechanical axis.[14]
- Assessment of the physis should occur to ensure adequate growth is available for guided growth. This would include checking for physeal bars and to identify whether the physis is normal or pathologic secondary to an underlying etiology.
- Secondary problems
  - Limb length discrepancy
  - Rotational problems
  - Osteochondritis dissecans
  - Angular problems resulting in subluxation
    - Hip—coxa valga
    - Patella—genu valgum

## PATHOGENESIS

- Physiologic
- Idiopathic genu valgum
- Heuter-Volkmann principle
  - Infantile and adolescent tibia vara
- Acquired (insult to the physis)—trauma, infection, radiation, iatrogenic, juvenile inflammatory arthritis, osteochondroma
- Congenital (condition affecting the health/growth of the physis)—skeletal dysplasia, focal fibrocartilaginous dysplasia, osteogenesis imperfecta, multiple hereditary exostosis, Ollier disease, Maffucci syndrome
- Metabolic bone disease (the physis is susceptible to the Heuter-Volkmann principle at the age of physiologic angulation, for example, onset before 2 years of age will lead to progressive varus, after 4 or 5 years of age will lead to progressive valgus)—rickets, renal osteodystrophy
- Adaptive response to a long bone deformity

## NATURAL HISTORY

- Physiologic = spontaneous resolution
- Progressive angular deformity can cause gait disturbance, limitations in function, and pain.
- There is no consistent evidence demonstrating what degree of malalignment could lead to osteoarthritis and at what age. Various biomechanical and gait studies describe increased force through the medial and lateral compartments with genu varum and valgum, respectively, but this has not been shown to cause osteoarthritis.[4,9,12,24]

## PATIENT HISTORY AND PHYSICAL FINDINGS

- History is important to identify underlying pathology and determine growth potential.
- Current symptoms
  - Pain, functional limitations, cosmetic concerns
- Observe gait
  - Thrust, instability, crouch, equinus
- Assess for limb length discrepancy and rotational profile.
- Joint examination
  - Range of motion of affected and adjacent joints
  - Joint instability and pain
- Foot deformities

## IMAGING AND OTHER DIAGNOSTIC STUDIES

- Plain radiographs (as indicated)
- Bone age
- Lower extremity
  - Standing, full-length anteroposterior (AP) alignment radiograph
  - Lateral views of the lower extremities and joints involved
  - Consider comparison views
  - Consider scanogram
  - Standing lateral foot film to assess foot height
- Computed tomography (CT)—most accurate assessment of rotational profile and best method to assess individual bone lengths in children with sagittal plane joint contractures
- CT or magnetic resonance imaging (MRI)—identifies a physeal bar

## DIFFERENTIAL DIAGNOSIS

- Physiologic
- Idiopathic genu valgum

- Infantile and adolescent tibia vara
- Acquired: trauma, infection, radiation, iatrogenic, juvenile inflammatory arthritis, osteochondroma, adaptive response to a long bone deformity
- Congenital: skeletal dysplasia, focal fibrocartilaginous dysplasia, osteogenesis imperfecta, multiple hereditary exostosis, Ollier disease, Maffucci syndrome
- Metabolic bone disease: rickets, renal osteodystrophy

## NONOPERATIVE MANAGEMENT

- Pathologic conditions by definition are progressive and therefore not commonly amenable to observation or bracing.
- Metabolic disorder—treat and optimize underlying condition first, then if progressive deformity remains, guided growth is indicated.

## SURGICAL MANAGEMENT

- Progressive angular deformity resulting in pain or functional limitation
  - Must have a physis with sufficient growth remaining (variable based on location of physis, patient, and pathology). It is important to remember that in some syndromes, the radiographic presence of an open growth plate does not ensure that the physis is growing sufficiently to correct deformity via guided growth.
- Surgical options
  - Temporary hemiepiphysiodesis
    - Rigid stapling
    - Percutaneous screw (Metaizeau)
    - Tension band plate and screws
      - Stainless steel or titanium
      - Cannulated or solid screws
      - One or two plates
  - Permanent hemiepiphysiodesis
    - Modified Phemister technique
- Percutaneous drilling

### Preoperative Planning

- Ensure physis has adequate growth remaining to allow guided growth.
- Consider placing an implant in an adjacent bone that is normal to accelerate correction of limb deformity. For example, in adolescent Blount disease, it may be necessary to guide growth of both the lateral tibia and lateral femur in an obese patient with less than 2 years of growth remaining.
- Identify the CORA and the corresponding growth plate(s) to affect correction of the deformity.
- Select the proper technique and implant. Specifically for tension band plates, options exist for metal (titanium or stainless steel) and screw type (cannulated or solid).

### Positioning

- Radiolucent operating table
- Tourniquet
- Fluoroscopy

### Approach

- Hemiepiphysiodesis (temporary or permanent) should be performed on the convex side of the deformity.
  - The implant should be placed midsagittal on the bone when attempting to correct pure coronal plane deformity to avoid causing unintended sagittal plane deformity.
  - Deformity may be in a plane that is not fully characterized by AP and lateral radiographs. Thus, the implant may need to be placed slightly anterior (to correct posterior slope) or posterior (to correct anterior slope).
- Open approach
  - Medial distal femur or proximal tibia for genu valgum (**FIG 2**)
  - Lateral distal femur or proximal tibia for genu varum (**FIG 3**)
  - Anterior distal femur (**FIG 4**)
  - Anterior distal tibia (**FIG 5**)
  - Medial distal tibia (**FIG 6**)
- Percutaneous approach (Metaizeau)
  - Medial distal tibia (**FIG 7**)
  - Lateral hip
  - Anterior knee (**FIG 8**)
  - Lateral distal femur and proximal tibia
  - Medial distal femur and proximal tibia

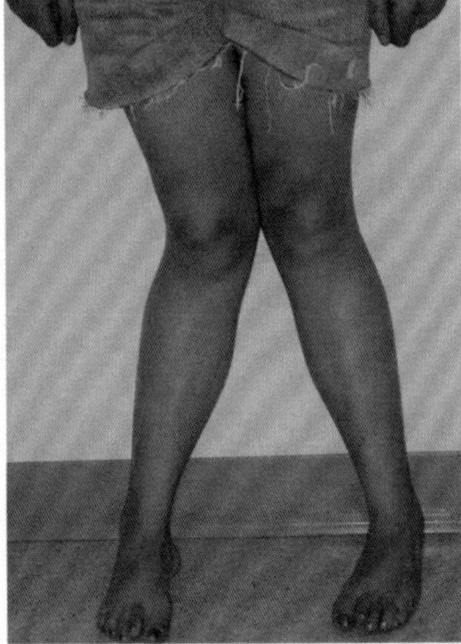
A

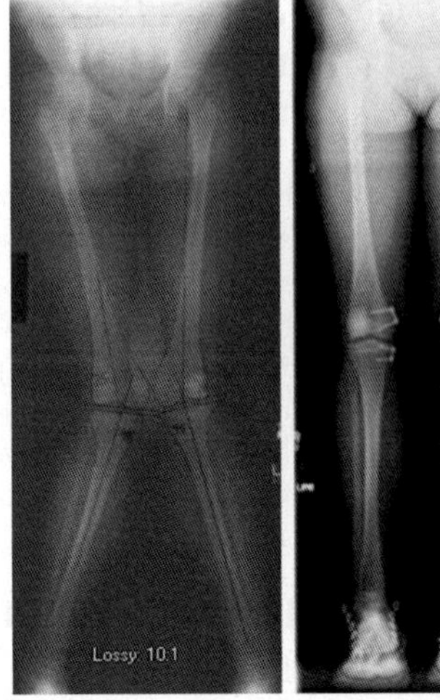


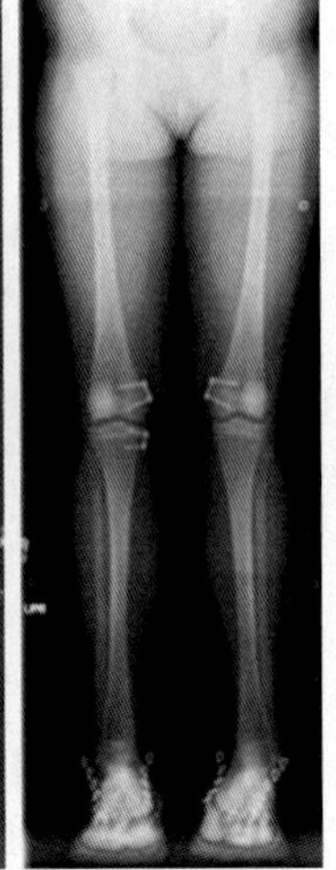
B,C

**FIG 2** • **A.** A 13-year-old girl with knee pain and difficulty with ambulation secondary to genu valgum. **B.** Standing AP radiograph of her lower extremities demonstrating bilateral genu valgum with abnormal LDFA bilaterally and an abnormal MPTA on the right tibia. She was indicated for bilateral medial distal femoral guided growth and right medial proximal tibia guided growth. **C.** Standing AP radiograph at 7 month postoperatively demonstrates normalization of her mechanical axis. (Courtesy of UW Pediatric Orthopaedics.)

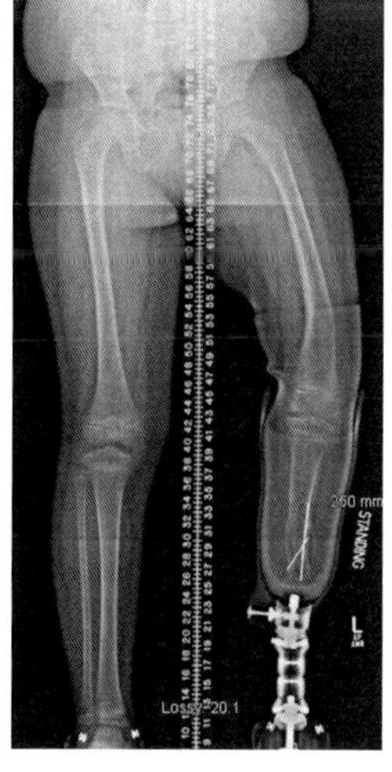


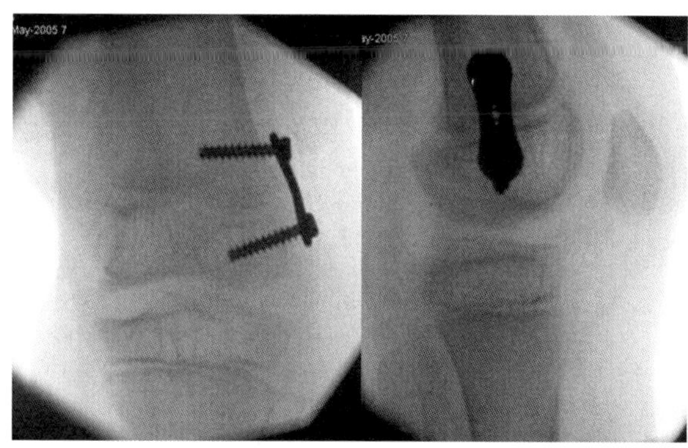


**FIG 3** • **A.** A 7-year-old boy with traumatic amputation from a lawn mower injury with varus deformity causing difficulty with prosthetic wear. **B,C.** Although the CORA was a result of fracture malunion proximal to the distal femoral physis, guided growth was chosen as an alternative to osteotomy to straighten the limb and to improve prosthetic wear.

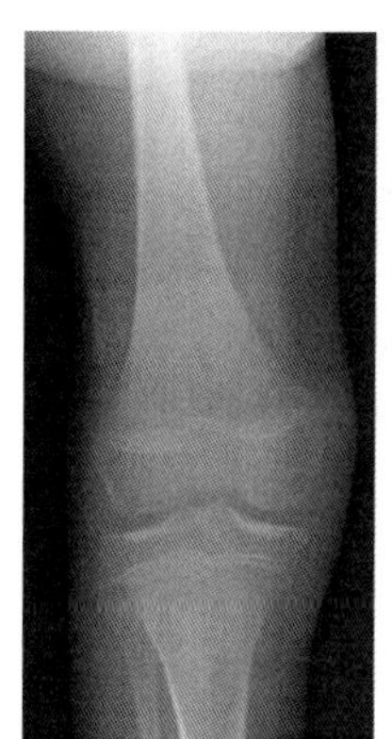
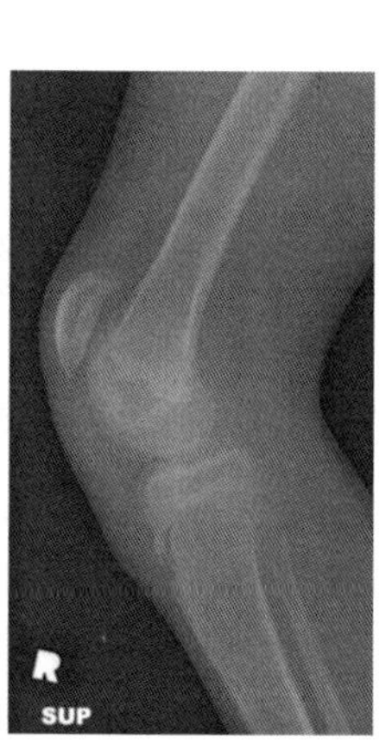


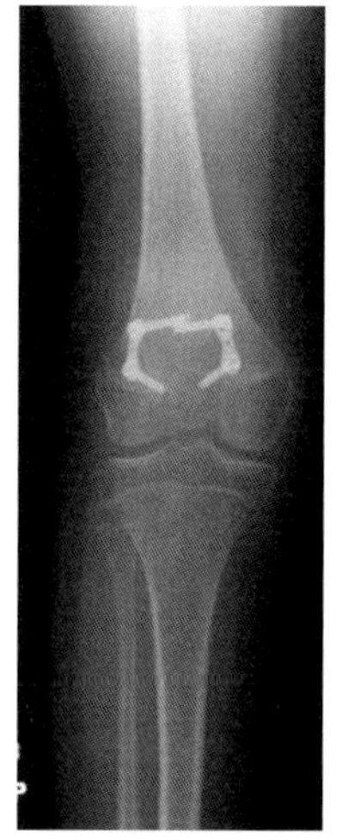


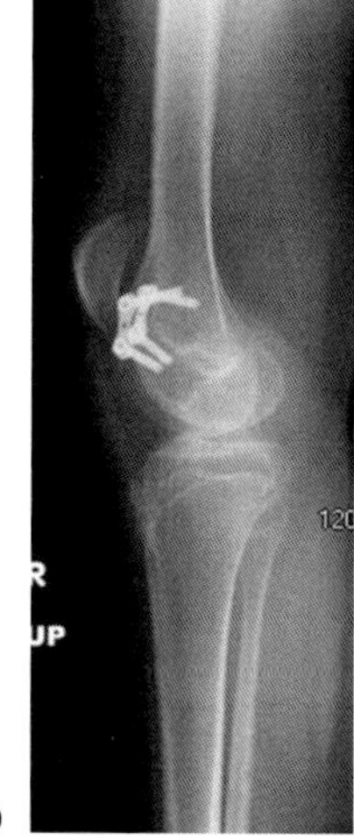


**FIG 4** • **A,B.** A 13-year-old boy with spastic diplegia who ambulates with a crouch knee gait, hamstring contracture, and knee flexion contracture. **C,D.** The patient was able to achieve full extension after hamstring release and anterior distal femoral guided growth with two modular implants placed next to the patella. To place these implants, two peripatellar incisions are needed to allow intra-articular placement of the devices across the physis and to ensure that no patellar contact ensues. (Courtesy of UW Pediatric Orthopaedics.)

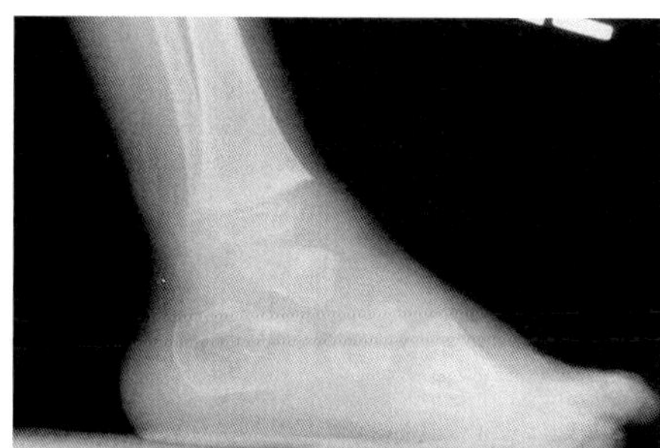


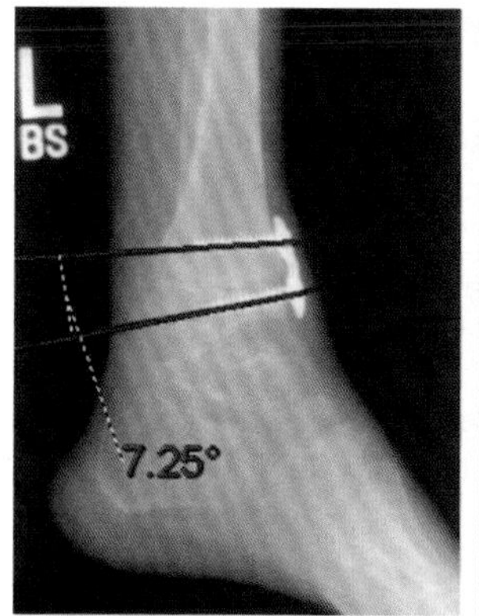


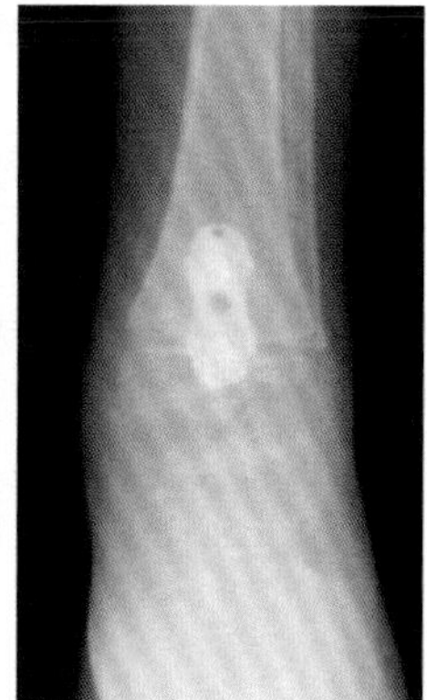


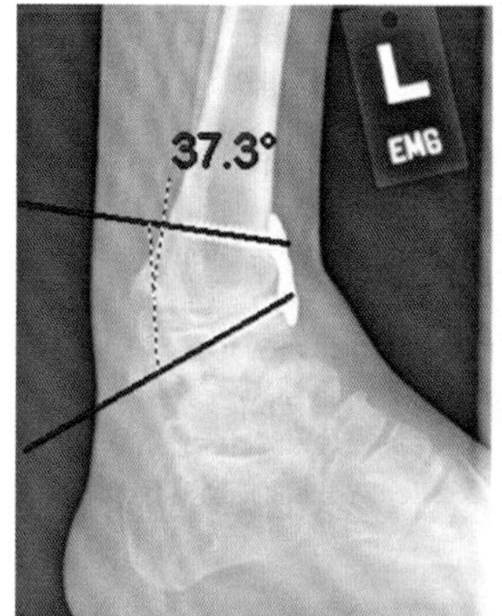


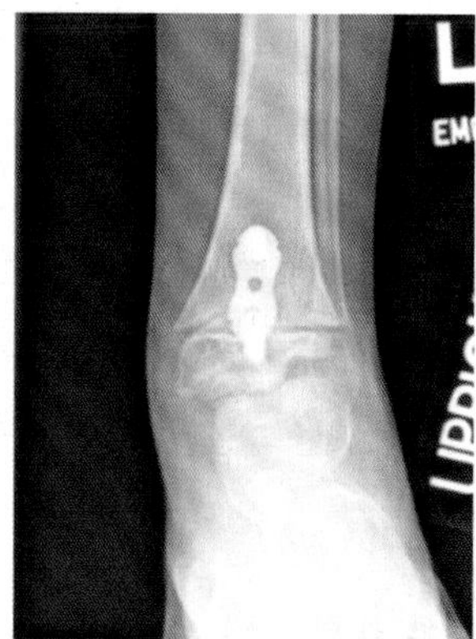


**FIG 5** • **A.** An 8-year-old boy with 20 degrees residual equinus and talus dysmorphology after revision posterior medial release. **B,C.** Anterior distal tibia guided growth was performed after a CT scan ensured appropriate sizing of the epiphysis. In this procedure, a modular implant is placed by putting a guide pin into the distal tibia epiphysis and then a cannulated screw is placed. **D,E.** Two years postoperatively, the patient now has 10 degrees of ankle dorsiflexion. (Courtesy of UW Pediatric Orthopaedics.)

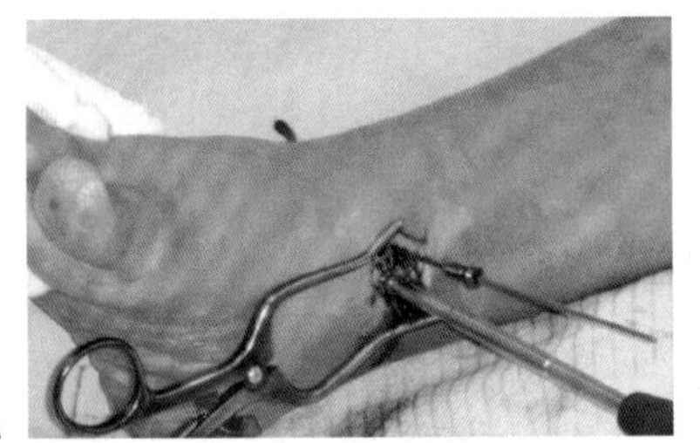
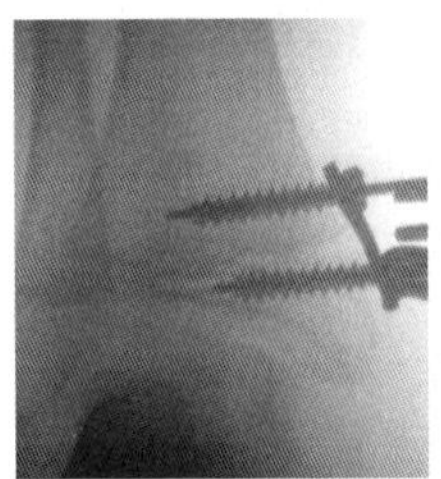

**FIG 6** • Open medial distal tibia guided growth for ankle valgus is performed with a modular implant.

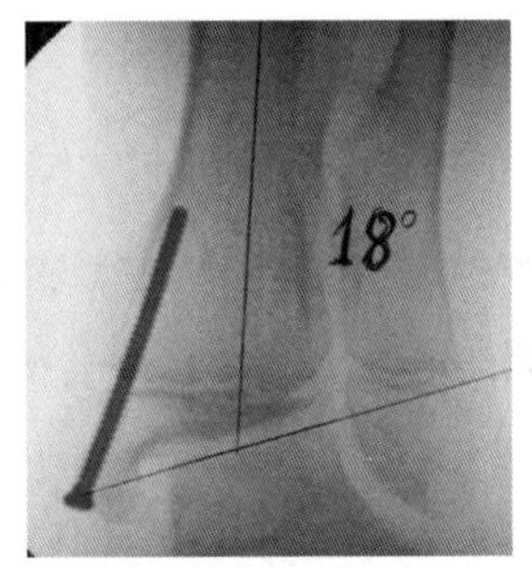

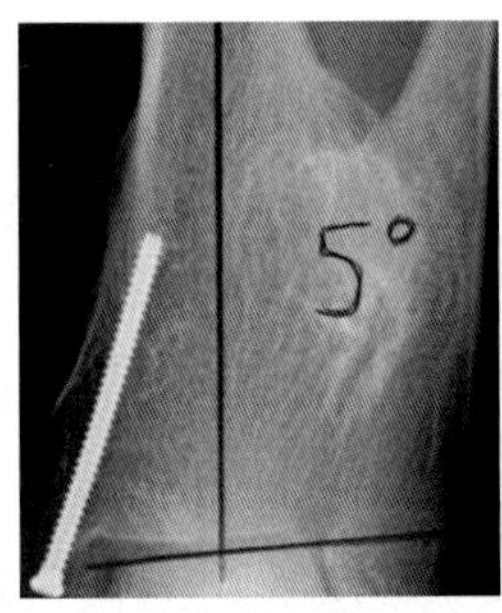


**FIG 7** • **A.** A 12-year-old boy with multiple hereditary exostosis who developed symptomatic ankle valgus underwent medial malleolus guided growth with a single percutaneously placed screw. **B.** AP radiograph at 3.5 years postoperatively demonstrates improvement in distal tibial articular alignment. (Courtesy of UW Pediatric Orthopaedics.)

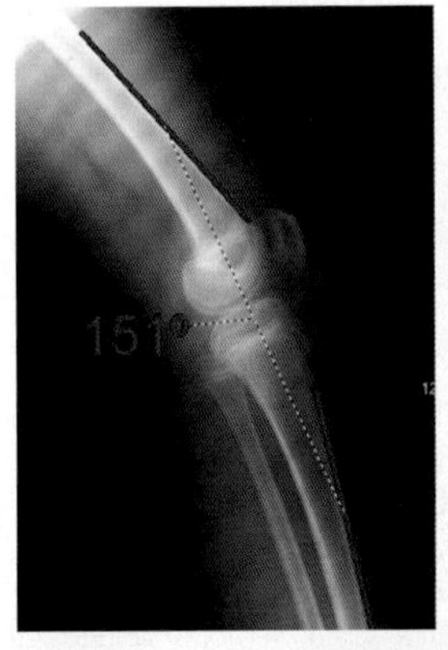

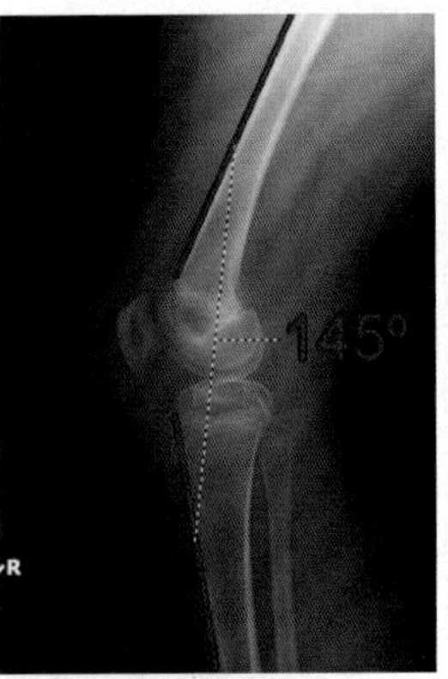

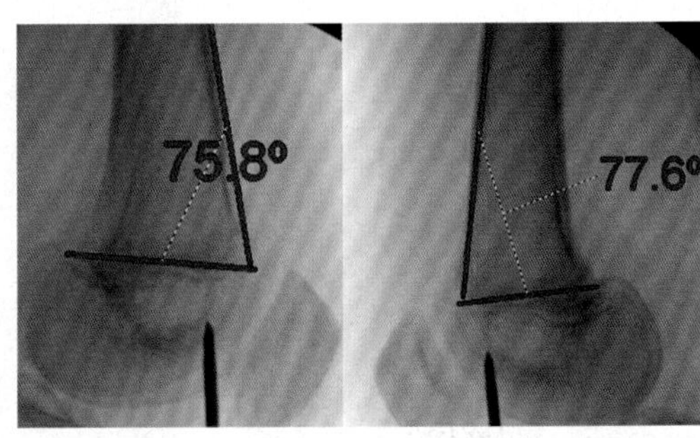

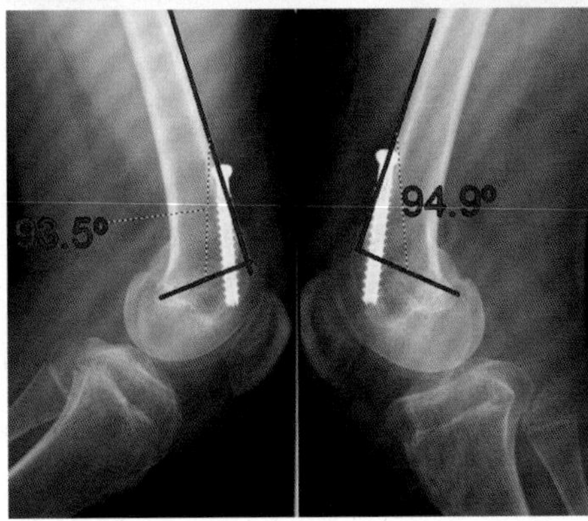


**FIG 8** • **A,B.** A 12-year-old boy with spastic diplegia who ambulates with a crouch gait, hamstring contracture, and knee flexion contracture. **C,D.** Intraoperative fluoroscopy demonstrating preoperative PDFA. The child underwent hamstring transfer and distal femoral guided growth with placement of 6.5-mm cannulated screw positioned anterior in the center of the distal femur. **E,F.** Postoperative lateral radiographs show improved PDFA and full extension on clinical examination. (Courtesy of UW Pediatric Orthopaedics.)



## Tension Band Plating for Pure Coronal Plane Deformity at the Knee

- The patient is positioned supine on a radiolucent table with a thigh tourniquet.
- Fluoroscopy is used to identify the distal femoral or proximal tibial physis (or both) and a 2- to 3-cm incision is made centered over the physis in the midsagittal plane.
  - Medial distal femur—the fascia of medial quadriceps mechanism and medial patella femoral ligament is incised and the vastus medialis muscle is retracted anteriorly.
  - Lateral distal femur: The iliotibial band is split longitudinally.
  - Medial proximal tibia: The pes anserine is split longitudinally.
  - Lateral proximal tibia: The anterior compartment may be left intact if the plate does not overlap or may need to be incised longitudinally and the muscle retracted.
- The dissection continues until periosteum is visualized but not violated.
- A guide pin is inserted into the physis, which serves to center the plate at the physis. Fluoroscopy is used to confirm proper position.
- A properly sized plate is chosen and placed over the guide pin through the center hole (**TECH FIG 1A**).

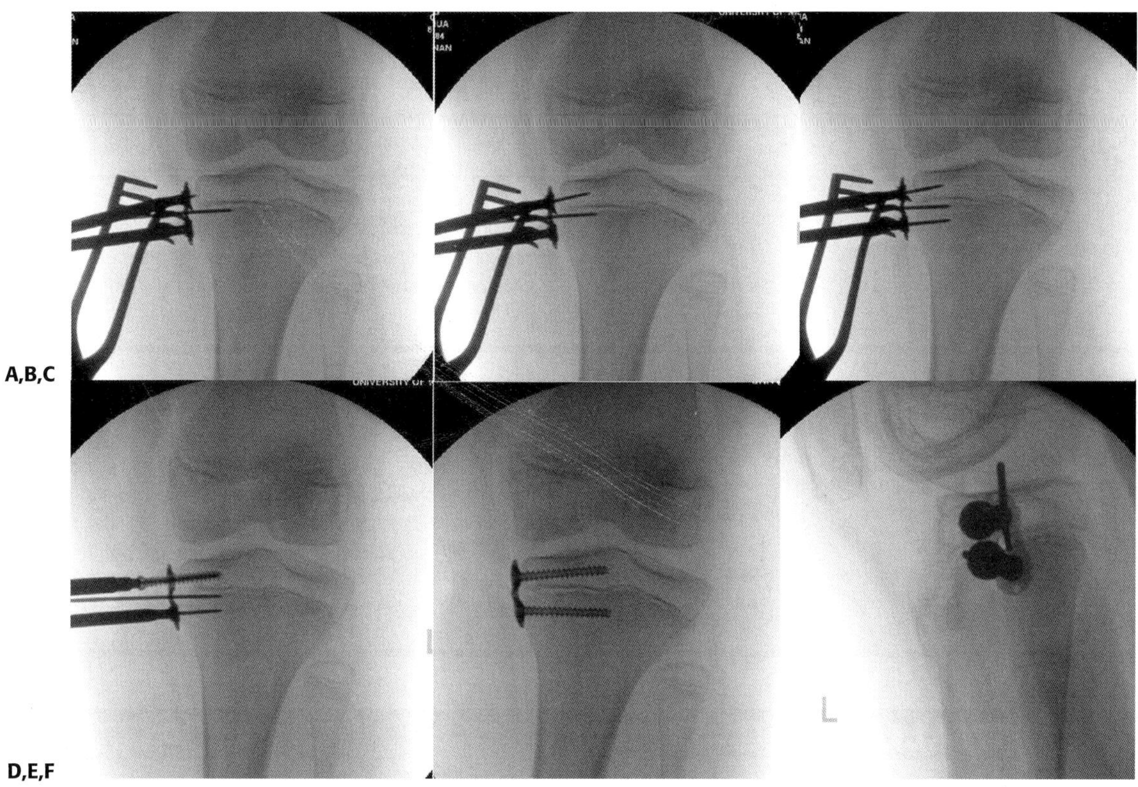

A,B,C

D,E,F

**TECH FIG 1** ● **A.** A guide pin has been placed into the physis and the plate slid over the guide pin to properly center it. **B.** An epiphyseal pin is placed parallel or slightly divergent to the physis. **C.** A metaphyseal pin is placed second aiming parallel or slightly divergent to the physis. **D,E.** The near cortex was drilled and then fully threaded cannulated screws were placed over the guide pins. **F.** Lateral fluoroscopic image of the proximal tibia demonstrating the midsagittal positioning of the plate.

- Guide pins are then inserted through the plate in a parallel to slightly divergent fashion from the physis, placing the epiphyseal pin first, followed by the metaphyseal pin. Confirm proper position with fluoroscopy and avoid inadvertent physeal or joint disruption (**TECH FIG 1B,C**).
- The near cortex is drilled and then a fully threaded screw is inserted (cannulated or solid screws depending on surgeon preference) (**TECH FIG 1D,E**).
- Confirm final screw positions with fluoroscopy (**TECH FIG 1E,F**).
- Finish with irrigation, routine wound closure, local anesthesia, dressing, and immobilization.

## Hemiepiphyseal Stapling

- The surgical approach is the same as tension band plating, with care taken not to disrupt the periosteum.
- The physis is marked with a guide pin and the proper position is confirmed with fluoroscopy.
- Usually, only one rigid staple is inserted, straddling the physis with one side of the staple in the epiphysis and the other in the metaphysis. Some surgeons use more than one staple.
- Confirm final position with fluoroscopy. Then irrigation, routine wound closure, local anesthesia, dressing, and immobilization.[2]

## Metaizeau Technique

- A percutaneous approach is used to place a transphyseal screw under fluoroscopic guidance.
- In the distal femur, the screw can be placed across the desired location in the physis from either the medial or lateral side of the bone.
- In the proximal tibia, a single screw is placed from the medial side to tether the lateral growth plate (genu varum) or placed from the lateral side to tether the medial growth plate (genu valgum). The screw passes from the metaphysis to the epiphysis and crosses the physis near its periphery.
- The goal is to place the tip of the screw into the epiphysis just across the physis at the peripheral aspect of the bone in order to maximally affect angular growth.
- Upon obtaining desired correction, the screw is able to be removed.[10]

## Modified Phemister Technique

- The surgical approach to the physis is the same as tension band plating. A headlamp or lighted sucker tip may help with visualization. The periosteum, however, is incised longitudinally with this technique.
- Periosteal flaps are made to allow visualization of the physis.
- A hemiepiphysiodesis is performed by removing a square block of bone that includes the physis (1 to 2 cm from anterior to posterior, 1 to 2 cm from superior to inferior, and 1 cm deep).
- Through the void left by the removed block of bone, the physis can be visualized and the exposed growth plate is then curetted anterior and posterior to allow a bony tether to occur. Care is taken to avoid to curette too much bone in order to effectuate a partial growth arrest as opposed to compete physeal arrest by extensive curettage across the physis.
- The bone block should be reinserted in an orientation 180 degrees from its original position to create a bone bridge.
- This technique is permanent and requires precise timing and calculation to ensure proper correction before growth plate closure.[6,17]

## Percutaneous Drilling

- Fluoroscopy is used to identify the physis and a 1-cm incision is made in the desired sagittal plane.
- A guide pin is inserted into the physis and proper position is confirmed with fluoroscopy.
- Anterior cruciate ligament (ACL) reamers are used to sequentially ream up to 1 cm to drill out the physis and curettes are able to be used to finalize the peripheral physeal removal. Similar to the open method, care is needed to avoid removing too much physis and thus limiting angular correction and resulting in complete arrest.
- Hemiepiphysiodesis is complete when a bone bridge is established. This technique is permanent and requires precise timing and calculation to ensure proper correction before growth plate closure.

## PEARLS AND PITFALLS

| | |
|---|---|
| **Ensure good indications, patient and family education** | ▪ Identify patients with a physis with adequate growth remaining to allow deformity correction.<br>▪ Consider advanced imaging (CT and MRI) to assess for bony bars that will diminish effectiveness.<br>▪ Educate families on expected rate of correction and the importance of close follow-up to ensure removal at the appropriate time to avoid undesired overcorrection. |
| **Prevent periosteal damage** | ▪ When performing instrumented hemiepiphysiodesis, avoid damaging the periosteum with implant insertion or removal to prevent damage to the physis. |
| **Avoid soft tissue tethering** | ▪ It is important to split and repair tendinous structures such as the pes anserinus and the medial patella femoral ligament during medial guided growth of the knee. Failing to place the implants under these structures can lead to painful tethering. |
| **Screw choice** | ▪ In obese patients, it may be desired to use stainless steel or solid screws to avoid fracture of the screw. This tends to happen at the metaphyseal location (**FIG 9**) |
| **Tension band plates** | ▪ Tension band plates may need to be prebent to maintain a low profile to the bone, especially at the lateral proximal tibia. |

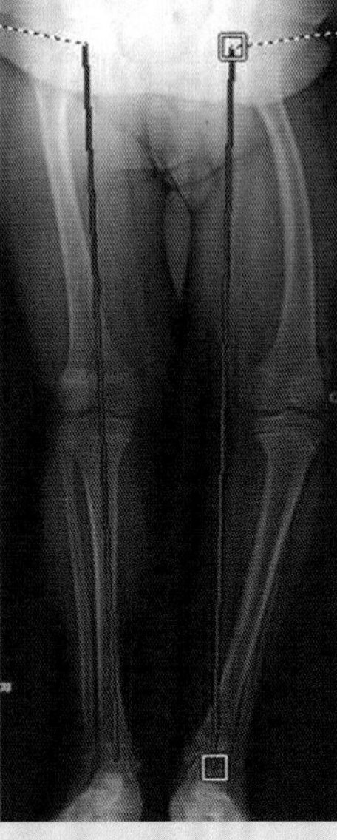

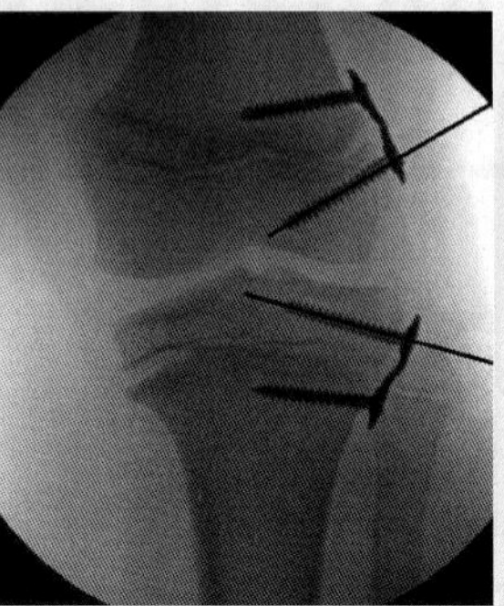

**FIG 9** • A 9-year-old boy with juvenile Blount disease and distal femoral and proximal tibia deformity was indicated for guided growth. In this method, lateral epiphysiodesis was performed by placing guide pins for cannulated screws into the epiphysis and solid screws were placed in the metaphysis. The metaphyseal screws are prone to failure, which is why solid screws were chosen. (Courtesy of UW Pediatric Orthopaedics.)

## POSTOPERATIVE CARE

- Local anesthetic or nerve block (use knee immobilizer for 24 hours in patients with femoral nerve block)
- Temporary immobilization for wound healing
- Activity as tolerated, physical therapy (PT) if necessary
- Follow-up
  - Standing AP lower extremity radiograph taken at 3- to 6-month intervals
  - Allow for slight overcorrection if there is growth remaining prior to implant removal (5 degrees).[5,7,10,11,13,19,21,22,25]
- Implant does not need to be removed if growth is finished and it is asymptomatic.

## OUTCOMES

- The rate of correction is variable between patients. A published calculation estimates angular correction of 7 degrees per year at the distal femur and 5 degrees per year at the proximal tibia.[3]
- Potential for 5 degrees of rebound once the plate is removed and if growth remains.

## COMPLICATIONS

- Implant failure—broken plate or screw with tension band plates; broken staples
- Implant loosening—staples may loosen; screws may lose purchase with tension band plates
- Wound complications in obese
- Infection
- Nerve damage
- Overcorrection or undercorrection

## REFERENCES


1. Ballock RT, O'Keefe RJ. Orthopaedic Basic Science, ed 3. Rosemont, IL: American Academy of Orthopaedic Surgeons, 2007.
2. Blount WP, Clarke GR. Control of bone growth by epiphyseal stapling; a preliminary report. J Bone Joint Surg Am 1949;31A(3): 464–478.
3. Bowen JR, Leahey JL, Zhang ZH, et al. Partial epiphysiodesis at the knee to correct angular deformity. Clin Orthop Relat Res 1985;(198):184–190.
4. Bruns J, Volkmer M, Luessenhop S. Pressure distribution at the knee joint. Influence of varus and valgus deviation without and with ligament dissection. Arch Orthop Trauma Surg 1993;113:12–19.
5. Cho TJ, Choi IH, Chung CY, et al. Hemiepiphyseal stapling for angular deformity correction around the knee joint in children with multiple epiphyseal dysplasia. J Pediatr Orthop 2009;29:52–56.
6. Green WT, Anderson M. Epiphyseal arrest for the correction of discrepancies in length of the lower extremities. J Bone Joint Surg Am 1957;39-A(4):853–72; discussion, 872; passim.
7. Inan M, Chan G, Bowen JR. Correction of angular deformities of the knee by percutaneous hemiepiphysiodesis. Clin Orthop Relat Res 2007;456:164–169.
8. Klatt J, Stevens PM. Guided growth for fixed knee flexion deformity. J Pediatr Orthop 2008;28:626–631.
9. McKellop HA, Llinas A, Sarmiento A. Effects of tibial malalignment on the knee and ankle. Orthop Clin North Am 1994;25:415–423.
10. Metaizeau JP, Wong-Chung J, Bertrand H, et al. Percutaneous epiphysiodesis using transphyseal screws (PETS). J Pediatr Orthop 1998;18:363–369.
11. Mielke CH, Stevens PM. Hemiepiphyseal stapling for knee deformities in children younger than 10 years: a preliminary report. J Pediatr Orthop 1996;16:423–429.
12. Morrison JB. The mechanics of the knee joint in relation to normal walking. J Biomech 1970;3:51–61.
13. Nouth F, Kuo LA. Percutaneous epiphysiodesis using transphyseal screws (PETS): prospective case study and review. J Pediatr Orthop 2004;24:721–725.
14. Paley D. Principles of Deformity Correction. Berlin: Springer, 2002.
15. Paley D, Herzenberg JE, Tetsworth K, et al. Deformity planning for frontal and sagittal plane corrective osteotomies. Orthop Clin North Am 1994;25:425–465.
16. Palocaren T, Thabet AM, Rogers K, et al. Anterior distal femoral stapling for correcting knee flexion contracture in children with arthrogryposis—preliminary results. J Pediatr Orthop 2010;30:169–173.
17. Phemister DB. Operative arrestment of longitudinal growth of bones in the treatment of deformities. J Bone Joint Surg Am 1933;15:1–15.
18. Salenius P, Vankka E. The development of the tibiofemoral angle in children. J Bone Joint Surg Am 1975;57:259–261.
19. Stevens PM. Guided growth for angular correction: a preliminary series using a tension band plate. J Pediatr Orthop 2007;27:253–259.
20. Stevens PM, Kennedy JM, Hung M. Guided growth for ankle valgus. J Pediatr Orthop 2011;31:878–883.
21. Stevens PM, Klatt JB. Guided growth for pathological physes: radiographic improvement during realignment. J Pediatr Orthop 2008;28:632–639.
22. Stevens PM, Maguire M, Dales MD, et al. Physeal stapling for idiopathic genu valgum. J Pediatr Orthop 1999;19:645–649.
23. Stevens PM, Novais EN. Multilevel guided growth for hip and knee varus secondary to chondrodysplasia. J Pediatr Orthop 2012;32:626–630.
24. Tetsworth K, Paley D. Malalignment and degenerative arthropathy. Orthop Clin North Am 1994;25:367–377.
25. Zuege RC, Kempken TG, Blount WP. Epiphyseal stapling for angular deformity at the knee. J Bone Joint Surg Am 1979;61:320–329.

61

CHAPTER

# Distal Tibial Osteotomy

J. Eric Gordon

## DEFINITION

- Angular deformities of the distal tibia can lead to varus or valgus malalignment of the ankle joint.
- Rotational deformities of the tibia include both internal and external tibial torsion.
- Additional sources of ankle malalignment include both bony and ligamentous disorders.

## ANATOMY

- The tibiotalar joint is normally oriented perpendicular to the long axis of the tibia. This is assessed by measuring the lateral distal tibial angle (LDTA), which has a normal value of 90 degrees (range, 88 to 95 degrees).
- Sagittal alignment of the ankle joint is in slight dorsiflexion and is assessed by measuring the anterior distal tibial angle (ADTA), which has a normal value of 80 degrees (range, 78 to 81 degrees).
- Rotational alignment of the tibia changes with age. Internal tibial torsion is common after birth and gradually corrects until approximately age 5 to 6 years. The normal thigh–foot angle after age 6 years is 0–15°.

## PATHOGENESIS

- Coronal plane deformities about the ankle are not uncommon and may occur secondary to congenital or acquired conditions.[1–3]
- Varus angular malalignment of the ankle is generally due to either a traumatic or infectious insult to the medial aspect of the distal tibial physis, with resultant premature closure of the injured area and relative overgrowth of the lateral distal tibial physis and fibula with resultant progressive varus.[2,3,7]
- Valgus deformity of the ankle in children is caused by a wide variety of congenital and developmental as well as posttraumatic conditions.
  - Neuromuscular conditions such as diplegic cerebral palsy can lead to foot pronation, and late ankle valgus and progressive ankle valgus with lateral wedging of the distal tibial epiphysis may be seen in patients with myelodysplasia.
  - Traumatic or postinfectious injury to the distal fibular or lateral distal tibial physis can produce distal tibial valgus.
  - Congenital fibular hemimelia is often associated with distal tibial valgus which can be exacerbated by hindfoot coalitions leading to severe hindfoot valgus.
  - Congenital pseudarthrosis of the fibula can often lead to ankle valgus as well.
  - Iatrogenic distal tibial valgus with fibular shortening can also occur following fibular harvest for vascularized or nonvascularized bone graft.
- Deformities occurring secondary to physeal injuries are progressive until skeletal maturity.
- Correction of deformities about the ankle is complicated by the fact that deformities are frequently centered about the distal tibial physis, very close to the ankle joint, and opening or closing wedge osteotomies performed proximal enough to allow fixation of the fragments can produce secondary deformities with unacceptable translation of the ankle joint.

## NATURAL HISTORY

- Angular deformity of the distal tibia leads to abnormal loading of the hindfoot, ankle joint, and knee and may lead to secondary deformities such as a planovalgus foot or hallux valgus. Long-term malalignment of the ankle joint may lead to the development of premature osteoarthritis of the ankle.[8,9]
- Initially, the limb may be treated with braces or orthotics relieving pain and correcting gait, but progression of the deformity with growth can lead to increased soft tissue pressure, bursa formation, and skin ulceration over the medial malleolus, lateral malleolus, or talonavicular region.

## PATIENT HISTORY AND PHYSICAL FINDINGS

- A detailed history should be obtained, including recent or remote trauma, infection, or congenital conditions. In addition, symptoms related to ankle malalignment or instability should be elicited.
- Physical examination should include gross inspection of both lower extremities with the patient standing, walking, and sitting to determine the location of deformity as well as the alignment of adjacent structures (in particular, the hindfoot and knee) that may contribute to perceived deformity as well as affect the surgical outcome.
- The orthopaedic surgeon should inspect standing foot and ankle alignment from behind the patient to determine the location of deformity (distal tibia, ankle, hindfoot).
  - Standing heel alignment in varus or valgus may indicate the presence of uncompensated distal tibial deformity. Normal alignment in the presence of known deformity should alert the surgeon to hindfoot compensation, which may be rigid or supple.
- The orthopaedic surgeon should check hindfoot passive inversion and eversion to evaluate the ability of the hindfoot to accommodate surgical changes.
  - Lack of hindfoot motion indicates that the patient may not be able to compensate for distal tibial osteotomies. Further procedures may be warranted to realign the hindfoot to correct fixed deformities.
- Single-limb toe rise: With the patient standing, viewed from posterior, the patient lifts one limb, then rises onto the toes

of the standing limb. This should result in prompt inversion of the heel, rising of the longitudinal arch, and external rotation of the supporting leg. Lack of hindfoot inversion should draw attention to the subtalar and transverse tarsal joints as possible sites of pathologic alignment.

- To check forefoot hindfoot alignment, the patient is seated, facing the examiner. The patient's hindfoot is grasped in one hand and the calcaneus is held in the neutral position, in line with the long axis of the leg. The examiner's other hand grasps the foot along the fifth metatarsal. The thumb of the hand grasping the heel is placed over the talonavicular joint, and the joint is manipulated by moving the hand holding the fifth metatarsal until the head of the talus is covered by the navicular. The position of the forefoot as projected by a plane parallel to the metatarsals is compared to the orientation of the long axis of the calcaneus. The forefoot will be in one of three positions relative to the hindfoot—neutral, forefoot varus, or forefoot valgus. The examiner should determine whether this relation is supple or rigid, especially when considering surgery because a fixed varus or valgus forefoot deformity will not allow the foot to become plantigrade after realignment of the tibiotalar or subtalar joints.
- Standing lower extremity alignment: If distal tibial deformity is present in conjunction with genu varum or valgum, the patient's entire deformity should be evaluated and a comprehensive plan developed.
- The patient's gait may show an antalgic pattern or may reveal limitations of functional motion in the hindfoot.

## IMAGING AND OTHER DIAGNOSTIC STUDIES

- Standing anteroposterior (AP) and mortise views of both ankle joints should be obtained (**FIG 1A–C**). The LDTA is measured from the intersection of a line drawn parallel to the long axis of the tibia and a second line drawn across the dome of the talus. The normal LDTA is 90 degrees as measured from the lateral side. The amount of deformity is calculated from the number of degrees that differ from 90 degrees.
- Lateral weight-bearing radiographs of both ankles should be obtained to detect any sagittal plane deformity (**FIG 1D**). The lateral tibiotalar angle is measured from the anterior side. The average ADTA is 80 degrees as measured from the anterior side.
- Foot radiographs, including standing AP, standing lateral, and oblique views, are used to evaluate hindfoot alignment to avoid over- or undercorrection at the time of surgery. The standing lateral view of the foot is used to evaluate talar–first metatarsal alignment; normally, the talus and first metatarsal are parallel. The standing AP view is used to evaluate the talocalcaneal angle; if the talocalcaneal angle exceeds 35 degrees, hindfoot valgus is present.
- A standing AP view of the pelvis is obtained to evaluate for leg length discrepancy.
- Computed tomography can be useful in assessing the presence and size of physeal bars.

## DIFFERENTIAL DIAGNOSIS

- In addition to distal tibial angular deformity, varus or valgus malalignment about the ankle joint may be due to other local bony or ligamentous disorders.
- Fixed hindfoot varus or valgus may simulate ankle deformity on clinical examination.
- Apparent ankle valgus may occur secondary to disorders such as angular deformity of the fibula with shortening and associated lateral shift of the talus hindfoot valgus, hindfoot valgus, or fixed forefoot varus.
- Apparent ankle varus may occur secondary to disorders such as hindfoot varus as seen in Charcot-Marie-Tooth disease, residual clubfoot, or fixed forefoot valgus.

## NONOPERATIVE MANAGEMENT

- Mild distal tibial angular deformity associated with ankle varus or valgus can be managed through the use of custom braces and orthotics or medial or lateral posting of the shoes.
- Surgery is the mainstay of treatment of bony deformity of the distal tibia.

## SURGICAL MANAGEMENT

- An opening or closing wedge supramalleolar osteotomy (SMO) may be performed for simultaneous correction of frontal and sagittal plane deformities of the ankle.
- SMOs allow for immediate correction of the deformity. However, they are considered technically demanding and relatively invasive and require a period of limited weight bearing or non–weight bearing and immobilization.

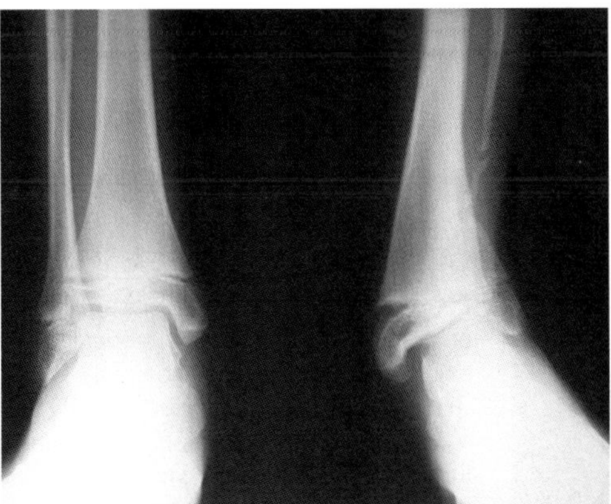
A

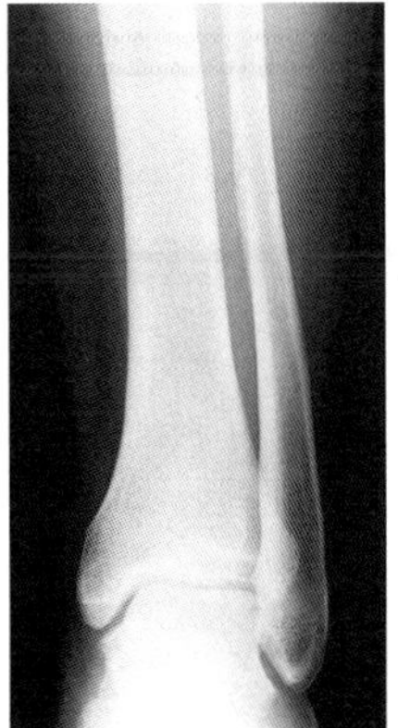
B

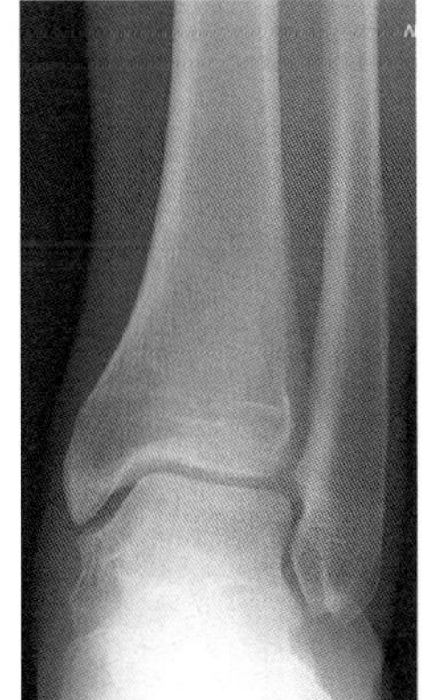
C

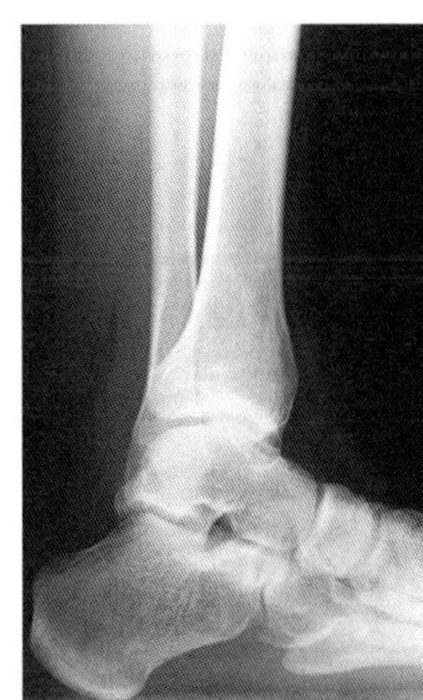
D

**FIG 1** • **A.** Standing AP view of both ankles in a 14-year-old boy with a left distal tibial valgus deformity due to congenital pseudarthrosis of the tibia. **B.** Standing AP radiograph of the left ankle in a 16-year-old boy showing a varus deformity after a healed physeal distal tibial fracture with medial physeal arrest. **C.** Standing lateral radiograph of the left ankle of the same patient. **D.** Standing mortise radiograph of the left ankle in the same patient showing a varus deformity after a healed physeal distal tibial fracture with medial physeal arrest.

- The challenge involved in correcting varus or valgus deformities of the ankle is to correct the deformity without introducing new secondary deformities. The mechanical axis of the tibia should pass through the center of the ankle perpendicular to the joint surface.
- Some SMO techniques may lead to the development of secondary deformities. For instance, a transverse closing wedge osteotomy performed 4 cm proximal to the joint surface to correct a valgus deformity causes lateral shift of the ankle and a prominent medial malleolus.
- In a child with growth remaining, physeal modulation via a hemiepiphysiodesis with an eight-hole plate, transphyseal screw, or staples can be used to correct distal tibial valgus deformities.
- Correction occurs gradually after hemiepiphysiodesis, so it is not ideal for patients requiring acute corrections such as those with skin breakdown or significant pain. Close follow-up after hemiepiphysiodesis is essential to avoid overcorrection.
- Currently, SMOs are the procedure of choice for correcting ankle valgus in the absence of adequate growth to correct the deformity by hemiepiphysiodesis techniques.

## Choosing the Technique

- Several techniques have been used and are described in the following text, including transphyseal SMO, transverse SMO with translation, and the Wiltse SMO.
- Oblique supramalleolar opening or closing wedge osteotomy
  - Lubicky and Altiok[3] described an oblique distal tibial osteotomy to correct varus and valgus deformity of the distal tibia.
  - This technique offers the advantage of placing the hinge of the osteotomy at the level of the deformity and thus performing the correction at the site of the deformity so that maximum correction can be obtained without creating a secondary translational deformity.
- Transverse SMO with translation: Concomitant fibular osteotomies are performed to allow for compression at the osteotomy site and translation of the tibial osteotomy.
- Wiltse osteotomy
  - Wiltse[10] noted that a simple wedge resection for correction of distal tibial valgus deformities will lead to malalignment and prominence of the medial malleolus.
  - The author developed and reported the results of resection of a triangular section from the distal tibia with rotation of the distal fragment in order to produce a normal-appearing ankle and improved weight-bearing alignment.
  - This procedure is effective because it creates a stable osteotomy and forces the surgeon to lateralize the osteotomy when correcting a valgus deformity, thereby bringing the ankle joint beneath the tibial shaft and preventing medial prominence of the medial malleolus.
- Screw hemiepiphysiodesis is used to address valgus deformities in children with sufficient growth remaining to correct the deformity.
- We have found that the oblique osteotomy allows for correction of the deformity and offers the advantage of improved bone healing, as minimal periosteal stripping is necessary and the deformity is corrected by hinging the osteotomy at a point along the bisector of the deformity.

## Preoperative Planning

- The principal issues to be addressed in surgical correction of distal tibial deformities are the magnitude and direction of the deformity, any rotational component, and length. The surgeon should address all of these components with a comprehensive plan.
- Length discrepancies in particular are critical because when the limb length discrepancy is greater than 2 cm, a lengthening or shortening procedure should be performed in conjunction with correction of the distal tibia. Either contralateral epiphysiodesis or shortening should be planned or lengthening of the index limb, which may make the entire procedure preferable to perform with circular external fixation.
- Weight-bearing radiographs of the ankle in the AP and lateral planes are essential to determine the extent of the deformity. In addition, it is important to thoroughly assess the hindfoot and forefoot.
- The magnitude and plane of the deformity to be addressed should be calculated preoperatively and noted in the preoperative plan (**FIG 2A**).
- After the deformity is assessed using the methods described by Paley and Tetsworth,[4,5] the position of the center of

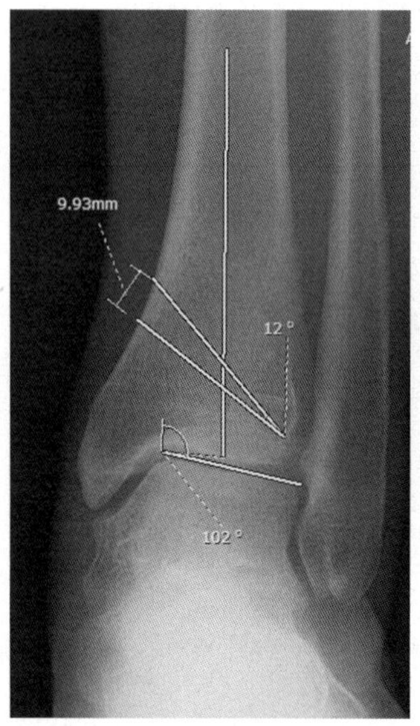


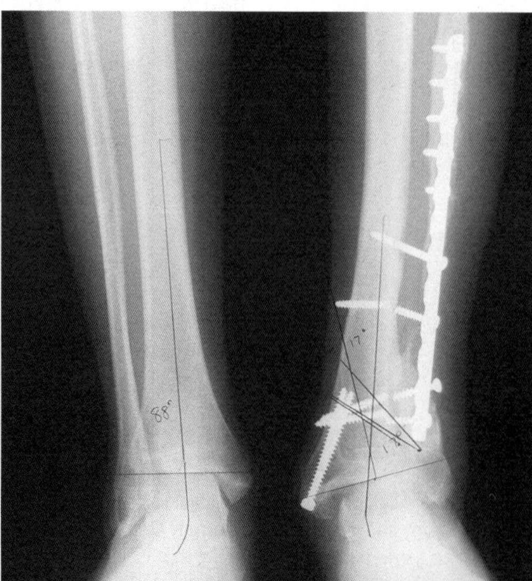


**FIG 2 • A.** Standing mortise radiograph of the left ankle showing preoperative planning. A 12-degree varus deformity is shown with planning for a 12-degree opening wedge oblique osteotomy with a 10-mm opening at the base. **B.** Standing AP view of both ankles in a different patient showing preoperative planning, revealing a 17-degree valgus deformity and plans for a 17-degree closing wedge osteotomy. The base of the wedge is planned as 14 mm along the medial tibial cortex.

rotation of angulation (CORA) is identified and a bisector is constructed. Most commonly, this point is very near the physis and articular surface (**FIG 2B**).

- Although the osteotomy can be performed at a level consistent with the biology of the bone and allowing for adequate fixation, the correction of the deformity should occur along the bisector.
- The goal of surgical correction should be to obtain an LDTA of about 90 degrees with a tibial mechanical axis that passes through the center of the ankle.
- Care should be taken to evaluate the hindfoot motion preoperatively. Patients with fixed varus or valgus hindfoot alignment may require additional procedures, such as a calcaneal osteotomy, or the surgeon may elect to compensate for a mild fixed deformity by leaving the ankle in mild varus or valgus alignment, thereby bringing the hindfoot into neutral alignment.

## Positioning

- The patient is placed in the supine position on a radiolucent operating table with or without a bolster placed under the ipsilateral hip. A well-padded nonsterile tourniquet is placed around the ipsilateral proximal thigh.
- Intraoperative fluoroscopy is essential. The C-arm should be placed on the opposite side of the table. The C-arm monitor should be placed with the image intensifier on the opposite side of the table from the limb to be corrected.

## Approach

- Distal tibial osteotomy is performed through either a medial incision centered over the medial malleolus or an anteromedial incision made slightly lateral to the anterior tibialis tendon.

TECHNIQUES

## Medial Approach

- The proximal extent of dissection is determined by the size of the bone wedge to be resected in a closing wedge osteotomy or by the extent of the fixation required in an opening wedge. If a simple derotational osteotomy is contemplated, a transverse osteotomy is planned.
- A medial incision is made directly along the medial border of the tibia extending from just proximal to the physis to as far proximal as needed based on the size of the wedge to be removed for correction of the valgus deformities (**TECH FIG 1A**).
- Care is taken to protect the saphenous vein and nerve (**TECH FIG 1B**). The distal tibia is exposed to a point just proximal to the physis. If the distal tibial physis is closed, the dissection can be extended beyond the physis and to the epiphysis if needed. The periosteum is divided sharply. This area is exposed subperiosteally anteriorly and posteriorly.
- After the tibia is exposed medially, a limited subperiosteal dissection is made anteriorly and posteriorly in an oblique direction down to the lateral aspect of the distal tibial physis (**TECH FIG 1C**). Crego or Chandler retractors are then placed to protect the soft tissues.

A 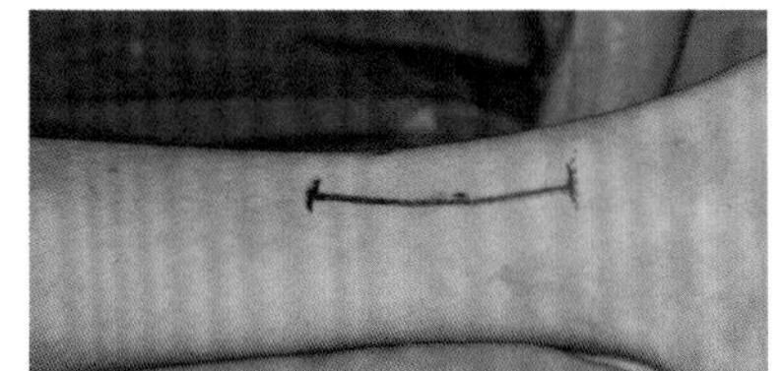
B 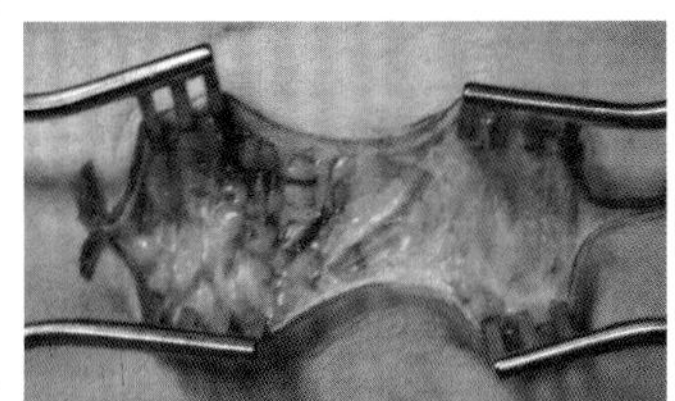
C 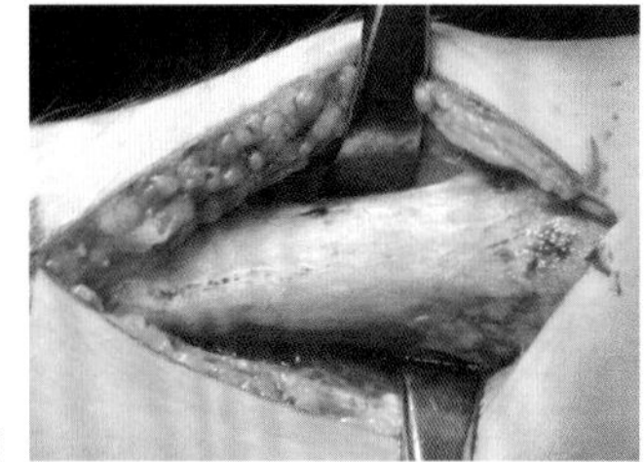

**TECH FIG 1** • **A.** Outlined incision over medial aspect of tibia prior to tibial derotational osteotomy. **B.** Superficial dissection to medial tibia showing branch of the saphenous vein. **C.** Medial subperiosteal dissection over distal tibia.

## Anterior Approach

- A longitudinal incision is made over the anterior aspect of the ankle extending distally to the ankle joint and proximally about 5 cm. The dissection should be carried down lateral to the anterior tibial tendon, protecting the anterior tibial artery and deep peroneal nerve laterally (**TECH FIG 2**).
- Subperiosteal dissection is carried out around the tibia distally to the level of the physis. Crego or Chandler retractors are then placed medially and laterally to protect the soft tissues.
- If necessary, the fibular osteotomy is performed using a separate 2-cm lateral incision that parallels the fibula and is centered over the point of the osteotomy.

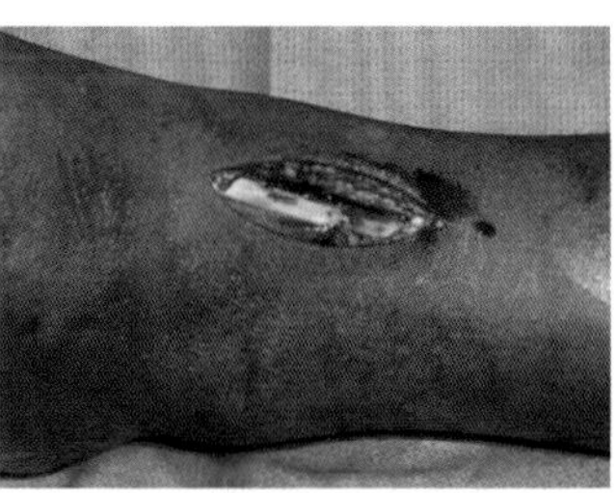

**TECH FIG 2** • Anterior incision over distal tibia showing interval lateral to the anterior tibialis tendon.

## Oblique Supramalleolar Opening or the Closing Wedge Osteotomy

- If the osteotomy is performed through a medial approach, the preplanned osteotomy is then performed with an oscillating saw to the physis, leaving the lateral cortex intact.

### Valgus Deformities

- For valgus deformities, a second osteotomy is made at an angle to the first corresponding to the amount of bone to be resected according to the preoperative plan. This is also done with a power saw, ending at the lateral extent of the first osteotomy, and the wedge is removed (**TECH FIG 3A,B**).
- The foot and ankle are then rotated into varus, closing the wedge while leaving the lateral hinge intact, and the correction is assessed using the image intensifier and if necessary plain radiographs. Additional bone can be removed from the proximal fragment if the amount of correction is insufficient.
- Once the osteotomy closes, the drill is passed through the medial malleolus in patients with a closed physis, securing the osteotomy. If the patient has an open physis, an oblique interfragmentary screw is passed across the osteotomy site beginning just proximal to the physis. The screw should be centered in the sagittal plane.
- If the fibula is an impediment to correction (it usually is not), an oblique osteotomy of the fibula is made and, if necessary, fixed with a plate and screws.

### Varus Deformities

- For varus deformities, an opening wedge is created along the same line. Once the osteotomy is made, the osteotomy site is distracted using a lamina spreader to the preplanned distance to correct the deformity (**TECH FIG 4A–C**).
- It is then held open by a wedge-shaped tricortical iliac crest graft or simply stabilized with a medial plate and screws (**TECH FIG 4D–H**), beginning with a screw passed from medial to lateral across the osteotomy site.
- After wound closure, a short-leg, non–weight-bearing cast is applied.

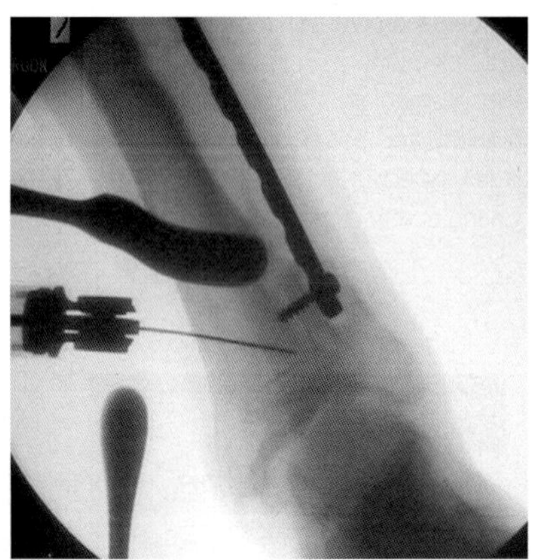
A

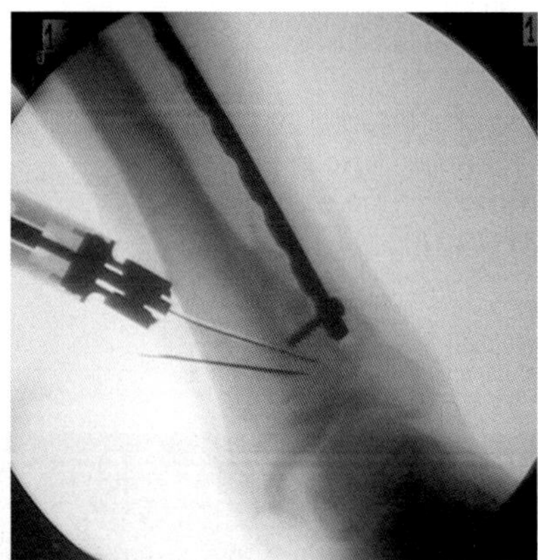
B

**TECH FIG 3** • **A.** AP intraoperative view of the ankle showing a Crego elevator in place with a saw blade performing the initial osteotomy. **B.** AP intraoperative view of the ankle with a saw blade placed into the initial cut and the saw completing the second cut.

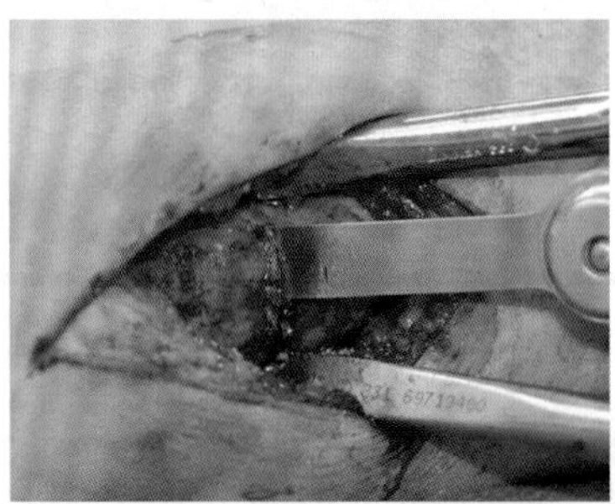
A

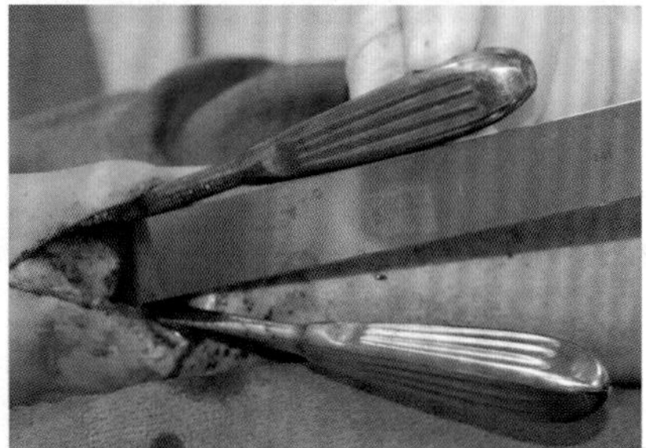
B

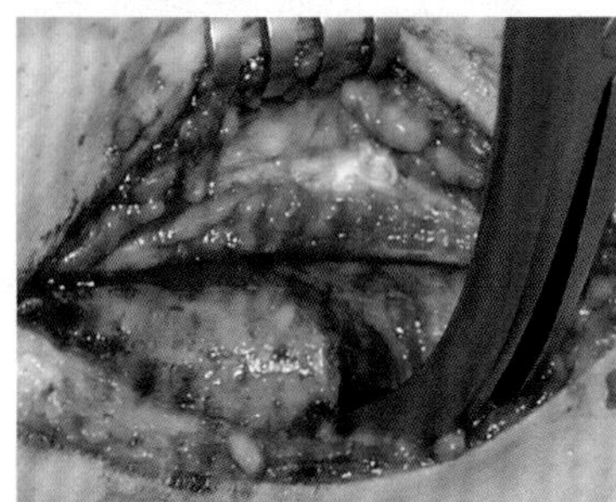
C

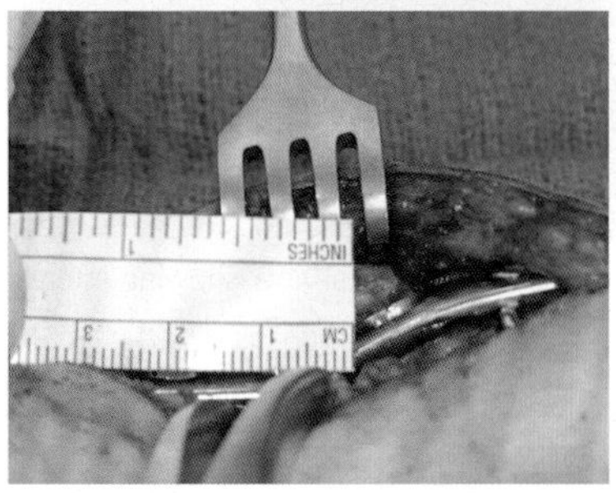

D

**TECH FIG 4** • **A.** Position of the two Crego elevators used to protect the soft tissues during the oblique osteotomy. An oscillating saw is used to create the oblique osteotomy. Fluoroscopy is used to confirm the angulation of the cut as well as to ensure that the lateral cortex remains intact. **B.** A large osteotome is placed into the osteotomy site and used to open the osteotomy. **C.** A laminar spreader is used to hold open the osteotomy site. **D.** The amount of medial opening needed for deformity correction is verified by measuring the medial opening in millimeters. *(continued)*

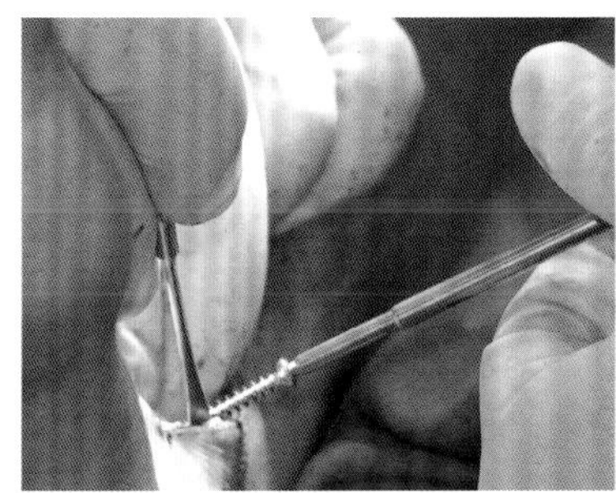
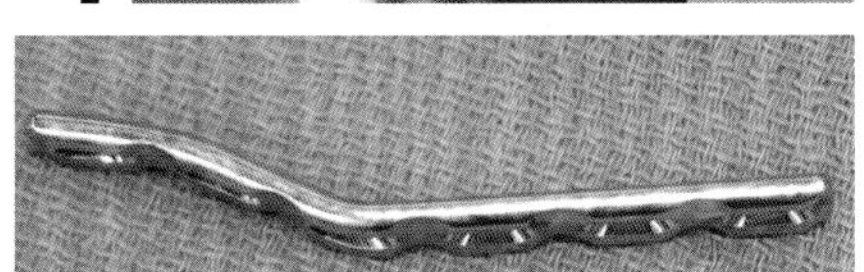
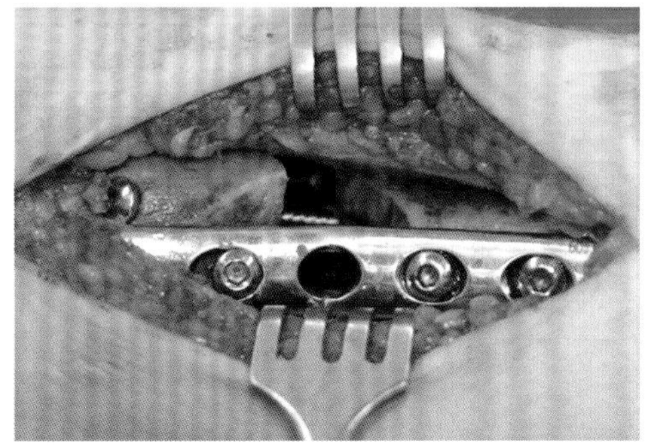
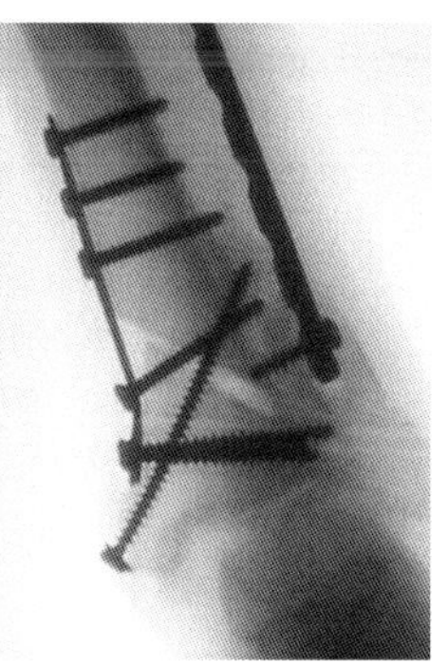

**TECH FIG 4** • *(continued)* **E.** A bicortical 3.5-mm screw (cortical) is inserted from the proximal to distal fragments to hold the osteotomy site open, allowing for removal of the laminar spreader. **F.** A 3.5-mm small fragment dynamic compression plate is contoured to the medial aspect of the distal tibia. **G.** The plate is secured to the distal tibia with 3.5-mm cortical bone screws. **H.** Intraoperative AP radiograph showing opening wedge osteotomy with internal fixation.

## Transverse Supramalleolar Osteotomy with Translation

- The tibiotalar joint should be corrected to neutral at the time of surgery.
- A wedge of bone is resected, apex medial in valgus ankles and apex lateral in varus ankles. The angle of the wedge is based on preoperative radiographs. The wedge of bone is harvested so that continuity of the apex is maintained and acts as a hinge.
- An anteromedial longitudinal incision is made over the distal tibial metaphysis. The periosteum is incised medial to the tibialis anterior tendon. The surgeon should avoid cutting into the physeal perichondral ring distally. The periosteum is elevated and retracted with Crego retractors placed medially and laterally. The level of the distal tibial physis is checked using fluoroscopy.
- When addressing valgus deformities, a closing wedge osteotomy is performed in the metaphyseal bone about 3 cm proximal to the ankle joint. The proximal cut is made first. It is aligned perpendicular to the long axis of the tibia. The second distal osteotomy cut is made obliquely. The triangle formed by the two cuts is medially based. Enough bone is removed to convert the preoperative LDTA to neutral.
- Preoperatively, a sterile template triangle can be prepared with a piece of paper and a goniometer. The paper is placed on the tibia, which is marked with an osteotome and then cut with an oscillating saw.
- The fibular osteotomy, if necessary, is performed at the same level as the tibial osteotomy. The fibular osteotomy is performed because it allows for sufficient compression at the tibial osteotomy site and it also allows for centralization of the distal tibial fragment to improve foot alignment.
- The tibial osteotomy may be fixed with a small fragment plate or Kirschner wires.
- The fibular osteotomy is made through a second incision, laterally over the fibula. The osteotomy is shaped in the form of a triangle. The proximal cut is oblique and ends proximal at the medial cortex. The distal cut is perpendicular to the shaft of the fibula.
- The extent of correction is checked with an intraoperative radiograph.
- Care is taken to avoid injury to the distal tibial physis when obtaining fixation of the osteotomy.
- Internal or external rotation deformities can be addressed at the same time.
- Alternatively, an opening wedge osteotomy may be performed about 2 to 3 cm proximal to the physis. An osteotomy is made parallel to the ankle joint, and an opening wedge correction is performed and filled with bone graft.

## Wiltse Osteotomy

- The osteotomy is performed through an anterior approach to the distal tibial metaphysis at the level of the metadiaphyseal junction.
- A triangular piece of bone is removed from the region of the distal tibial metadiaphyseal junction. The apex of the cut is centered on the longitudinal axis of the tibia.
- The magnitude of the angle of the lateral portion of the triangle should be equal in size to the magnitude of the deformity to be corrected.
- The osteotomy should be stabilized by a plate and screws or Kirschner wires and the wound is closed. A cast is placed as described in the following text.
- If growth is near completion, simple deformity correction should suffice. However, in children with growth remaining, the deformity can be overcorrected to avoid recurrent deformity.

## Derotational Osteotomy

- If a purely derotational osteotomy is planned, the incision should be slightly oblique to the long axis of the limb, such that after derotation, the resulting closed incision is oriented longitudinally.
- The proposed plate is placed onto the distal tibia and positioned on the bone with the distal end of the plate just proximal to the physis. A site for the osteotomy is selected at the metaphyseal–diaphyseal junction as distal as possible while still allowing for adequate fixation of the distal fragment.
- The plate is then removed and an oscillating saw is used to create an osteotomy perpendicular to the long axis of the tibia (**TECH FIG 5A**).
- The plate is then placed once again along the tibia and secured to the tibial shaft (**TECH FIG 5B**).
- The distal tibia is then derotated to a position where the thigh–foot angle is neutral (**TECH FIG 5C**).
- The distal fragment is then secured to the plate using screws. If a locking plate has been selected to stabilize the osteotomy, locking screws should be used to secure the distal fragment to the plate (**TECH FIG 5D**).
- Adequate fixation should be used to allow weight bearing for transfers.
- Wound closure is carried out in a routine fashion, and immobilization can be achieved using either a short-leg cast or a walking boot.

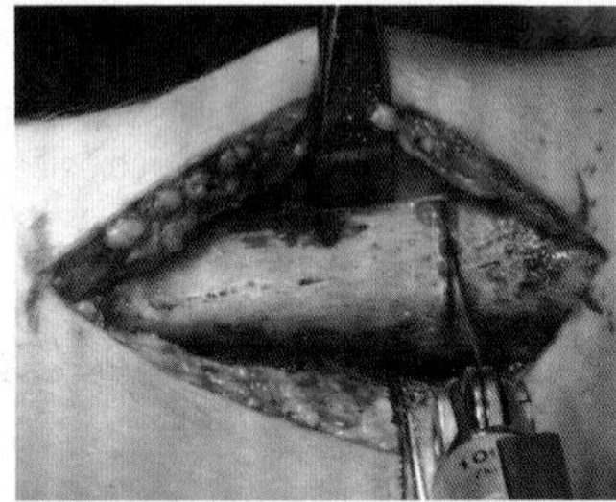
A

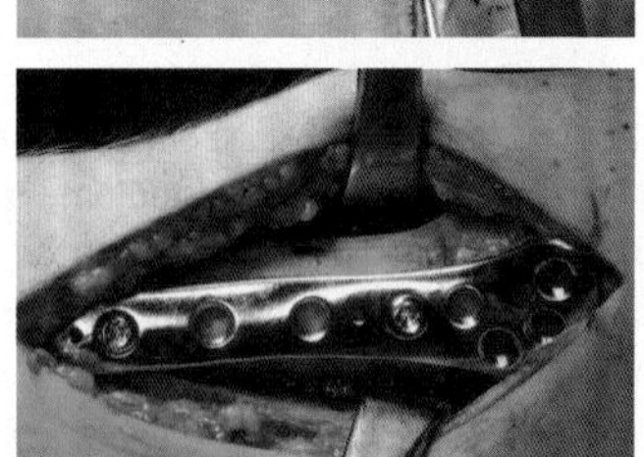
B

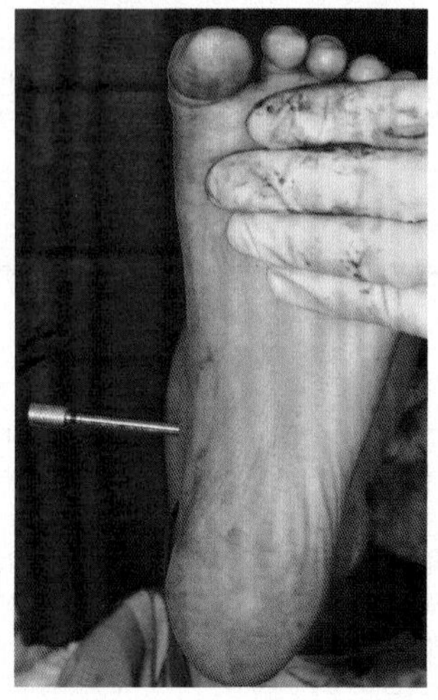
C

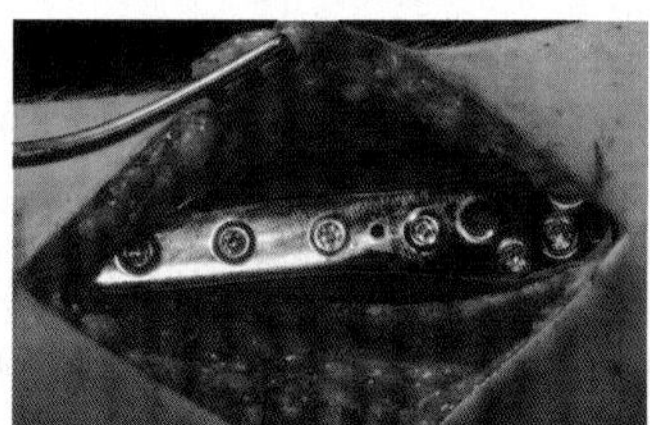
D

**TECH FIG 5** • **A.** Transverse osteotomy through distal tibia at metaphyseal–diaphyseal junction. **B.** Locking plate secured to the proximal fragment prior to derotation of the distal tibia. **C.** Image from distal of the thigh–foot angle showing correction of external tibial torsion prior to securing the distal fragment. **D.** Locking plate secured to distal tibia using combination of locking and nonlocking screws after correction of external tibial torsion.

## Screw Hemiepiphysiodesis

- Using image intensification, a drill bit is placed into the tip of the medial malleolus through a 3-mm stab wound.
- The drill is advanced under C-arm guidance proximally and medially across the distal tibial physis. Care is taken to avoid injury to the posterior neurovascular bundle, which passes inferior to the tip of the medial malleolus.
- The position of the drill bit is confirmed on AP and lateral fluoroscopic images. In the AP plane, the guide pin should be located as medially as possible. The guide pin should be centered in the sagittal plane.
- The drill bit is then withdrawn, and a 50- to 60-mm fully threaded cancellous screw is placed into the distal tibia. A second screw may be placed if necessary (**TECH FIG 6**).[6]
- The wound is closed, and a soft dressing is placed. The child is allowed full weight bearing as tolerated.

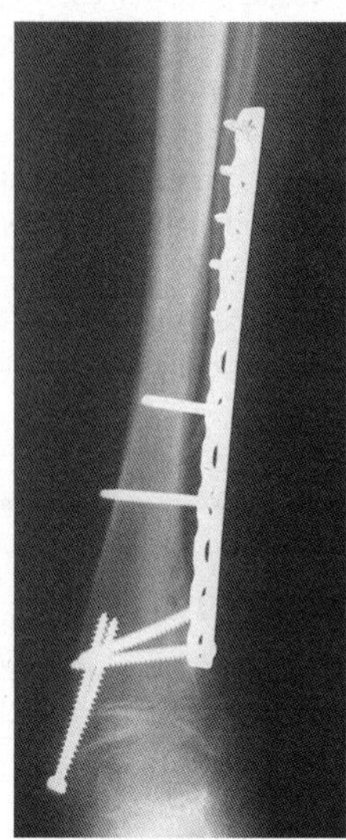

**TECH FIG 6** • Postoperative AP radiograph of the patient in **FIG 1A** after plate fixation and bone grafting of the fibula and screw hemiepiphysiodesis of the medial distal tibia.

## Staple or Eight-Hole Plate Hemiepiphysiodesis

- We currently prefer a hemiepiphysiodesis plate over hemiepiphyseal staples because of the lower incidence of failure due to backing out or breakage.
- A 1- to 2-cm incision is made directly over the medial distal tibial physis.
- Extraperiosteal dissection is carried out over the physis.
- The physis is localized using image intensification, and a guidewire is placed into the epiphysis.
- The appropriately sized two-hole plate is then selected and on end placed over the guidewire.
- A guidewire is then placed into the metaphysis parallel to the epiphyseal guidewire.
- Screws consistent with the anatomy are selected for use. Care must be taken to select screws long enough to provide purchase but not to penetrate the articular surface.
- Screws may be placed under power without drilling, or reaming may be performed over the guidewire and then the screws placed.

## PEARLS AND PITFALLS

| | |
|---|---|
| **Passive hindfoot motion** | ▪ Full preoperative evaluation of passive hindfoot motion is essential. Correction of a varus or valgus distal tibial deformity when the hindfoot does not have adequate motion to accommodate the correction requires either additional hindfoot procedures or modification of the procedure. |
| **Periosteal stripping** | ▪ The surgeon should avoid periosteal stripping whenever possible. Limited exposures, when possible, preserve soft tissue attachments and promote healing and stability. |
| **Lateral hinge** | ▪ When performing the oblique osteotomy, the surgeon must leave the lateral bony hinge intact, whether performing an opening or closing wedge osteotomy. This intact hinge is the key to stability in this osteotomy. If this principle is violated, stable fixation is difficult. |

## POSTOPERATIVE CARE

- After wound closure, a short-leg, non–weight-bearing cast is applied. Non–weight bearing is maintained for 4 to 6 weeks.
  - Closing wedge osteotomies are typically stable, and patients are allowed full weight bearing at 4 weeks.
  - Opening wedge osteotomies are stable based on fixation and grafting, and the patient is kept non–weight bearing for 6 weeks.
  - After 4 to 5 weeks, when weight bearing is initiated, the cast is removed and a CAM walker is applied.
- Physical therapy should be instituted to regain motion, strength, and proprioception before resuming activities.
- It is important to follow immature patients closely for the development of a limb length discrepancy, which can be addressed by performing an epiphysiodesis of the contralateral lower limb.

## OUTCOMES

- Lubicky and Altiok[3] reported their experience in 26 limbs with the oblique osteotomy and found rapid healing and few complications, with all patients resuming their preoperative level of activity.
- They noted that patients with preoperative hindfoot valgus had improved alignment with varus overcorrection of the distal tibia and recommended overcorrection by 5 degrees in these patients.
- We have not overcorrected patients with normal hindfoot alignment, particularly those with posttraumatic deformities.

## COMPLICATIONS

- Nonunions, wound healing problems, and loss of correction after surgery may be related to a number of factors.
- Historically, the distal tibia is associated with increased difficulty with both soft and hard tissue healing in the traumatized limb. Also, impaired tissue development and growth due to decreased innervation and physiologic stresses can create a barrier to normal healing.
- Leg length discrepancy can be seen after opening and closing wedge osteotomies in growing children.
- Delayed union may require prolonged immobilization with weight bearing as tolerated. Nonunion can be managed with improved fixation, autologous bone grafting, and further immobilization in a non–weight-bearing cast.
- Malunion can be due to inadequate fixation or slow healing and loss of fixation.
- Recurrence of the deformity can be due to continued growth with partial physeal arrest.
- Premature growth plate closure can occur with the oblique osteotomy. This can occur as a planned portion of the procedure or can be due to periosteal stripping at the level of the physis or fixation crossing the physis.
- Pseudarthrosis of the fibula can occur after fibular osteotomies. These are most often asymptomatic and can be observed. When painful, open reduction, plate fixation, and bone grafting should be considered.

## REFERENCES


1. Davids JR, Valadie AL, Ferguson RL, et al. Surgical management of ankle valgus in children: use of a transphyseal medial malleolar screw. J Pediatr Orthop 1997;17:3–8.
2. Kärrholm J, Hansson LI, Selvik G. Changes in tibiofibular relationships due to growth disturbances after ankle fractures in children. J Bone Joint Surg Am 1984;66(8):1198–1210.
3. Lubicky JP, Altiok H. Transphyseal osteotomy of the distal tibia for correction of valgus/varus deformities of the ankle. J Pediatr Orthop 2001;21:80–88.
4. Paley D, Tetsworth K. Mechanical axis deviation of the lower limbs. Preoperative planning of multiapical frontal plane angular and bowing deformities of the femur and tibia. Clin Orthop Relat Res 1992;(280):65–71.
5. Paley D, Tetsworth K. Mechanical axis deviation of the lower limbs. Preoperative planning of uniapical angular deformities of the tibia or femur. Clin Orthop Relat Res 1992;(280):48–64.
6. Stevens PM, Belle RM. Screw epiphysiodesis for ankle valgus. J Pediatr Orthop 1997;17:9–12.
7. Takakura Y, Takaoka T, Tanaka Y, et al. Results of opening-wedge osteotomy for the treatment of a post-traumatic varus deformity of the ankle. J Bone Joint Surg Am 1998;80(2):213–218.
8. Ting AJ, Tarr RR, Sarmiento A, et al. The role of subtalar motion and ankle contact pressure changes from angular deformities of the tibia. Foot Ankle 1987;7:290–299.
9. Wagner KS, Tarr RR, Resnick C, et al. The effect of simulated tibial deformities on the ankle joint. Foot Ankle 1984;5:131–141.
10. Wiltse LL. Valgus deformity of the ankle: a sequel to acquired or congenital abnormalities of the fibula. J Bone Joint Surg Am 1972; 54(3):595–606.

# Multiple Percutaneous Osteotomies and Fassier-Duval Telescoping Nailing of Long Bones in Osteogenesis Imperfecta

Paul W. Esposito and François Fassier

## DEFINITION

- Children with osteogenesis imperfecta (OI) and syndromes with congenital brittle bones sustain recurrent fractures and deformity, which cause chronic pain and limit their function.[24,25]
- Multiple percutaneous osteotomies and percutaneous telescoping intramedullary nailing can improve comfort and function with lower morbidity than previously was possible.
- The severity of bone disease, fracture incidence, degree of deformity, and functional level of the patient, as well as the patient's response to medical treatment, are more important in surgical decision making than the specific diagnostic type of OI or brittle bone disease.

## ANATOMY

- There is broad variation in anatomic findings in the different types of OI and other brittle bone diseases that resemble it.
- Some children have blue sclera, obvious dentinogenesis imperfecta, triangular faces, and ligamentous laxity, but this varies greatly, even within the same family, and many affected children have none of these findings.
- The defining characteristics of children with OI are a varying degree of bone fragility and recurrent fractures.
- Progressive anterior bowing of the long bones is quite common, especially in children with moderate to severe involvement, even with early treatment with bisphosphonates (**FIG 1**).
- Coxa vara, both apparent and true, can develop.[1,9]

## PATHOGENESIS

- OI is caused, in the great majority of cases, by dominant mutations in type I procollagen genes.
- In the remaining cases, children may have brittle bone disease with a similar presentation and problems that are not caused by mutations in the type I procollagen genes.[24,25]
- The flexors, such as the gastrocnemius muscles and hamstrings, contribute to the progressive bowing.
- Secondary joint contractures may be seen as a result of the long-standing deformities.
- Juxta-articular bone deformities can mimic joint contractures, and extra-articular osteotomies frequently will allow full joint motion.

## NATURAL HISTORY

- Historically, children with very severe OI, especially Sillence type II, rarely survived infancy, and children with types III and IV had severe disability secondary to recurrent fractures, bone pain, and deformities.[30,31]
- Before bisphosphonate therapy was available, ambulation and even functional, comfortable sitting were difficult if not impossible for many children with severe forms of OI.
- Even children with less severe forms of OI may have many significant fractures, which inhibit comfort, function, and quality of life.
- Scoliosis and vertebral flexion fractures with secondary kyphosis are common.
- Spondylolysis and spondylolisthesis are very common, especially in ambulatory children.[11]

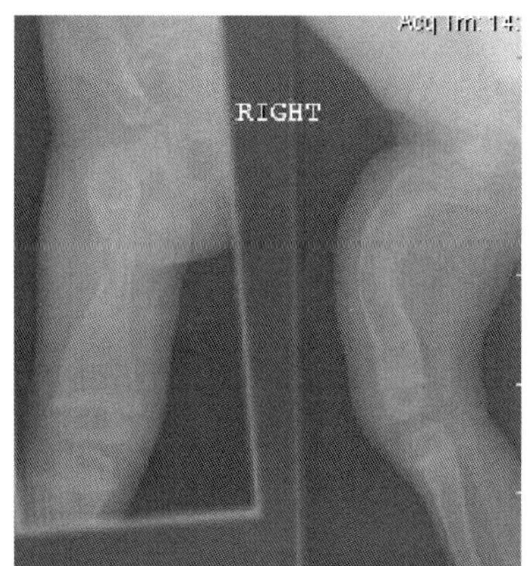


A

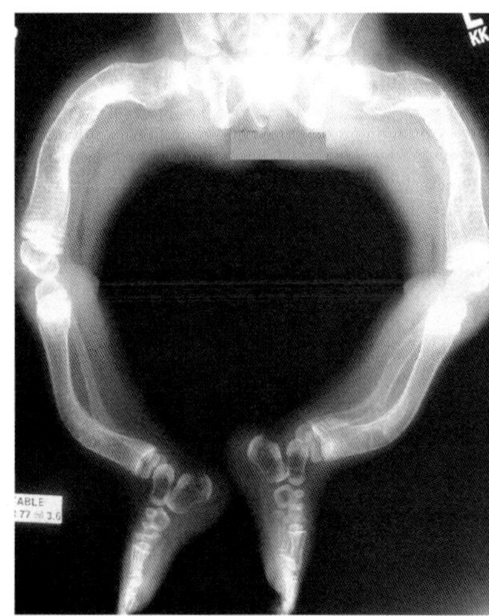

B

**FIG 1** • **A.** Radiographs of an infant with moderately severe OI, with the typical anterolateral bow most severe in the subtrochanteric region. **B.** At 16 months of age, bone strength is improved, but the deformity does not remodel.

- Progressive craniocervical abnormalities such as basilar invagination, cranial settling, as well as C2 fractures can occur and are not necessarily related to the overall severity of the OI.

## PATIENT HISTORY AND PHYSICAL FINDINGS

- Findings vary greatly depending on the type and severity of OI. In addition, findings on physical examination may change dramatically as children respond to treatment with bisphosphonates.
- Possible physical findings include blue sclera, triangular face, dentinogenesis imperfecta, joint laxity, bowing of the arms and legs, and flattening of the skull, especially in infants with severe involvement, but these findings vary greatly even within the same family, and many of the children have none of these classic physical findings.
- Flexible flat feet, lax joints, and externally rotated lower extremities are quite common.
- A variety of presentations are possible, and children with subtle forms of OI may appear totally normal on physical examination but present with multiple and recurrent fractures.
- The classic triad of bone fragility, blue sclera, and deafness is rarely present in infancy.

## IMAGING AND OTHER DIAGNOSTIC STUDIES

- There is no specific test for OI. The diagnosis is based primarily on clinical and radiologic basis.
- Plain radiographs are preferred as the initial study to evaluate children who have or may not have OI.
- Full-length radiographs of both legs on the same cassette from the hips to the ankles are ideal to assess areas of fractures and degree of deformity.
- Radiographs of the lower extremity should be performed with the patellas directly anterior and also with the legs maximally externally rotated. This helps assess the severity of the disease, can help predict risk of fracture, and is useful in preoperative planning for osteotomies and instrumentation (**FIG 2**).
- Standardized posteroanterior (PA) and lateral spine radiographs demonstrate spinal fractures, scoliosis, spondylolysis, and spondylolisthesis.
- Bone density (dual energy x-ray absorptiometry [DEXA]) scans, although not perfect, can be useful in monitoring changes in bone density, using age-matched Z-scores and consistently using the same techniques and machine type. The DEXA scan alone, however, cannot be used for diagnosis, especially in infants, for whom no standardized validated Z-scores have been established.
- The child's clinical course with regard to incidence of fracture and pain is a much more reliable indicator of successful medical treatment than a specific Z-score.

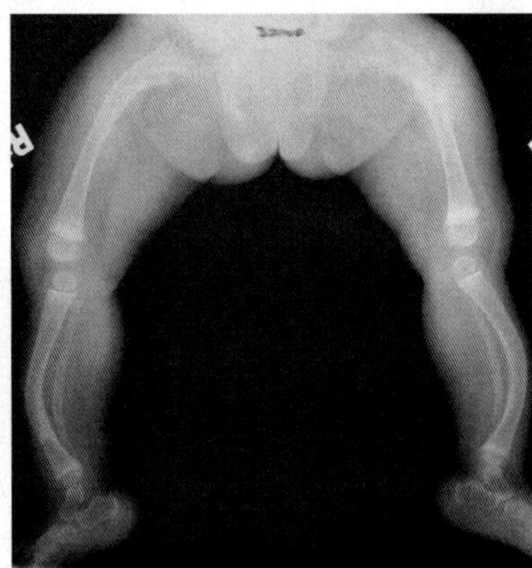

**FIG 2** • Typical bowing deformity of the femurs and tibias caused by preexisting deformity and recurrent fractures is accentuated by the pull of the flexors, including the hamstrings and gastrocnemius–soleus complex. Note sclerosis in the medullary canal of the right tibia.

## DIFFERENTIAL DIAGNOSIS

- Child abuse
- Metabolic bone disease (eg, hypophosphatasia, rickets)
- Idiopathic juvenile osteoporosis

## NONOPERATIVE MANAGEMENT

- Early diagnosis and treatment with bisphosphonates has significantly improved the lives of children with OI and potentially other disorders.[26] This treatment positively alters the mechanical properties of their bones, decreases their fracture rate and pain, and enhances their psychomotor development.[16,27]
- This improvement in bone density and strength often allows them to function at levels that previously were not possible by decreasing their bone fragility and pain.[2,6,13,16]
- Surgical treatment for these children is now possible, whereas previously in many cases, no surgical options existed because of the severity of their bone disease.
- It has, however, been suggested that treatment with pamidronate may be related to delayed healing of osteotomies—but not fractures—in children with OI.[20]
- It remains unclear whether the incidence of delayed healing will decrease with lower doses of bisphosphonates or discontinuing their use for a period of time postoperatively.[20,23]
- Casting, splinting, and bracing for many children with OI should be short-term temporizing measures only because residual deformities will not remodel, and osteoporosis is worsened by prolonged immobilization.

## SURGICAL MANAGEMENT

- Intramedullary fixation of long bones in children with OI required extensive soft tissue disruption with traditional techniques.[32]
- Insertion of many telescoping and nontelescoping rods requires extensive exposure and arthrotomies for insertion, and the reoperation rate is high.[3,4,6,10,34,35]
- Improved surgical treatment has been made possible by the development of percutaneous techniques,[17,18,29] as well as modification of existing nails and development of new nails for fixation, both telescoping[4,5,7–9,14,15,28,33] and nontelescoping.[6,10,14,17,29,34]

### Principles of Surgical Treatment

- Primary indications for surgical treatment include recurrent fractures, pain, and deformity.
  - These approaches should be considered, as children begin attempting to stand or crawl. There is no documented benefit to surgery performed before walking age.
  - There is no advantage to waiting until the child is older.
  - Surgical treatment should be considered in acute fracture with deformity, even with less severe OI.

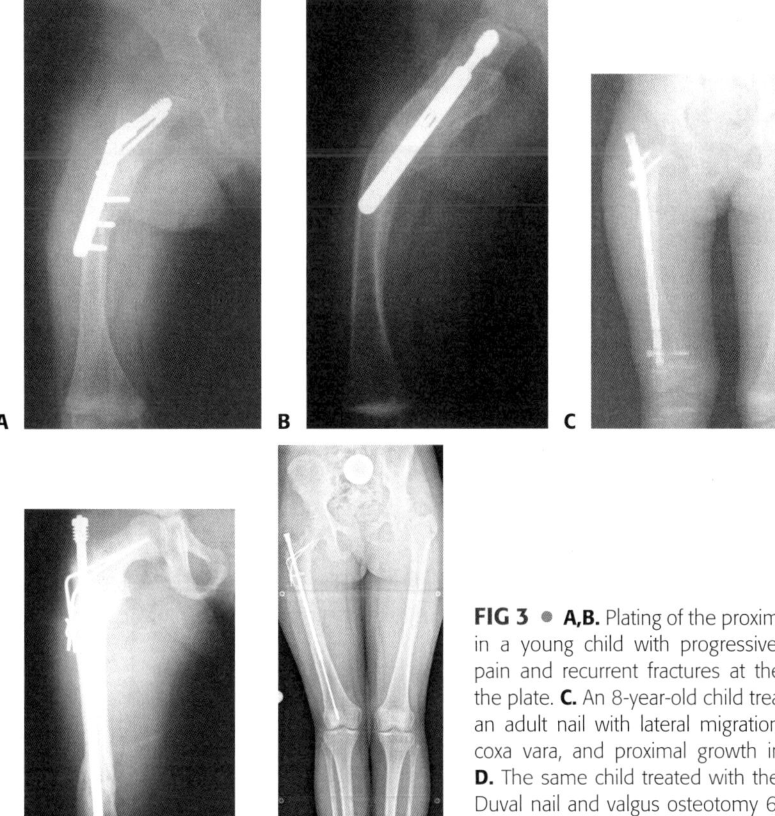

**FIG 3** • **A,B.** Plating of the proximal femur in a young child with progressive bowing pain and recurrent fractures at the end of the plate. **C.** An 8-year-old child treated with an adult nail with lateral migration distally, coxa vara, and proximal growth inhibition. **D.** The same child treated with the Fassier-Duval nail and valgus osteotomy 6 months postoperatively. **E.** Follow-up near maturity demonstrating telescoping of the nail, maintenance of the valgus neck–shaft angle but residual leg length discrepancy related to initial surgery.

- Correct deformity and axial alignment.
  - Residual bowing does not correct with growth and predictably leads to further fracture.
  - As many involved, symptomatic bones should be corrected at one setting as can be safely accomplished.
- Minimize soft tissue dissection and trauma.
  - Percutaneous technique provides more stability, less scarring, and earlier healing.
- Minimize immobilization.
  - Light splints only
  - Early weight bearing and motion as symptoms allow
  - The role of bracing for long bones is not proven, and bracing may inhibit function.
- Use telescoping intramedullary devices whenever possible.
  - Plating predictably leads to stress reaction, progressive deformity, and fracture (**FIG 3A,B**).
  - Use relatively small, flexible nails to share stress.
  - Excessively rigid nails may lead to disappearing bone (**FIG 3C,D**).
  - Do not remove nails electively.
- Indications in forearm are more limited.
  - Fixation in the forearm is less predictable and has higher risks and rate of complications.
  - Instrumentation and bone quality are not optimal.
  - Such fixation should be considered only when comfort, motion, and function are significantly limited by deformity.

## Preoperative Planning

- The keys to surgical success are careful selection of children with adequate bone strength, size, and availability of an experienced team and appropriate equipment (**FIG 4A**).
- Templates must be used to ensure that every appropriate size and type of device is available (**FIG 4B**).
- Radiographs can be used to estimate length and diameter of nails as well as to determine osteotomy sites (**FIG 5**).
- Measuring the Fassier-Duval nail
  - The distance from the greater trochanter to the distal femoral physis can be used to estimate the length of the female nail.
  - The female nail should be approximately 1 cm shorter than this distance.
    - Digital software and templates to determine length and diameter of the nails are available.
    - Angular correction can also be estimated on digital radiographs, but they can be deceiving because of the multiplanar nature of the angulation.
  - The female nail can be cut preoperatively, but the authors prefer to cut the female nail intraoperatively, after the osteotomies are completed, which allows more precise measurement after correction of the deformity. The long-threaded female nail is used in the femur and does not require a knee arthrotomy for placement. The "small bone" shorter threaded female nail does not require an ankle arthrotomy for insertion into the tibia and can also be used in the humerus.

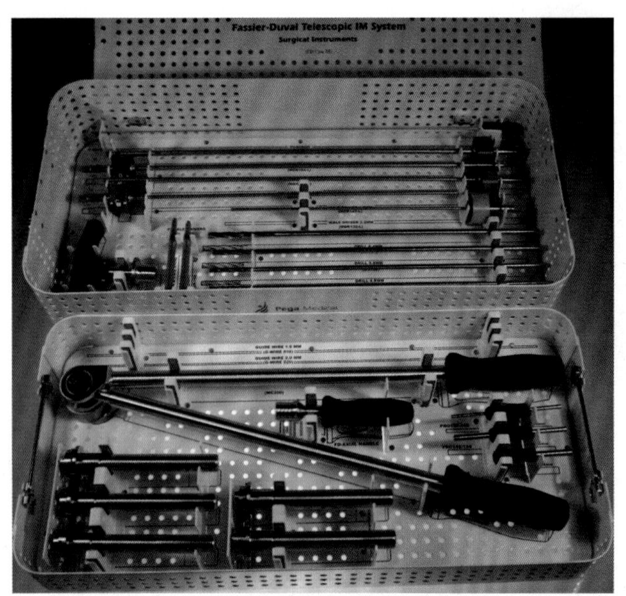


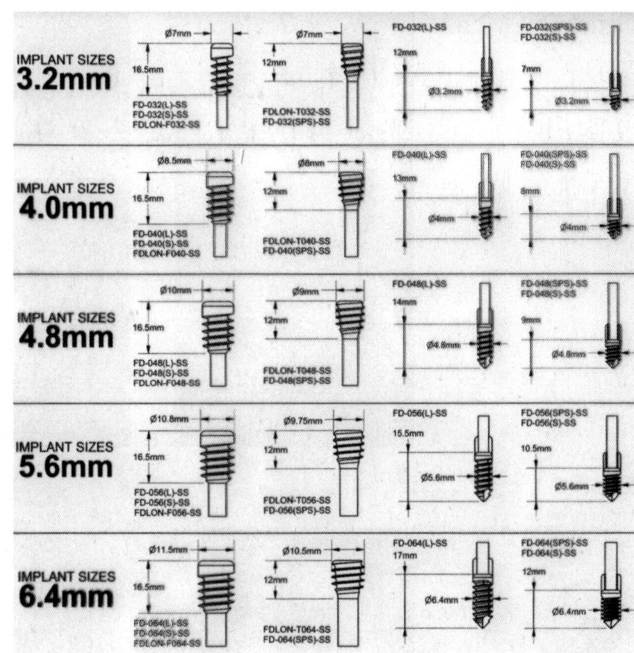


**FIG 4** • **A.** Fassier-Duval nail insertion tray. **B.** Templates for Fassier-Duval nail. (**B:** Courtesy of Pega Medical, Inc., Montreal, Canada.)

## Positioning

- For fractures and deformities of the tibia and femur, the patient is placed in the semilateral position with an axillary roll and a long, padded posterior roll near the edge of the radiolucent table.
- Take great care that the x-ray is not obscured by metal table parts.
- The leg can be gently rotated from the anteroposterior (AP) to the lateral position with the C-arm positioned on the opposite side of the table (**FIG 6**).
- Only one leg can be prepped at a time, especially if both the femur and tibia are being treated at the same surgical setting.
- Bilateral tibial surgery can be done supine but not femoral surgery.

## Approach

- For the femur, a 1.5-cm vertical incision is made, starting at the tip of the greater trochanter and extending proximally (**FIG 7A**).
- The tensor fascia is then incised, exposing the greater trochanter (**FIG 7B**).
- The tibia is approached through a medial peripatellar incision, bluntly dissecting behind the patellar tendon, when possible, without disrupting the synovium. If necessary, an arthrotomy can be used to expose the starting point for the tibial nail just anterior to the tibial spines.
- The humerus is approached through a small deltoid-splitting incision, or if there is severe proximal humeral bowing, through the supra clavicular fossa arthroscopic portal described by Neviaser.[21]

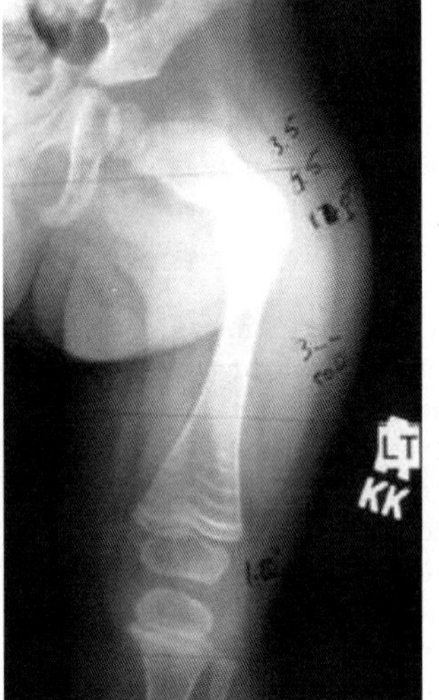

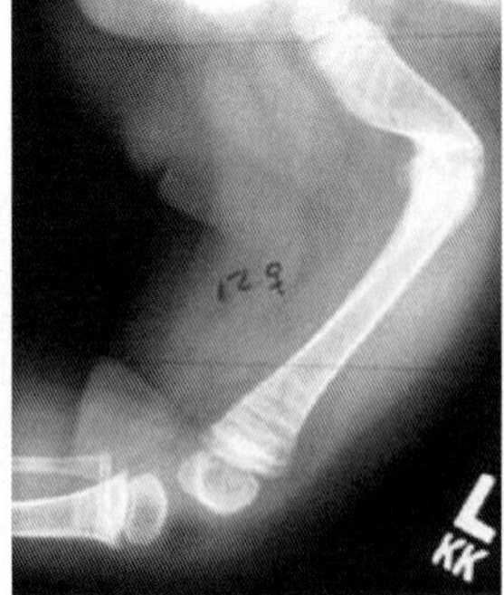

**FIG 5** • Common severe anterior (**A**) and lateral (**B**) femoral bowing. This is apparent rather than true coxa vara.

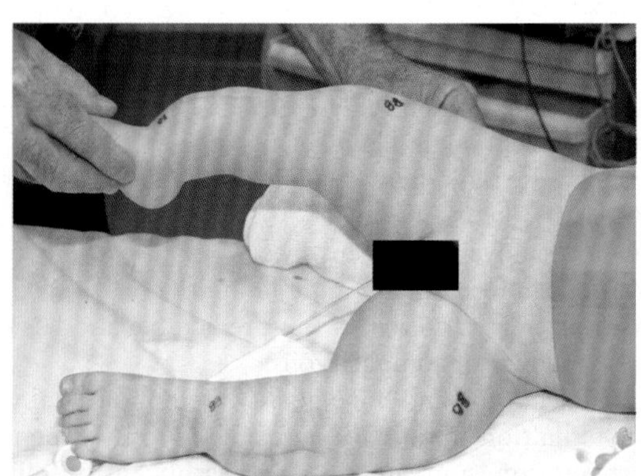

**FIG 6** • Positioning for lower extremity surgery.

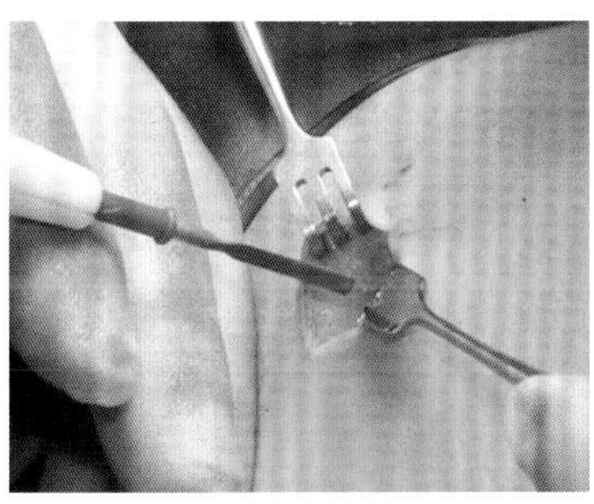

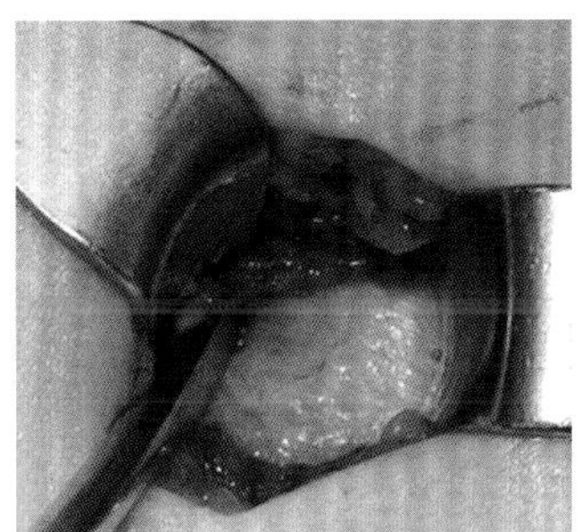

**FIG 7** • **A.** A 1.5-cm incision is made proximal to the greater trochanter. **B.** Greater trochanter is exposed.



# Surgical Approaches to Osteogenesis Imperfecta

## Percutaneous Osteotomy with Intramedullary Telescoping Fassier-Duval Nail

- The percutaneous technique described in this section is as described by Fassier and Duval[8,9] with only minor modifications, based on ongoing experience and equipment development.[22]
- The open technique, which is necessary for severe deformity and which is not described in this chapter, is performed in the same manner, with the following exceptions:
  - A larger incision at the osteotomy or fracture site is necessary.
  - Retrograde guidewire placement and reaming of the proximal fragment are used.
  - The wire is passed into the distal femur under direct vision.

## Guidewire Placement and Osteotomies in the Femur

- Short and long guidewires are available, depending on the length of the femur.
- Ideally, the tip of the guidewire is placed just medial to the center of the greater trochanter, in line with the shaft of the femur (**TECH FIG 1A**).
  - It may be difficult to visualize the greater trochanter in small children with poor bone density, and the insertion point may be necessarily in the piriformis fossa to avoid overreaming of the lateral cortex and to allow a straight line of advance to the femoral canal.
  - Lateral placement in the greater trochanter will lead to lateral migration of the rod and progressive varus.
  - Avascular necrosis has not been demonstrated in children in whom this technique has been used.
  - The relation between the entrance point and use of the nail and the development of coxa vara is not clearly defined at this point.[1]
- The wire is then advanced to the first osteotomy site.
  - In many cases, it is necessary to angle the wire markedly, both anteriorly and laterally, at first because of the very common severe anterior and lateral bowing of the femur in the subtrochanteric region.
- Osteotomy sites are marked on the skin after visualization with the C-arm, based on preoperative templating and intraoperative visualization (**TECH FIG 1B**).
- A 1-cm incision is made directly over the anterior lateral apex of the deformity.
- Blunt dissection then is performed with a hemostat down to the periosteum (**TECH FIG 1C**).
- The periosteum is incised longitudinally with a small osteotome, which is then rotated 90 degrees (**TECH FIG 1D**).
  - An incomplete osteotomy is performed while stability of the leg is maintained manually. The osteotomy is completed with gentle manual pressure, the guidewire is extended to the next osteotomy site, and the process is continued until all deformities are corrected. For severe deformities, an open segmental resection at the apex is necessary to avoid excessive soft tissue tension (see **FIGS 2** and **5**) on structures such as the sciatic nerve. Rarely are more than two osteotomies required.
- The guidewire is then passed into the distal femur (**TECH FIG 1E**).
  - Use of a longer guidewire can help to avoid capturing the guidewire in the reamer.
  - A subtle flexion deformity often is present distally, in both the femur and tibia, that is not always apparent on the preoperative radiographs and that will cause the nail to go too far anteriorly. An osteotomy in the distal femur allows appropriate central positioning of the nail in the distal epiphysis.

## Reaming and Placement of the Male Nail

- The reamers are 0.25 to 0.35 mm larger than the corresponding nails.
- The canal is reamed over the guidewire down to the distal femoral metaphysis, approximately 1 cm proximal to the physis in the center–center position on both AP and lateral radiographs (**TECH FIG 2A–C**).
- The guidewire is removed to insert the male nail driver and nail after verifying the distal male nail thread length while maintaining traction manually. The male nail driver will lock on the male nail if it is not precut, which allows for more secure manipulation. It must be unlocked (**TECH FIG 2D**) prior to removing the male nail driver.
  - Avoid bending the rod and driver to prevent impingement and damage to the nail.
  - The nail and driver cannot be used to forcefully manipulate the osteotomy or fracture site.
- The nail and driver are passed to the center–center position in the distal metaphysis (**TECH FIG 2C**).
  - If the male nail is precut and requires redirection, it should be retracted slowly while maintaining a gentle counterclockwise screwing motion to prevent dislodgment of the driver from the wing of the nail, which is not locked in the male nail driver (**TECH FIG 2E**).
  - On occasion, it may be necessary to remove the male nail and redirect.

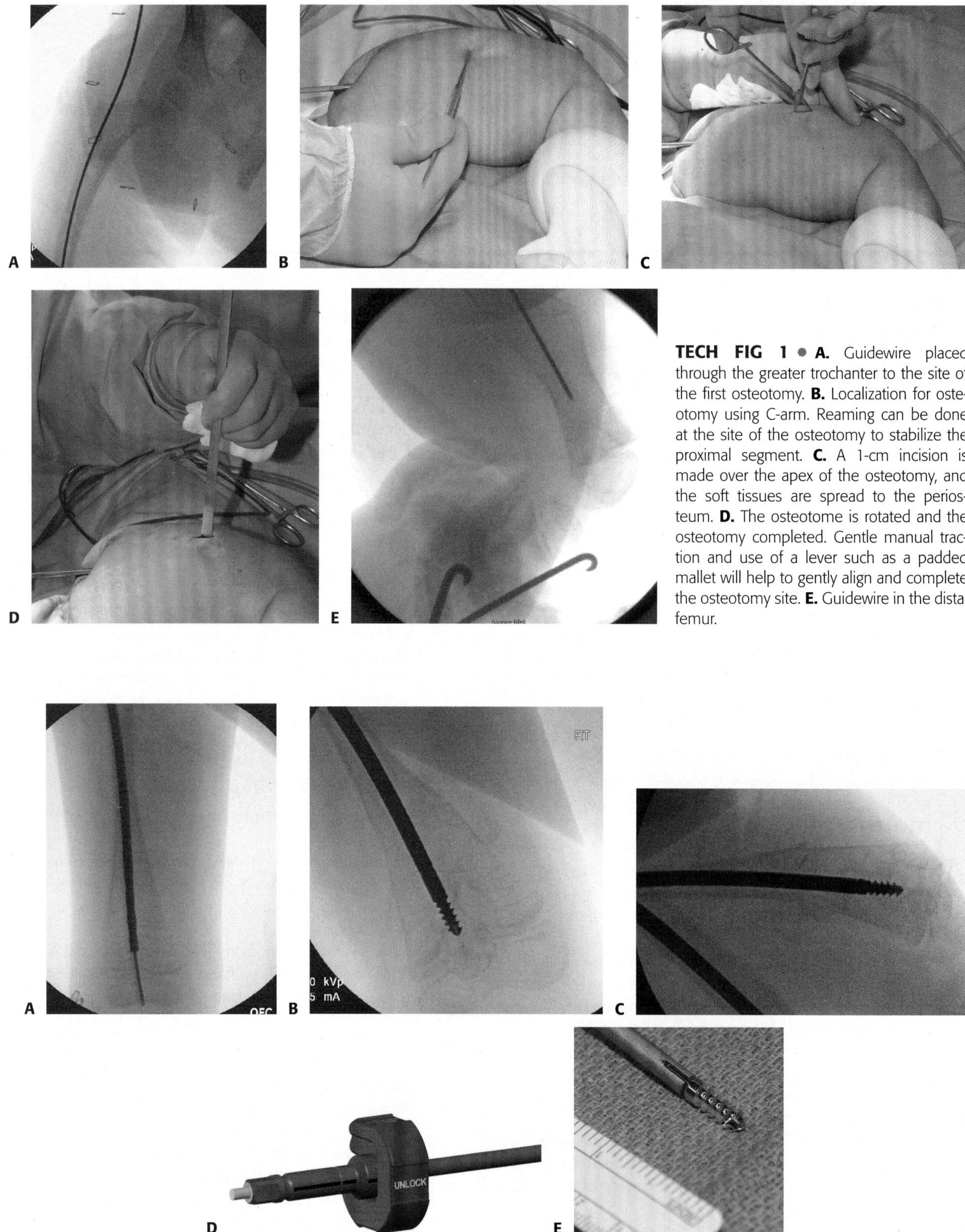


**TECH FIG 1 • A.** Guidewire placed through the greater trochanter to the site of the first osteotomy. **B.** Localization for osteotomy using C-arm. Reaming can be done at the site of the osteotomy to stabilize the proximal segment. **C.** A 1-cm incision is made over the apex of the osteotomy, and the soft tissues are spread to the periosteum. **D.** The osteotome is rotated and the osteotomy completed. Gentle manual traction and use of a lever such as a padded mallet will help to gently align and complete the osteotomy site. **E.** Guidewire in the distal femur.

**TECH FIG 2 • A.** The guidewire and reamer must be extended to the distal metaphysis in the central position on both the AP and lateral planes. The reamer can easily bind on the guidewire and be pushed distally. **B,C.** The male nail is then inserted to the center–center position at the distal metaphysis. At this point, valgus, varus, and distal flexion can be corrected. **D.** The male nail driver must be unlocked prior to removing the new locking male driver, if the male nail is not precut. The long probe or another male nail must be used to prevent backing out of the male nail, whether precut or full length. **E.** The male nail guides must be engaged with the male driver.

- Varus and valgus malalignment can be corrected with a distal osteotomy and correct placement of the nail in the center–center position in the distal femur.
- Correct positioning is checked using AP and lateral views with the C-arm just before passing the male nail across the center–center position of the physis.
- The threads are gently screwed into the epiphysis until the rounded portion of the rod located just proximal to the threads is bridging the physis.
  - Multiple transgressions of the physis are to be avoided.
- The rod pusher is then placed into the cannulated portion of the male nail driver, and a sharp backward blow is made on the T handle. The C-arm verifies that the male nail is still engaged in the epiphysis.

## Cutting and Insertion of the Female Nail

- To measure the length of the female rod intraoperatively, it is placed with the threaded portion just at the top of the ossified greater trochanter with C-arm verification using a metal marking device distally approximately 1 cm above the physis (**TECH FIG 3A**).
- The female nail is covered with K-Y Jelly (Johnson & Johnson, New Brunswick, NJ), then cut with a diamond-tip burr and cooled with sterile saline.
- The cannulated portion must be checked to ensure that no metal will impinge on the male nail to prevent it from lengthening and that any metal shards are rinsed off (**TECH FIG 3B,C**).
- A circular saw and rod holder are also available from the manufacturer to cut the female rod (**TECH FIG 3D**).
- The male nail driver is then removed, and the female nail is placed over the male nail.
- The female nail is then screwed into the greater trochanter with the T-handle screwdriver until just a few threads are engaging the bony portion of the proximal femur just distal to the greater trochanter (**TECH FIG 3E**).
- The female nail is checked distally to be sure there is some space between its distal end and the guide wings of the male nail to ensure that the male nail is not driven distally into the joint either acutely or with impaction of the osteotomy with weight bearing (**TECH FIG 3F,G**).
- If the female nail is too shallow proximally, it will back out, but if it is too deep, it is more likely to become overgrown and ultimately reside in the femoral canal.
- The male nail is then cut in situ with the male nail cutter (**TECH FIG 3H**).
- Cutting the male nail approximately 1 cm above the top of the female nail rarely causes persistent symptoms and allows for more growth.
- The probe is used to ensure that the cut male nail is smooth and not bent, which would prevent telescoping.
- Rarely, a diamond-tipped burr may be necessary to smooth the end of the male nail, but the soft tissues must be protected from debris and injury.

## Coxa Vara

- If true coxa vara is present, it should be corrected at the same setting by combining this femoral nail technique with the valgus osteotomy described by Fassier et al[9] (**TECH FIG 4**). Coxa vara can develop spontaneously, with or without weight bearing, or following osteotomy and intramedullary nailing.

## Revision

- When a rod system requires revision after maximal telescoping, it often can be retrieved through just a proximal incision.
- A guidewire is placed in the greater trochanter and into the cannulated portion of the female nail under fluoroscopic control.
- A reamer one size larger than the nail being removed is paced over the guidewire down to the top of the female nail.
- Specialized female and male retrievers, as shown, allow for intramedullary retrieval (**TECH FIG 5A–D**).
- Open osteotomy, cutting the rod and removing the segments, may be necessary to retrieve a broken or bent nail or one that has migrated laterally and distally. If the nail has overgrown into the bone, and open osteotomy can be performed, the rods cut,

A
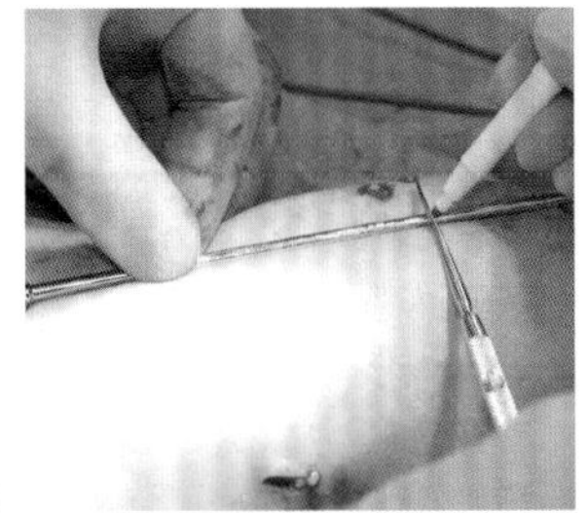
B
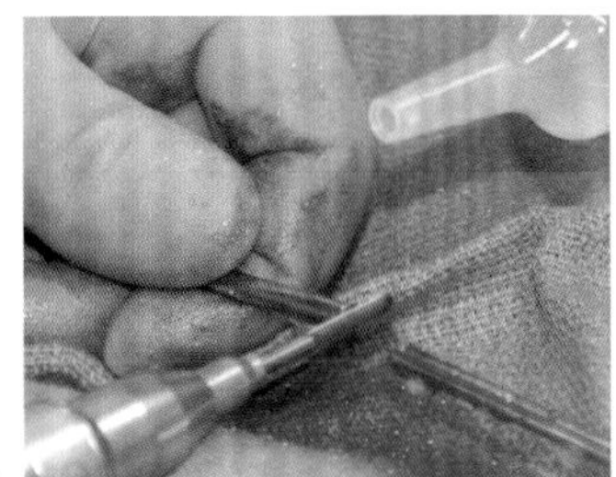
C
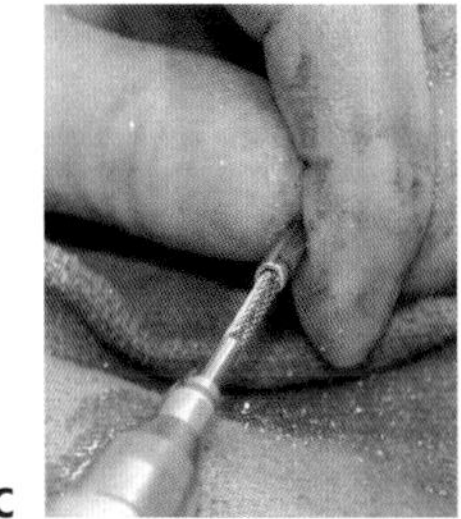
D
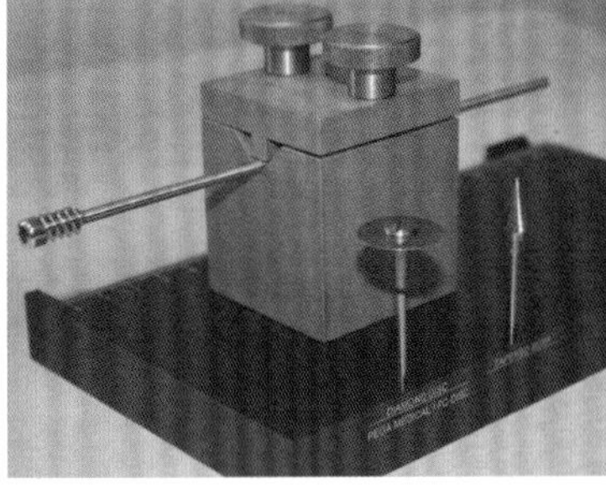

**TECH FIG 3** • **A.** Measuring the female nail length intraoperative with fluoroscopy. **B,C.** Cutting the rod with diamond burr. **D.** Manufacturer's female nail holder with cutting wheel and burr to smooth rough internal edges after cutting. *(continued)*

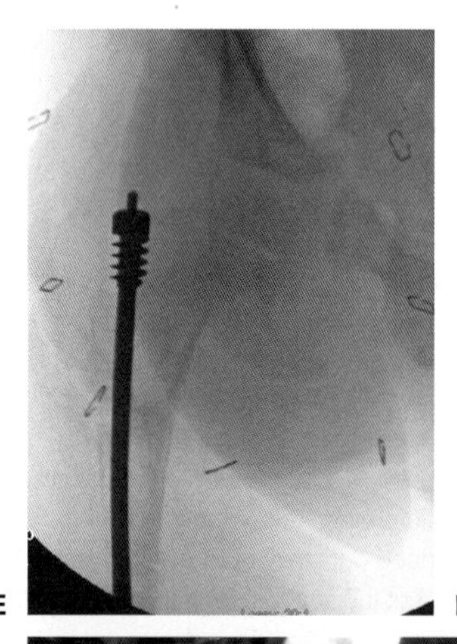
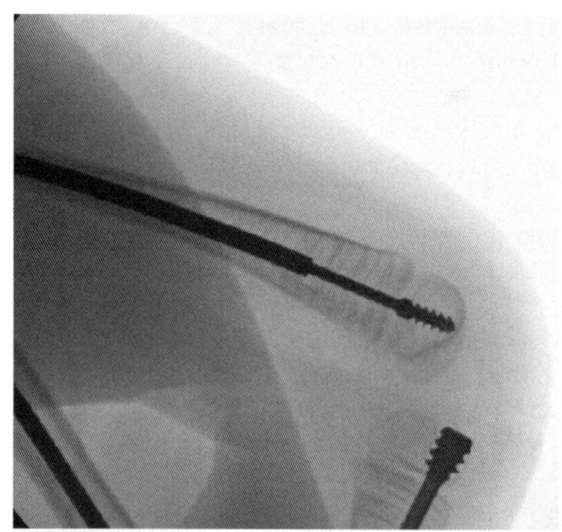
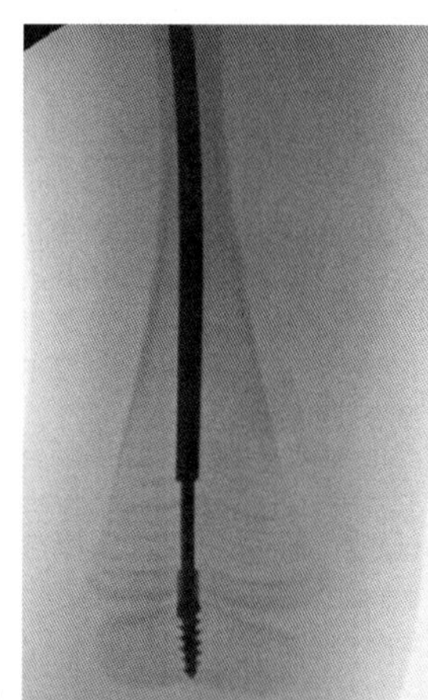
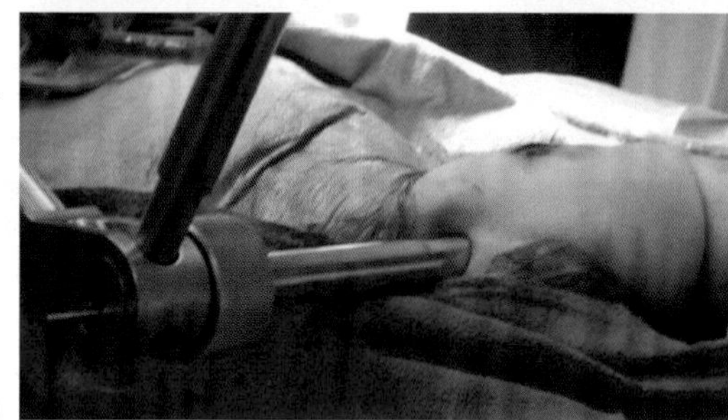

**TECH FIG 3** • *(continued)* **E.** The female threads are shown engaging the bone just distal to the greater trochanter to mitigate overgrowth of the trochanter apophysis but avoid proximal migration of the female nail. **F,G.** Distal placement of the male nail driver and nail in the center–center position is mandatory. The threads engage the epiphysis of the distal femur with the rounded, smooth portion traversing the physis. Ideally, the distal end of the female nail is as close as possible to the guide wings of the male nail for strength and growth but leave room for compression at the osteotomy. **H.** The male nail is cut in situ with the male nail cutter. (**D:** Courtesy of Pega Medical, Inc., Montreal, Canada.)

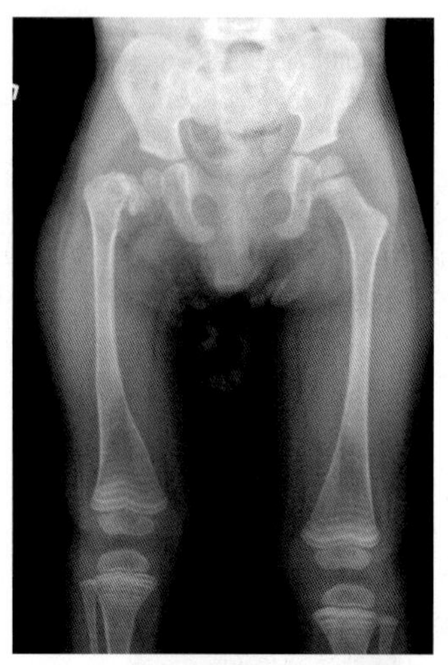
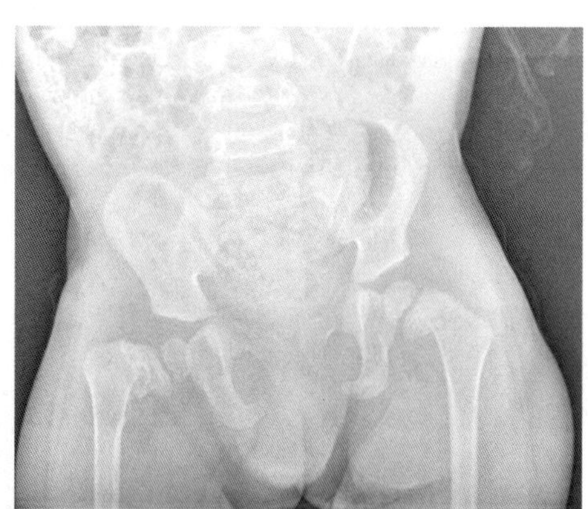
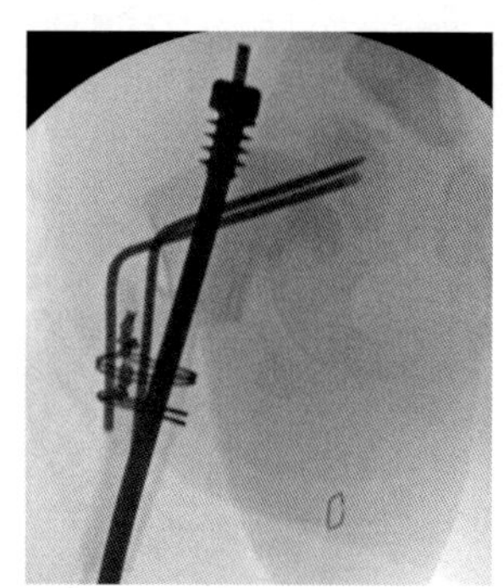
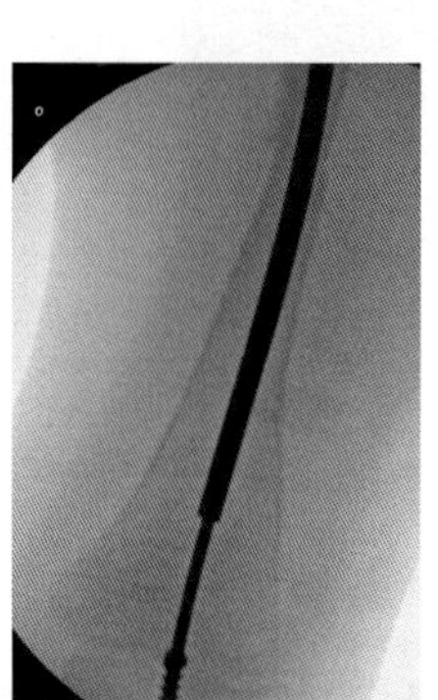
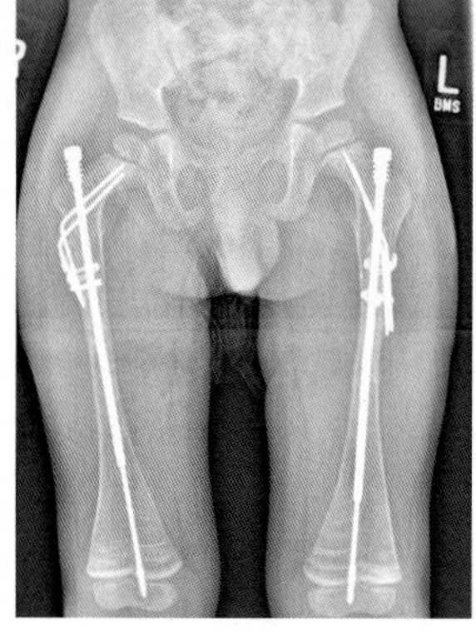


**TECH FIG 4** • **A.** A 2½ year-old boy with OI who developed progressive painful right coxa vara with walking. **B.** Age 3 developing coxa vara on left with progression in right hip. **C.** Age 3 bilateral valgus osteotomies. Note valgus correction and alignment of lateral cortex of the proximal segment with right femoral shaft. **D.** Distal femoral osteotomy to correct associated diaphyseal varus. **E.** At 13-month follow-up, maintenance of correction is demonstrated. The femoral head is growing away from the wires, and varus may recur.

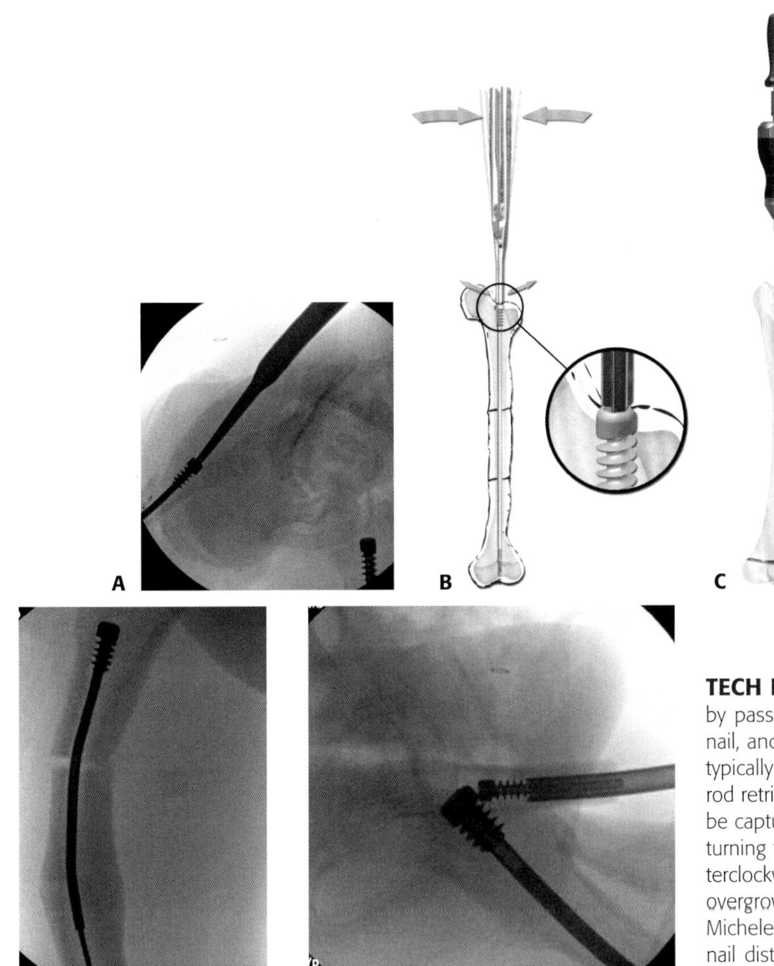

**TECH FIG 5 ● A.** The female nail can usually be removed by passing a guidewire into the nail, reaming to the female nail, and using the revised, thinner, female nail extractor. This typically works even if the nail is somewhat bent. **B.** Female rod retriever. **C.** Male nail rod retriever. **D.** The male nail must be captured above the hole in the male nail extractor prior to turning the torque head of the male nail extractor in a counterclockwise direction. **E.** Severely bent nail with female nail overgrown into femoral canal. **F.** Open osteotomy, rods cut, Michele trephine used to enlarge canal to allow passage of nail distally. (**B–D:** Courtesy of Pega Medical, Inc., Montreal, Canada.)

and it can be removed. A Michele trephine can be used if necessary to enlarge the canal to allow the passage of the female nail head (**TECH FIG 5E,F**).

## Tibial Technique

- Nails from the small bone set are used. These have a somewhat shorter female-threaded portion to avoid extension of the threads across the proximal tibial epiphysis.
- Injury to the anterior horn of the medial meniscus should be avoided, using an arthrotomy if necessary.
- A 0.62-inch K-wire is placed just lateral to the anterior horn of the medial meniscus and just anterior to the tibial spine in the non–weight-bearing surface. A soft tissue protector is helpful in directing the guidewire.
  - A slight bend can be placed in the tip of the wire to assist in advancing wire if necessary. This usually places the wire in the midportion of the tibial epiphysis on the AP view and at the junction of the anterior and middle thirds on the lateral view.
- With the knee kept flexed in excess of 90 degrees, the guidewire is passed into the center position of the proximal metaphysis and shaft.
  - Typically, the wire tends to go posteriorly and laterally so that the wire driver must be directed anteriorly and usually slightly medially.
  - Alternatively, the wire can be manually twisted and pushed into the epiphysis if this provides better control and visualization with the C-arm.
- Avoid repetitive injury to the physis by checking the direction of the wire with the C-arm while it is still in the proximal tibial epiphysis.
- While maintaining hip and knee flexion, the lateral radiograph can be done by simply abducting and externally rotating the leg.
- The guidewire is drilled down to the site of the first osteotomy, which often is the mid- to distal portion of the shaft of the tibia, although bowing of the proximal tibia also may be present.
- To perform the tibial osteotomy, a 1.5-cm incision is made. The periosteum is visualized and partially elevated. Multiple osteotomies may be necessary. However, in the vast majority of patients, a single incision with a segmental resection is preferable to multiple osteotomies (**TECH FIG 6A**).
- The key to the tibial osteotomy is to place the tibia in mild posterior bow to allow for anterior compression.
- Any residual anterior bow will lead to an increased risk of nonunion, progressive anterior bowing, and impede telescoping of the rod.
- A pure closed technique is more hazardous in the tibia.
  - When the medullary canal is obliterated by recurrent fracture and bowing, retrograde drilling is required to establish a medullary canal at the osteotomy site.

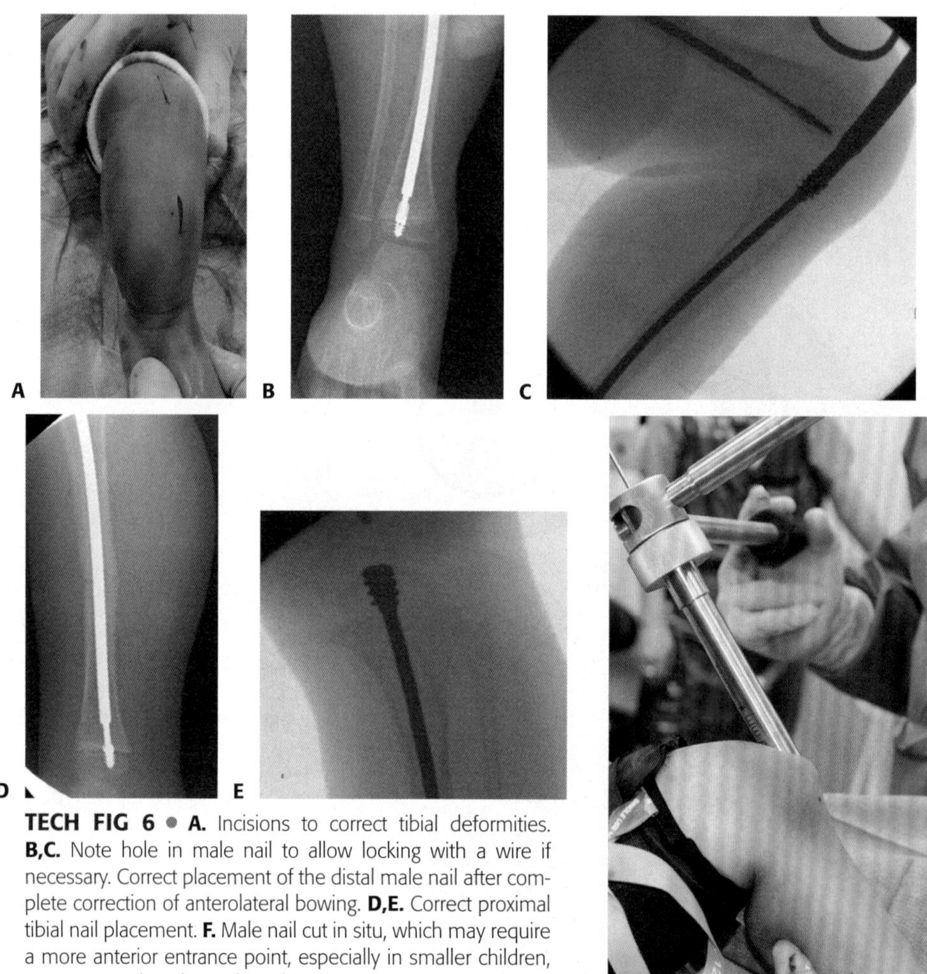

**TECH FIG 6** • **A.** Incisions to correct tibial deformities. **B,C.** Note hole in male nail to allow locking with a wire if necessary. Correct placement of the distal male nail after complete correction of anterolateral bowing. **D,E.** Correct proximal tibial nail placement. **F.** Male nail cut in situ, which may require a more anterior entrance point, especially in smaller children, to accommodate the male nail cutter.

- The guidewire is then passed beyond the osteotomy.
  - Ideally, the entrance point to the distal tibial epiphysis is slightly posterior on the lateral view and slightly lateral on the AP view. This helps to avoid the tendency to valgus and anterior cutout.
- Closed osteoclysis of the fibula often can be performed with minimal force after the tibial osteotomy, especially in younger children, but open osteotomy of the fibula may be necessary.
- The reamer is passed down to the distal metaphysis while maintaining the knee in flexion at all times.
  - Reaming should be done slowly, with frequent stops at the apex of the angular deformity. This bone typically is quite dense in response to recurrent fractures.
  - Extending the knee while the reamer is in place can impinge and injure the femoral condyles.
- The male nail is either cut after determining the length with the C-arm before placement into the tibia or inserted, removed, and then cut after the appropriate length is determined (**TECH FIG 6B–D**).
  - Alternatively, the rod can be placed in the standard fashion and cut in situ. However, this requires a somewhat more anterior entrance point to accommodate the male nail cutter.
  - There is a small hole in the distal male nail to allow interlocking with a small K-wire, if additional stability is required. A blocking screw or wire may be used if absolutely necessary but frequently migrates and requires early removal.
- The female nail is cut to length in the same manner as for the femoral technique and inserted until the threaded portion is fully seated into the epiphysis.
  - It usually is visible just a few millimeters deep to the articular cartilage, even when the C-arm suggests that the proximal nail is protruding into the joint (**TECH FIG 6D,E**).
  - If the male nail is protruding above the female nail, as occurs with in situ cutting with the male nail cutter, it is vital to ensure that the knee will fully extend without impingement of the nail into the femur. With growth, the male nail will migrate distally in the female nail (**TECH FIG 6F**).

## Humeral Nailing

- A bump is placed under the thorax. Placement of the endotracheal tube to the opposite side is helpful.
- The deltoid is spread in line with its fibers through a 1.5-cm incision, and the greater tuberosity is exposed.
- The guidewire is drilled down into the shaft.
- Alternatively, the guidewire is placed retrograde through an open osteotomy.

- In patients with a severe proximal bowing deformity, a percutaneous posterosuperior approach can allow a more medial entrance point in line with the shaft of the proximal humerus.[19,21]
- Typically, the diaphyseal deformity involves the mid- to distal shaft of the humerus. Nonunion of the distal humerus can be a difficult problem to resolve.[12]
- A distal anterolateral approach is used for mid- to distal deformity, and the radial nerve is identified and protected before the osteotomy is performed.
- If a proximal deformity is present, an open or percutaneous osteotomy can be considered.
- The guidewires are then drilled down into the ossified capitellum after correction of the varus and anterior bowing.
- The canal is then reamed to the size of the female nail down to the distal metaphysis.
- The male nail is then placed down into the capitellum, which commonly leaves a slight amount of varus, which is well tolerated (**TECH FIG 7A**).
- In older children, the nail can be placed into the superior segment of the ossified central trochlea, which allows better correction of the distal varus.
- The small bone female nail is used, cut to appropriate length before insertion. The upper end of the female nail should be deep to the articular cartilage to avoid impingement. This is verified by placing the shoulder through full range of motion (**TECH FIG 7B–D**).

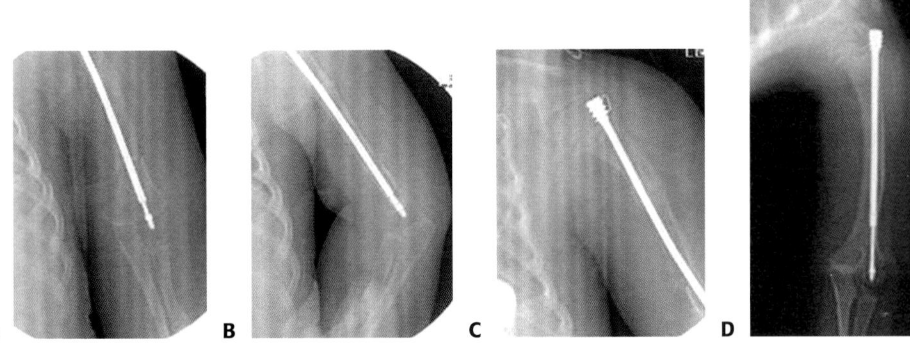

**TECH FIG 7 • A,B.** AP and lateral male nail in capitellum. **C.** Female nail appears to be protruding but is actually deep to the articular cartilage and is not causing impingement. **D.** Two years postoperatively. Note telescoping of nail. There is no clinical impingement.

## PEARLS AND PITFALLS

| | |
|---|---|
| **Multiple bone deformities** | ▪ Multiple bones can be safely treated at the same setting in most children if an experienced team is available.<br>▪ Transfusion may be necessary, especially if more than two bones are treated. Judicious use of tourniquets, such as the HemaClear, in carefully selected patients decreases the likelihood of transfusion. |
| **Postoperative immobilization** | ▪ Lightweight fiberglass lateral or posterior splints for 3 weeks typically are adequate. Casting rarely is necessary.<br>▪ Rotational control is present at 3 weeks.<br>▪ External rotation is common in most of these children and often improves over 12–24 months. |
| **Rod size** | ▪ The smallest rods available are 3.2 mm in diameter. Children with smaller canals can be treated with K-wires or rush rods.<br>▪ The length of the distal male nail threads also limits the ability to use these nails in some smaller children. |
| **Team approach** | ▪ It is mandatory to work with experienced anesthesia, operating room, physical therapy, occupational therapy, dietetics, and metabolic and nursing teams to safely and effectively treat these children.<br>▪ Blood pressure cuffs can be used for monitoring in many children treated with pamidronate if the pressure is set no higher than neonatal pressures.<br>▪ Fiberoptic intubation rarely is necessary when the anesthesiologist is experienced and the surgeon stabilizes the head and neck. |
| **Pain management** | ▪ Epidural analgesia is safe and extremely effective, especially when multiple lower extremity bones are treated at the same operative setting.<br>▪ Adequate analgesia upon awakening is necessary to avoid flailing and fracture.<br>▪ Treatment with Valium is significantly beneficial for spasm.<br>▪ Many children have high narcotic requirements for a short period of time when multiple exposures have been done. |

## POSTOPERATIVE CARE

- Postoperative immobilization can be accomplished safely with lightweight radiolucent fiberglass wrapped under the foot to resist equinus and avoid heel pressure.
- The splint can be extended up to the buttocks to support the femur and loosely overwrapped with an elastic wrap.
- Rarely, a percutaneous tendo Achilles tenotomy will be required.
- Floor activities can be increased whenever the child is comfortable.
- Weight bearing can begin in water approximately 4 weeks after the osteotomies achieve early healing and rotational control.
- Gentle passive range of motion of the hips, knees, and ankles can begin as soon as the child is comfortable.
- Hip, knee, ankle, and foot orthoses are a time-honored treatment and are used postoperatively in many centers.
  - Their effectiveness in avoiding recurrent fractures and deformity has not been demonstrated.
  - Many of the children are significantly more mobile without these orthoses, and healing is not impaired.
- Limit the use of orthoses to only those children with significant soft tissue laxity in the feet such that support is required for stability.

## OUTCOMES

- Improved comfort, a decreased rate of fracture, and an increased activity level are achieved in most children.
- Long-term monitoring of these patients and constant improvement in instrumentation are necessary to ensure optimal development, comfort, and function in this patient population.
- Revisions are still necessary as the children outgrow or damage the rods, but the instrumentation allows for a less traumatic experience for the patient and surgeon.

## COMPLICATIONS

- Complications include failure of telescoping of the rod, overgrowth of the greater trochanter, bending and breakage of the rods, as well as delayed union and nonunion.
- Fractures can occur even with satisfactory alignment, but recovery is typically rapid and requires short-term restriction of activities rather than long-term immobilization.

## REFERENCES


1. Aarabi M, Rauch F, Hamdy RC, et al. High prevalence of coxa vara in patients with severe osteogenesis imperfecta. J Pediatr Orthop 2006;26:24–28.
2. Amako M, Fassier F, Hamdy RC, et al. Functional analysis of upper extremity deformities in children with osteogenesis imperfecta. J Pediatr Orthop 2004;6:689–694.
3. Bailey RW. Further clinical experience with the extensible nail. Clin Orthop Relat Res 1981;(159):171–176.
4. Bailey RW, Dubow HI. Evolution of the concept of an extensible nail accommodating to normal longitudinal bone growth: clinical considerations and implications. Clin Orthop Relat Res 1981;(159): 157–170.
5. Birke O, Davies N, Latimer M, et al. Experience with the Fassier-Duval telescopic rod: first 24 consecutive cases with a minimum of 1-year follow-up. J Pediatr Orthop 2011;31(4):458–464.
6. Engelbert RH, Helders PJ, Keessen W, et al. Intramedullary rodding in type III osteogenesis imperfecta. Effects on neuromotor development in 10 children. Acta Orthop Scand 1995;66:361–364.
7. Esposito PW. Multiple osteotomies and telescoping intramedullary rodding in osteogenesis imperfecta. Presented at the Pediatric Orthopaedic Society of North America 2006 Annual Meeting, San Diego, May 3–6, 2006.
8. Fassier F, Esposito P, Sponseller P, et al. Multicenter radiological assessment of the Fassier-Duval femoral rodding. Presented at Pediatric Orthopaedic Society of North America 2006 Annual Meeting, San Diego, May 3–6, 2006.
9. Fassier F, Sardar Z, Aarabi M, et al. Results and complications of a surgical technique for correction of coxa vara in children with osteopenic bones. J Pediatr Orthop 2008;28(8):799–805.
10. Gamble JG, Strudwick WJ, Rinsky LA, et al. Complications of intramedullary rods in osteogenesis imperfecta: Bailey-Dubow rods versus nonelongating rods. J Pediatr Orthop 1988;8:645–649.
11. Hatz D, Esposito P, Schroeder B, et al. The incidence of spondylolysis and spondylolisthesis in children with osteogenesis imperfecta. J Pediatr Orthop 2001;31:655–660.
12. Hsiao CM, Mormino MA, Esposito PW, et al. Distal humerus atrophic nonunion in a child with osteogenesis imperfecta. J Pediatr Orthop 2013:33:725–729.
13. Huang RP, Ambrose CG, Sullivan E, et al. Functional significance of bone density measurements in children with osteogenesis imperfecta. J Bone Joint Surg Am 2006;88(6):1324–1330.
14. Joseph B, Rebello G, Chandra K. The choice of intramedullary devices for the femur and tibia in osteogenesis imperfecta. J Pediatr Orthop B 2005;14:311–319.
15. Laidlaw AT, Loder RT, Hensinger RN. Telescoping intramedullary rodding with Bailey-Dubow nails for recurrent pathologic fractures in children without osteogenesis imperfecta. J Pediatr Orthop 1998; 18:4–8.
16. Land C, Rauch F, Montpetit K, et al. Effect of intravenous pamidronate therapy on functional abilities and level of ambulation in children with osteogenesis imperfecta. J Pediatr 2006;148:456–460.
17. McHale KA, Tenuta JJ, Tosi LL, et al. Percutaneous intramedullary fixation of long bone deformity in severe osteogenesis imperfecta. Clin Orthop Relat Res 1994;(305):242–248.
18. Metaizeau JP. L'embrochage centro-médullaire coulissant. Application an traitement des formes graves d'ostéogenèse imparfaites. Chir Pédiatr 1987;28:240–243.
19. Meyer M, Graveleau N, Hardy P, et al. Anatomic risks of shoulder arthroscopy portals: anatomic cadaveric study of 12 portals. Arthroscopy 2007;23:529–536.
20. Munns CF, Rauch F, Zeitlin L, et al. Delayed osteotomy but not fracture healing in pediatric osteogenesis imperfecta patients receiving pamidronate. J Bone Miner Res 2004;19:1779–1786.
21. Neviaser TJ. Arthroscopy of the shoulder. Orthop Clin North Am 1987;3:361–372.
22. Pega Medical. Product instruction manual. Pega Medical website. Available at http://www.pegamedical.com. Accessed January 6, 2015.
23. Pizones J, Plotkin H, Parra-Garcia JI, et al. Bone healing in osteogenesis imperfecta treated with bisphosphonates. J Pediatr Orthop 2005;25: 332–335.
24. Plotkin H. Syndromes with congenital brittle bones. BMC Pediatrics 2004;4:16.
25. Plotkin H. Two questions about osteogenesis imperfecta. J Pediatr Orthop 2006;26:148–149.
26. Plotkin H, Coughlin S, Kreikmeier R, et al. Low dose pamidronate in children with severe cerebral palsy: a pilot study. Dev Med Child Neurol 2006;48:709–712.
27. Rauch F, Glorieux FH. Osteogenesis imperfecta. Lancet 2004;363 (9418):1377–1385.
28. Ruck J, Dahan-Oliel N, Montpetit K, et al. Fassier-Duval femoral rodding in children with osteogenesis imperfecta receiving bisphosphonates: functional outcomes at one year. J Child Orthop 2011; 5(3):217–224.
29. Ryöppy S, Alberty A, Kaitila I. Early semiclosed intramedullary stabilization in osteogenesis imperfecta. J Pediatr Orthop 1987;7: 139–144.

30. Sillence DO. Osteogenesis imperfecta: an expanding panorama of variants. Clin Orthop Relat Res 1981;159:11–25.
31. Sillence DO, Senn A, Danks DM. Genetic heterogeneity in osteogenesis imperfecta. J Med Genet 1979:16:101–116.
32. Sofield HA, Millare EA. Fragmentation, realignment, and intramedullary rod fixation of deformities of the long bones in children. A ten-year appraisal. J Bone Joint Surg Am 1959;41(8):1371–1391.
33. Wilkinson JM, Scott BW, Clarke AM, et al. Surgical stabilization of the lower limb in osteogenesis imperfecta using the Sheffield Telescopic Intramedullary Rod System. J Bone Joint Surg Br 1998;80(6):999–1004.
34. Williams PF. Fragmentation and rodding in osteogenesis imperfecta. J Bone Joint Surg Br 1965;47:23–31.
35. Zionts LE, Ebramzadeh E, Stott NS. Complications in the use of the Bailey-Dubow extensible nail. Clin Orthop Relat Res 1999;(348):286–287.

# Syme and Boyd Amputations for Fibular Deficiency

Anthony Scaduto and Robert M. Bernstein

## DEFINITION

- Fibular deficiency, previously known as *fibular hemimelia*, is a longitudinal deficiency of the fibula. It is the most common long bone deficiency and may be either partial or complete.[1]
- A wide spectrum of associated anomalies also may be seen on the affected limb. The extent of limb shortening and the degree of foot deformity are the most important components that determine treatment. Treatment options include use of a shoe lift, amputation, and limb lengthening.
- Delayed amputation should be avoided whenever possible. Ideally, amputation is performed at 10 to 18 months of age when the child is beginning to pull to stand.[4] Psychosocial adjustment to amputation and the adjustment to prosthetic wear are rapid at this age.
  - A common dilemma for parents and consulting physicians is an unwillingness to commit to a path of either multiple lengthenings or early amputation. It is generally agreed, however, that the least effective approach to fibular deficiency is "let's try lengthening and if it fails, do an amputation."
- The Syme amputation and the Boyd amputation are the two common amputations performed for fibular deficiency.
- The Syme amputation is an ankle disarticulation that preserves the heel pad as a weight-bearing surface. This procedure provides better energy efficiency than a transtibial amputation, may be self-suspending, allows weight bearing on the stump without the use of a prosthesis, and is cartilage capped, preventing terminal overgrowth.
- The Boyd amputation is a modified ankle disarticulation in which the calcaneus is preserved with the heel pad and fused to the distal tibia.
- The best indications for an amputation are a large leg length discrepancy (ie, a difference of more than 30%) at skeletal maturity and a nonfunctional foot.[2]
- The ideal candidate for lengthening has a smaller expected leg length discrepancy (<10%), a stable ankle, and a fully functional foot.
  - Because both amputation and multiple lengthenings have significant consequences, care must be individualized. This is especially important for patients with leg length discrepancies between 10% and 30%, for which both amputation and lengthening have been shown to be effective with excellent functional outcomes.

## ANATOMY

- Fibular deficiency is best considered an abnormality that affects the entire limb, not just the fibula (**FIG 1A**).
- The appearance of the leg can vary from nearly normal to severely deformed (**FIG 1B**).

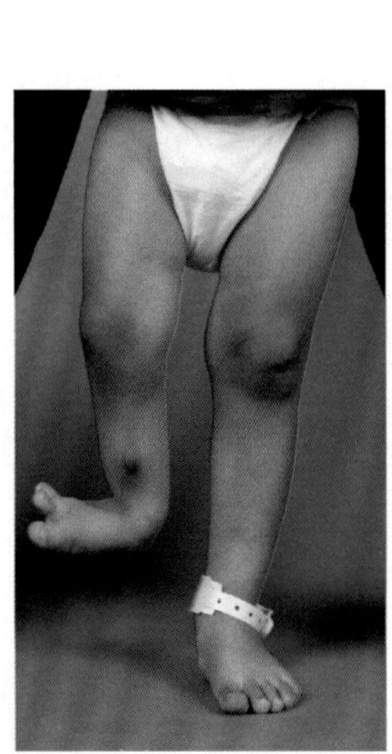


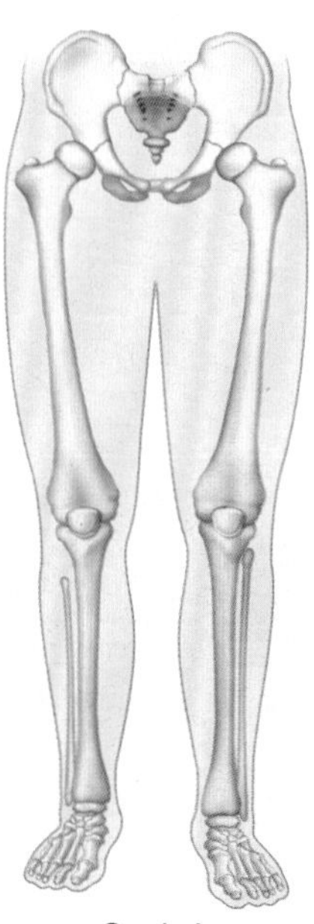


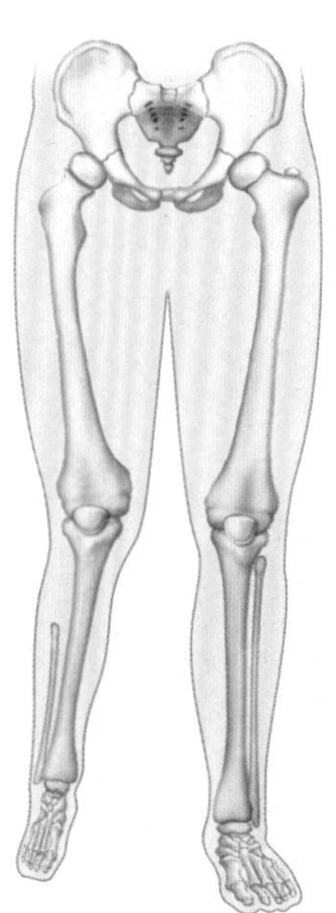


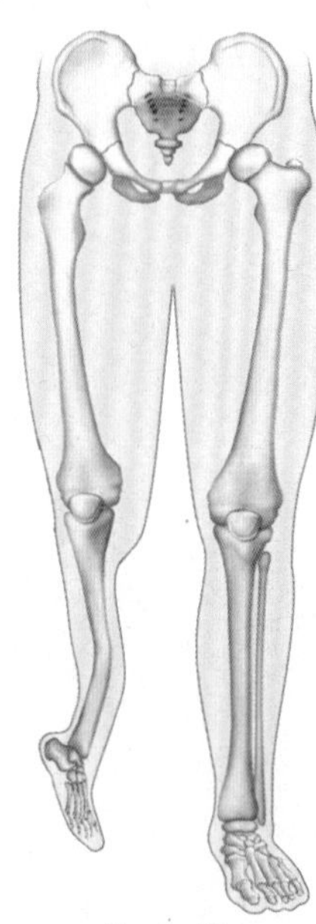


**FIG 1** • **A.** Clinical appearance of limb with fibular deficiency. **B.** Spectrum of fibular deficiency.

- Potential ipsilateral deformities associated with fibular deficiency are as follows:
  - Femur: mild femoral shortening, femoral retroversion, lateral femoral hypoplasia
  - Knee: cruciate ligament deficiency, valgus alignment, patellofemoral instability
  - Tibia: shortening, anteromedial diaphyseal bowing
  - Ankle: ankle valgus, absent lateral malleolus, ball-and-socket ankle
  - Foot: absent tarsal bones, tarsal coalitions, absence of one or more lateral rays
- The amount of fibula present does not aid treatment planning. For example, some patients with complete fibular absence have minimal leg length inequality and foot deformity.
- An understanding of the anatomy of the ankle and heel is necessary to perform either the Syme or Boyd amputation procedure.
  - The posterior tibial nerve and artery course posterior to the medial malleolus and split into the medial and lateral plantar nerves. These structures must be protected for the heel pad to maintain its sensation and viability.

## PATHOGENESIS

- Unlike tibial deficiency, fibular deficiency occurs sporadically with no inheritance pattern.
- No genetic defect has been identified, and no common teratogen is linked to fibular deficiency.
- Major limb malformations associated with fibular deficiency occur by the seventh week of fetal development.

## NATURAL HISTORY

- Without surgical intervention, the growth of the abnormal limb remains proportional to the normal side. Therefore, a final leg length discrepancy is predictable.
  - For example, if the short leg is 85% the length of the long side at age 2 years, the length of the short side at maturity also will be 85% of the estimated length of the long side at maturity.
- Tibial bowing is present in most cases of complete absence of the fibula. In some cases, this bowing will improve with age.
  - Unlike anterolateral bowing of the tibia, bowing associated with fibular deficiency does not increase the risk of fracture or pseudarthrosis.
- Knee valgus commonly worsens through childhood. It may require surgical treatment when prosthetic modifications are inadequate to compensate for the deformity.

## PATIENT HISTORY AND PHYSICAL FINDINGS

- Classically, the limb is short, with an equinovalgus foot and skin dimpling over the midanterior tibia.
- Because presentation varies widely, an examination to assess length, alignment, and function is critical to treatment.
- Hip range of motion: A common finding is limited internal rotation (<20 to 60 degrees) indicating femoral retroversion.
- Leg length assessment: There should be minimal shortening of the thigh. Otherwise, consider proximal femoral focal deficiency. Small leg length discrepancies can be corrected with a shoe lift or lengthening.
- Lachman test: Severe anterior/posterior laxity increases the risk of subluxation during lengthening.
- Valgus alignment and stability: Small angulation is accommodated through prosthetic adjustment, but larger angulation requires correction.
- Tibial bowing requires prosthetic adjustments or correction.
- Ankle alignment and stability: Amputation is preferred over lengthening when severe subluxation or instability exists.
- Hindfoot mobility: Suspect tarsal coalition if subtalar motion is reduced.
- Ray deficiency (number of missing rays): Amputation is indicated when the foot is nonfunctional.

## IMAGING AND OTHER DIAGNOSTIC STUDIES

- Anteroposterior (AP) and lateral radiographs of the leg (including the distal femur) should be obtained.
  - Absence of the anterior cruciate ligament and hypoplasia of the lateral femoral condyle with a valgus joint alignment are common (**FIG 2A,B**).
  - The amount of anterior bowing (tibial kyphosis) also can be assessed (**FIG 2C**).
- Additional radiographs of the affected limb (ie, femur, ankle, and foot) are obtained as necessary (**FIG 2D**).
- A full-length standing radiograph from hips to ankles should be obtained to check alignment in those children able to stand (**FIG 2E**).
- A scanogram and bone age should be obtained to determine the expected leg length discrepancy at maturity.
  - The desired limb length difference at maturity should be at least 3.5 cm to accommodate the height of the prosthetic foot. Epiphysiodesis may be necessary to achieve this and should be planned appropriately.
- An ankle and foot series should be obtained when abnormal position or motion is present at the ankle or subtalar joint or when lateral rays are absent. These views may reveal a ball-and-socket ankle (**FIG 2F**), tarsal coalitions, or absent or hypoplastic tarsal bones (**FIG 2G**).

## DIFFERENTIAL DIAGNOSIS

- Proximal femoral focal deficiency
- Tibial deficiency
- Tibial dysplasia

## NONOPERATIVE MANAGEMENT

- If the leg length discrepancy is small, the ankle is stable, and the foot is plantigrade, a shoe insert or lift may be all that is required.
- When amputation or lengthening is needed but must be deferred, an atypical prosthesis that accommodates the foot position can be used.

## SURGICAL MANAGEMENT

### Syme Amputation

- Meticulous care is needed to preserve the posterior tibial nerve and vessels to maintain a sensate stump.
- Care should be taken not to leave any cartilage remnants of the calcaneus during resection.
- The malleoli should not be resected in children.
- The heel pad may be proximal to the ankle joint and can be difficult to bring distally, even after sectioning the Achilles tendon.

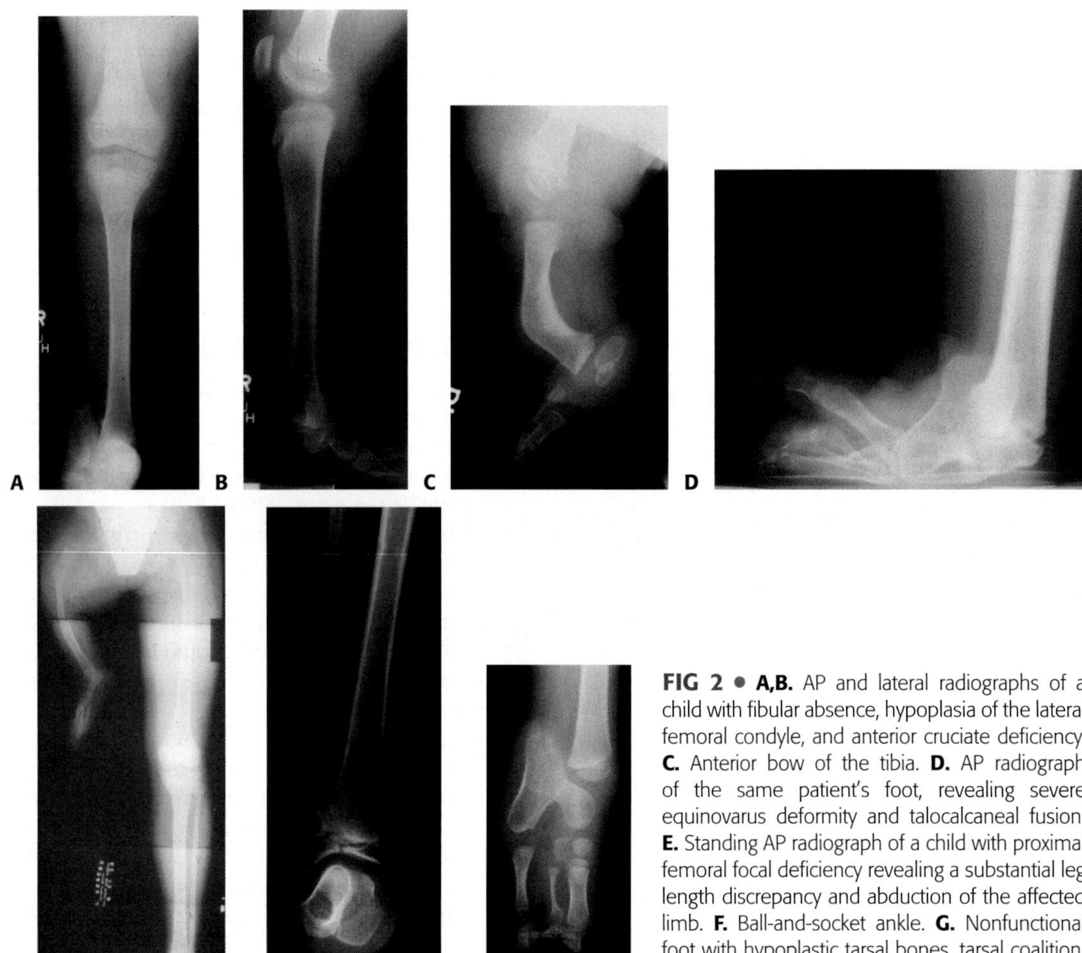

**FIG 2** • **A,B.** AP and lateral radiographs of a child with fibular absence, hypoplasia of the lateral femoral condyle, and anterior cruciate deficiency. **C.** Anterior bow of the tibia. **D.** AP radiograph of the same patient's foot, revealing severe equinovarus deformity and talocalcaneal fusion. **E.** Standing AP radiograph of a child with proximal femoral focal deficiency revealing a substantial leg length discrepancy and abduction of the affected limb. **F.** Ball-and-socket ankle. **G.** Nonfunctional foot with hypoplastic tarsal bones, tarsal coalition, and absent rays. (**E:** Courtesy of Hugh Watts, MD.)

- The Pirogoff modification maintains a portion of the calcaneus, which is fused to the distal tibia to better fix the heel pad.
  - Because in young children the distal tibial physis must be resected to obtain fusion of the calcaneus to the tibia, this is really a modification of the Boyd amputation because distal growth of the tibia will be lost.
- Advantages
  - Simple technique
  - Rapid prosthetic fitting
  - The stump is shorter and often tapered, which improves cosmesis (but also may inhibit end bearing)
- Disadvantages
  - Heel pad migration (**FIG 3**)
  - Less end-bearing potential

## Boyd Amputation

- Advantages
  - Maintains maximum length of limb
  - Eliminates heel pad migration
  - Flare at the end of the stump improves prosthetic suspension
  - Maximizes end-bearing potential. This may be especially important if it preserves end bearing without a prosthesis (eg, not having to put on a prosthesis to go from the bed to the bathroom).
  - The pin necessary for tibiocalcaneal fixation also can be used to stabilize the midtibia osteotomy when bowing of the tibia is corrected simultaneously.
- Disadvantages
  - Delays prosthesis fitting by several weeks while awaiting fusion
  - Excess length may leave less room for energy-storing prosthetic foot options, and the bulbous end may be difficult to hide if it is at the level of the opposite ankle.

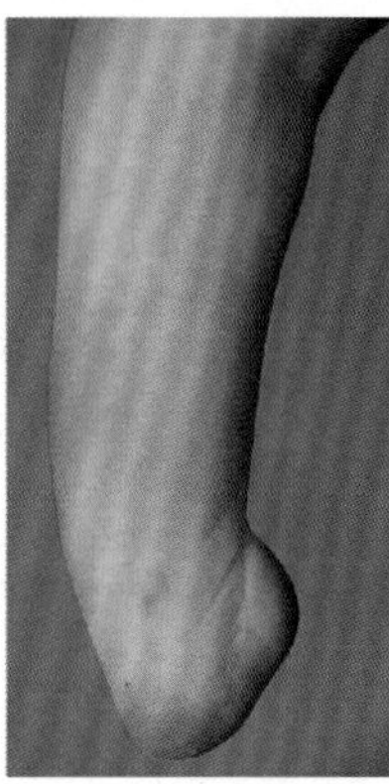

**FIG 3** • Posterior heel pad migration after Syme amputation.

## Preoperative Planning

### *Syme Amputation*

- In patients where the tibial length at skeletal maturity is expected to be equal to that of the opposite side, a Boyd amputation or timed epiphysiodesis should be considered to accommodate the height of the prosthetic foot to achieve equal limb lengths at maturity.
- It usually is not necessary to correct mild bowing (<30 degrees) of the tibia in a congenital deficiency in a skeletally immature patient. Bowing of more than 30 degrees should be addressed with osteotomy at the time of amputation.[6]

### *Boyd Amputation*

- If anterior tibial bowing is present, it is best to correct it at the same time as the Boyd amputation.
- The tarsal bones and distal tibia epiphysis are primarily cartilaginous in infancy.
  - If a Boyd amputation is performed early, it will be necessary to resect a significant portion of the superior calcaneus and distal tibia to achieve bone–bone contact for fusion.
- If maximum length of the tibia is a goal of treatment (eg, to allow occasional end bearing on the stump end without a prosthesis), consider waiting until the distal tibia epiphysis is ossified adequately to avoid resecting the distal physis.
- Some authors have suggested that routine resection of the distal tibia physis should be performed.
  - They observed that most children stop walking around the house without a prosthesis in early adolescence and that ideally the short limb should end in the middle fifth of the shank segment of the prosthesis to optimize cosmesis and allow room for a dynamic response foot–ankle unit.[2]

## Positioning

- The patient is positioned supine with a small bump under the greater trochanter. A tourniquet is placed around the upper thigh.
- Access to the entire leg from knee to toes is important (**FIG 4**).

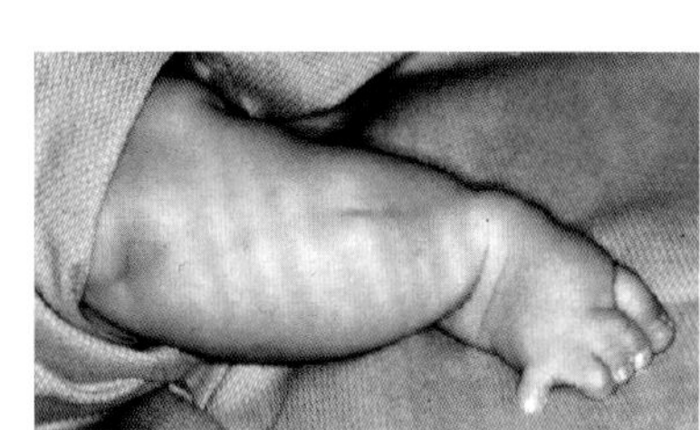
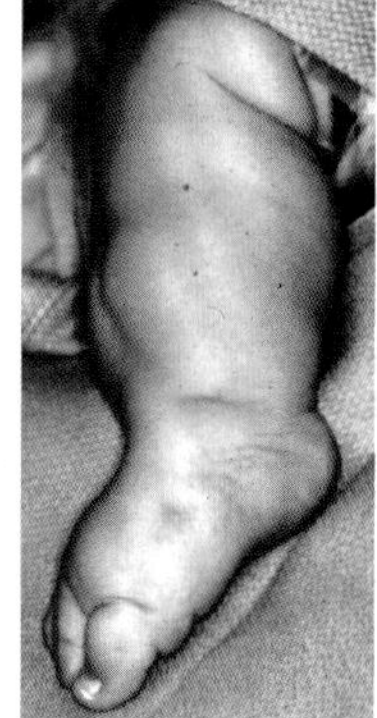

**FIG 4** • Intraoperative photos of patient position with tourniquet applied above the thigh. (Courtesy of Hugh Watts, MD.)

# Amputations for Fibular Deficiency

## Syme Amputation

### *Incisions*

- The dorsal incision is made at the tip of the lateral malleolus (or where it should be) across the ankle joint to end about 1 cm below the tip of the medial malleolus.
  - In children with congenital fibular absence, the lateral malleolus is not present, and the end of the first incision must be approximated.
- The Achilles tendon (often very tight in patients with congenital fibular absence) can be released through a separate, percutaneous incision posteriorly to improve exposure.
- The plantar incision is made at the midportion of the metatarsals and carried proximally up the medial and lateral sides of the foot to meet the anterior incision (**TECH FIG 1**).
  - The plantar incision can be cut directly down to bone, with care to be sure that the knife blade remains perpendicular to the skin. Vessels are ligated or cauterized.

### *Amputation*

- The foot is now plantarflexed (**TECH FIG 2A**). The anterior incision is deepened down to bone, again keeping the knife perpendicular to the skin.
- The anterior ankle joint is opened, and the deltoid and tibiofibular ligaments are cut sharply, with care not to injure the posterior tibial nerve and artery coursing behind the medial malleolus.
- The foot is further plantarflexed to expose the posterior ankle joint, which is released, exposing the posterior calcaneus and the Achilles tendon.
  - A bone hook or sharp retractor can be used to pull on the talus distally as the posterior joint is opened (**TECH FIG 2B**).
- The calcaneus is now released from the heel pad extraperiosteally. Care is taken not to separate the calcaneal apophysis from the body of the calcaneus.
- The Achilles tendon is now sectioned.
  - In very tight equinus, the Achilles can be released through a percutaneous incision posteriorly.
  - Once the tendon is easy to visualize, a 1-cm section of the tendon should be removed to prevent late migration of the heel pad.
- The tourniquet is deflated, and perfusion of the heel pad is checked and bleeding is controlled (**TECH FIG 2C**).
- The distal tibial cartilage and malleoli are left intact.
  - A Steinmann pin or Rush rod may be inserted through the heel pad into the distal tibia to affix the heel pad to the distal tibia (**TECH FIG 2D**).
- Closure is done over a drain using interrupted sutures.
  - In young children, an absorbable suture is used to avoid later removal.
- An antibiotic-impregnated gauze is applied followed by fluffs and Webril.

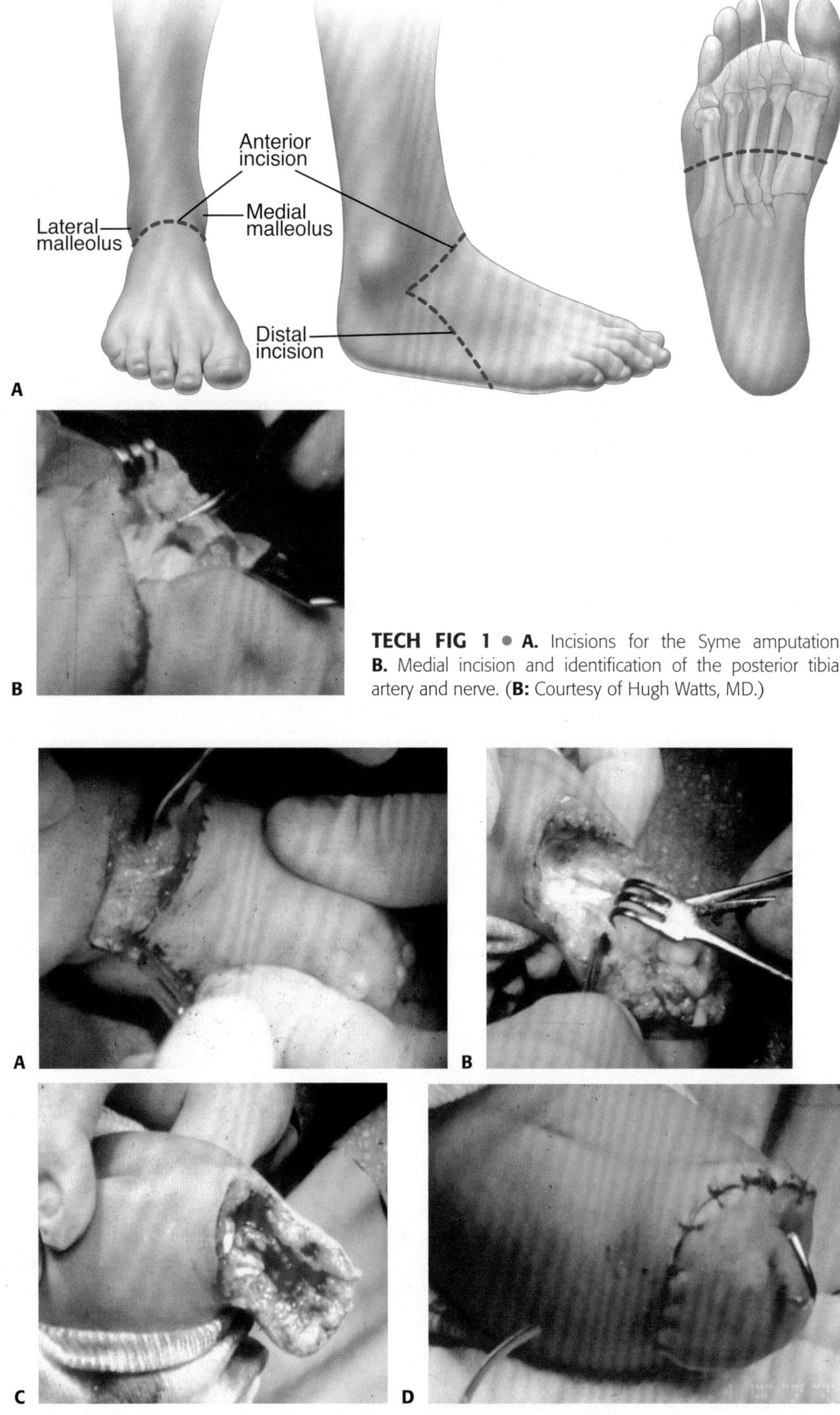


**TECH FIG 1** • **A.** Incisions for the Syme amputation. **B.** Medial incision and identification of the posterior tibial artery and nerve. (**B:** Courtesy of Hugh Watts, MD.)



**TECH FIG 2** • **A.** The foot is plantarflexed while the dorsal incision is completed. **B.** A retractor is placed in the talus to expose the posterior capsule and Achilles tendon. **C.** Intraoperative photograph after deflation of the tourniquet, illustrating a well-perfused heel pad. **D.** Stump closure with interrupted absorbable sutures after insertion of a Steinmann pin to stabilize the heel pad. (Courtesy of Hugh Watts, MD.)

# Boyd Amputation

## Incision and Dissection

- A fish-mouth incision is made (**TECH FIG 3**).
  - The plantar incision crosses the foot where the heel pad ends.
  - The dorsal incision crosses the foot at the level of the ankle joint.
  - The incisions meet medially about 1 cm distal to the medial malleolus and laterally in a similar location (the lateral malleolus often is absent in fibular deficiency).

## Midfoot and Forefoot Removal

- It is unnecessary to dissect layer by layer on the plantar side. Instead, sharply deepen the plantar incision down to the level of the bone (**TECH FIG 4A**).
  - Vessels can be ligated or cauterized (depending on their size) as they are cut or after the tourniquet is deflated before closure.
- While maximally plantarflexing the foot, transect the dorsal nerves and extensor tendons, which retract proximal to the incision (**TECH FIG 4B**).
- Do not remove the midfoot and forefoot at this time. They can serve as a handle to control the hindfoot when releasing the tibiotalar capsule and ligaments (**TECH FIG 4C**).
- Expose the tibiotalar joint by releasing the anterior capsule and then release the deltoid ligament medially and the talofibular ligament with the lateral capsule (**TECH FIG 4D,E**).
  - Use care to preserve the posterior tibial artery and vein while dividing the posterior ankle capsule.
  - A bone hook or skin rake on the talar dome will help expose the posterior tibiotalar capsule and Achilles tendon.
- Identify the flexor hallucis tendon and protect the neurovascular bundle that lies just medial to the tendon (**TECH FIG 4F**).
- Remove the talus after cutting through the talocalcaneal ligaments (**TECH FIG 4G**).
  - Removing the talus may be more difficult in the very young child, in whom the talus is primarily cartilaginous or when it has an irregular shape (**TECH FIG 4D,E**).
- The midfoot and forefoot are now removed.

## Completing the Amputation

- Use an oscillating saw (or, in very young children, a knife) to remove the anterior process of the calcaneus and enough of the superior articular surface to expose cancellous bone (**TECH FIG 5A–C**).
- Cut the distal tibia (**TECH FIG 5D**).
- Oppose the cancellous bone surfaces and stabilize with a retrograde K-wire placed through the heel pad and across the tibiocalcaneal surfaces (**TECH FIG 5E,F**).

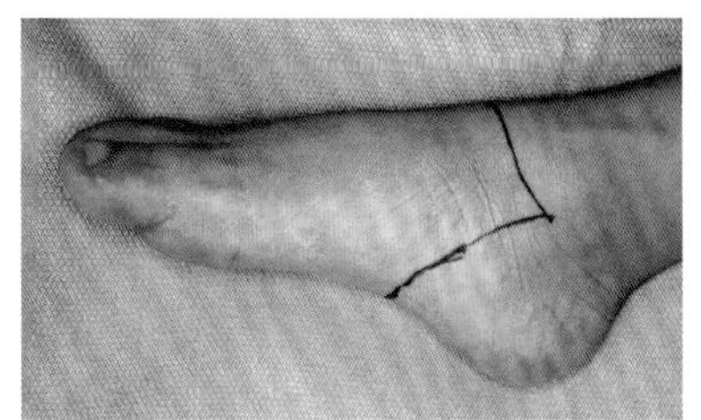
A

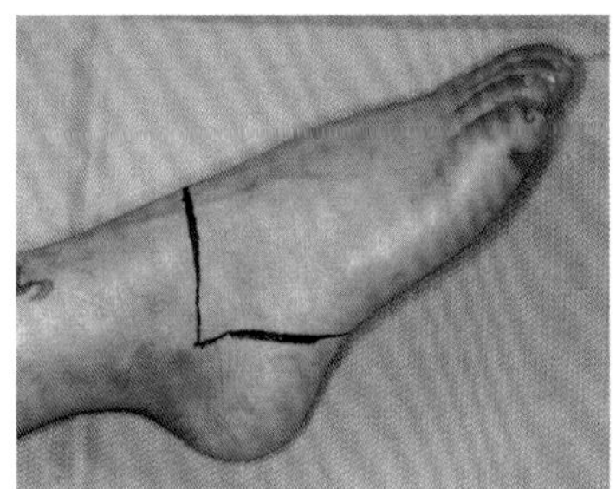
B

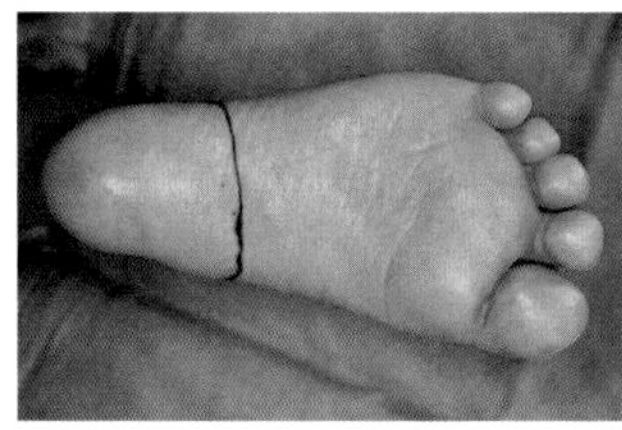
C

**TECH FIG 3 • A,B.** The dorsal and volar parts to the fish-mouth incision meet medially and laterally just distal to the malleoli. **C.** The plantar incision crosses the foot just distal to the heel pad.

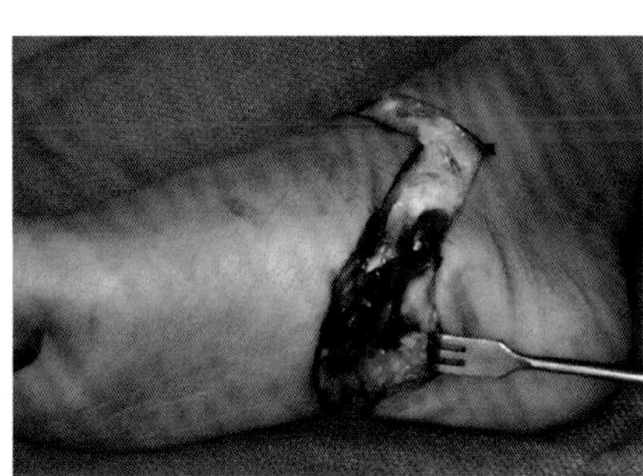
A

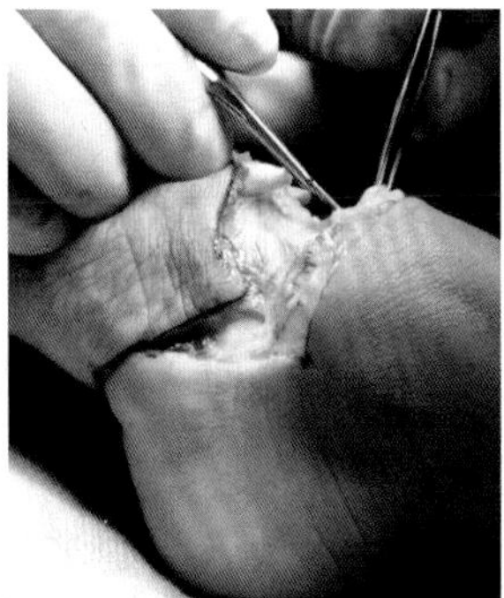
B

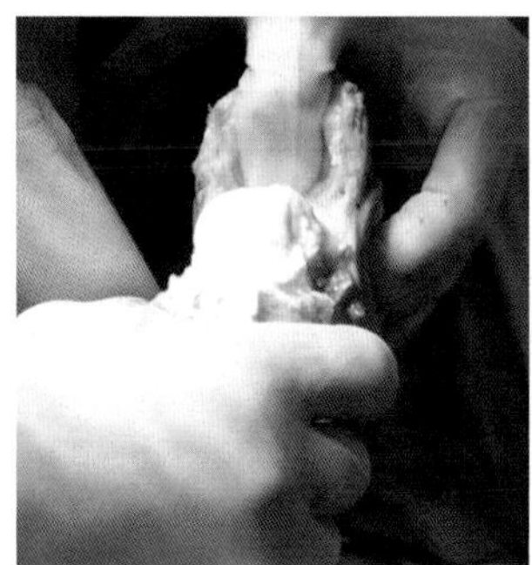
C

**TECH FIG 4 • A.** The plantar incision is carried down to the bone. **B.** Dorsal structures are transected with the foot in plantar flexion. **C.** Use the forefoot to control the hindfoot. *(continued)*

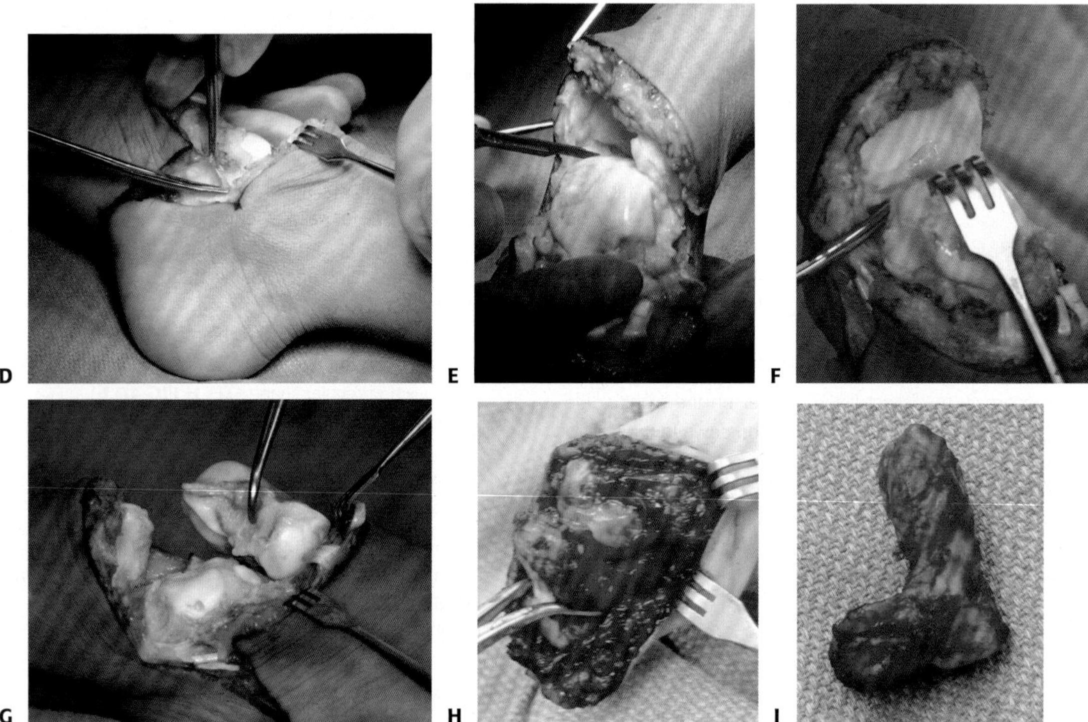

**TECH FIG 4** • *(continued)* **D,E.** Release the deltoid and lateral capsule. **F,G.** Carefully divide the posterior capsule and remove the talus. **H,I.** Sometimes, the talus is small and irregularly shaped, as seen in this case, in which the L-shaped talus hooked around the back of the distal tibia.

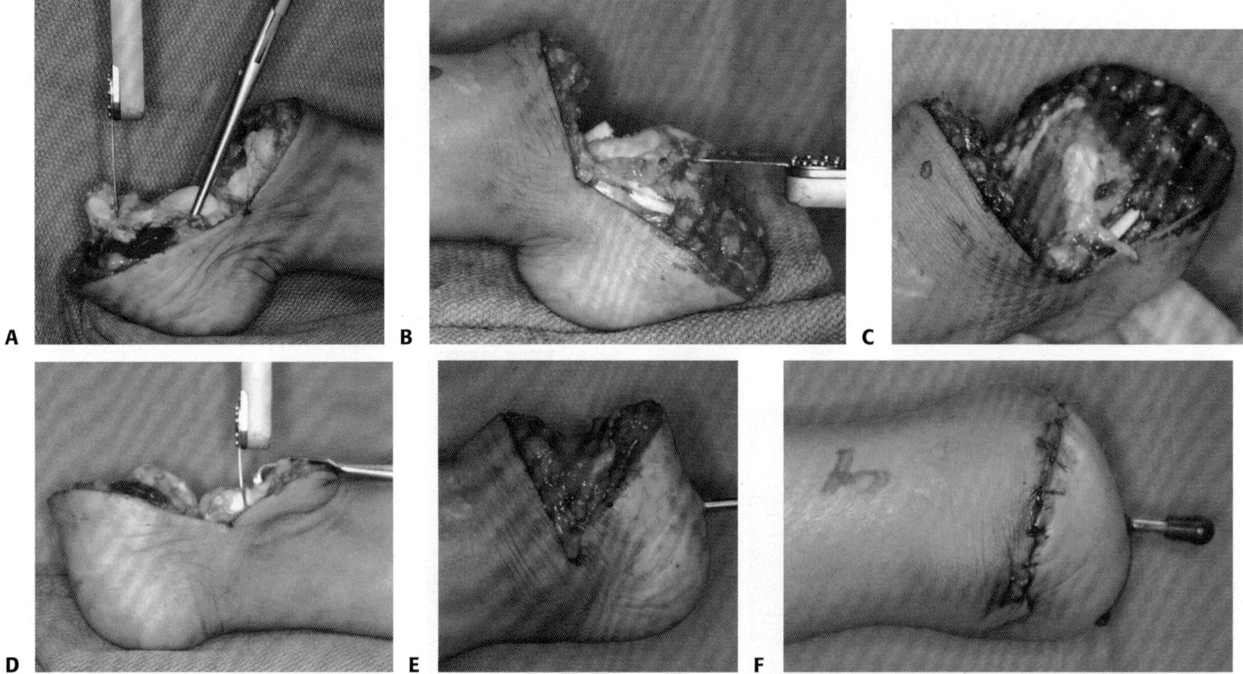

**TECH FIG 5** • **A–C.** Prepare the calcaneus by cutting the anterior and dorsal surfaces. **D–F.** Stabilize the calcaneus to the end of the tibia with a smooth K-wire.

### *Correction of Tibial Bowing*

- Make a longitudinal anterior incision at the apex of the bowing.
- Expose the tibia subperiosteally and place Chandler or Hohmann retractors to protect the soft tissues.
- The superior cut is made perpendicular to the long axis of the proximal tibia, whereas the distal cut is perpendicular to the long axis of the distal tibia, creating a bone wedge with its widest portion located anteromedially (**TECH FIG 6A**).
- The Steinmann pin used to stabilize the calcaneus as part of the Boyd amputation can be extended further into the proximal tibia fragment to simultaneously stabilize the osteotomy site.
  - Consider using a threaded pin if fixation is inadequate with a smooth pin (**TECH FIG 6B**).

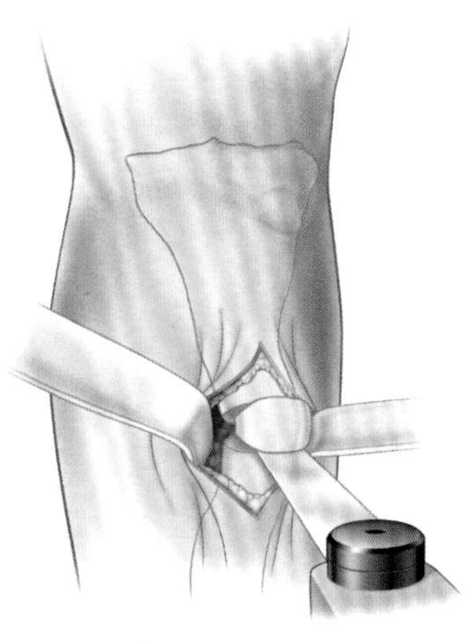


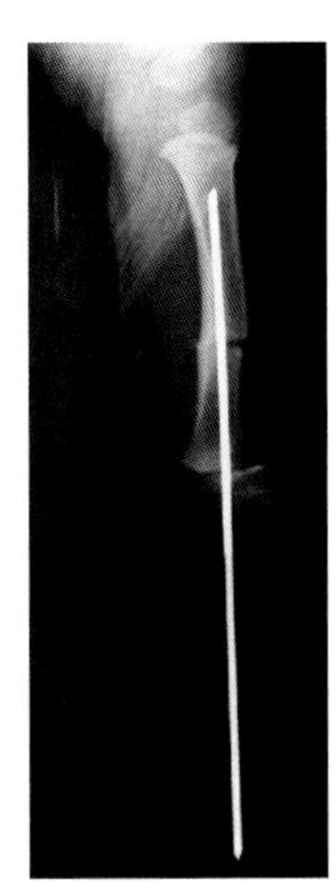


**TECH FIG 6 • A.** A saw is used to remove a wedge of bone to correct the anteromedial bow of the tibia. **B.** A retrograde pin stabilizes calcaneus to distal tibia and the midtibial osteotomy.

## PEARLS AND PITFALLS

| | |
|---|---|
| **Calcaneus excision (Syme)** | ▪ Remove the calcaneus extraperiosteally. This requires careful dissection but decreases the chance of reformation of the calcaneus. Any residual calcaneal cartilage left will result in painful pebbles of bone in the heel pad. |
| **Tibial bowing (kyphosis)** | ▪ Correct at the time of amputation if greater than 30 degrees, and fix with the transfixing Steinmann pin or Rush rod. |
| **Achilles tenotomy** | ▪ The Achilles tendon often is contracted and may make exposure of the calcaneus difficult. A percutaneous release posteriorly with a small tenotomy knife may make exposure easier. |
| **Talus excision (Boyd)** | ▪ Carefully assess the position and shape of the talus and calcaneus to ensure abnormalities of the talus and calcaneus are known in advance.<br>▪ In rare cases, a Boyd amputation will not be possible because of the severe posterior and proximal position of the calcaneus. If so, perform Syme amputation. |
| **Tibiocalcaneal fusion** | ▪ Carefully ensure that cancellous bone is evident on both the distal end of the tibia and the superior surface of the calcaneus. |
| **Skin closure** | ▪ The distal extent of the heel pad is difficult to identify in children who are not yet walking. Be sure the plantar part of the incision is distal enough to allow closure without tension.<br>▪ Cut the anterior process of the calcaneus to reduce the anterior prominence and skin tension. |
| **Angular deformities of leg** | ▪ Correct tibial deformity early to facilitate prosthetic fitting.<br>▪ Correct progressive genu valgum late (ie, in adolescence). |

## POSTOPERATIVE CARE

- Apply a long-leg cast with the knee flexed 90 degrees to prevent pin migration and keep the cast from slipping off.
- Postoperatively, the patient's leg is elevated for 24 hours.
  - The child should be non–weight bearing.
- The cast and pin are removed in the office at 4 to 6 weeks and, in the Boyd amputation, after radiographic healing is evident (**FIG 5A**).
- A stump wrap or shrinker is then applied.
- Once the swelling has resolved, the prosthetist can mold a socket (**FIG 5B,C**).

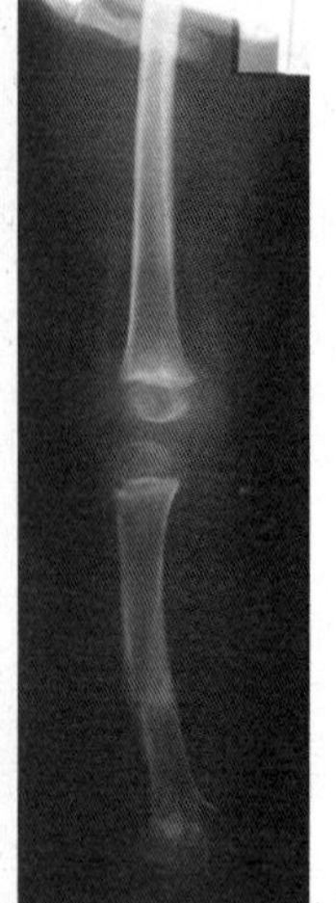
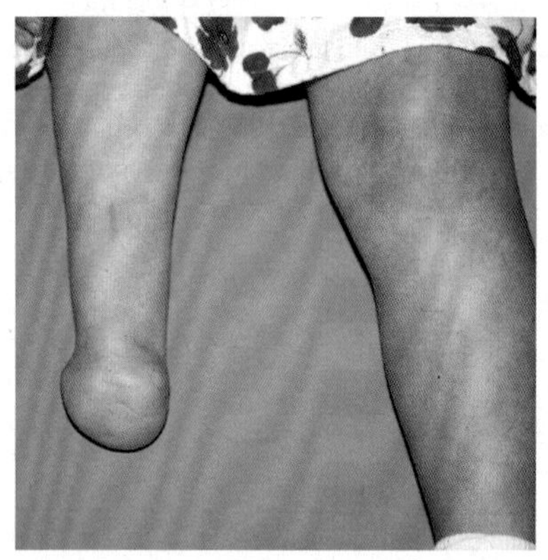
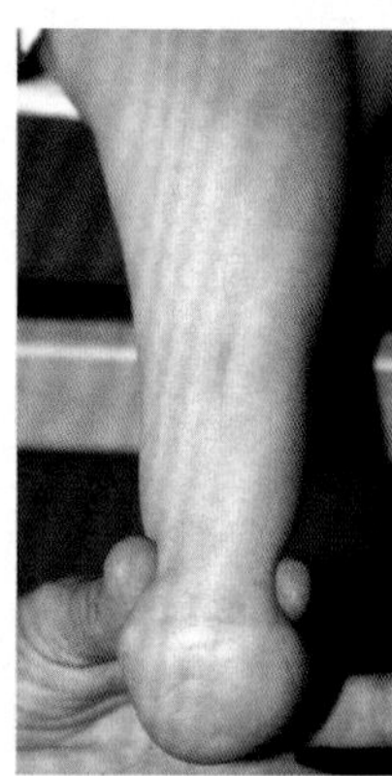

**FIG 5** • **A.** Healed osteotomy and calcaneus fused to tibia. **B,C.** Postoperative photographs demonstrate a good Syme stump with a bulbous end for possible self-suspending socket. (**B,C:** Courtesy of Hugh Watts, MD.)

## OUTCOMES

- McCarthy et al[5] reported on a comparison of amputation versus lengthening in the treatment of fibular hemimelia.
  - Patients who underwent amputation were more active, had less pain, were more satisfied, and had fewer complications than those who underwent limb lengthening.
- Fulp et al[3] reviewed 25 patients (31 extremities) with longitudinal deficiency of the fibula treated with either Syme amputation or Boyd amputation.
  - Patients who underwent Syme amputation had more problems with prosthetic suspension, reformation of the calcaneus, and migration of the heel pad.
- Late progressive genu valgum deformity requiring a stapling or osteotomy of the distal femur occurs in 29% to 58% of cases.

## COMPLICATIONS

- Wound slough/dehiscence
- Migration of the heel pad
- Penciling of the distal tibia
- Infection
- Pin migration
- Nonunion
- Excess length

## REFERENCES

1. Cummings D. General prosthetic considerations. In: Smith GS, Michael JW, Bowker JH, eds. Atlas of Amputations and Limb Deficiencies: Surgical, Prosthetic, and Rehabilitation Principles, ed 3. Rosemont, IL: American Academy of Orthopedic Surgeons, 2004:792–793.
2. Eilert RE, Jayakumar SS. Boyd and Syme ankle amputations in children. J Bone Joint Surg Am 1976;58(8):1138–1141.
3. Fulp T, Davids JR, Meyer LC, et al. Longitudinal deficiency of the fibula. Operative treatment. J Bone Joint Surg Am 1996;78(5):674–682.
4. Krajbich JI. Lower-limb deficiencies and amputations in children. J Am Acad Orthop Surg 1998;6:358–367.
5. McCarthy JJ, Glancy GL, Chang FM, et al. Fibular hemimelia: comparison of outcome measurements after amputation and lengthening. J Bone Joint Surg Am 2000;82-A(12):1732–1735.
6. Morrissey RT, Weinstein SL. Boyd amputation with osteotomy of the tibia for fibular deficiency. In: Morrissey RT, Weinstein LW, eds. Atlas of Pediatric Orthopaedic Surgery, ed 4. Philadelphia: Lippincott Williams & Wilkins, 2006:872–876.

# Neuromuscular Correction

# Adductor and Iliopsoas Release

Tom F. Novacheck

64 CHAPTER

## DEFINITION

- Psoas and adductor contractures are most common in cerebral palsy but can occur in any neuromuscular condition owing to disuse, muscular imbalance, or spasticity.
- The degree of contracture varies depending on the patient's age and the severity of neuromuscular dysfunction.
- Detecting hip flexion contracture (psoas) is challenging.
- The challenge for the adductors is deciding which muscles to lengthen and how much lengthening to do.

## ANATOMY

- The psoas is part of the primary hip flexor group, the iliopsoas.
- The psoas muscle originates from the transverse processes of the lumbar vertebrae. The muscle belly passes over the sacrum into the pelvis (**FIG 1A**).
- At the level of the pelvic brim (superior pubic ramus), the intramuscular tendon can be found.
- At this level, the psoas lies underneath the muscle belly of the iliacus. The femoral neurovascular bundle is superficial to the iliacus (**FIG 1B,C**).
- The psoas and iliacus tendons combine below the level of the pelvic brim to form a common tendon that inserts on the lesser trochanter.
- The adductor longus, adductor brevis, adductor magnus, and gracilis are clinically considered the adductor group of the hip. Their origins arise from the pubic and ischial rami as well as the pubic tubercle and they insert medially on the femur (adductors) and proximal tibia (gracilis) (**FIG 1D**).
- The adductor longus has a tendinous origin, the gracilis has a muscular fascia, and the adductor brevis and magnus have muscular origins.
- The anterior branch of the obturator nerve lies in the interval deep to the adductor longus and superficial to the adductor brevis, whereas the posterior branch of the obturator nerve lies in the interval deep to the adductor brevis and superficial to the adductor magnus.

## PATHOGENESIS

- Hip flexion and adduction contractures develop over time due to the following:
  - Lack of typical functional activities
  - Muscular imbalance between these muscle groups and their antagonists, the hip extensors and abductors, due to either weakness of the antagonists or spasticity of the agonists
- A hip flexion contracture is typical at birth and persists in infancy up until the time the child begins to stand and walk. In an older child who has not achieved standing and walking ability, a hip flexion contracture therefore may represent a persistence of the normal fetal alignment.
- At birth, the normal amount of hip abduction range of motion is 60 to 90 degrees, significantly greater than the expected range of motion of adults.
- Appropriate musculotendinous length develops during growth as the muscle responds to bone growth and stretch associated with typical childhood activities such as walking, running, and playing. Growth occurs at the musculotendinous junction through the addition of new sarcomeres.
- Contractures of these structures do not allow the joint to achieve normal positions for daily activities.

## NATURAL HISTORY

- Contractures, if severe and persistent, can lead to hip subluxation, hip dysplasia, and ultimately hip dislocation.
- Hip dysplasia and especially hip dislocation are most common with more severe cerebral palsy (quadriplegia, minimally ambulatory or nonambulatory, Gross Motor Function Classification System [GMFCS] IV and V) and in L2- or L3-level myelodysplasia because muscular imbalance at the hip is most severe (innervated hip flexors and adductors, paralyzed abductors and extensors).
- In more functionally mobile children with cerebral palsy (GMFCS I, II, and III), psoas and adductor contractures may lead to anterior pelvic tilt, excessive pelvic motion, and lack of hip extension in terminal stance and contribute to crouch.
- Although a scissoring gait is commonly considered to be due to adductor contractures, this visual appearance most commonly results from the combination of hip and knee flexion with internal hip malrotation due to excessive femoral anteversion.
- In long-standing cases, hip dysplasia can lead to degenerative arthrosis.

## PATIENT HISTORY AND PHYSICAL FINDINGS

- Physical examination methods include the following:
  - Hip flexion–extension range of motion: Normal walking function requires 7 degrees of extension beyond neutral pelvic position. Therefore, even small contractures limit functional range of motion, shorten step length, and induce compensatory movements.
  - Hip abduction–adduction range of motion: Maximum abduction range of motion during typical walking is only 5 degrees. Therefore, even moderate limitations of hip abduction range of motion may not have functional significance (unless spasticity is also present). Normal hip development may not occur if abduction range of motion is limited.
  - If resistance is felt as the hip is extended and abducted, spasticity is present. Increasingly severe spasticity increases

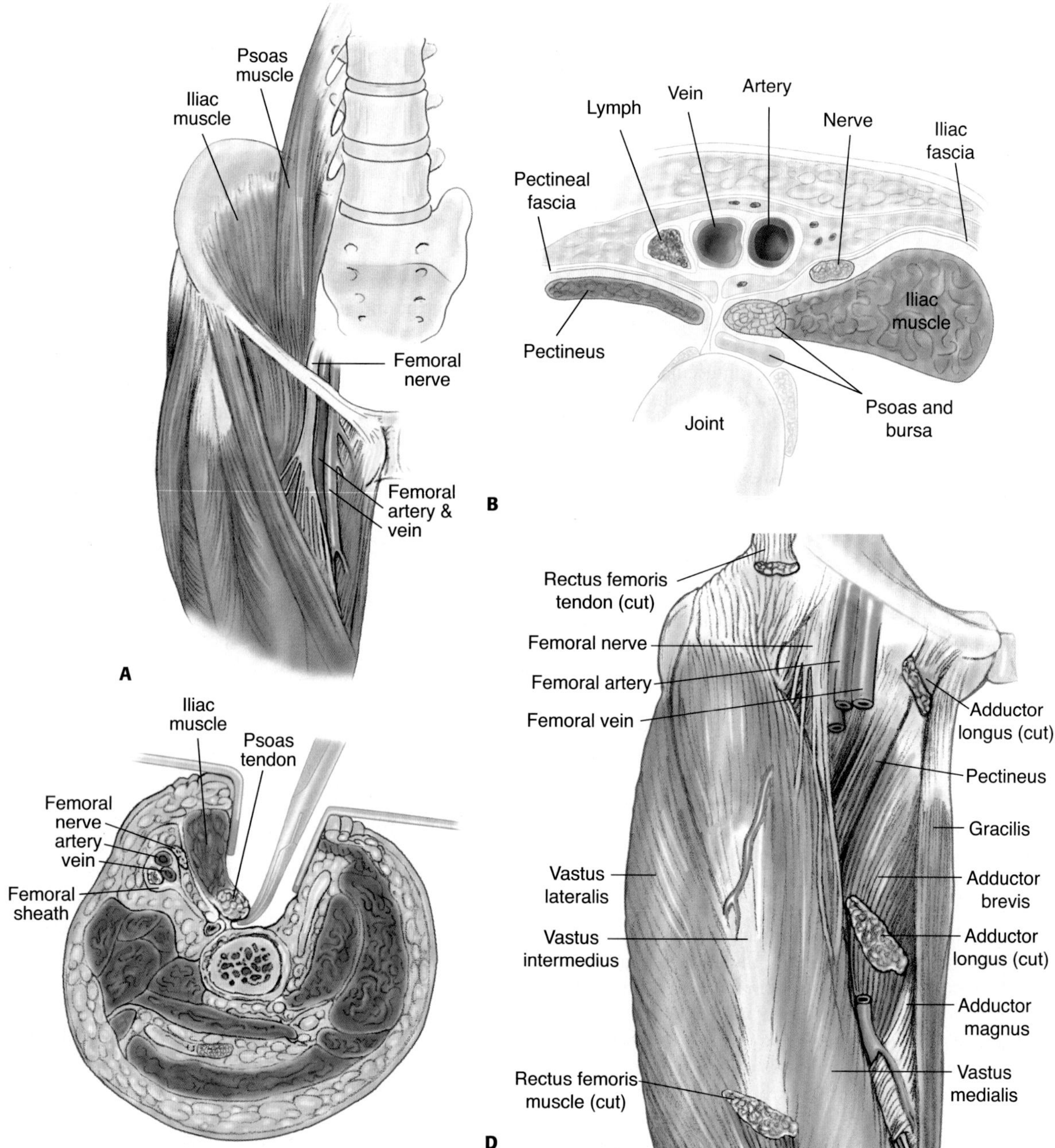


**FIG 1** • **A.** Hip flexor anatomy. The psoas arises from the lumbar spine transverse processes. At the level of the pubic ramus, as it exits the pelvis, it has an intramuscular tendon. Note the proximity of the femoral nerve and artery anteriorly. **B,C.** Transverse plane anatomy of the hip. **B.** Even though this cross-section is slightly distal to the pubic ramus, the reason for recommending an approach underneath (lateral) to the iliacus is clear. **C.** If the iliacus is retracted anteriorly and medially, the femoral neurovascular structures are protected by the muscle belly of the iliacus. The psoas muscle and tendon can be directly visualized. **D.** Adductor anatomy. The surgeon can orient himself or herself by identifying the tendinous adductor longus origin. The pectineus is lateral and the gracilis medial. The anterior branch of the obturator nerve lies on the anterior surface of the adductor brevis (deep to the adductor longus) after emerging from the obturator foramen just medial to the pectineus.

the risk of development of subsequent contracture. For ambulation, spasticity (even in the absence of contracture) can limit movement.

- Hip flexion and hip adduction strength are tested in the supine position. Lengthening a contracted and weak muscle may adversely affect function. Weak, antagonistic muscle groups (hip extensors, hip abductors) predispose to flexion and adduction contractures and contribute to muscle imbalance.
- When examining a child for hip flexion contracture, the examiner should not be misled by the presence of a knee flexion contracture that prevents full extension of the leg. This can be avoided by moving the patient to the side of the examination table and allowing the lower leg to drop off the side of the table.
- Femoral anteversion must also be examined for and ruled out.

- Accurately identifying and controlling pelvic position is crucial for evaluating hip extension and abduction range of motion.
- For the nonambulatory patient, the examiner should look for hyperlordosis and a flexed, adducted, internally rotated hip. For the ambulatory patient, observation of gait may show hyperlordosis, limited step length, scissoring gait, or crouch gait.

## IMAGING AND OTHER DIAGNOSTIC STUDIES

- Supine anteroposterior (AP) pelvis radiograph (**FIG 2**)
  - Pelvic obliquity
  - Adducted hip
  - Lordotic pelvis
  - Varying degrees of hip dysplasia
- Gait analysis may reveal the following:
  - Pelvic obliquity with affected side elevated
  - Limited hip abduction range of motion in late stance and during swing phase
  - Excessive anterior pelvic tilt with or without excessive pelvic range of motion
  - Limited hip extension range of motion in terminal stance

## DIFFERENTIAL DIAGNOSIS

- Hip dysplasia or dislocation
- Knee flexion deformity
- Hip abductor or extensor weakness

A

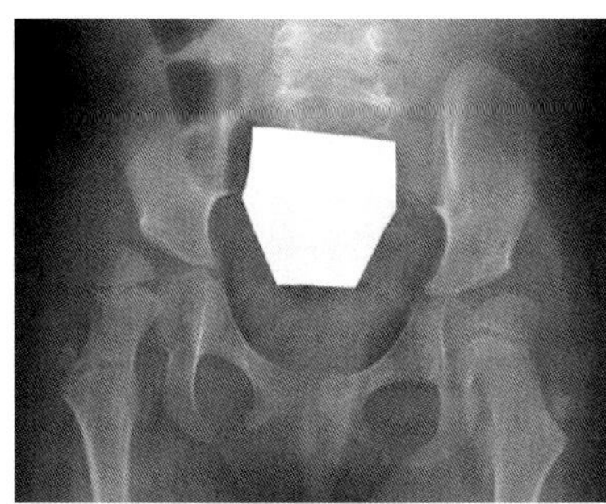

B

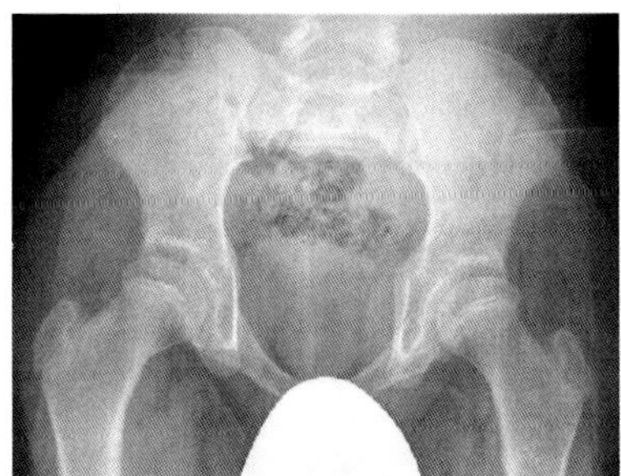

**FIG 2** • AP pelvis radiographs. **A.** Common findings of coxa valga (although femoral anteversion cannot be eliminated as a possibility): break in the Shenton line indicating subluxation, incomplete femoral head coverage, pelvic obliquity (right side elevated), mild windswept hips (right adducted), and mild acetabular dysplasia (right > left). **B.** In this case, severe hip flexion contractures result in anterior pelvic tilt. The AP pelvis radiograph results in an inlet view (obturator foraminae are not visible).

- Excessive femoral anteversion
- Contracture of secondary hip flexors (esp, myelodysplasia)

## NONOPERATIVE MANAGEMENT

- Physical therapy for range of motion and strengthening
- Positioning aids
  - Standers
  - Sleeping prone
  - Hip abduction pillow, Scottish Rite brace with thoracolumbar extension
- Botulinum toxin injections

## SURGICAL MANAGEMENT

### Preoperative Planning

- The AP pelvis radiograph is reviewed to rule out hip dysplasia.
- Examination under anesthesia is performed as described earlier. Under general anesthesia, hypertonicity is no longer present and the true difference between restricted range due to high muscle tone versus musculotendinous contracture can be appreciated.
- Also, the secondary hip flexors (tensor fascia lata and sartorius) can be palpated to rule out secondary contracture (uncommon in cerebral palsy but common in myelodysplasia).

### Positioning

- The patient is positioned supine.
- The leg is draped free to allow flexion and extension of the hip and knee joints as well as abduction of the hip.
- Care must be taken with draping to ensure access to the anterior pelvis up to the groin crease to allow adequate surgical exposure.

### Approach

- Various approaches have been described for psoas lengthening.
  - My preferred incision is a 3- to 4-cm oblique incision along the inguinal ligament that starts at the anterior superior iliac spine and is directed inferomedially.[3]
  - Surgeons less comfortable with dissecting the abdominal musculature near the inguinal ligament prefer a more proximal incision at the iliac crest with the abdominal musculature taken off the subcutaneous border of the ilium. The psoas tendon is approached at the same level (the pelvic brim) and therefore the exposure of the tendon is more difficult from this more proximal incision.
  - Sutherland et al[5] preferred an exposure distal to the inguinal ligament.
- All approaches use the same deep tissue plane underneath (lateral) to the iliacus muscle belly.
- The proximity of the femoral neurovascular structures has been well documented and is a cause for caution.[4]
- The surgical concept of psoas lengthening at the pelvic brim was adapted from Salter's description of lengthening the psoas tendon while performing a Salter pelvic osteotomy.

## Psoas Lengthening at the Pelvic Brim

### Incision and Dissection

- An oblique incision is made along the inguinal ligament starting at the anterior superior iliac spine and extending distal and medial along the course of the inguinal ligament (**TECH FIG 1A–C**).
- The external oblique fascia is identified and divided just above its attachment on the inguinal ligament (**TECH FIG 1D**).
- Blunt dissection through the internal oblique and transversus abdominis just medial and adjacent to the anterior superior iliac spine allows access to the inner table of the ilium extraperiosteally (**TECH FIG 1E**).
- The lateral femoral cutaneous nerve typically crosses the surgical wound and is identified and protected, but sometimes, it is medial and not encountered.

### Tendon Identification and Division

- With the hip flexed, a finger is passed down along the superior pubic ramus underneath the iliacus and psoas to identify the psoas tendon by palpation (**TECH FIG 2A**).
- The psoas tendon is visualized by retracting the iliacus medially with an Army-Navy retractor (**TECH FIG 2B**).
- A right-angled clamp is passed around the psoas tendon (**TECH FIG 2C**).
- By isolating it from the surrounding muscle, the structure is confirmed to be the psoas tendon.
- Muscle fibers are retracted, and the tendon is divided with electrocautery, leaving the muscle intact (**TECH FIG 2D**).
- Any inflexible (tendinous or myofascial tissues) should be divided. Many patients have a psoas minor tendon, which must also be identified and divided. Muscular tissues are left intact to maintain hip flexor function.

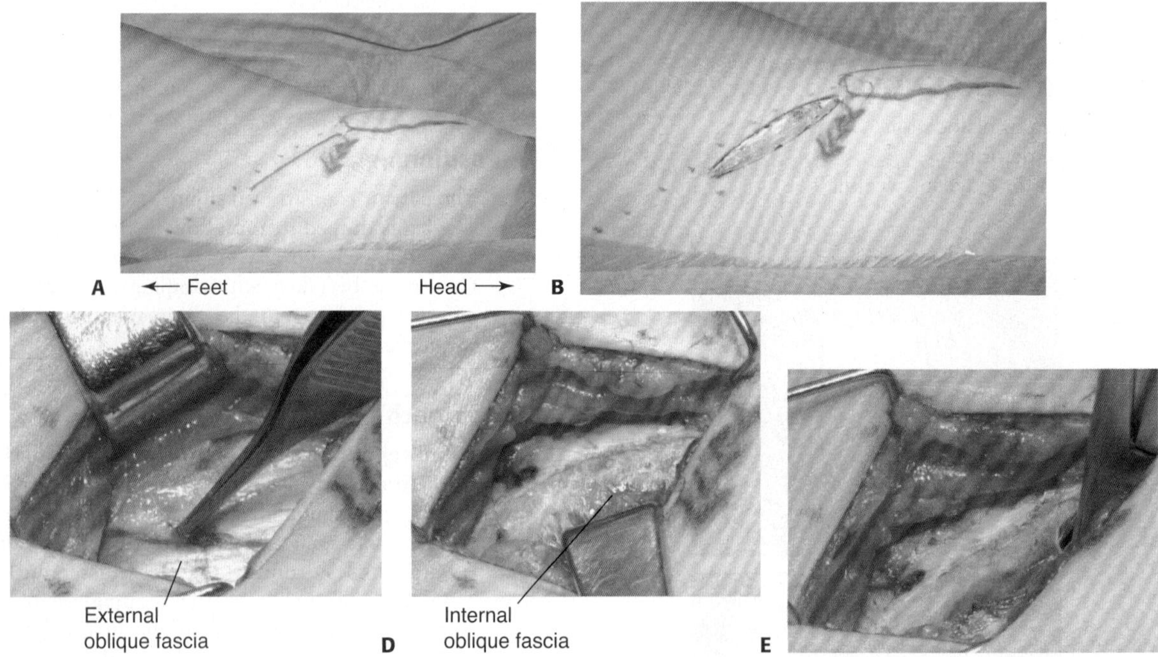


**TECH FIG 1** ● Incision and dissection for psoas lengthening. **A.** Right hip (patient supine, feet to the left); ilium and inguinal ligament are marked. **B.** Skin incision along inguinal ligament starting just distal to anterior superior iliac spine and extending distally 3 to 4 cm. **C.** Adson forceps identify the inguinal ligament with the external oblique fascia proximal and medial. **D.** External oblique fascia is divided along the inguinal ligament and retracted by Army-Navy retractors to visualize the internal oblique. **E.** A hemostat bluntly pierces the internal oblique and transversus abdominis just medial to the anterior superior iliac spine and is passed along the inner table of the ilium extraperiosteally (in this case, the lateral femoral cutaneous nerve was not encountered).

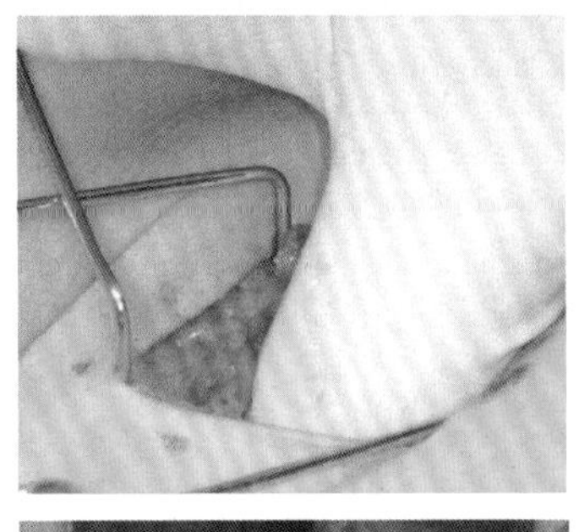
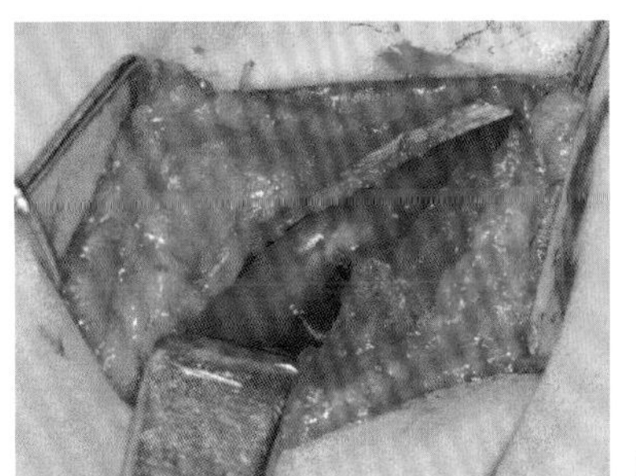
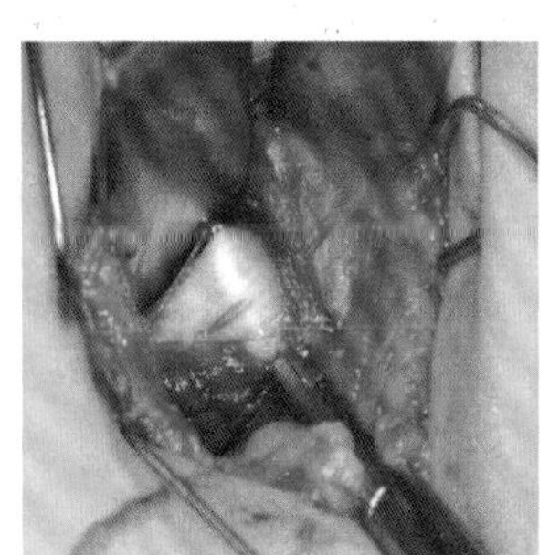
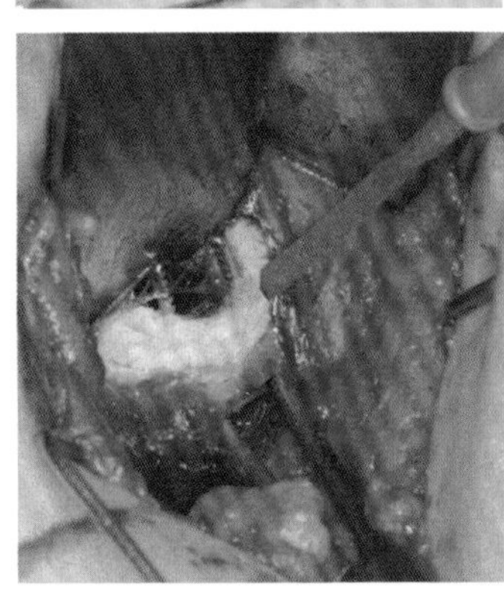

**TECH FIG 2** • **A.** With the hip flexed, the interval between the superior pubic ramus and the iliacus is developed with blunt finger dissection to palpate the psoas tendon. **B.** The psoas tendon is visualized by retracting the iliacus medially with an Army-Navy retractor. **C.** A right-angled clamp is passed around the psoas tendon. **D.** The tendon is divided with electrocautery, leaving the muscle intact.

## Adductor Lengthening

- For the adductors, a short transverse (most often) or longitudinal incision over the palpable origin of the adductor longus is used (**TECH FIG 3A**).
- The adductor longus tendon is separated from the surrounding tissues (pectineus laterally, gracilis medially [**TECH FIG 3B**], and adductor brevis and anterior branch of the obturator nerve deeply).
- The adductor longus tendon is divided as proximally as possible (**TECH FIG 3C,D**). For ambulatory patients, this is typically the only tissue that should be lengthened.
- If necessary, for nonambulatory patients and for more severe neuromuscular hip dysplasia, a partial or complete division of the adductor brevis and other contracted tissues can be performed.

← Proximal Distal →

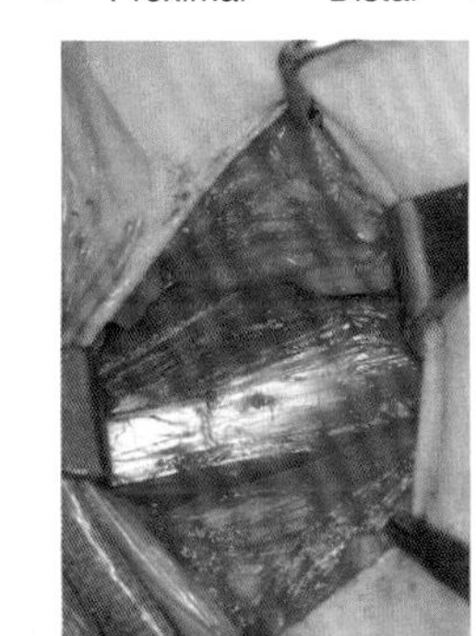
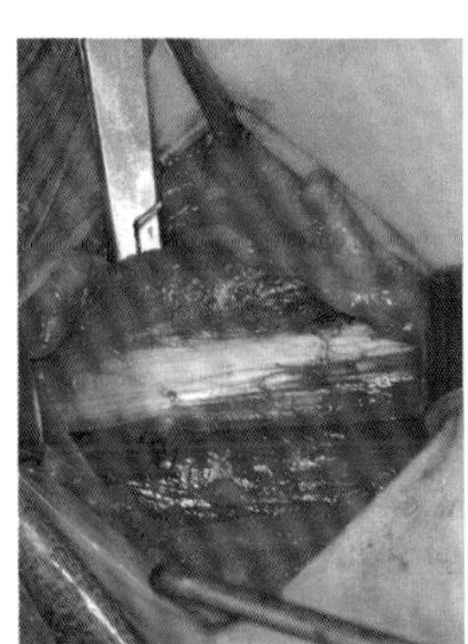
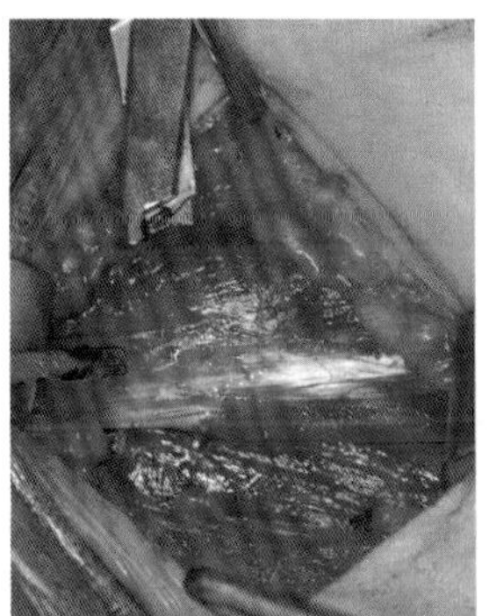
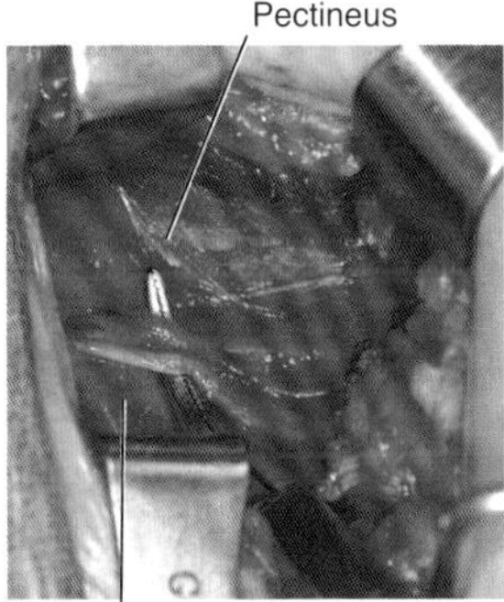


**TECH FIG 3** • Adductor longus tenotomy. **A.** A short transverse incision (pubis left, knee right) exposes the tendinous origin of the adductor longus (pectineus laterally, gracilis medially). **B.** A right-angled clamp isolates the adductor longus tendon and muscle. **C.** As proximally as possible, the origin is divided. **D.** The preserved anterior branch of the obturator nerve lies on the adductor brevis.

## PEARLS AND PITFALLS

| | |
|---|---|
| **Indications** | ■ In the nonambulatory cerebral palsy patient, hip flexor pathology is fairly routinely recognized and therefore not missed. On the other hand, identification of pathology and indications for psoas lengthening in the ambulatory cerebral palsy patient are less well agreed on. As a result, I believe that hip flexor pathology is not identified and as a result, psoas lengthening is too often not included in the surgical plan. |
| **Surgical site** | ■ In the 1970s, Bleck[1] recognized that release of the iliopsoas tendon at the lesser trochanter in the ambulatory patient resulted in excessive weakness. Release at that level must be avoided in ambulatory patients.<br>■ In nonambulators, the iliopsoas combined tendon can be released from the lesser trochanter, but care must be taken not to violate the apophysis of the lesser trochanter in order to avoid heterotopic bone formation along the iliopsoas tendon sheath postoperatively. |
| **Early recurrence** | ■ If significant spasticity is present, pain and spasm may lead to difficulty in maintaining postoperative positioning in extension and abduction, leading to recurrence of hip flexion or adduction contractures. Botulinum toxin injected into the hip flexors and adductors at the time of surgery, effective pain management, and meticulous care to avoid postoperative positioning in flexion and adduction are essential. |
| **Obturator neurectomy** | ■ Overcorrection resulting in abduction contracture is a high risk. Because of this iatrogenic risk with limited corrective options, this procedure should be abandoned. Safer, less aggressive procedures are favored. |
| **Femoral neurovascular injury** | ■ The femoral nerve, artery, and vein are very close to the psoas tendon but are anterior to the iliacus muscle. The iliacus muscle belly can provide protection for these structures if the surgical approach is deep to it. Other protection is afforded by performing the lengthening of the tendon with the hip in the flexed position to relax the neurovascular structures, directly visualizing the tendon within the muscle belly, and stimulating the tissue with electrocautery first before cutting (if the nerve is nearby, the knee will extend). |
| **Inappropriate adductor lengthening** | ■ The combination of femoral anteversion with hip and knee flexion deformity results in the visual appearance of a scissoring gait in ambulatory cerebral palsy patients and is more commonly the cause of scissoring. In ambulators, only adductor longus tenotomy should be performed, and it should be performed rarely.<br>■ The adductors are more commonly spastic and contracted in more severe hemiplegic cerebral palsy. Therefore, adductor longus tenotomy is more often necessary. |

## POSTOPERATIVE CARE

- Psoas lengthening
  - Postoperative elevation of the leg is avoided because it leads to a flexed hip position.
  - Prone positioning is done two or three times a day for at least 30 minutes.
  - A knee immobilizer promotes not only an extended knee but also an extended hip.
  - After 3 weeks, an active hip flexor strengthening program is instituted.
- Adductor lengthening
  - An abductor pillow is used full time for 3 weeks and part time for the next 3 weeks, and early range of motion is instituted.
  - After 3 weeks, an adductor strengthening program is instituted.
- For both procedures, weight bearing can be instituted as tolerated. These procedures are commonly performed in conjunction with osteotomy surgery, in which case weight bearing is typically begun 3 to 4 weeks postoperatively.

## OUTCOMES

- Psoas lengthening is commonly performed in conjunction with femoral osteotomy with or without pelvic osteotomy for treatment of hip dysplasia in nonambulatory patients. A redislocation rate of less than 10% can be expected.[2]
- In ambulatory cerebral palsy patients, psoas surgery improves dynamic hip dysfunction. There is no evidence that psoas lengthening causes hip flexor weakness.[3]
- Power production (H3 power burst) is maintained.
- When psoas lengthening is performed in conjunction with femoral derotation osteotomy, excessive anterior pelvic tilt may also improve.

## COMPLICATIONS

- Excessive hip flexor weakness with tendon release at the lesser trochanter[1]
- Femoral neurovascular injury
- Early recurrence of flexion–adduction deformity
- Worsened anterior pelvic tilt and forward trunk lean when hip flexion deformity is not recognized and treated
- Pelvifemoral instability if scissoring gait is treated with inappropriate adductor surgery

## REFERENCES

1. Bleck EE. Postural and gait abnormalities caused by hip-flexion deformity in spastic cerebral palsy. Treatment by iliopsoas recession. J Bone Joint Surg Am 1971;53(8):1468–1488.
2. McNerney N, Murbarak S, Wenger D. One-stage correction of the dysplastic hip in cerebral palsy with the San Diego acetabuloplasty: results and complications in 104 hips. J Pediatr Orthop 2000;20:93–103.
3. Novacheck TF, Trost JP, Schwartz MH. Intramuscular psoas lengthening improves dynamic hip function in children with cerebral palsy. J Pediatr Orthop 2002;22:158–164.
4. Skaggs DL, Kaminsky CK, Eskander-Rickards E, et al. Psoas over the brim lengthenings. Anatomic investigation and surgical technique. Clin Orthop Relat Res 1997;(339):174–179.
5. Sutherland DH, Zilberfarb JL, Kaufman KR, et al. Psoas release at the pelvic brim in ambulatory patients with cerebral palsy: operative technique and functional outcome. J Pediatr Orthop 1997;17:563–570.

# Rectus Femoris Transfer

Jon R. Davids

65 CHAPTER

## DEFINITION

- The gait pattern of children with cerebral palsy (CP) is frequently disrupted by dynamic overactivity of the rectus femoris muscle.
- This disruption is characterized by delayed and diminished peak knee flexion in swing phase.
- Surgical transfer of the rectus femoris muscle to the medial hamstrings is usually performed in conjunction with other surgical procedures selected to address all elements of soft tissue and skeletal dysfunction that compromise gait in children with CP.
- This surgical strategy, termed *single-event multilevel surgery* (SEMLS), requires a comprehensive assessment of gait dysfunction using quantitative gait analysis.
- Proper management (surgical, orthotic, and rehabilitative) in childhood can result in an improved gait pattern that will be sustainable in the adult years.

## ANATOMY

- The rectus femoris muscle is a portion of the quadriceps muscle group, which also includes the vastus lateralis, the vastus medialis, and the vastus intermedius muscles.
- The rectus femoris muscle is the only one of the quadriceps muscle group that is considered to be biarticular, as it crosses both the hip joint and knee joint. The remaining three muscles cross only the knee joint.
  - The rectus femoris muscle is innervated by the femoral nerve. It has its origin on the anterior inferior iliac spine (direct head) and the innominate portion of the pelvis just proximal to the superior margin of the acetabulum (reflected head) and its insertion on the superior pole of the patella.
    - The rectus femoris muscle fuses with the underlying vastus intermedius muscle several centimeters proximal to the superior pole of the patella.
    - The rectus femoris muscle and the other three portions of the quadriceps muscle group envelop the patella to form the patellar tendon, which inserts on the tibial tubercle apophysis of the proximal tibia. It serves as a hip flexor and knee extensor.
    - The rectus femoris muscle has a relatively small physiologic cross-sectional area and a relatively large ratio of tendon length to muscle fiber length, indicating that it is designed for maximal excursion and diminished force generation.[4,7]
- In normal gait, the rectus femoris muscle is active in the stance to swing phase transition, where it acts to control the magnitude of the flexion excursion of the knee as the gait velocity increases.[13] It is also active at the end of the swing phase to properly position the knee in the transition from swing to stance phase.[13]
  - The remaining three portions of the quadriceps muscle group are active during the loading response of stance phase, where they are essential in providing shock absorption function about the knee as the limb is loaded.[13]
  - From a functional perspective, the quadriceps muscle group is actually two groups, the first consisting of the rectus femoris muscle and the second consisting of the triceps femoris muscles (remaining three muscles).[9]

## PATHOGENESIS

- CP is the consequence of an injury to the immature brain that may occur before, during, or shortly after birth. The nature and location of the injury to the central nervous system (CNS) determines the components of the neuromuscular and cognitive impairments.
- Common functional deficits are related to spasticity, impaired motor control, and disrupted balance and body position senses.
- Although the injury to the CNS is not progressive, the clinical manifestations of CP change over time owing to growth and development of the musculoskeletal system.
  - The muscles typically exhibit a purely dynamic dysfunction during the first 6 years of life, characterized by a normal resting length and an exaggerated response to an applied load or stretch.
  - With time, between 6 and 10 years of age, the muscles develop a fixed or myostatic shortening, resulting in a permanent contracture.
- As such, it is best to consider CP not as a single specific disease process but rather a clinical condition with multiple possible etiologies.[18]

## NATURAL HISTORY

- Ambulatory children with CP whose gait is disrupted by overactivity of the rectus femoris muscle typically walk with delayed and diminished knee flexion in swing phase. This may be associated with decreased velocity of hip flexion in the stance to swing phase transition and increased ankle plantarflexion in swing phase, called a *stiff gait pattern*.[15,19]
- These dynamic gait deviations at the hip, knee, and ankle disrupt the normal limb segment coordination that contributes to functional shortening of the limb during the swing phase of the gait cycle.[17] As a result, children with CP who have a stiff gait pattern will exhibit compromised clearance of the limb in swing phase.[15,19]

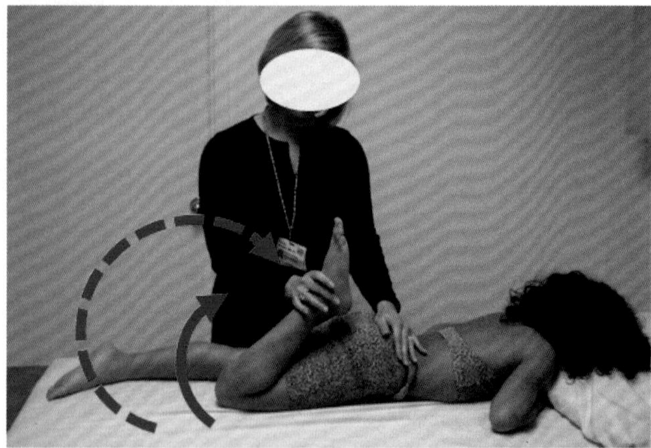

**FIG 1** • The Duncan-Ely or prone rectus test. The subject is placed in a supine position, with the hips and knees fully extended. The examiner stabilizes the pelvis with one hand and grasps the ankle of the side to be examined with the other hand. The knee is then flexed rapidly (*solid arrow*) until a "catch" is felt. The angle at which the catch is felt is measured with a goniometer and is referred to as the *R1* or *fast test*. The knee is then flexed slowly (slow test, *dashed arrow*) until the examiner feels the pelvis rise. The knee angle at which the pelvis begins to rise is measured with a goniometer and is referred to as the *R2* or *slow test*.

## PATIENT HISTORY AND PHYSICAL FINDINGS

- The clinical history, as provided by the child and the parents, usually contains complaints of toe dragging, tripping, abnormal shoe wear about the toes, and inability to keep up with peers in play and sports.
- A thorough examination will include the prone rectus femoris test (also known as the *Duncan-Ely test*) (**FIG 1**).
  - A positive slow rectus test indicates fixed shortening of the rectus femoris muscle.
  - A positive fast rectus test indicates the presence of spasticity of the rectus femoris muscle.

## IMAGING AND OTHER DIAGNOSTIC STUDIES

- Radiographic imaging is not required when determining the need for transfer of the rectus femoris muscle to improve gait in children with CP.
- Relevant data from quantitative gait analysis include temporospatial parameters, sagittal plane kinematics at the knee and hip, and dynamic electromyography (EMG) of the rectus femoris muscle.
  - Gait velocity should be greater than 60% of age-matched normal.[3] Children with CP who ambulate with a greatly diminished gait velocity will also exhibit disrupted sagittal plane knee kinematics in swing phase, which will not be corrected by a rectus femoris muscle transfer.
  - Sagittal plane knee kinematics will show decreased flexion range and velocity in the stance to swing transition, delayed and diminished peak knee flexion in swing phase, and diminished dynamic range of motion with a rounded or mounded wave form in swing phase (**FIG 2A**).[3,11,12]
  - Sagittal plane hip kinematics during the stance to swing phase transition should be evaluated when considering surgical transfer of the rectus femoris muscle (**FIG 2B**).
    - A poor transition at the hip is characterized by decreased flexion range and velocity and is a contraindication to rectus femoris muscle transfer.[3]

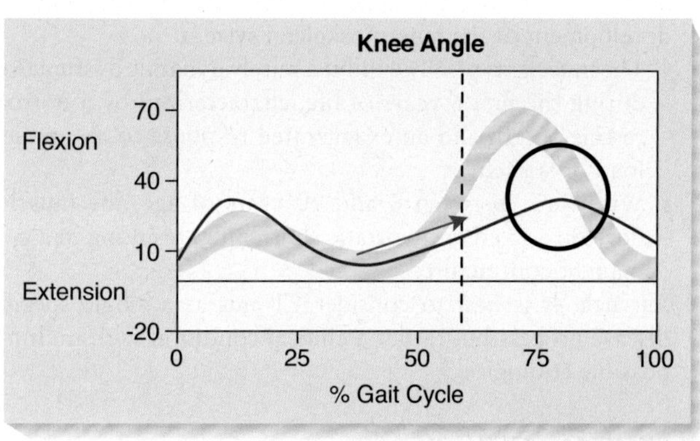


A

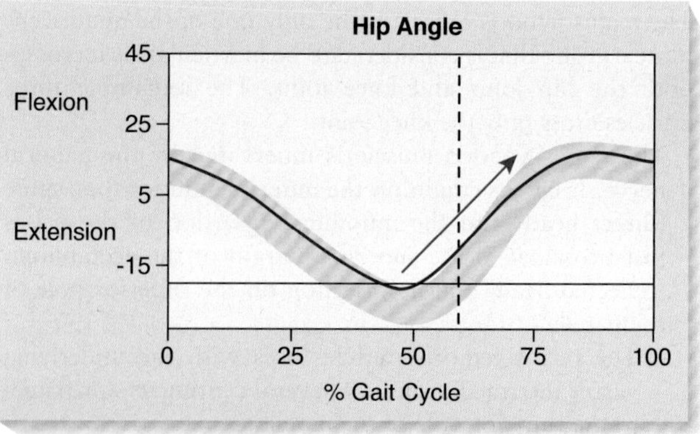


B

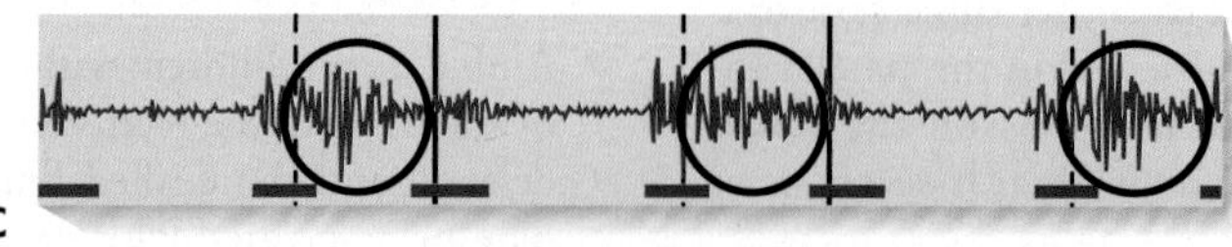

C

**FIG 2** • Sagittal plane knee (**A**) and hip (**B**) kinematic plots of a child with a jump gait pattern. The gait cycle appears on the horizontal axis, the direction of motion on the vertical axis. The age-matched normal motion (mean ± 2 SD) appears as a *purple band*, and the subject's data are indicated by a *blue line*. **A.** Kinematic indicators for transfer of the rectus femoris muscle are delayed and diminished peak knee flexion in midswing phase (*circle*) and decreased range and rate of knee flexion in the stance to swing transition (*arrow*). **B.** The kinematic contraindications at the hip for transfer of the rectus femoris muscle at the knee are decreased range and rate of hip flexion in the stance to swing transition (*arrow*). **C.** Dynamic EMG of the rectus femoris muscle in a child with CP. Three gait cycles are shown, separated by the *solid black lines*. The stance and swing phases of each cycle are separated by the *dashed black lines*. The normal timing of activation of the muscle is noted by the horizontal red lines at the bottom of the strip. The actual timing of activation of the muscle for the subject is shown by the oscillating *red line* at the middle of the strip. The dynamic EMG indicator for transfer of the rectus femoris muscle is prolonged and inappropriate activity in midswing phase (indicated by the *circles* in each gait cycle).

- Poor hip flexor function in the stance to swing transition will result in delayed and diminished peak knee flexion in swing phase, which will not be corrected by a rectus femoris muscle transfer.
- Dynamic EMG of the rectus femoris muscle will show prolonged, inappropriate activity into the middle subphase of swing phase (**FIG 2C**).[3,11,12]

## DIFFERENTIAL DIAGNOSIS

- Delayed and diminished peak knee flexion in swing phase may be the consequence of the following:
  - Inappropriate activity of the rectus femoris muscle in swing phase. Transfer of the rectus femoris muscle is indicated in this situation.
  - Diminished overall gait velocity. This circumstance is a contraindication for transfer of the rectus femoris muscle.
  - Poor hip flexor function in the stance to swing phase transition. This circumstance is a contraindication for transfer of the rectus femoris muscle.
  - Leg length inequality, when the reference limb is relatively short or the contralateral lower extremity is relatively long. In this situation, there is less need for functional shortening of the reference limb in swing phase. This circumstance is a contraindication for transfer of the rectus femoris muscle.

## NONOPERATIVE MANAGEMENT

- In the ambulatory child with CP who is younger than 6 years, neurodevelopmental therapy and gait training may be helpful in improving the stiff gait pattern due to inappropriate activity of the rectus femoris muscle in swing phase.
- In the ambulatory child with CP who is age 6 years or older, there is no effective nonsurgical management of the stiff gait pattern.

## SURGICAL MANAGEMENT

- Achieving optimal outcomes after transfer of the rectus femoris muscle requires careful patient selection, proper surgical technique, appropriate postoperative orthotic management, and adequate rehabilitation resources (primarily physical therapy for conditioning and gait training) in the months after the surgery.

### Preoperative Planning

- Proper clinical decision making and preoperative planning for surgery to improve gait in children with CP require the integration of data from five fields—clinical history, physical examination, diagnostic imaging, quantitative gait analysis, and examination under anesthesia—in a process described as a diagnostic matrix.[3]

### Positioning

- The child is placed on the operating table in the supine position.
- A tourniquet is placed about the most proximal portion of the thigh, and the extremity is carefully cleansed and draped to allow adequate exposure for the surgical approach to the rectus femoris muscle.

### Approach

- The rectus femoris muscle is usually exposed via a direct anterior approach at the distal third of the thigh.
- This approach is particularly appropriate when transfer of the rectus femoris muscle and lengthening of the medical hamstring muscles are to be performed at the same time as part of SEMLS.

TECHNIQUES

## Soft Tissue Dissection

- An 8- to 12-cm incision is made over the anterior aspect of the distal third of the thigh, ending one to two fingerbreadths onto the superior pole of the patella (**TECH FIG 1**).
- The dissection is carried down through the subcutaneous layers to the fascia overlying the quadriceps muscle group.
  - This fascial layer is incised for the full length of the incision, exposing the myotendinous portion of the rectus femoris muscle proximally and the superior pole of the patella distally.

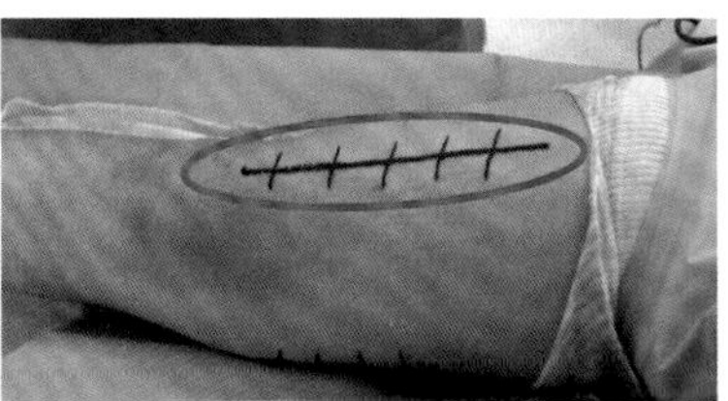

**TECH FIG 1** • Medial view of the right thigh, showing the anterior skin used for exposure of the rectus femoris muscle.

## Isolation of the Rectus Tendon

- The rectus femoris muscle is identified and isolated proximally from the surrounding muscles of the quadriceps muscle group (vastus lateralis muscle laterally, vastus medialis muscle medially, and the vastus intermedius muscle deeply) (**TECH FIG 2A**).
  - The rectus femoris muscle is dissected from proximal to distal, freeing it completely from the surrounding quadriceps muscle group.
  - The dissection is carried onto the superior pole of the patella for 1 to 2 cm, and the insertion of the rectus femoris muscle onto the patella is completely released (**TECH FIG 2B**).

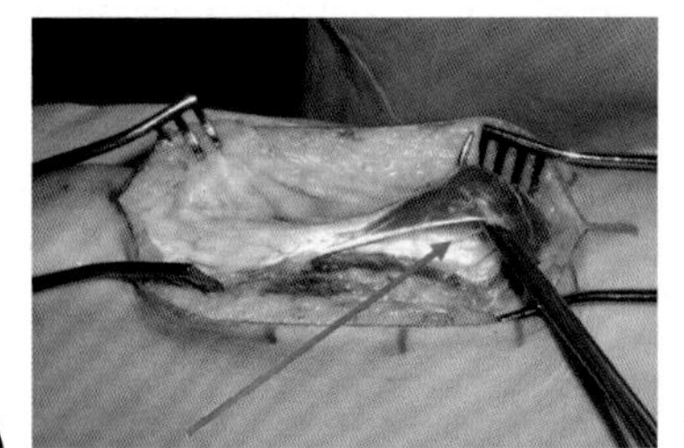

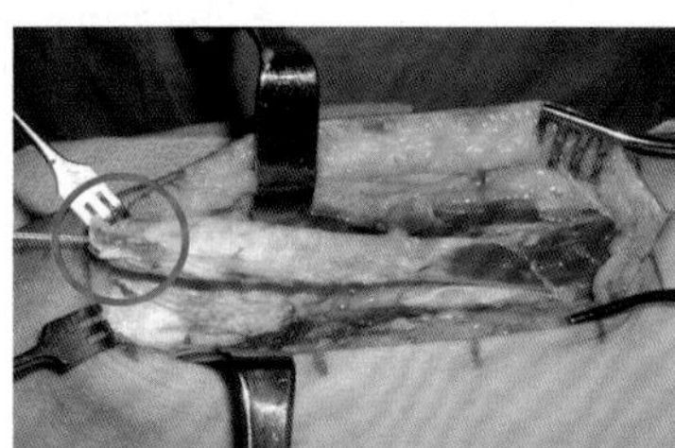

**TECH FIG 2** • Medial views of the right thigh (patella is to the left). **A.** Exposure of the quadriceps muscle group. The rectus femoris muscle is separated from the other muscles of the quadriceps muscle group proximally (*arrow*). **B.** Mobilization of the rectus femoris distally from its insertion on the superior pole of the patella (*circle*).

## Mobilization of the Rectus Femoris Tendon and Tunneling

- A transfer stitch is placed into the distal end of the rectus femoris tendon, and the muscle–tendon unit is mobilized from distal to proximal using intermuscular dissection with scissors.
  - The rectus femoris muscle should be completely mobilized proximally to the level between the proximal and middle thirds of the thigh (**TECH FIG 3A**).
- A subcutaneous tunnel is made between the proximal and medial margin of the incision used to expose the rectus femoris muscle and the distal and anterior margin of the incision used to expose the medial hamstring muscles (**TECH FIG 3B**).
  - This tunnel should be superficial to the quadriceps fascia and deep to the majority of the subcutaneous fat of the medial thigh and expanded to a width of two fingerbreadths.
- The rectus femoris muscle–tendon unit is passed through the subcutaneous tunnel and pulled into the incision overlying the medial hamstring muscles (**TECH FIG 3C**).
  - Tension is applied to the rectus femoris tendon using the transfer suture, and the line of pull of the rectus femoris muscle is assessed beneath the proximal margin of the anterior thigh incision.
  - Further proximal release may be necessary to optimize the line of pull of the rectus femoris muscle in its transferred position.

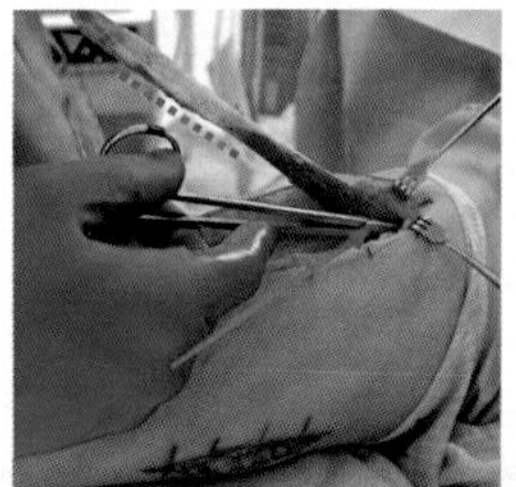

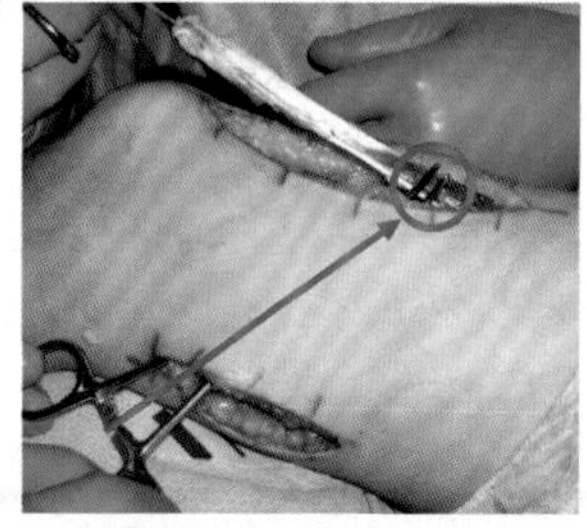

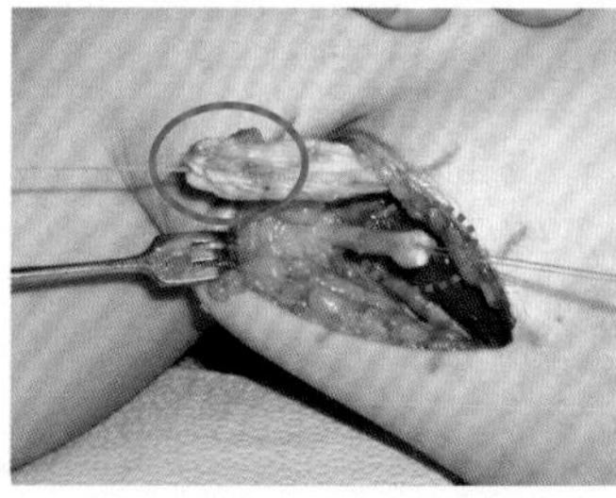

**TECH FIG 3** • Medial views of the right thigh. **A.** Hip is to the right. Proximal mobilization of the rectus femoris. The rectus femoris muscle is manipulated using the transfer suture (*dashed arrow*) and released proximally using the scissors (*solid arrow*). **B.** Patella is to the left. Orientation of the transfer tunnel between the medial and anterior skin incisions (*red arrow*). A clamp is placed into the tunnel from distal medial to proximal anterior and used to guide the rectus femoris muscle–tendon unit to its site of transfer insertion (*circle*). **C.** The rectus femoris tendon is delivered into the medial incision (*solid circle*), where it will be transferred to the distal portion of the semitendinosus muscle tendon (*dashed circle*).

## Transfer of the Rectus Tendon

- The distal aspect of the rectus femoris tendon is transferred to the distal segment of the semitendinosus muscle tendon, which was previously released in the medial hamstring muscle lengthening (see Chap. 63).
  - The transfer is performed using a single interweaving of the rectus femoris and semitendinosus tendons (modified Pulvertaft technique) (**TECH FIG 4**).
  - The transfer is tensioned so that the muscle belly of the rectus femoris muscle is slightly tighter to palpation than the muscle bellies of the remaining three muscles of the quadriceps muscle group, when the knee is held in full extension.
  - Three separate throws of a nonabsorbable suture are used to secure the transfer.

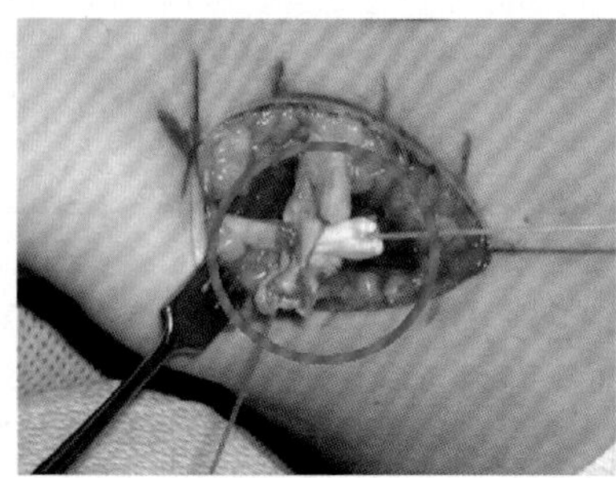

**TECH FIG 4** • Medial view of the right thigh (patella is to the left), showing the transfer of the rectus femoris tendon to the semitendinosus muscle tendon using a single interweaving (modified Pulvertaft technique; *circle*) that will be stabilized by three throws of a nonabsorbable suture.

## PEARLS AND PITFALLS

**Patient selection**

- Distal transfer of the rectus femoris muscle to the medial hamstring muscles should be considered only for children with delayed and diminished peak knee flexion in swing phase due to overactivity of the rectus femoris muscle. When gait velocity is diminished beyond 60% of normal, poor hip flexor function in the stance to swing transition is present, or there is an anatomic or functional leg length inequality (reference limb short), delayed and diminished peak knee flexion in swing phase will not be improved by transfer of the rectus femoris muscle.
- When there is spasticity of the rectus femoris muscle, and the proper kinematic and dynamic EMG indicators are present, failure to perform a rectus femoris transfer at the time of medial hamstring muscle lengthening will result in the development of a stiff gait pattern.[2,21]

**Release versus transfer**

- Distal transfer of the rectus femoris muscle is more effective than distal or proximal release of the muscle at improving the timing and magnitude of peak knee flexion in swing phase.[1,11,12,20]

**Medial versus lateral transfer (transverse plane kinematics)**

- Transfer to either the medial or the lateral hamstring muscle groups has no consequence on the dynamic rotational alignment of the hip or knee in stance phase.[11]

**Choice of medial transfer site**

- Transfer of the rectus femoris muscle to the sartorius, gracilis, semimembranosus, or semitendinosus muscles will have a comparable benefit on sagittal plane knee kinematics in swing phase.[1,8,11,12] Of the medial hamstring muscles, the semitendinosus muscle is preferred because of its myoarchitecture (long tendon length) and insertion site on the proximal tibia, which is the farthest from the knee joint center (optimizing the lever arm available for the transferred muscle).[4]

**Principles of tendon transfer**

- To achieve an optimal result after rectus femoris muscle transfer, the four principles of tendon transfer must be considered:
  - There must be adequate excursion of the transferred muscle–tendon unit. The rectus femoris muscle is a biarticular muscle and should be transferred to another biarticular muscle (such as the semitendinosus).
  - The line of pull of the transferred muscle–tendon unit should be as straight as possible. The long anterior thigh incision and intermuscular proximal release of the rectus femoris muscle must be performed. Adequate release of the rectus femoris muscle cannot be achieved through a small incision.
  - The transfer path should occur through a plane that minimizes scarring. The transfer tunnel for the rectus femoris muscle should be at the level of the subcutaneous fat, superficial to the quadriceps fascia.
  - The muscle transfer should be tensioned so the muscle belly is at a slight stretch to optimize the length–tension relationship of the transferred muscle. The rectus femoris muscle transfer should be tensioned so the muscle is slightly tighter than the other portions of the quadriceps muscle group.

## POSTOPERATIVE CARE

- Transfer of the rectus femoris muscle is rarely performed in isolation for children with CP but rather a component of SEMLS.
- If complete knee extension has been achieved after lengthening of the medial hamstring muscles and transfer of the rectus femoris muscle, then the knee is protected in a knee immobilizer after surgery. The knee immobilizer is worn full time, and the child is kept non–weight bearing for 2 weeks.
- Passive knee range of motion is initiated at 1 to 2 weeks after surgery.
- Weight bearing and gait training are begun 2 to 6 weeks after surgery, depending on which other surgeries have been performed as a part of SEMLS.
- Proper rehabilitation under the guidance of an experienced physical therapist is essential, as many children with CP who have undergone simultaneous lengthening of the medial hamstring muscles and distal transfer of the rectus femoris muscle as part of SEMLS will begin to ambulate with a quadriceps avoidance gait pattern. This should be corrected by appropriate gait training early in the rehabilitation phase.

## OUTCOMES

- The goals of surgical transfer of the rectus femoris muscle are to improve the timing and magnitude of peak knee flexion in swing phase in order to correct an existing stiff gait pattern or to avoid the development of such a pattern after inappropriate isolated lengthening of the medial hamstring muscles. Improved dynamic alignment at the knee during the swing phase of the gait cycle should result in improved gait efficiency and clearance of the swing limb.
  - Improvements in swing-phase knee kinematics after rectus femoris muscle transfer have been documented at 1 year after surgery and have been shown to be maintained at 5 and 10 years of follow-up.[1,5,6,8,10,11,14,16,20,22]
- Distal transfer of the rectus femoris muscle to the medial hamstring muscles has been shown to be superior to proximal or distal release alone.[1,11,12,20]
  - The site of transfer has been shown to have no impact on the dynamic transverse plane alignment of the hip or knee during stance phase.[11]

## COMPLICATIONS

- Theoretical complications, such as suprapatellar rupture of the knee extensor mechanism, lack of knee extension in stance phase due to excessive tightness of the transferred rectus femoris muscle, and weakening of the quadriceps muscle group after transfer of the rectus femoris muscle, have not been reported in the literature.
- The principal functional complication after transfer of the rectus femoris muscle is persistent quadriceps avoidance gait

pattern, which may occur in children with CP who have significant spasticity and anxiety.
  - Proper rehabilitation under the direction of an experienced physical therapist is effective in managing this problem.
- The principal cosmetic complication after transfer of the rectus femoris muscle is an unsightly scar that may develop at the incision site on the anterior aspect of the thigh. This is a consequence of the preferred incision crossing the skin lines of Langer.
  - Scar formation is minimized by proper incision wound management (pressure applied by massage) during the postoperative rehabilitation phase.

## REFERENCES


1. Chambers H, Lauer A, Kaufman K, et al. Prediction of outcome after rectus femoris surgery in cerebral palsy: the role of cocontraction of the rectus femoris and vastus lateralis. J Pediatr Orthop 1998;18:703–711.
2. Damron TA, Breed AL, Cook T. Diminished knee flexion after hamstring surgery in cerebral palsy patients: prevalence and severity. J Pediatr Orthop 1993;13:188–191.
3. Davids JR, Ounpuu S, DeLuca PA, et al. Optimization of walking ability of children with cerebral palsy. Instr Course Lect 2004;53:511–522.
4. Delp SL, Zajac FE. Force and moment generating capacity of the lower extremity muscles before and after tendon lengthening. Clin Orthop Relat Res 1992;(284):247–259.
5. Dreher T, Wolf SL, Maier M, et al. Long-term results after distal rectus femoris transfer as a part of multilevel surgery for the correction of stiff-knee gait in spastic diplegic cerebral palsy. J Bone Joint Surg 2012;94:e142(1–10).
6. Hadley N, Chambers C, Scarborough N, et al. Knee motion following multiple soft tissue releases in ambulatory patients with cerebral palsy. J Pediatr Orthop 1992;12:324–328.
7. Lieber RL. Skeletal Muscle Structure, Function, and Plasticity: The Physiological Basis of Rehabilitation, ed 2. Baltimore: Lippincott Williams & Wilkins, 2002.
8. Miller F, Cardoso Dias R, Lipton GE, et al. The effect of rectus EMG patterns on the outcome of rectus femoris transfers. J Pediatr Orthop 1992;12:603–607.
9. Nene A, Byrne C, Hermens H. Is rectus femoris really a part of the quadriceps? Assessment of rectus femoris function during gait in able-bodied adults. Gait Posture 2004;20:1–13.
10. Nene AV, Evans GA, Patrick JH. Simultaneous multiple operations for spastic diplegia. Outcome and functional assessment of walking in 18 patients. J Bone Joint Surg Br 1993;75(3):488–494.
11. Ounpuu S, Muik E, Davis RB III, et al. Rectus femoris surgery in children with cerebral palsy. Part I: the effect of rectus femoris transfer location on knee motion. J Pediatr Orthop 1993;13: 325–330.
12. Ounpuu S, Muik E, Davis RB III, et al. Rectus femoris surgery in children with cerebral palsy. Part II: a comparison between the effect of transfer and release of the distal rectus femoris on knee motion. J Pediatr Orthop 1993;13:331–335.
13. Perry J. Gait Analysis: Normal and Pathological Function. Thorofare, NJ: Slack Incorporated, 1992.
14. Rethelefsen S, Tolo VT, Reynolds RA, et al. Outcome of hamstring lengthening and distal rectus femoris transfer surgery. J Pediatr Orthop B 1999;8:75–79.
15. Rodda JM, Graham HK, Carson L, et al. Sagittal gait patterns in spastic diplegia. J Bone Joint Surg Br 2004;86(2):251–258.
16. Saraph V, Zwick EB, Zwick G, et al. Multilevel surgery in spastic diplegia: evaluation by physical examination and gait analysis in 25 children. J Pediatr Orthop 2002;22:150–157.
17. Saunders JR, Inman VT, Eberhart HD. The major determinants in normal and pathological gait. J Bone Joint Surg Am 1953;35-A(3): 543–558.
18. Stanley F, Blair E, Alberman E. Cerebral Palsies: Epidemiology and Causal Pathways. Clinics in Developmental Medicine, no. 151. London: MacKeith Press, 2000.
19. Sutherland DH, Davids JR. Common gait abnormalities of the knee in cerebral palsy. Clin Orthop Relat Res 1993;(288):139–147.
20. Sutherland DH, Santi M, Abel MF. Treatment of stiff-knee gait in cerebral palsy: a comparison of distal rectus femoris transfer versus proximal rectus release. J Pediatr Orthop 1990;10:433–441.
21. Thometz J, Simon S, Rosenthal R. The effect on gait of lengthening of the medial hamstrings in cerebral palsy. J Bone Joint Surg Am 1989;71(3):345–353.
22. Zwick EB, Saraph V, Linhart WE, et al. Propulsive function during gait in diplegic children: evaluation after surgery for gait improvement. J Pediatr Orthop B 2001;10:226–233.

# Proximal Hamstring and Adductor Lengthening

CHAPTER 66

Freeman Miller and Kirk W. Dabney

## DEFINITION

- Proximal hamstring lengthenings are primarily performed in the treatment of spastic hip subluxation, mainly in children prior to adolescence.
- Based on modeling studies, the hamstrings are a significant contribution to increasing the force in spastic hip disease, which causes hip subluxation. They are also a component that keeps the knees flexed and secondarily encourages flexion combined with spastic hip flexors, which causes the knee to fall into internal rotation and adduction, magnifying the influence of the concomitant spastic adductors.
  - This posture of hip flexion and internal rotation and adduction, with the addition of high muscle force, tends to drive the hip posterosuperiorly out of the acetabulum.
- The primary period during which spastic hip disease occurs is 2 to 8 years of age, although some children are still at risk through their adolescent growth spurt and need to be monitored.

## ANATOMY

- Hamstring attachments on the pelvis are very broad muscular attachments and do not have a substantial amount of tendon.
- The exception to this is that the semimembranosus tends to have a tendinous insertion and may be confused with the sciatic nerve if care is not taken.
- There tends to be some broad fascial insertion with both the biceps and the semitendinosus.

## PATHOGENESIS

- Spastic hip disease is a pathologic force that has both an abnormal direction of the vector and a force vector that is too high caused by spastic muscles.
- The muscles, in order of their importance, are the adductor longus, the gracilis, the proximal insertion of the hamstrings, and the iliopsoas.
- An important cause of spastic hip subluxation is positioning of the hip into internal rotation and hip flexion and adduction for a significant component of the child's daily posturing.

## NATURAL HISTORY

- Abnormal hip subluxation typically begins around 2 years of age and then has a progression of about 10% of migration every 6 months if the progression is occurring.
- Therefore, physical examination, monitoring of the hip in abduction, and an anteroposterior (AP) pelvis radiograph in which the Reimer migration index is measured every 6 months would be sufficient to pick up early spastic hip disease.

## PATIENT HISTORY AND PHYSICAL FINDINGS

- The concern for spastic hip disease is primarily present in children with spasticity, although some adolescents will be at risk.
- The primary physical examination finding is the limitation of hip abduction with hips extended and knees extended.
- Also, a child whose predominant posture both in sitting and lying is with hip flexion, adduction and internal rotation is at high risk.

## IMAGING AND OTHER DIAGNOSTIC STUDIES

- The primary radiographic investigation is a supine AP pelvic radiograph in which the Reimer migration index is measured.
  - Normal should be 25% or less at all ages. Abnormal is greater than 30%.
- If there is a question whether this is the standard hip subluxation predominantly occurring in the posterosuperior aspect of the acetabulum, a computed tomography (CT) scan may be obtained to fully evaluate the position of the hip joint. However, this is not routinely required.

## DIFFERENTIAL DIAGNOSIS

- Hip subluxation secondary to developmental hip dysplasia
- Congenital hip dislocation
- Hypotonic hip dislocation

## NONOPERATIVE MANAGEMENT

- No conservative treatment options have been documented to be efficacious.
- There have been several attempts at treating spastic hip subluxation with botulinum toxin injection; however, preliminary evidence suggests that the failure rate is high and the need for later reconstruction will be higher than with adequate surgical release.

## SURGICAL MANAGEMENT

### Preoperative Planning

- The indications for the procedure are a migration index of 30% to 60% in a child who is younger than 8 to 10 years of age and has limited hip abduction, meaning less than 30 degrees of hip abduction with hips and knees extended.
- This examination should be performed under anesthesia.

- The goal of the treatment is to have the child lie without any force or pushing with bilateral hip abduction of more than 45 degrees at the end of the operative procedure.
- The indication for proximal hamstring lengthening is a popliteal angle of greater than 45 degrees with the child under anesthesia.

## Positioning

- Proximal hamstring release combined with adductor lengthening is performed with the patient supine and with an adhesive drape placed over the groin.

## Approach

- There are two approaches to proximal hamstring release.
- One is a straight posterior approach. However, this approach has the negative consequences of going through the area of major weight bearing for sitting.
- For this reason, it is preferred to do an approach through the medial groin as part of an adductor lengthening going through the fascial compartment of the gracilis.
  - Only the approach to the gracilis as part of a full adductor lengthening is described here.



## Exposure

- An incision is made from the anterior border of the adductor longus for 2 cm posterior in a transverse plane (**TECH FIG 1A**).
- The adductor longus is identified with a longitudinal opening of the fascia realigning the adductor longus and is completely transected, with vigilance to ensure that the anterior branch of the obturator nerve is protected by visualizing it (**TECH FIG 1B**).

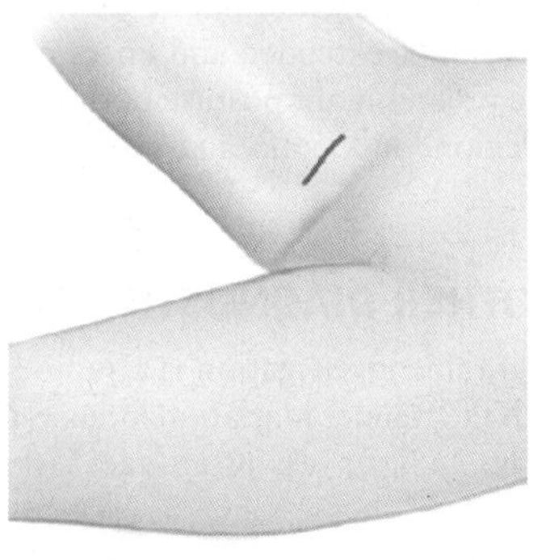

A

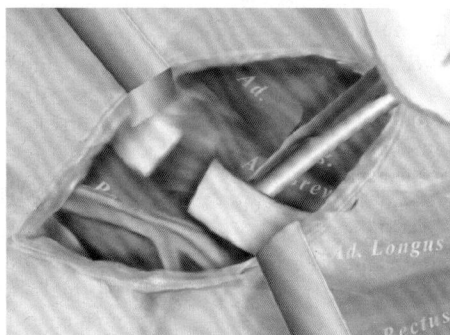


B

**TECH FIG 1** • **A.** The incision is made from the anterior border of the adductor longus for 2 cm posterior in a transverse plane. **B.** The adductor longus is exposed and completely transected, making sure the anterior branch of the obturator nerve is protected. (From Miller F. Cerebral Palsy. New York: Springer-Verlag, 2005. Copyright Springer Science and Business Media, Inc.)

## Myotomy

- The gracilis fascia is opened and a complete gracilis myotomy is performed (**TECH FIG 2A**).
- If the hip abduction with hip extended and under minimal force is now less than 45 degrees, the anterior branch of the obturator nerve is protected and the adductor brevis is identified, and sequential myotomy is performed until more than 45 degrees of abduction is obtained.
- If the child is not and will not be ambulatory and the hip migration is over 50%, the anterior branch of the obturator nerve is transected (**TECH FIG 2B**).

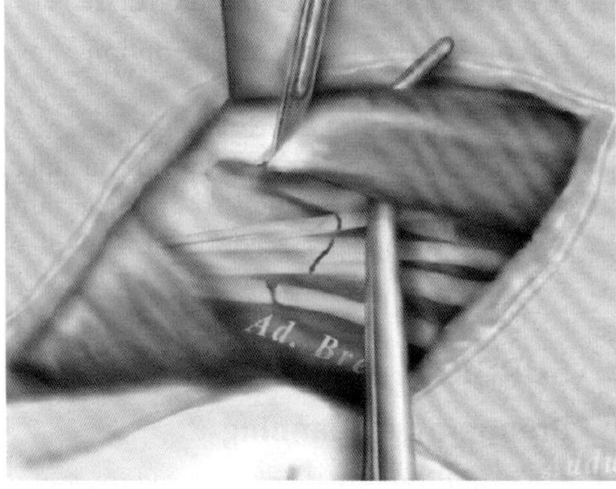


A

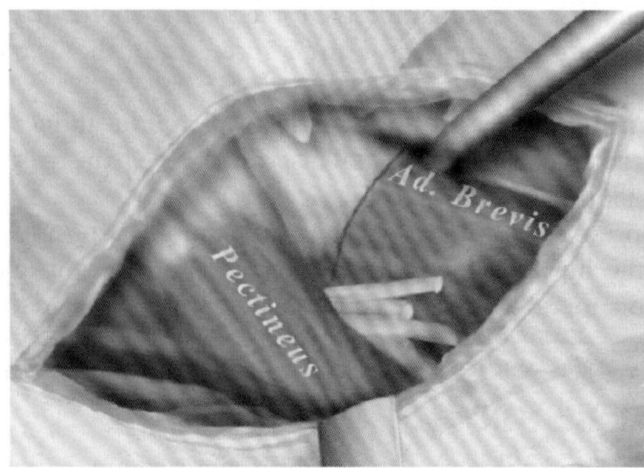


B

**TECH FIG 2** • **A.** The gracilis is identified and a complete gracilis myotomy performed. **B.** The anterior branch of the obturator nerve is protected and the adductor brevis identified. A sequential myotomy is performed of the adductor brevis until more than 45 degrees of abduction is possible with minimal force. If the child is not and will not be ambulatory and the hip migration is over 50%, the anterior branch of the obturator nerve is transected. (From Miller F. Cerebral Palsy. New York: Springer-Verlag, 2005. Copyright Springer Science and Business Media, Inc.)

## Iliopsoas Tenotomy

- The interval between the adductor brevis and pectineus or the interval between the pectineus and the neurovascular bundle is opened to the iliopsoas tendon.
- A complete tenotomy of the iliopsoas tendon is performed if the child is nonambulatory. If the child is ambulatory, the tendon is retracted proximally until only the fascia of the psoas is tenotomized, leaving intact the large muscular iliacus (**TECH FIG 3**).

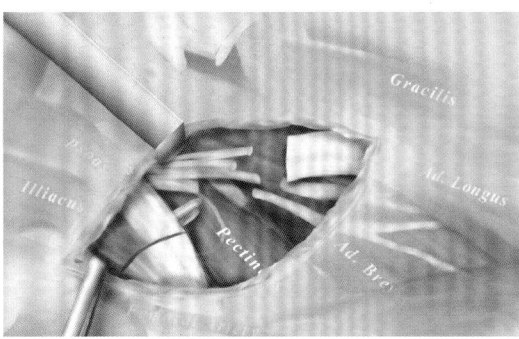


**TECH FIG 3** • The interval between the pectineus and the neurovascular bundle is opened to the iliopsoas tendon. A complete tenotomy of the iliopsoas tendon is performed if the child is nonambulatory. (From Miller F. Cerebral Palsy. New York: Springer-Verlag, 2005. Copyright Springer Science and Business Media, Inc.)

## Hamstring Lengthening

- The fascial compartment of the gracilis is opened posteriorly, and, with digital dissection, the posterior compartment muscles of the hamstrings are separated (**TECH FIG 4A**).
- The interval between the adductor magnus, which does not contract with knee flexion–extension, is separated from the semimembranosus and semitendinosus (**TECH FIG 4B**).
- The femur is palpated with the finger, and then the semimembranosus and semitendinosus and biceps muscles are all separated, leaving the sciatic nerve against the femur (**TECH FIG 4C**).
  - The sciatic nerve can be palpated on the posterior aspect of the femur along the linea aspera.
- A right-angled clamp is then placed around the muscle mass and it is pulled anteriorly into the surgical wound for visualization with the hip extended and the knees flexed (**TECH FIG 4D**).
  - Electrocautery is used and the muscle is transected.
  - Any fascial or tendinous material is carefully inspected and stimulated with a nerve stimulator to make absolutely sure that it is not the sciatic nerve.
  - It must be clear that the anesthesiologist has not had the child under paralysis, and there should be good muscle twitches documented by the anesthesiologist.

A
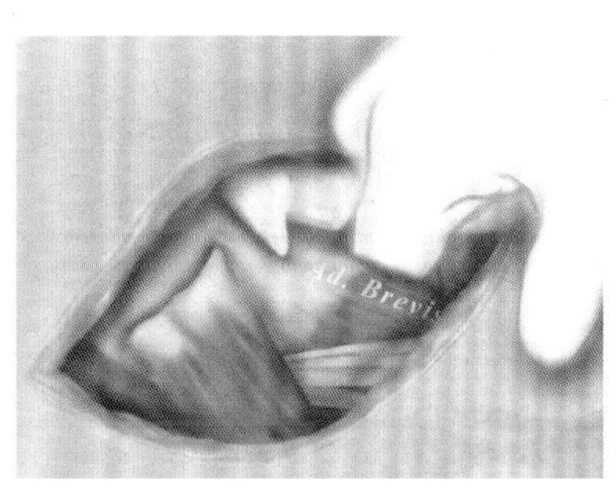

B
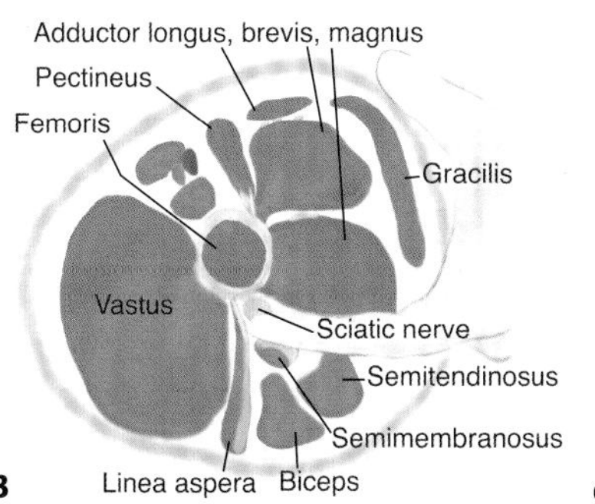


C
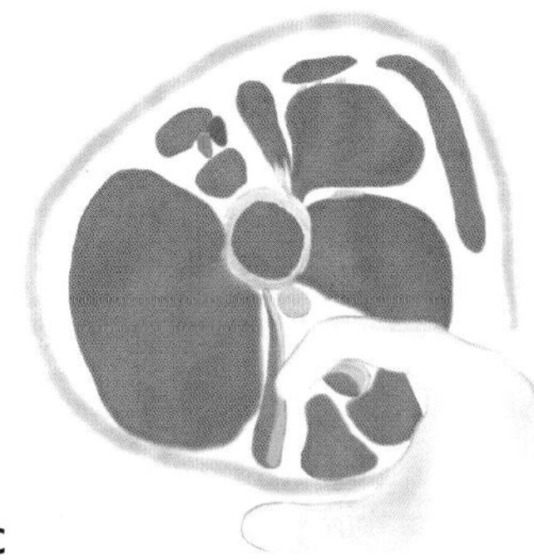

D
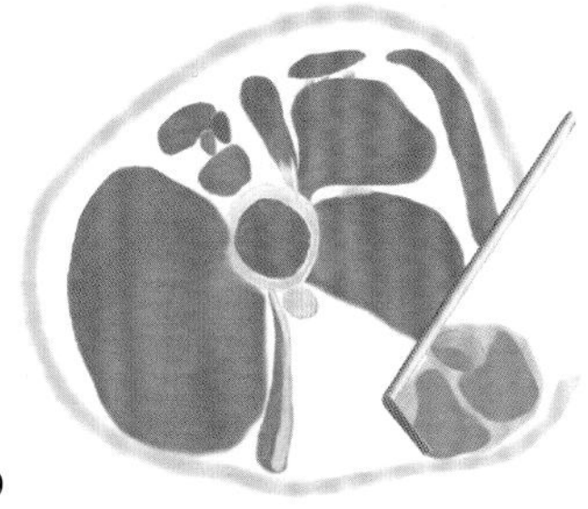

**TECH FIG 4** • **A.** The fascial compartment of the gracilis is opened posteriorly, and the posterior compartment muscles of the hamstrings are separated using digital dissection. **B.** The interval between the adductor magnus, which does not contract with knee–flexion extension, is separated from the semimembranosus and semitendinosus. **C.** The femur is palpated with the finger and then the semimembranosus and semitendinosus and biceps muscles are all separated, leaving the sciatic nerve against the femur. **D.** A right-angled clamp is then placed around the muscle mass and it is pulled anterior into the surgical wound for visualization with the hip extended and the knees flexed. Electrocautery is used and the muscle is transected. (From Miller F. Cerebral Palsy. New York: Springer-Verlag, 2005. Copyright Springer Science and Business Media, Inc.)

TECHNIQUES

## Completion and Wound Closure

- The popliteal angle is checked again.
  - It should have gone from greater than 45 degrees to about 20 to 30 degrees.
  - The surgeon should not stretch the popliteal angle without palpating the sciatic nerve, which tends to become very tight, and must be careful not to overstretch the hamstrings at this point for fear of causing sciatic nerve palsy.
- The wounds are closed with a longitudinal closure of the fascial wound and a transverse closure of the subcutaneous wound and skin wound.

## PEARLS AND PITFALLS

| | |
|---|---|
| **Avoiding paralytic anesthesia** | Ensure the child is not under paralytic anesthesia so you can use nerve stimulator to test the sciatic nerve or know that you are close to a nerve when you use electrocautery. |
| **Muscle release** | Ascertain that enough muscle is released. |
| **Indications for surgery completion** | When the surgery is complete, the hip should rest at 45 degrees of abduction with no force in full hip and knee extension. |
| **Avoiding heterotopic bone formation** | Do not do a complete release of the iliopsoas through the apophysis of the lesser trochanter, which will lead to heterotopic bone formation. |
| **The popliteal angle** | Ensure the hamstring release gets the popliteal angle to at least 20 degrees, but do not stretch hard because this will cause a sciatic nerve stretch. |

## POSTOPERATIVE CARE

- The patient is placed in knee immobilizers.
- Pain is controlled typically with morphine and spasticity with diazepam given orally or rectally. Diazepam should be used on a standing order for 48 hours.
- Care is taken not to overstretch the hamstrings, especially in the first 2 or 3 weeks, for fear of causing sciatic nerve palsy, particularly in individuals with severe contractures.
- Removable Velcro enclosed knee immobilizers are used 8 to 12 hours a day.

## OUTCOMES

- The goal of the surgical treatment is primarily to improve the child's standing ability, if the child is able, and secondly to treat the spastic hip disease. About two-thirds of patients whose migration index is 30% to 60% and who are 2 to 8 years old will not require further treatment for their spastic hip disease, and the hip subluxation will resolve either completely or to a major level.
- For children whose hip subluxation does not resolve, reconstruction with femoral and pelvic osteotomy may be required.
- It is important to monitor hip radiographs in individuals, even those who have responded well at an early age, throughout their whole adolescent growth because recurrent subluxation may occur as late as the adolescent growth period.
- After complete maturation of growth, hips should have a migration percentage of less than 40%. There does not need to be further monitoring or concern after the completion of skeletal growth.

## COMPLICATIONS

- The primary complication is sciatic nerve palsy. If it occurs, sciatic nerve palsy tends to occur from overstretching the nerve in the postoperative period.
- Wound infections are rare and can usually be treated with local care.
- Heterotopic ossification may occur, especially if the iliopsoas is released through the apophysis of the lesser trochanter.
- Proximal hamstring lengthenings during adolescence also run an increased risk of developing heterotopic ossification in the proximal muscle release site.

## SUGGESTED READINGS


1. Elmer EB, Wenger DR, Mubarak SJ, et al. Proximal hamstring lengthening in the sitting cerebral palsy patient. J Pediatr Orthop 1992;12:329–336.
2. Miller F, Cardoso Dias R, Dabney KW, et al. Soft-tissue release for spastic hip subluxation in cerebral palsy. J Pediatr Orthop 1997;17:571–584.
3. Miller F, Slomczykowski M, Cope R, et al. Computer modeling of the pathomechanics of spastic hip dislocation in children. J Pediatr Orthop 1999;19:486–492.
4. Presedo A, Oh CW, Dabney KW, et al. Soft-tissue releases to treat spastic hip subluxation in children with cerebral palsy. J Bone Joint Surg Am 2005;87(4):832–841.

# Distal Hamstring Lengthening

Jon R. Davids

67

CHAPTER

## DEFINITION

- The gait pattern of children with cerebral palsy (CP) is frequently disrupted by dynamic overactivity and shortening of the medial hamstring muscles.
- This disruption is characterized by increased knee flexion in stance phase and decreased knee extension at the end of swing phase.
- Surgical lengthening of the medial hamstrings is usually performed in conjunction with other surgical procedures selected to address all elements of soft tissue and skeletal dysfunction that compromise gait in children with CP.
- This surgical strategy, termed *single-event multilevel surgery* (SEMLS), requires a comprehensive assessment of gait dysfunction using quantitative gait analysis.
- Proper management (surgical, orthotic, and rehabilitative) in childhood can result in an improved gait pattern that will be sustainable in the adult years.

## ANATOMY

- The medial hamstrings consist of three muscles: the gracilis, the semimembranosus, and the semitendinosus. All three are considered biarticular muscles because they cross both the hip joint and knee joint.
  - The gracilis muscle is innervated by the obturator nerve and has its origin on the inferior pubic ramus and its insertion on the anteromedial aspect of the proximal tibia. It serves as a hip adductor and knee flexor. The gracilis muscle has a relatively small physiologic cross-sectional area and a relatively large ratio of tendon length to muscle fiber length, indicating that it is designed for maximal excursion and diminished force generation.[8,11]
  - The semimembranosus muscle is innervated by the sciatic nerve and has its origin on the inferolateral portion of the ischium and its insertion on the posteromedial aspect of the proximal tibia. It serves as a hip extensor and knee flexor. The semimembranosus muscle has a relatively large physiologic cross-sectional area and a relatively small ratio of tendon length to muscle fiber length, indicating that it is designed for minimal excursion and increased force generation.[8,11]
  - The semitendinosus muscle is innervated by the sciatic nerve and has its origin on the inferomedial portion of the ischium and its insertion on the anteromedial aspect of the proximal tibia. It serves as a hip extensor and knee flexor. The semimembranosus muscle has a relatively small physiologic cross-sectional area and a relatively large ratio of tendon length to muscle fiber length, indicating that it is designed for maximal excursion and diminished force generation.[8,11]
- The lateral hamstrings consist of the biceps femoris muscle, which is innervated by the sciatic nerve. The muscle is considered to be uniarticular, crossing only the knee joint, with its origin on the posterior aspect of the middle third of the femur and its insertion on the fibular head. It serves as a knee flexor. The biceps femoris muscle has a relatively large physiologic cross-sectional area and a relatively small ratio of tendon length to muscle fiber length, indicating that it is designed for minimal excursion and increased force generation.[8,11]

## PATHOGENESIS

- CP is the consequence of an injury to the immature brain that may occur before, during, or shortly after birth. The nature and location of the injury to the central nervous system (CNS) determines the neuromuscular and cognitive impairments.
- Common functional deficits are related to spasticity, impaired motor control, and disrupted balance and body position senses.
- Although the injury to the CNS is not progressive, the clinical manifestations of CP change over time because of growth and development of the musculoskeletal system. The muscles typically exhibit a purely dynamic dysfunction during the first 6 years of life, characterized by a normal resting length and an exaggerated response to an applied load or stretch. With time, between 6 and 10 years of age, the muscles develop a fixed or myostatic shortening, resulting in a permanent contracture.
- As such, it is best to consider CP not as a single specific disease process but rather a clinical condition with multiple possible causes.[16]

## NATURAL HISTORY

- Ambulatory children with CP whose gait is disrupted by overactivity and shortening of the medial hamstring muscles typically walk with increased knee flexion in stance phase and diminished knee extension in swing phase.
  - This is usually associated with increased ankle plantarflexion in stance phase and is called a *jump gait pattern*.[14,18]
  - Children with a jump gait pattern will have overactivity of the medial hamstring muscle group; the lateral hamstring muscle group is rarely involved.
- As the child gets older and heavier, ankle plantarflexor insufficiency (due to muscle weakness and foot segmental malalignment) will eventually occur. This will result in increasing ankle dorsiflexion and knee flexion in stance phase, which is called a *crouch gait pattern*.[14,18]
  - Teenagers with a severe crouch gait pattern will have involvement of both the medial and lateral hamstring muscle groups.
- As the ground reaction force falls further and further behind the knee during the stance phase in crouch gait, the demands

on the knee extensor muscles increase, eventually resulting in painful patellofemoral overload.

- For this reason, the crouch gait pattern is not sustainable, and by the late teenage or young adult years, individuals with this gait pattern frequently lose the ability to ambulate.

## PATIENT HISTORY AND PHYSICAL FINDINGS

- The clinical history, as provided by the child and the parents, usually contains complaints of inability to stand up straight, inability to keep up with peers in play and sports, inability to walk distances (such as at the grocery store or the mall), and anterior knee pain after walking activities or at the end of the day.
- A straight-leg raise of 60 degrees or less is indicative of shortening of the medial hamstrings.
- A popliteal angle of 45 degrees or greater is indicative of shortening of the medial hamstrings.

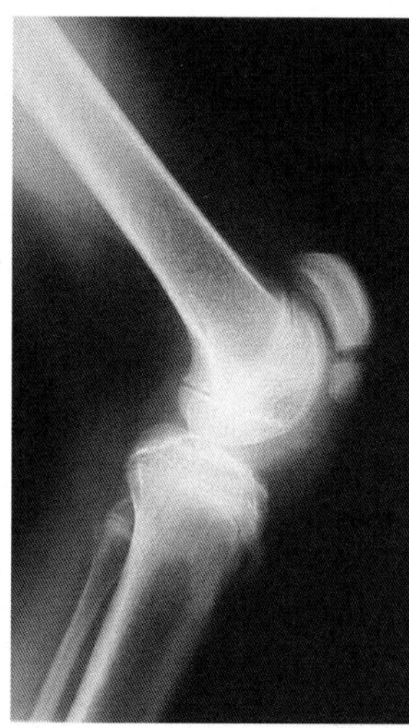

**FIG 1** • Standing lateral radiograph of the knee in a child with CP and a crouch gait pattern. There is a patella alta, with fragmentation of the inferior pole of the patella, indicating chronic overload of the knee extensor mechanism.

## IMAGING AND OTHER DIAGNOSTIC STUDIES

- Radiographic imaging is not required when determining the need for lengthening of the medial hamstrings to improve gait in children with CP.
  - If lateral radiographs of the knee are obtained, however, they will frequently show patella alta, with fragmentation of the inferior pole of the patella; these are the sequelae of chronic and progressive patellofemoral overload (**FIG 1**).
- Relevant data from quantitative gait analysis include sagittal plane kinematics and kinetics at the knee and dynamic electromyography (EMG) of the medial hamstrings.
  - Sagittal plane knee kinematics will show increased knee flexion of greater than 20 degrees at initial contact in loading response at the beginning of stance phase and diminished knee extension at terminal swing at the end of swing phase (**FIG 2A**).[5] Midstance alignment of the knee may be variable.
    - In jump gait pattern, full knee extension in midstance may occur. This is not a contraindication to lengthening of the medial hamstrings.
    - In crouch gait pattern, increased knee flexion will be of greater magnitude and is present throughout the stance phase.

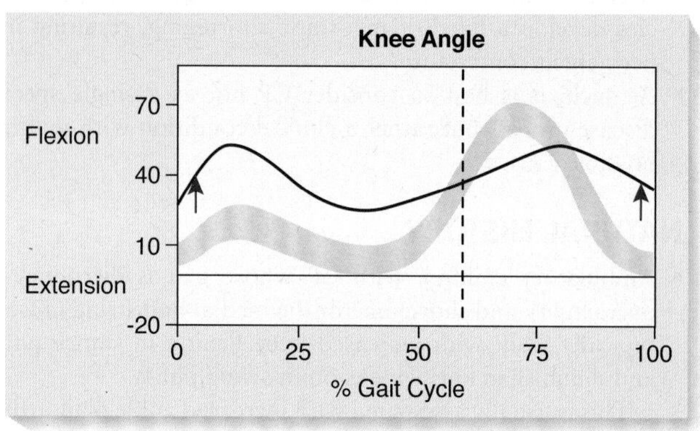


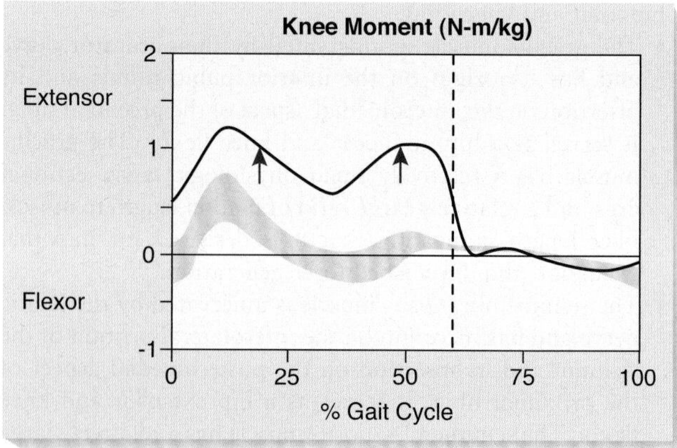


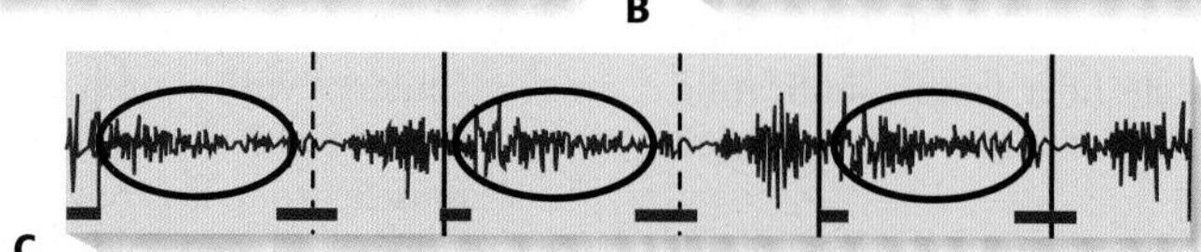


**FIG 2** • Sagittal plane knee kinematic plots of a child with a jump gait pattern (**A**) and kinetic plots of a child with crouch gait pattern (**B**). The age-matched normal motion (mean ± 2 standard deviations) appears as a *light purple band*, and the subject's data are indicated by a *blue line*. **A.** The gait cycle is on the horizontal axis, the direction of motion on the vertical axis. Kinematic indicators for lengthening of the medial hamstrings are increased flexion at initial contact and diminished extension at terminal swing (*arrows*). **B.** The gait cycle is on the horizontal axis, the internal moment on the vertical axis. Crouch gait pattern is characterized by an increased internal extension moment at the knee throughout stance phase (*red arrows*). **C.** Dynamic EMG of the medial hamstrings in a child with CP. Three gait cycles are shown, separated by the *solid vertical lines*. The stance and swing phases of each cycle are separated by the *dashed vertical lines*. The normal timing of activation of the muscle is noted by the *horizontal red lines* at the bottom of the strip. The actual timing of activation of the muscle for the subject is shown by the *oscillating red line* at the middle of the strip. The dynamic EMG indicator for lengthening of the medial hamstring muscles is prolonged activity in midstance (indicated by the *circles* in each gait cycle).

- Sagittal plane knee kinetics will show an increased internal knee extension moment in stance phase (**FIG 2B**).[12]
  - In jump gait pattern, the increased knee moment will occur in the loading response and terminal stance subphases of stance phase.
  - In crouch gait pattern, the increased knee moment will be of greater magnitude and will occur throughout the stance phase.
- Dynamic EMG of the medial hamstrings will show prolonged activity of the muscle group into the mid- and terminal stance subphases of stance phase (**FIG 2C**).

## DIFFERENTIAL DIAGNOSIS

- Increased knee flexion in stance phase may be the consequence of the following:
  - Overactivity or shortening of the medial hamstring muscles
    - Surgical lengthening of the medial hamstring muscles is appropriate.
- Ankle plantarflexor insufficiency, with disruption of the ankle plantarflexion–knee extension couple. This may be a consequence of muscle weakness or foot skeletal segmental malalignment, resulting in lever arm deficiency.[7,10,17]
  - The ankle plantarflexor insufficiency must be addressed directly to improve the gait deviation at the knee.
- Dyskinetic CP, with disrupted balance and body position sense. In such cases, mildly increased knee flexion in stance phase gives a sense of stability to the child and is habitual.
  - Surgical lengthening of the medial hamstring muscles will not correct the gait deviation in this situation.
- Increased knee flexion at the end of swing phase may be a consequence of the following:
  - Overactivity or shortening of the medial hamstring muscles
    - Surgical lengthening of the medial hamstring muscles is appropriate.
- Increased ankle plantarflexion at the end of swing phase. Increased knee flexion will occur in swing phase to promote limb clearance and improve the foot position in the transition from swing to stance phase.
- Decreased hip flexion in swing phase. Increased knee flexion will occur in swing phase to promote limb clearance.

## NONOPERATIVE MANAGEMENT

- In children younger than 6 years of age, with primarily dynamic deformity of the medial hamstrings, a community- or home-based stretching program may be effective at improving knee extension during gait for a limited period of time.
- Injection of botulinum toxin into the medial hamstrings, which decreases muscle spasticity via a reversible neuromuscular blockade, may also be effective for dynamic deformity in younger children.[3]
- Serial stretch casting of the knee has been shown to be effective for the treatment of mild myostatic deformity of the medial hamstrings, particularly after surgical lengthening.[20]
- Use of an ankle–foot orthosis may be effective treatment for increased knee flexion in stance phase that is the consequence of ankle plantarflexor insufficiency and disruption of the ankle plantarflexion–knee extension couple.[6]

## SURGICAL MANAGEMENT

- Achieving optimal outcome after lengthening of the medial hamstring muscles requires careful patient selection, proper surgical technique, appropriate postoperative orthotic management, and adequate rehabilitation resources (primarily physical therapy for conditioning and gait training) in the months after the surgery.

### Preoperative Planning

- Optimal clinical decision making and preoperative planning require the integration of data from five fields—clinical history, physical examination, diagnostic imaging, quantitative gait analysis, and examination under anesthesia—in a process described as a diagnostic matrix.[5]
- When considering lengthening of the medial hamstrings, the examination under anesthesia should include repeating the straight-leg raise and popliteal angle measurements as described earlier.
  - In children with CP that includes significant spasticity, it is frequently difficult to determine the relative contributions of dynamic overactivity and myostatic contracture to muscle deformity and dysfunction. When the child is under anesthesia, the spastic component is effectively removed, allowing the physician to perform a clinical examination to determine the presence or absence of myostatic or fixed muscle shortening.
  - Surgical lengthening of the muscle is most appropriate when significant myostatic or fixed shortening is present.
- Lengthening of the lateral hamstring muscle is not necessary for children with either jump or crouch gait patterns.
  - Lateral hamstring lengthening is indicated only for teenagers with a severe crouch gait pattern, whose popliteal angle measurement fails to improve adequately (as described in the following text) after lengthening of the medial hamstring muscles.

### Positioning

- The child is placed on the operating table in the supine position.
- A tourniquet may be placed about the most proximal portion of the thigh. The extremity is carefully cleaned and draped to allow adequate exposure for the surgical approach to the medial hamstring muscles. Use of a tourniquet to minimize blood loss and maximize the operative exposure is favored when performing SEMLS that includes both soft tissue and skeletal surgeries.

### Approach

- The medial hamstring muscles are usually exposed via a posteromedial approach at the distal third of the thigh.
- This approach is particularly appropriate when lengthening of the medial hamstring muscles and transfer of the rectus femoris muscle are to be performed at the same time as part of SEMLS.

## Lengthening of the Medial Hamstring Muscles (in Conjunction with Transfer of the Rectus Femoris Muscle)

- A 6- to 10-cm incision is made over the posteromedial margin of the distal third of the thigh, ending two or three fingerbreadths proximal to the posterior skin crease of the knee joint (**TECH FIG 1A**).
- The incision is carried down through the subcutaneous tissues, past the saphenous vein and the sartorius muscle, exposing the three muscles of the medial hamstring muscle group (**TECH FIG 1B**).
  - The gracilis and semimembranosus muscles are exposed at the level of their myotendinous junction, and the semitendinosus is exposed at the level of its distal tendon.
- A proximal tenodesis is performed between the gracilis (at its myotendinous junction) and the semitendinosus (at its proximal tendon), using two throws of a nonabsorbable suture (**TECH FIG 1C**).
- The semitendinosus muscle is then completely transected 1 cm distal to the tenodesis with the gracilis muscle (**TECH FIG 1D**).
- A fractional lengthening of the semimembranosus muscle is performed, using two transverse incisions, separated by 2 cm, through the broad and thin tendon overlying the muscle at the musculotendinous junction (**TECH FIG 1E**).
  - Care should be taken not to cut the muscle tissue underlying the tendon at this level.
- A fractional lengthening of the gracilis muscle is performed, using a single transverse incision located 1 cm distal to the tenodesis with the semitendinosus (**TECH FIG 1F**).
  - Care should be taken not to cut the muscle tissue underlying the tendon at this level.
- Repeat assessment of the popliteal angle is made after lengthening of the medial hamstring muscles.
  - The angle should be improved (ie, decreased) by 30 to 40 degrees.

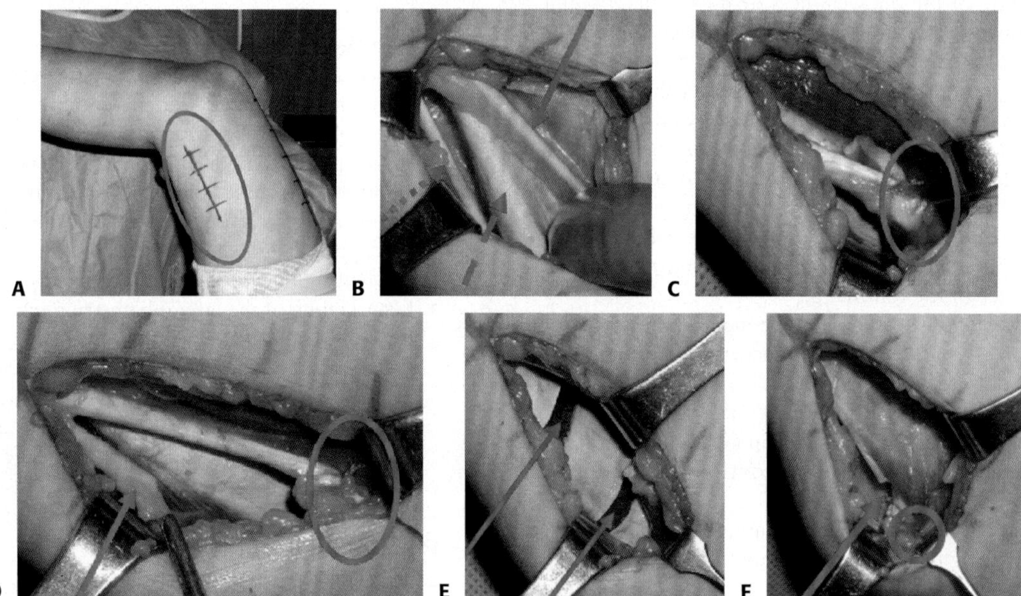

**TECH FIG 1** • Medial views of the right knee. **A.** The posteromedial skin incision used for exposure of the medial hamstring muscles. **B.** The three muscles of the medial hamstrings group—the gracilis (*solid arrow*), the semimembranosus (*dashed arrow*), and the semitendinosus (*dotted arrow*). Each has distinct myoarchitecture. **C.** Proximal tenodesis of the gracilis and the semitendinosus muscles (*circle*). **D.** The tendon of the semitendinosus has been transected (*arrow*) distal to the tenodesis (*red circle*). **E.** A two-level fractional lengthening (*arrows*) of the semimembranosus muscle has been performed. **F.** A fractional lengthening (*arrow*) of the gracilis muscle has been performed distal to the tenodesis of the gracilis and semitendinosus muscles (*circle*).

## Lengthening of the Lateral Hamstring Muscle

- A 3- to 5-cm incision is made over the posterolateral margin of the distal third of the thigh, posterior to the posterior margin of the iliotibial band, ending three to five fingerbreadths proximal to the head of the fibula (**TECH FIG 2A**).
- The incision is carried down through the subcutaneous tissues, past the posterior margin of the iliotibial band, exposing the biceps femoris at the level of its myotendinous junction (**TECH FIG 2B**).
  - The common peroneal nerve, which is located adjacent to the posteromedial margin of the biceps femoris muscle, should be identified and gently retracted away from the muscle before lengthening.
- A fractional lengthening of the biceps femoris muscle is performed, using a single transverse incision (**TECH FIG 2C**).
  - Care should be taken not to cut the muscle tissue underlying the tendon at this level.

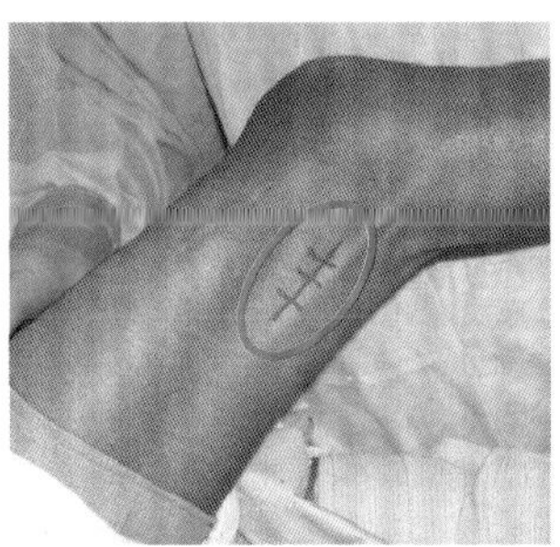
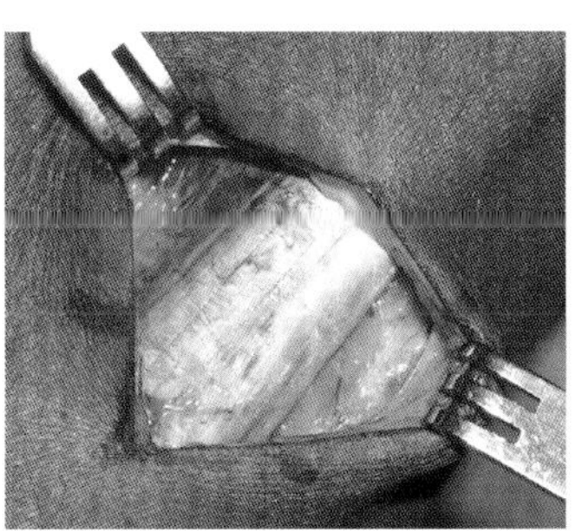
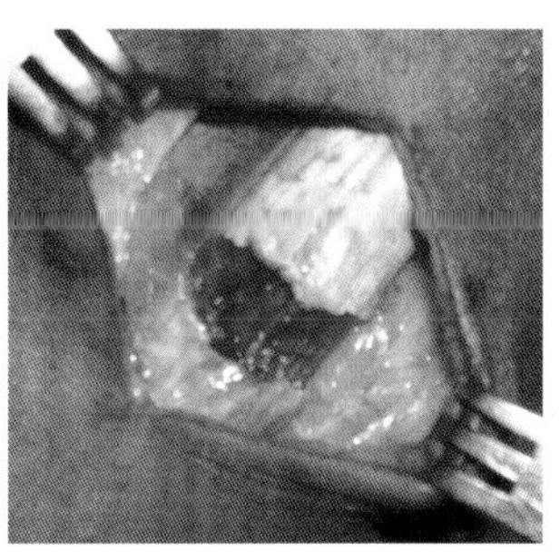

**TECH FIG 2** • Lateral views of the right knee. **A.** The posterolateral skin incision used for exposure of the lateral hamstring muscle. **B.** The lateral hamstring muscle is exposed at the myotendinous junction, which is relatively wide and long. The myoarchitecture of the biceps femoris muscle is similar to the semimembranosus muscle. **C.** A single-level fractional lengthening of the biceps femoris muscle has been performed.

## Fractional Lengthening of the Medial Hamstring Muscles (without Concomitant Transfer of the Rectus Femoris Muscle)

- A 6- to 10-mm incision is made over the posteromedial margin of the thigh, at the juncture between the middle and proximal thirds (**TECH FIG 3A**).
- The incision is carried down through the subcutaneous tissues, exposing the three muscles of the medial hamstring group.
  - The gracilis, semimembranosus, and semitendinosus muscles are all exposed at the level of their myotendinous junction (**TECH FIG 3B**).
- A fractional lengthening of each of the three muscles is performed, using two transverse incisions, separated by 2 cm, for the semimembranosus muscle, and a single incision each for the gracilis and semitendinosus muscles, through the broad and thin tendon overlying the muscle at the musculotendinous junction. The more distal the fractional lengthening, the greater the possible increase in anatomic lengthening of the muscle tendon unit.[4]
  - Care should be taken not to cut the muscle tissue underlying the tendon at this level (**TECH FIG 3C**).
- Repeat assessment of the popliteal angle is made after fractional lengthening of the medial hamstring muscles.
  - The angle should be improved (ie, decreased) by 15 to 30 degrees.

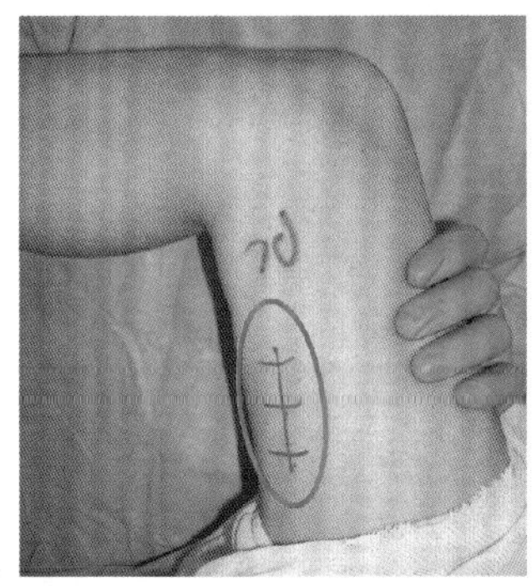
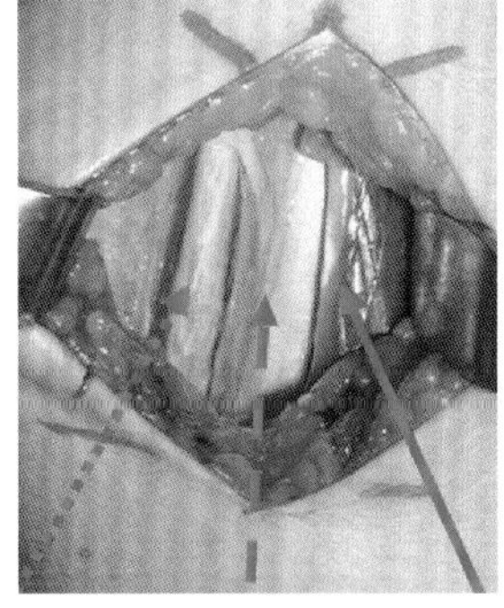
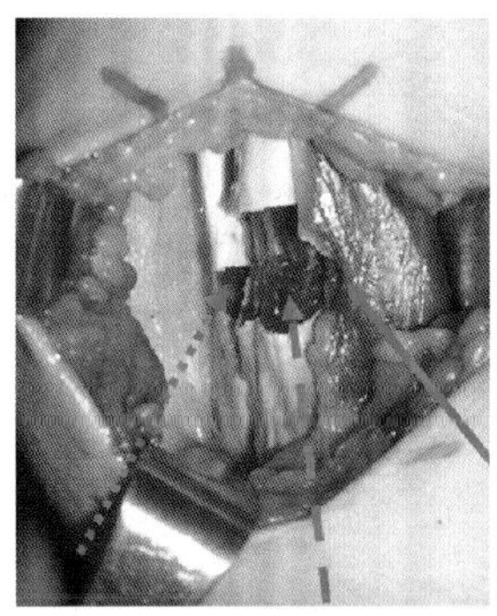

**TECH FIG 3** • **A.** Medial view of the right knee, showing the posteromedial skin incision used for exposure of the medial hamstring muscles. The incision is more proximal than that used for performing medial hamstring lengthening in conjunction with transfer of the rectus femoris muscle. **B.** Medial view of the incision in the right thigh, showing the three muscles of the medial hamstrings group—the gracilis (*solid arrow*), the semimembranosus (*dashed arrow*), and the semitendinosus (*dotted arrow*). All three muscles have been exposed at the level of their myotendinous junctions. **C.** Fractional lengthening has now been performed on each of the three muscles. Single-level fractional lengthening is sufficient for the gracilis (*solid arrow*) and semitendinosus (*dotted arrow*) muscles. A double-level fractional lengthening is usually necessary for the semimembranosus muscle (*dashed arrow*).

## Combined Fractional Lengthening and Transfer of Medial Hamstring Muscles (without Concomitant Transfer of the Rectus Femoris Muscle)

- A 6- to 10-cm incision is made over the posteromedial margin of the distal third of the thigh, ending two to three fingerbreadths proximal to the posterior skin crease of the knee joint (**TECH FIG 4A**).
- The incision is carried down through the subcutaneous tissues, past the saphenous vein and the sartorius muscle, exposing the three muscles of the medial hamstrings group.
  - The gracilis and semimembranosus muscles are exposed at the level of their myotendinous junction, and the semitendinosus is exposed at the level of its distal tendon.
- A clamp is placed on the proximal portion of the tendon of the semitendinosus muscle, and the tendon is transected distally (**TECH FIG 4B**).
- The gracilis muscle is transected proximally at the myotendinous junction, and the proximal portion of the muscle is released (**TECH FIG 4C**).
- The gracilis and semitendinosus muscles are retracted to expose the myotendinous junction of the semimembranosus muscle, where a two-level fractional lengthening is performed (**TECH FIG 4D**).
- The proximal portion of the semitendinosus muscle–tendon unit is transferred to the distal portion of the gracilis tendon and is secured with two throws of a nonabsorbable suture (**TECH FIG 4E**).
- Repeat assessment of the popliteal angle is made after combined fractional lengthening and transfer of the medial hamstring muscles.
  - The angle should be improved (ie, decreased) by 30 to 40 degrees.

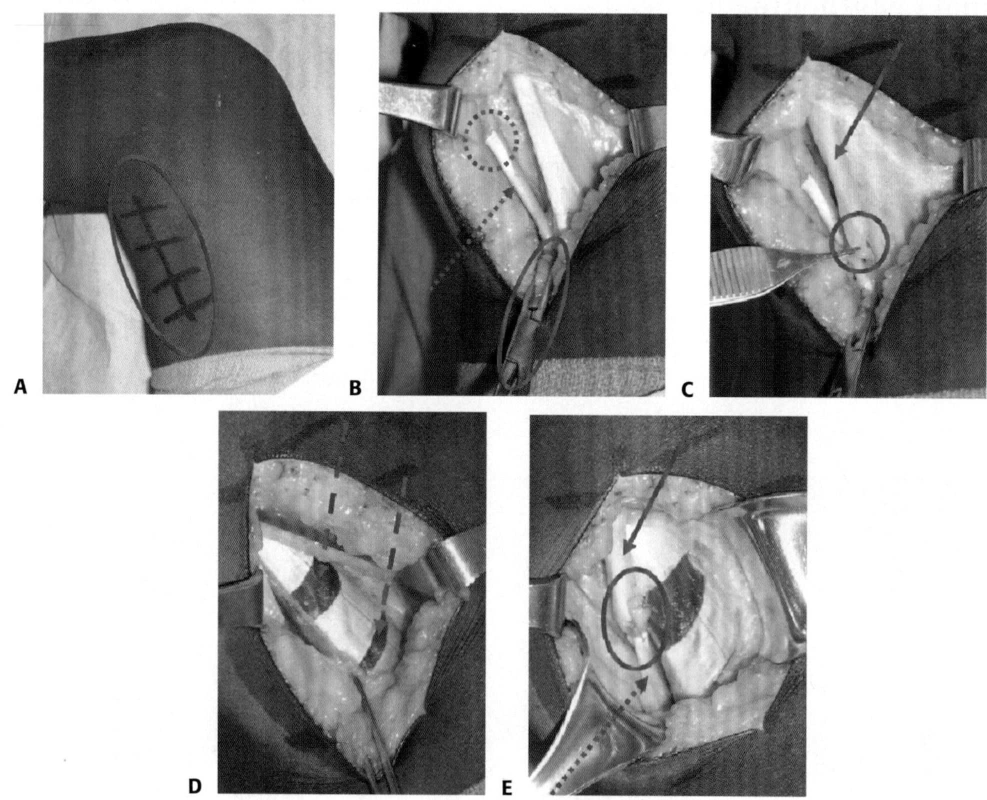

**TECH FIG 4** • Medial view of the right knee. **A.** The posteromedial skin incision used for exposure of the medial hamstring muscles. **B.** A clamp is placed on the proximal portion of the tendon of the semitendinosus muscle (*solid circle*), and the tendon (*dotted line*) is released distally (*dotted circle*). **C.** The tendon of the gracilis muscle (*arrow*) is released proximally at the muscle's myotendinous junction (*circle*). **D.** A two-level fractional lengthening (*arrows*) of the semimembranosus muscle has been performed. **E.** The proximal portion of the semitendinosus muscle–tendon unit (*dotted arrow*) is transferred to the distal portion of the tendon of the gracilis muscle (*solid arrow*). The transfer is secured with two throws of a nonabsorbable suture (*circle*).

## PEARLS AND PITFALLS

| | |
|---|---|
| **Patient selection** | ▪ Hamstring lengthening should be considered only for children with increased knee flexion in stance phase due to overactivity or fixed shortening (ie, contracture) of the hamstring muscles. Increased knee flexion due to ankle plantarflexor insufficiency (best managed by appropriate soft tissue and skeletal surgery at the foot and ankle and appropriate orthotic management) will not be improved by lengthening of the hamstrings. |
| **Excessive lengthening** | ▪ The popliteal angle should improve by 30–40 degrees on the examination after lengthening of the medial hamstring muscles. Aggressive lengthening to "improve" the popliteal angle closer to 0 degree may result in excessive lengthening, and subsequent weakness, of the medial hamstring muscles. It is the change in, not the absolute magnitude of, the popliteal angle that is the proper goal of the surgical lengthening. |
| **Indications for lengthening of the lateral hamstring muscle** | ▪ Lengthening of the lateral hamstring muscle is not necessary for children with either jump or crouch gait patterns. Lateral hamstrings lengthening is indicated only for teenagers with a severe crouch gait pattern whose popliteal angle measurement fails to improve adequately after lengthening of the medial hamstring muscles. Because of its myoarchitecture, the biceps femoris muscle is extremely sensitive to lengthening. Inappropriate lengthening of the lateral hamstring muscle may result in excessive weakness, resulting in a recurvatum gait pattern (characterized by rapid and excessive knee hyperextension in stance phase). |
| **Residual flexion deformity at the knee after lengthening of the hamstring muscles** | ▪ In older children and teenagers with a long-standing jump or crouch gait pattern, lengthening of the hamstring muscles alone may not result in complete knee extension when the hip is placed in extension. This finding indicates the presence of contracture due to deformity of the joint capsular and ligamentous structures and shortening of the neurovascular elements. Release of joint capsular and ligamentous structures to achieve full extension may result in a stretch injury (neurapraxia) of the sciatic nerve and knee instability. These procedures are no longer recommended. Serial stretch casting is preferred in this situation. |
| **Avoiding neurapraxia after lengthening of the hamstring muscles** | ▪ Forced immobilization of the extremity in extreme extension at the knee after lengthening of the hamstring muscles will be uncomfortable for the child and may also result in a neurapraxia to the sciatic nerve. Such an injury, which is painful and slow to recover, may significantly disrupt or prolong the rehabilitation phase following SEMLS. A neurapraxia is best avoided by immobilizing the extremity in a position of knee extension as achieved against gravity alone and performing gradual serial stretch casting to achieve complete knee extension in the weeks after surgery.[20] |

## POSTOPERATIVE CARE

- Lengthening of the hamstring muscles is rarely performed in isolation for children with CP; rather, it is usually a component of SEMLS.
- If full knee extension against gravity can be achieved immediately after surgery, use of a knee immobilizer is appropriate.
- Passive knee range of motion is initiated at 1 to 2 weeks after surgery.
- Weight bearing and gait training are begun 2 to 6 weeks after surgery, depending on which other surgeries have been performed as a part of SEMLS.
- If full knee extension cannot be achieved, a long-leg fiberglass cast is applied with the knee positioned in extension against gravity alone.
- The cast is univalved in the operating room to accommodate postoperative swelling and facilitate spreading of the cast in the first few days after surgery.
- Gradual serial stretch casting, correcting the residual knee flexion deformity at a rate of 5 degrees per week, is instituted.[20]

## OUTCOMES

- The early goals of surgical lengthening of the hamstring muscles are to improve knee extension at initial contact in stance phase and at terminal swing in swing phase.
- Improved dynamic alignment during gait (kinematics) should result in improved loading of the knee (kinetics) in stance phase.[1,9,10,13,15,19]
- Intermediate follow-up at 10 years after SEMLS has shown that kinematic and kinetic improvements after surgery are maintained despite deterioration in the static findings on physical examination.[2]

## COMPLICATIONS

- The most common and significant early complication after lengthening of the hamstrings is neurapraxia of the sciatic nerve, which is due to excessive stretching of the nerve after correction of the dynamic and static knee flexion deformities.
  - Neurapraxia of the sciatic nerve is characterized by pain and hypersensitivity about the foot. When this problem is encountered acutely in the immediate postoperative period, the position of immobilization of the knee should be adjusted toward increased flexion to relax the nerve.
  - If a neurapraxia develops during the period of serial stretch casting of a residual knee flexion contracture, the stretch casting should be terminated for 1 to 2 weeks, and then resumed at a slow rate.
  - If a neurapraxia is first appreciated during the rehabilitation period, management with medications such as gabapentin (mechanism of effect unknown) and physical therapy modalities for desensitization are appropriate.

- Recurrence of knee flexion deformity and increased knee flexion during the stance phase of gait may occur in the years after surgery due to a variety of factors.
  - As children grow, they pass through finite periods of accelerated rates of growth (growth spurts), where the longitudinal growth of the bones is greater than that of the muscles.
    - Muscle shortening may recur and is usually effectively treated with a period of home- or community-based stretching exercises.
  - As children grow, they get heavier, and as a result, greater muscle forces are required to balance external forces during gait. Weakness of the ankle plantarflexor, knee extensor, and hip extensor muscles is common and may result in development of a crouch gait pattern in the years after SEMLS.
    - Avoidance of obesity and ongoing muscle strength training and cardiovascular conditioning are important elements for maintaining optimal gait function in children with CP.

## REFERENCES


1. Abel MF, Damiano DL, Pannunzio PI, et al. Muscle-tendon surgery in diplegic cerebral palsy: functional and mechanical changes. J Pediatr Orthop 1999;19:366–375.
2. Bell KJ, Ounpuu S, DeLuca PA, et al. Natural progression of gait in children with cerebral palsy. J Pediatr Orthop 2002;22:677–682.
3. Corry IS, Cosgrove AP, Duffy CM, et al. Botulinum toxin A in hamstring spasticity. Gait Posture 1999;10:206–210.
4. Dagge B, Firth GB, Palamara JE, et al. Biomechanics of medial hamstring lengthening. ANZ J Surg 2012;82:355–361.
5. Davids JR, Ounpuu S, DeLuca PA, et al. Optimization of walking ability of children with cerebral palsy. J Bone Joint Surg Am 2003;85:2224–2234.
6. Davids JR, Rowan F, Davis RB. Indications for orthotics to improve gait in children with cerebral palsy. J Am Acad Orthop Surg 2007; 15:178–188.
7. Delp SL, Statler K, Carroll NC. Preserving plantar flexion strength after surgical treatment for contracture of the triceps surae: a computer simulation study. J Orthop Res 1995;113:96–104.
8. Delp SL, Zajac FE. Force- and moment-generating capacity of the lower extremity muscles before and after tendon lengthening. Clin Orthop Relat Res 1992;(284):247–259.
9. Dreher T, Vegvari D, Wolf SL, et al. Development of knee function after hamstring lengthening as a part of multilevel surgery in children with spastic diplegia: a long-term outcome study. J Bone Joint Surg 2012;94:121–130.
10. Gage JR. Surgical treatment of knee dysfunction in cerebral palsy. Clin Orthop Relat Res 1990;(253):45–54.
11. Lieber RL. Skeletal Muscle Structure, Function, and Plasticity: The Physiological Basis of Rehabilitation, ed 2. Baltimore: Lippincott Williams & Wilkins, 2002.
12. Lin CJ, Guo LY, Su FC, et al. Common abnormal kinetic patterns of the knee in gait in spastic diplegia of cerebral palsy. Gait Posture 2000;11:224–232.
13. Nene AV, Evans GA, Patrick JH. Simultaneous multiple operations for spastic diplegia. Outcome and functional assessment of walking in 18 patients. J Bone Joint Surg Br 1993;75:488–494.
14. Rodda JM, Graham HK, Carson L, et al. Sagittal gait patterns in spastic diplegia. J Bone Joint Surg Br 2004;86:251–258.
15. Saraph V, Zwick EB, Zwick G, et al. Multilevel surgery in spastic diplegia: evaluation by physical examination and gait analysis in 25 children. J Pediatr Orthop 2002;22:150–157.
16. Stanley F, Blair E, Alberman E. Cerebral Palsies: Epidemiology and Causal Pathways. Clinics in Developmental Medicine, No. 151. London: MacKeith Press, 2000.
17. Sutherland DH, Cooper L, Daniel D. The role of the ankle plantar flexors in normal walking. J Bone Joint Surg Am 1980;62:354–363.
18. Sutherland DH, Davids JR. Common gait abnormalities of the knee in cerebral palsy. Clin Orthop Relat Res 1993;(288):139–147.
19. Thometz J, Simon S, Rosenthal R. The effect on gait of lengthening of the medial hamstrings in cerebral palsy. J Bone Joint Surg Am 1989;71:345–353.
20. Westberry DE, Davids JR, Jacobs JM, et al. Effectiveness of serial stretch casting for resistant or recurrent knee flexion contractures following hamstring lengthening in children with cerebral palsy. J Pediatr Orthop 2006;26:109–114.

# Lengthening of Gastrocnemius Fascia

68

CHAPTER

James J. McCarthy and David A. Spiegel

## DEFINITION

- Lengthening of gastrocnemius fascia is commonly performed for conditions in which the patient positions their foot in equinus either while standing or walking.
- Equinus represents a loss of dorsiflexion and may be due to true shortening of the musculotendinous unit (myostatic contracture) and/or increased muscle tone or spasticity (dynamic contracture).
- The most common condition in which this procedure is performed is cerebral palsy; however, other conditions include idiopathic toe walking, traumatic conditions, complications of surgical procedures such as tibial lengthening, and a variety of neuromuscular disorders.
- Some disorders, such as Charcot-Marie-Tooth disease, may appear to have equinus, but the true deformity is plantar flexion of the midfoot on the hindfoot (midfoot cavus). Other disorders may have equinus that is less obvious due to a break in the midfoot and apparent dorsiflexion. The plantar flexion will be evident with correction of the midfoot.
- Ankle equinus and midfoot cavus may also be observed in selected conditions.

## ANATOMY

- The medial and lateral heads of the gastrocnemius muscles, the soleus, and the plantaris muscles form the triceps surae. Although all are part of the same muscle group, their structure and function differ.
- The larger medial head of the gastrocnemius arises from the popliteal surface of the femur just above the medial femoral condyle, and the lateral head originates from the superolateral surface of the lateral femoral condyle.
- The medial and lateral muscle bellies insert into a midline tendinous raphe that widens into the aponeurosis of the gastrocnemius at or just above the midcalf.
- This tendon unites with the soleus forms the conjoined tendon which inserts into the calcaneus by way of the tendo Achilles. A study of 40 cadavers indicated that there are five morphologic patterns identified at the "conjoint junction" or the place where the gastrocnemius tendon unites with the aponeurosis of the soleus. These include transverse (25%), oblique passing distally and medially (45%), oblique passing distally and laterally (5%), arcuate as an inverted U (17.5%), and a U-shape (7.5%).[5]
  - As far as the location of the conjoint junction, Elson et al[5] found that on the medial side, the gastrocnemius tendon could be located between 36% and 46% of the distance between the upper border of the calcaneus and the fibular head on the medial side, 45% to 58% in the midline, and 48% to 51% on the lateral side.
- Pinney et al[12] found that the gastrocnemius tendon was an average of 18 mm distal (20 to 57 mm) to the surface landmark of the distal aspect of the gastrocnemius muscle belly.
- The gastrocnemius spans the ankle and knee joint and therefore can plantarflex the ankle and/or flex the knee. It typically has fast twitch type II muscle fibers, allowing for short, powerful bursts of activity, important in activities such as running and jumping.
- The soleus lies deep (anterior) to the gastrocnemius muscle. It originates on the proximal tibia, fibula, and interosseous membrane, and its fascia blends with the tendon of the gastrocnemius to form the conjoined Achilles tendon or triceps surae. Contraction results in ankle plantarflexion. It is made up of primarily slow twitch type I muscle fibers. The soleus acts eccentrically to decelerate advancement of the tibia over the foot during the second rocker in stance phase and then concentrically during the push-off phase of gait.
- The plantaris arises just above the lateral head of the gastrocnemius and inserts into the calcaneus; it is largely vestigial and should be released at the time of surgery.

## PATHOGENESIS

- Equinus positioning of the foot can occur due to the following:
  - Increased tone or spasticity of the triceps surae muscles
  - Shortening of some or all of the muscles
  - Joint contracture
  - Bony deformity
- It is critical to differentiate the cause of the equinus because the treatment options differ in each circumstance.
- The initiating etiology of this disorder varies. Spasticity, weakness, and subsequent shortening of the muscle group can occur, secondary to neuromuscular disorders such as cerebral palsy. Relative shortening of the triceps surae, as occurs when the tibia is lengthened, or fixed positioning of the foot in equinus, such as prolonged casting in plantar flexion, can all result in equinus of the ankle. Bony changes at the ankle due to trauma or congenital disorders may also result in equinus.

## NATURAL HISTORY

- The natural history varies according to each disease process and prior treatment history.
- Equinus tends to progress in patients with cerebral palsy. The deformity begins as a dynamic loss of motion due to spasticity and then progresses to myostatic contracture. The contracted muscles may tether growth, resulting in skeletal deformities.
- Equinus is also likely to progress in the majority of neuromuscular disorders.
- Some disorders, such as idiopathic toe walking, often improve as the patient matures into adulthood.

## PATIENT HISTORY AND PHYSICAL FINDINGS

- Patients may complain of tripping/falling due to inability to easily clear the limb during swing phase and/or pain over the metatarsal heads or forefoot from increased stress distribution over the forefoot.
- Range of motion of the ankle should be assessed with the hindfoot inverted to lock the subtalar joint, avoiding spurious dorsiflexion through the transverse tarsal joints.
- The Silfverskiöld test assesses the degree of passive ankle dorsiflexion with the knee flexed and extended. If dorsiflexion is restricted with the knee flexed, then there is contracture of the soleus. Loss of dorsiflexion when the knee is in extension indicates a contracture of the gastrocnemius.
- Observational or instrumented gait analysis is important to correlate the physical finding with functional deficits during ambulation. The patient should be evaluated when walking and/or running.
- Small limitations in dorsiflexion range may have little functional deficit.
  - Silfverskiöld test: The ankle should be able to be dorsiflexed 10 degrees.
  - Observational gait analysis: rockers
    - First (heel): initial contact to loading response
    - Second (ankle): midstance foot flat
    - Third (forefoot): terminal stance

## IMAGING AND OTHER DIAGNOSTIC STUDIES

- Although not routinely required, standing lateral radiographs of the foot may help to evaluate equinus, especially when there may be a component of midfoot cavus (**FIG 1**).
- The angle between horizontal and a line drawn across the plantar aspect of the os calcis (calcaneal pitch) should be 15 degrees (0 and 30 degrees).
- The angle between the line drawn through the tibia and along the distal articular surface of the tibia parallel to the measure 80 degrees (distal articular surface is dorsiflexed).

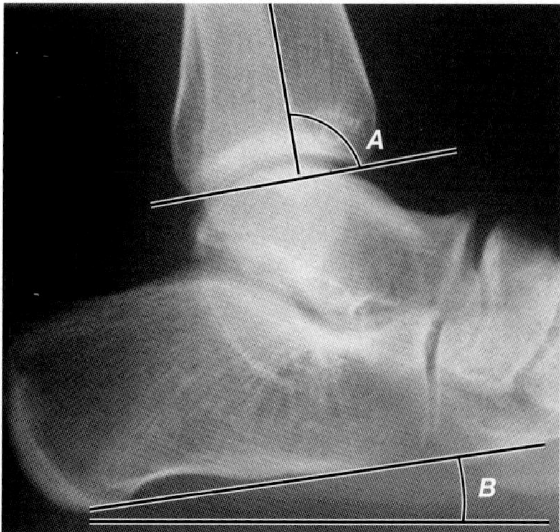


**FIG 1** • Radiographic measures. Standard standing lateral radiographs of the feet. Angle *A*, the angle between the line drawn through the tibia and along the distal surface of the tibia should measure 80 degrees. Angle *B*, the angle between horizontal and a line drawn plantar aspect of the os calcis should be 15 degrees (0 and 30 degrees).

- The contribution of the midfoot may be assessed by measuring the talo–first metatarsal angle (Meary angle).

## DIFFERENTIAL DIAGNOSIS

- Cerebral palsy, Duchenne muscular dystrophy, and other neuromuscular disorders
- Idiopathic toe walking
- Congenital limb deficiencies
- Bony deformity (posttraumatic, malalignment, asymmetric growth arrest)
- Postimmobilization
- Posterior tibial lengthening

## NONOPERATIVE MANAGEMENT

- Physical therapy and stretching is the most common form of treatment for mild deformities and used in an attempt to maintain range when gained by other methods. The knee must be extended and the hindfoot placed in an inverted position when stretching the ankle.
- Bracing and/or nighttime splinting can be used in combination with other techniques. It is primarily used to maintain gains or prevent worsening deformity.
- Botulinum toxin (BTX) causes a reversible neuromuscular blockade by blocking acetylcholine release at the neuromuscular junction and can be considered as an adjunct to physical therapy and/or casting especially in patients with spasticity. The effect lasts about 3 to 8 months.[1]
- Serial casting[10,13] can also be used, in which short-leg casts are typically placed. They are changed weekly or biweekly, each time with increasingly greater dorsiflexion.
  - Usually, three or four casts are used until satisfactory range is obtained.
  - Recurrence is common, and if not carefully performed, skin breakdown can occur.

## SURGICAL MANAGEMENT

- The gastrocnemius–soleus complex can be lengthened in a number of ways (**FIG 2**),[2–4,6,7,9,11,14,15] depending on the following:
  - The degree of fixed shortening
  - Whether there is contracture of the gastrocnemius or both the gastrocnemius and the soleus
- Isolated lengthening of gastrocnemius fascia is indicated if
  - The gastrocnemius is selectively tight.
  - This results in functional deficits.
  - Conservative (nonoperative) treatment has failed.
- The gastrocnemius can be released from its origin on the femoral condyles (Silfverskiöld procedure), but this is rarely performed.
- In this chapter, we focus on an isolated gastrocnemius recession, which is typically performed in zone 1 by either the Baumann-Koch technique[3,9,14] or by the Strayer technique.[12,14,15] The Baumann technique has also been referred to as an *intramuscular lengthening*, whereas the Strayer procedure has been termed a *distal gastrocnemius recession*.
- When the contracture involves both the gastrocnemius and the soleus muscles, techniques which lengthen both muscles are appropriate and these have also been termed *gastrocsoleus aponeurotic lengthening*. When the contracture is mild, either a zone 2 recession technique such as the

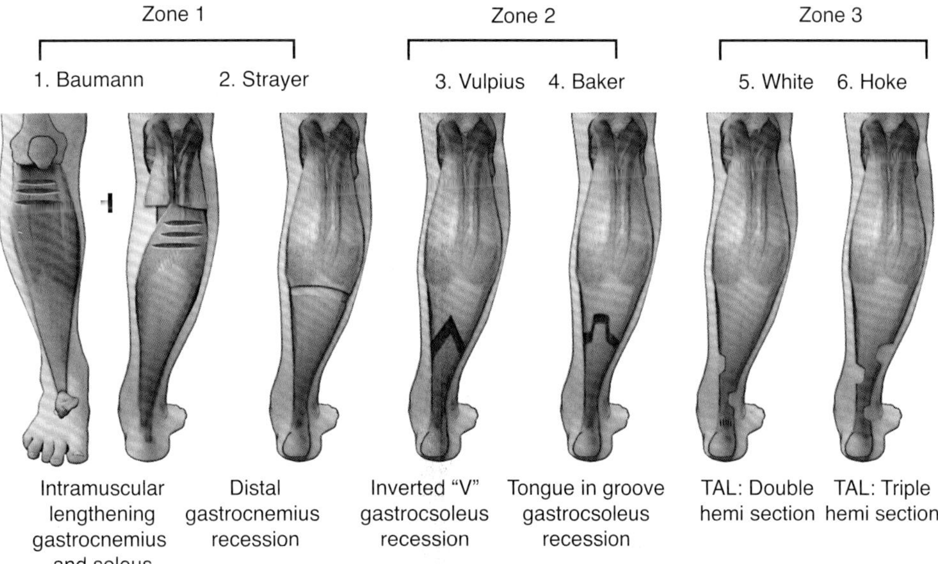


**FIG 2** • Procedures to lengthen the gastrocnemius–soleus complex can be described according to zones. Isolated gastrocnemius recession procedures are in zone 1 and include the Baumann and Strayer procedures. Recession techniques in which both the gastrocnemius and the soleus are lengthened, either selectively (Modified Strayer) or nonselectively (Vulpius, Baker), are in zone 2. Lengthening of the tendo Achilles itself occurs in zone 3 and involves either percutaneous or open techniques. (Adapted from Firth GB, Passmore E, Sangeux M, et al. Multilevel surgery for equinus gait in children with spastic diplegic cerebral palsy: medium-term follow-up with gait analysis. J Bone Joint Surg Am 2013;95:931–938.)

Baker or Vulpius, or a "modified Strayer" procedure (additional cuts are made in the soleus fascia in zone 1), allow for additional lengthening.

- Lengthening at or below the conjoined tendon (ie, the tendo Achilles), in zone 3, lengthens the entire triceps surae. These techniques afford the most correction but also have the greatest risk of overlengthening, especially when performed as an isolated procedure.
- Procedures in zone 2 carry a lesser risk of overlengthening but a greater chance of recontracture.
- Zone 1 procedures have a very low risk of overlengthening but also have a significant risk of recurrence of contracture.
- All of these recession techniques in which the gastrocnemius is lengthened, with or without the soleus, are commonly employed as part of a single-event multilevel surgery (SEMLS).
- The intraoperative goal is approximately 5 degrees of ankle dorsiflexion. Judicious lengthening coupled with multilevel surgery should drastically reduce the incidence of crouched gait complicating tendo Achilles lengthening surgery.

## Preoperative Planning

- Planning should involve assessment of the entire patient, especially in patients with underlying neuromuscular disorders. Lower limb pathology commonly involves multiple levels, and the most appropriate plan usually involves addressing all of the abnormalities under a single anesthetic.
- Isolated lengthening of gastrocnemius fascia in patients with cerebral palsy and tight hamstrings may be complicated by a crouch gait and should be avoided.
- The Silfverskiöld test should be repeated under anesthesia. The surgeon should be prepared for additional procedures if lengthening of the gastrocnemius fascia alone does not result in sufficient dorsiflexion range.

## Positioning

- The patient can be positioned either prone or supine, depending on what other procedures are planned and the preference of the surgeon.
  - In the supine position, the limb must be externally rotated to gain access to the posterior medial calf, and it is easier to place a posteromedial incision than to do a direct posterior approach.
- Similarly, some surgeons prefer a tourniquet, whereas others do not.

## Approach

- The incision for the Baumann procedure is made over the midcalf, about two fingerbreadths medial to the posteromedial edge of the tibia (**FIG 3**).
- For the Strayer procedure, either a posteromedial or a posterior midline incision is made over the midposition of the lower leg, centered approximately 2 cm distal to where the distal muscle fibers of the gastrocnemius can be palpated.
- The incision for the Vulpius and Baker are similar but should be centered several centimeters distal to that for the Strayer.

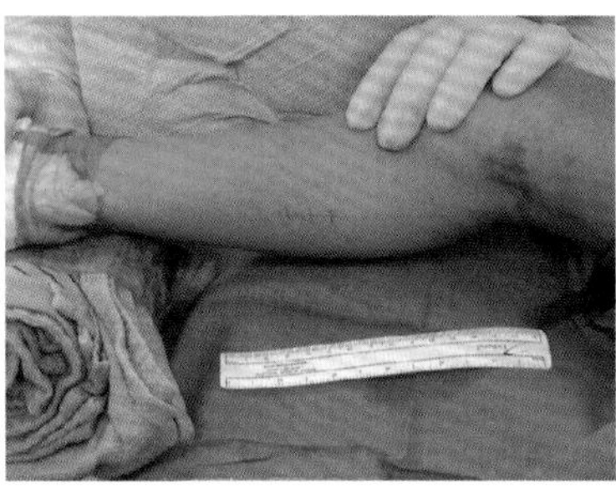

**FIG 3** • Location of the incision, with the patient in the supine position.

## Baumann Procedure

- The deep fascia is incised, exposing the gastrocnemius muscle, and the interval between the gastrocnemius and the soleus is developed bluntly (**TECH FIG 1A**).
- With a dorsiflexion force applied at the ankle, transverse cuts are made in the fascia overlying the gastrocnemius muscle until the desired degree of lengthening has been achieved (**TECH FIG 1B**).
- The subcutaneous tissues and skin edges are closed in layers.

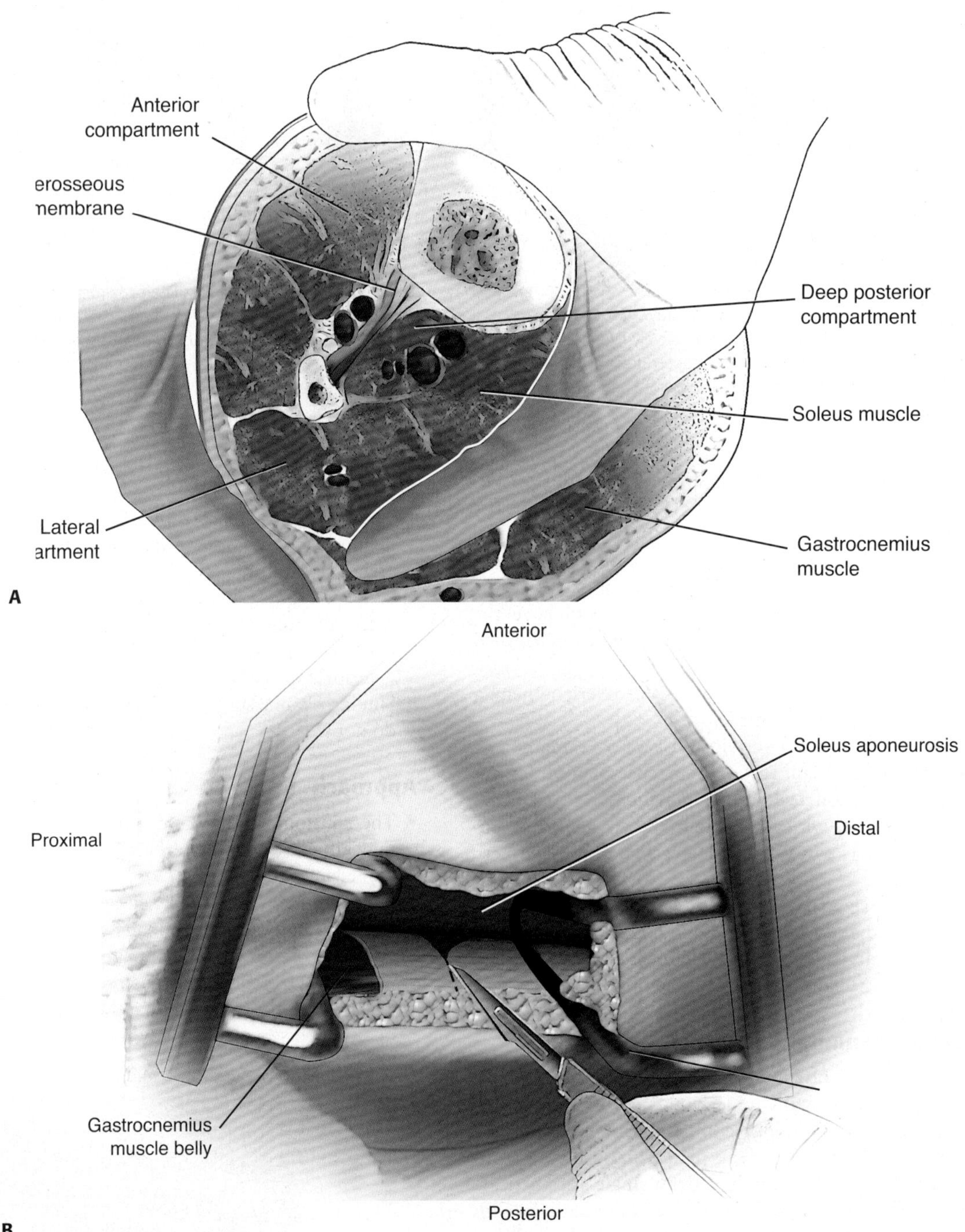


**TECH FIG 1** • **A.** Finger dissection is used to develop the plane in between the gastrocnemius and the soleus. **B.** Transverse cuts are made in the posterior fascia overlying the gastrocnemius muscle, whereas the ankle is dorsiflexed until normal Silfverskiöld test results are achieved. (Adapted from Herzenberg JE, Lamm BM, Corwin C, et al. Isolated recession of the gastrocnemius muscle: the Baumann procedure. Foot Ankle Int 2007;28:1154–1159.)

## Strayer Procedure

- Dissection is carried down to the posterior fascia, which should not be confused with the gastrocnemius tendon.
- The saphenous vein must be protected medially and the sural nerve laterally (**TECH FIG 2A**).
- The deep fascia is divided and the underlying tendon is identified; often, the muscle bellies of the medial and lateral head of the gastrocnemius overlie the tendon and need to be carefully retracted (**TECH FIG 2B**).
- The tendon of the gastrocnemius is identified proximal to the conjoined tendon and is isolated by blunt dissection and carefully divided, avoiding injury to the underlying soleus muscle (**TECH FIG 2C–F**).
- The foot is dorsiflexed to the desired degree of correction and the tendon is sutured down to the underlying soleus fascia in its lengthened position, with the ankle in 5 to 10 degrees dorsiflexion with the knee extended,
- If the soleus is also found to be tight, then a modified Strayer (or Strayer with soleal fascial lengthening) may be performed by making a cut in the soleus fascia in zone1.[7,8,11] In this scenario, a differential lengthening of both the gastrocnemius and the soleus is performed.
- The deep fascia can be repaired, followed by the subcutaneous tissue and a subcuticular closure on the skin. A short-leg cast is placed with the foot in neutral alignment.

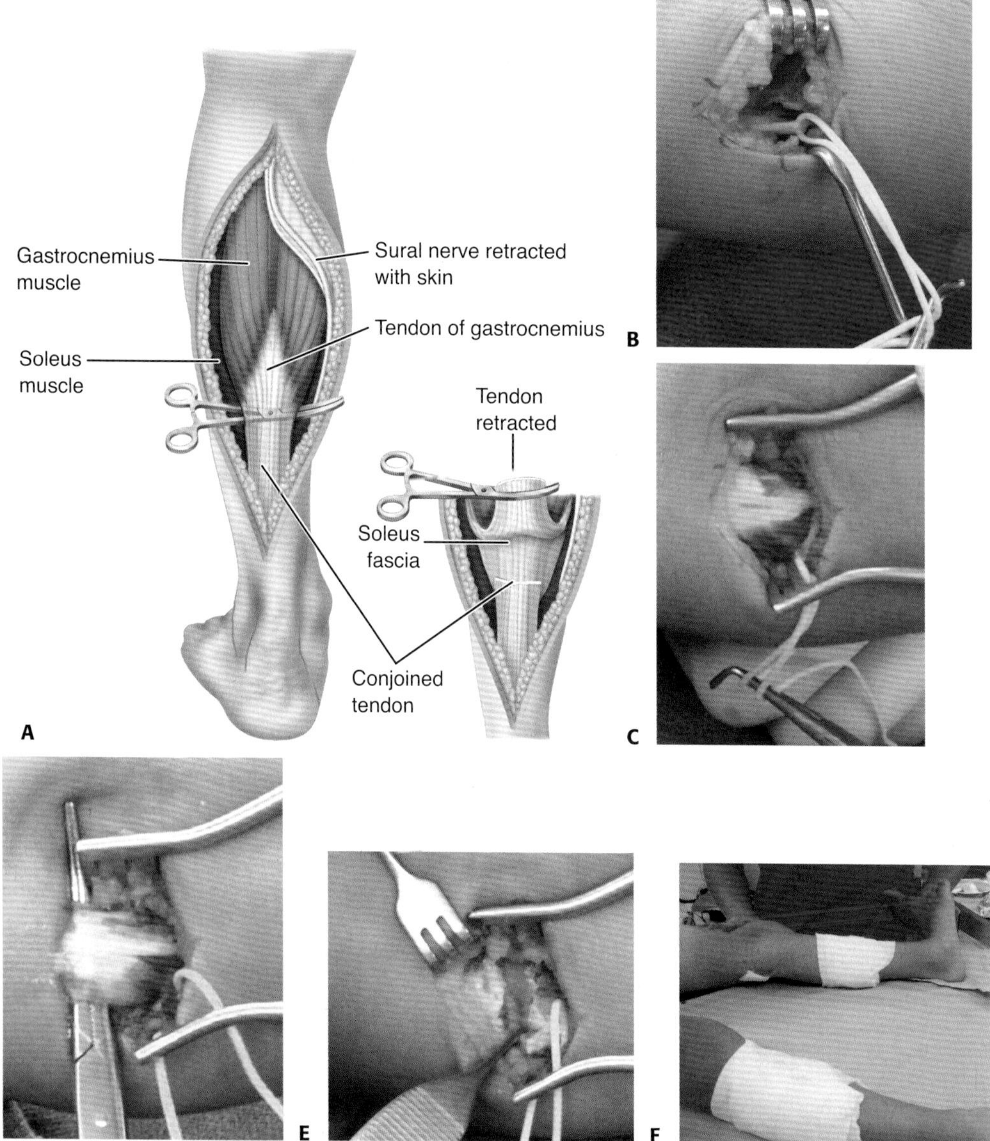


**TECH FIG 2** • The Strayer technique. **A.** Applied surgical anatomy. (Accurate incision size is shown in **FIG 3** and **TECH FIG 3A**.) **B.** Exposure with the sural nerve identified. **C.** The fascia of the gastrocnemius exposed below the muscle belly. The tendon of the gastrocnemius is isolated with a hemostat (**D**) and divided with the soleus muscle (and its overlying fascia intact; **E**). **F.** Ankle range of motion is now increased to 10 to 15 degrees of dorsiflexion with the knee extended.

## Baker Procedure

- This technique involves a recession of the conjoined fascia involving the gastrocnemius tendon and the soleus fascia in zone 2 (**TECH FIG 3A**).
- An inverted U incision is made through the aponeurosis, the lateral and medial portions remain intact with the underlying soleus muscle (**TECH FIG 3B**).
- The foot is then dorsiflexed to achieve correction, and the central "tongue" will slide distally (**TECH FIG 3C**).
- After lengthening, the four corners of the overlapping portion of the tendon are secured with sutures (**TECH FIG 3D**).
- The closure and postoperative care are similar to the Strayer procedure.

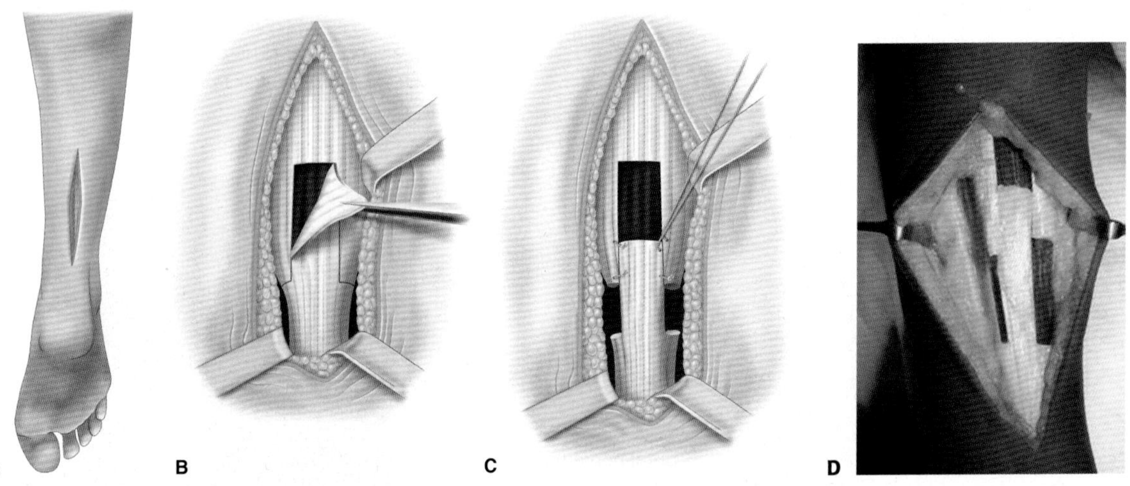


**TECH FIG 3** • The Baker technique. **A.** Incision. **B.** The "box" cut in the gastrocnemius fascia. **C.** The lengthened tendon, with sutures placed. **D.** Baker procedure with the fasciae of the gastrocnemius and soleus divided, the muscle of the soleus is exposed.

## Vulpius Procedure

- This technique is similar to the Baker technique, except that an inverted V incision is used to divide the conjoined fascia (**TECH FIG 4A**).
- More than one incision can be used if needed (**TECH FIG 4B**).

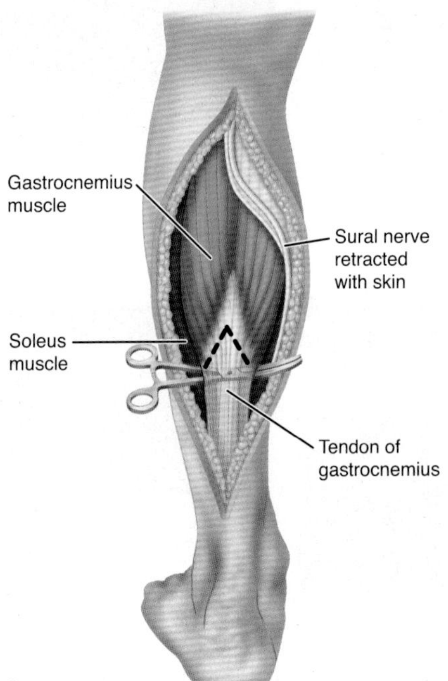


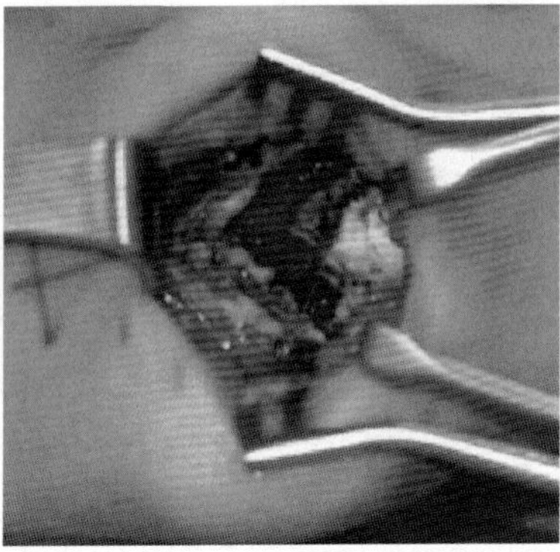


**TECH FIG 4** • The Vulpius technique. **A.** Applied surgical anatomy. (Accurate incision size is shown in **TECH FIG 3A**.) The incision in the gastrocnemius is indicated by the *dashed line*. **B.** With the fasciae of the gastrocnemius and soleus divided, the muscle of the soleus is exposed.

## PEARLS AND PITFALLS

| | |
|---|---|
| **Indications** | ▪ Carefully examine to ensure that this is isolated gastrocnemius tightness.<br>▪ Assess the soft tissue at the hip and knee and treat coexisting pathology at these levels to avoid a "crouch gait." |
| **Positioning** | ▪ Patient position depends on surgeon's preference and what other procedures may be needed.<br>▪ Tourniquet control is helpful. |
| **Avoid over- or underlengthening** | ▪ The goal should be approximately 5 degrees of passive dorsiflexion with the knee extended. If satisfactory dorsiflexion is not obtained, additional procedures may be required. |

## POSTOPERATIVE CARE

- Although Strayer and Baker originally described a "toe-to-groin cast," typically, a short-leg weight-bearing cast is worn for 4 to 6 weeks, with knee immobilizers to keep the knees extended when not ambulatory.
- Care must be taken to avoid skin irritation when applying the necessary dorsiflexion, especially over the anterior ankle and the region of the metatarsal heads.
  - Consideration can be given to placing foam padding over the anterior ankle, metatarsal heads, and/or heel.
- Bracing and nighttime splinting can be used to help maintain foot position.

## OUTCOMES

- Significant improvement in range of motion and dynamic joint motion during gait have been observed.
- Little difference has been demonstrated between the different techniques for lengthening the fascia of gastrocnemius.

## COMPLICATIONS

- Lengthening of gastrocnemius fascia is generally a safe procedure with few complications.
- Overlengthening of the triceps surae is considered to be less likely with this technique than by lengthening more distally at the Achilles tendon. Overlengthening may be complicated by a crouched gait pattern which is very difficult to treat.
  - Overlengthening is less likely when treatment of equinus is combined with other lower extremity procedures addressing soft tissue and bony pathology at multiple levels.
- Injury to the sural nerve or saphenous vein is possible but uncommon and carries little long-term consequences.
- Recurrence is the most common concern in the growing child especially when spasticity is present.

## REFERENCES


1. Baker LD. A rational approach to the surgical needs of the cerebral palsy patient. J Bone Joint Surg 1956;38-A(2):313–323.
2. Baker LD. Triceps surae syndrome in cerebral palsy; an operation to aid in its relief. AMA Arch Surg 1954;68:216–221.
3. Baumann JU, Koch HG. Lengthening of the anterior aponeurosis of the gastrocnemius muscle [in German]. Operat Orthop Traumatol 1989;1:254–258.
4. Dreher T, Buccoliero T, Wolf SI, et al. Long-term results after gastrocnemius-soleus intermuscular aponeurotic recession as a part of multilevel surgery in spastic diplegic cerebral palsy. J Bone Joint Surg Am 2012;94:627–637.
5. Elson DW, Whiten S, Hillman SJ, et al. The conjoint junction of the triceps surae: implications for gastrocnemius tendon lengthening. Clin Anat 2007;20:924–928.
6. Etnyre B, Chamber CS, Scarborough NH, et al. Preoperative and postoperative assessment of surgical intervention for equinus gait in children with cerebral palsy. J Pediatr Orthop 1993;13:24–31.
7. Firth GB, McMullan M, Chin T, et al. Lengthening of the gastrocnemius-soleus complex: an anatomical and biomechanical study in human cadavers. J Bone Joint Surg Am 2013;95:1489–1496.
8. Firth GB, Passmore E, Sangeux M, et al. Multilevel surgery for equinus gait in children with spastic diplegic cerebral palsy: medium-term follow-up with gait analysis. J Bone Joint Surg Am 2013;95:931–938.
9. Herzenberg JE, Lamm BM, Corwin C, et al. Isolated recession of the gastrocnemius muscle: the Baumann procedure. Foot Ankle Int 2007;28:1154–1159.
10. Kay RM, Rethlefsen SA, Fern-Buneo A, et al. Botulinum toxin as an adjunct to serial casting treatment in children with cerebral palsy. J Bone Joint Surg Am 2004;86-A(11):2377–2384.
11. Novacheck T. Orthopaedic treatment of muscle contractures. In: Gage JR, Schwartz MH, Koop SE, et al. The Identification and Treatment of Gait Problems in Cerebral Palsy, ed 2. London: MacKeith Press, 2009:458.
12. Pinney SJ, Sangeorzan BJ, Hanson ST Jr. Surgical anatomy of the gastrocnemius recession (Strayer procedure). Foot Ankle Int 2004;25:247–250.
13. Pohl M, Rückriem S, Mehrholz J, et al. Effectiveness of serial casting in patients with severe cerebral spasticity: a comparison study. Arch Phys Med Rehabil 2002;83:784–790.
14. Shore BJ, White N, Graham HK. Surgical correction of equinus deformity in children with cerebral palsy: a systematic review. J Child Orthop 2010;4:277–290.
15. Strayer LM Jr. Recession of the gastrocnemius; an operation to relieve spastic contracture of the calf muscles. J Bone Joint Surg 1950; 32-A(3):671–676.

CHAPTER

# Distal Femoral Osteotomy for Crouch Gait

Tom F. Novacheck

## DEFINITION

- Crouch gait is defined as walking with excessive knee flexion during stance.
- Crouch is a common walking pattern in neuromuscular conditions, particularly for individuals with cerebral palsy.
- Many potential abnormalities of bone alignment and joint flexibility can accompany or lead to crouch gait.
- Persistent crouch in adolescence frequently results in fixed knee flexion deformity and patella alta.
- Potential contributing factors include hamstring contracture, hip flexion deformity, foot deformity, loss of plantarflexion–knee extension couple, excessive femoral anteversion, and external tibial torsion. Weakness and impaired motor control are contributing factors. For some patients, disorders of balance or sensory impairments are major contributors.[1]
- Fixed knee flexion deformity is oftentimes associated with patella alta. Fixed knee contracture and patella alta are the components of the pathology that are treated with these procedures.

## ANATOMY

- Typical knee extension range is 0 degrees (full knee extension).
- Posterior capsular contracture can result from the imbalance between spastic or contracted hamstrings and knee extensor dysfunction (often associated with patella alta).
- Distal femoral anatomy is normal, although torsional deformity (excessive femoral anteversion) is commonly seen in neuromuscular conditions, especially cerebral palsy.

## PATHOGENESIS

- The pathogenesis of knee flexion deformity and crouch gait in cerebral palsy will be described, as it is the most common condition to be treated with this technique. However, other causes of knee flexion deformity and persistent crouch could be treated similarly.
- Preterm, perinatal, or infantile brain injury leads to static encephalopathy.
- This neurologic disorder causes hypertonia (commonly spasticity), impaired motor control, and weakness.
- Typical muscle growth results from the tension produced by normal bone growth and age-appropriate, typical gross and fine motor activities.
- Musculotendinous growth in children with cerebral palsy is delayed because spastic muscle does not grow normally in response to stretch and delays in attainment of typical functional activities.
- Bone growth and joint development are also adversely affected by a lack of normal functional activities as well as spasticity and musculotendinous contracture.

## NATURAL HISTORY

- Crouch gait is not uncommon at 5 to 7 years of age. At these ages, the primary causes are spasticity, weakness, and impaired balance mechanisms.
- If crouch persists during later childhood, musculotendinous contractures of the two-joint muscles (psoas, hamstrings, rectus femoris, and gastrocnemius) develop. Persistent alignment in a crouch position leads to excessive elongation of the one-joint muscles (gluteus maximus, quadriceps, and soleus), which are primarily responsible for normal upright posture.[1]
- The soleus, in particular, is responsible for restraining the forward movement of the tibia over the plantigrade foot (also known as the *plantarflexion–knee extension couple*).[1] As a result, the ground reaction force vector typically falls near the knee joint in midstance, minimizing the demand on the quadriceps to maintain knee extension.
- If weak or elongated, the ankle plantarflexors are no longer able to restrain the forward movement of the tibia over the plantigrade foot (loss of the normal plantarflexion–knee extension couple).
- Further growth leads to loss of knee joint mobility and the development of posterior capsular contracture.
- For some patients in adolescence, pain from stress fractures or from excessive stress in the patellofemoral joint itself can lead to a precipitous worsening of crouch.
- Knee pain, decreased ambulatory function, or the loss of walking ability in adulthood in individuals with cerebral palsy is common.[3]

## PATIENT HISTORY AND PHYSICAL FINDINGS

- Physical examination methods include the following:
  - Knee range of motion: Loss of extension indicates a posterior capsular contracture; loss of flexion could be due to quadriceps contracture and especially rectus femoris spasticity or contracture if the knee is flexed in the prone position. Normal upright walking requires full knee extension range of motion.
  - The examiner should palpate the inferior pole of the patella and tibial tubercle. This distance is typically equal to patellar length. The patella is pushed medial to lateral to detect patellar instability. Patella alta, which can be a cause of knee pain or can contribute to knee extensor dysfunction, is suspected if
    - The distance from the inferior pole of the patella to the tibial tubercle exceeds patellar height.
    - The patella is unstable medial to lateral.
    - The patellar tendon (as opposed to the patella) lies in the patellofemoral groove.
    - With the knees in extension, the superior pole of the patella is typically one fingerbreadth proximal to the adductor tubercle.

- Knee extension lag test: Normal extension lag is 0 degree. Terminal knee extension strength is required to control knee flexion during loading response.
- Hamstring contracture: Normal popliteal angle can be as much as 30 degrees during preadolescence. It is commonly greater in boys than in girls. For differential diagnosis purposes, it is important to identify all potential contributors to crouch gait.
- If resistance is felt as the popliteal angle is being assessed, hamstring spasticity is identified. If the knee is flexed with the patient prone and the hip extended, spasticity of the rectus femoris is identified.
  - Spasticity is one of the primary causes of the series of events that ultimately leads to crouch. If severe enough, direct spasticity treatment may be necessary.
- A complete examination of the patient should also include evaluation of associated abnormalities to identify all potential contributors to crouch gait, including hip flexion deformity, hamstring contracture, femoral anteversion, tibial torsion, foot deformity or instability, balance disorder, and visual or sensory disturbances.

## IMAGING AND OTHER DIAGNOSTIC STUDIES

- A plain lateral radiograph of the knee in maximum extension should be obtained to assess for fixed knee flexion contracture and patella alta (**FIG 1**).
- If the knee is held in maximum extension, the femoral–tibial angle on the lateral radiograph represents the degree of true knee flexion deformity.
- The knee is extended maximally with a bolster just below the patella to assess the true degree of patella alta. Patella alta can be documented using the Insall ratio or the Koshino index.[2]
- Inferior pole sleeve avulsion injuries of the patella are common in children with spastic cerebral palsy and can be identified on the lateral radiograph. The development of a stress fracture is typically painful and can lead to the rapid progression of crouch over a short period.
- Computerized gait analysis provides much needed insight to create a problem list to guide treatment decision making by identifying the numerous other contributors to crouch gait listed earlier.

## DIFFERENTIAL DIAGNOSIS

- Knee extensor lag with or without patella alta
- Hamstring spasticity or contracture
- Hip flexor spasticity or contracture
- Femoral anteversion
- Tibial torsion (typically external)
- Ankle plantarflexor insufficiency
  - Foot deformity
  - Excessive midfoot instability
  - Soleus weakness: primary versus iatrogenic from prior Achilles tendon lengthening

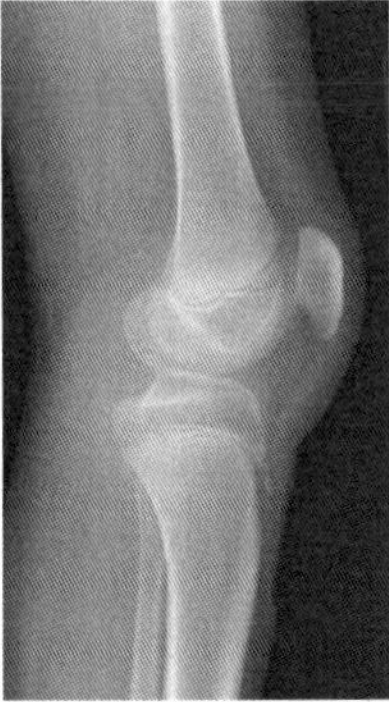

**FIG 1** • Lateral radiograph of knee in maximum extension. Patellar position and degree of knee contracture can be assessed from this view.

## NONOPERATIVE MANAGEMENT

- Physical therapy (stretching and strengthening) helps minimize the development of musculotendinous contracture secondary to spasticity and weakness.
- Botulinum toxin injections or oral spasmolytic agents can help manage spasticity.
- Functional strengthening of the muscle groups that contribute to crouch (ankle plantarflexors, knee extensors, and hip extensors) can help correct muscle imbalance.
- Nighttime knee extension splinting with knee immobilizers or bivalved casts can help prevent a flexed knee position during the night, thereby minimizing the development of knee capsular contracture.

## SURGICAL MANAGEMENT

### Preoperative Planning

- The lateral radiograph of the knee in maximum extension should be reviewed for the degree of knee contracture, patellar height, presence of a stress fracture at the inferior pole of the patella, and the status of skeletal maturation (see **FIG 1**).
- Gait analysis data should be reviewed to assess for knee extension lag, degree of crouch, presence of hip flexion contracture, spasticity or contracture of the rectus femoris, and hamstrings length and for the presence of tibial torsion, femoral anteversion, and foot deformity.
- Examination under anesthesia for femoral anteversion and coronal plane malalignment of the knee should be accomplished before positioning.
- Other deformities can be addressed concurrently under the same anesthetic.

### Positioning

- If severe femoral anteversion is present, a proximal femoral osteotomy may be required in addition to the distal osteotomy, as it may be difficult to correct more than 25 to 30 degrees of malrotation distally.
- Tibial torsion and foot deformity should also be addressed first. Although these can be done supine, prone positioning is preferred as it allows accurate examination and correction of rotational profile consistent with the physical examination methods used in the clinic.
- The extension osteotomy and patellar advancement are performed supine with the leg draped free (**FIG 2**).

### Approach

- The extension osteotomy of the distal femur is performed via a lateral distal femoral incision.
- The patellar advancement is performed through a direct anterior incision centered over the tibial tubercle.

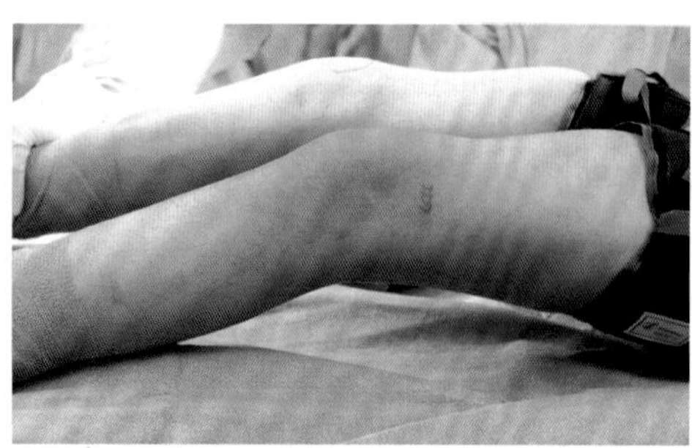

**FIG 2** • Positioning for distal femoral extension osteotomy. Supine position allows access for both extension osteotomy and patellar advancement. The procedures are performed under tourniquet control. Note the knee contracture and patella alta.



## Distal Femoral Extension Osteotomy

- The procedure is performed under tourniquet control.
- Through the lateral distal femoral incision, the fascia is opened and the vastus lateralis is reflected from its posterior origin and elevated to expose the distal femur subperiosteally.
- Circumferential subperiosteal retractors are placed.
- Typically, a 90-degree adolescent AO blade plate is used for fixation. If no varus or valgus deformity correction is required, the guidewire for chisel placement is placed at a 90-degree angle to the femoral shaft on an anteroposterior (AP) image in the plane of the tibia (as this will reflect final coronal plane alignment) (**TECH FIG 1A**).
- The guidewire entry point is through the anterior portion of the lateral femoral epicondyle in line with the femoral shaft to avoid anterior or posterior translation of the distal fragment. It is placed just proximal to the distal femoral physis if the patient is immature and at the physeal scar if growth is complete.
- Transverse plane position is in line with the axis from the lateral to the medial femoral condyle.
- The chisel is inserted exactly parallel and just proximal to the pin, with the angle guide for the AO chisel aligned parallel to the tibia (**TECH FIG 1B**). The angle between the AO chisel guide and the femoral shaft is equal to the degree of knee contracture and the extension to be obtained.
- Depending on preoperative assessment, a second pin can be placed proximal to the osteotomy site to assist with rotational control. It can be placed at a converging angle in the transverse plane to match the degree of derotation desired.
- The distal osteotomy is performed first. The oscillating saw blade is aligned exactly parallel and 10 to 15 mm proximal to the chisel (**TECH FIG 1C**).
- The second osteotomy is performed perpendicular to the femoral shaft, typically meeting the first osteotomy at the posterior cortex (although with more severe deformities, a cuneiform wedge including several millimeters of posterior cortex may also be removed to avoid postoperative neuropraxia).
- The anterior wedge of bone is removed (**TECH FIG 1D**).
- Varus–valgus deformities can be corrected by altering the guide pin placement in the coronal plane or bending the implant to match the desired correction.
- The osteotomy is realigned by derotating if necessary and extending the knee.
- The chisel is replaced with the Synthes AO blade plate.
- The femoral shaft is reduced to the plate and held with a Verbrugge clamp (**TECH FIG 1E**).
- After an initial screw is placed in compression to hold alignment, final coronal plane alignment is assessed. Proper mechanical axis alignment is confirmed if the electrocautery cord, aligned

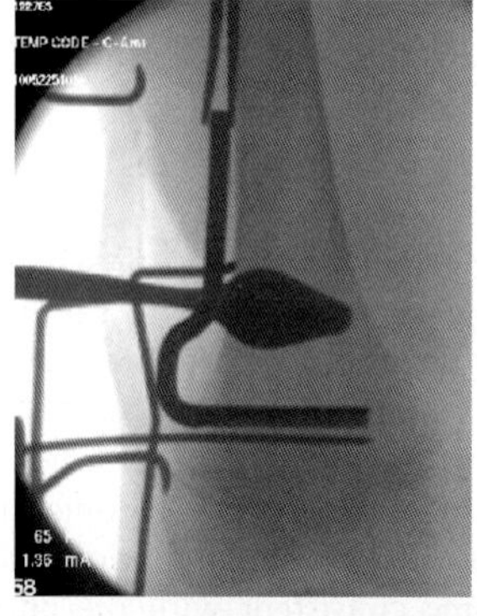

A

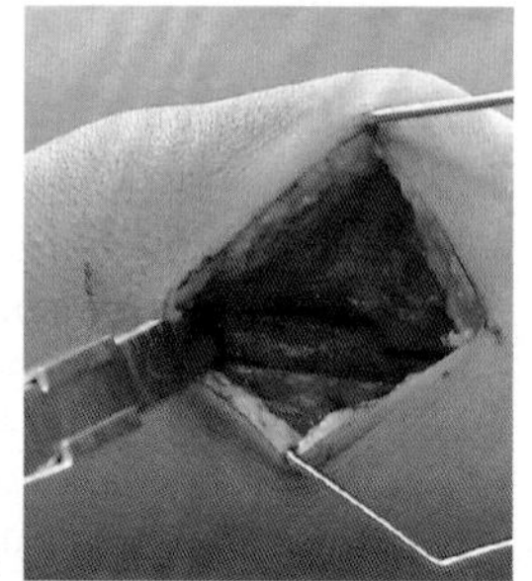

B

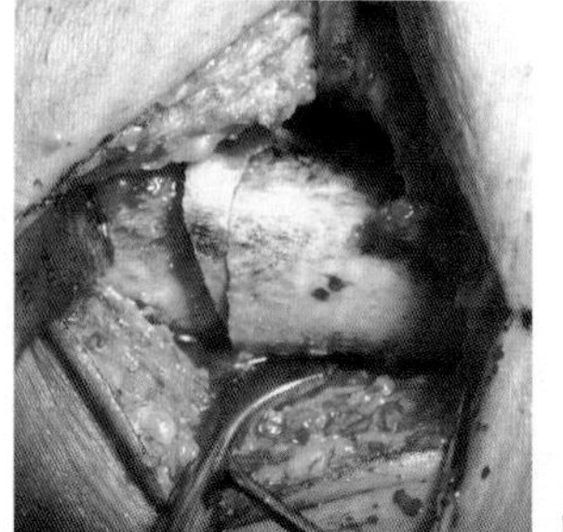

C

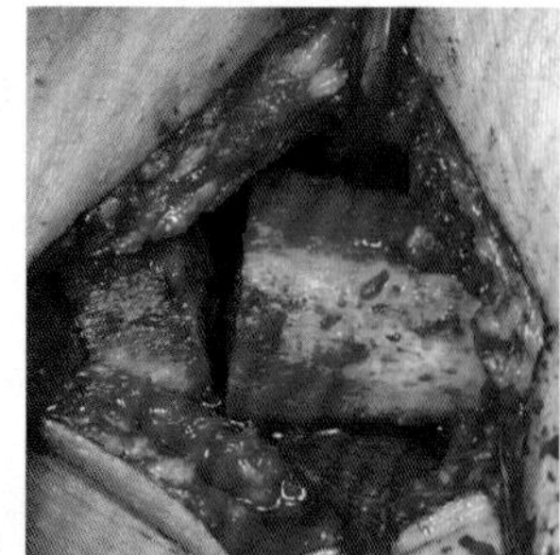

D

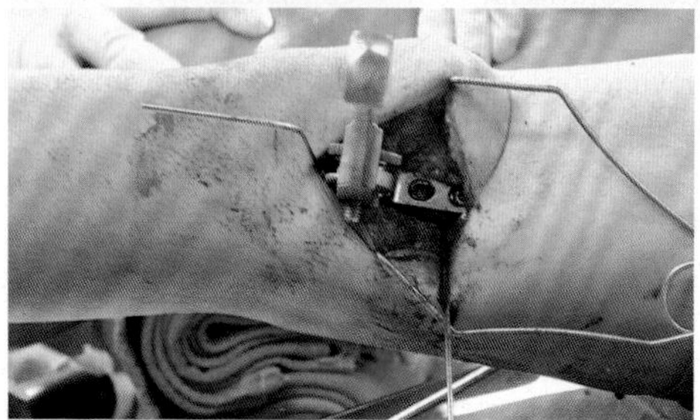

E

**TECH FIG 1** • Distal femoral extension osteotomy. **A.** Blade plate is held anteriorly over the leg to position guidewire 90 degrees to femoral shaft (C-arm view orthogonal to tibia, not femur). **B.** The chisel guide is parallel to the tibia. **C.** Distal osteotomy is parallel to chisel; proximal osteotomy is perpendicular to shaft. **D.** Anterior wedge of bone removed. **E.** Knee in full extension after blade plate is reduced to the femoral shaft.

directly over the hip and ankle joint centers, also passes directly over the knee joint center.

- Final coronal plane alignment can be adjusted if necessary by laterally displacing the distal fragment further by impacting the plate more completely or by removing the plate and adjusting its angle accordingly.

- The final screws are placed.
- Any significant posterior bone prominence should be resected with the oscillating saw.
- A Hemovac drain can be placed posteriorly.
- The wound is closed in layers.

## Patellar Advancement

- If the patient is skeletally immature, transposition of a tibial tubercle bone block would cause an anterior growth arrest. Instead, the patellar tendon is advanced without violating its insertion (**TECH FIG 2A**).
- A T-shaped periosteal incision is made just distal to the tibial tubercle apophysis.
- Medial and lateral flaps of periosteum are elevated (**TECH FIG 2B**).
- The tendon is separated from the cartilaginous tibial tubercle apophysis using a fresh scalpel, working at the junction of the fibers of the patellar tendon and the cartilage (**TECH FIG 2C**). It is best to err on the side of leaving a few fibers of tendon on the cartilage than to inadvertently injure the cartilage. Care must be taken to maintain an adequate thickness of tendon (about 2 mm) without defects.
- The next step is placement of a tension band from the patella to the tibia to protect the repair. A guidewire for the 2.7-mm cannulated AO drill bit is passed percutaneously transversely through the midportion of the patella.
- The cannulated drill bit is drilled across the patella from lateral to medial. The guidewire is removed, leaving the drill bit in place.
- A suture passer is passed retrograde through the drill bit from medial to lateral, and then the drill bit is removed.
- A 2-mm FiberTape suture is passed through the drill hole using the suture passer.
- Using a long, right angle clamp, the ends of the FiberTape suture are passed along the edges of the patellar tendon inside the patellar bursal sleeve to the anterior incision.
- A transverse drill hole (2–2.5 mm) is placed in the tibia and the suture is passed through it (**TECH FIG 2D**).

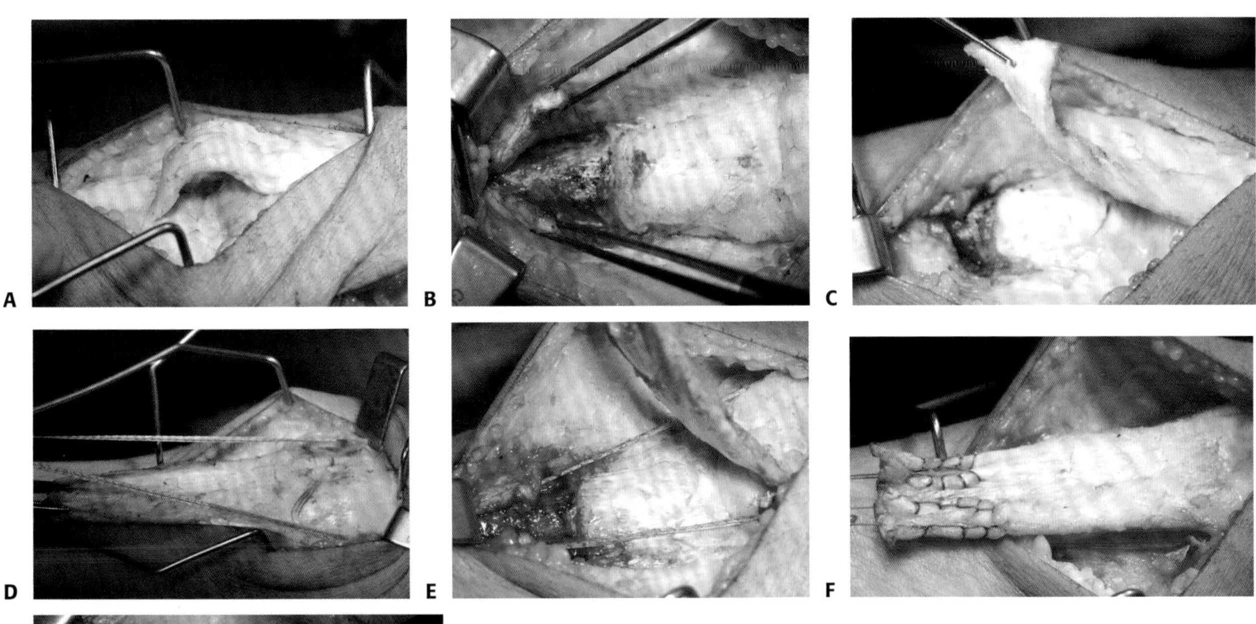

**TECH FIG 2** • Patellar advancement. **A.** Patellar tendon redundancy after extension osteotomy. **B.** Periosteal flaps distal to tibial tubercle apophysis. **C.** Patellar tendon after sharply dividing the tendon from the cartilaginous apophysis. **D.** FiberTape placed transversely across patella (here shown as open procedure, now performed percutaneously as described in the text). **E.** FiberTape tied to hold patella down in final position. **F.** Medial and lateral Krackow sutures in patellar tendon. **G.** Tendon advanced under periosteal flaps, flaps repaired over tendon, and FiberTape along medial and lateral edges of tendon.

- The patella is advanced distally by tensioning the FiberTape until the inferior pole of the patella is at the femoral–tibial joint line, at which point the knot in the FiberTape is tied (**TECH FIG 2E**).
- Two baseball (Krackow) stitches are placed in the patellar tendon, one medially and one laterally, using 0 Ethibond suture (**TECH FIG 2F**).
- These sutures are tied deeply under the periosteal flaps.
- The periosteal flaps are then sewn over the patellar tendon (**TECH FIG 2G**).
- The wound is closed in routine fashion.

## Tibial Tubercle Advancement

- For skeletally mature patients, the patellar tendon and tibial tubercle are exposed.
- A small tibial tubercle bone block with patellar tendon attached is created with an oscillating saw and completed with an osteotome. The typical size is the width of the patellar tendon, 2 to 2.5 cm in length and 7 to 10 mm thick.
- The 2-mm FiberTape is placed identical to the previous description.
- A receptacle site for the tibial tubercle bone block is created at the appropriate level.
- The distally excised bone block is impacted into the original tibial tubercle site.
- The tibial tubercle is inserted into its receptacle site and secured with a single 4.5-mm AO screw, overdrilling the tibial tubercle fragment to compress the bone block and countersinking to avoid screw prominence.
- The typical advancement is 2 to 2.5 cm.
- By keeping the tibial tubercle bone block relatively short in length, a small bridge of intact anterior cortical bone can provide a proximal buttress to resist proximal migration of the tibial tubercle bone block postoperatively.
- The knee should be able to flex 60 degrees at this point without excessive tension or disruption of the repair.
- The wound is closed in routine fashion.

## PEARLS AND PITFALLS

| | |
|---|---|
| **Recurrence of knee flexion deformity and persistence of crouch** | ▪ If a distal femoral extension osteotomy is performed without patellar advancement, there is a high risk of these postoperative problems. |
| **Patellar advancement in isolation** | ▪ The primary indication for patellar advancement is the finding of knee extensor lag on physical examination, not the finding of patella alta.<br>▪ This is effective to treat crouch in the presence of a knee extension lag without knee flexion contracture. |
| **Avoiding sciatic nerve palsy** | ▪ Postoperative immobilization in flexion during the time of acute swelling (first 3 days) and resection of the posterior bony prominence on the distal fragment have helped minimize this complication. |
| **Loss of patellar fixation** | ▪ Supporting patellar advancements with a FiberTape tension band has minimized this complication. |
| **Increased anterior pelvic tilt** | ▪ Detecting and treating hip flexion deformity as well as rectus femoris spasticity and contracture (simultaneous rectus femoris transfer) have been helpful, but this finding seems to be common with surgical intervention at this age. |
| **Miscellaneous** | ▪ Distal femoral osteotomy requires meticulous care to ensure optimal postoperative alignment in all three planes.<br>▪ Contractures between 10 and 25 degrees are typically appropriate for this compensatory osteotomy of the distal femur.<br>▪ In growing children with relatively small deformities, anterior distal femoral figure-8 plating may be a consideration.<br>▪ The treatment of flexion contractures of 30 degrees or greater introduces significant distal femoral deformity.<br>▪ Modest transverse plane deformities can easily be corrected, but again, this requires meticulous attention to detail.<br>▪ Malrotation greater than 30 degrees can be difficult to correct with this technique.<br>▪ Preoperative coronal plane deformities can be corrected, and care must be taken to avoid creation of postoperative varus–valgus deformities. |

## POSTOPERATIVE CARE

- AP and lateral radiographs are reviewed to confirm proper alignment (**FIG 3**).
- The knee is immobilized for 3 days in 20 to 30 degrees of flexion in a Robert Jones dressing to avoid sciatic nerve stretch.
- Then a knee immobilizer is used for 6 weeks.
- Use of a continuous passive motion (CPM) machine is begun on the third postoperative day; initially, the range is from 0 to 30 degrees, and it is advanced to 90 degrees by 6 weeks postoperatively.
- After 3 weeks, active range of motion and weight bearing are initiated. Once quadriceps strength and control are sufficient, the knee immobilizer can be discontinued.

## OUTCOMES

- Knee flexion deformity and terminal knee extensor insufficiency can reliably be corrected.[5]
- Preoperative stress fractures and knee pain are improved or resolved in the vast majority of patients.

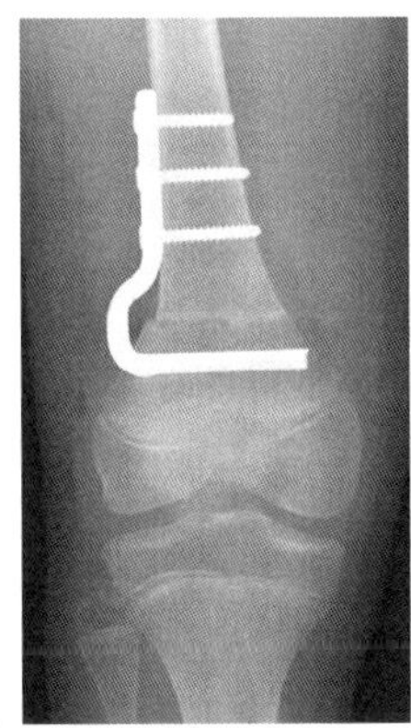


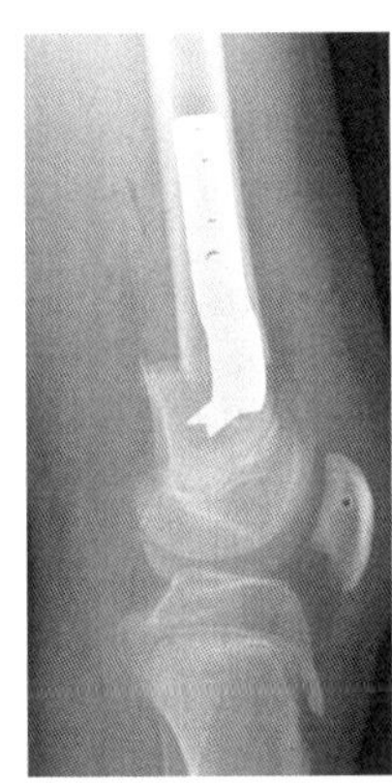


**FIG 3** • Postoperative radiographs. **A.** On the AP view, the blade can be seen just proximal to the growth plate and the osteotomy parallel to the blade. **B.** The lateral view shows the blade insertion anterior in the distal femur to avoid anterior translation of the distal fragment, the posterior bone prominence of the distal fragment (in this case, not felt to be large enough to warrant resection), the overcorrected patellar position (distal pole at femoral–tibial joint line), and the drill holes in the patella and proximal tibia for the FiberTape tension band.

- Worsened anterior pelvic tilt is commonly seen and does not seem to be a result of persisting contracture or weakness.
- Crouch gait is corrected effectively for those who have the combined procedure of extension osteotomy and patellar advancement. Crouch is also effectively treated in the absence of knee contracture with patellar advancement alone, as long as other musculotendinous contractures and bone or joint deformities are concurrently addressed.
- Distal femoral extension osteotomy without patellar advancement has a high risk of recurrence of contracture and typically results in only partial improvement in crouch.
- An overcorrection of patellar position compensates for weakness, impaired motor control, and spasticity and has been found to be safe (low rate of persisting anterior knee pain postoperatively) and necessary to treat crouch.
- The natural history of crouch gait is one of worsening. With these procedures, walking ability is either maintained or improved, as indicated by gait analysis and assessments of functional mobilty.[4]

## COMPLICATIONS

- Sciatic nerve palsy
- Loss of patellar fixation
- Recurrence of deformity
- Wound breakdown or infection
- Increased anterior pelvic tilt

## REFERENCES


1. Gage JR, ed. Treatment principles for crouch gait. In: Treatment of Gait Problems in Cerebral Palsy. London: MacKeith Press, 2004:382–397.
2. Koshino T, Sugimoto K. New measurement of patellar height in the knees of children using the epiphyseal line midpoint. J Pediatr Orthop 1989;9:216–218.
3. Murphy KP, Molnar GE, Lankasky K. Medical and functional status of adults with cerebral palsy. Devel Med Child Neurol 1995;37:1075–1084.
4. Novacheck TF, Stout JL, Tervo R. Reliability and validity of the Gillette Functional Assessment Questionnaire as an outcome measure in children with disabilities. J Pediatr Orthop 2000;20:75–81.
5. Stout JL, Gage JR, Schwartz MH, et al. Distal femoral extension osteotomy and patellar tendon advancement for the treatment of persistent crouch gait in cerebral palsy. J Bone Joint Surg Am 2008;90(11):2470–2484.

# Cysts

# Operative Management of Unicameral Bone Cyst, Aneurysmal Bone Cyst, and Nonossifying Fibroma

Alexandre Arkader

## UNICAMERAL BONE CYST

### DEFINITION

- Unicameral bone cyst (UBC) or simple bone cyst is a benign, active or latent, solitary fluid-filled cystic lesion that usually involves the metaphysis of long bones.

### PATHOGENESIS

- The cause is unknown; theories range from a reactive or developmental process to a true neoplasm. The most likely cause is perhaps an obstruction to the drainage of interstitial fluid, leading to the accumulation of fluid under pressure.
- Few isolated reports have shown cytogenetic abnormalities including the presence of translocation t(16;20)(p11.2;q13) and t(7;12)(q21;q24.3) and TP53 mutations in recurrent UBCs.
- UBCs are characterized by a fluid-filled cyst lined with a thin fibrous membrane without endothelial cell lining. However, owing to the high incidence of associated fractures, several nonspecific changes may be seen, such as hemorrhage, hemosiderin deposits, granulation tissue, new bone formation, and others.

### NATURAL HISTORY

- Active cysts are generally located near the growth plate and are usually asymptomatic. Approximately 85% of these cysts are diagnosed at the time of a pathologic fracture.
- Inactive or latent cysts tend to "migrate" away from the growth plate as longitudinal growth occurs and populate the midshaft or diaphyseal region.
- UBCs may regress spontaneously after skeletal maturity.

### PATIENT HISTORY AND PHYSICAL FINDINGS

- UBCs are usually asymptomatic; the usual presentation is with a pathologic fracture following a minor trauma.
- UBC is more often in boys (3:1), especially during the first two decades. The most common locations are the proximal humerus and the femur, accounting for 50% to 70% of the lesions. Calcaneal UBCs tend to occur in a slightly older group.

### IMAGING AND OTHER DIAGNOSTIC STUDIES

- Plain radiographs typically demonstrate a well-defined, centrally located, radiolucent lesion that may be associated with varying degrees of cortical thinning and mild expansion (**FIG 1**).
  - When UBCs are associated with bone expansion, it generally does not exceed the width of the nearest growth plate.
  - When a pathologic fracture occurs, there may be periosteal reaction, and occasionally, the typical "fallen leaf" sign is visualized (piece of fractured cortex "floating" inside the cavity). Most pathologic fractures are minimally displaced and stable.
- Computed tomography (CT) may be useful to characterize lesions that are of difficult visualization on plain films (eg, spine, pelvis) and to rule out fractures (nondisplaced or minimally displaced).
  - Noninvasive quantitative CT has been applied to evaluation of the risk of pathologic fractures through bone cyst and other benign bone lesions.
- Magnetic resonance imaging (MRI) is usually only needed for differential diagnosis of atypical UBCs.
  - Although the appearance may vary, they present as low to intermediate signals on T1-weighted images and bright and homogeneous signals on T2-weighted images.

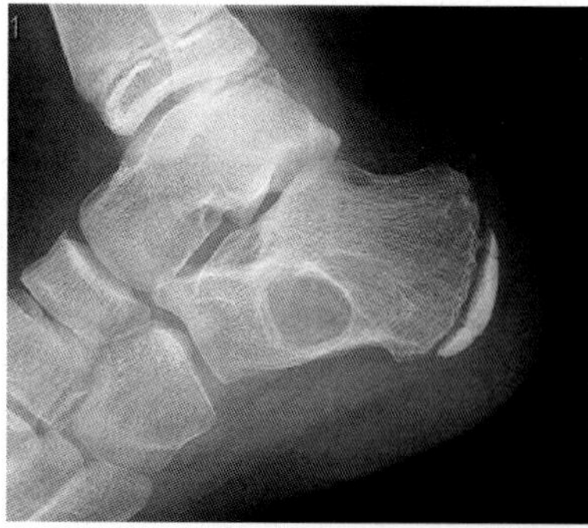

**FIG 1** • Lateral radiograph of the foot of a 12-year-old boy demonstrates a well-circumscribed, lucent lesion, consistent with unicameral bone cyst.

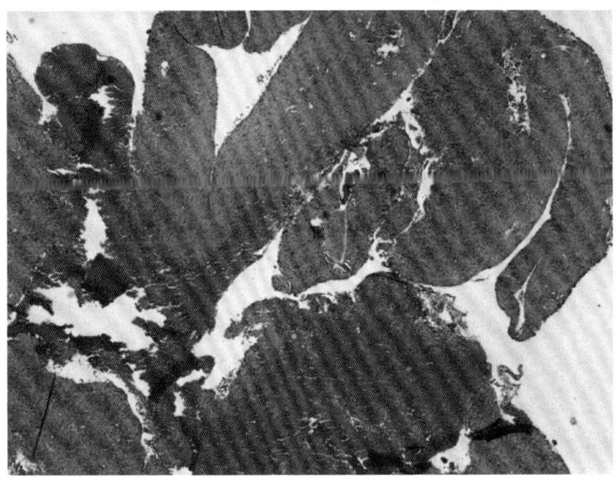


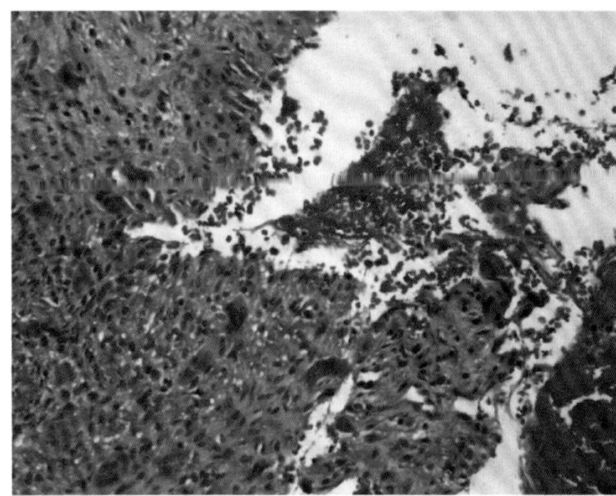


**FIG 2** • High-power (200× magnification; **A**) and low-power (40× magnification; **B**) photomicrographs of a lesion demonstrate blood-filled spaces surrounded by several focal giant cells as well as spindle-shaped cells lining the walls of these spaces. Some of the spaces are slit-like, whereas the other spaces are dilated. Hemosiderin is also seen.

## DIFFERENTIAL DIAGNOSIS

- Aneurysmal bone cyst (ABC)
- Nonossifying fibroma (NOF)
- Fibrous dysplasia (differential with latent/diaphyseal UBC)
- Brown tumor of hyperparathyroidism (usually presents with osteopenia and subcortical resorption)
- Osteomyelitis (commonly shows periosteal reaction)
- For calcaneus lesions, the differential also includes chondroblastoma and giant cell tumor.

## NONOPERATIVE MANAGEMENT

- Lesions with typical radiographic appearance involving non–weight-bearing bones, especially in the absence of significant cortical thinning, can be followed with serial radiographs.
- Small lesions (ie, those that involve less than one-third to half of the bone width) in weight-bearing bones that have low risk for fracture can also be observed.
- Following pathologic fracture, up to 15% of UBCs may spontaneously heal, and therefore an attempt for conservative treatment should be made. Exceptions include large lesions and unstable or displaced fractures of lower extremities, especially in older children.

# ANEURYSMAL BONE CYST

## DEFINITION

- ABC is a benign, active, and sometimes locally aggressive, solitary, expansile blood-filled cystic lesion, eccentric in location, most commonly seen in the metaphyseal region of long bones or posterior elements of the spine.

## PATHOGENESIS

- The neoplastic basis of primary ABCs has been, at least in part, demonstrated by the chromosomal translocation t(16;17)(q22;p13) that places the ubiquitin protease (UBP) *USP6* gene under the regulatory influence of the highly active osteoblast *cadherin 11* gene (CDH11), which is strongly expressed in bones. Abnormalities of the short arm of chromosome 17 appear to be recurrent.
- The lesion contains blood-filled cystic spaces that are not lined with vascular endothelium, divided by fibrous septa containing giant cells and immature bone (**FIG 2**).

## NATURAL HISTORY

- ABC can present as an active or locally aggressive lesion that tends to continue to grow and warrants intervention.
- They may also occur in association with other lesions such as giant cell tumor, osteoblastoma, chondroblastoma, or fibrous dysplasia.

## PATIENT HISTORY AND PHYSICAL FINDINGS

- ABCs often present with pain. Sometimes, swelling or a "mass" can be present.
- Pathologic fracture is not as prevalent as in UBC but it may occur following minor trauma.
- The most common locations are the metaphysis of long bones, particularly the femur and tibia, and the posterior elements of the spine.

## IMAGING AND OTHER DIAGNOSTIC STUDIES

- Plain radiographs show an eccentric, multilobulated, expansile (often expanding beyond the width of the nearest growth plate), radiolucent lesion with a narrow zone of transition.
  - Cortical thinning, disruption, and periosteal reaction are common.
- CT is helpful, for better characterization and treatment planning of axial lesions (**FIG 3A,B**).
  - CT demonstrates the typical ridges in the interior of the cyst.
  - Soft tissue extension can be appreciated, but there is no true soft tissue mass.
- MRI is useful to confirm the lobulated nature of the lesion and the cystic cavities filled with fluid; fluid levels on T2-weighted signal are characteristic but not pathognomonic (**FIG 3C,D**).
  - There is variable signal intensity in both T1- and T2-weighted images due to the nature of the cyst contents (fresh blood, mixed with degraded blood products).

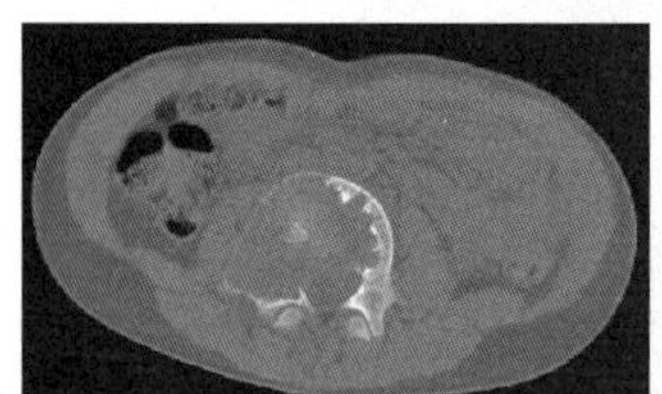
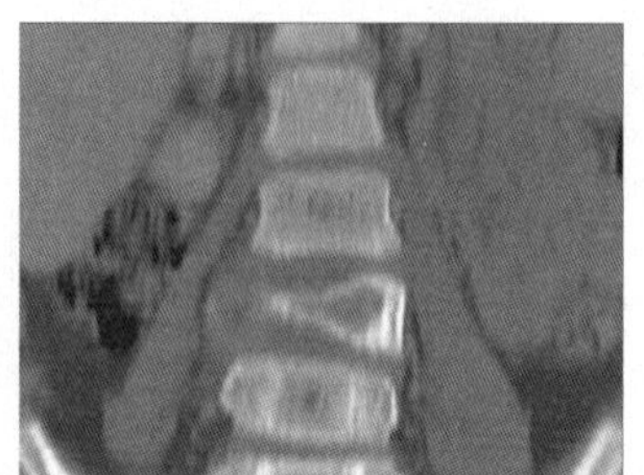
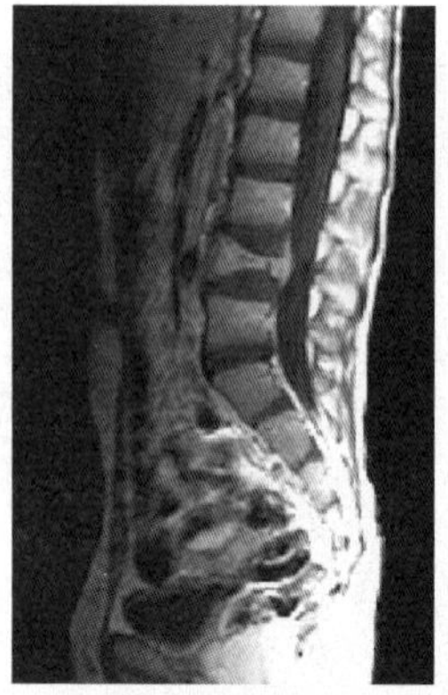
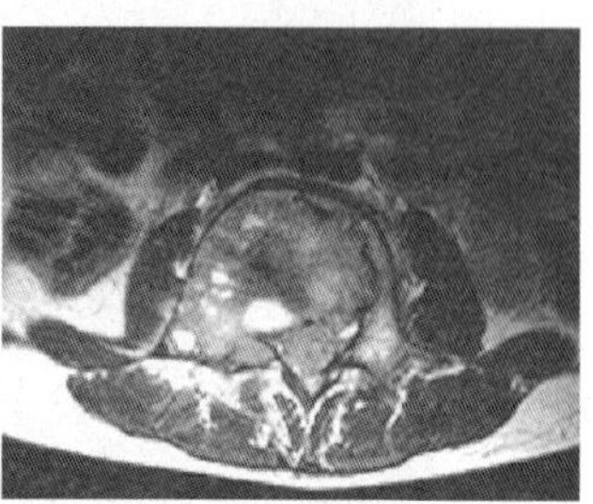

**FIG 3** • ABC of L4. **A.** Axial CT scan of the lower lumbar spine shows a destructive, lytic, expansile lesion, involving the body and posterior elements of L4 with disruption of the spinal canal. **B.** Three-dimensional reconstruction CT image demonstrates the asymmetric collapse of the vertebra. **C.** Sagittal T1 MRI shows the collapsed L4 with posterior disruption by the tumoral mass. **D.** Axial T2-weighted MRI shows the characteristic fluid–fluid level and disruption of the medullary canal.

## DIFFERENTIAL DIAGNOSIS

- UBC
- NOF
- Giant cell tumor
- Osteoblastoma
- Telangiectatic osteogenic sarcoma

## NONOPERATIVE MANAGEMENT

- There is little place for conservative treatment of ABCs. At least an incisional biopsy for diagnosis confirmation is recommended.
- For small, asymptomatic lesions located in non–weight-bearing bones, observation can be indicated.
- For lesions that are of difficult access/approach, serial embolization or sclerotherapy is another option.

# NONOSSIFYING FIBROMA

## DEFINITION

- NOF is a benign latent, cystic, eccentric, and cortical-based lesion that is most often found incidentally in the metaphyseal region of long bones. NOFs are the most common benign fibrous lesions, and it is estimated that up to 20% of all children have an NOF or the smaller counterpart, fibrous cortical defect. These lesions can be multicentric or synchronous.

## PATHOGENESIS

- NOF is part of a heterogeneous group of benign connective tissue tumors that are considered as reactive by many authors rather than a true neoplasm. Typically, they do not contain any bone and are characterized by a spindle cell proliferation with storiform arrangement of cells. Theories surround the notion that NOF is a developmental defect of the growth plate.
- There have only been three case reports demonstrating cytogenetic abnormalities in NOF, including a complex translocation involving chromosomes 3, 4, 11, and 14.

## NATURAL HISTORY

- The majority of NOF and fibrous cortical defects ossify (heal) spontaneously over time. At times, they can be associated with stress fractures, especially in very active children, or multicentric tumors.

## PATIENT HISTORY AND PHYSICAL FINDINGS

- The most common presentation is an incidental finding. At times, patients will report pain or discomfort, especially with physical activities; these cases are usually a reflection of a stress reaction or pathologic fracture. Most lesions are located around the knee and shoulder.

## IMAGING AND OTHER DIAGNOSTIC STUDIES

- Plain radiographs are usually diagnostic and demonstrate a well-defined, cortical-based/eccentric, lytic lesion with bubbly appearance, surrounded by a sharp sclerotic margin (**FIG 4A,B**).
- CT and MRI are usually not necessary for the diagnosis; however, they may be helpful for adequate evaluation of the lesion's size and extent as well as the presence of associated stress fracture (**FIG 4C,D**).

## DIFFERENTIAL DIAGNOSIS

- UBC
- ABC
- Osteofibrous dysplasia
- Chondromyxoid fibroma

## NONOPERATIVE MANAGEMENT

- Because NOF heals or ossifies over time, most lesions are amenable to conservative treatment. Large lesions in weight-bearing areas and/or associated with chronic pain or pathologic fracture may warrant surgical treatment.
- Unlike UBC, pathologic fracture associated to NOF will heal but the lesion will persist.

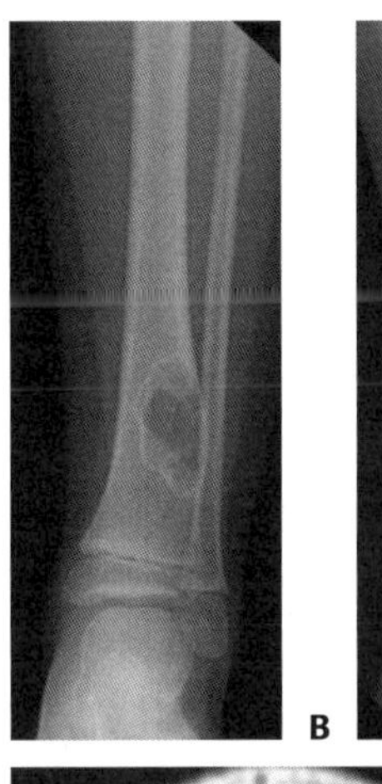
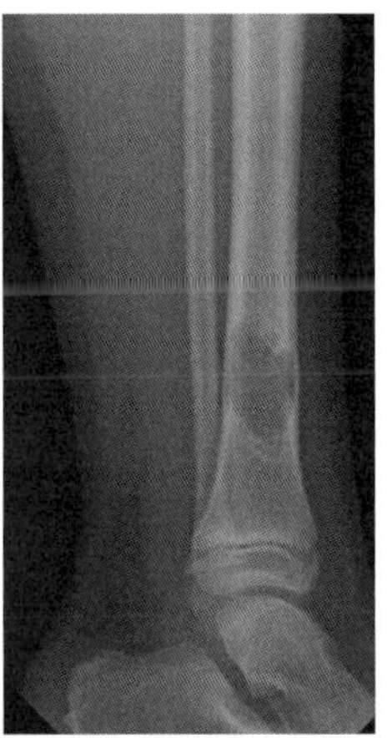
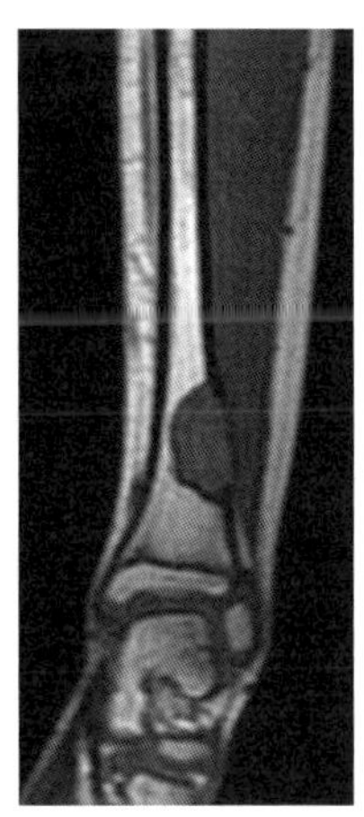
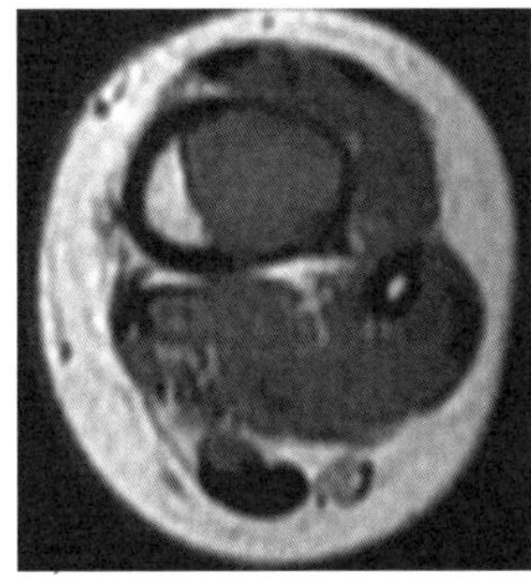

**FIG 4** ● NOF of the distal tibia. AP (**A**) and lateral (**B**) radiographs of a well-defined, cortical based, lytic lesion in the distal tibia metaphysis, surrounded by sharp sclerotic border, consistent with a NOF. MRI (**C,D**) shows low intensity on T1 and better defines the extent of the lesion and cortical involvement. There is no soft tissue extension or periosteal reaction.

# UNICAMERAL AND ANEURYSMAL BONE CYSTS AND NONOSSIFYING FIBROMAS

## SURGICAL MANAGEMENT

### Indications

- Diagnosis: The first indication for surgical treatment of these benign bone lesions is to confirm the diagnosis when the clinical and/or radiographic appearances are not classic.
- Symptoms: Although UBC and NOF are usually painless, ABC can be associated with significant pain that warrants treatment.
- Risk of fracture: Large lesions usually involving more than one-third to half of the bone width and lesions of weight-bearing bones are at a higher risk of pathologic fracture and may warrant surgery.
- Pathologic fracture: Although not an absolute indication for surgical treatment (especially in the upper extremities), fractures of weight bearing bones, especially around the hip, often need acute management. In general, it is preferred to wait for pathologic fractures to heal prior to treatment of the lesion.

### Preoperative Planning

- It is imperative to formulate the differential diagnosis and rule out a malignant process. If biopsy is planned, open biopsy yields best results, especially for ABC (filled with blood).
- Because most of these lesions are juxtaphyseal, it is important to rule out physeal involvement prior to any intervention.
- An image intensifier is useful for accurate localization of the lesion during percutaneous procedures and for intraoperative confirmation that the entire lesion is being addressed.
- Because most of these lesions are resected through a minimally invasive or limited approach, headlamps for illumination and loupes for magnification are recommended.
- Lesions in nonessential bones (eg, rib, fibula), in particular for locally aggressive ABC, can be treated with wide resection to avoid recurrence.

### Positioning

- Positioning depends on the lesion's location. For all extremity lesions, the entire affected extremity should be draped free. It is important to confirm that the extremity can be properly imaged by the image intensifier, especially for proximal lesions, such as around the shoulder and hip.

### Approach

- UBCs and NOFs are often latent lesions and therefore amenable to a percutaneous technique.
- ABCs are often locally aggressive, and a formal open approach with extensive curettage and adjuvants is recommended.
- Due to the risk involved with pathologic fractures and malunion around the hip, lesions in this region warrant a more aggressive approach, and often, open reduction and internal fixation is indicated (**FIG 5**).

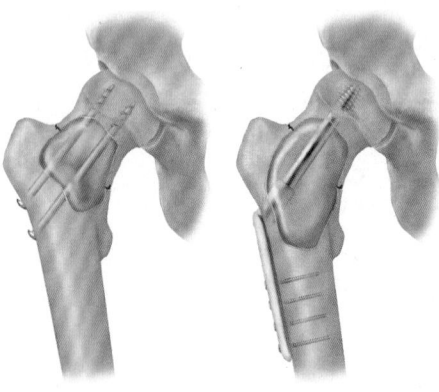

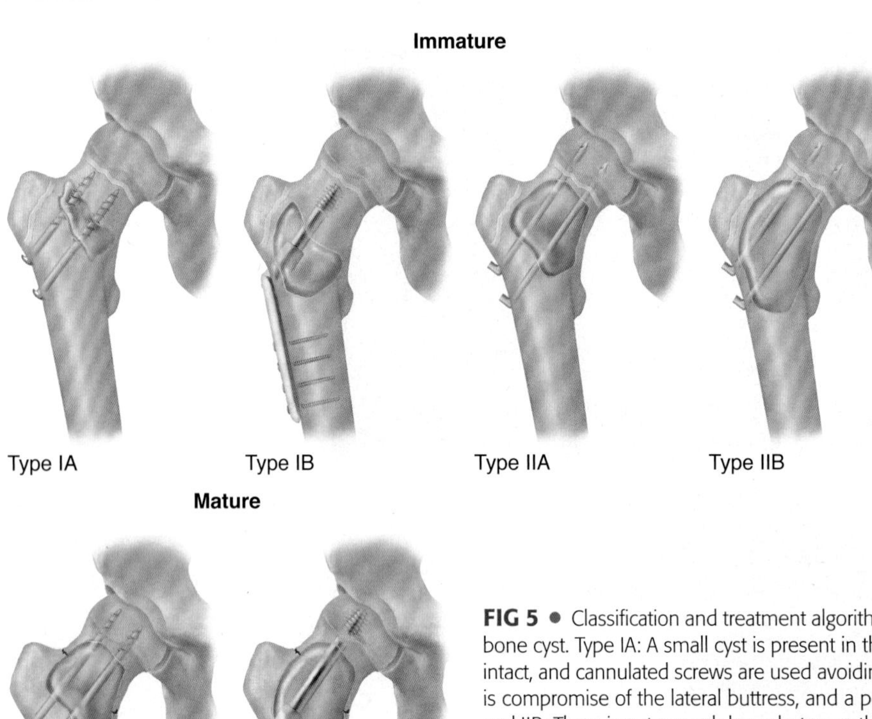


**FIG 5** • Classification and treatment algorithm for proximal femur pathologic fractures through a bone cyst. Type IA: A small cyst is present in the middle of the femoral neck, the lateral buttress is intact, and cannulated screws are used avoiding the physis. Type 1B: A larger cyst is present, there is compromise of the lateral buttress, and a pediatric dynamic hip screw (DHS) is used. Types IIA and IIB: There is not enough bone between the growth plate and the lesion; therefore, the patient can be kept in traction or a cast until initial healing occurs, or parallel Steinmann pins across the physis can be used. Type IIIA: Because the growth plate is closed, cannulated screws purchasing the femoral head are used. Type IIIB: Because of the loss of the lateral buttress, a pediatric DHS is recommended. A spica cast is generally recommended after the surgical treatment. Internal fixation should be preceded by a four-step approach. (Adapted from Dormans J, Flynn J. Pathologic fractures associated with tumors and unique conditions of the musculoskeletal system. In: Beaty JH, Kasser JR, eds. Rockwood and Wilkins' Fractures in Children, ed 5. Philadelphia: Lippincott Williams & Wilkins, 2001:151.)



## Percutaneous Intramedullary Decompression, Curettage, and Grafting with Medical-Grade Calcium Sulfate Pellets

- Under fluoroscopic guidance, a Jamshidi trocar needle (Cardinal Health, Dublin, OH) is percutaneously inserted into the cyst cavity/lesion.
- The cyst is aspirated to confirm the presence of straw-colored fluid, which is typical of previously untreated or unfractured UBCs; this step is not done for NOFs.
- Three to 10 mL of 50% diluted Renografin dye (E.R. Squibb & Sons, Princeton, NJ), or similar, is injected to perform a cystogram and confirm the single fluid-filled cavity (this step is not done for NOFs) (**TECH FIG 1A**).
- A 0.5-cm longitudinal incision is then made over the site of the aspiration and a 6-mm arthroscopy trocar is advanced into the cyst cavity through the same cortical hole, and the cortical entry (cortical window) is enlarged manually (**TECH FIG 1B**).
- Under fluoroscopic guidance, percutaneous removal of the cyst pseudo-lining or tumor contents is done, and curettage is performed using a pituitary rongeur and various-sized angled curettes (**TECH FIG 1C**).
- For UBCs, it's recommended to perform intramedullary decompression and this can be achieved using an angled curette or flexible intramedullary nail, in one direction (toward the diaphysis) or in both directions (when the growth plate is far enough away, avoiding penetration of the physis) (**TECH FIG 1D,E**).
  - For NOFs, curettage does not need to extend beyond the surrounding sclerotic bone into the medullary cavity, as this bone is structurally supportive.
- Medical-grade calcium sulfate pellets (Osteoset, Wright Medical Technology, Arlington, TN) are inserted through the same cortical hole and deployed to completely fill the cavity (**TECH FIG 1F,G**).
  - Angled curettes can be used to advance pellets into the medullary canal.
  - Tight packing of the cyst is preferred.
- The wound is closed in a layered fashion.

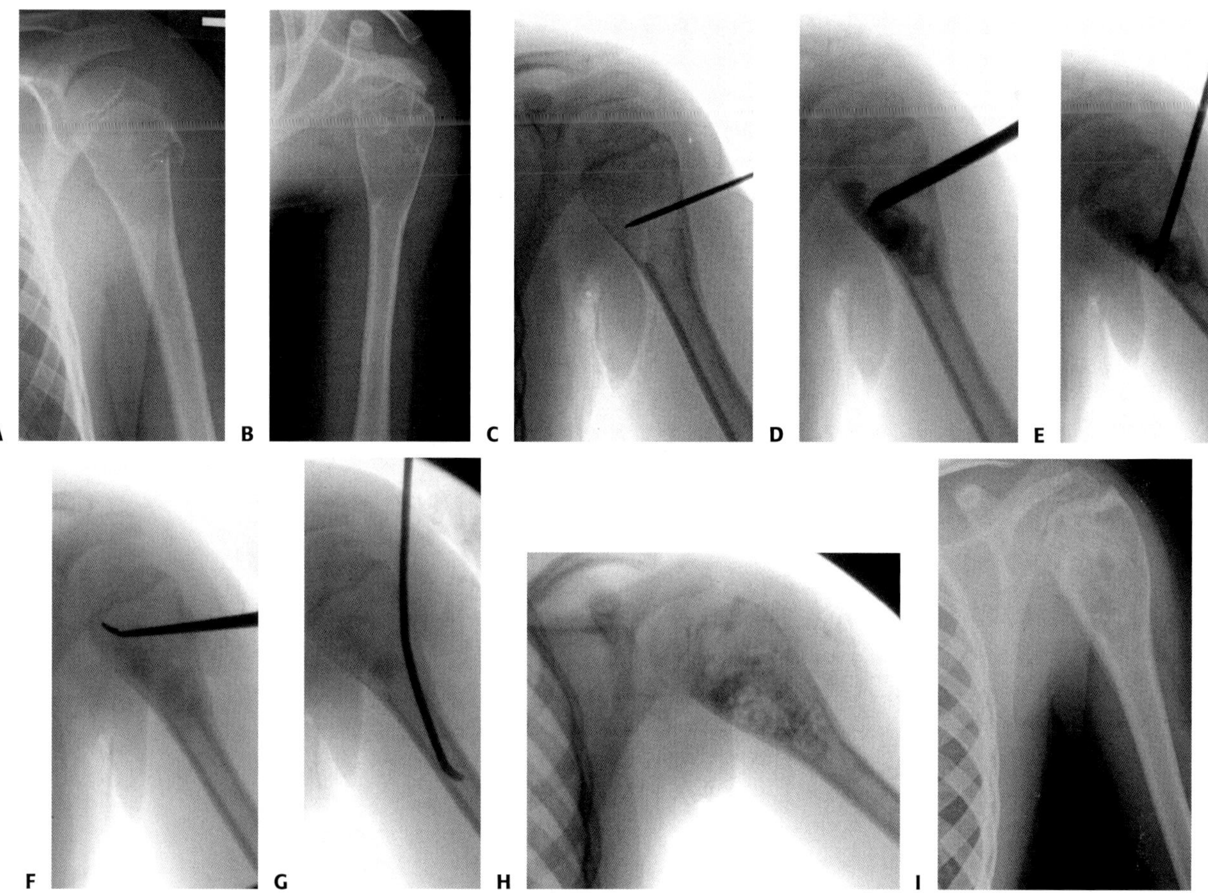

**TECH FIG 1** • UBC. **A.** Anteroposterior (AP) radiograph showing a pathologic fracture through a well-defined, lytic, central lesion in the proximal humerus metaphysis of a 6-year-old boy. **B.** At 4 weeks, the fracture has healed but the cyst persisted. **C.** Fluoroscopic image showing the placement of the Jamshidi needle. **D.** A 0.5-cm incision is made following the cystogram that showed some uneven filling, typical of postfractured cysts. The arthroscopy trocar is used to open a cortical window. **E,F.** The cyst is curetted using curettes and a pituitary rongeur. Material is then sent for pathology analysis. **G.** Intramedullary decompression of the cyst is done using flexible intramedullary nails or angled curettes. **H.** The cyst is filled with medical-grade calcium sulfate pellets. **I.** Three-month follow-up radiograph shows complete healing.

## Four-Step Approach with Open Curettage and Bone Grafting

- A more extensive, open approach is preferred for ABCs and for recurrent UBCs that have been previously treated with percutaneous techniques.
- Under fluoroscopic guidance, a Jamshidi trocar needle is percutaneously inserted into the cyst cavity.
- The cyst is aspirated to confirm the presence of blood-filled cavities or soft tissue septations typical of ABC.
- A longitudinal incision of roughly the same size of the cyst is made, the neurovascular structures are protected, and the periosteum is opened and retracted.
- Perforation of the thinnest part of the cyst wall is performed with a curette, burr, or drill.
- The fibrous lining of the lesion is completely curetted. Septations are opened and removed to access all components of the cyst.
  - The use of headlamps for illumination and loupes for magnification is recommended to ensure a thorough excision. Image intensifier may be helpful to ensure that all cavities were opened.
- A high-speed burr is used to improve the curettage and help with complete excision of any macroscopic tumor (extension of margins) (**TECH FIG 2A,B**).
- The cavity is then cauterized with electrocautery, and in selected cases, (eg, lesions distant from the growth plate and main neurovascular structures) phenol 5% solution is applied to the cyst wall with a cotton-tipped applicator to extend the margins.
  - Adjuvants are usually not needed for NOF; although recurrence is uncommon, incomplete excision will lead to persistence of the tumor.

- The cavity is now tightly packed with the bone graft of choice. For lesions that are not involving the subchondral bone, a combination of cancellous or corticocancellous allograft and demineralized bone matrix paste is usually preferred (**TECH FIG 2C–F**). For lesions that are juxta-articular and involving the subchondral bone, especially in the weight-bearing bones, a synthetic graft material, such as calcium sulfate/phosphate combo, is recommended for extra and acute structural support.
- The wound is closed in a layered fashion.

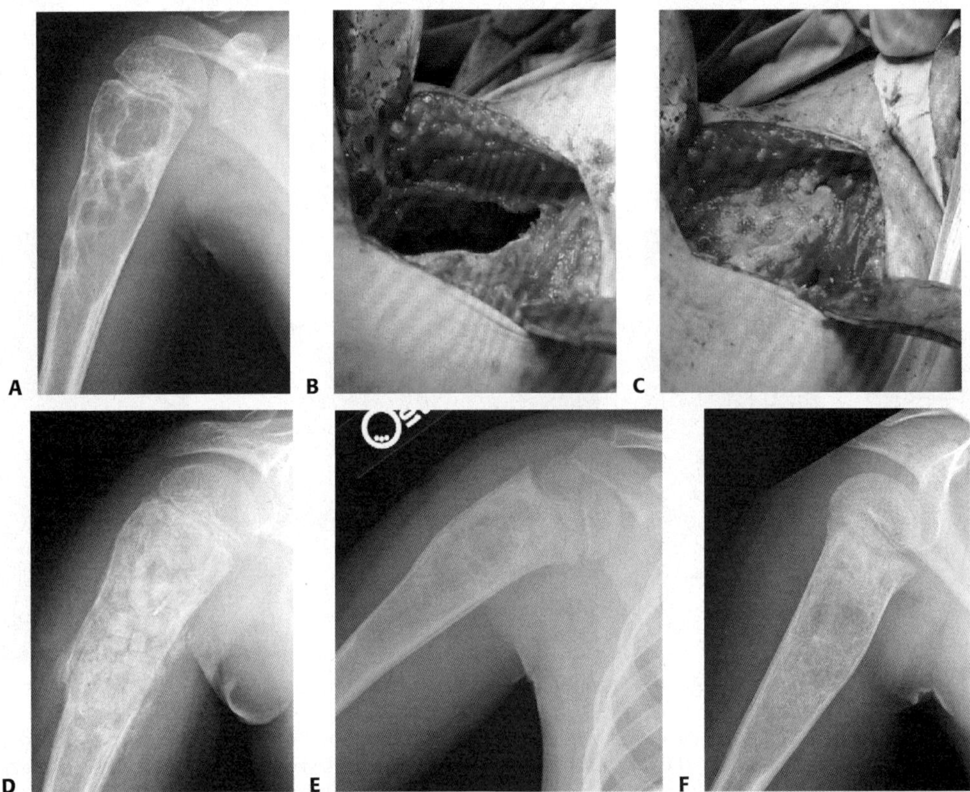

**TECH FIG 2** • **A.** Anteroposterior (AP) radiograph of the proximal humerus shows an expansile, lytic, loculated ABC. **B.** The cyst is thoroughly curetted, and a high-speed burr is used to remove any residual cyst lining. **C.** The cyst is completely filled with packed allograft chips and demineralized bone matrix. **D.** Radiographic aspect 2 weeks after the procedure; the cyst was entirely removed and the cavity was entirely grafted. **E,F.** At 4-month follow-up, AP radiographs of the right proximal humerus in internal and external rotation demonstrate that the lesion is completely healed, with good incorporation of the bone graft.

## PEARLS AND PITFALLS

| | |
|---|---|
| **Diagnosis** | ■ UBC and NOF diagnosis can be made solely based on radiographic findings.<br>■ The surgeon should always biopsy ABCs to rule out malignancies and other associated conditions. |
| **Growth arrest** | ■ Growth arrest can occur without or prior to the treatment. The family should be informed if there is a suspicion of growth plate damage before the treatment. MRI helps confirm physeal involvement. |
| **Pathologic fracture** | ■ UBCs may spontaneously resolve after fractures, so adopt a conservative treatment (if possible). |
| **Natural history** | ■ UBCs tend to grow away from the growth plate and will not grow after skeletal maturity. ABCs continue to grow beyond skeletal maturity. NOF heals over time and are most amenable to observation. |
| **Recurrent lesions** | ■ Bone cysts may "upgrade." UBCs may recur with an ABC component and ABCs may recur with a more aggressive behavior than the initial lesion. NOF may develop a secondary ABC.<br>■ Most recurrences following treatment occur in the first 24 months. |

## POSTOPERATIVE CARE

- In most cases, the extremity is protected from weight bearing for about 4 to 6 weeks. Before the patient is allowed to return to physical activity, radiographic evidence of bone healing is necessary, that can take up to 3 months.

## OUTCOMES

- The minimally invasive technique for UBC has shown promising results on a short-term evaluation, with reported success rate (eg, complete or partial healing or opacification) of about 95%; the intermediate- to long-term results (>2 years) show 80% complete or partial response following one surgical intervention.
  - Nonetheless, the success rate increases to 94% after a repeat surgery, reaching a 100% healing rate in patients who undergo more than two repeat surgeries.
  - These results compare favorably with outcomes after other surgical treatment of UBCs.
- The recurrence rate for any surgically treated ABC varies from 10% to 59% according to the reported results. In a large cohort including 45 children with primary ABC treated by the described four-step approach technique and at least 2 years of follow-up, the recurrence rate was only 18%.
  - Although the recurrence rate was slightly higher among younger children (younger than 10 years old), this difference did not show statistical significance.

## COMPLICATIONS

- Persistence or recurrence: varies from 10% to 20% for all techniques described
- Infection
- Allergic reaction to the graft (<5%)
- Fracture (intraoperative or postoperative)
- Intraoperative bleeding: For aggressive-looking ABCs and lesions in difficult locations such as the pelvis and spine, preoperative embolization is helpful.

## SUGGESTED READINGS


1. Althof PA, Ohmori K, Zhou M, et al. Cytogenetic and molecular cytogenetic findings in 43 aneurysmal bone cysts: aberrations of 17p mapped to 17p13.2 by fluorescence in situ hybridization. Mod Pathol 2004;17(5):518–525.
2. Boriani S, De Iure F, Campanacci L, et al. Aneurysmal bone cyst of the mobile spine: report on 41 cases. Spine 2001;26:27–35.
3. Brassesco MS, Valera ET, Engel EE, et al. Clonal complex chromosome aberration in non-ossifying fibroma. Pediatr Blood Cancer 2010;54:764–767.
4. Campanacci M, De Sessa L, Trentani C. Scaglietti's method for conservative treatment of simple bone cysts with local injections of methylprednisolone acetate. Ital J Orthop Traumatol 1977;3:27–36.
5. Cohen J. Etiology of simple bone cyst. J Bone Joint Surg Am 1970;52(7):1493–1497.
6. Dormans JP, Hanna BG, Johnston DR, et al. Surgical treatment and recurrence rate of aneurysmal bone cysts in children. Clin Orthop Relat Res 2004;(421):205–211.
7. Dormans JP, Sankar WN, Moroz L, et al. Percutaneous intramedullary decompression, curettage, and grafting with medical-grade calcium sulfate pellets for unicameral bone cysts in children: a new minimally invasive technique. J Pediatr Orthop 2005;25:804–811.
8. Garg S, Mehta S, Dormans JP. Modern surgical treatment of primary aneurysmal bone cyst of the spine in children and adolescents. J Pediatr Orthop 2005;25:387–392.
9. Mankin HJ, Hornicek FJ, Ortiz-Cruz E, et al. Aneurysmal bone cyst: a review of 150 patients. J Clin Oncol 2005;23:6756–6762.
10. Mik G, Arkader A, Manteghi A, et al. Results of a minimally invasive technique for the treatment of unicameral bone cysts. Clin Orthop Relat Res 2009;467(11):2949–2954.
11. Oliveira AM, Perez-Atayde AR, Inwards CY, et al. USP6 and CDH11 oncogenes identify the neoplastic cell in primary aneurysmal bone cysts and are absent in so-called secondary aneurysmal bone cysts. Am J Pathol 2004;165:1773–1780.
12. Ramirez AR, Stanton RP. Aneurysmal bone cyst in 29 children. J Pediatr Orthop 2002;22:533–539.
13. Richkind KE, Mortimer E, Mowery-Rushton P, et al. Translocation (16;20)(p11.2;q13), sole cytogenetic abnormality in a unicameral bone cyst. Cancer Genet Cytogenet 2002;137:153–155.
14. Shimal A, Davies AM, James SL, et al. Fatigue-type stress fractures of the lower limb associated with fibrous cortical defects/non-ossifying fibromas in the skeletally immature. Clin Radiol 2010;65:382–386.
15. Sullivan RJ, Meyer JS, Dormans JP, et al. Diagnosing aneurysmal and unicameral bone cysts with magnetic resonance imaging. Clin Orthop Relat Res 1999;(366):186–190.

# Upper Extremity

# Release of Simple Syndactyly

Donald S. Bae

## DEFINITION

- *Syndactyly* refers to the failure of separation between adjacent digits, resulting in "webbed" fingers.
- Congenital syndactyly is classified according to the extent of digital involvement and the character of the conjoined tissue.
  - *Complete syndactyly* extends to the digital tips (**FIG 1A**), whereas *incomplete syndactyly* ends proximal to the fingertips (**FIG 1B**).
  - *Simple syndactyly* refers to digits connected only by skin and soft tissue. *Complex syndactyly* denotes bony fusions between adjacent phalanges.
  - *Complicated syndactyly* refers to the interposition of accessory phalanges or abnormal bones between digits.

## ANATOMY

- Understanding of normal digital web space anatomy guides surgical reconstructive efforts.
- Typically, the index–long and ring–small finger commissures are U-shaped, whereas the long–ring web is V-shaped.
- The nonglabrous skin of the normal web space is sloped about 45 degrees from proximal–dorsal to distal–volar, extending to roughly the midpoint of the proximal phalanx.
- The natatory ligaments (or superficial transverse metacarpal ligament) help form the web contour and join adjacent lateral digital sheets.
- Normally, each digit is vascularized in part via a radial and an ulnar digital artery, which arise from the bifurcation of the common digital arteries.
- In simple syndactyly, adjacent digits are joined by varying amounts of skin and soft tissue.
  - The nail plates may or may not be fused.
  - The joints, ligaments, and tendons of the affected digits usually are normal.
- It is of critical surgical importance that the bifurcation of the digital arteries and nerves may be abnormally distal in cases of syndactyly.

## PATHOGENESIS

- Syndactyly represents a failure of differentiation and is so classified by the embryologic classification of congenital anomalies adopted by the International Federation for Societies for Surgery of the Hand.
- Embryologically, the digits arise from condensations of mesoderm within the rudimentary hand paddle of the developing upper limb.
- During the fifth and sixth weeks of gestation, interdigital clefts form through the process of apoptosis, or programmed cell death, beginning at the digital tips and proceeding in a distal to proximal direction.
- The apical ectodermal ridge regulates this embryologic process, in conjunction with fibroblast growth factors, bone morphogenetic proteins, transforming growth factors, homeobox gene products, and the sonic hedgehog protein.
- Interruption of this precise and highly regulated process results in syndactyly.

## NATURAL HISTORY

- There is no potential for spontaneous resolution.
- Given the importance of independent digit function in today's world, surgical release is recommended for simple complete syndactyly, with few exceptions.
- When digits of differing lengths are joined, the syndactyly may lead to deformity and growth disturbance, with the longer digit typically developing a flexion contracture and angular deviation toward the shorter digit.
- Simple complete syndactyly of the long–ring interspace may be well tolerated and may not significantly compromise growth or function in young patients.
- Simple incomplete syndactylies may be aesthetically subtle and cause little functional compromise. In these situations, observation may be considered.

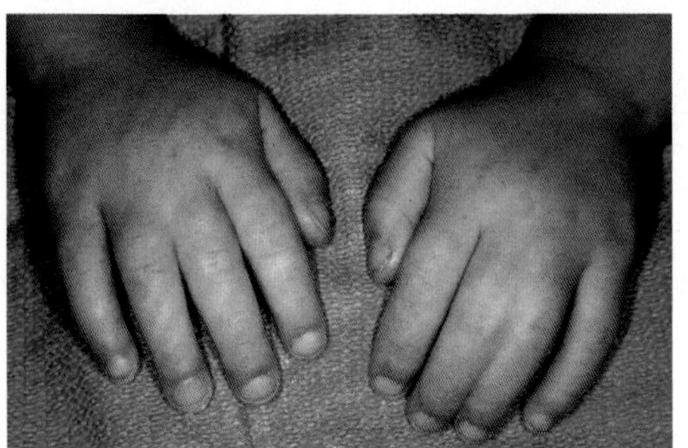

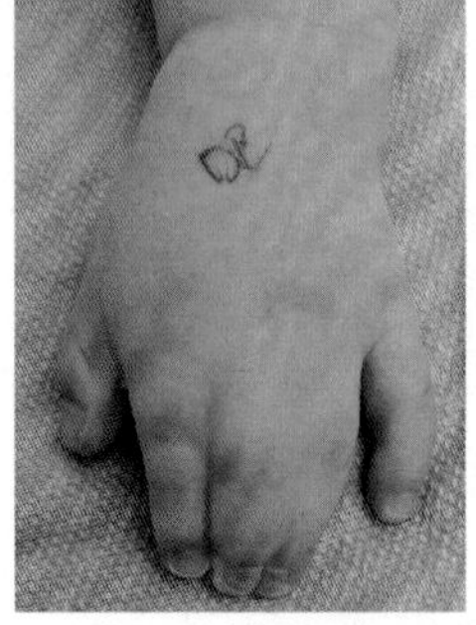

**FIG 1** • **A.** Simple incomplete syndactylies of the bilateral third web spaces, with the left hand more severely affected. **B.** Simple complete syndactyly of the second and third web spaces is seen in another patient. Observe the conjoined fingernail (synonychia) between the long and ring fingers. (Copyright © 2006 Children's Orthopaedic Surgery Foundation.)

## PATIENT HISTORY AND PHYSICAL FINDINGS

- The diagnosis of syndactyly usually is not subtle, and the extent of digital involvement typically is readily apparent.
- Syndactyly is the most common congenital hand anomaly, with an estimated incidence of 1 in 2000 to 2500 live births.
  - The true incidence of syndactyly is unknown, in part because of the difficulty distinguishing mild simple syndactylies from normal web spaces.
- The third web space is most commonly affected (50%), followed by the fourth (30%), second (15%), and first (5%) web spaces.
- Males tend to be more commonly affected than females and whites more than blacks or Asians.
- Inheritance is thought to be autosomal dominant with incomplete penetrance and variable expression.
- The absence of differential motion of the affected digits suggests a complex or complicated syndactyly.
- Because the joints and tendons usually are normal, patients typically have flexion and extension creases over the interphalangeal joints and active digital motion.
- Syndactyly may exist in isolation or may be seen in the context of associated clinical syndromes, including Poland syndrome, Apert syndrome, and constriction band syndrome. For this reason, careful evaluation of the entire upper extremity, contralateral upper limb, chest, and feet is advised.

## IMAGING AND OTHER DIAGNOSTIC STUDIES

- Plain radiographs of the affected digits or hand are routinely obtained to accurately classify the syndactyly and assess for bony fusions or interposed or accessory bones (**FIG 2**).
- Magnetic resonance imaging (MRI), angiography, or other diagnostic studies are not typically obtained because they do not assist surgical decision making or operative treatment.

## NONOPERATIVE MANAGEMENT

- Nonoperative management may be considered for mild, simple incomplete syndactyly.
- Nonoperative treatment also may be favored in cases of complicated syndactyly with the so-called "superdigit" or in cases of complex polysyndactyly because of the difficulty in achieving reproducible functional improvement with surgical release.

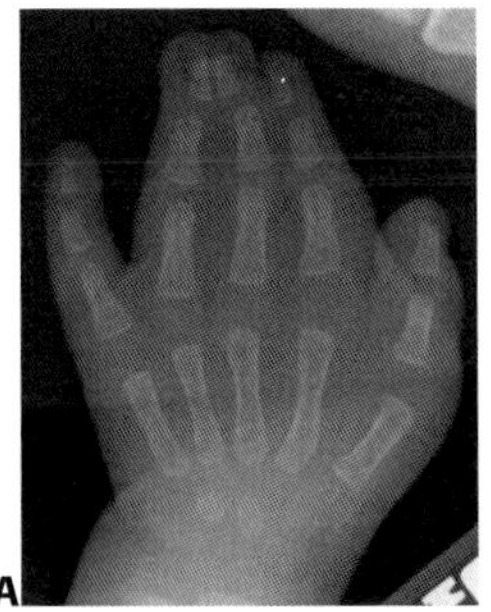

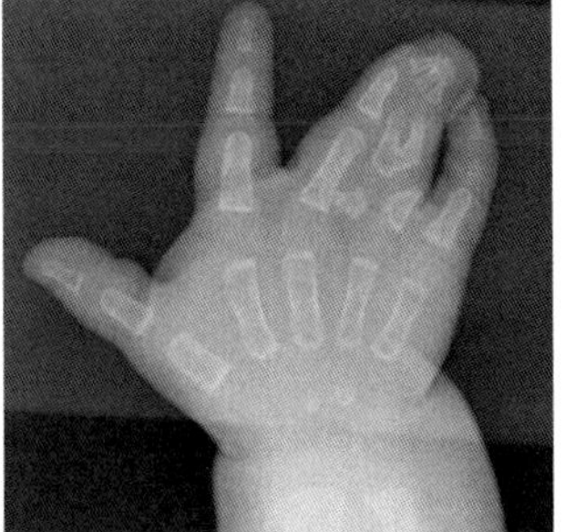

**FIG 2** • **A.** Anteroposterior (AP) radiograph of the patient depicted in **FIG 1B**. Note the simple complete syndactyly between the index and long fingers and a complex complete syndactyly between the long and ring fingers. **B.** AP radiograph depicting a complicated polysyndactyly in another patient.

- However, given the importance of independent digital motion—particularly in the current keyboard-driven digital age—nonoperative treatment of simple complete syndactyly is not recommended.

## SURGICAL MANAGEMENT

- General surgical principles include the following:
  - Digits of differing lengths should be released early to prevent deformity and growth disturbance of the affected digits.
  - Digits should be operated upon on only one side at the same time to avoid vascular embarrassment.
  - Local skin flaps should be used to recreate the commissure to avoid scar contracture and "web creep."
  - Zigzag lateral flaps should be created to avoid longitudinal scar contracture.
  - Judicious defatting of the skin flaps should be performed to facilitate skin closure, reduce tension across the flaps, and improve the aesthetics of the reconstructed fingers.
  - Full-thickness skin grafts typically are used to cover "bare areas" after syndactyly release. (In cases of simple complete syndactyly, the combined circumference of the separated digits is 22% greater than the original circumference of the syndactylized digits.)[7,8]

### Preoperative Planning

- The timing of surgery must be considered in preoperative planning.
- There is great variability in recommendations of when releases should be performed.
  - Flatt[8] wrote, "I believe one should ask not how soon the operation can be done but rather how late the functional demands of the hand will allow postponement of surgery."
  - In general, releases are performed between 6 and 24 months of age.
- As mentioned, digits of differing lengths (eg, thumb–index syndactyly) should be released earlier to avoid secondary deformity.
- There is some evidence that releases performed after 18 months have better long-term outcomes with lower incidence of web creep.[9,10]

### Positioning

- The patient is positioned supine with the affected limb supported on a hand table.
- Placement of a sterile or nonsterile tourniquet must be sufficiently proximal to allow access to the antecubital fossa, if full-thickness skin graft is to be taken from that site.
- If the skin graft is to be harvested from the inguinal region, the ipsilateral groin is prepared and draped to allow for easy access.
- Before draping, a surgical pen may be used to mark the inguinal skin fold when the hip is flexed; graft harvest along this axis will allow for a more aesthetic skin closure.
- Care should be taken to harvest the skin graft lateral to the femoral artery to avoid transfer of hair-bearing skin.

### Approach

- The principles of separation for simple complete syndactyly are well accepted; however, there is tremendous variation in the surgical incisions and skin flap designs used for these operations.

- All use local tissue to reconstruct the interdigital commissure, and all employ interdigitating zigzag lateral flaps. Dorsal skin flaps are preferred for commissure reconstruction because of their pliability and ability to recreate the normal dorsal–proximal to volar–distal slope of the web.
- When dorsal skin is used to create the commissure, the length of the dorsal flap should approximate two-thirds of the length of the proximal phalanx to create an appropriate slope to the web. The proximal extent of the volar incision will become the new palmodigital crease (**FIG 3A**).
- Furthermore, flaps are designed to interdigitate during closure; to achieve this, palmar triangular flaps are based at the level corresponding to the apex of the dorsal flaps. These flaps usually are fashioned to traverse between the midlines of the syndactylized digits.
- **FIG 3B** shows examples of skin incisions for simple complete syndactyly releases.[17]

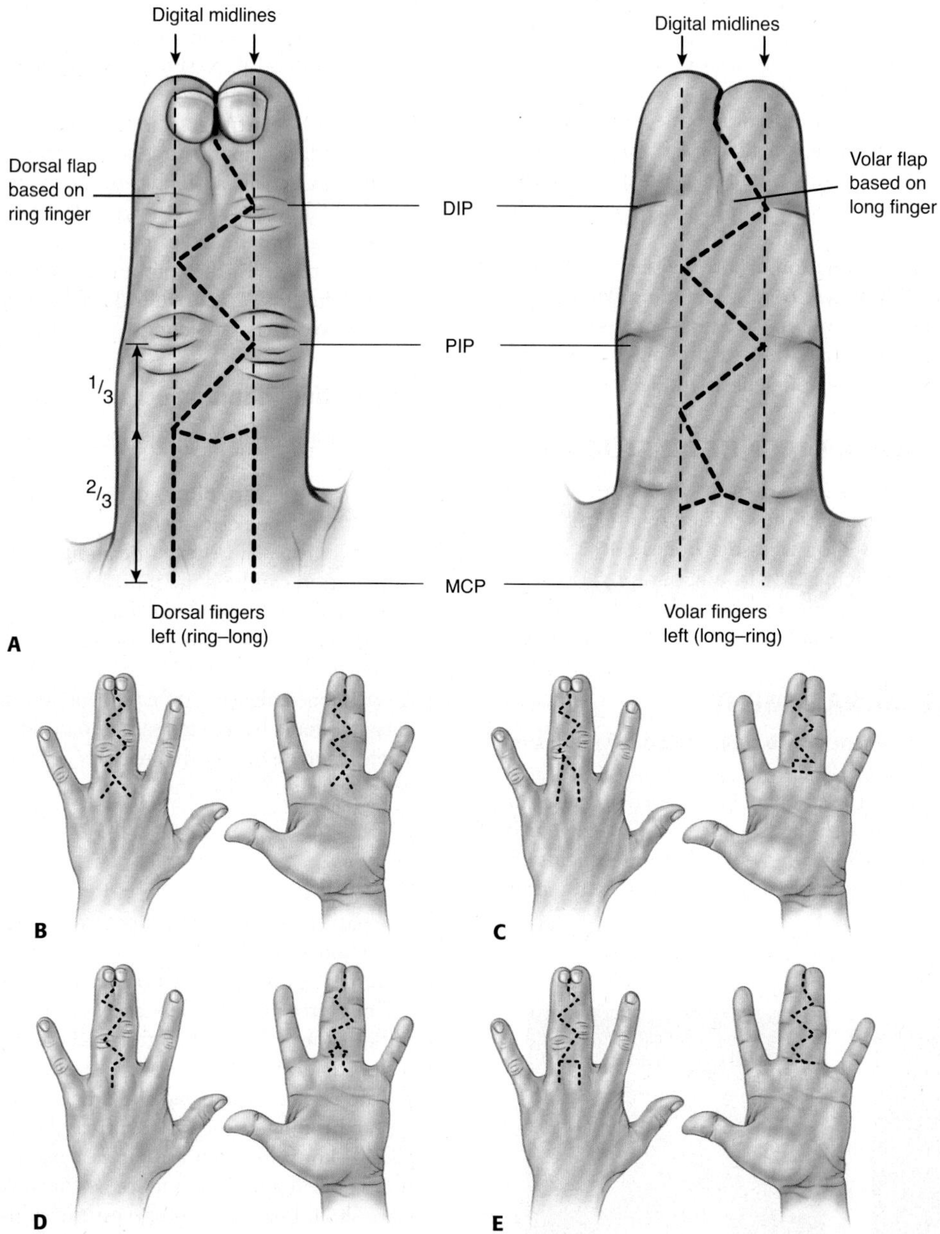


**FIG 3** • **A.** Skin incision design. The dorsal skin flap measures approximately two-thirds the length of the proximal phalanx, and the zigzag incisions are fashioned between the midlines of the syndactylized digits. **B–I.** Skin incisions used for release of simple complete syndactyly. (**B:** Cronin, 1943; **C:** Flatt, 1962; **D:** Blauth, 1970; **E:** Hentz, 1977; **F:** Upton, 1984; **G:** Gilbert, 1986; **H:** Wood, 1998; **I:** James, 2005.) *(continued)*

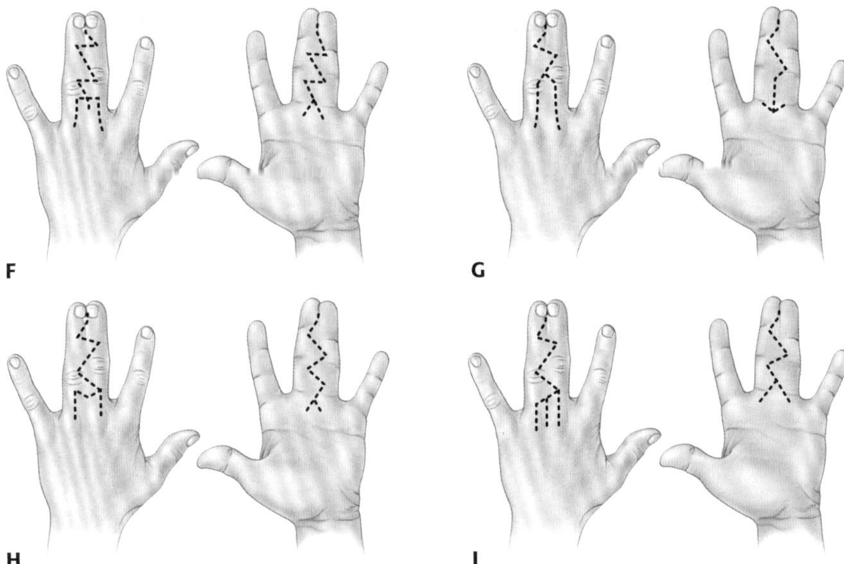

FIG 3 • *(continued)*



## Release of Simple Syndactyly

### Release of Simple Complete Syndactyly Using Full-Thickness Skin Graft

- After the tourniquet is inflated, the skin is incised, and hemostasis is achieved with bipolar electrocautery (**TECH FIG 1A,B**).
- Dorsal skin flaps are raised first, preserving the extensor paratenon.
- Volar skin flaps are then raised, and neurovascular bundles are identified.
- Digits are carefully separated distal to proximal, releasing the interdigital fascia that often connects the syndactylized digits (**TECH FIG 1C**). The transverse metacarpal ligament is not divided.
- The bifurcation of the common digital artery and nerve is identified; if there is a distal bifurcation precluding restoration of the commissure with the dorsal skin flap, consideration may be given to splitting the fascicles of the common digital nerve or ligating one of the proper digital arteries.
  - For isolated syndactyly release, the smaller caliber or nondominant artery may be taken.

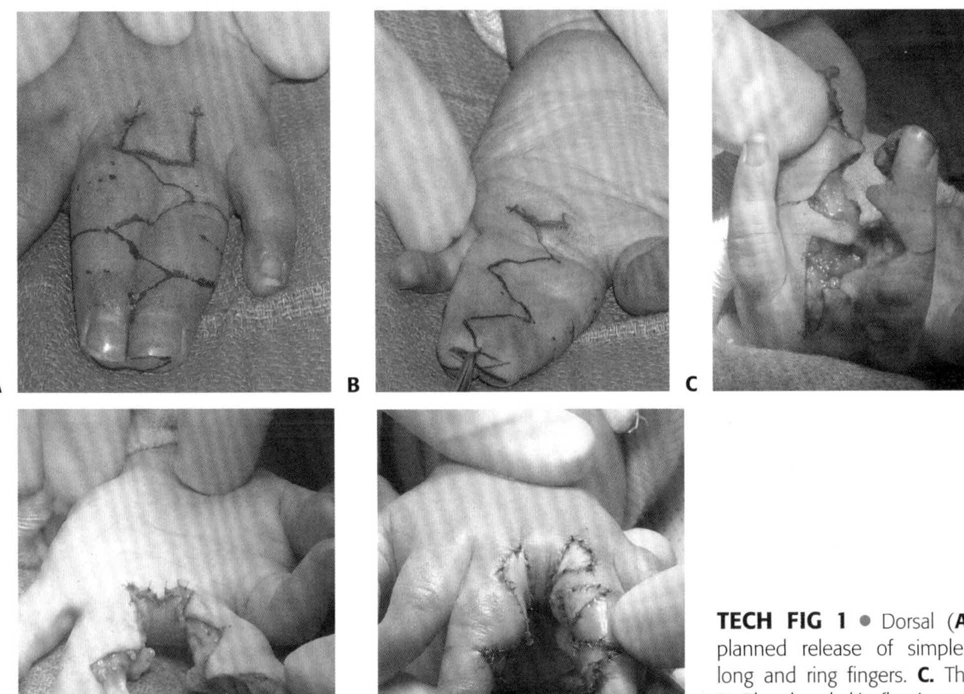

**TECH FIG 1** • Dorsal (**A**) and volar (**B**) incisions for planned release of simple complete syndactyly of the long and ring fingers. **C.** The digits have been separated. **D.** The dorsal skin flap is sewn in to recreate the interdigital commissure. **E.** Completion of the release with full-thickness skin grafting. (Copyright 2006 Children's Orthopaedic Surgery Foundation.)

- If a syndactyly release is planned on the other side of one of the digits, its proper digital artery should be preserved.
- Skin flaps are then defatted and allowed to interdigitate.
- The dorsal skin flap is then advanced to the palmodigital crease and secured with multiple interrupted 5-0 absorbable sutures (eg, chromic or polyglactin; **TECH FIG 1D**).
- Interdigitated skin flaps are similarly reapproximated with multiple interrupted 5-0 absorbable suture.
- Skin defects are identified and covered with full-thickness skin graft, which may be harvested from the hypothenar eminence, antecubital fossa, or inguinal region (**TECH FIG 1E**).
- The tourniquet is deflated, and vascularity of the digits and flaps is confirmed.
- A nonadherent gauze bolstered with moist cotton is then placed into the newly formed web space, applying gentle compression to the skin graft sites.
  - Care should be taken to place the dressing deep within the commissure to avoid resyndactylization during the healing process.
- An above-elbow cast is then applied with the elbow in 90 degrees of flexion, with liberal use of casting material to protect the surgical dressing.

## Reconstruction of the Paronychium

- In cases of simple complete syndactyly, the nail plates of the involved digits are conjoined, a phenomenon known as *synonychia*.
- Although division of the midportion of the nail plate is easily performed, care must be made to reconstitute the nail folds.
  - Ideally, this is performed using local tissue from the digital pulp.[2]
  - Laterally based flaps are incorporated into the skin incisions, raised from the shared hyponychium at the digital tips (**TECH FIG 2**).
  - The length of the flaps should equal the length of the nail plate.
  - Once these flaps are raised and the digits separated, the flaps are easily rotated and reapproximated adjacent to the new nail plates, recreating a paronychial fold.
  - Alternative solutions, including the use of skin graft, thenar or hypothenar flaps, or free composite toe grafts, are more involved and may provide less pleasing aesthetic results.

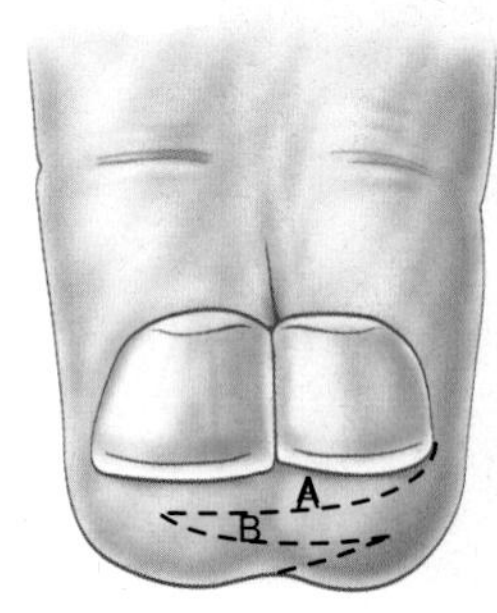


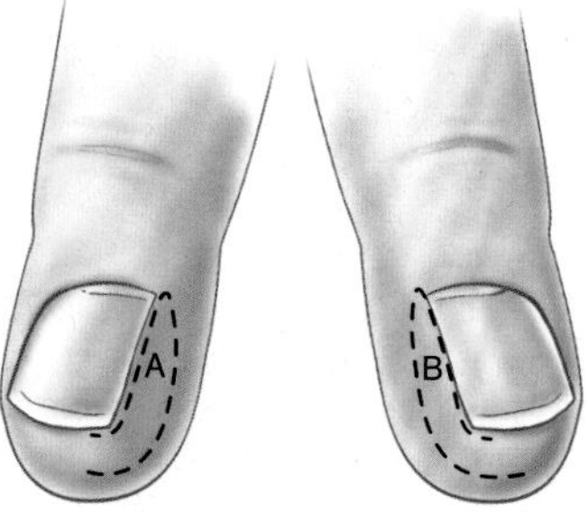


**TECH FIG 2** • Schematic diagram depicting the incisions used to release a synoncychia, using local tissue to reconstitute the nail folds.

## Technique of "Graftless" Syndactyly Release

- Simple complete syndactyly releases may also be performed without the need for full-thickness skin grafting.[1,5,11,12]
- In general, principles of syndactyly release mentioned earlier apply.
- In graftless techniques, however, dorsal skin is raised from the dorsum of the hand and advanced to recreate the interdigital commissure. The resulting defect is closed primarily in the fashion of a V-Y advancement flap (**TECH FIG 3**).
- Because proximal skin is used to recreate the web, more tissue is available to allow for primary closure of the digits following judicious defatting of the flaps, obviating the need for skin grafting.
- The use of preoperative tissue expansion to avoid the need for skin grafting for syndactyly release has been proposed. Results have been unpredictable at best, however, and this approach currently is not widely accepted.

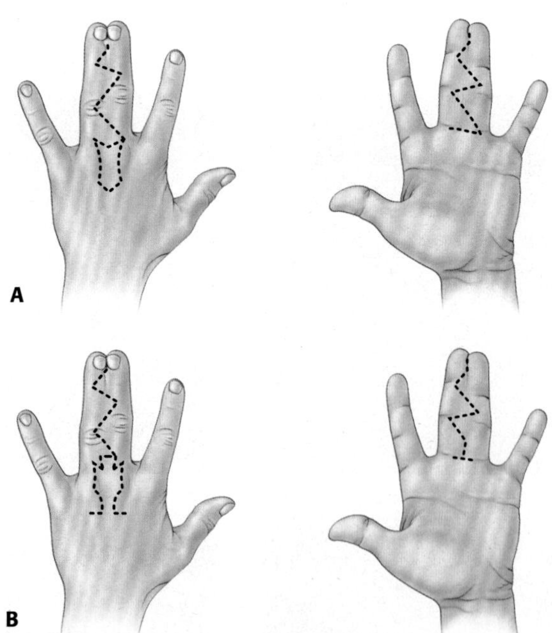


**TECH FIG 3** • **A,B.** Schematic diagram depicting incisions used to perform graftless syndactyly releases. (**A:** From Sherif MM. V-Y dorsal metacarpal flap: a new technique for the correction of syndactyly without skin graft. Plast Reconstr Surg 1998;101:1861–1866; **B:** From Niranjan NS, DeCarpentier J. A new technique for the division of syndactyly. Eur J Plast Surg 1990;13:101–104; Ekerot L. Syndactyly correction without skin-grafting. J Hand Surg Br 1996;21:330–337.)

## Local Skin Flaps for Simple Incomplete Syndactyly

- In cases of simple incomplete syndactyly in which the web does not extend beyond the level of the proximal interphalangeal joint (ie, the length of the syndactyly does not exceed the desired depth of the reconstructed interdigital commissure), release may be performed using local skin flaps without the need for full-thickness skin grafting.
- Multiple flap designs have been proposed, and, in general, all are variations of double opposing Z-plasties[13,15] (**TECH FIG 4**).
- In these situations, brief postoperative cast immobilization is recommended until skin flaps have healed.

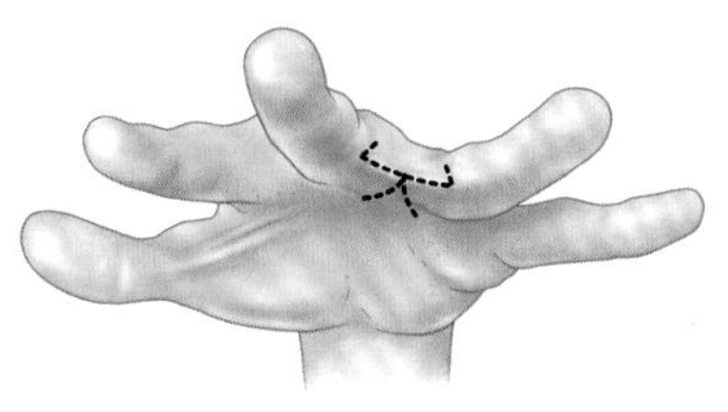
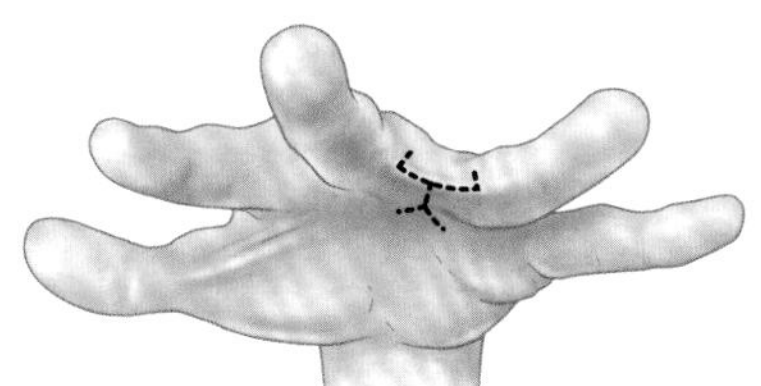
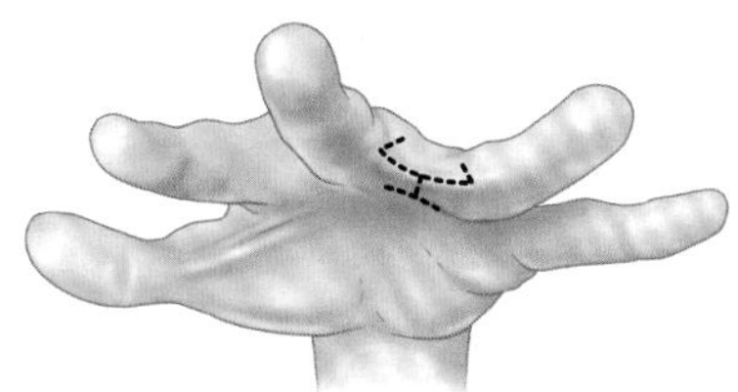
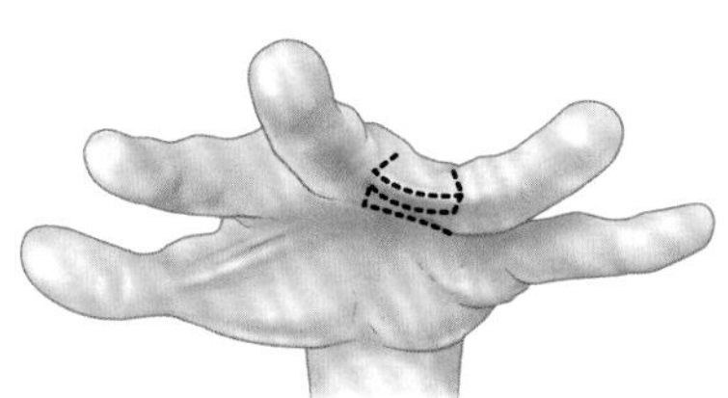
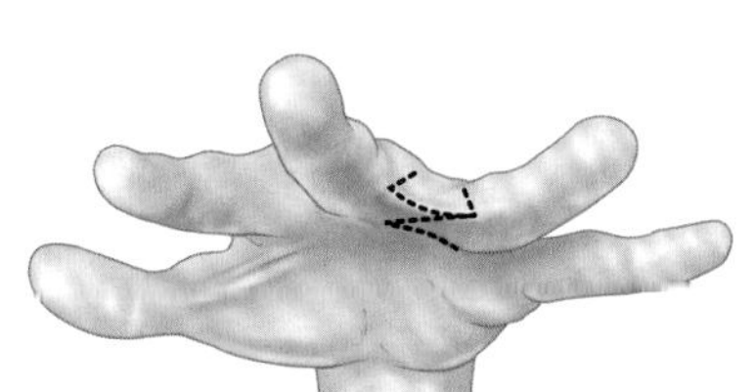
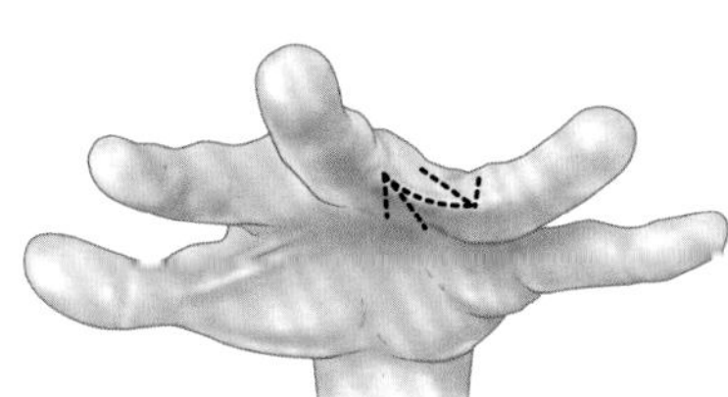

**TECH FIG 4** • Schematic diagram depicting incisions used to perform release of simple incomplete syndactyly.

## PEARLS AND PITFALLS

| | |
|---|---|
| **Patient selection** | ■ Caution should be used when considering release of the superdigit or polysyndactyly because functional results are mixed and postoperative deformity may ensue. |
| **Surgical approach** | ■ The proximal edge of the volar incision may be placed proximal to the palmodigital crease to account for possible late web creep. |
| **Commissure reconstruction** | ■ Zigzag closure of the interdigital commissure is preferred over transverse incisions to avoid scar contracture and subsequent narrowing of the web space. |
| **Interdigitating flaps** | ■ Judicious defatting of the triangular flaps will allow for tension-free closure and reduce the area of skin graft needed. |
| **Graft harvest** | ■ If skin graft is taken from the inguinal region, care should be taken to avoid transfer of hair-bearing skin. This is difficult to assess in the young child; however, harvest lateral to the femoral artery can serve as a helpful guide. |
| **Postoperative care** | ■ The importance of the postoperative dressing and immobilization cannot be overstated. Nonadherent gauze with appropriate bolsters placed over the skin grafts and deep into the reconstructed commissure will optimize skin graft "take" and lessen the risk of resyndactylization during the healing period. |

## POSTOPERATIVE CARE

- Cast immobilization usually is discontinued after 2 to 4 weeks.
- The wound is kept dry until the scabs desiccate and fall off.
- Silicone gel sheets, elastomer, or scar molds may be used to minimize hypertrophic scar formation.
- Formal occupational therapy for motion and strengthening is not typically required because most children will use their hands quite readily with activities of daily living.

## OUTCOMES

- Very little has been published regarding long-term outcomes following surgical release of syndactyly.
- Furthermore, interpretation of the available literature is difficult given the diversity of clinical presentations, surgical techniques, and methods of evaluation.
- In general, syndactyly release can be expected to provide excellent independent digital function with acceptable aesthetic results when performed according to the principles outlined in this chapter.
- Colville[3] reported the results of 57 simple syndactyly releases performed over a 10-year period with minimum 2-year follow-up.
  - Two patients required reoperation for early graft failure, and three others demonstrated slight angular deformity due to scar contracture, but they did not require additional surgery.
- D'Arcangelo et al[4] published their results of 122 releases in 50 patients with minimum 8 years of follow-up.
  - Satisfactory functional and aesthetic results were seen in most patients, but eight patients demonstrated web creep and three patients developed scar contractures.
- DeSmet et al[6] reported their results of 50 syndactyly releases in 24 patients.
  - A normal or near-normal web was seen in 74% of cases, and cosmesis was deemed satisfactory in 64%.
- In their review of 218 releases performed in 100 patients, Percival and Sykes[14] noted that 42 patients required secondary surgery for web creep (22%) and contracture (26%).
- Toledo and Ger[16] published their results of 176 releases performed in 61 patients with average 14-year follow-up.
  - Secondary procedures were performed in 30% of patients with simple syndactylies.
  - The need for secondary surgery was associated with operations performed before the age of 18 months, the use of split-thickness skin grafts, and the presence of complex or complicated syndactyly.

## COMPLICATIONS

- With adherence to the principles presented in this chapter and meticulous surgical technique, the risk of complications may be minimized; however, up to one-third of patients may require secondary procedures following simple complete syndactyly release.
- Digital necrosis is the most serious potential complication of syndactyly release. Careful identification and preservation of the digital arteries—in addition to avoidance of surgical release of both the radial and ulnar sides of a single digit at the same time—is critical to avoid vascular embarrassment and digital loss.
- Skin graft failure may result from hematoma formation beneath the graft or shear stresses imposed on the graft during the healing process.
  - This risk may be greater in younger patients, in whom appropriate graft tensioning is more difficult and in whom postoperative immobilization is a greater challenge.
  - If allowed to heal by secondary intention, subsequent hypertrophic scar formation may lead to suboptimal aesthetic and functional results.
- Skin flap failure due to devascularization is less common but also may lead to scarring and secondary contracture.
  - Triangular skin flaps should be designed with tip angles greater than 45 degrees to prevent tip necrosis.
  - Careful defatting of the flaps and primary closure without excess tension, in addition to assessment of flap viability after tourniquet release, will further aid in preventing skin flap complications.
- Contractures and angular deformity of the released digits may occur owing to linear scars on the radial or ulnar aspects of the fingers.
  - Use of zigzag incisions and interdigitating flap designs will minimize this risk.
- Nail plate deformity is common after simple complete syndactyly release in the presence of a synonychia.
  - Although techniques of nail fold reconstruction using distal pulp tissue will optimize aesthetic results, patients and families should be counseled in advance regarding this common occurrence.
- Web creep refers to the distal migration of the reconstructed interdigital commissure with continued growth and is a common occurrence following syndactyly release, with a variously reported incidence of between 7% and 60% of cases.
  - Some evidence suggests that the risk of web creep may be diminished if release is performed after 18 months of age.
  - Other factors that may contribute to web creep include inappropriate flap design for commissure reconstruction, the use of split-thickness rather than full-thickness skin grafts, skin graft loss, and creation of a transverse linear scar in the reconstituted web space.
  - In cases of clinically significant web creep, secondary releases may be required.

## REFERENCES


1. Aydin A, Ozden BC. Dorsal metacarpal island flap in syndactyly treatment. Ann Plast Surg 2004;52:43–48.
2. Buck-Gramcko D. Congenital malformations: syndactyly and related deformities. In: Nigst H, Buck-Gramcko D, Millesi H, et al, eds. Hand Surgery. New York: Thieme Medical Publishers, 1988:12.
3. Colville J. Syndactyly correction. Br J Plast Surg 1989;42:12–16.
4. D'Arcangelo M, Gilbert A, Pirrello R. Correction of syndactyly using a dorsal omega flap and two lateral and volar flaps. A long-term review. J Hand Surg Br 1996;21:320–324.
5. D'Arcangelo M, Maffulli N. Tissue expanders in syndactyly: a brief review. Acta Chir Plast 1996;38:11–13.
6. DeSmet L, Van Ransbeeck H, Deneef G. Syndactyly release: results of the Flatt technique. Acta Orthop Belg 1998;64:301–305.
7. Eaton CJ, Lister GD. Syndactyly. Hand Clin 1990;6:555–575.
8. Flatt AE. The Care of Congenital Ha nd Anomalies, ed 2. St Louis: Quality Medical Publishing, 1994:228–275.
9. Keret D, Ger E. Evaluation of a uniform operative technique to treat syndactyly. J Hand Surg Am 1987;12:727–729.

10. Kettelkamp DB, Flatt AE. An evaluation of syndactylia repair. Surg Gynecol Obstet 1961;113:471–478.
11. Niranjan NS, Azad SM, Fleming AN, et al. Long-term results of primary syndactyly correction by the trilobed flap technique. Br J Plast Surg 2005;58:14–21.
12. Niranjan NS, DeCarpentier J. A new technique for the division of syndactyly. Eur J Plast Surg 1990;13:101–104.
13. Ostrowski DM, Feagin CA, Gould JS. A three-flap web-plasty for release of short congenital syndactyly and dorsal adduction contracture. J Hand Surg Am 1991;16:634–641.
14. Percival NJ, Sykes PJ. Syndactyly: a review of the factors which influence surgical treatment. J Hand Surg Br 1989;14:196–200.
15. Shaw DT, Li CS, Richey DG, et al. Interdigital butterfly flap in the hand (the double-opposing Z-plasty). J Bone Joint Surg Am 1973;55(8):1677–1679.
16. Toledo LC, Ger E. Evaluation of the operative treatment of syndactyly. J Hand Surg Am 1979;4(6):556–564.
17. Upton J. Congenital anomalies of the hand and forearm. In: McCarthy JG, May JW, Littler JW, eds. Plastic Surgery. Philadelphia: WB Saunders, 1990:5279–5309.

# Preaxial and Postaxial Polydactyly

Robert Carrigan

## DEFINITION

- Polydactyly refers to having greater than the normal number of digits.
- Preaxial polydactyly is duplication or splitting of the thumb.
- Central polydactyly is duplication of the central digits (index, middle, and ring).
- Postaxial polydactyly is duplication of the small finger.

## ANATOMY

- In cases of digit duplication, one may observe duplication in some or all of the elements of the finger (bone, nail, joints, and tendon). The duplicate finger may be well formed and near normal in appearance or underdeveloped and rudimentary in appearance.
- Wassel published a classification of thumb duplication based on the work of Adrian Flatt, MD (Table 1).
- Postaxial polydactyly classification
  - Type A: well-formed duplicate small finger with bone or tendon attachments (**FIG 1**)
  - Type B: small pediculated nubbin

## PATHOGENESIS

- Duplication of the digits occurs early in embryogenesis.
- Patterning of the limb is demonstrated in three axis: proximodistal axis (modulated by the apical ectodermal ridge [AER]), anteroposterior axis (modulated by the zone of polarizing activity [ZPA]), and the dorsoventral axis regulated by the Engrailed 1 protein (EN1).
- Abnormal or ectopic presence of sonic hedgehog protein is implicated in preaxial polydactyly.
- Familial cases of postaxial polydactyly demonstrate a defect in the *GLI3* gene.

**Table 1 Wassel Classification of Thumb Duplication**

| Type | Description |
|---|---|
| I | Bifid distal phalanx |
| II | Duplicate distal phalanx |
| III | Bifid proximal phalanx |
| IV | Duplicate proximal phalanx |
| V | Bifid metacarpal |
| VI | Duplicate metacarpal |
| VII | Triphalangeal thumb |

From Wassel HD. The results of surgery for polydactyly of the thumb. Clin Orthop Relat Res 1969;64:175–193.

## PATIENT HISTORY AND PHYSICAL FINDINGS

- The diagnosis of polydactyly is straightforward, clinical examination and radiographs are sufficient to make the diagnosis.

## IMAGING AND OTHER DIAGNOSTIC STUDIES

- Standard radiographs (three views—anteroposterior, lateral, and oblique) of the hand and affected digit are sufficient to determine the area of involvement (**FIG 2**).
- Advanced imaging such as magnetic resonance imaging (MRI) and computed tomography (CT) is rarely needed.

## DIFFERENTIAL DIAGNOSIS

- Associated syndromes should be screened for, including trisomy 21 and Rubinstein-Taybi, Apert, and Russell-Silver syndrome.

## NONOPERATIVE MANAGEMENT

- Observation may be considered for duplicated digits that do not impair function of the hand.

## SURGICAL MANAGEMENT

### Preoperative Planning

- Timing of surgery is variable.
- Type B postaxial polydactyly may be removed in the office under local anesthesia, when the child is just a few weeks old.
- Preaxial polydactyly reconstruction and type A postaxial reconstructions are elective procedures and are generally performed after 1 year of age and before the start of school.

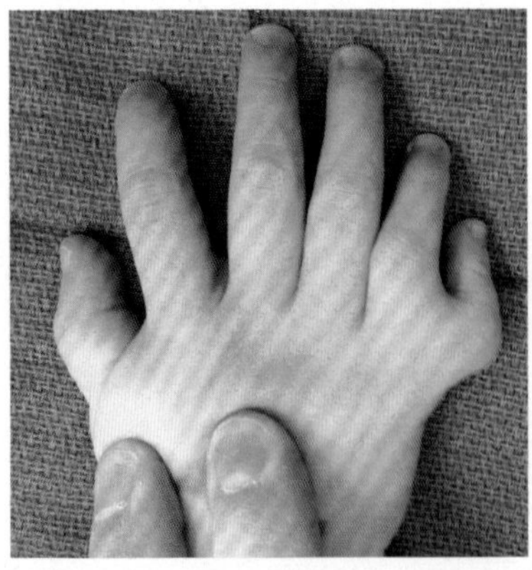

**FIG 1** • Type A postaxial polydactyly.

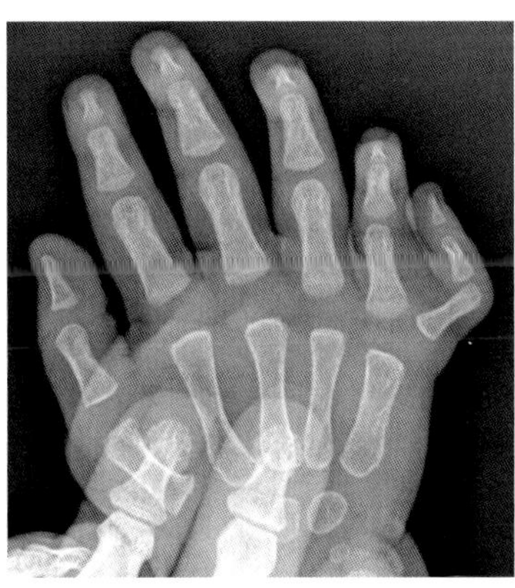

**FIG 2** • Preoperative radiograph of the patient in **FIG 1** with type A postaxial polydactyly, depicting the bifacet metacarpal head.

## Positioning

- The patient is positioned supine on the table and the body is pulled over to the affected side.
- The arm is placed on a radiolucent hand table and an arm tourniquet is applied.

## Approach

- Deletion and reconstruction of a polydactyly is not simply an amputation. The surgeon should be aware of protecting and preserving vital structures such as the collateral ligaments and tendon insertions for reattachment to the preserved digit.
- Several approaches may be considered for the management of pre- and postaxial polydactyly.
- Skin incisions must take in to consideration preservation of nail folds where appropriate.

TECHNIQUES

## Type A Postaxial Polydactyly

- A racquet-type incision is made around the digit to be deleted. Skin flaps are developed.
- The adductor digiti minimi (ADQ) is identified and detached from its insertion and tagged.
- The ulnar collateral ligament (UCL) from the metacarpophalangeal joint (MCP) is released from the proximal phalanx with a large sleeve of periosteum and tagged.
- The digital nerves and vessels are identified and ligated.
- The duplicated digit is removed (**TECH FIG 1**).
- The ADQ and UCL are reinserted with 4-0 nonabsorbable suture (Ethibond)
- Skin is closed with absorbable suture (5-0 fast absorbing chromic gut).
- The hand is dressed and casted with the fingertips exposed for 2 weeks.

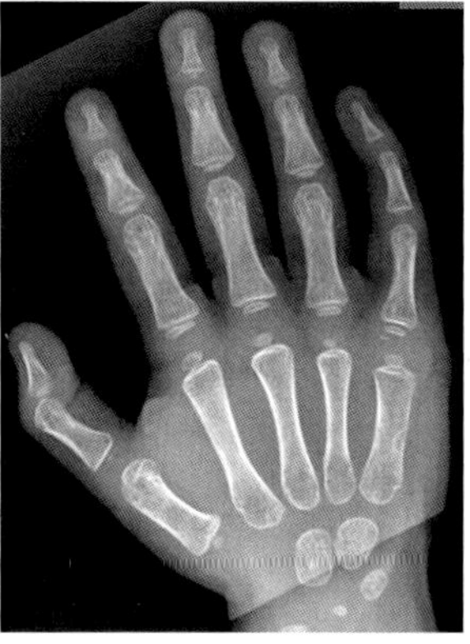

**TECH FIG 1** • Postoperative radiograph of the patient in **FIGS 1** and **2** demonstrating well-aligned MCP joint.

## Type B Postaxial Polydactyly

- These rudimentary supernumerary digits can be addressed by simple ligature or excision.
- Ligature of the rudimentary digit can be accomplished via a surgical tie such as 2-0 silk or hemaclip.
    - Application of the ligature should be tight enough to occlude the digital artery. A loose ligature will simple occlude the venous outflow and cause congestion, which can be painful for the child and prolong the time for the digit to become ischemic and fall off. A ligature placed too distal on the pedicle stalk will leave a stump and often a painful neuroma.
- Surgical excision can be performed in the office under local anesthetic.
- The child is placed in a papoose. A digital block is performed and the hand is prepped.
- The base of the supernumerary is pinched between the surgeon's index finger and thumb, and the stalk is cut with a pair of iris scissors. The vessel is identified and cauterized.
- The base is then sutured with interrupted locking absorbable 5-0 fast absorbing gut suture.
- Soft compressive dressings are applied with the tips available for the parents to observe.
- Dressings are removed in 3 days and bathing can be initiated after that.
- No follow-up is usually necessary.

## Wassel I or II Preaxial Polydactyly

- Reconstruction of the duplicated thumb involving the distal phalanx may be accomplished in one of two ways.

### Bilhaut-Cloquet Procedure

- The Bilhaut-Cloquet procedure has been historically advocated for treatment of Wassel I or II thumb duplication.
- This involves a central wedge resection and reapproximation of the radial and ulnar structures (**TECH FIGS 2** and **3**).
- This procedure has fallen out of favor due to residual nail irregularities.

### Removal of Duplicate Thumb

- Duplication of the thumb is rarely symmetric. One of the two duplicated thumb parts is usually larger. Deletion of the smaller thumb part is favorable.
- Racquet-shaped incisions are made about the thumb to excise the desired duplication. Careful attention is made to preserve the appropriate nail elements.
- Skin flaps are developed and the extensor tendons and flexor tendons are identified. Tendon insertions to the intended deleted digit are transected and tagged for reinsertion.
- The collateral ligament to the interphalangeal (IP) joint is elevated with a sleeve of periosteum.
- The duplicated digit is excised; if the head of the proximal phalanx has two facets, a chondroplasty (reshaping of the head) with a no. 15 blade may be necessary.
- The collateral ligament is reinserted and the joint is tested for stability.
- The flexor and extensor tendons are rebalanced.
- Skin is closed with 5-0 fast absorbing gut suture.
- Sterile dressings and a long-arm thumb spica cast are applied.
- Follow-up in 2 weeks for cast removal.

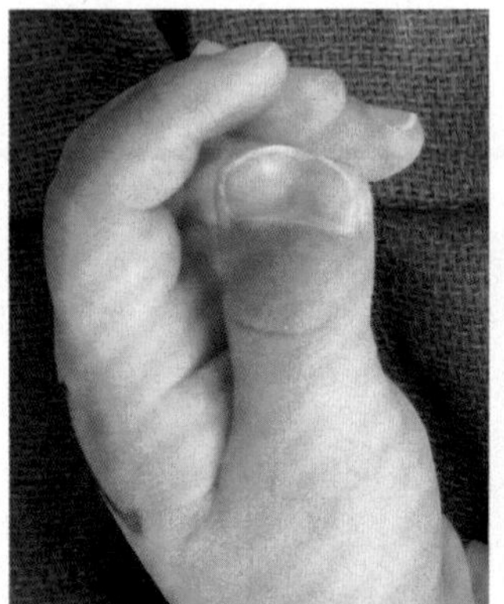
A

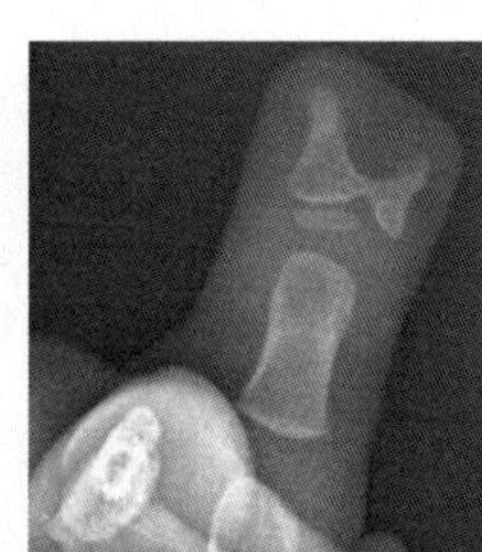
B

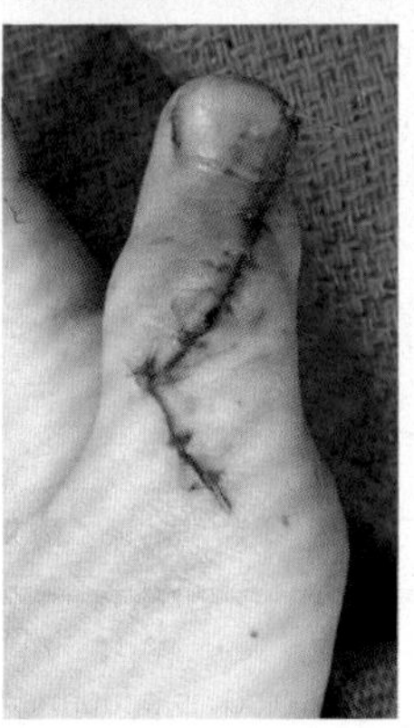
C

**TECH FIG 2** • **A.** Clinical photograph demonstrating conjoined nails in a Wassel I thumb. **B.** Preoperative radiograph. **C.** Postoperative photograph demonstrates normal IP alignment and nail fold following resection of small duplicated thumb.

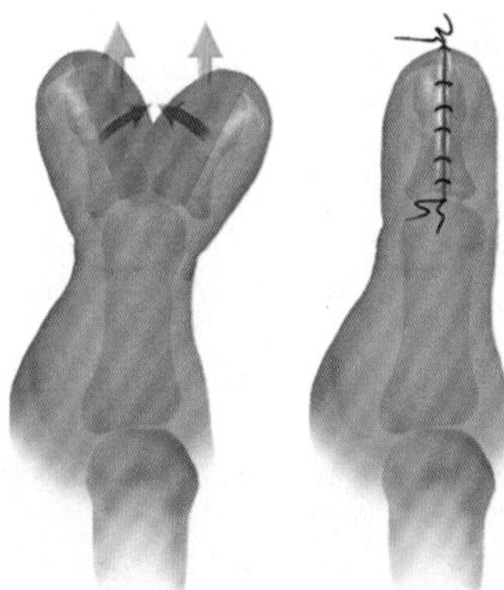

**TECH FIG 3** • Diagram depicting the Bilhaut-Cloquet procedure. (From Waters PM, Bae DS. Preaxial polydactyly. In: Pediatric Hand and Upper Limb Surgery: A Practical Guide. Philadelphia: Lippincott Williams & Wilkins, 2012:32–42.)

## Wassel Type III or IV Preaxial Polydactyly

- Duplication of the thumb is rarely symmetric. One of the two duplicated thumb parts is usually larger. Deletion of the smaller thumb part is favorable (**TECH FIG 4**).
- In most cases, the radial digit is the smaller of the two, and deletion is favored as it preserves the native UCL, which is important for pinch (**TECH FIG 5A,B**).
- Racquet-shaped incisions are made about the thumb to excise the desired duplication.
- Skin flaps are developed and the extensor tendons and flexor tendons are identified.
- Tendon insertions to the intended deleted digit are transected and tagged for reinsertion.

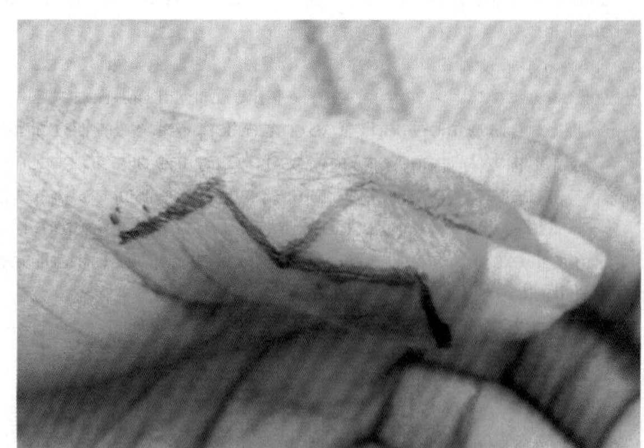

**TECH FIG 4** • Skin incisions for resection of Wassel III duplicate.

- The intrinsic musculature is elevated from its insertion and tagged.
- The collateral ligament to the MCP joint is elevated with a sleeve of periosteum.
- The duplicated digit is excised; if the head of metacarpal has two facets, a chondroplasty (reshaping of the head) with a no.15 blade may be necessary.
- If angulation of the thumb is present at the MCP joint, a closed wedge osteotomy of the metacarpal neck may be necessary to align the thumb. This can be accomplished with a small rongeur, removing bone on the radial side of the metacarpal, leaving the ulnar cortex intact, and closing the osteotomy and securing with wire.
- The collateral ligament is reinserted, and the joint is tested for stability.
- The intrinsic musculature is reinserted (**TECH FIG 5C**).
- The flexor and extensor tendons are rebalanced.
- Skin is closed with 5-0 fast absorbing gut suture (**TECH FIG 5D**).
- Sterile dressings and a long-arm thumb spica cast are applied.

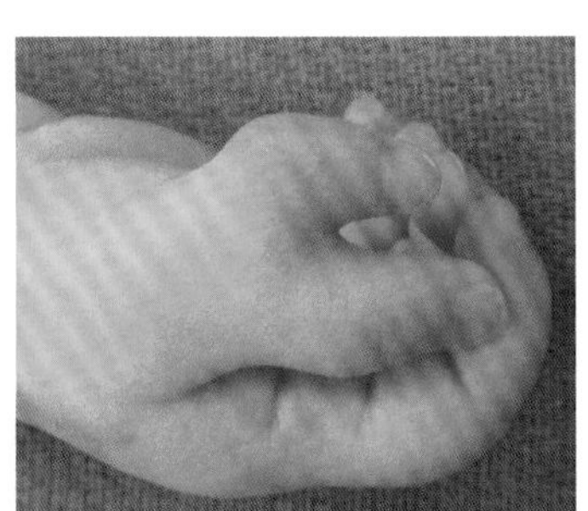
A

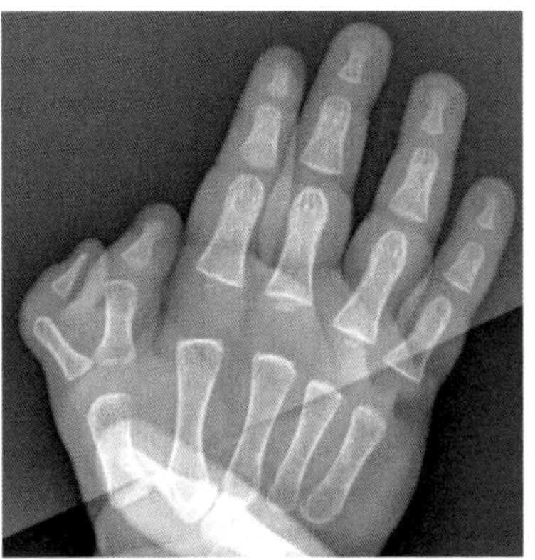
B

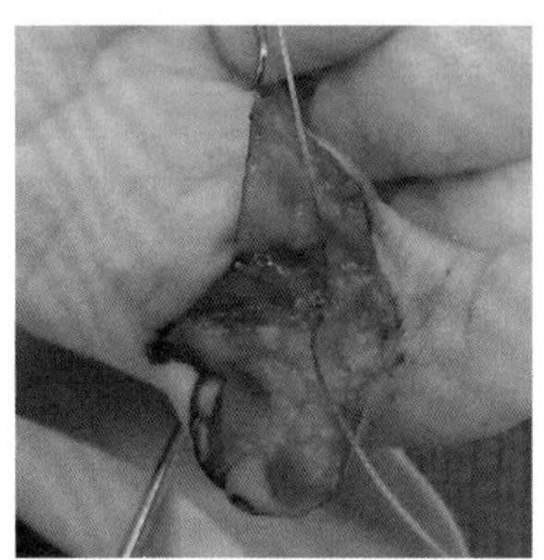
C

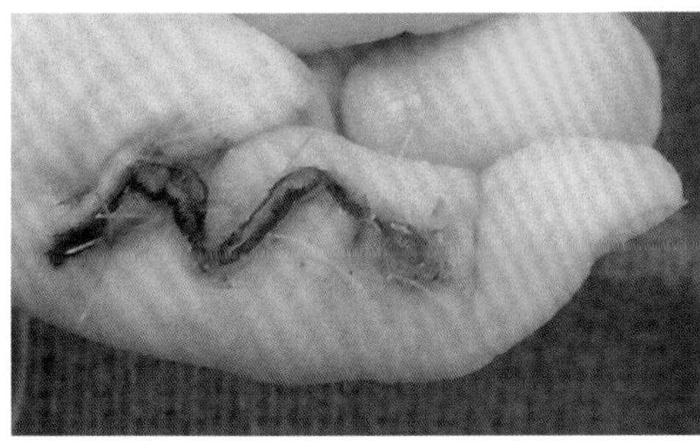
D

**TECH FIG 5** • **A,B.** Preoperative photograph and radiography, respectively, of Wassel IV duplicate thumb. **C.** Intraoperative photograph depicting reinsertion of intrinsic musculature following deletion of radial duplicate thumb. **D.** Postoperative skin closure following deletion of radial duplicate thumb.

## PEARLS AND PITFALLS

| | |
|---|---|
| **Persistent joint angulation** | ■ Failure to recognize deforming factors, such as misaligned tendons and residual bony deformity |
| **Persistent joint instability** | ■ Collateral ligaments must be properly reinserted. |
| **Painful neuromas (see FIG 3)** | ■ Digital nerves must be identified and cut short to retract away from the skin surface. |

## POSTOPERATIVE CARE

- The first postoperative visit is 2 weeks from surgery, 4 weeks if an osteotomy is performed.
- The cast is removed and digit is inspected.
- Radiographs are obtained to evaluate healing in the case of and osteotomy.
- Pins are pulled where appropriate.
- The family is instructed about wound care and scar massage.
- Occupational therapy is not instituted unless there is concern for persistent joint stiffness.

## OUTCOMES

- Outcomes from polydactyly reconstruction correction are generally good with most patients reporting good function and aesthetics.

## COMPLICATIONS

- Irregularities with the nail fold and residual IP joint angulation are common following thumb reconstruction.
- Neuroma sometimes occurs after suture ligation of postaxial polydactyly (**FIG 3**).

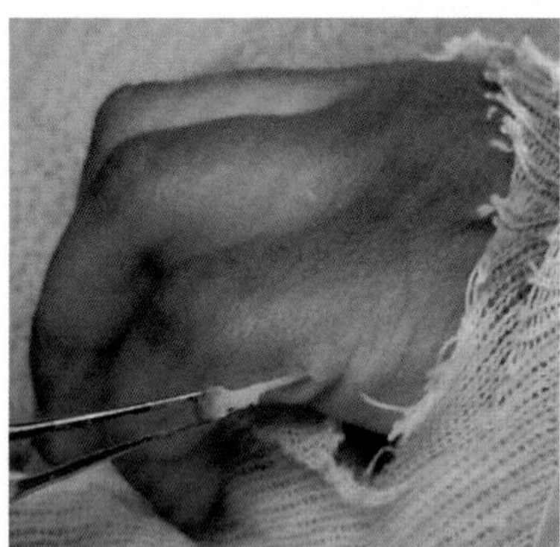

**FIG 3** ● Painful neuroma following suture ligation of postaxial polydactyly.

- Failure to reinsert collateral ligaments or intrinsic musculature may lead to joint incompetence or weakness, respectively.

## SUGGESTED READINGS

1. Al-Qattan MM, Kozin SH. Update on embryology of the upper limb. J Hand Surg Am 2013;38:1835–1844.
2. Dobyns JH, Lipscomb PR, Cooney WP. Management of thumb duplication. Clin Orthop Relat Res 1985:(195):26–44.
3. Ezaki M. Radial polydactyly. Hand Clin 1990;6:577–588.
4. Ganley TJ, Lubahn JD. Radial polydactyly: an outcome study. Ann Plast Surg 1995;35:86–89.
5. Goldfarb CA, Patterson JM, Maender A, et al. Thumb size and appearance following reconstruction of radial polydactyly. J Hand Surg Am 2008;33:1348–1353.
6. Manske PR. Treatment of duplicated thumb using a ligamentous/periosteal flap. J Hand Surg Am 1989;14:728–733.
7. Mih AD. Complications of duplicate thumb reconstruction. Hand Clin 1998;14:143–149.

# Amniotic Band Syndrome

**Joshua M. Abzug and Scott H. Kozin**

73

CHAPTER

## DEFINITION

- Amniotic band syndrome is a nonhereditary congenital difference. The entire fetal limb or a portion of it becomes entangled in amniotic membrane leading to partial or complete circumferential constriction, deformity, or amputation of the entire part.
- Multiple other terms are used to describe the condition including constriction band syndrome, Streeter dysplasia, and amniotic disruption sequence among others (Table 1).
- Bands affecting the upper extremities vary from mild with only appearance being an issue to severe with substantial deformity and functional limitations (**FIG 1**). The worst-case scenario is complete deletion or amputation of a part. Each case is different and requires individualized treatment.

## ANATOMY

- The bands may affect the soft tissue and involve partial or complete circumferential constriction of part or all of the following structures: skin, subcutaneous tissue, tendons/muscles, nerves, and bone.
- The bands may entangle any part of the upper or lower extremity. Proximal constricture can lead to loss of the entire arm or leg. Distal involvement is more common and presentation varies with degrees of constriction.
- The presence of a cleft proximal to acrosyndactyly (connection of the digit tips) is diagnostic of amniotic band syndrome as this represents normal apoptosis leading to development of the web and subsequent syndactylization due to scarring from the bands (**FIG 2**).

## PATHOGENESIS

- Numerous theories exist regarding the underlying cause of amniotic band syndrome. The most common theory is that amniotic disruption causes release of bands (free-floating strands of membrane) that encircle the affected part, causing circumferential constrictions that strangle the affected limb or digit.[5] Rupture also leads to oligohydramnios with resultant external compression on the developing limb.
- Protruding fetal structures are more likely to be involved due to entrapment by the bands.
  - Most common location is digits (56%), followed by hand/wrist (24%), then foot/ankle (10%).[3]
  - Most commonly affected digits are the central digits due to their increased length—long finger (28%), ring finger (27%), and index finger (23%).

**Table 1 Terms Used to Describe Amniotic Band Syndrome**

| |
|---|
| Constriction band syndrome |
| Streeter dysplasia |
| Amniotic disruption sequence |
| Constriction ring syndrome |
| Limb-body wall malformation complex |
| Annular band syndrome |
| Amniotic deformity, adhesions, and mutations complex |
| Simonart band |
| Early amnion rupture sequence |
| Intrauterine or fetal amputation |

## NATURAL HISTORY

- Amniotic band syndrome is nonprogressive.
- Recognition of the limb difference occurs either in utero via ultrasonography or is readily apparent at birth.
- Ultrasound will show a progressive enlargement of the digit distal to the band (Francisco).
- Peripheral nerve palsy, distal anesthesia, vascular insufficiency, venous congestion, or lymphedema may occur due to the presence of a band affecting the neurovascular structures.[8,10]

## PATIENT HISTORY AND PHYSICAL FINDINGS

- Examination of the child at birth will demonstrate the location and extent of the band(s).
- Digital constriction will dictate the clinical scenario.
  - Mild to moderate damage initiates an embryonic repair process and yields variable amounts of circumferential stricture with or without resultant distal lymphedema.
  - Inflammatory response may cause adjacent digits to merge distal to the rudimentary web.

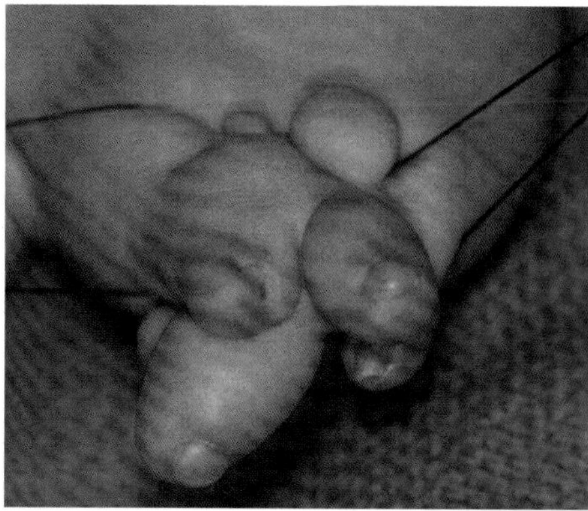

**FIG 1** • Photograph of a severe case of amniotic band syndrome that caused substantial deformity and functional limitations. (Courtesy of Shriners Hospital for Children, Philadelphia, PA.)

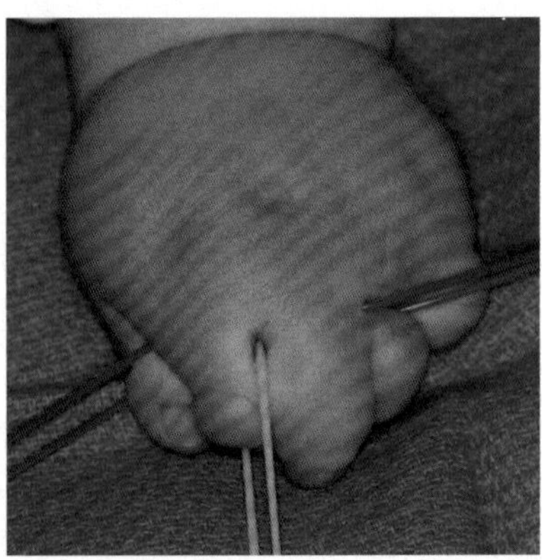

**FIG 2** • Dorsal view of brachysyndactyly that occurred due to amniotic band syndrome. The presence of the clefts proximally, that vessel loops are traversing is diagnostic of amniotic band syndrome. (Courtesy of Shriners Hospital for Children, Philadelphia, PA.)

- A large fusion mass may occur, making it difficult to decipher precise orientation of the digits.
- Severe constrictions may result in digit(s)/limb(s) amputation.
- Ulceration at the base of a ring or with firm skin protuberances on the dorsum of the finger may occur.[2]

## IMAGING AND OTHER DIAGNOSTIC STUDIES

- No imaging is required to manage simple bands or bands that are proximal.
- Plain radiographs are sufficient to evaluate digits when there are multiple digits fused.
  - Typically, only a posteroanterior (PA) view is needed (**FIG 3**).

## DIFFERENTIAL DIAGNOSIS

- Brachysyndactyly
- Transverse deficiency
- Apert syndrome
- Vasculocutaneous catastrophe of the newborn (also known as *neonatal gangrene*, *neonatal Volkmann contracture*)

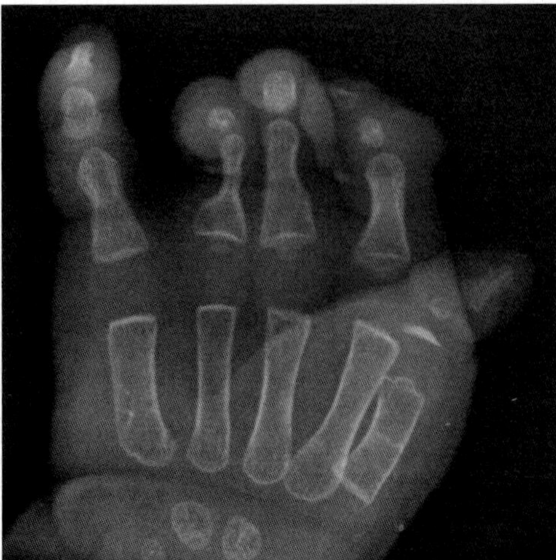

**FIG 3** • PA radiograph of a hand with multiple syndactylized digits due to amniotic band syndrome. Note the compression of the proximal phalanx of the ring and long fingers due to the band. (Courtesy of Shriners Hospital for Children, Philadelphia, PA.)

## NONOPERATIVE MANAGEMENT

- Observation is the nonoperative management of amniotic band syndrome.
- As with all congenital differences, priority should be given to function over appearance. In other words, function trumps form. Therefore, it may be better in certain circumstances to leave digits syndactylized if they function better together than apart.

## SURGICAL MANAGEMENT

- Surgical management is the most common management for amniotic band syndrome to maximize function and appearance. Once again, form trumps function in operative planning, and amputation of one or more digits may be the best course of action (**FIG 4**).
- Strategies are to prioritize the thumb, thumb–index web space, and digits with adequate separation, motion, and length.
  - Bands in sequence are released in stages beginning with release of the most distal band.[3,11]
- Release of bands requires complete excision of the invaginating band and subcutaneous tissue.
  - The void is covered with a Z-plasty, using the surrounding tissue.[11]
  - Traditional treatment is release of one-half of a circumferential band at a time; however, complete circumferential excision can be safely performed if the surgeon is confident that the artery and vein are preserved.[7,11,12]
- Timing is dictated by the depth of the band.
  - Mild to moderate bands and digital masses from amputations can be treated electively. However, bands causing tethering of adjacent digits should be released early following the principles of traditional syndactyly release (**FIG 5**).
  - A deep band jeopardizing limb viability requires immediate release if the limb is salvageable.
  - In utero release has been successfully performed, but there are noteworthy risks including the risk of spontaneous abortion.[9]

### Preoperative Planning

- Discussion with the family regarding the possibility of staged reconstruction and the need for skin grafting must occur.
  - In digits syndactylized, separate only one side of a digit at a time.

### Positioning

- Supine positioning on a standard operating room table.
  - A hand table can be used for older/larger children.
- A tourniquet is applied to the upper arm.

### Approach

- No standard approach is used, as the bands are circumferential and excision requires a circumferential incision.
  - Knowledge of the anatomy of the area is essential to avoid damaging neurovascular structures that may be tethered.
- Release of syndactylized digits uses a similar technique to traditional syndactyly release by typically using zigzag-type flaps as well as flaps to recreate the commissure.
- Synonychia release requires re-creation of paronychial folds with flaps such as Buck-Gramcko flaps.

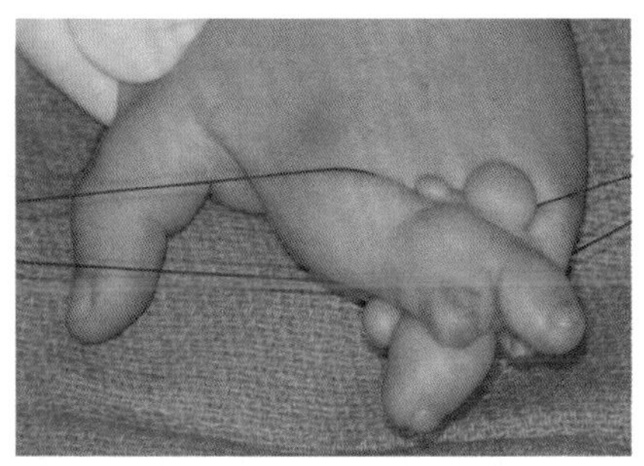
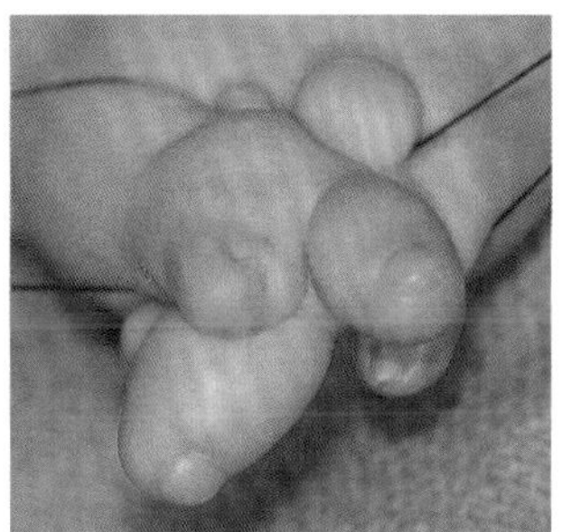
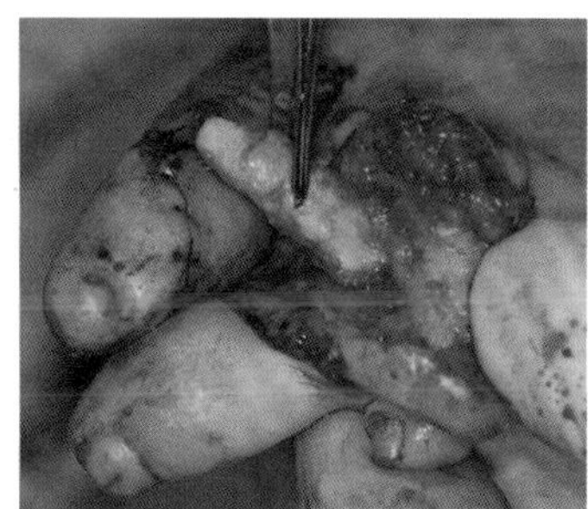
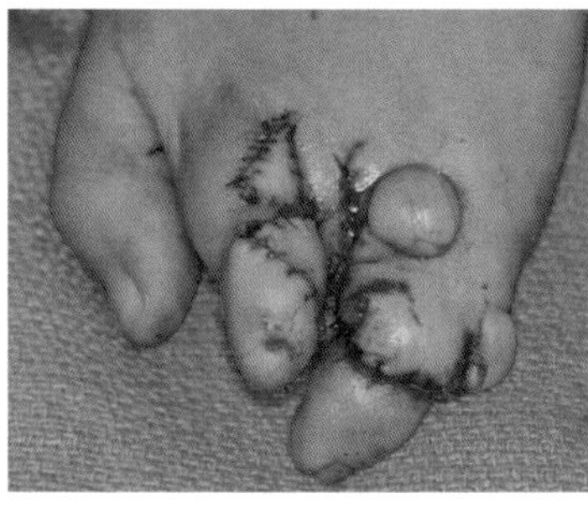

**FIG 4** • Three-year-old boy with complex banding of his left hand requiring long-finger amputation and commissure reconstruction. **A.** Preoperative dorsal view. **B.** Close-up of digital conglomeration. **C.** Amputation of long finger. **D.** Commissure reconstruction with flap and adjacent skin graft. (Courtesy of Shriners Hospital for Children, Philadelphia, PA.)

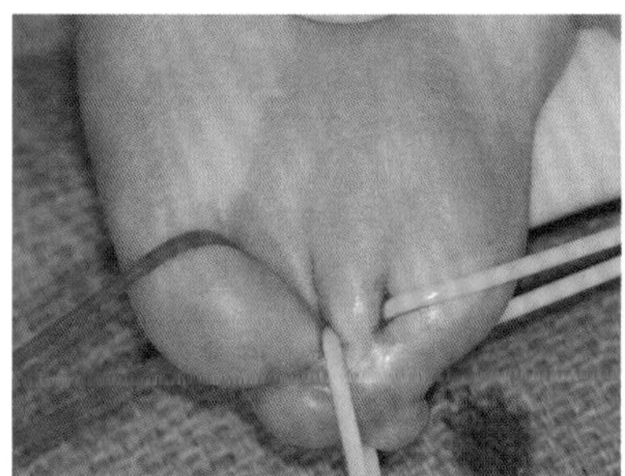
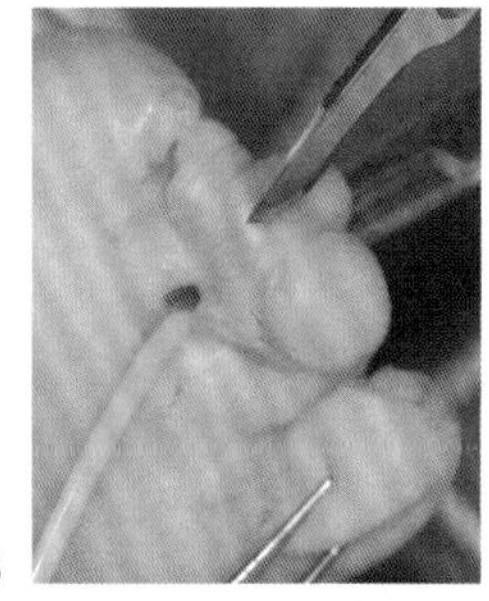
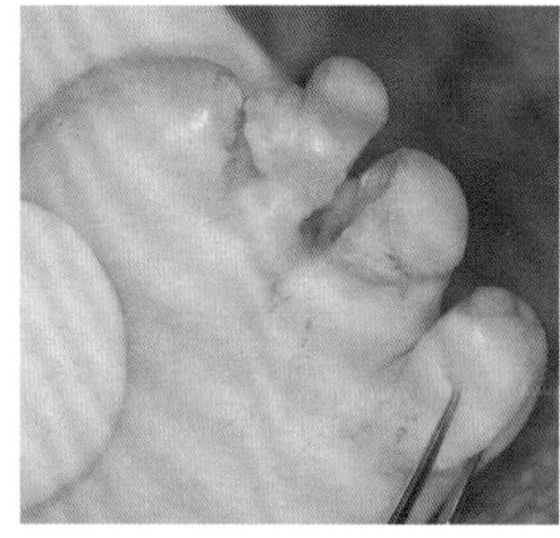

**FIG 5** • Three month-old boy with bands of his left hand requiring early release to prevent tethering. **A.** Preoperative dorsal view. **B.** Separation of connected fingertips with scalpel blade. **C.** Fingers liberated to allow unimpeded growth. (Courtesy of Shriners Hospital for Children, Philadelphia, PA.)



## Simple Constriction Ring Release

- Make a circumferential incision to excise band (**TECH FIG 1A,B**), including skin and subcutaneous adipose tissue.
  - Can mark sidewalls of band with marking pen and then bring proximal and distal skin edges together such that they touch. The painted area is the appropriate amount to excise.[11]
  - Failure to excise the entirety of a band, including the abnormal subcutaneous tissue, may result in scar contracture and "recurrence."
- Mobilize surrounding skin and subcutaneous adipose tissue (**TECH FIG 1C**).
  - Preserve deep subcutaneous veins and neurovascular bundles to prevent postoperative venous congestion.
- Reapproximate adipose tissue over muscle/fascia.
- Perform Z-plasty closure of band (**TECH FIG 1D**).

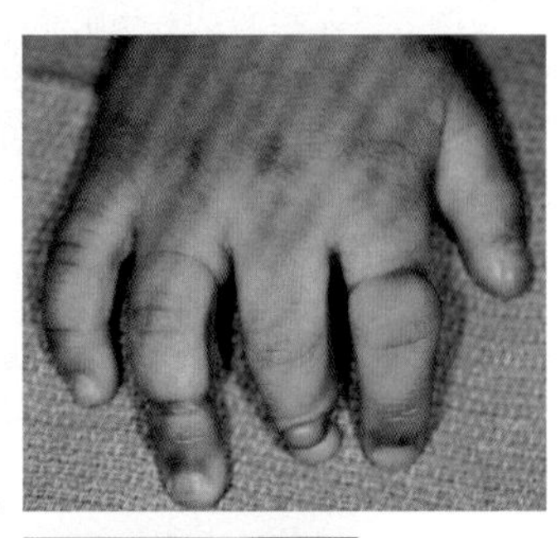
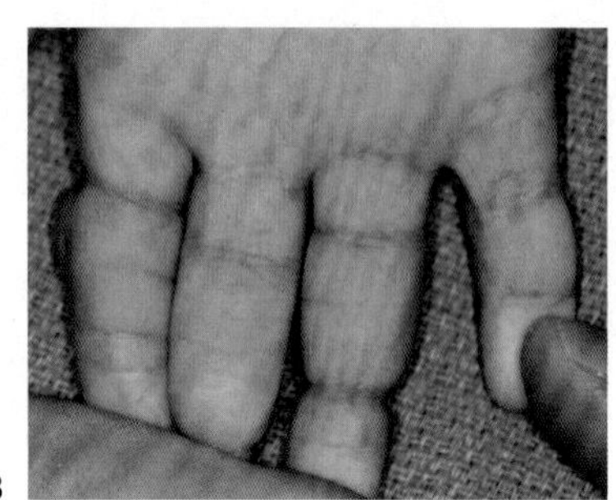
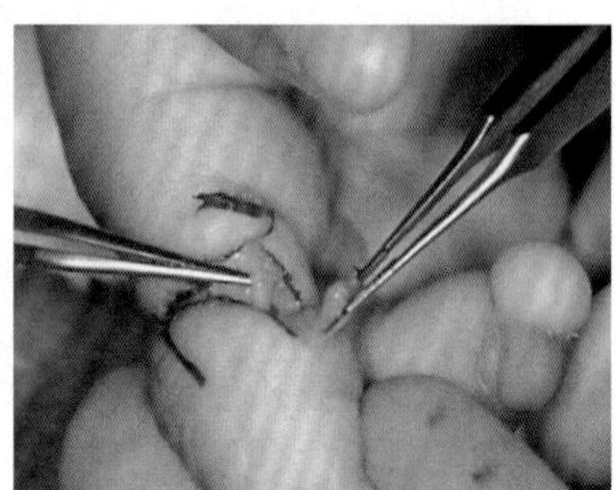
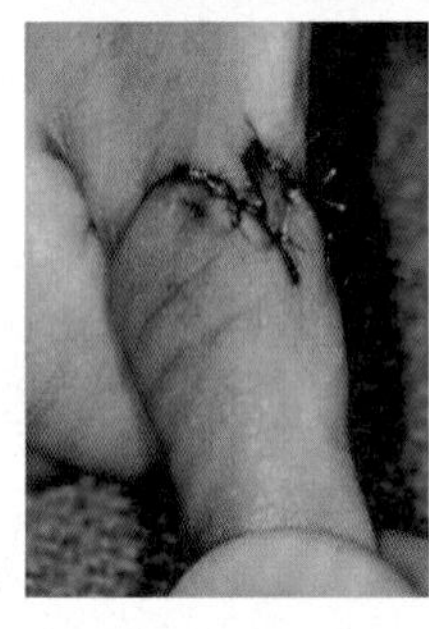

**TECH FIG 1** • Simple constriction rings present on multiple digits. **A.** Dorsal view. **B.** Palmar view. **C.** Elevation of skin flaps following excision of a band. Note the full-thickness nature of the flap by the presence of adipose tissue. **D.** Closure of the Z-plasty. (Courtesy of Shriners Hospital for Children, Philadelphia, PA.)

## Acrosyndactyly Release

- Draw flap designs.
  - Create new broad commissure using dorsal skin that ends approximately two-thirds of the way up the proximal phalanx from the metacarpophalangeal joint to the proximal interphalangeal joint (**TECH FIG 2A**).
  - Zigzag incisions to minimize the amount of necessary skin graft. The points of the zigzag should be opposite the base from the other side.
  - On the volar side, fashion a pattern such as a three-sided box to have a place for the commissure flap to set into (**TECH FIG 2B**).
  - In cases with a connected common nail, Buck-Gramcko flaps are needed to generate paronychial folds.
- Exsanguinate limb loosely and inflate tourniquet.
- Begin with dorsal skin incision to elevate commissure flap.
  - Start thin (full-thickness dermis) distally and progress to thick (full thickness including subcutaneous fat).

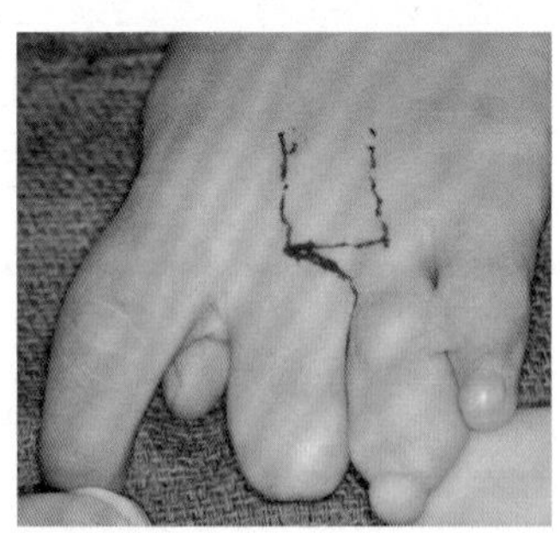
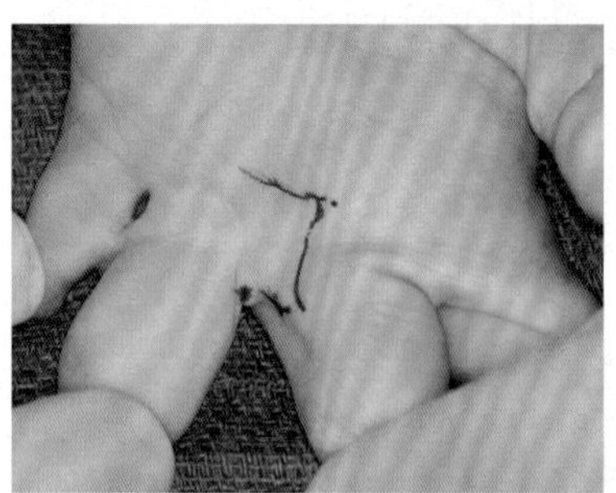
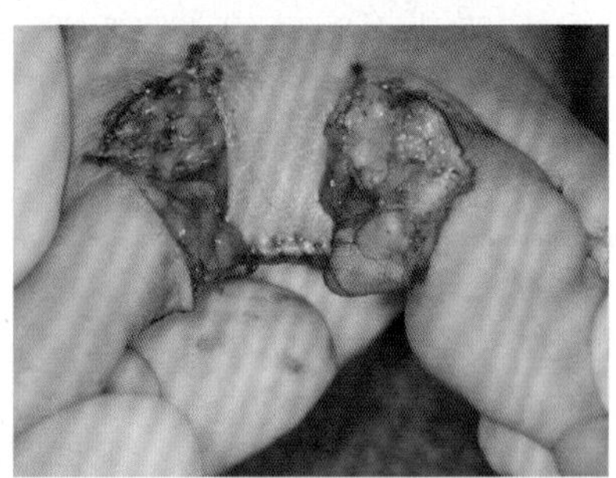
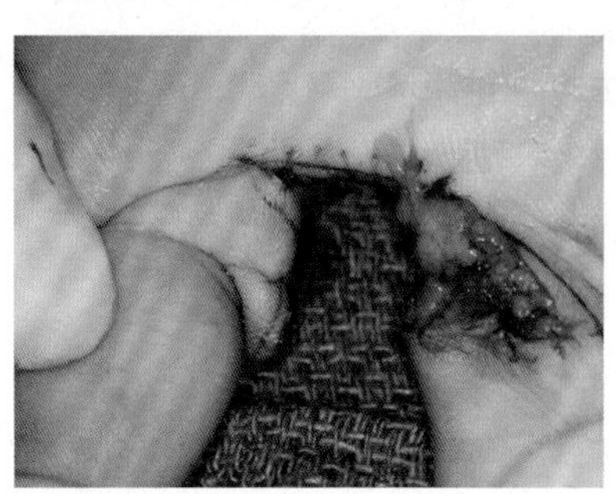
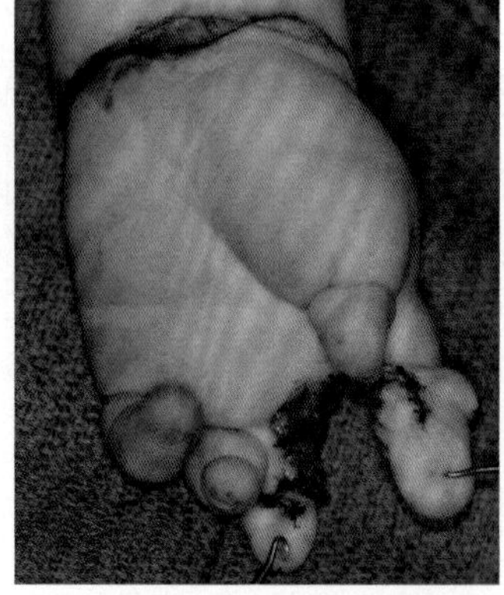

**TECH FIG 2** • **A.** Flap design of digital commissure using dorsal skin. **B.** Flap design on volar side to receive commissure. Note the ability of the three-sided box to wrap onto the ring finger. **C,D.** Dorsal and palmar views, respectively, of insertion of the commissure flap. **E.** Use of wrist flexion crease to obtain skin graft. Note the closure obtained which will leave a scar that is difficult to visualize. (Courtesy of Shriners Hospital for Children, Philadelphia, PA.)

- Incise dorsal zigzag template in a full-thickness skin manner.
  - Minimize fat present on this skin.
- Following raising of the flaps, spread transversally to separate digits.
- From dorsal side, identify neurovascular bundles.
- Raise volar flaps with minimal fat.
  - Ensure the Buck-Gramcko flaps are not damaged as you dissect distally.
- Raise Buck-Gramcko flaps.
- Separate bone/synonychia with knife as needed.
- Begin closing flaps by first insetting commissure flap (**TECH FIG 2C,D**).
  - Use 5-0 plain gut to close flaps.
- Obtain full-thickness skin graft to close remaining areas.
  - Make ellipse centered on wrist flexion crease.
  - Incise skin only and raise flap.
  - Can defat as you dissect with knife parallel to skin
  - Close donor site with subcutaneous and subcuticular closure (**TECH FIG 2E**).
- Deflate tourniquet and ensure brisk capillary refill is present.
  - Remove a few sutures if capillary refill is sluggish.
- Apply bulky dressing to prevent shear followed by a cast application.
- **TECH FIG 3** shows a complete acrosyndactyly release.

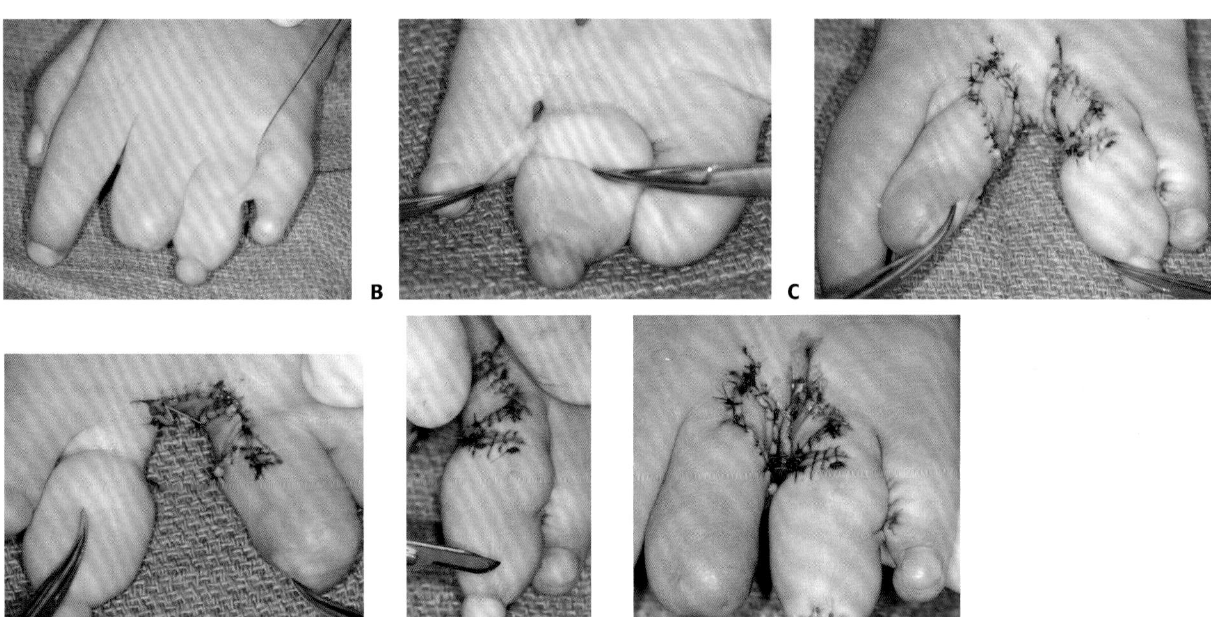

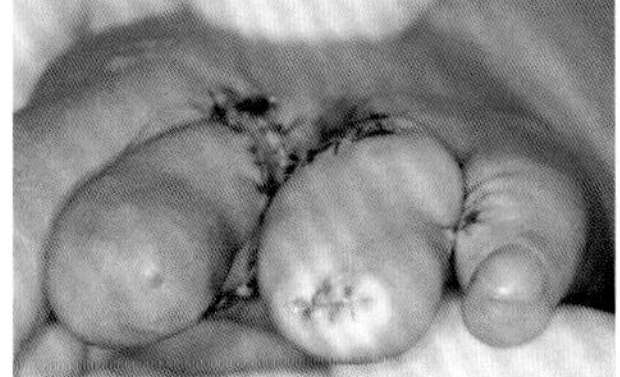

**TECH FIG 3** • A 5-year-old boy with amniotic band syndrome affecting his left hand. **A.** Dorsal view. **B.** Palmar view. **C.** Dorsal view following syndactyly release and skin grafting. **D.** Palmar view following syndactyly release and skin grafting. **E.** Presence of nonfunctional portion of distal ring finger. **F.** Excision of distal ring finger tip to improve appearance. **G.** Distal view following excision of tip of ring finger. (Courtesy of Shriners Hospital for Children, Philadelphia, PA.)

## Nonvascularized Toe Phalangeal Transfer

- Exsanguinate limb and inflate tourniquet.
- Dorsal zigzag incision on affected digit down to level of extensor mechanism
- Incise extensor mechanism longitudinally.
- Perform gentle longitudinal spreading to create a soft tissue pocket to accept toe.
- Attention now turned to foot where the proximal phalanx of second toe is now exposed through a chevron/longitudinal incision (**TECH FIG 4A**).
  - Proximal phalanx of third and fourth toes can be used if needed.
- Toe extensor mechanism is split longitudinally.
- Collateral ligaments released from distal extent of toe.
- Extraperiosteal dissection performed from distal to proximal.

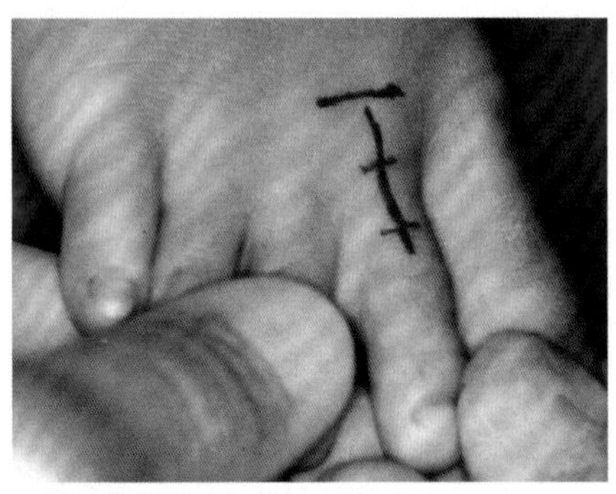
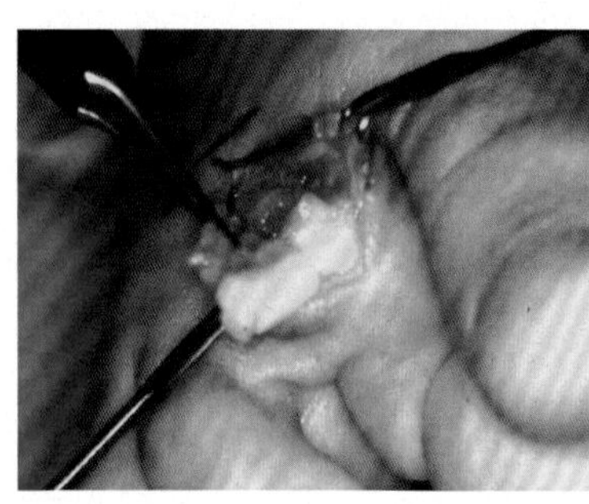
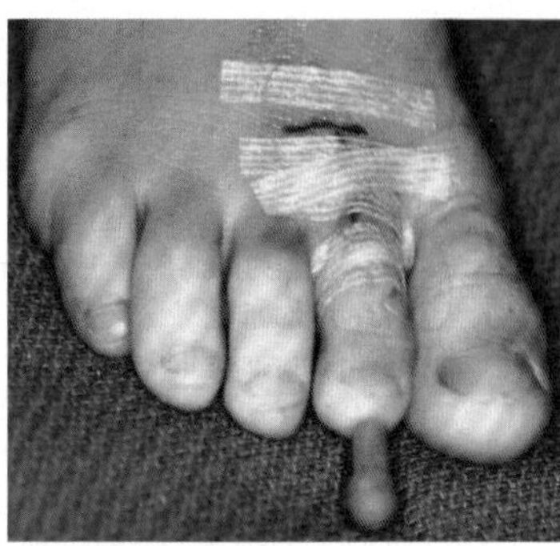

**TECH FIG 4** • **A.** Incision used to obtain proximal phalanx of second toe for nonvascularized toe transfer. **B.** Extraperiosteal excision of proximal phalanx. **C.** Appearance of second toe following excision of proximal phalanx and placement of a smooth wire. (Courtesy of Shriners Hospital for Children, Philadelphia, PA.)

- Plantar plate and then pulleys are released.
  - Be careful to protect and preserve the toe flexor tendons and neurovascular bundles.
- Toe phalanx now released while preserving the proximal collateral ligaments and plantar plate which are used for attachment to the metacarpal (**TECH FIG 4B**).
- Toe extensor tendon sewn to flexor tendon to close the defect and preserve length and alignment.[1]
- Smooth pin placed in a longitudinal direction across excised toe phalanx (**TECH FIG 4C**).
- Toe phalanx placed in finger soft tissue pocket and pin advanced antegrade out the tip of the soft tissue nubbin.
- Pin driven retrograde into metacarpal head.
- Collateral ligaments and plantar plate attached to metacarpophalangeal joint capsule and extensor mechanism attached to toe phalanx.
- Skin closed with simple interrupted sutures.
- Long-arm mitten cast applied over a bulky dressing.

## PEARLS AND PITFALLS

| | |
|---|---|
| **Timing** | ▪ If connected digits are unequal in length, early tip separation is warranted to prevent a tether and restricted growth. |
| **Skin graft** | ▪ Use of the volar wrist flexion crease skin allows for a hidden scar and avoids the potential for hair growth seen when using groin skin. |
| **Flap design** | ▪ If possible, wrap the three-sided box from the volar flap onto the ring finger to permit ring wear that does not overlie a potentially painful scar (see **TECH FIGS 2B** and **3C,D**). |
| **Postoperative care** | ▪ Use whirlpool to remove postoperative dressings at 2 weeks. |

## POSTOPERATIVE CARE

- Children are typically admitted for 24 hours for pain control and observation including regular neurovascular checks to ensure digit viability.
- Elevate limb for 48 hours to aid with venous return.
- Remove cast and dressings at 2 to 3 weeks postoperatively for band excisions or syndactyly releases.
- Remove cast and pins at 4 to 6 weeks for nonvascularized toe transfers.

## OUTCOMES

- Successful release of bands is the anticipated outcome following excision and Z-plasties. Specific results of band excision and syndactyly release are directly related to the extent of the constricture. Published results are limited.
- Nonvascularized toe transfers performed at young ages (before 12 to 18 months) yield good results exhibiting open physes that permits longitudinal and appositional growth.[1,5]
- Vascularized toe to hand transfers have been performed for amniotic band syndrome and can achieve 95% or greater success rates of viability in experienced hands.[4,6]
- However, this is a technically challenging procedure that requires substantial experience.

## COMPLICATIONS

- Flap/graft necrosis
- Hematoma formation
- Venous congestion
- Infection
- Web creep

- Circulatory compromise
- Stiffness
- Ugly/painful scar formation

## REFERENCES


1. Buck-Gramcko D. The role of nonvascularized toe phalanx transplantation. Hand Clin 1990;6:643–659.
2. Emmett AJ. The ring constriction syndrome. Handchir Mikrochir Plast Chir 1992;24:3–15.
3. Flatt AE. Constriction ring syndrome. In: The Care of Congenital Hand Anomalies. St. Louis: CV Mosby, 1977:214.
4. Foucher G, Medina J, Navarro R, et al. Toe transfer in congenital hand malformations. J Reconstr Microsurg 2001;17:1–7.
5. Goldberg NH, Watson HK. Composite toe (phalanx and epiphysis) transfers in the reconstruction of the aphalangic hand. J Hand Surg Am 1982;7:454–459.
6. Jones NF, Hansen SL, Bates SJ. Toe-to-hand transfers for congenital anomalies of the hand. Hand Clin 2007;23:129–136.
7. Miura T. Congenital constriction band syndrome. J Hand Surg Am 1984;9A(1):82–88.
8. Moran SL, Jensen M, Bravo C. Amniotic band syndrome of the upper extremity: diagnosis and management. J Am Acad Orthop Surg 2007;15:397–407.
9. Soldado F, Aguirre M, Peiró JL, et al. Fetoscopic release of extremity amniotic bands with risk of amputation. J Pediatr Orthop 2009;29:290–293.
10. Uchida Y, Sugioka Y. Peripheral nerve palsy associated with congenital constriction band syndrome. J Hand Surg Br 1991;16:109–112.
11. Upton J, Tan C. Correction of constriction rings. J Hand Surg 1991;(1695):947–953.
12. Wiedrich TA. Congenital constriction band syndrome. Hand Clin 1998;14:29–38.

# 74 CHAPTER

# Clinodactyly

Robert Carrigan

## DEFINITION

- *Clinodactyly* refers to an abnormal about of radioulnar angulation of a digit (>15 degrees).
- The small finger is most commonly observed.
- This condition is often bilateral.

## ANATOMY

- The finger consists of three phalanges (proximal, middle, and distal).
- The normal phalangeal physis is located at the proximal portion of each phalanx.

## PATHOGENESIS

- The angulation is result of abnormal development of one of the phalanges (most often the middle phalanx [p2]).
- Abnormal development of the phalanx may be due to an irregular physis (longitudinal bracket epiphysis). This may also be referred to as a *delta phalanx*.
- The tethering effect of the bracket epiphysis on the radial side of the finger causes abnormal growth of the phalanx resulting in a triangular or trapezoidal shape.
- Extra bones may be encountered.

## NATURAL HISTORY

- The natural history of clinodactyly is variable and poorly documented, owing to the great number of cases that are asymptomatic and do not require treatment.
- Angulation may be stable or rapidly progressive at times of growth, depending on the extent of the involvement of the physis and/or presence of extra phalanges.

## PATIENT HISTORY AND PHYSICAL EXAM FINDINGS

- Clinodactyly may be present at birth or develop during a period of growth (**FIG 1**).
- Clinodactyly is often bilateral in the small finger.
- Clinodactyly is an autosomal dominant condition with variable penetration.
- Involvement of the thumb is rare and is associated with varying syndromes.

## IMAGING AND OTHER DIAGNOSTIC STUDIES

- Standard radiographs (three views: anteroposterior[AP], lateral [LAT], and oblique [OBL]) of the hand and affected digit are sufficient to determine the area of involvement.
- Contralateral images are useful for comparison.
- Advanced imaging such as computed tomography (CT) is rarely needed. Magnetic resonance imaging (MRI) may be useful to delineate the shape of a bracket diaphysis.

## DIFFERENTIAL DIAGNOSIS

- The diagnosis of clinodactyly is straightforward; clinical examination and radiographs are sufficient to make the diagnosis.
- Associated syndrome should be screened for, these include Down, Rubinstein-Taybi, Apert, and Russell-Silver.

## NONOPERATIVE MANAGEMENT

- Observation may be considered for angulated digits that do not impair function. Splinting is not effective.
- Most cases can be treated nonoperatively; surgery should be considered for significant angular deformity that compromises hand function.

## SURGICAL MANAGEMENT

### Preoperative Planning

- Timing of surgery is variable, depending on the degree of angulation and how much growth potential remains.
- Small amounts of angulation with little remaining growth potential may be addressed when the child is older.
- Larger amounts of angulation or children with the potential for worsening angulation may consider earlier intervention.

### Positioning

- The patient is positioned supine on the operating room table and the body is pulled over to the affected side.

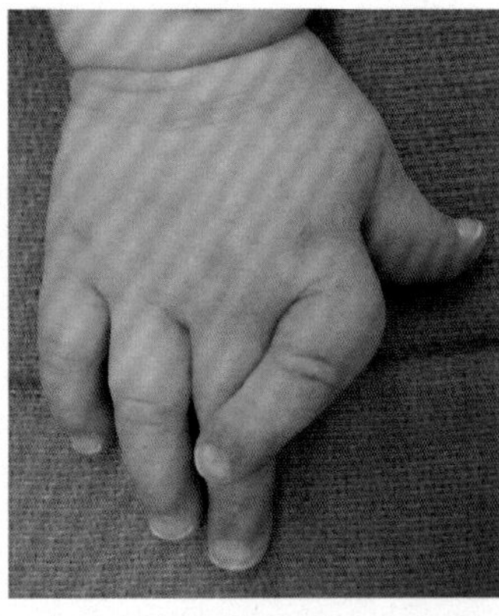

**FIG 1** • Clinodactyly of the index finger from osteochondroma in a child with multiple hereditary exostosis.

- The arm is placed on a radiolucent hand table and an arm tourniquet is applied.
- Prepping and draping are performed in the standard fashion.

## Approach

- Several approaches may be considered for clinodactyly correction, but the principles remain consistent regardless of surgical approach.
- Skin incisions must address the excess skin on the convex side of the angulation and the lack of skin on the concave side.
- Extensile incisions are preferred.
- Bony correction of the angulation can be accomplished via osteotomy, physiolysis of the bracket diaphysis, excision of extra phalanx, or a combination of all three.



## Physiolysis

- This technique is favored for the younger child with significant growth potential.
- Skin incisions are made over the radial aspect of the digit.
- Flaps are developed and the flexor and extensor tendons are identified and protected.
- Fluoroscopy is used to identify the physis.
- The physis is incised with a no. 15 blade transversely and the central portion of the physis is removed with a small curette. Local fat may be placed in the void but may not be necessary.
- The skin is closed and a cast is applied.

## Phalanx Excision

- Elliptical skin incisions along the convex side of the angulation are favored. These incisions allow for excision of redundant skin, aiding the cosmetic appearance on completion of the case (**TECH FIG 1**).
- The extensor tendons are protected and the extra phalanx is identified.
- The phalanx is excised and the collateral ligaments are preserved.
- The joint is inspected and reduced.
- The collateral ligaments are tightened with interrupted suture and the joint is pinned with a single K-wire along the long axis of the joint.
- Skin is closed with absorbable suture and a cast is applied.

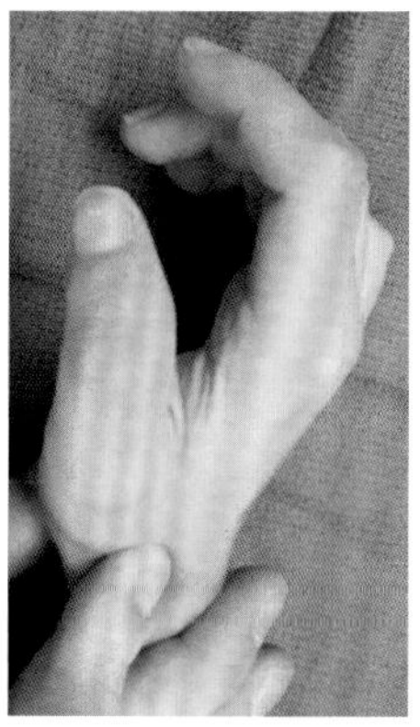

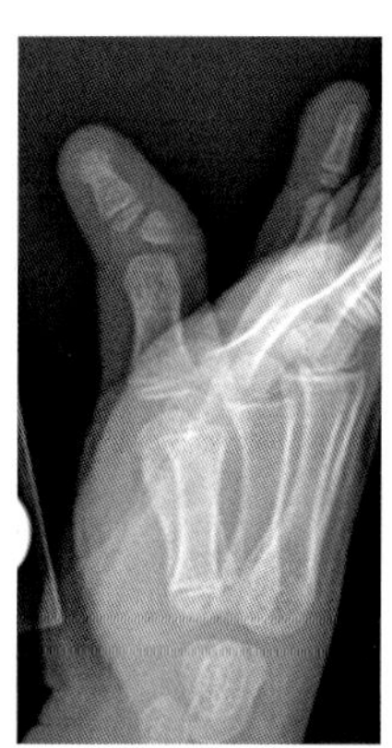

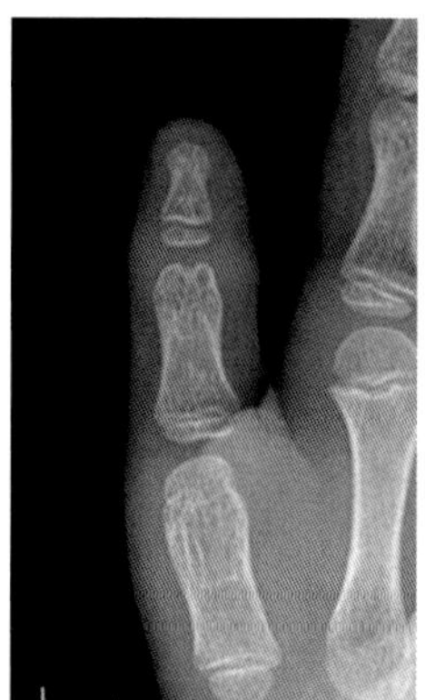

A B C

**TECH FIG 1** • Clinodactyly of the thumb. **A.** Clinical photograph. **B.** Radiograph demonstrating triangular phalanx. **C.** Postoperative photograph after excision of triangular phalanx and pinning.

## Osteotomy

- Closing wedge, opening wedge, or reverse wedge osteotomy can be strongly considered for large amounts of angulation in patients who are close to or skeletally mature (**TECH FIG 2**).
- Incisions are made along the convex side (ulnar side of the finger) for closing wedge osteotomies and along the concave side (radial side of the finger) for opening wedge ostetomies.
- Skin flaps are developed.
- The digital neurovascular bundles are protected as well as the extensor tendons.
- The periosteum is elevated off the phalanx and the osteotomy is templated.
- The closing wedge osteotomy can be performed with either thin narrow rongeur or oscillating saw.
  - A rongeur is favorable in smaller children where the bone is small.
  - Using this method, the far cortex is left in place and the finger is bent back to a neutral alignment using the far cortex as hinge.
  - The osteotomy is stabilized with one or two K-wires.

- The opening wedge osteotomy is performed in a similar fashion as the closing wedge, only the incision is made on the radial border of the digit; no wedge of bone is removed.
  - A single osteotomy is made in the radial aspect of the phalanx, leaving the ulnar cortex intact.
  - The osteotomy is opened and stabilized with one or two K-wires.
  - Bone graft is often not necessary in young children.
- The reverse wedge is useful when large amounts of angulation correction are necessary. This technique allows for correction of angulation with preservation of length.
  - This osteotomy is performed with an oscillating saw.
  - A wedge of bone is taken from the near side and flipped and inserted in the far side.
  - The osteotomy is stabilized with one or two K-wires.

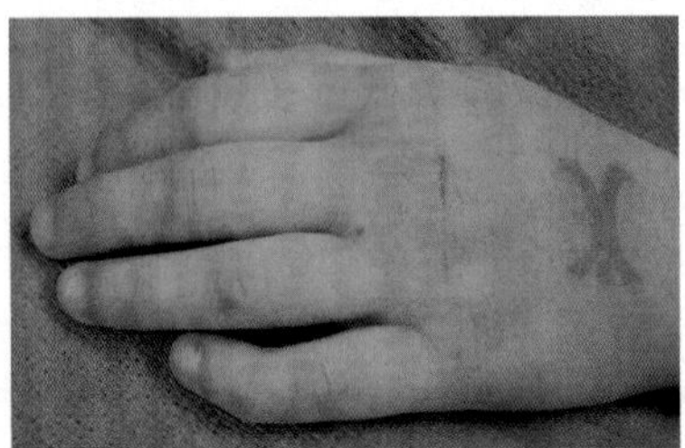
A

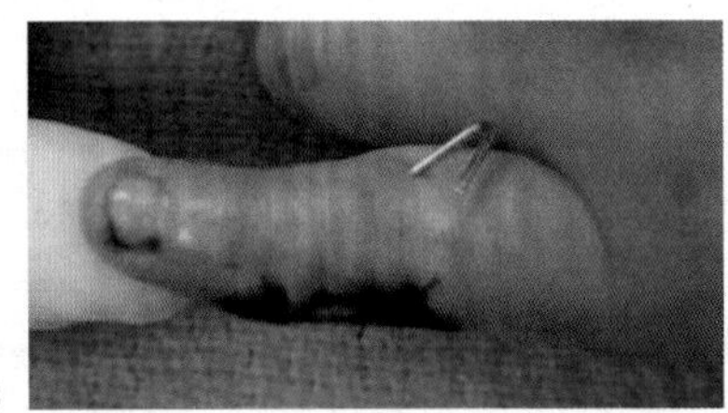
B

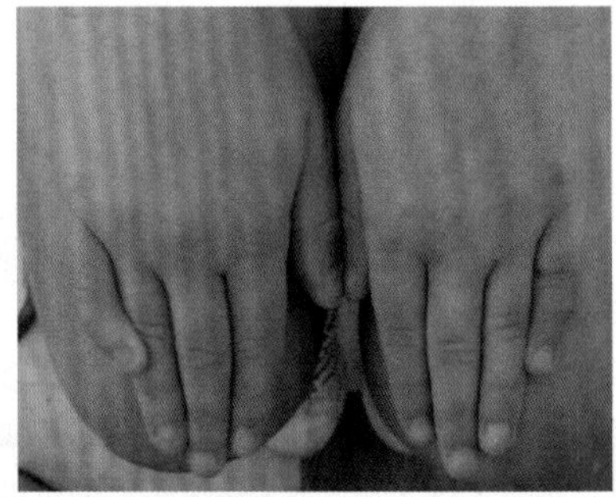
C

**TECH FIG 2** • Small finger clinodactyly. **A.** Preoperative clinical photograph. **B.** Intraoperative photograph after osteotomy and pinning. **C.** Postoperative photograph demonstrating surgical correction of the left and no correction on the right.

## PEARLS AND PITFALLS

| | |
|---|---|
| **Undercorrection or overcorrection of angular deformity** | ■ Precise surgical planning with good radiographs and measured correction |
| **Redundant skin causing uneven appearance of finger after phalanx excision** | ■ Elliptical skin incisions can reduce redundant skin on the convex side when excising a phalanx. |
| **Lack of motion after angular correction** | ■ Excessive periosteal stripping leading to tendon adhesions. Limit soft tissue dissection. |

## POSTOPERATIVE CARE

- Occupational therapy is started after the first postoperative visit. The parents are instructed to wash and clean the hand. A progressive active and passive range of motion program is initiated.
- In cases where an osteotomy is performed, the patient is placed in a cast until the osteotomy has healed (typically 4 weeks). At this time, the pins are removed and occupational therapy is initiated.
- Patients are followed until full range of motion has been achieved, typically 6 to 8 weeks.

## OUTCOMES

- Outcomes from clinodactyly correction are generally good.
- Patient satisfaction is correlated to the degree of preoperative angulation and degree of correction.

## COMPLICATIONS

- Residual angulation may persist, usually due to initial undercorrection or continued abnormal growth. This usually is not an issue especially when the amount of angulation is mild and when the magnitude of the correction is great.
- Digital stiffness may be encountered. Tendon adhesions and scar tissue are usually the cause. Occupational therapy and parental education are helpful to address a loss of full digital motion.

## SUGGESTED READINGS


1. Ali M, Jackson T, Rayan GM. Closing wedge osteotomy of abnormal middle phalanx for clinodactyly. J Hand Surg Am 2009;34: 914–918.
2. Al-Qattan MM. Congenital sporadic clinodactyly of the index finger. Ann Plast Surg 2007;59:682–687.
3. Bednar MS, Bindra RR, Light TR. Epiphyseal bar resection and fat interposition for clinodactyly. J Hand Surg Am 2010;35:834–837.
4. Strauss NL, Goldfarb CA. Surgical correction of clinodactyly: two straightforward techniques. Tech Hand Up Extrem Surg 2010;14: 54–57.
5. Ty JM, James MA. Failure of differentiation: part II (arthrogryposis, camptodactyly, clinodactyly, Madelung deformity, trigger finger, and trigger thumb). Hand Clin 2009;25:195–213.

# Correction of Thumb-in-Palm Deformity in Cerebral Palsy

Thanapong Waitayawinyu, Carley Vuillermin, and Scott N. Oishi

75 CHAPTER

## DEFINITION

- The thumb-in-palm deformity is a fixed adduction–flexion posture in the affected hand of the patient with spastic cerebral palsy. This influences both hand function and hygiene.

## ANATOMY

- Imbalance of the spastic thumb flexor–adductor and the paretic thumb extensor results in thumb-in-palm deformity (**FIG 1A**).
- The adductor pollicis (AP) is the most commonly involved muscle; the abductor pollicis brevis (APB) is usually not involved.[17]
- The spastic AP, the first dorsal interosseous muscle, or both adduct the thumb and index metacarpals and cause first web space contracture.
- If the flexor pollicis brevis (FPB) is spastic, the thumb metacarpophalangeal (MCP) joint will develop a flexion deformity.
- Involvement of both the AP and FPB results in a thumb flexion and adduction posture with the thumb lying across the palm.
- Involvement of the flexor pollicis longus (FPL) results in added thumb interphalangeal (IP) joint flexion (**FIG 1B**).
- Weak thumb extensor and abductor pollicis longus (APL) may also contribute to the deformity.
- Active function of the extensor pollicis longus (EPL) and extensor pollicis brevis (EPB) may result in hyperextension of the thumb MCP joint.

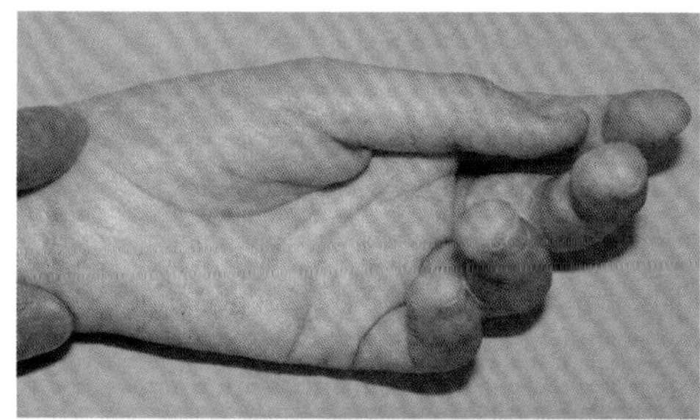

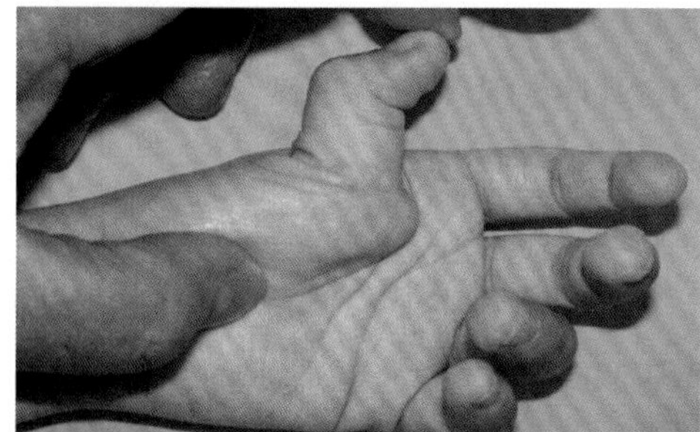

**FIG 1** • Thumb-in-palm deformity (**A**) demonstrating MCP laxity and hyperextension (**B**).

## PATHOGENESIS

- Cerebral palsy is permanent disorder of the development of movement and posture, causing activity limitation, attributed to a nonprogressive neurologic disturbance that occurred in the developing fetal or infant brain. The disorders of cerebral palsy are often accompanied by disturbances of sensation, perception, and cognition.[11]
- The musculoskeletal findings develop secondarily. Spasticity initially results in shortening of the myotendinous unit and ultimately secondary contractures.
  - Paresis of muscles may contribute to greater deformity when spastic muscles are unopposed. The ultimate deformity depends on the overall imbalance.

## NATURAL HISTORY

- A supple thumb-in-palm posture is a normal finding in infants during the first year. Persistence of a tightly closed thumb in palm longer than 1 year is abnormal and should be evaluated.[3]
- The deformity is usually correctable at first and then progresses to a fixed deformity as myostatic contracture develops.
- A progressive and variable-size discrepancy of the involved limb may develop, resulting in a smaller thumb.[1]
- The lack of thumb extension and abduction can impair hand grip, function, appearance, and hygiene.

## PATIENT HISTORY AND PHYSICAL FINDINGS

- A complete history and physical examination of a child with cerebral palsy should be done carefully and thoroughly.
- Input from other professionals such as neurologists and occupational therapists is often helpful.
- Associated deformities of the spastic upper extremity such as finger and wrist flexion, forearm pronation, elbow flexion, and shoulder adduction and internal rotation should also be evaluated. Surgical treatment of thumb-in-palm deformity may be only one part of surgical care of the involved extremity.
- Thumb muscle involvement, motion, and stability should be evaluated in the physical examination before organizing the treatment plan.
  - Individual muscle involvement is detected by observing thumb position and palpating spastic or contracted muscles (Table 1). As spasticity is rate-dependent tone, slow gradual stretch should be able to overcome this force, unlike a contracture which is a fixed shortening of a muscle tendon unit or joint.
  - Motion and stability are assessed by passive and active range of thumb abduction–adduction, flexion–extension, and palmar abduction and opposition.

**Table 1 Grading of Thumb-in-Palm Deformity**

| Degree of Deformity | Illustration | Classification: House (1981) | Tonkin (2001) | Description |
|---|---|---|---|---|
| Simple deformity | | Type I | | Spastic or contracted AP, first dorsal interosseous muscle, or both |
| Intrinsic deformity | | Type II | Type 1 | Spastic or contracted AP, first dorsal interosseous, or both<br>Spastic or contracted FPB |
| | | Type III | | Spastic or contracted AP, first dorsal interosseous, or both<br>Compensatory action of EPL and EPB to the unstable MCP joint<br>Absence of spastic FPL |
| Extrinsic deformity | | | Type 2 | Spastic or contracted FPL<br>Paretic EPL |
| Most severe: combined intrinsic and extrinsic deformity | | Type IV | Type 3 | Spastic or contracted AP, first dorsal interosseous, or both<br>Spastic or contracted FPB and FPL |

AP, adductor pollicis longus; FPB, flexor pollicis brevis; EPL, extensor pollicis longus; EPB, extensor pollicis brevis; MCL, metacarpophalangeal; FPL, flexor pollicis longus.

- The pattern of voluntary grasp and release of large objects and manipulation of small objects should be determined by observing the child during functional activities.
- Sensory deficits impair function. Assessment of sensation should include stereognosis.
- Repeated observation or videotaping of the child during various activities can also be useful for accurate evaluation. This can be particularly valuable in detecting dystonia.
- Lower extremity function and need for intervention should be considered and coordinated appropriately.

## IMAGING AND OTHER DIAGNOSTIC STUDIES

- Electrophysiologic testing and selective nerve blocks may help in localizing involved muscles and identifying muscles available for tendon transfers.
- Select nerve blocks may help differentiate between spastic, spared, and fibrotic muscles.
- Dynamic electromyography (EMG) with motion analysis may offer important information for planning tendon transfer surgery.[5]
- Radiographs may reveal thumb joint instability or growth disturbance.

## DIFFERENTIAL DIAGNOSIS

- Clasped thumb
- Distal arthrogryposis
- Apparent absence of thumb extensor (faux extensor agenesis)

## MANAGEMENT

- The goals of treatment need to be clearly defined.
- No peripheral intervention will overcome the fundamental central nervous system etiology.

- For many patients, the goal will be to improve thumb position for function; however, there is a subset of highly involved patients for whom improved hygiene alone may the goal.

## NONOPERATIVE MANAGEMENT

- Use of tone-reducing medication such as botulinum toxin to the AP can soften the deformities and improve joint range of motion for nonoperative management.[4]
- In mild, nonrigid deformity, nonoperative treatment with orthoses may help in maintaining thumb abduction and improve hand function,[13] but too-rigid splinting may result in limited thumb motion.

## SURGICAL MANAGEMENT

- The principles of surgery for thumb-in-palm deformity are the following[2]:
  - Release of spastic muscles or contractures
  - Augmentation of paretic muscles
  - Stabilization of unstable thumb joints
- Release of contracture with or without augmentation of weak muscles aims to rebalance the thumb muscles, depending on the pattern of motor dysfunction of the thumb and the patient's degree of voluntary control.
- Release of spastic muscle or myostatic contractures can be performed by intrinsic muscle release of the AP, FPB, APB, and first dorsal interosseous.
  - Extrinsic muscle release of the FPL may be considered if it is affected.
  - Secondary skin and fascial contracture of the first web space need to be addressed by four-flap or double-opposing Z-plasty.
- Augmentation of paretic thumb abduction and extension can be accomplished by a combination of tenodesis and tendon rerouting or transfers and depends on the specific deficit, the muscles available, and the extent of voluntary control of selected muscles.
- Thumb MCP joint arthrodesis or sesamoid capsulodesis should be considered for stabilizing the thumb MCP joints when the joint remains unstable.[2]
  - These joint stabilization procedures can also enhance tendon transfer procedures for extension–abduction.
- Thumb MCP joint arthrodesis is considered when tendon transfer fails to correct the deformities or when sesamoid capsulodesis cannot control the hyperextension of the MCP joint.[1]
- Thumb carpometacarpal (CMC) joint stabilization is indicated when metacarpal adduction cannot be controlled. CMC fusion, which preserves scaphotrapezial motion, is preferable to the rigid intermetacarpal fusion.[2]
- Thumb IP joint fusion is usually not necessary, but this procedure may be indicated when the IP joint flexion contracture is severe or in the rare event of an FPL rupture after lengthening.[2]
- Neurectomy may be an adjunct procedure for a clenched fist deformity in a hand with no active movement and difficulty with passive hand function including hygiene[9]; however, its role is limited.
- Table 2 lists surgical options for treating thumb-in-palm deformity.[14]

**Table 2 Surgical Options for Correcting Thumb-in-Palm Deformity**

| |
|---|
| **Releases** |
| Adductor release in palm |
| Adductor tenotomy |
| First dorsal interosseous release |
| FPB release |
| FPL slide |
| **First web skin and fascia release** |
| **Augmentation of APL, EPL, EPB using** |
| Brachioradialis |
| FDS |
| PL |
| EPL to EPB |
| FCR or FCU |
| ECRL |
| **APL tenodesis** |
| Through radius to brachioradialis, ECRL, FCR through first dorsal compartment |
| **Joint stabilization** |
| CMC joint fusion |
| MCP joint sesamoid capsulodesis |
| MCP joint fusion |
| IP joint fusion |

FPB, flexor pollicis brevis; FPL, flexor pollicis longus; APL, adductor pollicis longus; EPL, extensor pollicis longus; EPB, extensor pollicis brevis, FDS, flexor digitorum superficialis; PL, pollicis longus; FCR, flexor carpi radialis; FCU, flexor carpi ulnaris; ECRL, extensor carpi radialis longus; CMC, carpometacarpal; MCP, metacarpophalangeal; IP, interphalangeal. (Adapted from Tonkin MA. Thumb deformity in the spastic hand: classification and surgical techniques. Tech Hand Up Extrem Surg 2003;7:18–25.)

### Preoperative Planning

- Comprehensive evaluation is necessary with a multispecialty approach.
- Surgery should be done when the central nervous system has matured and the child is old enough to cooperate with postoperative therapy—usually at least 5 to 6 years old.[6]
- Associated abnormalities (eg, seizures, mental status problems) should be assessed and the management optimized before surgery is contemplated.
- Patient understanding and emotional readiness as well as family and social support should be addressed before surgery.
- Physical examination under anesthesia is crucial. This can differentiate spastic from myostatic conditions and can accurately evaluate the stability of thumb joints.

### Positioning

- The patient is placed in the supine position, and surgery is performed under general anesthesia and tourniquet control.

### Approach

- Surgical approaches for thumb-in-palm deformity depend on the objectives.
- Release of static or long-standing intrinsic contracture is usually performed through a curved incision located over the line of the thenar crease to release the origin of the AP with or without the origin of the FPB.[8]
- Release of a simple intrinsic contracture may be performed through the first web space approach to release the AP and the first dorsal interosseous muscle, combined with four-flap

or double-opposing Z-plasty to release the secondary web space contracture.[2]

- A surgical approach by a small incision over the volar aspect of the distal forearm is used for extrinsic release of the FPL tendon, if necessary.
- A dorsal approach to the thumb and a dorsoradial approach over the wrist is used for augmentation of thumb extensors, with a volar-radial approach being used for augmentation of the thumb abductor.



## Release of Contractures

### Release of Static Intrinsic Contracture

- A curved skin incision is performed next to the line of the thenar crease, extending distally from the carpal tunnel area (**TECH FIG 1A**).
- The superficial palmar arch and median nerve, including its motor branch to the thenar muscle, distal to the transverse carpal ligament are identified and protected. Careful dissection must be performed because occasionally, the motor branch comes through the transverse carpal ligament instead of being distal to this structure (**TECH FIG 1B**).
- The flexor digitorum sublimis and profundi are identified and retracted ulnarly with the neurovascular bundle.
- The transverse head of AP is identified and divided from its origin on the third metacarpal (**TECH FIG 1C,D**).
- The motor branch of the ulnar nerve and the deep palmar arch are identified and protected.
- Release of the oblique head of the AP from its origin at the bases of the second and third metacarpal, capitate, and trapezoid is performed.
- The FPB origin at the transverse carpal ligament and trapezium may also be released if this muscle limits abduction and extension of the thumb ray.
- The first dorsal interosseous may be released at the distal portion of the muscle from the ulnar aspect of the first metacarpal if needed to obtain adequate passive abduction and extension of the thumb.

### Release of Simple Intrinsic Contracture

- A four-flap Z-plasty over the contracted first web space is designed (**TECH FIG 2A,B**).
- After the skin incision, the dorsal fascia is incised while protecting the neurovascular bundles.
- The first dorsal interosseous is released at its origin from the thumb metacarpal.
- The AP is lengthened by release in an oblique cut at its intramuscular tendon; the surgeon should aim to preserve some adductor function (**TECH FIG 2C**).
- Four skin flaps are rearranged to increase the first web space (**TECH FIG 2D**).

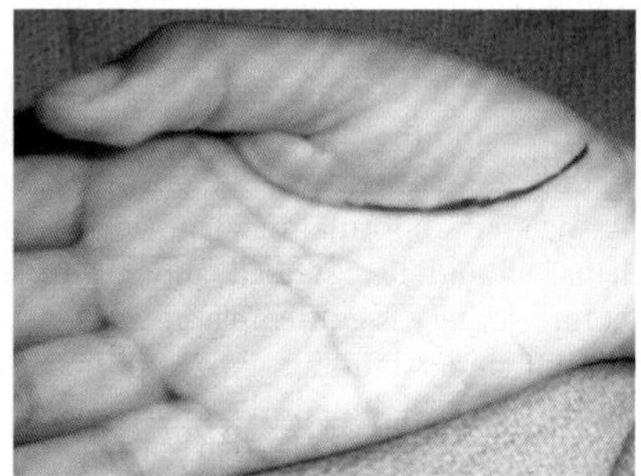
A

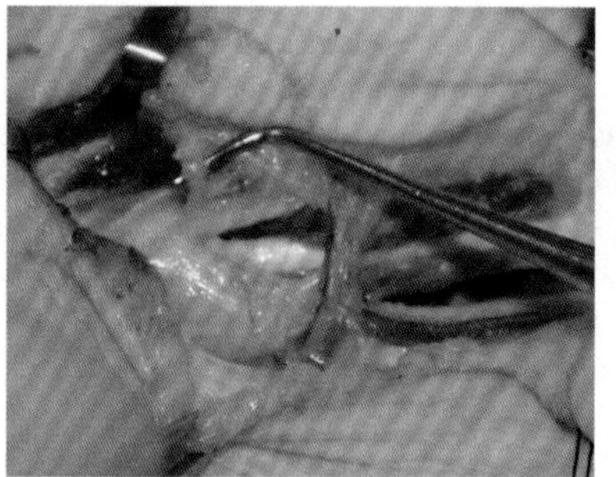
B

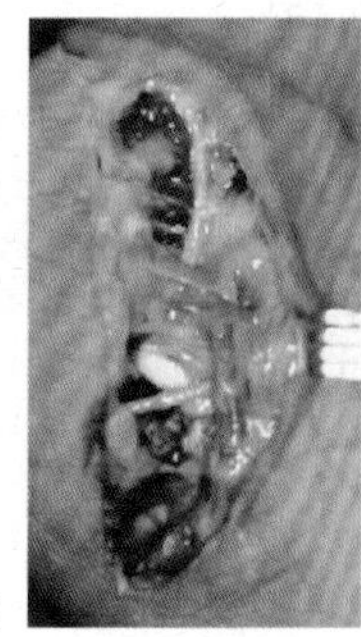
C

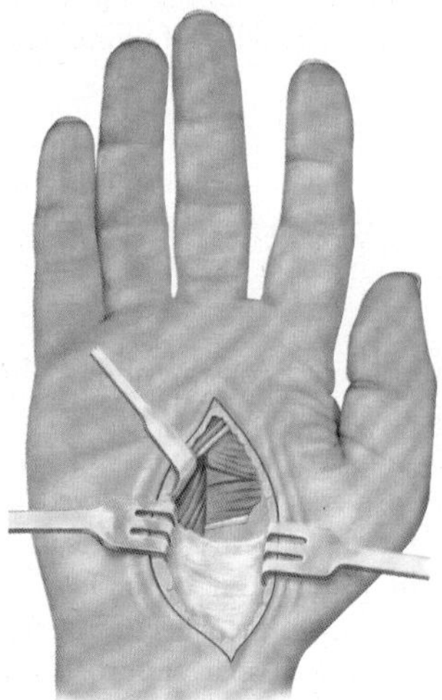
D

**TECH FIG 1** • Intrinsic release. **A.** A curved incision is made over the thenar crease. **B.** Thenar release showing motor branch. **C,D.** Thumb intrinsics are released.

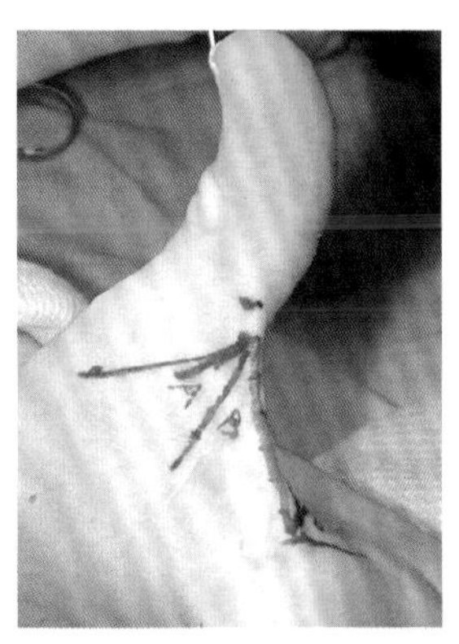
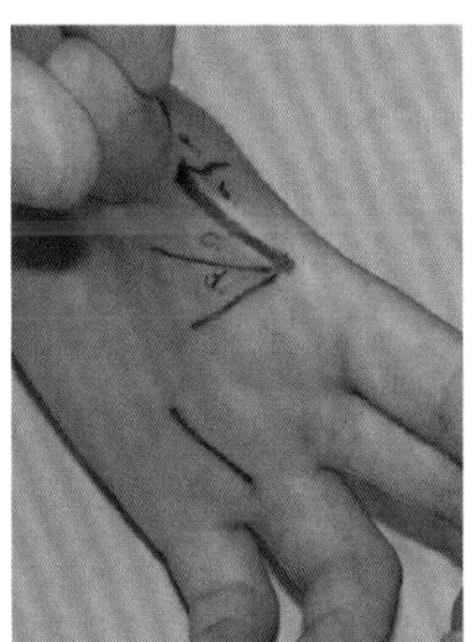
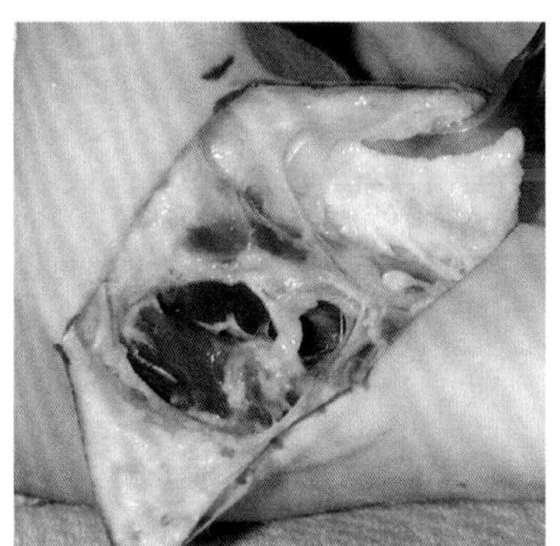
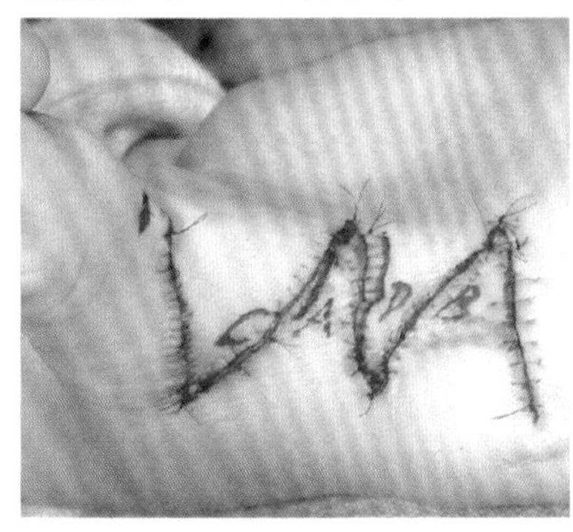

**TECH FIG 2** • Four-flap Z-plasty over first web space. **A,B.** Skin markings. **C.** Elevation of flaps and adductor exposure. **D.** After rotation of skin flaps.

## Release of Extrinsic Contracture

- A small longitudinal incision over the distal-volar aspect of the forearm is performed.
- The FPL tendon is exposed and incised over the musculotendinous portion.
- The thumb IP joint is hyperextended until 1 cm of distal sliding of the FPL tendon is identified.
- The FPL may be lengthened by Z-lengthening of the FPL tendon, with 0.5 mm of lengthening for each degree of correction.[1]

# Augmentation of Weak Muscles

## Abductor Pollicis Longus Augmentation

- Two small transverse incisions over the volar wrist crease and the first extensor compartment are made, aiming to expose the palmaris longus (PL) or flexor carpi radialis (FCR) and APL, respectively.
- The superficial branch of the radial nerve is identified and protected.
- The first extensor compartment is then opened, and the APL is identified. Each slip of the APL tendon should be pulled into tension to show the best slip for CMC joint abduction.
- At the volar incision, the palmar branch of the median nerve is identified and protected. The PL tendon is then divided.
- The selected APL tendon slip is translocated volarly until acceptable thumb metacarpal abduction is achieved.
- The PL tendon is passed through a subcutaneous tunnel to the volar-radial incision.
- End-to-side tendon weave of the PL to the translocated APL is then performed under sufficient tension to obtain appropriate thumb abduction (**TECH FIG 3A**).
- Alternatively, the APL tendon may be cut and the distal segment rerouted volarly and woven with end-to-end PL or end-to-side FCR. The proximal segment of the APL may be used to augment thumb MCP joint extension by end-to-side anastomosis with the EPB (**TECH FIG 3B**).

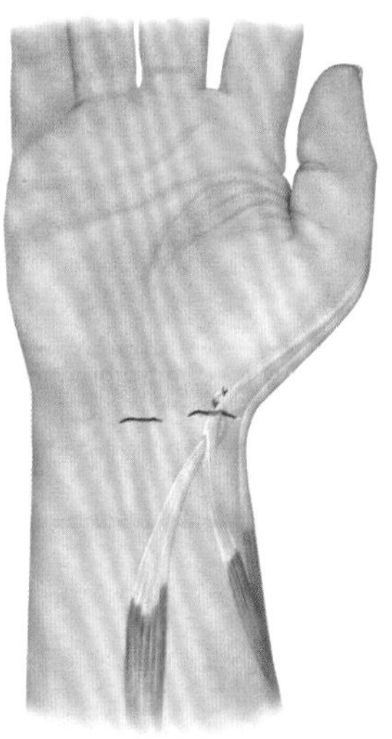
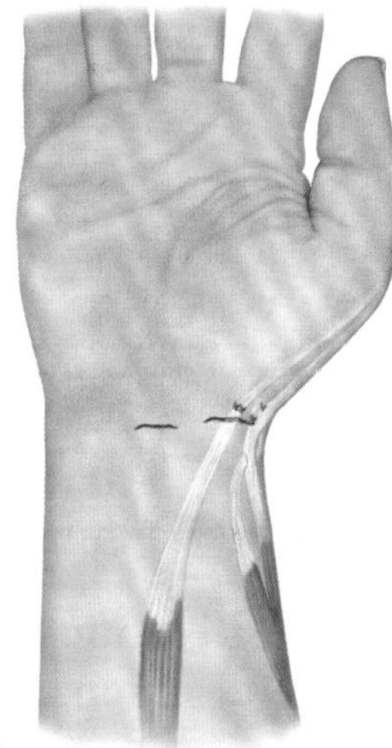

**TECH FIG 3** • **A.** Transfer of PL to translocated APL by end-to-side anastomosis. **B.** APL augmentation by rerouting of the distal segment and anastomosis with end-to-end pollicis longus or end-to-side FCR. Thumb MCP joint extension is augmented by anastomosis of the proximal segment of APL with end-to-side EPB.

### Extensor Pollicis Longus Rerouting

- A dorsal skin incision over the thumb MCP and IP joint and another small longitudinal incision just ulnar to the Lister tubercle are used for this procedure.[7]
- The EPL tendon is identified and divided 10 mm distal to the MCP joint. The tendon is then retracted out to the second incision (**TECH FIG 4A**).
- The EPL tendon is rerouted to the radial aspect of the Lister tubercle and passed subcutaneously around the APL and EPB tendon (**TECH FIG 4B**).
- The tendon is then passed through the MCP joint capsule (**TECH FIG 4C**).
- The thumb is set in appropriate abduction and IP extension. The rerouted EPL is sutured back to the extensor mechanism 10 mm distal to the defect.
- The rerouted EPL may be reinforced by the transfer of the PL, FCR, or brachioradialis.
- The EPL may be divided proximal to the Lister tubercle, leaving the tendon attached to its insertion. Rerouting is then performed from distal to proximal (**TECH FIG 4D**).[10]
- The EPL may be rerouted to the new pulley created from the extensor retinaculum (**TECH FIG 4E,F**).[1]

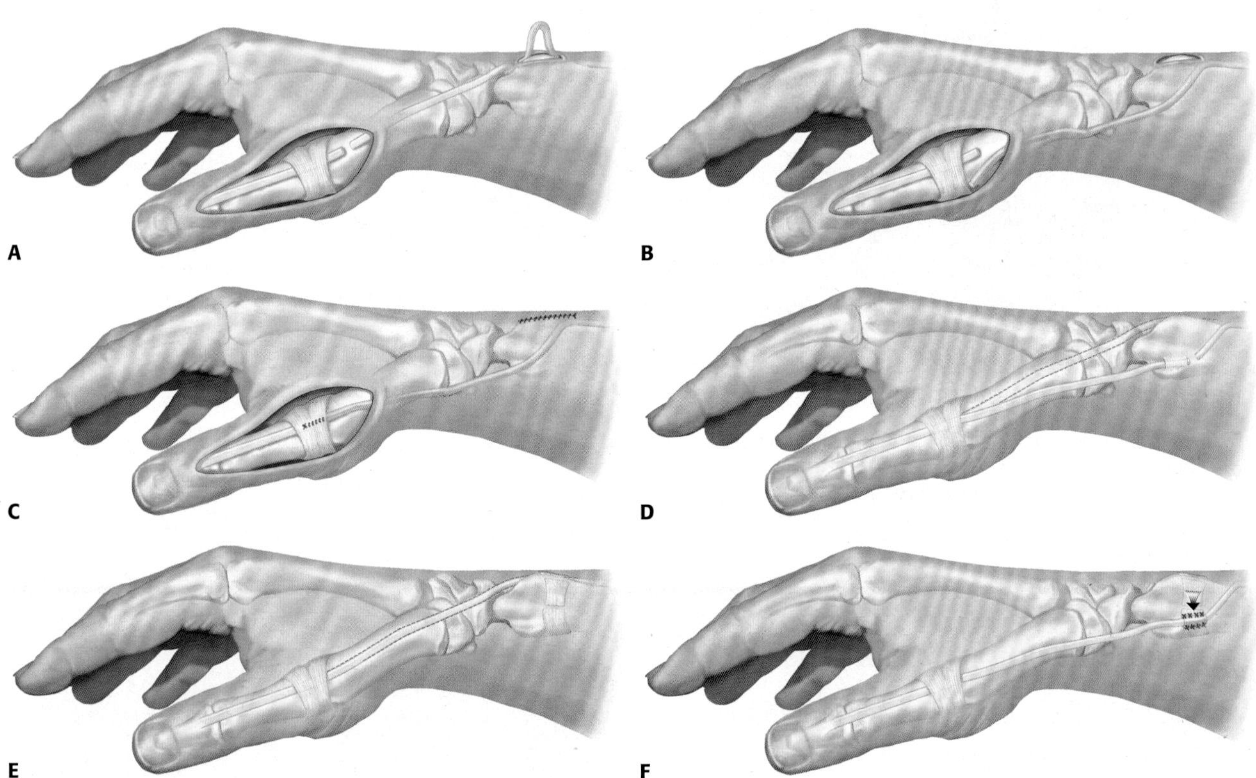


**TECH FIG 4** • EPL rerouting. **A.** EPL tendon is divided distally and mobilized. **B.** The tendon is rerouted to the radial aspect of the Lister tubercle and passed subcutaneously around the APL and EPB tendon. **C.** The rerouted EPL is sutured back to the extensor mechanism. **D.** Modified EPL rerouting technique. The EPL tendon is divided proximal to the Lister tubercle, rerouted to the first extensor compartment, and sutured back to the proximal stump. **E,F.** EPL routing to the retinaculum. **E.** The EPL tendon is released from the third extensor compartment and rerouted radially. **F.** The new pulley for the rerouted EPL is created from the extensor retinaculum.

## Stabilization of Thumb Metacarpophalangeal Joint

### Thumb Metacarpophalangeal Joint Arthrodesis

- A dorsoulnar incision is made over the thumb MCP joint.
- The extensor mechanism is split longitudinally, and the ulnar collateral ligament is then detached from the metacarpal head to expose the joint (**TECH FIG 5A**).
- The articular cartilage of the metacarpal head is removed with a scalpel, and the proximal phalanx epiphysis is shaved until the secondary center of ossification is exposed (**TECH FIG 5B**). This allows fusion of the epiphyses and preserves the physis.
- The joint is set in 10 degrees of flexion, 10 degrees of abduction, and slight pronation,[12] and a small (1 mm in diameter), smooth Kirschner wire is passed through the joint centrally to minimize epiphyseal damage (**TECH FIG 5C**).

### Sesamoid Capsulodesis

- A curved dorsoradial incision is made over the thumb MCP joint.[15]
- The accessory collateral ligament is divided at its insertion into the volar plate.

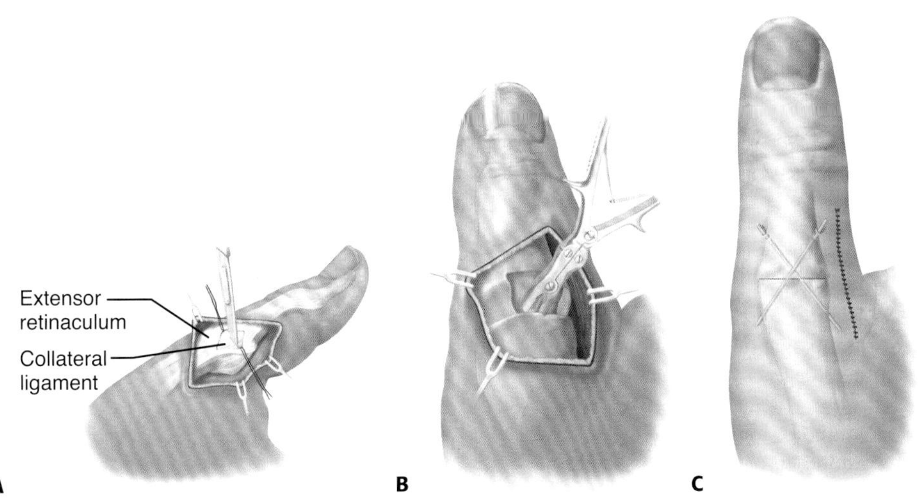


**TECH FIG 5** • Thumb MCP arthrodesis. **A.** After the extensor mechanism over the MCP joint is split longitudinally, the ulnar collateral ligament is detached from the metacarpal head. **B.** The articular cartilage of the metacarpal head is removed. The epiphyseal plate of the proximal phalanx is preserved. **C.** After the joint is set, smooth Kirschner wires are used to maintain the joint position.

- The volar plate is then mobilized to expose the radial sesamoid.
- The articular cartilage of the sesamoid is denuded. A cortical defect is created at the head–neck junction of the metacarpal.
- The suture is passed through the sesamoid–volar plate and metacarpal defect with straight needles by using a Kirschner wire driver (**TECH FIG 6A**).
- The MCP joint is set to 30 degrees of flexion. The intraosseous suture is then tied over the dorsal surface of the metacarpal under the extensor tendons to secure the sesamoid to the metacarpal neck.
- A Kirschner wire is passed through the joint to maintain the joint position for 6 weeks (**TECH FIG 6B**).

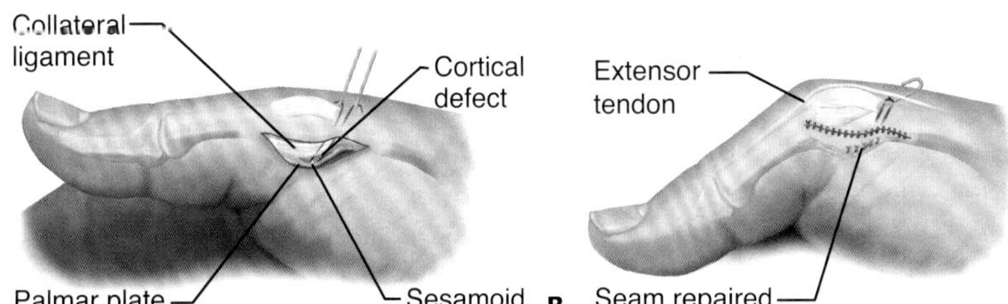


**TECH FIG 6** • Sesamoid capsulodesis. The volar plate is mobilized to expose the radial sesamoid. The articular cartilage of the sesamoid is denuded corresponding with the cortical defect created at the head–neck junction of the metacarpal. **A.** The suture is passed through the sesamoid–volar plate and metacarpal defect. **B.** The intraosseous suture is tied over the dorsal surface of the metacarpal under the extensor tendons. A Kirschner wire is used to maintain the joint position.

## PEARLS AND PITFALLS

| | |
|---|---|
| **General approach** | ■ A comprehensive history and physical examination, including appropriate investigations with other professionals, should be done for accurate diagnosis and treatment planning. |
| **Patient selection** | ■ Voluntary control of the selected muscle, which indicates the potential active use of the hand postoperatively, is important for selection of surgical candidates. |
| **Procedure selection** | ■ The procedures must be individualized because of variation in deformities in each patient. |

| | |
|---|---|
| **Release of spastic muscle and contractures** | ■ Selective release of the deforming forces is performed in sequential order to obtain adequate, functional thumb positions.<br>■ Adjacent neurovascular structures must be protected with care. |
| **Augmentation of paretic muscles** | ■ The muscle selected for transfer depends on the availability and the extent of voluntary control.<br>■ The stability of the MCP joint is evaluated before performing any augmentation procedures across it. |
| **Joint stabilization** | ■ Joint stabilization is the key to success of rebalancing the thumb-deforming forces.<br>■ The epiphyseal plate of the proximal phalanx must be preserved with care. |

## POSTOPERATIVE CARE

- Postoperative care for contracture releases includes immobilization in a short-arm thumb spica cast maintaining full thumb radial abduction and 20 degrees of palmar abduction for 4 weeks.
- Removable splinting is then continued for another 4 to 6 weeks.
- If tendon transfer has been done, immobilization should be extended to 6 weeks, followed by additional splinting for 6 weeks. Dynamic splinting may be considered.
- Immobilization of the MCP arthrodesis with a thumb spica cast should be continued until radiographic healing is detected.

## OUTCOMES

- The functional outcome of thumb-in-palm deformity should be assessed before and after surgery by the physician, therapist, parent, and patient.
- House et al[2] demonstrated improved functional grade in all 56 patients postoperatively. Half of patients improved three or more grades.
- Tonkin et al[16] found good results in 32 patients after surgical correction of thumb-in-palm deformity. The average follow-up was 32 months (range, 10 to 88 months).
  - The thumb was maintained out of palm in 29 of 32 patients (30 of 33 thumbs).
  - Patients could perform lateral pinch in 26 of 33 thumbs.
  - Many patients improved function, but no patient improved from dependent to independent functioning.

## COMPLICATIONS

- Inadequate release of contracted or fibrotic muscle may result in insufficient release of the thumb out of the palm.
- Adhesions along the transferred tendon may cause loss of excursion postoperatively.
- Improper techniques such as overlengthening and an incorrect vector of transfer may result in limited active abduction and extension of the thumb.
- Untreated or inadequate treatment of an unstable MCP joint may result in failed tendon transfer.
- Avoiding neurovascular injury is crucial. Care should be taken to properly identify and protect neurovascular bundles throughout surgery.
- An improper rehabilitation program and social support may result in failed treatment.

## REFERENCES


1. Goldner JL, Koman LA, Gelberman R, et al. Arthrodesis of the metacarpophalangeal joint of the thumb in children and adults. Adjunctive treatment of thumb-in-palm deformity in cerebral palsy. Clin Orthop Relat Res 1990;(253):75–89.
2. House JH, Gwathmey FW, Fidler MO. A dynamic approach to the thumb-in-palm deformity in cerebral palsy. J Bone Joint Surg Am 1981;63(2):216–225.
3. Jaffe M, Tal Y, Dabbah H, et al. Infants with a thumb-in-fist posture. Pediatrics 2000;105(3):E41.
4. Koman LA, Mooney JF III, Smith B, et al. Management of cerebral palsy with botulinum A toxin: preliminary investigation. J Pediatr Orthop 1993;13:489–495.
5. Kozin SH, Keenan MA. Using dynamic electromyography to guide surgical treatment of the spastic upper extremity in the brain-injured patient. Clin Orthop Relat Res 1993;(288):109–117.
6. Lawson RD, Tonkin MA. Surgical management of the thumb in cerebral palsy. Hand Clin 2003;19:667–677.
7. Manske PR. Redirection of extensor pollicis longus in the treatment of spastic thumb-in-palm deformity. J Hand Surg Am 1985;10(4):553–560.
8. Matev IB. Surgical treatment of flexion–adduction contracture of the thumb in cerebral palsy. Acta Orthop Scand 1970;41:439–445.
9. Pappas N, Baldwin K, Keenan MA. Efficacy of median nerve recurrent branch neurectomy as an adjunct to ulnar motor nerve neurectomy and wrist arthrodesis at the time of superficialis to profundus transfer in prevention of intrinsic spastic thumb-in-palm deformity. J Hand Surg Am 2010;35(8):1310–1316.
10. Rayan GM, Saccone PG. Treatment of spastic thumb-in-palm deformity: a modified extensor pollicis longus tendon rerouting. J Hand Surg Am 1996;21(5):834–839.
11. Rosenbaum P, Paneth N, Leviton A, et al. A report: the definition and classification of cerebral palsy April 2006. Dev Med Child Neurol Suppl 2007;109:8–14.
12. Swanson AB. Surgery of the hand in cerebral palsy. In: Flynn JE, ed. Hand Surgery. Baltimore: Williams & Wilkins, 1982:476–488.
13. Ten Berge SR, Boonstra AM, Dijkstra PU, et al. A systematic evaluation of the effect of thumb opponens splints on hand function in children with unilateral spastic cerebral palsy. Clin Rehabil 2012;26(4):362–371.
14. Tonkin MA. Thumb deformity in the spastic hand: classification and surgical techniques. Tech Hand Up Extrem Surg 2003;7:18–25.
15. Tonkin MA, Beard AJ, Kemp SJ, et al. Sesamoid arthrodesis for hyperextension of the thumb metacarpophalangeal joint. J Hand Surg Am 1995;20(2):334–338.
16. Tonkin MA, Hatrick NC, Eckersley JR, et al. Surgery for cerebral palsy part 3: classification and operative procedures for thumb deformity. J Hand Surg Br 2001;26(5):465–470.
17. Zancolli EA, Zancolli E Jr. Surgical rehabilitation of the spastic upper limb in cerebral palsy. In: Lamb DW, ed. The Paralyzed Hand. Edinburgh: Churchill Livingstone, 1987:153–168.

# Release of the A1 Pulley to Correct Pediatric Trigger Thumb

76

CHAPTER

Roger Cornwall

## DEFINITION

- Pediatric trigger thumb is a condition in which tightness of the first annular (A1) pulley of the thumb and an enlargement or nodule of the flexor pollicis longus tendon interact to prevent normal thumb interphalangeal joint motion.
- This condition appears distinct from pediatric trigger fingers and from adult trigger digits, although similarities in pathoanatomy and presentation have earned it its name.
- The term *congenital trigger thumb* is a misnomer, as it has yet to be detected at birth in several large series prospectively examining a combined 14,581 newborns in three countries.[14,19,22,24]

## ANATOMY

- The flexor pollicis longus tendon courses through a flexor sheath in the thumb composed of a series of pulleys that prevent bowstringing of the tendon during thumb flexion.
- The most proximal pulley is termed the *A1 pulley*, given its transverse annular nature. Division of this pulley does not cause bowstringing of the tendon during thumb flexion. The next pulley is the oblique pulley, although some authors have described an intervening distinct second annular pulley analogous to the A2 pulley in the fingers.[2] These pulleys are important constraints against bowstringing.
- The digital nerves to the thumb are in proximity to the flexor pollicis longus tendon sheath. The radial digital nerve obliquely crosses the tendon sheath just proximal to the A1 pulley, and the ulnar digital nerve runs parallel to the tendon immediately alongside the A1 pulley. Injury to these structures is possible during surgical release of the A1 pulley, so precise knowledge of the anatomy is important.

## PATHOGENESIS

- The pathogenesis of pediatric trigger thumb is unknown, although recent evidence implicates benign proliferation of myofibroblasts during growth.[13]
- In adults, the pathogenesis of trigger digits has a predominantly inflammatory nature. However, in pediatric trigger thumb, biopsies have been unable to detect signs of inflammation by gross morphology or light or electron microscopy.[3]
- A genetic predisposition has been considered, especially in cases of bilateral trigger thumb, but a genetic cause for the condition is not established.[28]
- Traumatic etiologies have been proposed but with no clear data to support this theory.

## NATURAL HISTORY

- The natural history of pediatric trigger thumb has been a focus of recent attention. The earliest reports of the condition described spontaneous resolution as rare, but newer reports have described spontaneous improvement rates of 24% to 63%.[1,5,20]
- A recent study[1] regarding the natural history of pediatric trigger thumb reported a 63% resolution rate, although the definition of resolution was improvement in passive interphalangeal joint extension to neutral, not to the normal hyperextension. Furthermore, the average time to reach this improvement was 48 months from diagnosis.
  - Therefore, when considering the use of observation to treat a pediatric trigger thumb, the clinician should inform the parents that the thumb motion may improve but not return to normal and that such improvement will take an average of 4 years.

## PATIENT HISTORY AND PHYSICAL FINDINGS

- Children typically present from late infancy through 5 years of age with painless loss of motion at the interphalangeal joint. The "triggering" phenomenon that so commonly occurs in adults is rare in children.
- Parents will usually be unable to determine how long the condition has been present. Some parents will describe a preceding traumatic injury to the thumb, although such an injury may simply call the parents' attention to the thumb closely enough to notice a preexisting trigger thumb.
- Functional impairment and pain are unusual complaints, except in the case of active triggering.
- The typical physical examination finding is a flexion contracture of the thumb interphalangeal joint, as the nodule in the flexor pollicis longus tendon typically lies proximal to the A1 pulley, preventing distal excursion of the tendon and extension of the interphalangeal joint (**FIG 1A**).
- In a few cases, the nodule lies distal to the A1 pulley and the thumb rests in an extended position with the child unable to actively flex the interphalangeal joint. In this case, the passive flexion of the interphalangeal joint is normal, but interphalangeal joint flexion will not occur by tenodesis with wrist extension.
- In even fewer cases, the child will be able to actively "trigger" the thumb with active flexion and passive extension.
- Regardless of the position of the thumb interphalangeal joint, a nodule is easily palpable (and even visible) in the flexor pollicis longus tendon in the region of the palmar digital crease (**FIG 1B**). The nodule can be felt to move proximally and distally with even the few available degrees of movement of the interphalangeal joint.
- In long-standing cases of fixed flexion deformity, thumb metacarpophalangeal joint hyperextension laxity is common.

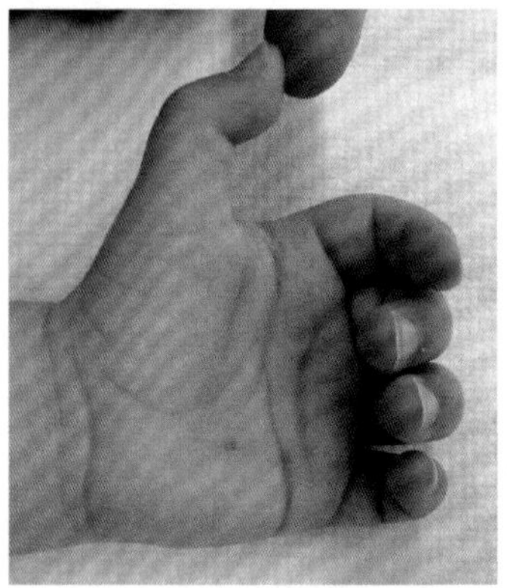
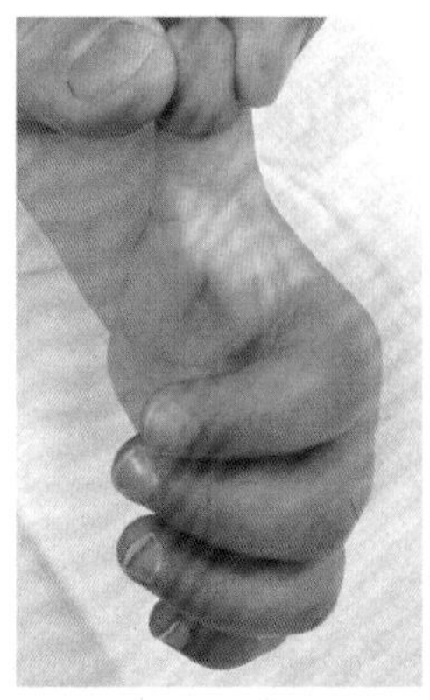
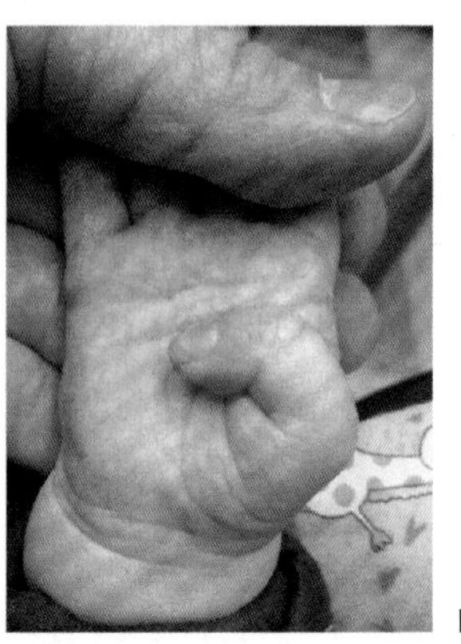
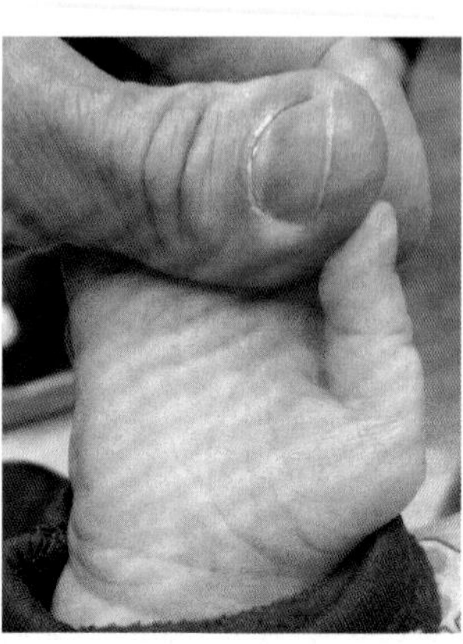

**FIG 1** • **A.** A typical pediatric trigger thumb locked in flexion. Note the inability to passively extend the interphalangeal joint. **B.** A typical trigger thumb locked in flexion. Note the visibly protruding nodule in the flexor pollicis longus tendon at the level of the palmar digital crease. **C,D.** Congenital clasped thumb. **C.** The flexed resting posture of both the interphalangeal and metacarpophalangeal joints. **D.** The interphalangeal joint typically has full passive range of motion, whereas the metacarpophalangeal joint is fixed in flexion, differentiating congenital clasped thumb from pediatric trigger thumb.

In other cases, a coronal plane deformity resembling clinodactyly may be present, although a causative relationship has yet to be established.

- Because of the possibility of bilateral involvement, both thumbs should be examined.
- An upper limb neurologic examination should be performed, including an assessment of tone in the intrinsic muscles of the hand because the thumb-in-palm deformity of cerebral palsy can be confused with trigger thumb.
- Pediatric trigger thumb should not be confused with congenital clasped thumb, in which the metacarpophalangeal joint is fixed in a flexed position, with normal interphalangeal joint motion (**FIG 1C,D**).

## IMAGING AND OTHER DIAGNOSTIC STUDIES

- Radiographs are unnecessary in the clinically obvious case; if obtained, they only confirm the resting position of the thumb interphalangeal joint.
- Radiographs may be misinterpreted as demonstrating a dorsal dislocation of the metacarpophalangeal joint due to its hyperextended posture, leading to attempts to "reduce" the dislocation. Often, these misguided attempts to reduce the dislocation involve traction on the thumb, which may pull the nodule through the pulley by extending the interphalangeal joint, satisfying the practitioner and parent that the problem has been solved. The flexed posture usually returns by the following morning, leading to a diagnosis of recurrent dislocation. Familiarity with the diagnosis of trigger thumb and its radiographic and clinical findings can prevent this cycle of intervention and anxiety.
- If the examination reveals signs of trauma (eg, swelling, ecchymosis), radiographs should be considered to rule out underlying skeletal injury.
- Advanced imaging is unnecessary.

## DIFFERENTIAL DIAGNOSIS

- Congenital clasped thumb
- Thumb-in-palm deformity (cerebral palsy)
- Arthrogryposis
- Thumb hypoplasia

## NONOPERATIVE MANAGEMENT

- Nonoperative management of pediatric trigger thumb has been described, including simple observation,[1] daily stretching by parents,[30] splinting,[16,21] and casting,[4] but it is unclear if any nonoperative treatment alters the natural history.
- A recent systematic review[7] summarized the results of conservative treatment of pediatric trigger thumbs as follows. Splinting was reported in 138 thumbs in 4 studies[15,16,21,26] with an overall success rate of 67% over 2.9 to 30 months, although the splinting was complicated by poor compliance and splint complications such as contact dermatitis. Many patients treated with splinting dropped out of the treatment to proceed with surgery. Passive stretching of the thumb was reported in 108 thumbs in 3 series,[8,12,30] with an overall success rate of 55% after 21 to 24 months of daily exercising. In addition, the success was even lower for thumbs locked in flexion. Therefore, the author discourages the use of nonoperative treatment, as it does not appear to alter the natural history despite long, arduous treatment regimens.
- In a series representative of splint treatment, Lee and associates[16] reported their results of splinting for passively correctable trigger thumbs (no locked flexion or extension deformities), finding a greater chance of improvement (decreased frequency of triggering) with splinting than with simple observation. Others[21] have reported improvement in triggering with nighttime splint treatment averaging 10 months, but in a series that included trigger fingers, there was a 24% dropout rate and there was no control group.
- In a series representative of passive stretching, Watanabe and colleagues[30] reported the results in 58 patients of passive stretching performed by the patient's mother 10 to 20 times daily for an average of 44 months. Despite claiming a 96% "satisfactory result," the authors describe only 25% of patients with locked flexion deformities experiencing improvement and none recovering normal interphalangeal joint hyperextension. Thus, it is unclear whether their results differ from other reports of natural history, even after years of stretching exercises.
- Percutaneous needle release of the A1 pulley as an office procedure under local anesthesia has been described for pediatric trigger thumb but with lower success rates than open surgical release; reported complications include incomplete release and patient intolerance of the procedure.[29]

## SURGICAL MANAGEMENT

- Surgical release of the A1 pulley has long been recognized as a safe and effective treatment for pediatric trigger thumb.
- When forming surgical indications, the surgeon must consider the available data regarding the natural history and the outcomes of conservative treatment outlined earlier and must discuss the options with the family. Nearly all reports of surgical treatment of trigger thumb describe complete resolution of the condition in the immediate postoperative period with a low complication rate, making surgical treatment an attractive option.
- The timing of surgery is controversial. Most authors recommend delaying surgery until 1 year of age; some recommend delaying surgery until after 3 or even 5 years of age; and others just recommend an undefined period of observation before surgery. No study has shown a clear detrimental effect of delaying surgery until 3 years or later, although compensatory metacarpophalangeal joint hyperextension laxity, permanent capsular contracture of the interphalangeal joint, and coronal plane deformity of the thumb have been cited as reasons to operate before 3 years of age. Anesthesia risk, although not completely elucidated in relation to age, should be considered in the decision regarding timing as well.

### Preoperative Planning

- Little preoperative planning is required other than preparing the child medically for the surgery and anesthesia and preparing the family for the surgery and early postoperative recovery period.

### Positioning

- The patient is positioned supine on the operating table with the affected arm (or arms) extended on a hand table or arm board.
- A pneumatic tourniquet is placed about the upper arm. The entire limb distal to the tourniquet is prepared and draped.
- The limb is exsanguinated with an Esmarch bandage, and the tourniquet is inflated to 100 mm Hg over systolic pressure.
- Alternatively, the Esmarch bandage can be used as a tourniquet about the forearm after exsanguinating the hand and wrist, although experience with this technique is necessary to avoid injury to the forearm from excessive pressure.

### Approach

- The approach to the A1 pulley is best performed through a transverse incision in or immediately parallel to the palmar digital crease. Longitudinal incisions can cause loss of metacarpophalangeal joint mobility by scar contracture long term.[18]
- As mentioned previously, great care must be taken in the volar approach to prevent injury to the digital nerves that lie in proximity to the A1 pulley.

TECHNIQUES

## Exposure

- A 7- to 10-mm transverse incision is planned in the region of the palmar digital crease. The exact location of the incision depends on the location of the A1 pulley relative to the crease. In the thumb with a fixed flexion posture, the proximal edge of the A1 pulley is immediately distal to the location of the palpable nodule when the interphalangeal joint is maximally extended.
  - The incision need not be in the skin crease to heal with an almost imperceptible scar.
  - Care must be taken to plan the incision directly over the thumb flexor sheath, which is pronated relative to the plane of the palm (**TECH FIG 1A**).
- The incision is made after exsanguination and tourniquet inflation. Great care must be taken to avoid incising the immediately adjacent digital nerves.
- The subcutaneous tissue is then spread bluntly to reveal the A1 pulley. The digital nerves need not be routinely dissected as long as the transverse fibers of the pulley are very clearly visualized under loupe magnification (**TECH FIG 1B**).

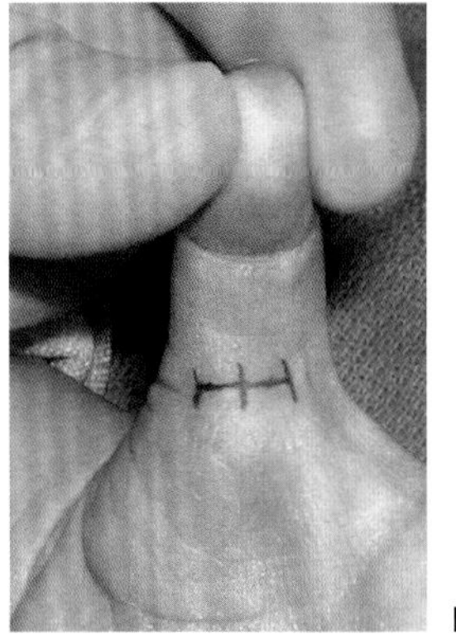
A

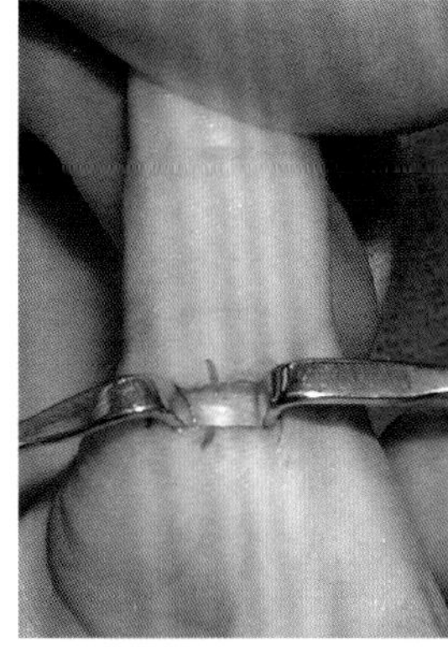
B

**TECH FIG 1** • **A.** Incision location for open release of pediatric trigger thumb. **B.** Exposure of the A1 pulley. Note the transversely oriented fibers without overlying subcutaneous tissue. The retractors on each side can be adjusted proximally and distally to allow visualization of the entire A1 pulley.

## Open Release of the A1 Pulley

- The distal and proximal edges of the A1 pulley are identified, and the A1 pulley is sharply incised longitudinally along its entire length (**TECH FIG 2A**). The oblique pulley is identified and protected distally. A gentle spread with a blunt scissor or hemostat in the proximal aspect of the sheath entering the thenar eminence will disrupt any remaining fibrous bands that can be a source of recurrent triggering.
  - The initial incision in the A1 pulley will produce an elliptical window in the pulley that may allow full extension of the interphalangeal joint (**TECH FIG 2B**), but the digit will still trigger postoperatively unless the entire pulley is divided.
- After adequate release, the distal edge of the A1 pulley should be separated by several millimeters, with the entire width of the flexor pollicis longus tendon clearly visible (**TECH FIG 2C**).

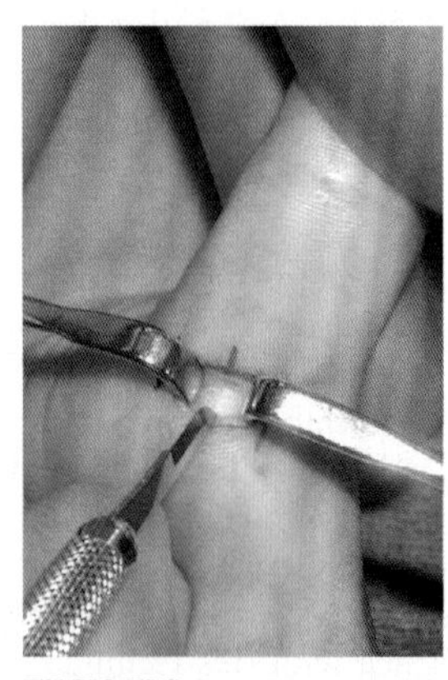
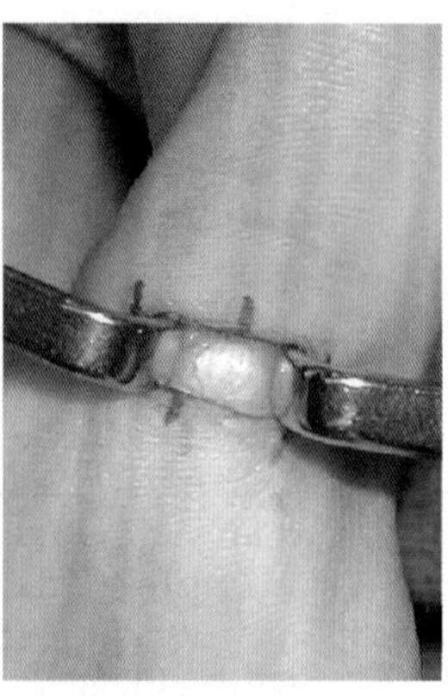
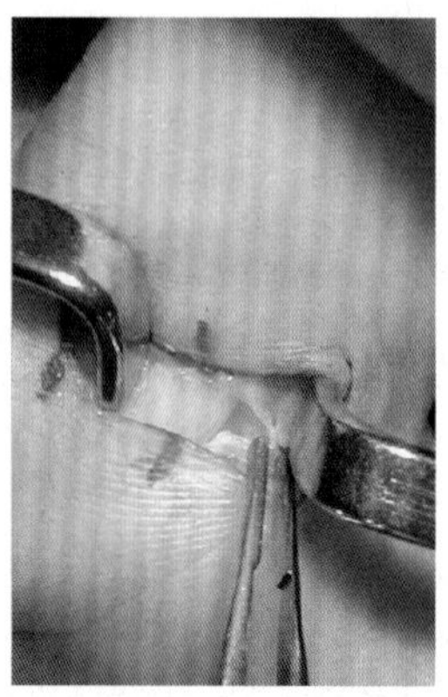
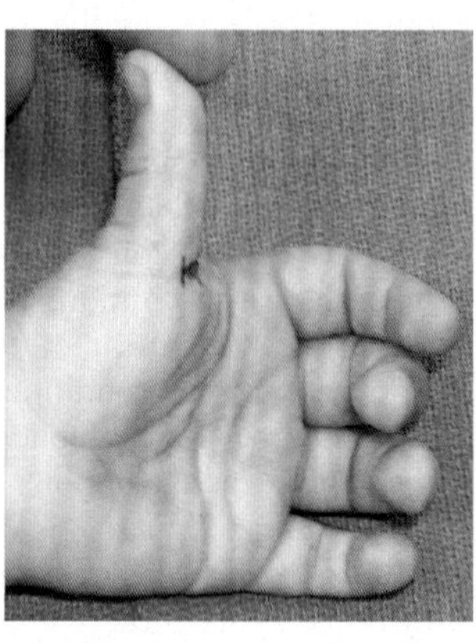

**TECH FIG 2** • **A.** Longitudinal division of the A1 pulley with a 6700 Beaver blade under direct visualization. **B.** Appearance of the A1 pulley after incomplete release. Note the elliptical cut edges of the pulley and the full extension of the interphalangeal joint. The intact proximal and distal ends of the pulley will be sources of recurrent triggering unless the entire pulley is released. **C.** Complete release of the A1 pulley. The flexor pollicis longus tendon is visible across its entire width. The forceps are holding one cut edge of the pulley. **D.** Full passive extension of the interphalangeal joint immediately after A1 pulley release of the patient in **FIG 1A**.

- After adequate release, the thumb interphalangeal joint should have full range of motion (**TECH FIG 2D**). In long-standing cases, that range of motion may not be much beyond neutral.
- If the thumb was locked in an extended position before tendon release, complete release can be confirmed by fully extending the wrist and compressing the distal volar forearm to provide proximal traction on the flexor pollicis longus tendon.
  - If the thumb does not have full flexion of the interphalangeal joint with these maneuvers, the release is incomplete.

## Closure and Dressing

- The wound is irrigated and closed with simple absorbable sutures.
- The wound is infiltrated with long-acting local anesthetic without epinephrine for postoperative analgesia.
- The wound is covered by a sterile dressing and cohesive bandage to prevent the child from removing the bandage (**TECH FIG 3**).

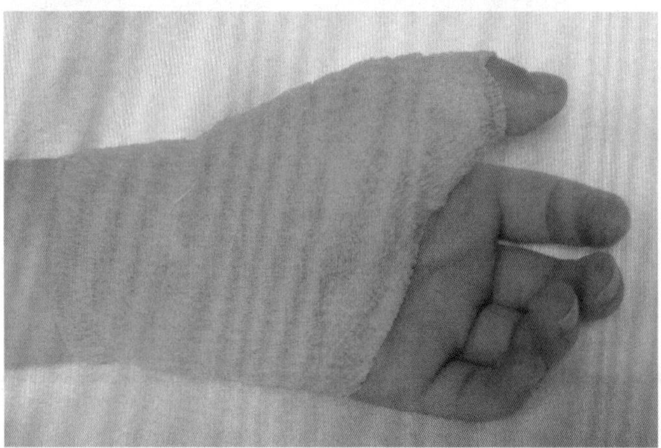

**TECH FIG 3** • Postoperative dressing for trigger thumb release. Loosely wrapped gauze is covered by a loosely wrapped cohesive bandage. Great care must be taken to keep the dressing loose to prevent excessive swelling or even ischemia distally.

## PEARLS AND PITFALLS

| | |
|---|---|
| **Indications** | ■ Given the recent literature regarding natural history and possible spontaneous improvement, parents must be made aware of the option of observation before recommending surgery, even if surgery can safely and effectively restore normal motion much faster and more reliably with very low risk. |
| **Anesthesia** | ■ Because of the close proximity of the digital nerves to the flexor sheath, the patient must be able to remain still during the entire procedure. Thus, although in experienced hands the entire procedure takes fewer than 5 minutes, general anesthesia or sedation is required, administered by an anesthesiologist. |
| **Incision placement** | ■ The thumb is pronated relative to the plane of the hand when the hand and thumb are held flat, making it easy to make the skin incision too radial with respect to the flexor sheath when the hand is held in this position for the surgery. Therefore, it is helpful to have an assistant hold the thumb in a vertical position to allow easier centering of the incision over the flexor sheath. |
| **Incomplete release** | ■ Cases of recurrence of triggering after surgical release have been attributed to incomplete release. After complete release at the distal end of the A1 pulley, the cut ends should be pointing palmarly and not toward each other. Proximally, fibrous bands in the thenar muscles can cause persistent triggering and can be divided by a gentle spread with a blunt scissor or hemostat in the flexor sheath after A1 pulley division. |
| **Digital nerves** | ■ The digital nerves need not be dissected and individually identified as long as the incision is well placed directly over the A1 pulley and subcutaneous dissection clearly reveals the A1 pulley with no overlying tissue. |

## POSTOPERATIVE CARE

- Cast or splint immobilization is not necessary postoperatively. However, protecting the incision for 7 days allows less inflamed wound healing and gives the absorbable sutures time to dissolve before the inquisitive toddler is allowed access to them.
  - A multilayer dressing of gauze and cohesive bandage is reliable and well tolerated.
  - Great care must be taken to prevent overtightening any elastic bandage and causing vascular compression.
- Dressings are removed in 7 days. If a determined child manages to escape the dressing prematurely, an adhesive bandage is used in its place until postoperative day 7.
- No activity restrictions are imposed postoperatively other than routine wound care.
- Postoperative analgesic medication beyond a single appropriate dose of acetaminophen is typically unnecessary, although children older than 8 to 10 years of age at the time of surgery tend to require more analgesics.
- Outpatient postoperative follow-up is scheduled for 1 to 2 weeks after the surgery. Full active range of motion and function of the thumb are typically achieved within 1 to 2 weeks of dressing removal. If parents perceive hesitance to use the thumb beyond that time period, a brief course of pediatric occupational therapy may be helpful.

## OUTCOMES

- Outcomes of open surgical release of trigger thumbs are excellent.
- Recovery of full range of motion is reported in all patients in many series.[6,9,10,23,25,31]
- A recent systematic review found a 95% success rate in 759 thumbs in 12 series.[7]
- Series that report less than 100% surgical cure describe recurrence due to incomplete pulley release as the most common reason for unsatisfactory outcome.[11,17] In these series, however, success rates exceed 93%, with 100% success after reoperation of the cases with incomplete release.
- Recovery of full range of motion after surgical correction is generally immediate. In long-standing cases, full hyperextension of the interphalangeal joint may take months to achieve despite achieving neutral extension immediately postoperatively. This phenomenon may represent a volar plate or capsular contracture of the interphalangeal joint from a prolonged locked flexion posture.
- A recent study of the long-term results of surgical treatment shows that despite obtaining normal motion postoperatively, 23% of patients followed at an average of 15 years postoperatively have mild loss of interphalangeal joint motion.[18]

## COMPLICATIONS

- Although rare, recurrence of the flexion posturing or triggering is attributed to incomplete pulley release.[11,17,27] Careful attention to surgical technique prevents this complication. If recurrence occurs, revision of the surgery with complete pulley release is curative.
- Longitudinal incisions are associated with scar contracture and patient complaints long term.[18] Wound complication was the most common reported complication in a systematic review of trigger thumb surgery,[7] although specific details regarding these complications were not described.
- Digital nerve injuries are exceedingly rare, being reported in only 1 of 759 thumbs reviewed in a recent systematic review.[7]
- Superficial wound infection has been reported[26] but is generally easily treated with oral antibiotics.

## REFERENCES


1. Baek GH, Kim JH, Chung MS, et al. The natural history of pediatric trigger thumb. J Bone Joint Surg Am 2008;90:980–985.
2. Bayat A, Shaaban H, Giakas G, et al. The pulley system of the thumb: anatomic and biomechanical study. J Hand Surg Am 2002;27:628–635.
3. Buchman MT, Gibson TW, McCallum D, et al. Transmission electron microscopic pathoanatomy of congenital trigger thumb. J Pediatr Orthop 1999;19:411–412.
4. Conners JJ, Obi LJ. Conservative treatment of trigger thumb in infants and children. J Fla Med Assoc 1968;55:819.

5. Dunsmuir RA, Sherlock DA. The outcome of treatment of trigger thumb in children. J Bone Joint Surg Br 2000;82:736–738.
6. Eyres KS, McLaren MI. Trigger thumb in children: results of surgical correction. J R Coll Surg Edinb 1991;36:197–198.
7. Farr S, Grill F, Ganger R, Girsch W. Open surgery versus nonoperative treatments for paediatric trigger thumb: a systematic review. J Hand Surg Eur Vol 2014;39(7):719–726.
8. Forlin E, Kaetsu EY, Vasconcelos JEE. Success of conservative treatment of trigger thumb in children after minimum follow-up of five years. Rev Bras Ortop 2012;47:483–487.
9. Ger E, Kupcha P, Ger D. The management of trigger thumb in children. J Hand Surg Am 1991;16:944–947.
10. Herdem M, Bayram H, Togrul E, et al. Clinical analysis of the trigger thumb of childhood. Turk J Pediatr 2003;45:237–239.
11. Hudson DA, Grobbelaar AO, Bloch CE. Trigger thumb in children—results of simple surgical treatment. S Afr J Surg 1998;36:91–92.
12. Jung HJ, Lee JS, Song KS, et al. Conservative treatment of pediatric trigger thumb: follow-up for over 4 years. J Hand Surg Eur Vol 2012; 37:220–224.
13. Khoshhal KI, Jarvis JG, Uhthoff HK. Congenital trigger thumb in children: electron microscopy and immunohistochemical analysis of the first annular pulley. J Pediatr Orthop B 2012;21:295–299.
14. Kikuchi N, Ogino T. Incidence and development of trigger thumb in children. J Hand Surg Am 2006;31:541–543.
15. Koh S, Horii E, Hattori T, et al. Pediatric trigger thumb with locked interphalangeal joint: can observation or splinting be a treatment option? J Pediatr Orthop 2012;32:724–726.
16. Lee ZL, Chang CH, Yang WY, et al. Extension splint for trigger thumb in children. J Pediatr Orthop 2006;26:785–787.
17. Marriott FP. Trigger thumb in infancy and childhood. A survey of 80 patients. Ulster Med J 1967;36:53–61.
18. McAdams TR, Moneim MS, Omer GE Jr. Long-term follow-up of surgical release of the A(1) pulley in childhood trigger thumb. J Pediatr Orthop 2002;22:41–43.
19. Moon WN, Suh SW, Kim IC. Trigger digits in children. J Hand Surg Br 2001;26:11–12.
20. Mulpruek P, Prichasuk S. Spontaneous recovery of trigger thumbs in children. J Hand Surg Br 1998;23:255–257.
21. Nemoto K, Nemoto T, Terada N, et al. Splint therapy for trigger thumb and finger in children. J Hand Surg Br 1996;21:416–418.
22. Rodgers WB, Waters PM. Incidence of trigger digits in newborns. J Hand Surg Am 1994;19:364–368.
23. Skov O, Bach A, Hammer A. Trigger thumbs in children: a follow-up study of 37 children below 15 years of age. J Hand Surg Br 1990;15:466–467.
24. Slakey JB, Hennrikus WL. Acquired thumb flexion contracture in children: congenital trigger thumb. J Bone Joint Surg Br 1996;78:481–483.
25. Sprecher EE. Trigger thumb in infants. Clin Orthop 1953;1:124–128.
26. Tan AH, Lam KS, Lee EH. The treatment outcome of trigger thumb in children. J Pediatr Orthop B 2002;11:256–259.
27. Taylor BA, Waters PM. A case of recurrent trigger thumb. Am J Orthop 2000;29:297–298.
28. Vyas BK, Sarwahi V. Bilateral congenital trigger thumb: role of heredity. Indian J Pediatr 1999;66:949–951.
29. Wang HC, Lin GT. Retrospective study of open versus percutaneous surgery for trigger thumb in children. Plast Reconstr Surg 2005;115:1963–1970.
30. Watanabe H, Hamada Y, Toshima T, et al. Conservative treatment for trigger thumb in children. Arch Orthop Trauma Surg 2001;121: 388–390.
31. White JW, Jensen WE. Trigger thumb in infants. AMA Am J Dis Child 1953;85:141–145.

# Transfer of Flexor Carpi Ulnaris for Wrist Flexion Deformity

77 CHAPTER

Ann E. Van Heest

## DEFINITION

- Cerebral palsy is a primary central nervous system dysfunction that leads to significant functional impairment due to its secondary peripheral manifestations in the upper extremity.
- The upper motor neuron lesion in the brain leads to loss of normal inhibition of tone (ie, spasticity), loss of motor control in the limb (ie, weakness), or impaired coordination of muscle activity (ie, athetosis).
  - The most common manifestation is spasticity.
  - Spastic hemiplegia is the main type of cerebral palsy for which upper extremity surgery is indicated.
- In spastic hemiplegia due to cerebral palsy, the most common peripheral manifestations in the upper limb are shoulder internal rotation, elbow flexion, forearm pronation, wrist flexion and ulnar deviation, finger clenching or swan necking, and thumb-in-palm deformity.
  - Increased muscle spasticity causes muscle imbalance across joints, which leads to impaired function and over time can lead to joint contractures with skeletal deformation.
  - The wrist is the most commonly affected joint and will be the focus of this chapter.

## ANATOMY

- Five primary wrist motors control wrist joint position.
- The three wrist extensor muscles are the extensor carpi radialis brevis (ECRB), the extensor carpi radialis longus (ECRL), and the extensor carpi ulnaris muscles (ECU).
- The two wrist flexor muscles are the flexor carpi radialis (FCR) and the flexor carpi ulnaris (FCU).
- The finger and thumb flexor muscles (flexor digitorum profundus [FDP], flexor digitorum superficialis [FDS], and flexor pollicis longus [FPL]) cross the wrist joint and exert a wrist flexion force. The finger and thumb extensor muscles (extensor pollicis longus [EPL], extensor indicis proprius [EIP], extensor digitorum communis [EDC], and extensor digiti quinti [EDQ]) also cross the wrist joint and exert a wrist extension force.
- Each of the muscles that crosses the wrist joint exerts a vector force for wrist extension and flexion as well as radial and ulnar deviation.[3] These vector force graphs can be used to help determine which muscles are the major deforming force for wrist flexion posturing.
- In cerebral palsy, the most common deformity is wrist flexion associated with ulnar deviation.
  - The muscle with the greatest flexion and ulnar deviation vector is the FCU.
  - The FCU is most commonly the deforming force, particularly because it may be coupled with a weak wrist extensor–radial deviator (ECRL and ECRB).

## PATHOGENESIS

- In the early stages of spastic hemiplegia, the joints and muscles will be supple, with full passive range of motion.
- With skeletal growth, the muscle imbalance across joints over time leads to muscle–tendon unit shortening and joint contractures, eventually leading to skeletal deformity.
- Increased FCU tone overpowers the decreased strength of the ECRL and ECRB, leading to a wrist flexion posture.

## NATURAL HISTORY

- In spastic hemiplegia due to cerebral palsy, the FCU is the most common deforming force, pulling the wrist into flexion and ulnar deviation.
  - Over time, the overpull of the FCU leads to contracture of the muscle, which may lead to fixed contracture of the wrist joint.
  - Ultimately, a fixed skeletal deformity can occur by the time of skeletal maturity.
  - Initial management involves exercises to keep the FCU stretched and to prevent contracture of the muscle.
- If muscle contractures develop, splinting may be necessary to prevent worsening of wrist joint contractures.
- Tendon transfer surgery is best performed before fixed contractures develop.
- If fixed joint contractures and muscle contractures exist, a salvage procedure with muscle lengthenings, wrist fusion, or both may be necessary.

## PATIENT HISTORY AND PHYSICAL FINDINGS

- Patient evaluation begins with interviewing the parents regarding use of the affected limb.
- Most commonly, children with spastic hemiplegia will show premature hand dominance, favoring the unaffected side even as young as 6 months of age.
  - This may be the presenting complaint leading to the diagnosis of cerebral palsy.
- Delay of normal pinch and grasp function patterning at 1 year of age is evident.
- Generalized patterns of upper extremity use for activities of daily living, commensurate with the child's age, are discussed with the parents and child. The clinician also observes for bimanual skills such as doing zippers and buttons, cutting food, and tying shoes.
- The child's functional use of the hand can be quantified using House classification of upper extremity functional use:
  - In this nine-level classification, functional use is assessed as follows: does not use, passive assist (poor, fair, good), active assist (poor, fair, good), and spontaneous use (partial, complete).

- This provides a baseline that the physician can use to help communicate the functional goals of treatment with the parents.
- Agreement with the parents on the child's present overall level of limb function serves as a baseline for comparing the outcome of treatment.

- Examinations and tests to perform include the following:
  - Passive range of motion of each joint. If a joint is passively stiff, a joint contracture exists. Tendon transfer surgery is best performed in patients with full passive mobility of all joints.
  - Volkmann angle test. This test indicates muscle contracture, as the finger flexors are biarticular, crossing both the wrist joint and the finger joints.
  - Active range of motion of the wrist. This indicates whether this patient has control to be able to actively extend the wrist. If this is absent, a tendon transfer surgery may be indicated to provide better active wrist extension.
  - Active range of motion of the fingers with the wrist held in a neutral position. This test indicates whether a wrist extensor tendon transfer surgery would be helpful. If the patient has better digital control with the wrist in an extended position, then a wrist extensor tendon transfer surgery would be helpful. If the patient has no digital extension, then an FCU tendon transfer should be considered to the EDC. If the patient develops a clenched fist with wrist neutral position, then a wrist extensor tendon transfer would be contraindicated.
  - If a patient has full passive mobility of the joints and no muscle contractures of the finger flexors but positions the wrist in significant flexion, leading to impairment with grasp and release or fine motor tasks, then a wrist extensor tendon transfer surgery to improve wrist position would be indicated.
  - Stereognosis testing. Impaired stereognosis does not preclude surgical intervention, but it is important to identify it preoperatively as a part of the disability present.

## IMAGING AND OTHER DIAGNOSTIC STUDIES

- Motion laboratory analysis has been used to assist in determining the position of the joints of the upper extremity during tasks.
- A fine needle electrode can be used to determine whether phasic control of the muscle occurs during grasp and release.
  - A muscle that is well controlled with phasic activity, without significant or continuous spasticity, is the best candidate for muscle–tendon transfer surgery.[6]

## DIFFERENTIAL DIAGNOSIS

- Wrist flexion posturing due to ineffective wrist extensors
- Flexor contracture or spasticity
- Wrist or carpal abnormalities

## NONOPERATIVE MANAGEMENT

- Occupational therapy includes the use of splints, stretching and strengthening programs, and active functional use activities.
- Two types of splints can be used: nighttime serial static splinting for treatment of muscle or joint contractures and daytime splints for prepositioning the hand to improve active function.
  - The indication for nighttime splinting is contractures.
    - If no contractures of the muscles or joints exist, nighttime splinting is not necessary and is a waste of time and money for the child and family.
    - If contractures exist at the wrist or fingers and thumb, a nighttime forearm-based wrist–hand orthosis is indicated.
  - Daytime splints are usually used to preposition the wrist in a neutral to slight "cock-up" position to help improve grasp and to preposition the thumb out of the palm to help improve pinch.
    - If the splint is bulky or cumbersome, it will interfere with rather than enhance function, defeating its purpose.
    - Care should be given to ensure proper fit of the splint so that its purpose can be achieved.
    - Stretching and strengthening programs, along with active functional use activities, are carried out by the therapist as well as taught to the parents and child as a home program.
- For patients with more focal muscle tone imbalance, botulinum toxin type A injections have been shown to be effective in reducing spasticity in the muscles injected and in improving hand function.[1,5,9]
  - Botulinum toxin locally blocks the release of acetylcholine at the neuromuscular junction, with a reversible action lasting on average 3 to 4 months. During this period, antagonist muscles can be strengthened and spastic muscles can be stretched, with the benefits lasting beyond the direct effects of the medication.
  - For the mildly involved child, treatment with Botox injections may obviate the need for surgical intervention.

## SURGICAL MANAGEMENT

- The most common deformity of the wrist is flexion, often with ulnar deviation as well. This is the most functionally disabling deformity in hemiplegia, as it significantly interferes with grasp and release function.
  - Several surgical options exist, with the choice depending on the degree of deformity and the extent of volitional control of each muscle involved.
- The three main options for treatment of a wrist flexion deformity are the following:
  - Release or lengthening of the deforming spastic muscles (FCU, FCR)
  - Transfer of tendons to augment the weak wrist extension
  - Wrist fusion to stabilize the joint for the severe, fixed, nonfunctioning wrist
- If the wrist flexor deformity is significant and the patient does not have active control of wrist extension, then tendon transfer surgery to augment wrist extension may be necessary.
  - Using the FCU as a transfer to wrist extension has the advantage of removing its force as a spastic wrist flexor and ulnar deviator and transferring its forces into wrist extension.
  - Care must be taken to prevent overcorrection if the deformity is not severe or if the transfer is tensioned too tightly, particularly in the younger child.

## Preoperative Planning

- In all cases of transfer into the wrist extensors, the finger function must be assessed preoperatively with the wrist in neutral, the desired postoperative position.
- If the finger flexors are too tight when the wrist is brought into neutral, a finger flexor lengthening will be necessary as part of the procedure.
- If the patient does not have finger extensor control to allow for release of grasped objects, then a transfer into the finger extensors (EDC) may be indicated.

## Positioning

- The patient is positioned supine on the operating room table, with an arm board to support the upper limb during the procedure (**FIG 1**).
- A tourniquet is applied above the elbow.

## Approach

- A volar–ulnar approach to the forearm is used to harvest the FCU tendon, and a dorsal approach to the distal forearm and wrist is used for inserting the tendon transfer.

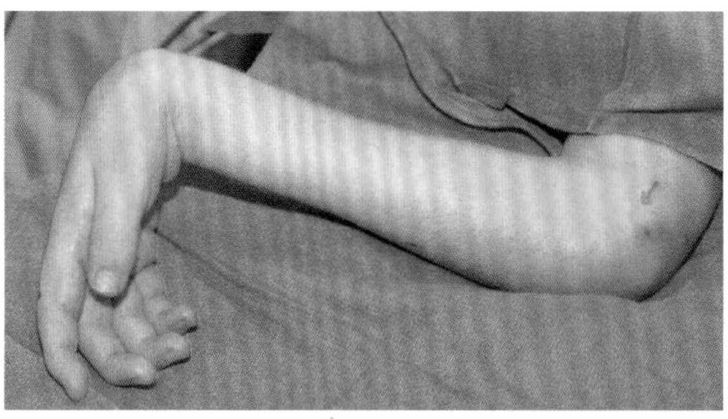

**FIG 1** • The patient is positioned supine on the operating room table with the arm extended on an arm board. A tourniquet is applied proximally on the arm.



# Mobilization of the Flexor Carpi Ulnaris

- The incision for exposure of the FCU is a longitudinal one on the volar and ulnar aspect of the forearm from the proximal third of the forearm to its distal insertion on the pisiform (**TECH FIG 1A**).
- Dissection is carried out through the subcutaneous layer and the forearm fascia, onto the muscle belly proximally and onto the tendon insertion distally.
  - The ulnar nerve and artery lie radial to the tendon and are carefully identified and protected, including the dorsal ulnar sensory branch in the distal aspect of the wound.
- The tendon is transected at its distal insertion on the pisiform, and a grasping suture is placed (**TECH FIG 1B**).
- The FCU is then freed of its fascial insertion back to the most proximal aspect of the wound to allow full mobilization of the muscle to its dorsal position (**TECH FIG 1C**).
- Full mobilization of the muscle to the proximal third of the forearm has been shown to increase its vector as a forearm supinator, in addition to its wrist extension moment arm.[8]

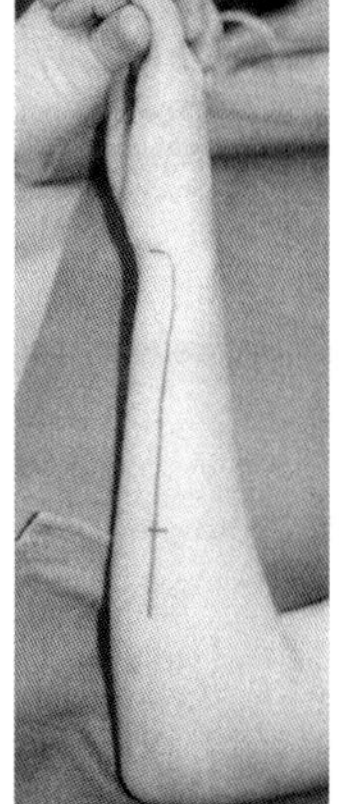

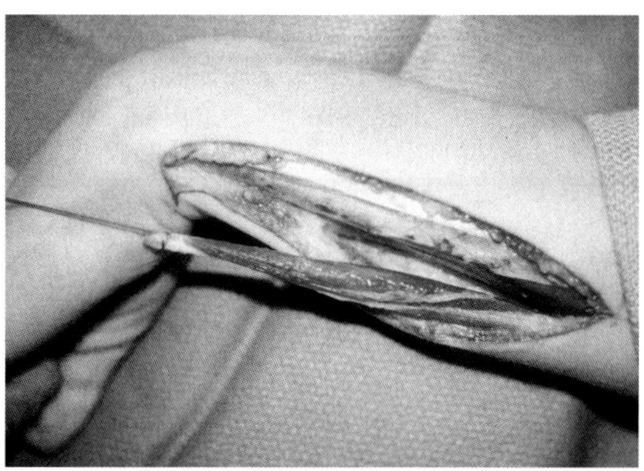

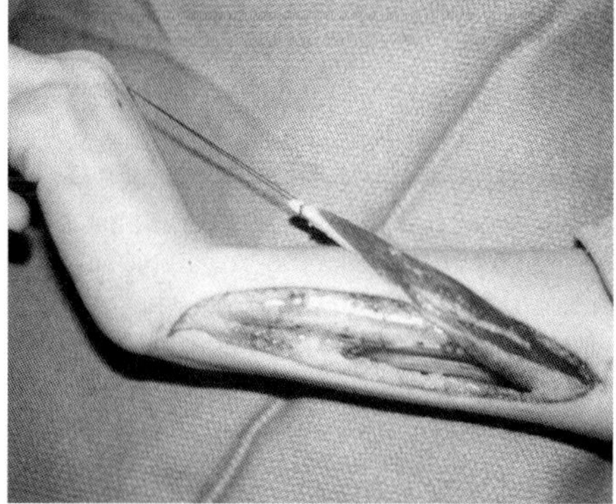

**TECH FIG 1** • **A.** A longitudinal incision is made down the ulnar aspect of the forearm from the proximal third of the forearm to the pisiform, with a small distal curve to allow visualization of the ulnar nerve and artery, which are just radial to the FCU at the level of the pisiform. **B.** The FCU tendon is transected distally at its insertion on the pisiform, with a grasping suture placed through the distal end of the tendon. **C.** The tendon is fully mobilized back to the proximal third of the muscle belly to allow the muscle to be transferred to the dorsal wrist with a straight line of pull.

## Transfer of the Flexor Carpi Ulnaris to the Extensor Carpi Radialis Brevis Tendon

- A second incision is made over the dorsal radial aspect of the wrist diagonally over the second dorsal compartment (ECRB, ECRL) of the wrist (**TECH FIG 2**).
- Just distal to where the first dorsal compartment tendons (abductor pollicis longus and extensor pollicis brevis) cross the second dorsal compartment, a generous fascial window over the second dorsal compartment is made to fully expose the ECRB and ECRL tendons.
- A subcutaneous tunnel is then made in direct line from the proximal end of the ulnar incision to the radial incision to allow a straight line of pull for the tendon transfer.
- The FCU tendon is then woven into the ECRB tendon using the Pulvertaft weave technique and tensioned so that the wrist sits at rest against gravity in a neutral position.
- Standard wound closure is performed after the tourniquet is deflated.

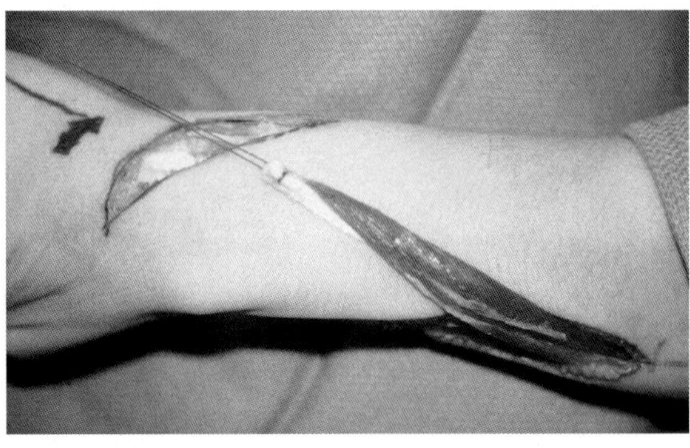

**TECH FIG 2** • A second incision made dorsally allows dissection of the ECRB as a recipient tendon. The FCU tendon is passed through a subcutaneous tunnel and woven into the ECRB tendon.

## PEARLS AND PITFALLS

| | |
|---|---|
| **Tensioning of the tendon transfer** | ▪ If the tendon transfer is tensioned too tightly, the wrist will sit in extension at rest and too much wrist extension will occur with active range of motion. A careful assessment of tendon transfer tensioning is necessary to avoid this pitfall.<br>▪ However, if the tendon transfer is tensioned too loosely, the wrist will not achieve as much wrist extension as desired. If one is to err, one would prefer too little tension than too much, as the transfer tends to tighten over time, particularly if performed in a young child with significant remaining growth potential. |

## POSTOPERATIVE CARE

- The postoperative rehabilitation regimen is imperative to maximize surgical results.
- The limb is immobilized in a cast for 1 month after tendon transfer surgery.
- After 1 month, the cast is removed and a custom splint is used holding the wrist in a neutral position (as well as protecting any other procedures that were done concomitantly).
- The splint is worn full time for an additional month but is removed three to five times a day for active range of motion and light functional activities.
- After 1 month of full-time splinting, the patient then progresses to nighttime splinting only with active functional use of the hand during the day, including lifting and strengthening exercises.
- Individualized sessions with a therapist experienced in tendon transfer rehabilitation are very helpful to maximize use of the limb and incorporate the wrist into activities of daily living, but success may be limited by the overall extent of the patient's cerebral palsy involvement.

## OUTCOMES

- The greatest functional benefit in upper extremity surgery has been reported with correction of the wrist flexion deformity, regardless of the transfer used.
- Beach et al,[2] as an example of the correction achieved, reported a postoperative arc of motion of almost 50 degrees, centered around the neutral axis, at greater than 5 years of follow-up.
  - Significant aesthetic improvement was noted as well in 90% of patients.
  - A functional outcome study of 134 cerebral palsy patients treated surgically showed that the average functional improvement was from use of the hand as a poor passive assist to use of the hand as a poor active assist.[7] This article advocates performing multiple procedures simultaneously for correction of the elbow, forearm, wrist, and thumb in a single surgical setting.

## COMPLICATIONS

- All surgical procedures carry risk, and this must be weighed against the potential benefits that most commonly are achieved.

- Preoperatively, patients must be screened for anesthetic complications as follows:
  - A bleeding screen for patients on long-term Depakote antiseizure medications
  - Screening for bladder and lung infections, particularly for patients with poor urinary or pulmonary control
  - Nutritional status (height and weight percentiles for age)
- Intraoperative attention to wound care is imperative to avoid wound healing problems.
- Wounds may need a postoperative drain to prevent hematoma formation.
- Nerve and artery injury can be avoided with appropriate planes of dissection and a thorough knowledge of the pertinent anatomy.
- Postoperatively, the splint or cast should be adequate to allow for postoperative swelling and should be split if excessive swelling is encountered.
  - Many children with spasticity do not have normal preoperative sensory or motor findings and may not have normal mentation, so normal parameters cannot be used to monitor for compartment syndrome.
  - Premature removal of the cast or splint, as well as overzealous patient activities, can lead to tendon rupture or attenuation.
  - Excessive immobilization can lead to excessive adhesion formation, diminishing the eventual functional use.
- Long-term problems most commonly involve loss of the muscle balance achieved at the time of the surgery.[4]
  - Many children have tendon transfers as young as 7 years old; with continued skeletal growth, they may have recurrent deformity.
  - Overcorrection can also occur, with the "opposite" deformity occurring. "Fine-tuning" surgery may be necessary to address complications that develop after correction of the original deformity.
- Several principles will help prevent these complications.
  - Do not overcorrect deformity, particularly in the younger child.
  - Leave options to reverse the surgical correction if necessary.
  - Keep functional grasp and release as the highest priority in surgical planning.
  - Avoid wrist arthrodesis, as this precludes the tenodesis effect of the wrist for finger use.

## REFERENCES


1. Autti-Rämö I, Larsen A, Peltonen J, et al. Botulinum toxin injection as an adjunct when planning hand surgery in children with spastic hemiplegia. Neuropediatrics 2000;31:4–8.
2. Beach WR, Strecker WB, Coe J, et al. Use of the Green transfer in treatment of patients with spastic cerebral palsy: 17–year experience. J Pediat Orthop 1991;11:731–736.
3. Brand PW, Hollister A, eds. Operations to restore muscle balance to the hand. In: Clinical Mechanics of the Hand, ed 2. St. Louis: Mosby, 1993:179–222.
4. Carlson MG. Cerebral Palsy. In: Green DP, Hotchkiss RN, Pederson WC, et al, eds. Green's Operative Hand Surgery, ed 5. Philadelphia: Elsevier Churchill Livingstone, 2005:1197–1234.
5. Van Heest AE. Applications of botulinum toxin in orthopedics and upper extremity surgery. Tech Hand Up Extrem Surg 1997;1:27–34.
6. Van Heest AE. Functional assessment aided by motion laboratory studies. Hand Clin 2003;19:565–571.
7. Van Heest AE, House JH, Cariello C. Upper extremity surgical treatment of cerebral palsy. J Hand Surg Am 1999;24(2):323–330.
8. Van Heest AE, Murthy NS, Sathy MR, et al. The supination effect of tendon transfer of the flexor carpi ulnaris to the extensor carpi radialis brevis or longus: a cadaveric study. J Hand Surg Am 1999;24(5):1091–1096.
9. Wall SA, Chait LA, Ternlett JA, et al. Botulinum A chemodenervation: a new modality in cerebral palsied hands. Br J Plast Surg 1993;46:703–706.

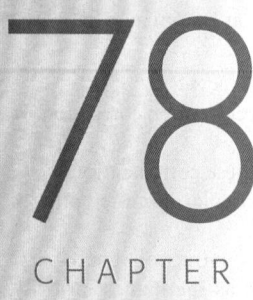


# Radial Dysplasia Reconstruction

**Carley Vuillermin, Marybeth Ezaki, and Scott N. Oishi**

## DEFINITION

- Radial dysplasia represents a spectrum of longitudinal deficiency in radial growth.
- This deficiency can be mild or severe based on the deficiency in the radius.

## ANATOMY

- The anatomic relations of the radial aspect of the wrist are altered due to the variable absence of the radius.
  - The higher the degree of radial dysplasia, the more divergent from normal anatomic relationships the findings will be. This is critically important when undertaking surgical intervention.
  - A consistent but highly abnormal brachiocarpalis muscle has been described in thrombocytopenia–absent radius (TAR) syndrome.[14] This muscle spans from just distal to the deltoid insertion directly into the radial side of the carpus and inserts as a broad aponeurotic fan into the carpus, joint capsule, and tendons of the radial wrist.
- Many patients have associated thumb hypoplasia.[10]
- Bayne and Klug[2] have provided a classification based on radiographic findings (Table 1).
  - Several authors have proposed alterations to this classification in order to better describe the spectrum of presentation. James et al[12] added N and 0 categories. N represents patients with a normal radius and carpus but hypoplastic thumb and 0 for patients with carpal abnormalities and

**Table 1 Bayne and Klug Classification of Radial Dysplasia**

| Type | Radiograph | Description |
|---|---|---|
| I | | Short distal radius; distal epiphysis present, delayed; mild radial deviation |
| II | | Defective growth proximal–distal epiphyses; radius in miniature |
| III | | Partial absence of radius; wrist unsupported |
| IV | | Total absence of radius |

Adapted from Bayne CG, Klug MS. Long-term review of the surgical treatment of radial deficiencies. J Hand Surg Am 1987;12(2):169–179.

normal radial length. Goldfarb et al[9] proposed a type V for more proximal deficiencies.

## PATHOGENESIS

- Radial dysplasia develops during the period of embryogenesis. During this period, other organ systems are developing and may also be affected, as discussed later in this chapter.

## NATURAL HISTORY

- The natural history of patients with radial dysplasia clearly depends on the type of dysplasia present and the associated conditions.
  - Patients with isolated type I or II radial dysplasia usually do not require surgical intervention to address the wrist and radial deformity.
  - Patients with more severe dysplasia can frequently benefit from surgical intervention.
- Many times radial dysplasia is part of a syndrome, and the associated sequelae clearly affect these patients more than the underlying radial dysplasia. The most common associations are with Holt-Oram syndrome, TAR syndrome, Fanconi anemia, and VACTERL (vertebral anomalies, anal atresia, cardiovascular anomalies, tracheoesophageal fistula, esophageal atresia, renal or radial anomalies, limb anomalies).[10,11]
- An association with several craniofacial syndromes has been well documented.[8]
- No matter what procedure is used for treating the radial dysplasia, the patients all have a high incidence of recurrent deformity as they get older.[2,4,17]

## PATIENT HISTORY AND PHYSICAL FINDINGS

- The most significant finding is radial deviation at the wrist (**FIG 1**).
- If the patient is older, the affected forearm will also be short.
- Assessment of adjacent joints is essential. Frequently, there will be associated thumb hypoplasia or absence, and in more severe cases (especially Holt-Oram syndrome), the other digits may be stiff. Elbow range of motion is important and the ability to bring the hand to the mouth once the wrist is in a corrected position should be assessed. Radioulnar synostosis is also sometimes present especially in children with Holt-Oram syndrome.
- Because of its frequent association with systemic conditions, all patients require careful examination of their spine and cardiac, renal, and hematologic systems.

## IMAGING AND OTHER DIAGNOSTIC STUDIES

- Radiographs should be taken of both forearms to assess stage of radial dysplasia (see Table 1).
- In addition, all patients warrant a workup for syndromes and associated conditions, such as Holt-Oram syndrome, Fanconi anemia, TAR syndrome, and VACTERL.
  - This may require echocardiogram, renal ultrasound, hematologic studies (complete blood count [CBC] and chromosomal fragility studies), and spinal evaluation.
  - Each treating physician should consider these associations and not assume they have already been worked up, especially if surgical care of the limb is contemplated.

## NONOPERATIVE MANAGEMENT

- All patients warrant stretching and splinting before consideration of any surgical intervention.
  - The splints should be large enough to be effective and also to minimize any choking hazard.

## SURGICAL MANAGEMENT

- Patients with type I or II radial dysplasia usually do not require surgical intervention.
- Surgical treatment has generally ranged from soft tissue rebalancing alone to full centralization of the wrist with or without external fixation.
  - Before any procedure is contemplated, the surgeon must remember that the patient must maintain the ability to get his or her fingers to the mouth with the wrist in the surgically altered position.
  - Very severe radial dysplasia associated with poor elbow function or poor fingers is a contraindication to surgical intervention. The patient may rely on the radial deviation to reach their mouth or use radial wrist pinch for function.
- Many different surgical procedures have been described (**FIG 2**).
  - Soft tissue procedures have traditionally been combined with skeletal rearrangement. Local rotational flaps allow for redistribution of tissue from the ulnar side of the wrist. Evans et al[7] first described the bilobed flap in 1995.

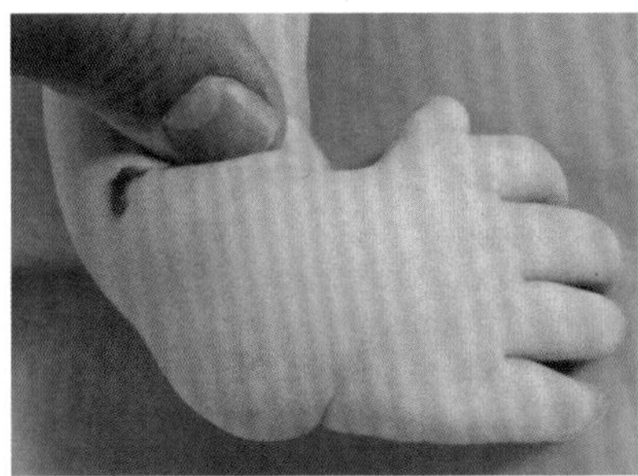

A

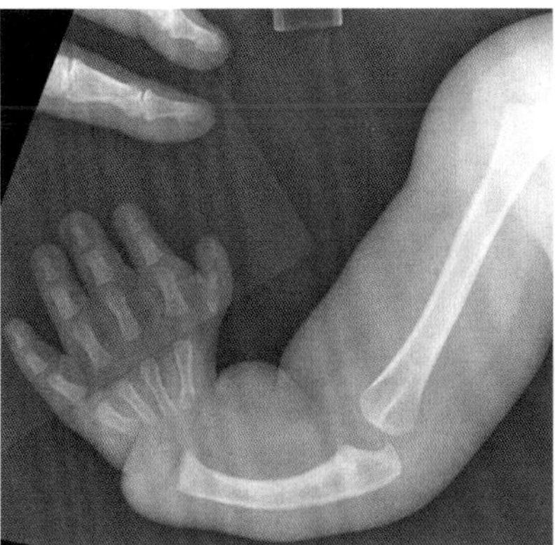

B

**FIG 1** • **A.** Preoperative photo showing radial deviation of the wrist. **B.** Anteroposterior (AP) radiograph of the same child demonstrating type IV radial deficiency.

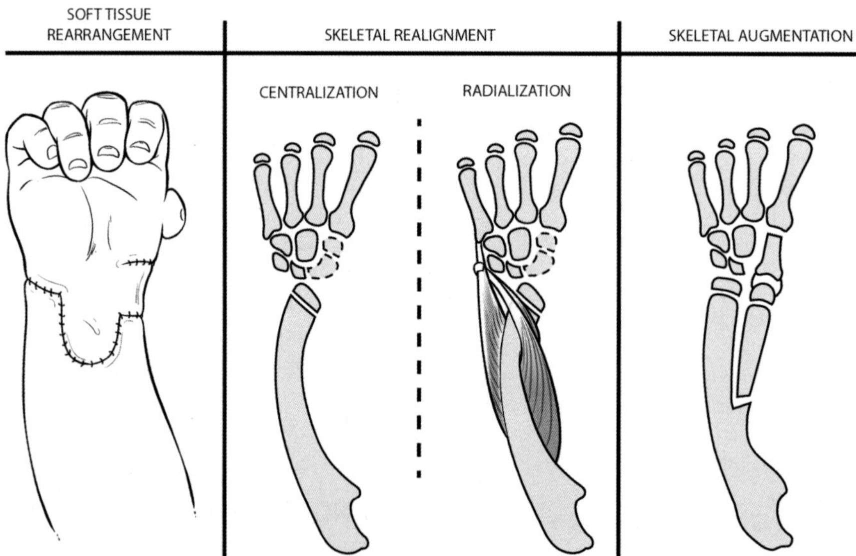


**FIG 2** • Surgical options for correction of radial dysplasia.

Manske and others[13] previously described simple excision of the ulnar redundancy without the addition of tissue to the radial side.

- Centralization has been the most common procedure and was first described by Sayre in 1893.[15] These procedures bring the carpus in line with the distal ulna and many create a notch to stabilize the carpus in a mortise and tenon fashion. Buck-Gramcko[3] described radialization, where the carpus is brought across to the ulnar side of the ulna and the extensor carpi radialis (ECR) and flexor carpi radialis (FCR) muscle are transposed. This was proposed to improve balance and limit the recurrence seen after centralization.
  - Ulnar growth disturbance has been found to be increased in patients who have undergone centralization procedures.[16]
- Nonvascularized bone transfer has been tried with or without epiphyseal transfer[1,18] and largely abandoned due to a lack of ongoing growth leading to recurrent deformity.
- Vascularized bone transfer can be used in selective cases to provide stabilization of the radial side of the wrist.[19] A vascularized second toe metatarsophalangeal (MTP) joint as described by De Jong et al[5] and Vilkki[20] or proximal fibular transfer, provide structural support to the deficient radial side of the wrist and allow for continued growth with the growth of the child. These potentially limit recurrence while maintaining wrist motion.
- The long-term problem for any surgical procedure is the recurrence rate.
- Interventions should aim to minimize risk of further growth abnormality and preserve motion. Total range of motion of the fingers and wrist are more important to activity and participation than the angulation at the wrist.[6] Preservation of range of motion should be the goal of any selected surgical procedure.
- We have had experience with various procedures for the treatment of radial dysplasia, including centralization, free toe MTP transfer for stabilization of the radial wrist, and soft tissue release alone. We no longer use formal centralization procedures, as we have found the recurrence rate to be similar to our soft tissue release procedure. In addition, this procedure jeopardizes the ulnar epiphysis, which can lead to an extraordinarily short forearm. Also, loss of mobility results when a centralization procedure is successful.
- For our patients, soft tissue release with a bilobed flap reconstruction has provided the most reliable, effective results. This maintains motion, improves position, and minimizes injury to the distal ulnar physis. This does not preclude vascularized free joint transfer or other procedures at a subsequent juncture.

## Preoperative Planning

- Timing of surgery. Younger patients have the most to gain from soft tissue release with bilobed flap. Our preference is to perform this procedure between 12 months and 2 years of age; however, older patients will also benefit.
  - May be combined with other indicated surgical procedures, including flexor digitorum superficialis (FDS) opponensplasty
  - We prefer to perform pollicization or thumb reconstructive procedures for associated types IIIB to V thumb hypoplasia in a staged manner.
  - Others have combined centralization procedures with bilobed flaps.
- Radiographs are performed to confirm clinical findings (see **FIG 1B**).
- Clearance of associated comorbidities—appropriate consultation or investigation in particular to exclude cardiac and hematologic abnormalities that may influence safety of anesthesia and surgical complications.
- Before surgery, the patient must have undergone adequate soft tissue stretching.
  - In the first few months, this is accomplished by splinting. In severe cases, serial casting may be necessary.

- After about 6 months of age, active stretching is started by the parents with use of nighttime splinting.
- External fixator–assisted soft tissue distraction is reserved for the most severe cases and, in our experience, is uncommonly indicated prior to a bilobed flap; it may be beneficial in older children.

## Positioning

- The patient is placed in the standard supine position, and a general anesthetic is used in all cases.
- We do not use a standard tourniquet, as we have found this to be inadequate in young children. Instead, we use the elastic Esmarch bandage as a tourniquet on the upper arm.



## Approach

- The bilobed flap design must be drawn appropriately to take advantage of the redundant tissue on the ulnar side of the wrist.
- A dorsal or volar surgical approach and flap design may be used, our experience with the volar approach is that it allows more direct access and release of the tight structures on the volar radial aspect of the wrist and places the scars in an aesthetically less prominent position without compromising the surgical outcome.

## Volar Bilobed Flap

- After induction of general anesthesia, the upper extremity is prepared and draped to allow access to the entire arm.
- The volar bilobed flap is then carefully designed using a marking pen (**TECH FIG 1**).
  - Key points in marking out the flap:
    - Point for insetting of the flap on the radial side of the wrist is at the maximal concavity of the deformity. This is the point of maximal tension when the wrist is ulnarly deviated.
    - Mark the first lobe of the flap on the volar surface of the wrist with the apex proximal (starting at the inset point). The base of the flap is perpendicular to the long axis of the forearm.
    - The second lobe of the flap is identical in geometry to the first however perpendicular to it on the ulnar side of the wrist. This flap uses the redundant ulnar skin.
    - Finally, the inset incision on the radial side of the wrist is marked to correspond to the height of the lobes.
- The Esmarch bandage is used to exsanguinate the limb; it is then wrapped three times around the upper arm for use as a tourniquet.

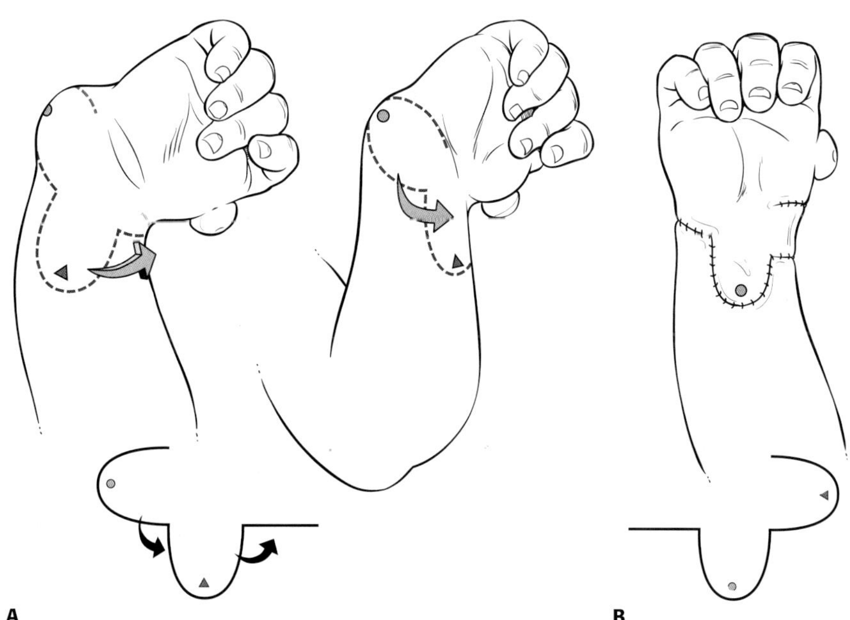


**TECH FIG 1** • **A.** Flap design. **B.** Flap rotation and final positioning. *(continued)*

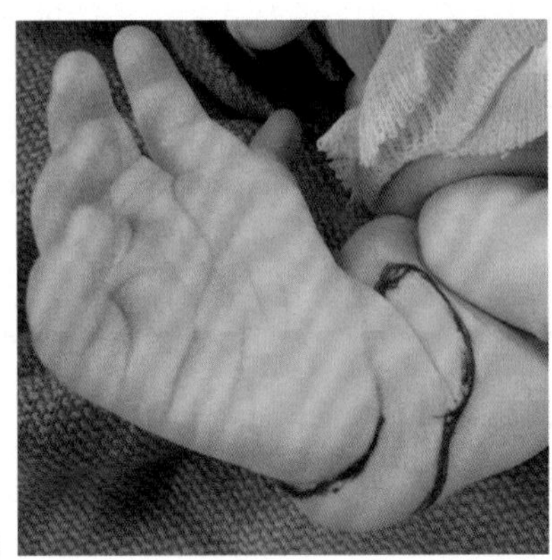
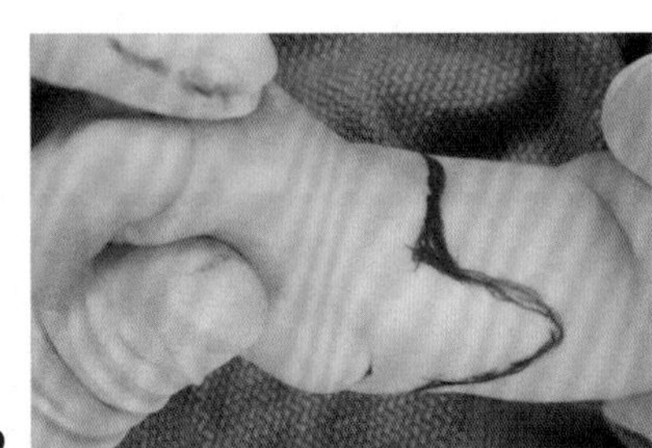
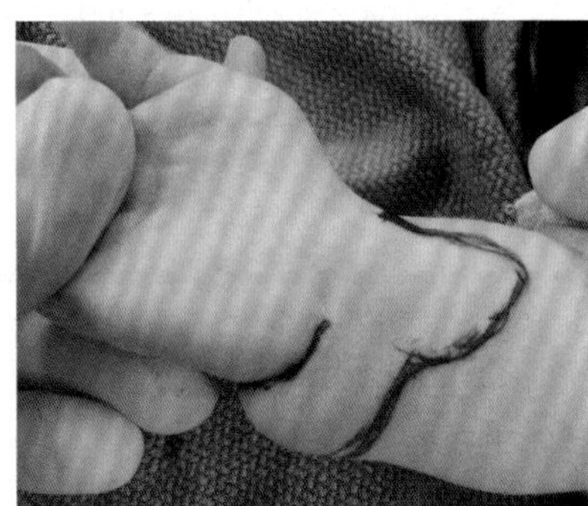

**TECH FIG 1** • *(continued)* **C–E.** Markings for bilobed flap.

## Release of the Radial Deviation of the Wrist

- After careful incision and elevation of full-thickness skin flaps, the finger and flexor tendons, as well as the median and superficial radial nerves, are carefully identified and preserved. A vascular loop may be used for protection (**TECH FIG 2A**).
- All other tissues in the radial wrist are released including fascial bands and tendons with pure radial deviation wrist moments.
  - Rebalancing of radial wrist flexors to an ulnar insertion or extensor may be performed.
  - Care must be taken not to dissect excessively near the ulnar epiphysis to prevent injury to the vascular supply to this area.
- After release is accomplished, the wrist is placed in a neutral position and pinned with a 0.062-inch Kirschner wire.
  - The Kirschner wire is temporary and is put across the joint from either direction (ie, there is no specific location for the exit or entrance site). Our preferred trajectory is one which avoids crossing the ulnar physis.
- The flaps are then rotated and sutured in place (**TECH FIG 2B–E**).
- The tourniquet is removed to ensure perfusion to the fingers, and a long-arm cast is placed.

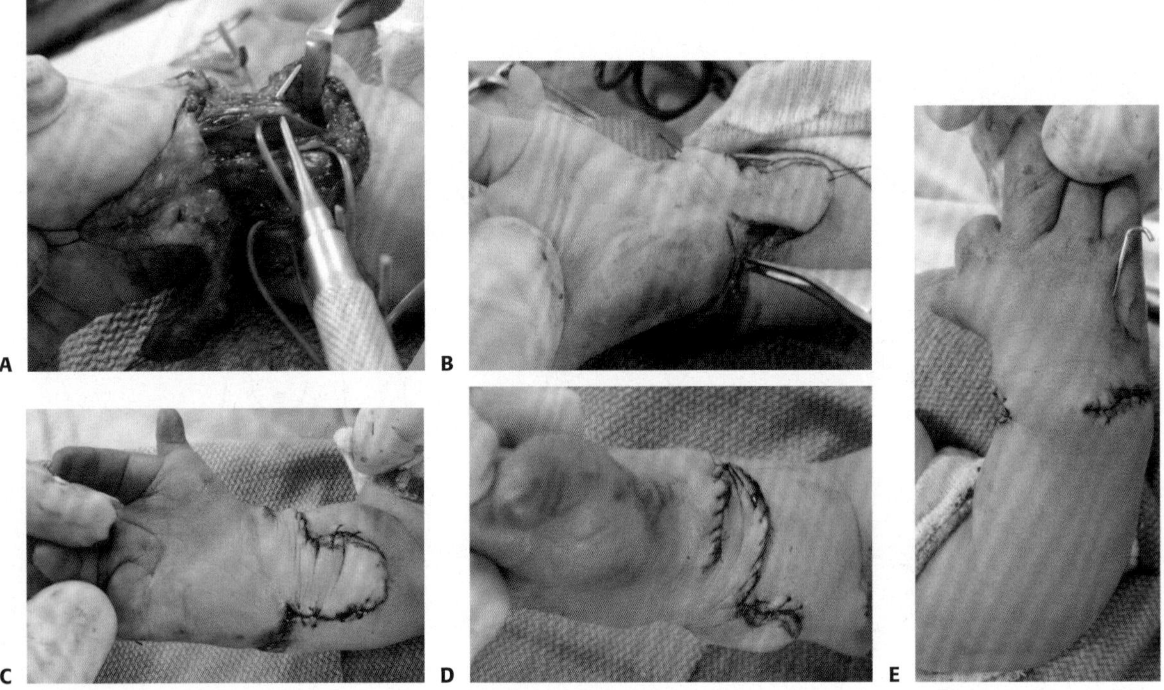

**TECH FIG 2** • **A.** After release of radial tethering tissue, protection of finger flexors, extensors, and neurovascular structures. **B.** Rotation of flaps. **C,D.** Skin is sutured. **E.** Dorsal view with protective pin.

## PEARLS AND PITFALLS

| | |
|---|---|
| **Adequate preoperative stretching of soft tissues** | ■ If not adequate, this may lead to a suboptimal result. |
| **Identification of median nerves and tendons, as these structures tend to be in very aberrant locations** | ■ There is the potential for injury to nerve or tendon during soft tissue release if this is not done. |
| **Careful dissection around the distal ulna** | ■ If too aggressive, it can lead to injury to the epiphyseal region, leading to growth problems in the ulna. |
| **Pinning of ulnocarpal joint after release** | ■ Failure to do this can lead to partial flap loss because of motion at the joint. |

## POSTOPERATIVE CARE

- The long-arm cast is left on for 3 to 4 weeks.
- At that point, the pin is removed and the patient is changed to a removable splint.

## OUTCOMES

- The bilobed flap procedure is an effective procedure for treating radial dysplasia (**FIG 3**).
- Deformity tends to recur, although the incidence of this appears to be similar to that for other procedures used to treat radial dysplasia.

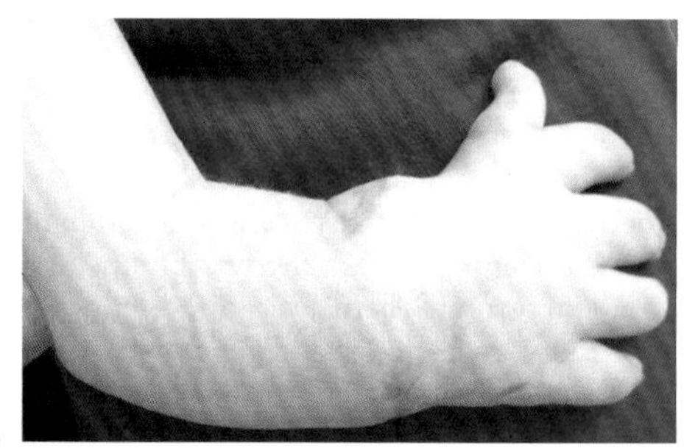

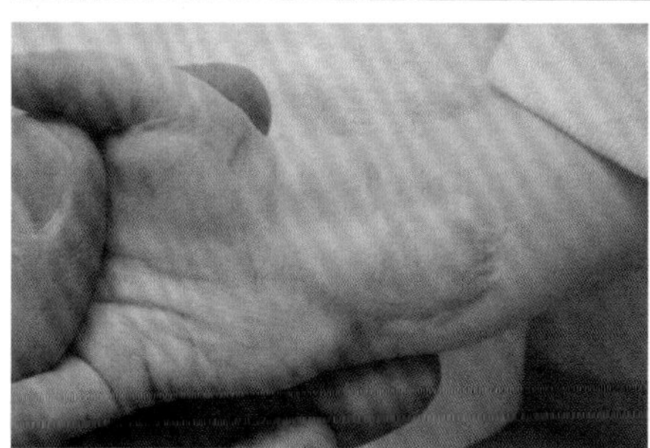

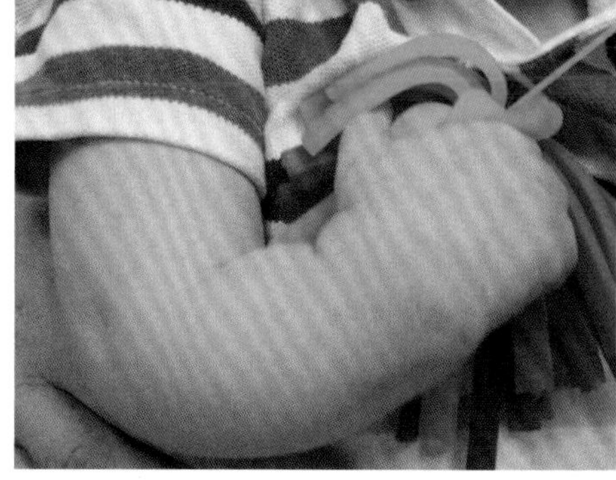

**FIG 3** ● Postoperative results. **A.** Early healing and resting wrist position. **B.** Volar bilobed flap, post staged pollicization procedure. **C.** Functional positioning post pollicization.

## COMPLICATIONS

- Few complications are associated with this procedure.
- Partial flap loss can occur, but the risk seems to be minimized by appropriate flap design, transfixion with a Kirschner wire, and immobilization after the procedure.

## REFERENCES


1. Albee FH. Formation of radius congenitally absent: condition seven years after implantation of bone graft. Ann Surg 1928;87(1):105–110.
2. Bayne LG, Klug MS. Long-term review of the surgical treatment of radial deficiency. J Hand Surg Am 1987;12(2):169–179.
3. Buck-Gramcko D. Radialization as a new treatment for radial club hand. J Hand Surg Am 1985;10(6 pt 2):964–968.
4. Damore E, Kozin SH, Thoder JJ, et al. The recurrence of deformity after surgical centralization for radial clubhand. J Hand Surg Am 2000;25(4):745–751.
5. De Jong JP, Moran SL, Vilkki SK. Changing paradigms in the treatment of radial club hand: microvascular joint transfer for correction of radial deviation and preservation of long-term growth. Clin Orthop Surg 2012;4(1):36–44.
6. Ekblom AG, Dahlin LB, Rosberg HE, et al. Hand function in children with radial longitudinal deficiency. BMC Musculoskelet Disord 2013;14:116.
7. Evans DM, Gateley DR, Lewis JS. The use of a bilobed flap in the correction of radial club hand. J Hand Surg Br 1995;20(3):333–337.
8. Goldberg MJ, Bartoshesky LE. Congenital hand anomaly: etiology and associated malformations. Hand Clin 1985;1(3):405–415.
9. Goldfarb CA, Manske PR, Busa R, et al. Upper-extremity phocomelia reexamined: a longitudinal dysplasia. J Bone Joint Surg Am 2005;87(12):2639–2648.
10. Goldfarb CA, Wall L, Manske PR. Radial longitudinal deficiency: the incidence of associated medical and musculoskeletal conditions. J Hand Surg Am 2006;31(7):1176–1182.
11. James MA, Green HD, McCarroll HR, et al. The association of radial deficiency with thumb hypoplasia. J Bone Joint Surg Am 2004;86-A(10):2196–2205.
12. James MA, McCarroll HR Jr, Manske PR. The spectrum of radial longitudinal deficiency: a modified classification. J Hand Surg Am 1999;24(6):1145–1155.
13. Manske PR, McCarroll HR Jr, Swanson K. Centralization of the radial club hand: an ulnar surgical approach. J Hand Surg Am 1981;6(5):423–433.
14. Oishi SN, Carter P, Bidwell T, et al. Thrombocytopenia absent radius syndrome: presence of brachiocarpalis muscle and its importance. J Hand Surg Am 2009;34(9):1696–1699.
15. Sayre RH. A contribution to the study of club-hand. Trans Am Orthop Assn 1893;6:208–216.
16. Sestero AM, Van Heest A, Agel J. Ulnar growth patterns in radial longitudinal deficiency. J Hand Surg Am 2006;31(6):960–967.
17. Shariatzadeh H, Jafari D, Taheri H, et al. Recurrence rate after radial club hand surgery in long term follow up. J Res Med Sci 2009;14(3):179–186.
18. Starr DE. Congenital absence of the radius: a method of surgical correction. J Bone Joint Surg Am 1945;27(4):572–577.
19. Vilkki SK. Distraction and microvascular epiphysis transfer for radial club hand. J Hand Surg Br 1998;23(4):445–452.
20. Vilkki SK. Vascularized metatarsophalangeal joint transfer for radial hypoplasia. Semin Plast Surg 2008;22(3):195–212.

# Forearm Osteotomy for Multiple Hereditary Exostoses

Carley Vuillermin, Carla Baldrighi, and Scott N. Oishi

## DEFINITION

- Multiple hereditary exostoses (MHE), first described by Boyer[3] in 1814, is a familial disorder with an autosomal dominant mode of inheritance exhibiting very high penetrance and variable expressivity.[12]
- Also known as *multiple osteochondromatosis*, *multiple osteochondromata*, *multiple cartilage exostoses*, *diaphyseal aclasis*, or *metaphyseal aclasis*[5,23]

## ANATOMY

- Knowledge of the normal anatomy and biomechanics of the forearm in the immature individual is instrumental in understanding the pathogenesis of the deformity and ultimately in planning appropriate treatment.
- During forearm pronation–supination, the relationship between the radius and ulna changes. This rotational movement requires near-anatomic alignment of both as well as integrity of the proximal and distal radioulnar joints and the interosseous membrane. Minimal axial or rotational bone deformity, asymmetric bone shortening, or ligament instability can hinder this function.
- The ulna acts like a swivel hinge around which the radius rotates. The axis of forearm rotation is oblique.

## PATHOGENESIS

- The most common genetic mutations are in the *EXT-1* and *EXT-2* genes.[6]
- Approximately 10% of individuals with manifestations of multiple exostoses have no family history of MHE.[22]
- The prevalence of MHE in the general population is estimated to be at least one in 50,000, with a median age of first diagnosis of 2 to 3 years of age (exostoses rarely develop before age 2 years).[22] An average of five or six exostoses, involving both upper and lower extremities, is found at the time of the first consultation.[9]
  - The presence of exostoses is almost always evident by the age of 12 years.
- Osteochondromas develop at numerous sites in the immature skeleton, they may affect any bone except the skull. They most commonly affect the ends of long bones and flat bones including the scapula and pelvis.
- Osteochondromas consist of a base or stalk covered by a cartilaginous cap. They arise from the peripheral aspect of the growth plate of bones that undergo endochondral ossification.[14]
  - They are the product of abnormal proliferation of chondroblasts and subsequent defective remodeling of the metaphysis. This leads to the two main characteristics of this condition: skeletal metaphyseal exostoses and retardation of longitudinal bone growth.
  - They migrate away from the physis with longitudinal growth.[14]
- In MHE, the exostoses vary greatly in number, location, size, and configuration. They tend to have a more irregular and bizarre shape than solitary osteochondromas.
  - Should always be continuous with the medullary cavity of the bone from which they arise
  - Once skeletal maturity is reached, the lesions will become quiescent.[22] Lesions that enlarge after skeletal maturity should be investigated to exclude malignant change.

## NATURAL HISTORY

- Deformity of the forearm is seen in 30% to 60% of the individuals with MHE.[22] The forearm deformities can be progressive and result in a variable amount of weakness, pain,[4] functional limitation, and aesthetic deformity.
  - The deformities are almost always accompanied by discrepancy in length between the two bones. Asynchronous longitudinal growth between paired bones leads to a greater risk of anatomic distortion. Most of the longitudinal growth of the ulna occurs at the distal physis,[15] which is also the more commonly affected physis (30% to 85% of the cases).[22,23]
  - The affected ulna typically remains relatively shortened and curved, and this often leads to significant bowing of the radius. When the ulna is shorter, the ulnar-sided soft tissue acts as a tether, causing bowing of the radius. In addition, the local presence of the exostosis itself causes radial bowing by disturbing hemiepiphyseal growth.[15]
- A serious risk associated with MHE is the potential for malignant transformation of an exostosis into chondrosarcoma. This can occur at any age, but it is exceedingly rare during childhood.[22]
- Patients affected by MHE have a normal life expectancy unless malignant degeneration and metastasis develop.[9] The risk of malignant degeneration in adults with MHE has been reported to range from 0.57% to 5%.[12,22,31]
- MHE can have a serious influence on the quality of life of affected individuals, affecting sporting participation, occupation, and daily activities.[8]

## HISTORY AND PHYSICAL FINDINGS

- The diagnosis is rarely difficult as 90% of affected individuals have a positive family history, and therefore initial history taking should focus on the symptoms and functional impairment that exist.

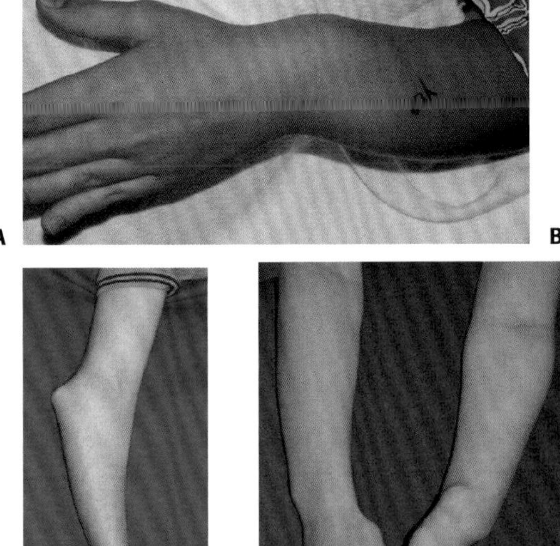

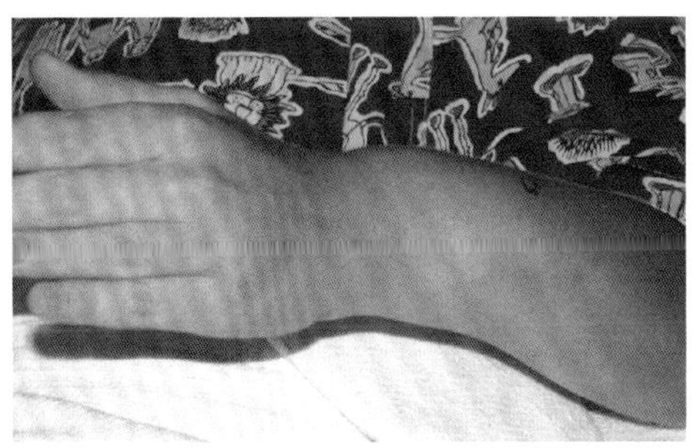

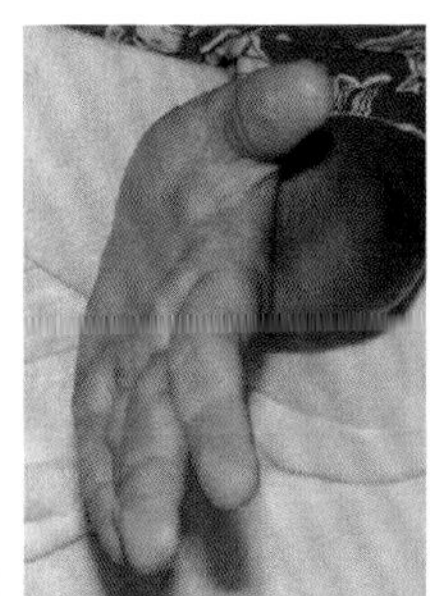

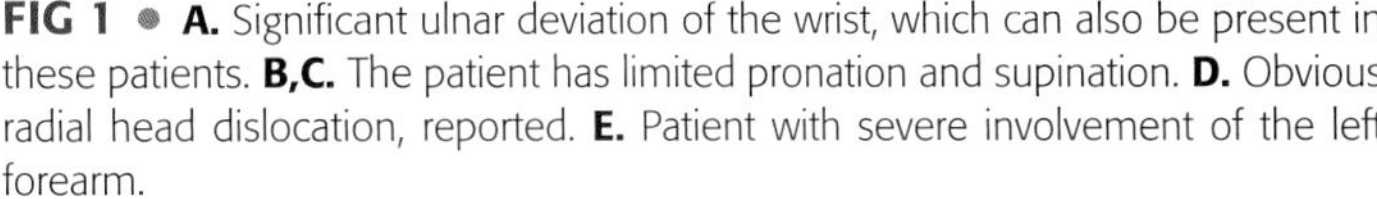

**FIG 1** • **A.** Significant ulnar deviation of the wrist, which can also be present in these patients. **B,C.** The patient has limited pronation and supination. **D.** Obvious radial head dislocation, reported. **E.** Patient with severe involvement of the left forearm.

- Physical examination of the upper extremity should assess for location of disease burden and common associated findings.
  - It is a common finding that the deformity is quite asymmetric. One forearm may be heavily affected, whereas the other relatively spared.
- Shortening of the forearm, specifically relative shortening of the ulna, increased radial bow and possible radial head dislocation.
- A mild flexion deformity of the elbow is often present.
- At the wrist level, an increased ulnar tilt of the radial epiphysis, ulnar deviation of the hand, and progressive ulnar translocation of the carpus are often present. These deformities can lead to a loss of radial deviation of the hand and loss of pronation–supination of the forearm (**FIG 1**).
- The loss of forearm pronation–supination may develop early and become progressively more severe as the child ages.[26] Pronation–supination may be limited due to altered mechanical alignment, osteochondroma blocking motion, or radial head dislocation. The greater the number of osteochondromas and shorter the ulna, the greater the loss of motion.[10,32]
- Radial head dislocation is reported to occur in 22% of the affected forearms.[23] It may present as pain, a mass on the lateral side of the elbow, altered carrying angle, decreased elbow range of motion or decreased pronation–supination, or catching.
- It is possible to have neurologic impingement from either direct compression by an osteochondroma or through deformity including radial head dislocation.

## IMAGING AND OTHER DIAGNOSTIC STUDIES

- Plain radiographic evaluation is usually sufficient to confirm the diagnosis and to determine the number, location, and morphology of the exostoses (**FIG 2**).
- Like solitary osteochondromas, the exostoses may be described as sessile or pedunculated; they nearly always point away from the physis, however in the hand they may not. In MHE, the lesions tend to be larger and have a more bizarre shape (see **FIG 2**).
- At least two full views of the forearm (true anteroposterior and lateral containing both the elbow and the wrist) are necessary to properly assess the ulnar variance, the radial articular angle (RAA), the carpal slip, and the relative radial bow. These radiographic measurements are useful in the surgical planning phase (**FIG 3**).[2]

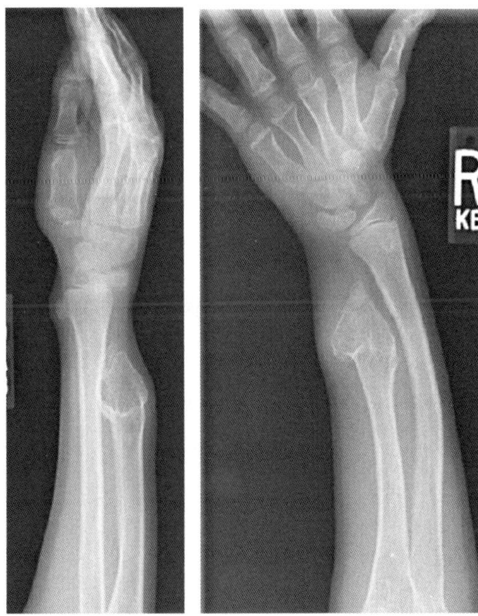

**FIG 2** • Radiographs showing large osteochondroma of distal ulna affecting the epiphysis and causing significant tethering of the radius. Characteristically, the distal ulna is narrow with a pointed end.

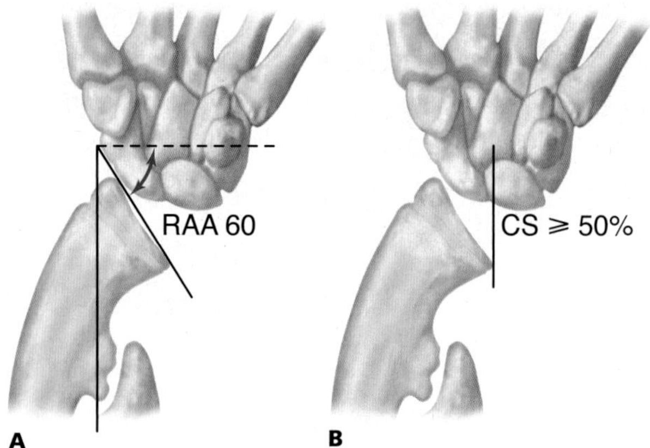


FIG 3 • The RAA and carpal slip (CS). **A.** The RAA is defined as the angle between a line running along the articular surface of the radius and another line that is perpendicular to a line joining the center of the radial head to the radial border of the distal radial epiphysis (the radial styloid in skeletally mature individuals). The normal range of the angle is 15 to 30 degrees. **B.** CS is measured by determining the percentage of the lunate that is in contact with the radius. First, a line is drawn from the center of the olecranon through the ulnar border of the radial epiphysis (the radial articular surface in skeletally mature individuals).[1] This line normally bisects the lunate. An abnormal CS is defined as being present when ulnar displacement of the lunate exceeds 50%. (Adapted from Akita S, Mursae T, Yonenobu K, et al. Long-term results of surgery for forearm deformities in patients with multiple cartilaginous exostoses. J Bone Joint Surg Am 2007;89:1993–1999.)

- Alterations of the radial head on radiographs must always be assessed. They range from flattening to subluxation and complete radial head dislocation.
- Masada et al[15] morphologically classified the involvement of the forearm in MHE into three types (**FIG 4**). This classification is also used for treatment planning.
- Computed tomography (CT), magnetic resonance imaging (MRI), and magnetic resonance angiography are performed at times for specific and symptomatic lesions. These can be especially helpful to detail the anatomic position relative to soft tissue structures or when malignant transformation is suspected.[27]
  - In older children and teenagers, irregular areas of calcification of the cartilaginous cap may be present. Extensive calcification with changes in the shape, thickness of the cartilaginous cap, or a lesion enlarging more rapidly than the growth of the child should raise suspicion of possible chondrosarcoma transformation.

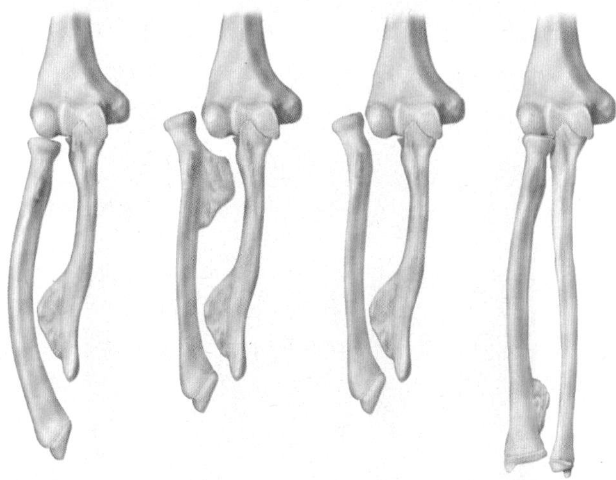


FIG 4 • Masada classification of the involvement of the forearm in MHE. (Adapted from Masada K, Tsuyuguchi Y, Kawai H, et al. Operations for forearm deformity caused by multiple osteochondromas. J Bone Joint Surg Br 1989;71:24–29.)

## DIFFERENTIAL DIAGNOSIS

- Langer-Giedion syndrome
- Madelung deformity
- Chondrosarcoma

## NONOPERATIVE MANAGEMENT

- Patients with MHE can often be managed successfully using a conservative approach.
  - Exostoses alone can often be surprisingly well tolerated and result in minimal loss of function.[26] It has been reported that forearm function in untreated adults with MHE is subjectively greater than the one objectively measured.[17]
  - The conspicuous number of lesions and the fact that they are mostly asymptomatic warrant a cautious surgical approach.
  - A dislocated radial head that is not symptomatic should be left alone.
    - Attempts at relocating a dislocated radial head have been unsuccessful.[2,19]

## SURGICAL MANAGEMENT

- Surgical treatment of forearm deformities in MHE remains controversial. A number of operative techniques have been proposed.[5,10,15,20,24]
- The main surgical indications are to
  - Improve forearm function (pronation–supination)[2]
  - Relieve pain from external trauma or irritation of the surrounding soft tissue[4]
  - Improve appearance[10]
  - Exclude malignancy when there is a rapid increase in size of a lesion[18]
- When evaluating the surgical indications in an individual patient, it is important to distinguish between the functional deficit and the cosmetic appearance.
  - The postoperative appearance of the forearm has been shown to be unrelated to the functional outcome.[17]
- Despite many maintaining good function even without treatment,[2,17] a percentage of patients find the appearance of the shortening, angulation, and deformities unacceptable.[17] If surgery is being undertaken for aesthetic rather than functional purposes, the hopes, concerns, and expectations of patient and parents must be thoroughly discussed and accurately outlined.
  - A mass or deformation may be removed; however, a scar shall be added.
  - Restoration of range of motion and improvement of radiographic parameters are unpredictable but may occur.[2,11]
- Some[5,15,18] advocate an aggressive approach based on the rationale that forearm deformities may lead to functional impairment especially if radial head dislocation occurs.[2,26]

Surgical treatment employed includes excision of the exostoses and ulnar lengthening and associated radial osteotomy when indicated.

- Radiographic indications cited include relative ulnar shortening (with or without bowing) of more than 1.5 cm, RAA of greater than 30 degrees, carpal slip of more than 60%, and bowing of the radius or the ulna (or both).[5]
- Predication of radial head dislocation has remained one of the most difficult aspects of MHE forearm care.
  - The most common association with radial head dislocation is isolated distal ulnar osteochondromas.[7]
- However, our approach reflects that the presence of forearm deformities alone is relatively unrelated to functional impairment,[2,17,26] and therefore we do not recommend surgical correction of the deformities only to prevent a possible, but not predictable, future functional impairment.

- Symptomatic dislocation of the radial head is an indication for surgical intervention when it interferes with joint motion or causes significant pain.

## Procedures

- Exostosis excision alone is indicated when a lesion becomes symptomatic or when it directly causes limitation of forearm pronation–supination.
  - This procedure alone does not necessarily correct the forearm deformity.
  - Excision of a distal ulnar osteochondroma may lead to remodeling of the radius.[11]
- Ulnar tether release is indicated when there is significant wrist deformity present secondary to ulnar shortening.
  - When the distal epiphyseal plate of the ulna has lost its growth potential and resultant significant radial bowing exists, extensive ulnar tether release is our preferred technique to improve wrist position and potentially decrease the risk of radial head subluxation/dislocation. Lengthening may temporarily level the joint; however, the physis will not provide growth and recurrent deformity is common.
  - May be combined with osteochondroma excision or radial osteotomy
  - If the patient has significant growth potential remaining, ulnar tether release alone can lead to radial correction.
- Ulnar lengthening with or without radial osteotomy remains a common procedure.
  - Acute[10,30] and gradual[1,13,16,20,28] lengthenings have been used.
  - Ulnar lengthening levels the joint and relieves tension on the ulnar-sided soft tissues.
  - Anatomic structure, alignment, and potential for remodeling of the DRUJ needs to be considered prior to lengthening the ulna.
  - Lengthening will not restore growth to the distal ulna, the remaining growth potential and possible recurrence of deformity needs to be considered.
  - There are incumbent risks associated with lengthening procedures. The risks and benefits must be considered. The time to union or consolidation of bone regenerate is commonly 2 to 3 months.
- Radial osteotomy is performed in the skeletally mature or nearly skeletally mature patient.
  - Significant remodeling of the radius is unlikely in the older patient.
  - Radial osteotomy acutely corrects the radial deformity.
  - Combination with osteochondroma excision and ulnar-sided procedures is common.
  - Consider staging procedures if the level of surgery is similar on the radius and ulna to minimize the risk of synostosis or loss of correction.
- Distal radial hemiepiphysiodesis with stapling has been used in the past.[15,25] It has not gained widespread use.
- Treatment for symptomatic radial head dislocation is usually limited to salvage procedures.
  - Surgical excision may be performed once the patient is skeletally mature. Excision before this time may lead to instability, growth disturbance, and possible worsening of the wrist or elbow deformity.
- Formation of a single-bone forearm has been successfully used in the skeletally immature and skeletally mature patient.[19,21,29]
- In rare instances, exostosis excision with osteotomy or ulnar lengthening may be effective in relocating the radial head.[16]

TECHNIQUES

## Exostosis Excision and Ulnar Tethering Release

- The location of the incision in the distal forearm varies depending on where the osteochondroma is located. Planning of this is important, as the ability to access the distal ulna is imperative whether the osteochondroma is located on the distal ulna or radius.
  - If the patient has ulnar involvement only, the incision can be placed on the subcutaneous border of the ulna between the flexor carpi ulnaris and the extensor carpi ulnaris (ECU). Care must be taken to identify and preserve the dorsal branch of the ulnar nerve.
  - If the patient has osteochondroma of both the radius and ulna, the incision has to be modified to allow exposure of both bones as well as the distal ulna.
- A tourniquet of appropriate size is used.
- Once the initial incision is made, the soft tissues are cleared from around the base, and the osteochondroma is carefully exposed and excised, ensuring that the cartilage cap is not breeched.
  - If near the physis, resection should proceed from the base nearest the physis and away from it (**TECH FIG 1**). Care must be taken to preserve satisfactory bony cortex for stability.
  - Bone wax is applied to the base of the resected osteochondroma to minimize bleeding and potential for bone regrowth.
- Next, the distal ulna is exposed and the ulnar tethering force is released.
  - This is usually done by transecting the distal ulna through the ulna styloid or epiphyseal area, leaving the triangular fibrocartilage complex attached to the distal fragment.
  - The ECU subsheath needs to be released for a maximal correction.
  - A radiocarpal wire can be used to maintain radiocarpal alignment in addition to a long-arm cast in the early postoperative period.

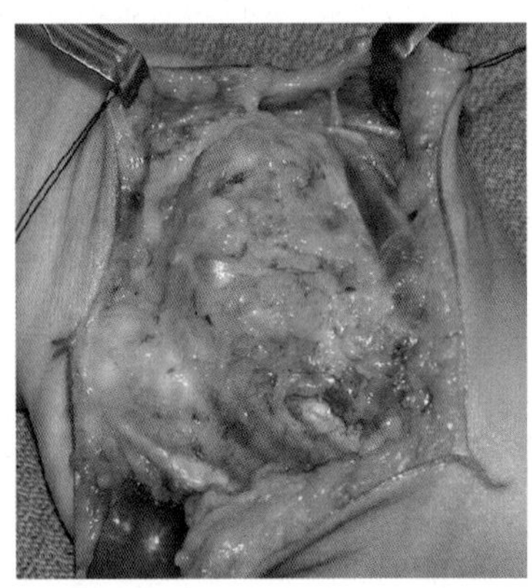

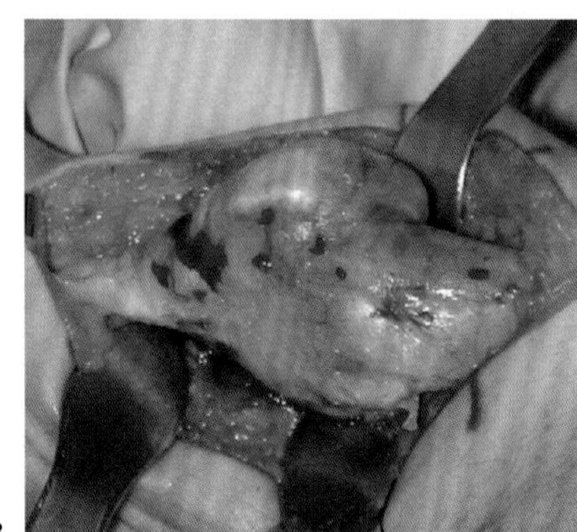

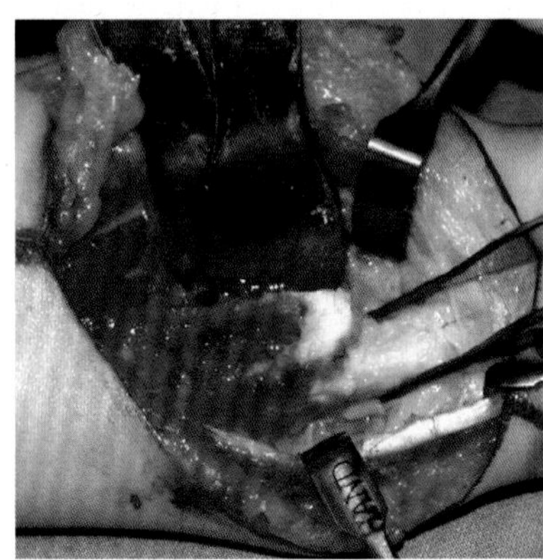

**TECH FIG 1** • **A.** Exposure of large osteochondroma of the distal ulna. **B.** Dissection and exposure of the osteochondroma. Significant tethering is present distally. **C.** After excision of osteochondroma and release of ulnar tethering.

## Distal Radial Osteotomy

- Radial osteotomy can be performed if the forearm bowing and deformity is severe, especially close to skeletal maturity (**TECH FIG 2A**).
- Preoperative radiographs are used for osteotomy planning. The site and magnitude of correction are determined, aiming for normalization of the RAA.
- A volar flexor carpi radialis (FCR) bed approach is made (unless another appropriate approach has been used for osteochondroma excision).
- Pronator quadratus is reflected, leaving a small cuff of tissue along the radial border for later repair.
- A closing wedge osteotomy is normally selected. A closing wedge osteotomy reduces radial height; however, this is not problematic when ulnar shortening has occurred.
  - A dome osteotomy is selected when there is no significant ulnar shortening.
  - Wire fixation is usually adequate for the osteotomy (either two stout K-wires or multiple smaller caliber wires).
    - Wires may be preplaced in the radial styloid before completion and displacement of the osteotomy. They are inserted percutaneously into the radial styloid.
  - Once the osteotomy is displaced, the wires are driven across until they obtain bicortical fixation.
- Adequacy of correction and final alignment is checked using fluoroscopy (**TECH FIG 2B,C**).
- Pronator quadratus is repaired using interrupted absorbable sutures.

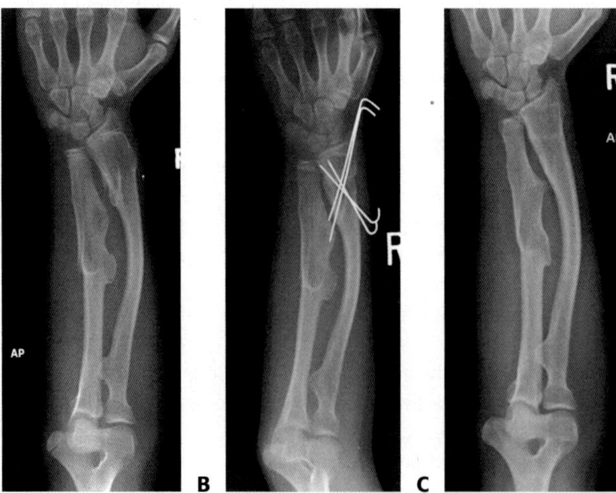


**TECH FIG 2** • **A.** Prior to distal radial dome osteotomy. **B.** Early postoperative radiograph. **C.** Postoperative outcome at skeletal maturity.

## Radial Head Excision

- An incision is made over the prominent radial head with the forearm in pronation to protect the posterior interosseous nerve.
- Dissection is then carried down in the interval between the anconeus muscle and ECU.
- The radial head is then exposed and excised (**TECH FIG 3**).
- Layered closure is then performed and the extremity is immobilized for 2 weeks, followed by institution of range-of-motion exercises.

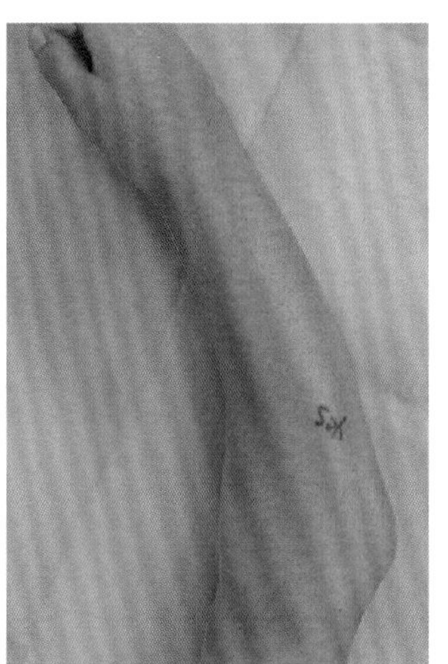
A

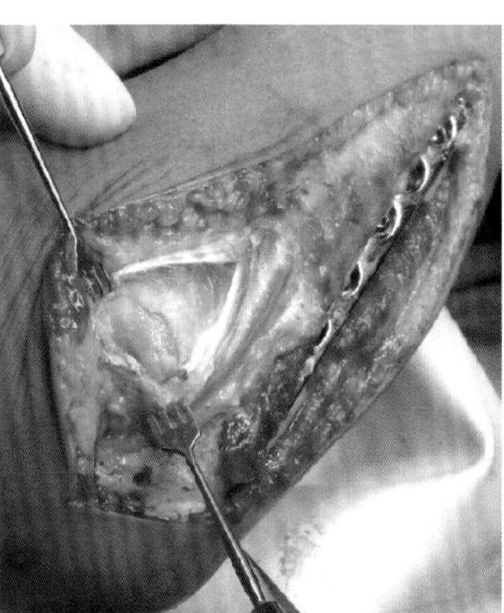
B

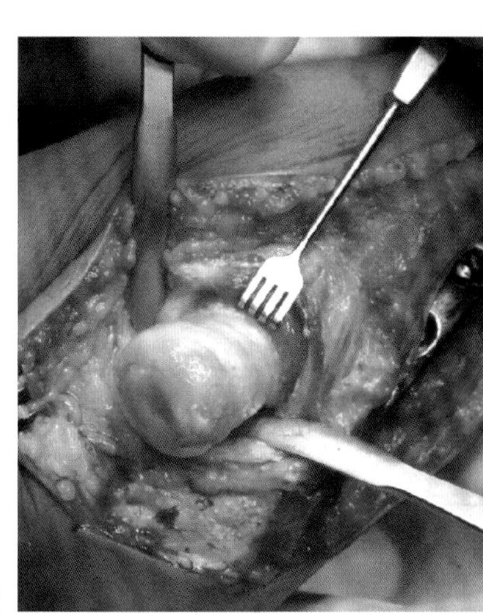
C

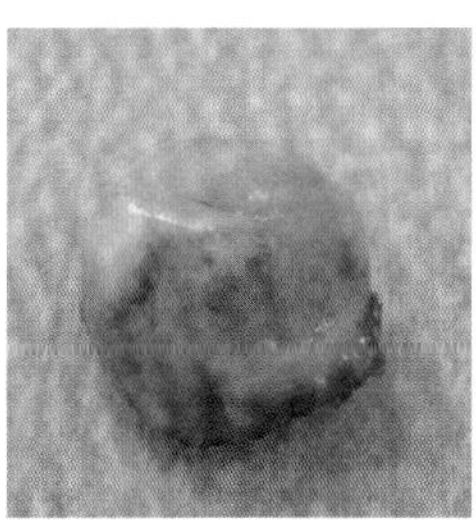
D

**TECH FIG 3** • **A.** Patient with painful radial head dislocation. **B.** Exposure of the radial head. Forearm is in a pronated position to protect the posterior interosseous nerve. **C.** Radial head exposed before excision. **D.** Excised radial head. Significant degenerative changes are present.

## PEARLS AND PITFALLS

| | |
|---|---|
| **Surgical approach** | ■ Be aware of the risk of creating a synostosis. Use separate approaches or staged procedures if both sides of the distal radius and ulna require surgical treatment. |
| **Excision of osteochondromas** | ■ When resecting pedunculated osteochondromas, ensure that the axilla is clear of soft tissue—this is particularly so in the proximal radius as the radial nerve may become entrapped. Cutaneous nerves are also commonly draped over the surface of symptomatic lesions around the wrist.<br>■ Be aware of the physis when resecting osteochondromas. Minimize any additional trauma. |
| **Ulnar tether release** | ■ Ensure that the ECU subsheath is completely released for maximal correction. |
| **Radial osteotomy** | ■ Preplaced K-wires need to be almost parallel to the radial cortex to be correctly aligned once the osteotomy is displaced.<br>■ If using a dome osteotomy for correction of increased radial inclination, orient the concavity of the dome toward the joint to avoid excess translation.<br>■ Have a low threshold for a limited fasciotomy if a forearm osteotomy has been performed. |
| **Radial head excision** | ■ Distorted anatomy means the radial/posterior interosseous nerve may be in a location that you do not expect it to be.<br>■ Avoid posterior dissection and further disruption of the lateral ulnar collateral ligament (LUCL). Repair the soft tissue envelope to minimize secondary instability. |

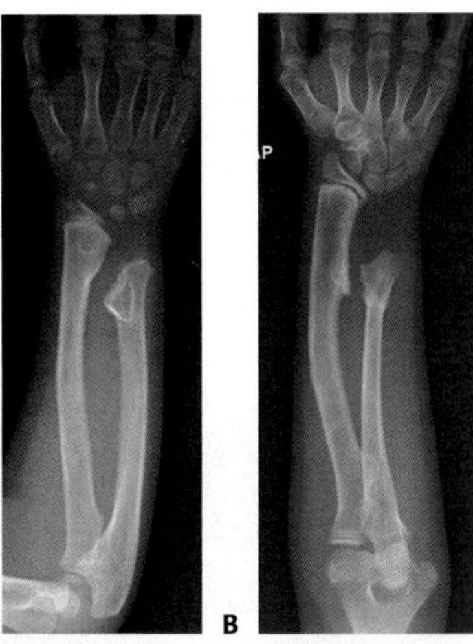


**FIG 5** • **A.** Radiograph of a 5-year-old child prior to ulnar tether release with increased radial slope and severely affected distal ulnar physis. **B.** Seven years after ulnar tether release.

## POSTOPERATIVE CARE

- Exercises to maintain the range of motion of the fingers are encouraged immediately after surgery regardless of the technique used.
- In cases of ulnar tethering release, casting is performed for 4 weeks, followed by range-of-motion exercises and splinting.
- If an osteotomy was performed, casting is continued until radiographic evidence of healing is seen.

## OUTCOMES

- Many MHE patients do not need surgery. In patients who require surgery, ulnar tether release, with or without exostoses excision, with or without radial osteotomy, provides reliable results with the few complications (**FIG 5**). In selected patients, this can greatly improve function in addition to the improved cosmesis of the extremity.
- Ulnar lengthening is reserved for select patients.
- For symptomatic radial head dislocations, radial head excision usually leads to a consistent, reproducible result; however, formation of single-bone forearm can certainly be beneficial, especially in the skeletally immature patient.

## REFERENCES

1. Abe M, Shirai H, Okamoto M, et al. Lengthening of the forearm by callus distraction. J Hand Surg Br 1996;21:151–163.
2. Akita S, Murase T, Yonenobu K, et al. Long-term results of surgery for forearm deformities in patients with multiple cartilaginous exostoses. J Bone Joint Surg Am 2007;89:1993–1999.
3. Boyer A. Traite des Maladies Chirurgicales et des Operations qui Leur Conviennent. Paris: Chez l'Auteur, 1814.
4. Darilek S, Wicklund C, Novy D, et al. Hereditary multiple exostoses and pain. J Pediatr Orthop 2005;25:369–376.
5. Fogel GR, McElfresh EC, Peterson HA, et al. Management of deformities of the forearm in multiple hereditary osteochondromas. J Bone Joint Surg Am 1984;66:670–680.
6. Francannet C, Cohen-Tanugi A, LeMerrer M, et al. Genotype–phenotype correlation in hereditary multiple exostoses. J Med Genet 2001;38:430–434.
7. Gottschalk HP, Kanauchi Y, Bednar MS, et al. Effect of osteochondroma location on forearm deformity in patients with multiple hereditary osteochondromatosis. J Hand Surg Am 2012;37:2286–2293.
8. Goud AL, de Lange J, Scholtes VA, et al. Pain, physical and social functioning, and quality of life in individuals with multiple hereditary exostoses in The Netherlands: a national cohort study. J Bone Joint Surg 2012;94:1013–1020.
9. Herring JA. Tachdjian's Pediatric Orthopaedics. ed 4. Philadelphia: WB Saunders, 2007.
10. Ip D, Li YH, Chow W, et al. Reconstruction of the forearm deformities in multiple cartilaginous exostoses. J Pediatr Orthop B 2003;12:17–21.
11. Ishikawa J, Kato H, Fujioka F, et al. Tumor location affects the results of simple excision for multiple osteochondromas in the forearm. J Bone Joint Surg Am 2007;89:1238–1247.
12. Legeai-Mallet L, Munnich A, Maroteaux P, et al. Incomplete penetrance and expressivity skewing in hereditary multiple exostoses. Clin Genet 1997;52:12–16.
13. Mader K, Gausepohl T, Pennig D. Shortening and deformity of radius and ulna in children: correction of axis and length by callus distraction. J Pediatr Orthop B 2003;12:183–191.
14. Mansoor A, Beals RK. Multiple exostosis: a short study of abnormalities near the growth plate. J Pediatr Orthop B 2007;16:363–365.
15. Masada K, Tsuyuguchi Y, Kawai H, et al. Operations for forearm deformity caused by multiple osteochondromas. J Bone Joint Surg Br 1989;71:24–29.
16. Matsubara H, Tsuchiya H, Sakurakichi K, et al. Correction and lengthening for deformities of the forearm in multiple cartilaginous exostoses. J Orthop Sci 2006;11:459–466.
17. Noonan KJ, Levenda A, Snead J, et al. Evaluation of the forearm in untreated adult subjects with multiple hereditary osteochondromatosis. J Bone Joint Surg Am 2002;84:397–403.
18. Peterson HA. Deformities and problems of the forearm in children with multiple hereditary osteochondromata. J Pediatr Orthop 1994;14:92–100.
19. Peterson HA. The ulnius: a one-bone forearm in children. J Pediatr Orthop B 2008;17:95–101.
20. Pritchett JW. Lengthening the ulna in patients with hereditary multiple exostoses. J Bone Joint Surg Br 1986;68:561–565.
21. Rodgers WB, Hall JE. One-bone forearm as a salvage procedure for recalcitrant forearm deformity in hereditary multiple exostoses. J Pediatr Orthop 1993;13:587–591.
22. Schmale GA, Conrad EU III, Raskind WH. The natural history of hereditary multiple exostoses. J Bone Joint Surg Am 1994;76:986–992.
23. Shapiro F, Simon G, Glimcher MJ. Hereditary multiple exostoses. Anthropometric, roentgenographic, and clinical aspect. J Bone Joint Surg Am 1979;61:815–824.
24. Shin EK, Jones NF, Lawrence JF. Treatment of multiple hereditary osteochondromas of the forearm in children: a study of surgical procedures. J Bone Joint Surg Br 2006;88:255–260.
25. Siffert RS, Levy RN. Correction of the wrist deformity in diaphyseal aclasis by stapling. Report of a case. J Bone Joint Surg Am 1965;47:1378–1380.
26. Stanton RP, Hansen MO. Function of the upper extremities in hereditary multiple exostoses. J Bone Joint Surg Am 1996;78:568–573.
27. Vanhoenacker FM, Van Hul W, Wuyts W, et al. Hereditary multiple exostoses: from genetics to clinical syndrome and complications. Eur J Radiol 2001;40:208–217.
28. Vogt B, Tretow HL, Daniilidis K, et al. Reconstruction of forearm deformity by distraction osteogenesis in children with relative shortening of the ulna due to multiple cartilaginous exostosis. J Pediatr Orthop 2011;31:393–401.
29. Waters PM. Forearm rebalancing in osteochondromatosis by radioulnar fusion. Tech Hand Up Extrem Surg 2007;11:236–240.
30. Waters PM, Van Heest AE, Emans J. Acute forearm lengthenings. J Pediatr Orthop 1997;17:444–449.
31. Watts AC, Ballantyne JA, Fraser M, et al. The association between the ulnar length and the forearm movement in patients with multiple osteochondromas. J Hand Surg Am 2007;32(5):667–673.
32. Wicklund CL, Pauli RM, Johnston D, et al. Natural history study of hereditary multiple exostoses. Am J Med Genet 1995;55:43–46.

# Modified Woodward Repair of Sprengel Deformity

80 CHAPTER

J. Richard Bowen

## DEFINITION

- Sprengel deformity is a congenital anomaly of the shoulder characterized by a high elevation of a hypoplastic scapula and medial rotation of its inferior pole.[6,7,22] The exact cause of the deformity is unknown.
- Associated anomalies include Klippel-Feil syndrome, rib deformities, omovertebral bone formation, muscleanomalies, clavicle hypoplasia, tracheoesophageal fistula, anal stenosis, kidney anomalies, diastematomyelia, and scoliosis.[1,2,5,14,17,25]
- Eulenberg[6,7] first described three cases of congenital "high dislocation of the scapula" in 1863, and in 1880, Willet and Walsham[25] were the first to describe the omovertebral bone—a broad osseous band of bone connecting the scapula with the spinous process of C6.

## ANATOMY

- The normal scapula forms in the fifth week of fetal development adjacent to the level of C5 and then descends to the dorsal thoracic area at a level between T2 and T8.
- The scapula in Sprengel deformity is abnormally high, has a decreased vertical diameter, and is deformed in shape.
  - The supraspinous region is rotated anteriorly in a convexity near the shape of the dorsal thorax.
  - The inferior aspect of the scapula is rotated medially.
- The scapula in Sprengel deformity may be attached to the lower cervical vertebrae (usually C6) by an abnormal band of tissue, which may be fibrous, cartilage, or bone (ie, omovertebral bone).[25]
- The musculature of the shoulder girdle may be hypoplastic, absent, or weak.
  - The trapezius muscle, the levator scapulae muscle, and the rhomboid muscles often are hypoplastic.
  - The trapezius is the most commonly affected muscle. Other muscle groups that attach to the scapula occasionally are affected.
- Associated bony congenital anomalies include Klippel-Feil syndrome, fused ribs, cervical ribs, congenital scoliosis, cervical spina bifida, hypoplastic clavicle, and short humerus.[2,10]

## PATHOGENESIS

- The normal scapula develops in the cervical region and then descends to the upper posterior area of the thorax by the end of the third month of fetal development.
- Sprengel deformity occurs as a result of interruption of the normal caudal migration of the scapula during fetal development.[10]
- The etiology of Sprengel deformity is unknown, but the following theories have been proposed[5,21,24]:
  - Cerebrospinal fluid escapes through a "bleb" in the membrane of the roof of the fourth ventricle into the adjacent tissue of the neck to cause malformations.
  - Heredity (there have been several reports of familial occurrence)
  - Increased intrauterine pressure
  - Abnormal articulation of the scapula to the cervical vertebrae and defective musculature formation

## NATURAL HISTORY

- The Sprengel deformity is present at birth, and the location of the scapula in relation to the neck and thorax remains constant as the child grows.
- The abnormal scapula appears to grow proportionally to the growth of the child.
- Associated congenital anomalies such as congenital scoliosis may progress, thereby changing the appearance of the deformity.

## PATIENT HISTORY AND PHYSICAL FINDINGS

- At birth, the shoulder with a Sprengel deformity appears to be displaced upward and forward.
  - In unilateral cases, shoulder asymmetry is evident.
    - The left scapula is involved more commonly than the right (**FIG 1A**).
  - In bilateral cases, both shoulders appear to be high, and the neck may appear thick and short.
- The scapula may be tilted upward.
- Motion of the shoulder is reduced in abduction and elevation (**FIG 1B**).
- Muscle weakness or hypoplasia can be observed in the shoulder area.
- Torticollis may be present.
- Scoliosis and kyphosis as well as deformities of the chest from rib anomalies may be observed.

## IMAGING AND OTHER DIAGNOSTIC STUDIES

- Radiographs of the shoulder and neck show the bone deformities (**FIG 2**).
- Sonography of the spinal cord is helpful in infants younger than about 4 months of age who have congenital spine anomalies.
  - Sonography can be performed through the cartilage of the lamina and spinous process, but after about 4 to 5 months of age, ossification blocks the views.
  - Congenital spine anomalies have a high association with intraspinal abnormalities.

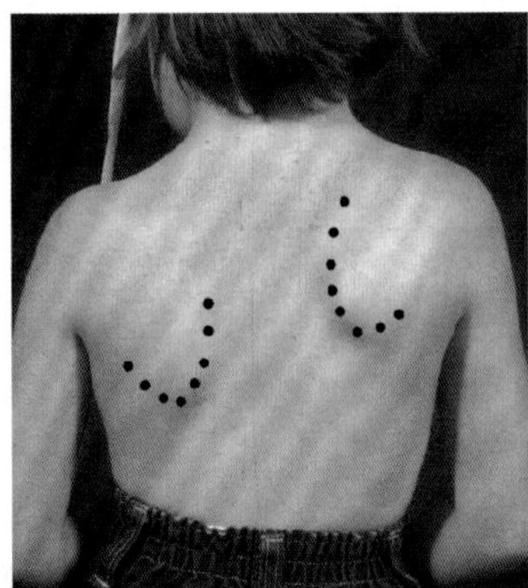

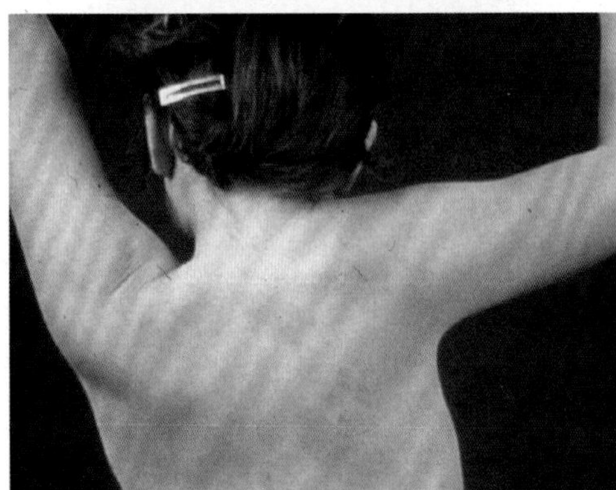

**FIG 1** • **A.** Sprengel deformity of the right shoulder. **B.** Appearance of Sprengel deformity when the right arm is held in maximum abduction.

- Sonography of the kidneys is helpful in cases associated with congenital spine anomalies.
- Magnetic resonance imaging (MRI) is extremely helpful for evaluating muscle and soft tissue development.
- Computed tomography (CT) (with three-dimensional [3-D] reconstruction) is helpful to define the extent of bone deformity. CT provides excellent visualization of the omovertebral structure.
- Both still and video photography are helpful to record pre- and postoperative appearance and to document function.

## DIFFERENTIAL DIAGNOSIS

- No other abnormality resembles Sprengel deformity.

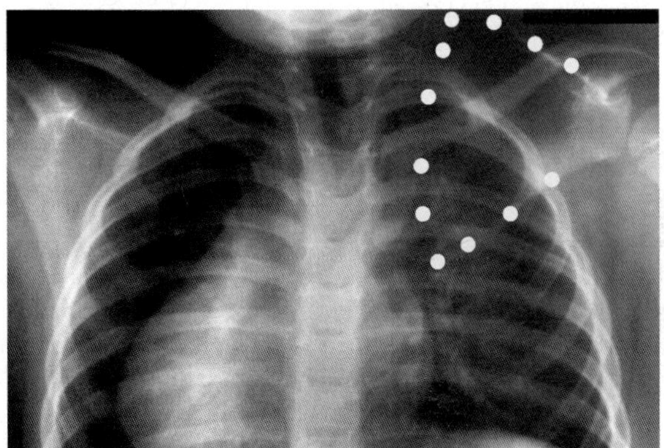

**FIG 2** • Anteroposterior (AP) radiograph of the right shoulder of a child with Sprengel deformity.

## NONOPERATIVE MANAGEMENT

- In infants and young children, passive and active stretching exercises may be performed daily to maintain motion of the shoulder.

## SURGICAL MANAGEMENT

- Operative procedures are designed to improve the appearance of the elevated shoulder and, to a limited extent, improve its function.[3,8,9,11–13,15,18–20,23]
  - Operative treatment can be considered in cases in which the deformity is disfiguring and shoulder function is impaired.
  - In children with mild deformities in which the appearance of the shoulder is acceptable, operative treatment probably is not indicated.
  - The recommended age for surgery is 3 to 8 years.

### Preoperative Planning

- Preoperative evaluation of the appearance of the deformity with photographs is advised.
  - The author prefers full-profile photographs taken from the frontal, posterior, and both side views.
  - Motion can be documented by a series of photographs taken with the arms extended, elevated, and abducted.
  - Videos of the patient performing motion activities of the shoulder are helpful to determine the degree of deformity and whether or not the appearance is acceptable.
    - "Gait laboratory" analysis of the upper extremities is helpful; it quantifies kinetic and kinematic functions, electromyography, postural equilibrium, and energy expenditure.
- The Cavendish grading scale is helpful in evaluating appearance[4]:
  - Grade I (very mild): Shoulder joints are level, and the deformity is not obvious when the patient is dressed.
  - Grade II (mild): Shoulder joints are level, but the deformity is visible when the patient is dressed.
  - Grade III (moderate): The involved shoulder is elevated 2 to 5 cm, and the deformity is obvious.
  - Grade IV (severe): The involved shoulder is greatly elevated, and the superior angle of the scapula is near the occiput.
- Preoperative evaluation of shoulder motion
  - Occupational therapy measurement of combined abduction of both shoulders (combined glenohumeral and scapulothoracic movement) as well as other shoulder motion is useful.
  - Shoulder functional testing also may be useful.
  - The author uses radiographs at the extremes of motion and gait laboratory analysis to verify the degree of measurements.
- The anomalies of the shoulder, spine, and rib cage need to be evaluated radiographically.
- CT scanning and MRI are helpful to determine both bone and soft tissue abnormalities.
- Currently, the author uses somatosensory evoked potentials and transcranial electrical motor evoked potentials to evaluate the brachial plexus nerve function during surgery.
  - Baseline values are obtained after the induction of anesthesia, and monitoring is continued during the procedure.

### Positioning

- The patient is placed in the prone position with the head positioned as if facing forward. (Patients with congenital cervical spinal anomalies may require individualized head positioning to prevent undue stress on the neck.)

- The entire arm, the shoulder, and the posterior thorax back area (ie, superiorly from the high cervical area, inferiorly to the lumbar area, and laterally to the contralateral scapular area) are prepared and draped.
  - The arm and scapular girdle are left free for manipulation during the operation.
- Leads for the somatosensory evoked potentials and transcranial electrical motor evoked potentials are positioned on the skin and muscles in a sterile fashion.

## Approach

- The Woodward procedure consists of detaching the origins of the trapezius and rhomboid muscles from the spinous process and moving them downward after resection of the omovertebral bone and any fibrous bands from the scapula.[21,26]
- The procedure described by Green[8] involves division of the muscles connecting the scapula to the trunk, excision of the omovertebral bone, excision of the supraspinous portion of the scapula, and reattachment of the muscles to hold the scapula reduced.
- The modification described by the author[2] is performed as originally described by Woodward,[26] with the addition of excision of the medial border of the scapula and resection of the supraspinous portion of the scapula.
  - The muscles attached on the medial and superior borders of the scapula are reflected extraperiosteally to facilitate bony resection.
  - Bone resection superiorly is medial to the suprascapular notch, and about 1 cm of the medial border of the scapula is excised.
- The author does not usually recommend routine osteotomy of the clavicle, but it is indicated if neurologic issues arise during surgery. The procedure may be performed at the discretion of the surgeon to diminish the risk of neurologic problems.

TECHNIQUES

# Modified Woodward Procedure[2]

## Incision and Dissection

- A midline incision is made that extends from the spinous process of the C4 distally to the spinous process of T9 (**TECH FIG 1A**).
- The skin and subcutaneous tissue are undermined on the involved side laterally to the medial border of the scapula and the lateral border of the trapezius muscle.
- The trapezius muscle is bluntly dissected from the underlying latissimus dorsi muscle.
  - To achieve this, bluntly dissect the lateral border of the trapezius muscle in the inferior aspect of the operative area from the latissimus dorsi muscle.
  - Continue the dissection medially to the origin of the trapezius muscle at the spinous process of T9. The fibers of the trapezius muscle blend into the fibers of the other muscles that originate from the spinous processes.
- Detach the trapezius muscle distally and proceed superiorly by detaching the remainder of the trapezius and then the rhomboid muscles to the level of the spinous process of C4 (**TECH FIG 1B**).
- Retract the trapezius and rhomboid muscles laterally.
  - The levator scapulae muscle is identified as it originates from the superior medial aspect of the scapula and courses toward the spinous process of the cervical vertebra.
  - Occasionally, the muscles are fibrotic, which makes identification and dissection more difficult.
- The omovertebral structure (which may be fibrotic, cartilage, or bone) is under the levator scapulae muscle.
  - The omovertebral structure is excised extraperiosteally by sharp dissection.
  - Any fibrotic bands in the area that may limit inferior mobility of the scapula are incised.
- During the dissection, the spinal accessory nerve and the nerve to the rhomboids must be protected as they course beneath the trapezius muscle.
  - The spinal accessory nerve is in line with the vertebral border of the scapula.
  - In cases involving significant fibrosis of muscles, the nerves may be difficult to identify, and the use of spontaneous or electrical triggered electromyography may be helpful.

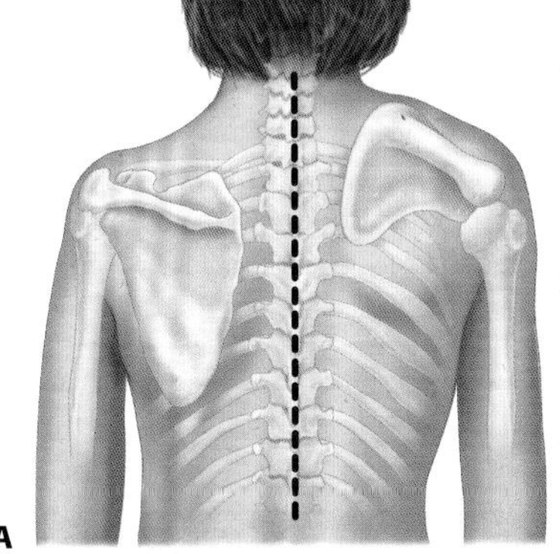


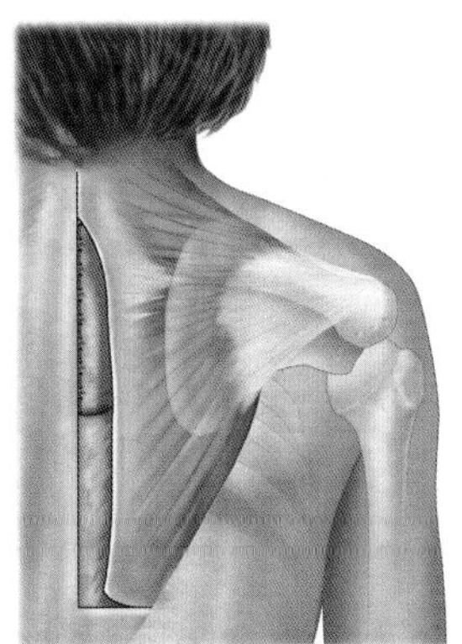


**TECH FIG 1** • **A.** Location of the incision. **B.** Dissection of the trapezius and rhomboid muscles from the spinous processes of the vertebrae.

- The levator scapulae muscle is divided at the superior medial corner of the scapula.
- The transverse cervical artery, which is deep to the levator scapulae muscle, needs to be protected at the superomedial area of the scapula because bleeding occasionally can be problematic.

## Scapular Resection and Reduction

- Superiorly, the scapula is excised medially to the suprascapular notch, after which approximately 1 cm of the medial border of the scapular is excised (**TECH FIG 2**).

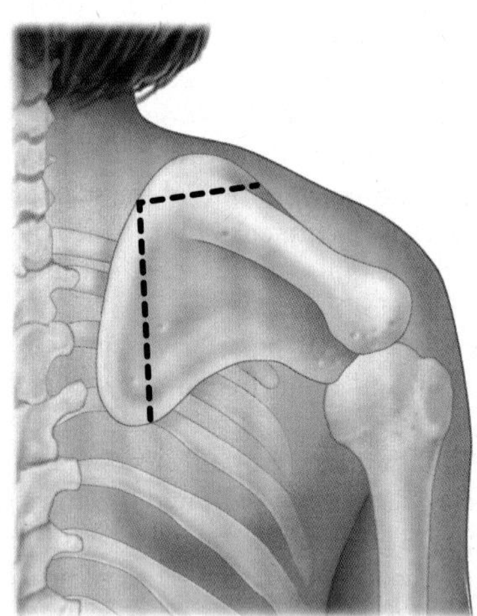

**TECH FIG 2** • Areas of resection of the scapula.

- The scapula can be lifted, and any fibrotic bands between the undersurface of the scapula and chest wall are incised.
- The scapula can now be drawn inferiorly and reduced to a more normal anatomic level.
  - Any fibrotic bands that prevent the reduction may be incised.
- As the scapula is reduced, the somatosensory evoked potentials and the transcranial electrical motor evoked potentials may be used to verify the function of the nerves to the arm.
  - During reduction, the nerves of the brachial plexus may become entrapped between the clavicle and the chest wall.
  - If the evoked potentials become abnormal, the scapula is elevated to relieve tension on the nerves, and a clavicular osteotomy[16] is recommended to alleviate compression on the nerves that may have developed between an intact clavicle and the chest wall.

### Clavicular Osteotomy[16]

- A 2-cm incision is made over the middle clavicle area.
- Beneath the platysma muscle, the periosteum is incised longitudinally, and the clavicle is exposed by subperiosteal elevation.
  - The author incises the mid-area of the clavicle with a rongeur to make chips of cortical bone over a length of approximately 1 cm.
- The incised bone chips are used as graft in the osteotomy.
- The periosteum and operative wound are closed in layers.
- The scapula is reduced, and the rhomboid muscles (and fascia) and the trapezius muscle are reattached in a more caudal position at the midline to the ligaments between the spinous processes.
- The latissimus dorsi muscle can be lifted to allow the inferior wing of the scapula to be positioned beneath it.
- The inferior tip of the scapula wing can be sutured to the latissimus dorsi muscle.
- The operative wound is closed in layers, and wound suction drainage may be used at the surgeon's discretion.

## PEARLS AND PITFALLS

| | |
|---|---|
| **Somatosensory evoked potentials and transcranial electrical motor evoked potentials are helpful to monitor the neurologic status of the arm.** | ■ May indicate brachial plexus compromise and the need for a clavicular osteotomy |
| **Resection of the prominent superior and the medial border of the scapula** | ■ Offers the opportunity to improve both appearance and functional outcomes |
| **Osteotomy of the clavicle** | ■ May prevent brachial plexus palsy |

## POSTOPERATIVE CARE

- Postoperatively, the arm is maintained in a Velpeau bandage for about 4 weeks.
- Physical therapy is initiated after removal of the Velpeau bandage, with emphasis on glenohumeral motion and muscle strengthening.

## OUTCOMES

- Operative treatment of Sprengel deformity generally improves the appearance of the elevated shoulder and, to a limited extent, improve its function.[3,8,9,11–13,15,18–20,23]
- In the author's cases,[2] at an average of 8 years postoperatively, the glenohumeral/scapulothoracic motion was 150 degrees (range, 100 to 180 degrees). This represents 45-degree improvement from preoperative measurements. All children improve their appearance by at least on Cavendish grade and most returned to grade I or II. One out of 14 case was grade III and that child had multiple spinal deformities and scoliosis adjacent to the Sprengel deformity.[2]

## COMPLICATIONS

- Brachial plexus palsy
- Nerve palsy
- Persistent scapular winging
- Incomplete correction
- Vascular problems
- Wound infection
- Operative scar appearance

## REFERENCES


1. Banniza von Bazan U. The association between congenital elevation of the scapula and diastematomyelia: a preliminary report. J Bone Joint Surg Br 1979;61:59–63.
2. Borges JL, Shah A, Torres BC, et al. Modified Woodward procedure for Sprengel deformity of the shoulder: long-term results. J Pediatr Orthop 1996;16:508–513.
3. Carson WG, Lovell WW, Whitesides TE Jr. Congenital elevation of the scapula. Surgical correction by the Woodward procedure. J Bone Joint Surg Am 1981;63(8):1199–1207.
4. Cavendish ME. Congenital elevation of the scapula. J Bone Joint Surg Br 1972;54(3):395–408.
5. Engel D. Etiology of multiple deformities. Am J Dis Child 1940;60:562.
6. Eulenberg M. Beitrag zur dislocation der scapula. Amtlicher Bericht über die Versammlung deutscher Naturforscher und Artze 1863;37:291–294.
7. Eulenberg M. Casuistische Mittheilungen aus dem Gebiete der Orthopadie. Arch Klin Chir 1863;4:301.
8. Green WT. The surgical correction of congenital elevation of the scapula (Sprengel's deformity). J Bone Joint Surg 1957;39A:1439–1448.
9. Grogan DP, Stanley EA, Bobechko WP. The congenital undescended scapula. Surgical correction by the Woodward procedure. J Bone Joint Surg Br 1983;65:598–605.
10. Horwitz AE. Congenital elevation of the scapula: Sprengel's deformity. Am J Orthop Surg 1908;6:260–311.
11. Inclan A. Congenital elevation of the scapula or Sprengel's deformity: two clinical cases treated with Ober's operation. Circ Ortop Traum 1949;15:1.
12. Jeannopoulos CL. Congenital elevation of the scapula. J Bone Joint Surg Am 1952;34-A(4):883–892.
13. Khairouni A, Bensahel H, Csukonyi Z, et al. Congenital high scapula. J Pediatr Orthop B 2002;11:85–88.
14. Pinsky HA, Pizzutillo PD, MacEwen GD. Congenital elevation of the scapula. Orthop Trans 1980;4:288–289.
15. Ross DM, Cruess RL. The surgical correction of congenital elevation of the scapula. A review of seventy-seven cases. Clin Orthop 1977;(125):17–23.
16. Robinson RA, Braum RM, Mark P, et al. The surgical importance of the clavicular component of Sprengel's deformity. J Bone Joint Surg Am 1967;49A:1481.
17. Schrock RD. Congenital abnormalities at the cervicothoracic level. Instr Course Lect 1949;6:228.
18. Schrock RD. Congenital elevation of the scapula. J Bone Joint Surg 1926;8:207–215.
19. Shea KG, Apel PJ, Showalter LD, et al. Somatosensory evoked potential monitoring of the brachial plexus during a Woodward procedure for correction of Sprengel's deformity. Muscle Nerve 2010;41:262–264.
20. Siu KK, Ko JY, Huang CC, et al. Woodward procedure improves shoulder function in Sprengel deformity. Chang Gung Med J 2011;34:403–409.
21. Smith AD. Congenital elevation of the scapula. Arch Surg 1941;42:529.
22. Sprengel O. Die angeborene Verschiebung des Schulterblattes nach oben. Arch Klin Chir 1891;42:545–549.
23. Walstra FE, Alta TD, van der Eijke JW, et al. Long-term follow-up of Sprengel's deformity treated with the Woodward procedure. J Shoulder Elbow Surg 2013;22:752–759.
24. Weed LH. The Development of the Cerebro-spinal Spaces in Pig and Man. Washington, DC: Carnegie Institute of Washington, 1916.
25. Willet A, Walsham WJ. An account of the dissection of the parts removed after death from the body of a woman the subject of congenital malformation of the spinal column, bony thorax, and left scapular arch; with remarks on the probable nature of the defects in development producing the deformities. Med Chir Trans 1880;63:257–302.
26. Woodward JW. Congenital elevation of the scapula. Correction by release and transplantation of muscle origins: a preliminary report. J Bone Joint Surg Am 1961;43A:219–228.

CHAPTER 81

**Spine**

# Release of the Sternocleidomastoid Muscle

Gokce Mik, Denis S. Drummond, and B. David Horn

## DEFINITION

- The term *torticollis* comes from the Latin words *tortus* (twisted) and *collum* (neck). It refers to a clinical deformity where the head tilts in one direction and the neck rotates to the opposite side involuntarily.
- Congenital muscular torticollis (CMT) associated with a contracture of the sternocleidomastoid (SCM) muscle is the most common etiology of torticollis in infants.
- CMT is the third most common congenital deformity, next to developmental dysplasia of the hip (DDH) and congenital clubfoot. The incidence of CMT ranges from 0.4% to 1.3%.[4,6,10]
- Shortening and contracture of the SCM muscle results in tightness that gives the typical clinical appearance, which is detected at birth or shortly thereafter.
- Cheng et al[4] subdivided the CMT patients into three groups:
  - Clinically palpable sternomastoid "tumor" or pseudotumor
  - Muscular torticollis group without palpable or visible tumor but with clinical thickening or tightness of the SCM on the affected side
  - All the clinical features of torticollis with neither a palpable mass nor tightness of the SCM muscle

## ANATOMY

- On each side, the SCM muscle passes obliquely across the side of the neck and divides the neck into anterior and posterior triangles.
- It originates from two heads:
  - Sternal head: superior and anterior surface of manubrium sterni
  - Clavicular head: superior surface of medial third of clavicle. With the two heads combining, the muscle ascends laterally and posteriorly to insert in the mastoid process of the temporal bone.
  - The clavicular origin of the SCM muscle can vary in size. In some cases, the width of the clavicular attachment may extend to the midpoint of the clavicle.
- It inserts on the lateral aspect of the mastoid process.
- The functions of SCM are multiple:
  - With unilateral contraction, it
    - Flexes the head and cervical spine ipsilaterally
    - Laterally rotates the head to the contralateral side
  - With bilateral contraction, it
    - Protracts the head
    - Extends the incompletely extended cervical spine
- The SCM is innervated by the following:
  - Spinal accessory nerve (XI)
  - Ventral ramus of second cervical nerve (C2)
- Erb point is located roughly in the middle of the posterior border of the SCM muscle. At this point, the anterior branch of the great auricular nerve crosses the SCM.
- The spinal accessory nerve penetrates the deep surface of the SCM muscle, giving off a branch that supplies it. It passes deep to Erb point at the posterior aspect of the SCM.
- The external jugular vein is located anterior to the SCM muscle at the proximal part. It crosses the SCM muscle obliquely at its midpoint and ends at the subclavian vein posteroinferior to the SCM muscle.
- The SCM protects the carotid artery and internal jugular vein, both of which lie deep to it.
- The anatomy of the SCM muscle and important surrounding structures is shown in **FIG 1**.

## PATHOGENESIS

- The etiology of CMT in infants is contracture or shortening of the SCM muscle.

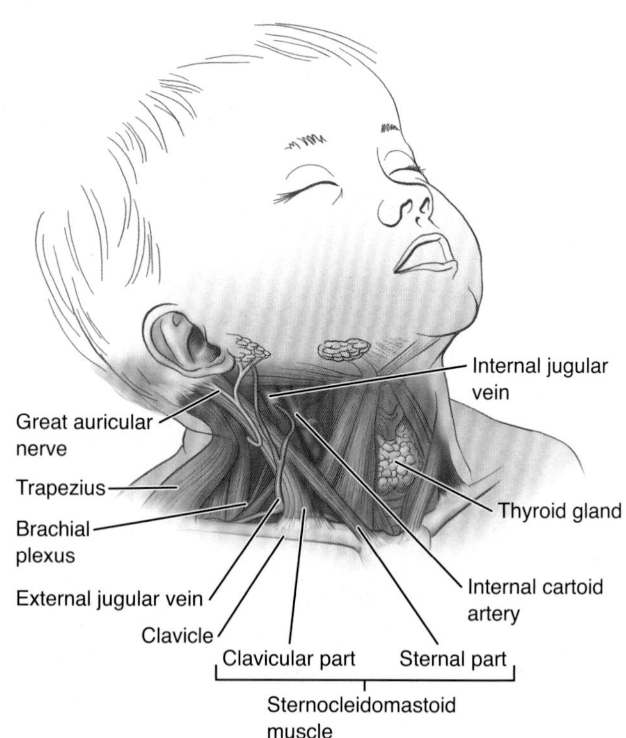


**FIG 1** • Anatomy of SCM muscle and important surrounding structures. Note the course of the external jugular vein and greater auricular nerve; the carotid artery and internal jugular vein lie deep to the SCM muscle.

- Infants with CMT may have a history of difficult or traumatic delivery.
- Davids et al[7] reported that the position of the head and neck in utero or during labor or delivery can lead to local trauma to the SCM muscle.
- Progressive fibrosis and contracture of the SCM muscle may be the sequelae of an intrauterine or perinatal compartment syndrome.[7]
- CMT may occur in association with oligohydramnios, multiple births, firstborn children, and DDH.[9]
  - These associated conditions support the theory that CMT is related to restricted fetal motion and malpositioning of the head and neck. These conditions may also be associated with more difficult and traumatic deliveries.
- About 50% of patients with CMT are born with a clinically palpable SCM mass (pseudotumor).[1,3] This pseudotumor is believed to be a hematoma that undergoes subsequent fibrosis and may result from either birth trauma or intrauterine malposition.
- Torticollis may also result from many other diseases such as ophthalmologic problems (eg, Duane syndrome), congenital cervical anomalies, and neurologic problems (eg, posterior fossa tumors).

## NATURAL HISTORY

- Diagnosis of CMT is usually made at or near birth. Other causes of torticollis generally present later (4 months to 1 year).
- A mass (SCM tumor) or fullness in the SCM muscle usually presents within a few weeks or months after delivery.
- Typically, the mass decreases in size and disappears between 6 and 12 months of age.
- If untreated, contraction and fibrosis of the muscle can occur.
- Flexion and rotation deformity of the neck begins in infancy.
  - Typically, the head turns toward the involved side and the chin points to the opposite shoulder.
  - Plagiocephaly and facial asymmetry may be present early on; they increase with time.
- Flattening of the skull and facial bones can develop on the affected or normal side depending on the sleeping position of the child.
- In older children with persistent deformity, radiographic abnormalities can also occur; they include asymmetry of the articular facets of the axis, tilt of the odontoid process to the side of the torticollis, and possibly cervicothoracic scoliosis.[2,12]

## PATIENT HISTORY AND PHYSICAL FINDINGS

- A complete history and physical examination should be done in newborns with torticollis.
  - The incidence of the breech presentation and birth trauma in children with CMT is higher than the general population.
- There is known coexistence of DDH with torticollis.
  - The reported incidence of DDH with CMT varies from 8% to 20%.[9,14,15]
  - A clinical examination of the hip and ultrasonography screening are thus warranted for children with CMT.
  - A previous belief that CMT was associated with metatarsus adductus and clubfoot is not supported by the literature.
- Typically, children with CMT hold their head laterally flexed to the affected side and rotated to the opposite side.
- Neck range of motion can initially be normal in infants with CMT. This gradually decreases as the muscle contracture becomes tighter. Later, the typical deformity can usually be observed.
  - Any restriction of neck motion should be noted during the examination.
- The facial bones and cranium are observed for asymmetry. Any flattening of the skull bones should also be noted.
- With palpation, a nontender, soft mass 1 to 2 cm in diameter may be found in the lower or middle third of the SCM muscle. With time, this mass changes to a fibrous bundle, and the SCM tendon can then be identified as a tight band that resists correction (**FIG 2**).
- The flexible deformity seen in the early stage can be corrected by gentle stretching.

## IMAGING AND OTHER DIAGNOSTIC STUDIES

- Radiographs
  - Standard cervical spine anteroposterior (AP) and lateral views and open mouth odontoid views can be obtained to rule out bony abnormalities such as atlantoaxial rotary subluxation, cervical fusion, cervical scoliosis, and odontoid anomalies.
  - In older children, radiographic abnormalities such as asymmetry of the articular facets of the axis, tilt of the odontoid process to the side of the torticollis, and sometimes cervicothoracic scoliosis may be observed.[2,12]

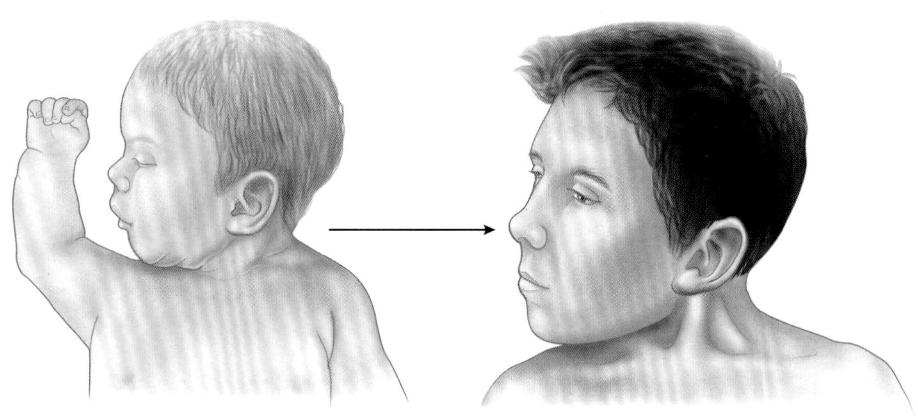

**FIG 2** • A nontender, soft mass of 1 to 2 cm can be found in the lower or middle third of the SCM muscle within weeks or a few months after delivery. At later ages (usually after 6 to 12 months of age), the mass changes to a fibrous bundle and the SCM tendon then can be identified as a tight band.

- Ultrasound examination in children with a palpable SCM mass will demonstrate the fibrotic lesion within the SCM muscle and differentiate the mass from other pathologies in the neck such as neoplasms, cysts, and vascular malformations.
  - In a recent study, Tang et al[13] presented their observations with the use of ultrasound for the long-term follow-up of CMT. They noticed that CMT is a polymorphic and dynamic condition rather than a fixed presentation. The alterations of the fibrosis in muscle can affect the type of treatment.
- Hip imaging should be routinely done in patients born with CMT because there is a high incidence of coexistence of DDH with CMT.[9,14]
  - Patients younger than 6 months of age should have a hip ultrasound performed; children older than 6 months should have an AP pelvis radiograph performed.
- Some investigators have advised magnetic resonance imaging (MRI) to evaluate the SCM muscle for thickening and fibrosis; however, it does not provide additional information. Furthermore, for infants, MRI requires a general anesthetic, with its associated risks.
  - If a posterior fossa tumor is suspected, MRI is indicated.

## DIFFERENTIAL DIAGNOSIS

- Nucci et al,[11] in a multidisciplinary study, reported 25 ocular and 4 neurologic causes in 65 children with abnormal head posture.
- Ophthalmologic torticollis occurs with oculomotor imbalance, which is usually observed after the development of focusing skills (3 months). Ophthalmologic torticollis is caused by a weakness of one of the oculomotor muscles of the eye (typically the superior oblique). This causes a strabismus that can be observed if the head tilt is manually corrected. (This maneuver is useful in providing a diagnosis.) Other causes are strabismus, nystagmus, and paralysis of the sixth cranial nerve resulting in paralysis of the lateral rectus muscle of the eye (Duane syndrome).
- Neurologic causes such as posterior fossa tumors must be ruled out.
  - About 10% of posterior fossa tumors initially present with torticollis.
  - Postural head tilt may be seen with posterior fossa tumors and this may mimic recurrent or relapsed CMT.
- Other orthopaedic causes of torticollis include congenital cervical vertebral anomalies (scoliosis, Klippel-Feil syndrome) and atlantoaxial rotational subluxation.
- Grisel syndrome is torticollis secondary to neck inflammation and is associated with retropharyngeal abscess or post-tonsillectomy status.
- Sandifer syndrome (neck posturing secondary to reflux)
- Other neurologic diseases such as dystonia

## NONOPERATIVE MANAGEMENT

- The initial treatment of CMT is nonoperative and is successful in the vast majority of infants when treatment is initiated before 1 year of age.
- A program of gentle stretching exercises should include flexion–extension, lateral bending away from the involved side, and rotation toward it.
- Stretching exercises can be done by a physical therapist or by the parents with a home program.
  - In our experience, a supervised home program monitored by a physical therapist has been successful.
- Manual stretching should be continued until full neck rotation is achieved.
- In children 1 year of age or younger, the plagiocephaly and facial asymmetry usually will correct spontaneously after the child regains full range of motion of the neck.
- Cervical orthoses may be an adjunct and support for children whose lateral head tilt does not resolve with exercises or for older children who no longer tolerate stretching. These, however, are frequently poorly tolerated.
- Children who present with an SCM pseudotumor may require more prolonged treatment and have less success with stretching than those children without an SCM tumor.[5]
- Surgery is recommended for recalcitrant deformity or when adequate correction is not achieved by 12 to 18 months of age.
- Children who present after 1 year of age with or without previous treatment are candidates for surgery if they have the following:
  - Significant head tilt with tight band or contracture of the SCM muscle
  - Limitation of passive head rotation and lateral flexion by more than 10 to 15 degrees

## SURGICAL MANAGEMENT

- Surgical intervention is indicated for children who have not responded to nonoperative treatment applied for a minimum of 6 months and for children who present with a significant deformity after 12 to 18 months of age.
- The optimal age for surgery is controversial.
- The hypothesis is that the sooner the CMT is corrected, the better the chance for correction of the plagiocephaly and facial asymmetry.[10]
- If the diagnosis of CMT is in doubt, surgery is contraindicated until a workup has been completed because the torticollis could be caused by conditions other than a tight SCM muscle, such as ocular or neurogenic pathologies.
- The operative techniques described for CMT are based on release or lengthening of the tight and shortened SCM muscle.
- The most commonly described procedures are either an unipolar release of the SCM or a bipolar release with or without Z-plasty lengthening of the sternal head.
  - Open, percutaneous, and endoscopic techniques have been described for these procedures. We have no experience with percutaneous or endoscopic techniques and strongly prefer an open approach.

### Authors' Preferred Treatment

- For infants, a home stretching program is taught and supervised by a physical therapist for 6 months.
- In children with appropriate surgical indications, an open unipolar or bipolar release (with or without Z-plasty lengthening) is performed.

### Preoperative Planning

- Cervical spine radiographs should be reviewed before surgery to look for bony anomalies or cervical scoliosis.

- In fixed deformities, positioning of the head can be difficult for the anesthesiologist. Flexible fiberoptic intubation should then be considered.
- The ear is taped anteriorly, and hair around the mastoid process is shaved.

## Positioning

- The procedure is performed under general anesthesia in the supine position. A sandbag is placed in the midline between the scapulae.
- The endotracheal tube should be kept at the unaffected side so as not to interfere with the operative field.
- Draping should allow the correction to be evaluated by bending the neck intraoperatively. This determines the adequacy of the release.
- The neck is bent toward the unaffected side and the head is rotated to the affected side so that the SCM muscle is kept under tension and the origin and insertion can be clearly identified (**FIG 3**).

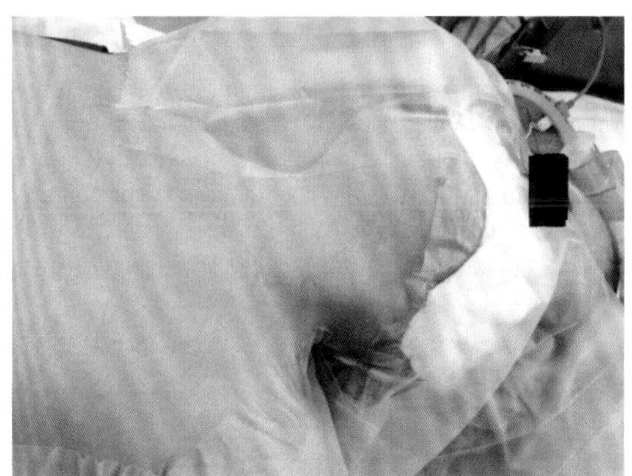

**FIG 3** • The neck is bent toward the unaffected side and the head is rotated to the affected side so that the SCM muscle is kept under tension and the origin and insertion can be clearly identified.

TECHNIQUES

## Incision and Dissection

- For the release of the distal pole of the SCM muscle, a transverse, 3- to 4-cm long incision is made 1 cm superior to the clavicle and between the two heads of the SCM muscle (**TECH FIG 1**).
- The subcutaneous tissue and platysma muscle are divided in line with the incision, and the tendon sheaths of the clavicular and sternal heads are exposed.
- For the proximal pole exposure, a 2- to 3-cm horizontal incision is made just distal to the tip of the mastoid process.
- The dissection is carried deeper until the periosteum of the mastoid process is exposed. The insertion of the muscle is then exposed subperiosteally.

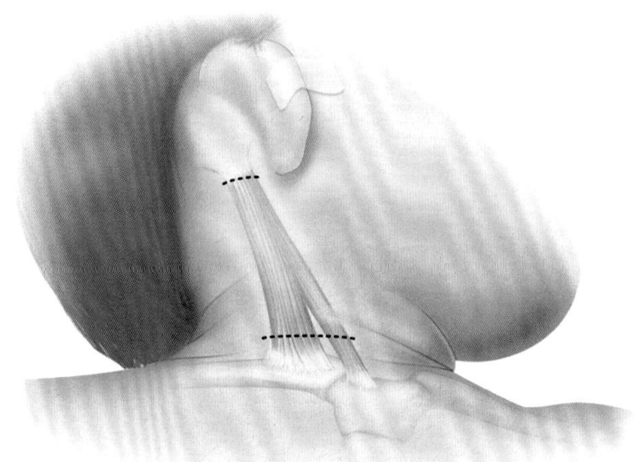

**TECH FIG 1** • Proximal and distal incisions (*dotted lines*).

## Distal Unipolar Release

- Distal unipolar release includes the release of the sternal and the clavicular heads of the SCM muscle. It is commonly used for mild deformities and in younger children.
- A 3- to 4-cm long transverse incision is placed parallel and 1 cm proximal to the clavicle between the clavicular and sternal heads of the SCM.
- The incision should incorporate a Langer line in the neck. An incision that overlies over the clavicle may result in a hypertrophic scar. A higher incision may jeopardize the external jugular vein and may also lead to an unsightly scar.
- The two heads of the SCM muscle are then identified.
- Surrounding fascia is cleared and both heads are undermined and dissected off of the underlying deep cervical fascia with spreading dissection.
- The muscles are elevated with the help of a clamp and divided using electrocautery (**TECH FIG 2**).

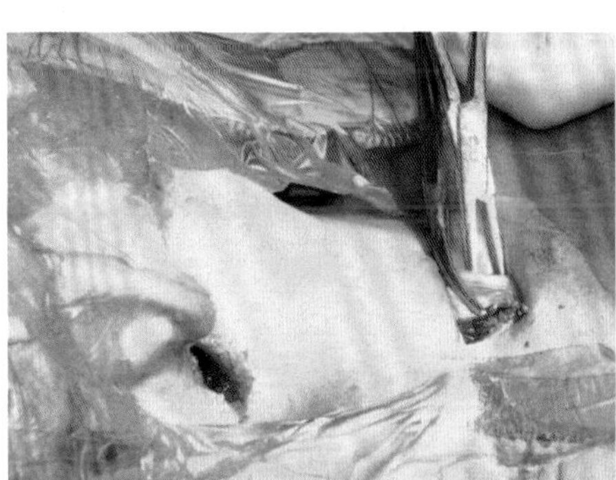

**TECH FIG 2** • The origin of the muscle is elevated with the help of a clamp and divided using electrocautery. About 5 to 10 mm of muscle–tendon segment is divided to prevent further contracture and fibrous adhesions.

- About 5 to 10 mm of the muscle–tendon segment is excised to prevent further contracture and fibrous adhesions.
- Alternatively, the sternal head can be lengthened by Z-plasty.
- The adequacy of the release is checked by bending the neck to the contralateral side and rotating it to the ipsilateral side while palpating the area with a fingertip to identify any remaining tight bands. Any remaining tight bands should then be divided. The neck should have a full range of motion after the procedure.
- The incision is closed with subcuticular suture after careful hemostasis. The platysma muscle should be closed as a separate layer in order to preserve the appearance of the neck.



## Bipolar Release

- Bipolar release includes the release of the mastoid insertion of the SCM muscle along with the distal release described earlier.
- The procedure starts with a distal incision (see discussion earlier).
- The two heads of the SCM muscle are identified. After undermining the tendons, a small Penrose drain is passed underneath them and clamped.
- The Penrose drain can be used to gently retract the (intact) SCM muscle and by applying tension to the muscle facilitate proximal exposure and identification of the insertion of the SCM (**TECH FIG 3A**).
- Attention is directed to the proximal insertion and the incision is placed as described before.
- The insertion of the muscle is identified anteriorly and posteriorly. Dissection starts subperiosteally from the mastoid process to avoid the facial nerve anteriorly and the anterior branch of the great auricular nerve inferiorly.
- A curved clamp is passed just deep to the tendon to elevate it. It can then be safely divided (**TECH FIG 3B**).
  - There is no need to resect a segment of muscle proximally.
- After the proximal release is performed, attention is then directed back to the distal incision and a distal release is completed as described earlier.
  - Release of the clavicular head with the lengthening of the sternal head by Z-plasty may be appropriate in older children to help provide a symmetric appearance postoperatively (**TECH FIG 3C**).[8]
- The neck is rotated and bent with the help of the anesthesia team while sequentially palpating both incisions in order to identify any remaining tight bands; any remaining tight bands or fascia is then completely released.
- Subcutaneous and subcuticular skin closure is then performed after hemostasis. Distally, care should be taken to repair the platysma, as this helps preserve the cosmesis of the neck.

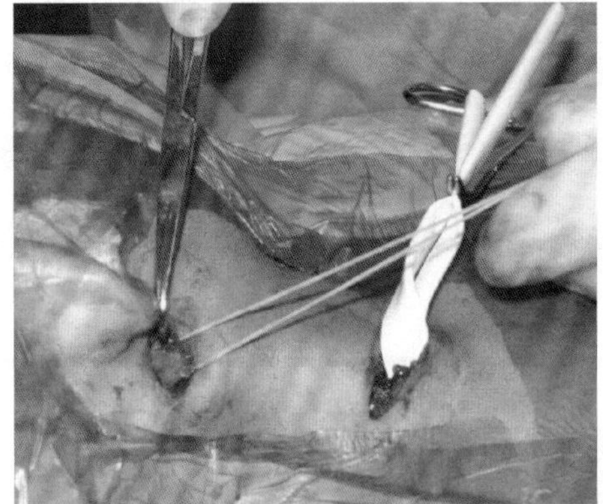


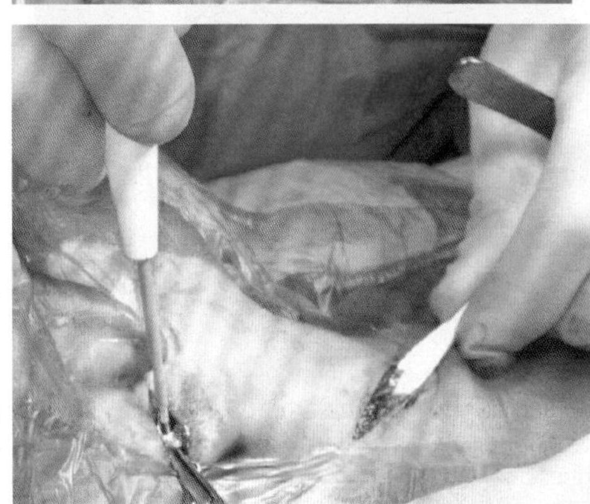


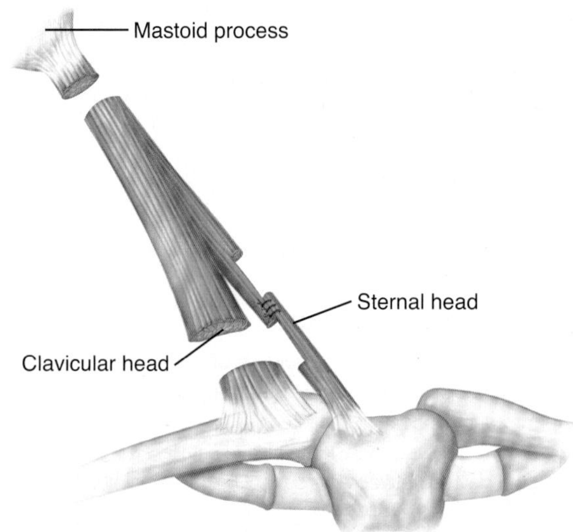


**TECH FIG 3** • **A.** With tension applied to the tendon at the distal exposure, a safe identification of the origin has been simplified. Furthermore, the limited exposure avoids the important anatomy. **B.** A curved clamp is passed just deep to the tendon to elevate it for complete sectioning. **C.** Bipolar release with the lengthening of the sternal head by Z-plasty. (**C:** Modified from Ferkel RD, Westin GW, Dawson EG, et al. Muscular torticollis. A modified surgical approach. J Bone Joint Surg Am 1983;65:894–890.)

## PEARLS AND PITFALLS

| | |
|---|---|
| **Approach** | ■ The distal pole incision is made about 1 cm superior and parallel to the clavicle.<br>■ Incisions made over the clavicle may result in a hypertrophic scar and unacceptable cosmesis.<br>■ Incisions close to the midpoint of SCM may compromise the external jugular vein and neurologic structures and may lead to an unacceptable scar.<br>■ To avoid complications, the proximal horizontal incision is placed just distal to the tip of the mastoid process. Applying tension to the SCM distally simplifies safe identification of its insertion. |
| **Unipolar release** | ■ Unipolar release is used only in younger patients with mild deformities. |
| **Bipolar release** | ■ A bipolar release may be more likely to avoid residual and recurrent deformity.<br>■ The SCM tendon is first exposed at the origin in the distal wound. Both origins of the SCM are elevated to provide tension, the proximal release is then performed, and finally, the distal release is completed. |

## POSTOPERATIVE CARE

- Postoperative management includes immobilization of the head and neck in a slightly overcorrected position with a rigid cervical collar, custom-made brace, or pinless halo for 2 to 3 weeks (**FIG 4**).
  - The purpose of the brace immobilization is to avoid the preoperative habitual posture which could result in postoperative scarring. It might also help to reprogram the corrected posture as a norm for the child.
- The brace is removed in 2 to 3 weeks and physical therapy is begun consisting of passive stretching is recommended as well as active strengthening exercises.
  - Exercises are continued at home for 3 to 6 months.

## OUTCOMES

- Early conservative management is successful in over 90% of children with CMT who are younger than 1 year.[4,6]
- In resistant cases, there is still controversy between unipolar and bipolar release.
- Cheng et al[3–5] reported excellent results in children operated on at age 6 months to 2 years with unipolar release.
- Canale et al[1] found better results after bipolar release, although the difference was not statistically significant.
- Wirth et al[16] reported satisfactory results in 48 of 55 patients who had undergone bipolar release, with low recurrence rates (1.8%).

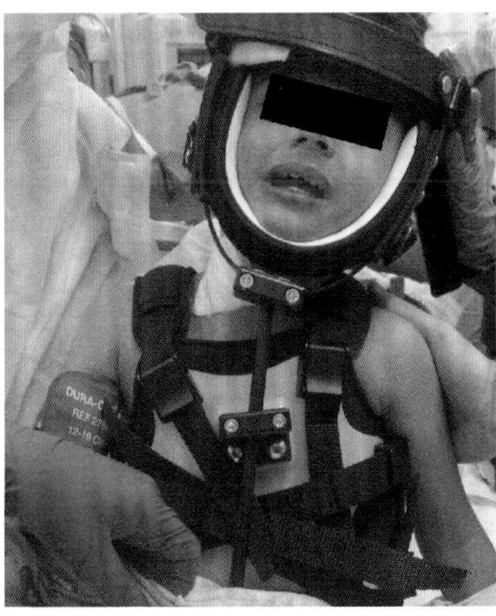

**FIG 4** • Pinless halo device for postoperative management.

- Ferkel et al[8] described a modified bipolar release technique that includes release of the mastoid and clavicular attachments of the SCM muscle and Z-plasty lengthening on the sternal origin to maintain a V contour of the neck distally for cosmesis. They reported 92% satisfactory results with this technique.
- Lee et al[10] reported improvement in the craniofacial deformity after surgical release of the SCM, with greater correction when the surgery was performed before 5 years of age.

## COMPLICATIONS

- Wound breakdown
- Hematoma
- Incomplete correction
- Neurovascular damage
  - Spinal accessory nerve
  - Anterior branch of the great auricular nerve
  - External jugular vein
- Carotid artery
- Hypertrophic scar

## REFERENCES


1. Canale ST, Griffin DW, Hubbard CN. Congenital muscular torticollis: a long-term follow-up. J Bone Joint Surg Am 1982;64:810–816.
2. Chen CE, Ko JY. Surgical treatment of muscular torticollis for patients above 6 years of age. Arch Orthop Trauma Surg 2000;120:149–151.
3. Cheng JC, Tang SP, Chen TM. Sternocleidomastoid pseudotumor and congenital muscular torticollis in infants: a prospective study of 510 cases. J Pediatr 1999;134:712–716.
4. Cheng JC, Tang SP, Chen TM, et al. The clinical presentation and outcomes of treatment of congenital muscular torticollis in infants—a study of 1086 cases. J Pediatr Surg 2000;35:1091–1096.
5. Cheng JC, Wong MW, Tang SP, et al. Clinical determinants of the outcome of manual stretching in the treatment of congenital muscular torticollis in infants. A prospective study of eight hundred and twenty-one cases. J Bone Joint Surg Am 2001;83:679–687.
6. Coventry MB, Harris LE. Congenital muscular torticollis in infancy: some observations regarding treatment. J Bone Joint Surg Am 1959;41:815–822.
7. Davids JR, Wenger DR, Mubarak SJ. Congenital muscular torticollis: sequela of intrauterine or perinatal compartment syndrome. J Pediatr Orthop 1993;13:141–147.
8. Ferkel RD, Westin GW, Dawson EG, et al. Muscular torticollis. A modified surgical approach. J Bone Joint Surg Am 1983;65:894–900.
9. Hummer CD, MacEwen GD. The coexistence of torticollis and congenital dysplasia of the hip. J Bone Joint Surg Am 1972;54:1255–1256.
10. Lee JK, Moon HJ, Park MS, et al. Change of craniofacial deformity after sternocleidomastoid release in pediatric patients with congenital muscular torticollis. J Bone Joint Surg Am 2012;94:e93.

11. Nucci P, Kushner BJ, Serafino M, et al. A multi-disciplinary study of the ocular, orthopaedic, and neurologic causes of abnormal head postures in children. Am J Opthalmol 2005;140:65–68.
12. Oh I, Nowacek CJ. Surgical release of congenital torticollis in adults. Clin Orthop Relat Res 1978;(131):141–145.
13. Tang S, Liu Z, Quan X, et al. Sternocleidomastoid pseudotumor of infants and congenital muscular torticollis: fine-structure research. J Pediatr Orthop 1998;18:214–218.
14. Tang SF, Hsu KH, Wong AM, et al. Longitudinal follow-up study of ultrasonography in congenital muscular torticollis. Clin Orthop Relat Res 2002;(403):179–185.
15. Walsh JJ, Morrissy RT. Torticollis and hip dislocation. J Pediatr Orthop 1998;18:219–221.
16. Wirth CJ, Hagena FW, Wuelker N, et al. Biterminal tenotomy for the treatment of the muscular torticollis. J Bone Joint Surg Am 1992;74:427–434.

# Posterior Cervical Arthrodeses: Occiput–C2 and C1–C2

82
CHAPTER

Jaime A. Gomez and Daniel J. Hedequist

## DEFINITION

- The occipitocervical articulation is formed by the occiput, the atlas (C1), and the axis (C2). This functional unit provides a large degree of mobility and range of motion through the strong ligamentous structures and cup-shaped joints.
- Over 50% of the total axial rotation occurs between C1 and C2, whereas flexion–extension movement predominantly occurs at the occipitoatlantal junction which allows approximately 20 degrees of extension.[1]
- Cervical spine range of motion is significantly decreased in children after posterior occipitocervical arthrodesis. Axial rotation is the most affected, decreasing 30 degrees in each direction, flexion and extension each decrease by 13 degrees, and lateral bending by 7 degrees in each direction.[25]
- Excessive movement at this junction due to either bony or ligamentous abnormalities causes instability. A wide variety of pathologies such as genetic and congenital developmental abnormalities, trauma, tumors, and inflammatory and degenerative conditions can lead to upper cervical spine instability.
- Depending on the degree of displacement and spinal canal compromise, cord compression and myelopathy may occur.
- Major instability is usually addressed with surgical occipitocervical or C1–C2 arthrodesis. Since Foerster first described a technique for occipitocervical arthrodesis using fibular strut graft in 1927, several procedures have been reported with variable rates of fusion and techniques of stabilization.
- In this chapter, brief information on upper cervical spine instability is given and general principles of occipitocervical and C1–C2 arthrodesis are discussed. Also, different techniques developed for posterior occipitocervical fusion are described in detail.
- Modern instrumentation techniques have dramatically changed the instrumentation potential and wiring strategies are being replaced for screw instrumentation techniques. These techniques can decrease the risk of cord damage from wire passage, increase biomechanically fixation, and improves fusion rates.[13,16]

## ANATOMY

- It is important to understand that the pediatric upper cervical spine is not a "miniature model" of the adult spine. The cervical spine approaches adult size and shape by ages 8 to 12 years, as growth cartilage fuses and vertebral bodies gradually lose their oval or wedge shape and become more rectangular.
- The upper cervical spine has unique development, anatomy, and biomechanics.
  - The C1 develops from three ossification centers, a body and two neurocentral arches, which become visible by age 1 year (**FIG 1A**).
  - The neurocentral synchondroses fuse with the body at about 7 years of age and may be mistaken for fractures on radiographs.[18]
- The C2 is derived from five primary ossification centers: the two neural arches or lateral masses, the two halves of the dens, and the body.
  - There are two secondary centers: the ossiculum terminale and the inferior ring apophysis (**FIG 1B**).
  - The two halves of the odontoid are generally fused at birth but may persist as two centers, known as the *dens bicornis*.[19]
- The dentocentral synchondrosis, which separates the dens from the body, closes between the ages of 5 and 7 years (**FIG 1B**). Until the ossification is complete, it gives the appearance of a "cork in a bottle" on an open mouth odontoid view.
  - The tip of the dens appears at age 3 years and is fused by age 12 years.
  - Occasionally, it remains as a separate ossiculum.[11,19]
- After skeletal maturity, the C1 does not have a body as such and is shaped like a ring. The flat, cup-shaped articular surface under the occipital condyle allows for flexion, extension, and some bending. The dens articulates with C1 through the dorsal facet of the anterior arch. C1–C2 articulation allows for rotation.[1] The vertebral artery passes through the foramen that is located in the transverse processes.
- The ligamentous structure allows for a wide range of motion of the upper cervical spine while maintaining stability. The short ligaments at the base of the skull are as follows (**FIG 1C**):
  - The tectorial membrane anteriorly from the foramen magnum is a continuation of the posterior longitudinal ligament that provides considerable support.
  - Cruciate ligament, which includes transfer ligaments, restrains against atlantoaxial anteroposterior (AP) translation.
  - Alar and apical ligaments, which run from foramen magnum to the odontoid, act as secondary stabilizers.
- Posterior atlanto-occipital ligaments are the continuation of the ligamentum flavum.
- Vertebral artery anatomy can also be different in children compared to adults. Younger patients have vertebral arteries that are significantly closer to the midline over the superior border of C1 than older patients. Ninety-seven percent of vertebral arteries are greater than a centimeter lateral to the midline.[12]

## PATHOGENESIS

- Fundamentally, upper cervical spine instability can develop from osseous or ligamentous abnormalities resulting from acquired or congenital disorders. As a result of instability, excessive motion and spinal cord compression may occur at the occipitoatlantal and/or atlantoaxial joint.

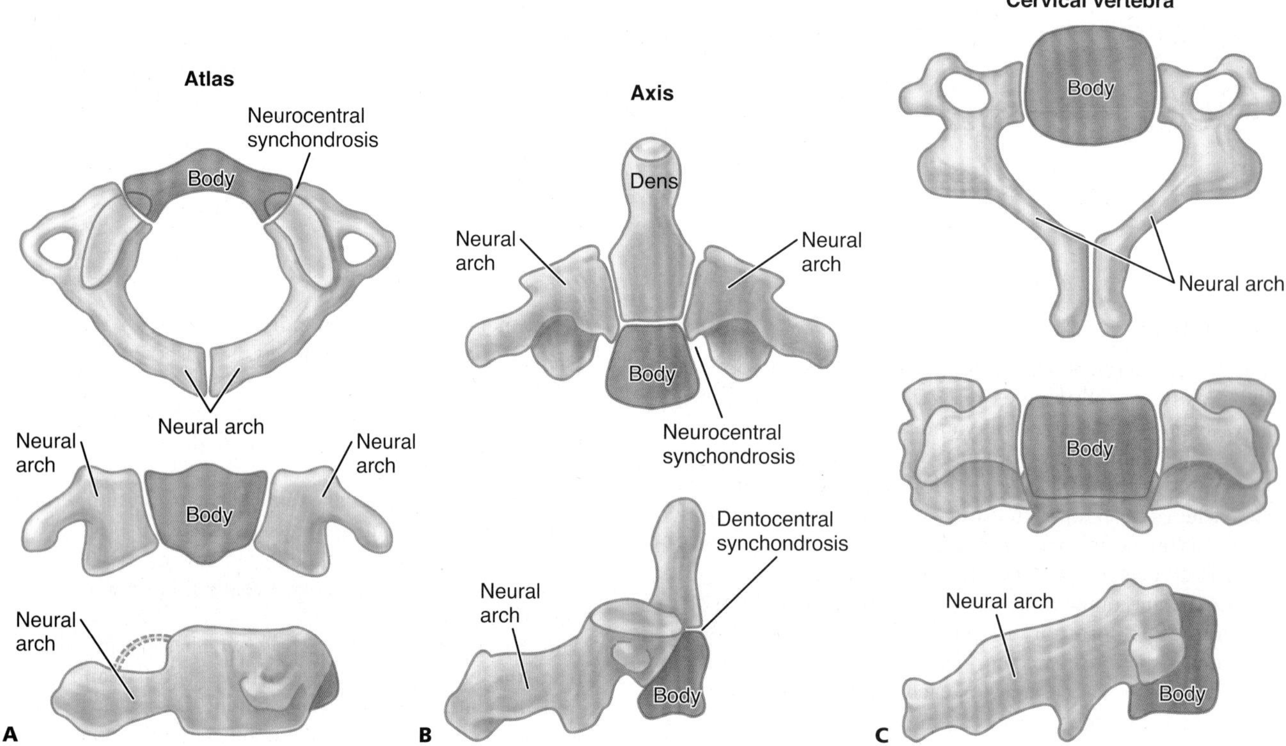


**FIG 1** • **A–C.** Anatomy ossification centers of the C1, C2, and cervical vertebrae during development.

- In nontraumatic conditions, ligamentous laxity (particularly in the transverse ligament) or abnormalities of the odontoid cause instability.
- In Grisel syndrome, a type of atlantoaxial rotatory displacement, inflammation of the retropharyngeal space, caused by upper respiratory tract infections or by adenotonsillectomy, spreads through the pharyngovertebral veins to the ligaments of the upper cervical spine. This results in impairment of the transverse atlantal ligament and instability.[27]
- In Down syndrome, the main cause of atlantoaxial instability is the laxity of the transverse ligament, which holds the dens against the posterior border of the anterior arch. Also, malformation of the odontoid can be observed in this condition.[8]
- Klippel-Feil syndrome is associated with congenital cervical anomalies, such as occipitocervical synostosis, basilar impression, and anomalies of the odontoid, and can be associated with instability, stenosis, or both.
- Odontoid anomalies include aplasia, hypoplasia, duplication, third condyle, persisting ossiculum terminale, and os odontoideum.

## NATURAL HISTORY

- Patients with upper cervical instability frequently have other associated pathologic conditions in the occipitocervical region such as spinal stenosis, basilar impression, cervical fusions, occipitalization, or congenital anomalies of the C1 or C2 (dens), and central nervous system abnormalities.
  - When one encounters one of these conditions, others should be sought also.
- Instability of the upper cervical spine and stenosis often are two major factors in the development of myelopathy.
- Patients who are symptomatic at initial presentation are often at risk for progressive neurologic symptoms. Once cervical myelopathy develops, it rarely resolves entirely.
- Paralysis and death are rare but may be encountered in patients with upper cervical spine instability.

## PATIENT HISTORY AND PHYSICAL FINDINGS

- Upper cervical spine instability is rare in patients without predisposing conditions or trauma.
- The instability is usually determined in radiographic examination of the children with syndromes or conditions known to have frequent involvement of the musculoskeletal system.[24] An orthopaedic surgeon is usually consulted for children with such conditions.
- Clinical presentation can vary because of the associated syndromes and anomalies.
- Patients may present with symptoms such as loss of range of motion, stiffness, mechanical pain of the head or neck, and torticollis.
- It is not uncommon to see patients presenting with neurologic symptoms, which can vary from minor sensory or motor disturbances to established myelopathy. Neurologic symptoms or signs result from mechanical compression of the spinal cord or nerve roots.
- Torticollis may be the presenting symptom of rotatory or postinfectious atlantoaxial instability.
- According to the degree of compression and the affected site of the spinal cord, signs and symptoms can vary. They may include loss of physical endurance, difficulty walking, weakness, and upper motor neuron signs (spasticity, hyperreflexia, clonus, Babinski sign), which can be seen with anterior spinal column involvement.

- Pain deficits and proprioception and vibratory sense deficits can be seen with posterior spinal column involvement.
- Increased nasal resonance may also be observed. It may occur because of the decreased size of the nasopharynx resulting from anterior displacement of the C1.
- Vertebral artery distortion and insufficiency may lead to bizarre symptoms such as syncopal episodes, sudden postural collapse without unconsciousness, change in behavior, dizziness, and seizures.
- In cerebellar involvement, nystagmus, ataxia, and incoordination are the common findings.
- Neurogenic bladder and bowel, cranial nerve involvement, paraplegia, hemiplegia, and quadriplegia should be kept in mind; sometimes, the patient presents with only one of these findings.

## IMAGING AND OTHER DIAGNOSTIC STUDIES

- Standard radiographs include AP, open mouth odontoid, and lateral (neutral and flexion–extension) cervical spine views.
- Instability can be identified on the lateral flexion–extension view. Atlantoaxial instability is diagnosed on the basis of an increased atlantodental interval (ADI).
  - The ADI is measured from the anterior aspect of the dens to the posterior aspect of the anterior ring of the C1 (**FIG 2A**).
  - In children older than 8 years and in adults, the ADI should be 3 mm or less, whereas in younger children, the ADI should be 4 mm or less (some consider 4.5 to 5 mm acceptable).[14]
  - In children, we consider an ADI of 4 mm or more as evidence of atlantoaxial instability. This measurement does not always correlate with the degree of brainstem or cord compression (as seen on magnetic resonance imaging [MRI]), however. An asymptomatic patient may have instability.
- Space available for the spinal cord (SAC) is measured from the posterior border of the dens to the anterior border of the posterior tubercle. According to Steel's rule of thirds,[22] SAC should be about one-third of the diameter of the ring of C1 (see **FIG 2A**).
  - This safe zone allows for some degree of pathologic displacement. Displacement of more than one-third of the diameter causes cord compression.
  - This measurement directly describes the SAC, which is highly associated with the neurologic involvement.
- The relationship between the foramen magnum, C1, and odontoid can be determined in lateral radiographs.
- The line of McRae connects the anterior rim of the foramen magnum to the posterior rim (see **FIG 2A**).
  - The upper tip of the odontoid should normally be 1 cm below the anterior margin of the foramen magnum.
  - If the effective sagittal diameter of the canal (length of the line) is less than 19 mm, neurologic symptoms occur.
- The line of Chamberlain is drawn from the posterior margin of the hard palate to the posterior margin of the foramen magnum (see **FIG 2**).
  - The tip of the odontoid should be 6 mm below this line. It bisects the line in basilar invagination. However, determination of the landmarks can be difficult on plain radiographs.
- The McGregor line is drawn from the most caudal point of the occipital projection to the posterior edge of the hard plate (see **FIG 2A**).
  - This line is one of the best for detecting basilar impression because the osseous landmarks can usually be seen at all ages. If the tip of the odontoid process lies more than 4.5 mm above this line, the finding is consistent with basilar impression.
- The line of Wackenheim is drawn parallel to the posterior surface of the clivus (see **FIG 2A**).
  - The inferior extension of the line should be in touch with the posterior tip of the odontoid. In basilar invagination, it is over that line.
- The Wiesel-Rothman line is drawn connecting the anterior and posterior arches of the C1. Two lines are drawn perpendicular to this line, one through the basion and the

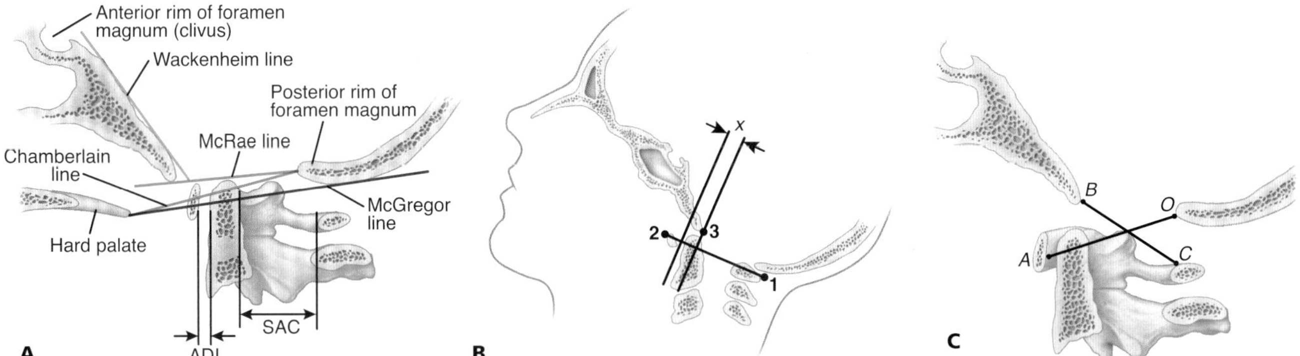


**FIG 2** • **A.** Lateral craniometry of the craniocervical junction with landmarks, commonly used lines, and methods for examining the relationship between the C1, odontoid, and foramen magnum and measuring the SAC. The ADI is measured from the anterior aspect of the dens to the posterior aspect of the anterior ring of the C1. The McRae line connects the anterior rim of the foramen magnum to the posterior rim. The Chamberlain line is drawn from the posterior margin of the hard palate to the posterior margin of the foramen magnum. The McGregor line is drawn from the most caudal point of the occipital projection to the posterior edge of the hard palate. The Wackenheim line is drawn parallel to the posterior surface of the clivus. **B.** Method for calculating the Wiesel-Rothman line for atlanto-occipital instability. A line is drawn connecting the anterior and posterior arches of the C1 (*line 1* to *2*). Two lines are drawn perpendicular to this line, one through the basion and the other through the posterior margin of the anterior arch of the C1 (*line 3*). A change in the distance (*x*) between these lines of more than 1 mm in flexion and extension indicates increased abnormal translational motion. **C.** Lines used to calculate the Power ratio. A line is drawn from the basion (*B*) to the posterior arch of the C1 (*C*) and a second line from the opisthion (*O*) to the anterior arch (*A*) of the C1. The length of the first line is divided by the length of the second.

other through the posterior margin of the anterior arch of the C1 (**FIG 2B**).
  - A change in the distance ($x$) between these lines of more than 1 mm in flexion and extension indicates increased abnormal translational motion.
- The ratio of Power is calculated from a line drawn from the basion to the posterior arch of the C1 and a second line from the opisthion to the anterior arch of the C1 (**FIG 2C**). The length of the first line is divided by the length of the second.
  - A ratio of less than 1.0 is normal.
  - A ratio of 1.0 or more is abnormal and is diagnostic of anterior occipitoatlantal dislocation.
- MRI is useful to identify pathologic changes at the dura mater and spinal cord as well as additional soft tissue pathologies.
  - Functional MRI scans performed in flexion and extension can be used to assess dynamic brainstem or cord compression.
- CT scan is essential for screw trajectory planning and it can also provide additional information regarding the bony anomalies.
  - Two-dimensional (2-D) and three-dimensional (3-D) reconstructions can clarify the course of the vertebral artery and careful attention should be paid to the location of the artery through the foramen transversarium of C2, where is most likely to be injured.
  - In atlantoaxial rotational displacement, pathoanatomy is determined by fine-cut dynamic CT scan with left–right rotation of the head.
- CT or magnetic resonance (MR) angiogram can be useful to evaluate the vertebral artery anatomy prior to instrumentation of C1–C2.

## DIFFERENTIAL DIAGNOSIS

- Pseudosubluxation
- Os odontoideum
- Congenital muscular torticollis
- Ankylosing spondylitis

## NONOPERATIVE MANAGEMENT

- Children with known risk of upper cervical instability should be evaluated carefully. Especially patients with congenital syndromes associated with upper cervical spine instability should have periodic clinical and radiographic examinations until maturity.[24]
- Upper cervical spine radiographs including AP, lateral (neutral and flexion–extension views), and open mouth odontoid views are obtained periodically to assess and detect any trends and changes.
- Patients and parents should be educated about the diagnosis and natural history of the disorder and encouraged to report any symptoms as soon as they occur.
- Because of bone and ligament abnormalities, patients with upper cervical spine instability have a greater risk of spinal cord injury even with minor trauma and even when they are asymptomatic.
- As previously described, periodic observation should be done, and if any progression is noticed, the patient should be prepared for appropriate surgical stabilization when indicated.
  - In children, we consider an ADI of 4 mm or more as evidence of atlantoaxial instability. Documented significant instability at the atlanto-occipital or atlantoaxial joints is an indication for posterior arthrodesis of occiput–C2 and C1–C2 arthrodesis, respectively.
- In some congenital disorders such as Morquio syndrome, progression of the instability is frequent; in these cases, prophylactic fusion should be considered before neurologic symptoms occur.[24]
- However, in Down syndrome, the patients with instability are usually asymptomatic, and in most cases, signs and symptoms progress slowly. Restriction of high-risk activities usually is appropriate. If the clinical symptoms persist or neurologic symptoms are starting to occur in the setting of significant instability, surgical treatment is indicated.[8,21]
- Children with congenital fusion of cervical vertebrae (mostly in Klippel-Feil syndrome) should be restricted from high-risk sports. Patients with progressive symptomatic segmental instability or neurologic compromise are candidates for surgical stabilization.[23]

## SURGICAL MANAGEMENT

- The main indication for the posterior occiput–C1 or C1–C2 arthrodesis is instability of the atlanto-occipital or atlantoaxial joint.
- Many techniques of atlantoaxial fusion using cables, transarticular screws, plates, and bone graft materials have been described.
- For isolated atlantoaxial instability, we describe the Gallie technique, the Mah modified Gallie technique, and the Brooks sublaminar wire technique.
  - The authors currently preferred instrumentation method which includes occipital plating and Harms (C1 lateral mass with C2 pedicle screw) or Magerl (C1–C2 transarticular screw) techniques are also described.

### Preoperative Planning

- Plain radiographs and CT scans are reviewed and any osseous findings noted.
- MRI evaluation for the spinal cord compression is recommended.
- CT scans and MR images should be reviewed to evaluate the course of the vertebral arteries, the dimensions of the C1 lateral mass, the trajectories and sizes of the C2 pedicles, and the thickness of the keel of the occipital bone.
- Occipital screws risk dural sinus injury. The safe zone for occipital screw placement is a triangular region created by connecting two dots 2 cm lateral to the midline just distal to the external occipital protuberance (EOP) and a midline point 2 cm inferior to the EOP[9,17](**FIG 3**).
- An appropriate halo ring is measured for the patient.
- Somatosensory evoked potentials, transcortical motor evoked potentials, and electromyography are the preferred neurologic monitoring modalities.
- Flexible fiberoptic intubation with manual in-line axial stabilization should be considered to minimize cervical motion during intubation maneuvers.

### Positioning

- After induction of general anesthesia in the supine position, a halo ring is applied, and the patient is carefully turned to the prone position.

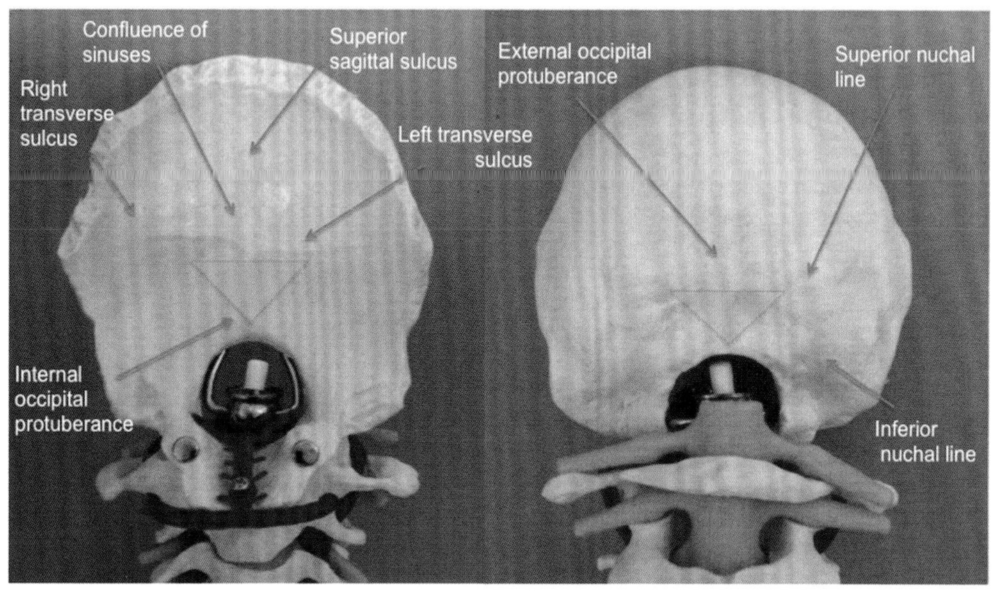


**FIG 3** • Pertinent intracranial (**A**) and extracranial (**B**) occipital anatomy. Highlighted are the safe zones for screw instrumentation. (From Roberts DA, Doherty BJ, Heggeness MH. Quantitative anatomy of the occiput and the biomechanics of occipital screw fixation. Spine 1998;23:1100–1108.)

- Head is adjusted with the halo device supported by a head positioner, which is securely fixed to the operating table. A Mayfield positioning device can also be used (**FIG 4**).
- The table is placed on slight reverse Trendelenburg position to facilitate venous drainage and reduce facial swelling.
- The shoulders are taped to improve radiographic visualization, and the patient's hair is shaved 2 cm above the EOP.
- Lateral fluoroscopy or radiography should be done before starting the procedure to confirm the alignment of the occiput and cervical spine.
- Donor sites (rib or iliac crest) are also prepared for graft harvesting.

## Approach

- A posterior midline incision is made from the occiput to the intended distal fusion site (usually C2) for occipitocervical arthrodesis.
- Proximally, midline dissection up to the EOP is performed for occipitocervical instrumentation.
- Through an exact midline split of the nuchal ligament, the paraspinal muscles are elevated with electrocautery and Cobb elevators and retracted laterally. Excessive lateral dissection should be avoided to prevent injury to the vertebral artery, which runs in a serpentine course in relationship to the C2 vertebra.
- For atlantoaxial arthrodesis, the dissection is started from the lower occiput and the surgeon identifies the posterior arch of the C1, the bifid spinous processes, and the lamina of the C2. The C2–C3 interval should not be exposed.
- Care should be taken during exposure to avoid dissection immediately superior to the arch of C1 where the vertebral artery can be found in children 1 cm lateral to the midline.
- The surgical exposure of vertebra is limited up to the intended level of fusion to prevent unintentional inclusion of the adjacent level in the fusion mass.

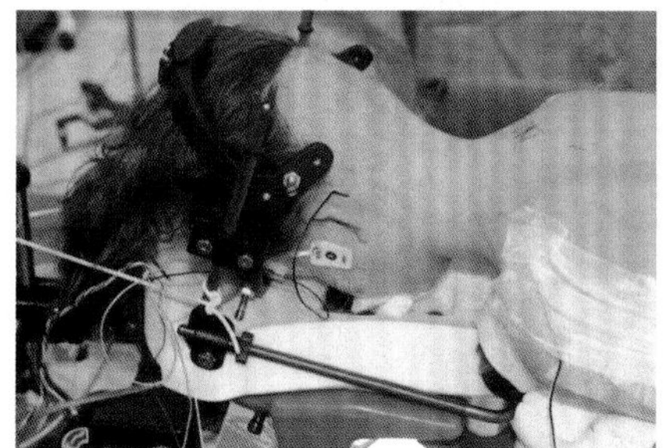
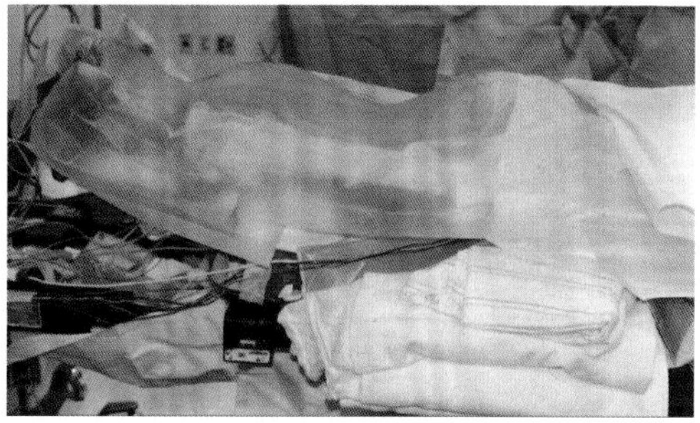

**FIG 4** • **A.** Patient's head positioning with halo device supported by a head positioner, which is securely fixed to the operating table. **B.** Prone positioning on radiolucent table, shoulders are taped distally to improve x-ray visualization.

## Occipital Plating and C1–C2 Harms Screws Instrumentation

- Subperiosteal exposure proximally to the level of the EOP is performed; bone wax can be used to control bony bleeding.
- A 4.5-mm screw placement is planned over the occipital safe zone as described earlier. A precontoured plate is chosen and appropriately placed below the EOP.
- Occipital drill holes are hand drilled through the plate with an appropriate drill guide with fixed depths (starting at 6 mm depth) (**TECH FIG 1A**).
- 4.5-mm bone screws can be kept unicortical, and preoperative CT scan measurement can aid in the length calculation because pediatric occiput width is variable. The midline keel will allow the surgeon to place the longer and stronger screws.
- If bicortical purchase is required (in cases of poor bone quality or thin occiput), progressive hand drilling should be made in 2-mm increments, with frequent blunt palpation until the inner table is breached, avoiding dural penetration and cerebrospinal fluid leak.
- Screw holes should be tapped because of the hard nature of the occipital tables.
- If a foramen magnum decompression is to be performed in conjunction with instrumentation, care should be taken to leave enough occipital safe zone bone for screw placement.
- The occipital plate is secured with uni- or bicortical 4.5-mm bone screws (**TECH FIG 1B**).

### C1 Lateral Mass Screw

- The lateral mass of C1 is covered by the C2 dorsal root ganglion.
- C1 lateral mass is approached with careful detachment of the paraganglious tissue from the underside of the posterior arch of C1, this can be performed with fine-tipped bipolar cautery.
- Bleeding is frequently encountered from the C1 to C2 epidural venous plexus (**TECH FIG 2A**) and should be controlled with bipolar cautery and thrombin-soaked Gelfoam sterile sponge (Pfizer). A Penfield no. 4 retractor can be used to gently retract the C2 dorsal root ganglion caudally exposing the inferior border of the lateral mass (**TECH FIG 2B**).
- C1 screw entry point is located in the center of the C1 lateral mass (**TECH FIG 2C**). Overhanging bone form the posterior arch of C2 sometimes requires removal with a Kerrison rongeur without disrupting the integrity of the C1 arch (**TECH FIG 2D**).
- A 2-mm high-speed burr can be used to mark the entry point and avoid slippage with the hand drill. The screw on the coronal plane is directed 0 to 5 degrees medially and parallel to the inferior border of the C2 lateral mass (20 to 30 degrees cranial) on the sagittal plane (**TECH FIG 2E,F**).
  - The screw is tapped, and we recommend bicortical placement of a 3.5-mm polyaxial of the appropriate length. Although the lateral mass will be 10 to 15 mm deep, the C1 screw should be a longer partially threaded screw that will allow for the unthreaded segment to be proud posteriorly and in contact with the C2 nerve root avoiding irritation of the greater occipital nerve.
  - The proud polyaxial head of the C2 screw will also allow for symmetric alignment with the C2 screw in order to permit rod fixation between the two segments.

### C2 Pedicle Screw

- Various C2 instrumentation techniques are valid and available but the surgeon should evaluate individual anatomy for proper instrumentation technique. C1 pars interarticularis can be performed, but in children, the pars is usually small and we prefer the use of a pedicle-type screw.
- A transarticular screw C1–C2 can be performed, but distal exposure or percutaneous incision need to be done to achieve the steep angle for insertion of such a screw. For these reasons, we favor the use of C2 pedicle screws.
- The exposure of C2 is carried out to the lateral edge of the lateral mass and not past this point because the vertebral arteries lie lateral to it. Complete visualization of the dorsal isthmus as well as the medial and lateral borders is possible and necessary in pediatric patients. Given the smaller anatomy, it is necessary to ensure safety of screw placement via thorough exposure.
- The starting point for the C2 pedicle screw is the intersection of a horizontal line through the midline of the lamina and a vertical line through the center of the pars interarticularis (see **TECH FIG 2C**).
- The medial border of the pedicle as well as the superior articular facet of C2 can be palpated with a Penfield no. 4 elevator and the starting point marked with a 2-mm burr. A hand drill is used, and the screw hole trajectory should be 20 to 30 degrees medially and cephalad; this angulation should be individualized for each patient with evaluation of the CT scan (**TECH FIG 3A**).

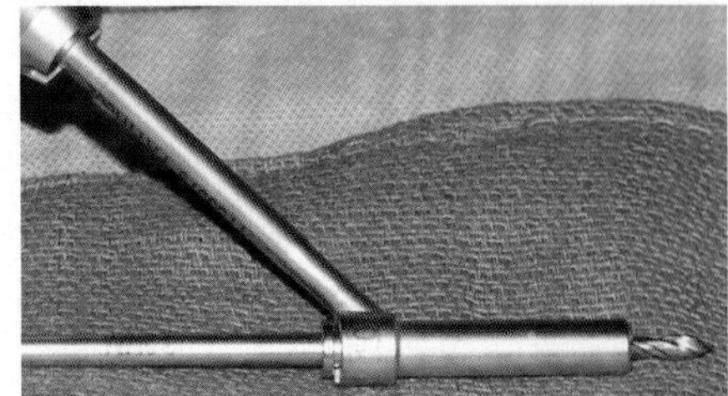
A

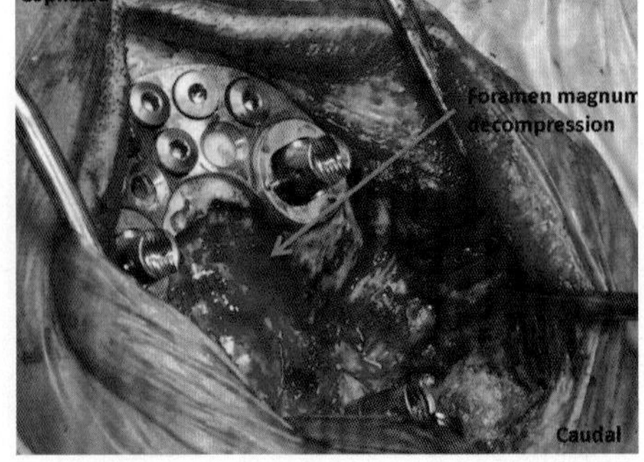

B

**TECH FIG 1** • **A.** Occipital drill holes are hand drilled through the plate with an appropriate drill guide with fixed depths (starting at 6 mm depth). **B.** Appropriate occipital plate positioning. In this case, a foramen magnum decompression was performed distal to the plate location.

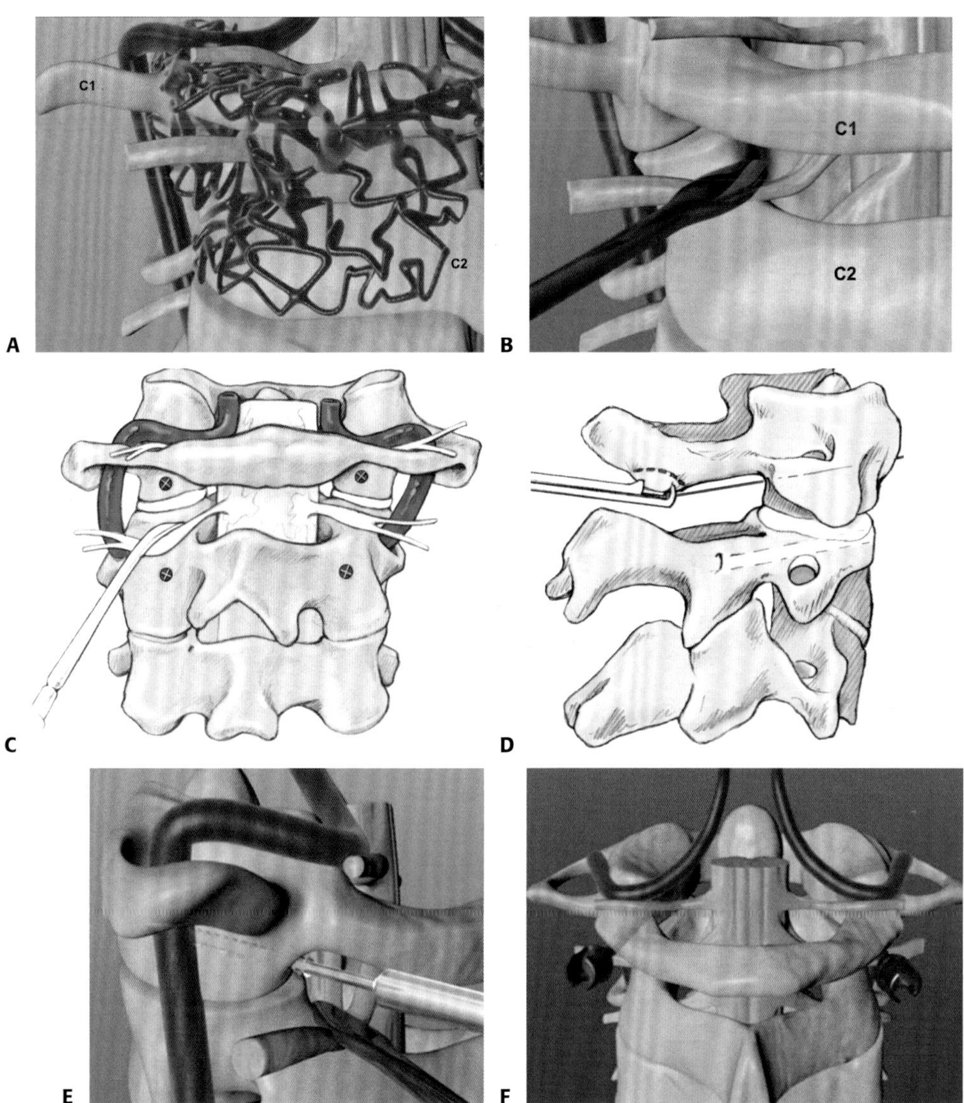


**TECH FIG 2** • **A.** Diagram demonstrating the C1–C2 epidural venous plexus. Bleeding is frequently encountered and bipolar cautery should be used for control. **B.** Penfield no. 4 retractor can be used to gently retract the C2 dorsal root ganglion caudally exposing the inferior border of the lateral mass. **C.** The posterior entry points for C1 and C2 screws. **D.** Overhanging bone from the posterior arch of C2 sometimes requires removal with a Kerrison rongeur without disrupting the integrity of the C1 arch. **E,F.** Orientation of C1 lateral mass screw. The screw on the coronal plane is directed 0 to 5 degrees medial and parallel to the inferior border of the C2 lateral mass (20 to 30 degrees cranial) on the sagittal plane. (**C,D:** From Melcher RP, Harms J. C1-C2 posterior screw rod fixation In: Bradford DS, Zdeblick T, eds. Master Techniques in Orthopaedic Surgery: The Spine, ed 2. Philadelphia: Lippincott Williams & Wilkins, 2004:129–145.)

- The screw hole should be bicortical, and a ball-tipped probe can be used to palpate anterior breech. The hole is tapped, and measurement of the appropriate length with a depth gauge is performed and checked on fluoroscopy.
- Decortication of the lamina and pars of C2 is done followed by placement of a 3.5-mm screw of appropriate length. The polyaxial head of the C2 screw should be in line with the C1 screw head.
- After C1–C2 instrumentation is completed, a 3.5- or 4.5-mm rod is contoured to provide neutral sagittal occipitocervical alignment. The surgeon must contour the rod carefully to avoid kyphosis. Radiographic assessment of positioning should be performed with fluoroscopy or final x-rays (**TECH FIG 3B**).
- If further reduction is required (occasionally, reduction is obtained with positioning), the screw heads can be used to generate anterior translation of the posteriorly dislocated facet. The bony stock of C1 and C2 will not allow for major manipulation in a young child and the surgeon should be careful to not plow a screw. Traction and gentle manipulation can also be helpful when reduction is required. The rod can be placed loosely and tightened once successful reduction is achieved.
- Biomechanically plating with six occipital screws connected to a C2 pedicle or a C1–C2 transarticular construct has proven to be the most rigid occipitocervical fixation (**TECH FIG 3C**).[20]
- Occiput, C1, and C2 decortication is performed.

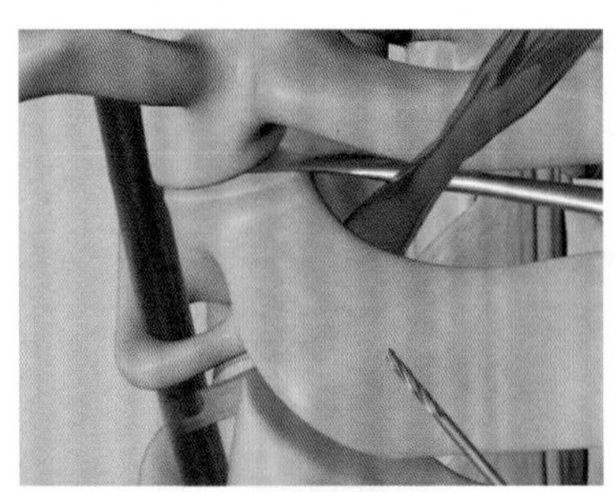

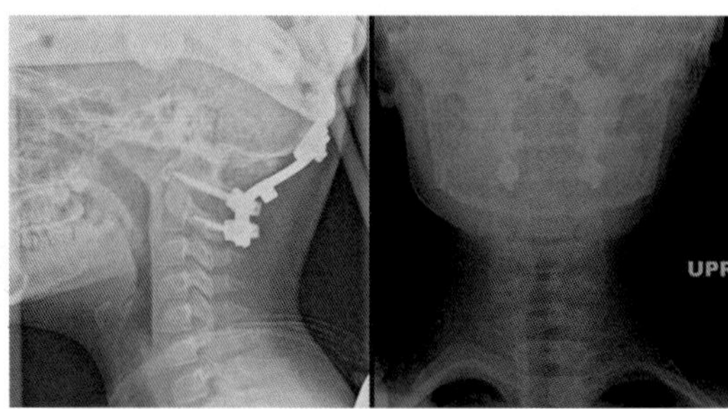

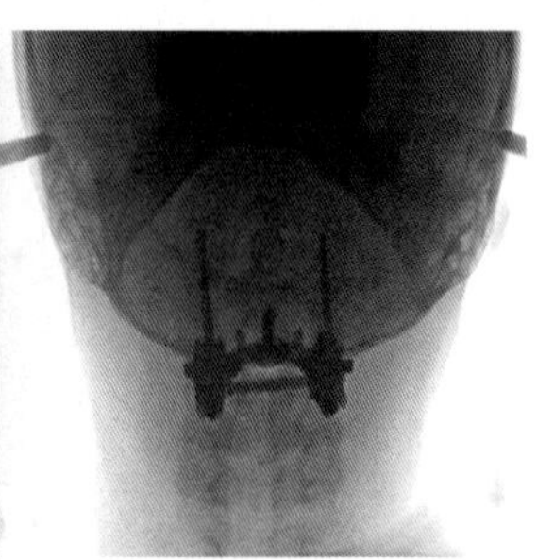


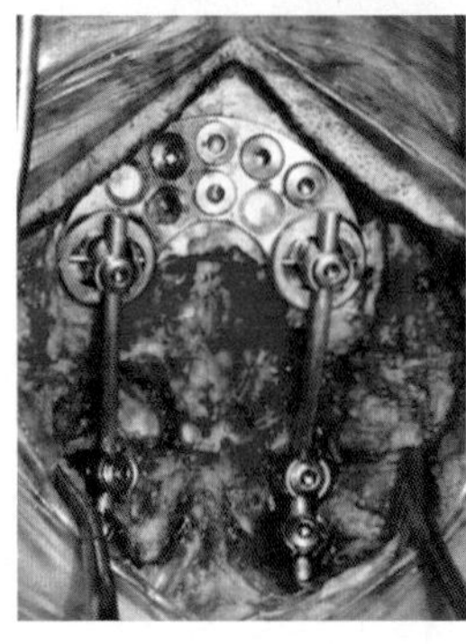

**TECH FIG 3** • **A.** C2 pars screw direction, the medial border of the pedicle as well as the superior articular facet of C2 can be palpated with a Penfield no. 4 elevator and the starting point marked with a 2-mm burr. A hand drill is used and the screw hole trajectory should be 20 to 30 degrees medially and cephalad. **B.** Postoperative radiograph demonstrating final occiput–C1–C2 construct. **C.** Final occiput–C1–C2 construct. A foramen magnum decompression was performed in this case for a Chiari decompression in conjunction with instrumentation.

- Morcellized posterior superior iliac spine (PSIS) iliac crest autograft and allograft are packed into the fusion area to add additional support.
- The surgical area is irrigated, hemostasis is obtained, and the incision is closed in three layers: The supraspinous ligament can be sutured to the spinous process of C2, then watertight fascial closure is performed with 1-0 Vicryl; subcutaneous tissue is closed with interrupted 3-0 Vicryl; and a 3-0 running Monocryl subcuticular is used for the skin.
- Additional halo immobilization is only necessary if the surgeon encounters poor bone quality or if there is concern for wound complications secondary to prominent occipital hardware.

## C1–C2 Transarticular Screws and C2 Translaminar Screws

- The technique is similar to a pedicle screw. A cannulated system can be used to help with the increased precision required for this instrumentation technique.
- A threaded guidewire is used to cannulate the pars, making sure that the borders remain well visualized and defined by the assistant.
- The lateral fluoroscopic view is frequently checked, as the inclination of the pars screws in the cephalocaudal direction is paramount. The most frequent error in trajectory would be aiming to anterior and either missing C1 or only catching the anteroinferior edge of C1.
- A Penfield in the C1–C2 joint can help confirm position both by direct feel and radiographically. When reached with the guidewire, the Penfield is removed and the wire advanced into C1 (**TECH FIG 4A,B**).
- After confirmation of the appropriate positioning, drill and tap over the guidewire. Decortication of the lamina and pars of C2 is done followed by placement of a 4.0-mm screw ranging from 32 to 40 mm (**TECH FIG 4C,D**).
- Translaminar C2 screws are not described in detail but can be a salvage option when other fixation methods are not possible (**TECH FIG 4E,F**).

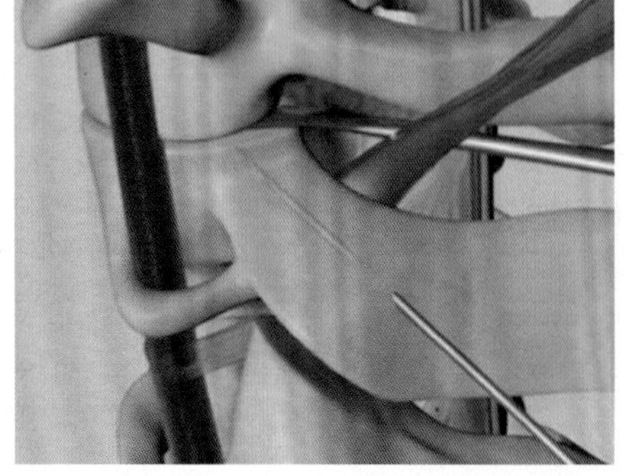

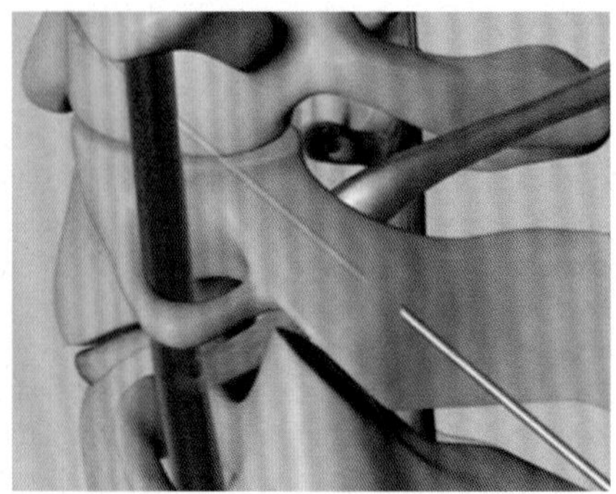

**TECH FIG 4** • C1–C2 transarticular screw. **A.** Penfield in the C1–C2 joint can help confirm position both by direct feel and radiographically. **B.** When reached with the guidewire, the Penfield is removed and the wire advanced into C1. *(continued)*

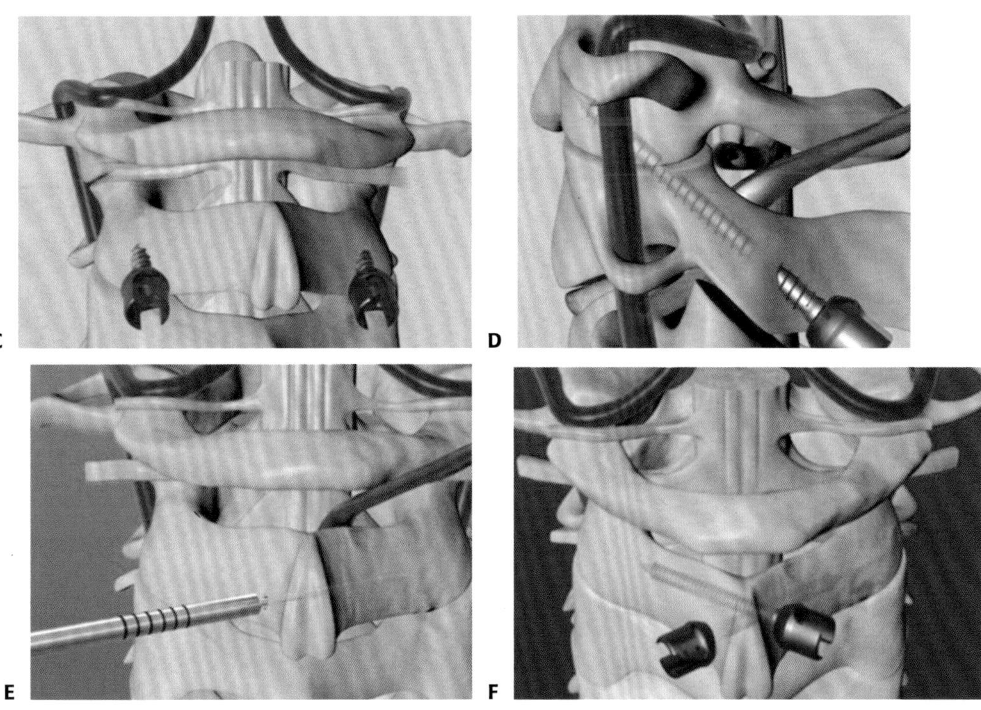


**TECH FIG 4** • *(continued)* **C.** C1–C2 transarticular screw AP direction. **D.** The polyaxial head of the C2 screw should be in line with the C1 screw head on sagittal plane and coronal plane as well. **E,F.** Placement of translaminar screws.

## Occipitocervical Arthrodesis with Iliac Graft

- At the level below the transverse sinus, four transverse-oriented holes are drilled through both cortices of the occiput with a high-speed diamond drill.[6]
  - The holes are aligned transversely with two on each side of the midline. At least 1 cm of intact bone should be left between the holes to prevent wire pullout through the skull (**TECH FIG 5A**).
  - Surgical loupes and a headlamp are recommended for this procedure.
- Using a high-speed diamond burr, the surgeon makes a transverse-oriented trough into the base of the occiput to fit the rectangular superior part of the iliac autograft.
- A single corticocancellous autograft (3 × 4 cm) is harvested through an oblique incision over the PSIS.
- A rectangular graft is taken. The surgeon creates a notch in the inferior base of the graft to be suitable for the base of the spinous process of the second or third vertebra (**TECH FIG 5B**).
- A 16- or 18-gauge wire is passed through the burr holes on each side of the midline and the wire is looped on itself (**TECH FIG 5C,D**).
- A sublaminar wire is placed under the ring of C2 or C3 (or passed through the base of the spinous process, if structurally sufficient, or if there is canal stenosis).
  - The left side of the graft accepts the left end of the wire and the right end of the graft accepts the right end of the wire (**TECH FIG 5E**).
- The edges of the graft are contoured to fit appropriately into the occipital trough and around the base of the spinous process (**TECH FIG 5F**).
- The wires are tightened over the graft in figure-8 shape. After satisfactory tightening, the edges of the wire are cut and bent away from skin (**TECH FIG 5G,H**).
- Intraoperative fluoroscopy or radiography is used to confirm the alignment of the occiput and cervical spine, stability, and the position of the graft and wires.
- The graft should be structurally stable at the end of the procedure.
- Flexion–extension of the halo frame, better contouring of the graft, and appropriate tightening of the wires can be used to make adjustments in reduction and alignment.

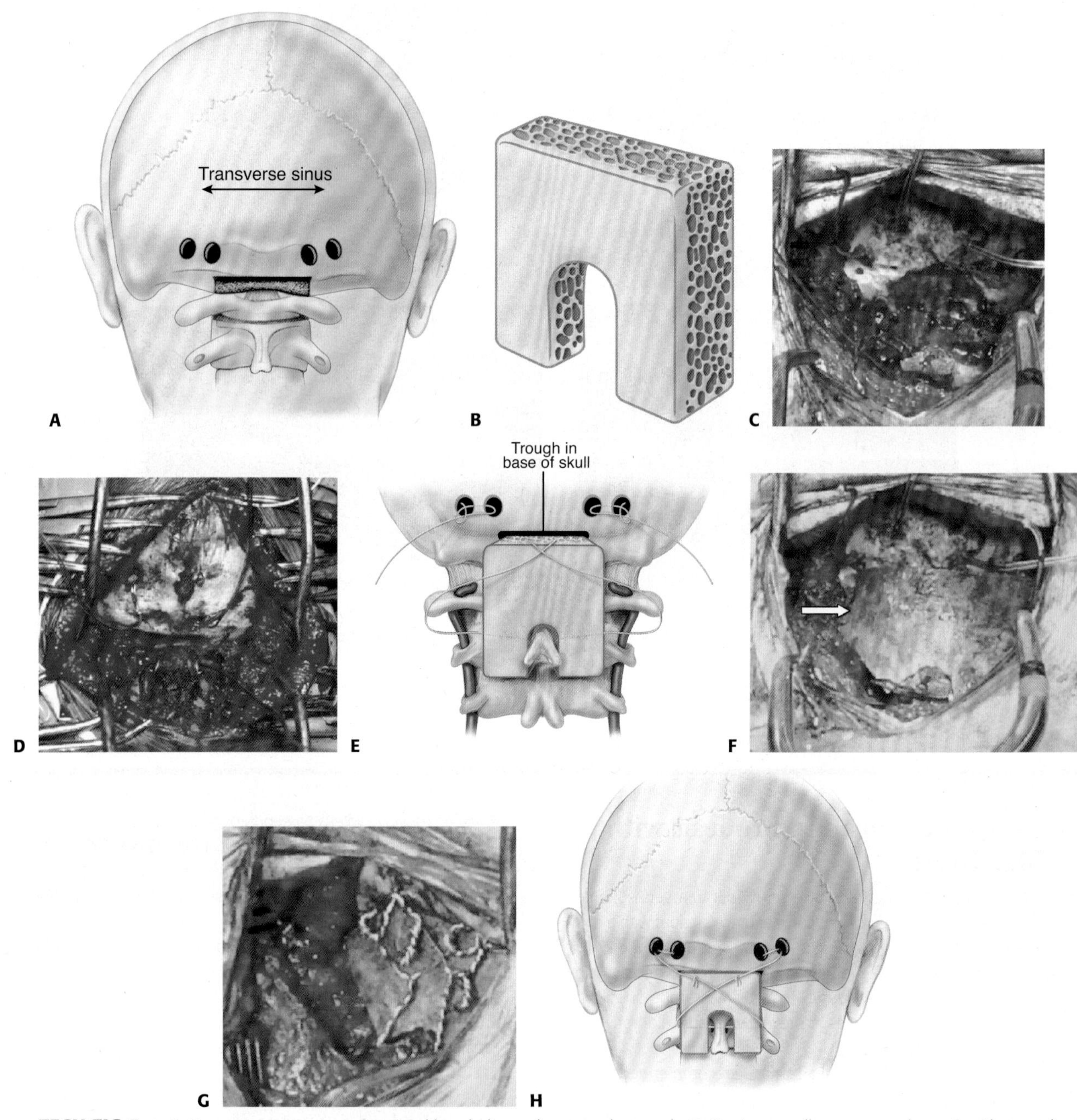


**TECH FIG 5** • **A.** Four transverse-oriented occipital burr holes and rectangular trough. **B.** Corticocancellous rectangular graft with a notch at the inferior base of the graft. **C.** A Luque wire is passed through the occipital burr hole and another wire is passed sublaminarly under the arch of C2 or through the base of the C2 spinous process. **D.** Occipital wire is looped on itself. **E.** Schematic drawing showing occipital wire looped on itself and the wire passed through the base of the C2 spinous process. **F.** Graft (*arrow*) placed between the occiput and C2. **G.** The wires are tightened over the graft in a figure-8 shape, twisted, and cut. **H.** Schematic drawing showing the graft placement and securing with wires.

## Occipitocervical Arthrodesis with Rib Graft

- An oblique incision overlying the posterior rib allows for adequate exposure.[3]
  - The muscle fibers are separated, and dissection is carried down to the periosteum of the rib.
- Adequate rib is exposed and cut.
  - The size of the rib graft is greater than the area to be fused because part of the rib is used as morcellized graft.
  - Using a rib cutter, the graft is cut distally and proximally and removed (**TECH FIG 6A**).
- Irrigation fluid is placed in the surgical site and positive pressure applied to check for pleural leaks.
- If a pleural tear is detected, air can be removed from the chest cavity by using a red rubber tube and suction.
- A larger leak may require placement of a thoracostomy drainage tube.
  - In all patients, a chest radiograph should be taken after rib harvest to rule out pneumothorax.
- Two full-thickness structural grafts are prepared to fit the arthrodesis site.
- The rib grafts can span large defects and fit nicely into large or abnormally shaped skull, and we find this best for young infants.
- A 16- or 18-gauge wire is looped through the burr holes on each side of the midline (see **TECH FIG 5C**).
  - The burr holes are drilled and aligned similarly to the ones described for the iliac graft technique.
  - There is no need to create a groove at the base of the occiput.
- Braided cable or no. 5 Mersilene sutures may be used instead of wire.
  - With Mersilene sutures, there is a reduced risk of cutting out in thin bone of poor quality.
- After this, purchase of two wires is made to the posterior elements of most caudal vertebra on each side of the midline by sublaminar wiring.
- Suitable grafts on either side are then secured to the occiput and lamina of the most caudal vertebra by wires.
  - The stability of the grafts is checked under radiographic control and the wires are then crimped and cut (**TECH FIG 6B,C**).
- Adjustments are made by flexion–extension of the halo frame, contouring of the graft, and appropriate tightening of the wire.
  - Intraoperative radiographs are obtained to confirm acceptable reduction, alignment, and placement of the graft.
- For both techniques, morcellized autograft is packed into the arthrodesis site. The wound is closed in layers.
- The halo vest is worn for 8 to 12 weeks after both techniques to maintain postoperative stability (**TECH FIG 6D,E**).

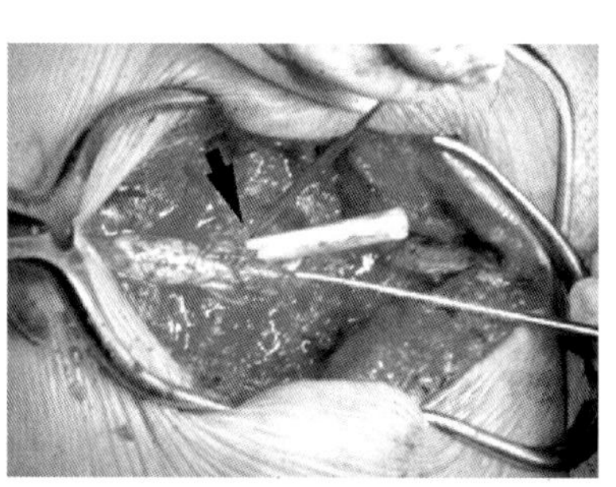
A

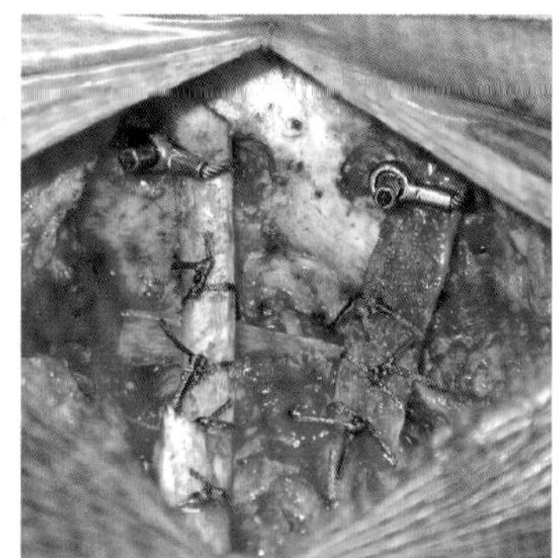
B

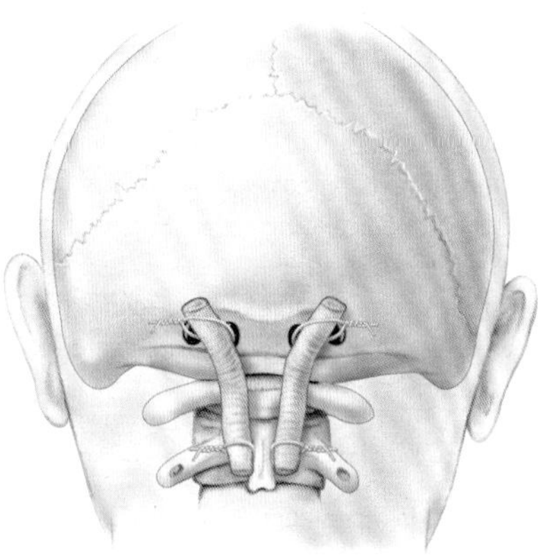
C

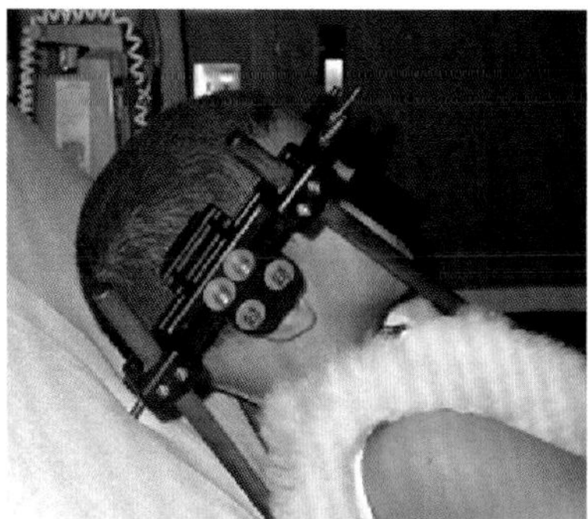
D

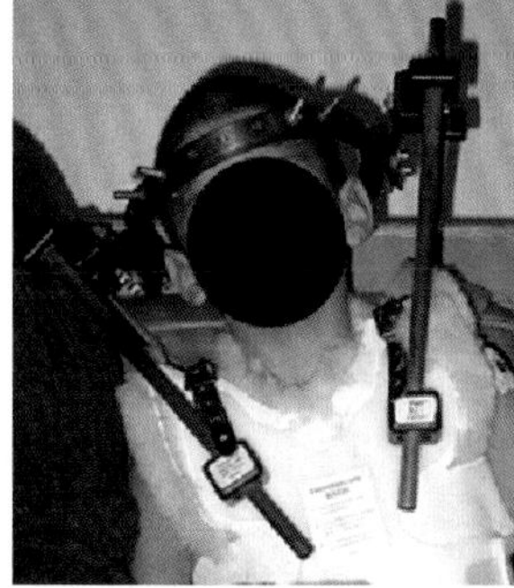
E

**TECH FIG 6** • **A.** Adequate rib is exposed and harvested. **B.** Rib graft is placed and fixed with braided cables and no. 5 Mersilene suture. **C.** Schematic drawing showing the rib graft fixed with wire. **D,E.** A 5-year-old-boy immobilized with a halo vest postoperatively. (**C:** Adapted from Cohen MW, Drummond DS, Flynn JM, et al. A technique of occipitocervical arthrodesis in children using autologous rib grafts. Spine 2001;26:825–829.)

## Posterior C1–C2 Arthrodesis

- The preoperative planning is similar to that for the occipitocervical arthrodesis described earlier in the section.

### Gallie Technique

- After exposing the posterior arch of the C1 and spinous process of the C2, the two free ends of a single 16- or 18-gauge wire are passed beneath the posterior arch of the C1 from a superior to inferior direction.[10]
- The free ends are passed beneath the posterior arch and are brought around superiorly to loop on themselves.
- A rectangular corticocancellous autograft is harvested from the posterior iliac spine.
  - A notch is created at the distal part of the graft. This part will be placed across the spinous process of C2.
- The notched graft is placed between the posterior portion of the arch of C1 and the posterior spinous process of C2.
- Now the free ends of the looped wire are brought down over the graft and passed below the spinous process.
- The free ends of the wire are tightened and twisted over the graft (**TECH FIG 7**).
- Morcellized bone grafts may be packed into the fusion area to add additional support.
- Intraoperative fluoroscopy is necessary to check for satisfactory reduction and alignment of C1–C2.

### Mah Modified Gallie Technique

- In 1989, Mah described a modification of the Gallie technique.[15]
- All the steps of the Mah technique are similar to the Gallie technique, except that a threaded Kirschner wire is placed through the spinous process of the C2 and both ends of the Kirschner wire are cut, leaving about 2.5 cm of the total wire.
- The free ends of the looped wire are brought down below the free ends of the threaded Kirschner wire (**TECH FIG 8**).
- The free ends of the wire are tightened, secured, and crimped over the graft.

### Brooks Technique

- A standard posterior midline incision is used to expose the posterior arch of C1 and the lamina of C2.[2]
- Two sublaminar wires are passed under both C1 and C2 laminas, one on each side of the midline.

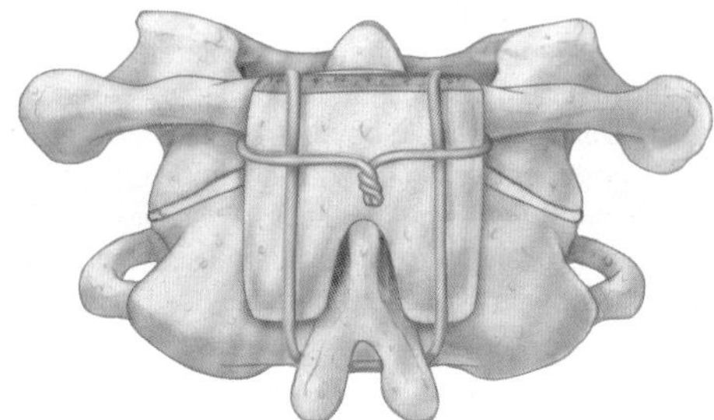

**TECH FIG 7** • Gallie technique for atlantoaxial arthrodesis.

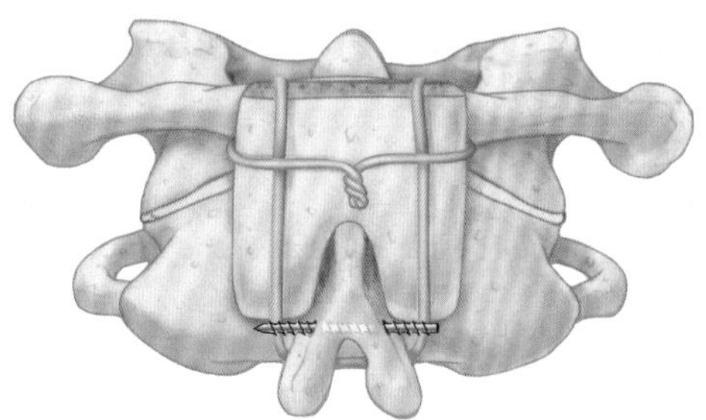

**TECH FIG 8** • Mah modified Gallie technique for atlantoaxial arthrodesis.

- Unlike the Gallie technique, two separate corticocancellous grafts are required in this technique. A single rectangular iliac crest graft is harvested; it can be separated into two equal parts.
- Each iliac crest graft is cut into a trapezoid-like shape (one end is narrower than the other) so that they can be wedged between the C1 and C2 posterior arches (**TECH FIG 9A**).
- The grafts are snugly wedged into place. The wires are then tightened around the grafts, twisted, and cut (**TECH FIG 9B**).

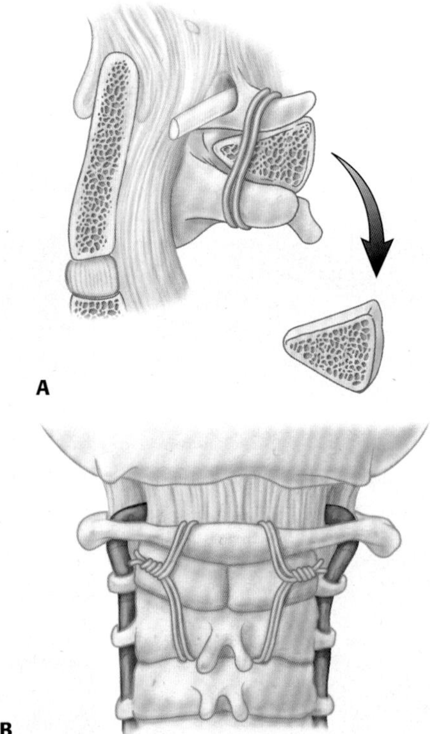


**TECH FIG 9** • Brooks arthrodesis. **A.** Lateral view demonstrating a wedge-shaped graft between the spinous processes to prevent hyperextension. The graft is shaped so that one end is narrower than the other to achieve a good fit. **B.** The grafts are snugly wedged between the C1 and C2 posterior arches, and the wires are tightened around the grafts.

## PEARLS AND PITFALLS

| | |
|---|---|
| **Approach** | ■ Excessive lateral dissection should be avoided so as not to damage the vertebral arteries and major venous junctions.<br>■ In the case of an open posterior arch, meticulous and blunt dissection should be used to keep from injuring the dura mater and the cord.<br>■ Excessive dissection and extended dissection time are avoided.<br>■ This may increase the risk of inadvertent extension of the fusion mass. |
| **Occipital plating and C1–C2 Harms screw instrumentation** | ■ CT imaging and evaluation of vertebral artery anatomy is mandatory.<br>■ Instrumentation is possible in majority of pediatric patients with manageable complications.[7]<br>■ Reports have shown that this technique is safe and feasible to use in children older than 6 years of age.<br>■ Clinical union rates of 90%–100% have been reported.[26] |
| **Occipitocervical arthrodesis with iliac graft technique** | ■ This technique is associated with stable internal fixation and high fusion rates.[3,11] |
| **Occipitocervical arthrodesis with rib graft technique** | ■ A large occipitocervical segment can be spanned.<br>■ Rib grafts can be shaped easily because of their elastic structure.<br>■ This technique is best for infants, small children, or patients with an abnormally shaped skull. |
| **C1–C2 arthrodesis with Gallie technique** | ■ This procedure is more suitable in older children who have a competent spinous process.<br>■ It is not always necessary to pass wire or cable underneath the lamina of C2.<br>■ This technique provides good stability in flexion and extension but may be insufficient in rotational maneuvers. |
| **C1–C2 arthrodesis with Mah modification** | ■ The wire can securely hold behind an insufficiently ossified spinous process with the help of a transverse Kirschner wire. |
| **C1–C2 arthrodesis with Brooks technique** | ■ This technique provides more rotational stability than the Gallie technique.<br>■ Disadvantages include the need to pass bilateral sublaminar cables beneath both C1 and C2. |

## POSTOPERATIVE CARE

- Postoperative management can include halo vest immobilization for 8 to 12 weeks. In cases of screw fixation, the halo is not necessary. If there are concerns regarding stability of the construct, poor bone quality or hardware prominence immobilization with halo can be maintained postoperatively.
- Using a standardized method of halo application reduces the rate of complications associated with halo use in children.[4]
  - The rate of pin tract infection with prolonged use of a halo device in children is similar to that in adults. Particular care should be taken to keep the pin tract sites clean.[5]
    - Short-term antibiotic treatment is usually satisfactory in decreasing inflammation at the pin site.
- When a bony union is documented radiographically, the halo device is removed.
  - Patients can gradually return to their daily activities.
  - Special care should be taken to avoid excessive flexion or extension of the neck.
- Long-term follow-up is necessary for evaluation of potentially progressing junctional instability below the level of fusion.
  - The additional stress placed on the adjacent vertebrae below the level of fusion may result in instability with time.[7]

## OUTCOMES

- Screw fixation techniques in children have demonstrated excellent outcomes.
- Several reports have demonstrated a better than 90% fusion rates and normal alignment on postoperative imaging studies.[26]
- Occipitocervical fusions with plates and screws have proven to be relatively safe and effective in treating pediatric patients.[26]
- Reports of wiring techniques for occipitocervical arthrodesis in 38 children with more than 2 years of follow-up have been reported.
  - Thirty-eight patients were treated with autograft and posterior wiring.
  - Thirty-four patients had bony union, three patients had fibrous union, and one patient had nonunion.
  - Ninety-seven percent of the patients (37 children) showed baseline or improved neurologic status at the most recent follow-up.
  - Complications
    - Superficial infection, postoperative pneumonia (1 patient), and pin tract infections from halo pins
    - In 11 patients (29%), we had a distal extension of the fusion mass, 7 patients had fusion at one additional level and 4 patients had fusion at two additional levels.

## COMPLICATIONS

- Graft or wire breakage
- Nonunion, insufficient fusion
- Additional fusion levels and loss of motion
- Junctional instability distal to the fusion mass
- Infection
  - Deep wound infection
  - Meningitis
  - Pin tract infections (halo)
- Neurologic injury
- Donor site morbidity

## ACKNOWLEDGMENTS

- Thanks to John P. Dormans, Gokce Mik, and Purushottam A. Gholve, who authored this chapter in the first edition, which provided the basis for this revision.

## REFERENCES

1. Bogduk N, Mercer S. Biomechanics of the cervical spine. I: normal kinematics. Clin Biomech 2000;15:633–648.
2. Brooks AL, Jenkins EB. Atlanto-axial arthrodesis by the wedge compression method. J Bone Joint Surg Am 1978;60:279–284.
3. Cohen MW, Drummond DS, Flynn JM, et al. A technique of occipitocervical arthrodesis in children using autologous rib grafts. Spine 2001;26:825–829.
4. Copley LA, Dormans JP, Pepe MD, et al. Accuracy and reliability of torque wrenches used for halo application in children. J Bone Joint Surg Am 2003;85-A(11):2199–2204.
5. Dormans JP, Criscitiello AA, Drummond DS, et al. Complications in children managed with immobilization in a halo vest. J Bone Joint Surg Am 1995;77:1370–1373.
6. Dormans JP, Drummond DS, Sutton LN, et al. Occipitocervical arthrodesis in children: a new technique and analysis of results. J Bone Joint Surg Am 1995;77:1234–1240.
7. Dormans JP, Wills B. Junctional instability and extension of fusion mass associated with posterior occipitocervical arthrodesis in children. Presented at POSNA 2004 Annual Meeting. St. Louis, MO, April 2004.
8. Doyle JS, Lauerman WC, Wood KB, et al. Complications and long-term outcome of upper cervical spine arthrodesis in patients with Down syndrome. Spine 1996;21:1223–1231.
9. Ebraheim NA, Lu J, Biyani A, et al. An anatomic study of the thickness of the occipital bone. Implications for occipitocervical instrumentation. Spine 1996;21:1725–1729; discussion 9–30.
10. Gallie WE. Skeletal traction in the treatment of fractures and dislocations of the cervical spine. Ann Surg 1937;106:770–776.
11. Ganey TM, Ogden JA. Development and maturation of the axial skeleton. In: Weinstein SL, ed. The Pediatric Spine, ed 2. Philadelphia: Lippincott Williams & Wilkins, 2001:3–54.
12. Goldstein R, Sunde C, Assad P, et al. Location of the Vertebral Artery at C1: How Far Out Laterally Can You Safely Dissect? In: POSNA Annual Meeting. Los Angeles, CA, 2013.
13. Hwang SW, Gressot LV, Rangel-Castilla L, et al. Outcomes of instrumented fusion in the pediatric cervical spine. J Neurosurg Spine 2012;17:397–409.
14. Locke GR, Gardner JI, Van Epps EF. Atlas-dens interval (ADI) in children: a survey based on 200 normal cervical spines. Am J Roentgenol Radium Ther Nucl Med 1966;97:135–140.
15. Mah JY, Thometz J, Emans J, et al. Threaded K-wire spinous process fixation of the axis for modified Gallie fusion in children and adolescents. J Pediatr Orthop 1989;9:675–679.
16. Melcher RP, Harms J. C1-C2 posterior screw rod fixation. In: Bradford DS, Zdeblick T, eds. Master Techniques in Orthopaedic Surgery: The Spine, ed 2. Philadelphia: Lippincott Williams & Wilkins, 2004: 129–145.
17. Nadim Y, Lu J, Sabry FF, et al. Occipital screws in occipitocervical fusion and their relation to the venous sinuses: an anatomic and radiographic study. Orthopedics 2000;23:717–719.
18. Ogden JA. Radiology of postnatal skeletal development. XI. The first cervical vertebra. Skeletal Radiol 1984;12:12–20.
19. Ogden JA. Radiology of postnatal skeletal development. XII. The second cervical vertebra. Skeletal Radiol 1984;12:169–177.
20. Puttlitz CM, Goel VK, Traynelis VC, et al. A finite element investigation of upper cervical instrumentation. Spine 2001;26:2449–2455.
21. Segal LS, Drummond DS, Zanotti RM, et al. Complications of posterior arthrodesis of the cervical spine in patients who have Down syndrome. J Bone Joint Surg Am 1991;73:1547–1554.
22. Steel HH. Anatomical and mechanical considerations of the atlanto-axial articulation. J Bone Joint Surg Am 1968;50:1481–1482.
23. Tracy MR, Dormans JP, Kusumi K. Klippel-Feil syndrome: clinical features and current understanding of etiology. Clin Orthop Relat Res 2004;(424):183–190.
24. Wills BP, Dormans JP. Nontraumatic upper cervical spine instability in children. J Am Acad Orthop Surg 2006;14:233–245.
25. Wills BP, Jencikova-Celerin L, Dormans JP. Cervical spine range of motion in children with posterior occipitocervical arthrodesis. J Pediatr Orthop 2006;26:753–757.
26. Wills BPD, Drummond DS, Schaffer A, et al. Posterior occipitocervical arthrodesis in children: intermediate and long-term outcomes. Presented at AAOS 2005 Annual Meeting, Washington, DC, February 2005.
27. Wilson BC, Jarvis BL, Haydon RC III. Nontraumatic subluxation of the atlantoaxial joint: Grisel's syndrome. Ann Otol Rhinol Laryngol 1987;96:705–708.

# Posterior Cervical Fusion with Lateral Mass Screws

83

CHAPTER

Jonathan H. Phillips and Lindsay Crawford

## DEFINITION

- The lateral mass is a quadrangular area of bone lateral to the lamina and between borders of superior and inferior facets as seen from posteriorly. Seen in three dimensions, the lateral mass is a skewed box. Its appearance on lateral radiographic projection is that of a parallelogram whose anterosuperior corner points cephalad (**FIG 1**).
- Roy-Camille first described the use of lateral mass screw fixation for cervical spine stabilization. Posterior cervical fusion with rigid constructs provides better deformity correction and stability for arthrodesis.
- Cervical instability and/or deformity are indications for posterior cervical arthrodesis in the pediatric population.

## ANATOMY

- Each segment from C3 to C7 is made up of a centrum (body) and two posterior arches that form from mesenchymal tissue migrating around each side of the neural tub.
  - The arches fuse posteriorly by age 2 or 3 years, and they fuse to the body between 3 and 6 years.
  - Secondary ossification centers for the superior and inferior ring apophyses ossify during late childhood and fuse to the vertebral bodies by 25 years of age.
  - Other ossification centers for the transverse and spinous processes generally fuse by 3 years of age.
- The facet joints initially are relatively horizontal and, during growth, gradually become more vertical, which enhances stability in flexion and extension. The vertebral bodies initially have an oval or wedge shape but gradually become fully ossified in a more rectangular configuration.[4] The spinal nerve exits the canal through the interpedicular foramen. The ventral ramus travels anterolaterally on the transverse process. The spinal nerve sits anteromedial to the anterior aspect of the superior facet. The dorsal ramus runs posteriorly against the anterolateral corner of the base of the superior articular process. When the lateral mass is divided into quadrants, the superolateral quadrant is away from the spinal nerve.
- The vertebral artery enters the transverse foramen of the sixth cervical vertebra and courses cephalad through the foramina. The vertebral artery is anterior to the lateral mass but is also anterior to the spinal nerve (**FIG 2**).
- A study by Al-Shamy et al[1] of computed tomography (CT) scans of the pediatric cervical spine found that in children age 4 years and older, the size of the lateral mass would allow for lateral mass screw fixation from C3 to C7.

## PATHOGENESIS

- Trauma
  - Although spine injuries are rare in children, cervical spine injuries are the majority of spine injuries in children
  - Children younger than 10 years of age are more likely to sustain upper cervical injuries (occiput to C2), whereas older children have a preponderance of lower cervical injuries (maximally at C4 or C5).
- Tumor: Aneurysmal bone cyst, osteoblastoma, and osteochondroma involving posterior elements are the tumors most likely to be encountered in the first and second decades of life.
- Iatrogenic: posterior instability after tumor decompression or postlaminectomy

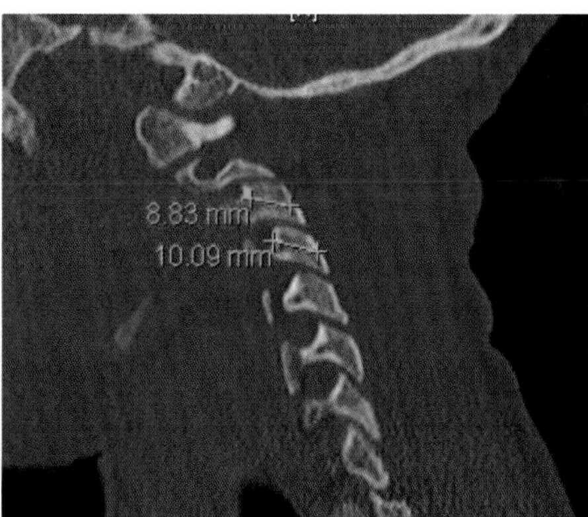


**FIG 1** • Sagittally reformatted CT scan through the lateral masses of a 12-year-old boy with short stature bone dysplasia and paraparesis due to cervical stenosis. Note the templating lines for preoperative planning (see text).

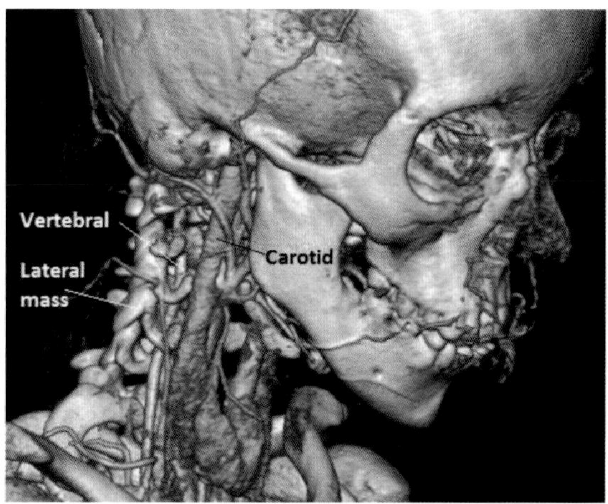


**FIG 2** • Preoperative CT angiogram of an 11-year-old girl with Down syndrome and paraparesis due to C1–C2 instability. Note the relationship of the vertebral artery to the lateral masses.

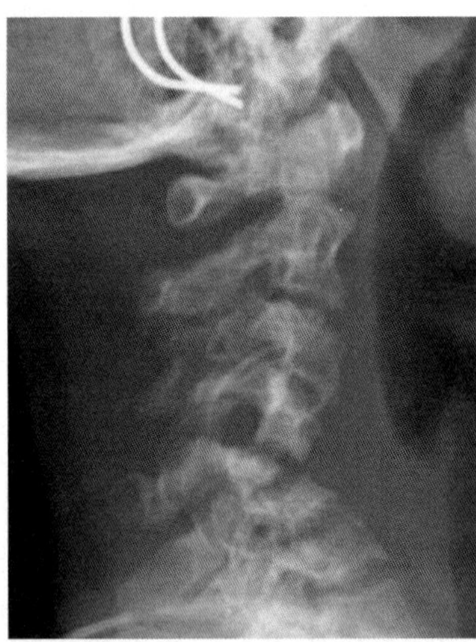

**FIG 3** • Lateral radiograph of an 11-year-old boy with neurofibromatosis. Despite the extent of the kyphosis, he was neurologically intact except for lower extremity hyperreflexia.

- Congenital/syndromic: Anomalous cervical spine anatomy can be seen with VACTERL (vertebral, anal atresia, cardiac, tracheoesophageal fistula, renal anomalies, and limb defects) and Klippel-Feil syndrome.
- Cervical kyphosis
  - This can be posttraumatic, postlaminectomy (tumor decompression), or syndromic.
  - Congenital or developmental cervical kyphosis is associated with Larsen syndrome, diastrophic dysplasia, chondrodysplasia punctata (Conradi syndrome), camptomelic dysplasia, and neurofibromatosis (**FIG 3**).

## NATURAL HISTORY

- Instability of the subaxial spine can present with or develop myelopathy.
- There is risk of progressive neurologic symptoms and/or progressive deformity of the cervical spine.
- Paralysis or death are rare but may occur.

## PATIENT HISTORY AND PHYSICAL FINDINGS

- A thorough history for traumatic injury, conditions that are associated with cervical instability, or history of posterior cervical surgery
- Patients may present with complaints of neck pain or decreased range of motion. Patients may have neurologic symptoms on presentation, which may be radicular in nature from cervical nerve root compression or myelopathic from spinal cord compression.
- Examination should include a thorough neurologic evaluation including motor and sensory examinations and assessment for myelopathy (hyperreflexia, clonus, pathologic reflexes).
- Assess for possible associated abnormalities including a cardiac examination (for congenital/syndromic etiologies).

## IMAGING AND OTHER DIAGNOSTIC STUDIES

- Standard radiographs including anteroposterior (AP) and lateral views in neutral, flexion, and extension. An open mouth view should also be taken to ensure that concomitant O/C1/C2 instability is not present.
- Lateral views allow for assessment of true instability from *pseudosubluxation*, which occurs most commonly between the second and third cervical vertebrae and between the third and fourth cervical vertebrae.
- The spinolaminar line of Swischuk is helpful to differentiate between pseudosubluxation and true subluxation. This line is drawn along the posterior arch from the first cervical vertebra to the third. It should pass within 1.5 mm of the anterior cortex of the posterior arch of the second cervical vertebra during forward flexion. As long as Swischuk line is maintained, as much as 4 mm of vertebral body subluxation can be accepted.
- Fine-cut CT scan of the cervical spine to assess for anomalies of the cervical anatomy including location of the vertebral artery and for preoperative planning of screw lengths and trajectories
- Magnetic resonance imaging (MRI) to evaluate for spinal cord or nerve root involvement

## DIFFERENTIAL DIAGNOSIS

- Posttraumatic instability
- Infection/tumors involving the posterior elements
- Postlaminectomy instability/kyphosis (post-tumoral decompression)
- Congenital/syndromic cervical abnormalities
  - Cervical kyphosis (Larsen syndrome, diastrophic dysplasia, chondrodysplasia punctata [Conradi syndrome], camptomelic dysplasia, and neurofibromatosis)
  - Cervical abnormalities of segmentation/formation (VACTERL, Klippel-Feil syndrome)

## NONOPERATIVE MANAGEMENT

- Stable cervical spine deformity with no neurologic involvement can be treated with observation and serial imaging.
- Unstable cervical spine, neurologic involvement, or progressive deformity would be indications for surgical management.

## SURGICAL MANAGEMENT

- Many techniques of posterior cervical fusion including wiring, plate and screw, and rod and screw constructs have been described.
- Lateral mass screw fixation provides benefits compared to nonrigid fixation including fixation of patients with posterior laminar element deficiency, providing immediate stability, and allowing for greater deformity correction.

### Preoperative Planning

- Fine-cut CT evaluation to preoperatively plan screw lengths and trajectories, note any anomalous anatomy and assess location of the vertebral artery.
  - CT angiography can be performed at the same time as assessment of the bony anatomy.
  - Flexion and extension CT can also be helpful.
- The measured angle of 35.9 degrees seen in **TECH FIG 1A** is the most extreme lateral angulation that can be achieved with a more medial starting point in this particular patient. This maximally protects the vertebral artery but impinges against the spinous process in drill placement. In practice, a compromise between vertebral artery safety and easy access of drilling is ideal.

- MRI evaluation for any spinal cord or nerve root compression
- Neuromonitoring, including somatosensory evoked potentials and transcortical motor evoked potentials of upper and lower extremities
- Fiberoptic intubation minimizing cervical motion.

## Positioning

- While supine, placement of halo or Mayfield tongs followed by careful turning of patient into a prone position with surgeon stabilizing the cervical spine (**FIG 4**)
- Fixation of Mayfield device to operating room (OR) table with careful attention to cervical spine flexion–extension
- Padding of all bony prominences, positioning of upper extremities to avoid nerve stretch or compression, ensuring patient is secure on table
- Take AP and lateral fluoroscopy images to ensure all anatomy can be seen and assess cervical alignment.
- Prepare autograft donor site.
- Ensure that good baseline neuromonitoring is present once positioned.

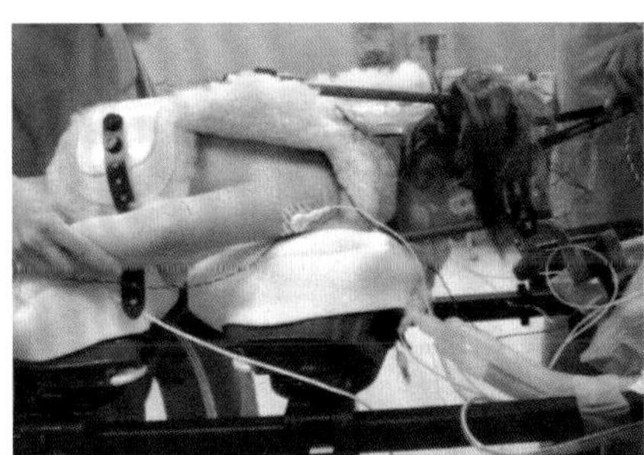

**FIG 4** ● A halo vest has been placed in this patient with Down syndrome and paraparesis to maximize spinal control during the turn to prone position. The posterior half of the vest is removed for surgical access.

## Approach

- A standard posterior cervical approach is used.
- A midline approach posteriorly, dissecting midline through the muscle down to the spinous process
- Subperiosteal dissection to expose the posterior vertebra to the lateral border of the lateral mass

TECHNIQUES

# Lateral Mass Screw Placement

### Starting Point Identification

- Define the medial and lateral borders of the lateral mass as well as superior and inferior borders as defined by the facets. Outline the lateral mass as a rectangular box.
- Divide the rectangular box of the lateral mass into quadrants and identify the center point.
- Entry point[2,5,6]
  - Roy-Camille technique: Entry point is at the center point of the four quadrants.
  - Magerl technique: Entry point is 1 mm superior and 1 mm medial to the center point.
  - Anderson technique: Entry point is 1 mm medial to center point.
  - Our technique: In smaller children, often the simplest starting point is in the center of the lateral mass (Roy-Camille). The smallest screws (usually 3.5 mm) fill much of the lateral mass, and maximal containment is the most desirable technical goal.

### Lateral Mass Screw Hole Creation

- Make a small burr hole at your entry point. Confirm this starting point on AP fluoroscopy if there is much congenital deformation or bone dysplasia.
- Use a hand-powered drill with a stop mechanism at desired depth to create screw hole. Start with a conservative depth stop and deepen the hole after probing for bone integrity.
  - Roy-Camille technique: Direct the drill 10 degrees laterally and perpendicular to the posterior cortex of the lateral mass.
  - Magerl technique: Direct the drill 30 degrees laterally and parallel to the facet joint.
  - Anderson technique: Direct the drill 10 degrees laterally and parallel to the facet joint.
  - Our technique: Direct the drill in the sagittal plane parallel to the facets on lateral fluoroscopy projection and angled away from the midline at an angle approaching the preoperative CT scan templating lines (**TECH FIG 1A**). This usually results in a larger lateral angulation (more than 10 degrees) (**TECH FIG 1B**).

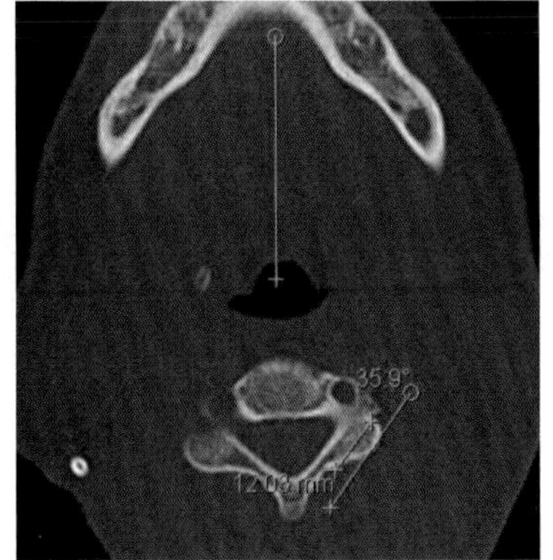


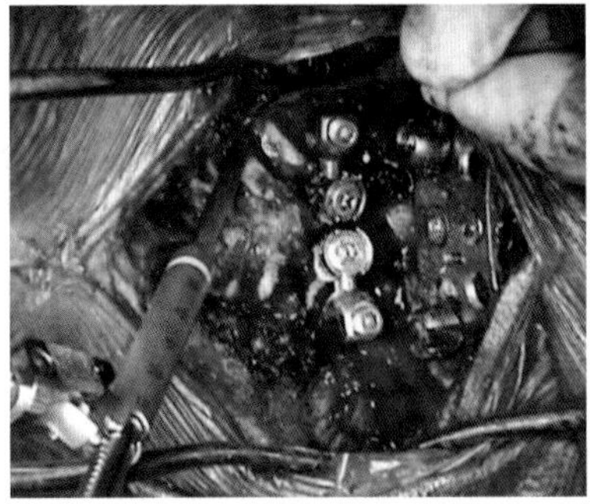


**TECH FIG 1** ● **A,B**. Same patient as **FIG 1**. **A.** Axial CT scan. The depth and angle of screw insertion are derived from these two CT formats and the live fluoroscopic lateral projection intraoperatively. **B**. There has been an occipital plate placed and translaminar screws with lateral connectors at C2. *(continued)*

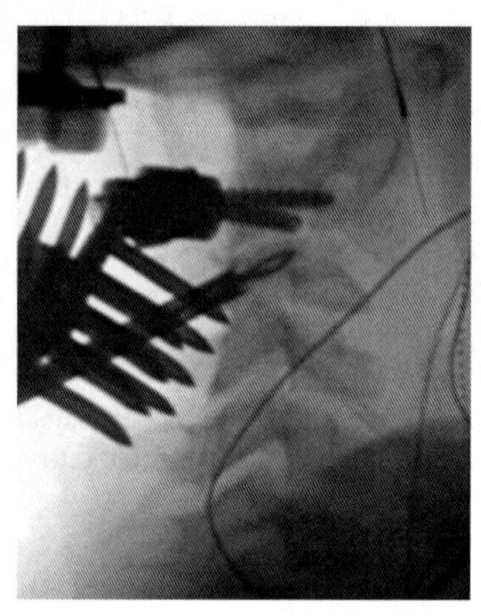

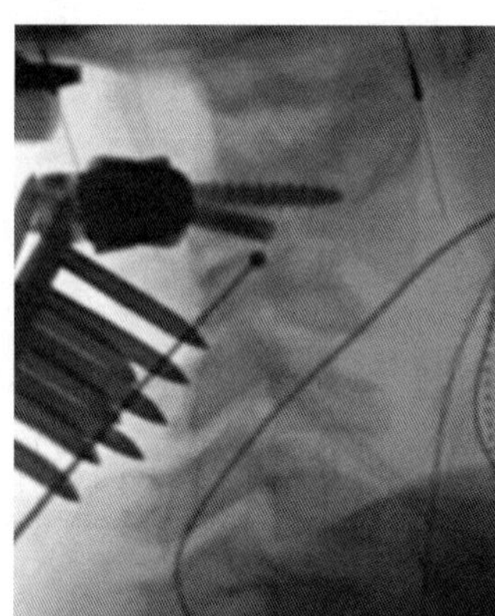

**TECH FIG 1** • *(continued)* **C,D.** Same patient as in **FIG 1**. **C.** This is the lateral fluoroscopic projection of the left C3 lateral mass being drilled. **D.** The probe has bottomed out in the anterior wall of the drilled hole. Depth measurement followed by screw placement ensues.

- The head is to the right. Note the measured depth stop sleeve and drill guide. The drill is angled laterally greater than 10 degrees, approaching the preoperative templated angle of 36 degrees. A more medial starting point necessitates greater lateral angulation, whereas a more lateral starting point allows a more "straight back" approach but puts the vertebral artery at greater risk (**TECH FIG 1C**).
- Check trajectory with fluoroscopy in the lateral view to confirm your position (see **TECH FIG 1**).
- Once you have drilled, probe the screw hole to ensure there are intact walls on all sides (**TECH FIG 1D**).

## Screw Placement

- Tapping the dorsal cortex can be helpful in hard bone, followed by placement of a 3.5-mm polyaxial screw.
- Usual screw lengths are between 10 and 14 mm. Given the trajectory of the screw hole, the screw head will not be flush to the bone but rather angled. The polyaxial nature of the head allows rod placement despite screw head angulation.
- Check screw position with fluoroscopy in the lateral view.

## Rod Placement

- Measure and cut rods to appropriate length.
- Precontour rods with rod benders, then place rods and set screws (**TECH FIG 2**).
- Perform any compression or distraction then final tightening.

## Fusion Bed Preparation

- Decorticate in area of fusion with a small burr.
- Obtain posterior iliac crest autograft and place along fusion.
- Perform standard layered closure.

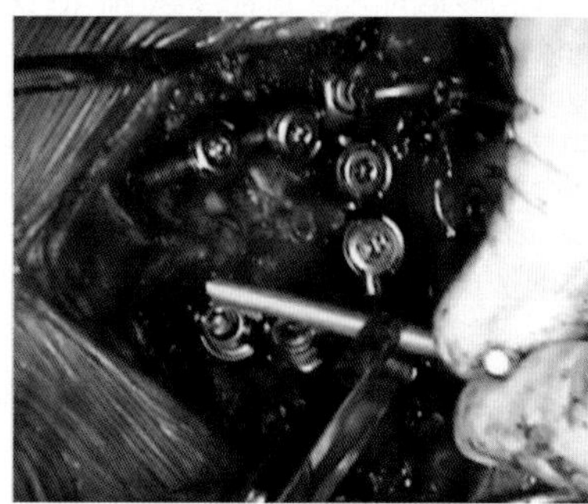

**TECH FIG 2** • The *left* rod has been bent and placed in two lateral mass screws at C3 to C4, a translaminar screw at C2 and attached to a lateral connector at C2 occipital plate. The *right* rod is being manipulated into position. Final tightening follows.

## PEARLS AND PITFALLS

| | |
|---|---|
| **Positioning** | ■ Careful positioning of the cervical spine to avoid cord compression as well as to allow for fusion in appropriate position; this can be confirmed clinically and with lateral fluoroscopy. |
| **Approach** | ■ Avoid lateral dissection which will increase bleeding.<br>■ Ensure you have extended the incision caudal enough to allow for appropriate hand position to achieve the trajectory of the lowest instrumented level. |

| | |
|---|---|
| **Screw positioning** | ■ Several anatomic structures at risk with screw placement: Screws that are too high put the facet at risk, screws that are too low put the spinal nerve at risk, and screws too lateral (straight back) put the spinal nerve and vertebral artery at risk. However, a more medial approach (exaggerated Magerl or Anderson) makes the drill guide impinge on the spinous process.<br>■ CT of the levels to be instrumented should be reviewed to determine appropriate screw trajectories and lengths. |
| **C7 level** | ■ C7 vertebra has a thinner lateral mass; studies have advocated screw placement directed more superior and lateral.<br>■ If unable to place a lateral mass screw at C7, a pedicle screw may be placed instead. |
| **Screw length** | ■ Studies have supported both unicortical and bicortical screw purchase. Although bicortical has a biomechanical advantage, screw lengths must be carefully assessed to avoid too long screws that may place neurovascular structures at risk. Oblique views can help assess screw length (**FIG 5**). |

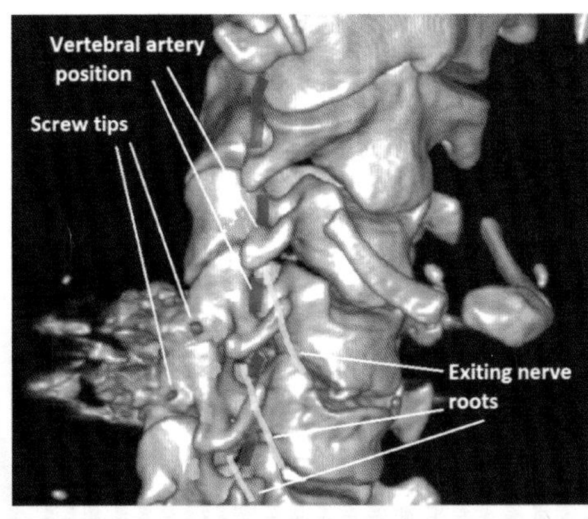


**FIG 5** • A 15-year-old female suffered a flexion distraction injury at C4–C5. Lateral mass instrumention and fusion was performed achieving bicortical purchase over just one level. Note the tips of the screws safely away from neurovascular structures.

| | |
|---|---|
| **Rod placement** | ■ Perform careful rod precontouring to avoid screw loosening or pullout during rod placement. |

## POSTOPERATIVE CARE

- Postoperative CT scan is obtained to assess screw positioning (**FIG 6**)
- Immobilization in halo vest or rigid cervical orthosis until bony union is achieved.
- Long-term follow-up with radiographs to assess for any development of junctional sagittal imbalance

## OUTCOMES

- Radiographic and cadaveric studies of the different techniques of screw placement have shown that the Magerl technique allows for longer screw lengths and has a larger margin of safety than the Roy-Camille technique. Studies have shown that a modified Anderson technique with 20 to 30 degrees of lateral angulation is safer with regard to avoidance of the nerve root and artery. Our technique approximates to this. The standard Roy-Camille technique did pose risk to neurovascular structures at C4–C7 levels, whereas Magerl posed a risk to the spinal nerve at C7.
- Hedequist et al[3] reported on 36 patients that had undergone posterior cervical fusion with lateral mass screw fixation. On postoperative CT scans, it was noted that 100% of the screws were contained in the lateral mass. (Our technique occasionally results in bicortical purchase but with anterolateral penetration safely away from the nerve root and vertebral artery; see **FIG 5**.)
- Complications included one infection, one seroma, and one pseudarthrosis. There were no neurologic complications and no surgery revisions.
- Studies reporting results from lateral mass cervical fixation in adults have shown 85% to 100% fusion rates.

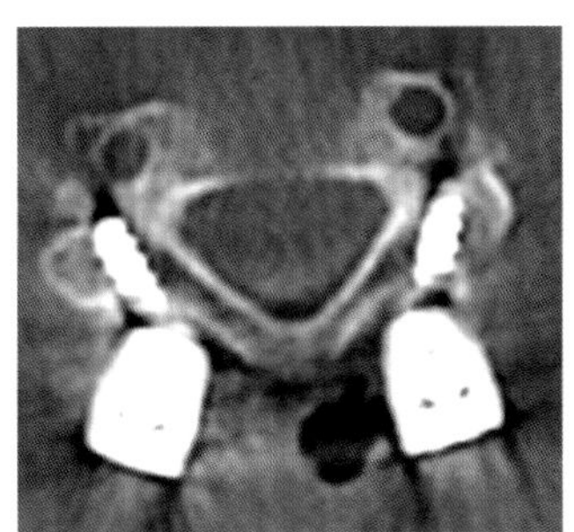

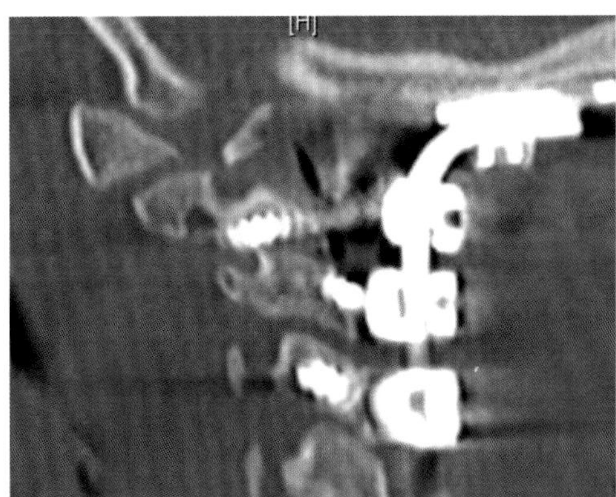

**FIG 6** • Same patients as **TECH FIGS 1** and **2**. **A.** Postoperative axial CT scan. Two lateral mass screws have been placed at C3 with a significant lateral angulation. They are unicortical. The vertebral artery is safe. **B.** Sagittal reformatted CT scan. Note the cephalad trajectory of the lateral mass screws at C3 and C4. The polyaxial attributes of the screws allow for accommodation of the contoured rod without pullout stresses. Note again the occipital plate and C2 laminar screws.

## COMPLICATIONS

- Neurologic injury to spinal cord or spinal nerves
- Injury to vertebral artery
- Screw penetration of the facet joint
- Infection
- Implant failure (screw loosening or pullout)
- Pseudarthrosis
- Junctional sagittal imbalance (kyphosis/lordosis)

## REFERENCES

1. Al-Shamy G, Cherian J, Mata JA, et al. Computed tomography morphometric analysis for lateral mass screw placement in the pediatric subaxial cervical spine. J Neurosurg Spine 2012;(17):390–396.
2. Ebraheim N. Posterior lateral mass screw fixation: anatomic and radiographic considerations. Univ Penn Ortho J 1999;12:66–72.
3. Hedequist D, Proctor M, Hresko T. Lateral mass screw fixation in children. J Child Orthop 2010;4(3):197–201.
4. Lustrin ES, Karakas SP, Ortiz AO, et al. Pediatric cervical spine: normal anatomy, variants, and trauma. Radiographics 2003;23(3): 539–560.
5. Merola AA, Castro BA, Alongi PR, et al. Anatomic consideration for standard and modified techniques of cervical lateral mass screw placement. Spine 2002;2(6):430–435.
6. Stemper BD, Marawar SV, Yoganandan N, et al. Quantitative anatomy of subaxial cervical lateral mass: an analysis of safe screw lengths for Roy-Camille and magerl techniques. Spine 2008;33(8): 893–897.

CHAPTER 84

# Posterior Exposure of the Thoracic and Lumbar Spine

Wudbhav N. Sankar and John M. Flynn

## DEFINITION

- Scoliosis is a three-dimensional deformity of the spine and rib cage.
- The hallmark of scoliotic spines is curvature in the coronal plane along with abnormal curvature in the sagittal plane (eg, lordoscoliosis in adolescent idiopathic scoliosis) as well as abnormal vertebral rotation in the transverse plane.
- A Cobb angle measurement of greater than 10 degrees distinguishes minor spinal asymmetry from true scoliosis.
- The posterior approach to the thoracic and lumbar spine takes advantage of the segmental innervation of the posterior spinal musculature to obtain an internervous and intermuscular plane to provide access to the posterior elements of the spine.
- The posterior approach is the most commonly used route for spinal fusion and instrumentation in the scoliotic spine.

## ANATOMY

- Surface landmarks in the prone position
  - The vertebra prominens (C7) is typically the most prominent bony structure palpated at the base of the neck.
  - The superior angle of the scapula is at the level of the T3 spinous process.
  - The scapular spine is at the level of the T4 spinous process.
  - The inferior angle of the scapula is at the level of the T7 spinous process.
  - With the patient in the prone position, the iliac crests are palpated with the fingers and the thumbs brought together at the midline, where they typically overlie the L4–L5 interspace.
  - The posterior superior iliac spines are at the level of the L5–S1 interspace.
- Posterior spinal musculature is divided into superficial and deep layers. The superficial layer, also known as the *erector spinae*, is composed of the iliocostalis, longissimus, and sacrospinalis muscles. The deep layer consists of the short rotators (multifidus and rotatores) as well as the intertransversarii and interspinous muscles (**FIG 1A,B**).
- Segmental innervation of spinal musculature
  - Provided by the dorsal rami of the thoracolumbar nerve roots
- Segmental blood supply
  - The posterior intercostal arteries branch from the aorta and subsequently send a dorsal branch posteriorly to the spinal musculature. On its way past the neural foramina, the spinal artery branches off and is sent through the foramina. The spinal artery then divides into anterior and posterior radicular branches within the spinal canal, ultimately supplying the anterior and posterior spinal arteries. Care should be taken to cauterize the branches that lie adjacent to the lateral aspect of the facet (**FIG 1C**).
- In the scoliotic spine, there is rotation of the vertebral bodies in the transverse plane with the spinous processes rotating toward the concavity of the curve.
- In the scoliotic spine, the pedicles on the concave side are shorter and have a smaller diameter.[5]
- In scoliosis, the dural sac hugs the concavity of the spinal canal[2] and the aorta is posterolateral to its normal position.[8]

## PATHOGENESIS

- Idiopathic
- Congenital
  - Failure of formation or segmentation of vertebral precursors leading to asymmetric vertebral growth with subsequent abnormal curvature
- Neuromuscular
  - Variety of etiologies, such as cerebral palsy, muscular dystrophy, polio, spinal muscular atrophy, and myelomeningocele
  - Related to an inability to provide muscular support to the spinal column

## NATURAL HISTORY

### Idiopathic

- Infantile (0 to 3 years of age)
  - Less than 1% of all cases of idiopathic scoliosis
  - More common in boys
  - Left thoracic curves predominate
  - Most resolve spontaneously
- Juvenile (3 to 10 years of age)
  - Eight percent to 16% of all cases of idiopathic scoliosis
  - More even female–male ratio
  - Bracing may correct some curves.
  - Curves of more than 30 degrees usually progress to surgery.
- Adolescent (10 to 18 years of age)
  - Most common form of idiopathic scoliosis
  - Etiology and pathogenesis are not well understood.
- Family history is positive in 30% of cases but does not predict curve magnitude or progression.
- More common in girls. The female–male ratio is 1.4:1 for curves 11 to 20 degrees and increases to 5:1 for curves greater than 20 degrees.
- Curves have the greatest chance of progression in the period of peak growth velocity leading up to skeletal maturity (prior to menses in females), after which the potential decreases significantly.[1]
- Scoliotic curves measuring less than 20 degrees are at lower risk for progression.

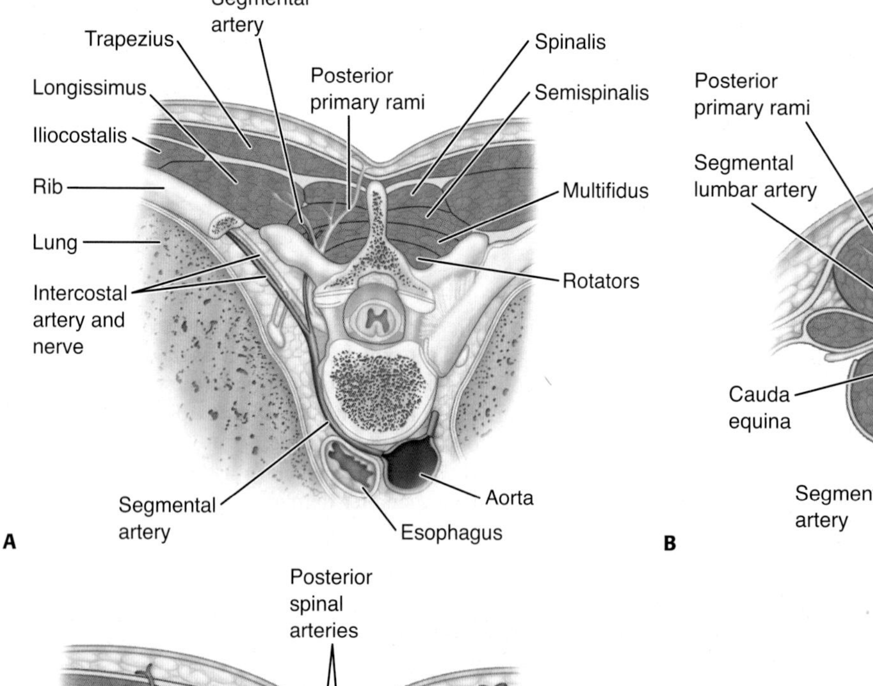


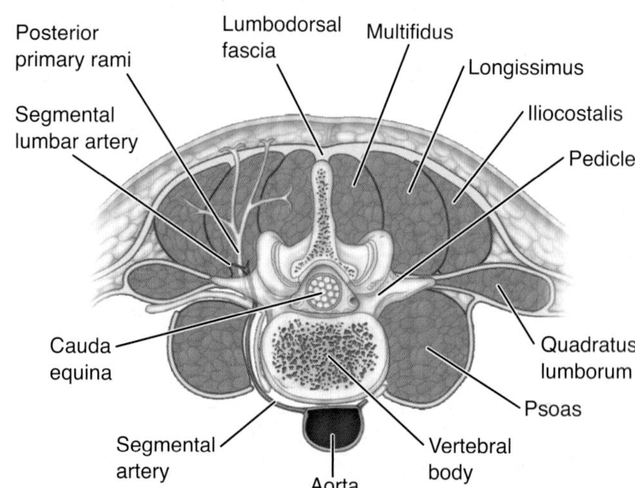


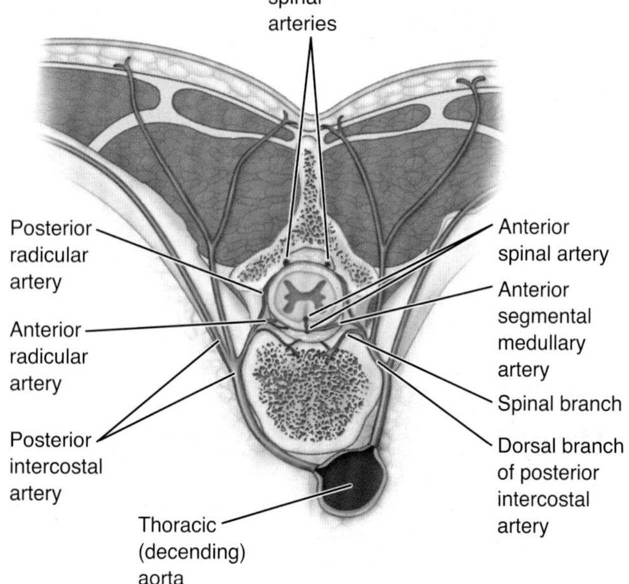


**FIG 1** • **A,B.** Cross-sections of paraspinal musculature. **C.** Overview at the level of the lumbar spine. The segmental artery courses posteriorly, adjacent to the vertebral body toward the posterior spinal musculature. On passing the neural foramen, the vessel sends a branch through the neural foramen to supply the spinal cord. The vessel continues toward the posterior spinal musculature arising between the transverse processes during the surgical approach where it is prone to bleed.

- Scoliotic curves measuring greater than 50 degrees are at higher risk for further progression during adult life (with a percentage of these progressing at a rate of about 1 degree per year).[9]
- There are no significant differences in the prevalence of back pain between adults with scoliotic spines and the general population.[7,10]
- Scoliotic curves measuring greater than 100 degrees have an increased prevalence of cardiopulmonary compromise (eg, cor pulmonale, restrictive lung disease).[6]

### Congenital

- Severity of deformity related to type and location of anomaly
- Highest chance of curve progression with unilateral unsegmented bar with contralateral hemivertebrae (nearly 100%), followed by a lone unilateral unsegmented bar, double convex hemivertebrae, single convex hemivertebrae, and finally the block vertebrae[3]

### Neuromuscular

- Most curves are progressive and are more difficult to manage nonoperatively.
- Curves can cause pelvic obliquity and sitting problems in nonambulatory individuals.

## PATIENT HISTORY AND PHYSICAL FINDINGS

- Complete history, including age at onset, timing of growth spurts, menses, presence of pain, family history of scoliosis, nerve, or muscle diseases
- A complete examination is important to obtain a diagnosis because certain etiologies can predispose the patient to increased operative risk (eg, cardiac abnormalities in patients with Marfan syndrome).
- The skin is inspected for café-au-lait spots, the axilla for freckling, and the lumbosacral area for sinus tracts, hairy patches, or dimples. Axillary freckling and multiple café-au-lait spots are associated with neurofibromatosis. Sinus tracts,

hairy patches, or dimples in the lumbosacral area are associated with intraspinal anomaly.
- The Adams forward bending test detects curvatures by physical examination. Abnormalities in vertebral rotation become apparent as an asymmetric rib hump, prominence, or fullness, leading to possible identification of patients at risk for having scoliosis.
- Any shoulder or scapular asymmetry is noted. It is important to point out to parents that this is not always corrected by surgery.
- Pelvic obliquity can indicate a possible leg length discrepancy that can mimic a lumbar scoliosis.
- Trunk shift and sagittal profile are noted; these indicate coronal balance and sagittal balance, respectively.

## IMAGING AND OTHER DIAGNOSTIC STUDIES

- Plain radiographs, including standing posteroanterior (PA) and lateral views of the entire spine, should be obtained to determine the degree of scoliosis, to identify any skeletal abnormalities (eg, hemivertebra), and to evaluate overall alignment.
  - PA views are obtained to decrease exposure of sensitive breast tissue to ionizing radiation in girls.
  - Side-bending supine views of the thoracolumbar spine are useful to determine the flexibility of the primary and secondary curves. This information is useful during preoperative planning in choosing fusion levels and determining the approach.
- Risser staging system for gauging skeletal maturity (**FIG 2**)
  - Ossification of the iliac apophysis proceeds along the iliac crest from the anterior superior iliac spine to the posterior superior iliac spine. When ossification is complete, fusion of the apophysis to the iliac crest occurs.
    - Risser 0 = no ossification
    - Risser 1 = 25% excursion
    - Risser 2 = 50% excursion
    - Risser 3 = 75% excursion
    - Risser 4 = 100% excursion
    - Risser 5 = fusion of iliac apophysis to the iliac crest
  - In girls, the end of spinal growth corresponds to Risser stage 4.
  - In boys, spinal growth can occur after Risser stage 4 and is less well defined.
- Magnetic resonance imaging (MRI) should be obtained for patients with an onset before age 10 years; left thoracic curves, kyphoscoliotic curves, or rapidly progressive curves; patients with moderate to severe back pain; patients with congenital or neuromuscular scoliosis; and patients with abnormal findings on the physical examination.

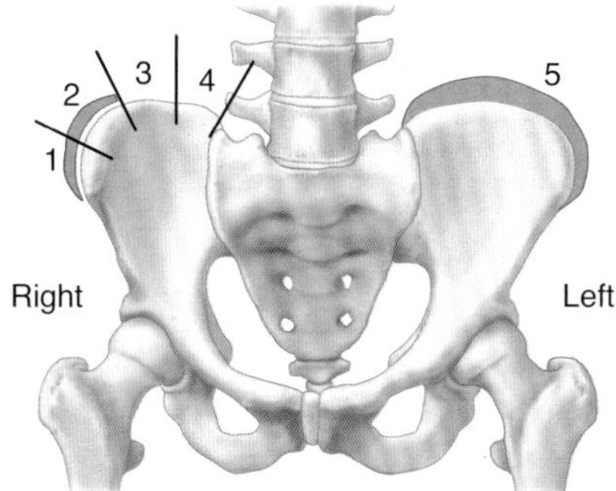


**FIG 2** • Risser staging system. Ossification proceeds from the anterior superior iliac spine to the posterior superior iliac spine.

## DIFFERENTIAL DIAGNOSIS

- Scoliosis
  - Idiopathic
  - Congenital
  - Neuromuscular
- Limb length discrepancy
- Osteoid osteoma
- Sprengel deformity

## NONOPERATIVE MANAGEMENT

- Observation for progression for curves of 0 to 20 degrees. Patients are followed with serial clinical and radiographic examinations.
- Bracing for progressive curves of 20 to 40 degrees if the patient is skeletally immature. Braces cannot correct curves; their purpose is to prevent curve progression.

## SURGICAL MANAGEMENT

### Preoperative Planning

- Preoperative radiographs with supine side-bending films are obtained to determine fusion levels according to the Lenke criteria.
- Cobb angles (**FIG 3A**)
  - Quantitates the degree of curvature
  - Method
    - Determine apex of curve to be measured.
    - Select the most tilted vertebra above the apex of the curve and draw a line along the top of the vertebral endplate.
    - Select the most tilted vertebra below the apex of the curve and draw a line along the bottom of the vertebral endplate.
    - Drop perpendicular lines to these previous two lines.
    - The angle subtended by the two lines is the Cobb angle.
    - The intraobserver intrinsic error in Cobb angle measurements is about 5%; interobserver validity is about 7%.[4]
- Center sacral vertical line (**FIG 3B**)
  - Used to help determine distal extent of fusion
  - The vertebral body most closely bisected by the center sacral line is the stable vertebra.
  - Fusion is usually extended to the stable vertebra or the one immediately cephalad.

### Positioning

- Patient is intubated in the supine position on the stretcher.
- Neurologic monitoring leads are placed cranially, on the intercostal and abdominal musculature, and on all four extremities.
- Multiple large-bore intravenous access is obtained for fluid management, and an arterial line is placed for intraoperative blood pressure monitoring.
- The patient is transferred to the prone position on a well-padded operating room table such as a Jackson frame (Mizuho Osi, Orthopaedic Systems, Union City, CA).
- Care should be given to the degree of hip flexion–extension, as this can affect the amount of lordosis in the lumbar spine.
- Bolsters underneath the chest and anterior superior iliac spines prevent abdominal compression and allow epidural venous return, thus decreasing epidural bleeding.
- All bony prominences are well padded, including medial elbows, knees, pretibial areas, and ankles.

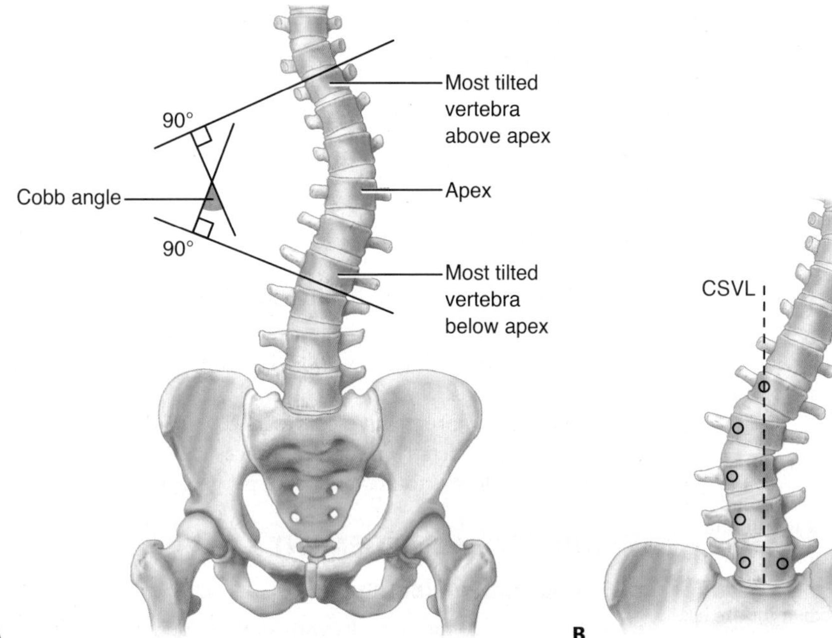


**FIG 3** • **A.** Cobb angle is a quantitative measure of the coronal curvature. Lines parallel to the vertebral endplates of the end vertebrae are drawn. Perpendiculars to these two lines are drawn. The angle subtended is the Cobb angle. **B.** Center sacral vertical line (*CSVL*) is the vertical line in a PA radiograph that passes through the center of the sacrum, identified by suitable landmarks, preferably on the first sacral segment (SRS terminology). The vertebra most closely bisected by the CSVL is considered the stable vertebra.

- Care is taken to avoid abduction and forward flexion past 90 degrees at the shoulder and flexion past 90 degrees at the elbow (**FIG 4**).
- Skin is shaved if necessary.
- Clear adhesive surgical drapes (3M Steri-Drape towel drapes) are placed around the perimeter of the surgical site, extending from the hairline to the top of the gluteal crease (regardless of levels to be fused, the entire spine should be draped).

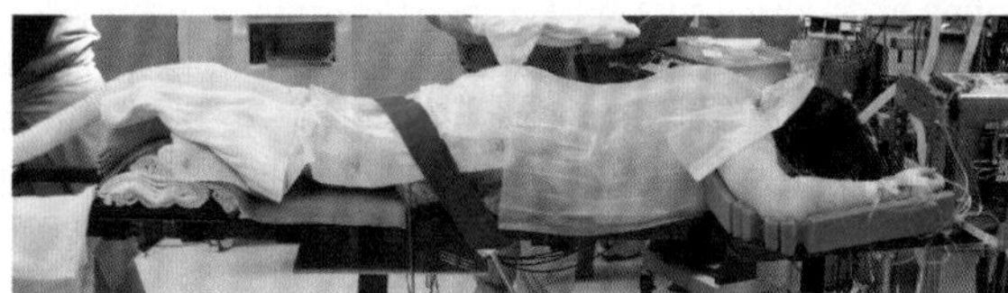

**FIG 4** • Patient positioning. All bony prominences are well padded. Note the positioning of the upper extremities.

TECHNIQUES

## Incision

- A Bovie electrocautery cord is centered over the back using the vertebra prominens and the gluteal crease as landmarks, and the line for the straight midline back incision is marked based on the extent of the intended fusion (**TECH FIG 1A**).
- The skin is sharply incised with a scalpel, and electrocautery is then used to dissect through the subcutaneous fat until the thoracolumbar fascia is reached.
- Weitlaner retractors are placed.
- The spinous processes are identified via palpation (**TECH FIG 1B**).
- Electrocautery is used to split the apophyses along the tips of the spinous processes. A clamp can be used to isolate each spinous process sequentially (**TECH FIG 1C–E**).
  - These incisions are connected (**TECH FIG 1F**).
  - This proceeds throughout the extent of the incision.
- Care is taken at the cephalad and caudal aspects of the dissection to preserve the interspinous ligaments.

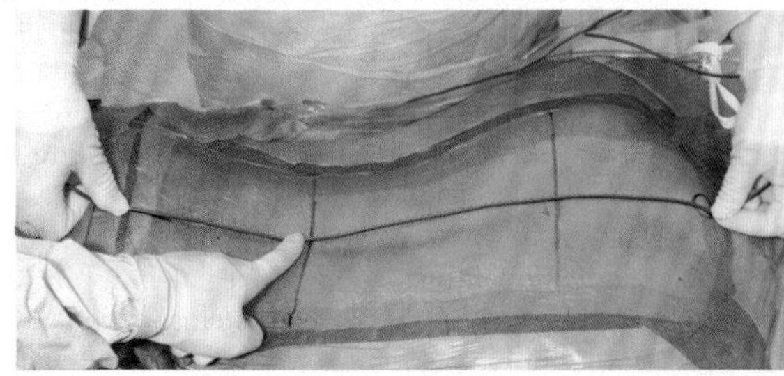

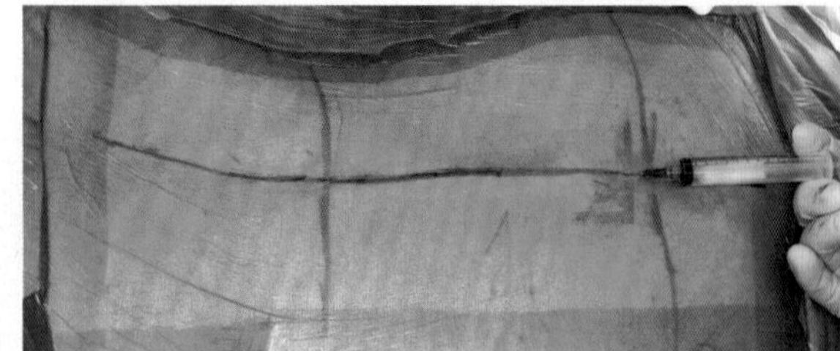

**TECH FIG 1** • **A.** Bovie electrocautery cord centered over back using vertebra prominens and gluteal crease as cephalad and caudal landmarks. **B.** Mixture of local anesthetic and epinephrine being injected along the course of incision. *(continued)*

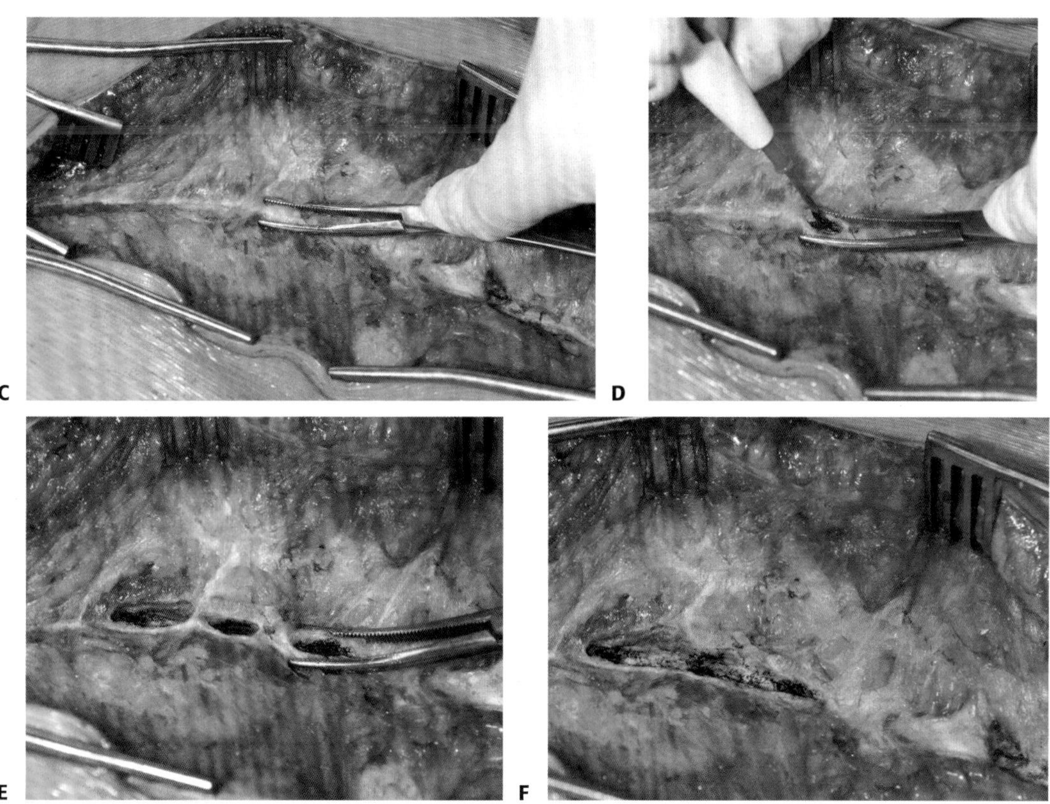

**TECH FIG 1** • *(continued)* **C.** Spinous process identified via palpation after dissection down to the thoracodorsal fascia. **D.** Splitting of the spinous process apophysis with electrocautery. **E.** A clamp can be used to define the spinous process. **F.** Dissection at three adjacent spinous processes are connected.

## Subperiosteal Dissection

- Dissection then proceeds subperiosteally.
- In skeletally immature individuals, the apophyses of the spinous processes are further dissected with a Cobb elevator. It is often helpful to peel subperiosteally with one Cobb elevator on each spinous process/lamina to put the soft tissues on tension while the exposure is advanced with electrocautery (**TECH FIG 2A,B**).
- Electrocautery is used to advance the dissection deep along the spinous processes until the laminae are reached and the retractors are repositioned (**TECH FIG 2C**).

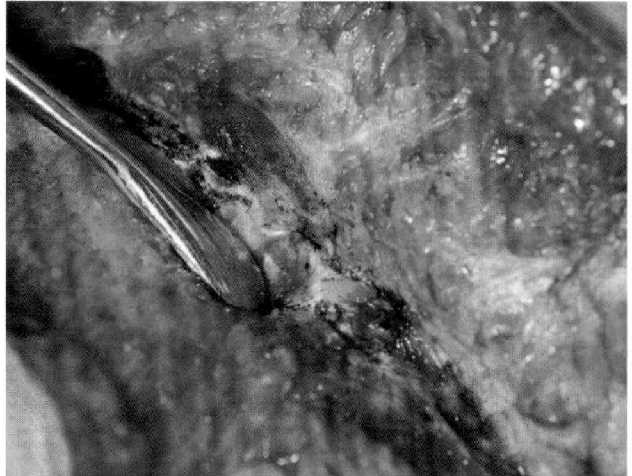

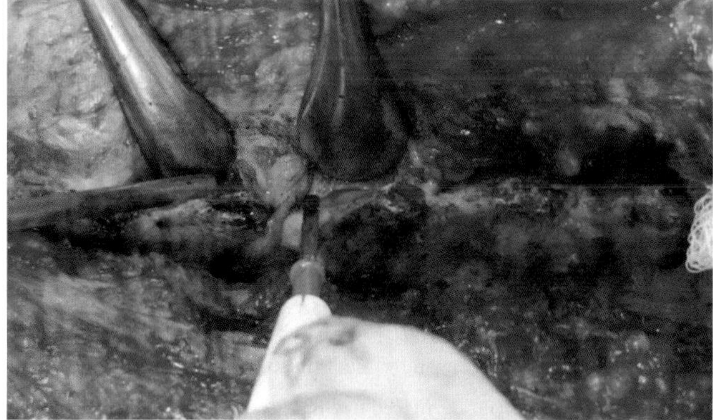

**TECH FIG 2** • **A.** Further dissection of spinous process apophysis with a Cobb elevator. **B.** Placing a Cobb elevator on each spinous process/lamina and putting the soft tissues on tension allows the exposure to be advanced with electrocautery. *(continued)*

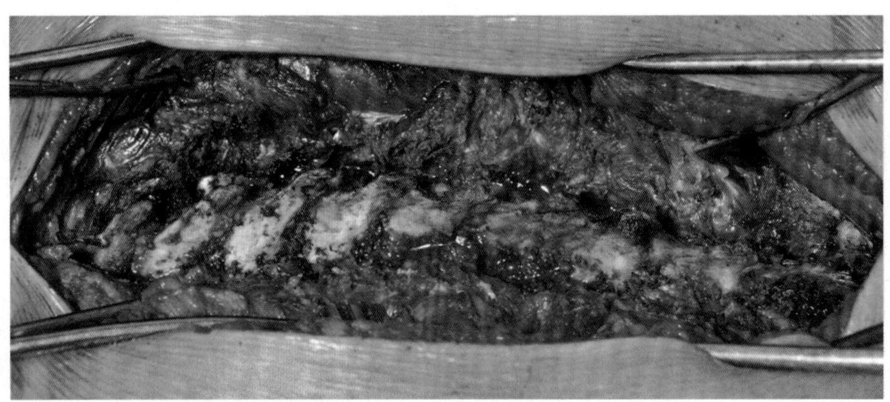

**TECH FIG 2** • *(continued)* **C.** Dissection is advanced down the laminae out to the tips of the transverse processes.

- In the thoracic spine, dissection proceeds until the tip of the transverse process is fully exposed.
- In the lumbar spine, dissection proceeds until the facet joint, pars interarticularis, and transverse process are exposed.
- Once the exposure is completed, it is vital that one check to be sure that the appropriate levels have actually been exposed.
- By convention, we typically place a pedicle marker in what we believe to be the left T12 pedicle and check a C-arm image to confirm that the correct levels have been exposed. It is important to compare the presence/size of the T12 rib on the C-arm image to the preoperative radiographs to reduce the risk of making a mistake. If T12 is not going to be included within the fusion segments, a different level can be chosen for the marker.
- At this point, the spine is instrumented and the correction is performed (see Chap. 85).

## Closure

- Before closure, the wound is assessed for any frank bleeding vessels.
- All exposed areas of bone are decorticated using a burr in order to facilitate fusion.
- The wound is now irrigated with 3 L of normal saline via low-pressure cystoscopic tubing.
- The spine is bone grafted using a mixture of locally harvested autograft and cancellous allograft.
- At our institution, vancomycin powder is mixed with the bone graft for all patients. In certain neuromuscular patients, gentamicin can be used as well.
- Fascia is closed with a running braided absorbable suture (no. 1 Vicryl). The goal is a watertight closure.
- A medium Hemovac drain is placed superficial to the fascia exiting at the inferior extent of the wound.
- Subcutaneous layers are closed with running braided absorbable suture (no. 0 and 2-0 Vicryl). The goal is to decrease wound tension.
- The subcuticular layer of skin is closed with a running single filament absorbable suture (4-0 Monocryl). The goal is cosmetic closure.
- Skin closure is reinforced with 1-inch Steri-Strips.
- A silver-impregnated dressing is used (Mepilex Border, Mölnlycke Health Care, Göteborg, Sweden).

## PEARLS AND PITFALLS

| | |
|---|---|
| **Decreasing blood loss** | ■ Subperiosteal dissection<br>■ Bovie electrocautery on high power<br>■ Traction with self-retaining retractors<br>■ Topical thrombin (FloSeal)<br>■ Mean arterial pressure is 60 to 70 mm Hg during exposure but is increased to more than 70 mm Hg during correction to maintain spinal cord perfusion. |
| **Determining vertebral level intraoperatively** | ■ Marker placed in what is believed to be left T12 pedicle and a C-arm image is taken to confirm that the appropriate levels have been exposed. It is important to compare the presence/size of the T12 rib on the C-arm image to the preoperative radiographs to reduce the risk of making a mistake. |
| **Exposure** | ■ Neuromuscular blockade during exposure allows for ease of retraction of paralyzed spinal musculature. |

## POSTOPERATIVE CARE

- No postoperative immobilization is required with modern pedicle screw fixation.
- Postoperative restrictions include limitations with lifting, bending, and twisting.
- Intravenous antibiotics are used based on local protocol.
- Neurovascular checks are made every 2 hours for the first 8 hours, then every 8 hours.
- Patients are out of bed on postoperative day 1.
- The Foley catheter and Hemovac are typically removed on postoperative day 2.
- Diet is advanced as tolerated.
- Patient-controlled analgesia is used for appropriate patients. Continuous narcotic infusion with demand for the first 24 hours is followed by demand only for the next 24 hours, followed by oral pain medications when tolerating diet.
- A 3–4 day hospital course is typical.
- Routine follow-up is done at 6 weeks and 6 months and at 1, 2, and 5 years.
- Activity is increased based on the degree of fusion.

## OUTCOMES

- With meticulous attention to detail with regard to instrumentation and fusion techniques, excellent outcomes in terms of correction and fusion of the scoliotic spine can be expected.
- Long-term outcomes are variable and depend on the underlying diagnosis and the extent of retained spinal mobility.

## COMPLICATIONS

- Early or late infection: less than 5%
- Wound dehiscence
- Hematoma
- Instrumentation failure
- Pseudarthrosis: 1% to 12% depending on type of fusion and underlying diagnosis
- Neurologic injury
  - Spinal cord injuries: consider initiating steroid protocol
  - Nerve root injuries
- Wrong-level surgery

## ACKNOWLEDGMENT

- The authors would like to acknowledge James T. Guille and Reginald S. Fayssoux for their contributions to the previous edition.

## REFERENCES

1. Dimeglio A. Growth in pediatric orthopaedics. J Pediatr Orthop 2001;21:549–555.
2. Liljenqvist UR, Allkemper T, Hackenberg L, et al. Analysis of vertebral morphology in idiopathic scoliosis with use of magnetic resonance imaging and multiplanar reconstruction. J Bone Joint Surg Am 2002; 84-A(3):359–368.
3. McMaster MJ, Ohtsuka K. The natural history of congenital scoliosis. A study of two hundred and fifty-one patients. J Bone Joint Surg Am 1982;64:1128–1147.
4. Morrissy RT, Goldsmith GS, Hall EC, et al. Measurement of the Cobb angle on radiographs of patients who have scoliosis. Evaluation of intrinsic error. J Bone Joint Surg Am 1990;72(3):320–327.
5. Parent S, Labelle H, Skalli W, et al. Thoracic pedicle morphometry in vertebrae from scoliotic spines. Spine 2004;29:239–248.
6. Pehrsson K, Bake B, Larsson S, et al. Lung function in adult idiopathic scoliosis. Thorax 1991;46:474–478.
7. Ramirez N, Johnston CE, Browne RH. The prevalence of back pain in children who have idiopathic scoliosis. J Bone Joint Surg Am 1997;79(3):364–368.
8. Sucato DJ, Duchene C. The position of the aorta relative to the spine: a comparison of patients with and without idiopathic scoliosis. J Bone Joint Surg Am 2003;85-A(8):1461–1469.
9. Weinstein SL, Ponseti IV. Curve progression in idiopathic scoliosis. J Bone Joint Surg Am 1981;65(4):447–455.
10. Weinstein SL, Zavala DC, Ponseti IV. Idiopathic scoliosis: long-term follow-up and prognosis in untreated patients. J Bone Joint Surg Am 1981;63(5):702–712.

# Posterior Spinal Fusion for Idiopathic Scoliosis

Peter O. Newton and Vidyadhar V. Upasani

## DEFINITION

- Idiopathic scoliosis is a progressive three-dimensional spinal deformity in the absence of any congenital spinal anomaly or associated musculoskeletal condition.
- Categorized as early onset (before the age of 5 years) or late onset (after the age of 5 years).[3]

## ANATOMY

- The spinal deformity is divided into three areas: proximal thoracic, main thoracic, and thoracolumbar/lumbar.
- A proximal thoracic curve has an apex between T2 and T5. A main thoracic curve has and apex between T5 and T12 and a thoracolumbar/lumbar curve has an apex between T12 and L4.
- Vertebral definitions (**FIG 1**)
  - The end vertebrae define the extent of each curve and are most tilted from horizontal in the coronal plane.
  - The stable vertebra is defined as the vertebra most closely bisected by the center sacral vertical line (CSVL).
  - The neutral vertebra is defined as the least rotated vertebra in the axial plane based on the radiographic symmetry of its pedicles.

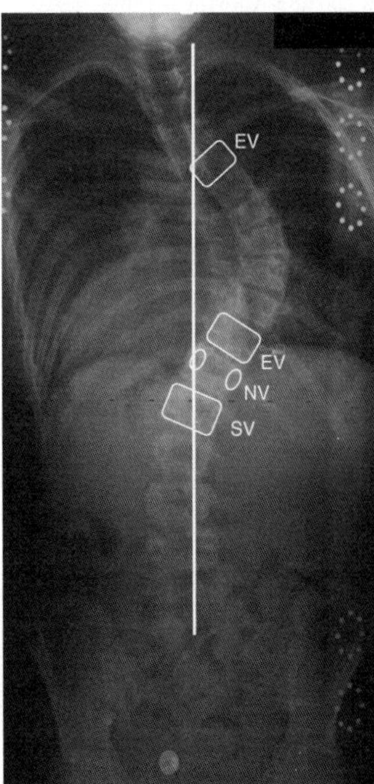


**FIG 1** • Vertebral definitions: The end vertebrae (*EV*) define the extent of each curve and are most tilted from horizontal in the coronal plane; the stable vertebra (*SV*) is defined as the vertebra most closely bisected by the CSVL; the neutral vertebra (*NV*) is defined as the least rotated vertebra in the axial plane based on the radiographic symmetry of its pedicles. (©SD PedsOrtho.)

## PATHOGENESIS

- Twin studies and observations of familial aggregation reveal significant genetic contributions to deformity progression.[1,13]
- Increased calmodulin (which regulates the contractile properties of muscles and platelets) and decreased melatonin (a calmodulin antagonist) levels have been found in patients with progressive scoliosis.[7,11]
- Differential growth rates in the anterior and posterior spinal column may cause imbalance in the sagittal plane with subsequent buckling of the vertebral column.[5]

## NATURAL HISTORY

- Risk factors for deformity progression include female gender, greater growth potential, thoracic curve location, and larger curve magnitude.[6,15]
- Radiographic markers of skeletal maturity (state of the triradiate cartilage, Risser sign, carpal ossification, growth centers around the elbow) can be used to define a patient's remaining growth potential.
- After skeletal maturity, curves less than 30 degrees tend not to progress, whereas curves greater than 50 degrees tend to progress about 1 to 2 degrees per year.[19,21]
- Thoracic lordosis and severe scoliosis (>80 degrees) result in restrictive lung disease and decreased pulmonary function.[14,22]

## PATIENT HISTORY AND PHYSICAL FINDINGS

- Document medical history, developmental milestones, growth history, and family history.
- Observation should assess for asymmetries of the neck, shoulders, ribs, waist, and hips. Cutaneous lesions such as hairy patches or sinuses may suggest spinal dysraphism, whereas café-au-lait spots or axillary freckling may suggest neurofibromatosis.
- Adams forward bend test is used to identify a unilateral prominence of the thoracic rib cage or lumbar paraspinal muscles due to axial rotation of the spine.
- Coronal decompensation can be identified as lateral translation of the C7 spinous process in relation to the gluteal cleft.
- Clinical assessment of maturity based on Tanner stage. Peak growth velocity occurs approximately 6 to 12 months prior to the onset of menses in girls and the onset of axillary and facial hair in boys.[17]
- Assessment of functional capacity is performed by analyzing gait, stance, motor and sensory function, and reflexes.

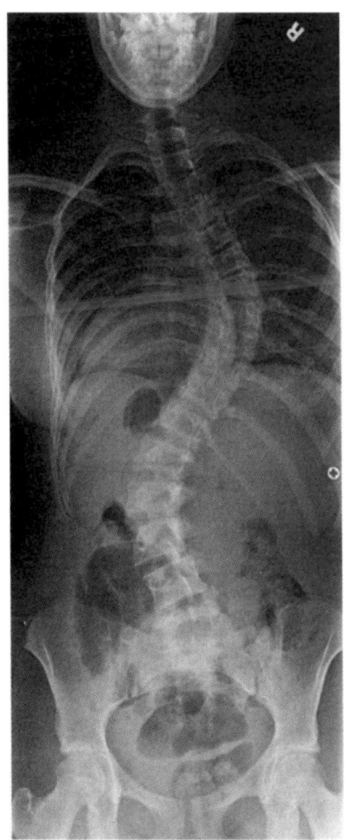

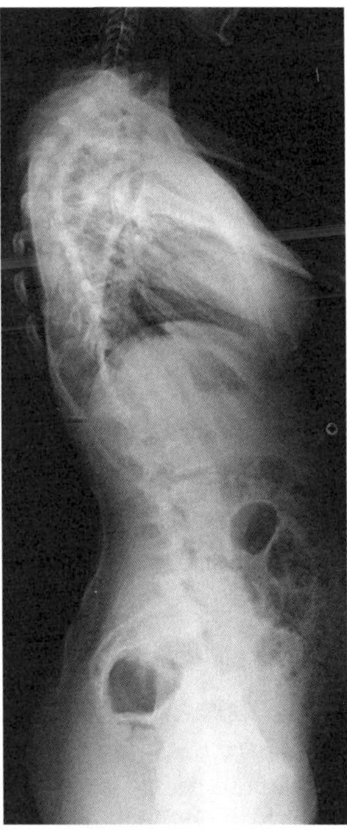

**FIG 2** • Posteroanterior (**A**) and lateral (**B**) radiographs demonstrating a typical right thoracic deformity with apical lordosis. (©SD PedsOrtho.)

- Abdominal reflexes should be assessed to rule out intramedullary lesions. Unilateral absence of the reflex suggests the need for a spine magnetic resonance imaging (MRI).
- Limb length discrepancy can result in apparent scoliosis.

## IMAGING AND OTHER DIAGNOSTIC STUDIES

- Full-length, upright posteroanterior (**FIG 2A**), and lateral (**FIG 2B**) spinal radiographs are adequate for routine assessment.
- Three-dimensional reconstructions using advanced, low-radiation imaging technology can provide important insights into the true scoliotic deformity (**FIG 3**).[4]
- Lateral bending radiographs are important for preoperative planning to determine curve flexibility but are not required otherwise.
- Advanced imaging studies including computed tomography and MRI can be used to identify neurologic or congenital abnormalities.

## DIFFERENTIAL DIAGNOSIS

- Congenital scoliosis (failure of vertebral formation or segmentation)
- Neuromuscular scoliosis (cerebral palsy, spinal muscular atrophy, Duchenne muscular dystrophy)
- Syndromic scoliosis (osteochondrodystrophies, neurofibromatosis, Marfan syndrome)

## NONOPERATIVE MANAGEMENT

- Periodic observational monitoring is appropriate for skeletally immature patients with curves between 11 and 25 degrees. During periods of peak growth, more frequent evaluations (every 4 to 6 months) should be performed.
- Skeletally immature patients (less than Risser 2) with documented curve progression to greater than 25 degrees or 30 degrees on initial presentation can be treated with a rigid thoracolumbosacral orthosis.[2]

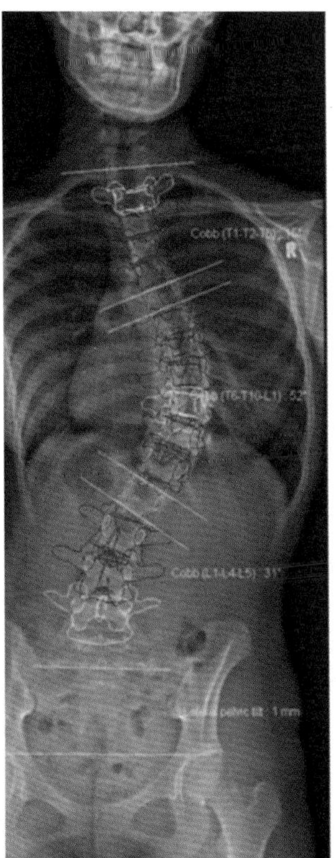


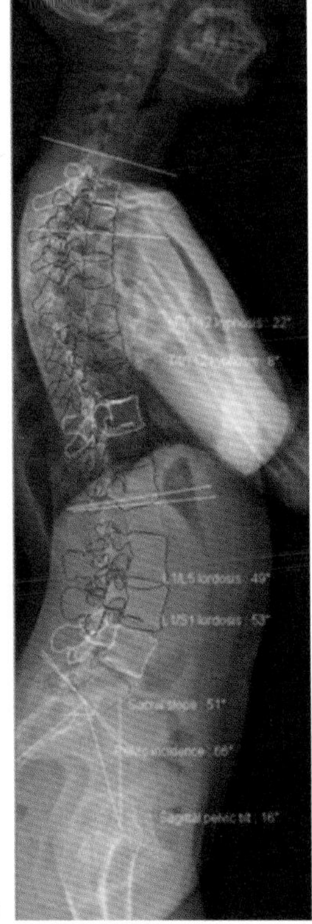


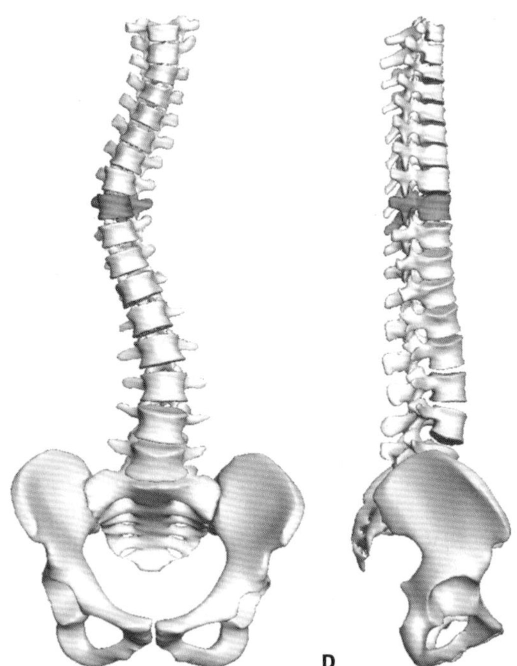

**FIG 3** • Posteroanterior (**A**) and lateral (**B**) EOS images with representative coronal (**C**) and sagittal (**D**) three-dimensional (3-D) reconstructions. (©SD PedsOrtho.)

- Bracing has been shown to successfully decrease the progression of high-risk curves during the adolescent growth spurt. A dose-dependent relationship between hours of brace wear and success with bracing has been identified.[16,20]
- A coordinated effort between the patient, the treating physician, and the orthotist is required to optimize success with bracing.

## SURGICAL MANAGEMENT

- Surgical goals are as follows:
  - Obtain three-dimensional and well-balanced deformity correction while fusing as few motion segments as possible.
  - Obtain a solid arthrodesis to prevent deformity progression.

### Indications

- The decision to proceed with surgical treatment is based on curve magnitude, the clinical deformity, and the risk for further progression.
- In general, skeletally immature patients with progressive curves greater than 45 or 50 degrees or skeletally mature patients with curves greater than 50 degrees can be considered for surgical intervention.

### Preoperative Planning: Fusion Levels

- The primary driver of the scoliotic deformity is either the thoracic curve or the thoracolumbar/lumbar curve.
- Compensatory curves occur adjacent to the primary deformity (major curve) seemingly in an attempt to maintain coronal or sagittal balance.

#### *Thoracic Major Curves*

- The main decision is to selectively fuse the thoracic spine or fuse both the thoracic and lumbar spine. The Lenke classification system can be used to guide this decision.[8]
  - For 1AR curves (main thoracic curve with L4 tilt to the right), the lowest instrumented vertebra (LIV) should be the vertebral body whose concave pedicle is last touched by the CSVL (**FIG 4A**).
  - For 1AL/1B curves (main thoracic curves with L4 tilt to the left), the LIV should be the stable vertebra or one proximal to the stable vertebra but never short of the end vertebra (**FIG 4B**).
  - 1C curves
    - For a selective thoracic fusion, the LIV should be the stable vertebra or one distal to the stable vertebra.
    - With a significantly rotated compensatory lumbar curve, an effort should be made to counter-rotate the distal vertebral body to allow for maximum spontaneous lumbar curve correction.
- Upper instrumented vertebral (UIV) body selection in thoracic primary curves.
  - If the left shoulder is higher than the right shoulder, the UIV should be T1 or T2.
  - If the shoulders are level, the UIV should be T3.
  - If the left shoulder is lower, the UIV should be T4 or T5.
  - The sagittal plane should also be analyzed when selecting the UIV. The instrumented fusion should include any proximal areas of focal hyperkyphosis.

#### *Thoracolumbar/Lumbar Major Curves*

- For thoracolumbar/lumbar and structural thoracolumbar/lumbar curves with major thoracic curves (double major pattern), LIV should be the end vertebra.

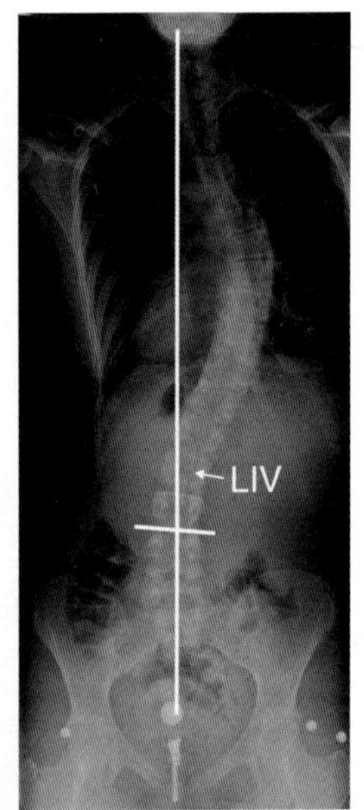


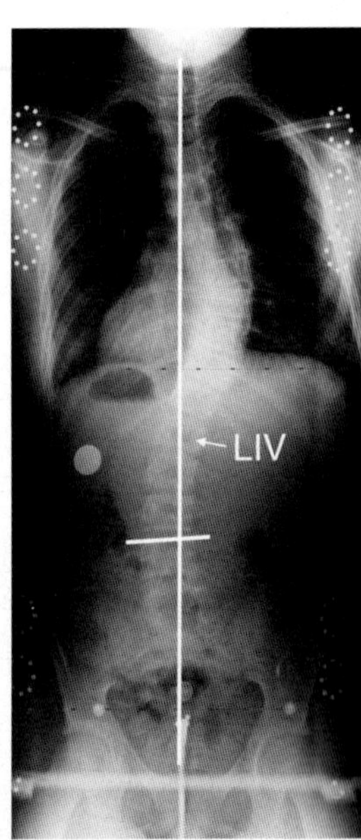


**FIG 4** • **A.** Lenke 1AR curve (L4 tilt to the right) with LIV of L2 (vertebral body whose pedicle is last touched by the CSVL). **B.** Lenke 1B curve (L4 tilt to the left) with LIV of L1 (stable vertebra). (©SD PedsOrtho.)

- Main decision is to fuse to L3 or L4.
  - The LIV should be L3 if the L3–L4 disc is parallel or wedged open opposite to the side of the apex of the curve.
  - The LIV should be L4 if the L3–L4 disc is wedged open in the same direction as the apex of the curve (ie, L4 is the end vertebra) (**FIG 5**).
- The UIV should be the end vertebra or more proximal if thoracolumbar junctional kyphosis is present. Use the thoracic curve UIV criteria if both thoracic and lumbar curves are being fused.

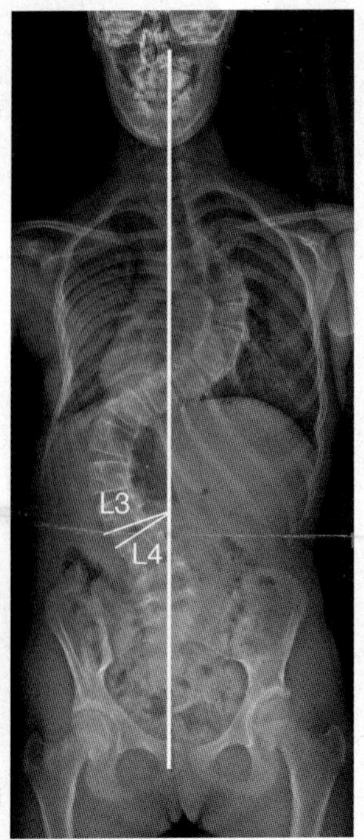


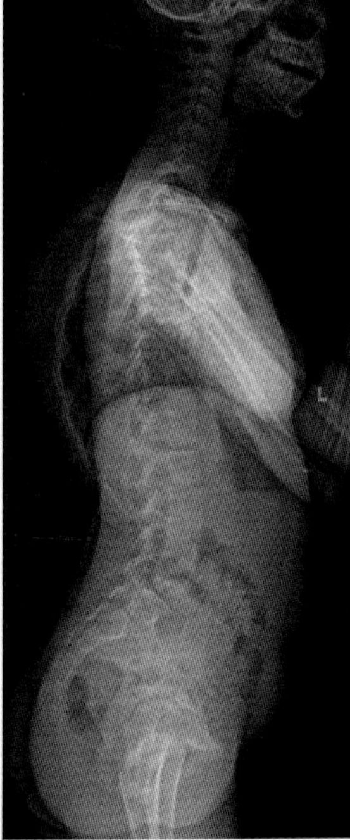


**FIG 5** • Posteroanterior (**A**) and lateral (**B**) radiographs of a double major curve with the L3–L4 disc open toward the apex. (©SD PedsOrtho.)

## Posterior Spinal Exposure and Instrumentation

- Standard posterior spinal exposure with segmental facetectomies and pedicle screw placement (detailed description in Chap. 84) (**TECH FIG 1A–C**).
- Proximal foundation of four fixation points
  - We prefer to use hooks at the most proximal level to limit soft tissue dissection and provide a less rigid transition to the uninstrumented spine in an effort to minimize proximal junctional kyphosis.
- High-density fixation on the concavity of the deformity to resist the posteriorly directed loads involved in correcting the lordotic thoracic spine.
  - Fewer fixation points are required on the convexity, as the deformity correction forces are anteriorly directed at the apex (**TECH FIG 1D,E**).
- Distal foundation of four fixation points.
- What if proximal pedicle screw fixation is limited secondary to anatomic deformity or missed screw placement?
  - Hooks can be used to create a claw construct on the right proximal end of construct (proximal transverse process hook and adjacent pedicle hook) and upgoing hooks can be used on the left proximal end (pedicle hooks).

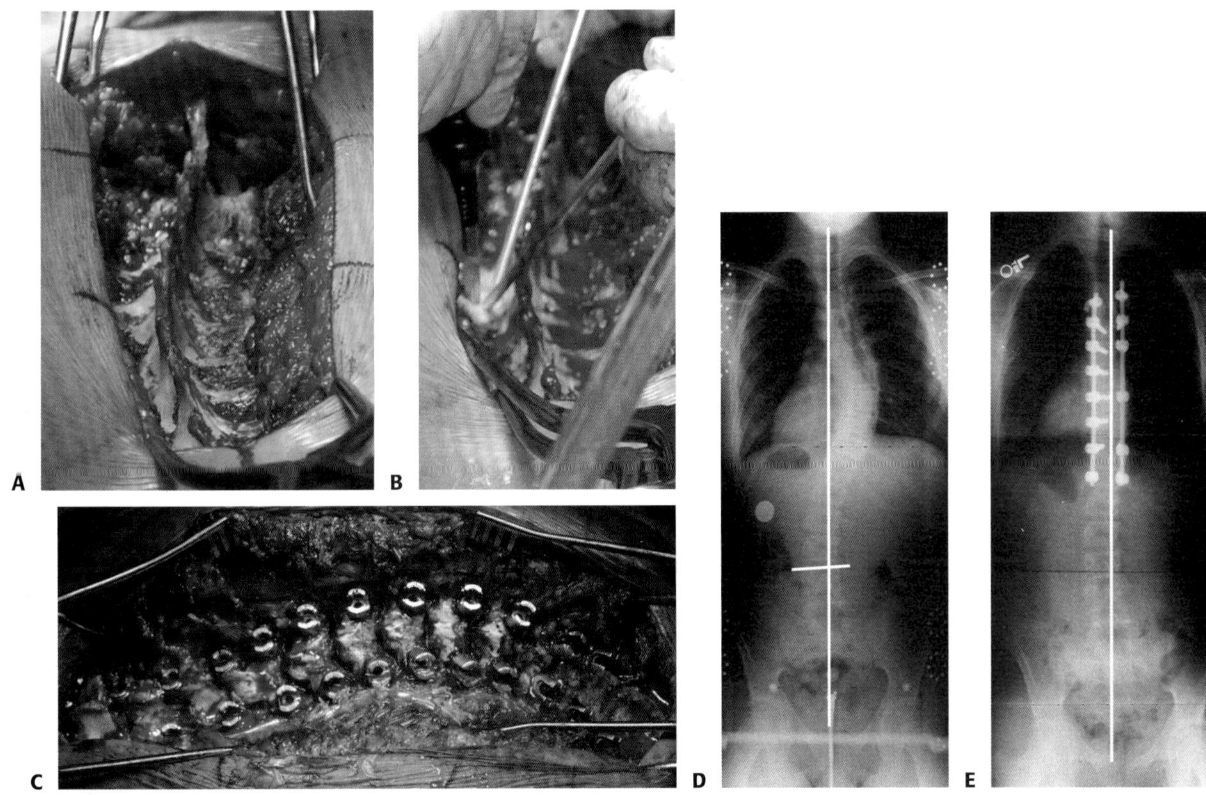

**TECH FIG 1** • **A.** Posterior spinal exposure. **B.** Ultrasonic bone scalpel (Misonix, Inc., Farmingdale, NY) used to perform facetectomies. **C.** Uniplanar pedicle screws placed segmentally using freehand technique. **D.** Posteroanterior radiograph of a Lenke 1AL curve (L4 tilt to the left). **E.** After posterior instrumented spinal fusion from T5 to T12. LIV is one proximal to stable. High-density fixation used on the concavity of the deformity and low density on the convexity. (**A–C:** ©SD PedsOrtho.)

## Deformity Correction Technique

- Posterior spinal releases (Ponte-type osteotomy) should be performed at the apex of the deformity based on the amount of sagittal plane correction required (**TECH FIG 2**).

### Aggressive Differential Rod Contouring

- Overbend kyphosis in concave rod and underbend kyphosis on convexity (**TECH FIG 3A,B**)
- Change in rod shape (unbending during rod approximation) determines the force of correction (**TECH FIG 3C**).
- Rod shape, material, and diameter are the primary determinants of correction (**TECH FIG 3D**):
  - High-strength rods: stainless steel or cobalt chromium
  - Low-strength rods: titanium

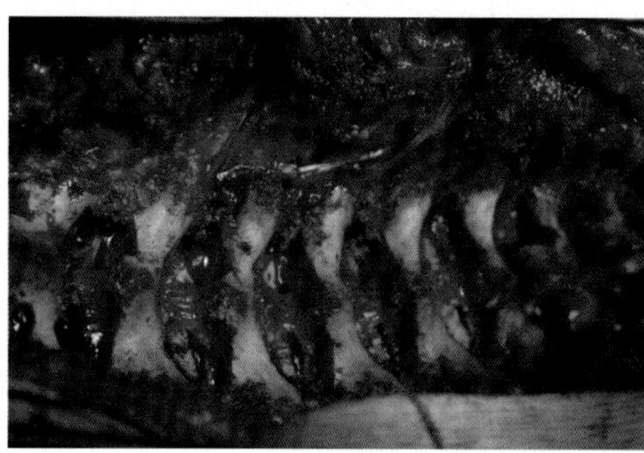

**TECH FIG 2** • Ponte-type osteotomies with excision of the spinous process, intraspinous ligaments, superior articulating facet, capsule, and ligamentum flavum. (©SD PedsOrtho.)

### Rod Insertion

- Concave rod is inserted first and rotated into position to obtain initial deformity correction (**TECH FIG 4A**). Anteriorly directed counterforce applied to the convex rib hump to limit increasing rotational deformity (**TECH FIG 4B**).
- Convex rod is inserted proximally and cantilevered into distal fixation points (**TECH FIG 4C**). This second rod applies anteriorly directed force on the convexity of the spine and results in axial derotation of the vertebral bodies (**TECH FIG 4D**).

### Segmental Vertebral Manipulation and Completion

- The rods are then locked into proper sagittal plane only at the neutral vertebra.
- Starting at the neutral vertebra, each segment is then manipulated (moving proximal one level at a time up to the apex of the deformity) in three-dimensional space to assist the rod in regaining some of its original shape (**TECH FIG 5**).
- Segmental distraction in the concavity and compression on the convexity are used to increase kyphosis and improve coronal plane deformity.
- Decortication of the posterior elements is performed. Vancomycin powder, local bone autograft and allograft are placed to achieve a midline arthrodesis.

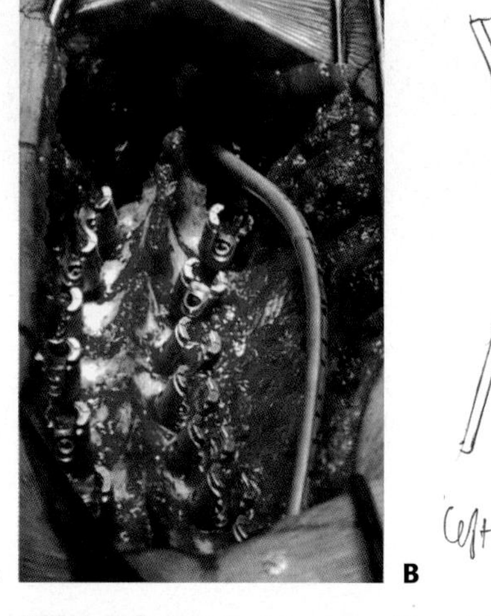


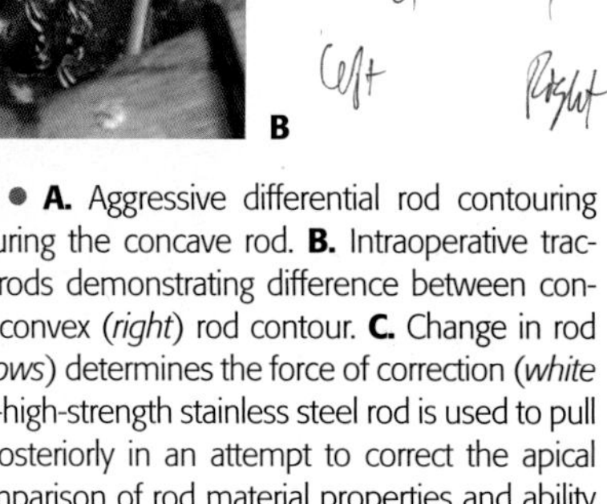


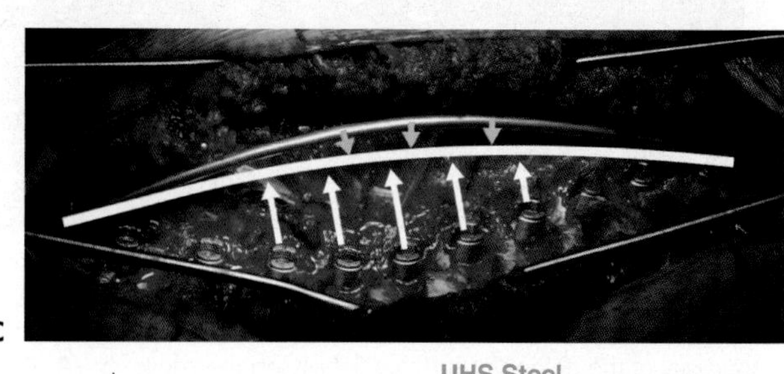


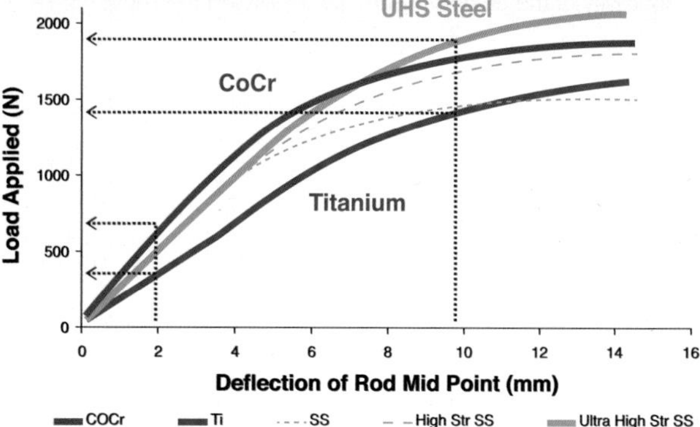

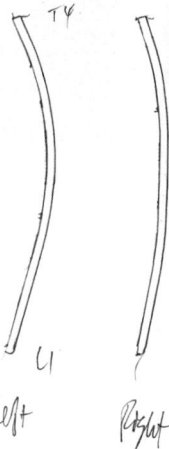

**TECH FIG 3** • **A.** Aggressive differential rod contouring with overcontouring the concave rod. **B.** Intraoperative tracing of the two rods demonstrating difference between concave (*left*) and convex (*right*) rod contour. **C.** Change in rod shape (*blue arrows*) determines the force of correction (*white arrow*). An ultra-high-strength stainless steel rod is used to pull the concavity posteriorly in an attempt to correct the apical lordosis. **D.** Comparison of rod material properties and ability to withstand plastic deformation. (**A,C:** ©SD PedsOrtho.)

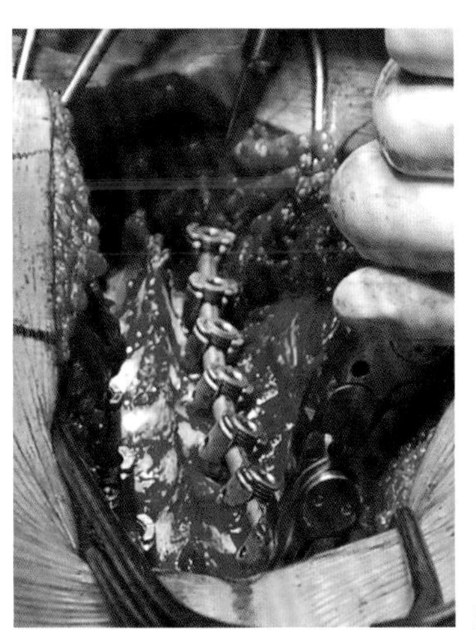
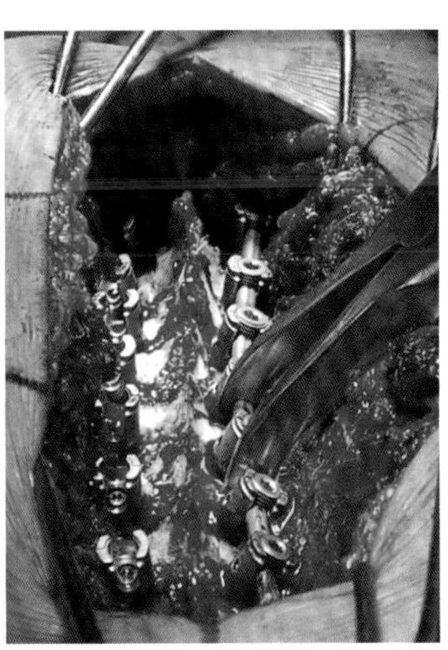
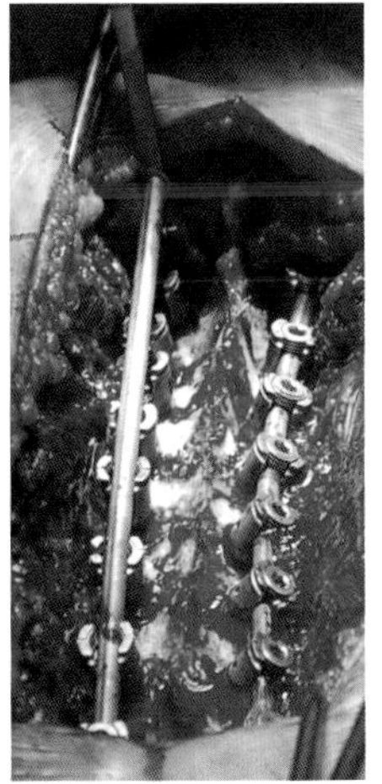
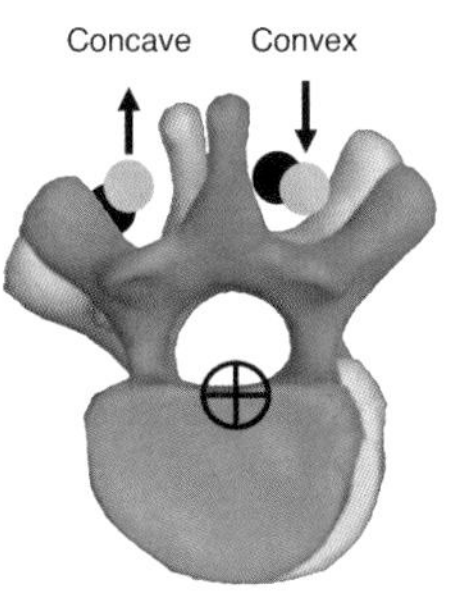


**TECH FIG 4** • **A.** The concave, overcontoured rod is inserted first and rotated into position while applying an anteriorly directed force on the contralateral ribs. **B.** Distraction is used to lengthen the posterior column, correct the apical lordosis, and allow the rod to spring back and regain some of its precontoured shape. **C.** The convex rod is then inserted and cantilevered into the distal fixation. **D.** Differential rod contouring indirectly enables vertebral derotation about a point in the posterior vertebral body (typical center of axial rotation). (©SD PedsOrtho.)

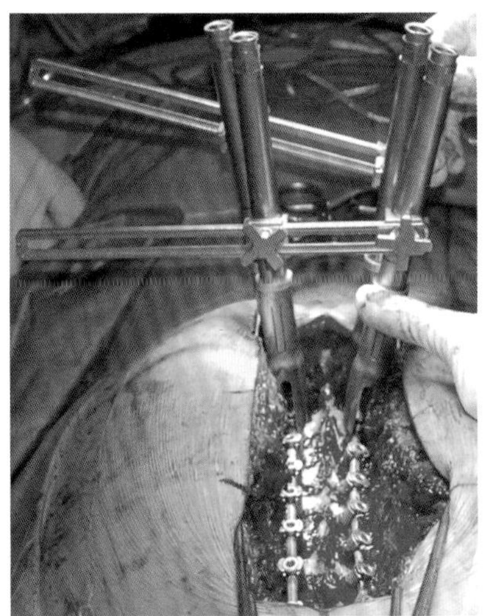
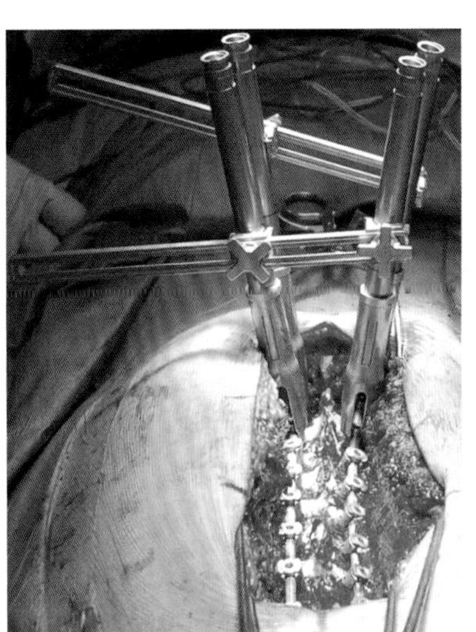
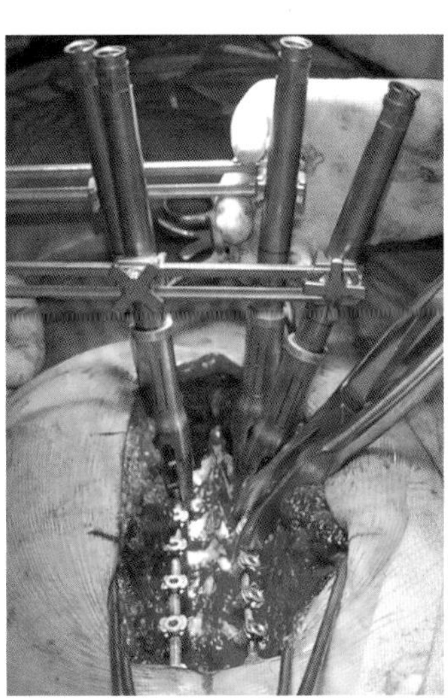
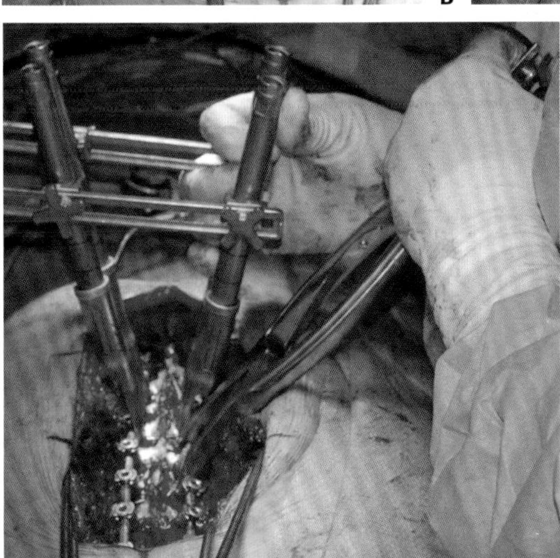

**TECH FIG 5** • Segmental vertebral manipulation is performed starting at the neutral vertebra and working proximal one level at a time toward the apex of the deformity. **A.** Premanipulation at T11–T12 (neutral vertebra). **B.** Postmanipulation at T11–T12. **C.** Premanipulation at T10–T11. **D.** Postmanipulation at T10–T11. Simultaneous distraction in the concavity allows further three-dimensional deformity correction. (©SD PedsOrtho.)

## PEARLS AND PITFALLS

| | |
|---|---|
| **Perform a closing timeout to ensure all essential steps are completed.** | ▪ Final set screw tightening, decortication, bone graft and antibiotic powder placement, and post-deformity correction neuromonitoring. |
| **Overcorrection of the thoracic curve** | ▪ Iatrogenic elevation of the left shoulder can occur.<br>▪ Nonstructural upper thoracic curves based on the Lenke classification guidelines (bend to <25 degrees) may need to be included in the instrumentation and fusion to control postoperative shoulder height. |
| **Immature patients with open triradiate cartilage** | ▪ Deformity progression and/or crankshaft may occur.<br>▪ Consider concomitant anterior fusion procedures to avoid this complication. |
| **Axial plane correction (vertebral derotation)** | ▪ Iatrogenic thoracic flatback can occur without posterior column lengthening.<br>▪ Ponte-type osteotomies allow correction of thoracic lordosis to achieve three-dimensional deformity correction. |
| **Wide posterior releases (Ponte-type osteotomies)** | ▪ Should be covered with long strips of autograft to protect the neural elements and avoid bone graft in the canal. |

## POSTOPERATIVE CARE

- The patient is admitted to the orthopaedic floor postoperatively.
- Patient-controlled analgesia used postoperatively and transitioned to oral narcotic medication once tolerating fluids.
- Physical therapy begins on the first postoperative day to sit and stand with assistance. Progression to ambulation on subsequent days.
- No postoperative bracing is required.
- Upright postoperative radiographs can be used to assess three-dimensional deformity correction (**FIG 6**).
  - Axial plane correction can be approximated by assessing the position of bilateral pedicle screw tips in relation to the rods on a posteroanterior radiograph[18] or the projection of the rods in relation to one another on the lateral radiograph.[9]

## OUTCOMES

- Expect 50% to 70% correction of the coronal plane deformity. May consider undercorrection in a selective thoracic fusion to balance the lumbar coronal plane deformity.
- Expect about 50% rib hump correction despite advanced techniques to axially derotate vertebral bodies (likely secondary to rib deformity).
- Preservation of a greater number of vertebral motion segments allows for greater distribution of functional motion across the remaining unfused levels.[12]

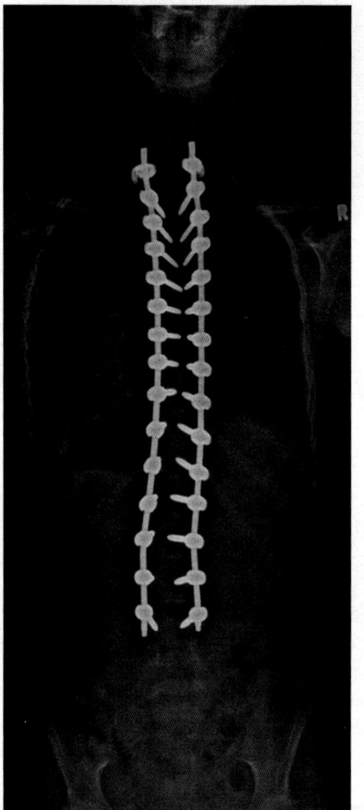


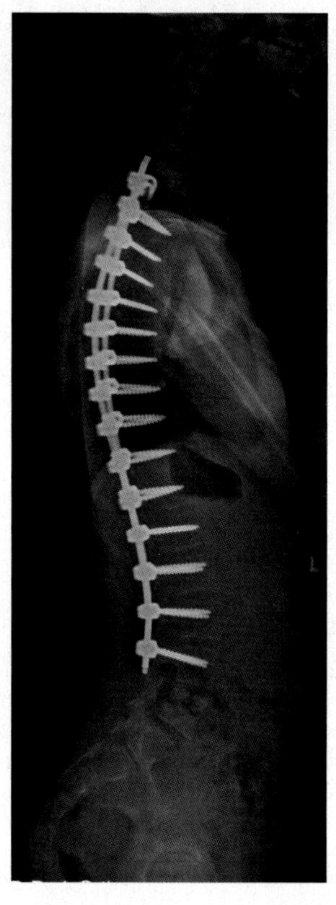


**FIG 6** • Posteroanterior (**A**) and lateral (**B**) radiographs after a T2–L4 posterior instrumented spinal fusion in the patient in **FIG 5**. (©SD PedsOrtho.)

- Recent meta-analysis of mid- to long-term outcomes (average 14.9 year follow-up) after three commonly used posterior spinal instrumentation and fusion techniques demonstrated that Harrington rods had a detrimental effect on the sagittal alignment. Cotrel-Dubousset constructs resulted in a greater degree of correction in the coronal and sagittal planes; however, all-pedicle screw constructs showed lower risk of complications or need for revision surgery.[10]

## COMPLICATIONS

- Most common complications of posterior procedures for idiopathic scoliosis are instrumentation related (1.6%) and wound related (1.2%).
- Instrumentation complications: broken rods/screws, misplaced screws, proximal junctional kyphosis, screw loosening, pseudarthrosis
- Wound complications: erythema, hypertrophic scar, pain, dehiscence, hematoma, seroma, abscess/deep infection
- Balance complications: deformity progression, adding-on, crankshaft
- Medical complications: blindness, death, myocardial infarction, vocal cord paresis, gastrointestinal complications
- Pulmonary complications: aspiration, atelectasis, hemithorax, pneumonia, pleural effusion
- Neurologic complications: decreased neuromonitoring signals, paresthesias, femoral cutaneous neuralgia, lower extremity weakness, pain
- Hematologic complications: require blood transfusion, excessive blood loss, transfusion reaction

## REFERENCES


1. Andersen MO, Thomsen K, Kyvik KO. Adolescent idiopathic scoliosis in twins: a population-based survey. Spine 2007;32:927–930.
2. Blount WP. Use of the Milwaukee brace. Orthop Clin North Am 1972;3:3–16.
3. Dickson RA. Conservative treatment for idiopathic scoliosis. J Bone Joint Surg Br 1985;67:176–181.
4. Glaser DA, Doan J, Newton PO. Comparison of 3-dimensional spinal reconstruction accuracy: biplanar radiographs with EOS versus computed tomography. Spine 2012;37:1391–1397.
5. Guo X, Chau WW, Chan YL, et al. Relative anterior spinal overgrowth in adolescent idiopathic scoliosis: results of disproportionate endochondral-membranous bone growth. J Bone Joint Surg Br 2003;85:1026–1031.
6. Karol LA, Johnston CE II, Browne RH, et al. Progression of the curve in boys who have idiopathic scoliosis. J Bone Joint Surg Am 1993;75:1804–1810.
7. Kindsfater K, Lowe T, Lawellin D, et al. Levels of platelet calmodulin for the prediction of progression and severity of adolescent idiopathic scoliosis. J Bone Joint Surg Am 1994;76:1186–1192.
8. Lenke LG, Betz RR, Harms J, et al. Adolescent idiopathic scoliosis: a new classification to determine extent of spinal arthrodesis. J Bone Joint Surg Am 2001;83:1169–1181.
9. Liu RW, Yaszay B, Glaser D, et al. A method for assessing axial vertebral rotation based on differential rod curvature on the lateral radiograph. Spine 2012;37:E1120–E1125.
10. Lykissas MG, Jain VV, Nathan ST, et al. Mid- to long-term outcomes in adolescent idiopathic scoliosis after instrumented posterior spinal fusion: a meta-analysis. Spine 2013;38:E113–E119.
11. Machida M, Dubousset J, Imamura Y, et al. Melatonin. A possible role in pathogenesis of adolescent idiopathic scoliosis. Spine 1996;21:1147–1152.
12. Marks M, Newton PO, Petcharaporn M, et al. Postoperative segmental motion of the unfused spine distal to the fusion in 100 patients with adolescent idiopathic scoliosis. Spine 2012;37:826–832.
13. Ogilvie JW, Braun J, Argyle V, et al. The search for idiopathic scoliosis genes. Spine 2006;31:679–681.
14. Pehrsson K, Bake B, Larsson S, et al. Lung function in adult idiopathic scoliosis: a 20 year follow up. Thorax 1991;46:474–478.
15. Peterson LE, Nachemson AL. Prediction of progression of the curve in girls who have adolescent idiopathic scoliosis of moderate severity. Logistic regression analysis based on data from The Brace Study of the Scoliosis Research Society. J Bone Joint Surg Am 1995;77:823–827.
16. Rowe DE, Bernstein SM, Riddick MF, et al. A meta-analysis of the efficacy of non-operative treatments for idiopathic scoliosis. J Bone Joint Surg Am 1997;79:664–674.
17. Sanders JO, Little DG, Richards BS. Prediction of the crankshaft phenomenon by peak height velocity. Spine 1997;22:1352–1356.
18. Upasani VV, Chambers RC, Dalal AH, et al. Grading apical vertebral rotation without a computed tomography scan: a clinically relevant system based on the radiographic appearance of bilateral pedicle screws. Spine 2009;34:1855–1862.
19. Weinstein SL. Idiopathic scoliosis. Natural history. Spine 1986;11:780–783.
20. Weinstein SL, Dolan LA, Wright JG, et al. Effects of bracing in adolescents with idiopathic scoliosis. N Engl J Med 2013;369:1512–1521.
21. Weinstein SL, Ponseti IV. Curve progression in idiopathic scoliosis. J Bone Joint Surg Am 1983;65:447–455.
22. Winter RB, Lovell WW, Moe JH. Excessive thoracic lordosis and loss of pulmonary function in patients with idiopathic scoliosis. J Bone Joint Surg Am 1975;57:972–977.

CHAPTER

# Posterior Osteotomies of the Spine

Daniel Grant, Leok-Lim Lau, and Suken A. Shah

## DEFINITION

- Spinal osteotomies encompass a range of techniques involving resection of bone from the spinal column to induce flexibility and correct rigid pediatric spinal deformity. These osteotomies can resect the deformity or create more mobility in the spine to allow for deformity correction.
- The types of spinal osteotomies include the following:
  - Ponte osteotomy
  - Smith-Petersen osteotomy (SPO)
  - Pedicle subtraction osteotomy (PSO)
  - Vertebral column resection (VCR)
- The aim of correction varies from a balanced correction to complete correction in the coronal, sagittal, and axial planes.
  - A balanced correction improves the deformity by maintaining the skull and trunk over the pelvis without a straight spine while keeping the spine in an acceptable sagittal position.
  - A complete correction aims to achieve a straight spine in coronal plane with the skull and trunk over the pelvis both in the coronal and sagittal planes.
- Achieving good sagittal alignment correlates with improved quality of life in adults. In children, its usefulness is desirable but less obvious because children and young adults can compensate for regional malalignment to maintain balance.
- Spinal osteotomies have inherent risks, particularly neurologic deficit and bleeding.
  - Neurologic deficits can come about directly or indirectly; care must be taken to avoid direct spinal cord contusion, manipulation, or spinal column subluxation in the course of the osteotomy and destabilization procedure. Excessive distraction and conversely significant spinal cord shortening can cause ischemia and neurologic deficit.
  - Below the conus medullaris, attention should be focused on prevention of nerve root injury.
  - Multimodality intraoperative neurologic monitoring (IONM) should be employed to detect impending neurologic deficit in real time and allow proper intraoperative intervention and reduce risk of permanent deficit.
  - Risk of complications is high and should be discussed with the patient's family to manage expectations.
  - Blood loss may be significant and involve transfusion of blood and/or components. The use of antifibrinolytics such as tranexamic acid (TXA) may reduce intraoperative blood loss.
  - Transcranial motor evoked potential (TcMEP) monitoring allows direct surveillance of the anterior motor pathway, whereas somatosensory evoked potential (SSEP) allows surveillance of the posterior columnar sensory pathway. The loss of MEP data with normal SSEP registration has been reported to occur with an incidence up to 20%.[2]
- Ponte osteotomy: wide resection of the posterior elements involving removal of the superior and inferior articular facets, the interspinous ligament, the cephalad spinous process with a portion of the lamina, and the ligamentum flavum. Thought to hinge at the posterior longitudinal ligament (PLL) as the fulcrum of correction and may open the disc space anteriorly. Up to 5 to 10 degrees of angular correction is possible for each level where this is performed.
  - Originally described for kyphosis correction by Alberto Ponte, this technique is now used for scoliosis and lordosis as well as kyphosis due to its versatility.
- SPO: wedge-shaped osteotomy through the posterior elements of a previously fused or autofused spine
  - Frequently, this term is used interchangeably with a Ponte osteotomy, but the definition is clear.
- PSO: Three-column resection in which the posterior elements, the pedicles, and a vertebral wedge are resected and the fulcrum is at the anterior portion of the vertebral body. This allows for the generation of approximately 30 degrees of lordosis and is commonly used for fixed sagittal imbalance or focal, rigid kyphosis.
- VCR: involves complete resection of a vertebra with discs above and below, resulting in three-column destabilization, allowing for significant deformity correction not obtainable by any other means.
- A classification of spinal osteotomies (Table 1) is a useful aid to understand the degrees of the spinal releases, destabilization, and power of correction.
  - Ponte osteotomy or SPO is a grade 2 spinal osteotomy.
  - PSO is graded as 3 or 4, whereas VCR is graded as 5 or 6, depending on the extent of the resection.

## ANATOMY

- Kyphosis of the thoracic spine is normally between 10 and 40 degrees.[6]
- Lordosis of the lumbar spine averages around 40 to 60 degrees.[6]
- Lordosis is also present in the cervical spine.
- The C7 plumb line, which is a measure of overall sagittal balance, is a straight line drawn vertically through the center of the C7 vertebral body that should cross the S1 vertebral body at its posterosuperior edge.[6] This is called the *sagittal vertical axis* (SVA).
- Vertebral anatomy
  - The spinous processes of the thoracic vertebrae are shingled and cover the interlaminar space. The spinous processes of the lumbar vertebrae are more horizontal in profile, especially, at the caudal part of the spinal column. This makes the interlaminar space more uncovered and accessible.
  - The laminae are thicker laterally than medially.

**Table 1 Spinal Osteotomy Classification**

| Grade | Anatomic Resection | Description |
|---|---|---|
| 1 | Partial facet joint | Resection of inferior joint facet and joint capsule |
| 2 | Complete facet joint | Both superior and inferior facets at a spinal segment are resected with complete ligamentum flavum removal; other posterior elements including lamina and spinous process may be resected (Ponte osteotomy). |
| 3 | Pedicle/partial body | Partial wedge resection of the posterior vertebral body and posterior elements with pedicles (PSO) |
| 4 | Pedicel/partial body/disc | Wider wedge resection of a substantial portion of the vertebral body, posterior elements with pedicles, and includes resection of one endplate and adjacent intervertebral disc |
| 5 | Complete vertebra and discs | Complete removal of a vertebra and both adjacent discs (VCR) |
| 6 | Multiple vertebrae and discs | Resection of more than one entire vertebra and adjacent discs (VCR+) |

Adapted from Schwab F, Blondel B, Chay E, et al. The comprehensive anatomical spinal osteotomy classification. Neurosurgery 2014;74:112–120.

  - Facet joint orientation (supine position) in the thoracic spine is more horizontal to facilitate lateral bending and rotation; in the lumbar spine, the facets are oriented vertically to promote flexion and extension.
  - The ligamentum flavum originates from the superior margin of a lamina and extends cephalad to attach to the inner surface of the lamina above it. The attachment at the cephalad lamina is more lateral compared to the attachment at the caudal lamina which is more medial. Ligamentum flavum is deficient at the midline as it meets at the raphe.
- The thoracic pedicles origination and orientation vary based on their location in the spine.[8]
  - Proximal thoracic spine (T1–T2): The starting point is at the junction between the midpoint of the transverse process and the lamina at the region of the lateral pars. Twenty-five to 30 degrees of medial angulation exists.
  - Middle thoracic spine (T7–T9): The origin of the pedicle is at the junction of the proximal transverse process and lateral to the middle of the base of the superior articular facet. About 5 degrees of medial angulation is present.
  - Lower thoracic spine (T11–T12): The pedicles start at the midpoint of the transverse process and medial to the lateral aspect of the pars. They are perpendicular in the transverse plane to the vertebral body.
  - In deformities such as scoliosis, considerable rotational variability and dysmorphism of thoracic pedicles are encountered.
- The lumbar superior and inferior articular facets are oriented approximately 45 degrees from the coronal plane with the articular surface facing posterior medially and anterior laterally, respectively. The lumbar pedicle starting point is at the lateral aspect of the pars and the midpoint of the transverse process at the inferior edge of the articular process.
  - The upper lumbar vertebral pedicles are perpendicular to the vertebral body in the transverse plane, but the pedicles gradually angle laterally to medial in the lower lumbar region to reach a transverse pedicle angle of 25 to 30 degrees at L5.[17]
- Spinal cord and spinal column growth
  - There is differential growth between spinal column and spinal cord. For most of the period of fetal development, the spinal cord ends at the lower lumbar spine, but the spinal column grows faster than the neural elements. The spinal cord terminates at the L1 vertebra, which is its final position 2 months after birth.
  - The most rapid growth rate happens in utero. After birth, the first peak growth period of the spine occurs in the first 5 years of life. The second growth peak occurs just prior to and includes puberty.
  - In boys, the remaining growth at age 5 years before the onset of puberty is 18 cm and at the onset of puberty is 13 cm.
  - In girls, the remaining growth at age 5 years before the onset of puberty is 14 cm and at the onset of puberty is 12 cm.
  - Spinal canal achieves 95% of its adult size and 70% of the spinal height at the age of 5 years. The neurocentral synchondrosis closes at the age of 9 years.[1,4]
- The effect of posterior spinal fusion on an immature spine
  - Lung growth continues until the age of 9 years. This is supported by a rib-sternal-vertebrae housing. A thoracic spine height of at least 18 to 22 cm is necessary to avoid thoracic insufficiency syndrome.[7]
  - Assuming growth ceases at 14 years in girls and 16 years in boys, 0.7 mm per year of longitudinal growth per vertebra is lost after spinal fusion in the immature spine for thoracic vertebrae and up to 1.2 mm per year of remaining growth per lumbar level.[4]
  - Crankshaft phenomenon—continued anterior growth with a posterior tether (fusion) may cause deformity recurrence through rotation of the previously fused spine.
  - It is postulated that the loss of correction postimplant removal after posterior spinal fusion is less of a problem, as some late anterior column growth helps to buttress the spine against kyphosis.[3]

## PATHOGENESIS

### Scoliosis

- Scoliosis is a spinal curvature with a Cobb angle of greater than 10 degrees measured in the coronal plane. It is typically a three-dimensional (3-D) deformity involving the coronal, sagittal, and transverse planes.
- Congenital
  - This occurs as a result of malformation of vertebral elements due to a failure of formation, failure of segmentation, or a combination of the two.

- Failure of formation includes hemivertebra and wedged vertebra.
- Failure of segmentation includes block vertebrae and unilateral bars.
- There can be mixed deformities with bizarre combinations of the previously discussed as well as rib deformities.
- Idiopathic
  - Three different subtypes were described by James:
    - Infantile scoliosis develops between 2 months and 3 years of age.
    - Juvenile scoliosis develops between 3 and 10 years of age and is often associated with intraspinal pathology.
    - Adolescent (adolescent idiopathic scoliosis [AIS]) develops after 10 years of age and prior to skeletal maturity.
  - This classification has now been supplanted by early (usually before age 5 years) and late-onset idiopathic scoliosis, reflecting the velocity of growth prior to age 5 years.
  - Idiopathic scoliosis appears to be a multifactorial process for which the etiology is not yet clearly understood, although may be related to genetics, abnormalities of skeletal growth or the nervous system, biomechanical or biochemical factors, and environmental factors.
- Neuromuscular
  - This is a broad category representing multiple etiologies with various presentations with spastic and paralytic conditions.
  - Some of these conditions include cerebral palsy, Freidreich ataxia, myelomeningocele, and spinal cord injury.
- Syndromic scoliosis includes causes such as neurofibromatosis, skeletal dysplasias, osteogenesis imperfecta, and Down syndrome.
- Neurogenic scoliosis includes causes such as Chiari malformation, syringomyelia, and tethered cord.

### Kyphosis

- Kyphosis describes flexion of the spine in the sagittal plane beyond 40 degrees in the thoracic spine.
- Scheuermann kyphosis involves at least 5 degrees of anterior wedging of three consecutive vertebrae, Schmorl nodes, and endplate irregularities (Sorensen criteria).
- Congenital kyphosis can occur due to failure of formation of the vertebral body, failure of separation of the anterior vertebral body, or a combination of these.

## NATURAL HISTORY

- Idiopathic scoliosis
  - Progression has been noted to be associated with growth, with the highest risk at or just after peak height velocity and in large curves.
  - Curves of less than 30 degrees in the thoracic spine do not typically continue to progress after maturity.
  - Curves of 50 to 75 degrees at skeletal maturity, especially thoracic curves, have been noted to consistently progress, with rates of progression of around 1 degree per year. Large deformities in adulthood can cause pain, coronal and/or sagittal imbalance, concerns about appearance, and significant disability.
  - A trend toward increased back pain exists in patients with AIS in adulthood, although most patients stated this pain was moderate or less.[14]
- Congenital scoliosis: The greatest rate of progression is seen in patients having a unilateral bar with a contralateral hemivertebra, followed by a unilateral bar, and then by two unilateral hemivertebrae.
- Scheuermann kyphosis: Patients have a tendency for some increase in kyphosis when followed into adulthood and increased back pain when compared to age-matched cohorts.[16]
- Congenital kyphosis: These vertebral malformations have the potential to progress rapidly and result in neurologic compromise, especially the posterolateral quadrant failure of formation type of anomaly.

## PATIENT HISTORY AND PHYSICAL FINDINGS

- The initial onset of the spinal deformity can be important for assessing the etiology of the condition (ie, congenital, infantile, juvenile, or adolescent scoliosis).
- Symptoms such as pain may be related to the spinal deformity or may be a sign of other intraspinal pathology and thus should be evaluated.
- It is important to assess for symptoms of neurologic compromise, such as bowel or bladder incontinence, numbness, tingling, asymmetric reflexes, or weakness.
- Evaluate for truncal shift, shoulder height asymmetry, and waist asymmetry, as well as the patient's sagittal alignment for kyphosis and lordosis.
- On the Adams forward bend test, lumbar or thoracic prominences can be evaluated and provide insight in the rotational deformity of the spine.
- Understanding the underlying medical conditions of the patient is essential when evaluating the risks and goals of these procedures, for example, presence of congenital heart disease or prior thoracotomy or radiation can increase the risk of scoliosis.

## IMAGING AND OTHER DIAGNOSTIC STUDIES

- Full-length posteroanterior (PA) and lateral spine erect x-rays are essential to the evaluation and surgical planning for spinal deformities.
- Bending, traction, and/or bolster films are helpful in determining the flexibility index of the spine and thus the likelihood that osteotomies may need to be done.
- With complex congenital abnormalities or deformity, computed tomography (CT) scans with 3-D reconstruction provide additional information about the morphology of the spine.
- A magnetic resonance imaging (MRI) can reveal intraspinal pathology and further anatomic details. Frequently, these are obtained in individuals requiring significant spinal osteotomies due to concern for intraspinal pathology (eg, syrinx, tethered cord).
- A dual energy x-ray absorptiometry (DEXA) scan may be valuable if there is concern for underlying osteopenia.
- Consider echocardiogram and renal ultrasound in patients with congenital scoliosis.

## DIFFERENTIAL DIAGNOSIS

- Congenital scoliosis or kyphosis
- Idiopathic scoliosis: infantile, juvenile, or adolescent
- Neuromuscular scoliosis
- Scheuermann kyphosis
- Prior spinal fusion

## NONOPERATIVE MANAGEMENT

- Nonoperative management typically consists of observation or bracing.
- Observation is typically indicated for scoliotic curves less than 25 degrees in skeletally immature patients and for thoracic kyphosis of less than 60 degrees.
- Bracing is indicated in skeletally immature children with scoliotic curves of 25 to 40 degrees. Brace use of 13 to 22 hours per day results in a 90% to 93% success rate in avoiding surgical intervention.[15]
- Bracing and physical therapy for Scheuermann kyphosis may be used to assist with pain reduction.

## SURGICAL MANAGEMENT

- The main goal of spinal osteotomies is to increase the mobility of the spine to aid with deformity correction.
- The aim of the correction varies from a complete correction in both the coronal and sagittal planes to a balanced correction. A complete correction aims to achieve a straight spine in the coronal plane with the skull over the pelvis both in the coronal and sagittal planes. A balanced correction improves the deformity by maintaining the skull over the pelvis without a straight spine coronally while keeping the spine in an acceptable sagittal position.
- Determining which osteotomy to perform largely depends on the anatomy, magnitude of the deformity, underlying cause of the spinal deformity, and the experience of the surgeon.
- A focal deformity over fewer vertebral segments often requires osteotomies that can create more acute correction such as PSO or VCR.
- A global deformity over more vertebral levels may be adequately addressed using Ponte osteotomies.
- Preoperative halo-gravity traction may improve some of the severe spinal deformities to the extent that a VCR is averted.
- Spinal osteotomies typically involve a learning curve. A pathway in developing the skillset of the spinal osteotomies is shown in **FIG 1**.

### Preoperative Planning

- Review of all medical imaging and understanding of the patient's spinal deformity and anatomy is essential.
- Determining the osteotomies to be performed and the levels at which they will be performed is important as well as the type and levels of spinal fixation. Identifying levels intraoperatively can be difficult.

**Pathway in Spinal Osteotomies**

1. Multilevel posterior (Ponte) osteotomy
2. Anterior Surgery
   - corpectomy vs. discectomy
3. Hemivertebra excision
   - Anterior vs. posterior
4. PSO
5. VCR
   - Anterior vs. posterior

Deformity correction = Spinal instability

**FIG 1** ● There is a graduated progression of spinal osteotomies in that with increasing spinal destabilization comes increased correction power (and risk).

- A preoperative hemoglobin and hematocrit should be drawn. Autologous donor blood may be obtained. The patient should be typed and screened for potential transfusion. Intraoperative cell salvage machine (cell saver) is used to decrease transfusions. TXA is used intraoperatively to reduce blood loss.
- A preoperative urinalysis evaluating for an active urinary tract infection should be obtained.
- Metabolic panels and clotting profiles should also be evaluated.
- Skin of the back is evaluated for possible dermatologic conditions (ie, acne or eczema) preoperatively. In patients with myelomeningocele, soft tissue closure with the aid of a plastic surgeon may be required.
- Preoperative prophylactic antibiotics are administered according to local hospital guidelines.

### Positioning

- For posterior exposures, the patient is positioned prone; intubated; gastric tube, esophageal temperature probe, and Foley catheter placed; blood pressure cuff, electrocardiogram (ECG) leads, and pulse oximetry device applied; and neuromonitoring needles inserted. Baseline neuromonitoring signals may be obtained prior to positioning the patient prone on the operative table.
- A rolled sponge is placed on the mouth as a guard to prevent laceration to the tongue during TcMEP muscle stimulation.
- The patient is placed on a translucent table in a prone position to allow unobstructed radiographic visualization (**FIG 2**).
- It is important to pad pressure areas including the chest, anterior superior iliac spines (ASIS), and patella. A chest bolster is placed in the area of the expected sagittal apex while ensuring the abdomen is hanging free.
- Care must be taken with positioning of the face. The eyes are checked throughout the case to ensure no external force is being placed on them.
- The arms are positioned in 90 degrees of external rotation and shoulder abduction less than 90 degrees with the elbows flexed.

### Approach

- Typically, these osteotomies are performed with a posterior midline approach to the spine, although they are also used with combined anterior and posterior approaches.
- A posterior midline skin incision is made over the levels to be exposed.

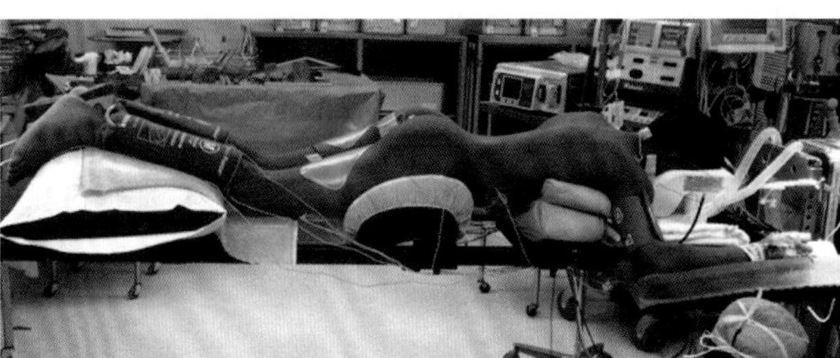

**FIG 2** ● Patient positioned for spinal osteotomy surgery in the prone position on a radiolucent frame. The face and orbits are protected, and chest, hips, knees, and feet are padded. The abdomen should hang free to decrease epidural venous bleeding.

- Anatomic landmarks
  - The iliac crest demarcates L4–L5 in most patients.
  - T4 is at the level of the scapular spine.
  - C7 is the vertebra prominens, the most prominent spinal process.
- Dorsal thoracolumbar fascia is incised at the midline along the length of the skin incision.
- The spinous processes are identified. The unossified apophysis can be easily identified with either a Kelly clamp or hemostat. It is cut sharply down to the bone either with a scalpel or Bovie. A Cobb elevator is used to separate multifidus from the spinal processes and laminae subperiosteally to the lateral edge of the facet joints laterally. The landmarks are identified in a dry operative field.
- Ensure the cephalad interspinal and intraspinal ligaments are well preserved to minimize the risk of proximal junctional kyphosis.
- Facet joints capsules are denuded once the spinal level is confirmed with an intraoperative fluoroscopy.
- Partial facetectomy is performed with either an osteotome or ultrasonic bone scalpel.

## Ponte Osteotomy

- This named osteotomy was described by Alberto Ponte in 1987.
- The osteotomy was classically described as posterior column shortening procedure in a mobile, nonossified spine for Scheuermann kyphosis. Closed wedge osteotomy is performed segmentally.
- The osteotomy pivots on the mobile anterior disc and anterior longitudinal ligament that acts as a tension band in assisting closure in the posterior element of the spine. The closing force is created by the moment arm of the instrument used which includes pedicle screws, pedicle hooks, laminar hooks, or transverse hooks. Improved pedicle screw extenders can magnify the corrective force exponentially. In pediatric patients, anterior column lengthening with the discs "open" anteriorly are observed.[13]
- It allows an estimated 5- to 10-degree correction at a spinal unit in the sagittal plane. It is indicated when the deformity is global, long, gradual, and sweeping. It is less useful when the deformity is focal in the sagittal plane.
- It has also been used in hypokyphotic AIS to recreate normal kyphosis in a reversed manner.[11]
- SPO is similar to Ponte osteotomy and sometimes used interchangeably. It was classically described for ankylosing spondylitis patients with the anterior spinal ligaments ossified and fused. Its extended use includes posterior osteotomy in any adjoining vertebra with fusion seen at the posterior elements.
- Indications
  - Stiff AIS with flexibility of less than 50%
  - Hypokyphotic AIS
  - Scheuermann kyphosis
  - Revision surgery for junctional kyphosis

## Pedicle Subtraction Osteotomy/ Hemivertebra Excision

- Types of PSO
  - Unilateral PSO
  - Asymmetric PSO
  - Symmetric PSO
- Indications
  - Hemivertebra resection is similar in technique to unilateral PSO and most common in congenital scoliosis (**FIG 3A,B**).
  - Asymmetric PSO is indicated in a stiff scoliosis (flexibility of 20% to 40%) with Cobb over 90 degrees.
  - Symmetric PSO is indicated for the following:
    - Severe, rigid Scheuermann kyphosis (**FIG 3C,D**)
    - Revision scoliosis with significant hypokyphotic thoracic deformity or hyperkyphotic lumbar deformity with fixed sagittal imbalance

## Vertebral Column Resection

- Indications
  - Stiff scoliosis curve with severe curvature (over 80 degrees) with flexibility of less than 25%.[12]
  - Fully segmented hemivertebra in which full correction is desirable by resection of entire hemivertebra, discs above and below, and concave disc (**FIG 4**).
  - Circumferentially fused spine (congenital or iatrogenic)
  - Tumor resection for solitary metastasis or primary tumor

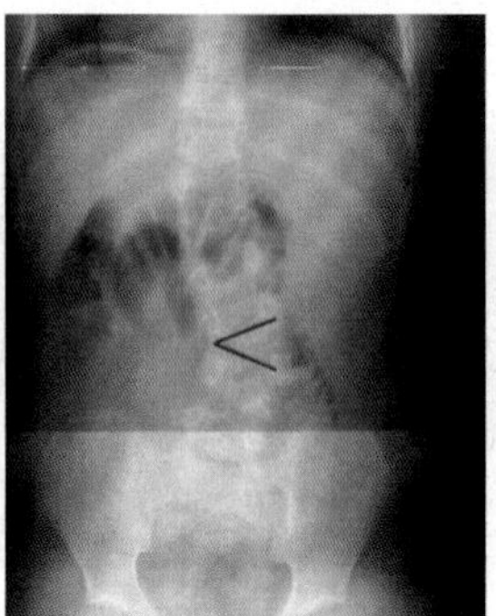
A

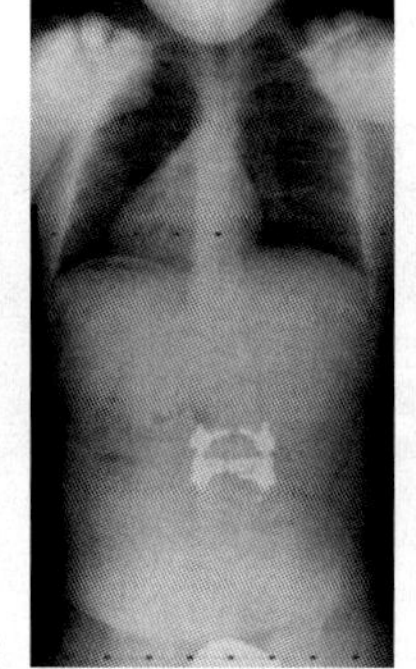
B

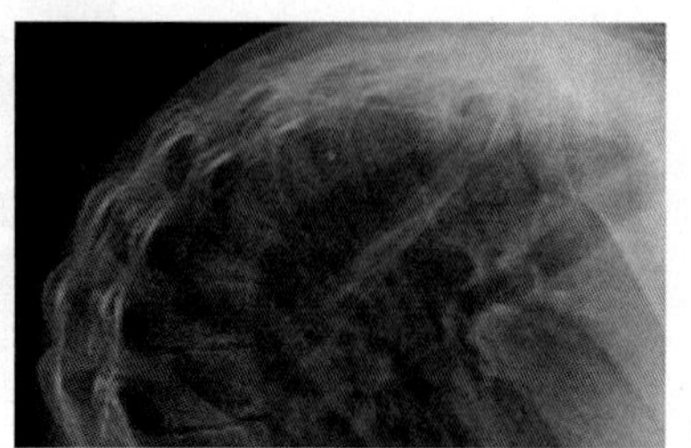
C

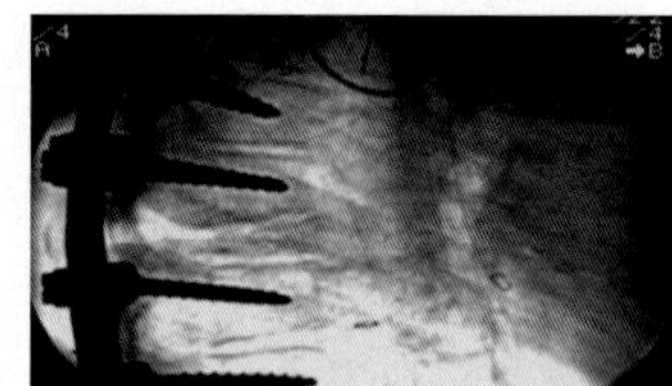
D

**FIG 3** • **A,B.** Preoperative and postoperative radiographs, respectively, of a patient with congenital scoliosis who underwent a hemivertebra resection. **C,D.** Preoperative and postoperative radiographs, respectively, of a patient with severe, rigid kyphosis who underwent a PSO and instrumented correction and fusion.

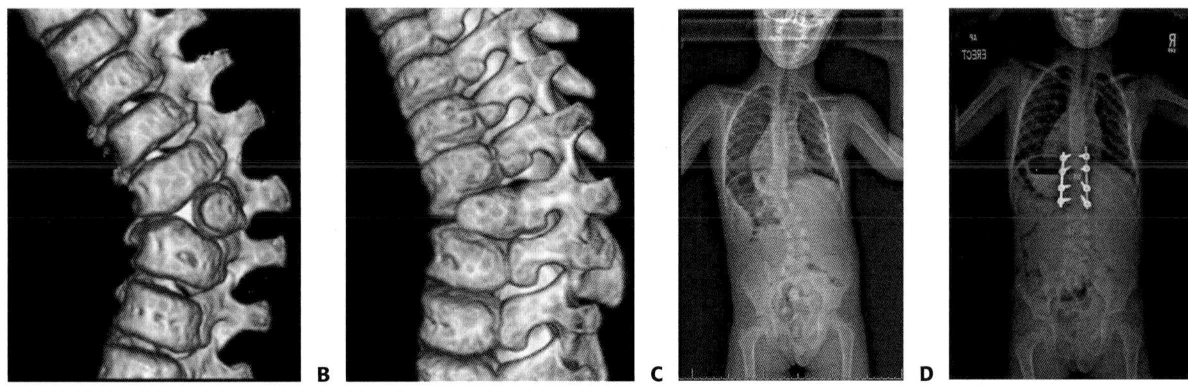

**FIG 4** ● **A,B.** 3-D CT reconstructions of a patient with a fully segmented hemivertebra and kyphoscoliosis. **C,D.** Pre- and postoperative erect X-rays of the patient after posterior hemivertebra resection, reconstruction and short-segment fusion with instrumentation.



## Ponte Osteotomy

- A standard midline approach is used (**TECH FIG 1A**).
- Resect the inferior articular facets by using an ultrasonic scalpel or chisel bilaterally. Then, extend the resection along the inferior lamina to create a chevron-shaped osteotomy (**TECH FIG 1C–E**).
- Create an interlaminar window by removing interspinal and intraspinal ligaments (**TECH FIG 1B**).
- Remove the spinous process with bone cutter to expose the interlaminar space. Keep this bone for use as autologous bone graft.
- Excise the ligamentum flavum with a double-action Leksell rongeur and/or a Kerrison rongeur to expose the underlying epidural fat.
- Place a Woodson dural separator deep to the superior articular facet to protect the exiting nerve root. Use an ultrasonic osteotome or Kerrison rongeur to osteotomize the superior articular facet.
- An epidural vein is commonly present at the lateral edge of the facetal resection. Bleeding is controlled by a combination of bipolar cautery, thrombin-soaked patty, or Gelfoam.
- The exiting nerve roots are decompressed completely.
- Multiple symmetric V-shaped gutters are formed, with complete resection of the articular facets bilaterally and spinous processes (**TECH FIG 1F–J**). In patients with scoliosis, crowding of structures at the concavity of the curve will result in an asymmetric V-shaped gutters; this will aid in coronal correction with distraction.
- In an AIS patient with hypokyphosis, the thoracic segment typically has a more lordotic appearance (**TECH FIG 1K**).
- Undercut the osteotomized lamina margin to avoid dural impingement during the closure of the osteotomy.
- Pedicle instrumentation is performed at all levels of the Ponte osteotomy. The entry point is created with a burr. In our practice, the freehand technique for pedicle screw insertion is used.
- In Scheuermann kyphosis, cantilever reduction technique is used to assist in reduction. Reduction pedicle screws are placed

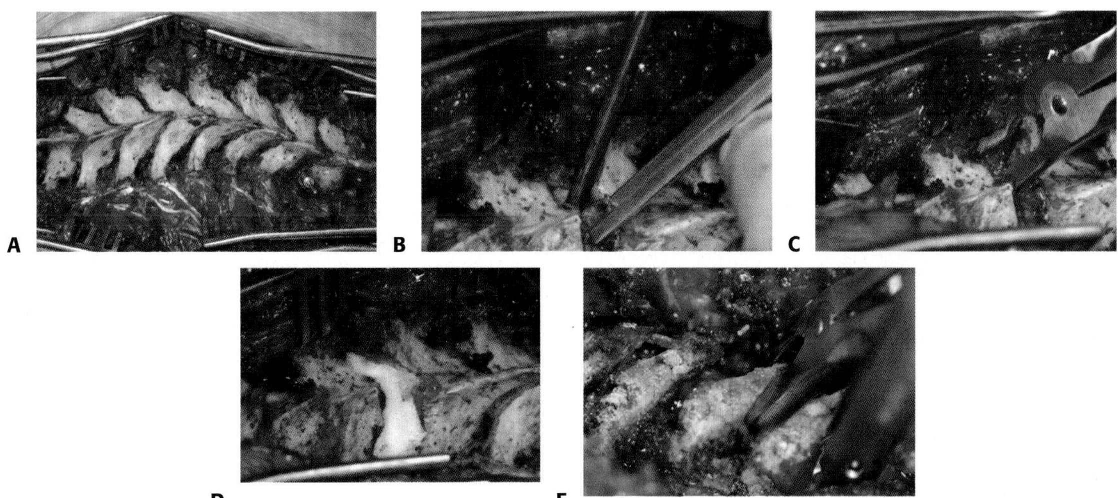

**TECH FIG 1** ● Ponte osteotomy. **A.** The posterior elements of the spine are shown after soft tissue exposure and hemostasis. **B.** Creating interlaminar window in Ponte osteotomy. **C.** Removal of the ligamentum flavum with a Kerrison rongeur. **D.** Removal of the facet with a narrow, double-action Leksell rongeur. **E.** Completed osteotomy with Gelfoam in vertebral interspace. *(continued)*

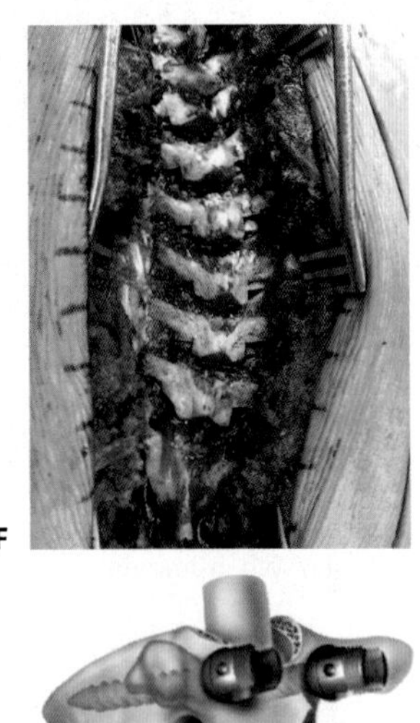
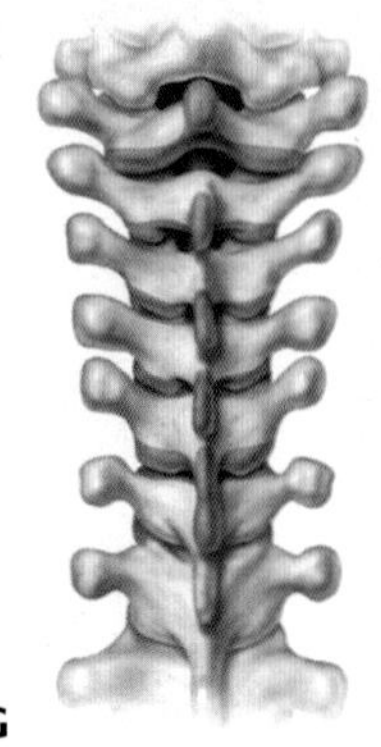
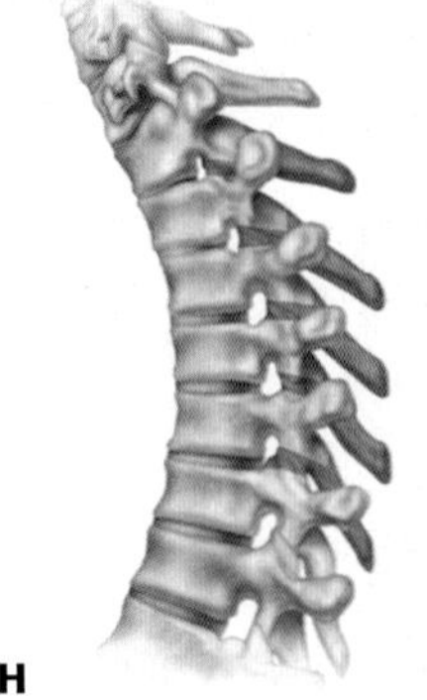
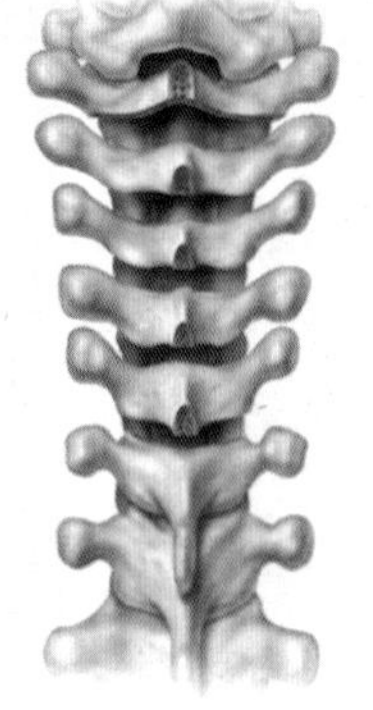
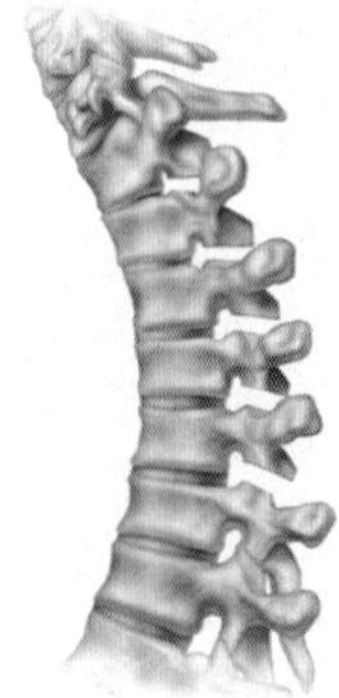
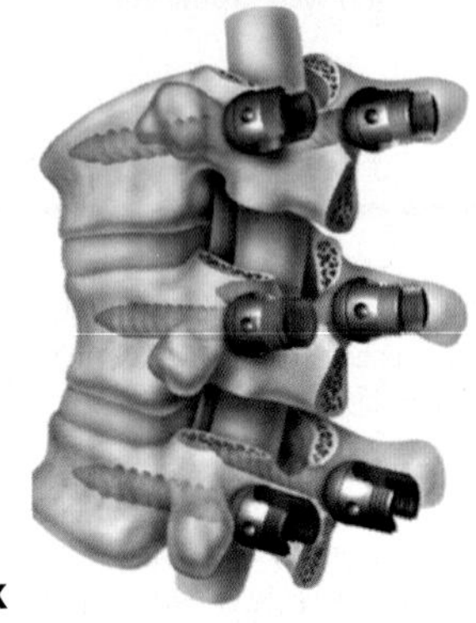

**TECH FIG 1** • *(continued)* **F.** Multiple chevron-shaped Ponte posterior column osteotomies used in this case of Scheuermann kyphosis. **G,H.** Spinous process and inferior facet resection. **I,J.** Completion of facetectomies with superior articular process and pars interarticularis resection. **K.** Oblique view of pedicle screw insertion after multiple Ponte osteotomies and distraction for a typical AIS case. (**G–K:** Courtesy of James Millerick.)

strategically at the most caudal levels. Load-sharing principle is followed during reduction.

- In a patient with AIS with hypokyphotic thoracic sagittal alignment, the reduction is achieved first by insetting the concave rod, which is contoured hyperkyphotically. The rod is captured by the pedicle screws mainly by translation. The convex rod, which is contoured hypokyphotically, is reduced by cantilever technique. Differential rod contouring helps to restore the sagittal alignment while achieving derotation. Segmental derotation is performed for further correction in the axial plane if needed.
- Negatively charged tricalcium phosphate silica bone graft substitute is placed over the sites of Ponte osteotomy to prevent unwanted ossification in the spinal canal while encouraging fusion externally at the posterior elements.
- Decortication of the remaining spinal processes and posterior elements is performed followed by bone grafting. Vancomycin powder is mixed in with the bone graft.
- Layered closure is performed with the goal of a watertight closure.
- Placement of drain is controversial and is not part of our practice.

## Hemivertebra Excision

- Patient is positioned and a midline posterior approach performed.
- Pedicle screws instrumentation is performed with the freehand technique one or two levels cephalad and caudad to the level of interest depending on the indications. (Longer fusions to span the deformity are needed in patients with contralateral bar formation and rib synostosis.)
- Perform a partial facetectomy with either chisel or ultrasonic osteotome at the level above and below the hemivertebra to expose the underlying superior articular facets.
- The pedicle of the hemivertebra at the level of interest is cannulated with a pedicle probe prior to further releases.
- Ponte osteotomy is performed at the level of interest and one or two levels above and below it.
- Remove the caudal half of the hemilamina above and cephalad half of the hemilamina below.
- Complete hemilaminectomy at the hemivertebra level is done by thinning the lamina with a small rongeur and burr and finally resecting it piecemeal with a Kerrison rongeur.
- A temporary rod is inserted on the opposite array of pedicle screws prior to further destabilization.
- The pedicle is disconnected from all the posterior elements.
- At the thoracic level, costotransversectomy is performed for one or two levels depending on the size of the hemivertebra.
  - Sharp dissection along the axis of the rib for about 2 to 3 cm on the bony surface 2 to 3 cm laterally from the costotransverse joint.
  - Subperiosteal dissection using Alexander elevator around the rib segment, taking care to preserve the neurovascular bundle along the inferior costal margin of the rib.
  - The rib is resected with a Giertz-Stille rib cutter or ultrasonic osteotome.

- The transverse process of the thoracic rib is amputated using ultrasonic osteotome or conventional osteotome.
- The costotransverse joint and costovertebral joint are dissociated with a combination of sharp and blunt dissection.
- The extracavitary approach allows extrapleural approach to the lateral aspect of the pedicle and lateral part of the vertebral body.

- At the lumbar region, the transverse process is amputated at the base. The exiting nerve root from the hemivertebral level is protected. The psoas muscle is separated from the vertebral body with periosteal elevator subperiosteally. The retroperitoneal plane is developed into the ventral aspect. The plane is kept opened with a pair of specialized angled retractors or malleable retractors.
- Decancellation of the vertebral body using eggshell technique
  - The pedicle track is expanded with a series of curettes while maintaining the integrity of the pedicle walls. This allows access to the vertebral body. The cancellous bone at the vertebral body is shelled out with curettes of various sizes and angles without breaching the cortex.
  - The lateral wall of the pedicle is intentionally breached. This facilitates the lateral angulation of the curette to reach the medial limit of the hemivertebra.
  - The concavity of the deformity acts as a pivot for closure. A curette is placed as medially as possible intraosseously at the hemivertebra. This is confirmed with an intraoperative fluoroscopy.
- Care is taken to preserve the posterior cortex of the vertebral body and medial and inferior walls of the pedicle until the last stage of the operation. The former two protect the dura, whereas the latter protects the exiting nerve root.
- The discs cephalad and caudad to the hemivertebra are removed.
- The inferior wall of the pedicle is removed with Kerrison rongeur while protecting the exiting nerve root. This is followed by the medial wall.
- A posterior tamp is used to collapse dorsal cortex of the vertebral body anteriorly to the shell-out vertebral body. The fracture wall is then removed.
- A temporary rod is placed at the ipsilateral pedicle screws.
- Gradual compression is performed across the osteotomy site to close it.
- The temporary rods are exchanged out with permanent rods and final compression/distraction is performed for correction (see **FIG 4C,D**).

## Symmetric and Asymmetric Pedicle Subtraction Osteotomy

- Patient is prepared, exposed as discussed earlier.
- Ponte osteotomy is performed at the apex of the deformity.
- Pedicles are cannulated with the freehand technique spanning two or three levels cephalad and caudad to the level of interest.
- The pedicles at the level of interest are disconnected from the posterior element as detailed earlier. Caudal half of the lamina above the level of interest is resected to avoid impingement during closure.
- At the thoracic level, two-level costotransversectomy centered at the level of PSO is performed. Extracavitary approach is developed.
- At the lumbar region, the transverse processes are amputated at the base. The exiting nerve roots from the cephalad level are protected. The psoas muscles are separated from the vertebral body with periosteal elevator subperiosteally. The plane is developed into the ventral aspect bilaterally. The plane is kept opened with a specialized retractor or a malleable retractor.
- Decancellation of the vertebral body is performed bilaterally from the pedicles with series of curette of different sizes. Ensure the posterior wall is thinned with reverse curette.
- A symmetric wedge of bone or asymmetric wedge of bone is removed with small osteotome bilaterally. The first cut is at the superior roof of the foramen parallel to the superior endplate. The second cut is wedge-shaped. Asymmetric wedge is created in patient with concurrent coronal deformity.
- The posterior wall is fractured with a posterior tamp anteriorly.
- The wedge of bone is removed piecemeal with curettes, reverse curettes, and pituitary rongeurs.
- The temporary rods are compressed sequentially. Dura is inspected and palpated gently for buckling.
- The temporary rods are sequentially exchanged out for full-length, precontoured, permanent rods.
- The dura is covered.
- Bridging autologous rib grafts are placed across the resection site.
- A layered closure is performed.

## Vertebral Column Resection

- Patient is positioned and exposed as described in the previous section.
- Ponte osteotomy is performed at the apical region of the deformity as detailed previously.
- Pedicles spanning three or four levels cephalad and caudad to the level of interest are cannulated with pedicle gearshift via the freehand technique, taking care to preserve the medial wall of the pedicles especially at the level of VCR.
- At the thoracic level, three-level costotransversectomy centered at the level of VCR is performed (**TECH FIG 2A**).
- At the lumbar region, the transverse processes are amputated at the base. The exiting nerve roots from the cephalad level are protected. The psoas muscles are separated from the vertebral body with periosteal elevator subperiosteally.
- Pedicle screws are inserted at the levels both cephalad and caudad to the level of resection.
- Complete laminectomy is performed at the level of interest. The caudad portion of the lamina above and the cephalad portion of the lamina below are also resected (**TECH FIG 2B**).

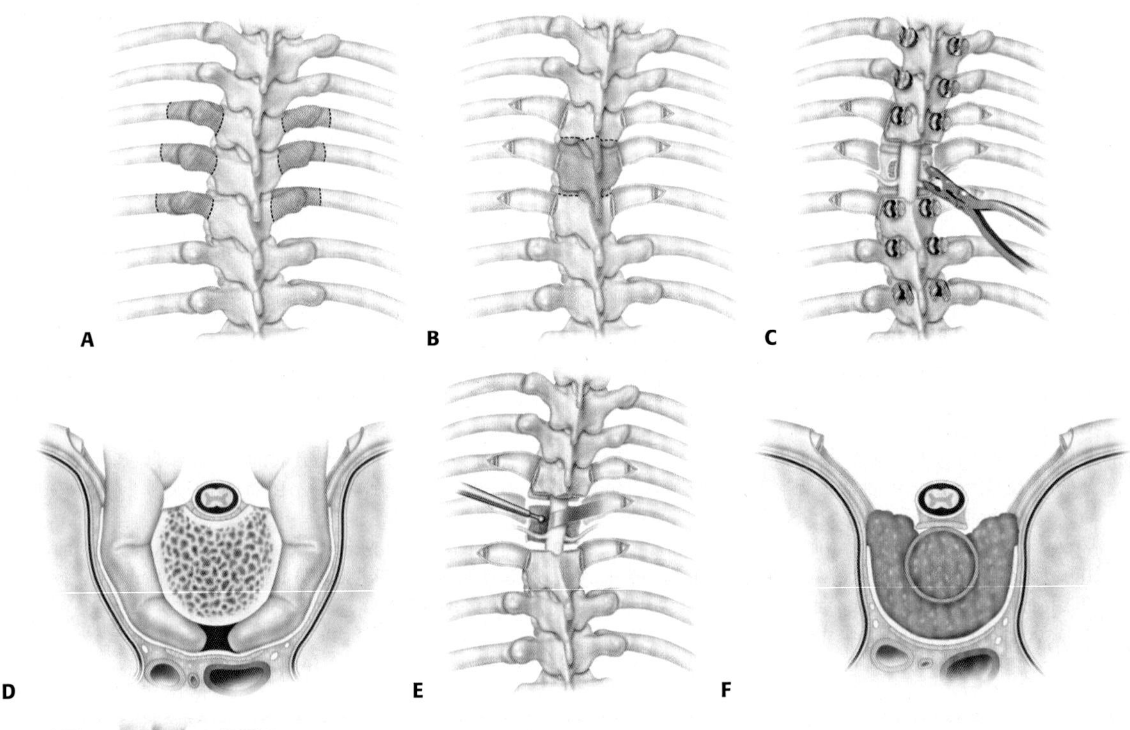


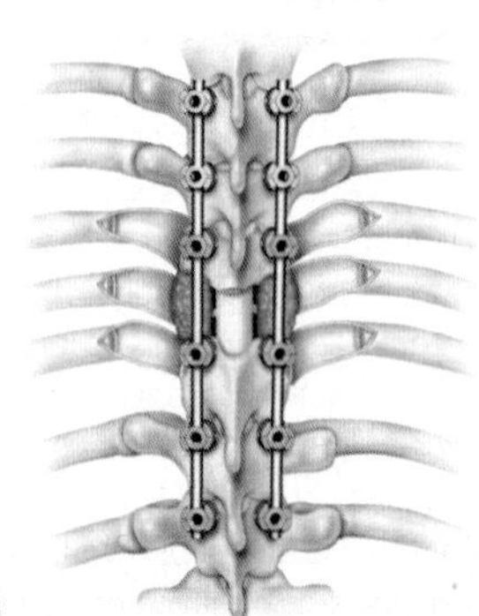


**TECH FIG 2** • Important sequential steps in VCR in the thoracic spine. **A.** Bilateral transverse process and rib head resection to allow exposure of the lateral vertebral walls. **B.** Shaded area indicates laminectomy needed for dural exposure. **C.** Pedicles are resected and thoracic nerve roots are tied off. **D.** Blunt finger dissection of lateral and anterior vertebral body prior to retractor placement. **E.** With the dura protected and temporary rods implanted to prevent spinal instability, the vertebral body is resected with a burr, rongeurs, or ultrasonic device. **F.** A structural cage filled with autologous bone is placed anteriorly to provide anterior column support and prevent excessive spinal shortening; additional autograft cancellous bone is placed around the cage and laterally. **G.** The temporary stabilizing rods are replaced with the final rods, and compression/distraction is performed as needed for correction; dura is inspected for compression or buckling. (Courtesy of James Millerick.)

- Thoracic roots may be sacrificed and ligated sharply between ties to improve the working space.
- The pedicles are disconnected from the posterior elements (**TECH FIG 2C**); TcMEPs are reconfirmed, and the mean arterial pressure (MAP) is raised to over 80 mm Hg.
- A single temporary rod is placed on the convexity of the curve to maintain stability.
- Lateral vertebral walls are dissected.
  - The dissection is completed with blunt dissection using index fingers from the subperiosteal plane developed, aiming to meet the tips of fingers at the ventral aspect of the vertebral body (**TECH FIG 2D**).
  - This plane is kept open with specialized retractors.
- Vertebral body is decancellated with a series of curettes, reverse curettes, and pituitary rongeurs via the pedicle (**TECH FIG 2E**). Posterior wall of the vertebral body is thinned out with the reverse curettes. Pedicle is then removed leaving the medial wall of the pedicle and posterior wall of the vertebral body intact to protect the dura and spinal cord.
- Cephalad and caudal discectomies are performed bilaterally.
- Medial wall of the pedicle is carefully removed with 2-mm Kerrison rongeur, whereas the posterior wall is pushed anteriorly with a posterior tamp.
- The convex temporary rod is compressed.
- A cage filled with morselized autologous graft is inserted into the void (**TECH FIG 2F**). Additional tricortical autograft from the resected rib can be placed.
- Both temporary rods are secured.
- The temporary rods are compress sequentially. Dura is inspected and palpated gently for buckling with a Penfield elevator.
- The temporary rods are sequentially exchanged out for full-length, permanent rods (**TECH FIG 2G**).
- The dura is covered.
- Bridging autologous rib grafts are placed across the resection site.
- A layered closure is performed (**TECH FIG 3**).

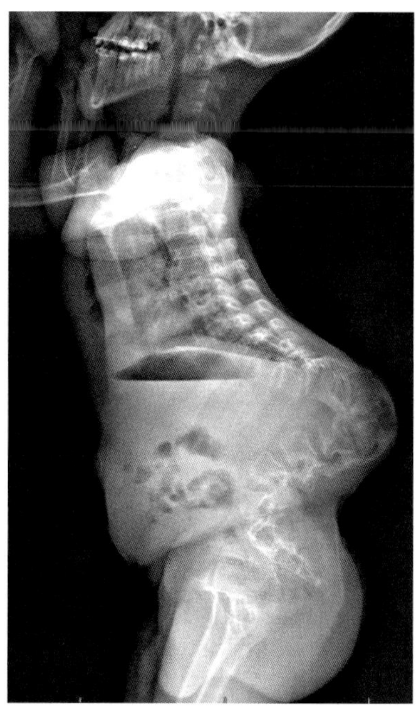

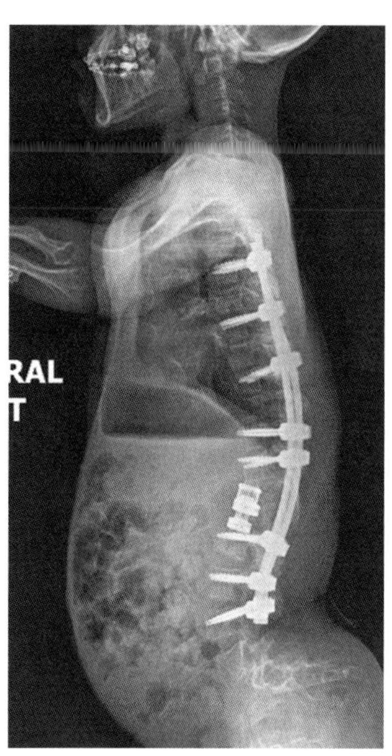

**TECH FIG 3** • **A.** Achondroplastic patient with severe thoracolumbar kyphosis. **B.** This was corrected with posterior VCR at T12, L1, and L2 (grade 6 osteotomy) and posterior instrumented fusion.

## PEARLS AND PITFALLS

| | |
|---|---|
| **All spinal osteotomies** | ▪ Exposure at a wrong level may result in premature autofusion in pediatric patients.<br>▪ Maintain normotensive anesthesia with MAP of at least 75–80 mm Hg during osteotomy.<br>▪ On table traction with skull tong and femoral skin or skeletal traction assist in spinal reduction.<br>▪ Neuromonitoring is essential throughout the procedure. Prepositioning baseline is needed in patients with large curve. Monitoring should not cease till the closure of the skin. |
| **Ponte osteotomy** | ▪ Ultrasonic osteotome resection minimizes epidural bleeding during facet resection. It is particularly useful in the concave part of the scoliosis where there is often crowding of dysplastic structures.<br>▪ Symmetric resection of the articular facet processes is essential to preserve coronal balance in Scheuermann kyphosis. |
| **Pedicle subtraction osteotomy—unilateral** | ▪ Temporary rods can be overbent at the coronal plane at the concavity of the curve to improve the working space at the hemivertebra. |
| **VCR** | ▪ Thoracic exiting nerve roots could be sacrificed to create more working space. The nerve is sharply ligated between ties.<br>▪ Temporary rod is necessary to prevent translation during destabilization.<br>▪ Care is taken to avoid spinal translation during reduction. The caudal segment often translates posteriorly, whereas the rostral segment often translates anteriorly. |
| **What do you do when the neuromonitoring signals disappear?** | ▪ Check neuromonitoring equipment.<br>▪ Reverse the last step in the reduction.<br>▪ Increase the patient's blood pressure.<br>▪ Ensure patient is normothermic.<br>▪ Transfuse patient to maintain hemoglobin.<br>▪ Ensure adequate decompression at the site of osteotomy.<br>▪ Loosen the set screws.<br>▪ Remove the reduction rods if needed (in a stable spine).<br>▪ Ensure proper decompression and avoid dural buckling.<br>▪ Order a Stagnara wake-up test. |

## POSTOPERATIVE CARE

- Postoperative care may vary based on the patient's preoperative status and intraoperative findings.
- Bracing is usually not necessary with stable spinal instrumentation and fusion. The ultimate plan should be individually tailored according to patient's demand and situation.
- Perioperative antibiotics are continued for 24 hours postoperatively.
- The patients are mobilized to a chair on postoperative day 1 and begin walking on postoperative day 2. They are allowed to weight bear as tolerated and ambulate as tolerated.
- At 6 months, patients are allowed to return to most sports.

## OUTCOMES

- Spinal osteotomies have considerable morbidity with increased operative time and blood loss.
- Geck at al[5] reported an average correction of 9.3 degrees per osteotomy for Ponte osteotomy at 2-year follow-up. There were no reoperations for nonunion or instrumentation failure. None of the patients had neurologic complications. One case of delayed infection in the cohort of 17 patients was reported. Two (12%) of the patients had junctional kyphosis.
- In hemivertebra resection, 70% main curve correction rate can be expected in children aged 1 to 6 years.[10] In this cohort of 28 patients, Ruf and Harms[10] reported one case of infection, two pedicle fractures, and three implant failures.
- A recent study evaluating the complications of VCR by a group of experienced surgeons from multiple centers was reported by Lenke et al.[9] The average operative time was 545 minutes and estimated blood loss averaged 1610 mL. Six of the 147 patients underwent an operative irrigation and débridement for wound infection. Overall, the complication rate was 58% and a third of the cases had IONM changes; fortunately, there were no permanent neurologic deficits in this series.
- These techniques should be used by individuals familiar with the procedures and the inherent complications.

## COMPLICATIONS

- Neurologic injury
- Pseudarthrosis
- Hardware failure
- Loss of correction
- Infection
- Proximal or distal junctional kyphosis or progressive scoliosis
- Pneumothorax
- Great vessel injury
- Pancreatitis
- Superior mesenteric syndrome

## REFERENCES


1. Canavese F, Dimeglio A. Normal and abnormal spine and thoracic cage development. World J Orthop 2013;4:167–174.
2. Cheh G, Lenke LG, Padberg AM, et al. Loss of spinal cord monitoring signals in children during thoracic kyphosis correction with spinal osteotomy: why does it occur and what should you do? Spine 2013; 33:1093–1099.
3. Cook SM, Asher M, Lai S, et al. Reoperation after primary posterior instrumentation and fusion for idiopathic scoliosis. Toward defining late operative site pain of unknown cause. Spine 2000;25:463–468.
4. Dimeglio A. Growth of the spine before age 5 years. J Pediatr Orthop B 1992;1:102–107.
5. Geck MJ, Macagno A, Ponte A, et al The Ponte procedure: posterior only treatment of Scheuermann's kyphosis using segmental posterior shortening and pedicle screw instrumentation. J Spinal Disorders Techniques 2007;20:586–593.
6. Joseph SA Jr, Moreno AP, Brandoff J, et al. Sagittal plane deformity in the adult patient. J Am Acad Orthop Surg 2009;17:378–388.
7. Karol LA, Johnston C, Mladenov K, et al. Pulmonary function following early thoracic fusion in non-neuromuscular scoliosis. J Bone Joint Surg Am 2008;90:1272–1281.
8. Kim YJ, Lenke LG, Bridwell KH, et al. Free hand pedicle screw placement in the thoracic spine: is it safe? *Spine* 2004;29:333–342.
9. Lenke LG, Newton PO, Sucato DJ, et al. Complications after 147 consecutive vertebral column resections for severe pediatric spinal deformity: a multicenter analysis. Spine 2013;38:119–132.
10. Ruf M, Harms J. Posterior hemivertebra resection with transpedicular instrumentation: early correction in children aged 1 to 6 years. Spine 2003;28:2132–2138.
11. Shah SA, Dhawale AA, Oda JE, et al. Ponte osteotomies with pedicle screw instrumentation in the treatment of adolescent idiopathic scoliosis. J Spine Deformity 2013;1:196–204.
12. Suk SI, Chung ER, Kim JH, et al. Posterior vertebral column resection for severe rigid scoliosis. Spine 2005;30:1682–1687.
13. Tsutsui S, Pawelek JB, Bastrom TP, et al. Do discs "open" anteriorly with posterior-only correction of Scheuermann's kyphosis? Spine 2011; 36:E1086–E1092.
14. Weinstein SL, Dolan LA, Spratt KF, et al. Health and function of patients with untreated idiopathic scoliosis: a 50-year natural history study. JAMA 2003;289:559–567.
15. Weinstein SL, Dolan LA, Wright JG, et al. Effects of bracing in adolescents with idiopathic scoliosis. N Engl J Med 2013;369:1512–1521.
16. Wood KB, Melikian R, Villamil F. Adult Scheuermann kyphosis: evaluation, management, and new developments. J Am Acad Orthop Surg 2012;20:113–121.
17. Zindrick MR, Knight GW, Sartori MJ, et al. Pedicle morphology of the immature thoracolumbar spine. Spine 2000;25:2726–2735.

# Kyphectomy in Spina Bifida

Richard E. McCarthy

87 CHAPTER

## DEFINITION

- Kyphosis in the patient with myelomeningocele can occur at the thoracolumbar junction, the midlumbar spine, or the lumbosacral junction.
- The different types of kyphosis have some bearing on the treatment needed for the repair, but whether the origin is congenital, developmental, or paralytic, the consequences can be devastating for the child with this condition.
- Skin breakdown over the apex of the kyphosis can cause deep wound infections and lead to central nervous system infections.
- Secondary changes in other organ systems can create compromise in the gastrointestinal or genitourinary systems or even potentially disastrous kinking of the great vessels due to compromise in the abdominal height. Diminished absorption frequently occurs in the gastrointestinal tract, and renal calculi may develop from poor urinary drainage.
- Secondary effects on the pulmonary capacity produce thoracic insufficiency syndrome because the abdominal contents are pushed into the thoracic cage. Further worsening the respiratory compromise is a thoracic lordosis cephalad to the kyphosis.
- Bracing generally leads to problems from skin pressure and ultimately does not solve the problem.

## ANATOMY

- The kyphotic angle can be a gradual slope or an acute gibbus.
- The paraspinal musculature is segmentally innervated, thus partially active in a flexion position lateral to the bony ridges owing to lack of posterior migration from an embryologic origin. In this position, they contribute to forward flexion of the spinal column.
  - The bony ridges laterally in the area of the diastasis leave meager bone for fusion mass on the posterior side of the vertebral column.
- The midline defect from the original myelomeningocele characteristically is covered by a fragile dura separated from the overlying skin by a thin layer of subcutaneous tissue.
  - The soft tissue coverage is made worse by poorly vascularized scarred skin.
- One of the most reliably formed vertebral structures is the sacral ala.
- The great vessels generally do not follow the kyphotic contours into the kyphotic apex.

## PATHOGENESIS

- Embryologically, the notochord is covered dorsally by closure of the ectoderm, progressing in a cephalad to caudal direction. In myelomeningocele, the closure is incomplete, usually at the caudal end.
- Less common types of myelomeningocele occur in the thoracic and cervical area. Thoracolumbar, lumbar, and lumbosacral kyphosis is the most commonly seen type and occurs because of lack of posterior migration of the ectoderm surrounding the notochord, leaving the neural placode in a vulnerable position resulting in an exposed myelomeningocele sac at birth.
  - Congenital bony defects occurring in this area lead to an early-onset kyphosis that can pose significant problems for the neurosurgeon's closure at birth. This has led some experts to encourage neonatal correction of the kyphosis.
- With further growth and an upright sitting posture, the paraspinal musculature, which has formed in a lateral and anterior position, pulls the upper torso into a more kyphotic position, both actively through muscle contracture and secondarily from gravity.
  - This can lead to further skin compromise and pressure in the soft tissues overlying the kyphosis.
  - Skin breakdown can be a serious problem over the apex of the kyphosis.
- The C7 lateral plumb line shows the upper torso to be far out of balance in a forward flexed posture, leading to thoracic insufficiency from the abdominal contents pressing under the diaphragm.
  - This can render the child a "functional quadriplegic" because he or she uses the upper extremities for balance and to unweight the diaphragm by pivoting on the extended arms for breathing purposes (marionette maneuver; **FIG 1**).
  - From a developmental standpoint, this can further limit the young child's upper extremity interaction with his or her environment, which is essential for the development of normal intelligence.

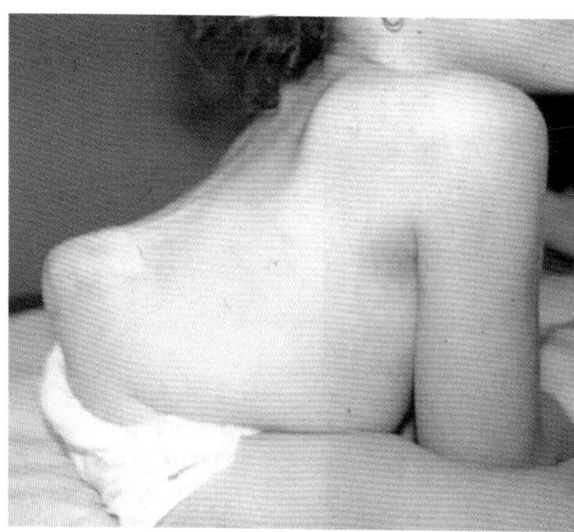

**FIG 1** • Functional quadriplegia supporting position with arms in myelokyphosis; lumbar kyphosis with thoracic lordosis.

## NATURAL HISTORY

- The natural history of unpublished cases of severe kyphosis is one of respiratory compromise from thoracic insufficiency syndrome, progressive decline in pulmonary capacity, and death.

## PATIENT HISTORY AND PHYSICAL FINDINGS

- A careful history and physical examination should elicit possible signs and symptoms of associated anomalies, including the following:
  - Chiari malformation
  - Tethered cord
  - Respiratory compromise
  - Gastrointestinal malabsorption
  - Urinary hydrostasis and lithiasis
- Physical examination of the child should include flexibility tests of the curve by physically supporting the child under the armpits to suspend him or her against gravity. Bending back supine on the examining table can also indicate the extent of lumbar flexibility.

## IMAGING AND OTHER DIAGNOSTIC STUDIES

- Standard radiographs, anteroposterior (AP) and lateral views of the full spine, in the upright sitting posture assess the effects of gravity on the curve (**FIG 2A,B**).
  - Supine radiographs are helpful for visualization of bony definition.
  - Flexibility films with traction, manual push, or back bending over a bolster with a shoot-through lateral film are helpful adjuncts.
- Computed tomography (CT) scans, especially three-dimensional CT scans, offer the best delineation of the anatomy.

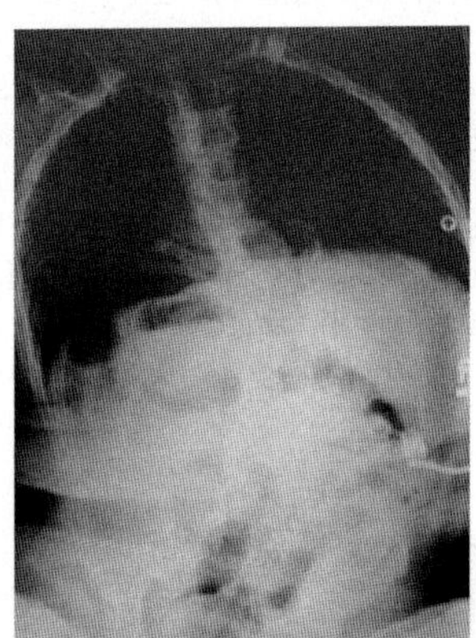

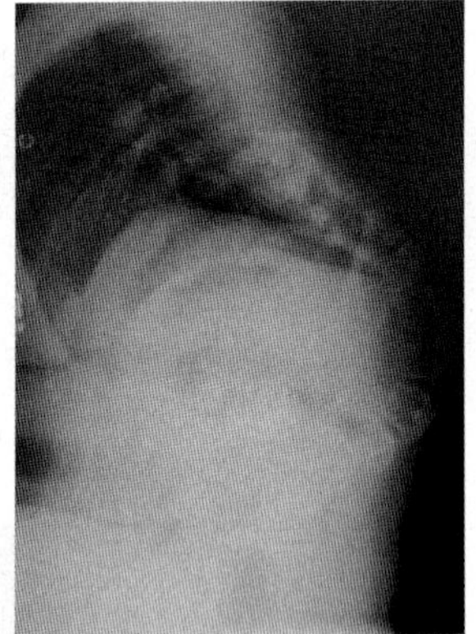

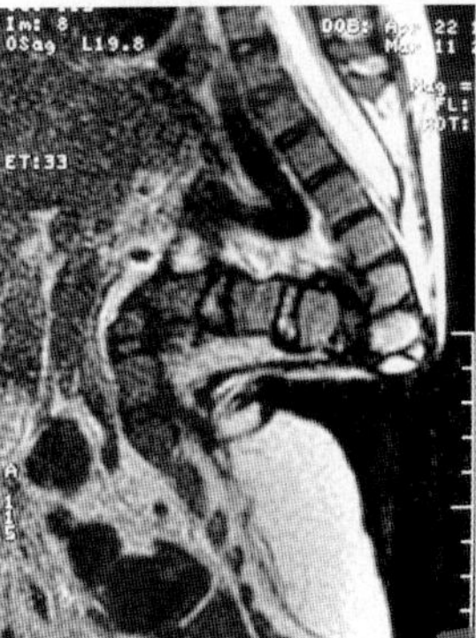

**FIG 2** • **A,B.** A 13-year-old child with myelokyphosis with diastasis beginning at T6 with 127 degrees of kyphosis. **C.** Preoperative MRI in a 9-year-old child with myelomeningocele before undergoing kyphectomy with growing construct.

- Magnetic resonance imaging (MRI) is critical for assessment of the intrathecal structures and assessing for Chiari malformation, syringomyelias, and tethering (**FIG 2C**).

## DIFFERENTIAL DIAGNOSIS

- Congenital versus developmental kyphosis
- Sacral agenesis
- Charcot joints secondary to vertebral column breakdown across the apex of the kyphosis

## NONOPERATIVE MANAGEMENT

- Bracing has no place in the treatment of this disorder.
- Occasionally, traction is helpful to stretch the kyphosis, especially in a developmental type, to aid in correction at the time of surgery.
- This can be done with cervical traction or halo traction, and some authors have promoted the use of this traction during surgery to aid in the correction.

## SURGICAL MANAGEMENT

### Preoperative Planning

- Vascular monitoring devices are an important adjunct during surgery, and either arterial lines or pulse oximeters on both feet are important to monitor blood supply to the lower extremities at the time of correction.
- A great deal of tension can come to bear on the aorta at the time of kyphosis realignment. Thus, arterial and central venous lines are necessary to monitor central pressure and allow for rapid administration of medication and fluids.
- Areas of skin breakdown should be addressed prior to kyphectomy.
  - Preoperative planning may include consultation with a plastic surgeon and possible placement of tissue expanders in the posterolateral axillary margins to aid in skin closure at surgery (**FIG 3**).
- As a part of the preoperative planning, all imaging studies are carefully reviewed to assess flexibility, the adequacy of the vertebral bodies to tolerate pedicle screws, and planning for which levels will need to be decancellized or removed.
  - It is recommended that these plans be recorded on a "blueprint" that can be placed on the operating room wall outlining the location of implants, osteotomies, and order of progression for the surgical plan.
- Assessment by neurosurgery is necessary preoperatively regarding shunt functioning and review of the MRIs.

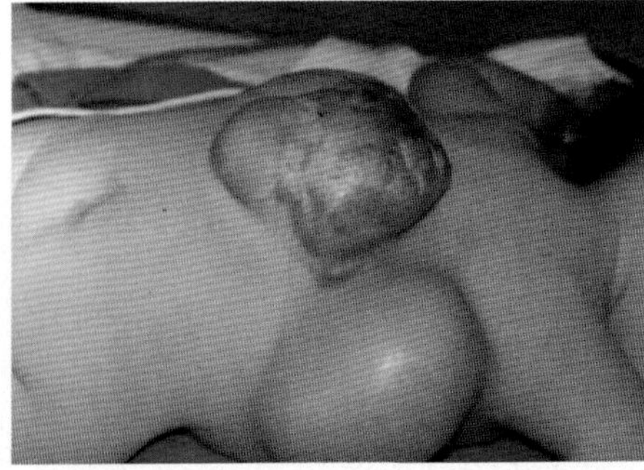

**FIG 3** • Myelomeningocele in an 11-month-old child with tissue expanders placed bilaterally before delayed closure and kyphectomy.

- Preoperative antibiotics are essential, including gram-negative coverage for urinary pathogens. These are continued postoperatively for 6 to 12 weeks.
- Nutritional status is maximized and may require hyperalimentation via a gastrostomy tube button months ahead of surgery to maximize postoperative healing.

## Positioning

- During positioning, careful padding with extra foam is essential to protect delicate skin during a prolonged operation.
- Eye protection to guard against intraoperative ocular compromise and a spinal frame that allows for suspension of the abdominal structures will diminish the epidural vascular pressure.
- Preoperative assessment of the hips is important to anticipate the intraoperative positioning, and if the flexion contractures about the hips are too severe, a preliminary release of contractures done a few weeks ahead of time may be necessary to allow for proper positioning of the legs at the time of the kyphectomy.

## Approach

- The surgical incision may involve excision of compromised skin lesions or scars, although this is best addressed before surgery.
- The previous incisions on a myelomeningocele back may not be midline or ideally placed.
  - The best skin incision for kyphectomy should follow the previous skin incisions to maximize blood supply to the skin edges at closure. Maximum skin and subcutaneous tissue coverage is important for good closure.
- If soft tissue quality is poor, then previously placed tissue expanders may be removed from the midline at closure and the expanded tissue brought to the midline.
- There may be times when the poorly healed, convoluted scars from previous neurosurgical interventions may be source of bacteria that can impair healing or may contribute toward postoperative infection. Preliminary excision of the scars by plastic surgery may afford the best defense against outside-in infections.

TECHNIQUES

# Incision and Lumbar Dissection

- The incision—either straight or curvilinear—follows the previous scars. It is extended deep to the spinous processes in those sections where they exist.
  - The caudal portion of the incision is made to the level of the dura, with care taken to avoid laceration of the fragile dura.
- The surgical plane is then deviated to the right and left side superficial to the dura while palpating for the lateral bony elements. The deep portion of the incision is directed toward the bone.
  - It is desirable to maintain as much subcutaneous thickness as possible.
- If there are lacerations of the dura, it is best to stop and sew them as one proceeds because the thinned dura may require a flap of adjacent tissue for a watertight closure. Sometimes, it is necessary to sew in a piece of Duragen sealant to ensure a watertight closure.
  - A 4-0 Nurolon on a small tapered needle works quite well for an incidental durotomy repair.
- As one proceeds from distal to proximal in the lumbar spine, the lateral elements are palpated, and with the use of electrocautery, the soft tissues are incised to bone.
- The muscle and soft tissue attachments to the laterally positioned lumbar bones are released to reveal the underlying bony elements that embryologically should have progressed posteriorly to become the lamina and facets (**TECH FIG 1A–C**).
  - The rudiments of these bones can be visualized along with a transverse process at each level in the bony ridge of the diastasis.
- The medial neural placode is left intact because it acts as third-space filler and padding for the implants.
- There may be instances in which the neuroplacode has to be mobilized, and this is done by releasing nonfunctioning roots on one side and reflecting the dura laterally to gain access to the disc space and underlying vertebrae (**TECH FIG 1D**).

A
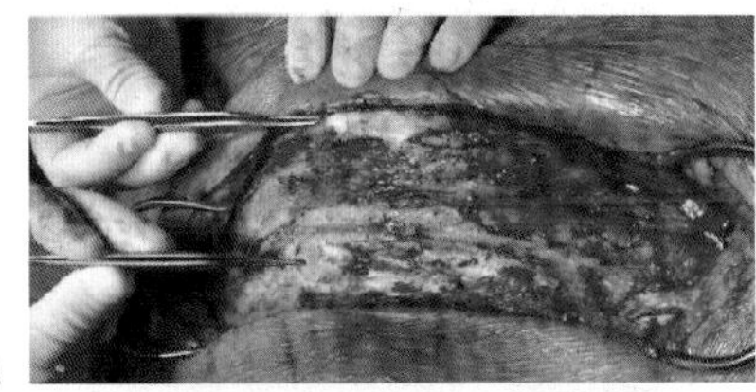

B
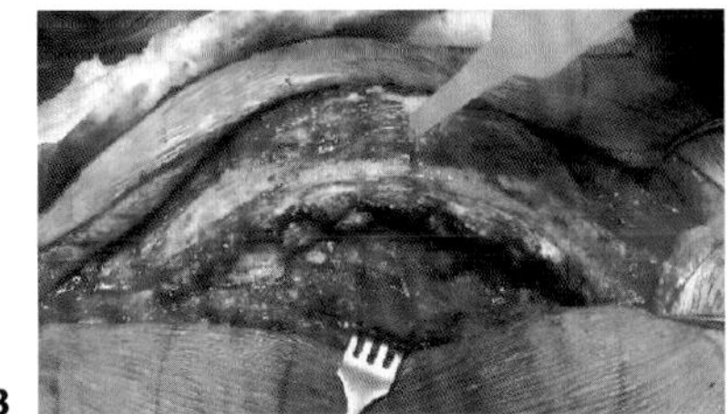

C
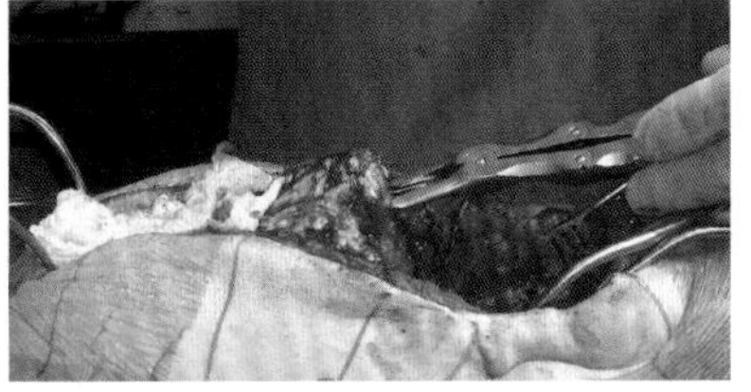

**TECH FIG 1** • **A.** Intraoperative dissection with neuroplacode left in place and forceps placed on bilateral bony ridges. **B.** Paraspinal muscles are dissected away from the kyphosis, with frequent irrigation of neural elements. **C.** In a different patient, the kyphosis has been dissected out. *(continued)*

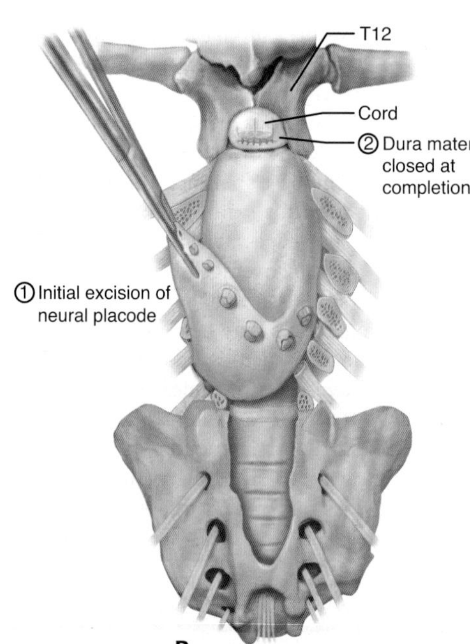


**TECH FIG 1** • *(continued)* **D.** The neuroplacode can be left in place, mobilized to one side by releasing nonfunctioning nerve roots over four levels, or resecting to the level of the diastasis and oversewing.

## Thoracic Dissection

- Once the lumbar spine is dissected, the thoracic area is approached.
  - If one is contemplating a fusion of the thoracic spine, such as in a child older than 8 years of age, full dissection out to the tips of the transverse processes should be accomplished.
- If a growing rod construct is being used, such as in a child younger than 8 years, this is done with minimal dissection in order to preserve growth.
  - In these cases, the muscle and soft tissue attachments are cleaned from the sides of the spinous processes as far as the facet joints.
- One needs to be able to visualize the ligamentum flavum sufficiently to pass sublaminar wires for the Luque trolley portion of the "growing" construct.
  - Generally, four thoracic levels for wires are all that is necessary.
- In the lumbar spine, soft tissues should be cleaned from bone sufficiently to allow for fusion between the lateral elements and to the sacrum.

## Pedicle Screw Placement

- At this point in the operation, radiographic C-arm guidance is helpful for placement of pedicle screws.
- The entrance point for the lumbar dysplastic pedicles is in a lateral position, with the pedicles directed obliquely toward the vertebral body (**TECH FIG 2**).
  - Bilateral screws can be obliquely placed for fixation.
- Fixation to the pelvis can be done with multiple types of fixation devices, including S rods, S hooks, and iliac threaded bolts.
  - Fusion to the sacrum is essential to firmly plant the rod on the pelvis and allow for growth off the top of the rods in the thoracic spine.
- The C-arm is used in both AP and lateral positions to confirm satisfactory placement of the screws in bone. Bicortical fixation is generally not necessary because of the strong fixation supplied by the triangulation of the screws.
- Polyaxial screws are desirable through the lumbar segments.

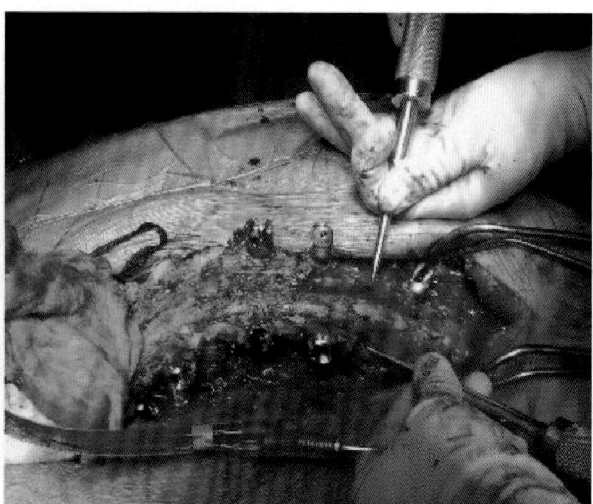

**TECH FIG 2** • Screws in place and bilateral curettes in pedicles to decancellize at L3 before doing the same at T12.

## Decancellization

- Decancellization can be accomplished at multiple levels, leaving adequate vertebral levels for fixation and correction. Ideally, it is accomplished at one or two levels in a location that will leave sufficient midlumbar fixation points to push the vertebrae forward to create lordosis.
  - The levels chosen for decancellization are approached after screw placement, based on the preoperative planning.
- The decancellization begins with a burr at the entrance to the pedicle. It continues with enlarging sizes of curettes, saving the bone for the fusion.
- The inside of the vertebral body is completely cored out, and when bleeding points are encountered, the pedicle can be filled with FloSeal and, if necessary, further packed with some rolled Gelfoam to stop the bleeding.
- Care is taken to avoid violating the posterior cortex of the vertebral body until the very end because this is where the epidural vessels are most prolific.
  - The lateral margins of these vertebral bodies are removed, including the transverse process and posterolateral bone.
- The decancellization should be thorough, leaving only the cortex. This is carried out bilaterally, followed by implosion of the posterior cortex with an Epstein curette, pushing the bone fragments into the cavity of the vertebral body (**TECH FIG 3**).
  - Bleeding points are stabilized.
- In most instances, decancellization alone at select levels is all that is necessary to gain the mobility for correction.

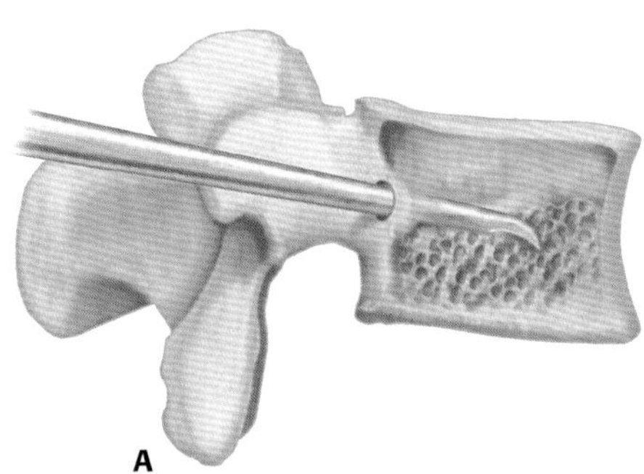


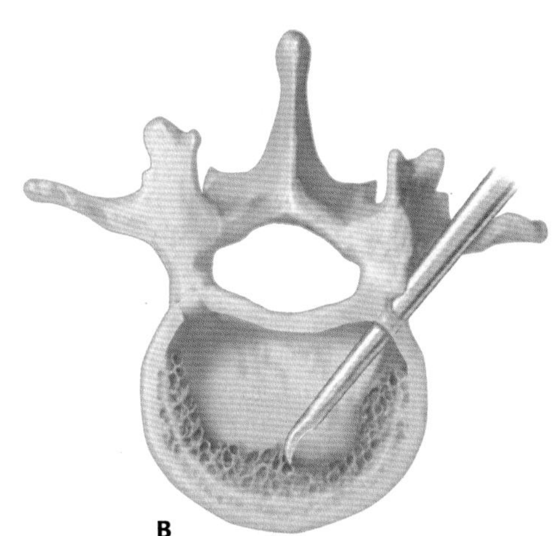


**TECH FIG 3** • Decancellization. **A.** Lateral view. **B.** Cross-sectional view.

## Horizontal Resection

- Occasionally, removal of a vertebral segment may be indicated. If so, it can be accomplished while maintaining the neuroplacode.
- The vertebral section for removal in that instance would be taken from that section of the curve that is horizontal and cephalad to the apex of the kyphosis (**TECH FIG 4**).

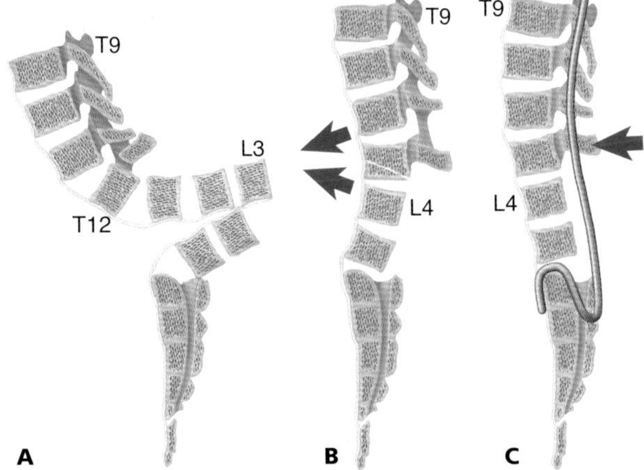


**TECH FIG 4** • **A.** If bone is to be resected (due to extreme stiffness), this should be done in the horizontal section at the top of the kyphosis, not at the apex. **B.** After horizontal resection, the bone is pushed forward to realign. **C.** After resection, realignment and fixation are accomplished.

## Rod Placement

- Once these corrective maneuvers have been completed, rods linked to the sacrum can then be placed bilaterally to push the vertebral bodies anteriorly into a straight or preferably a lordotic position (**TECH FIG 5A**).
- Through gradual approximation of the rod forward toward the thoracic fixation points, the lumbar segments are brought into alignment and the rods gradually tightened to the wires of the thoracic spine (**TECH FIG 5B,C**).
  - Physiologic kyphosis can be contoured into the thoracic component of the rods to correct the thoracic lordosis.
  - Generally, the rods are left one level long at the top to allow for growth in the thoracic spine.
- The final tightening should produce some distraction between the lowest lumbar segment fixation point and the S hooks pushed against the sacral ala (**TECH FIG 5D,E**). This will set the S hooks in place securely.
- Final contouring with the in situ benders can allow for further lordosis of the lumbar spine if desired.

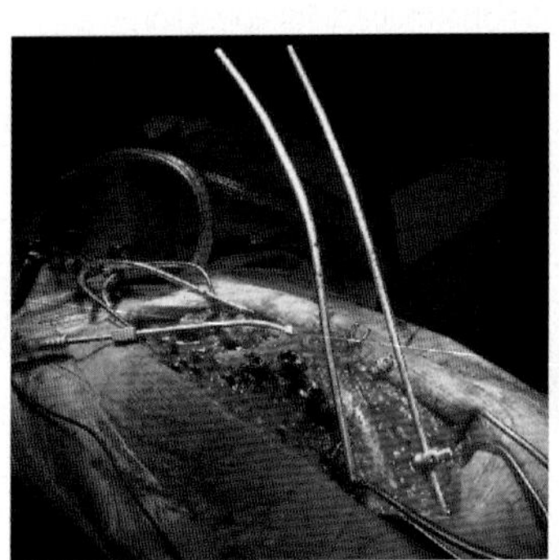
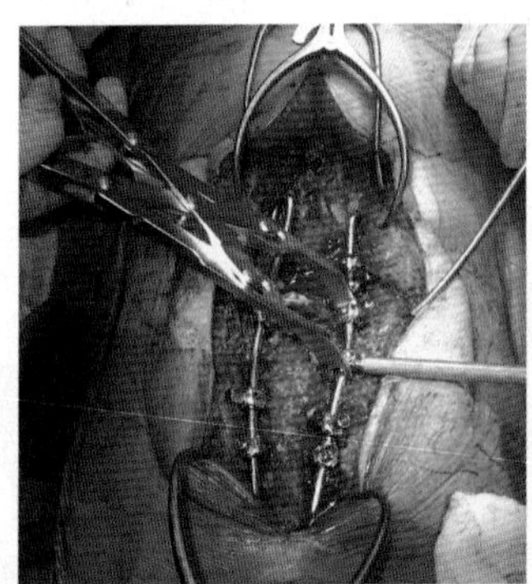
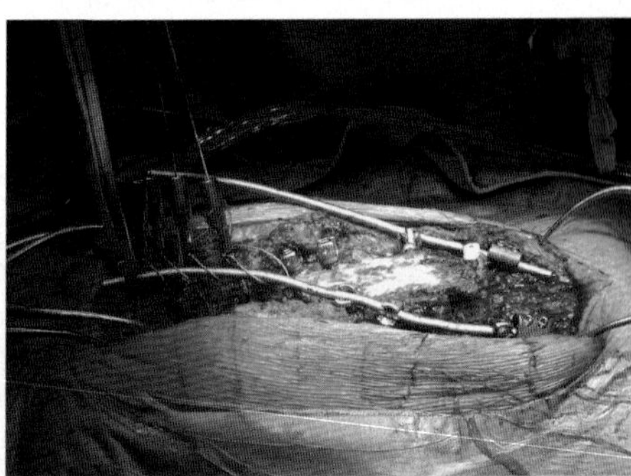
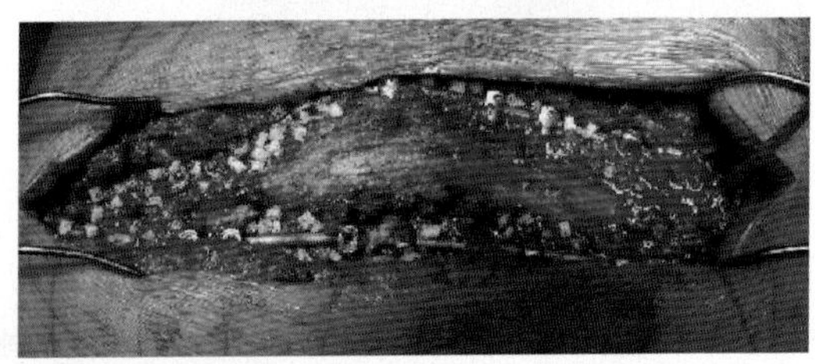
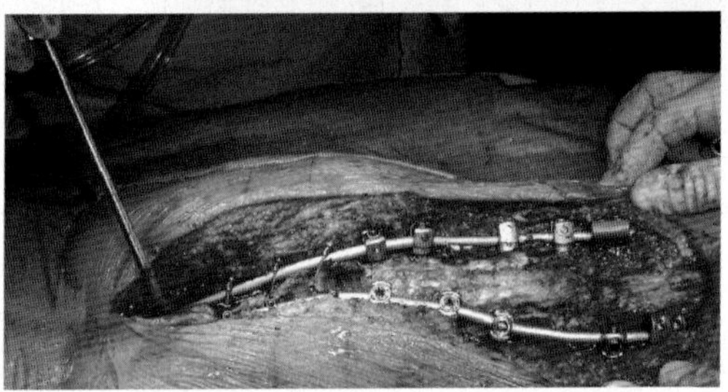

**TECH FIG 5** • **A.** Bilateral rods are anchored to L4 and S hooks in preparation for reduction. **B.** Decancellized levels are crushed by compressing adjacent screw heads. **C.** In a different patient, gradual reduction with wires and provisional tightening are accomplished using a growing construct. **D.** Completed reduction in patient in **A** and **B**. Allograft and autograft have been applied to decorticated bone for fusion. **E.** Completed reduction in patient with growing construct in **C**.

## Assessing and Managing Lower Extremity Hypoperfusion

- Frequently, the initial maneuvers for correction across the kyphosis are accompanied by a decrease in blood flow to the lower extremities. Therefore, it is important to do this corrective maneuver gradually in small increments.
- The baroreceptors in the aorta can accommodate to the change in alignment and stretch. If the blood flow to the feet is unable to accommodate to the new position of the spine, further decancellization or vertebral body removal will be necessary.
  - This decision is based on the flow to the lower extremities reflected in the pulse oximeter or arterial catheters in the feet.

## Closure

- As part of the closure, it is important to grasp the paraspinal musculature with clamps to pull the muscles toward the midline by elevating and mobilizing the muscle layer with a Cobb elevator.
  - Sometimes, release of the fascia on the posterior side of the musculature is necessary, and this is best done in the posterior axillary line with a vertical cut in the fascia.
- The paraspinal musculature should be brought as close as possible toward the midline on both sides and sewn down (**TECH FIG 6**).
- At least one and more likely two Hemovac drains should be left, one in the deep and one in the superficial layers, for drainage over 1 week to 10 days postoperatively.
- Subcuticular closures can be used, but they should be reinforced with external suture of some kind, either clips or interrupted nylon sutures on a temporary basis.

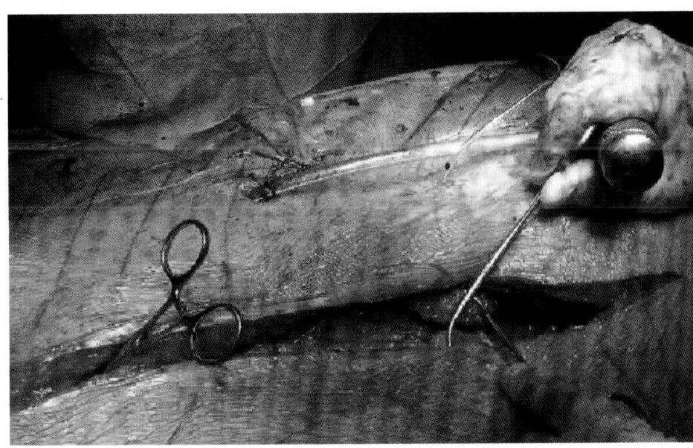

**TECH FIG 6** • The paraspinal muscle flaps are brought to midline for final closure.

## PEARLS AND PITFALLS

| | |
|---|---|
| **Evaluation** | ■ The surgeon can assess flexibility of the curve by physically supporting the child under the armpits to suspend him or her against gravity. Bending back supine on the examining table can also indicate the extent of lumbar flexibility. |
| **Preoperative preparation** | ■ Areas of skin breakdown should be addressed and healed before kyphectomy. |
| **Intraoperative monitoring** | ■ Vascular monitoring of the lower extremities is a critical part of the intraoperative monitoring. |
| **Preoperative preparation** | ■ Preoperative antibiotics are essential, including gram-negative coverage for urinary pathogens. These are continued postoperatively for 6–12 weeks. |
| **Managing incidental dural tears** | ■ A 4-0 Nurolon on a small taper needle in a running fashion works quite well for an incidental durotomy repair. Duragen can be sewn over the repair, and occasionally, the use of a sealant (Tisseel) is necessary. |
| **Preventing epidural bleeding** | ■ Care is taken to avoid violating the posterior cortex of the vertebral body until the very end because this is where the epidural vessels are most prolific. |
| **Setting the S hook** | ■ The final tightening should produce some distraction between the lowest lumbar segment fixation point and the S hooks pushed against the sacral ala. This will set the S hooks in place securely. |
| **Postoperative care** | ■ All reasonable measures must be taken to avoid any pressure on the wound or extremities in the postoperative period. All areas of insensate skin must be protected from excessive pressure with frequent change in position on a soft surface. The dressings should be covered with a waterproof covering to protect against secondary contamination from stool. |

## POSTOPERATIVE CARE

- For recovery, patients are placed on their back with an extra-thick foam on top of the mattress to avoid excessive skin pressure.
- Logrolling is instituted 6 hours postoperatively and repeated every 2 hours.
- Recovery occurs in the intensive care unit until the patient is sufficiently stable.
- Although postoperative immobilization is not necessary, if desired, it can be accomplished with careful molding of a bivalved jacket with a Plastazote soft lining.

## OUTCOMES

- Improved sitting
- Improved respiratory function
- Better blood supply to skin

## COMPLICATIONS

- Skin breakdown
- Infection, superficial or deep
- Vascular compromise to feet with stretch on aorta
- Loosening of spinal implants
- Pseudarthrosis

## SUGGESTED READING

1. McCarthy RE. Myelokyphosis. Shriners Hospitals for Crippled Children, Symposium on Caring for the Child with Myelomeningocele. Rosemont, IL: American Academy of Orthopaedic Surgeons, 2002.

# Anterior Interbody Arthrodesis with Instrumentation for Scoliosis

Janay E. Mckie and Daniel J. Sucato

## DEFINITION

- Thoracic scoliosis and thoracolumbar–lumbar scoliosis are typical curves seen in idiopathic scoliosis and can be treated anteriorly.
- Anterior arthrodesis refers to the fusion of the anterior part of the vertebral bodies, usually with instrumentation for these curve patterns.

## ANATOMY

- Thoracic idiopathic scoliosis usually has an apex at T8 or T9. It is most commonly a right convex curve pattern and has axial plane rotational deformity as well as hypokyphosis.
- Thoracolumbar–lumbar scoliosis has an apex of the curve at T12 or below and is most commonly a left-sided curve, with or without a compensatory thoracic curve.
- The vertebral bodies are nearly normal in their shape, although some distortion of the vertebral body and pedicles is seen, with thin, long pedicles on the concavity and shorter, wider pedicles on the convexity.

## PATHOGENESIS

- The cause of idiopathic scoliosis is not yet known.

## NATURAL HISTORY

- Idiopathic scoliosis progresses with continued growth of the spine, especially during the peak growth periods and when the curve magnitudes are "large" at the completion of growth.
- Thoracic curves tend to progress at skeletal maturity when the curve is greater than 45 to 50 degrees.
- Thoracolumbar–lumbar curves tend to progress when the curve is greater than 35 to 40 degrees at the time of skeletal maturity.

## PATIENT HISTORY AND PHYSICAL FINDINGS

- Patients with thoracic scoliosis and thoracolumbar scoliosis should be evaluated for their perception of spine and body deformity to include asymmetric shoulder elevation, trunk shift, waistline asymmetry, and rib or flank prominence.
- Pain in the axial spine and pain radiating into the lower extremities should be ascertained with a good history; such symptoms warrant a magnetic resonance imaging (MRI).
- Neurologic symptoms such as paresthesias, hyperesthesia, or bowel or bladder symptoms are relevant and require further imaging with an MRI.
- Physical examination should assess the trunk imbalance in the coronal plane, which can be seen with isolated thoracic or thoracolumbar–lumbar curves.
- The Adams forward bend test characterizes the axial plane deformity seen in scoliosis and is used to assess rotational deformity of the thoracic rib prominence or the flank prominence. The rotational deformity of the thoracic and lumbar spine is graded using a scoliometer with the patient bending forward. The rotational deformity seen in scoliosis can be very prominent and the most obvious deformity seen by patient and families.
- Cutaneous manifestations of dysraphism should also be analyzed.

## IMAGING AND OTHER DIAGNOSTIC STUDIES

- Anteroposterior (AP) and lateral radiographs of the spine should be obtained to review the coronal and sagittal plane deformities, respectively (**FIG 1**).
- On the AP radiograph, the coronal plane deformity is measured using the Cobb method. Truncal imbalance can be measured using the Floman method (bisecting the distance between the lateral rib margins and comparing this point to the center sacral vertical line [CSVL]).
- The decompensation of the head relative to the pelvis is measured by the distance between the C7 plumb line and the CSVL.
- The Risser sign should be evaluated by assessing the ossification of the iliac apophysis, giving it a grade between 0 and 5.
- The triradiate cartilage status should be assessed as either open or closed.
- The lateral radiograph is used to measure thoracic kyphosis (measured from T5 to T12) and lumbar lordosis (from L1 to S1) as well as the sagittal balance (comparing a C7 plumb bob line to the front edge of S1).

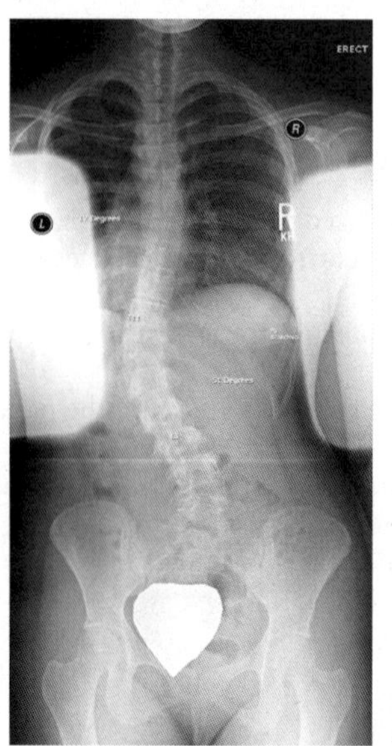


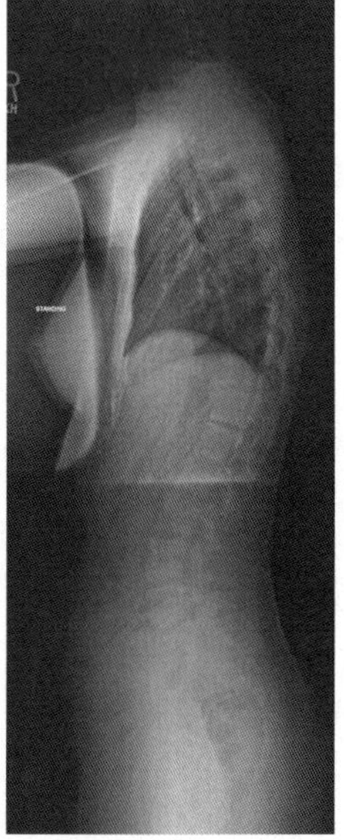


**FIG 1** • **A,B.** AP and lateral radiographs of a 51-degree left lumbar curve.

- Supine best-bend radiographs can be used to determine the flexibility of the spine and are especially useful to determine whether the thoracolumbar–lumbar curve is flexible when a primary thoracic curve is present or if the thoracic curve is flexible and compensatory when the primary thoracolumbar–lumbar curve is present.

## DIFFERENTIAL DIAGNOSIS

- Idiopathic scoliosis should be differentiated from other types of scoliosis in which congenital abnormalities are not seen in ambulatory patients. This list includes, but is not limited to, neurofibromatosis, Marfan syndrome, type 3 spinal muscular atrophy, scoliosis associated with syringomyelia, or tethered cord.

## NONOPERATIVE MANAGEMENT

- Adolescent thoracic and thoracolumbar scoliosis can be treated with bracing when curve magnitudes are between 25 and 45 degrees during peak growth periods.
- Bracing is used for these curve magnitudes to prevent curve progression and is indicated in Risser grade 0 to 2 patients.
- Nonoperative management is primarily indicated when the cosmetic appearance of the patient is acceptable to him or her.

## SURGICAL MANAGEMENT

- Surgical indications for thoracic idiopathic scoliosis are curves exceeding 45 to 50 degrees with unacceptable cosmetic deformity.
- Surgical indications for thoracolumbar–lumbar curves are curves exceeding 40 to 45 degrees with unacceptable cosmetic deformity with a compensatory thoracic curve.

### Preoperative Planning

- A careful physical examination as noted earlier is necessary to ensure that there are no neurologic signs or symptoms, which would indicate neural axis abnormalities. If these are present, MRI of the neural axis is indicated.
- Radiographic imaging should be used to ensure the curve is characteristic of an idiopathic curve. For thoracic curve patterns, this should demonstrate apical lordosis. The atypical curves, such as left-sided thoracic curves or those with significant decompensation despite minimal rotational deformity, or patients who have excessive thoracic kyphosis should be further evaluated with an MRI.
- The AP radiograph, the lateral standing radiograph, and the supine best-bend radiograph should be used to determine the Lenke classification.
- Specific detailed analysis of the compensatory curves should be performed to fine-tune a surgical plan to ensure that postoperative decompensation does not occur. This is especially important to determine the flexibility of the lumbar curve and the lumbar modifier for primary thoracic curves as well as the flexibility of the compensatory thoracic curve for primary thoracolumbar–lumbar curves.
- Anterior fusion levels for thoracic scoliosis are, in general, proximal end vertebra to distal end vertebra. Occasionally, a parallel disc is noted at the distal segment. It is controversial whether this disc should be included in the fusion levels. When the curve is relatively small (50 to 60 degrees) and flexible (>50% flexibility index) and the patient is skeletally mature (triradiate cartilage is closed and Risser grade 1 or higher), inclusion of the parallel disc is not often necessary (**FIG 2A,B**).
- Anterior fusion levels for thoracolumbar–lumbar curves in general are proximal end vertebra to distal end vertebra. When the disc below the planned lowest instrumented vertebra is reversing and opening into the fractional lumbosacral curve, then disc wedging is not seen postoperatively. However, a disc below the lowest instrumented vertebra that is parallel preoperatively will often be wedged postoperatively (**FIG 2C,D**).

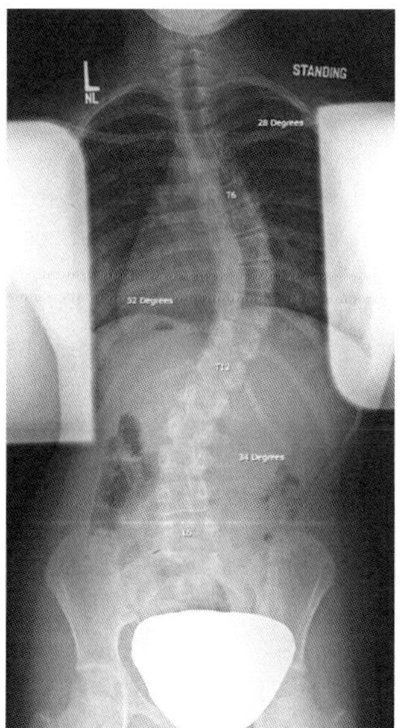

A

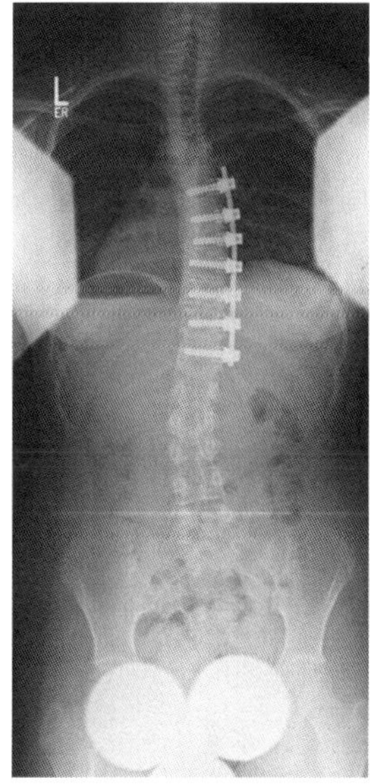
B

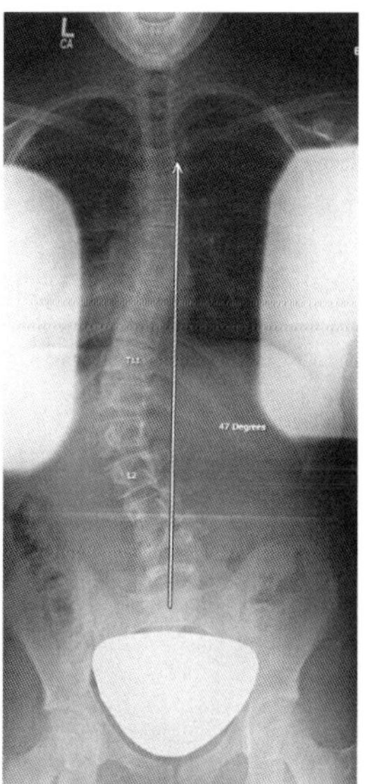
C

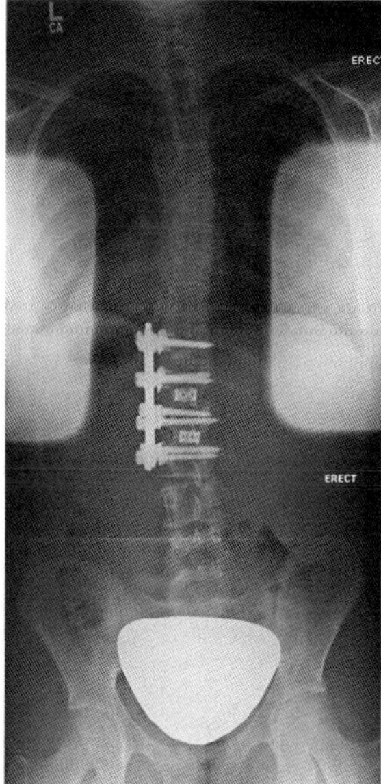

D

**FIG 2** • **A.** Preoperative radiograph of a 13-year-old girl with a right thoracic curve measuring 52 degrees from T6 to T12. The disc at T11–T12 is open into the right thoracic curve while the disc at T12–L1 is parallel. **B.** Thoracoscopic anterior spinal fusion and instrumentation from T6 to T12 demonstrating excellent correction of the main thoracic curve with excellent response of the proximal thoracic and lumbar curves. **C.** A left thoracolumbar curve measured between T11 and L2 with a trunk shift to the left. **D.** Two-year postoperative radiographs following an open anterior fusion and instrumentation from T11 to L2 with dual rod–dual screw system and anterior cages placed at the T12–L1 and L1–L2 levels with excellent coronal plane correction.

## Positioning

- Positioning for anterior surgery for either the thoracic or thoracolumbar curves is fairly similar. Patients are placed in the lateral decubitus position with the convex side of the curve up.
- An axillary roll is used for safe upper extremity neurologic function (**FIG 3**).
- An inflatable beanbag is used to position the patient, and body positioners can be added for further patient stabilization.
- For thoracolumbar–lumbar curves, a table that can be flexed allows for greater access to the abdomen and spine. It should be centered over the apex of the curve.
- For thoracic scoliosis surgery, the patient can be placed on a flat radiolucent table.

## Approach

- The anterior approach is used for thoracic scoliosis.

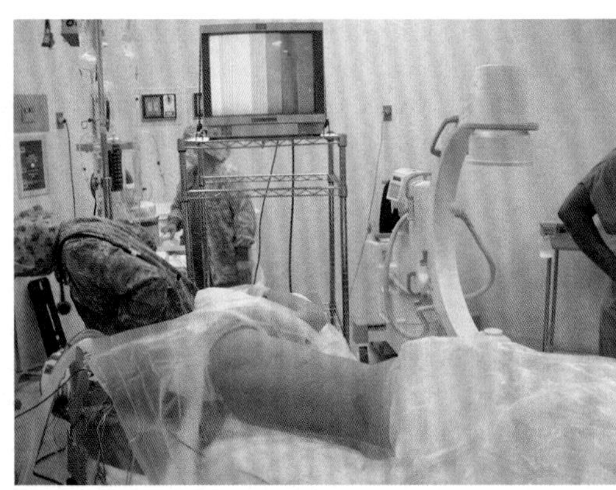

**FIG 3** • Positioning for access for a thoracoscopic anterior spinal fusion and instrumentation in the left lateral decubitus position. The arms are positioned at 90 degrees, axillary rolls are placed on the left axilla, and the patient is secured with a beanbag.



# Open Thoracic Anterior Instrumentation and Arthrodesis

- A curved incision is made over the proximal rib corresponding to the proximal fusion level (ie, commonly T5 with the fifth rib). The incision is carried through the thoracic and abdominal musculature to the periosteum of the rib.
- Subperiosteal dissection of the rib is performed circumferentially, and the rib is cut posteriorly and anteriorly.
- The parietal pleura is incised in a longitudinal fashion over the vertebral bodies across the intended levels of instrumentation and fusion.
- The segmental vessels can be temporarily ligated and spinal cord monitoring should be observed during temporary ligation.
- Permanent ligation can be performed after 20 minutes of normal spinal cord monitoring.
- Discectomy is performed (see the section on the thoracoscopic technique).
- Instrumentation is placed (see the following text).
- For the remaining procedures, see details under the thoracoscopic approach.

# Thoracoscopic Anterior Instrumentation and Arthrodesis

## Positioning, Preparation, and Draping

- After true lateral positioning is confirmed, fluoroscopy is used to mark the skin for the proximal end vertebra and distal end vertebra on the AP view. The skin markings are made to identify the angle of the proximal end vertebra on the AP view (**TECH FIG 1**).
- The anterior and posterior edges of the vertebral bodies are then marked using the lateral fluoroscopy view.
- The chest and flank are prepared and draped in the normal sterile fashion.

## Thoracoscopic Portal and Guidewire Placement

- An anterior portal is placed, bisecting the distance between the proximal and the distal intended instrumented vertebra, in the anterior axillary line. This portal is used for placement of the camera (**TECH FIG 2A**).
- A guidewire is then placed directly over the vertebral bodies over the intended second most proximal portal and is visualized

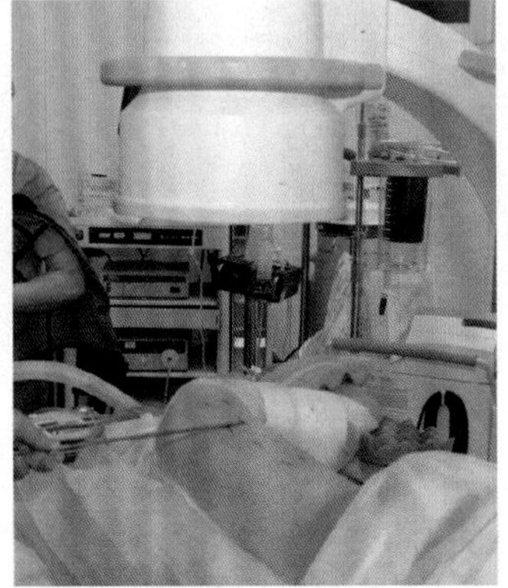

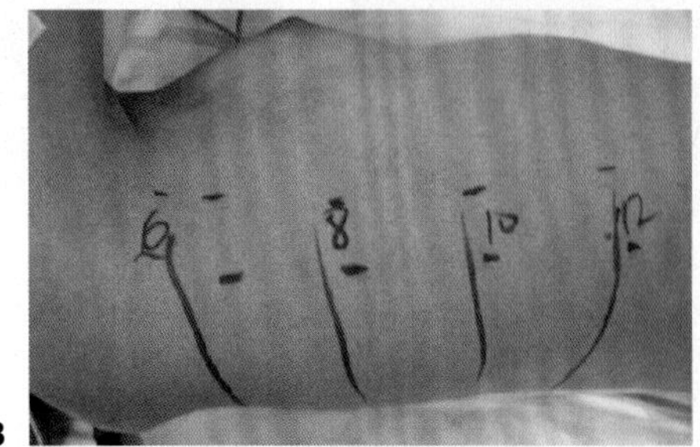


**TECH FIG 1** • Fluoroscopic imaging of the spine prior to surgery. **A.** The lateral radiograph is used to identify the anterior and posterior edges of the vertebral body. **B.** The AP radiograph is used to mark the skin over the intended fusion levels to direct portal placement. This example demonstrates a T6–T12 fusion.

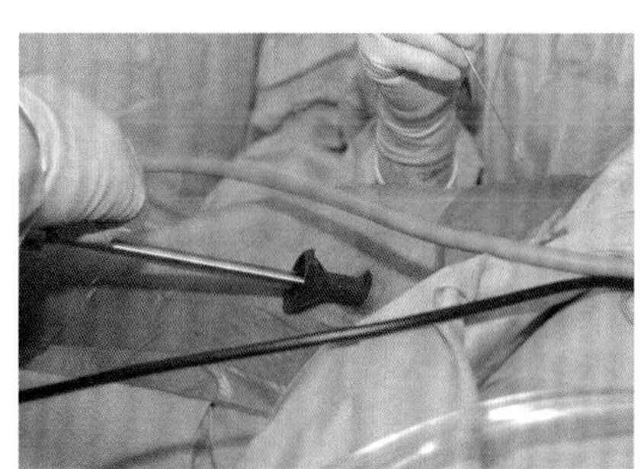

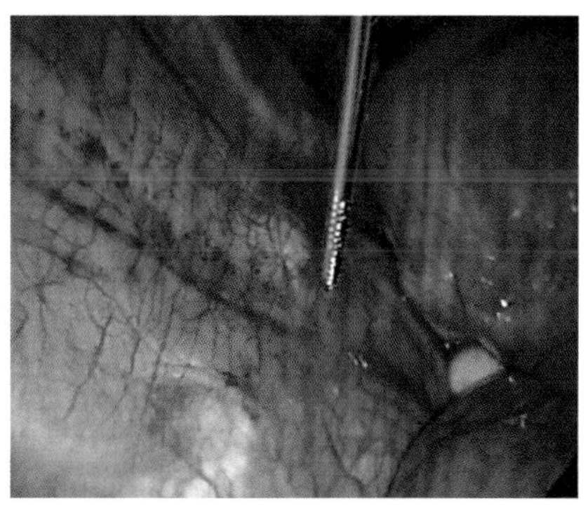

**TECH FIG 2** • **A.** The anterior portal is placed in the anterior axillary line with the camera inserted in the portal. The patient is in the left lateral decubitus position: proximal to the right and distal to the left. **B.** A guidewire is placed before placing the posterolateral portals. The guidewire is directed just anterior to the rib heads and marks a good position for the posterolateral portal.

with the thoracoscope placed in the anterior portal (**TECH FIG 2B**).

- After good placement of the guidewire (directly over the rib head), the portal is placed with a transverse incision centered over the rib. This portal can be used for visualization with a thoracoscope to place the remaining portals.
- The most proximal posterolateral portal is placed after the intended second posterolateral portal to ensure exact location of the proximal portal. The proximal portal position is most important because the most proximal two screws are often placed in small vertebral bodies and have significant coronal angulation, and retraction of the scapula makes this portal difficult.
- The remaining portals are placed in the posterolateral line.
- The portals will house the camera, a fan retractor to retract the lung, a suction device, a working portal, and then a free portal.

## Discectomy Technique

- The pleura is incised in the midvertebral line in a longitudinal fashion, keeping the segmental vessels intact (**TECH FIG 3A**).
- The segmental vessels are then ligated two or three at a time (normotensive anesthesia is used for anterior surgery).
- The parietal pleura is retracted anteriorly, all the way to the opposite side, and access to the anterior longitudinal ligament and the contralateral annulus is allowed (**TECH FIG 3B**).
- Posterior retraction allows for identification of the rib heads (**TECH FIG 3C**).
- The disc is incised from the convex rib head to the opposite annulus (**TECH FIG 3D**).
- The periosteum for the proximal and distal vertebra is incised to allow for subperiosteal dissection when the discectomy is performed.

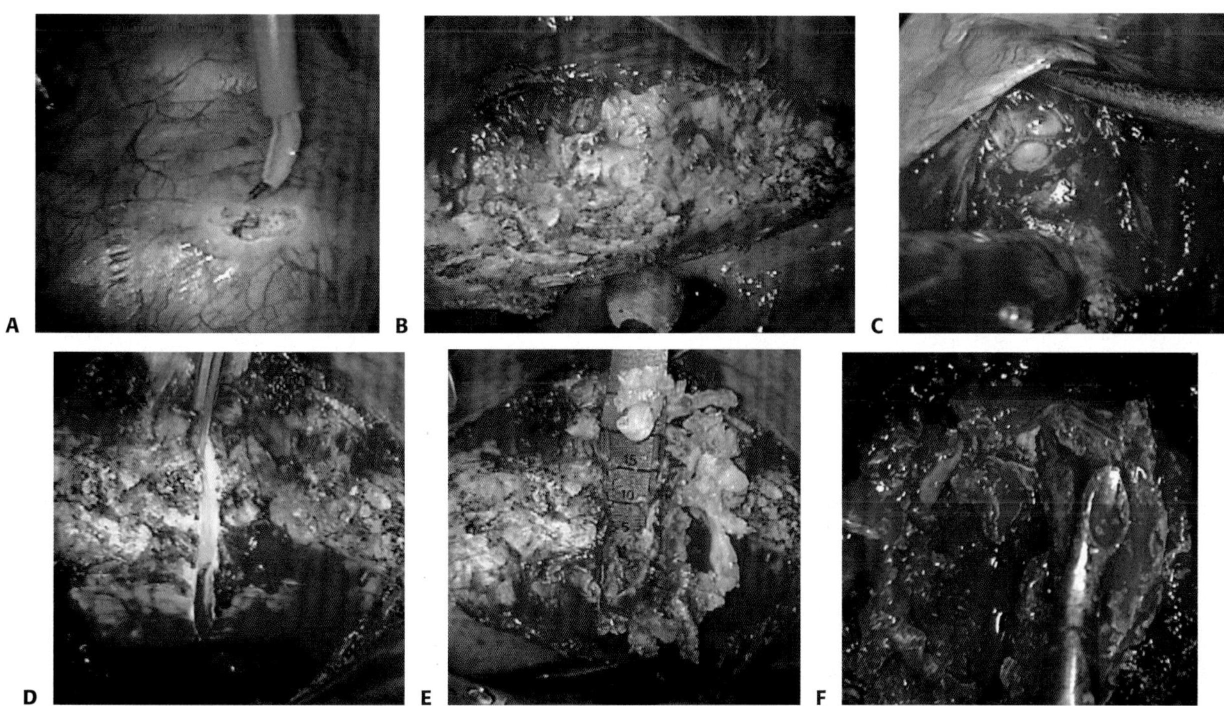

**TECH FIG 3** • **A.** Electrocautery is used to incise the parietal pleura longitudinally, starting over the disc to avoid the segmental vessels. The segmental vessels are left intact on the first pass. **B,C.** After ligation of the segmental vessels, the pleura is bluntly retracted. **B.** Anterior dissection circumferentially to the opposite side of the pleura. **C.** Posterior retraction of the parietal pleura beyond the rib head. **D.** A scalpel blade is used to incise the annulus from rib head posteriorly all the way to the opposite annulus. Shown here is the incision up against the rib head after incising the annulus and the anterior longitudinal ligament. **E.** Disc shavers are used to break up the disc material. **F.** An angled curette is used to take down the endplate and tease the periosteum around the corner to get full access to the bone. *(continued)*

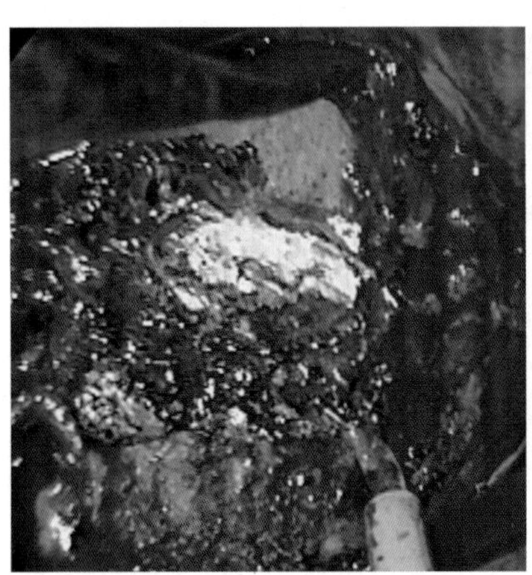

**TECH FIG 3** • *(continued)* **G.** The most anterior aspect of the rib head is being removed. Electrocautery is used to loosen the soft tissues attaching the rib head to the vertebral body. Part of the rib head has been removed in this photo.

- Disc shavers are used to break up the disc material, using shavers of increasing width (**TECH FIG 3E**).
- A rongeur is used to remove the annulus and nucleus pulposus.
- An angled curette is used to take down the endplate circumferentially (**TECH FIG 3F**).
- The rib head is removed at the T4–T7 levels. Because it is positioned relatively anterior on the vertebral bodies, it allows for good discectomy and good placement of the screws at these levels (**TECH FIG 3G**).
- After discectomy, Gelfoam or Surgicel is placed in the disc space to prevent endplate bleeding.

## Implant Placement and Grafting

- Screw placement is performed beginning at the apex of the curve.
- The proper screw position starts just anterior to the rib head and is angled in line with the midaxial plane of the vertebral body (angled anteriorly at the apex, especially with less angulation at the proximal distal levels) (**TECH FIG 4A**).
- Screw position should be parallel to the endplate, and the proximal and distal levels should be angled toward the apex of the curve so that during correction, any screw plow will not loosen screws. Visualization of adjacent screws should confirm good alignment (**TECH FIG 4B**).
- After screw placement, the screw height should be visualized to ensure that rod seating will occur without difficulty (**TECH FIG 4C**).
- Autologous bone is packed into the disc space after removal of Gelfoam or Surgicel.
- Rod placement is performed; rods can be seated either proximally or distally. Depending on rod flexibility and size, a straight rod is placed on the end and the set screws are engaged to secure the rod (**TECH FIG 4D**).
- Compression across the initial levels is then performed to improve the coronal and sagittal plane deformity (**TECH FIG 4E**).
- The rod is then cantilevered down to the remaining screws, and compression is sequentially performed over those levels. Often, the rod cannot be cantilevered down to all of the screws, so sequential cantilever and compression are performed (**TECH FIG 4F**).

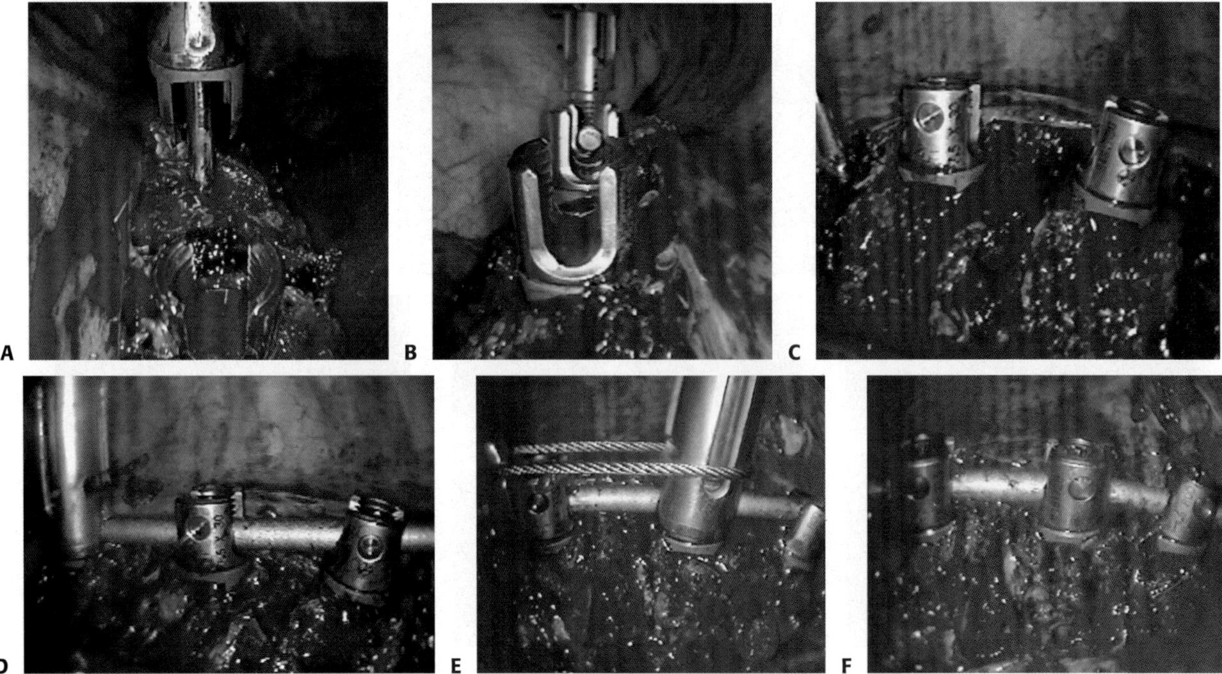

**TECH FIG 4** • **A.** The screw awl device is placed while visualizing a previously placed screw. The starting point is just anterior to the rib head in this photo. **B.** Final placement of a distal screw while visualizing the more proximal screws. The diaphragm is seen in the background. **C.** After screw placement, the height of the screws should be consistent to allow easy seating of the rod. **D.** The rod is inserted into the most distal screws. **E.** Compression across the most distal segment is first performed using the cable compressor. **F.** After distal compression, the rod is cantilevered to the remaining screw heads. *(continued)*

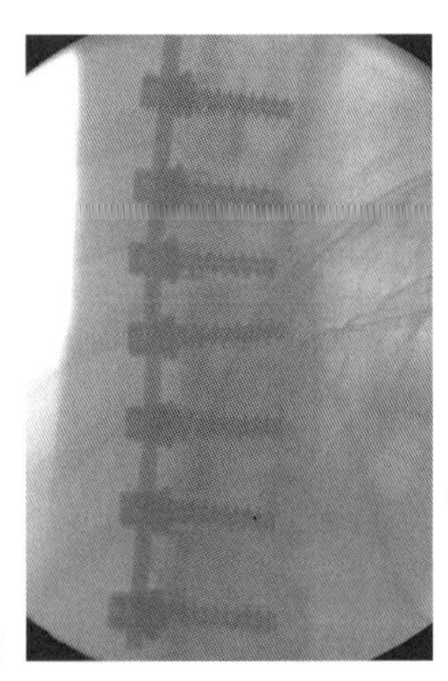
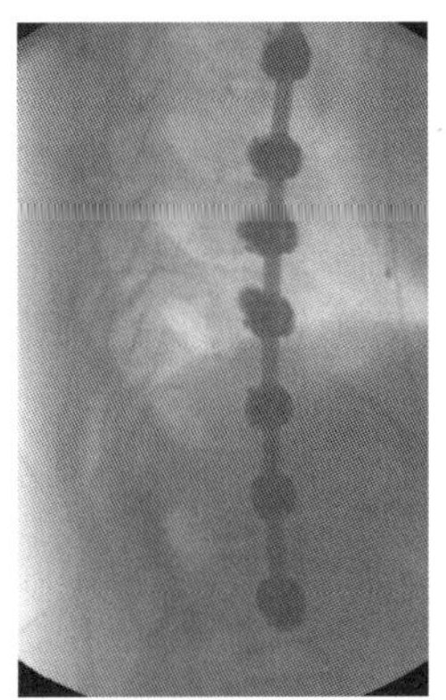
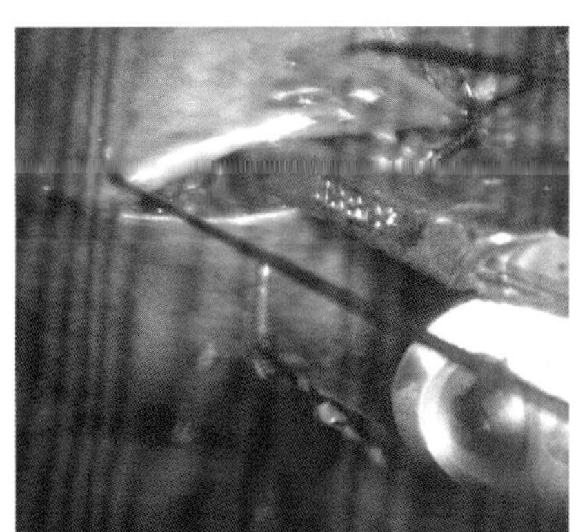
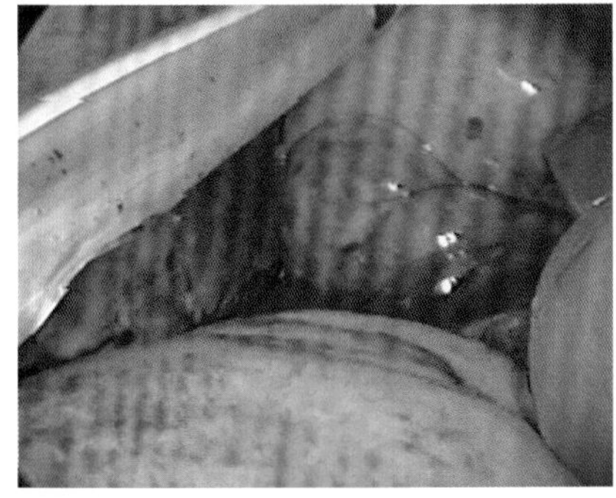

**TECH FIG 4** • *(continued)* **G.** AP intraoperative fluoroscopic image confirms good correction of the spine with maintenance of screw position. **H.** Lateral fluoroscopic image demonstrates good position of the screws with restoration of thoracic kyphosis. Rotational correction is also seen with rib margins symmetric. **I.** Closure of the parietal pleura over the instrumentation. **J.** Placement of chest tube under direct visualization while the lung is still deflated.

- Radiographs are obtained at this point, and the desired correction is compared with the radiographs. Further compression is performed as needed. Care should be taken to ensure that screw plow or loosening is not occurring radiographically or visually (**TECH FIG 4G,H**).
- Set screws are completely torqued down.
- The pleura is closed over the instrumentation to ensure correct bone graft positioning, decrease chest tube drainage, and improve long-term pulmonary function (**TECH FIG 4I**).
- The lung is inflated under direct visualization.
- A chest tube is placed through the distal portal incision and tunneled to the proximal portal (**TECH FIG 4J**).
- The incisions are closed in the normal fashion.

## Open Instrumentation and Arthrodesis of the Thoracolumbar–Lumbar Spine

### Preparation and Exposure

- The patient is placed in the lateral decubitus position with the convex side of the spine up.
- An axillary roll is placed.
- The bed can be flexed to allow for easier access to the flank (**TECH FIG 5A**).
- A curved linear incision is made in line with the rib just proximal to the planned upper instrumented vertebra (**TECH FIG 5B**).
- The incision is carried down through the subcutaneous layer through the various muscle layers down over the rib. The incision can be carried out distally lateral to the umbilicus.
- Subperiosteal dissection is carried out around the rib. The rib is transected posteriorly near its insertion to the spine (**TECH FIG 5C**).
- The costochondral junction is then incised. A marking suture is placed at the costochondral junction for later reapproximation (**TECH FIG 5D**).
- Usually at the costochondral level at the 10th rib, access into the retroperitoneal space is quite easy, with retroperitoneal fat evident. The peritoneal contents are then bluntly dissected off the abdominal wall and the undersurface of the diaphragm (**TECH FIG 5E**).
- The diaphragm is then incised just proximal to its insertion, and marking sutures are placed to ensure proper reapproximation (**TECH FIG 5F**).
- A pleural incision is made longitudinally in line with the spine, leaving the segmental vessels intact (**TECH FIG 5G**).
- Segmental vessel ligation is then carried out, maintaining good blood pressure to ensure good spinal cord perfusion (**TECH FIG 5H**).

### Discectomy

- Discectomies are performed with incision of the annulus fibrosus (**TECH FIG 6A**).
- Endplate dissection is carried out using a Cobb elevator to remove the entire endplate disc material back to the posterior aspect of the annulus and to the posterior longitudinal ligament if necessary (for severe curves; **TECH FIG 6B**).
- The disc material is removed completely using rongeurs and curettes (**TECH FIG 6C**).
- The disc space is packed with Surgicel.

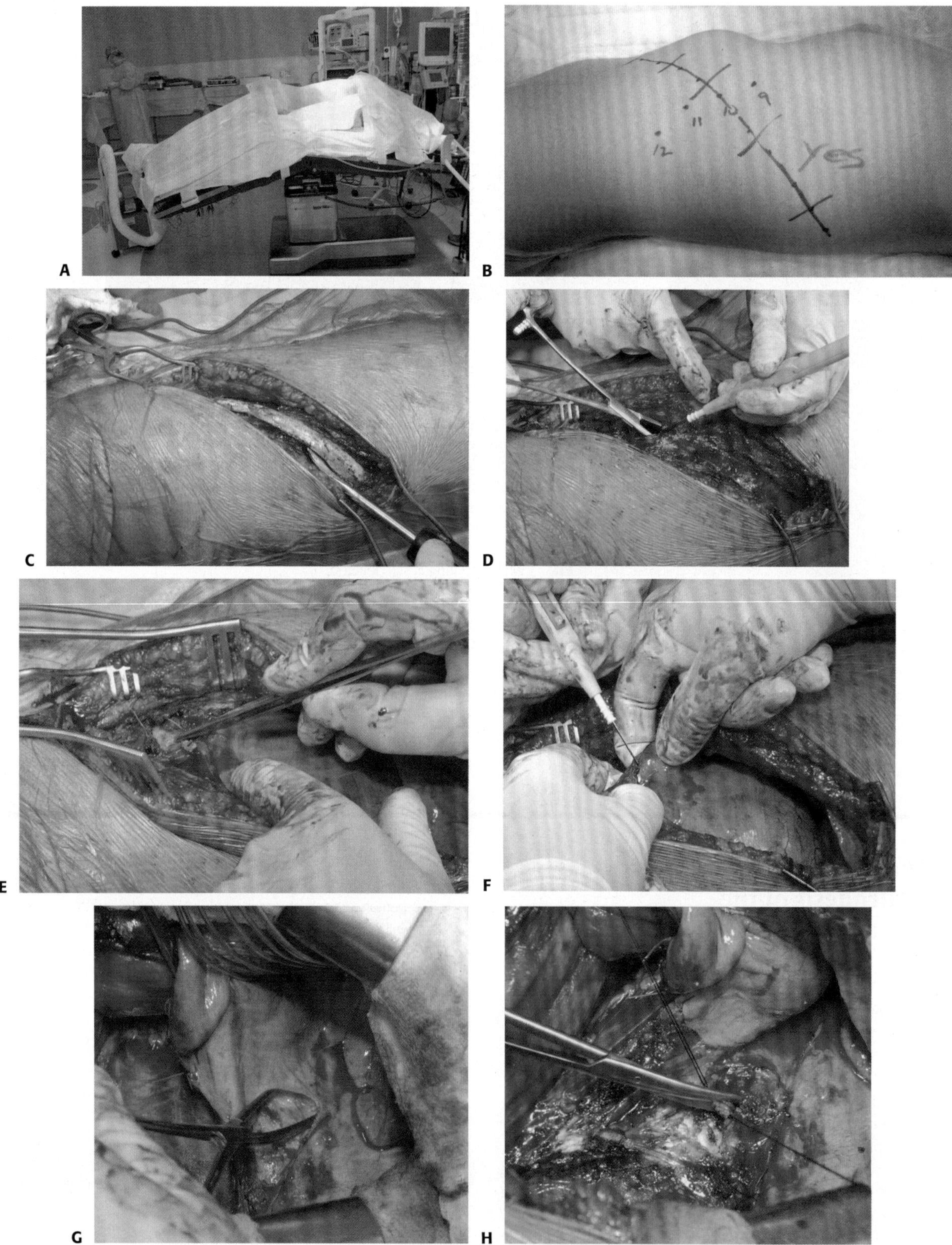


**TECH FIG 5** • **A.** Positioning for thoracoabdominal approach to the spine. The table is flexed to allow full access to the thoracoabdominal region. **B.** Skin incision is marked. This example is centered over the 10th rib for a T11–L3 fusion. **C.** The incision is made over the rib and subperiosteal dissection is carried out circumferentially around the rib after sequential dissection through the musculature. **D.** The posterior aspect of the periosteum is then incised and the chest is entered. **E.** After incision of the costochondral junction, the retroperitoneal fat is visualized and the retroperitoneal cavity is entered. **F.** The diaphragm is incised a fingerbreadth proximal to its insertion. **G.** The parietal pleura is incised proximally. **H.** Ligation of segmental vessels after suture tying.

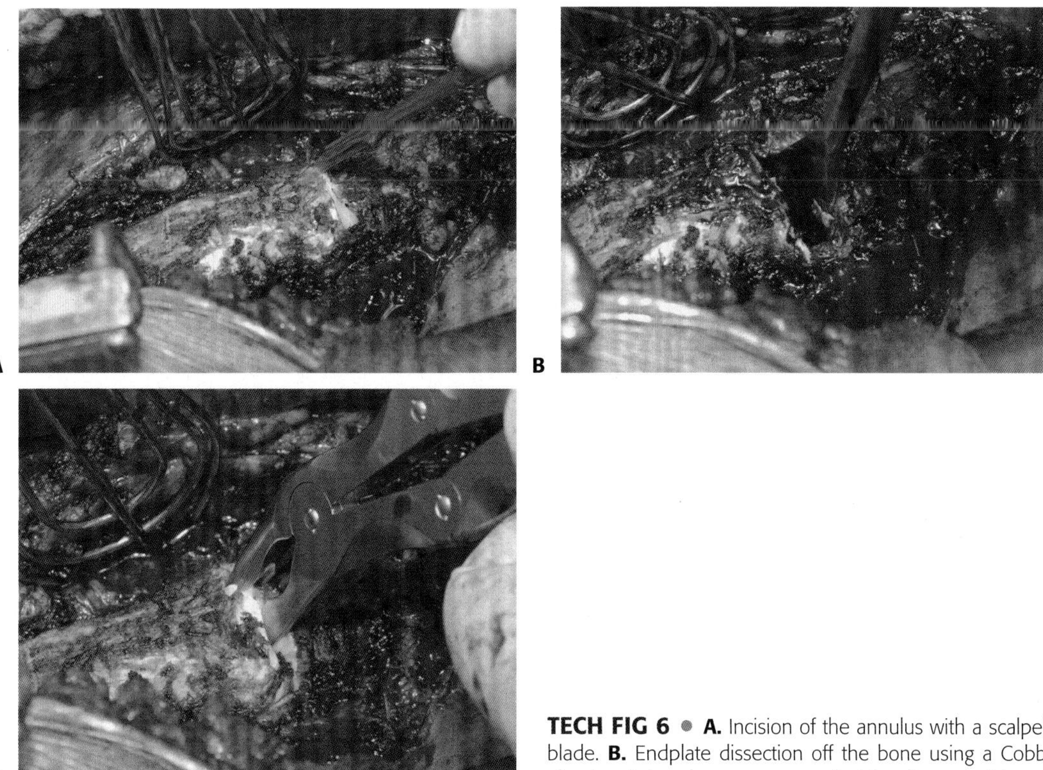

**TECH FIG 6** • **A.** Incision of the annulus with a scalpel blade. **B.** Endplate dissection off the bone using a Cobb elevator. **C.** Lexel rongeur removal of the disc material.

## Implant Placement, Correction, and Fusion

- The instrumentation is then placed using single large screws with a quarter-inch single-rod implant system or a dual rod with a 5.5-mm rod (shown here).
- Screws are initially placed at the apex in the middle to posterior third of the vertebral body in the midaxial plane (**TECH FIG 7A**).
- When using a dual-rod system, the posterior screws are initially placed angled in the midaxial plane, whereas the anterior screws are directed slightly posteriorly. A staple is often used when both the single- and dual-rod screws are used (**TECH FIG 7B**).
- Once screws are placed, the bone graft material is placed as far back toward the posterior longitudinal ligament as possible or the posterior rim of the annulus fibrosus.
- The operating table should now be leveled to allow for correction of the spine.
- The posterior rod is initially placed with the dual-rod system, and a 90-degree rod rotation removal can be performed (**TECH FIG 7C**).
  - Alternatively, directed force on the anterior screws to correct the coronal and axial plane is achieved, and then the posterior rod is inserted (**TECH FIG 7D**).
- After rod rotation with a dual-rod system or single-rod system, or correction with pressure on the anterior screws and fixation

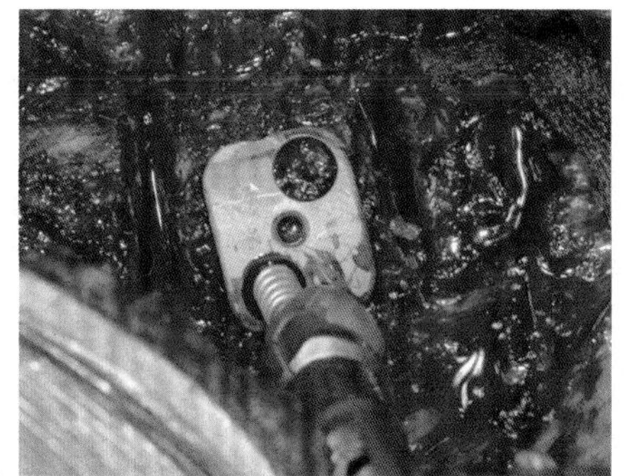

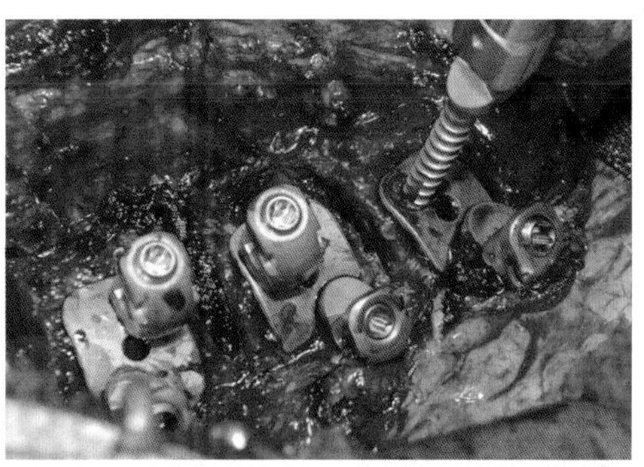

**TECH FIG 7** • **A.** Placement of the posterior screw directed slightly anteriorly with direct visualization of the endplates after complete disc removal. **B.** Anterior screw placement after placement of the posterior screws. The anterior screws are directed slightly posteriorly. *(continued)*

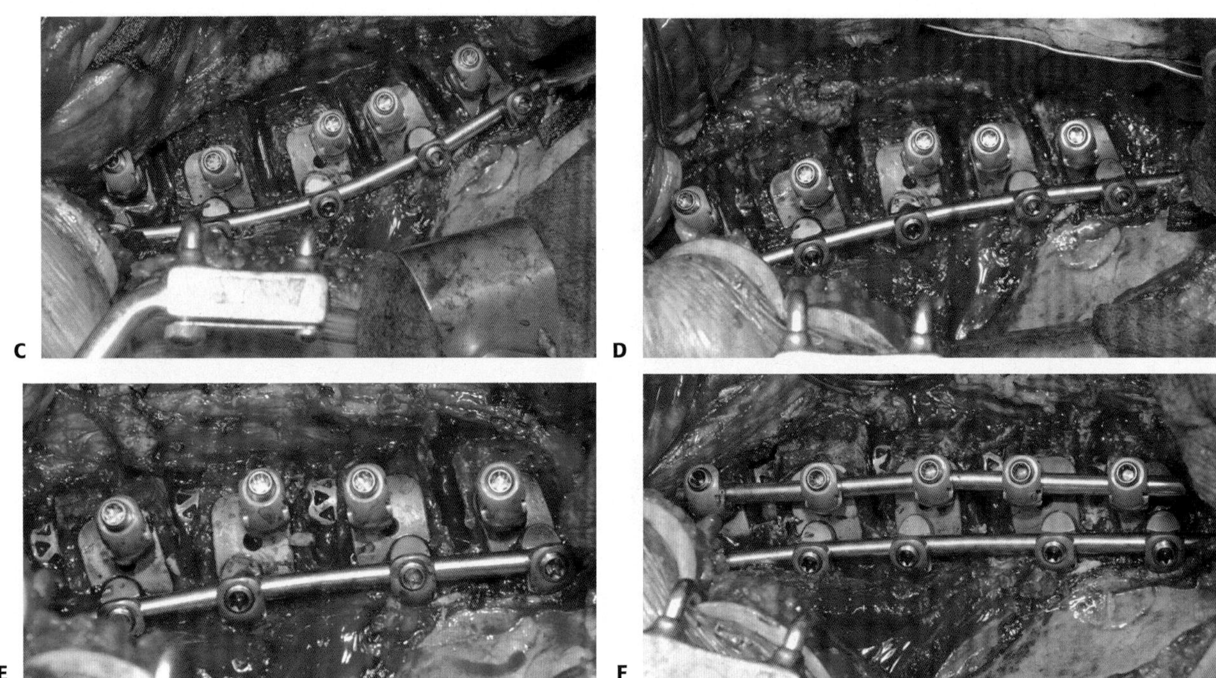

**TECH FIG 7** • *(continued)* **C.** Insertion of the posterior rod with lumbar lordosis built into the rod. **D.** After 90 degrees of rod rotation, scoliosis correction is achieved while restoring lumbar lordosis, as shown here. **E.** After rod rotation, the anterior structural support is placed anteriorly and toward the concavity of the deformity. **F.** The anterior rod is seated into the anterior screws.

with the posterior rod, the anterior structural support is placed. This is most commonly at levels distal to T12 or alternatively at all instrumented levels (**TECH FIG 7E**).

- Compression can then be performed to further correct coronal plane deformity.
- The anterior structural support should be placed anteriorly and onto the concavity to ensure maintenance of the lordosis and improvement of coronal plane correction.
- The second anterior rod should be then placed with a dual-rod system and all set screws completely tightened (**TECH FIG 7F**).
- The remaining bone graft material is then placed in the remaining disc space.

## Closure

- The pleura is closed as far distally as possible (**TECH FIG 8A**).
- The diaphragm is reapproximated with interrupted Nurolon sutures (**TECH FIG 8B**).
- The costochondral junction is reapproximated, and the periosteum of the rib is reapproximated (**TECH FIG 8C**).
- A chest tube of fairly large diameter is then placed.
- The abdominal wall is reapproximated in layers (**TECH FIG 8D**).
- The remaining muscle layers are closed as well as the skin and subcutaneous layers (**TECH FIG 8E**).
- The postoperative radiographs are shown in **TECH FIG 8F,G**.

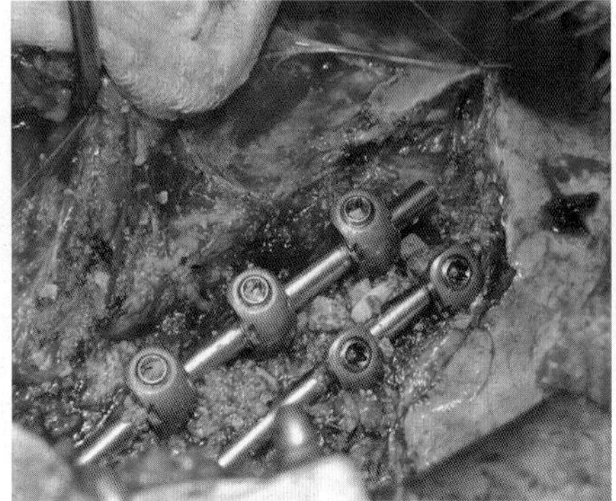

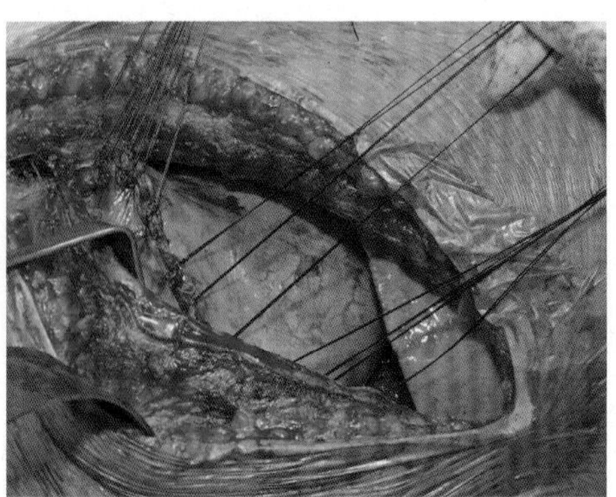

**TECH FIG 8** • **A.** The parietal pleura is closed beginning proximal to the implants. **B.** Interrupted Nurolon sutures are used to close the diaphragm in an anatomic fashion. *(continued)*

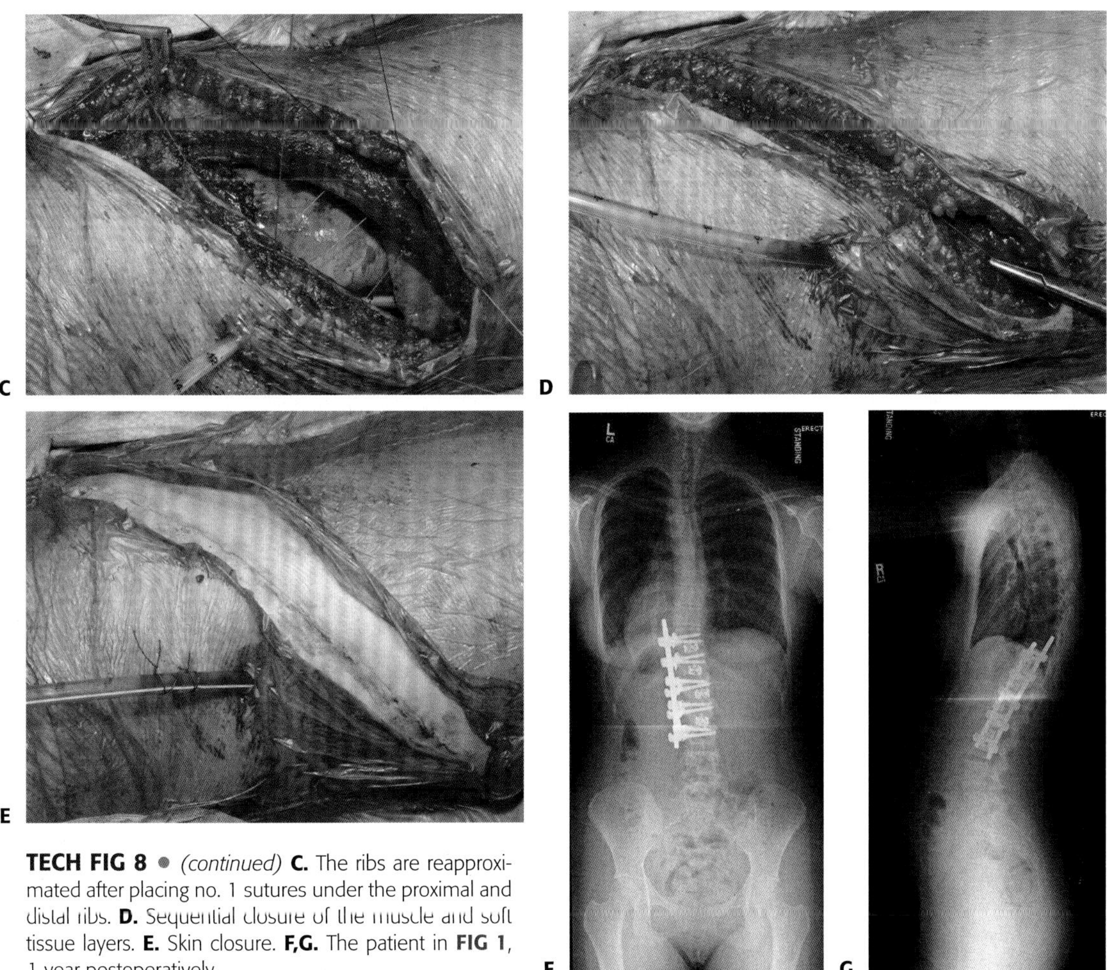

**TECH FIG 8** • *(continued)* **C.** The ribs are reapproximated after placing no. 1 sutures under the proximal and distal ribs. **D.** Sequential closure of the muscle and soft tissue layers. **E.** Skin closure. **F,G.** The patient in **FIG 1**, 1 year postoperatively.

## PEARLS AND PITFALLS

| | |
|---|---|
| **Anesthesia** | ■ During anterior surgery, normotensive anesthesia should be performed to maintain spinal cord perfusion, especially when segmental vessel ligation is performed.<br>■ Complete discectomy is necessary to achieve fusion because pseudarthrosis rates continue to be higher with anterior surgery than with posterior surgery. |
| **Camera performance** | ■ Thoracoscopy requires outstanding visualization and camera performance to ensure safe and effective discectomy as well as instrumentation. |
| **Rib head removal** | ■ Rib head removal during thoracic instrumentation from T4 to T7 is necessary to ensure screws are placed posteriorly enough to achieve good purchase. |
| **Discectomy** | ■ This is the most important aspect of the procedure to mobilize the spine for correction and to achieve a solid arthrodesis. |
| **Screw placement** | ■ Screw placement is always challenging at the proximal and distal levels. Screw trajectories should always be parallel to the endplate, or if anything angled toward the apex of the curve, so that during correction, plowing does not result in loosening of the screw. |
| **Deformity correction** | ■ Thoracic curve: compression at sequential levels, followed by cantilever of an undercontoured rod, followed by further compression<br>■ Thoracolumbar–lumbar curve: rod rotation followed by compression |

## POSTOPERATIVE CARE

- The chest tube should be placed to wall suction and can usually be removed between 48 and 72 hours, when the drainage decreases below 80 mL per shift and when it turns more straw-colored.
- Serial hemoglobin and hematocrit levels should be obtained in the first 48 hours.
- Advancing activities: Sitting in a chair the first postoperative day and walking on the second postoperative day ensures good postoperative pulmonary status and normal bowel function.
- Postoperative bracing is used for 3 months for single-rod anterior thoracoscopic thoracic arthrodesis and instrumentation. No bracing is necessary with single quarter-inch rod instrumentation or dual-rod instrumentation when anterior structural support is used.
- Normal activities are resumed when arthrodesis is visualized (best seen on the lateral radiograph).

## OUTCOMES

- Thoracoscopic anterior instrumentation and fusion achieves a good radiographic and functional outcome.
- Thoracoscopic anterior instrumentation and fusion continues to have a fairly high pseudarthrosis rate of 5% to 6%.
- Pulmonary function is somewhat decreased early in the postoperative period with anterior surgery, but then it can return to baseline at 1 to 2 years.
- Thoracolumbar–lumbar anterior instrumentation and fusion results in excellent coronal, axial, and sagittal plane realignment, especially when dual-rod and large single-rod instrumentation systems with anterior structural support are used.

## COMPLICATIONS

- Acute complications
  - Infection is rare in anterior spine deformity surgery.
  - Atelectasis and mucous plugs can be seen, especially with single-lung ventilation with anterior instrumentation. Aggressive pulmonary toilet and resuming activities minimize this risk.
- Late complications
  - Pseudarthrosis: The incidence is 4% to 10% for thoracic scoliosis (usually occurs at the apex of the curve) and 4% to 12% for thoracolumbar scoliosis (usually occurs at the distal fusion level).
  - Loss of correction with kyphosis is seen for thoracolumbar–lumbar curves treated anteriorly when anterior structural support is not used.

## SUGGESTED READINGS


1. Bernstein RM, Hall JE. Solid rod short segment anterior fusion in thoracolumbar scoliosis. J Pediatr Orthop B 1998;7:124–131.
2. Betz RR, Shufflebarger H. Anterior versus posterior instrumentation for the correction of thoracic idiopathic scoliosis. Spine 2001;26:1095–1100.
3. Bitan FD, Neuwirth MG, Kuflik PL, et al. The use of short and rigid anterior instrumentation in the treatment of idiopathic thoracolumbar scoliosis: a retrospective review of 24 cases. Spine 2002;27:1553–1557.
4. Bridwell KH. Indications and techniques for anterior-only and combined anterior and posterior approaches for thoracic and lumbar spine deformities. Instr Course Lect 2005;54:559–565.
5. Bullmann V, Halm HF, Niemeyer T, et al. Dual-rod correction and instrumentation of idiopathic scoliosis with the Halm-Zielke instrumentation. Spine 2003;28:1306–1313.
6. Fricka KB, Mahar AT, Newton PO. Biomechanical analysis of anterior scoliosis instrumentation: differences between single and dual rod systems with and without interbody structural support. Spine 2002;27:702–706.
7. Kaneda K, Shono Y, Satoh S, et al. New anterior instrumentation for the management of thoracolumbar and lumbar scoliosis. Application of the Kaneda two-rod system. Spine 1996;21:1250–1261.
8. Lenke LG, Newton PO, Marks MC, et al. Prospective pulmonary function comparison of open versus endoscopic anterior fusion combined with posterior fusion in adolescent idiopathic scoliosis. Spine 2004;29:2055–2060.
9. Lonner BS, Kondrachov D, Siddiqi F, et al. Thoracoscopic spinal fusion compared with posterior spinal fusion for the treatment of thoracic adolescent idiopathic scoliosis. J Bone Joint Surg Am 2007;89(suppl 2, pt 1):142–156.
10. Lowe TG, Alongi PR, Smith DAB, et al. Anterior single rod instrumentation for thoracolumbar adolescent idiopathic scoliosis with and without the use of structural interbody support. Spine 2003;28: 2232–2242.
11. Newton PO, Parent S, Marks M, et al. Prospective evaluation of 50 consecutive scoliosis patients surgically treated with thoracoscopic anterior instrumentation. Spine 2005;30:S100–S109.
12. Ouellet JA, Johnston CE II. Effect of grafting technique on the maintenance of coronal and sagittal correction in anterior treatment of scoliosis. Spine 2002;27:2129–2135.
13. Picetti GD III, Pang D, Bueff HU. Thoracoscopic techniques for the treatment of scoliosis: early results in procedure development. Neurosurgery 2002;51:978–984.
14. Reddi V, Clarke DV Jr, Arlet V. Anterior instrumentation thoracoscopic instrumentation in adolescent idiopathic scoliosis: a systematic review. Spine 2008;33:1986–1994.
15. Sanders AE, Baumann R, Brown H, et al. Selective anterior fusion of thoracolumbar/lumbar curves in adolescents: when can the associated thoracic curve be left unfused? Spine 2003;28:706–713.
16. Saraph VJ, Krismer M, Wimmer C. Operative treatment of scoliosis with the Kaneda anterior spine system. Spine 2005;30:1616–1620.
17. Satake K, Lenke LG, Kim YJ, et al. Analysis of the lowest instrumented vertebra following anterior spinal fusion of thoracolumbar/lumbar adolescent idiopathic scoliosis: can we predict postoperative disc wedging? Spine 2005;30:418–426.
18. Sucato DJ, Kassab F, Dempsey M. Analysis of screw placement relative to the aorta and spinal canal following anterior instrumentation for thoracic idiopathic scoliosis. Spine 2004;29:554–559.
19. Sucato D, Kassab F, Dempsey M. Thoracoscopic anterior spinal instrumentation and fusion for idiopathic scoliosis: a CT analysis of screw placement and completeness of discectomy. Scoliosis Research Society, Cleveland, Ohio, 2001.
20. Sweet FA, Lenke LG, Bridwell KH, et al. Prospective radiographic and clinical outcomes and complications of single solid rod instrumented anterior spinal fusion in adolescent idiopathic scoliosis. Spine 2001;26:1956–1965.
21. Watkins RG IV, Hussain N, Freeman BJ, et al. Anterior instrumentation for thoracolumbar adolescent idiopathic scoliosis: do structural interbody grafts preserve sagittal alignment better than morselized rib autografts? Spine 2006;31:2237–2342.
22. Wong HK, Hee HT, Yu Z, et al. Results of thoracoscopic instrumented fusion versus conventional posterior instrumented fusion in adolescent idiopathic scoliosis undergoing selective thoracic fusion. Spine 2004;29:2031–2039.

# Thoracoscopic Release and Fusion for Scoliosis

89

CHAPTER

Daniel J. Sucato and Matthew D. Abbott

## DEFINITION

- Thoracoscopy provides the ability to gain access to the thoracic spine via small incisions (portals).
- Anterior release includes removal of the annulus fibrosus, anterior longitudinal ligament, nucleus pulposus, and, if necessary, the rib head.
- Scoliosis is a lateral curvature of the spine with axial plane rotation.
- Fusion is the healing of two vertebral bodies together, usually fused by bone graft or bone graft substitute.

## ANATOMY

- The thoracic spine spans from the first thoracic vertebra (T1) to the 12th thoracic vertebra (T12).
- The rib head attachment to the vertebral body is more anterior in the proximal thoracic spine than the distal thoracic spine.
- The annulus fibrosus is the circumferential fibrous tissue that surrounds the nucleus pulposus, which is in the center of the disc.
- The anterior longitudinal ligament, which runs on the anterior aspect of the vertebral body, is a strong fibrous tissue that is contiguous throughout the spine. The segmental arteries and veins originate from the aorta and vena cava, respectively, and traverse the vertebral body. The parietal pleura of the chest surrounds the thoracic spine, covering the segmental vessels and the disc and vertebral bodies. The anterior, middle, and posterior axillary lines run (in reference to the axilla) in the anterior, middle, and posterior aspects of the axilla. Scoliotic deformity in the thoracic spine is lateral curvature with axial plane rotation as well as hypokyphosis (idiopathic scoliosis).
- The arch of the aorta and the arch of the azygos vein typically are located at the T4–T5 levels.

## PATHOGENESIS

- Scoliosis can be grouped into many categories based on pathogenesis.
- The most common type of scoliosis seen is idiopathic, in which the etiology and pathogenesis are unknown.
- Theories of pathogenesis include hormonal influences, growth disturbance, genetic factors, muscle imbalance, and proprioception and balance abnormalities.
- Other types of scoliosis include the following:
  - Congenital: abnormal vertebra due to failure of formation or segmentation
  - Neuromuscular: for example, cerebral palsy, Duchenne muscular dystrophy, spinal muscular atrophy
  - Neurogenic: for example, neurofibromatosis, spinal cord injury

## NATURAL HISTORY

- An idiopathic scoliosis curve may progress in two ways:
  - With continued spine growth
  - When curve magnitude is greater than 50 degrees at skeletal maturity
- Curve progression can be rapid during spine growth or slow following skeletal maturity (approximately 1 degree per year).
- Curve magnitudes above 80 to 90 degrees in the thoracic spine may result in symptomatic pulmonary issues.
- Large curves in adulthood can result in pain.

## PATIENT HISTORY AND PHYSICAL FINDINGS

- The examination for spine deformity should include standing visualization of the spine to look for shoulder height differences, waist asymmetry, overall trunk balance, or coronal head imbalance (**FIG 1**).
- Further information is obtained as to the character of the pain (eg, sharp, dull, aching), when the pain occurs (eg, during activity, while attempting to sleep, pain waking from sleep), and the location of the pain (eg, upper, middle, lower back) as well as whether it radiates into the lower extremities.
- Other history should include any information on other neurologic symptoms such as bowel or bladder incontinence.
- Sensory symptoms should be elicited, especially with hyperesthesias along the chest wall or upper or lower extremities.
- Cutaneous manifestations of dysraphism should be analyzed.

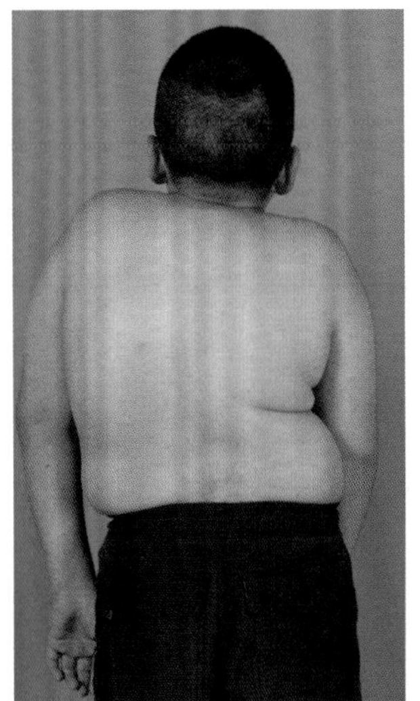
A

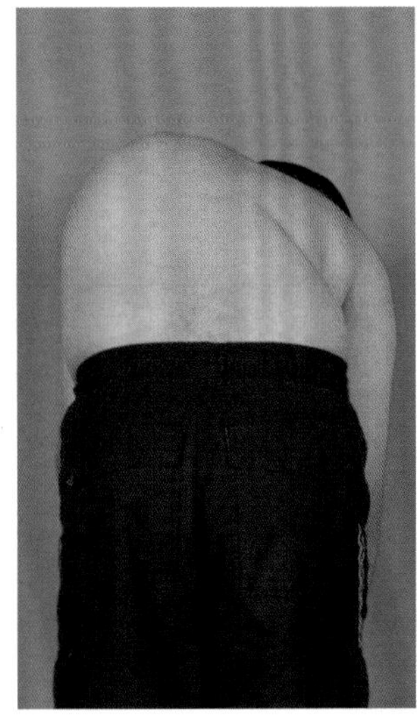
B

**FIG 1** • **A,B.** This 9-year-old boy has a left-sided large thoracic scoliosis but no evidence of neural axis abnormalities on preoperative MRI.

- The neurologic examination should include motor strength and a sensory examination of the upper and lower extremities.
- The abdominal reflexes are the most important neurologic assessment. They are assessed by stroking the skin adjacent to the umbilicus on the left and right and upper and lower quadrants and should be symmetrically absent or present. When asymmetric, magnetic resonance imaging (MRI) is necessary to evaluate for neural axis abnormalities.
- The lower extremities should be carefully examined for asymmetry with respect to size and strength of the legs as well as foot deformities (eg, cavovarus foot deformities) as an indication for the presence of neural axis abnormalities.
- Deep tendon reflexes and the Babinski reflex should be investigated.

## IMAGING AND OTHER DIAGNOSTIC STUDIES

- Plain radiography should include a standing posteroanterior (PA) and lateral radiograph of the spine to include the cervical spine to the pelvis and hips.
- The PA radiograph (**FIG 2A**) should be evaluated for the following:
  - Coronal plane deformities using the Cobb method
  - The C7–center sacral vertebral line (CSVL) placement
  - A trunk shift using Floman method (the distance between the CSVL and the mid-distance between the lateral rib margins)
  - Evaluation for any congenital abnormalities (eg, hemivertebra, congenital bar)
  - The Risser stage (0 through 5)
  - The status of the triradiate cartilage (open or closed)
- The lateral radiographs (**FIG 2B**) should be analyzed to determine the following:
  - Thoracic kyphosis and lumbar lordosis
  - Presence of associated spondylolisthesis or spondylolysis
  - Sagittal balance (distance between C7 plumb line and the posterior edge of the first sacral vertebral body)

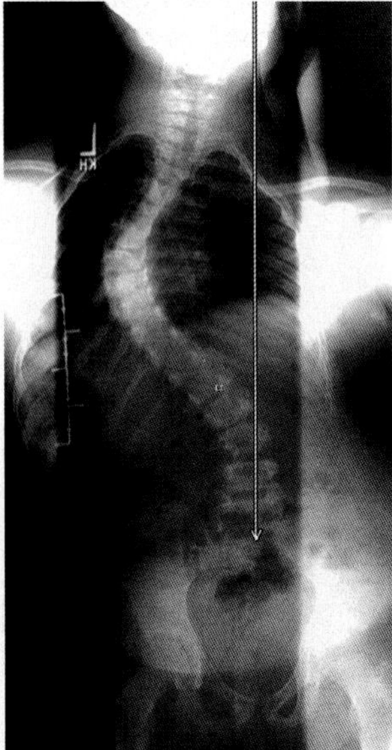
A

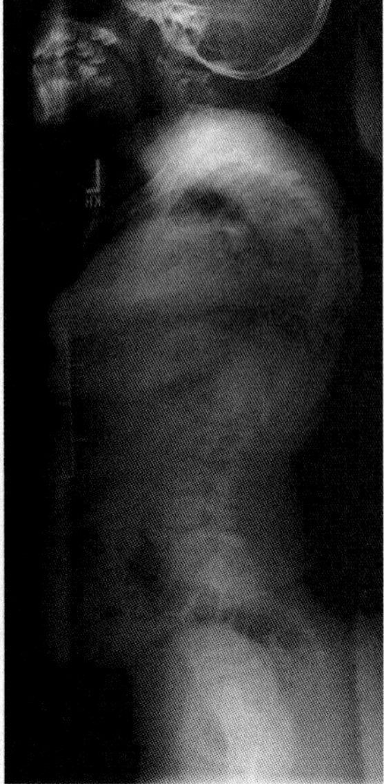
B

**FIG 2 • A,B.** Preoperative anteroposterior (AP) and lateral radiographs demonstrate a 93-degree left thoracic scoliosis with a large trunk shift and open triradiate cartilage in the patient shown in **FIG 1**.

  - The Stagnara view is an oblique view to the patient, but an orthogonal view to the coronal curve that is used in severe spinal deformities to better visualize the spine.
- Indications for MRI include neurologic abnormalities, significant back pain associated with scoliosis, atypical curve patterns such as a left thoracic curve, very young age, congenital scoliosis, neurofibromatosis, Marfan disease.
- Computed tomography (CT) scanning may be useful to fully define the osseous anatomy, especially for extremely large curves and congenital curves.

## DIFFERENTIAL DIAGNOSIS

- Idiopathic scoliosis
- Congenital scoliosis
- Neurofibromatosis
- Scoliosis associated with Marfan disease

## NONOPERATIVE MANAGEMENT

- Nonoperative management has little or no role for severe deformity.
- Patients who are very young with moderate deformity may be treated with a brace to buy time to allow the patient to grow.
  - Bracing can be effective to prevent curve progression for smaller idiopathic curves (ie, 25 to 40 degrees).

## SURGICAL MANAGEMENT

- Anterior thoracoscopic release for spinal deformity has many technical considerations, which are discussed later in this chapter.
- Indications for an anterior release/fusion
  - Severe spinal deformity: scoliosis greater than 80 to 90 degrees with significant rotational deformity or kyphosis greater than 100 degrees with flexibility index less than 50%
  - Skeletal immaturity, to avoid the crankshaft phenomenon. Usually performed for children younger than 10 years of age with open triradiate cartilage and Risser grade 0. Thoracoscopy has been shown to be safe in children less than 20 kg weight.
  - Deficient posterior elements, so that a posterior fusion may be difficult. Such deficiencies occur secondary to previous surgery with laminectomies for tumors or the treatment of neural axis abnormalities.

### Preoperative Planning

- Each patient should be carefully analyzed with respect to those curves that will undergo an anterior release.
- The radiograph should be viewed to determine preoperatively which levels should be released. Release always includes the apical levels and usually includes all of the levels within the Cobb measurement.
- For severe curves, traction in the operating room may be helpful in assisting curve correction.

### Positioning and Approach

#### *Lateral Position*

- Advantages
  - More familiar and traditional approach
  - Conversion to open procedure is easy.

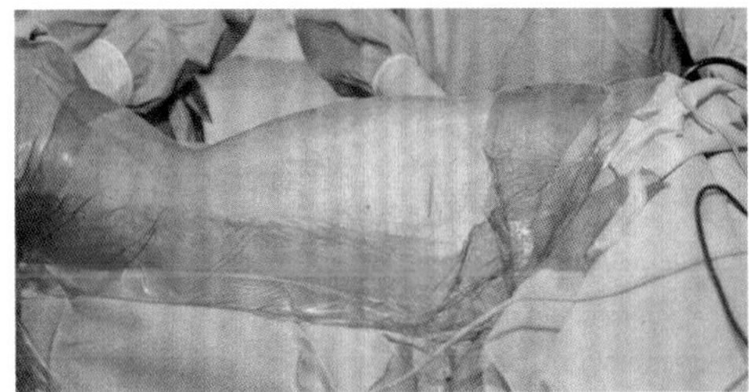

**FIG 3** • Lateral positioning. The patient is positioned in the lateral decubitus position with the surgical side up (left in this case). An axillary roll was placed and the patient is in the direct lateral position to assist in surgeon orientation. Proximal is to the right and distal is to the left. A single anterior portal and four posterolateral portals are planned.

- All thoracic levels can be accessed.
- One can effectively obtain access to the T1–T5 levels, which are not accessible when the patient is in the prone position.
- Disadvantages
  - Repositioning is necessary for the posterior approach.
  - Single-lung ventilation is required.
- Approach
  - Single-lung ventilation is achieved with a double-lumen endotracheal tube or a Univent tube.
  - Position the patient in the lateral decubitus position.
  - Check the endotracheal tube position and the single-lung ventilation status.
  - Prepare and drape the chest and side (**FIG 3**).
  - Place four portals in the anterior axillary line.

### Prone Position

- Advantages
  - Not necessary to reposition patient for the posterior procedure
  - No need for single-lung ventilation
  - Significantly decreased respiratory complications. Single double-lung ventilation is used.
- Disadvantages
  - Difficult to obtain an anterior release proximal to T5.
  - Conversion to open procedure is difficult.
- Approach
  - Placement of regular endotracheal tube
  - Double-lung ventilation with decreased tidal volumes (about 50% to 60% of normal) and increased ventilatory rate which allows the lung to fall away from the spine
  - Place prone on a spine frame (**FIG 4A,B**)
  - Ensure access to the flank and chest.
  - Prepare and drape the back and the chest and flank (**FIG 4C,D**).

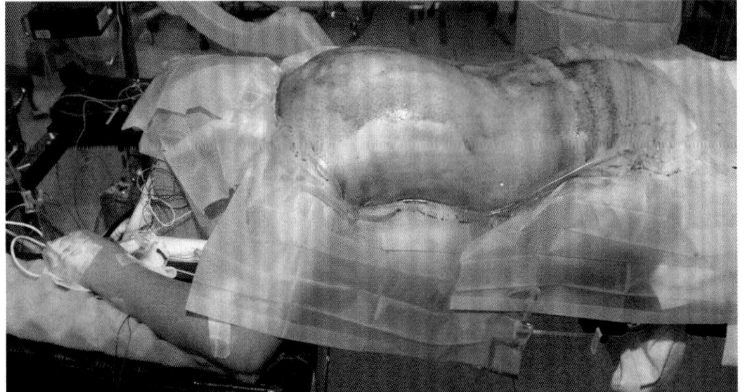

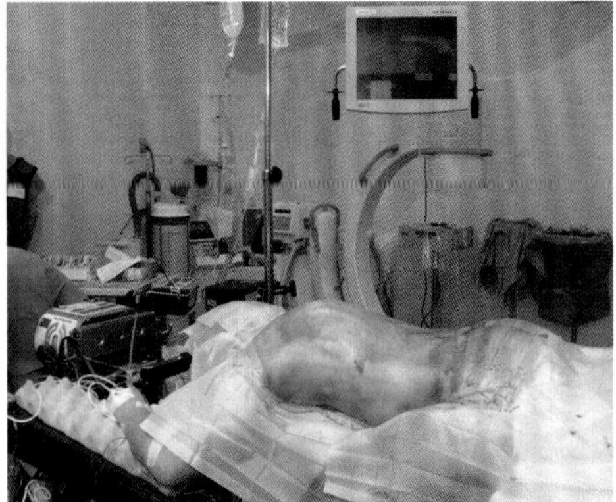

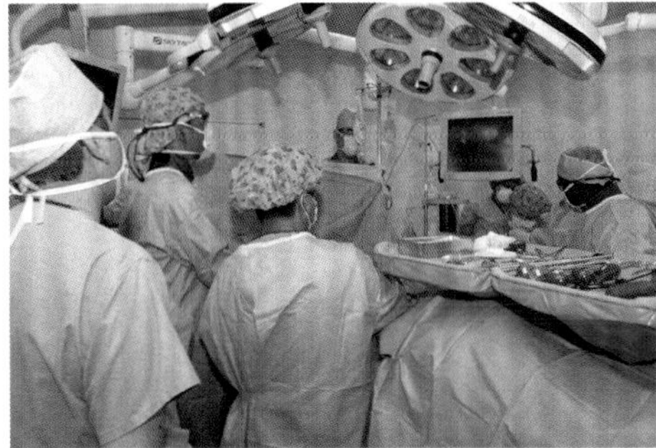

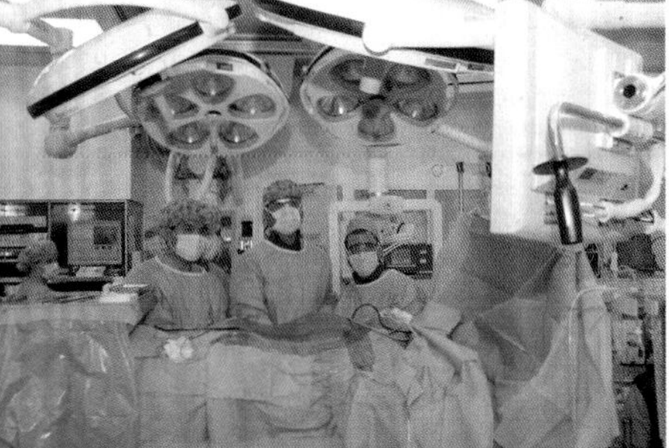

**FIG 4** • Prone positioning. **A.** Close-up view of the patient who has a left thoracic scoliosis. The left flank and spine have been prepared. **B.** The position of the monitor on the opposite side of the patient is shown. **C,D.** Surgical setup for a prone endoscopic release. **C.** View from behind the surgeons. The surgical assistant is on the opposite side of the operating table along with the monitor. The surgeon and first assistant are on the convex side of the patient—in this case, the left side. **D.** View from the opposite side: The surgeons are viewing the monitor. The primary surgeon and two assistants are operating.

## Thoracoscopic Release and Fusion for Scoliosis

### Placement of Portals and Visualization

- Place portals as anteriorly as possible, usually in the midaxillary line (**TECH FIG 1A,B**).
- Insert the camera into the initial portal with the lens directed posteriorly (**TECH FIG 1C**).
- Find a clear space between the posterior chest wall and the lung and advance the thoracoscope.
- Place a small, blunt-tipped cottonoid to retract the lung to identify the spine and other anatomic structures.
- Place a fan retractor to fully retract the lung, if necessary (**TECH FIG 1D**).
- Place suction into the chest.
- Place working portal.
- Visualize the spine in the horizontal plane with the segmental vessels intact (**TECH FIG 1E**).

### Exposure and Disc Removal

- Incise the pleura along the midvertebral body line (**TECH FIG 2A**).
- Spare the segmental blood vessels to preserve perfusion to the spinal cord.
- Bluntly retract the pleura anteriorly and posteriorly (**TECH FIG 2B**).
- Incise the annulus fibrosus with the scalpel blade circumferentially from lateral rib head to near-opposite rib head (**TECH FIG 2C**).
- Break up the disc with disc shavers (**TECH FIG 2D**).
- Remove the disc material with a rongeur (**TECH FIG 2E**).
- Take down the endplate with a curved curette (**TECH FIG 2F**).
- Place Surgicel (Ethicon, Inc., Somerville, NJ) or other thrombotic agent.
- Remove the disc from all levels planned.
- Place bone graft if desired (**TECH FIG 2G**).
- Close the pleura using the Endostitch device (US Surgical, Warsaw, IN), running one suture from proximal and one from distal (**TECH FIG 2H–J**).
- Place a chest tube (**TECH FIG 2K**).
- Close the portal incisions.

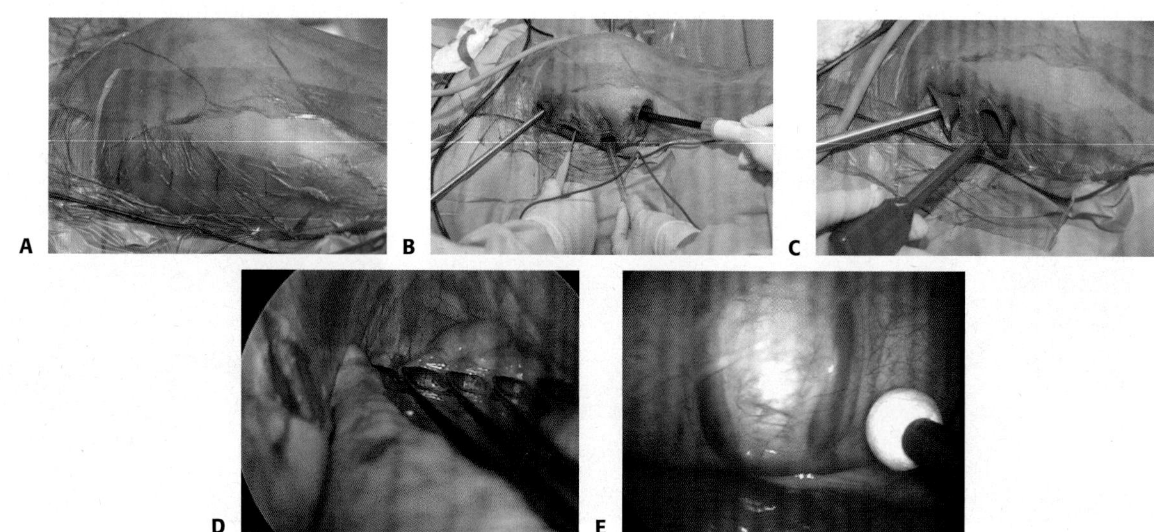

**TECH FIG 1** • Prone anterior release. **A.** Skin markings are made to identify the left scapula and the four lateral portals. To the left is proximal. The most proximal portal usually gains access to the T5–T6 disc when it is in the midscapular region, as shown. **B.** Following placement of the four portals, the thoracoscope is placed in the most proximal working portal with an electrocautery in the second portal, suction is in the third portal, and the fan retractor in the fourth portal. **C.** The first portal is placed first, as shown; in this illustration, it is the most proximal portal, to the left. The secondary portal is then placed approximately two fingerbreadths distally and in line with the first. **D.** A fan retractor is placed to gently push down on the atelectatic lung. Visualized here is the superior most aspect of the chest. **E.** The spine is visualized in the horizontal plane. The segmental vessels are easily seen.

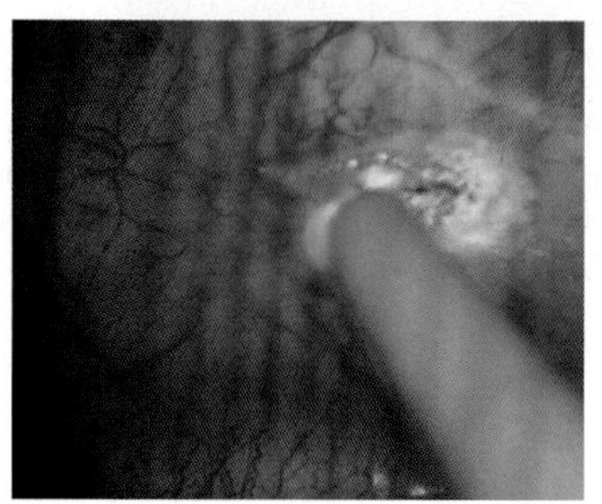

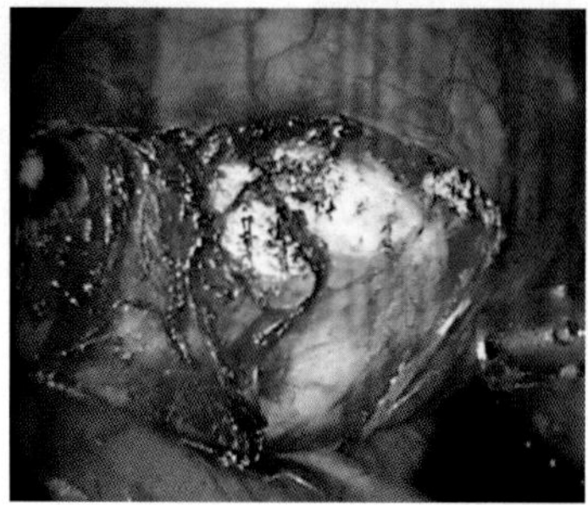

**TECH FIG 2** • **A.** Using a curved electrocautery blade, the pleura is incised in the longitudinal fashion, sparing the segmental vessels. **B.** The parietal pleura is retracted anteriorly, as shown, to allow for complete access to the anterior longitudinal ligament as well as the opposite annulus. The posterior pleura is also retracted. *(continued)*

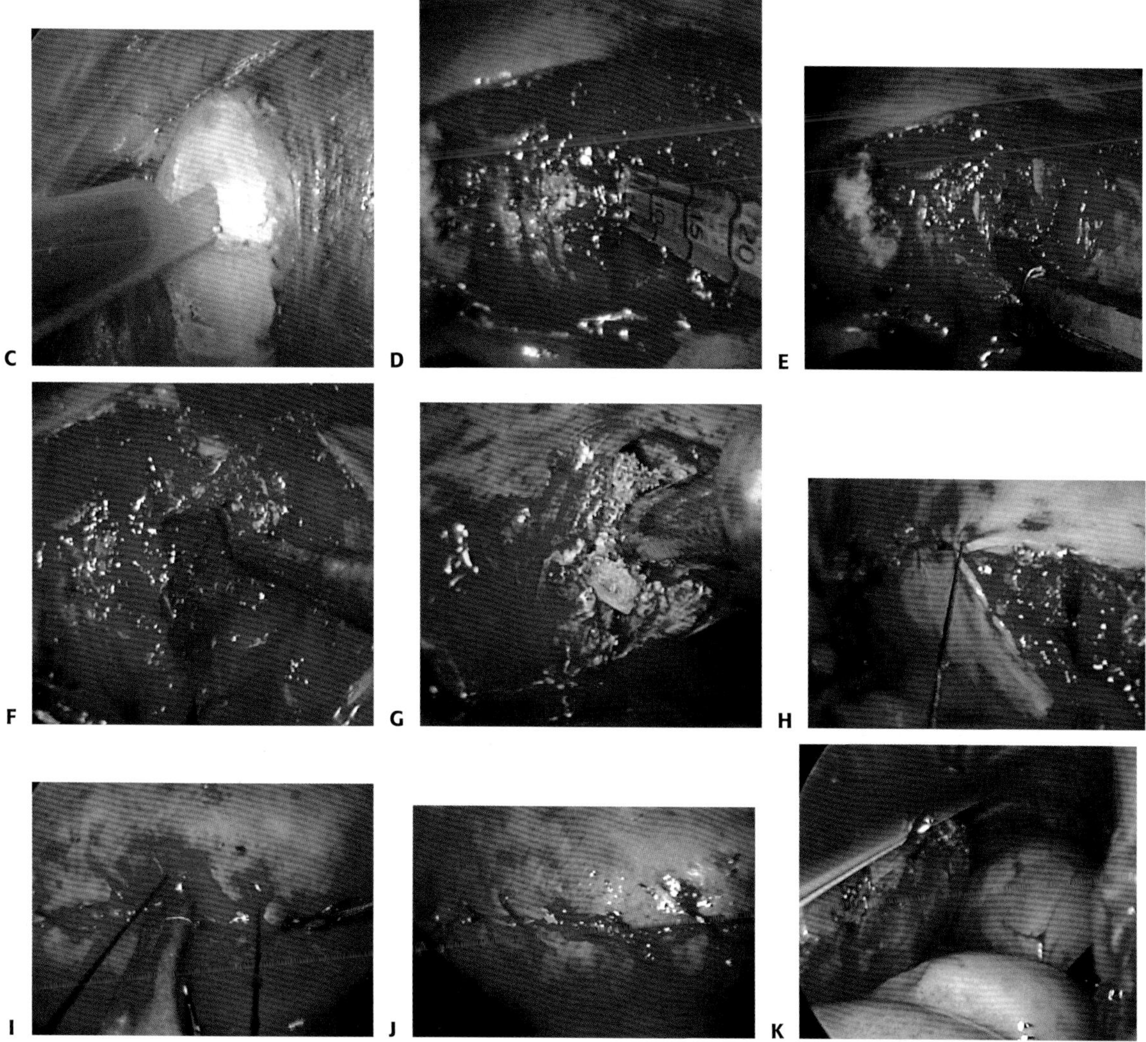

**TECH FIG 2** • *(continued)* **C.** The annulus is incised parallel to the disc. **D.** Disc shavers are used to break up the disc material. **E.** The disc material is removed with a rongeur. **F.** The endplate is taken down to bone with an angled curette. **G.** Bone graft is placed. **H–J.** The pleura is closed with an Endostitch device. **H.** Closure is started distally with a running suture. **I.** Final closure of the pleura, in which the proximal suture is brought to the distal suture. **J.** The pleura is closed nicely with a running suture. **K.** Placement of the chest tube at the completion of the procedure, from distal to proximal. The lung is still deflated. The pleura, seen in the background, has been closed previously.

## PEARLS AND PITFALLS

| | |
|---|---|
| **Portal placement** | ■ Placement of portals is key for visualization and achieving good discectomy.<br>■ Place the skin incision for the portal over a rib to allow the portal to be placed above and below the rib (two portals per skin incision).<br>■ Ensure that portals are neither too posterior nor too anterior. |
| **Preservation of segmental blood vessels** | ■ Incise the pleura in a longitudinal fashion, staying superficial to the segmental vessels.<br>■ Use a curved harmonic scalpel or electrocautery.<br>■ Incise any adventitial tissue adherent to the pleura over the disc to free up the parietal pleura.<br>■ Bluntly retract the pleura to gain access to the disc. |

| | |
|---|---|
| **Complete removal of the disc** | ■ Develop the same sequence for disc removal:<br>■ Incise the disc with a scalpel blade.<br>■ Break up disc material with shavers.<br>■ Remove loosened disc material.<br>■ Take down the endplates of the vertebral bodies with a curved curette.<br>■ Remove excess endplate material. |
| **Pleural closure** | ■ Use the Endostitch device with 2-0 Vicryl suture.<br>■ Use two sutures: The first begins in the proximal aspect and is run distally, and the second is started distally and is run proximally. |

## POSTOPERATIVE CARE

- Chest tube management
  - Connect chest tube to wall suction.
  - Obtain daily chest radiographs.
  - The chest tube may be removed when drainage is less than 80 mL over 12 hours and serous color returns (with good pleural closure, removal usually is done on the first day).
- Mobilize the patient to chair on postoperative day 1.
- Mobilize the patient to ambulation when the chest tube is removed (usually postoperative day 2).
- Serial hemoglobin and hematocrit on postoperative days 1 and 2
- Advance activities as tolerated to daily activities in the initial 6 weeks.
- For the following 6 weeks, physical activities are advanced, depending on posterior constructs.

## OUTCOMES

- The addition of a thoracoscopic anterior release and fusion results in a decrease in pulmonary function in the first 6 weeks; however, at 1 to 2 years, it is 30% to 45% above baseline. Thoracoscopy has been shown to have less effect on pulmonary function compared tothoracoplasty.

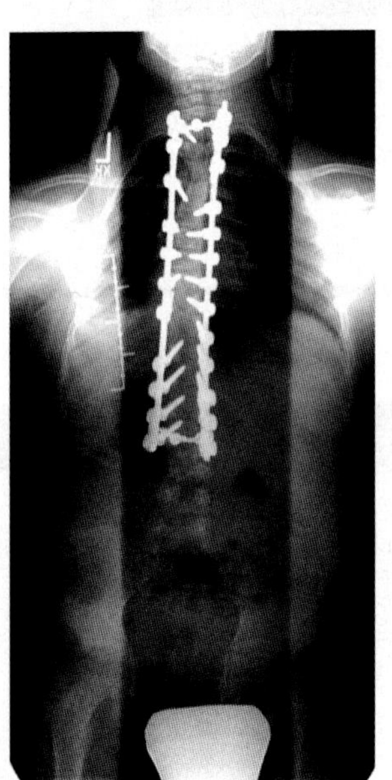

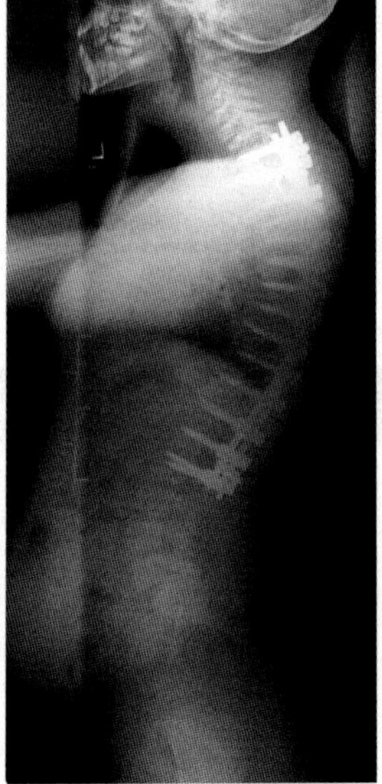

**FIG 5** ● The 2-year postoperative AP (**A**) and lateral (**B**) radiographs of the patient shown in **FIGS 1** and **2** demonstrated outstanding coronal and sagittal plane correction after prone thoracoscopic anterior release and fusion followed by a posterior spinal fusion and instrumentation from T2 to L2.

- Anterior release increases the flexibility of the spine and allows for great coronal, axial plane, and sagittal plane correction.
- With good surgical technique, an outstanding anterior release can be achieved and will allow for exceptional three-dimensional correction of the spine with posterior instrumentation and fusion (**FIG 5**).

## COMPLICATIONS

- Single-lung ventilation
  - Intraoperative complications: inability to ventilate adequately secondary to ventilation–perfusion mismatches, high airway pressures and barotrauma, and underlying pulmonary issues
  - Postoperative complications: atelectasis secondary to barotrauma or mucous plugs
  - Continuous chest tube drainage, especially when the parietal pleura has not been closed
- Pneumothorax following chest tube removal
- Intraoperative injury to the segmental blood vessels or the great vessels
- Intraoperative injury to the thoracic duct, which usually occurs on the right side at the T11–T12 area. This can be avoided by dissection deep to the parietal pleura.
- Chylothorax is treated with total parenteral nutrition and avoidance of a fatty diet.
- Intraoperative excessive bleeding secondary to inadvertent segmental vessel injury. Strategies to coagulate the vessel are used.
- Long-term complications secondary to a thoracoscopic anterior release and fusion are limited.

## SUGGESTED READINGS


1. Al-Sayyad MJ, Crawford AH, Wolf RK. Video-assisted thoracoscopic surgery: the Cincinnati experience. Clin Orthop Relat Res 2005;(434):61–70.
2. Cheung KM, Wu JP, Cheng QH, et al. Treatment of stiff thoracic scoliosis by thoracoscopic anterior release combined with posterior instrumentation and fusion. J Orthop Surg Res 2007;2:16.
3. Crawford AH. Anterior surgery in the thoracic and lumbar spine: endoscopic techniques in children. Instr Course Lect 2005;54:567–576.
4. Huang EY, Acosta JM, Gardocki RJ, et al. Thoracoscopic anterior spinal release and fusion: evolution of a faster, improved approach. J Pediatr Surg 2002;37:1732–1735.
5. Lefevre Y, Ilharreborde B, Huot O, et al. Thoracoscopy in children less than 20 kg for the management of spinal disorders: efficacy of long-term follow-up. J Pediatr Orthop 2011;31:170–179.
6. Newton PO, Cardelia JM, Farnsworth CL, et al. A biomechanical comparison of open and thoracoscopic anterior spinal release in a goat model. Spine 1998;23:530–535.
7. Newton P, Shea K, Granlund K. Defining the pediatric spinal thoracoscopy learning curve: sixty-five consecutive cases. Spine 2000;25:1028–1035.

8. Niemeyer T, Freeman BJ, Grevitt MP, et al. Anterior thoracoscopic surgery followed by posterior instrumentation and fusion in spinal deformity. Eur Spine J 2000;9:499–504.
9. Picetti GD III, Pang D, Bueff HU. Thoracoscopic techniques for the treatment of scoliosis: early results in procedure development. Neurosurgery 2002;51:978–984.
10. Sucato DJ, Elerson E. A comparison between the prone and lateral position for performing a thoracoscopic anterior release and fusion for pediatric spinal deformity. Spine 2003;28:2176–2180.
11. Sucato DJ, Erken YH, Davis S, et al. Prone thoracoscopic release does not adversely affect pulmonary function when added to a posterior spinal fusion for severe spinal deformity. Spine 2009;34:771–778.
12. Sucato DJ, Welch RD, Pierce B, et al. Thoracoscopic discectomy and fusion in an animal model: safe and effective when segmental blood vessels are spared. Spine 2002;27:880–886.
13. Verma K, Lonner BS, Kean KE, et al. Maximal pulmonary recovery after spinal fusion for adolescent idiopathic scoliosis: how do anterior approaches compare? Spine 2011;36:1086–1095.

# Spinal Fusion for Neuromuscular Scoliosis

Kirk W. Dabney and Freeman Miller

## DEFINITION

- Neuromuscular diseases are heterogeneous between and within diseases and are due to a vast number of pathologies involving the brain, spinal cord, peripheral nervous system, and muscle.
- Neuromuscular spinal deformity is a result of neuromuscular disease which occurs during childhood, including cerebral palsy, muscular dystrophy, spinal muscular atrophy, etc. It may be related to a pathologic abnormality in muscle tone, motor control, weakness, or a combination.
- Although neuromuscular scoliosis (coronal deformity) is the most common neuromuscular spinal deformity, sagittal plane deformity (hyperlordosis and hyperkyphosis) may also occur.

## ANATOMY

- The curve patterns of neuromuscular scoliosis are most commonly lumbar and thoracolumbar with associated pelvic obliquity (**FIG 1**).
- Because many children are nonambulatory, associated pelvic obliquity affects sitting balance.
- Ambulatory neuromuscular patients often have decompensation, with the inability to center their head over the center sacral line.

## PATHOGENESIS AND NATURAL HISTORY

- The biologic basis of both scoliosis and sagittal plane spinal deformity in neuromuscular disorders differs depending on the specific neuromuscular disease. In general, however, most neuromuscular spinal deformities are largely due to muscle imbalance (high tone or low tone) and abnormal postural reflexes.
- The natural history of neuromuscular scoliosis is typically that of progression, beginning with the development of a flexible scoliosis, often in middle childhood, and the more rapid progression to a more rigid scoliosis during the adolescent growth spurt. Some neuromuscular conditions are associated with a more progressive scoliosis than others.
- The pathogenesis and natural history of some of the more common neuromuscular disorders associated with spinal deformity and the spinal deformity itself within the disease follow.

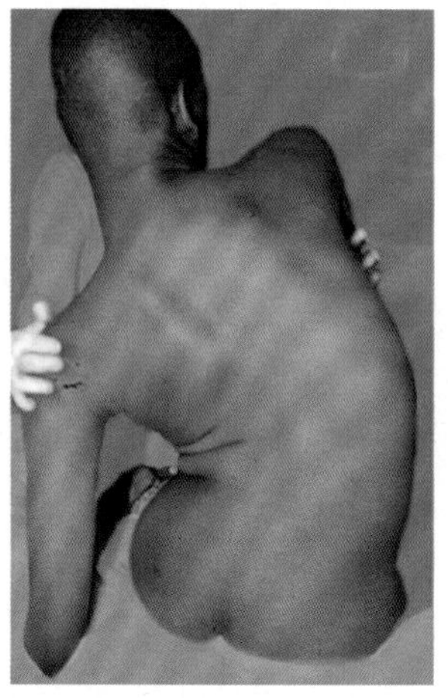

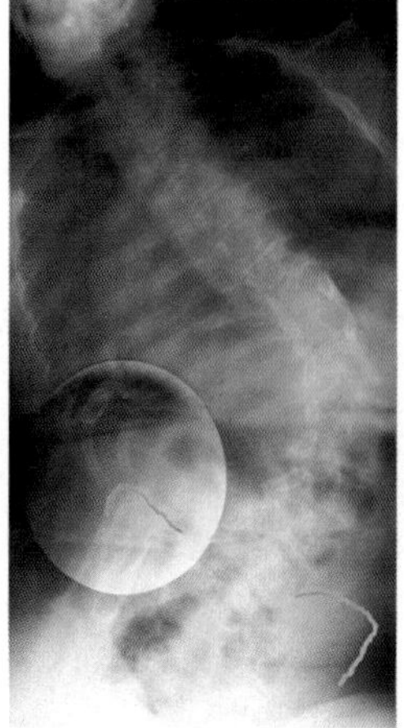

**FIG 1** • Typical neuromuscular curve pattern in a child with quadriplegic-pattern cerebral palsy. **A.** Child with poor sitting balance. **B.** Radiograph showing long thoracolumbar curve with pelvic obliquity.

### Cerebral Palsy

- Cerebral palsy is a heterogeneous disorder that is characterized by a static lesion (eg, injury, congenital defect) to the immature motor cortex of the brain.
- The natural history of neuromuscular scoliosis in cerebral palsy is relentless progression. Progression is most common in spastic quadriplegic cerebral palsy. The rate of progression can be severe in adolescent years (2 to 4 degrees per month).
- Progression also occurs after skeletal maturity. In curves greater than 40 degrees, it may occur at a rate of 2 to 4 degrees per year.[25]
- Curves in the 60- to 90-degree range begin to effect sitting balance, arm control, and head control. Further progression may prevent the child from sitting in an upright position.
- Conservative treatment with chair modifications and bracing is only a temporary treatment and does not stop curve progression. Conservative treatment is especially helpful in the younger child with a flexible scoliosis to temporarily maintain upright sitting posture. This will allow the spine to grow to its maximum size (to achieve maximum sitting height) so that the resulting fusion can correct the spinal deformity without limiting growth.

### Muscular Dystrophy

- Duchenne muscular dystrophy is a sex-linked recessive disorder involving a defect on the Xp21.2 locus of the X chromosome resulting in a marked decrease or absence of the protein dystrophin.[11]
- Affected children become progressively weaker with age, eventually becoming nonambulatory.
- Death typically occurs in the second or third decade secondary to pulmonary or cardiac failure.
- Scoliosis is almost universal when the child becomes nonambulatory, and curve progression correlates strongly with a decline in respiratory function.
- In the past, the prevalence of scoliosis approached 100%.[22] For this reason, surgery was previously recommended soon after the child became nonambulatory before an irreversible

decline in forced vital capacity occurred. Now with the advent of corticosteroids, the life expectancy of children with Duchenne muscular dystrophy is extended with a reported delay or prevention of the severity of scoliosis with long-standing use of corticosteroids.[1,13,15] The risk of progression decreases if the scoliosis develops after 14 years of age.[31] Pulmonary function decreases as the natural history of the disease and scoliosis magnitude progresses. Scoliosis surgery should be done before the forced vital capacity decreases to less than 30%.

## Myelomeningocele

- Myelomeningocele, a congenital malformation of the nervous system, is due to a neural tube defect and results in a spectrum of sensory and motor deficits.
- Although the level of the spinal cord defect influences the clinical presentation of the condition, neurologic deterioration may occur at any age owing to hydrocephaly, hydrosyringomyelia, Arnold-Chiari deformity, and tethered cord syndrome.
- In general, the higher the level of the defect, the higher the prevalence of scoliosis. Almost 100% of thoracic level paraplegic patients develop scoliosis.[26]
- A long C-shaped curve is associated with a high level of paralysis and usually occurs at a young age.
- Hydromyelia and tethered cord syndrome may also be associated with scoliosis and should be suspected if the scoliosis onset is more sudden and associated with other symptoms of acute neurologic deterioration.
- Bracing in younger children can be attempted to slow progression, but it does not stop eventual progression.

## Spinal Muscular Atrophy

- Spinal muscular atrophy is an autosomal recessive disorder resulting in spinal cord anterior horn cell degeneration. Two genes on the chromosome 5q locus have been found to be associated with this disorder: survival motor neuron (*SMN*) gene and neuronal apoptosis inhibitory (*NAIP*) gene.[24]
- Clinically, progressive muscular weakness occurs and eventual pulmonary compromise is common.
- Three forms of the disease exist:
  - Type 1: early, acute Werdnig-Hoffman
  - Type 2: intermediate, chronic Werdnig-Hoffman
  - Type 3: late, Kugelberg-Welander type
- Most children with the early form of the disease die at an early age and therefore do not require treatment.
- Most children with the intermediate and late type who survive into adolescence develop a progressive spinal deformity. The curvature typically develops in the first decade. Thoracolumbar and thoracic patterns are most common.
- One-third of patients have an associated kyphosis in the sagittal plane. Bracing is ineffective at preventing curve progression but may delay progression in the very young patient to allow further growth of the spine.[2]

## Freidreich Ataxia

- This autosomal recessive disorder results in a slowly progressive spinocerebellar degeneration. A defect on chromosome 9 has been identified.
- The incidence of scoliosis is 100%, and progression is related to the age of disease onset. When disease onset is prior to age 10 years and scoliosis onset is before 15 years, scoliosis progression is usually greater than 60 degrees.
- Progressive scoliosis requiring surgery occurs in about 50% of patients.[14]
  - Curve patterns are similar to idiopathic scoliosis: double major, single thoracic, and thoracolumbar.
- Orthotic treatment may slow but usually does not prevent progression.

## Rett Syndrome

- This is an X-linked disorder that affects females almost exclusively. Some children have a mutation on the *MECP2* gene.[21] The child's development is normal until 6 to 18 months of age, followed by rapid deterioration in cognitive and motor function.
- After the initial deterioration in function, the neurologic picture may become relatively static for years. The clinical spectrum is variable, with some children remaining ambulatory and others becoming wheelchair bound.
- Rett syndrome may be mistaken for cerebral palsy.
- Scoliosis has been reported in up to 80% of patients.[12]
- A long C-shaped thoracolumbar pattern is common. Bracing is usually ineffective, and curve progression is common. Surgical stabilization allows maintenance of sitting balance.

## Spinal Cord Injury

- Spinal cord injury in the skeletally immature child is associated with a nearly 100% incidence of scoliosis.[7]
- The predominant curve type is a long C-shaped curvature. The younger the child, the higher the progression.
- Prophylactic bracing may be effective in smaller curves (under 20 degrees). There are no data to support that bracing is effective in preventing progress in established curves greater than 20 degrees.

# PATIENT HISTORY AND PHYSICAL FINDINGS

- An accurate medical history is crucial for patients with neuromuscular disease.
  - In patients with cerebral palsy, the medical comorbidities strongly correlate with postoperative complications.[17] This appears to also be true in patients with Duchenne muscular dystrophy, spinal muscular atrophy, and other neuromuscular disease.
- Important historical information includes respiratory status, cardiac status, gastrointestinal status (eg, gastroesophageal reflux, nutritional intake), bone health (low bone density and history of fracture), and the presence of seizure disorder.
- Physical examination should assess sitting or standing balance, the pelvic obliquity, curve magnitude, and stiffness (including the curve's coronal, sagittal, and rotational components).
  - Coronal stiffness is best assessed by performing the side-bending test (**FIG 2**).
- The physician should also assess for the possible coexistence of hip subluxation or dislocation, common in many neuromuscular diseases.
- A complete neurologic examination should also be performed.

# IMAGING AND OTHER DIAGNOSTIC STUDIES

- Anteroposterior (AP) and lateral radiographic views should be obtained to assess the Cobb angle and pelvic obliquity in the coronal plane and lumbar lordosis and thoracic kyphosis in the sagittal plane.

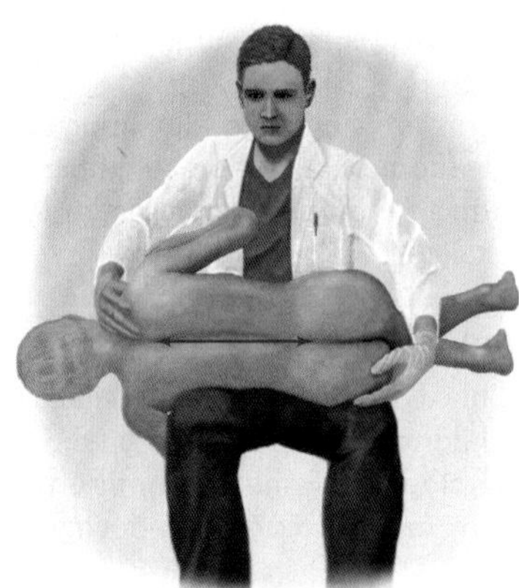

**FIG 2** • Side-bending test. Patient is being bent over the examiner's thigh at the apex of the curve. If the patient's curve reverses and the pelvis levels to perpendicular to the trunk, the curve is still flexible enough to correct through posterior fusion and instrumentation alone. If not, an anterior release is performed.

- If intraspinal pathology is suspected, especially in the ambulatory patient, a preoperative magnetic resonance imaging (MRI) scan should be obtained.
- If severe low bone density is suspected (history of multiple fractures), dual energy x-ray absorptiometry (DEXA) scan is recommended to assess bone density and potential need to treat.

## DIFFERENTIAL DIAGNOSIS

- Some neurologic diseases can look similar.
- It is important to diagnose progressive neurodegenerative in which mortality from the disease is more rapid than the progression of the spinal deformity.

## NONOPERATIVE MANAGEMENT

- Although there was initially some historical enthusiasm for the treatment of neuromuscular scoliosis with casting or bracing, orthotic management is rarely able to halt progression of neuromuscular scoliosis.
- Flexible curves in younger children may require seating modifications (hip guides and offset lateral seatback supports) or a sort thoracolumbar orthosis to maintain balanced seating until the child is at optimal sitting height.

## SURGICAL MANAGEMENT

### Indications

- The indications for spinal fusion in neuromuscular scoliosis depend largely on the natural history of the specific neuromuscular disease and the natural history of the scoliosis within the specific disorder.
- Examples of two neuromuscular diseases with different indications are Duchenne muscular dystrophy and cerebral palsy.

#### *Duchenne Muscular Dystrophy*

- The major comorbidity in Duchenne muscular dystrophy is restrictive lung disease, with forced vital capacity dropping dramatically with scoliosis progression.
- Due to the natural history, the indication for fusion is a scoliosis curvature greater than 25 degrees and forced vital capacity above 35%.

#### *Cerebral Palsy*

- The indications for spinal fusion in children with cerebral palsy are a scoliosis curve magnitude approaching 60 degrees in the older child, especially if the curve is becoming stiff by physical examination.
- Surgical correction is indicated when the child is not tolerating seating with a combination of either seating adjustments or a soft orthosis. This is usually done before the curvature reaches 70 degrees when the risk of complications increases.[17]
- Less commonly, sagittal plane spinal deformity, hyperlordosis, and kyphosis will cause seating problems or back pain. Cerebral palsy patients with sagittal plane spinal deformity of 70 degrees or more causing seating difficulties or back pain can benefit from surgical correction.[16]
- Typically during the middle part of adolescent growth, the scoliosis becomes much larger and begins to stiffen. Surgical instrumentation and fusion are recommended at this time.

### Preoperative Planning

#### *Technical Considerations*

- Three main technical preoperative considerations require careful consideration:
  - Is fusion to the pelvis necessary?
  - Is there a significant rotational component to the scoliosis that is contributing to difficulty in seating?
  - Is anterior release (discectomies around the stiff portion of the curve) necessary?
- The only treatment that has made a definitive impact on neuromuscular spinal deformity is instrumentation and fusion.
- The standard surgical procedure for neuromuscular scoliosis is a posterior spinal fusion with segmental instrumentation from T1 to T2 down to the pelvis if there is a significant pelvic obliquity.
- Even if the pelvis is not involved in a severely involved nonambulatory patient or an ambulatory patient with a poor "righting reflex," the surgeon should consider fusion to the pelvis to prevent the development of late pelvic obliquity. However, with modern pedicle screw instrumentation, complete correction of the lumbar spine to L5 may prevent subsequent development of pelvic obliquity or so that in the era sublaminar wire fixation.
- The unit rod incorporates these concepts into one instrumentation system (**FIG 3**) as well as the concept of cantilever correction.[3,9,18,20]
- Newer methods of instrumentation allow modularization of the unit rod concept and cantilever correction by combining pelvic screws, precontoured rods, and a proximal connector (**FIG 4**).
- Both the unit rod and the precontoured rods (in the modular unit rod construct) have prebent sagittal contour.
  - The unit rod comes in lengths from 250 to 450 mm.
  - Both 3/16- and 1/4-inch diameter rods are available. The 1/4-inch rod is used whenever possible, reserving the 3/16-inch rod for patients with a very thin gracile pelvis.
  - With the modular system, precontoured rods are connected with a proximal connector, in addition to pelvic screw with diameter (7 to 10 mm) and length (65 to 100 mm) that can be selected according to pelvic size.
- Some surgeons are using pedicle screws instead of wires for segmental fixation, especially if there is a severe rotational

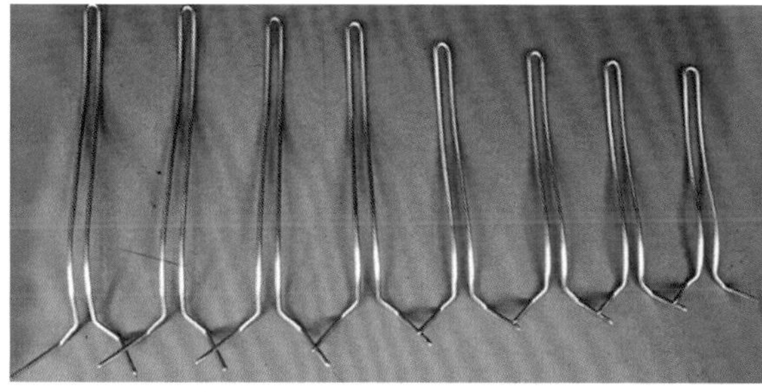

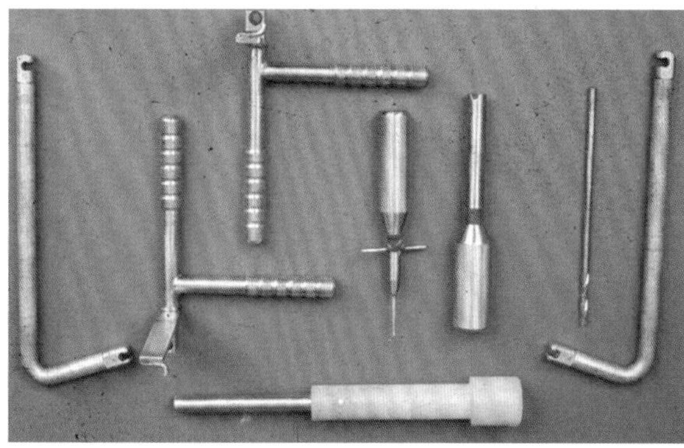

**FIG 3** • **A.** The unit rod is available commercially in a range of sizes. **B.** Drill guides are provided for placement of the pelvic limbs as well as the impactor and pusher for the rod.

component to the curvature or pelvis. Caution should be taken when the bone is severely osteopenic, as the pedicle screws may pull out of the bone. Screws can be supplemented by wires or sublaminar cables as necessary.

- The unit rod (**FIG 5A–C**) and the modular unit rod (see **FIG 4**) are especially powerful as cantilevers to correct pelvic obliquity.
- Anterior release for scoliosis is required for larger stiff curves that do not bend out on the bending test (generally >90 degrees) (**FIG 5D**).
  - Anterior release is also recommended for severe hyperlordotic and hyperkyphotic spinal deformities.[16]

### Other Preoperative Considerations

- The general medical condition of the child should always be considered first. Many children with neuromuscular conditions will have comorbidities such as pulmonary disease, cardiac disease, seizure disorder, poor nutrition, and so forth.
  - All patients with complex preoperative medical conditions should have the appropriate preoperative workup.
- The surgeon and anesthesiologist should plan for the possibility of large intraoperative blood loss.
  - Type and cross-matched blood (up to twice the patient's blood volume), fresh frozen plasma, and platelets should be available. In addition, consider the use of cell-saver blood.
  - The use of antifibrinolytic such as tranexamic acid or Amicar can successfully decrease overall blood loss.[8]
  - Good vascular access is required, often through central venous access.
- Another consideration is the use of spinal cord monitoring. Most children with neuropathies, myopathies, and mild to moderate cerebral palsy (without severe motor cortex involvement) can be monitored using a combination of somatosensory and motor evoked potentials.[10] On the other hand, only about 40% of children with severe quadriplegic cerebral palsy and poor motor function can be monitored. In addition, it is difficult to justify removing implant hardware if there are signal changes in the child with minimal motor function because the risk of repeat operation to reimplant hardware is quite high in this population.
  - As a general rule, any child with ambulatory or functional standing (able to assist with standing transfers) should have somatosensory and motor evoked potential monitoring attempted. There may also be some efficacy in monitoring neuromuscular patients with intact sensation and bowel and bladder control.
  - Any child with neurogenic bladder should be carefully evaluated for urinary tract infection preoperatively, and if present, should be treated to clear the urine prior to surgery.
- A final preoperative consideration is the bone density of the child undergoing spinal fusion. The child who is nonambulatory, poorly nourished, and on seizure medication is at highest risk. Children with low bone density may be difficult to instrument owing to the possibility of sublaminar wires pulling through or pedicle screws pulling out of osteopenic bone.
  - Any nonambulatory child with low-impact long bone fracture should be checked for low bone density using DEXA scan.
  - Children on seizure medication should have calcium, phosphorous, and vitamin D levels measured.
  - Patients with bone density two or more Z scores below the mean should be considered for treatment using intravenous pamidronate.

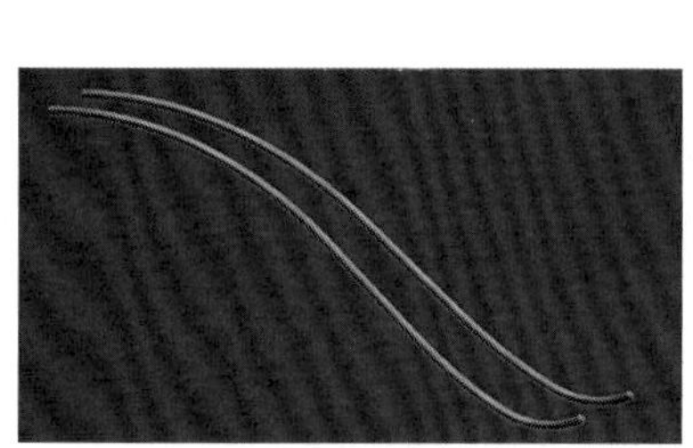

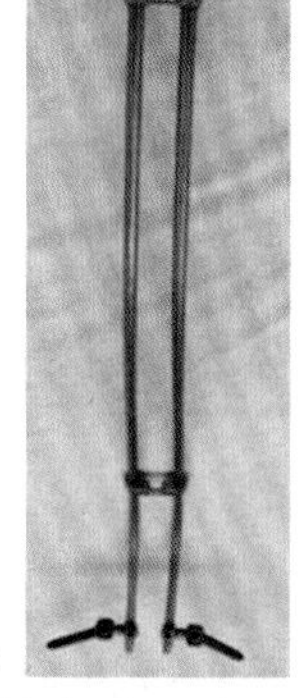

**FIG 4** • **A.** Lateral profile of the prebent rods with built-in thoracic kyphosis and lumbar lordosis. **B.** AP profile of the prebent rods connected via the lateral connectors to the iliac screws. (**B:** Courtesy of DePuy Synthes Spine.)

## Positioning

- The patient is positioned prone on a Jackson table (a Relton Hall frame can also be used) with the abdominal area free (**FIG 6**).
- We have adapted special radiolucent posts for the table that can be spaced at a narrower distance compared to the standard posts.
- Some surgeons prefer intraoperative traction, using a combination of skin traction, halo traction, or halo femoral traction depending on surgeon preference and experience. Establishing good deformity correction with preoperative traction can dramatically improve results especially when bone density is very low and indirect correction is safer.

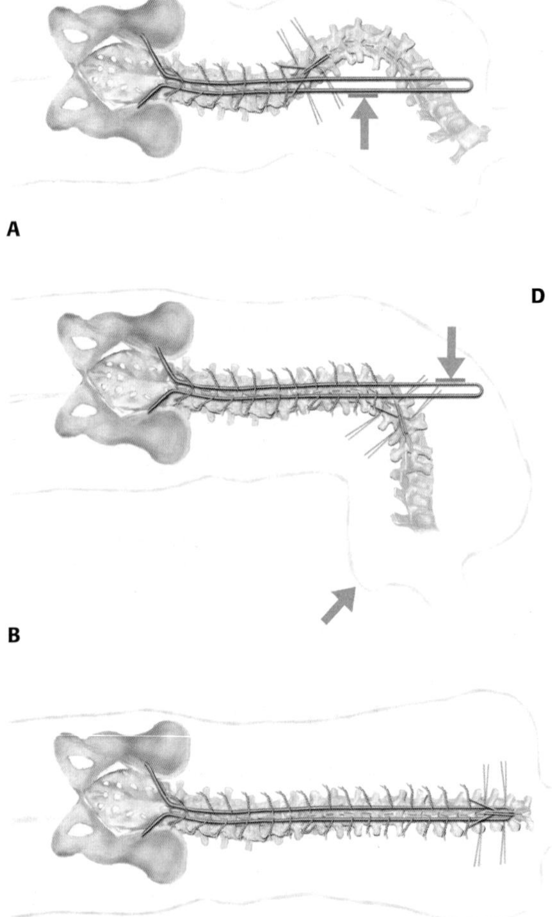

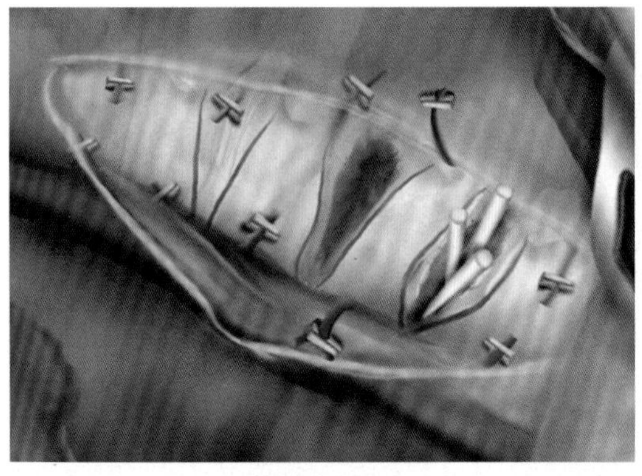

**FIG 5** • **A–C.** Cantilever effect of the rod correcting pelvic obliquity and scoliosis. The rod is gradually pushed to each vertebra, and each wire is tightened, progressively correcting the deformity using transverse forces. **D.** Anterior release. Wedge resections of the discs are performed around the apical vertebra if the spinal deformity is stiff.

- The hips and knees are bent to minimize lumbar lordosis and to optimize insertion of the limbs of the rod into the pelvis when using the unit rod. All bony prominences should be well padded.
- Many children with cerebral palsy have significant contractures, making their extremities hard to position. They should be positioned with minimal tension on the joints.
- Urinary catheters should be free flowing, especially children with neurogenic bladder with a vesicostomy or other bladder reconstruction.

## Approach

- A posterior approach to the spine is performed from T1 to T2 to the sacrum.
- A complete subperiosteal exposure of each vertebra is performed followed by exposure of the outer wing of the iliac crest down to the sciatic notch and the bottom tips of the posterior superior iliac spine (PSIS).
- Alternatively, if using iliac screws, exposure of S2 to prepare for an S2 iliac approach can also be performed.[6,23]

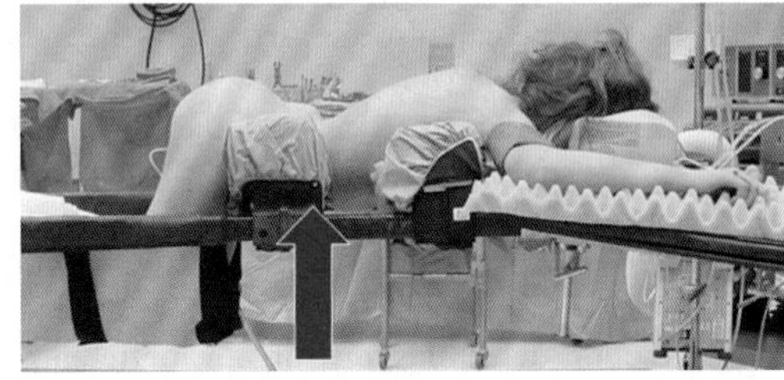

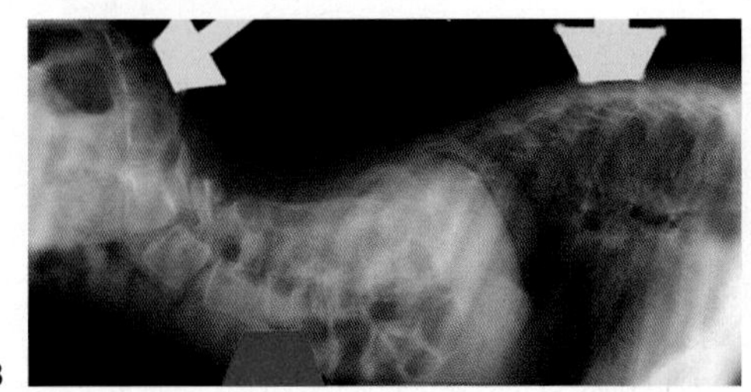

**FIG 6** • **A,B.** Positioning the patient should leave the abdomen free and minimize lumbar lordosis by allowing the knees to hang low to optimize pelvic limb placement. If necessary, an unscrubbed assistant can push up on the abdomen (*arrow* in **A**) to aid in the pelvic limb insertion with severe lordosis.

## Pelvic Preparation

### Posterior Superior Iliac Spine Placement

- A drill hole is made between the outer and inner cortex of the ilium with a drill bit. Before drilling, the drill bit is marked 10 mm past the drill guide's hook for the sciatic notch in children who weigh less than 45 kg and 15 mm past the hook in children heavier than 45 kg.
- The right and left drill guide is next inserted into the right and left sciatic notch, respectively.
  - The lateral handle of the drill guide is placed parallel to the pelvis (iliac crests), whereas the axial handle is held parallel to the sacrum.
- The pelvis is drilled from the inferior tip of the posterior iliac spine in a line just superior and anterior to the sciatic notch, where the bone is densest.[19]
  - To confirm proper placement, a fluoroscopic view is taken with drill bit or pedicle probe in place parallel with its trajectory (**TECH FIG 1**).
- The hole is probed to ensure that the pelvic cortex or sciatic notch is not penetrated.
- The drill hole is countersunk if a pelvic screw will be used so as to prevent prominence of the screw.
- Pelvic screw fixation of largest diameter possible (usually a 7- to 10-mm diameter) is placed in this trajectory and should be of sufficient length to pass the sciatic notch by at least 1 cm.
  - We prefer to use a closed polyaxial screw head to maximize the rigidity of the final rod–pelvic screw construct.
  - Typically, we use pelvic screws alone, but when additional fixation is needed to improve the rigidity of pelvic fixation, we add S1 screws. We prefer this over sacral screw fixation alone because pelvic screw fixation provides a better lever arm to correct both pelvic obliquity and sagittal plane pelvic deformity.
- The drill hole can be temporarily packed with Gelfoam to control bleeding if the unit rod is to be placed.

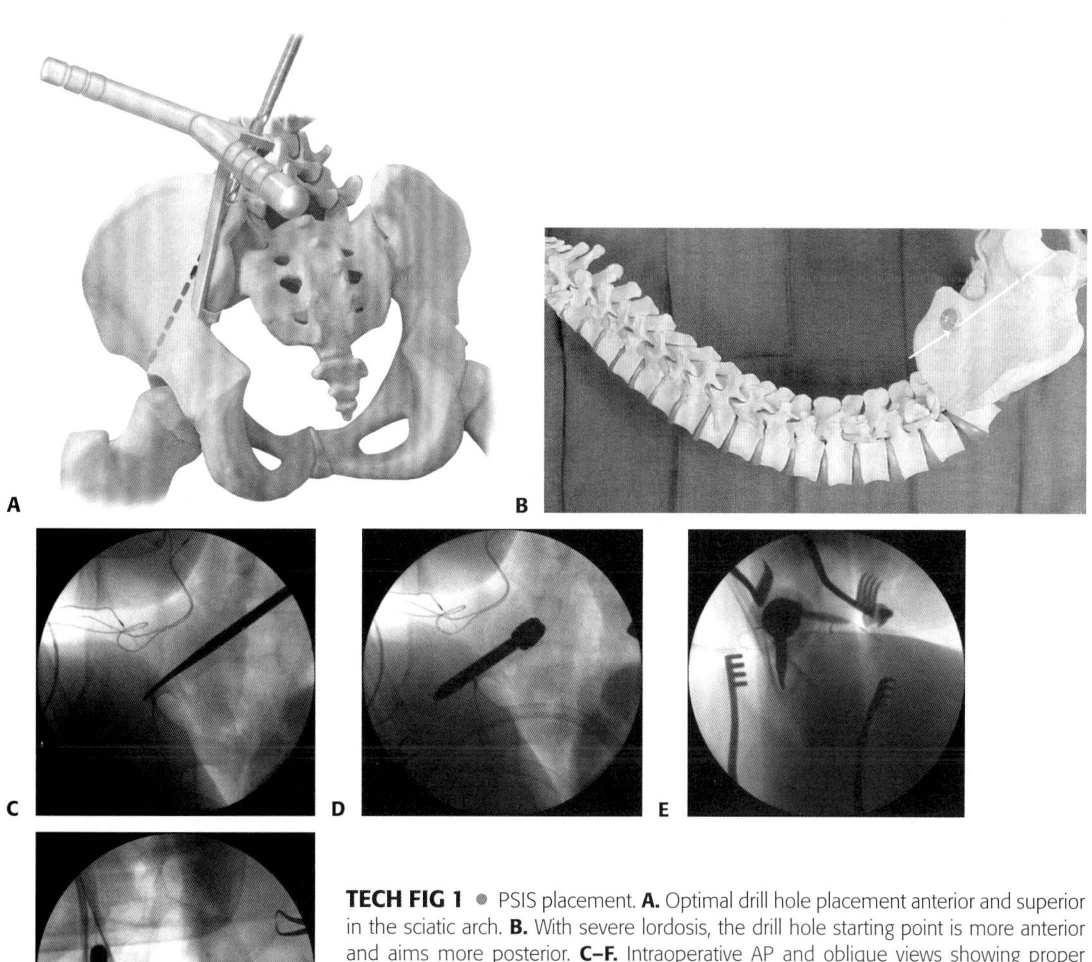


**TECH FIG 1** • PSIS placement. **A.** Optimal drill hole placement anterior and superior in the sciatic arch. **B.** With severe lordosis, the drill hole starting point is more anterior and aims more posterior. **C–F.** Intraoperative AP and oblique views showing proper placement of pelvic screw. **C,D.** The AP views show the trajectory of the pedicle probe from the PSIS to just superior and adjacent to the sciatic notch and the final screw position at least 1 cm lateral to the notch. **E,F.** The oblique views are taken parallel with the probe and show the probe and the final screw position between the inner and outer cortex just superior to the sciatic notch, which appears as a teardrop. (**C–F:** Courtesy of DePuy Synthes Spine.)

## S2 Alar Iliac Placement

- Alternatively, pelvic screws can be placed using the medial portal as described by Chang et al[6] and Sponseller et al.[23] The start point approximately 1.5 cm deeper than the traditional entry from the PSIS placement.
  - Advocates for this method state that there is less exposure time, less bleeding, and that the screw head is less prominent. Also, because the start point is in line with L5 and S1 pedicle screws, offset rod connection can be avoided if pedicle screw instead of wire fixation is being used.
- The starting point for the screw is 2 to 4 mm lateral and 4 to 8 mm inferior to the S1 foramen (**TECH FIG 2A–E**); minimal muscle stripping and dissection is needed.
  - A sharp awl or burr is used to mark the starting point and penetrate the cortical bone.
  - Then, a drill or pedicle gearshift is used to enter the cancellous bone of the sacrum directed toward the dorsal aspect of the sacroiliac joint into the ilium.
- The trajectory is lateral (approximately 40 degrees to the horizontal plane) and 20 to 30 degrees caudal (this depends on pelvic tilt), and fluoroscopy is helpful to guide this trajectory as described in the PSIS approach earlier.
- Once in the ilium, the pathway is 1 to 2 cm above the sciatic notch directed toward the anterior inferior iliac spine (**TECH FIG 2F,G**).
- The hole is probed with a pedicle probe to ensure that the pelvic cortex or sciatic notch is not penetrated.
- A pelvic screw (65 to 100 mm long; 7 to 10 mm diameter) is placed at this time.

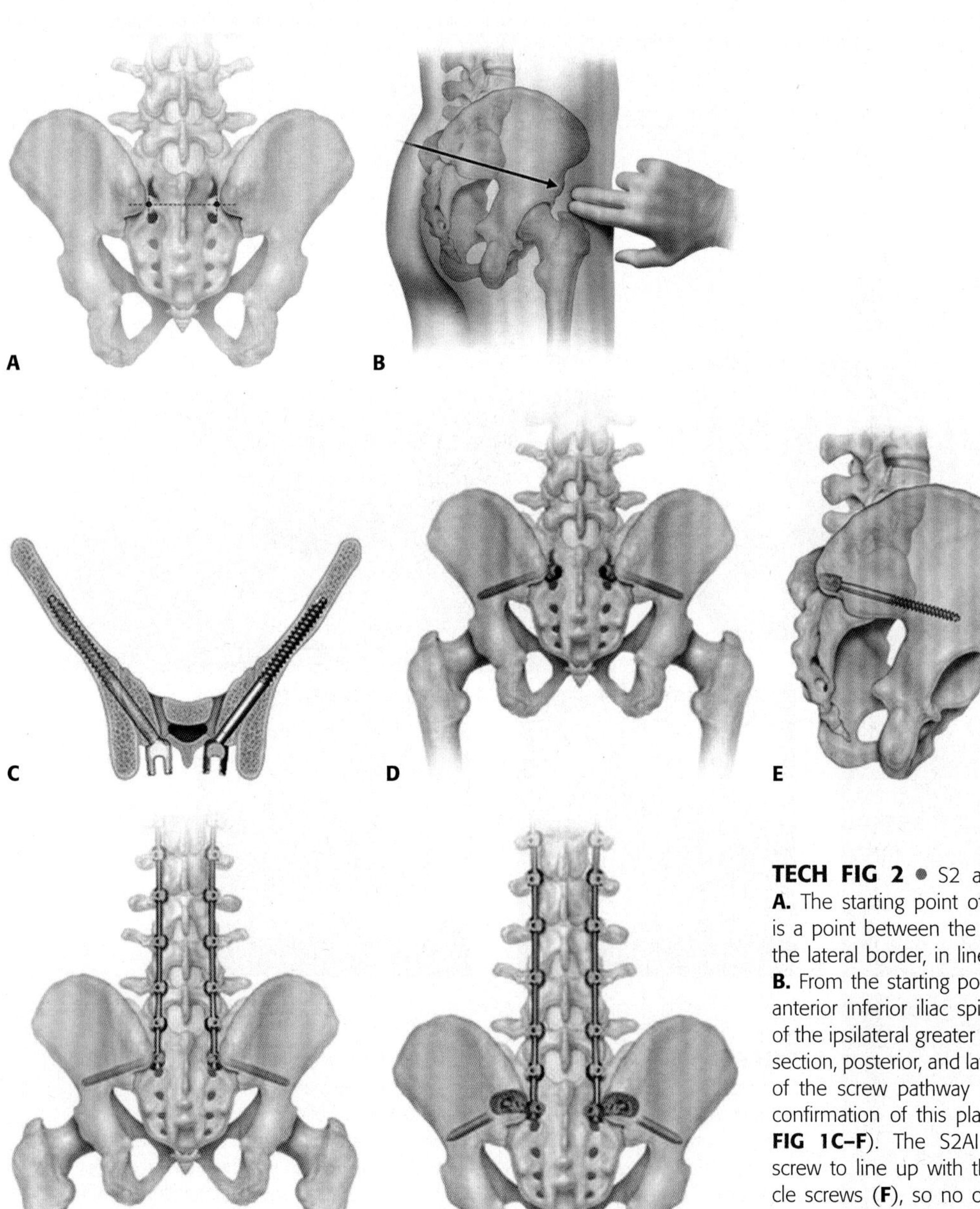


**TECH FIG 2** • S2 alar iliac (S2AI) placement. **A.** The starting point of the sacroiliac (SAI) screw is a point between the S1 and S2 foramen, along the lateral border, in line with an S1 pedicle screw. **B.** From the starting point, one should aim for the anterior inferior iliac spine (AIIS), palpating the tip of the ipsilateral greater trochanter. **C–E.** Axial cross-section, posterior, and lateral iliac views, respectively, of the screw pathway in the ilium. (Radiographic confirmation of this placement is similar to **TECH FIG 1C–F**). The S2AI pathway allows the iliac screw to line up with the lumbar and sacral pedicle screws (**F**), so no offset connection is needed when securing the longitudinal rods as is needed using the PSIS placement (**G**). (Courtesy of DePuy Synthes Spine.)

## Luque Wire Passage

- After the spine is completely exposed and the pelvis is prepared, the spinous processes are completely removed and the ligamentum flavum is carefully removed to expose the sublaminar spaces.
- Double Luque wires are bent (prebent wires are also available) and passed under the lamina from the lamina of L5 up to and including the T1 or T2 lamina.
    - The radius of curvature for the wire bend must approximate the width of the laminae to allow safe passage of the wire.
- Two double wires are passed at the L5 and the proximal most vertebra (T1 or T2) only, whereas a single wire is passed at each of the other levels (**TECH FIG 3A–E**).
- Wires are pulled to equal length and next bent, with the midline bent flat down onto the spinous process beds and the beaded end flat down onto the paraspinous muscles (**TECH FIG 3F**).
    - This helps the wires from getting inadvertently pushed into the spinal canal and allows for easier wire organization.

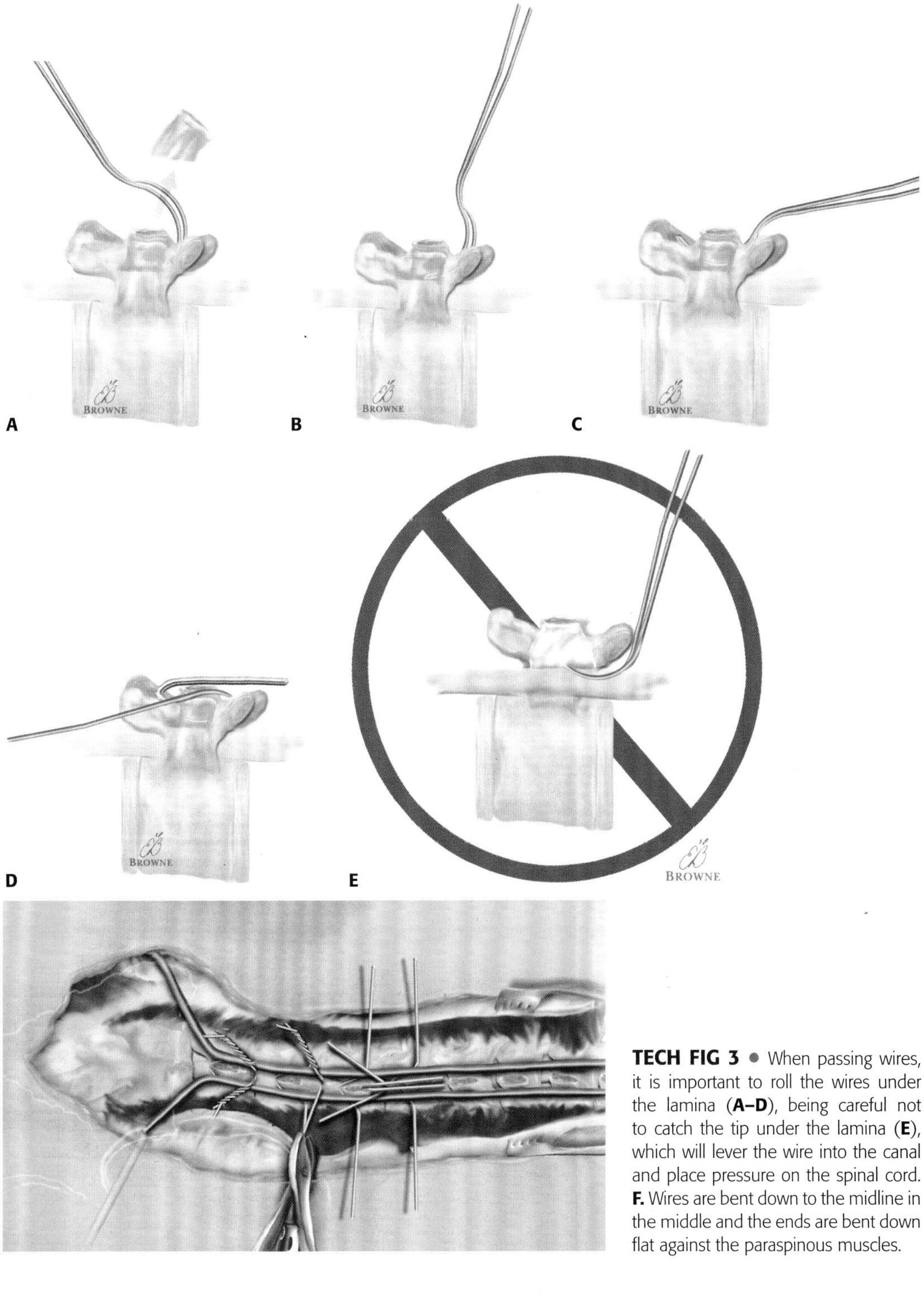

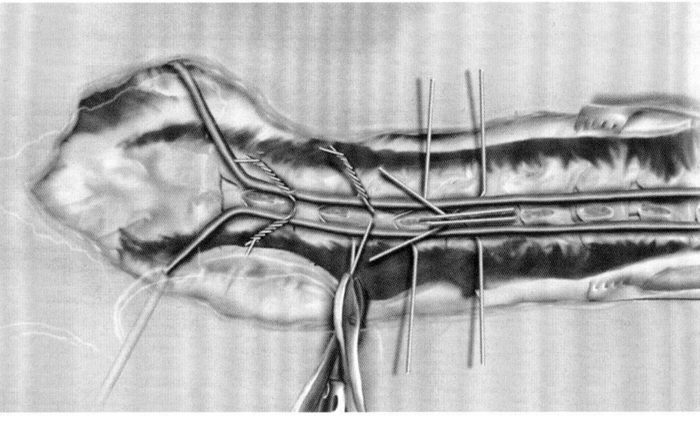

**TECH FIG 3** • When passing wires, it is important to roll the wires under the lamina (**A–D**), being careful not to catch the tip under the lamina (**E**), which will lever the wire into the canal and place pressure on the spinal cord. **F.** Wires are bent down to the midline in the middle and the ends are bent down flat against the paraspinous muscles.

## Rod Selection and Insertion

### Unit Rod

- After the wires are passed, the length of the unit rod is selected.
- This is done by placing the rod upside down with the corner of the rod placed at the drill hole on the elevated side of the pelvis (**TECH FIG 4A**).
  - The proper length rod should reach either T1 or T2 (the selected proximal end point) (**TECH FIG 4B**).
  - A rod one length shorter should be chosen if there is severe kyphosis because the spine shortens with correction.
  - With severe lordosis, a rod length longer should be chosen because the spine lengthens with correction.
- It is best to err on the side of the rod being too short because the wires can be brought down to the rod two or three levels if necessary.
- If the rod is more than 2 cm long, it may become too prominent under the skin.
  - In such cases, cutting the rod and cross-linking the rod may be advisable.
- Facetectomy and decortication of the transverse processes are performed. Corticocancellous allograft (crushed) bone is added (180 to 240 mL).
- Insertion of the rod involves crossing the pelvic limbs of the rod to insert them into the previously drilled pelvic holes (**TECH FIG 4C**).
- In patients with pelvic obliquity, the pelvic limb of the rod is placed into the drill hole on the low side of the pelvic obliquity first, with this side crossed underneath the other limb.
- With the rod impactor, the surgeon inserts three quarters to half of this pelvic limb first and then insert the opposite pelvic limb, using a rod holder to direct it into the correct direction of the previously drilled hole.
- The rod impactor is next used to drive the rod limbs into the pelvis, alternatively impacting each pelvic leg and making certain to direct each of the legs into the previously drilled holes.

### The Modular Unit Rod Construct

- After the right and left pelvic screws are placed, the fixed lateral rod connector is connected to each pelvic screw, the wires are

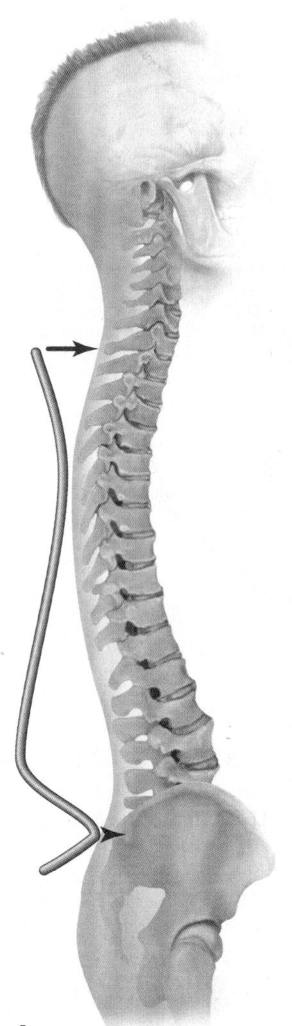


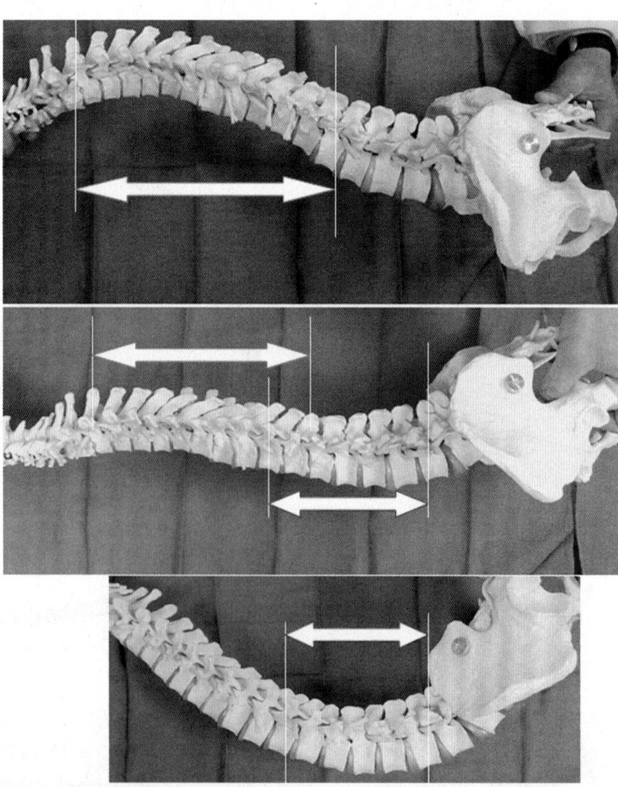


**TECH FIG 4 • A.** Measuring for the proper rod length is one of the most difficult aspects of the surgery and is done by turning the rod upside down and placing the top of the rod at T1 and the bottom corner of the rod at the drill hole in the pelvis. **B.** The spine shortens (*top*) as kyphosis is corrected and lengthens (*bottom*) as excessive lordosis is corrected to normal (*center*). *(continued)*

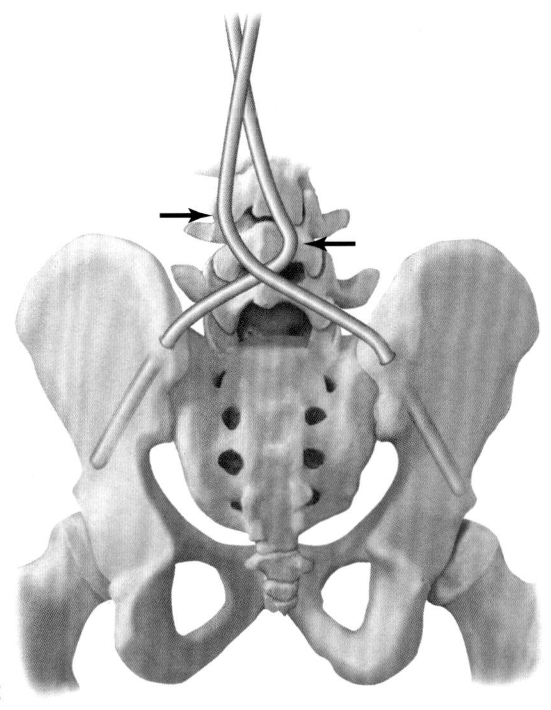

C

**TECH FIG 4** • *(continued)* **C.** The pelvic limbs of the unit rod are crossed to insert them into the drill holes into the pelvis. They are gradually impacted 1 cm at a time, alternating between the right and left limbs, until each is completely within the pelvis.

passed, the precontoured rods are connected to the fixed lateral connectors, and the proximal closed connector is placed at the proximal end of the rods (**TECH FIG 5A**).

- Critical to the correction is to attach and secure each of the precontoured rods to the iliac screws with the fixed lateral connectors so that each of the rods is perfectly perpendicular to the horizontal axis of the pelvis and that the sagittal contour of the rods is aligned with the sacrum.

- The sagittal bend (**TECH FIG 5B,C**) should be identical on each rod and should also be aligned so that the contour matches from proximal to distal. If these steps are not meticulously done, the pelvic obliquity will not be fully corrected with the cantilever maneuver. Once this is done, the set screws at each connection (the pelvic screws, lateral connectors, and proximal connector) are tightened and torqued down onto the rod.
- If the top of the rod is too long, it can be cut in situ and the proximal connector adjusted. A drop entry cross-connector can be added at the thoracolumbar junction to augment the stability of the construct. This foundation from the pelvic screws up to the proximal connector serves as modular constructed unit rod which is now ready to serve as a cantilever to correct the spinal deformity.

## Cantilever Correction

- The surgeon should not try to see if the rod fits by pushing it down into the wound completely in one move, as this may cause the pelvic limbs of the rod or the pelvic screws to pullout of the pelvis or fracture the ilium.
- The surgeon should push the rod to line up with the lamina only (**TECH FIG 6A,B**) and then twist the wires being careful not to overtighten (we suggest a jet wire twister). It is important that the remaining spinous process lies in the midline. The wires are cut 10 to 15 mm long.
- The rod is pushed to L4 and the wires are twisted and cut.
  - Then, the rod is pushed to L3 and the wires are twisted and cut.
- This process continues one level at a time until the surgeon reaches T1 or T2 (**TECH FIG 6C,D**).

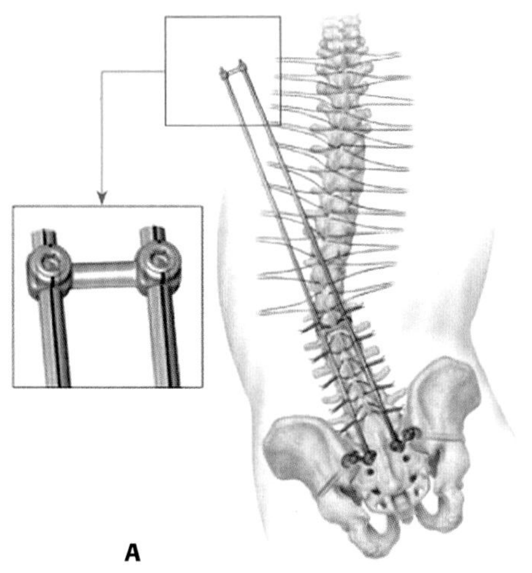

A

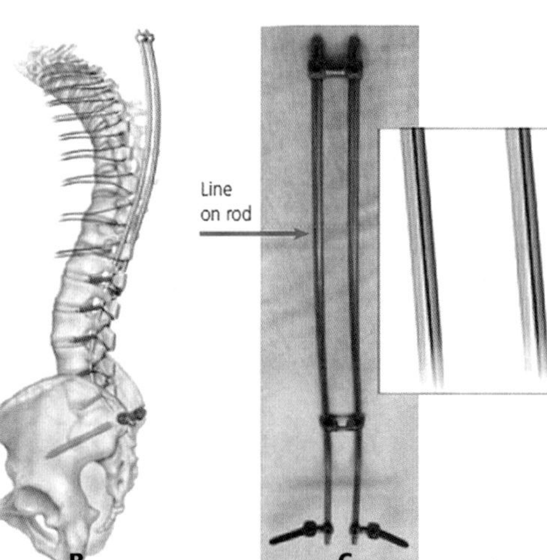


B C

**TECH FIG 5** • **A.** AP profile of the modular unit rod construct with precontoured rods connected to the pelvic screws in the PSIS position (S2AI pathway can also be used after the wires have been passed). The connection should make the rods perpendicular to the horizontal axis of the pelvis to maximize cantilever correction. A distal cross-connector and proximal closed connector make the construct rigid. The rods should match in both length and contour with rotation matched before final tightening of the connectors. **B.** Lateral contour of the prebent rods in line with the sagittal profile of the sacrum. **C.** There is a line on the posterior contour of the rod to help line it up with the sacrum. (Courtesy of DePuy Synthes Spine.)

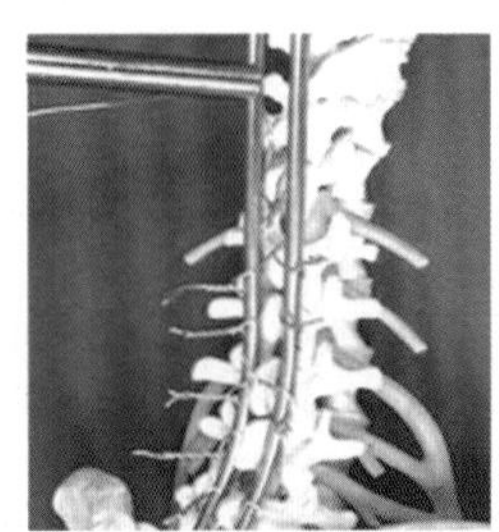
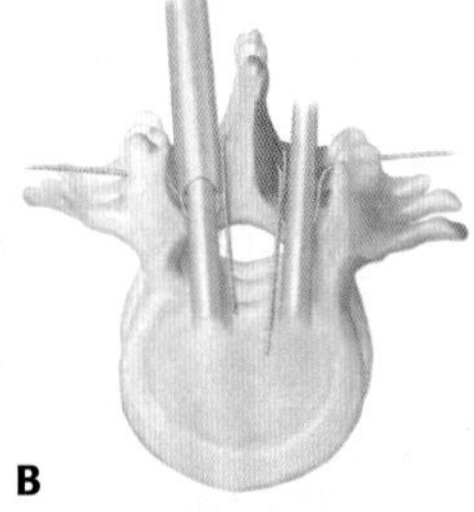
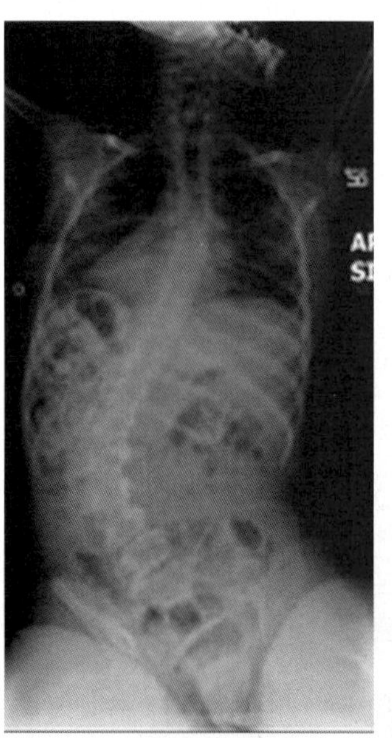
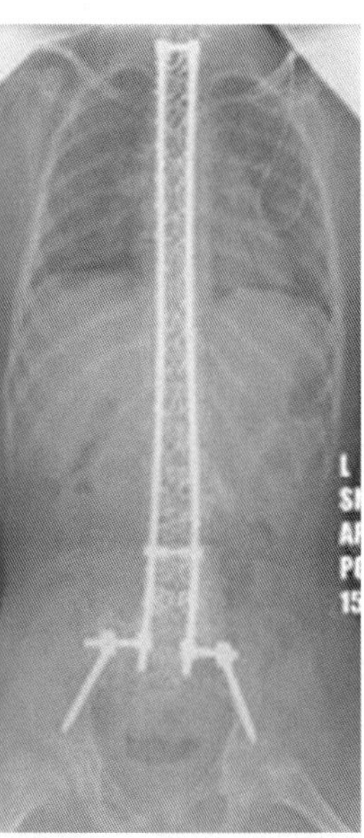

**TECH FIG 6 • A.** Once the foundation is instrumented, the rod construct is manually pushed down at each level with a rod pusher (similar to the unit rod) at each level before tightening wires (if sublaminar wires are to be used). **B.** The rod is manually pushed down at each level with a rod pusher before tightening the wires. This is important to prevent wire breakage or cutout through the lamina. It is important to keep the center of the unit rod at the spinous process. **C,D.** Preoperative and postoperative AP radiographs. (**A,C,D:** Courtesy of DePuy Synthes Spine.)

## Thoracic Scoliosis and Kyphosis

- Spinal curvatures in the thoracic region are more difficult to correct with cantilever correction.
- In such cases, starting distally at the pelvis or in the lumbar spine leaves a short lever arm at the proximal end of the rod by the time one reaches fixation in the thoracic spine, making it difficult to center the head over the remainder of the thorax and pelvis.
- This type of curvature is difficult to correct with the traditional unit rod because the unit rod requires distal fixation into the pelvis first (**TECH FIG 7A**).
  - With this type of curvature, a reverse cantilever (proximal to distal) can be performed (**TECH FIG 7B–D**).
- After exposing the spine and pelvis, pelvic screws and sublaminar wires are placed as previously described.

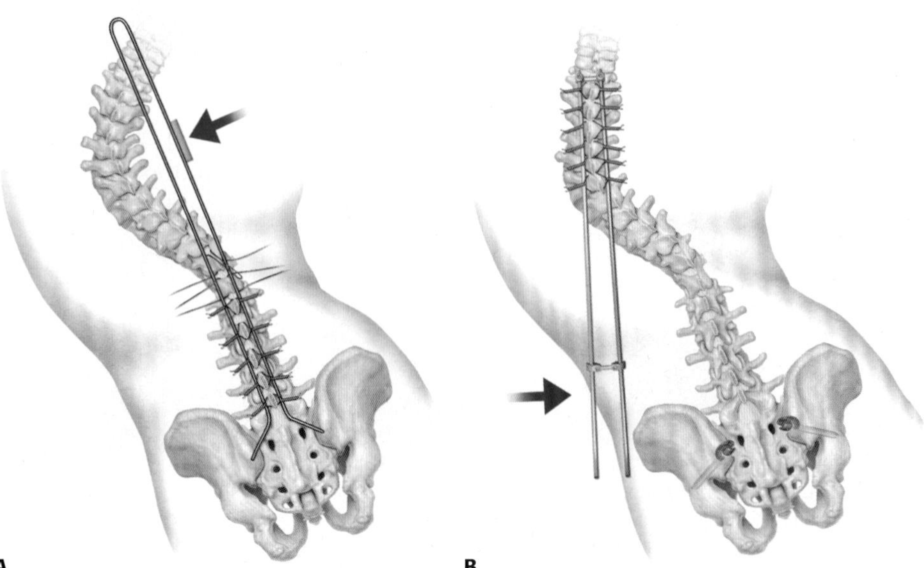

**TECH FIG 7 • A.** It is difficult to cantilever this type of thoracic curvature using the unit rod due to insufficient lever arm. **B.** This diagram shows proximal to distal cantilever technique that can be used for thoracic scoliosis. *(continued)*

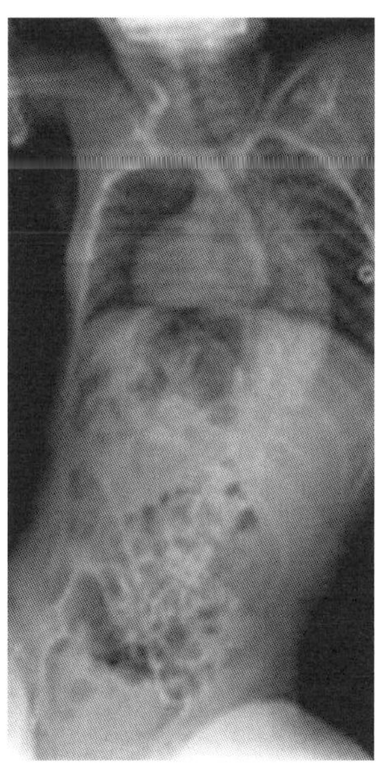

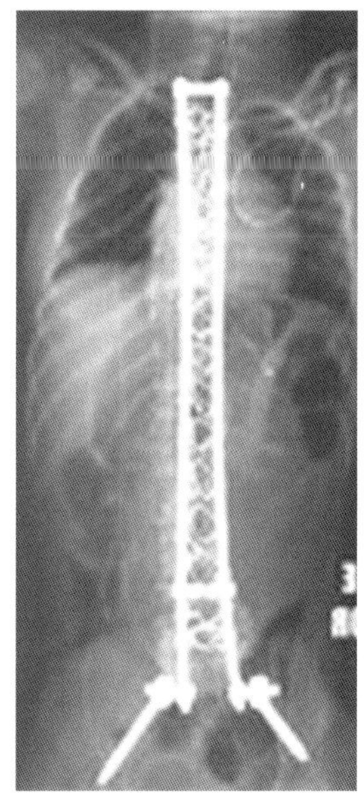

**TECH FIG 7** • *(continued)* **C,D.** Preoperative and postoperative AP radiographs. (Courtesy of DePuy Synthes Spine.)

- The rod construct is then preassembled by first connecting the precontoured rods with the proximal closed rod connector at the top and placing a cross-connector in the lumbar region. The rods should be parallel from proximal to distal with respect to their contour.
- Next, the top of the rod construct is secured using sublaminar wires from T1 down to the apex of the curvature.
- After the apical vertebra is secured to the rod, cantilever correction can be performed by gradually pushing the rod down to the next more distal vertebra, tightening the sublaminar wire, pushing the rod down to the next more distal vertebra, and then tightening the wire, performing the same maneuver progressively down the spine until the pelvis screws are reached.
- The fixed rodded lateral connectors are then used to connect the rod to the pelvic screws.
- Using this "proximal to distal" cantilever technique for cantilever correction allows for a better lever arm to correct thoracic scoliosis as well as thoracic kyphosis (**TECH FIG 8**) and to center the head over the trunk.

**TECH FIG 8** • **A,B.** The proximal to distal cantilever technique can be used for thoracic kyphosis. **C,D.** Preoperative and postoperative radiographs. (Courtesy of DePuy Synthes Spine.)

## Completion and Wound Closure

- All wires are bent down into the midline of the rod and directly caudally. This allows easier exposure of the rod and wires if reoperation should ever become necessary.
- The remaining bone graft is applied (**TECH FIG 9A**).
  - We mix the remaining 60 mL of allograft with either gentamicin (three or four 80-mg vials)[4] and, more recently, vancomycin (500 mg for smaller children, 1000 mg for larger children [>50 kg]). This has lessened the postoperative infection rate.
- If the child is thin and the sacrum is prominent, the sacral spinous processes and lateral processes are trimmed.
  - The sacral lamina and lateral processes can be completely removed if they are severely prominent.
- The fascia is closed tightly (any leakage may predispose to infection, especially in the lower part of the spine and if the child is incontinent of urine and stool).
  - No drain is used.
- The subcutaneous tissue and skin are meticulously closed.
- Final radiographs are taken to confirm coronal and sagittal alignment (**TECH FIG 9B–D**).
- In patients with hyperlordosis, pedicle screws with reduction posts are useful in the apex of the sagittal plane deformity to aid in the correction (**TECH FIG 9E,F**).
- If plastic surgery expertise is available, flap closure by a plastic surgery reconstructive team may lead to lower rates of wound breakdown and deep infections.

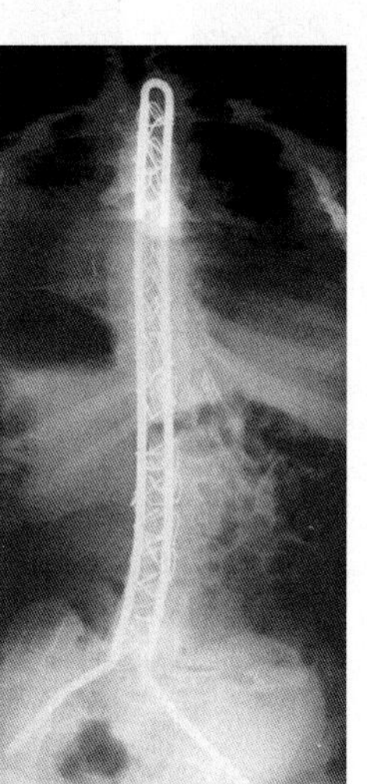
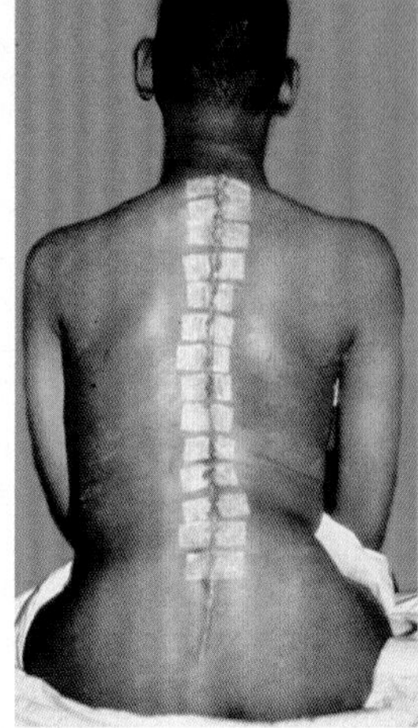
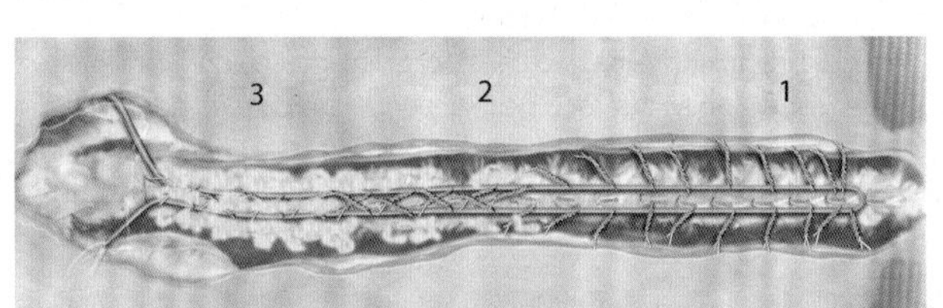

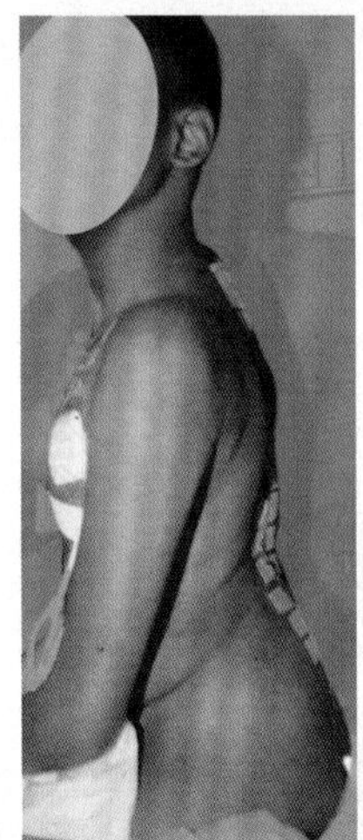

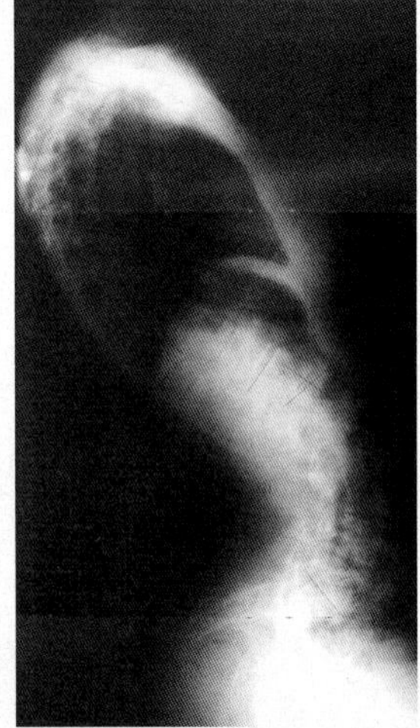

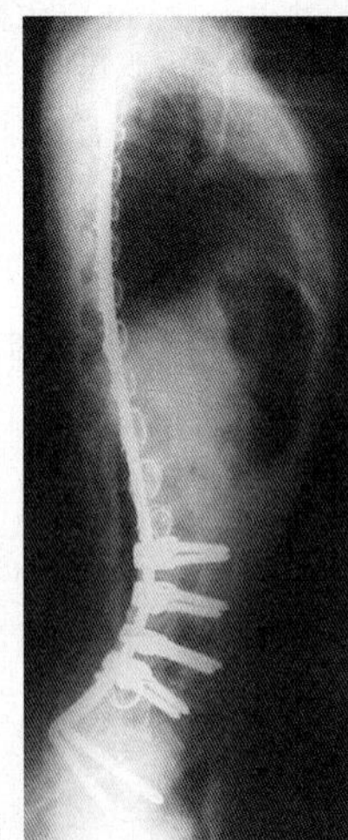


**TECH FIG 9** • **A.** Wires are passed and then twisted in a clockwise direction (*1*). Wires are cut about 1 cm and then bent to the midline (*2*). Allograft bone (*yellow*) is placed out laterally along the transverse processes and is impacted into the facet joints after facetectomy (*3*). **B.** AP radiograph of the patient in **FIG 1** shows postoperative correction of coronal plane deformity. Clinical photographs show correction of pelvic obliquity (**C**) and good sagittal plane alignment (**D**). **E,F.** Preoperative and postoperative lateral radiographs of patient with severe hyperlordosis corrected with unit instrumentation and pedicle screws used to correct lordosis in the apex of the deformity.

## PEARLS AND PITFALLS

| | |
|---|---|
| **Severe intraoperative hypotension may suddenly occur, especially after decortication.** | ▪ Constant communication between the surgeon and the anesthesiologist is critical. Type and cross-matched packed red blood cells (1.5–2 times blood volume), fresh frozen plasma, and platelets should be available. |
| **Hypothermia** | ▪ Hypothermia can be avoided by keeping the room temperature high and using a heated ventilator, a warmer for intravenous fluids and blood, and an airflow heating device. |
| **Excessively stiff scoliosis or accompanying sagittal plane deformity (hyperkyphosis or hyperlordosis)** | ▪ The surgeon should recognize stiffness preoperatively on the physical examination or bending radiographs to plan for anterior release. |
| **Rod insertion** | ▪ Using the wires to pull the rod down to the lamina may cause the wires to cut through the lamina.<br>▪ Relaxing the push on the rod between levels while correcting the major curve may cause an "unzipper" effect, with several wires tearing through lamina or breaking from too much force on the end vertebra.<br>▪ The surgeon should use a rod holder to prevent the pusher from slipping off the rod as the top of the rod is approached.<br>▪ The force from pushing may become large, preventing the patient from being ventilated or causing a drop in blood pressure. If this occurs, the surgeon should relax the push on the rod just enough to allow ventilation and return of pressure. |
| **Pelvic insertion of rod limb in severe lordosis** | ▪ Difficulty occurs as the surgeon attempts to insert the pelvic limb of the rod and cannot get the rod anterior enough to steer the rod into the drill holes. This may allow the rod to perforate into the sciatic notch or through the inner pelvic table.<br>▪ Intraoperative fluoroscopy should be used to check proper placement of the pelvic limbs. If pelvic penetration of the rod occurs, the penetrated rod limb should be cut, reinserted into the pelvis, and reconnected with an end-to-end or side-to-side connector.<br>▪ Alternatively, if severe lordosis is present, the modular unit rod concept with separate insertion of pelvic screws may be performed instead of the unit rod which allows easier placement of the pelvic portion of the instrumentation with separate attachment of the rods. |
| **Misjudgment of rod length** | ▪ If the rod is too long and prominent, both rods can be cross-linked together and then cut at the T1 vertebra. If the rod length is misjudged too short by more than two levels, the top of another unit rod can be connected with end-to-end connectors. This is important when there is excessive kyphosis to prevent drop-off of the spine over the top of the rod. |
| **Wires cut through lamina** | ▪ Only enough bone should be removed to allow wires to pass through the sublaminar space. Wires should not be used to pull the rod to the lamina. This may also be due to inadequate anterior release in a stiff deformity. |
| **Pedicle screw pulling out of bone** | ▪ A larger diameter screw may be placed or a sublaminar wire may be added at the level where the screw is beginning to back out to add to the fixation. |

## POSTOPERATIVE CARE

- Neuromuscular patients are managed in the intensive care unit postoperatively in most cases in most centers
- If blood loss is not excessive and the anesthesiologist feels the child can be extubated, the breathing tube is removed. Some children remain intubated and are ventilated for 2 to 5 days. This latter group of children requires more intensive respiratory management.
- Pain management consists of short-acting narcotic (fentanyl) drip and management of spasticity using diazepam. Oral pain management can be started on the third or fourth postoperative day.
- Core body temperature should be increased to 37° C and maintained. Blood clotting is impaired by low body temperature below 33° C, which can easily develop in this patient population.
- Hypotensive episodes are avoided by maintaining increased fluid intake and pressor support as needed. Urine output should be maintained at a minimum of 0.5 mL/kg/hour.
- Most children require aggressive postoperative nutritional support.
  - Gastrostomy tube feedings can be started as soon as bowel sounds are present.
- If bowel sounds are not present, gastrojejunostomy or nasojejunostomy feedings are attempted.
- Central hyperalimentation is started if feeding through the gut is not tolerated. A tunneled central venous catheter (Hickman) is placed at the time of surgery. This is discontinued as soon as central access is no longer needed to avoid the risk of line infection.
- Pancreatic enzyme levels are monitored carefully postoperatively, as elevated amylase and lipase levels are common and indicative of subclinical pancreatitis.[5]
  - Oral and gastrostomy feedings should be delayed if these values are increasing above normal.
  - Adequate nutritional intake for optimal wound healing usually requires about 1.5 times the child's normal preoperative requirements and is continued up to 1 month postoperatively.
- Proper wheelchair assessment postoperatively is also important.

## OUTCOMES

- Unit rod instrumentation achieves a scoliosis correction of 70% to 80% of the preoperative curve magnitude and an 80% to 90% correction of pelvic obliquity.[9,30]
- In a subset of 24 ambulatory cerebral palsy patients who underwent posterior spinal fusion with unit rod instrumentation, all patients have preservation of ambulatory status.[29]
- Sagittal plane spinal deformity is also well corrected with unit rod instrumentation. Lipton et al[16] showed relief of symptoms and correction of sagittal plane deformity in 24 cerebral palsy patients with hyperlordosis and kyphosis after unit rod instrumentation.
- In one survey of 190 parents and caretakers assessing functional improvement of children with cerebral palsy after posterior spinal fusion, 95.8% of parents and 84.3% of caretakers would recommend spinal surgery again.[27] Positive responses included improved appearance, overall function, quality of life, and ease of care.
- Overall life expectancy of the cerebral palsy child after posterior spinal fusion is critically important. A survival analysis showed that the presence of severe preoperative thoracic hyperkyphosis and the number of postoperative days in the intensive care unit correlated with decreased life expectancy after evaluating a number of variables.[28]

## COMPLICATIONS

- Complications are common but usually not life-threatening and range from minor to major. They include excessive intraoperative bleeding, neurologic complications, atelectasis, pneumonia, prolonged postoperative ileus pancreatitis, wound infection, and so forth.
- Mechanical or technical complications also occur and include rod or wire prominence, pseudarthrosis, rod penetration through the pelvis, curve progression after fusion due to crankshafting, and so forth.
- In one study, the curve magnitude, preoperative pulmonary status, and degree of neurologic involvement had the highest correlation with postoperative complications.
- Infection rates vary but should be expected in about 10% of cases, even when all conditions are optimized. Family should be counseled and prepared for high rate of perioperative problems.

## REFERENCES


1. Alman BA, Raza SN, Biggar WD. Steroid treatment and the development of scoliosis in males with Duchenne muscular dystrophy. J Bone Joint Surg Am 2004;86-A(3):519–524.
2. Aprin H, Bowen JR, MacEwen GD, et al. Spine fusion in patients with spinal muscular atrophy. J Bone Joint Surg Am 1982;64:1179–1187.
3. Bell DF, Mosely CF, Koreska J. Unit rod segmental spinal instrumentation in the management of patients with progressive neuromuscular spinal deformity. Spine 1989;14:1301–1307.
4. Borkhuu B, Borowski A, Shah SA, et al. Antibiotic-loaded allograft decreases the rate of acute deep wound infection after spinal fusion in cerebral palsy. Spine 2008;33:2300–2304.
5. Borkhuu B, Nagaraju D, Miller F, et al. Prevalence and risk factors in postoperative pancreatitis after spine fusion in patients with cerebral palsy. J Pediatr Orthop 2009;29:256–262.
6. Chang TL, Sponseller PD, Kebaish KM, et al. Low profile pelvic fixation: anatomic parameters for sacral alar-iliac fixation versus traditional iliac fixation. Spine 2009;34:436–440.
7. Dearolf WW III, Betz RR, Vogel LC, et al. Scoliosis in pediatric spinal cord-injured patients. J Pediatr Orthop 1990;10:214–218.
8. Dhawale AA, Shah SA, Sponseller PD, et al. Are antifibrinolytics helpful in decreasing blood loss and transfusions during spinal fusion surgery in children with cerebral palsy scoliosis? Spine 2012;37:E549–E555.
9. Dias RC, Miller F, Dabney K, et al. Surgical correction of spinal deformity using a unit rod in children with cerebral palsy. J Pediatr Orthop 1996;16:734–740.
10. DiCindio S, Theroux M, Shah S, et al. Multimodality monitoring of transcranial electric motor and somatosensory-evoked potentials during surgical correction of spinal deformity in patients with cerebral palsy and other neuromuscular disorders. Spine 2003;28:1851–1855.
11. Karol LA. Scoliosis in patients with Duchenne muscular dystrophy. J Bone Joint Surg Am 2007;89:155–162.
12. Keret D, Bassett GS, Bunnell WP, et al. Scoliosis in Rett syndrome. J Pediatr Orthop 1988;8:138–142.
13. King WM, Ruttencutter R, Nagaraja HN, et al. Orthopedic outcomes of long-term daily corticosteroid treatment in Duchenne muscular dystrophy. Neurology 2007;68(19):1607–1613.
14. Labelle H, Tohme S, Duhaime M, et al. Natural history of scoliosis in Friedreich's ataxia. J Bone Joint Surg Am 1986;68:564–572.
15. Lebel DE, Corston JA, McAdam LC, et al. Glucocorticoid treatment for the prevention of scoliosis in children with Duchenne muscular dystrophy: long-term follow-up. J Bone Joint Surg Am 2013;95(12):1057–1061.
16. Lipton GE, Letonoff EJ, Dabney KW, et al. Correction of spinal plane deformities with unit rod instrumentation in children with cerebral palsy. J Bone Joint Surg Am 2003;85:2349–2357.
17. Lipton GE, Miller F, Dabney KW, et al. Factors predicting postoperative complications following spinal fusions in children with cerebral palsy. J Spinal Disord 1999;12:197–205.
18. Maloney WJ, Rinsky LA, Gamble JG. Simultaneous correction of pelvic obliquity, frontal plane and sagittal plane deformities in neuromuscular scoliosis using a unit rod and sublaminar wires: a preliminary report. J Pediatr Orthop 1990;10:742–749.
19. Miller F, Moseley C, Koreska J. Pelvic anatomy relative to lumbosacral instrumentation. J Spinal Disord 1990;3:169–173.
20. Rinsky LA. Surgery of spinal deformity in cerebral palsy. Twelve years in the evolution of scoliosis management. Clin Orthop Relat Res 1990;(253):100–109.
21. Smeets E, Schollen E, Moog U, et al. Rett syndrome in adolescent and adult females: clinical and molecular genetic findings. Am J Med Genetics A 2003;122:227–233.
22. Smith AD, Koreska J, Moseley CF. Progression of scoliosis in Duchene muscular dystrophy. J Bone Joint Surg Am 1989;71:1066–1074.
23. Sponseller PD, Zimmerman RM, Ko PS, et al. Low profile pelvic fixation with sacral alar iliac technique in the pediatric population improves results at two-year minimum follow-up. Spine 2010;35:1887–1892.
24. Sucato DJ. Spinal deformity in spinal muscular atrophy. J Bone Joint Surg Am 2007;89:148–154.
25. Thometz JG, Simon SR. Progression of scoliosis after skeletal maturity in institutionalized adults who have cerebral palsy. J Bone Joint Surg Am 1988;70:1290–1296.
26. Trivedi J, Thompson JD, Slakey JB, et al. Clinical and radiographic predictors of scoliosis in myelomeningocele. J Bone Joint Surg Am 2002;84:1389–1394.
27. Tsirikos AI, Chang WN, Dabney KW, et al. Comparison of parents' and caregivers' satisfaction after spinal fusion in children with cerebral palsy. J Pediatr Orthop 2004;24:54–58.
28. Tsirikos AI, Chang WN, Dabney KW, et al. Life expectancy in pediatric patients with cerebral palsy and neuromuscular scoliosis who underwent spinal fusion. Dev Med Child Neurol 2003;45:677–682.
29. Tsirikos AI, Chang WN, Shah SA, et al. Preserving ambulatory potential in pediatric patients with cerebral palsy who undergo spinal fusion using unit rod instrumentation. Spine 2003;28:480–483.
30. Tsirikos AI, Lipton G, Chang WN, et al. Surgical correction of scoliosis in pediatric patients with cerebral palsy using unit rod instrumentation. Spine 2008;33:1133–1140.
31. Yamashita T, Kanaya K, Yokogushi K, et al. Correlation between progression of spinal deformity and pulmonary function in Duchenne muscular dystrophy. J Pediatr Orthop 2001;21(1):113–116.

CHAPTER 91

# Pelvic Fixation for Neuromuscular Scoliosis

Jaysson T. Brooks and Paul D. Sponseller

## DEFINITION

- Neuromuscular scoliosis (NMS) is a spinal deformity in the coronal plane in patients with abnormal myoneural pathways of the body.[16]
- Pelvic fixation refers to the anchorage of spinal fixation to the sacrum or ilium or both.

## ANATOMY

- The pelvis can accommodate large screws that aid in the correction of pelvic obliquity while also providing a stable base in long fusion constructs.
- In adolescents, the mean length of the sacral alar iliac (SAI) screw pathway is 106 mm, whereas that of the posterior superior iliac spine (PSIS) to anterior inferior iliac spine pathway (for standard iliac screws) is 123 mm (**FIG 1**).
- The narrowest mean width of the ilium is 12 mm for the right or left side, indicating that the SAI pathway can accommodate large-diameter screws for increased bone purchase.
- The average depth below the skin of the SAI screw insertion point is 52 mm, whereas that for the PSIS insertion point[7] is 37 mm. This difference of 1.5 cm is important for the patient with neuromuscular deformity who has vulnerable skin because he or she spends most of the time in a recumbent position.
- It has been shown that intrapelvic asymmetry between the right and left side is common in patients with NMS.[12] A firm grasp not just of normal anatomy but also of the patient's individual anatomy is vital in placing screws in the right trajectory.

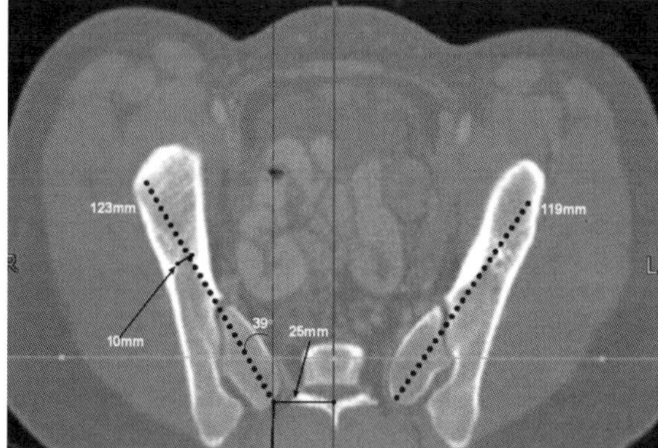


**FIG 1** • In space, three-dimensional CT imaging of SAI pathway. (Modified from Chang TL, Sponseller PD, Kebaish KM, et al. Low profile pelvic fixation: anatomic parameters for SAI fixation versus traditional iliac fixation. Spine 2009;34:436–440.)

- The sacroiliac joint is composed of hyaline cartilage anteriorly and fibrocartilage posteriorly. An SAI screw traverses the hyaline cartilage of the sacroiliac joint 60% of the time.[21]

## PATHOGENESIS

- The Scoliosis Research Society has classified the abnormal myoneural pathways that cause NMS into the following categories[6]:
  - Neuropathic
    - Upper motor neuron: cerebral palsy, spinocerebellar degeneration (Friedreich ataxia, Charcot-Marie-Tooth disease, Roussy-Lévy disease), syringomyelia, spinal cord tumors, spinal cord trauma, Rett syndrome
    - Lower motor neuron: poliomyelitis, traumatic, spinal muscular atrophy, dysautonomia
    - Combined upper and lower pathologies: myelomeningocele
  - Myopathic
    - Arthrogryposis
    - Muscular dystrophy
    - Fiber-type disproportion
    - Congenital hypotonia
    - Myotonia dystrophica

## NATURAL HISTORY

- The rates of spinal deformity are high in patients with NMS, including 20% to 70% of patients with cerebral palsy (depending on the amount of trunk control), 60% of patients with Friedreich ataxia, 80% of patients with spinal muscular atrophy, 86% of patients with familial dysautonomia, 50% to 90% of male patients with Duchenne muscular dystrophy, and nearly 100% of patients with traumatic quadriplegia or thoracic level paraplegia before skeletal maturity.[4]
- Unlike adolescent idiopathic scoliosis, most curves in patients with NMS tend to progress.
- Pelvic obliquity of 15 degrees or more in patients with NMS will likely worsen after spinal fusion if pelvic fixation is not included as part of the instrumentation construct.[18]

## PATIENT HISTORY AND PHYSICAL FINDINGS

- The importance of understanding a patient's baseline function cannot be understated.
- Patients with NMS have a wide range of motor and sensory function. Knowledge of this fact is important for postoperative comparison. This baseline should be recorded in the chart, and the patient should be reexamined immediately before surgery. Does he or she move the toes to command or only spontaneously? Is he or she able to ambulate? These questions should be answered by physical examination before surgery begins.

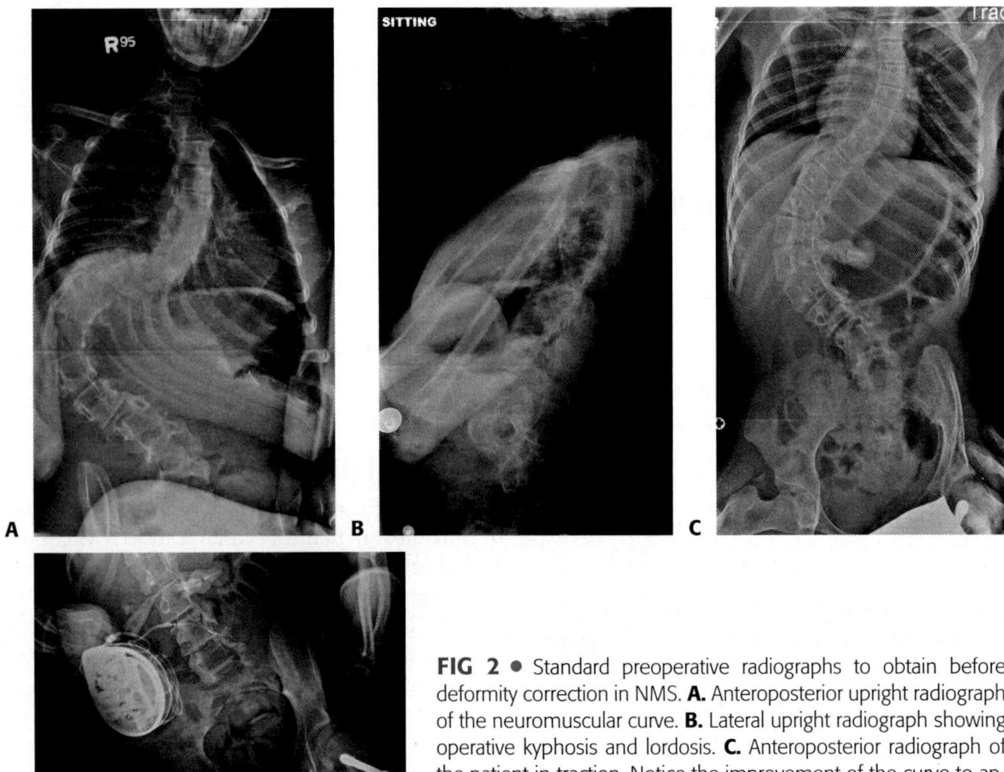


**FIG 2** • Standard preoperative radiographs to obtain before deformity correction in NMS. **A.** Anteroposterior upright radiograph of the neuromuscular curve. **B.** Lateral upright radiograph showing operative kyphosis and lordosis. **C.** Anteroposterior radiograph of the patient in traction. Notice the improvement of the curve to approximately 75 degrees in the coronal plane as compared with the anteroposterior radiograph in **A**. **D.** Anteroposterior radiograph of the pelvis revealing the degree of pelvic obliquity and the location of the baclofen pump.

## IMAGING AND OTHER DIAGNOSTIC STUDIES

- Standard posteroanterior and lateral 3-foot upright scoliosis radiographs (**FIG 2A,B**) should be obtained.
- The rigidity of the curve is assessed by obtaining traction or fulcrum radiographs (**FIG 2C**).
- Pelvic obliquity, sagittal alignment, and the status of the patient's hips are assessed to help with positioning of the patient on the day of surgery (**FIG 2D**).
- If a baclofen pump is present, the side it is on should be identified to help with the surgical approach.

## DIFFERENTIAL DIAGNOSIS

- It is important to make sure that the patient's scoliosis is truly neuromuscular and does not fall in other categories such as congenital, idiopathic, or syndromic scoliosis.
- Congenital scoliosis is caused by a failure of vertebral formation or segmentation during the fourth to fifth week of gestation. Syndromic scoliosis is discerned by certain pathognomonic features of the suspected diagnosis such as the ligamentous laxity, arachnodactyly, and dolichostenomelia seen in Marfan syndrome.

## NONOPERATIVE MANAGEMENT

- Bracing
  - Bracing in patients with NMS is ineffective in preventing progression of the curve and resultant pelvic obliquity.[22]
  - If bracing is used, it is often a soft thoracolumbosacral orthosis to help with sitting balance for a flexible curve.
- Additional nonoperative interventions include sitting supports, custom seating, and functional sitting programs.[9]

## SURGICAL MANAGEMENT

- Posterior spinal fusion has not been shown to prolong the life of patients with NMS, but it often increases the quality of life through improving trunk balance, sitting position, and comfort; through correction of pelvic obliquity; and by prevention of further progression of their curve.[20,24]
- Historically, fusion to the pelvis was thought to be difficult with associated poor outcomes; however, major advances in spinal fusion techniques have improved outcomes significantly.
  - In the 1980s, Luque[14] introduced segmental spinal instrumentation using sublaminar wires to better control progressive deformity in patients with postpoliomyelitic scoliosis.
  - The Cotrel-Dubousset instrumentation system[8] further expounded on Luque's findings by adding hooks and pedicle screws to the construct and introducing the concept of derotation of the spinal deformity.
  - In 1988, Allen and Ferguson[1] introduced the Galveston technique, involving fixation to the pelvis using an L-shaped rod inserted at the PSIS and placed between the inner and outer tables of the ilium. The Galveston technique improved caudal fixation in long fusions and brought to the forefront the importance of pelvic fixation.
  - In 1989, Bell et al[3] built on the Galveston technique with the unit rod, which was one continuous rod with precontoured bends for kyphosis and for fixation to the pelvis. It was developed to counteract translation of one rod with

respect to the other and to resist rotation of the pelvis around the caudal ends.

- The iliosacral screw[11] was a natural progression and provided increased caudal purchase because it traversed both cortices of the ilium before entering the S1 pedicle. Its main disadvantage was the extensive soft tissue dissection required to place it in the correct position.

- The most recent development in pelvic fixation is the SAI screw.
  - Its start point is on the sacrum, avoiding the extensive soft tissue dissection needed to use the PSIS as a start point.
  - As described by McCord et al,[17] the stiffness of a construct connected caudally to SAI screws is greatly increased because of the marked anterior extension past the lumbosacral pivot point.
  - The start point for the SAI screw is 1.5 cm deeper than that the unit rod, avoiding many of the complications associated with the latter, such as prominence and backout.
  - Implants used for SAI fixation may include standard large screws, cannulated screws, and favored-angle screws. Some have a smooth shank and others have a dual-lead thread.

## Preoperative Planning

- The decision to fuse to the pelvis depends on the curve pattern and preoperative trunk control. Curves with an apex above the thoracolumbar junction and an end vertebra above L4 may not require fusion to the pelvis. Patients with NMS who have a reasonable ability to sit independently with a balanced pelvis may not require fusion to the pelvis, especially if it would limit their function.
- Preoperative traction radiographs help to determine the flexibility of the curve, but the curves of most patients with NMS progress caudally if left unfused, so extension down to S2 is common.
- Another variable is from how far cephalad to fuse. As a general rule, all vertebrae within the main coronal and sagittal curves, as well as any proximal thoracic curve larger than approximately 30 to 35 degrees, should be included in the fusion.
- The decision on whether or not to use traction via Gardner-Wells tongs should be made during preoperative planning. It is our preference to use proximal traction via Gardner-Wells tongs for all patients with NMS undergoing primary posterior spinal fusion.
- Some degrees of pelvic obliquity can be corrected with distally in addition to proximal traction. The senior author prefers to use skin traction when distal traction is required. A prerequisite for use of distal extremity traction is the absence of hip or knee flexion contractures greater than 30 degrees.
- The use of antifibrinolytic agents such as tranexamic acid, aprotinin, or epsilon-aminocaproic acid should be decided on preoperatively.
  - Tranexamic acid has been shown to decrease blood loss and the need for transfused blood products in patients requiring vertebral column resections for the correction of their deformity.[19]
  - Tranexamic acid works by competitively binding to and inhibiting plasminogen and plasmin, which would otherwise break down fibrin, the principle component of clot formation in the body.

## Positioning

- Starting 1 cm superior to the pinna, the skin is injected down to the skull with approximately 1 mL of lidocaine. While the patient is supine, Gardner-Wells tongs are placed at the anesthetized sites and the screws are tightened to the appropriate torque.
- The patient is turned, and the pads are adjusted on the modified Jackson table so that the superior pad is three fingerbreadths below the sternal notch, the middle pad is under the anterior superior iliac spine, and the inferior pad is under the midthigh (**FIG 3A**).
- The distal legs are placed in a padded sling, which can be tightened or loosened to affect the amount of lordosis assumed intraoperatively after the posterior elements have been released (**FIG 3B**).
- Once the patient is properly positioned, weight is attached to the Gardner-Wells tongs (**FIG 3C**).

**A**

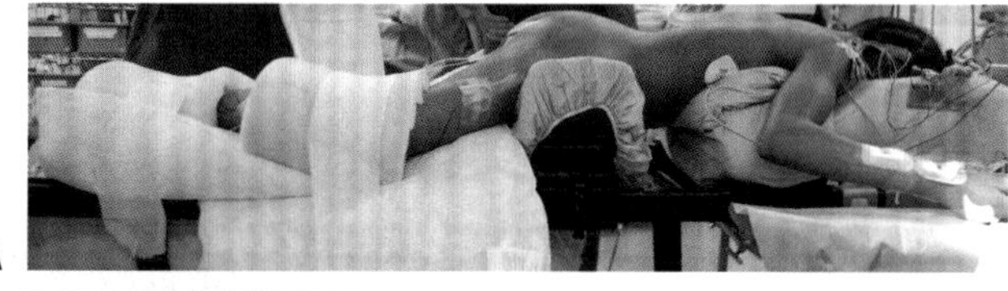

**B**

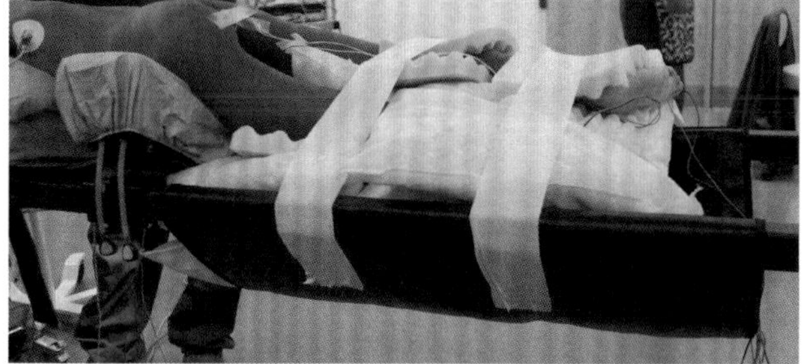

**C**

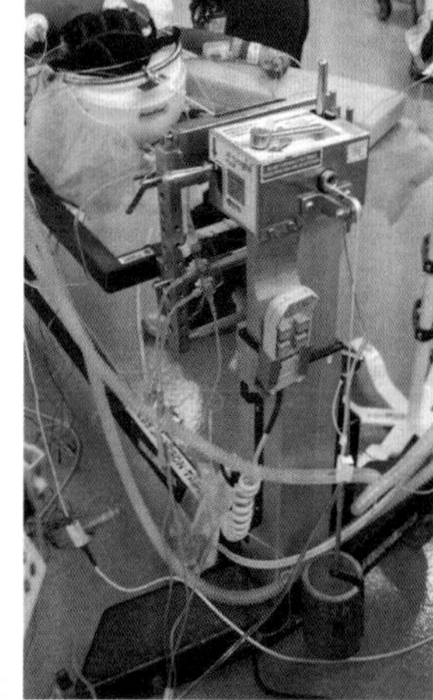

**FIG 3** • Positioning the patient for surgery. **A.** When positioning the patient on the modified Jackson table, the clinician should place the superior pad three fingerbreadths below the sternal notch, the middle pad under the anterior superior iliac spine, and the inferior pad under the midthigh (not pictured). **B.** The patient's legs can be placed in a padded sling, which can be tightened or loosened to affect the amount of lordosis assumed intraoperatively after the posterior elements have been released. **C.** Once the patient is turned to the prone position, the desired amount of weight is added to the rope attached to the Gardner-Wells tongs.

## Approach

- The approach is performed by standard technique with a midline incision down to the spinous processes, with subperiosteal dissection.
- When exposing the sacrum, it is often helpful to place a bend in the electrocautery to assist in removing the soft tissues from the sacral surface. The clinician should be alert for spina bifida occulta in the sacrum, which occurs in up to 12.4% of the population.[10]
- Before any pedicle screws are placed, it is important to decide whether correction of the patient's deformity will be made from distal to proximal or from proximal to distal. The senior author prefers to correct from distal to proximal; however, the other approach is used if the patient has substantial proximal thoracic kyphosis or focal proximal thoracic scoliosis.



## Placement of S1 Screws

- Once the sacrum is exposed, a distractor is placed between the spinous processes of L5 and S1. If it is truly at the correct level, the sacrum will move as one complete unit during gentle distraction.
- The start point for the S1 screw is at the base of the superior articular process of S1 (**TECH FIG 1A**).
- The path is initially made with a starting awl and then widened with a dilator or tapped. The trajectory should be angled 25 degrees medially and toward the sacral promontory, which has been shown to increase insertional torque by up to 99%.[13] The ideal position for the tip of the screw is in the cortical bone at the acute angle of the anterior sacrum with its endplate. The screw at this level is typically 7 to 8 mm in diameter (**TECH FIG 1B**).
- Finally, the S1 pedicle screw is inserted and the head is turned until the opening for the rod is in line with the future position of the rod (**TECH FIG 1C**).

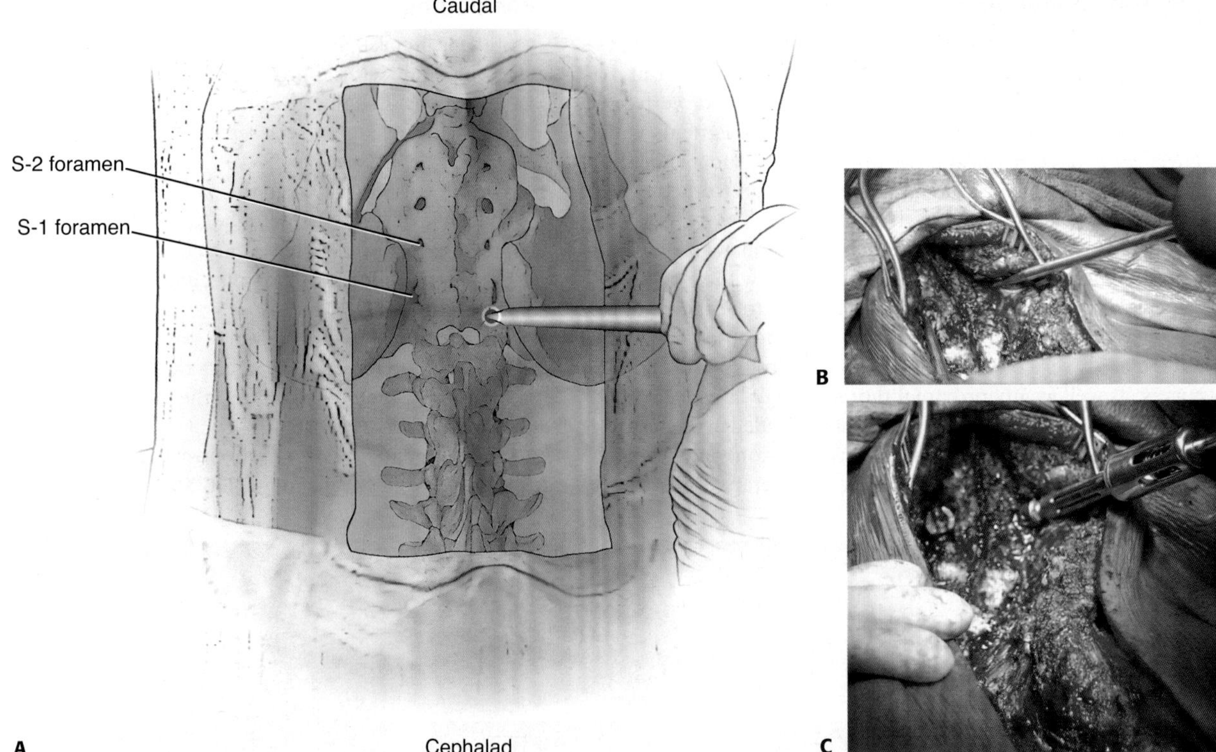


**TECH FIG 1** • Technique for placement of S1 screw. **A.** The start point for the S1 screw (*red dot*) is at the base of the superior articular process of S1. **B.** With a start point at the base of the superior articular process of S1, a starting awl is used to create the screw pathway, aiming 25 degrees medially and toward the sacral promontory. **C.** Final position of S1 screws.

## Placement of Sacral Alar Iliac Screws

- The typical start point for the SAI screw is 25 mm inferior to the S1 endplate and 22 mm lateral from the midpoint of the S2 body (**TECH FIG 2A**).
- With the starting awl and a trajectory angled 40 degrees laterally and 40 degrees caudally, the desired screw pathway is created (**TECH FIG 2B**).
- Mild resistance will be felt crossing the sacroiliac joint with the awl. If too much resistance is felt after passing the sacroiliac joint, it is from the lateral table of the ilium. If this occurs, the awl should be backed out and the trajectory should be made more vertical to avoid hitting the lateral wall.
- Fluoroscopy is used to confirm that the awl is in the desired position in the ilium. The awl should cross the sacroiliac joint and the ilium just cranial to the sciatic notch (**TECH FIG 2C**).

- A depth gauge is used to measure the length of the screw pathway. The senior author prefers to place screws 90 mm in length, with diameters of 8, 9, or 10 mm. Doing so allows the pelvis to be manipulated when correcting pelvic obliquity, even in the presence of osteoporosis.
- A guidewire is inserted, and fluoroscopy is used to confirm it is still in the desired screw trajectory (**TECH FIG 2D,E**).
- The screw is inserted over the guidewire, and another fluoroscopic image is obtained to confirm that the guidewire is not bending (**TECH FIG 2F,G**). Before the screw is advanced completely, a sternal needle driver is used to partially pull out the guidewire.
- The SAI screw should be advanced until the top of the screw is at the same height as, and in line with, the S1 and L5 pedicle screws.

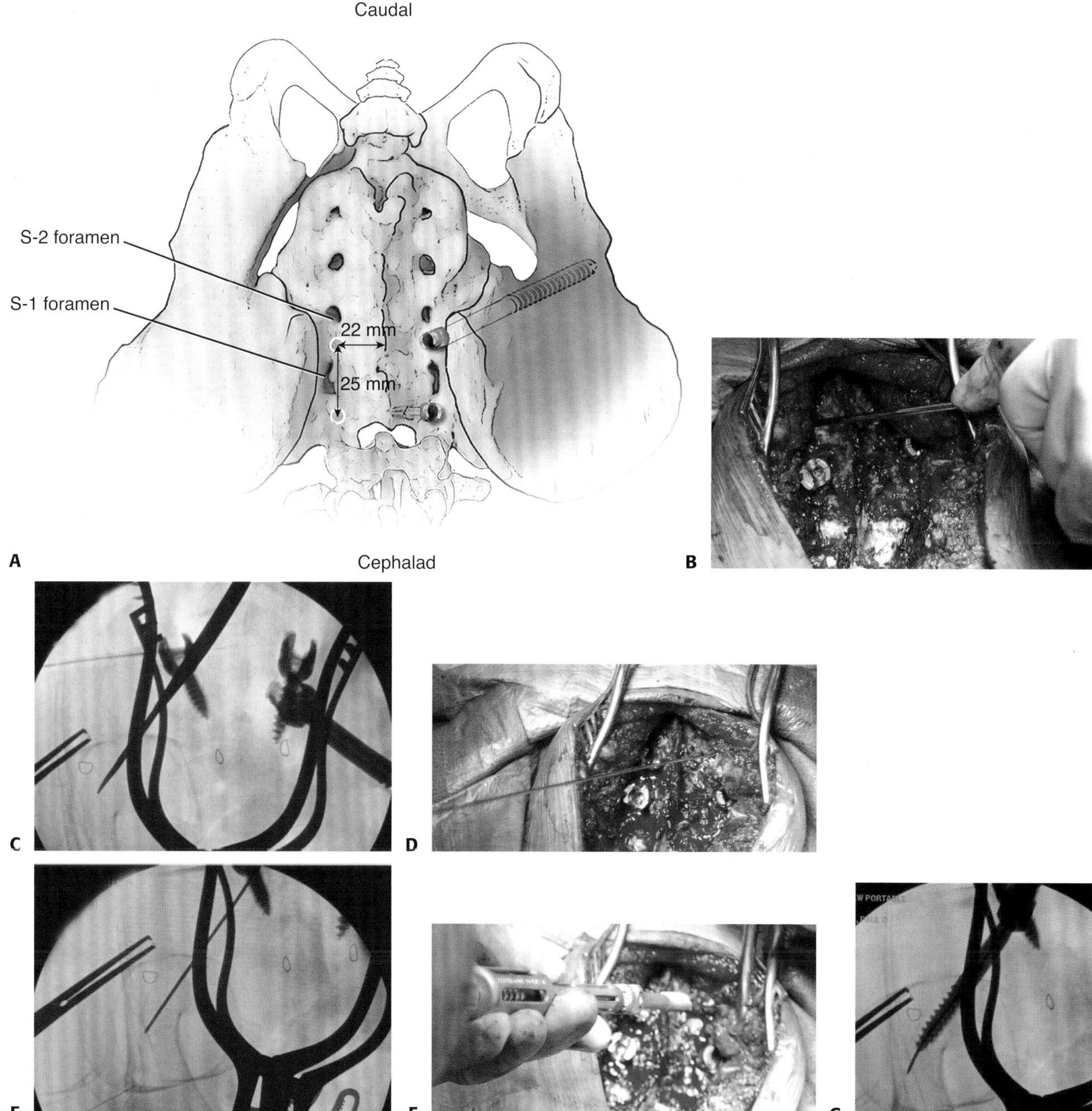


**TECH FIG 2** • Technique for placement of SAI. **A.** The start point for the SAI screw (*red dot*) is 25 mm inferior to the S1 endplate and 22 mm lateral from the midpoint of the S2 body. **B.** The starting awl is used to create the desired screw pathway with a trajectory angled 40 degrees laterally and 40 degrees caudally. **C.** The desired trajectory is confirmed while advancing the starting awl under fluoroscopy. **D.** The guidewire is inserted and impacted into the anterolateral bone of the SAI screw pathway. **E.** It is confirmed under fluoroscopy that the guidewire is still in the desired trajectory. **F.** The SAI screw is inserted over the guidewire and advanced into the sacrum and ilium. **G.** It is confirmed fluoroscopically that the guidewire is not bending while the SAI screw is advanced.

## Confirmation of Sacral Alar Iliac Screw Position

- With time and repetition, it is possible to know by tactile feel alone that the SAI screw is within the column of bone in the ilium.
- If radiographic confirmation is desired, the C-arm should be positioned for a "teardrop view."
  - The C-arm is advanced 30 degrees over the top of the patient.
  - Then, the radiology technician lowers the top of the C-arm 30 degrees closer to the patient's body (**TECH FIG 3**).

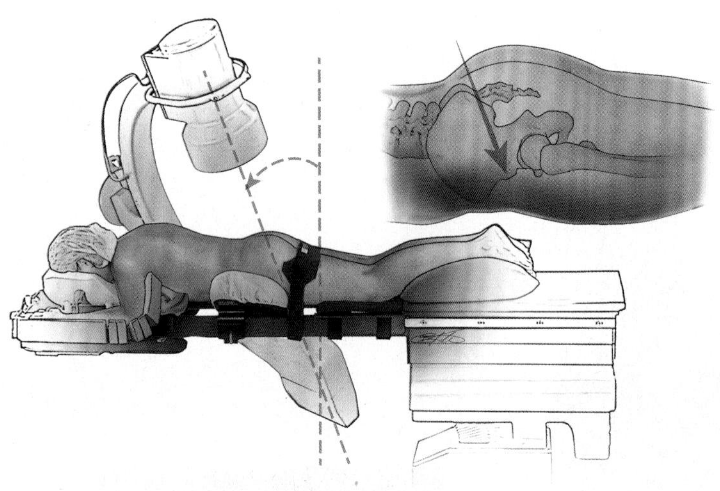

**TECH FIG 3** • A teardrop view is obtained to confirm the placement of the SAI screw by advancing the C-arm 30 degrees over the top of the patient so that it is colinear with the head of the SAI screw. Then the top of the C-arm is lowered 30 degrees closer to the patient's body.

## Correction of Pelvic Obliquity

- The length of the instrumented spine is measured, and the rods are cut accordingly.
- At least 2 cm of the rod must extend distally below the SAI screw to allow space for any distraction or compression required.
- A T-square instrument is placed on top of the spine with the horizontal arms parallel to the superior dome of the acetabulum bilaterally and the vertical arm in line with the center sacral vertebral line (**TECH FIG 4A**). If adequate balance has been achieved, the top of the T-square instrument will cross the vertebral body of T1.[2]
- If pelvic obliquity is present, the top of the T-square instrument will not cross the T1 vertebral body. Confirmation that the T-square is sitting in the appropriate position should be obtained fluoroscopically.
- Once there is fluoroscopic confirmation of the direction in which the pelvis is guiding the spine, the concavity should be distracted or the convexity should be compressed directly off of the SAI screws to obtain a full correction. Additional options are to distract, compress, or contour the spine in situ.
- After correction, the clinician should recheck that the spine is balanced over the pelvis with the T-square instrument.

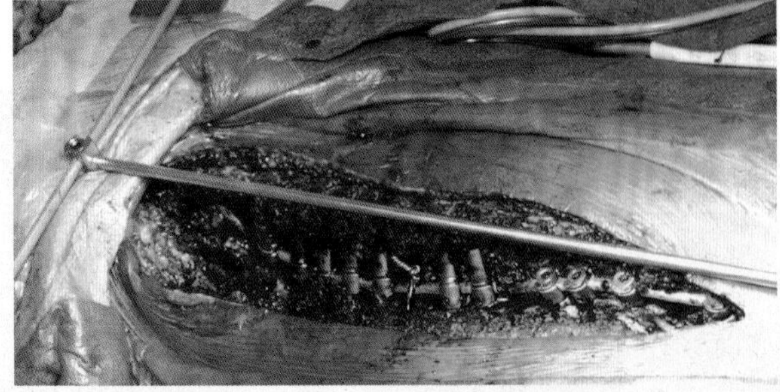

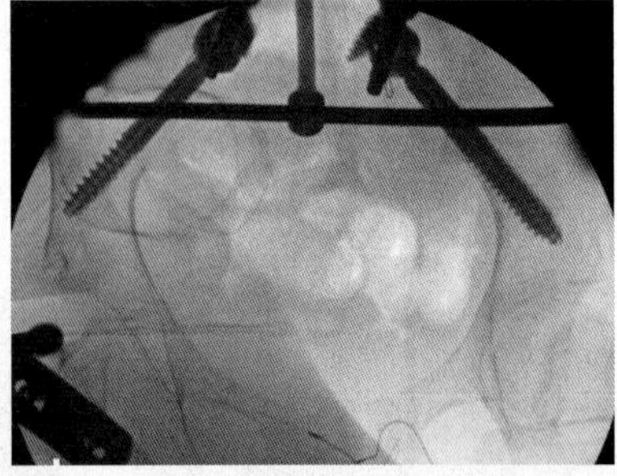

**TECH FIG 4** • **A.** A T-squared instrument is placed with the horizontal arms parallel with the pelvis and the vertical arm in line with the assumed central sacral vertebral line. **B.** It is confirmed with fluoroscopy that that horizontal arms of the T-squared instrument are parallel with the superior dome of the acetabulum. Then the C-arm is moved to the top of the spine and, if the deformity has been adequately corrected, the top of the T-squared instrument will cross the vertebral body of T1.

TECHNIQUES

## Working Around a Baclofen Pump

- Many patients with NMS have increased muscular tone that requires baclofen pumps to keep them functional. It is important to work around these pumps while still achieving the desired correction of the deformity.
- Preoperative evaluation should note on which side the baclofen pump is located.
- Once dissection reaches the spinous processes, subperiosteal dissection of the soft tissues should be started on the side with the baclofen pump.
- Once the baclofen pump catheter is identified, it can be followed superficially to release it from the surrounding soft tissues. The goal is to get enough slack in the catheter to safely place the pedicle screws and slide the rod underneath it (**TECH FIG 5**).

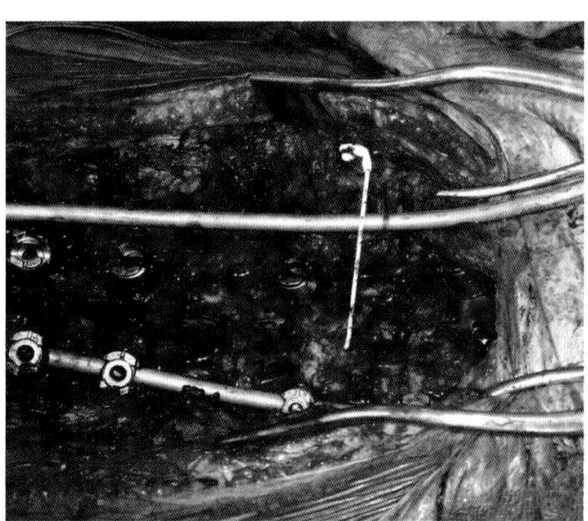

**TECH FIG 5** • The baclofen pump is isolated as it exits the spine then dissected from the surrounding tissues to allow insertion of the pedicle screws and corresponding rods.

## PEARLS AND PITFALLS

| | |
|---|---|
| **Approach** | ■ Patients with NMS with long fusion constructs are at risk for proximal junctional kyphosis. Attempts should be made to avoid this complication by not disrupting the soft tissue attachments of the most cephalad instrumented levels. |
| **Choosing levels to instrument** | ■ The L5 level in patients with NMS is often difficult to instrument secondary to the severe curves and dysplastic pedicles in this patient population.<br>■ In such cases, it is the senior author's preference to instrument the L4, S1, and S2 levels.<br>■ S1 screws are much more useful in osteoporotic bone where more points of fixation are needed caudally. They should engage the "tricortical portion" of the sacrum. |
| **Placement of SAI screws** | ■ When cutting the rod, the clinician should leave 2 cm of rod distal to the SAI screw to allow for any subsequent distraction or compression.<br>■ When advancing the SAI screw over the guidewire, the clinician should fluoroscopically check that the wire is not bending as the screw head begins to seat into sacrum.<br>■ Marked resistance is felt while advancing the SAI screw usually indicates that the screw is hitting the lateral cortex of the ilium. The screw should be reversed and the trajectory made more vertical and less oblique.<br>■ The SAI screw should be torqued before any correction of pelvic obliquity is attempted. |
| **Fusion** | ■ While decorticating the spine to ensure a fusion, it is important to decorticate the area where the sacral ala meets the ilium.<br>■ Our practice is to partially release the muscle from the undersurface of the iliac tuberosity, which relaxes the posterior paraspinous muscle and eases the closure. It also allows for fusion mass to bridge to the ilium as well as the sacrum, strengthening the fusion at the level of the SAI screw. |
| **Postoperative imaging** | ■ It is rare to see mild lucency around the SAI screws. However, if present, it does not necessarily indicate loosening and as of yet does not have clinical significance. |

## POSTOPERATIVE CARE

- When the patient is extubated and alert, the neurologic examination is repeated to make sure there has been no worsening from preoperative evaluation levels.
- Packed red blood cells are transfused as necessary; our threshold for transfusion is a hemoglobin less than 7 g/dL.
- If the patient is nonambulatory, we obtain supine scoliosis radiographs once the patient is transferred to the floor.
- Dressings are changed on the second postoperative day and then as needed thereafter.

## OUTCOMES

- In one study, the 2-year outcomes of patients with NMS who underwent spinal fusion with SAI pelvic fixation were compared with those of control patients who underwent spinal fusion with pelvic fixation involving sacral and iliac screws through a PSIS insertion.[23]

- There was no statistically significant difference in correction of Cobb angle between the SAI and control groups.
- There was a greater improvement of pelvic obliquity in the SAI than in the control group.
- Patients in the SAI group experienced no episodes of deep surgical site infections, whereas the control group had three cases.
- In the SAI group, there were no cases of screw prominence, late skin breakdown, or anchor migration.

- To date, more than 200 patients have undergone pelvic fixation with SAI screws at our institution, and there is a trend overall to less skin breakdown secondary to screw prominence, less cases of screw backout, and less cases of deep surgical site infection as compared with patients with iliosacral screws and other forms of pelvic fixation.[23]

## COMPLICATIONS

- It has been estimated that the risk of surgical site infection is between 3.7% and 8.5% in patients with NMS.[15]
- At our institution, numerous steps are taken to prevent infection.
  - After the spine has been fully instrumented, povidone-iodine is poured into the incision and is allowed to sit for 20 seconds (**FIG 4A**).
  - Before the incision is finally closed, vancomycin powder is sprinkled onto the hardware and the surrounding soft tissues (**FIG 4B**).
  - If allograft is used, it is soaked in gentamicin.[5]
  - A one-quarter–inch Hemovac drain (Zimmer, Warsaw, IN) is usually placed on straight drain to prevent pooling of blood.
  - The incision is closed with interrupted figure-of-eight sutures to ensure a watertight closure.
- Because of the changed body alignment, the clinician should watch for pressure concentration in the ischium or coccyx when the patient first sits.

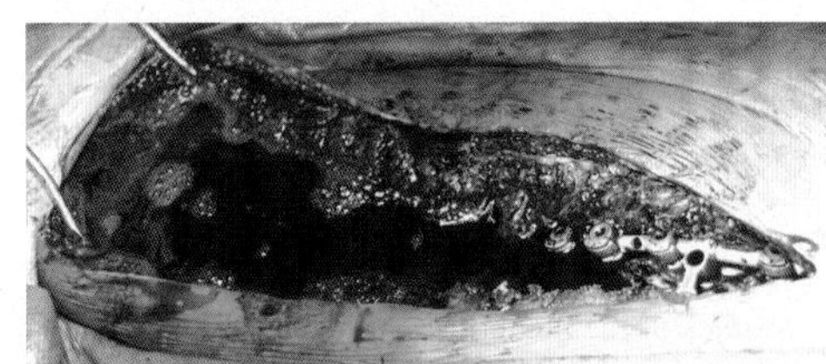

A

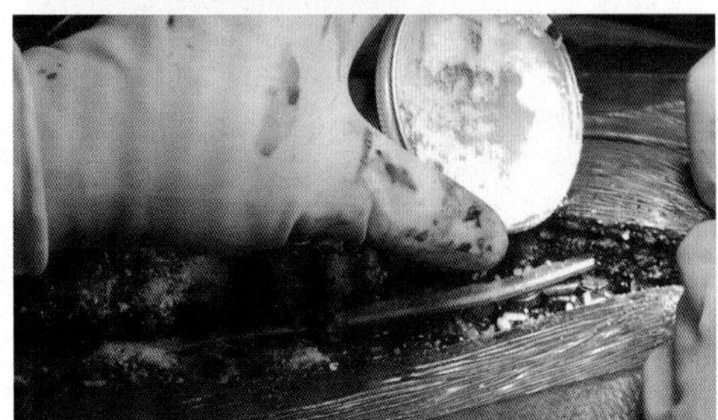

B

**FIG 4** ● **A.** In addition to standard measures, a povidone-iodine solution is poured into the incision as prophylaxis against deep surgical site infection. **B.** Vancomycin powder is poured into the surgical site as prophylaxis against surgical site infection.

## REFERENCES


1. Allen BL Jr, Ferguson RL. The Galveston experience with L-rod instrumentation for adolescent idiopathic scoliosis. Clin Orthop Relat Res 1988;(229):59–69.
2. Andras L, Yamaguchi KT Jr, Skaggs DL, et al. Surgical technique for balancing posterior spinal fusions to the pelvis using the T square of Tolo. J Pediatr Orthop 2012;32:e63–e66.
3. Bell DF, Moseley CF, Koreska J. Unit rod segmental spinal instrumentation in the management of patients with progressive neuromuscular spinal deformity. Spine 1989;14:1301–1307.
4. Berven S, Bradford DS. Neuromuscular scoliosis: causes of deformity and principles for evaluation and management. Semin Neurol 2002;22:167–178.
5. Borkhuu B, Borowski A, Shah SA, et al. Antibiotic-loaded allograft decreases the rate of acute deep wound infection after spinal fusion in cerebral palsy. Spine 2008;33:2300–2304.
6. Bradford DS. Neuromuscular spinal deformity. In: Bradford DS, Lonstein JE, Moe JH, et al, eds. Moe's Textbook of Scoliosis and Other Spinal Deformities, ed 2. Philadelphia: WB Saunders, 1987:271.
7. Chang TL, Sponseller PD, Kebaish KM, et al. Low profile pelvic fixation: anatomic parameters for sacral alar-iliac fixation versus traditional iliac fixation. Spine 2009;34:436–440.
8. Cotrel Y, Dubousset J. A new technic for segmental spinal osteosynthesis using the posterior approach [article in French]. Rev Chir Orthop Reparatrice Appar Mot 1984;70:489–494.
9. Driscoll SW, Skinner J. Musculoskeletal complications of neuromuscular disease in children. Phys Med Rehabil Clin North Am 2008;19:163–194.
10. Eubanks JD, Cheruvu VK. Prevalence of sacral spina bifida occulta and its relationship to age, sex, race, and the sacral table angle: an anatomic, osteologic study of three thousand one hundred specimens. Spine 2009;34:1539–1543.
11. Farcy JP, Rawlins BA, Glassman SD. Technique and results of fixation to the sacrum with iliosacral screws. Spine 1992;17(6 suppl):S190–S195.
12. Ko PS, Jameson PG II, Chang TL, et al. Transverse-plane pelvic asymmetry in patients with cerebral palsy and scoliosis. J Pediatr Orthop 2011;31:277–283.
13. Lehman RA Jr, Kuklo TR, Belmont PJ Jr, et al. Advantage of pedicle screw fixation directed into the apex of the sacral promontory over bicortical fixation: a biomechanical analysis. Spine 2002;27:806–811.
14. Luque ER. The anatomic basis and development of segmental spinal instrumentation. Spine 1982;7:256–259.
15. Mackenzie WGS, Matsumoto H, Williams BA, et al. Surgical site infection following spinal instrumentation for scoliosis: a multicenter analysis of rates, risk factors, and pathogens. J Bone Joint Surg Am 2013;95:800–806.
16. McCarthy RE. Management of neuromuscular scoliosis. Orthop Clin North Am 1999;30:435–449.
17. McCord DH, Cunningham BW, Shono Y, et al. Biomechanical analysis of lumbosacral fixation. Spine 1992;17:S235–S243.
18. Modi HN, Suh SW, Song HR, et al. Evaluation of pelvic fixation in neuromuscular scoliosis: a retrospective study in 55 patients. Int Orthop 2010;34:89–96.
19. Newton PO, Bastrom TP, Emans JB, et al. Antifibrinolytic agents reduce blood loss during pediatric vertebral column resection procedures. Spine 2012;37:E1459–E1463.
20. Obid P, Bevot A, Goll A, et al. Quality of life after surgery for neuromuscular scoliosis. Orthop Rev (Pavia) 2013:5:e1.
21. O'Brien JR, Yu WD, Bhatnagar R, et al. An anatomic study of the S2 iliac technique for lumbopelvic screw placement. Spine (Phila Pa 1976) 2009;34:E439–E442.
22. Olafsson Y, Saraste H, Al-Dabbagh Z. Brace treatment in neuromuscular spine deformity. J Pediatr Orthop 1999;19:376–379.
23. Sponseller PD, Zimmerman RM, Ko PS, et al. Low profile pelvic fixation with the sacral alar iliac technique in the pediatric population improves results at two-year minimum follow-up. Spine 2010;35:1887–1892.
24. Watanabe K, Lenke LG, Daubs MD, et al. Is spine deformity surgery in patients with spastic cerebral palsy truly beneficial?: a patient/parent evaluation. Spine 2009;34:2222–2232.

# Casting for Early-Onset Scoliosis

James O. Sanders

92

CHAPTER

## DEFINITION

- Early-onset scoliosis is defined as scoliosis occurring by age 5 years. The term was developed because it is more likely associated with long-term pulmonary compromise than in children with later onset scoliosis.[2,16]
- Infantile scoliosis is another term referring to scoliosis detected by age 3 years. It usually refers to idiopathic scoliosis unlike "early-onset scoliosis" which can include congenital and neuromuscular curves. Occasionally, the term *infantile scoliosis* will include syndromic children because of the difficulty in identifying many syndromes in young children. Practically, infantile and early-onset scoliosis are often used synonymously.

## ANATOMY

- Infantile scoliosis is a deformity of the discs, vertebral bodies, and the chest wall. The ribs articulate with the vertebra at both the transverse processes (costotransverse joints) and the vertebral bodies (costovertebral joints).
- The spine is usually rotated about the longitudinal axis with the lateral convex side more posterior than the concave side (**FIG 1**).

## PATHOGENESIS

- The pathogenesis of idiopathic or most syndromic early-onset scoliosis is unknown. Early-onset scoliosis may have an underlying neurologic or muscular abnormality.

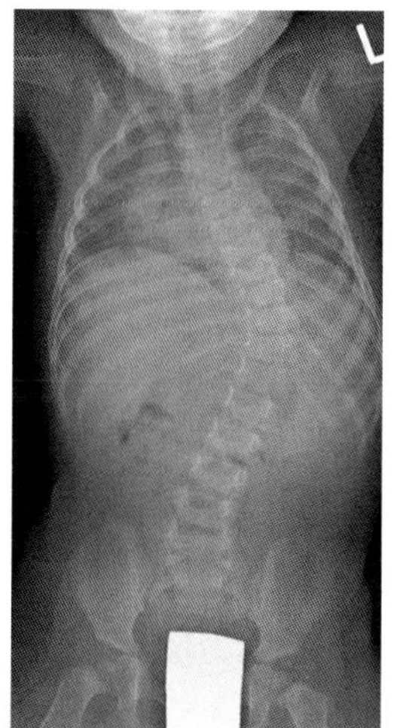


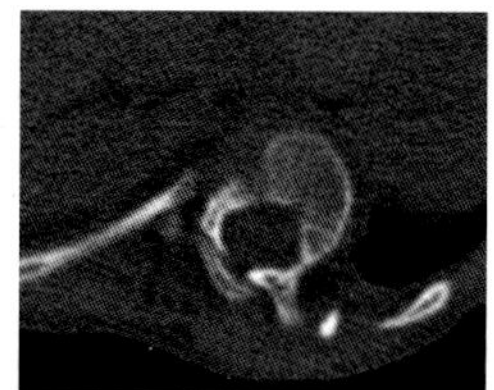

**FIG 1** • **A.** An AP radiograph of a 12-month-old child with a typical left lower thoracic infantile scoliosis. **B.** A computed tomography (CT) scan at the apex of an infantile scoliosis showing the rotation with the anterior spine rotated toward the concavity and the posterior spine toward the convexity.

## NATURAL HISTORY

- Infantile curves may be either resolving or progressive with resolving curves being far more common.
- Scoliosis presenting during the first year of life has a greater likelihood of resolving spontaneously, whereas curves developing after 1 year of age have a worse prognosis.[12,13]
- Both the rib–vertebral angle difference (RVAD) and rib phase are important for predicting which curves will progress[15] (**FIG 2**).
  - The RVAD is the difference of the angles made between each rib and the corresponding vertebral body. This is measured at the vertebral level with the greatest angular difference between the concave and convex rib.
  - Rib phase is classified as phase 1 or 2, depending on whether or not spinal rotation causes the rib head to overlap the vertebral body (phase 1, no overlap; phase 2, overlap).
  - Eighty-three percent of resolving curves have a RVAD of less than 20 degrees and 83% of progressing curves have a RVAD of greater than 20 degrees.
  - In progressive curves, the RVAD increases and the phase gradually transitions from 1 to 2.
  - Phase 2 ribs are the hallmark of progressive curves, as all phase 2 curves progress.
  - Double curves present a special problem as most of them progress.
- The RVAD in double curves may be quite low, but an oblique 11th or 12th convex rib with lumbar rotation is a poor prognostic sign.
- Generally, the RVAD and phase are reliable, but the measurement error may make discernment difficult in marginal cases,[4] in which case, close observation, typically with repeat radiographs in 3 months, is the best course.
- Left untreated, the prognosis for curves that do progress is invariably poor: By age 5 years, 57% of untreated children

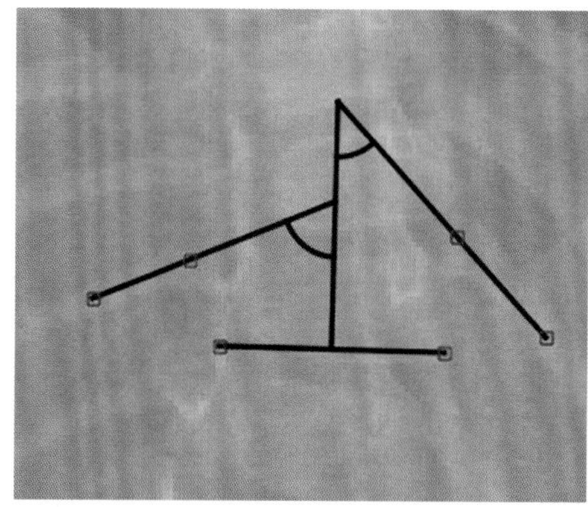

**FIG 2** • The RVAD from the same child shown in **FIG 1A**.

will have a curve greater than 70 degrees.[15] These large thoracic curves can cause restrictive lung disease or thoracic insufficiency syndrome (TIS) characterized by decreased thoracic growth and lung volume, inhibiting alveolar development and lung function, which may cause respiratory failure and death at an early age.[7] The thoracic deformity can also lead to pulmonary hypertension and cor pulmonale, with respiratory failure and death occurring at a later age.[3,10,15,18] Curves of greater than 70 degrees are sufficient to cause cor pulmonale and have a higher mortality rate than smaller curves.[10,16]

- Patients with progressive curves progress by about 5 degrees per year reaching 70 degrees or more by age 10 years.[9,17] Thoracic curves greater than 70 degrees in adolescence are associated with significantly lower forced expiratory volume in 1 second (FEV1) and forced vital capacity (FVC) values compared to patients with smaller deformities.
- EOS patients have greater pulmonary function test (PFT) impairment than adolescent idiopathic scoliosis patients.[11]

## PATIENT HISTORY AND PHYSICAL FINDINGS

- Typically, parents have noticed the deformity before their physicians. It is important to ask about a family history of nerve or muscle disorders. Unlike adolescent scoliosis, early-onset scoliosis is not often familial except in neuromuscular disorders. Because young children cannot cooperate with a manual motor examination or an Adams forward bend test, one must rely on close observation to identify the curve and any evidence of neurologic issues or myopathies.
- The neurologic examination should include an assessment of gait, upper and lower extremity motor strength where feasible, tone, deep tendon reflexes including abdominal reflexes, clonus, Hoffman, and Babinski signs. Foot deformities, particularly any equinus, cavus, varus, or foot size difference may be the only neurologic signs seen.
- Common syndromes associated with early-onset scoliosis include Marfan syndrome, characterized by arachnodactyly (**FIG 3**) and often having more severe aortic involvement in young children, and Ehlers-Danlos syndrome, characterized by marked ligamentous laxity.

## IMAGING AND OTHER DIAGNOSTIC STUDIES

- The diagnosis of infantile scoliosis is made on plain anteroposterior (AP) or posteroanterior (PA) and lateral radiographs of the spine. In infants and young children who cannot stand, the radiographs are obtained supine. Once children can stand reliably, they are obtained in a standing position.
- Congenital vertebral anomalies such as unpaired pedicles, rib anomalies, and spina bifida are identified on plain radiographs. Because the spine is not fully ossified, the posterior elements may not be fully visualized on the AP view at a young age.
- Disorders such as syringomyelia and Arnold-Chiari are sufficiently common that they should be sought with a spinal magnetic resonance imaging (MRI).[6,8]

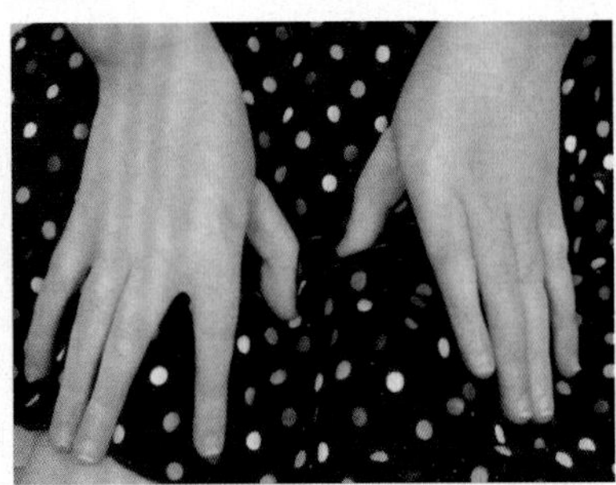

**FIG 3** • Arachnodactyly in a 2-year-old child with infantile scoliosis and Marfan syndrome.

## DIFFERENTIAL DIAGNOSIS

- Idiopathic scoliosis
- Syndromic scoliosis particularly Marfan syndrome, Prader-Willi, and Ehlers-Danlos
- Congenital scoliosis
- Spinal cord anomalies, particularly tethered cord, syringomyelia, and Arnold-Chiari
- Myopathies and neuropathies such as congenital myopathies and spinal muscular atrophy
- Cerebral palsy

## NONOPERATIVE MANAGEMENT

- Bracing is the most common nonoperative treatment of early-onset scoliosis with variable success.[1] Bracing is an important adjunctive treatment in cast treatment for early-onset scoliosis and plays an important role in delaying the need for surgery. Braces are difficult to fit in young patients. Young children have more pliable ribs than adolescents, and braces using a three-point bend on the apical rib can create a chest wall deformation by pushing the ribs toward the spine. Bracing may be difficult to properly apply each time to a young child's cylindrical shape. This is compounded by the need to make the brace sufficiently flexible for donning and doffing.

## SURGICAL MANAGEMENT

- Casting works best in younger patients with idiopathic smaller curves, but it can still help in older patients, those with larger curves, and syndromic curves. Be wary of neuromuscular and congenital curves.
- Because of the problem with diminishing returns in growing instrumentation, if casting does not cure the curve, it will, ideally, delay growing rod surgery until at least age 6 or 7 years.
- Begin casting when the child is diagnosed with progressive infantile scoliosis, is safe for anesthesia, and the goals are either cure or delay surgery.
- The family must agree to minimum 1 year of casting and understand that even if the curve is not cured, delay for surgery is important.

### Preoperative Planning

- Because the derotation must be applied to each curve at its apex, it is important to review the patient's radiographs, determine the apices of each curve, and have a plan to properly rotate the spine stabilized against the pelvis and either the right or left pectoral region.

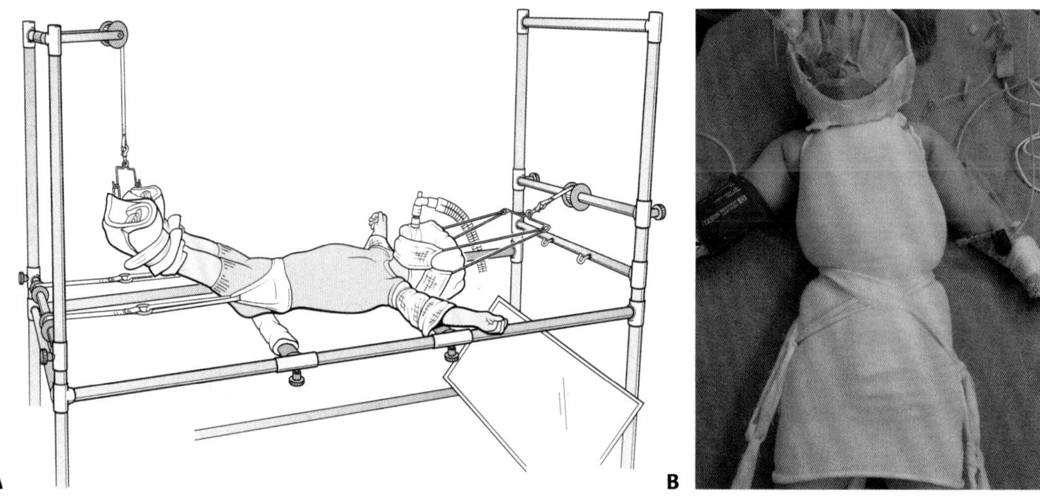

FIG 4 ● **A.** The child is intubated and prepared on the Mehta casting table with head halter–pelvic traction. **B.** Covering over the face and mouth, Boston brace shirt, abdominal pad, head halter, and pelvic straps are applied before positioning on the casting frame. (**A:** From Sanders JO, D'Astous J, Fitzgerald M, et al. Derotational casting for progressive infantile scoliosis. J Pediatr Orthop 2009;29:581–587.)

## Positioning

- A proper table that allows secure positioning of the patient with head and pelvic traction, as well as full access to the torso, shoulder girdle, and pelvis, is required.
  - Although it is possible to cast with either Risser or a Cotrel adult-sized frame, they are quite large for small children and are now rarely available.
  - A mirror slanted under the table is useful for visualizing the rib prominence, the posterior cast, and the molds.
  - We use a table designed for young children by Min Mehta, which supports the head, arms, and legs while the shoulders, torso, and pelvis remain free (**FIG 4A**).
  - Salt Lake City Shriners Hospital designed a custom table, which performs a similar function of supporting the child in traction while leaving the body free for the cast application.
- Patients are intubated rather than using a laryngeal mask airway (LMA) because thoracic pressure during the cast molding can make ventilation temporarily difficult. A bite block prevents teeth from constricting the tube during head halter traction. Cover the head and neck to prevent plaster or fiberglass irritation.
- A silver-impregnated shirt is used as the innermost layer and can either be custom-made or one made for scoliosis bracing such as a Boston brace shirt.
- An abdominal pad made of stockinette prevents excessive abdominal pressure during the casting (**FIG 4B**).

## Approach

- Plaster is preferred for correction because it is highly moldable and expands slightly when setting unlike fiberglass, which shrinks.
- In select patients, typically those with supine curves have been corrected to less than 20 degrees or those who are in casts which are holding rather than obtaining further correction, we use fiberglass with a waterproof liner and waterproof padding allowing the children to bathe and get in a swimming pool. The Gore-Tex pantaloon designed for spica casts works well as a shirt undergarment with the pantaloon legs used as the arms.

# Head Halter–Pelvic Traction

- Head halter–pelvic traction assists in stabilizing the patient and in narrowing the body. Even though traction can correct the curve while applied, the position cannot be retained in the cast once traction is released and the body recoils unless the cast also supports the occiput or the mandible (**TECH FIG 1**).
- If the patient has a lumbar curve, the hips are slightly flexed to decrease lumbar lordosis and facilitate curve correction.

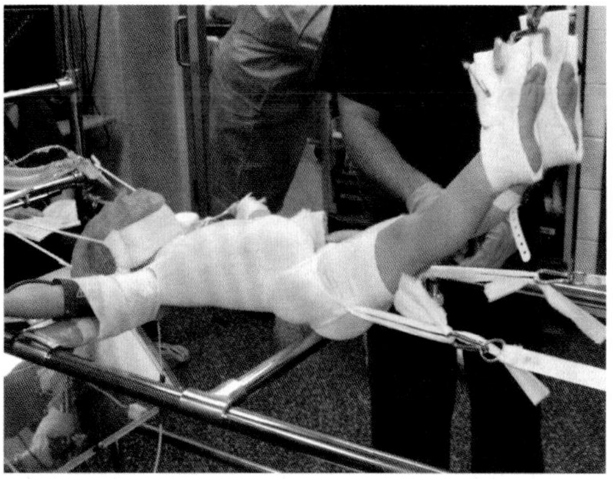

**TECH FIG 1** ● Child positioned on the frame for the casting.

## Padding and Plaster Application

- A thin layer of cotton padding is applied with occasional felt on significant bony prominences such as the iliac crest or rib prominence (**TECH FIG 2A**).
- For curves with an apex above T8, the shoulders are incorporated, and high thoracic curves may require an occipital–mandibular extension.
- It is a well-molded and snug cast rather than more padding that prevents sores as it is less likely to rub and cause pressure sores than an excessively padded, poorly molded, or loose cast.
- As the plaster is applied, it is important to obtain a good mold over the iliac crests, as the pelvis is the foundation of the cast (**TECH FIG 2B**).

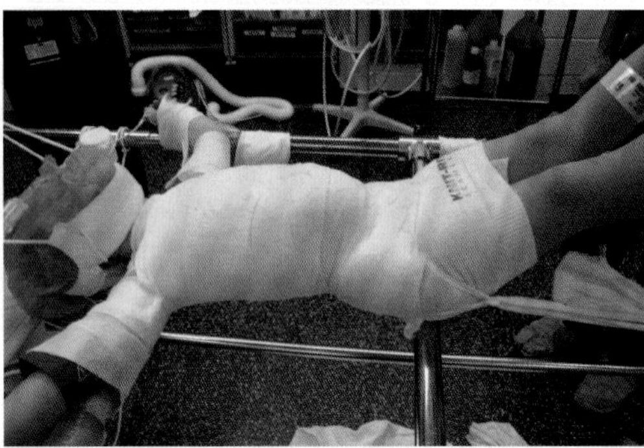

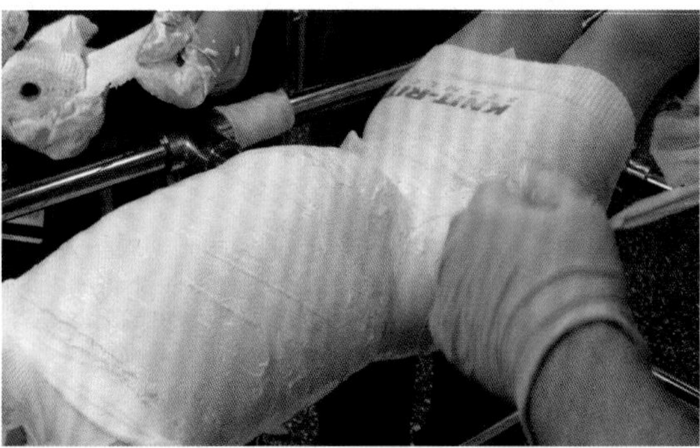

**TECH FIG 2** • **A.** Only a thin layer of padding is applied because it is the mold which prevents sheer and skin breakdown. **B.** The pelvis is molded well just above the iliac crests as the foundation of the cast against which everything else rotates.

## Curve Correction

- Although the Cotrel and Morel[5] elongation-derotation-flexion (EDF) technique and Mehta[14] both use an over-the-shoulder cast, we have had excellent success staying below the shoulders because most infantile curves have low apices, typically at T10–T11 with results nearly identical to Mehta's.
- For a typical left thoracic curve, the pelvis is carefully molded and stabilized while the left posterior thorax is rotated anteriorly, the right anterior thorax is rotated posteriorly and stabilized against the left pectoral girdle.
  - It is important that the cast does not compress the convex ribs toward the spine and consequently narrow the space available for the lung. Rather, the posteriorly rotated ribs are rotated anteriorly to create a more normal chest configuration with counter rotation applied through the pelvic mold and upper torso (**TECH FIG 3**).
- Proper casting corrects the curve through the rotation and a shift toward the midline without deforming the ribs toward the spine.
  - If the cast is found to be pushing the ribs toward the spine, we recommend it be removed and either reapplied or abandoned.
- We cover the plaster with a layer of fiberglass both for color and strength.

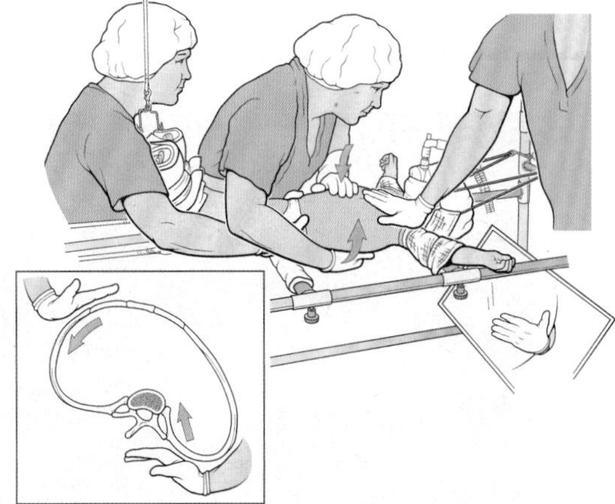

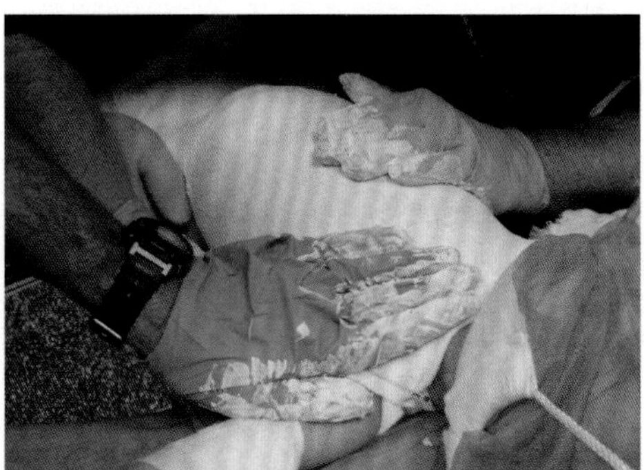

**TECH FIG 3** • **A.** The technique of curve manipulation, which rotates the spine posteriorly and stabilized against both the pectoral girdle and the pelvis. It is important not to displace the ribs laterally into the spine and chest. **B.** Application of the plaster mold. (**A:** From Sanders JO, D'Astous J, Fitzgerald M, et al. Derotational casting for progressive infantile scoliosis. J Pediatr Orthop 2009;29:581–587.)

## Windows, Trim, and Cast Edges

- An anterior window is made to relieve the chest and a large abdominal window created to allow for abdominal distention and breathing because younger children are diaphragmatic (belly) breathers while still preventing the lower ribs from rotating.
  - We have changed over time to larger abdominal windows trimmed to the inferior rib level because the abdomen does not provide additional support and it allows better breathing (**TECH FIG 4A**).
- A posterior window is made on the concave side allowing the depressed concave ribs or transverse processes and spine to move posteriorly (**TECH FIG 4B**).
- For under-the-shoulder casts, the superior trim line is at the manubrium. This is not as important for over-the-shoulder casts as long as the upper thorax is captured.
- The lower trim line should be low enough to hold the pelvis securely while high enough to allow the hips more than 90 degrees flexion.
  - Lower trims prevent hip flexion and cause the cast to ride up when sitting, particularly in car seats that require significant hip flexion.
- Once the child is awakened, the fit should again be assessed as it will shift slightly in an upright position. The child should be comfortable and find it easy to get around afterward (**TECH FIG 4C**).

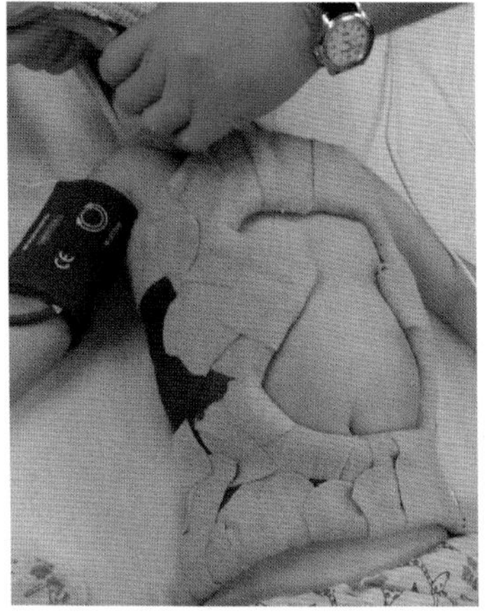
A
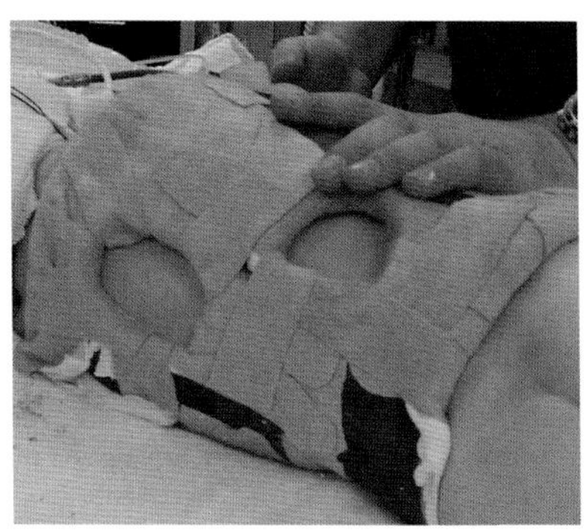
B
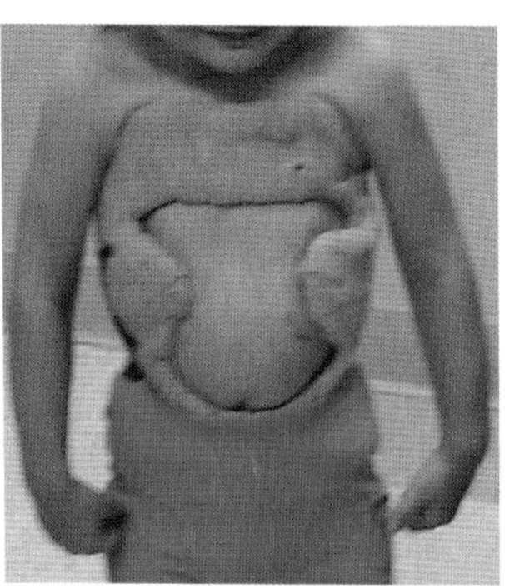
C

**TECH FIG 4** • **A.** The anterior window captures the inferior ribs to keep them from protruding and leaves the abdomen as free as possible. **B.** The posterior windows allow the spine to rotate and help relieve excessive pressure. This particular patient had a double curve. **C.** A well-fitting cast in the patient when upright.

## PEARLS AND PITFALLS

| | |
|---|---|
| **Difficulty ventilating during surgery** | ▪ Make sure the patient is intubated and has a bite block. |
| **Troubles with trims** | ▪ Work with a cast technician who can do any final trimming once the child is awake and up after their body returns to a more normal configuration. |
| **Skin irritation at cast removal** | ▪ Leaving off the cast overnight before recasting makes a big difference. A little light hydrocortisone cream can also help. |
| **Patients sometimes need the cast removed for asthma or other respiratory issues.** | ▪ In patients where this is likely, have a brace made from an intraoperative mold that the child could use if the cast has to be urgently removed. |
| **Parents expect a cure when the curve only decreases or stabilizes.** | ▪ The parents must be educated in what to expect. |
| **Cast sores** | ▪ Use broad distribution of forces during correction and leave no sharp edges. |

## POSTOPERATIVE CARE

- Casting is done more frequently in younger than older children because they are growing faster. We typically change the cast every 2 months for children 2 years and younger, 3 months for those 3 years of age, and every 4 months for those 4 years and older.
- Children are seen the day before cast application where the prior cast is removed and they are allowed to swim and bathe.
- Casting continues until the curve is gone (<10 degrees) or has stabilized. Parents are informed before casting that the casting will continue for a minimum of a year. Radiographs

are not necessary at every visit, as these children will often have large cumulative radiation doses.

- Once the child is placed into a brace, the first brace is molded under anesthesia just like the casts by the surgeon.

## OUTCOMES

- In our patients, we found that 27% of casted patients resolved their scoliosis, 56% improved but did not resolved, 14% remained stable, and 3% progressed during casting.
- Only 10% have had surgery, although this increases to 28% if considering only curves 50 degrees or more at the start of casting.
- Among those who have had surgery, it was delayed by an average 2.7 years after the start of casting.

## COMPLICATIONS

- During casting, the major complications are pulmonary with increased pressures during plaster molding and setting. This is usually relieved once the plaster has set but is the reason intubation is important. The anesthesiologist must often apply positive pressure during the molding and plaster setting.
- Postcasting pressure sores, although rare, are the major complication.
- Many patients experience minor skin irritation which resolves overnight with cast removal.
- Some patients, particularly those with asthma or other pulmonary disease, may require cast removal urgently to provide more chest expansion and access to their thorax.

## REFERENCES


1. Akbarnia BA, Yazici M, Thompson GH. The Growing Spine: Management of Spinal Disorders in Young Children. New York: Springer, 2010.
2. Branthwaite MA. Cardiorespiratory consequences of unfused idiopathic scoliosis. Br J Dis Chest 1986;80(4):360–369.
3. Ceballos T, Ferrer-Torrelles M, Castillo F, et al. Prognosis in infantile idiopathic scoliosis. J Bone Joint Surg Am 1980;62:863–875.
4. Corona J, Sanders JO, Luhmann SJ, et al. Reliability of radiographic measures for infantile idiopathic scoliosis. J Bone Joint Surg Am 2012; 94(12):e86.
5. Cotrel Y, Morel G. The elongation-derotation-flexion technic in the correction of scoliosis [in French]. Rev Chir Orthop Reparatrice Appar Mot 1964;50:59–75.
6. Dobbs MB, Lenke LG, Szymanski DA, et al. Prevalence of neural axis abnormalities in patients with infantile idiopathic scoliosis. J Bone Joint Surg Am 2002;84-A(12):2230–2234.
7. Ferreira JH, de Janeiro R, James JI. Progressive and resolving infantile idiopathic scoliosis. The differential diagnosis. J Bone Joint Surg Br 1972;54(4):648–655.
8. Gupta P, Lenke LG, Bridwell KH. Incidence of neural axis abnormalities in infantile and juvenile patients with spinal deformity. Is a magnetic resonance image screening necessary? Spine 1988;23(2):206–210.
9. James JI. Idiopathic scoliosis. The prognosis, diagnosis, and operative indications related to curve patterns at the age of onset. J Bone Joint Surg Br 1954;36-B(1):36–49.
10. James JI. The management of infants with scoliosis. J Bone Joint Surg Br 1975;57(4):422–429.
11. Johnston CE, Richards BS, Sucato DJ, et al. Correlation of preoperative deformity magnitude and pulmonary function tests in adolescent idiopathic scoliosis. Spine 2011;36(14):1096–1102.
12. Lloyd-Roberts GC, Pilcher MF. Structural idiopathic scoliosis in infancy: a study of the natural history of 100 patients. J Bone Joint Surg Br 1965;47:520–523.
13. McMaster MJ. Infantile idiopathic scoliosis: can it be prevented? J Bone Joint Surg Br 1983;65(5):612–617.
14. Mehta MH. Growth as a corrective force in the early treatment of progressive infantile scoliosis. J Bone Joint Surg Br 2005;87(9): 1237–1247.
15. Mehta MH. The rib-vertebra angle in the early diagnosis between resolving and progressive infantile scoliosis. J Bone Joint Surg Br 1972; 54(2):230–243.
16. Pehrsson K, Larsson S, Oden A, et al. Long-term follow-up of patients with untreated scoliosis. A study of mortality, causes of death, and symptoms. Spine 1992;17(9):1091–1096.
17. Scott JC, Morgan TH. The natural history and prognosis of infantile idiopathic scoliosis. J Bone Joint Surg Br 1955;37-B(3):400–413.
18. Thompson SK, Bentley G. Prognosis in infantile idiopathic scoliosis. J Bone Joint Surg Br 1980;62-B(2):151–154.

# Growing Rod Instrumentation for Early-Onset Scoliosis

CHAPTER 93

Christine M. Goodbody and John M. Flynn

## DEFINITION

- Early-onset scoliosis (EOS) is defined by the diagnosis of scoliosis at or before the age of 5 years.
- The many etiologies of EOS include the following:
  - Congenital vertebral or spinal anomalies: for example, vertebral bars, hemivertebrae
  - Neuromuscular diseases: for example, cerebral palsy, spinal dysraphism, muscular dystrophy
  - Syndromes associated with scoliosis: for example, neurofibromatosis
  - Idiopathic causes
- Progressive and severe curves can be associated with deformity, thoracic insufficiency, restrictive pulmonary disease, pulmonary hypertension, cardiac disease, and increased mortality.

## ANATOMY

- Two periods of increased growth velocity are associated with increased incidence of curve progression. T1 to S1 growth velocity is greatest from birth until the age of 5 years (more than 2 cm per year), and by the age of 5 years, two-thirds of the final sitting height is achieved. Growth rate slows between ages 5 and 10 years (1 cm per year) before increasing again during puberty and the adolescent growth spurt (1 to 2 cm per year).[5,14]
- The increased spinal growth during the first years of life is paralleled by an increase in thoracic and lung dimensions. Thoracic volume at birth is about 5% of the adult volume; by 5 years of age, it equals 30% of adult volume. A slower rate of thoracic growth occurs from 5 to 10 years of age, by which time it has reached 50% of the adult volume. The final 50% of adult volume is achieved during the adolescent growth spurt from 10 to 15 years of age.

## PATHOGENESIS

- The pathogenesis of EOS depends on its etiology.
  - Vertebral anomalies cause scoliosis by an imbalance in bone growth, secondary to either an increase in growth on a side associated with a hemivertebrae or growth retardation on the side associated with a vertebral bar.
  - In neuromuscular and central nervous disorders, an imbalance in muscular forces is pathogenic, likely following the Heuter-Volkmann principle that the physeal growth rate is related to the forces it is exposed to, with compression inhibiting growth and tension promoting it.
  - The etiology and pathogenesis of infantile idiopathic scoliosis (IIS) (0 to 3 years of age) is, by definition, unknown, but there is likely a component of genetic susceptibility. The external factors resulting in scoliosis are not yet clearly delineated but may include intrauterine molding as well as infant positioning. The etiology of IIS most likely differs from that of adolescent idiopathic scoliosis (AIS).

## NATURAL HISTORY

- The natural history of EOS also depends on the etiology.
  - The natural history of EOS due to IIS is favorable when compared with late-onset scoliosis (LOS). Spontaneous resolution occurs in a large number of patients. Progression of congenital curves depends on the type of anomaly and growth potential.
  - EOS due to neuromuscular etiologies usually follows the natural history of said neuromuscular disease, in addition to specific problems associated with progressive curves in this age group.
  - Regardless of the etiology, progression of scoliosis during the first 5 years of life adversely affects growth as well as pulmonary function.
    - A history of EOS is associated with a higher risk of cardiopulmonary decompensation in middle-aged patients, which can lead to disabling and even fatal respiratory failure.

## PATIENT HISTORY AND PHYSICAL FINDINGS

- Evaluation of the patient with EOS includes a complete history, including the family history, prenatal history, birth history, and developmental history.
  - IIS has been associated with breech presentation and, in boys, with premature birth.
- Physical examinations includes observation of gait (if patient is ambulatory), respiration, truncal and pelvic balance in the coronal and sagittal planes, cutaneous lesions, and any prominence on Adams forward bending test.
- Any deficits in motor, sensory, or reflex function, including abdominal reflexes, may indicate central nervous system pathology and should be thoroughly evaluated with advanced diagnostic studies.
- Flexibility of the curve can be assessed either by the manual application of traction through the cervical spine or by applying a three-point bending force at the apex of the curve.
- Examination techniques unique for EOS include the thumb excursion test for thoracic expansion and sitting height measurement.

## IMAGING AND OTHER DIAGNOSTIC STUDIES

- All patients should have full-length standing anteroposterior (AP) and lateral radiographs (**FIG 1**) covering the cervical spine to the pelvis, including the entire thorax. For patients who are unable to stand, supine radiographs encompassing the same area should be taken.
  - The cervical spine, lumbosacral spine, pelvis, and hips all may need to be studied to elicit whether or not developmental hip

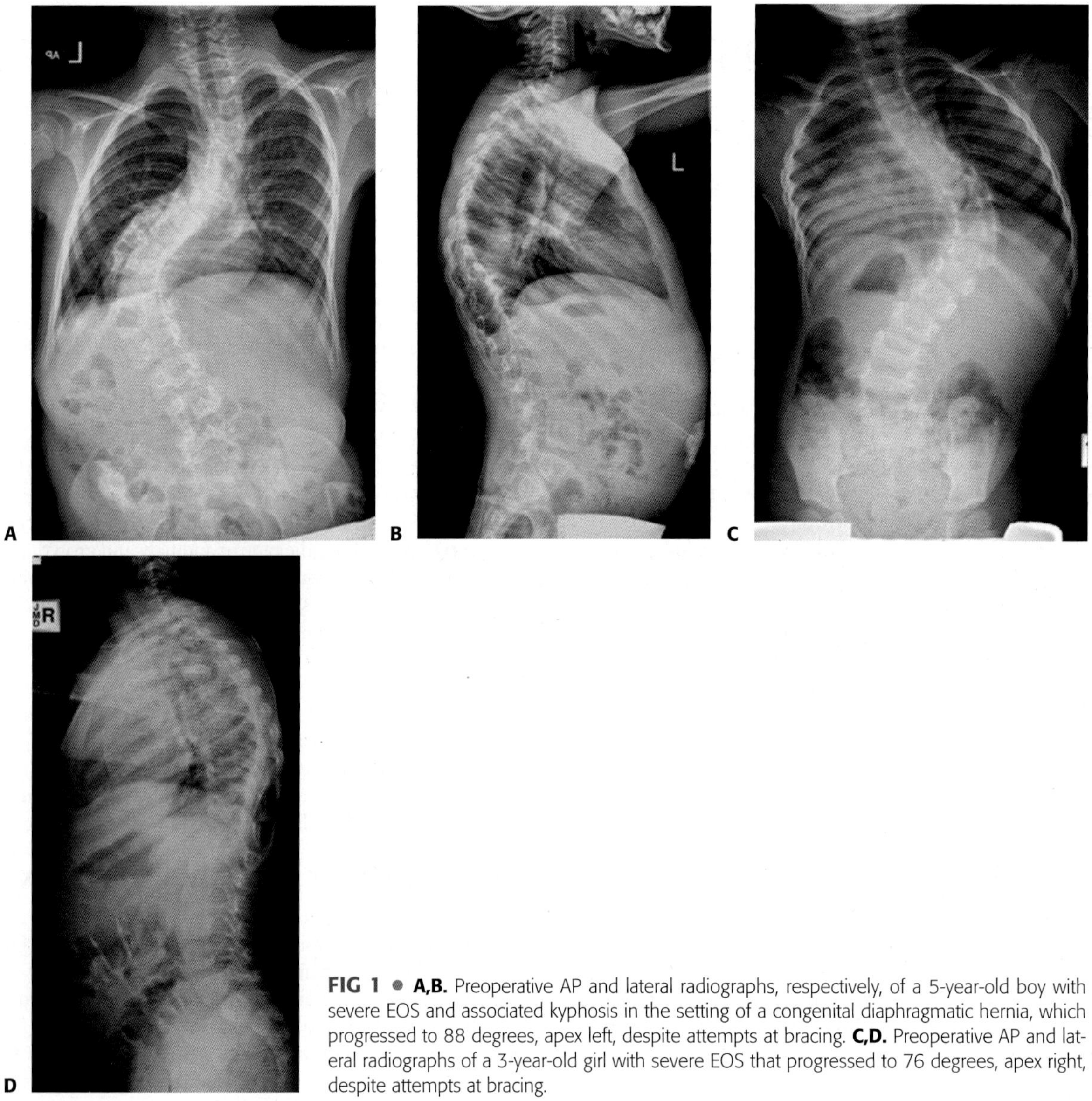

**FIG 1** ● **A,B.** Preoperative AP and lateral radiographs, respectively, of a 5-year-old boy with severe EOS and associated kyphosis in the setting of a congenital diaphragmatic hernia, which progressed to 88 degrees, apex left, despite attempts at bracing. **C,D.** Preoperative AP and lateral radiographs of a 3-year-old girl with severe EOS that progressed to 76 degrees, apex right, despite attempts at bracing.

dysplasia or other vertebral anomalies are contributing to the scoliosis.

- Bolster bending, side-bending, or traction radiographs are necessary to help delineate the degree of flexibility of the curves.
- The Cobb angle is used to assess initial curve severity and is followed over successive visits to evaluate for curve progression.
- Spinal height is obtained by measuring the distance from the top of T1 to the top of S1 on the AP view of the spine.
- Coronal balance is measured by the distance from the center of C7 to a line drawn up from S1.
- The sagittal balance is measured from the posterior cranial corner of S1 to a line drawn down from the center of C7.
- All of these measurements should be recorded and compared on successive visits to document any change in curve magnitude or growth of the spine.

- The rib–vertebral angle difference (RVAD) of Mehta (**FIG 2**), first described in 1972, measures the amount of rotation at the apex vertebra and has some prognostic value.[10]

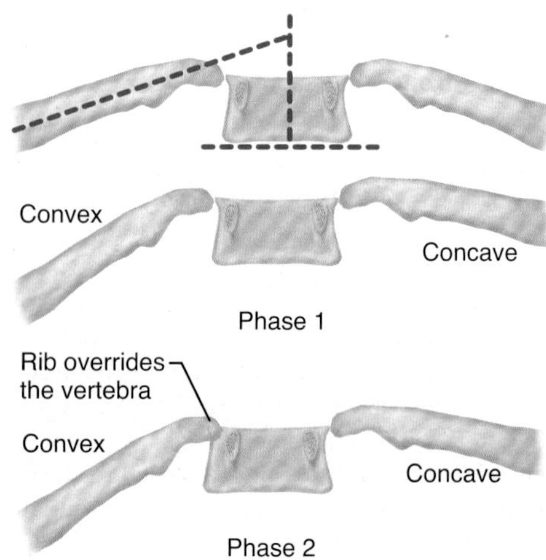


**FIG 2** ● The RVAD measures the angle of a line drawn perpendicular to the apical thoracic vertebra endplate and a line drawn down the center of the concave and convex ribs. The difference is calculated by subtracting the convex from the concave angle.

- The angles formed by a line perpendicular to the vertebra and a line drawn down the center of the rib is compared between the convex and concave side. If the difference calculated by subtracting the convex angle to the concave angle is 20 degrees or less, there is an 85% to 90% chance the curve will resolve; when there is a difference of 21 degrees or more, it will likely progress.
- The phase of the rib head is determined by whether or not the head of the convex rib overlaps the vertebral body.
  - If there is no overlap (phase 1), then the RVAD is calculated as previously mentioned.
  - If there is overlap (phase 2), the risk of progression is high, regardless of RVAD.
- The space available for the lung (SAL) is calculated by taking the ratio of the distance from the apex of the most cephalad rib to the highest point of the hemidiaphragm of the concave side divided by the convex side.
  - A lower SAL points toward a poorer prognosis for lung function.
- Magnetic resonance imaging (MRI) is recommended to evaluate for spinal cord anomalies in children with rapidly progressive spinal deformities, clinical findings concerning for spinal cord anomalies, or preoperative patients. Before embarking on a repetitive distraction technique such as growing rods, it is particularly valuable to know whether there is a tethered spinal cord.
  - MRI is also used to measure lung volume and assess thoracic architecture when thoracic insufficiency is an issue.
  - In severe congenital deformity, the ribs may spiral around the vertebrae, causing the thoracic volume on one side to be severely diminished while the other is larger, creating what Campbell[4] calls a "windswept thorax."
- Computed tomography (CT) scanning is not routinely used, particularly in an era where we are increasingly concerned about high levels of medical radiation in very young patients.

## DIFFERENTIAL DIAGNOSIS

- Congenital vertebral or spinal anomalies
  - Vertebral bars
  - Hemivertebrae
  - Syrinx
  - Tethered cord
- Neuromuscular diseases
  - Cerebral palsy
  - Myelodysplasia
  - Muscular dystrophy
- Syndromes associated with scoliosis
  - Beel syndrome
  - Trisomies
- IIS

## NONOPERATIVE MANAGEMENT

- Nonoperative treatment for EOS is indicated in curves that are not expected to progress.
  - Patients with a curve of less than 25 degrees and RVAD less than 20 degrees may be followed with serial radiographs every 4 to 6 months to document any progression.
  - Active treatment is warranted in the following:
    - Progression greater than 10 degrees
    - Phase 2 rib–vertebral relationship, RVAD greater than 20 degrees, or a Cobb angle greater than 25 degrees in any skeletally immature patient
  - Nonoperative treatment generally starts with casting or bracing.
    - Brace treatment should be abandoned in favor of surgical management when unacceptable curve magnitude or progression is seen.

## SURGICAL MANAGEMENT

- Surgical treatment of EOS attempts to stop progression of the scoliosis, allowing improvements in growth of the spine, thorax, and lungs.
- Surgery is recommended for progressive curves with a Cobb angle greater than 45 degrees.
- The age of the patient helps to determine the type of surgery needed.
  - Adolescents and more skeletally mature patients may do well with spine fusions, which stabilize the spine but also stop growth.
  - Younger patients with substantial growth potential suffer from the "crankshaft" phenomenon if fusion is performed early in life from an isolated posterior approach. They suffer from severe growth retardation in height and thoracic volume if fusion is performed using a combined anterior and posterior technique.
- The growing rod technique for EOS was developed to correct spinal deformity while allowing spinal growth to continue or even enhancing that growth.

### Preoperative Planning

- Careful evaluation of radiographic studies allows planning of surgical levels. Typically, the cranial level of the construct includes T2 and extends two or three levels caudal to the end vertebra of the curve.
- Medical and subspecialty consultations should be obtained before operation if the patient has any history of medical comorbidities.
  - Pulmonary function tests may be obtained in children who are able to cooperate if thoracic insufficiency is suspected.

### Positioning

- The patient is placed under general anesthesia on the stretcher and then placed on the operating room table in the prone position on two longitudinal chest rolls or tightly rolled blankets.
- Neurologic monitoring is used during the procedure for neurologically intact patients. Leads should be placed before prone positioning, as should a Foley catheter.
- Care must be taken to be sure all bony prominences and compressible nerves are well padded.

### Approach

- The growing rod technique is performed posteriorly through either a single long midline incision or two smaller incisions cranially and caudally.

## Placing the Foundation Anchors

- Unlike traditional exposures used for thoracolumbar fusions, placement of growing rods begins by only exposing the two anchor clusters, first distally for pedicle screw placement then proximally for hook and sublaminar cable placement.
- After radiographically localizing the exposure sites for the two sets of anchor clusters, the distal anchor site is exposed subperiosteally (**TECH FIG 1A,B**).
- Pedicle screws are generally placed bilaterally at two or three adjacent vertebra (**TECH FIG 1C**), optimal placement of the screws is confirmed radiographically, and the wound is packed and attention turned to placing the proximal anchors.
- The proximal anchor site is exposed subperiosteally. Generally, we use bilateral transverse process hooks at the upper instrumented vertebrae and bilateral pedicle hooks at the level below, protected with bilateral sublaminar cables at the level of the pedicle hook (**TECH FIG 1D**). In the past, pedicle screws were used for proximal rod fixation, but recent literature has revealed the potential for significant complications.[12]

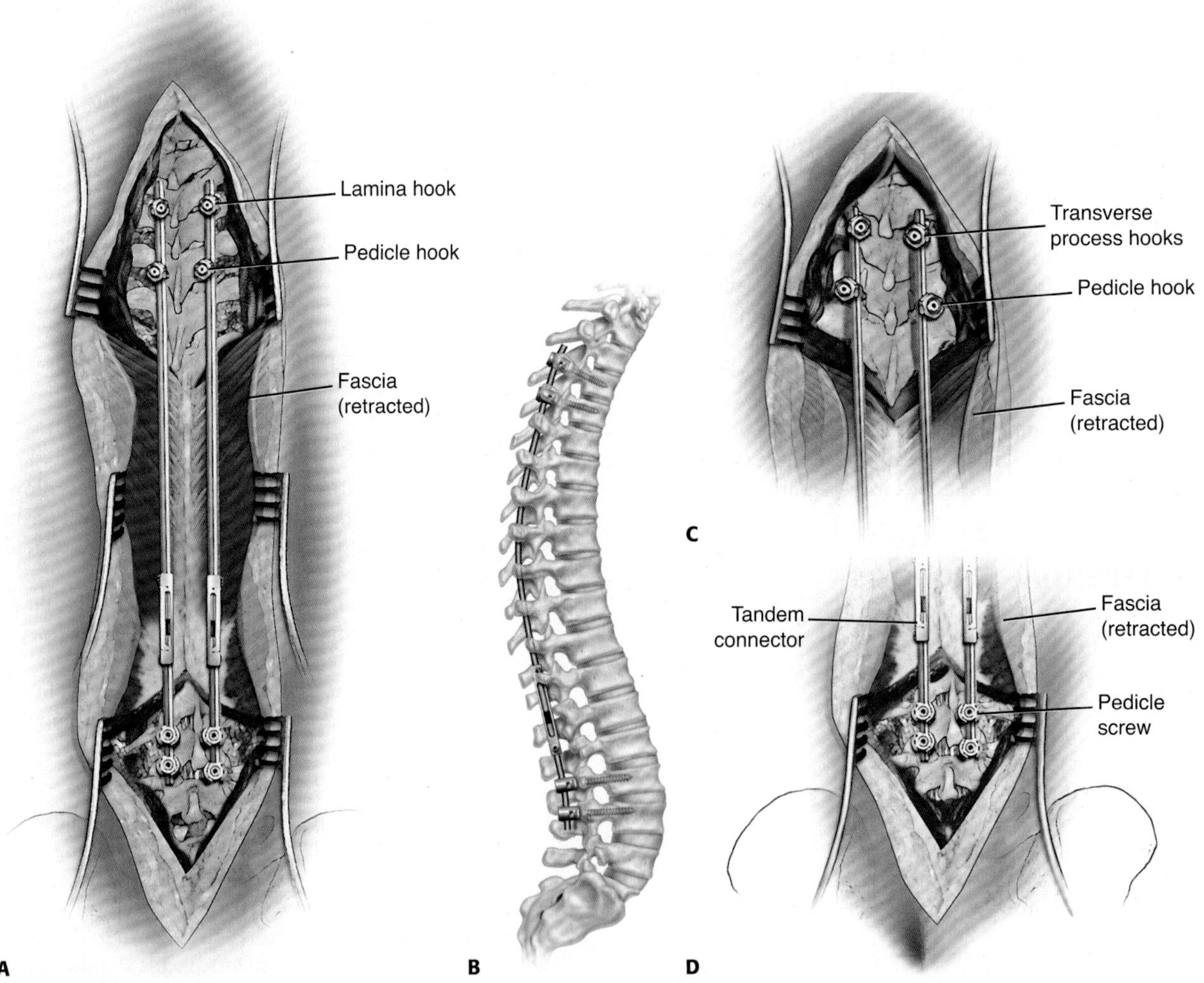


**TECH FIG 1** • **A.** A single skin incision may be used with subperiosteal exposure of the cranial and caudal foundation sites. The rods and tandem connectors are placed under the fascia in a bed of paraspinal muscle. Pedicle hooks have been used as anchors for the cranial foundation and pedicle screws for the caudal foundation. **B.** The lateral view shows the straight tandem connector placed in the thoracolumbar region. The trajectory of the pedicle screws can also be seen and varies by patient. **C.** Close-up of the cranial foundation shows two transverse process hooks and two pedicle hooks spanning two levels in the thoracic region. **D.** Close-up of the caudal foundation shows four pedicle screws spanning two levels in the lumbar spine. Hooks may also be used for this foundation.

## Placing the Rods and Rod-to-Rod Connectors

- The next step is to place the concave rod. The fascia on the concave side is divided, and a bed is created in the paraspinous muscle for the rod. To avoid unwanted autofusion, care is taken to avoid exposure of the posterior elements of the spine (as is done in a normal spine exposure).
- Either of two types of connectors may be used: a tandem connector, which houses the cranial and caudal rods inside a rectangular box so the ends meet end-to-end, or side-to-side connectors, which allow the rods to overlap.
- Tandem connectors are used most commonly. Because these connectors are straight and cannot be contoured, the rods are measured so that they meet inside the tandem connector in the relatively straight thoracolumbar region.
- The ends of the rods that fit inside the connector also must be straight. If any contouring is necessary in the region where the cranial and caudal rods meet, closed dual connectors must be used, with an overlap of 2 to 4 inches to allow future lengthening.
- After the concave rod is placed, the spine is manually corrected to its maximum amount, then the concave rod is tightened. For the initial implant, it is best to correct the spine and let the rod hold that correction passively rather than try to drive the correction by distracting the rod at a time when the anchor sites are not yet fused.
- Next, the convex rod is placed. Generally, it must be contoured with increased kyphosis.
- After the rods are placed in the hooks or screws of each foundation, transverse connectors are often placed between the two cranial rods and the two caudal rods, preferably between the points of fixation on each foundation.
- If distraction is required, the caudal set screw is tightened, a distractor is implemented in the slot of the tandem connector between the two rods, and the cranial set screw is tightened (**TECH FIG 2A**).
- Similarly, a rod clamp can be used to distract against if a closed dual connector, or even a tandem connector, is used (**TECH FIG 2B**).
- The surgical area is then irrigated, followed by a limited arthrodesis, decorticating and applying autograft bone or other graft extenders between the vertebrae making up each foundation.
- Before final closure, AP and lateral radiographs are taken to confirm alignment and proper position of the implants (**TECH FIG 2C–F**).
- The wound is then closed in standard fashion.

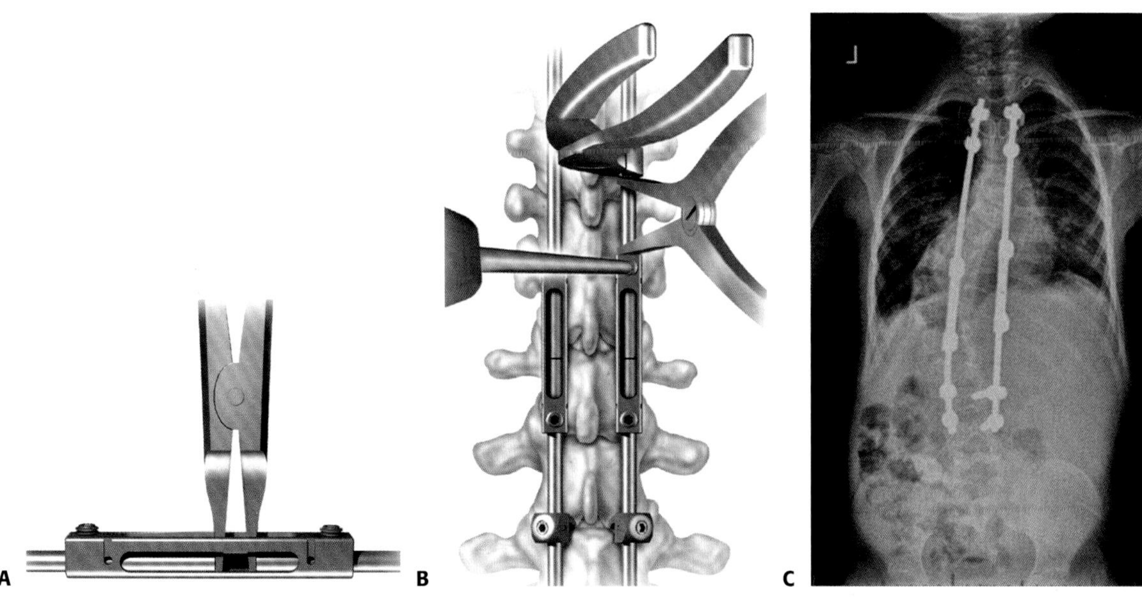


**TECH FIG 2** • **A.** Lengthening can be performed by inserting the distractor between the rods through the slot of the tandem connector. One set screw is loosened, distraction is performed, and the set screw secured. **B.** Alternatively, a rod clamp can be placed on the rod a few centimeters from the connector and the distractor placed between the rod clamp and the end of the connector. The set screw nearest the rod clamp is then loosened, the distractor employed, and the screw retightened. **C,D.** AP and lateral radiographs, respectively, after the dual growing rod procedure using tandem connectors was performed on the patient shown in **FIG 1A,B**. *(continued)*

D 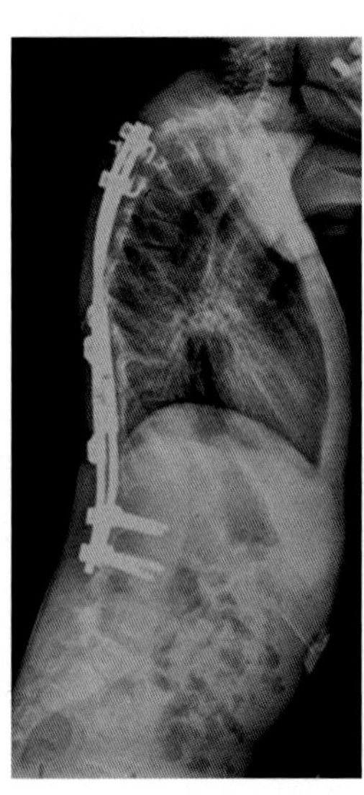
E 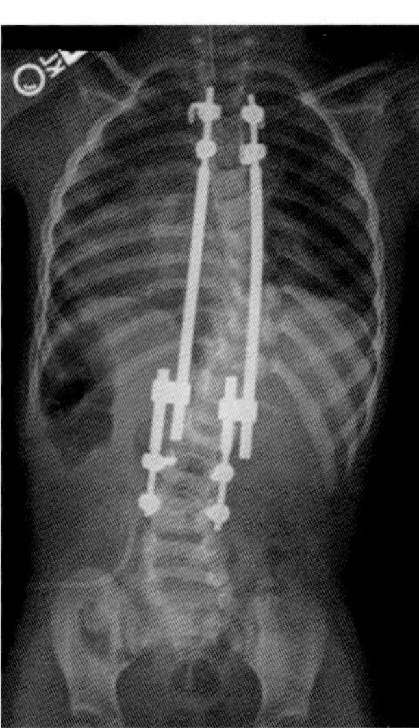
F 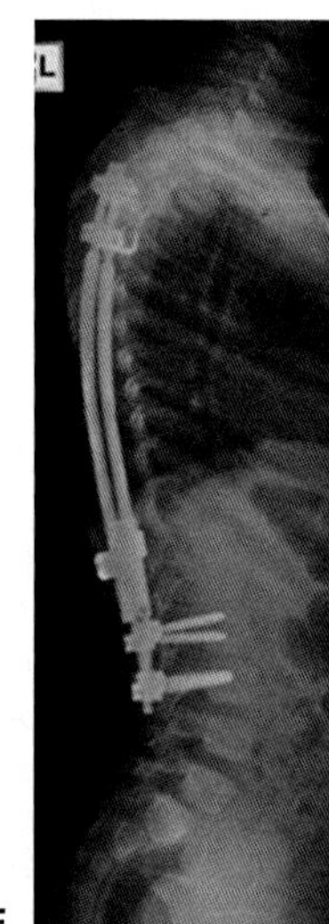

**TECH FIG 2** • *(continued)* **E,F.** AP and lateral radiographs, respectively, after the dual growing rod procedure using side-to-side connectors was performed on the patient in **FIG 1C,D**. (**A,B:** From Bagheri R, Akbarnia BA. Pediatric ISOLA (DePuy Spine) instrumentation. In: Kim DH, Vaccaro AR, Fessler RG, eds. Spinal Instrumentation: Surgical Techniques. New York: Thieme, 2005:640,642.)

## Lengthening and Exchange

- Lengthening of the dual rod construct may be performed as either an inpatient or outpatient procedure with neural monitoring for patients with normal neurologic function.
- The connector is located through palpation or fluoroscopy, and a small incision is made over that area where the lengthening is planned.
- After dissection of the connector is performed, lengthening similar to that performed during the index procedure is carried out by loosening the set screw (mostly cranial), distracting between the two rods, and then tightening the set screw again.
- Lengthening is generally performed every 6 months initially and in children with long constructs and a flexible spine. Over time, the interval is usually lengthened to 8 to 12 months as diminishing returns are noted.
- Once further distraction is no longer achievable, final correction and arthrodesis are performed.

## Changing the Connector or Rod

- Exchange of the tandem connector or the rod may be needed if the amount of lengthening exceeds the initial length of the tandem connector.
  - In such a case, both set screws should be loosened and the tandem connector slid cephalad until full clearance of the caudal rod is achieved.
  - The connector can then be removed off the cranial rod, replaced by a longer connector, and slid onto the caudal rod again.
  - Connectors longer than 70 mm are rarely used to minimize the adverse effect on sagittal balance.
- If the needed length exceeds the longest connector or if the longest connector is too long, it is necessary to fashion new rods and remove the old ones.
  - This entails exposing and removing the tandem connectors, exposing the foundation, removing the rods, and replacing them with longer rods, creating a construct similar to the initial procedure.
  - Replacement of the cephalad rods is most common.

## PEARLS AND PITFALLS

| | |
|---|---|
| **Exposure** | ■ Avoid subperiosteal dissection anywhere except the foundation to avoid premature fusion. |
| **Implants** | ■ Perform a careful radiographic examination or use image-guided navigation if pedicle screws are desired.<br>■ Use proper rod contouring to correct both coronal and sagittal deformity. Perhaps the most common pitfall is to attempt to overcorrect a kyphotic deformity. Over time, overcorrection leads to frequent anchor failure, especially at the proximal anchors.<br>■ Tandem connectors are straight and should be placed in the thoracolumbar region, which also is straight. |
| **Lengthening** | ■ Do not be too aggressive with lengthenings, especially at the index procedure and first lengthening, to avoid implant issues. |
| **Indications** | ■ Growing rods may not be indicated in very stiff curves, poor bone quality, older children with limited growth potential, or children too young to allow internal fixation. |

## POSTOPERATIVE CARE

- Patients are braced postoperatively with a thoracolumbosacral orthosis for up to 6 months to facilitate fusion of the foundations. Rehabilitation proceeds according to the patient's tolerance and ability.

## OUTCOMES

- The available literature on growing rods for EOS shows it to be a safe and effective method for correcting spinal curves while preserving growth.[1,2,6,13,15]
  - In a retrospective series of 23 patients with EOS of any etiology, Akbarnia and colleagues[2] demonstrated an improvement in the mean curve from 82 degrees preoperatively to 38 degrees after the initial implantation procedure. Patients in this study saw a mean T1–S1 length increase of 1.2 cm per year and an increase in lung space ratio from 0.87 to 1.
  - A more recent series by Akbarnia and coworkers[1] showed Cobb angle improvement from 81.0 degrees to 35.8 degrees after the initial procedure and to 27.7 degrees after final fusion.
- Complications, while similar in frequency to other growth preserving spinal procedures,[11] are frequent[1,2,15] and must be anticipated and thoughtfully managed. Complication risk worsens with increased number of surgical procedures and younger age at first surgery.[3] However, more frequent lengthenings are also associated with improved curve correction and T1–S1 growth.[1]
  - In a study of 140 growing rod patients, Bess and coworkers[3] found that 81 (58%) experienced at least one complication. Improved complication profiles were associated with dual rods as opposed to single ones and in submuscular rod placement versus subcutaneous placement.
  - Another study by Watanabe and colleagues[16] of 88 patients with EOS and growing rods found that 50 patients had complications (57%). Complications occurred in 119 of 538 procedures and included 86 implant-related failures (72%), 19 infections (16%), 3 neurologic impairments (3%), and 11 other complications. The most frequent implant-related failure was dislodgement (71%), with 95% of the dislodgements occurring at the proximal foundation.
  - Also of concern is the psychosocial toll of repeat operative procedures, and physicians treating these patients should be vigilant for possible adverse psychological outcomes in this population.[8,9]
- Final fusion is usually performed in late childhood or early adolescence and involves a similar number of levels as the growing rod instrumentation, achieves some additional correction in most cases, and has a similar complication rate to other spinal fusion procedures.[7]

## COMPLICATIONS

- Wound breakdown
- Infection
- Junctional kyphosis
- Crankshaft phenomenon
- Curve progression
- Implant failure
- Patients with more frequent lengthenings have fewer implant problems but more wound problems, whereas patients with less frequent lengthenings have more implant problems and fewer wound complications. Implant complications often can be treated during scheduled lengthenings, but wound infections should be treated urgently.

## ACKNOWLEDGMENTS

- We would like to acknowledge Victor Hsu and Behrooz Akbarnia for their work in writing the previous edition of this chapter.

## REFERENCES

1. Akbarnia BA, Breakwell LM, Marks DS, et al. Dual growing rod technique followed for three to eleven years until final fusion: the effect of frequency of lengthening. Spine 2008;33(9):984–990.
2. Akbarnia BA, Marks DS, Boachie-Adjei O, et al. Dual growing rod technique for the treatment of progressive early-onset scoliosis: a multicenter study. Spine 2005;30(17 suppl):S46–S57.
3. Bess S, Akbarnia BA, Thompson GH, et al. Complications of growing rod treatment for early-onset scoliosis: analysis of one hundred and forty patients. J Bone Joint Surg Am 2010;92(15):2533–2543.
4. Campell RM Jr, Smith MD, Mayes TC, et al. The characteristics of thoracic insufficiency syndrome associated with fused ribs and congenital scoliosis. J Bone Joint Surg Am 2003;85-A(3):399–408.
5. DiMeglio A. Growth of the spine before age 5 years. J Pediatr Orthop B 1993;1:102–107.
6. Elsebai HB, Yazici M, Thompson GH, et al. Safety and efficacy of growing rod techniques for pediatric congenital spinal deformities. J Pediatr Orthop 2011;31(1):1–5.
7. Flynn JM, Matsumoto H, Torres F, et al. Psychological dysfunction in children who require repetitive surgery for early onset scoliosis. J Pediatr Orthop 2012;32(6):594–599.
8. Flynn JM, Tomlinson LA, Pawelek J, et al. Growing-rod graduates: lessons learned from ninety-nine patients who completed lengthening. J Bone Joint Surg Am 2013;95(19):1745–1750.
9. Matsumoto H, Williams BA, Corona J, et al. Psychosocial effects of repetitive surgeries in children with early-onset scoliosis: are we putting them at risk? J Pediatr Orthop 2014;34(2):172–178.
10. Mehta MH. The rib-vertebra angle in the early diagnosis between resolving and progressive infantile scoliosis. J Bone Joint Surg Br 1972;54:230–243.
11. Sankar WN, Acevedo DC, Skaggs DL. Comparison of complications among growing spinal implants. Spine 2010;35(23):2091–2906.
12. Skaggs KF, Brasher AF, Johnston CE, et al. Upper thoracic pedicle screw loss of fixation causing spinal cord injury: a review of the literature and multicenter case series. J Pediatr Orthop 2013;33(1):75–79.
13. Thomspson GH, Akbarnia BA, Kostial P, et al. Comparison of single and dual growing rod techniques followed through definitive surgery: a preliminary study. Spine 2005;30:2039–2044.
14. Tis JE, Karlin LI, Akbarnia BA, et al. Early onset scoliosis: modern treatment and results. J Pediatr Orthop 2012;32:647–657.
15. Wang S, Zhang J, Qiu G, et al. Dual growing rods technique for congenital scoliosis: more than 2 years outcomes: preliminary results of a single center. Spine 2012;37(26):E1639–E1644.
16. Watanabe K, Uno K, Suzuki T, et al. Risk factors for complications associated with growing-rod surgery for early-onset scoliosis. Spine 2013;38(8):E464–E468.

94

# Hemivertebra Excision

CHAPTER

Daniel J. Hedequist and Michael P. Glotzbecker

## DEFINITION

- A hemivertebra is a congenital anomaly of the spine that forms during the 8th to 12th weeks of embryologic development. It is characterized by the formation of half of a vertebral body, a corresponding pedicle, and a corresponding hemilamina.
- Hemivertebra are classified as a congenital failure of formation.
- A hemivertebra may be classified as fully segmented (ie, separated from the bodies above and below by discs), partially segmented (ie, separated from one adjacent body by a disc and fused to the other adjacent body), or unsegmented (ie, fused to the body above and below; **FIG 1**).[1]
- Progressive curvatures of the spine caused by a hemivertebra result from unbalanced growth. Full-segmented hemivertebra have a much higher rate of progression because the presence of an intact disc space above and below signifies the presence of growth plates and potential asymmetric spinal growth.

## ANATOMY

- The hemivertebra has a partial vertebral body, a pedicle, and a hemilamina.
- Anatomically, it may be joined to the level above or below at either the body, the hemilamina, or both. If the hemivertebra is not fused to either adjacent segment, the potential for asymmetric spinal growth is high.
- A local kyphotic or lordotic deformity may occur with hemivertebra if the associated failure of formation is greater anteriorly or posteriorly.

## PATHOGENESIS

- Progressive spinal curvatures due to hemivertebra are a result of disordered growth.

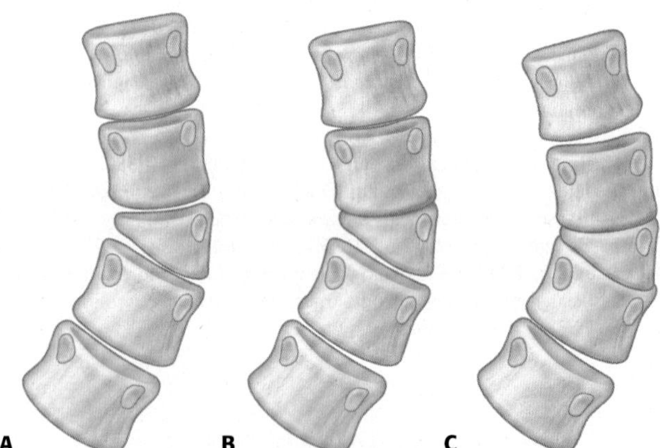


**FIG 1** ● Schematic of a hemivertebra. **A.** Fully segmented hemivertebra. **B.** Partially segmented hemivertebra. **C.** Unsegmented hemivertebra.

- The hemivertebra is a wedge on the convex side of a curve. In the presence of healthy growth plates above and below (ie, a fully segmented hemivertebra), convex growth is faster than contralateral concave growth, causing a progressive scoliosis.
- In cases of hemivertebra, if the vertebral body lies in the posterolateral quadrant, a progressive kyphosis may arise in association with the scoliosis.
- The disordered growth eventually may cause curvature to such a degree that normally segmented areas of the spine become involved in the curve, causing deformity and spinal imbalance.

## NATURAL HISTORY

- The natural history of a hemivertebra depends on its location and the potential for growth and curve progression.
- Hemivertebrae that are fully segmented progress at approximately 2 degrees a year and can exceed over 45 degrees at maturity.[3] These require treatment to prevent deformity and also to prevent adjacent spinal curvature.
- Partially segmented hemivertebrae have much less growth potential (<1 degree per year), rarely exceeding 40 degrees at maturity. They usually do not require treatment. Unsegmented hemivertebrae generally require no treatment.
- Hemivertebra at the lumbosacral junction almost always require treatment because the lumbar spine takes off obliquely from the sacrum, causing a long compensatory curve in normally segmented regions of the lumbar spine, with resultant cosmetic deformity and spinal imbalance.

## PATIENT HISTORY AND PHYSICAL FINDINGS

- Embryologic development of the spine occurs between the 8th and 12th weeks of gestation; hence, other organ systems developing at the same time also may have a congenital anomaly.
- A complete musculoskeletal examination looking for diagnoses such as clubfoot, developmental dysplasia of the hip, and limb anomalies is warranted.
- A complete neurologic examination should be performed because as many as 40% of patients with congenital scoliosis have a corresponding spinal dysraphism. This examination includes sensory, motor, and reflex testing.
- Occult signs of spinal dysraphism include cutaneous manifestations such as midline spinal hemangiomas, penetrating sacral dimples, or midline hairy patches. Foot anomalies such as vertical talus or asymmetric cavus feet can signify spinal dysraphism.
- Cardiac auscultation should be done because 20% of patients with congenital scoliosis have congenital heart anomalies.

- Observe shoulder position, trunk position, and waist symmetry. Truncal imbalance is an indicator of curvature.
- Observe the flexibility of the patient's spine.
- Rotation of the spine during the Adams forward bend test is indicative of deformity and points to its location.

## IMAGING AND OTHER DIAGNOSTIC STUDIES

- Standing 36-inch posteroanterior (PA) and lateral radiographs are mandatory to define the deformity and assess the Cobb measurement. Apparent progression may be seen from supine radiographs to standing radiographs (**FIG 2A**).
  - Bending radiographs, in which the patient is directed to bend in a concave and then in a convex direction, are useful to assess the flexibility of curves above and below the hemivertebra.
- Magnetic resonance imaging (MRI) scanning of the brainstem and spinal cord is mandatory before any surgical intervention, given the high association (30% to 40%) of congenital scoliosis with spinal dysraphism.[1]
- Computed tomography (CT) scans with three-dimensional (3-D) reconstructions should be obtained to delineate the anatomy of the anterior and posterior elements as an aid in planning the operation and to avoid intraoperative problems such as unexpected posterior element deficiencies or fusions (**FIG 2B**).[2]
  - A pediatric protocol should be used for CT scans to avoid the significant radiation exposure that results when adult protocols are used for children.
- Preoperative evaluation of the genitourinary system with a screening ultrasound and evaluation of the cardiac system with an echocardiogram are necessary if these have not been performed, given the rate of anomalies associated with congenital scoliosis.

## DIFFERENTIAL DIAGNOSIS

- Failure of vertebral formation
- Failure of vertebral segmentation
- Sequela of infection causing partial vertebral body destruction
- Tumor

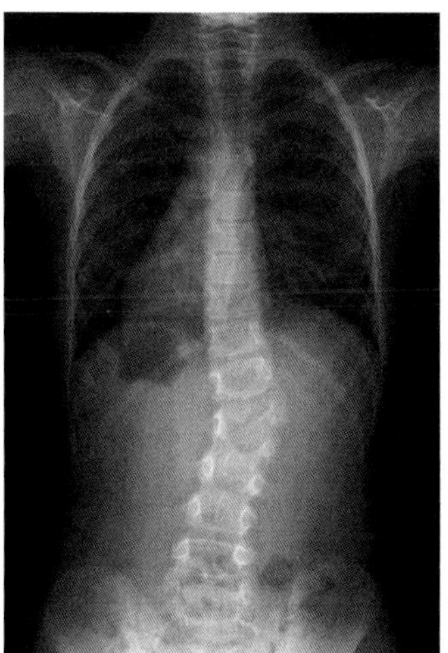
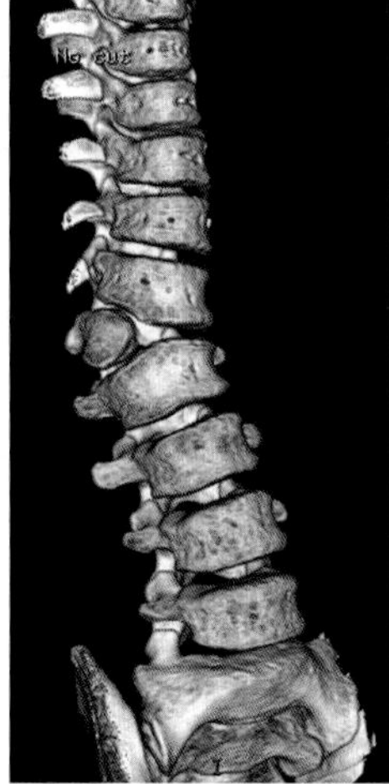

**FIG 2** • **A.** Standing PA radiograph of a 5-year-old patient with a fully segmented hemivertebra at the thoracolumbar junction. **B.** A 3-D reconstructed CT scan of a fully segmented hemivertebra in a different patient.

## NONOPERATIVE MANAGEMENT

- Nonoperative management is reserved for nonprogressive curves caused by hemivertebra.
- Hemivertebra associated with little or no curve progression (unsegmented or partially segmented) may be followed during growth with radiographs every 6 to 12 months, depending on the degree of deformity and age of the patient.
- Bracing has no role in the management of a hemivertebra.

## SURGICAL MANAGEMENT

- The classic indication for a hemivertebra resection is a patient with a progressive curve secondary to a fully segmented hemivertebra in the thoracolumbar, lumbar, or lumbosacral regions with a resultant deformity.
- We have found that excision is best performed between the ages of 18 months and 4 years.
  - Patients younger than this may be more difficult to instrument, and waiting until this age rarely has caused irrevocable deformity.
  - Excision in older patients is feasible; we have found, however, that if diagnosed early, there is no reason to wait past the age of 4 years given the progression of curvature and its effect on normally segmented regions of the spine.
  - Instrumentation at these ages is technically feasible.

### Preoperative Planning

- Review of the preoperative MRI of the spine
  - If spinal dysraphism is present, referral to a neurosurgeon is mandatory.
  - If the patient requires neurosurgical intervention for dysraphism, that procedure should precede the hemivertebra excision, either at the same setting or in a staged setting, at the discretion of the spine surgeon and neurosurgeon.
- Review of the 3-D CT scans
  - A complete understanding of the anatomy of the hemivertebra is crucial to avoid intraoperative confusion, especially because associated posterior element fusions or absences can make identifying levels difficult.
  - Studying the pedicle anatomy (ie, length and diameter) of the levels above and below is efficacious given the smaller size of these patients.
- Neurologic monitoring is important and should be done using somatosensory evoked potentials and motor evoked potentials.
  - Communication between the monitoring and anesthesia teams should be facilitated to prevent any change in neurologic function brought on by anesthetics, hypotension, or low blood volume.

### Positioning

- We perform hemivertebra excisions with the patient in the prone position.
  - This is done on a radiolucent operating frame with chest and pelvic support, which leaves the abdomen free.
  - We also have found it useful to slightly "airplane" the table or bolster the patient so that the convex side is slightly higher than the concave side. This helps with visualization anteriorly, control of bleeding, and retraction of the dura and its contents (**FIG 3**).

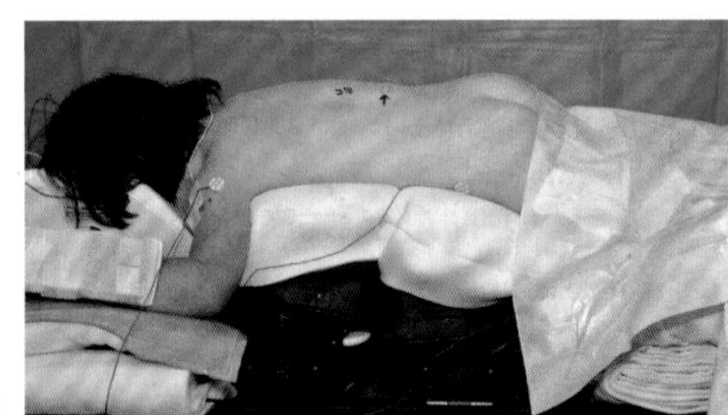

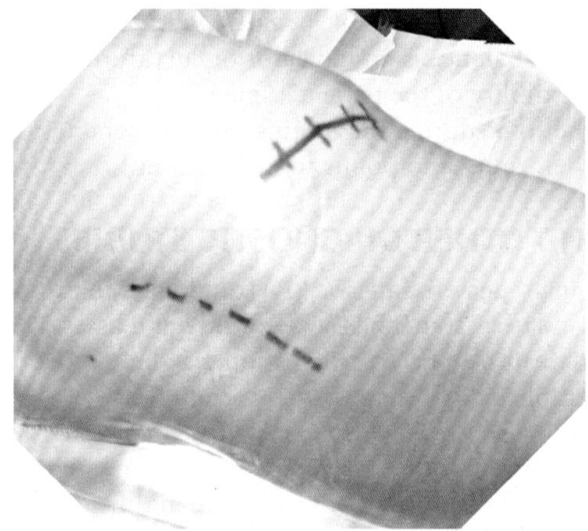

**FIG 3** • Positioning for a hemivertebra resection. **A.** Prone positioning. Observe the paper clip placed for radiographic marking before incision. **B.** Positioning for simultaneous anteroposterior (AP) excision.

- Before draping the patient, we place a marker over the hemivertebra region and obtain a radiograph.
  - This both confirms the side of the hemivertebra and helps limit excessive incisions and dissections.
- In the past, we recommended that hemivertebra excision be performed as a simultaneous anteroposterior procedure.[2]
  - If the surgeon elects to do this, the patient is placed in the lateral decubitus position with the anterior and posterior fields being prepped into the fields. The patient should be placed at the edge of the bed to facilitate retractor placement in the posterior field.
  - The anterior approach is on the convex side and should be marked before the patient goes to the operating room.
- Although we advocate for posterior-only surgery for most hemivertebra, we still recommend considering an anteroposterior procedure when medical conditions (eg, congenital heart disease) caution against excessive bleeding, when a lordotic component renders access to the vertebral body difficult, and when the surgeon is unfamiliar with posterior-only approaches.

## Approach

- If an anteroposterior procedure is being performed, the anterior procedure should be a standard transthoracic, transthoracic–retroperitoneal, or retroperitoneal approach, depending on the location of the hemivertebra. The anterior approach often can be a limited one because the only exposure needed is of the hemivertebra and the discs above and below.
- The posterior approach is a standard posterior midline incision with subperiosteal dissection out to the tips of the transverse processes.
  - Diathermy aids in keeping blood loss to a minimum during dissection.
  - Preoperative review of the CT scan should forewarn the surgeon of posterior element fusions and, more importantly, posterior element deficiencies.
  - Dissection should proceed with caution over areas of laminar deficiency.
  - Once completely dissected, a spot radiograph or fluoroscopic view should be obtained to confirm the appropriate level.



# Hemivertebra Excision

## Pedicle Screw Placement

- Implant anchors should be placed before excision because blood loss at this point should be at a minimum.
  - Where possible, we prefer bilateral pedicle screws as a basis for fixation. Pedicle screws may be placed in patients as young as 1 year of age.
  - Preoperative CT scans can help assess the feasibility of screw placement.
- Implants should be titanium, and either 3.5- or 4.5-mm rod systems should be used in younger patients.
  - Screw diameter and length can be at least estimated based on the preoperative CT scan.
- Screws should be placed in a stepwise manner, beginning with obtaining a cancellous blush with a burr at the appropriate starting position.
  - Starting positions in normally segmented areas of the spine are well documented.
- A pedicle awl can then be used to obtain access down the pedicle into the vertebral body.
- Once the pedicle has been accessed, probing of the four walls of the pedicle and floor of the body is necessary to confirm accurate position. We then use the probe as a depth gauge to determine screw length.
  - The hole is then tapped 0.5 mm under the expected screw diameter, and the pedicle walls and floor are reprobed.
  - A fixed-angle screw of the appropriate diameter and length is then placed (**TECH FIG 1A**). Use of fixed-angle screws helps minimize implant prominence.
- Appropriate screw position is confirmed using triggered electromyography (EMG) stimulation of all screws (**TECH FIG 1B**) and then checking PA and lateral radiographs and fluoroscopic views (**TECH FIG 1C**).

## Hemivertebra Excision

- The first step in excision is dissecting over the edge of the transverse process and down the lateral wall of the body using a

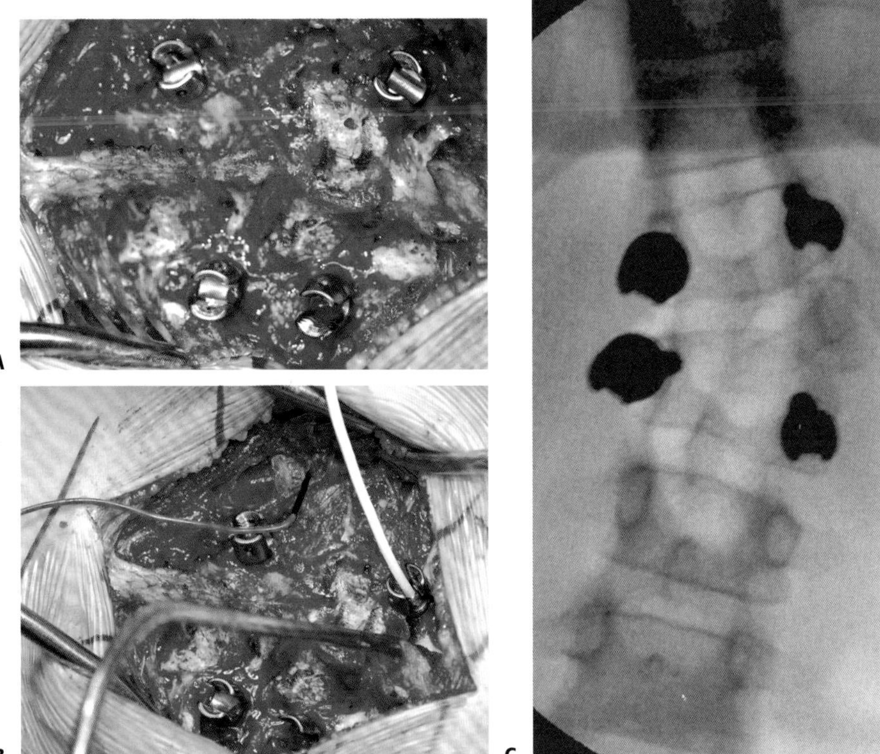


**TECH FIG 1** • Pedicle screw placement. **A.** Exposure of the spine with placement of screws. **B.** Triggered EMG stimulation of the pedicle screws. **C.** Fluoroscopic view confirming correct screw placement.

Cobb elevator and curved-tip device, followed by curved retractor placement (**TECH FIG 2A**).

  - This step aids in protection of structures lateral and anterior to the wall on the hemivertebra. If the hemivertebra is in the thoracic region, it will be necessary to resect the rib head first to obtain access.

- The cartilaginous surfaces of the concave facet should be resected to encourage fusion.
- Resection then begins in the midline with the ligamentum flavum using a Kerrison rongeur (**TECH FIG 2B,C**), followed by resection of the hemilamina.
  - Resection should extend over to the facet while the exiting nerve roots above and below the hemivertebra are identified and protected.
  - The transverse process and dorsal cortical bone over the pedicle can be resected in similar fashion until the cancellous bone of the pedicle and cortical outlines of its wall are visualized (**TECH FIG 2D,E**).
    - Care should be taken to avoid nerve roots, which are present rostral and caudal to the pedicle walls of the hemivertebra.
  - Gelfoam (Pfizer Inc., New York, NY) and cottonoids should be used judiciously to protect the dura and create a space between dura and bone to be resected.
- The subperiosteal plane down the lateral wall of the pedicle and body is then developed, with a Cobb elevator used to facilitate retraction and protection. The dural contents can be protected by a nerve root retractor.
  - Bipolar sealing of epidural vessels that lie on the medial aspect of the pedicle and down on the inner wall of the body will aid in controlling blood loss and improving visualization.
  - Continued resection down the pedicle and into the hemivertebra body can be done by a diamond-tipped burr, which helps protect against unwanted injury to soft tissue structures.
- Working stepwise within the walls of the pedicle and down within the confines of the body helps protect surrounding vital structures and makes removal of the cortical shells easier (**TECH FIG 2F**). The walls of the pedicle can then be easily resected with a curette or pituitary rongeur, as can the remaining walls of the body of the hemivertebra.
  - Protection lateral and anterior to the confines of the hemivertebra wall is necessary to avoid injury to vital structures such as the aorta. Generally, the dorsal cortex of the vertebral body is removed last (**TECH FIG 2G**).
- This resection is a wedge resection, which includes the discs above and below as well as the concave area of the disc.
  - The disc material should be removed with a pituitary rongeur and curettes; the dura and its contents are protected with a nerve root retractor.
  - If the disc material above and below is not removed, correction will be limited, and anterior fusion will be less reliable.

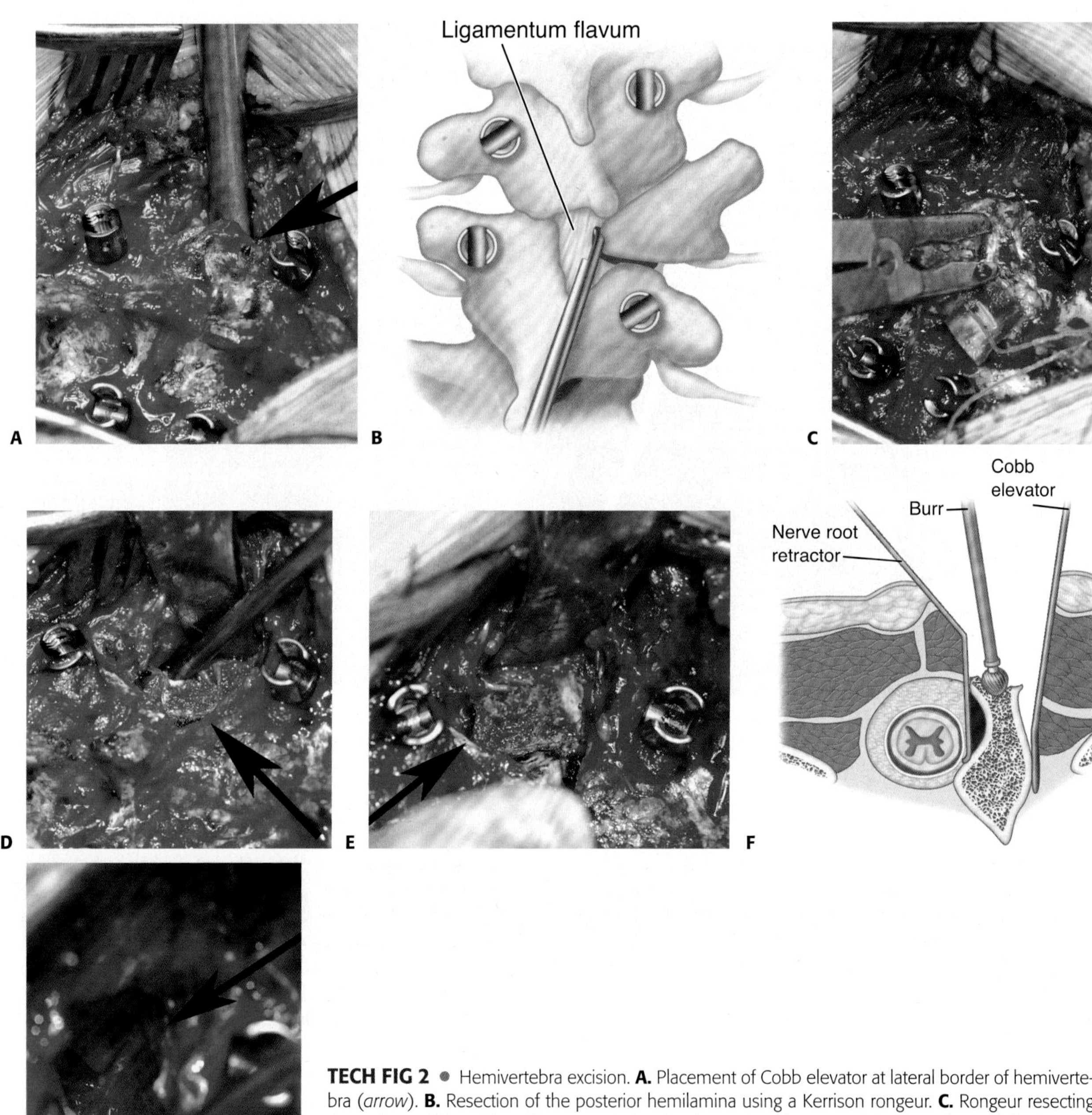


**TECH FIG 2** • Hemivertebra excision. **A.** Placement of Cobb elevator at lateral border of hemivertebra (*arrow*). **B.** Resection of the posterior hemilamina using a Kerrison rongeur. **C.** Rongeur resecting down the pedicle, with Gelfoam protecting the dura. **D.** Further resection down the pedicle (*arrow*), with lateral structures protected. **E.** Complete visualization of the vertebral body (*arrow*), with anterolateral protection. **F.** Axial schematic illustration of working down the pedicle with medial and lateral protection. **G.** *Arrow* points to the area of complete resection.

## Closure of Wedge Resection

- We place resected vertebral cancellous bone as well as allograft clips into the wedge resection site anteriorly.
- We have found that it is beneficial to compress and close the resection site with laminar hooks and by external three-point pressure on the body (**TECH FIG 3A**).
  - We place a downgoing supralaminar hook at the superior level and an upgoing infralaminar hook on the inferior level.
  - We place a rod and compress with closure of the resection site and correction of the deformity. Using this rod avoids having to place large compression forces across pedicle screws. This allows the screws to maintain correction without possible plowing of the screws into the immature bone or pedicles.
- The compression should be slow and controlled, with the dura directly visualized so that it is not caught in the closure of the posterior elements (**TECH FIG 3B,C**).
  - If insufficient correction is achieved or if the adjacent laminae abut prematurely, it may be necessary to resect further along the edges of the laminae.

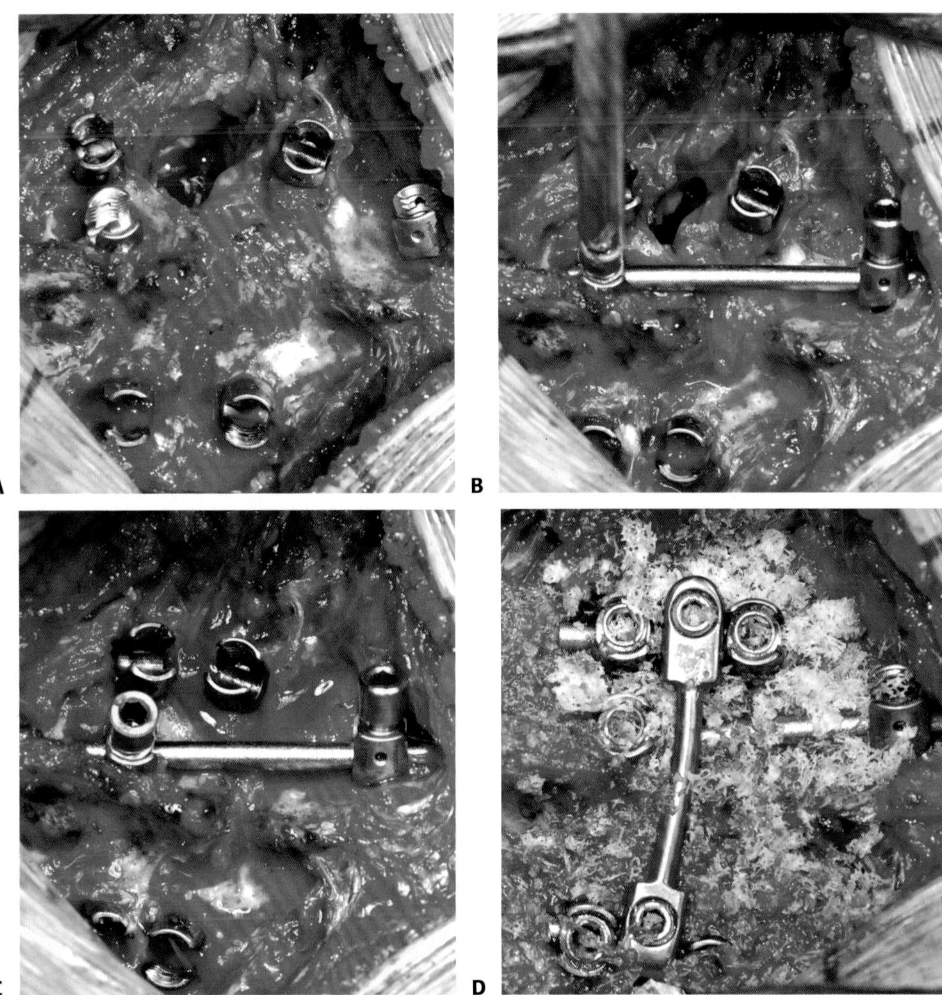

**TECH FIG 3** • Closure of wedge resection. **A.** Laminar hooks in place. Note the spacing between pedicle screws. **B.** Compression of laminar hooks with closure of the excision site. **C.** Complete closure of the excision site. The convex screws have now come together, representing wedge closure. **D.** The three-rod system in place, plus the cross-link that should be applied if technically feasible.

- Two additional rods are then placed, one on either side of the spine, connected to the corresponding screws. A cross-link should be applied if at all possible (**TECH FIG 3D**).
- The spine is then decorticated. We prefer to place corticocancellous allograft because it is effective and avoids harvesting the iliac crest.

## Anteroposterior Excision

- We routinely place our posterior implant anchors before performing any resection. Once complete exposure (both anterior and posterior) has been performed (**TECH FIG 4A**), posterior screws are placed.
- Anterior resection begins by creating a full-thickness subperiosteal flap over the hemivertebra after localization is confirmed (**TECH FIG 4B**).
- Starting at the inferior endplate of the adjacent superior body and the superior endplate of the adjacent inferior body, we create longitudinal full-thickness cuts in the periosteum.
  - At the endplate region, we make anteroposterior cuts in the periosteum and start a full-thickness periosteal flap, working anteriorly to the contralateral side.
  - We move posteriorly until we can visualize the hemivertebra pedicle.
- The discs above and below the hemivertebra are resected all the way posteriorly to the posterior longitudinal ligament.
- We then start resection of the hemivertebra vertebral body back to the posterior cortical wall of the body with rongeurs and a diamond-tipped burr.
  - The posterior wall can be resected and peeled off the posterior longitudinal ligament with a rongeur, obtaining access by starting at the level of the disc resections.
  - Part of the visualized pedicle can be resected.
- Posterior resection can then begin, starting with the hemilamina and proceeding to the pedicle (**TECH FIG 4C**).
- With both incisions open and fields exposed, resection of the pedicle can be done by working through both regions (**TECH FIG 4D**). This allows complete visualization and maximum control of the surgical field.
- Once the hemivertebra has been resected, correction of the deformity is the same as described earlier, using a three-rod technique if possible (**TECH FIG 4E**).
  - With this technique, correction is aided by unbreaking the table (or removing any lateral bolster) and pushing down on the convex spine to facilitate closure of the wedge resection.

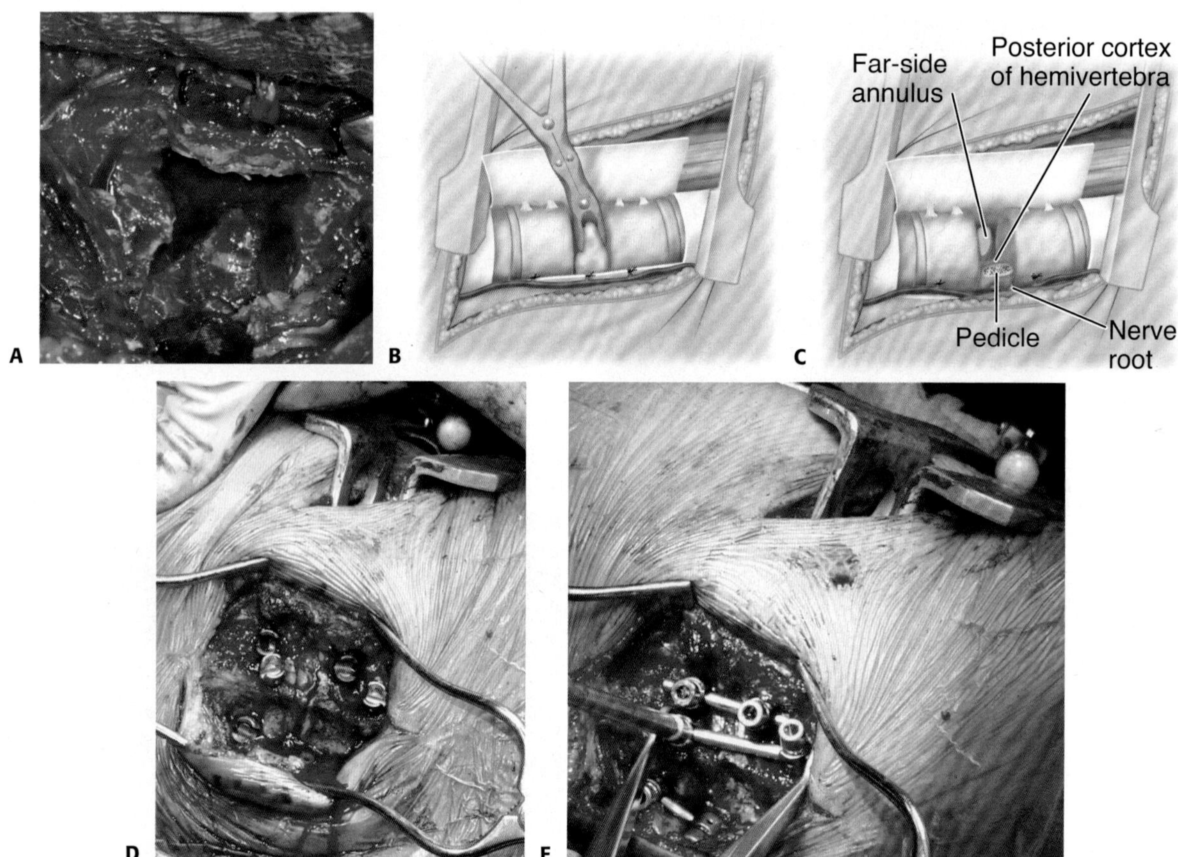


**TECH FIG 4** • AP excision. **A.** Hemivertebra isolated anteriorly with removal of discs above and below. **B.** Anterior resection. **C.** Resection back to the pedicle. **D.** Photograph of surgeon working through both operative sites simultaneously. **E.** Compression to close wedge resection site.

## PEARLS AND PITFALLS

| | |
|---|---|
| **Localization of the hemivertebra** | ▪ The intraoperative anatomy can be confusing. A thorough understanding of the patient's anatomy can be gained by studying the preoperative 3-D CT scans. |
| **Implant placement** | ▪ It is useful to place implant anchors first because the resection may make this difficult owing to blood loss and possible instability of the spine following resection. |
| **Blood loss** | ▪ Blood loss may be minimized by sealing the epidural veins on the inner aspect of the hemivertebral wall and pedicle with a bipolar cautery before resecting these areas. |
| **Inadequate correction** | ▪ Can be avoided by resection of the far-side concave disc and complete resection of the hemivertebra |

## POSTOPERATIVE CARE

- The immediate postoperative hospitalization and care are similar to that for most patients being treated for spinal deformity.
- When fixation is adequate, we place the patients in a custom-molded thoracolumbosacral orthosis for 3 months.
- In patients who are younger than 2 years of age, or in cases where fixation is not adequate, we recommend a Risser-type cast, to include a shoulder or both thighs for 2 months, followed by a brace for up to a total of 6 months postoperatively.
- The removal of spinal implants is not mandatory; however, given the young age of the patients and individual body habitus, occasionally, it is necessary to remove the implants after a year secondary to prominence.

## OUTCOMES

- Hemivertebra excision may be performed as a posterior-only technique or as a combined anteroposterior technique, with excellent curve correction of approximately 70% (**FIG 4**).[4]

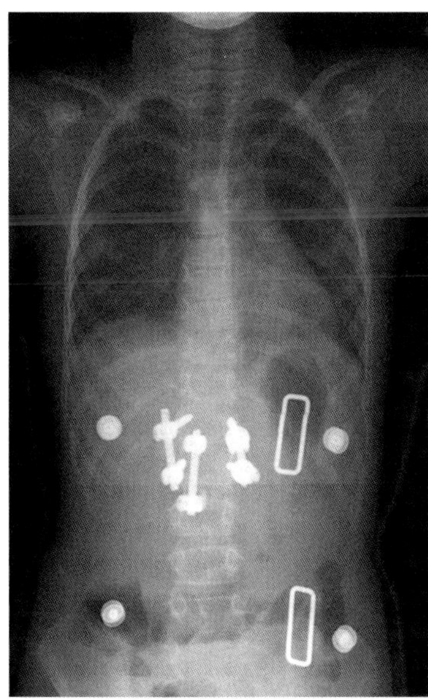


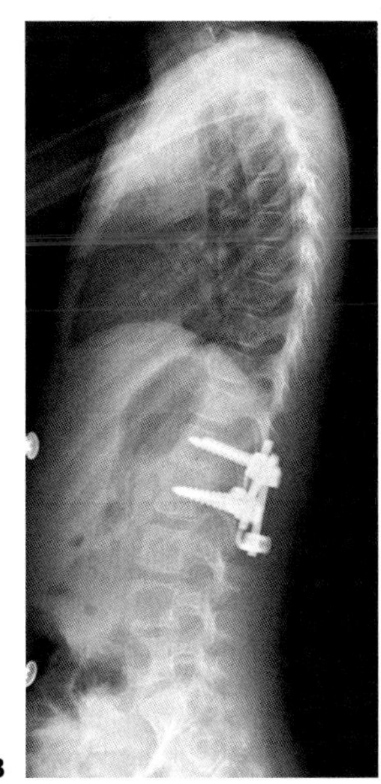


**FIG 4** • Correction of deformity. **A.** Postoperative standing radiograph after excision and curve correction of patient shown in **FIG 2A**. **B.** Standing lateral radiograph of the same patient showing excellent sagittal balance after excision.

- The rate of union for this procedure is near 100% in pediatric patients.
- The procedure may be performed safely using either technique with no neurologic complications.

## COMPLICATIONS

- Inadequate correction
- Dural injury
- Neurologic injury
- Loss of fixation
- Implant failure
- Excessive blood loss
- Nonunion
- Infection

## REFERENCES


1. Hedequist D, Emans J. Congenital scoliosis. J Am Acad Orthop Surg 2004;12:266–275.
2. Hedequist DJ, Hall JE, Emans JB. Hemivertebra excision in children via simultaneous anterior and posterior exposures. J Pediatr Orthop 2005;25:60–63.
3. McMaster MJ, David CV. Hemivertebra as a cause of scoliosis. A study of 104 patients. J Bone Joint Surg Br 1986;68(4):588–595.
4. Ruf M, Harms J. Hemivertebra excision by a posterior approach: innovative operative technique and first results. Spine 2002;27:1116–1123.


## SUGGESTED READINGS


1. Belmont PJ Jr, Kuklo TR, Taylor KF, et al. Intraspinal anomalies associated with isolated congenital hemivertebra: the role of routine magnetic resonance imaging. J Bone Joint Surg Am 2004;86-A(8):1704–1710.
2. Hedequist DJ, Emans JB. The correlation of preoperative three-dimensional computed tomography reconstructions with operative findings in congenital scoliosis. Spine 2003;28:2531–2534.

# Decompression, Posterolateral, and Interbody Fusion for High-Grade Spondylolisthesis

Nanjundappa S. Harshavardhana, Dino Colo, and John P. Dormans

## DEFINITION

- *Spondylolisthesis* is derived from the Greek words (spondylo = spine and olisthesis = to slip). It is the forward displacement of a vertebra relative to its neighboring vertebra (ie, adjacent caudal vertebral segment).
- In children and adolescents, spondylolisthesis most commonly occurs due to a pars defect (ie, nonunion of the pars interarticularis). Wiltse called this an isthmic type of spondylolisthesis. It may also occur in the presence of inherent spinal anomalies such as deficient or maloriented lumbar and lumbosacral facets (ie, dysplastic or congenital type).[2,11,12,16,27,29]
- It has been grouped into five different types under the Wiltse-Newman classification[28]:
  - Type I: dysplastic
  - Type II: isthmic
  - Type III: degenerative
  - Type IV: traumatic
  - Type V: pathologic
- Pars interarticularis is "the place between two joints".[17] Most spondylolisthesis cases are of dysplastic (congenital), isthmic, and degenerative types. Degenerative listhesis is common in adults and most commonly seen at L4–L5 level. The dysplastic and isthmic types most commonly affect L5–S1 level and are usually seen in children (**FIG 1A**).
- The Meyerding classification is used to quantify the severity of slippage (**FIG 1B**) and has five grades[19]:
  - Grade I: 0% to 25% slip
  - Grade II: 26% to 50% slip
  - Grade III: 51% to 75% slip
  - Grade IV: 76% to 100%
  - Grade V: corresponds to spondyloptosis

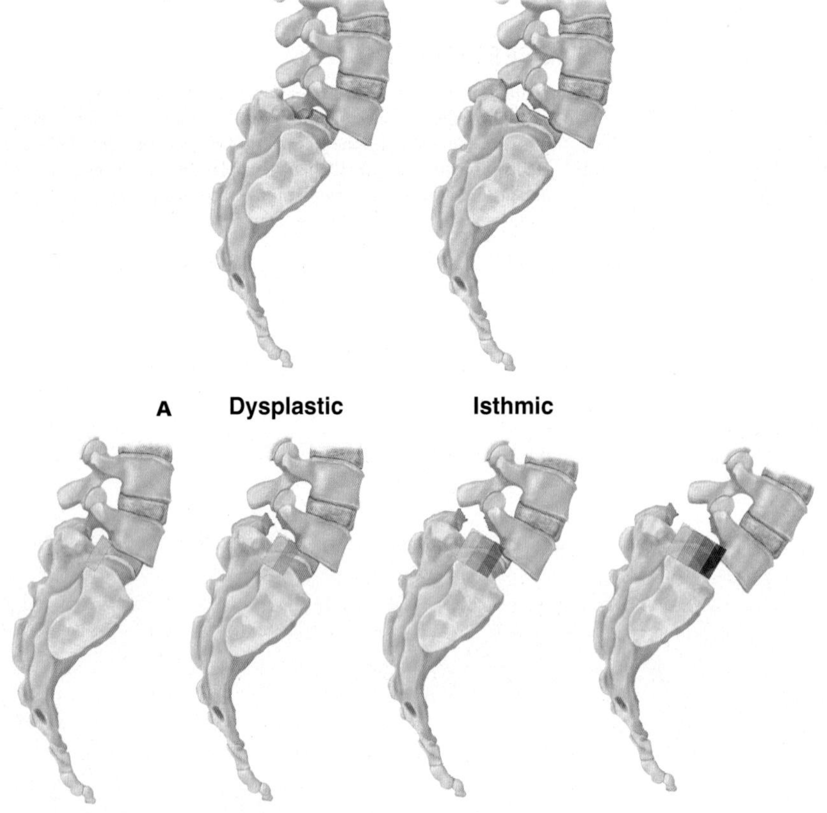


**FIG 1** • **A.** The dysplastic and isthmic types of spondylolisthesis. **B.** The Meyerding classification is based on degrees of slippage: grade I, 0 to 25%; grade II, 26% to 50%; grade III, 51% to 75%; grade IV, 76% to 100%.

- Marchetti and Bartolozzi divided spondylolisthesis into low- and high-grade slips irrespective of underlying etiology.[17] Anterior slippage of 50% or more (Meyerding grade III and above) of the transverse width of the caudal segment is termed a *high-grade slip*.

## ANATOMY

- The vertebral bodies increase in size and dimensions with progression caudally from the cervical spine. This increase is believed to be related to the demands of increased stress and weight bearing placed on the lumbosacral spine.
- The lumbar vertebrae have a wider transverse diameter in comparison to the anteroposterior (AP) diameter. The lumbar foramina appear trefoil-like. The spinous processes have a larger surface area and have an oblong appearance. Transverse processes are long, slender, project laterally, and are more oriented in the sagittal plane allowing for flexion and extension motion.[24,30]
- The neurovascular structures in the lumbar spine run a similar course as in the thoracic spine. The segmental vasculature arises directly from the aorta and runs dorsally around the lateral aspect of each vertebral body. Branching occurs near the pedicles, wherein one branch supplies the spinal canal and the other supplies the paraspinal musculature. These vessels run between the transverse processes and are susceptible to bleeding in lateral dissection while performing a posterolateral fusion.
- The spinal cord usually ends at the upper border of L1 or L1–L2 disc. The conus medullaris extends from the most distal portion and innervates the bowel and bladder. Beneath the conus, the lumbar and sacral nerve roots are arranged to form the cauda equina. Each of these roots exits below the pedicle of the corresponding vertebrae from the neural foramen and form the lumbar/lumbosacral plexus that innervates the lower extremities.[6]
- The pedicles are cylindrical structures with a cortical shell that bridge the posterior elements of the spine with the vertebral body.
  - The height and diameter as well as the transverse diameter of the pedicles increases from the thoracic to the lumbar spine. T5 has the narrowest and L5 has the widest transverse diameter.
  - They are directed medially in the transverse plane, increasing gradually from L1 to L5.
    - The sagittal plane orientation of the lumbar spine pedicles is neutral at L2 and L3.
    - It has a mild cephalad angulation at L1 and caudal angulation at L4 and L5.[24,30]
- The spinal cord and the dural sac lie within the vertebral canal protected by vertebral body ventrally, pedicles laterally, and posterior elements dorsally. The exiting nerve roots are in proximity with the inferior aspect of the pedicle.[24]
- The orientation of the facet joints in the lumbar and lumbosacral spine is related to function. In the upper part of the lumbar spine, the orientation of the joints allows for multidirectional stabilization. This is in contrast to the lumbosacral facet joint, which is flat and more coronally oriented and acts to resist shearing forces through the joint.[10]

## PATHOGENESIS

- Spondylolisthesis is a disorder related to upright posture and seen in bipedal mammals due to increasing forces acting on the lower segments of the spine. It is never seen in quadrupeds and nonambulatory individuals.
- The lumbar spine is subject to high shear forces and compressive loads. The "bony hook," consisting of the pedicle, pars interarticularis, intervertebral disc, and the facet joints, provides stability by resisting these shear forces by preventing forward slippage.
- Gravity, paraspinal, and anterior abdominal muscle contraction on the lordotic lumbar spine and pelvis apply forces to the lower lumbar vertebra with a caudal–ventral vector. If left unchecked, these forces would cause the lower lumbar vertebrae to slip and rotate forward relative to the sacrum.
- Congenital anomalies of the posterior elements in spina bifida (ie, dysplastic spondylolisthesis) can significantly compromise their normal buttressing function and stability offered by the facet joints. The spine has a tendency to slip even if the posterior elements are intact. This is brought about by the structural abnormality in the facet joint's inability to resist the load and shear forces.
- In the isthmic type of spondylolisthesis, secondary to a pars defect, there is loss of posterior restraint. The high shear and compressive forces occurring through the lumbar spine and lumbosacral joint are less well resisted.[11–13]
- Observing the spectrum of spondylolisthesis developing owing to such dysplastic elements prompted Marchetti and Bartolozzi to further subdivide this category into low and high-grade dysplasias.[17] Of the high-grade spondylolisthesis, they identified mainly two subtypes: (1) with elongation and (2) with lysis.
- In low-grade spondylolisthesis, the L5 vertebral body maintains its rectangular shape. The superior endplate of the sacrum is flat and lumbar lordosis remains within the normal range. However, high-grade spondylolisthesis has a trapezoidal L5 body and rounding of the superior sacral endplate (dome-shaped sacrum). The sacrum tends to be vertical with loss of lumbar lordosis (flat back). This distinction between high and low dysplasia also has prognostic value, as high-grade dysplasias lead to progressive deformity and predisposition for lumbosacral kyphosis with worsening of symptoms over time.[17]
- Some of the changes seen in high-grade slips are secondary to forward displacement of vertebrae. They are mainly seen as Modic endplate changes in discs with degeneration. High-grade slips may already occur by adolescence and the severity of deformity makes it highly unlikely that these teenagers remain asymptomatic or progress into adulthood without progressive worsening of symptoms.

## NATURAL HISTORY

- Harris and Weinstein[13] reviewed 38 cases with high-grade spondylolisthesis treated nonoperatively and with in situ fusion with a mean follow-up of 24 years and showed that 36% of patients treated nonoperatively were asymptomatic, 55% had back pain, and 45% had neurologic symptoms.
- Beutler et al[2] in a 45-year follow-up study of 30 patients diagnosed with spondylolysis, screened in the 1950s from

a pool of 500 first-grade children, showed that no patients with unilateral pars defects developed spondylolisthesis. They also showed that cases with bilateral pars defects and low-grade slips follow a course similar to that seen in the general population. Slowing of slip progression was observed with each decade.[2]

- In a comparison of patients with dysplastic and isthmic spondylolisthesis, it was found that dysplastic spondylolisthesis progressed more rapidly and to a greater Meyerding grade than isthmic spondylolisthesis.[18]

## PATIENT HISTORY AND PHYSICAL FINDINGS

- In symptomatic patients, the most common clinical manifestation is low back pain, with or without radicular pain radiating through the L5 or S1 dermatome. Onset of pain is usually chronic and insidious, but acute episodes do occur. Pure radiculopathy in the absence of back pain is uncommon. Adolescents and teenagers most often complain of back pain with little or no leg pain.[16]
- In patients with radicular symptoms, unilateral involvement is more common.
- Flattening of the lumbar lordosis is commonly seen on physical examination (**FIG 2**).
- A palpable step in the spinous processes is often seen in isthmic spondylolisthesis.
- Abnormal gait exemplified by a flexion at hips and knees gait pattern and tight hamstrings may be present (Phalen-Dickson gait).
- Hamstring tightness is recorded by measuring the popliteal angle. Many patients with high-grade slips will have a tendency to develop tight hamstrings owing to the development of abnormal biomechanics in the lumbar spine.
- Straight-leg raise should be done to test for nerve root compression or hamstring tightness. A positive examination with radicular pain denotes either an L5 or S1 nerve root compression. Radicular pain elicited between 30 and 70 degrees is indicative of nerve root compression, whereas that elicited above 70 degrees might denote extraspinal compression of the sciatic nerve. Pain in the posterior thigh denotes hamstring tightness.

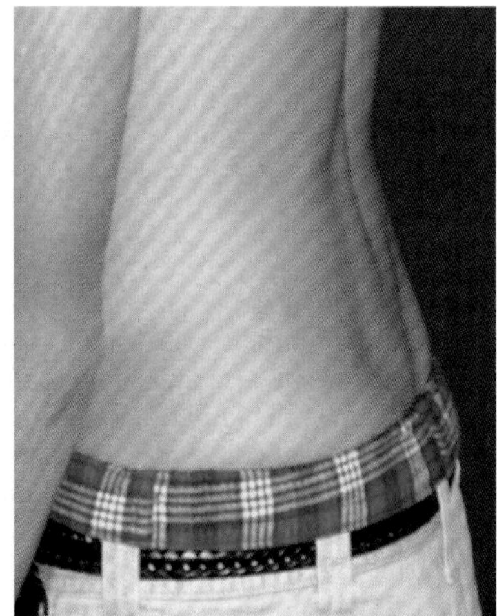

**FIG 2** • A 14-year-old boy diagnosed with spondylolisthesis with flattening of the lumbar lordosis.

- Examination should also include the Lasegue test. Exacerbation of the pain is suggestive of nerve root tension (most commonly L5). Femoral nerve stretch test might be positive in degenerative listhesis (L4 being most commonly affected).
- A digital rectal examination should be done in suspected cases of bladder and bowel dysfunction as a part of preoperative neurologic assessment.

## IMAGING AND OTHER DIAGNOSTIC STUDIES

- Initial imaging includes standing posteroanterior and lateral radiographs of the spine (**FIG 3A,B**). Oblique views (**FIG 3C**)

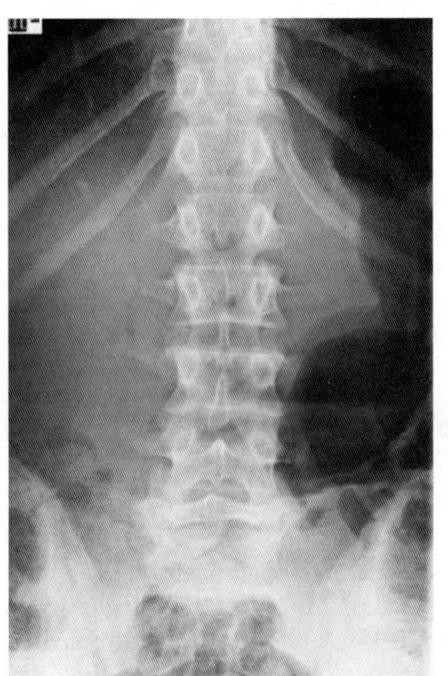

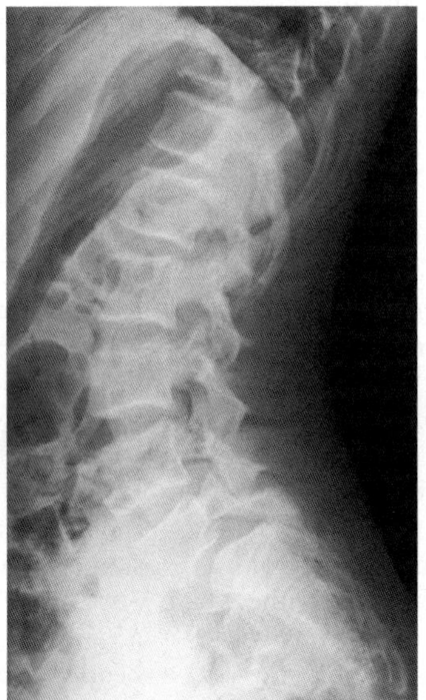

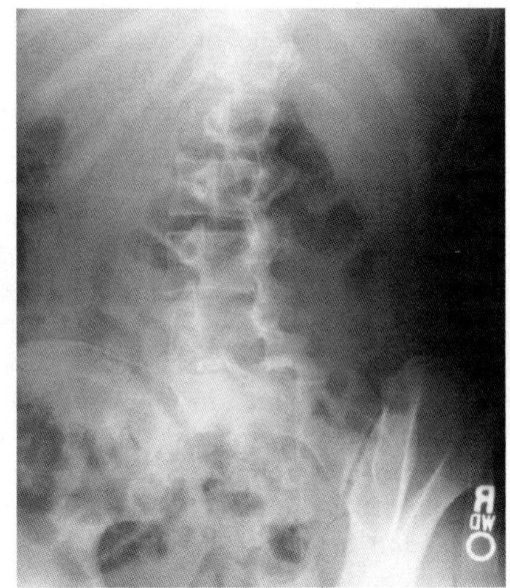

**FIG 3** • Posteroanterior (PA) (**A**), lateral (**B**), and oblique (**C**) radiographs demonstrating high-grade spondylolisthesis. *(continued)*

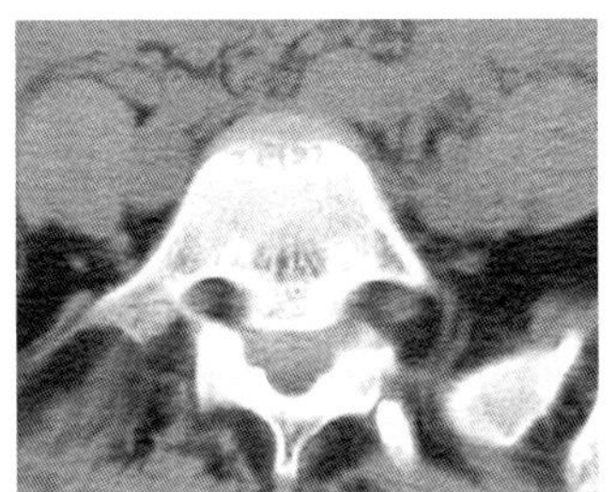
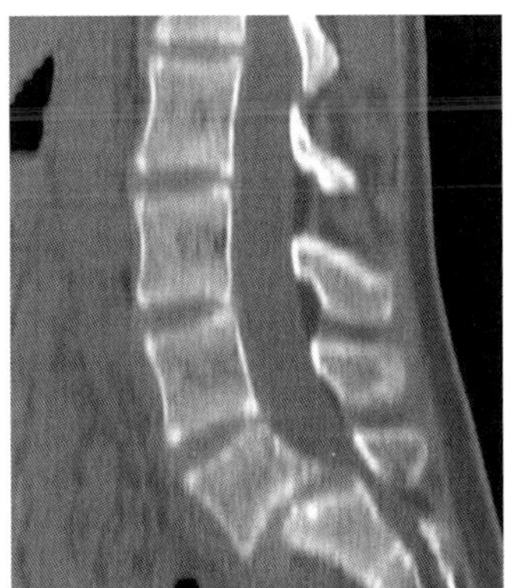
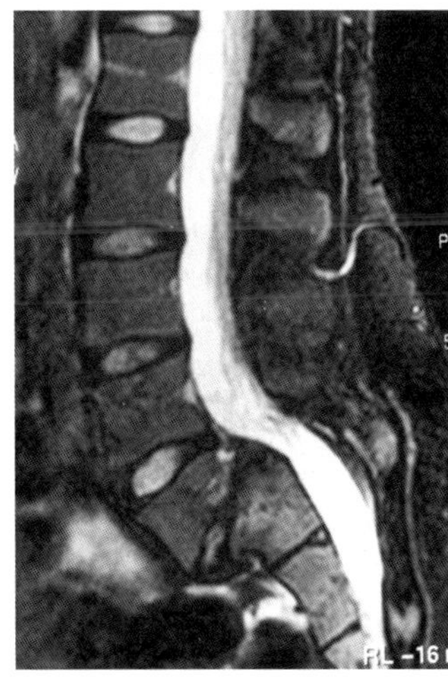

**FIG 3** • *(continued)* Axial (**D**) and sagittal (**E**) CT scan sections demonstrating bony deformity. **F.** MRI demonstrating high-grade spondylolisthesis.

may provide additional information in certain cases, but their use for diagnosing spondylolysis without listhesis in adolescents is controversial.[1]

- Plain radiographs are used to establish the overall alignment of the spine in both the coronal and sagittal plane. The sagittal alignment should be noted, particularly the degree of lumbar lordosis above the lumbosacral kyphosis. Any structural abnormalities in the spine in addition to the slip should be noted. These abnormalities include the presence of spina bifida occulta, scoliosis, or sagittal plane abnormalities. Other spinal problems should be treated as per individual merits.
- Coned down view of lumbosacral junction and Ferguson view (20-degree cranially angulated AP x-ray centered over lumbosacral junction) may also be performed to rule out coexistent far out syndrome.
- Computed tomography (CT) scans with three dimensional (3-D) reconstruction are valuable in defining the exact bony abnormality and will help in preoperative planning (**FIG 3D,E**).
- Magnetic resonance imaging (MRI) studies are indicated when there is evidence of neurologic compromise. MRI provides good visualization of nerve roots, spinal stenosis, and cauda equina compression (**FIG 3F**).

## DIFFERENTIAL DIAGNOSIS

- Mechanical disorders: trauma, overuse syndromes, herniated disc, and slipped vertebral apophysis
- Developmental disorders: Scheuermann kyphosis
- Inflammatory disorders: discitis, vertebral osteomyelitis, calcific discitis, rheumatologic conditions
- Neoplastic disorders

## NONOPERATIVE MANAGEMENT

- Surgery is generally recommended for the treatment of high-grade spondylolisthesis in adolescents and teenagers. Even in asymptomatic cases, the risk of progression or the development of cauda equina syndrome warrants surgical intervention.
- Asymptomatic adults with high-grade stable slips may be treated conservatively under close supervision. They have been reported to autofuse in an acceptable, good sagittal balance.[13]

## SURGICAL MANAGEMENT

- The first goal of surgical management is to avoid complications.
- Surgical management is indicated in high-grade slips, with or without the presence of neurologic compromise, or in refractory symptomatic patients.
- The reduction techniques for high-grade spondylolisthesis are associated with high risk of complications. Distorted anatomy, stretched nerve roots, prolonged surgery, and a challenging biomechanical environment with a deep or hidden trajectory for L5 pedicle screw insertion increase the potential for nerve root injuries, nonunion, and other perioperative complications.[21]
- A growing consensus is evolving that the priority of high-grade spondylolisthesis is restoration of lumbosacral lordosis (ie, reduction in slip angle), not complete correction of AP translation. Although anatomic correction of AP translation offers restoration of lumbosacral biomechanics with increased surface area for interbody fusion (and hence enhanced fusion rates), slip translational reduction is associated with a high incidence of lumbar nerve root injury and cauda equine syndrome.
- Selecting the appropriate surgical intervention for each patient requires:
  - A thorough evaluation of the deformity
  - An in-depth understanding of the nature of the pathology
  - An understanding of the indications for treatment
  - Awareness of the limitations of each procedure and its possible complications

### Preoperative Planning

- A detailed assessment of the history and physical and neurologic examinations should be performed.

- All imaging studies must be carefully reviewed and analyzed with attention aiming to correlate physical and neurologic findings with those found in special examinations.
- The degree of the slip as seen on the lateral standing spine radiographs is assessed and graded according to the Meyerding classification.[2]
  - Slippage of 50% or more is considered a high-grade slip.
- The *slip angle* measures the degree of lumbosacral kyphosis.
  - A slip angle greater than 50 degrees is associated with progression, instability, and pseudarthrosis (**FIG 4A**).
- *Pelvic incidence* (PI) is a fixed anatomic parameter that estimates the position of the sacral endplates and overall pelvic morphology. It helps to determine the overall sagittal profile of the spine and is constant for a particular individual. Pelvic incidence is defined as the sum of the pelvic tilt and sacral slope.[14,15]
  - The PI increases with age and stabilizes in adulthood.
  - The mean PI is 47 degrees in children and 57 degrees in adults.
  - Increased PI is indicative of increased lumbar lordosis and increased shear forces (**FIG 4B**). Increased PI may predispose to the development of spondylolisthesis.[14,15]
  - In the presence of spondylolisthesis, an increased PI may be indicative of an unbalanced pelvis and is a risk factor for slip progression. Slip reduction is required in these cases to restore proper spinopelvic biomechanics and stabilize the spine. In cases where the spine is balanced and PI is low, a fusion in situ may be all that is required for treatment.[15]

## Positioning

- The patient is positioned prone on the operative frame.
- Two operative positions are commonly used for posterior approaches to the spine.
  - The first is the knee-chest position, where both the hips and knees are flexed.
  - The second position is with the use of a four-poster frame, where the lower extremities are fairly parallel to the trunk. In this position, the patient is supported under the anterior superior iliac spines and pectoral muscles bilaterally. The abdomen is free to reduce venous engorgement and intraoperative bleeding.
  - Our preference is to place the patient in the Jackson spinal table with the hips and knee in the flexed position, allowing for easier access to the lumbar spine.
- The position of the face and arms is important.
  - The face should be adequately supported in a head holder, making sure that no excessive pressure is applied, especially around the orbits.
  - The neck should be in neutral position.
  - The upper extremities should also be in 90–90 position, in which the arms are in 90 degrees of abduction and the elbows are in 90 degrees of flexion. The upper extremities should be adequately padded to allow for venous and arterial access. Hyperabduction is avoided to minimize the risk of brachial plexopathy and traction injury to the brachial plexus. Adequate padding, support, positioning, and monitoring of the upper extremities likewise prevents undue neurologic injury due to stretch or excessive pressure.

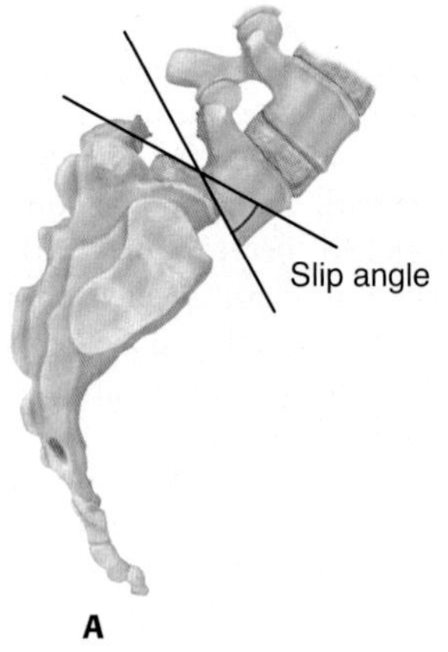


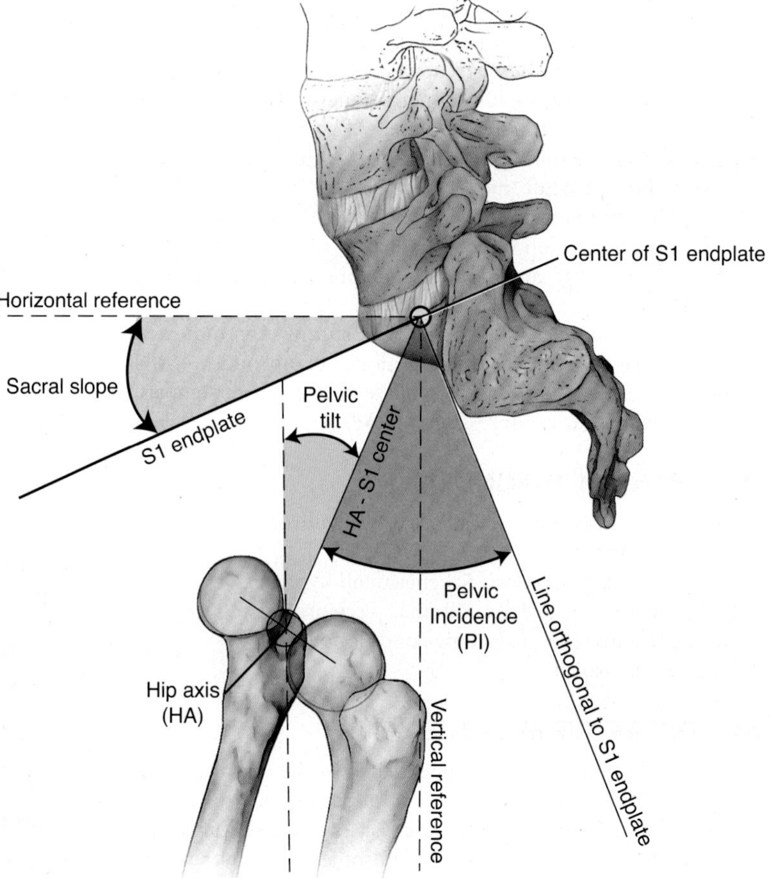


**FIG 4** ● **A.** Slip angle is a measure of lumbosacral kyphosis. A slip angle greater than 50 degrees is associated with progression, instability, and pseudarthrosis. **B.** PI (PI = pelvic tilt [PT] + sacral slope [SS]) is the angle formed between a line perpendicular to the center of the sacral endplate and a line connecting this point to the center of the femoral heads (equal to hip axis). In contrast to PI, PT and SS are positional spinopelvic parameters, which can change with the position and orientation of the subject. PT is the angle between the line connecting the midpoint of the sacral endplate to the hip axis and the vertical reference line. SS is the angle between the superior endplate of S1 and the horizontal reference line.

## Incision and Dissection

- The lumbar spine is approached posteriorly through a direct midline incision extending from L2 to S2 (**TECH FIG 1A**).
- The midline incision is carried down to the fascia through sharp dissection of the skin and subcutaneous tissue.
- The midline dissection is carried down subperiosteally, exposing the posterior elements of the spine, with care taken to protect the most proximal intact facets (**TECH FIG 1B,C**).
- In isthmic spondylolisthesis, removal of loose bodies (the *rattler*) and the posterior elements of L5 (the *Gill fragment*) is done.[9]

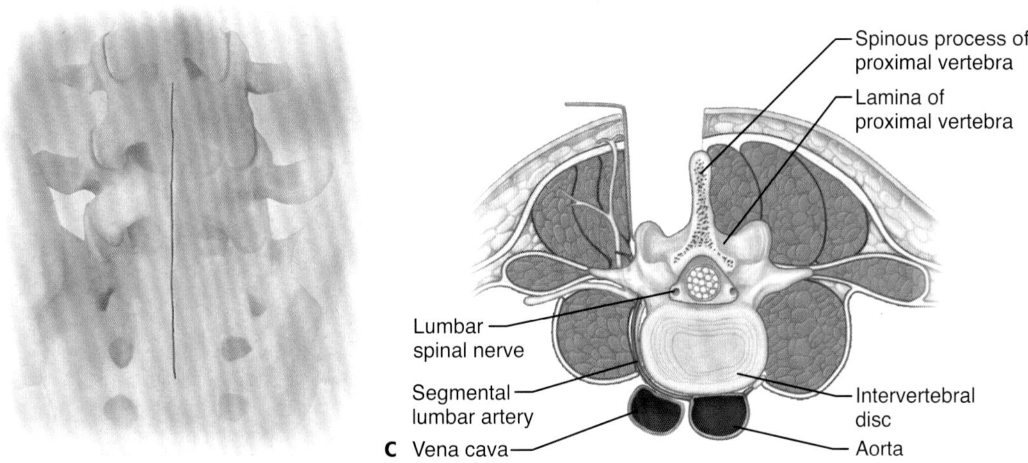


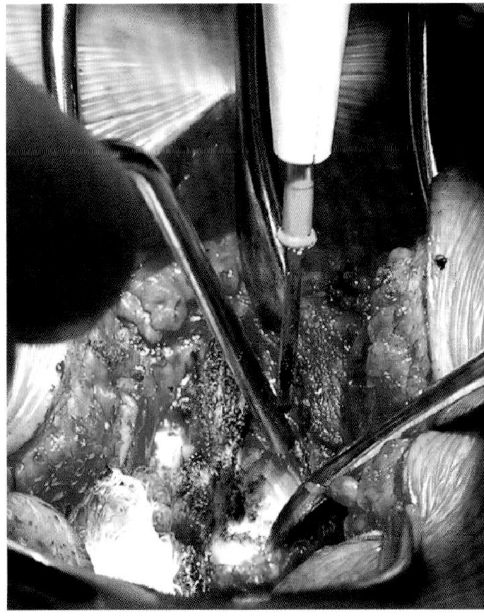


**TECH FIG 1** • **A.** A direct midline posterior skin incision along the spine is made, extending from L4 to S2. **B,C.** The fascia is incised along with the skin incision, and the paraspinal muscles are dissected off of the posterior elements subperiosteally.

## Decompression

- The nerve roots of L5 and S1 are identified, and a wide decompression of the L5/S1 roots is carried out bilaterally (**TECH FIG 2A**).
- The dura and neural elements over the sacrum are gently retracted, and a sacroplasty is done using an osteotome or a high-speed diamond burr (**TECH FIG 2B**).

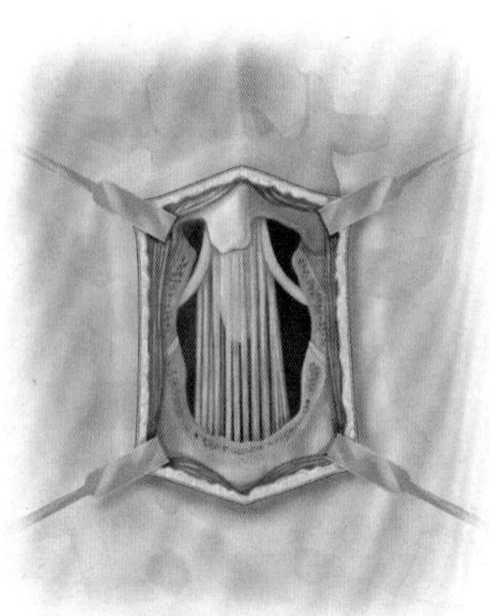

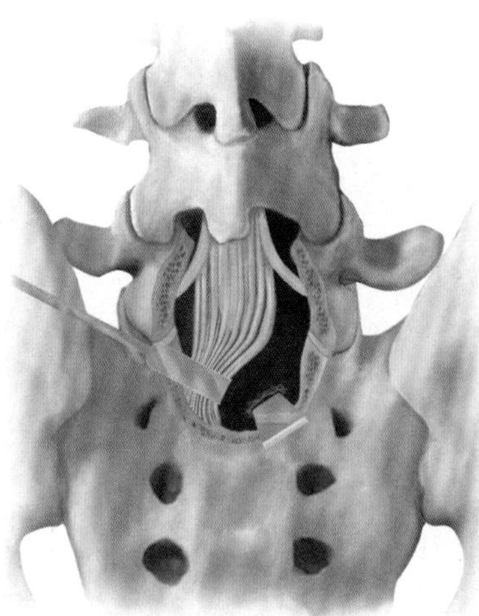

A B

**TECH FIG 2** • **A.** A wide laminectomy is performed by removing the posterior elements of L5 and S1, and adequate decompression of the nerve roots is done. **B.** The dura is retracted gently, and a sacroplasty is then performed to take pressure off of the dura by using an osteotome.

## Reduction and Fusion

- Pedicle screws are placed into the L4, L5, S1, and S2 pedicles (**TECH FIG 3A**). Use of intraoperative navigation increases the chances of first-time accurate and safe pedicle screw, especially in the distorted anatomy of the L5–S1 junction.
- Alternatively, iliac screws (7.5- to 8.5-mm diameter long cancellous screws inserted into iliac wings) can be used for enhanced fixation and pull-out strength.
- The anesthetic and spinal monitoring team is informed before any corrective maneuvers are performed.
- The reduction is performed under fluoroscopic guidance, avoiding overcorrection. With the use of reduction tools attached to the pedicle screws, the slip angle is gradually reduced under fluoroscopic guidance by applying a dorsal extension maneuver to the lumbar pedicle screws (**TECH FIG 3B**).
  - The reduction is performed slowly and maintained over time to allow for stretch of the soft tissue. Once a satisfactory correction of the slip angle has been achieved, gradual, partial reduction of the slip may performed by applying force to the sacrum while a counterforce is applied to the lumbar spine (**TECH FIG 3C**). As mentioned, this slip correction is associated with neurologic injury, especially to the L5 root.
  - Reduction of the slip angle is much more important than reduction of the slip itself. Frequent, accurate spinal cord monitoring is crucial during the entire reduction maneuver.
- The rods are templated, cut, and contoured and then attached to the construct while reduction is maintained.
- Final tightening of the entire construct is done and checked with fluoroscopy or plain radiographs (**TECH FIG 3D**).
- The L5–S1 disc is identified and removed, a fusion is performed, and the L5–S1 disc space is filled with cancellous autograft or allograft.
- An anterior cage is placed to provide adequate anterior column support (**TECH FIG 3E**).
- As an alternative, a fibular strut graft (modified Bohlman technique)[3,26] can be inserted from the sacrum to the body of L5 to add anterior column support. The dura is gently retracted to one side, and a guide pin is inserted from the sacrum to the body of L5 (**TECH FIG 3F**).
  - A 6-mm cannulated reamer is then used to ream this channel.

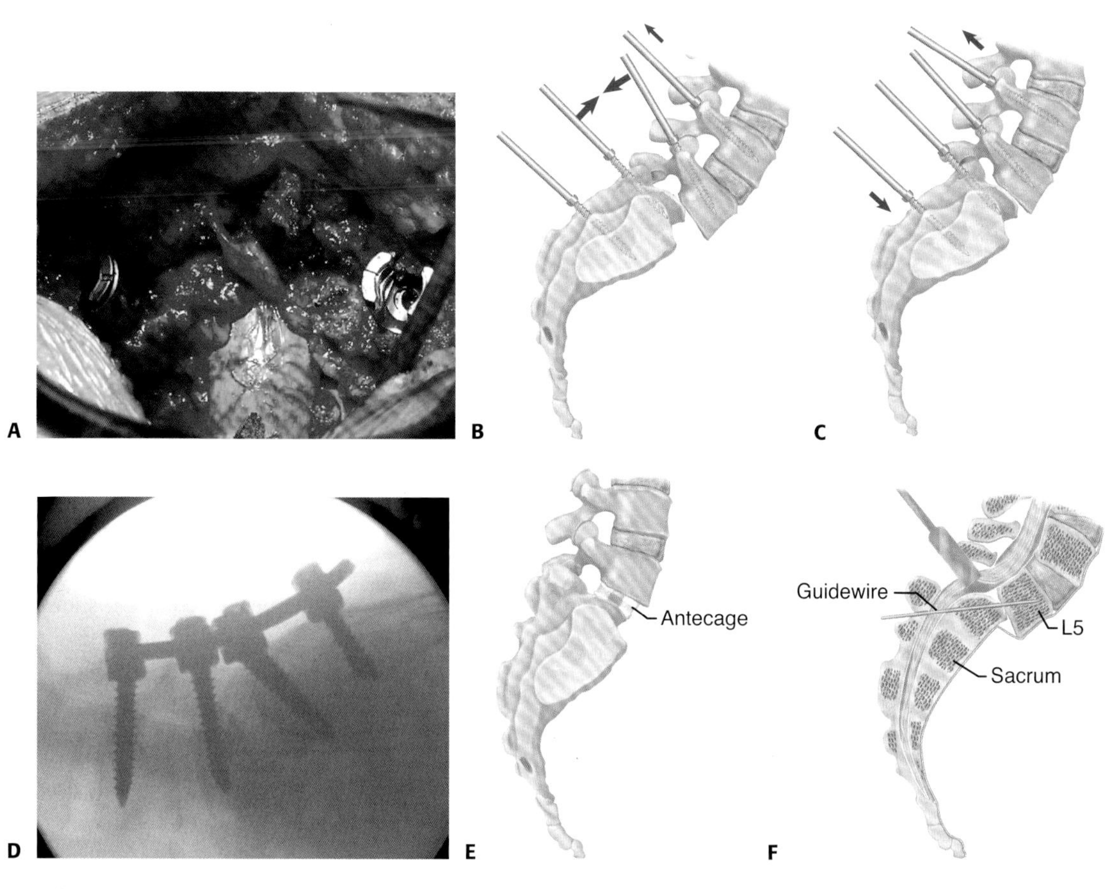


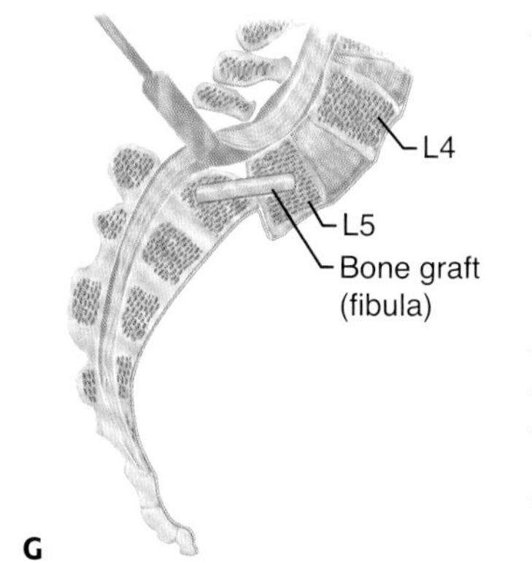


**TECH FIG 3** • **A.** Pedicle screws are placed from L4 to S2. Once all of the pedicle screws have been placed, a gentle reduction is performed, aimed at correcting the slip angle. **B.** Using reduction tools attached to the pedicle screws, a dorsal extension force is applied to the lumbar spine while a counterforce is applied to the sacrum. This maneuver gently corrects the slip angle and restores lumbar lordosis. Attention to spinal cord monitoring is crucial at this point in the operation to avoid undue neurologic injury. **C.** Following correction of the slip angle, gradual correction of the slip is performed by applying pressure on the sacrum while the lumbar spine is held and a gentle force is applied in the opposite direction, affording reduction. Overcorrection of the slip should be avoided. **D.** The entire construct is checked after reduction under fluoroscopy to ensure proper implant placement and adequate correction of the spondylolisthesis, and final tightening is done. **E.** The dura is gently retracted, and a cage is placed to add anterior column support. **F.** Alternatively, fibular strut grafting may be used to provide anterior column support. This is done by inserting a guide pin through the sacrum to the body of L5. **G.** A split fibular graft is fashioned and countersunk into each drill hole bilaterally.

- A fibular auto- or allograft is then placed through the channel and countersunk (**TECH FIG 3G**).
  - The same procedure is repeated on the contralateral side.
- The procedure is completed by placing bone graft lateral to the implants along the transverse processes from L4 to the sacrum.
- Meticulous hemostasis is carried out, and a layer-by-layer closure of the operative site is performed with sprinkling of vancomycin powder over the instrumentation and soft tissues deeper to deep fascia. A drain is placed superficial to deep fascia.

## PEARLS AND PITFALLS

| | |
|---|---|
| **Indications** | ▪ A complete history and physical and neurologic examination must be performed before surgery.<br>▪ All needed and appropriate imaging studies must be evaluated carefully to identify all aspects of the deformity—including the degree of the deformity and the type (eg, isthmic vs. congenital)—as well as any other coexistent spinal deformity that may be present (eg, spina bifida occulta). |
| **Surgical exposure** | ▪ Careful and meticulous technique must be observed. Care should be taken, especially when pathologies such as spina bifida occulta are present, to prevent iatrogenic neurologic injury.<br>▪ Decompression of at-risk nerve roots (ie, L5 and S1) is a key component to exposure and operation. |
| **Instrumentation** | ▪ Careful preparation should be undertaken before performing instrumentation and reduction.<br>▪ Adequate decompression of all neurologic structures at risk should be ensured to prevent iatrogenic injury.<br>▪ Close attention must be paid to neurophysiologic monitoring during both instrumentation and reduction. |
| **Reduction** | ▪ Slow, gentle force is applied during the reduction maneuver. This procedure should be done over time to allow for relaxation of the soft tissue structures.<br>▪ Avoid excessive reduction of the translation. Reduction of the slip angle is more important than reduction of AP vertebral translation. Excessive reduction may result in neurologic compromise. |

## POSTOPERATIVE CARE

- High-quality radiographs are taken immediately postoperatively to ensure proper graft and instrumentation placement before the patient is taken out of the operative room (**FIG 5**).
- In the immediate postoperative period, the hips and knees are flexed and elevated using pillows to alleviate pain and immediate tension on the L5 root.
- Pain control is instituted (eg, intrathecal analgesia and intravenous [IV] patient-controlled analgesia), and the patient is fitted with a thoracolumbosacral orthosis for comfort. The patient is then encouraged to stand and ambulate as tolerated. Postoperative posteroanterior and lateral standing spine radiographs are taken before discharge.
- Activity restriction (ie, avoidance of bending and rotational motion) is carried out until fusion has occurred (at about 4 to 6 months).
- The patient may return to sports and strenuous physical activity after 1 year as long as spinal fusion has been confirmed. Adequate precautionary measures should be taken before engaging in any contact sport.
- Full-contact sports, which may entail collision, should still be avoided.

## OUTCOMES

- In high-grade spondylolisthesis treated with in situ fusion techniques, clinical improvement in back pain symptoms has been reported in 74% to 100% of cases. Solid fusion rates have also been reported to be 71% to 100%.[7,11,13,20,21]
- A study on 18 adolescents with high-grade spondylolisthesis treated with instrumented reduction and fusion reports complete resolution of preoperative neurologic symptoms with 100% fusion rates. No loss of fixation or instrument-related failures were reported at a minimum follow-up of 2 years.[25]
- Another series[21] comparing in situ fusion, decompression, reduction with instrumented posterior fusion, and circumferential fusion techniques in treating high-grade spondylolisthesis

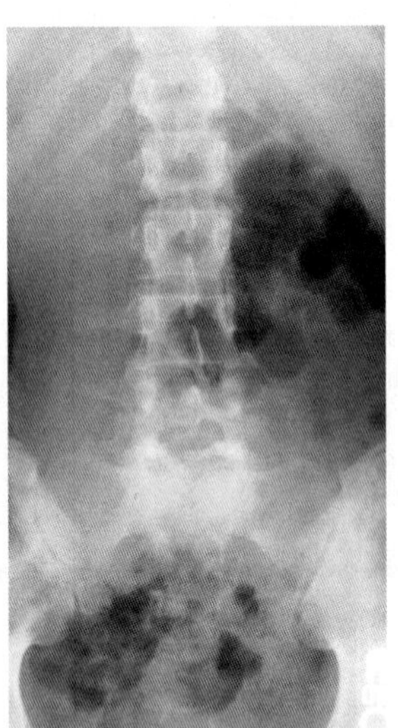
A

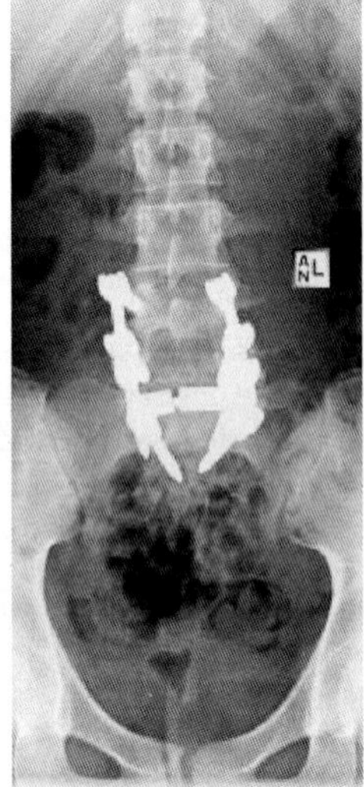
B

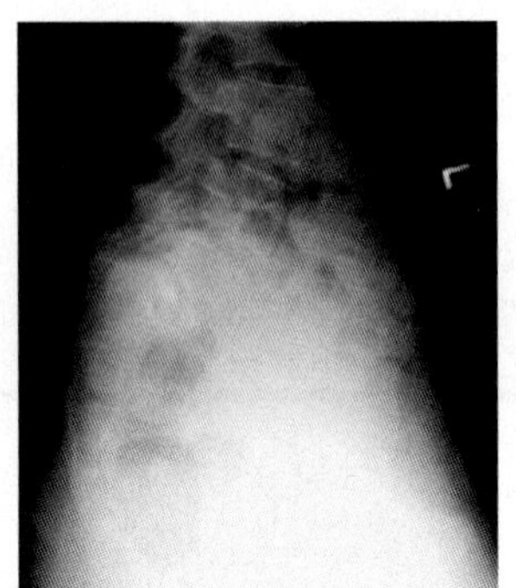
C

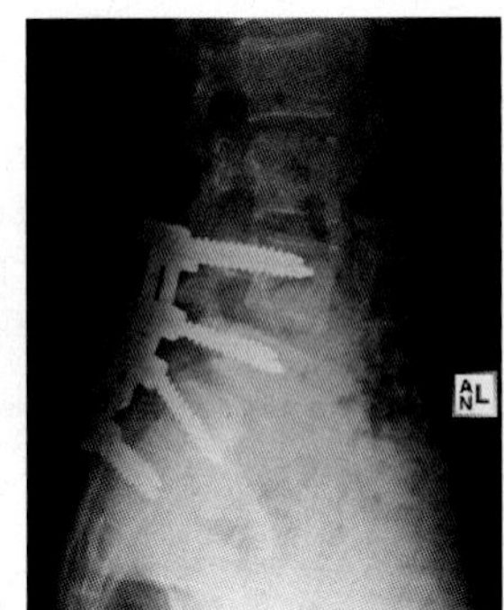
D

**FIG 5** • Radiographs from a 17-year-old girl with high-grade isthmic spondylolisthesis who underwent decompression, reduction, and instrumented fusion. **A,C.** Initial PA and lateral radiographs showing the preoperative deformity. **B,D.** PA and lateral films showing postoperative correction using the CHOP technique.

**Table 1 Scoliosis Research Society Morbidity and Mortality Database Summary for High-Grade Spondylolisthesis (Meyerding III to V)[a]**

| Age Groups | No. of Patients | Overall Complication Rate | Neurodeficit | Mortality | Visual Loss |
|---|---|---|---|---|---|
| **Pediatric** | 127 | 10.4% | 11.3% | 0/605 | 0/605 |
| **Adult** | 67 | 9.2% | 22.9% | 10/10,242 cases (0.10%) | 5/10,242 cases (0.05%) |

[a]Scoliosis Research Society started collecting info on the grade of slip only w.e.f. 2007 onward.
From Fu KM, Smith JS, Polly DW Jr, et al. Morbidity and mortality in the surgical treatment of six hundred five pediatric patients with isthmic or dysplastic spondylolisthesis. Spine 2011;36(4):308–312; Sansur CA, Reames DL, Smith JS, et al. Morbidity and mortality in the surgical treatment of 10,242 adults with spondylolisthesis. J Neurosurg Spine 2010;13:589–593.

reported a 45% (5 of 11 patients) pseudarthrosis rate in patients treated with in situ fusion and a 29% (2 of 7 patients) pseudarthrosis rate in cases treated with posterior decompression, instrumentation, and fusion. All of these cases had small transverse processes (surface area of <2 cm$^2$). Circumferential techniques achieved the highest fusion rates. Excellent functional outcomes were observed in those cases where a solid fusion was achieved. Final outcomes, however, did not differ amongst the three groups.

- The posterior lumbar interbody fusion (PLIF) is an attractive alternative in the treatment of high-grade spondylolisthesis. It allows for satisfactory decompression and circumferential arthrodesis by a single approach. There are mixed results in the literature for this procedure. Cloward[5] reported on 100 patients using uninstrumented PLIF without posterolateral fusion. He found a 93% fusion rate and 90% clinical satisfaction. Fabris et al[7] reported on 12 patients with 100% fusion rate with instrumented fusion.
- Poussa et al[22] compared 22 pediatric patients treated with in situ fusion or reduction with pedicle screw posterior fixation and circumferential fusion. The reduction group had better radiographic correction of slip angle and improvement in Meyerding grade, but no differences were seen in terms of function or pain. Boxall et al[4] reported on 39 pediatric patients treated with either in situ fusion, decompression and fusion, or reduction and posterior fusion. Twenty-six percent of patients with solid fusion had a slip angle of greater than 50 degrees preoperatively. The authors concluded that a high-slip angle is predictive for slip progression and recommended reduction and fusion in such patients. Molinari et al[20,21] reviewed 32 patients treated with either in situ L4 to sacrum fusion, posterior decompression with instrumented reduction and fusion, or reduction and circumferential fusion. No patient in the circumferential fusion subgroup had pseudarthrosis, whereas the in situ fusion and instrumented fusion groups had 45% and 29% pseudarthrosis rates, respectively. Outcomes were excellent in those patients who attained fusion regardless of the surgical procedure performed.

## COMPLICATIONS

- Pseudarthrosis
  - Pseudarthrosis is the most common complication.
  - Signs include lucency around implants, implant breakage, and slip progression.
  - Pseudarthrosis may be minimized by using meticulous technique and proper preparation of the graft site.[21]
- Neurologic complications
  - Neurologic complications
  - Root lesions (L5 root)
    - From direct trauma, manipulation of nerve roots or compression from an epidural hematoma
  - Cauda equina syndrome
    - Autonomic dysfunction
    - Chronic pain
    - Immediate release of the correction should be done when necessary.
    - Must be thoroughly evaluated with proper imaging techniques
    - May be minimized by good preoperative planning and meticulous surgical technique and by using multimodal spinal cord monitoring
  - A review of 605 cases of pediatric spondylolisthesis from the Scoliosis Research Society identified 127 cases of high-grade slips and reduction was attempted in 76% of the cases. The incidence of neurologic deficit was 11.3% as against to 1.4% for low-grade slips. The overall postoperative neurologic deficit was 5% (31/605 cases). 29/31 patients had neurologic recovery (15 complete and 14 partial recovery). Dural tears were seen in 1.3% of the cases (8/605).[8]
  - A review of 10,242 cases of adult spondylolisthesis from the same database identified 67 cases of high-grade slips and 1700 low-grade slips. The overall complication rate for high-grade spondylolisthesis was 22.9% in comparison to 8.3% for low-grade spondylolisthesis. The overall mortality rate was 0.1% (10 deaths) and visual loss was 0.05% (5 cases). The complication rate was similar for various approaches and instrumentation preferences, that is, combined AP, PLIF and TLIF, and anterior fusions at 7% to 8% (Table 1).[23]
- Transition syndromes
  - Spondylolisthesis acquisita
  - Adjacent segment degeneration
  - S1–S2 deformity
- Instrument-related complications
- Wound infections

## REFERENCES


1. Beck NA, Miller R, Baldwin K, et al. Do oblique views add value in the diagnosis of spondylolysis in adolescents? J Bone Joint Surg Am 2013;95(10):e65.
2. Beutler WJ, Fredrickson BE, Murtland A, et al. The natural history of spondylolysis and spondylolisthesis: 45-year follow-up evaluation. Spine 2003;28:1027–1035.

3. Bohlman HH, Cook SS. One-stage decompression and posterolateral and interbody fusion for lumbosacral spondyloptosis through a posterior approach: report of two cases. J Bone Joint Surg Am 1982;64:415–418.
4. Boxall D, Bradford DS, Winter RB, et al. Management of severe spondylolisthesis in children and adolescents. J Bone Joint Surg Am 1979;61(4):479–495.
5. Cloward RB. Spondylolisthesis: treatment by laminectomy and posterior interbody fusion. Clin Orthop Relat Res 1981;(154):74–82.
6. Ebraheim NA, Xu R, Darwich M, et al. Anatomic relations between the lumbar pedicle and the adjacent neural structures. Spine 1997;22:2338–2341.
7. Fabris DA, Costantini S, Nena U. Surgical treatment of severe L5-S1 spondylolisthesis in children and adolescents. Results of intra-operative reduction, posterior interbody fusion, and segmental pedicle fixation. Spine 1996;21(6):728–733.
8. Fu KM, Smith JS, Polly DW Jr, et al. Morbidity and mortality in the surgical treatment of six hundred five pediatric patients with isthmic or dysplastic spondylolisthesis. Spine 2011;36(4):308–312.
9. Gill GG. Long-term follow-up evaluation of a few patients with spondylolisthesis treated by excision of the loose lamina with decompression of the nerve roots without spinal fusion. Clin Orthop Relat Res 1984;(182):215–219.
10. Grobler LJ, Robertson PA, Novotny JE, et al. Etiology of spondylolisthesis. Assessment of the role played by lumbar facet joint morphology. Spine 1993;18:80–91.
11. Grzegorzewski A, Kumar SJ. In situ posterolateral spine arthrodesis for grades III, IV, and V spondylolisthesis in children and adolescents. J Pediatr Orthop 2000;20:506–511.
12. Hammerberg KW. New concepts on the pathogenesis and classification of spondylolisthesis. Spine 2005;30(6 suppl):S4–S11.
13. Harris IE, Weinstein SL. Long-term follow-up of patients with grade III and IV spondylolisthesis. Treatment with and without posterior fusion. J Bone Joint Surg Am 1987;69:960–969.
14. Labelle H, Roussouly P, Berthonnaud E, et al. Spondylolisthesis, pelvic incidence, and spinopelvic balance: a correlation study. Spine 2004;29:2049–2054.
15. Legaye J, Duval-Beaupère G, Hecquet J, et al. Pelvic incidence: a fundamental pelvic parameter for three-dimensional regulation of spinal sagittal curves. Eur Spine J 1998;7:99–103.
16. Lonstein JE. Spondylolisthesis in children. Cause, natural history, and management. Spine 1999;24:2640–2648.
17. Marchetti PC, Bartolozzi P. Classification of spondylolisthesis as a guideline for treatment. In: Bridwell KH, DeWald RL, eds. The Textbook of Spinal Surgery, ed 2. Philadelphia: Lippincott-Raven, 1997:1211–1254.
18. McPhee IB, O'Brien JP, McCall IW, et al. Progression of lumbosacral spondylolisthesis. Australas Radiol 1981;25:91–95.
19. Meyerding HW. Spondylolisthesis. J Bone Joint Surg Am 1931;13(1):39–48.
20. Molinari RW, Bridwell KH, Lenke LG, et al. Anterior column support in surgery for high-grade, isthmic spondylolisthesis. Clin Orthop Relat Res 2002;(394):109–120.
21. Molinari RW, Bridwell KH, Lenke LG, et al. Complications in the surgical treatment of pediatric high-grade, isthmic dysplastic spondylolisthesis. A comparison of three surgical approaches. Spine 1999;24:1701–1711.
22. Poussa M, Remes V, Lamberg T, et al. Treatment of severe spondylolisthesis in adolescence with reduction or fusion in situ: long-term clinical, radiologic and functional outcome. Spine 2006;31(5):583–590.
23. Sansur CA, Reames DL, Smith JS, et al. Morbidity and mortality in the surgical treatment of 10,242 adults with spondylolisthesis. J Neurosurg Spine 2010;13:589–593.
24. Senaran H, Yazici M, Karcaaltincaba M, et al. Lumbar pedicle morphology in the immature spine: a three-dimensional study using spiral computed tomography. Spine 2002;27:2472–2476.
25. Shufflebarger HL, Geck MJ. High-grade isthmic dysplastic spondylolisthesis: monosegmental surgical treatment. Spine 2005;30(6 suppl):S42–S48.
26. Smith MD, Bohlman HH. Spondylolisthesis treated by a single-stage operation combining decompression with in situ posterolateral and anterior fusion. An analysis of eleven patients who had long-term follow-up. J Bone Joint Surg Am 1990;72:415–421.
27. Wiltse LL, Jackson DW. Treatment of spondylolisthesis and spondylolysis in children. Clin Orthop Relat Res 1976;(117):92–100.
28. Wiltse LL, Newman PH, Macnab I. Classification of spondylolysis and spondylolisthesis. Clin Orthop Relat Res 1976;(117):23–29.
29. Wiltse LL, Winter RB. Terminology and measurement of spondylolisthesis. J Bone Joint Surg Am 1983;65:768–772.
30. Zindrick MR, Knight GW, Sartori MJ, et al. Pedicle morphology of the immature thoracolumbar spine. Spine 2000;25:2726–2735.

# Rib to Pelvis Vertical Expandable Prosthetic Titanium Rib Insertion to Manage Neuromuscular Scoliosis

96 CHAPTER

Anish G. R. Potty and John M. Flynn

## DEFINITION

- Vertical expandable prosthetic titanium rib (VEPTR) has gained enormous worldwide popularity in the last decade as an effective method to manage potentially lethal chest and spine deformity in children.
- Initially, VEPTR was used primarily to expand the congenitally abnormal chest, particularly in circumstances where there were fused, absent, or hypoplastic ribs.
- As surgeons gained familiarity with the technique, the VEPTR device was adopted as a very effective nonfusion method to manage severe early-onset neuromuscular scoliosis in conditions such as spinal muscular atrophy (SMA), spina bifida, and cerebral palsy.
- With refinement, the rib to pelvis bilateral VEPTR technique has become one of the most commonly used initial implant strategies for these conditions because the technique can be done through a few small incisions, the spine is left untouched (and thus hopefully, unfused), and the expansions for growth are simple and of low morbidity.[7]

## ANATOMY

- The thoracic cage is composed of 12 pairs of ribs, the sternum, and 12 thoracic vertebrae. The ribs are interspaced with intercostal muscles. The external intercostals arise from the inferior border of one rib and attach to the superior border of the caudal rib with the external intercostal membrane lying posterior to it. Below this is the internal intercostal which has its fibers running at right angles to the external intercostal and the internal intercostal membrane deeper to the internal intercostal.
- The neurovascular structures which are composed of the intercostal vein, artery, and nerve live beneath the internal intercostal muscle. It is important to understand that the vein lies superior to the subcostal groove, whereas the artery and the nerve reside inferior to the subcostal groove. This nerve innervates the adjacent intercostal muscles. Further deeper to the internal intercostal but above the parietal pleura is the innermost intercostal muscle, which becomes the transversus thoracic muscle anteriorly.
- A normal thoracic development during childhood is essential for lung growth. Hence, respiratory function will depend on the lung growth and ability of the thorax to act as a dynamic pump to facilitate inhalation and exhalation.
  - The complexity of thoracic growth is not well understood but it is believed that the thoracic spine plays a critical role and contributes to vertical growth of the rib cage.
- The thoracic spine grows 1.4 cm per year from birth to 5 years of age, 0.6 cm per year from 6 to 10 years of age, and 1.2 cm per year from 11 to 15 years of age.[1,3]
  - The expected shortening of the thoracic spine can be calculated in congenital scoliosis or early spine fusion but the complex relationship between loss of thoracic volume and thoracic spine shortening and its indirect adverse effect on lung volume and expansion has yet to be quantified and remains unclear.
  - However, studies done on a natural history model of spondylothoracic dysplasia (Jarcho-Levin syndrome),[4] in which the thoracic spine is only one-fourth of normal height in adults, have shown most surviving adults to have restrictive lung disease with an average vital capacity of only 27%.
- Symmetric growth and the correct orientation of the ribs for the age of the child contributes to the width and depth of the rib cage and helps to maximize volume expansion and make respiration more effective. The thoracic cross-sectional volume is directly proportional to the length of the ribs and the degree of rib obliquity. At birth, infants have a square shaped thoracic cross-section, which becomes a more rectangular-shaped thoracic cross-section in adults.
- The ribs are oriented horizontally and the growth of the ribs occurs primarily at the anterior physis. At birth, the thoracic volume is only 6.7% of the adult volume. By 2 years of age, the ribs grows downward more obliquely and the thoracic cross-section changes to an oval shape. By 5 years of age, the thoracic volume increases to 30% of the adult size and to 50% of the adult size by 10 years of age. From age 10 years to skeletal maturity, the thorax grows rapidly and doubles itself to the adult size.
- Almost 85% of lung alveolar cells are formed immediately after birth, with only slight increase in the first 2 years of life. The end age of alveolar cell formation is controversial and so is the concept of alveolar cell hypertrophy. The lungs still continue to increase in size even if the alveolar cell formation ceases due to compensatory lung growth triggered by a lung "stretch reflex." Experimental pneumonectomy in young animals and partial pneumonectomy in children aged 30 months to 5 years showed compensatory lung growth by alveolar cell multiplication.

## PATHOGENESIS

- VEPTR is currently widely accepted treatment for volume depletion deformities of the thorax (VDD). VDD can be classified into three main types:
  - Type I: absence of ribs and exotic scoliosis
  - Type II: ribs that are fused and exotic scoliosis

- Type IIIa: hypoplastic and foreshortened thoracic cavity as in Jarcho-Levin syndrome
- Type IIIb: transverse constricted as in Jeune thoracic dystrophy or the windswept thorax of scoliosis

## NATURAL HISTORY

- Thoracic insufficiency may initially present with early occult respiratory deficiency when the child begins to show signs of limited pulmonary capacity. They fatigue easily with play activities and compensate with an increased respiratory rate at rest but do not yet require oxygen support. The final sequela of progressive thoracic insufficiency syndrome is respiratory insufficiency.
- An increase in the ventilation requirements reflects an exponential clinical deterioration in respiratory function with important consequences for the family and the child.
- Early-onset scoliosis in neuromuscular conditions such as SMA begins in the first decade of life due to truncal weakness. It then progress steadily unless managed surgically and can become lethal. It occurs in 100% of the type I SMA and most of the type II SMA when they become nonambulators.

## PATIENT HISTORY AND PHYSICAL FINDINGS

- Physical examination should include careful evaluation of the spinal deformity, pelvic obliquity, sitting balance, and shoulder balance.
- Respiratory effort is assessed by determining the rate of respiration, lung auscultation for abnormal breath sounds, anthropomorphic measurements (height, weight, chest circumference at the nipple line, and limb length) looking for failure to thrive, and the thumb excursion test to evaluate thoracic wall expansion during respiration.

## IMAGING AND OTHER DIAGNOSTIC STUDIES

- The radiographic assessment includes standard posteroanterior (PA) (**FIG 1**) and lateral views of the spine with rib cage. The Cobb angle is measured for the scoliosis, and the head and truncal decompensation is assessed. The space available for the lungs to expand is measured by the ratio between the concave heights to the convex height.
- If cervical spine instability is a possibility, a cervical spine series including flexion and extension views is performed.
- A formal consultation with a pediatric pulmonologist, including pulmonary function testing, is very valuable to establish baseline function and counsel the family appropriately regarding risk of postoperative pulmonary complications.
- Magnetic resonance imaging (MRI) of the entire spine should be ordered to evaluate the spinal cord and those children who have any physical findings concerning for tethered cord.
- Computed tomography lung volumes can be compared with normative values to provide more information but such results may not be available.
- Dynamic MRI may be performed to assess the function of the diaphragm, and a screening MRI is routinely performed to look for abnormalities such as cord tethering or syrinx.
- Echocardiogram can be done to detect early-onset cor pulmonale.

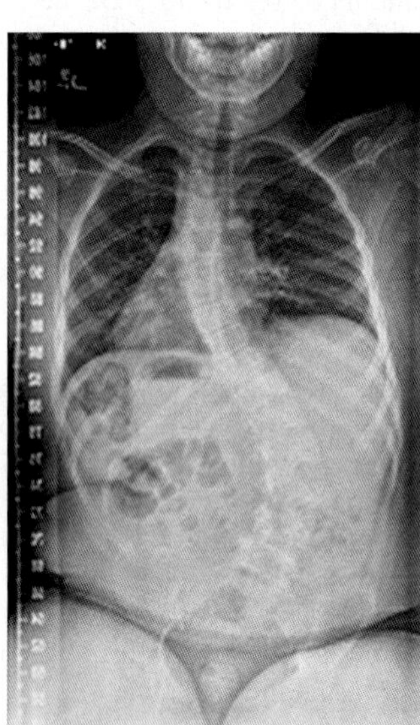

**FIG 1** • Preoperative radiograph of a 10-year-old boy with SMA and progressive scoliosis. The preoperative Cobb angle was 56 degrees and a 3.5-cm pelvic tilt.

## NONOPERATIVE MANAGEMENT

- The primary nonoperative option is observation, with serial radiographs and close monitoring of pulmonary function.
- In some cases, braces or serial casting can be offered, although it is often impractical in children with neuromuscular spinal deformity at risk for thoracic insufficiency.

## SURGICAL MANAGEMENT

- Bilateral rib to pelvis VEPTR technique offers a relatively minimally invasive way to manage early-onset neuromuscular scoliosis associated with thoracic insufficiency. The technique can be performed with relatively low blood loss and morbidity and with much less risk of autofusion as is seen in standard dual growing rod techniques.
- The bilateral rib to pelvis VEPTR technique is generally contraindicated in ambulatory children because a recent report shows a significant incidence of crouched gait, likely due to mechanical factors at the lumbosacral junction.[7]

### Indications

- A rapidly progressive curve with pelvic obliquity and nonambulatory patients. Thoracic insufficiency may or may not be present.
- A greater than 10% reduction in the height of the hemithorax on the concave side of the curve compared with the height of the contralateral hemithorax (space available for the lung is <90%)
- Progressive thoracic insufficiency syndrome
- An age of at least 6 months up to skeletal maturity. The younger the patient, the more likely there will be beneficial lung growth with thoracic expansion.
- Concurrent approval of the previously mentioned indications by a pediatric orthopaedist, a pediatric general surgeon, and a pediatric pulmonologist

### Contraindications

- Inadequate soft tissue coverage for the devices. Generally, this correlates clinically with a child with a body weight below the 25th percentile.

- Inadequate rib bone stock for device attachment, such as in a patient with severe osteogenesis imperfecta
- Absence of cephalad osseous ribs for attachment of the devices
- Inability to undergo repetitive episodes of general anesthesia because of cardiac disease, pulmonary disease, or other medical conditions
- Active pulmonary infection
- Absent diaphragm function

## Preoperative Planning

- At our institution, all patients with possible thoracic insufficiency syndrome are evaluated by a multidisciplinary team of clinicians including a pediatric orthopaedic surgeon, a pediatric general surgeon, and a pediatric pulmonologist.
- Preoperative full-length spinal radiographs should be reviewed, with careful attention to the anatomy of the ribs and pelvis, which will become anchor fixation sites.
- Preoperative nutritional evaluation is valuable for children with very low body mass index (BMI).

## Positioning

- The patient is placed in the prone position over gel bolsters. The upper extremities are draped out of the field with the shoulders flexed no more than 90 degrees.
- Upper and lower extremity intraoperative multimodal spinal cord monitoring is performed.
- A pulse oximeter is placed on the hand on the side of the operation. Both an arterial line and a central venous line are established. Prophylactic antibiotics are given intravenously.

TECHNIQUES

## Exposure

- The C-arm image intensifier is used to mark out four longitudinal incisions.
- As in all cases of VEPTR surgery, it is critically important to avoid placing the actual incision directly over the anchor site. Incision should always be either medial or lateral to the anchor site by a centimeter or two.
  - This fundamental principle of VEPTR surgery will markedly decrease the risk of postoperative wound breakdown for your patients, especially those with poor nutrition and limited subcutaneous tissue.
- The two proximal longitudinal paraspinous incisions are for the proximal cradles to the right and left upper thoracic rib segments.
- Two longitudinal distal incisions are placed for the pelvic hooks on the right and left ilium (**TECH FIG 1**).

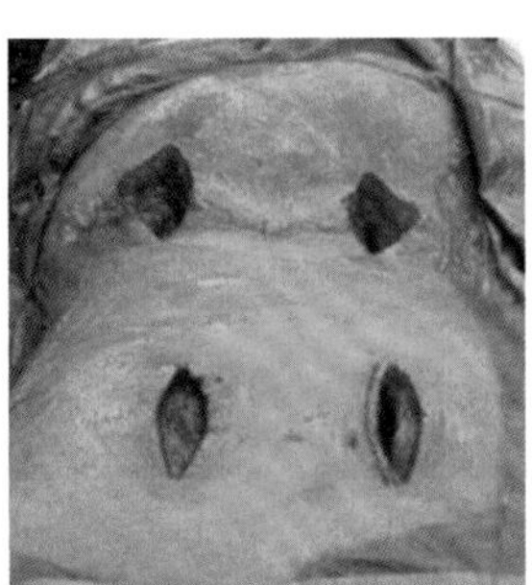

**TECH FIG 1** ● Ten-year-old boy with a history of SMA and progressive scoliosis. He was placed in prone position over gel bolster and incision sites marked under C-arm. Two proximal incision on either side of T4–T5 rib segments at the top of the picture and two distal incisions over the right and left ilium for the pelvic hooks is seen at the *bottom* of the picture.

## Rib Cradle Insertion

- The two upper rib cradles are placed first. Optimal positioning is about 2 cm lateral to the costotransverse junction. A narrow window in the trapezius and rhomboid muscles is made and the rib is exposed.
- Care should be taken not to divide the blood supply of the rib by stripping it of surrounding soft tissue.
- In most cases, we use two adjacent ribs with a double rib cradle. Depending on the sagittal contour, this can be T4–T5, T3–T4, or even in some cases T2–T3.
  - Because implant migration is so common after prolonged distraction in medically fragile children, the surgeon should plan for the next step if there is migration. Therefore, using more caudal ribs (T4–T5) allows the surgeon to simply move the cradle to the next most cephalad pair of ribs (T2–T3) if there is bone failure at the initial anchor site.
  - It is always easier to reattach more cephalad than more caudad because the latter requires collapsing the device rather than expanding the device.
- The first rib should never be used, as cephalad migration of this device places the brachial plexus at risk.
- Once the rib is exposed, a towel clip is placed on some adjacent soft tissue (do not place the towel clip on the rib, it may damage smaller, more fragile ribs) and image intensifier is used to confirm the site where the rib cradle will be placed.
- The narrow entry point for the curved Freer elevator is over the intercostal space proximal and distal to the rib (**TECH FIG 2A**).
  - The Freer elevator is used to carefully create an entry point for the rib cradle anteriorly and guide it along the curve of the rib, carefully protecting the pleura beneath it (**TECH FIG 2B**).
  - The rib trial is inserted, and the superior rib cradle is then encircled around the rib by sweeping it from medial to lateral. The cradle is finally locked into place by the cap (**TECH FIG 2C**).

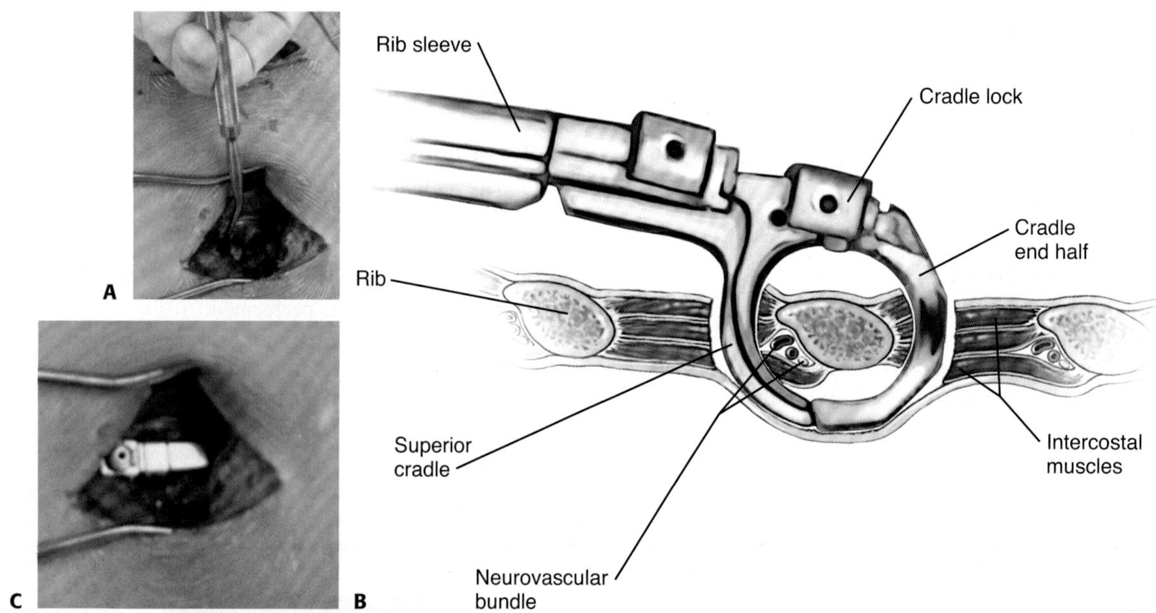


**TECH FIG 2** • **A.** A curved narrow Freer is passed around the rib surface before a rib cradle trial to free the periosteum around the rib and to prevent puncturing the pleura. **B.** Cross-sectional anatomy of the rib with the intercostal muscles and the neurovascular bundle. Placement of the rib cradle is demonstrated. **C.** A cephalad rib cradle was placed over the right T4 rib segment. A similar construct was placed over the left side corresponding rib segment. The placement was finally checked with C-arm.

## Insertion of Pelvic Hooks

- A longitudinal incision is made and carried down to the paraspinous muscles to the iliac crest. A small window is made in the paraspinous muscle and fascia at its insertion on the iliac crest and gentle digital dissection is used along the inner table of the crest at this location, which will later be the site of the internal portion of the pelvic hook.
  - Every effort should be made to keep the soft tissue window as small as possible, helping to minimize the risk of immediate migration of the hook to an unsatisfactory location.
- The optimal location on the pelvis is just a few millimeters medial to the most cephalad crest of the pelvis (**TECH FIG 3A**).
  - Placing the hook lateral to the crest will cause it to ride off the lateral edge into the soft tissues and placing it medially risks the sacroiliac joint and perhaps the lumbar nerve root.
- The hook is then inserted through small window in the fascia, coming to rest on the iliac crest, with cartilage left intact on the ilium. The portion of the iliac apophysis caudad to the hook prevents acute inferior drift into the pelvis.
- After all four anchors are in place, image intensifier should be used to confirm optimal position of both rib cradles and both pelvic hooks, before proceeding to implant placement (**TECH FIG 3B,C**).

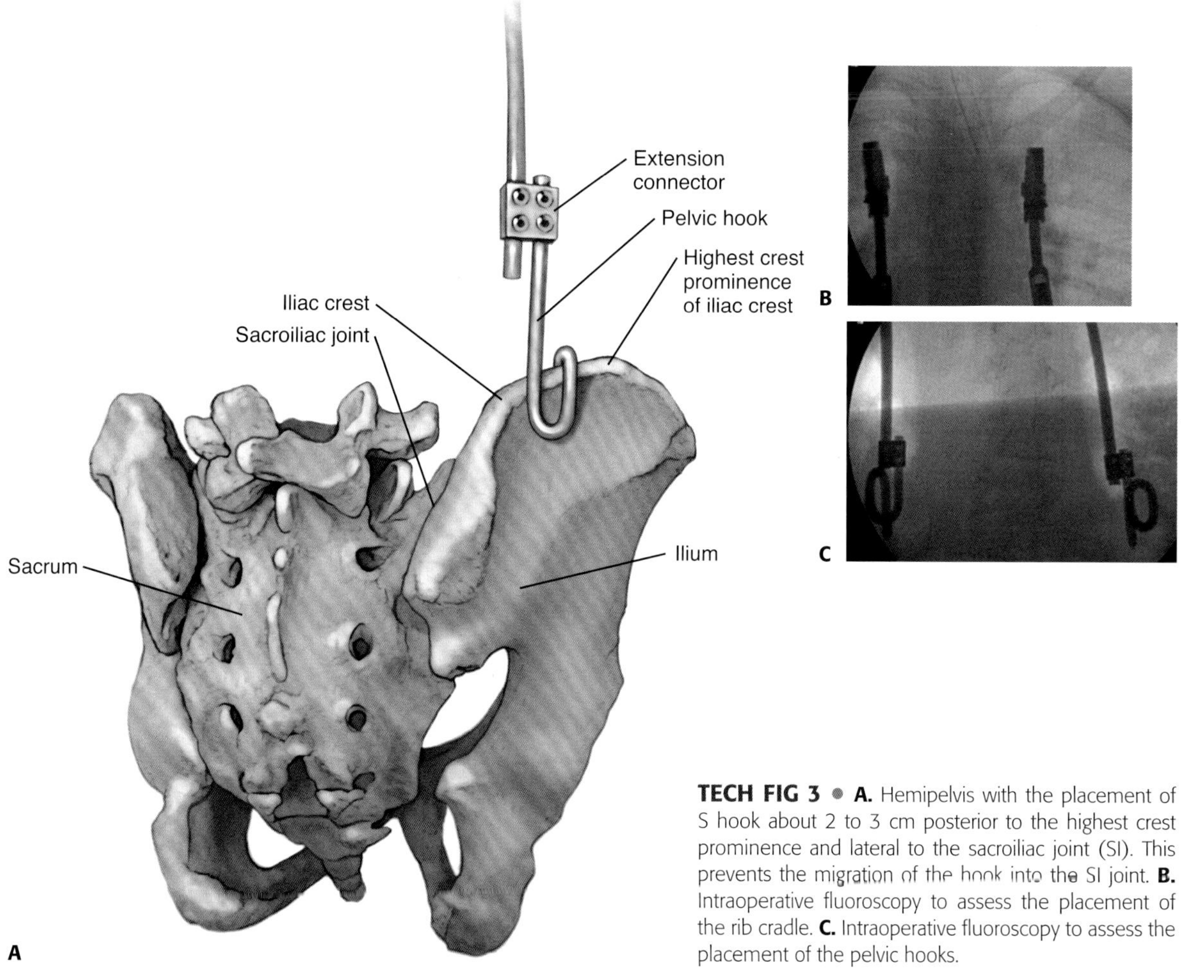

**TECH FIG 3** • **A.** Hemipelvis with the placement of S hook about 2 to 3 cm posterior to the highest crest prominence and lateral to the sacroiliac joint (SI). This prevents the migration of the hook into the SI joint. **B.** Intraoperative fluoroscopy to assess the placement of the rib cradle. **C.** Intraoperative fluoroscopy to assess the placement of the pelvic hooks.

## Concave Device Creation and Insertion

- The concave VEPTR is placed first.
- Gentle digital dissection and uterine forceps are used to develop a subcutaneous tunnel between the proximal rib cradle site and the distal pelvic hooks site.
- The direction of this dissection, and the subsequent placement of devices, should always be proximal to distal to avoid inadvertent abdominal or chest intrusion, which can be lethal (**TECH FIG 4**).

### Sizing

- Perhaps the most challenging aspect of building the construct is getting the length correct.
  - Only through a good understanding of the deformities flexibility and a significant amount of experience can the surgeon create a properly sized device consistently.
  - It is generally wise to plan a device several centimeters longer than measured with the rod template because it is always easier to remove a centimeter of the rod than to realize that the construct is much too small and needs to be discarded for a larger device.

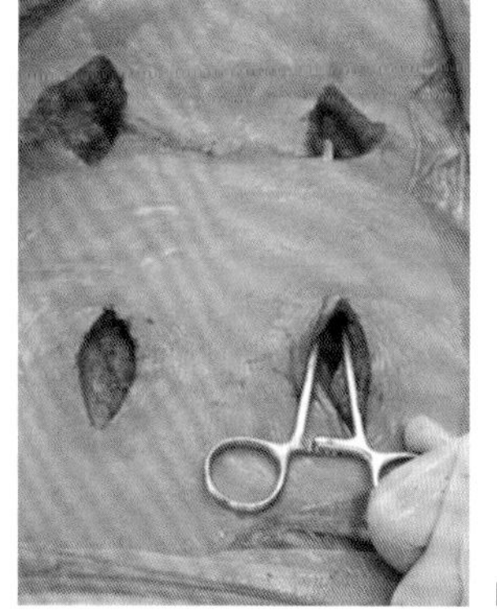


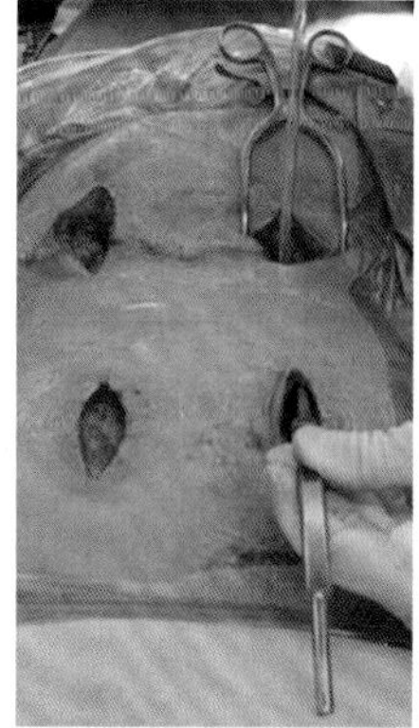


**TECH FIG 4** • **A.** Submuscular tunneling of the uterine artery forceps. Note the pointed end of the forceps always faces the skin and should be palpated throughout the tunneling process. **B.** A size 20F chest tube is clamped to the uterine artery forceps caudally and pulled out cephalad. The rod is then placed submuscular through the tunnel by gently pulling and rotating the chest tube from the caudal end.

- Begin estimating the concave construct length by placing a rod template into the proximal rib cradle, through the subcutaneous tunnel and down to the pelvic hook.
  - Be certain that the pelvic hook is fully seated on the iliac crest.
- Once the template is in place, manually maximally correct the deformity to get a better estimation of the length. Then add a couple centimeters to your measurement to account for the additional length that invariably is needed.
- Select a VEPTR size that allows the lengthening portion of the device to sit appropriately based on the sagittal contour of the deformity (ie, avoid having the lengthening portion of the VEPTR device over sharp kyphosis).
- Allow 2 to 3 cm of rod proximal to the lengthening portion of the device.
  - It is wise to contour this proximal portion into kyphosis, as it will diminish the forces that will, over time, cause the rib cradle to erode through the rib.

### Contouring

- Distally, a large portion of the rod can be contoured into satisfactory lumbar lordosis.
- Creating proper lordosis is essential, and can diminish postoperative hip flexor spasms and other problems, especially in children with spasticity associated with their neuromuscular scoliosis.

### Insertion

- After the construct is created, attached by an expansion clip, and properly contoured, it is threaded through the subcutaneous tunnel with the aid of a chest tube as a shuttle. After attaching the device to the proximal rib cradle, a side-to-side connector is attached to the end of the device and to the pelvic hook. This may be somewhat challenging unless the deformity is corrected as the concave device is inserted; until the deformity is corrected, the concave device will be much too long and it will be difficult to fit it in the distal portion of the incision.
- Ideally, after the concave device is inserted with maximal manual deformity correction, there will still be 2 to 3 cm of rod distal to the rod-to-rod connector. This is the site where further correction can be obtained during this initial insertion.
  - With distraction, and manual correction of the deformity, this last bit of rod is brought up through the rod-to-rod connector, ideally leaving it flush.
  - It is imperative that the communication be maintained with their monitoring team during this aggressive distraction and correction.
- After the first device is inserted and fully lengthened, the surgeon should visually inspect both anchor sites to assure that the rib is intact proximally and the pelvic hook is not subsiding into the pelvis (rare).

## Convex Device Creation and Insertion

- Once the concave device is in place, a similar technique is used to build the convex device.
- There are two important considerations for the convex device: sagittal contour and length.
  - The sagittal contour of the convex device may need to be a bit more kyphotic, and this should be built into the sagittal contour. Sometimes, the lengthening segment needs to be a bit shorter on this side to accommodate convex kyphosis.
  - The convex device should be built to be only slightly longer than original templates because at this point, most of the deformity is already corrected.
  - Inevitably, the pelvic hook is not completely seated and there is flexibility in the ribs proximally, so the surgeon should still make the convex device a little bit longer than indicated by the template measurement.
- Once both devices are inserted and fully seated and out to length, and monitoring is normal, the anchor sites are again visually inspected to ensure their integrity.

## Completion and Wound Closure

- After final tightening, all incisions are aggressively irrigated with both Betadine solution and normal saline solution.
- We prefer the use of vancomycin powder in all patients who weigh more than 30 kg. We do this as an adjunct to our intravenous antibiotics that are designed to cover both gram-positive and gram-negative in these neuromuscular cases.
- Meticulous soft tissue handling and wound closure is essential. We do not use drains for these incisions, which generally are very dry. We use Dermabond and a silver-impregnated dressing to give us maximal protection against surgical site infection, which is known to be a high risk in these cases.
- Full-length, high-quality intraoperative radiographs (both PA and lateral) should be taken in the operating room (OR) and reviewed carefully prior leaving the OR (**TECH FIG 5**).

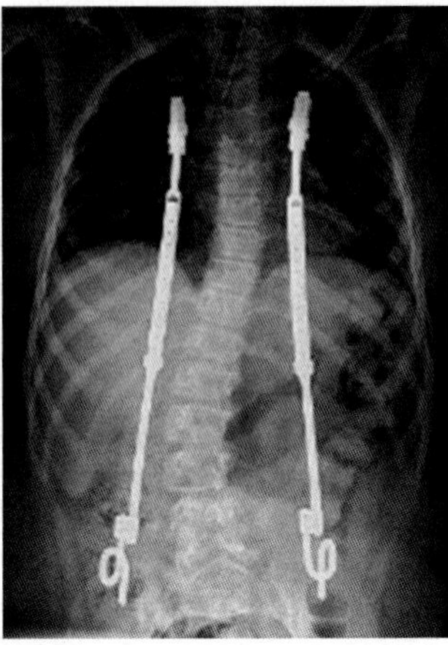

**TECH FIG 5** • Postoperative radiograph of the patient in **FIG 1** shows excellent correction of the scoliosis. Cobb angle is 16 degrees and a fully corrected pelvic tilt.

## PEARLS AND PITFALLS

| | |
|---|---|
| **Indications** | ■ Avoid this technique in ambulatory children. |
| **Clinical assessment and preoperative evaluation** | ■ A multidisciplinary approach, especially with pulmonary medicine and nutrition, makes the surgery safer for these children. |
| **Anchor placement** | ■ Optimize incision placement by marking out sites guided by intraoperative fluoroscopy.<br>■ Never make a VEPTR incision directly over the anchor insertion site. Incision should always be a centimeter or two medial or lateral to the anchor insertion site.<br>■ Avoid placing superior rib cradle above second rib to prevent brachial plexus injury.<br>■ The pelvic hook should be placed a few millimeters medial to the crest of the pelvis. |
| **Construct creation** | ■ The concave construct should always be made several centimeters larger than templated after deformity correction.<br>■ Do not place the lengthening portion of the VEPTR over kyphotic segment.<br>■ Contour kyphosis into the small segment of rod near the rib anchor.<br>■ Contour satisfactory lumbar lordosis. |
| **Construct insertion** | ■ Place the concave construct first, using maximal manual correction of the deformity as it is inserted.<br>■ Use a uterine forceps with a size 20F chest tube to pass the rod from cephalad to caudad. |

## POSTOPERATIVE CARE

- Most patients are extubated, and ventilator support is not needed unless they have significant comorbidities.
- In cases with a pleural tear, a chest tube is used and it is removed when drainage is less than 20 to 25 mL/day.
- Weight-bearing anteroposterior and lateral radiographs are made postoperatively. No external bracing is necessary after surgery. Patients are allowed to return to full activities 6 weeks after hospital discharge.

## OUTCOMES

- The outcomes for rib to pelvis VEPTR as reported by Smith[7] provides good insight that VEPTR can give excellent correction of scoliosis as the mean Cobb values of the primary and secondary curves including the kyphosis were shown to be significantly corrected.
  - In a series of 37 patients, 18 ambulatory patients underwent 139 procedures and the 19 nonambulatory patients underwent 100 procedures with an average follow-ups of 84 and 64 months, respectively. The nonambulators did significantly better than their ambulatory counterparts who developed crouch gait (7/18) and often needed conversion to rib–spine constructs (39%).
  - The overall rate of adverse events per procedure was reported to be 13%. The rate of adverse events in the nonambulatory group was 15%.

## COMPLICATIONS

- Complications for VEPTR include infection, skin sloughing, displacement and migration of devices through the rib, fatigue fracture, and neurologic issues such as brachial plexus neurapraxia or spinal cord injury. Sankar et al,[5] in a retrospective series, compared the complication rates of different systems. Dual growing rods had an average of 0.52 per year complications, "hybrid growing rods" had 0.36 per year complications, and VEPTR patients had 0.52 per year complications.
- Campbell and Smith[2] in 201 VEPTR patients (1412 surgeries) reported 3.3% infection rate per surgery. Skin slough rate was 8.5% and 27% rib cradle migration rate with complete cutout in 3 years.
- Upper extremity neurologic injury is more common during VEPTR surgery than the lower extremity. The rates of potential neurologic injuries during primary implantation of the VEPTR are 2.8% and during exchange of the VEPTR is 1.3%.[6]

## REFERENCES

1. Butler JP, Loring SH, Patz S, et al. Evidence for adult lung growth in humans. N Engl J Med 2012;367:244–247.
2. Campbell RM Jr, Smith MD. Thoracic insufficiency syndrome and exotic scoliosis. J Bone Joint Surg 2007;89(suppl 1):108–122.
3. Davies G, Reid L. Effect of scoliosis on growth of alveoli and pulmonary arteries and on the right ventricle. Arch Dis Child 1971;46:623–632.
4. Ramírez N, Cornier AS, Campbell RM Jr, et al. Natural history of thoracic insufficiency syndrome: a spondylothoracic dysplasia perspective. J Bone Joint Surg Am 2007;89(12):2663–2675.
5. Sankar WN, Acevedo DC, Skaggs DL. Comparison of complications among growing spinal implants. Spine 2010;35(23):2091–2096.
6. Skaggs DL, Choi PD, Rice C, et al. Efficacy of intraoperative neurologic monitoring in surgery involving a vertical expandable prosthetic titanium rib for early-onset spinal deformity. J Bone Joint Surg Am 2009;91(7):1657–1663.
7. Smith JT. Bilateral rib-to-pelvis technique for managing early-onset scoliosis. Clin Orthop Relat Res 2011;469(5):1349–1355.

# Opening Wedge Thoracoplasty and Vertical Expandable Prosthetic Titanium Rib Insertion for Congenital Scoliosis and Fused Ribs

Robert M. Campbell, Jr.

## DEFINITION

- This procedure lengthens the concave constricted hemithorax through a vertical expandable prosthetic titanium rib (VEPTR) expansion thoracoplasty with indirect correction of congenital scoliosis to maximize the potential for thoracic growth in order to benefit the growth of the underlying lungs.

## ANATOMY[2]

- Congenital scoliosis and fused ribs is a severe variant of congenital scoliosis.
- Long unilateral unsegmented bars are common on the concave side of the curve with multiple contralateral hemivertebrae (**FIG 1**).
- The extent of rib fusion is commonly extensive, usually concentrated on the concave side of the curve, and, when adjacent to the spine, can contribute to curve progression through tethering.
- Mixed deformities are also seen, with areas of absent ribs adjacent to areas of fused ribs.

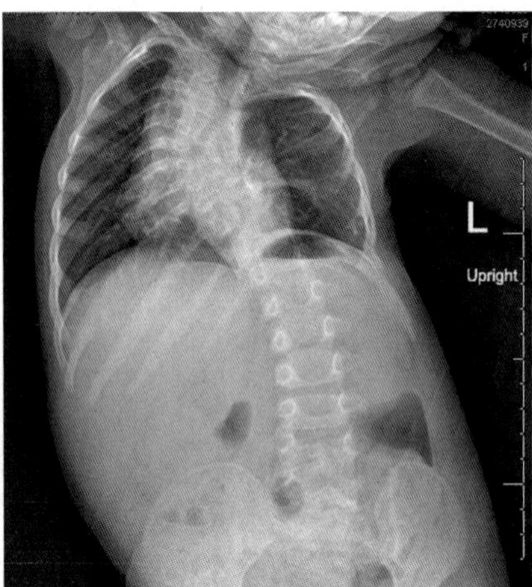


**FIG 1** • A 2 1/2-year-old girl with rapidly progressing congenital scoliosis and fused ribs. A long, unilateral, unsegmented bar is seen on the concave side and multiple hemivertebrae are seen on the convex side. The height of the concave hemithorax is considerably decreased compared to the convex side.

- Both the height and width of the concave fused hemithorax is often diminished, with reduction in height of the entire thorax common from multiple congenital anomalies of the thoracic spine.
- All these anomalies combine to reduce overall thoracic volume.
- This variant is classified as a type II volume depletion deformity of the thorax.[1]

## PATHOGENESIS

- Congenital scoliosis is associated with haploinsufficiency of the Notch signaling pathway genes[8] and the more severe variant spondylocostal dysostosis is associated with DLL3 mutations.[4]
- Fused ribs and congenital scoliosis is a widespread "failure of segmentation" involving both spine and rib cage and is most commonly seen in conditions such as VACTERL (vertebral anomalies, anal atresia, cardiovascular anomalies, tracheoesophageal fistula, esophageal atresia, renal or radial anomalies, limb anomalies) syndrome or spondylocostal dysostosis but can also occur as an isolated anomaly.

## NATURAL HISTORY

- Severe congenital scoliosis with fused ribs often progresses rapidly without treatment, with growth inhibition of the lung on the concave side of the curve.
- Early extrinsic restrictive lung disease from the constrictive effects of the severe spine and rib cage anomalies may be clinically masked in the young child by elevation in resting respiratory rate and reduction in play activities to aid overall body oxygenation, but as the youngster becomes older, a high respiratory rate becomes difficult to sustain and early respiratory insufficiency develops.
- Clinically, sleep disturbances are usually first seen, then frank clinical daytime dyspnea may develop with the need for respiratory assistance such as nasal oxygen, continuous positive airway pressure (CPAP)/bilevel positive airway pressure (BIPAP), or even ventilator support. Untreated infantile scoliosis patients begin to experience increased mortality from respiratory failure after age 20 years, with a death rate three times normal by age 60 years,[6] but the long-term mortality in untreated congenital scoliosis and fused ribs is unknown.

## PATIENT HISTORY AND PHYSICAL FINDINGS

- The clinical assessment should include both general and pulmonary health.
  - Onset of radiologic and clinical scoliosis should be determined; clinical course and response to treatment recorded.
  - Details about any prior spine surgery are important to note because that may affect growth potential of the spine.
  - A respiratory history should include determination of the frequency of colds, bronchitis, and pneumonias due to bacterial origins or viral etiology such as respiratory syncytial virus (RSV). Increasing frequency of respiratory illnesses, need for hospitalization for them, or the need for ventilatory assist to recover from them is worrisome and suggests developing respiratory insufficiency.
  - Voluntary reduction in play activities by the child, gradually lowering them to the point where aerobic demands are minimal, also is an early sign of respiratory insufficiency. An extensive review of related body systems is important.
  - Congenital heart disease can contribute to clinical respiratory insufficiency and cor pulmonale can be life-threatening.
  - Gastrointestinal (GI) abnormalities such as gastroesophageal reflux disease (GERD) may cause aspiration pneumonia.
  - Congenital renal abnormalities are seen in a third of congenital scoliosis patients.
  - Abnormal bowel and urinary incontinence should be documented and neural cause investigated.
- Physical examination should include measurement of percentile weight/height and resting respiratory rate.
  - Low weight is common in children with thoracic insufficiency syndrome and may be related to the increased work of rapid breathing.[7]
  - Normal respiratory rate is 60 to 80 breaths per minute in the first year of life, declining to 20 to 24 breaths per minute by age 4 to 6 years.[5]
    - Nasal flaring suggests labored breathing.
    - Perioral cyanosis or clubbing of the fingertips implies hypoxia.
  - Unequal shoulder heights, head and truncal decompensation as well as any leg limb inequality are measured.
  - Adams forward bend test is used to observe rotation of the back on the convex side of the curve. Isolated rib prominences and any generalized abnormal shape of the chest is noted, including pectus carinatum or excavatum.
  - Rib defects are measured, and clinical instability is estimated by degree of collapsing inward paradoxical motion with respiration. Areas of stiff chest wall over fused ribs are measured and location recorded. Chest circumference at the nipple line is measured and normal percentile determined.
  - A thumb excursion test (**FIG 2**) is done. From the back, the hands are placed lightly on each side of the chest with the thumbs extended medially, equidistant from the spine. The patient takes a deep breath, with chest expansion moving each hand outward with the tips of the thumbs moving away from the spine.
    - In normal individuals, the thumbs move out symmetrically with deep respiration, but with chest wall stiffness, the thumbs barely move with breathing.
    - The motion is graded: +3 is greater than 1 cm motion outward, +2 is 1 to 0.5 cm motion, +1 is less than 0.5 cm, and +0 is no movement. The patient is also assessed for a marionette sign.[1]

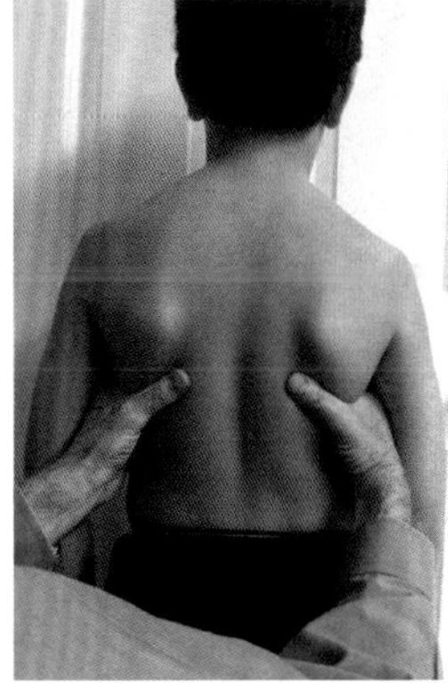
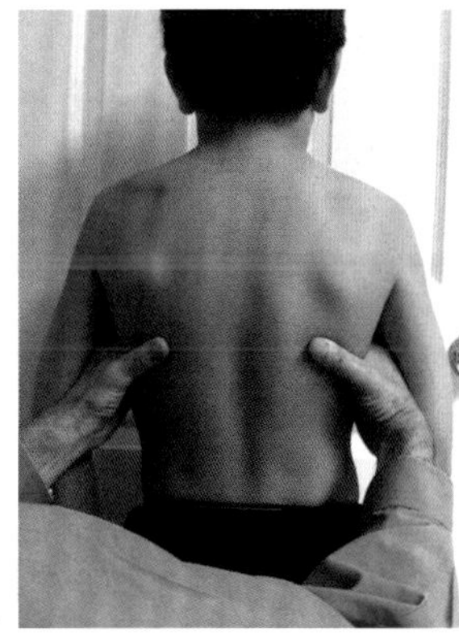

**FIG 2** • **A.** The thumb excursion test in a normal 9-year-old boy. The hands are placed loosely around the trunk, with the thumbs equidistant from the spine. **B.** The patient is asked to take a deep breath and the outward motion of the medial tip of the thumb is graded for each side: +3 is more than 1 cm of motion outward, +2 is 1 to 0.5 cm of motion, +1 is less than 0.5 cm, and +0 is no movement. The lower the score, the more stiff the chest is clinically, reflecting diminished ability to contribute to respiration. Note the large movement of the thumbs away from the spine in this normal child.

  - With respiration, the patient's head bobs up and down, much like that of a marionette puppet.
    - This is a positive sign, suggesting that the diaphragm is encountering resistance to downward excursion with inspiration, common in spine deformity, and in essence, the diaphragm is doing a "push-up" against body weight to fully expand the lung.
    - This is a high-energy expenditure and is not sustainable over time, leading to respiratory failure.

## IMAGING AND OTHER DIAGNOSTIC STUDIES

- Weight-bearing anteroposterior (AP) and lateral radiographs of the spine, including the entire chest as part of the radiographs should be obtained, along with supine lateral bending films of the spine.
- AP and lateral radiographs of the C-spine with flexion/extension laterals should be obtained. Computed tomography (CT) scan of the chest and lumbar spine, 5-mm intervals, and an unenhanced magnetic resonance imaging (MRI) of the entire spinal cord is obtained.
- Dynamic lung MRI (**FIG 3**) is helpful in visualizing functional impairment of the thorax.
- Pulmonary function tests by spirometry for patients older than age 6 years and infant pulmonary function tests for younger patients, if available. Complete blood count (CBC), sedimentation rate, C-reactive protein (CRP), electrolytes, prothrombin time (PT), and partial thromboplastin time (PTT) are also obtained.

## DIFFERENTIAL DIAGNOSIS

- Infantile scoliosis
- Congenital scoliosis without rib fusion
- Scoliosis associated with arthrogryposis

## NONOPERATIVE MANAGEMENT

- Observation with serial radiographs is indicated for mild or even moderate curves.
- Bracing is ineffective for congenital scoliosis.
- Progression requires operative intervention.

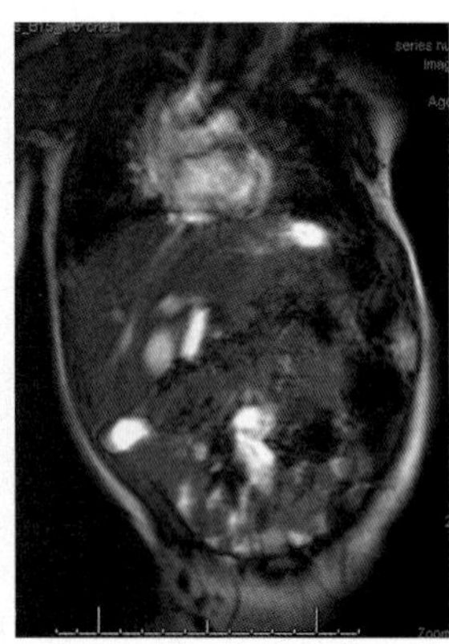

**FIG 3** • A dynamic lung MRI was performed and showed complete absence of rib cage expansion in inspiration and marked decrease in downward excursion of each respective hemidiaphragm during respiration.

## SURGICAL MANAGEMENT

- VEPTR expansion thoracoplasty is indicated for patients skeletally immature, as young as age 6 months, with progressive congenital scoliosis associated with fused ribs when the space available for lung (SAL) is less than 90%.
- Patients unable to tolerate repetitive surgeries for later expansion of devices may not be suitable candidates for this procedure.
- Absence of proximal ribs for device attachment also may be a contraindication for this procedure.

### Preoperative Planning

- For operative candidates, a trispecialty approach is highly recommended, with evaluation by not only by an orthopaedist but also a pediatric general surgeon and a pediatric pulmonologist, to best evaluate the multisystem abnormalities common for these complex congenital scoliosis cases.
  - The central question to address is whether expansion of the thorax with the likelihood of lung growth will provide a clinical benefit for the patient.
  - Anesthesia consultation preoperatively is also recommended. Any concerns raised by any of the consultants should be addressed preoperatively.
- Spinal cord abnormalities, such as tethers and diastematomyelia, should be addressed neurosurgically at least 6 weeks prior to VEPTR surgery to minimize the risk of traction to the spinal cord during the VEPTR procedure.
- Significant gastric reflux may require fundoplication before VEPTR surgery.
- Any coagulation disorders diagnosed that need treatment for surgery should be monitored by hematology services. Upper airway abnormalities may need scope-assisted operative intubation.

### Positioning

- The patient is placed in a prone position with longitudinal chest rolls. The knees and ankles are padded by foam pads.
- A 2-inch strip of cloth adhesive tape is placed transversely across the pelvis (**FIG 4**), with a folded hand towel underneath it to protect the skin, and the ends of the tape are secured beneath the operating room (OR) table to provide gentile stabilization of the torso.
- Arms are extended 90 degrees anteriorly and padded with foam pads.

### Approach

- Approach is through a modified thoracotomy incision.

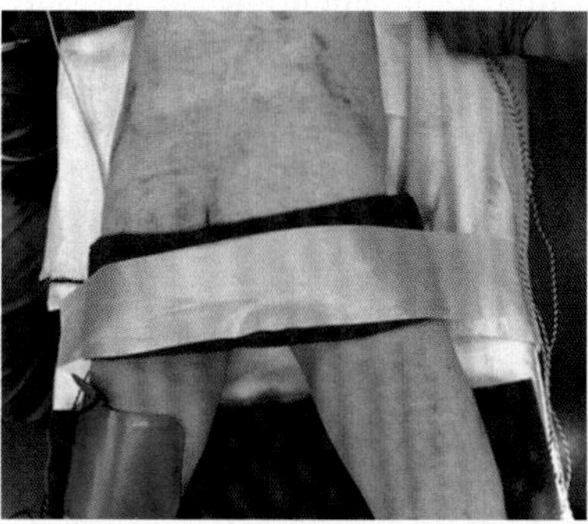

**FIG 4** • The patient is placed in a prone position, with longitudinal chest rolls to support the torso. Knees and ankle are supported by rolls and foam pads. Stabilization is through cloth tape over the buttocks across a hand towel secured under the OR table.

TECHNIQUES

## Opening Wedge Thoracoplasty

### Exposure

- A modified thoracotomy incision is made with the distal portion carried anteriorly in line with the 10th rib.
- Dissection with cautery continues through the muscle in line with the skin incision.
- The interval between the ribs and the scapula is opened by blunt dissection.
- The insertion of the middle and the posterior scalene muscles on the second rib is identified. The neurovascular bundle is just anterior to this landmark and should be avoided.
- The paraspinal muscles are reflected medially to the tips of the transverse processes, with care taken not to damage the rib periosteum.
- The proximal ribs for VEPTR attachment are assessed by palpation for strength, usually the second and third ribs are adequate.

### Implantation of the Proximal Rib Cradle

- The superior rib cradle of the VEPTR II (Depuy-Synthes Spine Co., Raynham, MA) is now ready for insertion.
- Cautery is used to place shallow 1-cm transverse incisions in the midportion of the intercostal muscles above and below the ribs of attachment.
  - For best mechanical advantage, it should be placed adjacent to the tips of the transverse processes of the spine, around at least two ribs or a fused rib mass.
- A Freer elevator is used to encircle the rib attachment to strip away the medial periosteum/pleural layer. The VEPTR trial is used to widen the soft tissue tunnel.

- The VEPTR cradle cap is inserted in the superior incision facing laterally to avoid mediastinum structures then turned distally.
- The VEPTR II rib cradle is next inserted, the two mated, and then locked by a distraction lock.
  - When the two ribs or the fused rib mass is somewhat large, the extended cradle cap is used.
  - The multiple rib attachment VEPTR II "stacked cradles" construct is seldom practical for this procedure.
  - For very small children, the small stature rib cradles can be used.
- The attached cradle is tested for stability.
- If doubtful, include another rib distally to enhance strength.
- Never extend to include the first rib because this may increase the risk of impingement of the device on the brachial plexus.

## Thoracostomy

- Once the superior attachment site is complete, the opening wedge thoracostomy can be performed at the apex of the fused chest wall.
- Usually, there is a fibrous cleft present anteriorly in the fused ribs in line with the planned thoracostomy.
  - This is released with cautery, with a no. 4 Penfield retractor inserted to protect the underlying pleura, and then the thoracostomy is continued with a Kerrison rongeur, cutting a channel transversely through the rib fusion mass up to the transverse processes of the spine (**TECH FIG 1A**).
- The osteotomized interval is then expanded with small lamina spreaders, and a Kittner sponge in a clamp is used to gently strip the pleura down proximal and distal.
- Any bone bridge remaining medial is carefully resected with a rongeur with fused bone adjacent to the spine carefully pulled out laterally with a curved curette to avoid trauma to the spinal cord.
- A second opening wedge thoracostomy, paralleling the first more distally, may be necessary when there is broad expanse of fused ribs.
- The opening wedge thoracostomy is held open with a VEPTR II set rib retractor and the distal attachment sites are selected (**TECH FIG 1B**).

## Distal Attachment Site

- In patients older than 18 months, the spinal canal is adequate for a laminar hook, so either a proximal lumbar spine hook insertion is chosen for primary thoracic curves or an iliac crest S-hook insertion when there is lumbar spinal curve/pelvic obliquity.
- In patients younger than 18 months, a hybrid VEPTR II use is not practical because the spinal canal is too small for a spinal hook,

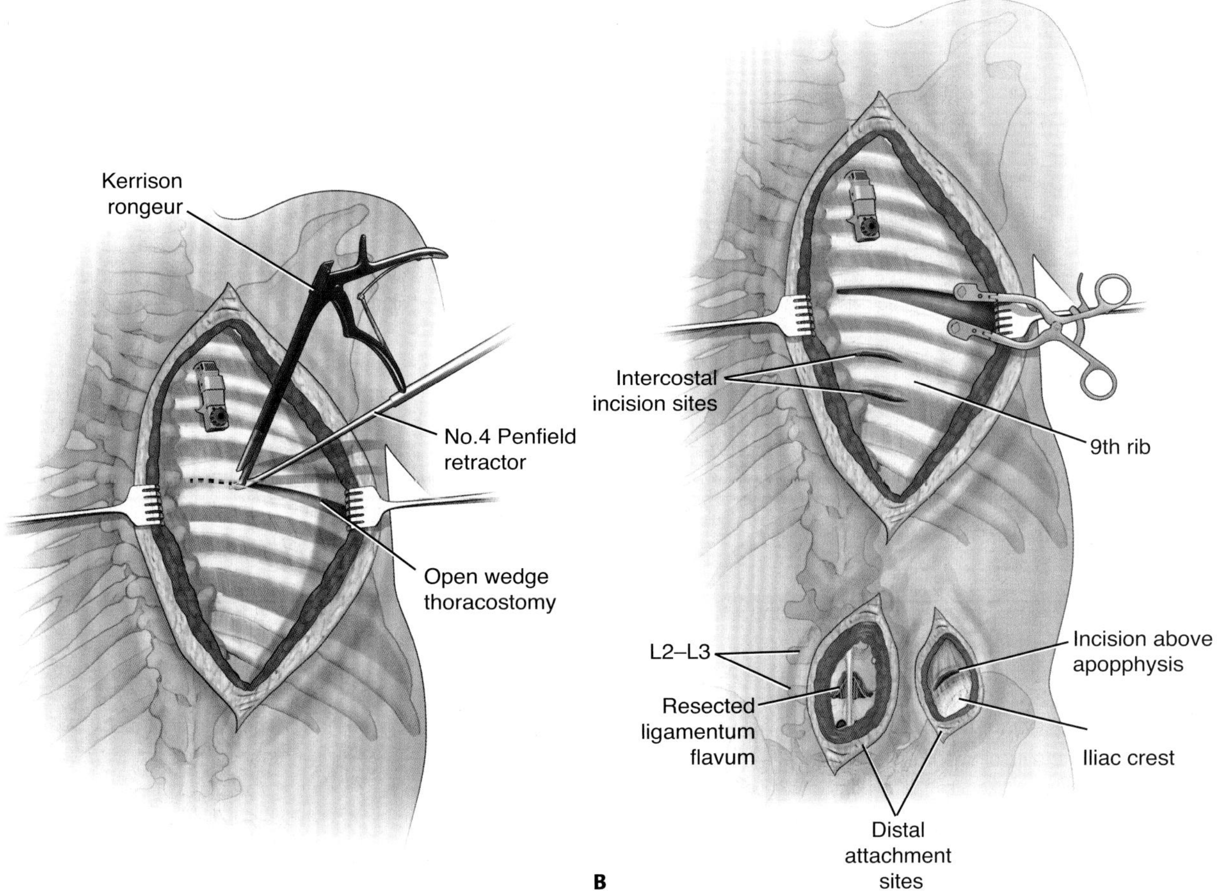


**TECH FIG 1** • **A.** The opening wedge thoracostomy is cut from lateral to medial, with a no. 4 Penfield underneath protecting the lung. **B.** Distal attachment sites can be the lower ribs in a rib-to-rib VEPTR construct or to the proximal lumbar spine or the iliac crest for a VEPTR hybrid.

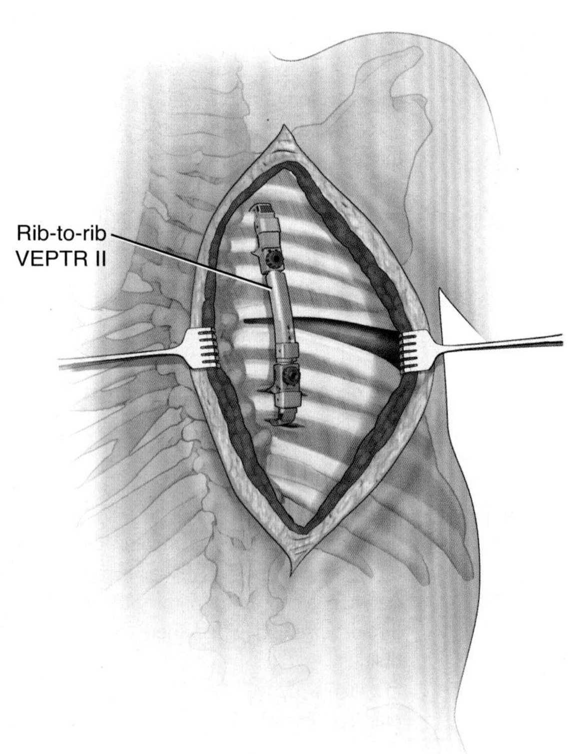


**TECH FIG 2** • A rib-to-rib VEPTR II construct.

so a single rib-to-rib VEPTR II device is implanted on the distal ribs just adjacent to the spine.

- An inferior VEPTR II cradle site is prepared on a stable, relatively horizontal rib, usually the 9th or 10th rib, and then the VEPTR II is implanted and tensioned (**TECH FIG 2**).
- In patients older than 18 months, a hybrid VEPTR II from ribs to proximal lumbar spine is used for more robust correction.
- For the distal hook site, a longitudinal skin incision is made at the selected level of the lumbar spine, usually L2–L3, and a two-level unilateral exposure is made for insertion of a single lamina hook.
- Care is taken to be below any areas of junctional kyphosis.
- If there is considerable pelvic obliquity/lumbar curve, extending the hybrid VEPTR to the iliac crest is recommended.

## Rib Sleeve and Lumbar Extension Implantation

- With the hemithorax deformity corrected by the rib retractors across the thoracostomy, the hybrid VEPTR II size is chosen.
- In general, 2 cm of proximal rod of the VEPTR II rib sleeve is needed to mate with the superior cradle, but if there is considerable kyphosis, a longer proximal rod segment is needed so that it can be bent to accommodate the deformity.
- The expandable portion of the hybrid rib sleeve should end at the lower end of T12 and the lumbar extension spinal rod should be cut to extend distally 1.5 cm past the lumbar hook.
- To form a tunnel in the paraspinal muscles for the device between incisions, a Kelly clamp is threaded from the proximal incision into the lumbar incision and used to pull a no. 20 chest tube back into the proximal wound.
- The assembled and sized VEPTR II, distraction lock in place, is threaded into the chest tube proximally, and the tube is used to guide the device into the distal wound through the soft tissue tunnel.
- The distal rod is then threaded through the closed hook, and the proximal rod attached to the superior cradle, and the device is distracted.
- The rib retractors are then removed.
  - The thoracostomy interval should remain distracted apart.
- A second rib-to-rib VEPTR device, if needed, is usually placed in the posterior axillary line (**TECH FIG 3A**).
- The medial hybrid VEPTR II device is distracted a final time.
- Extending the lumbar extension to the iliac crest is performed in a similar fashion (**TECH FIG 3B**).

## Closure

- Closure is in the usual thoracotomy fashion, but first, the musculocutaneous flaps are stretched to perform closure without tension (**TECH FIG 4A**).
- A chest tube can be used if there is a large pleural leak on Valsalva maneuver with irrigant in the chest, but this is seldom the case.
- Two round Jackson-Pratt drains are placed, along with a deep pain catheter for ropivacaine infusion postoperatively.
- Weight-bearing AP and lateral spine radiographs are taken within the week after surgery (**TECH FIG 4B**).

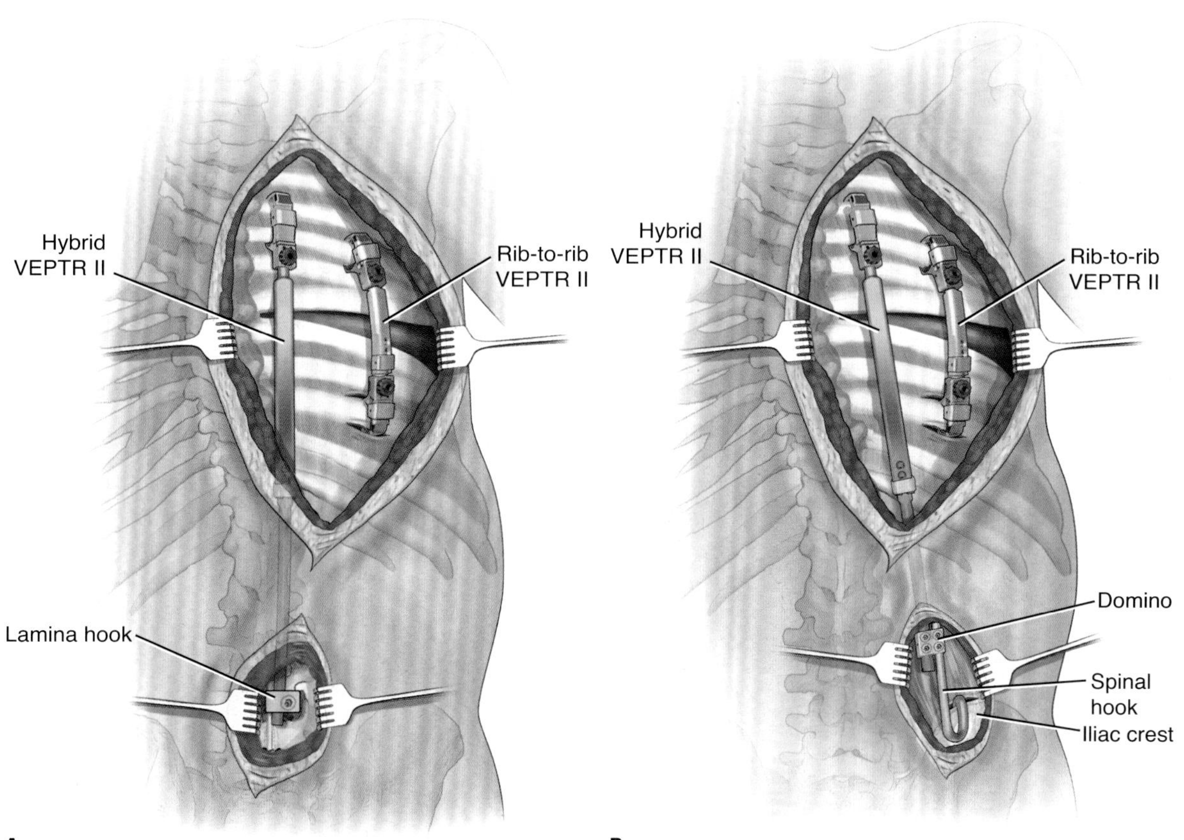


**TECH FIG 3** • **A.** Implantation of rib sleeve/lumbar extension. **B.** Implantation of VEPTR II hybrid to pelvis.

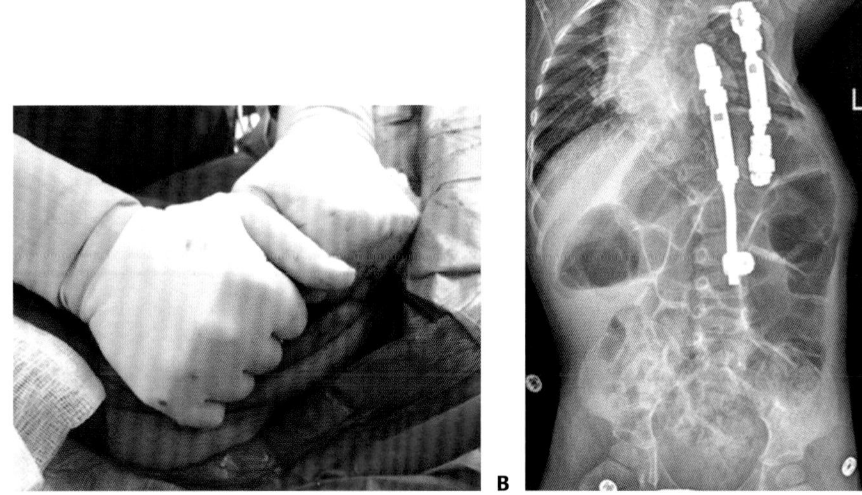


**TECH FIG 4** • **A.** The skin/muscle flaps are stretched vigorously for at least 10 seconds. **B.** Immediate postoperative radiograph of the 2 1/2-year-old female treated with opening wedge thoracostomy and a hybrid VEPTR I, which had more expansion capability than a VEPTR II for the limited area where it had to be placed, and a rib-to-rib VEPTR II. The medial hybrid VEPTR could not be placed more proximally because of poor bone stock.

## Vertical Expandable Prosthetic Titanium Rib Lengthening

- The devices are lengthened on schedule at least twice a year in outpatient surgery (**TECH FIG 5A**).
- Device expansion access is through 3-cm skin incisions, the distraction locks are removed, and the devices are extended slowly over several minutes, stopping when the reactive force is excessive.
  - A new distraction lock is inserted.
  - Expansion can be as minimal as 0.5 cm in a very tightly constricted chest and as much as 2.0 cm when the patient has had a growth spurt.
- Lengthening continues through skeletal maturity, with replacement as needed of completely expanded device through limited incisions proximal and distal.
- Infrequently, a second opening wedge thoracostomy may be needed (**TECH FIG 5B**).

### Kyphosis Correction

- When the proximal rods of the VEPTR II are bent to accommodate kyphosis, during lengthening procedures, the rods can be accessed through separate incisions and straightened slightly by in situ benders to reduce the kyphosis (**TECH FIG 6**).
  - This can be repeated as much as needed.

A
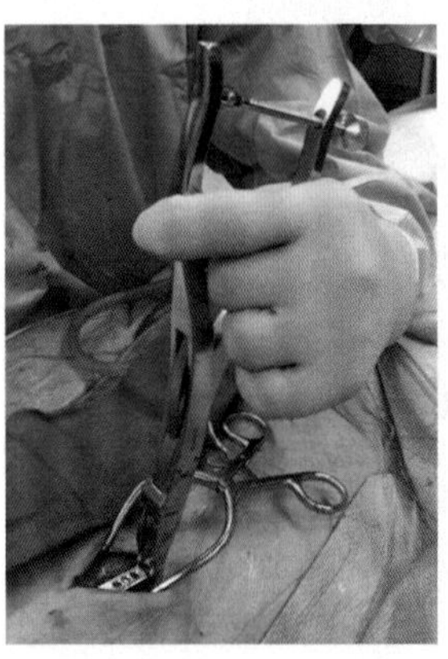
B
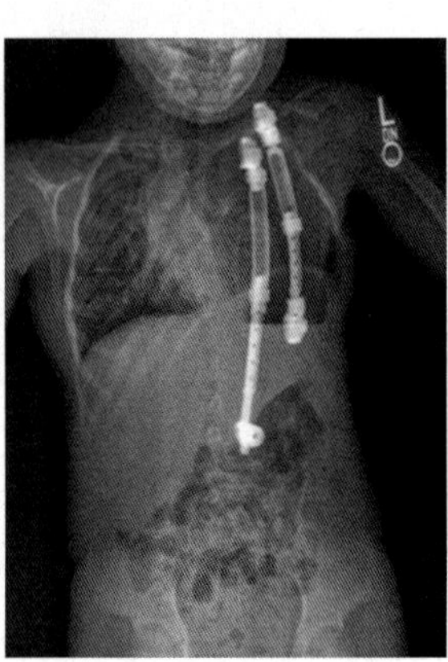

**TECH FIG 5** • **A.** VEPTR lengthening. A 3-cm incision is made parallel to the distraction lock, the lock removed, and the device lengthened until the reactive force mounts rapidly, then the device is locked. **B.** Five-year follow-up. To improve longitudinal expansion of the constricted hemithorax, a second opening wedge thoracostomy was performed 2 years after implant with more proximal positioning of the rib cradle because of improved bone stock.

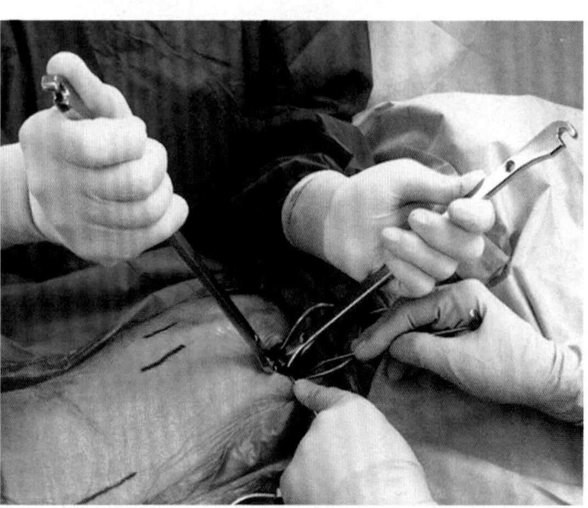

**TECH FIG 6** • Kyphosis correction. During a lengthening procedure, separate 2-cm incisions are made parallel to the middle of the proximal rods of the VEPTR II; the rods bent into kyphosis are gently straightened until the reactive force increases significantly. This can be done at each lengthening until the kyphosis is substantially reduced.

## PEARLS AND PITFALLS

| | |
|---|---|
| **Inadequate correction of the thoracic deformity** | ■ Correction in the initial implant surgery cannot be addressed by expanding the devices later, so every effort should be made to completely correct the asymmetry between the concave and convex hemithorax with the initial procedure. |
| **Poor soft tissue coverage for devices preoperative** | ■ Diet supplementation, along with an oral appetite stimulant such as Periactin, may be adequate. If not, tube feedings or gastric percutaneous endoscopic gastrostomy (PEG) feedings are useful. A body weight at the 25th percentile of normal, or greater, reduces the risk of skin slough over devices. |
| **Iatrogenic proximal compensatory curves** | ■ The superior VEPTR cradle site should be placed at the superior aspect of the curve but not into the flexible spine above it because of the risk of a proximal compensatory curve. |
| **Acute thoracic outlet syndrome** | ■ Rare but can be encountered with closure because of the altered proximal thoracic anatomy, so both pulse oximeter and upper extremity evoked potentials are monitored for loss of signal, and any changes are addressed by altering closure to let the scapula retract itself more proximal. |

## POSTOPERATIVE CARE

- Most patients can be extubated soon after surgery.
  - There is a 50% risk of a transfusion because of the dead space beneath the large flaps created.
  - The chest tube, if present, is removed when drainage is less than 1 mL/kg/day, and the round Jackson-Pratt drains are removed when the drainage for each is 20 mL or less per day.
- No bracing is necessary.
- Patients are mobilized to ambulation as soon as tolerated.
- Postoperative assessment should include standing AP and lateral radiographs of the spine.

## OUTCOMES

- For VEPTR treatment of fused ribs and congenital scoliosis, the average scoliosis curve was 74 degrees preoperatively and 49 degrees at postoperative follow-up.[3]
  - The ratio of the radiographic height of the concave lung divided by the height of the convex lung, the SAL, improved from 63% to 80%.
  - Mean increase in height of the thoracic spine was 0.71 cm per year. Patients who underwent surgery before age 2 years did best in percentage of predicted forced vital capacity (FVC).
  - Complications included device infection (1.9 % per procedure), skin slough (18 % of patients), and asymptomatic migration of devices (32% of patients).
- Once the patients have reached skeletal maturity, the VEPTRs controlling the spinal deformity can be removed and a definitive spine fusion performed.
  - VEPTR devices stabilizing rib cage deformity should be retained.
  - Yearly follow-up with radiographs and pulmonary function studies are recommended.
  - Magnetic expansion capabilities for the VEPTR device, much like the MAGEC growing rod, will likely be available in the near future.

## COMPLICATIONS

- Infections can be resolved most of the time by débridement and irrigation with loose approximation of the wound to allow granulation tissue to cover devices and wound vacuum-assisted closure (VAC) treatment.
  - Recurrent infections are best addressed by temporary removal of the central portion of the devices, with reinsertion done once the infection is resolved.
- Skin slough is treated by débridement, usually rotational muscle grafts, and primary closure.
  - Sometimes, it is necessary to use soft tissue expanders to provide skin coverage over the devices.
- Upward migration of the superior rib cradle can usually be addressed by reanchoring it to the reformed rib of original attachment through a limited exposure, often done during regularly scheduled procedures.
  - Spinal hooks that have migrated distally can be reseated at a lower level. Spinal hooks migrating distally into the iliac crest can be removed and then reanchored onto the reformed iliac crest.

## REFERENCES


1. Campbell RM Jr, Smith MD. Thoracic insufficiency syndrome and exotic scoliosis. J Bone Joint Surg Am 2007;89(suppl 1):108–122.
2. Campbell RM Jr, Smith MD, Mayes TC, et al. The characteristics of thoracic insufficiency syndrome associated with fused ribs and congenital scoliosis. J Bone Joint Surg Am 2003;85:399–408.
3. Campbell RM Jr, Smith MD, Mayes TC, et al. The effect of opening wedge thoracostomy on thoracic insufficiency syndrome associated with fused ribs and congenital scoliosis. J Bone Joint Surg Am 2004;86:1659–1674.
4. Maisenbacher MK, Han JS, O'Brien ML, et al. Molecular analysis of congenital scoliosis: a candidate gene approach. Hum Genet 2005;116: 416–419.
5. Oakes DF. Neonatal/Pediatric Respiratory Care: A Critical Care Pocket Guide, ed 2. Old Town, ME: Health Educator Publications, 1994.
6. Pehrsson K, Larsson S, Oden A, et al. Long-term follow-up of patients with untreated scoliosis. A study of mortality, causes of death, and symptoms. Spine 1992;17:1091–1096.
7. Skaggs DL, Sankar WN, Albrektson J, et al. Weight gain following vertical expandable prosthetic titanium ribs surgery in children with thoracic insufficiency syndrome. Spine 2009;34:2530–2533.
8. Sparrow DB, Chapman G, Smith AJ, et al. A mechanism for gene-environment interaction in the etiology of congenital scoliosis. Cell 2012;149:295–306.

# Vertebral Column Resection for Severe Rigid Spinal Deformity through an All Posterior Approach

Michael P. Kelly, Lukas P. Zebala, and Lawrence G. Lenke

## DEFINITION

- Posterior vertebral column resection (VCR) entails the removal of the anterior, middle, and posterior columns of the vertebra(e) through a posterior-alone approach.
- VCR is often performed at the apex of a deformity for severe, rigid scoliotic and kyphotic spinal deformities.

## ANATOMY

- A thorough understanding of the anatomy of the vertebral segment and spinal cord is needed to safely perform this procedure. This includes understanding the peculiarities of rotated vertebral segments in severe scoliotic deformities. The morphologic and iatrogenic changes of the posterior elements must be appreciated, as must the course of the spinal cord and nerve roots.

## PATHOGENESIS

- The origins of these deformities are multiple and varied, including congenital, idiopathic, neoplastic, traumatic, and iatrogenic causes.

## NATURAL HISTORY

- The natural history of the diseases leading to severe scoliotic, kyphotic, or combined deformities are variable.
- Those that do progress to severe, rigid deformities may present with intolerable deformity, severe pain, decreased ability to perform activities of daily living, myelopathy/spinal cord compression, and pulmonary dysfunction.
- Those fixed deformities that are asymptomatic (ie, a well-balanced patient without complaint) may be managed nonoperatively. However, one must obtain careful follow-up to assess for possible deformity progression over time.

## PATIENT HISTORY AND PHYSICAL FINDINGS

- The overall coronal and sagittal plane balance should be observed with the patient standing upright.
- The deformity should be assessed for any flexibility by placing the patient prone and supine on the examination table. Several minutes of supine positioning will allow one to assess the flexibility of a kyphotic deformity. Often, we will have the patient lie supine on the examining table, turn the lights off, and return in 15 to 20 minutes for repeat evaluation.
- The history should include a careful assessment of current pain medication usage as preoperative narcotic usage may complicate the perioperative care. Additionally, any medications that may confer a risk of increased bleeding (eg, aspirin) should be noted and the patient cautioned to stop them prior to surgery.
- The use of nicotine-containing products, particularly cigarettes, is a relative contraindication to this procedure as the risk of pseudarthrosis is increased as well as perioperative complications.
- Those patients with diabetes mellitus must have well-controlled blood glucose levels before surgery as uncontrolled blood glucose levels are associated with increased risk of perioperative infection.
- A patient's nutritional status should be assessed and optimized prior to surgery. In addition, a bone density test should be performed to diagnose presence of osteoporosis and initiate preoperative treatment of any deficiencies.
- The patient's gait should be assessed for evidence of myelopathy (eg, wide based, shuffling gait).
- A detailed neurologic examination must be performed and documented, including examination for pathologic reflexes such as asymmetric abdominal reflexes, Babinski response, and sustained clonus. Pathologic reflexes must alert the surgeon to possible intraspinal pathologies (eg, Chiari II, syrinx, tethered cord) that may need to be addressed prior to the deformity correction.
- Preoperative examinations by a primary care physician, a cardiologist (including stress testing as indicated), and an anesthesiologist is mandatory to mitigate any risks of perioperative morbidity and mortality.
- A review of systems should include a review of the respiratory system and any history of respiratory compromise or distress. Preoperative pulmonary function tests should be obtained in all patients with a deformity severe enough to be considered for a VCR procedure.

## IMAGING AND OTHER DIAGNOSTIC STUDIES

- A radiographic spinal deformity series is obtained, which includes standing anteroposterior (AP) and lateral long-cassette radiographs, left and right side bending, full AP, and lateral supine or prone images (**FIG 1**).
- Flexibility radiographs include push-prone and axial traction x-rays and help assess coronal plane rigidity.
- Hyperextension radiographs (bolster placed at apex of kyphosis) and hyperflexion radiographs (bolster at apex of lordosis) help assess sagittal plane rigidity.
- A three-dimensional (3-D) computed tomography (CT) scan is obtained to evaluate the entire anterior and posterior spinal column. This aids in the identification of important vertebral landmarks (**FIG 2**).
- Skull to sacrum magnetic resonance imaging (MRI) is necessary to evaluate the entire neural axis (eg, Chiari malformation, syringomyelia, tethered spinal cord) (**FIG 3**).

## DIFFERENTIAL DIAGNOSIS

- Severe scoliosis
- Global kyphosis

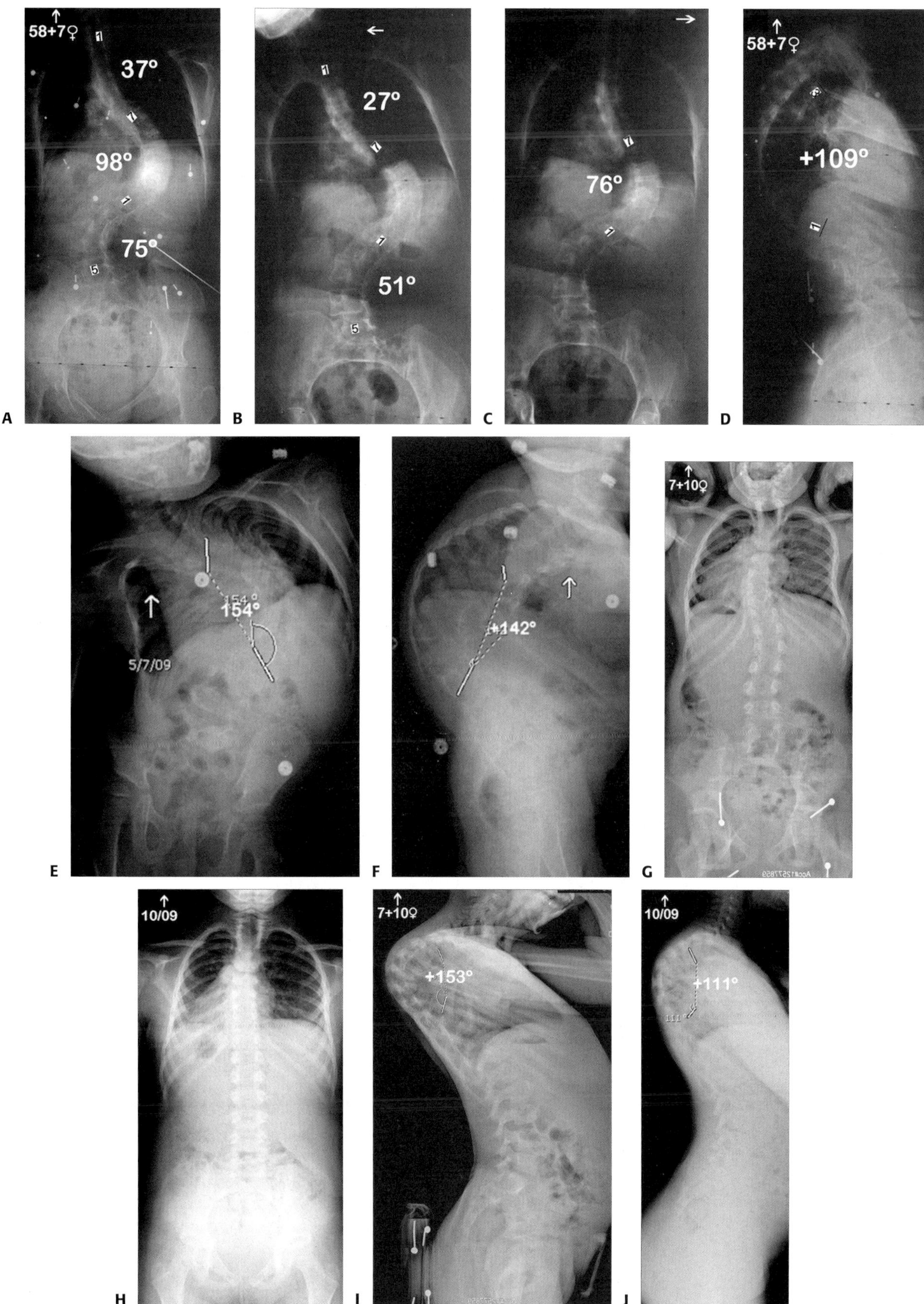


**FIG 1** • **A–D.** Case 1. Fifty-eight-year-old woman with adult idiopathic thoracic kyphoscoliosis. **E,F.** Case 2. Six-year-old boy with severe congenital kyphoscoliosis. **G–J.** Case 3. Seven-year-old girl with a severe 153-degree postlaminectomy kyphosis with myelopathy. She was placed in preoperative halo-gravity traction.

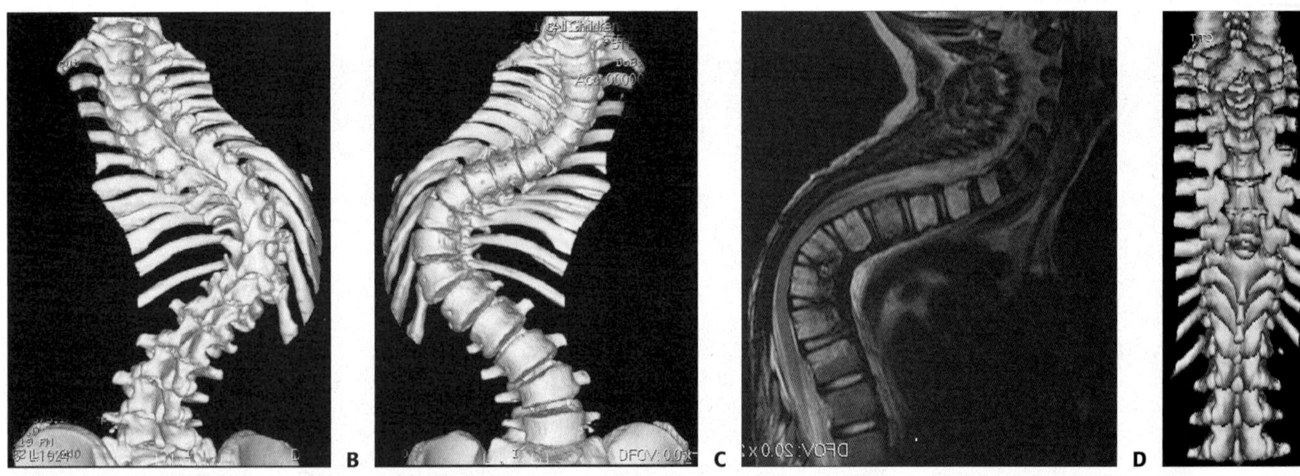

**FIG 2** • **A,B.** Posterior and anterior 3-D CT scans, respectively, of a patient with severe idiopathic scoliosis. **C.** Case 3. Preoperative sagittal MRI scan shows postlaminectomy kyphosis with draping of the spinal cord. **D.** Case 3. Preoperative 3-D CT scan shows the laminectomy defect.

- Angular kyphosis
- Kyphoscoliosis
- Fixed coronal and sagittal imbalance syndrome (eg, status post-Harrington rod instrumentation)

## NONOPERATIVE MANAGEMENT

- Patients with static deformities and only mild pain or physical impairment should be managed with a trial of nonoperative therapy.
- This includes a directed physical therapy program, to include cardiovascular conditioning, postural training, and abdominal strengthening.
- For those patients with moderate to severe pain, a referral to a pain specialist, most notably for those patients with complaints of pain not consistent with their presenting pathology or other signs of nonorganic causes of pain
- As with nerve root compression, epidural and transforaminal steroid injections offer a less invasive, potentially diagnostic and/or therapeutic intervention.

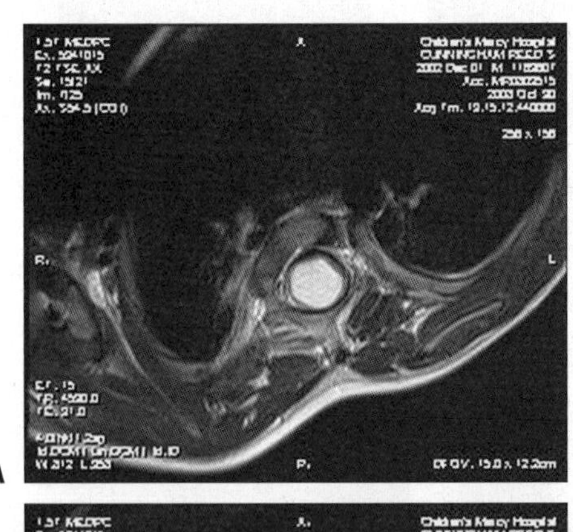

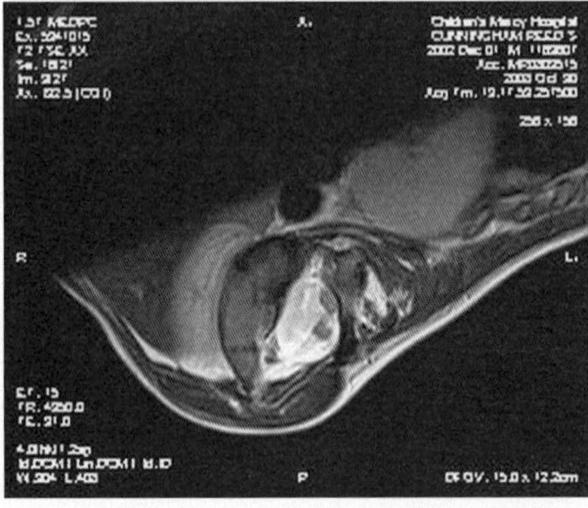

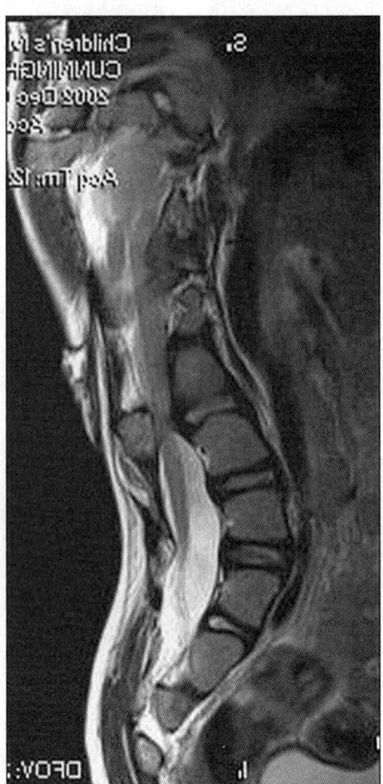

**FIG 3** • **A–C.** Case 2. Patient's total spine MRI demonstrated a syringomyelia, diplomyelia, and a tethered spinal cord.

## SURGICAL MANAGEMENT

- Classically, rigid deformities were treated with staged anterior and posterior procedures to resect and reconstruct the spine through the rigid segment.[2–4] The posterior VCR allows a similar correction of deformity, with the benefits of shorter total operative time and lower blood loss.[6]
- Location of the deformity often determines whether a VCR (thoracic) or pedicle subtraction osteotomy (lumbar) will assist in correction of sagittal imbalance. For less severe and flexible deformity with mobile disc spaces, multilevel Ponté/Smith-Petersen osteotomies may be adequate for deformity correction.[1]
  - Flexibility films will help determine whether a three-column osteotomy is needed versus posterior column osteotomies alone. Posterior column osteotomies may on average correct 10 degrees of kyphosis per level of osteotomy dependent on the spinal level being osteotomized. For large, angular deformities, a three-column osteotomy allows for greater correction in the coronal and sagittal planes.
  - We perform VCR in place of anterior and posterior procedures, electing to perform the correction through one single approach.
  - The VCR is almost invariably performed at the apex of the deformity.

### Preoperative Planning

- A multidisciplinary team approach is often necessary in the treatment of patients with complex deformity that requires a VCR.
- Preoperative assessment of the patient's cardiovascular, pulmonary, nutritional, hematologic, and metabolic systems is required to maximize the patient's preoperative reserve.
- Careful examination of the preoperative CT scan should alert the surgeon to areas of bony deficiency in the posterior elements to prevent incidental durotomies (see **FIG 2C,D**).

### Positioning

- The patient is positioned prone on an OSI Jackson frame with six pads, which are placed strategically to allow the abdomen to rest free, reducing intra-abdominal pressure and intraoperative bleeding.
- We prefer to place a halo or Gardner-Wells tongs with 5 to 15 pounds of traction that allows for rigid positioning of the skull with the face free.
- The arms are placed in a 90–90 position with care to position the axillae free and elbows well padded to decrease the risk of brachial plexopathy or ulnar nerve neuropathy.
- Pressure areas are carefully padded as the length of the procedure increases the risk of position-related complications (eg, skin macerations, plexopathies).
- The hips are gently extended and the knees slightly flexed with the use of multiple pillows.
- Spinal cord monitoring leads are placed to monitor the sensory and motor function of the lower extremities.

### Approach

- The standard posterior, subperiosteal approach is used.

TECHNIQUES

## Exposure

- A subperiosteal approach is undertaken from the transverse processes of the most superior instrumented level to the most distal vertebra or ilium to be instrumented/fused (**TECH FIG 1**).
- Thoracoplasties may be necessary at apical vertebrae to obtain adequate exposure of the transverse processes at the apex of a severe scoliosis or kyphoscoliosis deformity.
- Intraoperative radiographs or fluoroscopy should always be used to confirm vertebral levels.
- An efficient, meticulous exposure is necessary to minimize blood loss.

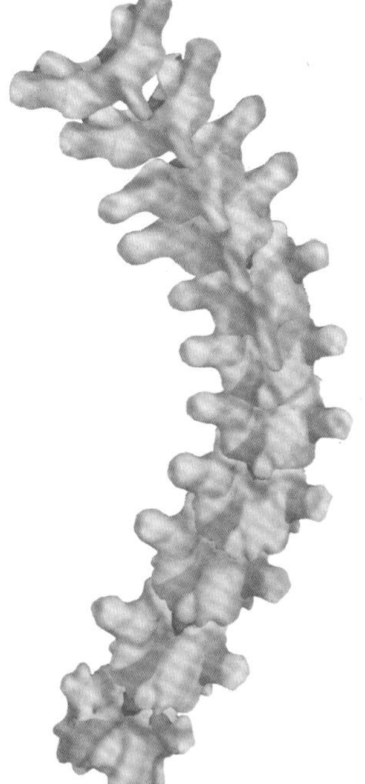

A

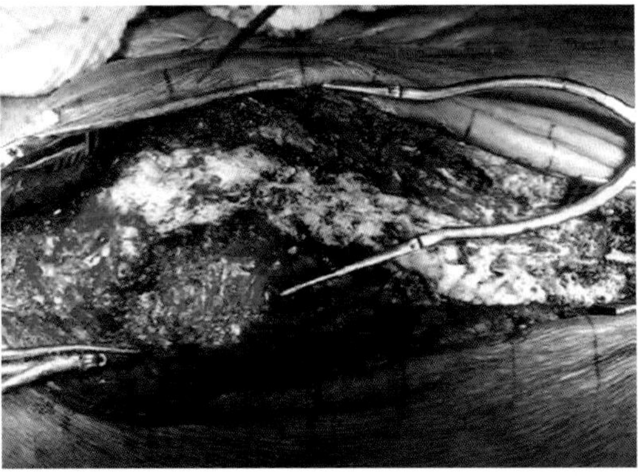

B

**TECH FIG 1** • **A.** Schematic of posterior exposure. **B.** Intraoperative view of posterior exposure of fusion mass in preparation for VCR.

## Facet Osteotomies

- Inferior facetectomies are performed at every level where motion exists, resecting approximately 3 to 4 mm of the inferior facet joint.
- Ponté or Smith-Petersen osteotomies are performed around the apex of the deformity, usually from the upper end vertebra to one level below the lower end vertebra. The ligamentum flavum and facet joints are excised.
  - These osteotomies allow for more harmonious correction of the deformity as well as offering access to the medial pedicle to aid in screw placement at the concavity of the deformity.
  - In those patients with severe apical kyphosis, we will place pedicle screws prior to any osteotomies. A temporary rod is placed prior to any osteotomy to prevent sagging of the vertebral column, which can put the spinal cord at risk of neurologic impairment.

## Pedicle Screw Placement

- We employ a modified anatomic freehand technique with a straight-ahead screw trajectory to increase pedicle pullout strength.[5] Assessment of preoperative imaging allows for assessment of pedicle screw diameter and length at each vertebra (**TECH FIG 2**).
- Pedicle screw placement is performed in a sequential fashion from distal to proximal.
- Placement of segmental apical screws is important to ensure rigid stabilization of the VCR site.
- Intraoperative use of fluoroscopy, CT scan, or navigation may be used in assisting the placement of screws, especially through areas of prior fusion with distorted anatomy.
- Multiaxial screws (or multiaxial reduction screws) are most commonly used.
  - Reduction screws are used when cantilever bending is needed for reduction of the rod and deformity. This is often at the distal end of a construct and in areas of hyperlordosis, where rod reduction may be difficult.

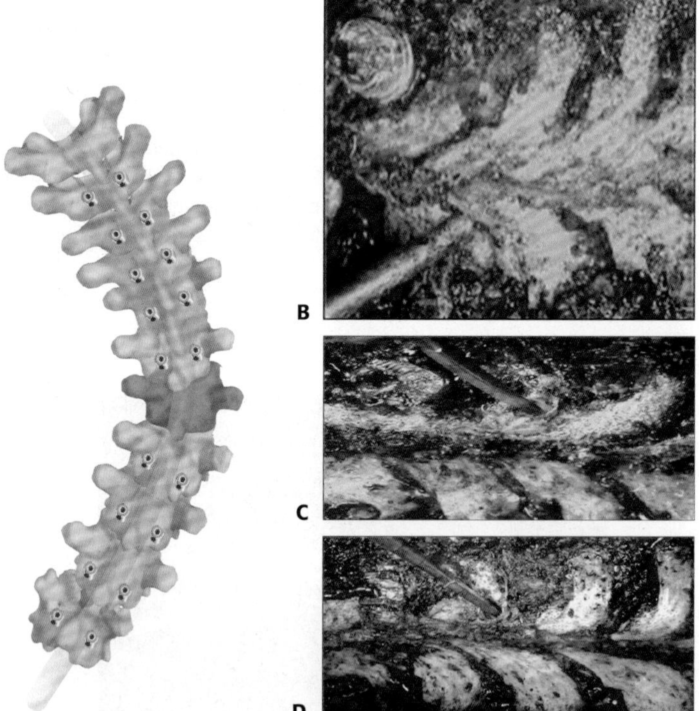

**TECH FIG 2** • **A.** Pedicle screws placed segmentally except at shaded apical level where resection is planned. **B–D.** Freehand pedicle screw placement.

## Vertebral Column Resection

### Costotransversectomy and Laminectomy

- In the thoracic spine, bilateral costotransversectomies are performed at the level of resection (**TECH FIG 3A**).
  - Five to 6 cm of medial rib is resected prior to the laminectomy to minimize the risk of canal intrusion.
  - After subperiosteal dissection, the medial rib fragment is removed, ideally with the rib head attached. Often, however, the rib head remains attached at the vertebral body and can be removed later during the corpectomy.
- The ribs are kept intact, not morselized, and are used as structural grafts to bridge the laminectomy site after osteotomy closure. Next, a wide laminectomy is performed extending from the cranial vertebral pedicles of the level(s) of resection to the caudal vertebra pedicles (**TECH FIG 3B,C**).
- A thorough central decompression is necessary to prevent dorsal dural compression with osteotomy closure. Exiting nerve roots are isolated by removing the facet joints and pedicles bilaterally.
- The nerve roots at the level of the osteotomy are temporarily clamped with a bulldog-type vascular clamp for 5 to 10 minutes and attention is turned to any spinal cord, monitoring data changes.
  - In the thoracic spine, we prefer to ligate the nerve roots medial to the dorsal root ganglion.
    - If spinal cord monitoring data remains stable, then the nerve root is ligated with two 2-0 silk sutures.
    - In our experience, two or three contiguous, unilateral thoracic roots can be sacrificed without neurologic deficits, except for occasional chest wall numbness.
  - In the lumbar spine, the nerve roots are preserved.

### Stabilizing Rod Placement

- In preparation for the vertebral body resection, a unilateral stabilizing rod is placed with pedicle screws two or three levels above and below the level of resection (**TECH FIG 4**).
  - For extreme angular kyphotic or kyphoscoliotic deformities, bilateral rods are used to prevent subluxation of the vertebral column.

### Vertebral Body Removal and Discectomy

- The cancellous bone of the vertebral body is accessed via a lateral pedicle body window. Subperiosteal dissection on the lateral vertebral body is done with a combination of blunt dissection tools and electrocautery. The paraspinal structures are carefully peeled away until access to the anterior vertebral body is gained. Special retractors may help protect these structures during the corpectomy (**TECH FIG 5A**).
  - The cancellous bone is then curetted and saved for use as local bone graft.
  - Resecting the concave pedicle poses a challenge, as it is very cortical.
    - In a pure scoliosis deformity, the dural sac and cord rest on the medial pedicle, with no ventral body due to rotation.
  - We prefer to use a matchstick burr to remove this cortical bone in these situations.
    - In these deformities, most of the vertebral body will be removed from the convexity.
    - The concave pedicle is removed first as blood may obscure the field if the convexity is removed first. This also allows the cord to drift medially, away from the majority of the resection.

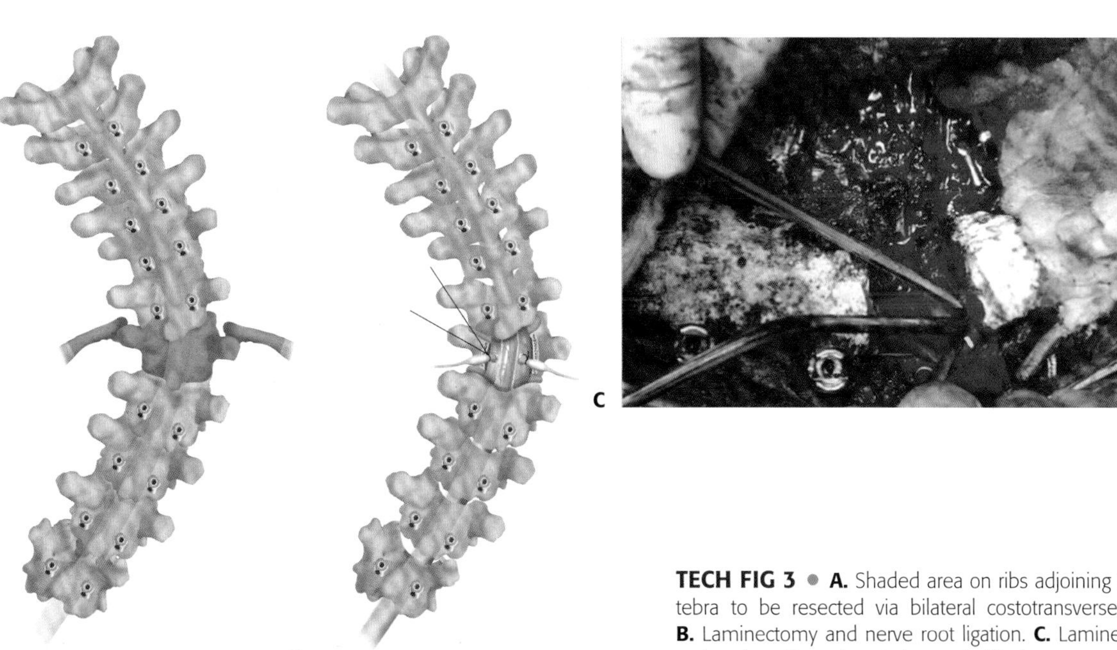


**TECH FIG 3** • **A.** Shaded area on ribs adjoining to vertebra to be resected via bilateral costotransversectomy. **B.** Laminectomy and nerve root ligation. **C.** Laminectomy and undercutting of ventral aspect of fusion mass.

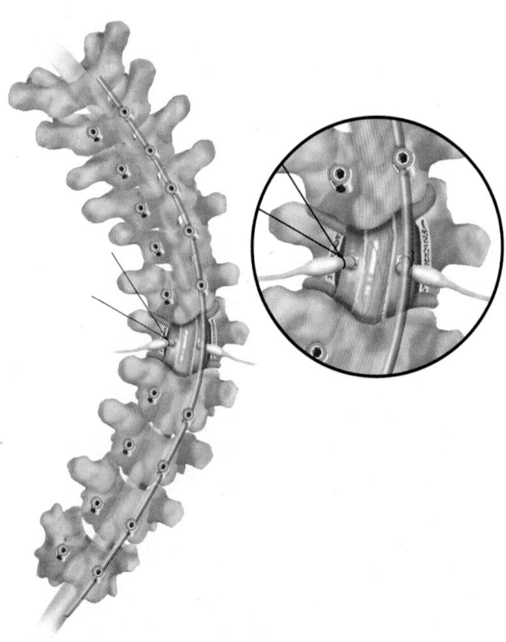

**TECH FIG 4** • Stabilizing rod placement.

- The entire vertebral body is removed except for a thin section preserving the anterior longitudinal ligament (ALL) (**TECH FIG 5B,C**).
- Discectomies are performed at the levels above and below the vertebral body resection (**TECH FIG 5D,E**).
  - Care must be taken to preserve the endplates for cage placement.
  - The last section of the vertebral body, which is removed by impaction, is the posterior vertebral body wall or ventral spinal canal (**TECH FIG 5F**).
  - The dural sac must be freed from the posterior longitudinal ligament.
  - The posterior body wall is removed with reverse-angled curettes, Woodson elevators, or a specialized posterior wall resector (PSO tool set; Medtronic Spinal and Biologics, Memphis, TN).
  - Care must be taken to remove any posterior osteophytes to prevent cord impingement during the correction.

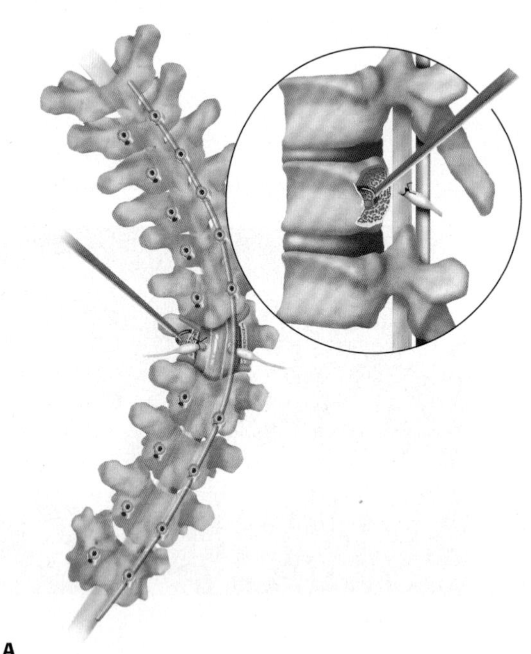

A

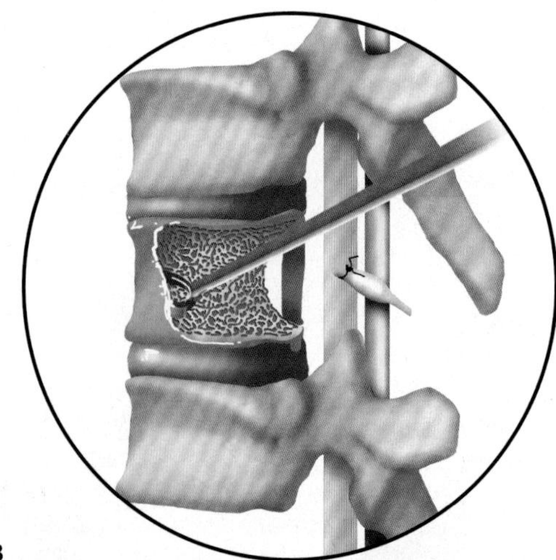

B

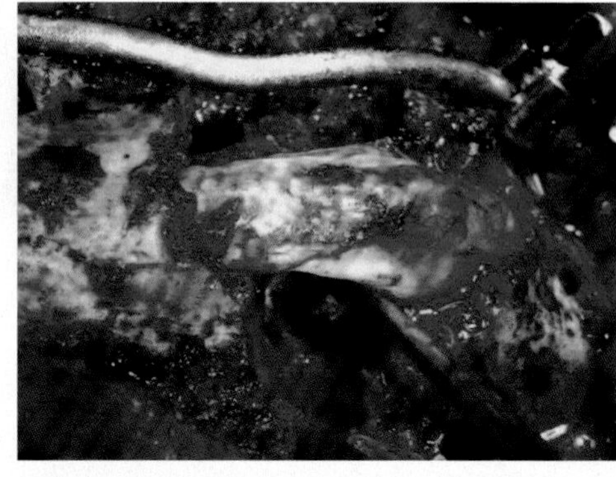

C

**TECH FIG 5** • **A.** Lateral vertebral body access. **B.** Vertebral body removal beginning at posterolateral edge of vertebra. **C.** Vertebral body removal continued. *(continued)*

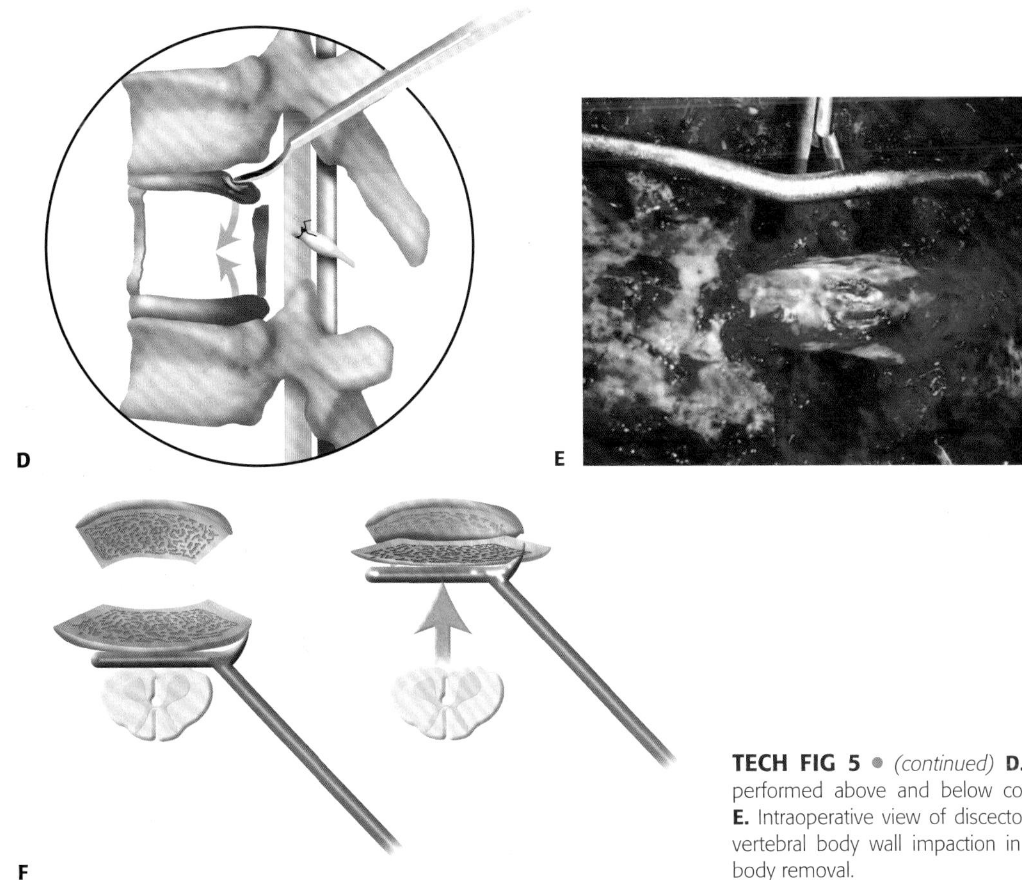


**TECH FIG 5** • *(continued)* **D.** Discectomy is performed above and below corpectomy level. **E.** Intraoperative view of discectomy. **F.** Posterior vertebral body wall impaction in final aspect of body removal.

## Closure of Resection Site

- Closure of the resected area is now performed with compression (**TECH FIG 6A**). Compression of the convexity allows for shortening of the spinal column. Sequential compression on the convexity and distraction of the concavity, performed in an alternating fashion, allows for safe reduction of the deformity through a shortening procedure. Distraction is not an initial technique as this may put traction on the spinal cord and cause a neurologic deficit.
  - In cases with large degrees of kyphosis, a structural cage is placed anteriorly. This prevents overshortening and acts as a hinge for greater correction of the kyphotic deformity (**TECH FIG 6B,C**).
    - To choose the cage height, close the osteotomy approximately 50%. Ensure that no excessive dural buckling has occurred and that neurological monitoring data are unchanged. After using trial sizers, place a cage that fits approximately endplate to endplate and compress around the cage.
  - In cases with good pedicular fixation, compression is applied through the screws.
  - In cases with less rigid pedicular fixation, a closure is performed, with dominoes at the level of the resection.
    - Care must be taken to watch for subluxation or dural sac impingement during closure.
    - To create a configuration, rods are cut and contoured to fit the deformity above and below the level of resection. These rods are then fixed in place with set screws, which are tightened. The rods are connected to each other via domino connectors. Thus, compression and distraction forces are applied to the rods through the domino and a rod gripper, with the forces distributed across the multiple pedicle screws above or below the domino connector.
  - After the closure is performed, a contralateral rod is placed. The temporary stabilization rod is removed, and a final rod is placed (**TECH FIG 6D,E**).
  - In situ contouring of the rods is performed, again with care taken to watch for subluxation at the resection or dural sac impingement.
- Intraoperative radiographs are obtained to check alignment.
- Decortication of dorsal laminae and transverse processes is performed with a matchstick burr.
- The laminectomy defect at the site of resection is covered with the resected rib sections (from the previously performed costotransversectomy) (**TECH FIG 6F**).
  - The ribs are split longitudinally, and placed, cancellous side down, from the lamina above to the lamina below.
  - The ribs may be secured with sutures or a cross-link, if space allows.
  - A final circumferential check of the dura is performed to ensure no dural sac impingement.

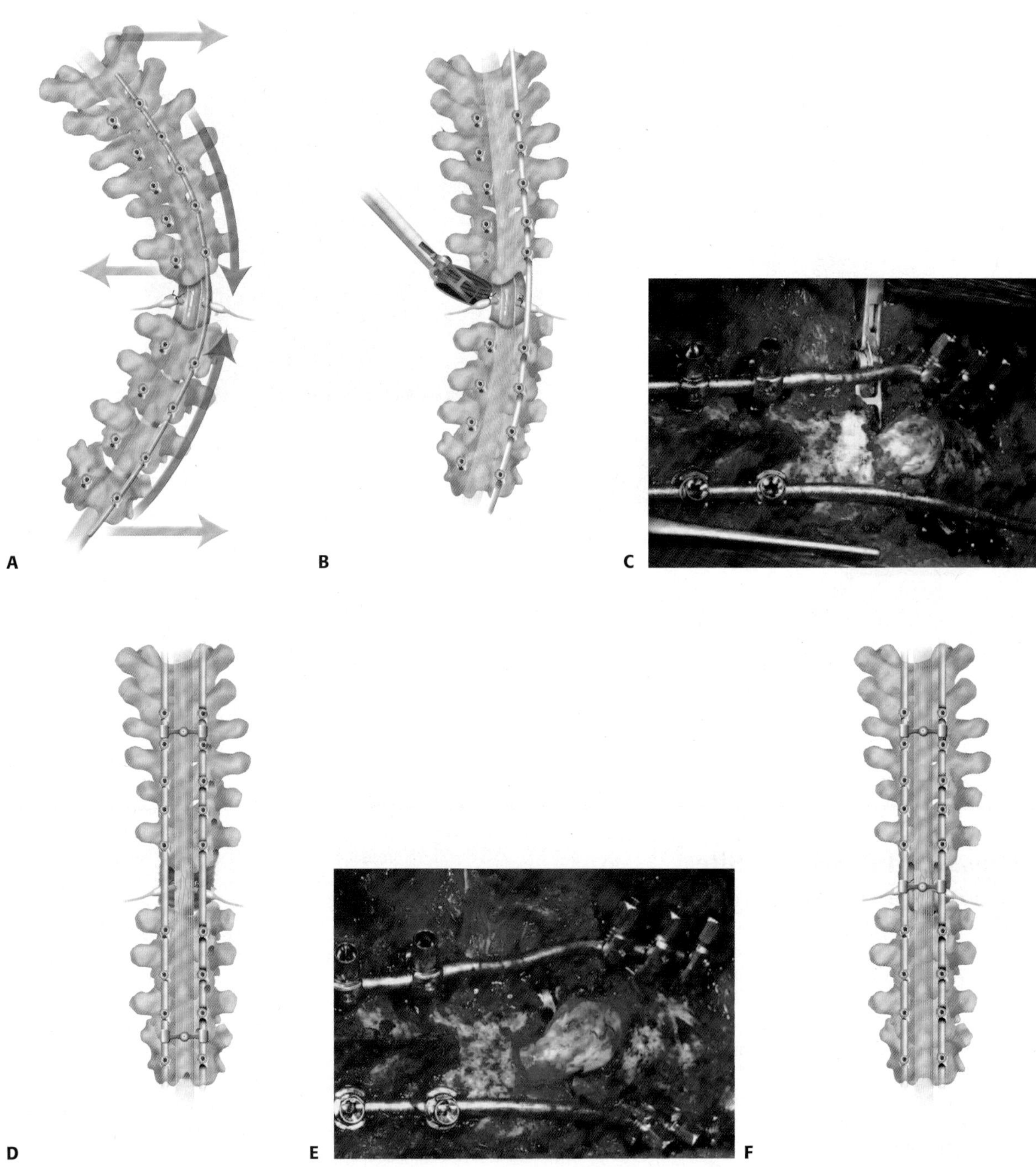


**TECH FIG 6** • **A.** Posterior shortening is always the initial corrective maneuver. **B,C.** Cage placement is performed before final closure. **D,E.** Final correction with both rods placed. **F.** Rib grafts placed over laminectomy defect.

## Wound Closure

- Deep drains are placed, and the fascial layer closed using 0 Vicryl (Ethicon, Somerville, NJ). A suprafascial drain is placed and the subcutaneous layer closed using 2-0 Vicryl suture. The skin is closed using absorbable 3-0 Vicryl suture.
- A rehearsed wake-up test is performed prior to extubation. Deleting an intraoperative wake-up test is performed.
- Final radiographs are obtained to confirm implant position and overall alignment.

## PEARLS AND PITFALLS

| | |
|---|---|
| **Preoperative planning** | ■ A multispecialty approach to preoperative surgical clearance should include cardiac, pulmonary, hematologic, and bone mineral density workups.<br>■ Use of neuromonitoring of motor and sensory pathways is mandatory. |
| **Vertebral column resection** | ■ Prior to starting VCR, mean arterial pressure should be kept at 80 mm Hg to help with spinal cord perfusion, hemoglobin should be close to 30, and room should be warmed.<br>■ Subperiosteal dissection of lateral vertebral body wall with careful attention to save segmental vessels will minimize blood loss.<br>■ Temporary rod placement prior to decompression to prevent subluxation<br>■ Wide laminectomy from superior to inferior level pedicles with complete facetectomies<br>■ Identification of bilateral nerve roots. In the thoracic spine, often, only one nerve root needs to be sacrificed. Tieing off nerve root should be done medial to dorsal root ganglion.<br>■ Resection of vertebral body should be accomplished as much as possible from one side to minimize the number or exchanges necessary of the temporary rods.<br>■ The spinal cord should be free from the posterior longitudinal ligament/dorsal vertebral body prior to removal of the posterior vertebral body wall.<br>■ Osteotomy closure should be done slowly with constant neuromonitoring.<br>■ Limit osteotomy closure to approximately 2.0–2.5 cm to prevent overshortening of spinal cord.<br>■ Use of an anterior intervertebral cage will limit amount of spine shortening and should be placed after initial round of osteotomy closure. |
| **After resection complete** | ■ Neuromonitoring is followed for up to 1 hour after final osteotomy compression, and a formal neurologic examination is performed prior to leaving the operating room.<br>■ Rib autograft should be used as a bridge over osteotomy site to protect neural elements.<br>■ Deep and superficial drains may reduce postoperative hematoma/seroma formation. |

## POSTOPERATIVE CARE

- Patients are often sent to the intensive care unit for close monitoring (for 24 to 48 hours as needed), then transitioned to the hospital ward.
- Patients are mobilized on postoperative day 1.
- Drains are retained until recorded output is less than 30 mL per 8-hour shift.
- Diet is advanced slowly with the return of bowel sounds.
- Deep vein thrombosis prophylaxis is provided with sequential compressive devices and thromboembolic deterrent hose.

## OUTCOMES

- **FIGS 4** and **5** show postoperative results in two of the patients in **FIG 1**.
- One of the authors (L.G.L.) has performed 107 consecutive posterior VCRs:
  - Sixty-three pediatric and 44 adult
  - Forty-seven primary and 60 revision
  - Ninety-nine in the spinal cord region and 8 in the lumbar spine
  - Seventy-three were one-level, 28 were two-level, and 6 were three-level

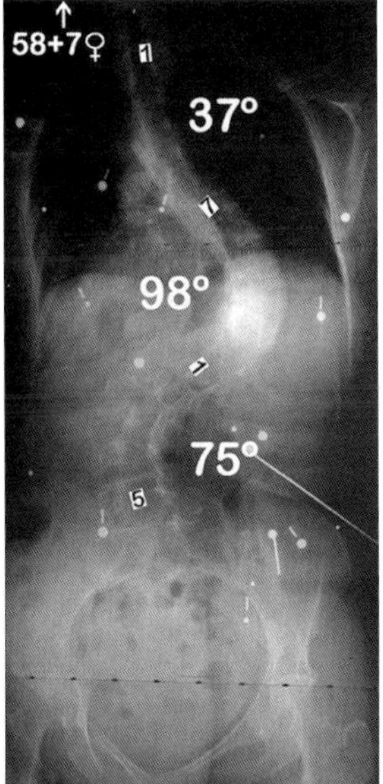

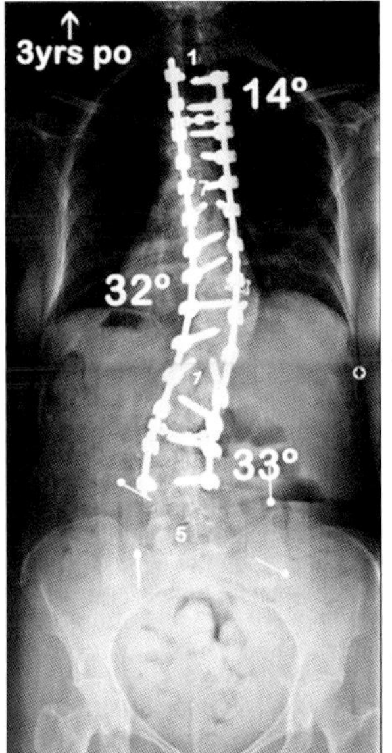

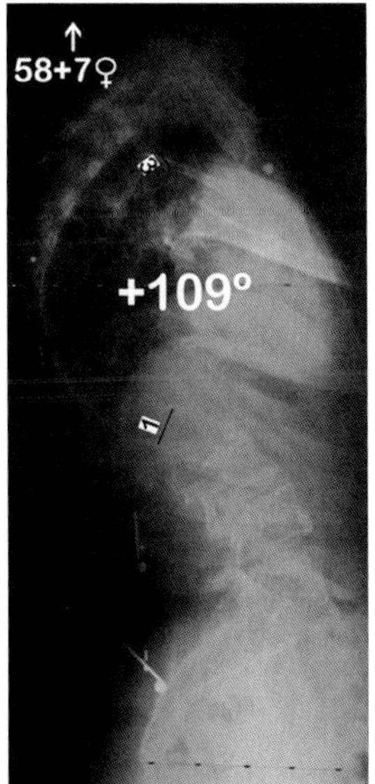

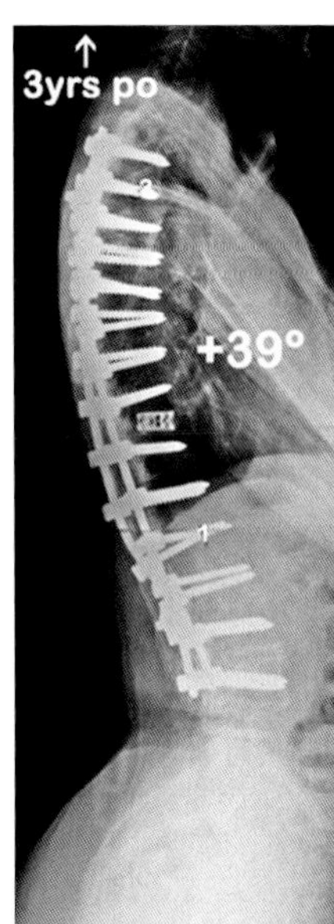


**FIG 4** • **A–D.** Case 1. Patient underwent a posterior spinal fusion T2–L4 with a T10 VCR with radiographs demonstrating excellent alignment at 3 years postoperatively. *(continued)*

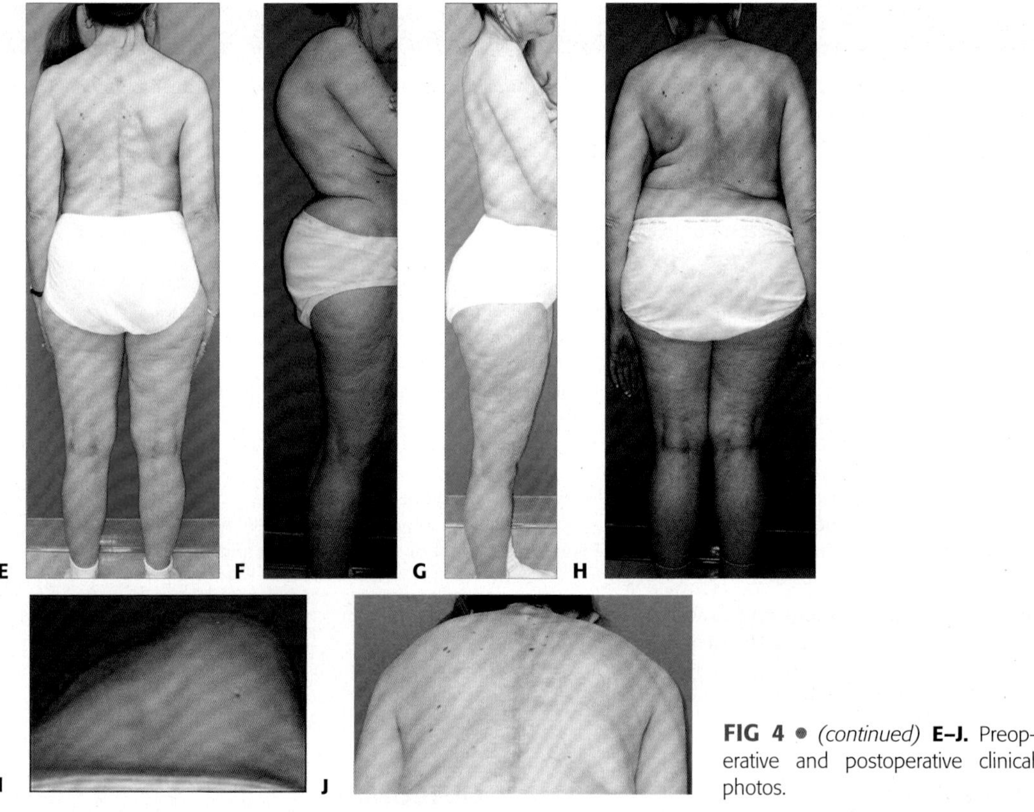


**FIG 4** • *(continued)* **E–J.** Preoperative and postoperative clinical photos.

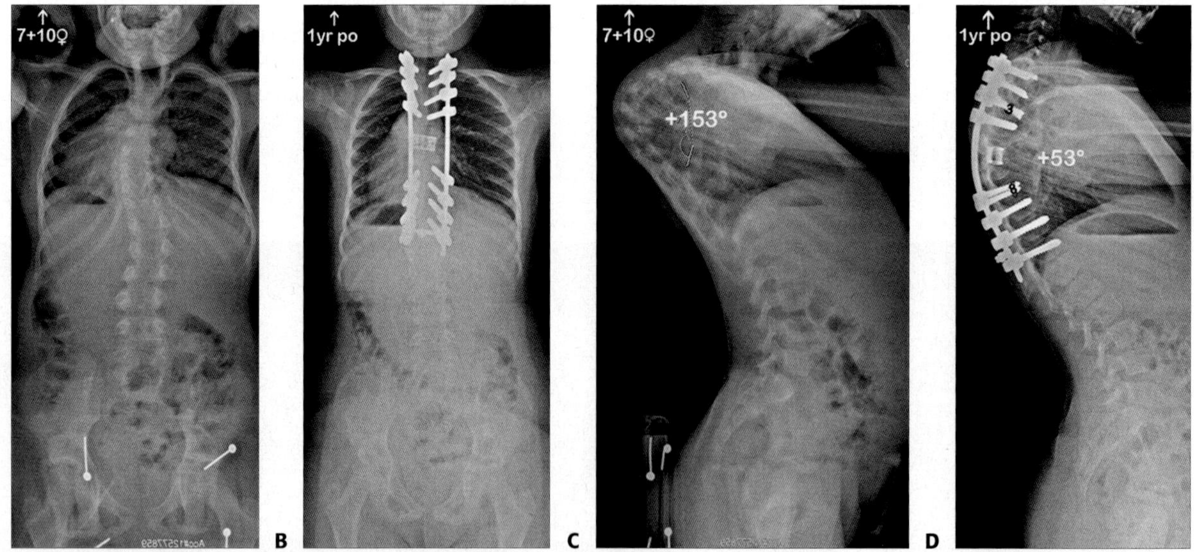


**FIG 5** • **A–D.** Case 3. Patient underwent a two-level posterior VCR and posterior spinal fusion T1–T11 with complete relief of her myelopathy *(continued)*.

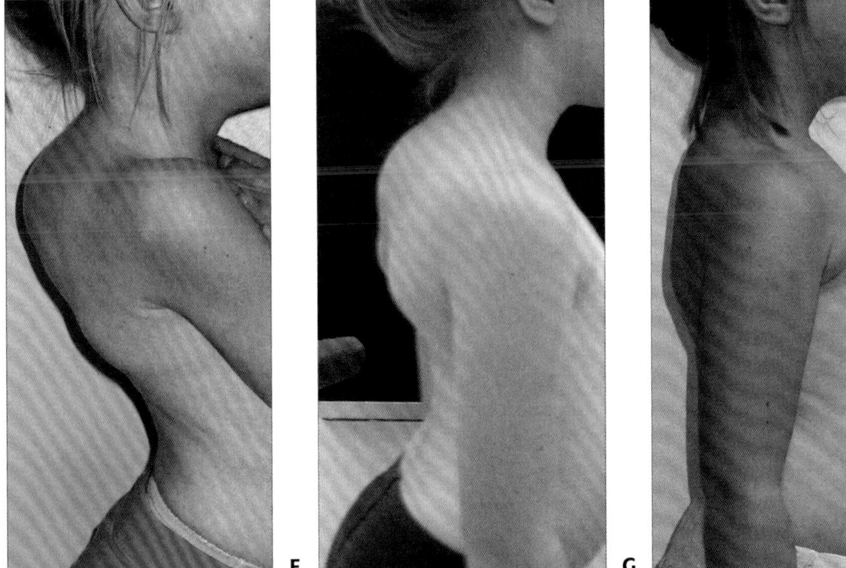

**FIG 5** • *(continued)* **E–G.** Preoperative, traction, and 1-year postoperative clinical photos, respectively.

- Diagnoses: severe scoliosis (29), global kyphosis (16), angular kyphosis (25), kyphoscoliosis (37)
- Average correction: severe scoliosis (69%), global kyphosis (54%), angular kyphosis (63%), kyphoscoliosis (56%)
- Mean estimated blood loss: 1300 mL; mean operative time: 9 hours, 37 minutes

## COMPLICATIONS

- Twelve spinal cord monitoring changes: All reversed with intraoperative measures to restore spinal cord blood flow (increased mean arterial pressure, wider decompression, larger interbody cage, reduced subluxation). No neurologic deficits upon wake up.
- Two neurologic deficits: Spinal cord monitoring is not available on either because of preexisting severe myelopathic disease. Both awoke paraplegic with intact sensation. Both have improved and are able to walk.

## REFERENCES

1. Cho KJ, Bridwell KH, Lenke LG, et al. Comparison of Smith-Petersen versus pedicle subtraction osteotomy for the correction of fixed sagittal imbalance. Spine 2005;30(18):2030–2037.
2. Dick J, Boachie-Adjei O, Wilson M. One-stage versus two-stage anterior and posterior spinal reconstruction in adults. Comparison of outcomes including nutritional status, complications rates, hospital costs, and other factors. Spine 1992;17(8 suppl):S310–S316.
3. Johnson JR, Holt RT. Combined use of anterior and posterior surgery for adult scoliosis. Orthop Clin North Am 1988;19(2):361–370.
4. Leatherman KD, Dickson RA. Two-stage corrective surgery for congenital deformities of the spine. J Bone Joint Surg Br 1979;61-B(3): 324–328.
5. Lehman RA Jr, Polly DW Jr, Kuklo TR, et al. Straight-forward versus anatomic trajectory technique of thoracic pedicle screw fixation: a biomechanical analysis. Spine 2003;28(18):2058–2065.
6. Lenke LG, Sides BA, Koester LA, et al. Vertebral column resection for the treatment of severe spinal deformity. Clin Orthop Relat Res 2010;468(3):687–699.

CHAPTER 99

# Lumbar Discectomy

**Bradley K. Weiner and Ronald Mitchell**

## DEFINITION

- Clinically significant lumbar disc herniations are characterized by a focal distortion of the normal anatomic configuration of discal material resulting in compression *and* subsequent dysfunction of the lumbar nerve roots.

## ANATOMY

- The functional components of the intervertebral disc are the annulus fibrosus (fibrous concentric rings, type I collagen) enclosing the central nucleus pulposus (gelatinous, type II collagen, proteoglycans) and the vertebral endplates (hyaline cartilage).
- The anatomic unit of the lumbar spine is the vertebral body with its attached posterior elements and the disc below (**FIG 1A**).
- The nerve roots travel within the common dural sac (the cauda equina) and then exit at each level. They are numbered according to the pedicle beneath which they pass.
- The spinal canal is divided into zones from medial to lateral: central canal, subarticular zone, foraminal zone, and extraforaminal (far lateral) zone (**FIG 1B**).
- Disc herniations are best classified based on the following ways:
  - Based on the integrity of the annulus fibrosus and whether there is a connection of herniated discal material with the disc space (**FIG 2**)
  - Based on the anatomic location of the herniated material relative to the disc space, the canal, and the compressed nerve root using the nomenclature mentioned earlier (**FIG 3**)
- Accurate anatomic classification of disc herniations facilitates preoperative planning and can minimize the risk of surgical complications such as missed pathology and iatrogenic nerve root injury.
- The importance of a complete knowledge of spinal anatomy and understanding of the particular patient's pathoanatomy cannot be overstated.

## PATHOGENESIS

- In the normal disc, the nucleus pulposus imbibes and releases water to balance mechanical loads. The annulus fibrosus converts these loads to hoop stresses, thereby containing the nuclear material. The endplates allow diffusion of nutrition into, and waste products out of, the nucleus.
  - Together, they allow for the three basic spinal segmental functions: mobility, stability, and protection of the nearby neurologic structures.
- With early or intermediate disc degeneration (natural aging with or without minor repetitive trauma), the endplates fail to allow adequate diffusion, the nucleus fails to replace degraded proteoglycans, and annular support weakens (failure of cross-linking, development of clefts). Biomechanical dysfunction occurs, with possible herniation of nuclear material.
- Many disc herniations do not cause pain or neurologic symptoms. A combination of herniation, nerve root compression, and an inflammatory interface is required for nerve root dysfunction and associated radiculopathy and sciatica.

## NATURAL HISTORY

- Many studies have shown that with time and nonoperative treatment, over 90% of patients with a first-time lumbar disc herniation will get better without surgery. Accordingly, to propose surgery requires clear indications.

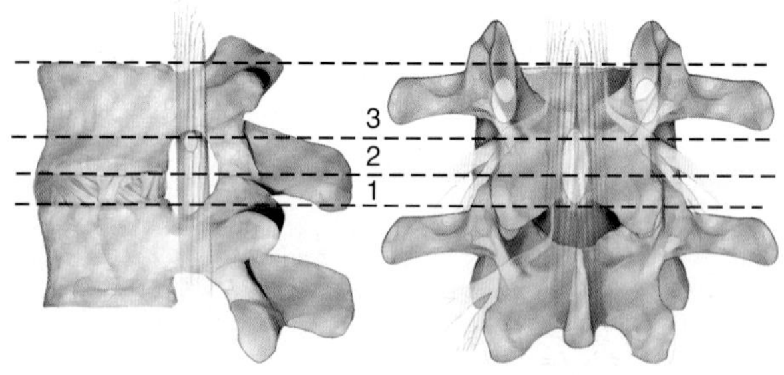


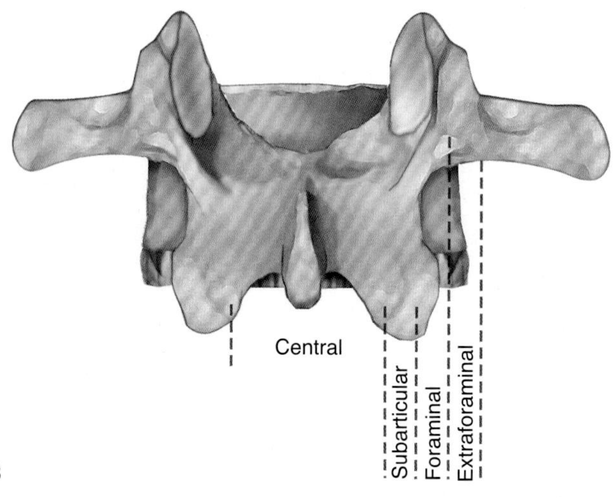


**FIG 1** • **A.** Anatomic unit. The first floor is the disc level, the second floor is the foraminal level, and the third floor is the pedicle level. **B.** Regions of the canal.

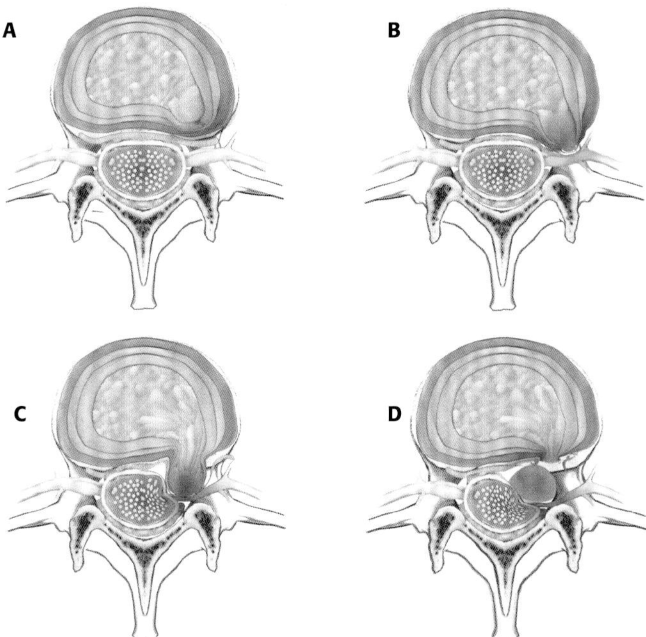


**FIG 2** • Classification of disc herniations based on relation to outer annulus: (**A**) protrusion, (**B**) subannular extrusion, (**C**) transannular extrusion, and (**D**) sequestration.

- Absolute indications
  - Bladder or bowel involvement secondary to a massive disc herniation and cauda equina syndrome: immediate surgical intervention
  - Progressive (ie, worsening) neurologic deficit: the earlier, the better prognostically
- Relative indications
  - Failure of conservative measures greater than 6 weeks to 3 months
  - Multiply recurrent sciatica
  - Significant neurologic deficit
- In each case, the properly informed patient must clearly understand the current best evidence: Most patients get better quickly with nonoperative care. For those with significant symptoms that are not better within 6 weeks, short-term and long-term (8 years) outcomes are better in patients treated with discectomy as compared with continued nonoperative care.

## HISTORY AND PHYSICAL FINDINGS

- The most common complaint is pain with or without associated paresthesias or weakness in a specific monoradicular anatomic distribution.

## IMAGING AND OTHER DIAGNOSTIC STUDIES

- Magnetic resonance imaging (MRI) is the imaging study of choice for the diagnosis and anatomic classification of lumbar disc herniations. It is highly sensitive and specific and provides, along with the clinical picture, adequate information for detailed preoperative planning.
- Computed tomography (CT) myelography is invasive and less specific than MRI but provides excellent sensitivity when MRI is unavailable or contraindicated.
- Plain radiographs may show disc space narrowing, early formation of osteophytes, or a "sciatic scoliosis." Although providing no direct evidence of a herniated disc, they may be helpful to rule out unexpected destructive pathology (eg, infection, tumor, fracture) in patients who have failed to respond to nonoperative intervention or those with red flags. They also allow excellent delineation of bony anomalies that may prove vital to preoperative planning and intraoperative localization, such as transitional lumbosacral articulations or spina bifida occulta.

## DIFFERENTIAL DIAGNOSIS

- Intraspinal, extrinsic compression, or irritation at the level of the nerve root: spinal stenosis, osteomyelitis or discitis, neoplasm, epidural fibrosis (scar)
- Intraspinal, extrinsic compression, or irritation proximal to the nerve root: conus and cauda lesions such as neurofibroma or ependymoma
- Intraspinal, intrinsic nerve root dysfunction: neuropathy (diabetic, idiopathic, alcoholic, iatrogenic [chemotherapy]), herpes zoster, arachnoiditis, nerve root tumor
- Extraspinal sources distal to the nerve root: pelvic or more distal neoplasms with associated sciatic or femoral nerve compression, sacroiliac disease (eg, infection, osteoarthritis), osteoarthritis of the hip, peripheral vascular disease

## NONOPERATIVE MANAGEMENT

- The evidence base is still a bit unclear, but the following are commonly recommended.
  - Rest: bed rest (no more than 2 or 3 days), activity or job modification, weight loss
  - Medication: analgesics (very short term for severe pain only), nonsteroidal anti-inflammatories, tapered doses of oral steroids
  - Exercise: physical therapy (McKenzie program)
  - Injections: epidural or selective root blocks (may provide some temporary relief while the natural history takes over)—no impact on long-term outcomes
  - Time: 6 weeks to 3 months (unless absolute indications for surgery exist as noted earlier)

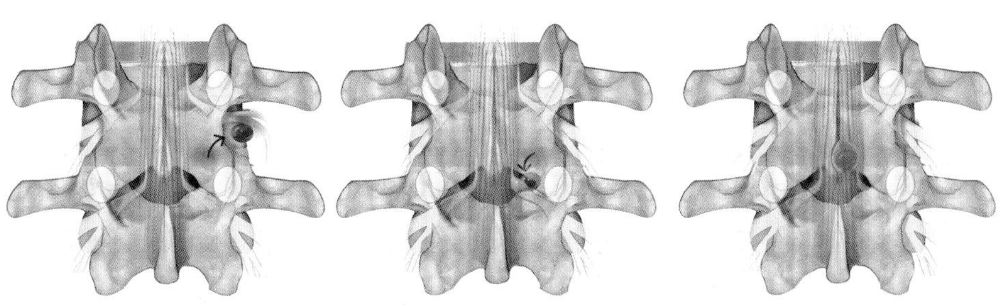

**FIG 3** • The patterns of disc migration can be characterized relative to the structures of the anatomic unit (eg, at the disc level or at the pedicle level). The area of root compression can be described relative to the nerve root anatomy (eg, at the shoulder of the traversing root, in the axilla of the exiting root).

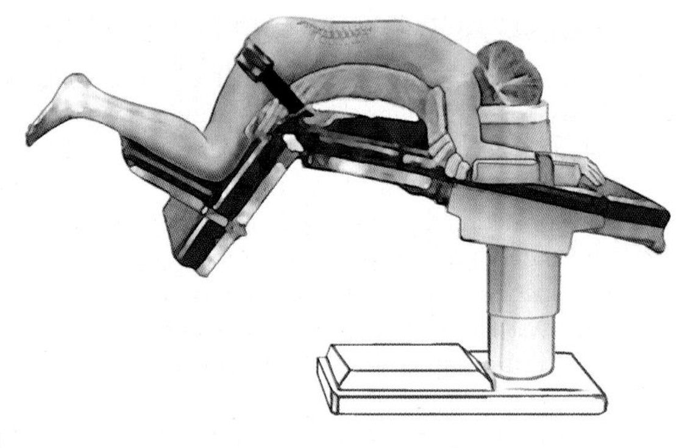

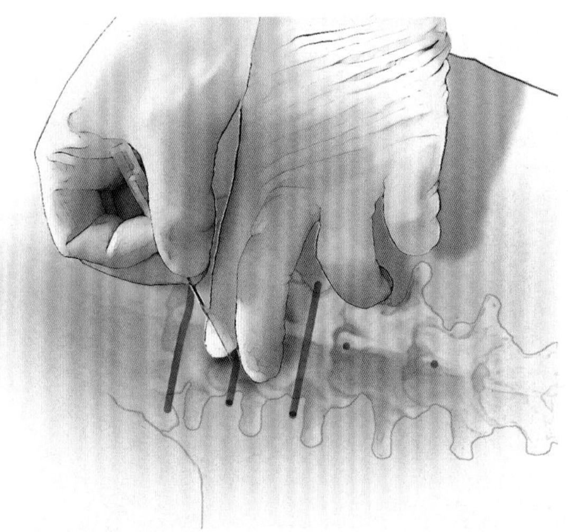

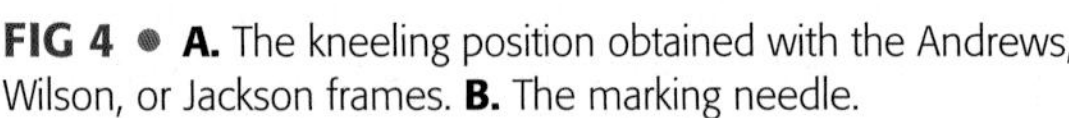

FIG 4 • A. The kneeling position obtained with the Andrews, Wilson, or Jackson frames. B. The marking needle.

## SURGICAL MANAGEMENT

- The evidence base is clear: Open discectomy and microdiscectomy are the operative techniques with the best-documented short-term and long-term outcomes and are the gold standards of surgery for lumbar disc herniations.

### Preoperative Planning

- This is *vital* and should aim to answer three questions:
  - What nerve root is involved (answered by history and physical examination)?
  - Where is the herniated material relative to the disc space, the canal, and the nerve root (answered by MRI)?
  - What approach will afford the best visualization and access to the herniated material while minimizing injury to tissues not directly involved in the pathologic process?

### Positioning

- A "kneeling" position is generally used, with the patient stabilized on an Andrews frame, a Wilson frame, or the Jackson table (**FIG 4A**).
  - Some hip and knee flexion will decrease lumbar lordosis and facilitate an approach through the interlaminar window.
  - The abdomen must be free to decrease intra-abdominal pressure and venous backflow through the plexus of Batson into the spinal canal.
- Shoulders should be abducted less than 90 degrees and with some flexion. The neck should be neutral or gently flexed.
- Eyes must be protected and elbows, knees, and feet well padded.
- A needle is passed between and lateral to the spinous processes at the involved level, and C-arm imaging is used to confirm that the proper level will be approached (**FIG 4B**). The needle is removed, and the level is marked and labeled on the skin.
- The involved side will be determined preoperatively by patient complaint and location of herniation on MRI but should also be marked on the patient's skin at this point.

### Approach

- The interlaminar window approach is used in about 90% of lumbar disc herniations requiring surgery. It is appropriate for herniations within the central canal or subarticular zones from L1 to S1 and for herniations within the foramen at L5–S1.
- The intertransverse window approach is used in about 10% of lumbar disc herniations requiring surgery. It is appropriate for herniations within the foraminal and extraforaminal zones from L1 to L5.
- For each step in the procedure, incision, excision, and retraction of tissues should be minimized. The goal is to *get the job done completely and safely with minimal trauma to tissues not directly involved in the pathologic process.*

TECHNIQUES

## Incision and Dissection

- The skin incision is made directly midline posteriorly and extends from the top of the cephalad spinous process to the bottom of the caudal spinous process, about 1.5 inches for single-level pathology.
- The subcutaneous tissues are then gently and bluntly mobilized and retracted to allow visualization of the dorsolumbar fascia.
- From here, one of two windows of approach will be undertaken based on the location of the disc herniation: the interlaminar window or the intertransverse window.

## Interlaminar Window

- The dorsolumbar fascia is incised just off the midline in a gentle curvilinear fashion on the involved side at a length to match the skin incision.
- A Cobb elevator is used to gently elevate the muscle (multifidus) from the spinous processes to the midportion of the facet joint laterally.
  - The degree of muscle elevation should be limited to what is necessary to allow adequate laminar exposure for laminotomy.
- A retractor is then placed. We prefer a retractor with a medial hook for the interspinous ligament and a blade for gentle lateral muscular retraction (**TECH FIG 1A**).
  - An intraoperative C-arm image is then obtained to confirm the level. Alternatively, a lateral radiograph can be taken.
  - A cylindrical retractor, placed transmuscularly using a sequential dilation technique, is a reasonable alternative as long as great care is taken to expose the correct portion of the interlaminar window (there is a tendency to be "pushed" too far laterally).

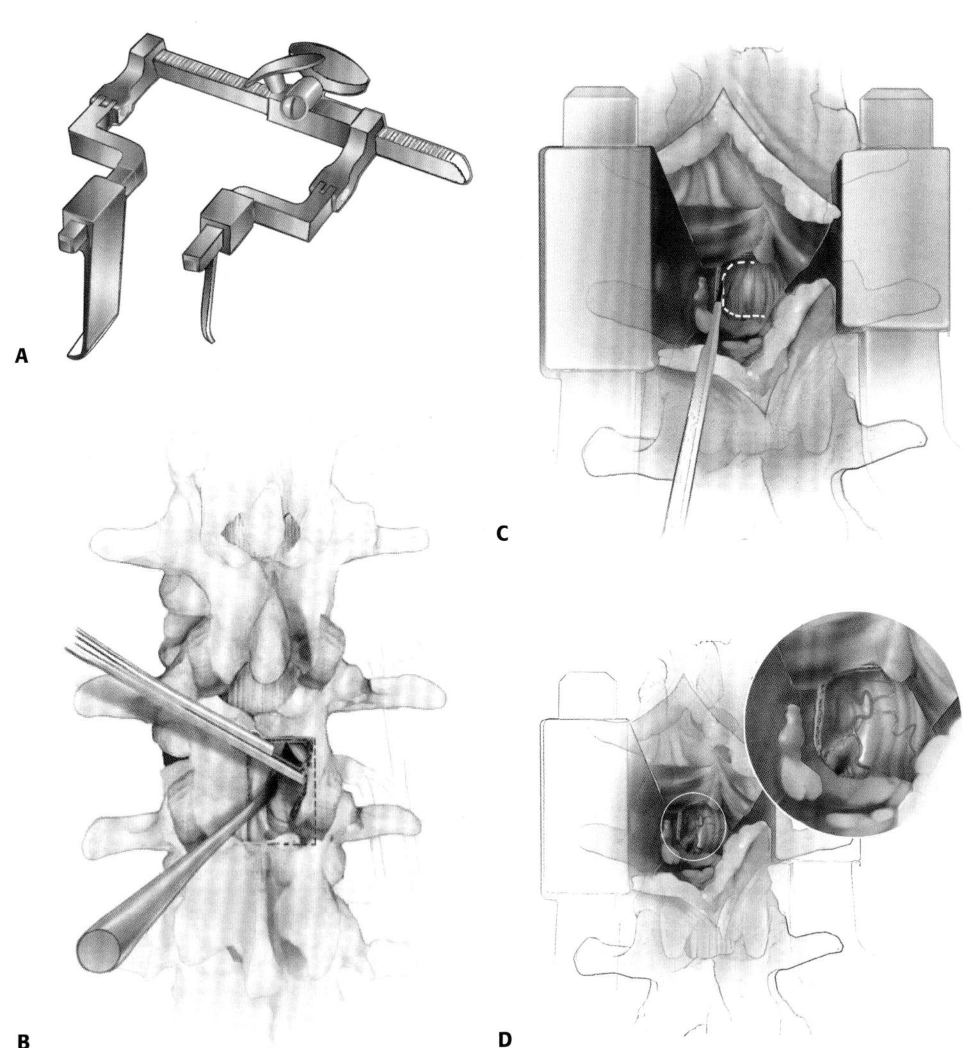


**TECH FIG 1** • **A.** Muscle retractor. **B.** Laminotomy. **C.** Laminotomy and the ligamentum. Bony excision used for the typical disc herniation in the canal or subarticular zones. It may need to be extended cephalad for herniations extending upward into the second story or may need to include the upper portion of the caudal lamina for herniations extending downward into the third story of the level below. The ligamentum is either freed from its insertions on the undersurface of the lamina above and the undersurface of the facet capsule laterally using a sharp curette, creating a flap, or is incised and split as depicted. **D.** Identifying the lateral edge of the root. The traversing root is readily identified by vessels that travel along its lateral edge longitudinally, rise up onto its shoulder, and form a plexus in its axilla. Further caudally, the root is closely associated with the medial border of the pedicle.

- At this point, illumination and magnification are gained by the use of the operative microscope (our preference) or a headlamp and loupes.
  - Outcomes are similar for the two when used properly, and the surgeon should decide on his or her preference based on experience and comfort level.
- A laminotomy on the undersurface of the cephalad lamina and minimal medial facetectomy is then performed using a Kerrison rongeur (**TECH FIG 1B**).
  - The degree of laminotomy and facetectomy should be enough to allow full visualization of the underlying nerve root at the area of compression and to allow access for excision of herniated disc material—no more and no less.
    - For small disc herniations in the canal or subarticular zones (the "typical disc herniation"), minimal bony excision is required at lower lumbar levels.
    - For larger disc herniations and those extending cephalad into the second story, a larger laminotomy or even hemilaminectomy may be required. The key in these situations is to preserve at least 5 mm of the lateral pars interarticularis and at least 50% of the medial facet.
- Laminotomy of the upper surface of the caudal lamina is generally not needed unless the herniated material has migrated caudally to the third story of the level below adjacent to the pedicle.
- The ligamentum flavum is then addressed. One of two techniques is used: the Rick Delamarter and John McCulloch flap or the Rob Fraser split (**TECH FIG 1C**).
  - The former preserves the ligamentum flavum as a complete barrier to minimize scar formation from posterior, whereas the latter offers a little less coverage but preserves the ligament's biomechanical integrity.
- The lateral edge of the traversing nerve root is then identified.
  - This is readily identified by consistent lateral veins and the root's association with the pedicle (**TECH FIG 1D**).
  - These veins can then be gently mobilized to allow exposure of the underlying annulus.
  - Occasionally, anomalous roots lateral to the traversing root may be present. Again, safety is ensured by identifying the veins directly overlying the annulus and using these to provide a window to access.

## Herniation Exposure

- For herniations within the canal or subarticular zones and in the first or second story (85% of encountered discs), the traversing nerve root is gently mobilized medially, allowing exposure of the herniated disc.
  - If the root is immobile, the surgeon should excise more bone within the subarticular region (medial facetectomy) to afford visualization and palpation of the medial border of the pedicle associated with the traversing root.
  - Access to the disc cephalad to this will be within a safe zone lateral to the traversing root and within the axilla of the exiting root.
  - Once larger fragments are teased out, the traversing root will become mobile, allowing greater access.
  - Retraction should be minimal at upper levels (L1–L3 due to presence of the conus) and limited to about 40%—that is, to less than half the width of the unilateral hemilaminotomy below this (**TECH FIG 2**).
    - Retraction should be relaxed during periods in which no active work is undertaken in or near the disc space: The nerve is rested while the pituitary rongeur is being cleaned and gently reretracted when it returns. This will minimize trauma to the root.
  - Hemostasis is then obtained by gently tucking small pieces of Gelfoam or thrombin cephalad and caudally to the exposed disc space. These are to be removed at the end of the case.
    - If bipolar cautery is used, it should be done with caution to avoid root injury.
- Herniations extending caudally to the third story of the level below (uncommon, 5%) are most often within the "axilla" of the traversing root. Retraction of the root is not used; rather, the herniation (usually sequestered) is gently teased out.

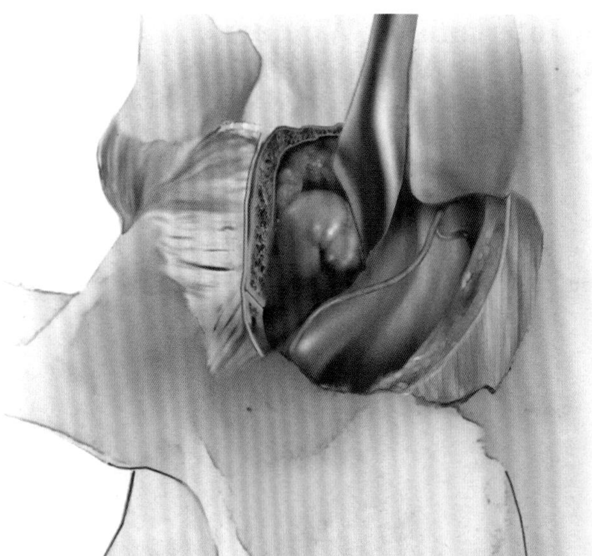

**TECH FIG 2** • Root retraction is minimal and intermittent.

## Discectomy

- Once visualized, any free disc material is removed with a pituitary rongeur. A ball-tipped probe is used to tease out any additional free fragments hiding further out in the subarticular zone or under the common dural sac or root.
- The disc space is then entered (this will be the first step in "contained" herniations) by annulotomy. A long-handled no. 15 blade facing away from the traversing root is used, preferably with a longitudinal orientation.
- Within the disc space, any loose fragments are removed with the pituitary rongeur (**TECH FIG 3**), and the disc space is irrigated.
  - More aggressive excision ("complete discectomy") may slightly decrease the risk of recurrence but at the price of increased back pain and a potential for accelerating the degenerative process.
  - Depth of work should be limited to avoid anterior perforation and potential vascular injury. The surgeon should respect the anterior portion of the annulus and avoid perforating it with an instrument.

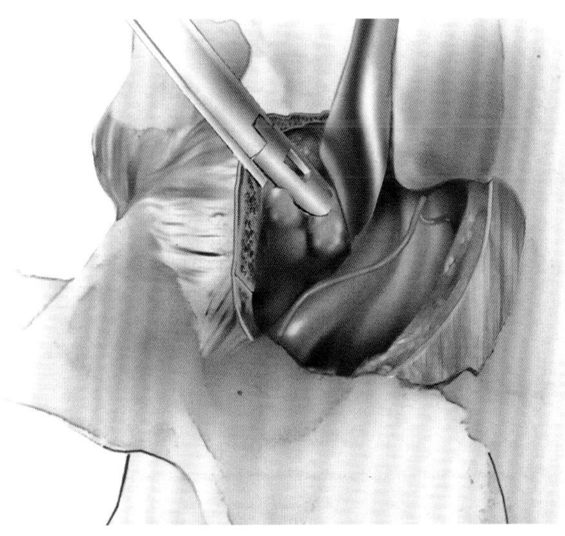

- Discectomy is complete when no additional loose fragments can be removed from the disc space and free mobility of the nerve root is confirmed.
- The root retractor is then removed, along with the pieces of Gelfoam.
- The wound is thoroughly irrigated. This "washing," coupled with removing the root retractor, is usually adequate to stop any epidural bleeding.
  - If it persists, temporarily placing Gelfoam again is almost always adequate.
- Unless there is still a bit of oozing, drains are generally not indicated, and the wound is closed in three layers (fascia, subcutaneous tissue, and skin [absorbable, subcuticular]).

**TECH FIG 3** ● Discectomy. After annulotomy, the pituitary rongeur is used to remove the herniation and loose fragments within the disc space.

## Intertransverse Window

- The dorsolumbar fascia is incised 1.5 fingerbreadths off the midline longitudinally (**TECH FIG 4A**).
- The plane between the multifidus medially and the longissimus laterally is freed by finger dissection, allowing palpation of the facet joint.
- A retractor is placed within this plane (**TECH FIG 4B**) and an intraoperative C-arm image is obtained to confirm the level.
- The tip of the superior articular process and the lateral pars interarticularis are exposed with electrocautery and partially resected (**TECH FIG 4C,D**).
- The intertransverse membrane is gently retracted laterally using a ball-tipped probe.
- Gentle blunt dissection is used to identify the exiting nerve root and the underlying herniated material. Gentle technique, patience, and really good lighting and magnification are required here (again, we prefer the operative microscope but outcomes are similar regardless). There is plenty of adipose tissue and a venous plexus surrounding the dorsal root ganglion of the root that must be identified before introducing the pituitary rongeur.
- A ball-tipped probe and pituitary rongeur are used to gently tease out the loose fragment, with minimal to no retraction applied to the root. This can be traced back into the disc space as necessary and any loose fragments are removed.
- The wound is irrigated, hemostasis is obtained, and closure is performed as described earlier.

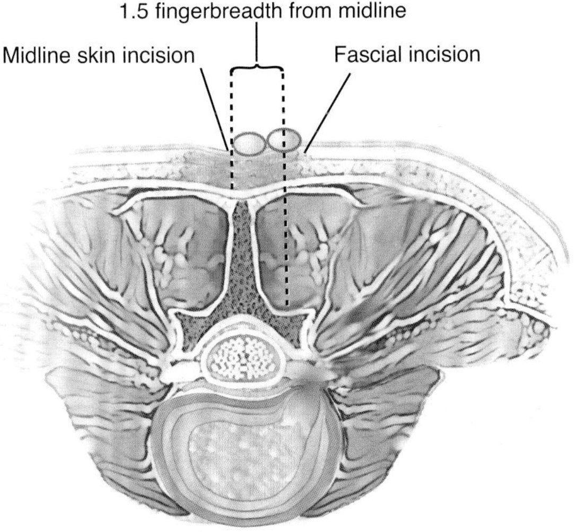


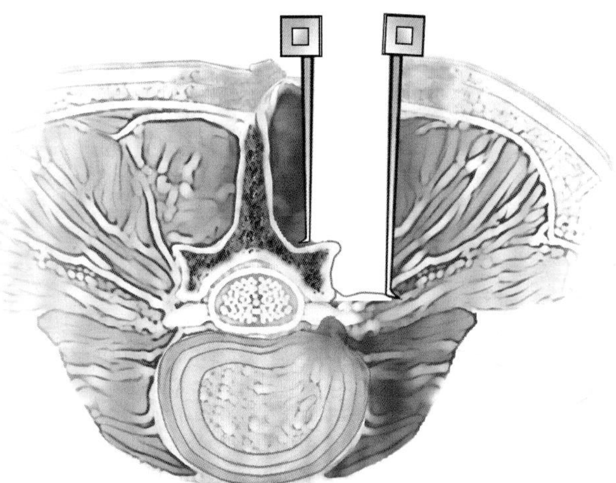


**TECH FIG 4** ● **A.** The fascial incision is made 1.5 fingerbreadths from the midline. **B.** Retraction. *(continued)*

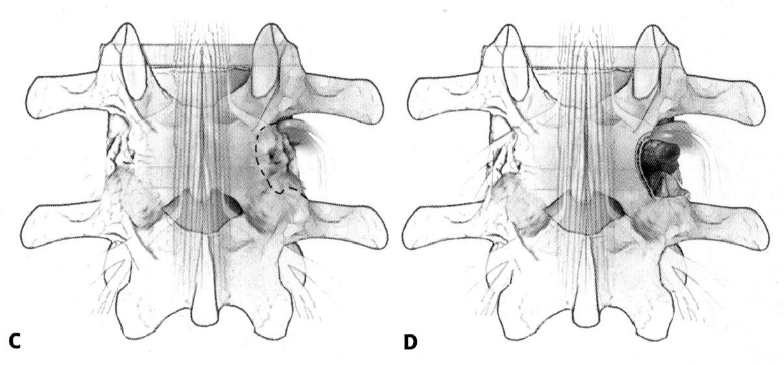


**TECH FIG 4** • *(continued)* **C.** The *shaded areas* represent the area of bony excision during discectomy. **D.** The intertransverse membrane is then gently mobilized laterally, allowing exposure and excision of the herniated disc.

## PEARLS AND PITFALLS

| | |
|---|---|
| Wrong-level exposure, exploration, or surgery is always a risk. The level is marked preoperatively and intraoperatively as noted earlier. | ■ The surgeon should beware of obese patients with a significant lumbar lordosis. It is very common to expose the wrong level despite proper localization of the skin incision. Thus, the correct level must be ensured radiographically before entering the spinal canal.<br>■ The surgeon should also beware of patients with "transitional" lumbar vertebrae (sacralization or lumbarization). Here, it is often best to correlate the level on intraoperative images with the preoperative MRI, which will clearly show the disc herniation as well as the immobile, uninvolved transitional levels (narrow disc space with maintained bright signal intensity on T2 with or without poorly developed facet joints). |
| Certain differences exist between revision discectomy via the interlaminar window and primary surgery. | ■ In revision surgery, the laminotomy and facetectomy should be extended cephalad and laterally to allow exposure of "normal" dura (above and lateral to areas of epidural fibrosis [scar]).<br>■ Identification of the traversing root may be difficult (scar, loss of characteristic veins), but it will still *always* be associated with its pedicle. The medial border of the pedicle is readily identified, and tissues medial to it (scar, root) are gently mobilized to identify the fragment and disc space.<br>■ If the root is completely immobile, further medial facetectomy will be required, and the disc space should be entered in line with the subjacent pedicle to ensure being lateral to the traversing root and medial to the exiting root. |
| Revision discectomy via the intertransverse window for foraminal or extraforaminal disc herniations is not recommended as the planes will be distorted and safe surgery is difficult. | ■ Using the interlaminar window instead, with resection of the inferior articular process of the cephalad vertebra with or without arthrodesis, is safer and affords excellent visualization. |
| Anomalous neural anatomy can be best identified preoperatively on MRI. | ■ The surgeon should beware of large, perfectly round soft tissue masses within the foramen on parasagittal imaging or in the canal on axial imaging. If it does not look like the other roots (mimicking a large round disc herniation) but has their signal intensity, it is likely an anomalous or conjoined root. |

## POSTOPERATIVE CARE

- After surgery, patients may be fitted with a light lumbar corset if desired and are encouraged to walk once anesthesia has worn off and pain permits. About 85% are discharged as outpatients. Fifteen percent who are older (less mobile) or have nausea and vomiting require an overnight stay and 23-hour observation.
- Once home, patients engage in a program of progressive walking, stretching, and corset use for comfort. For those progressing slowly, physical therapy may be introduced. Heavy lifting and excessive bending and twisting should be avoided in the first few weeks.
- If all is well, they may drive in about a week and return to light work once they feel up to it. Heavy labor should be avoided for 6 to 12 weeks to ensure proper soft tissue healing (skin, muscle, annulotomy). Long-term activities are not restricted.

## OUTCOMES

- There is an 85% likelihood of an excellent or good outcome 8 years postoperatively.

- Patients with significant medical or social comorbidities (eg, diabetes, heavy smoking), worker's compensation or litigation, and psychological problems (depression) are less likely to do well. The same is true for patients who receive no care for more than 6 months before presentation.
- Anatomically, patients with larger disc herniations (sac compression one-third or more) and those at higher levels (L2–L3 or L3–L4) have a better prognosis. Those with a retrolisthesis at L5–S1 do not do as well.
- Truly informed consent is mandatory.

## COMPLICATIONS

- Surgeon-dependent: wrong level, wrong side, missed pathology, iatrogenic instability, "battered root syndrome," dural tear, hemorrhage, positioning (eg, eyes, ulnar nerve)
- Operative environment or patient-dependent: wound infection, disc space infection, urinary retention, thrombophlebitis, or pulmonary embolism

## SUGGESTED READINGS


1. Atlas SJ, Deyo RA, Keller RB, et al. The Maine Lumbar Spine Study, Part II. 1-year outcomes of surgical and non-surgical management of sciatica. Spine 1996;21:1777–1786.
2. Boden SD, Davis DO, Dina TS, et al. Abnormal magnetic-resonance scans of the lumbar spine in asymptomatic subjects. A prospective investigation. J Bone Joint Surg Am 1990;72(3):403–408.
3. Lurie J, Weinstein J, Lurie JD, et al. Surgical versus nonoperative treatment for lumbar disc herniation: eight-year results for the spine patient outcomes research trial. Spine 2014;39:3–16.
4. McCulloch JA. Microdiscectomy. In: Frymoyer JW, ed. The Adult Spine: Principles and Practice. New York: Raven Press, 1991:1765–1783.
5. McCulloch JA, Weiner BK. Microsurgery in the lumbar intertransverse interval. Instr Course Lect 2002;51:233–241.
6. Spangfort EV. The lumbar disc herniation. A computer-aided analysis of 2,504 operations. Acta Orthop Scand 1972;142:1–95.
7. Weber H. Lumbar disc herniation. A controlled prospective study with ten years of observations. Spine 1983;8(2):131–140.
8. Weiner BK, Dabbah M. Lateral lumbar disc herniations treated with a paraspinal approach: an independent assessment of longer-term outcomes. J Spinal Disord Tech 2005;18(6):519–521.

Hip

# Anterior Approach for Open Reduction of the Developmentally Dislocated Hip

Richard M. Schwend

## DEFINITION

- Developmental dysplasia or dislocation of the hip (DDH) is a disorder that may affect the development and stability of the hip joint during the critical period of growth, either in utero or after birth.
- This may lead to dysplasia, subluxation, or frank dislocation of the hip joint.

## ANATOMY

- Growth of the hip joint is genetically and mechanically determined.
  - In the first trimester, the structures of the joint begin as a single mass of scleroblastema with a globular femoral head that becomes cartilage at 6 weeks.
  - By 8 weeks' gestation, the start of the fetal period, vascular invasion leads to endochondral ossification.
  - The joint space develops by degeneration at 7 to 8 weeks, and the structure of the joint is well apparent by week 11.
  - A round and reduced femoral head influences the concave shape of the acetabulum to develop.
- Acetabular growth depends on interstitial, appositional, periosteal new bone and secondary centers of ossification growth.
  - In the first two trimesters of fetal life, the acetabulum is a hemisphere with a depth 50% of its diameter. However, by the time of birth, the depth is only 40% of its diameter, which may contribute to instability at birth.
  - The acetabular labrum, which resembles an O ring (**FIG 1A**), contributes considerable mechanical stability and proprioceptive feedback (**FIG 1B**).
  - By 8 years of age, the acetabular shape is for the most part determined and thus surgical reduction is less advised, especially if the dislocation is bilateral.
  - There is continued growth into adolescence, with the triradiate cartilage fusing by 13 years in girls and 15 years in boys.
  - Closure of the triradiate cartilage may occur earlier in the dysplastic hip.
  - By adulthood, the acetabular depth is 60% of its diameter.
- The proximal femur is formed initially as a single chondroepiphysis (**FIG 1C**), with the ossific nucleus typically appearing in infancy at 2 to 8 months of age.
- There may be some side-to-side size discrepancy in appearance.
- The greater trochanter nucleus appears at about 3 years in girls and 5 years in boys, with the lesser trochanter appearing by age 6 to 11 years.
- The femoral head vascularity is mostly from the medial and somewhat from the lateral femoral circumflex arteries. Because it is an intra-articular dome-shaped structure, this blood supply is susceptible to injury.

## PATHOGENESIS

- Around the time of birth, capsular laxity, a normally shallow acetabulum, and abnormal mechanical forces, such as those seen in breech presentation, may cause the hip capsule to be lax and to dislocate.
- An absent or subluxated femoral head eventually leads to a flat, egg-shaped acetabulum, which is a consistent finding on three-dimensional computer modeling performed of the acetabulum (**FIG 2A**).

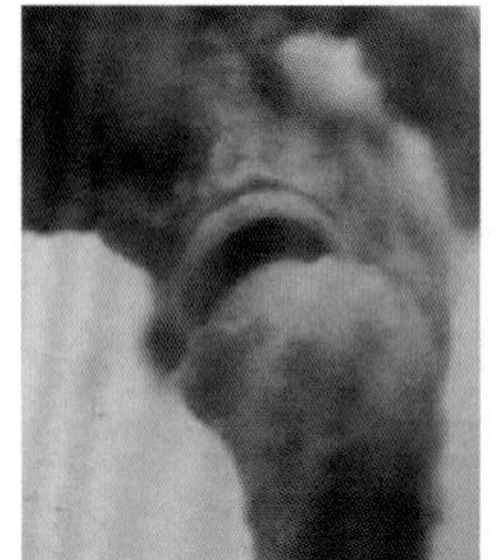
A
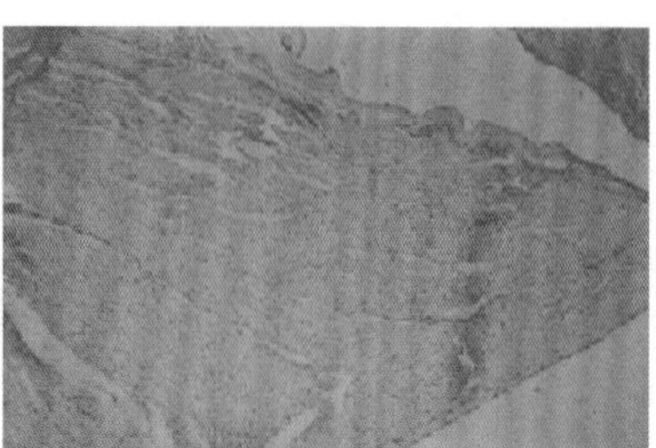
B
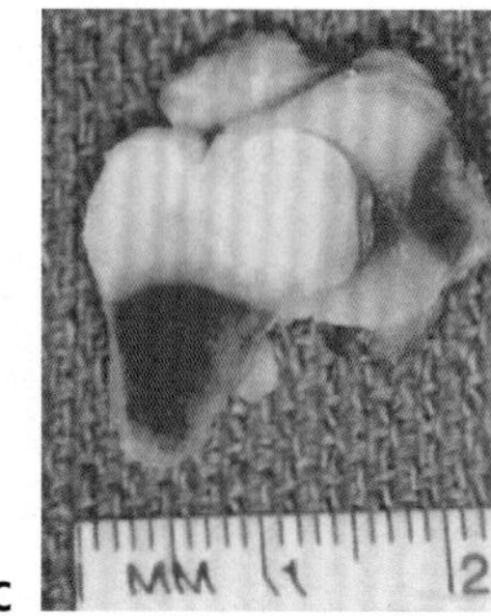

C

**FIG 1** • **A.** Femoral head and acetabulum of newborn hip. Note the concentric nature of the acetabular labrum, resembling in form and function an O ring. **B.** Acetabular labrum in a second trimester human fetus. S100 stain shows nerve tissue extending to the tip of the labrum. This is evidence of the proprioceptive function of the labrum. **C.** Coronal section of a third trimester fetal hip joint showing the extensive cartilaginous nature of the femoral chondroepiphysis and the acetabular cartilage. (**A:** Courtesy of Gene Mandell, MD.)

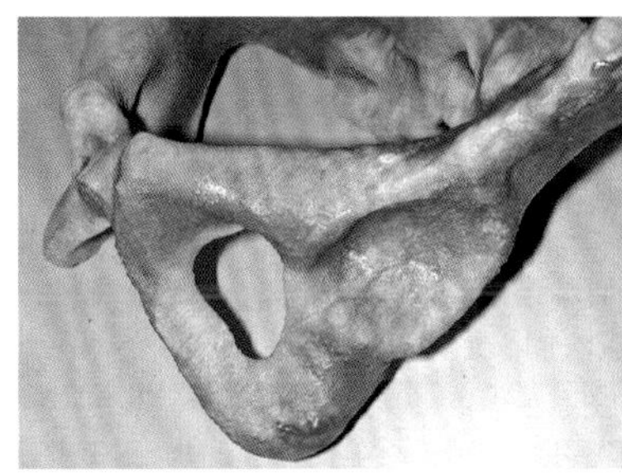

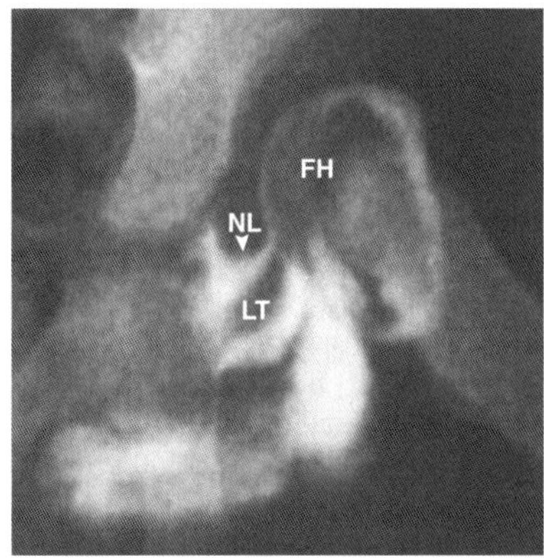


**FIG 2** • **A.** Three-dimensional computer-generated hip model of adolescent with long-standing left hip developmental dysplasia. The acetabulum is shallow and elongated in its superior aspect, resembling an egg. **B.** Intraoperative left hip arthrogram of a dislocated femoral head (*FH*). *Arrowhead* shows the neolimbus (*NL*) contributing to blocking the reduction of the femoral head. *LT*, ligamentum teres.

- With time, the neolimbus, which is abnormally formed articular cartilage, can develop at the edge of the acetabulum. It can be a barrier to reduction (**FIG 2B**).[8]
- A steep, maloriented growth plate; intra-articular obstructions; and stunting of periosteal new bone formation all in time contribute to further deformity.
- Mechanical blocks to reduction include the anteromedial capsule, ligamentum teres, psoas tendon, neolimbus, transverse acetabular ligament (which is an inferior medial extension of the acetabular labrum), and intra-articular pulvinar tissue.
  - An inverted labrum is rarely a block to reduction.
  - The average unit load of human and animal joint cartilage is 25 kg/cm$^2$.
  - Hips with acetabular dysplasia, and particularly with subluxation, have about 25% less contact area and more unit load (stress) per area of contact.
  - There is an inverse relationship between greater contact pressures and the onset of osteoarthritis.

## NATURAL HISTORY

- Newborn period
  - About 1 in 60 infants have instability at birth, with 60% of cases resolving in the first week of life and 88% by the first 2 months. Thus, about 1.5 in 1000 have a true dislocation.[2]
  - Muscle activity is considered important for recovery and is the basis of the Pavlik harness success.
- Untreated acetabular dysplasia with subluxation or dislocation
  - The natural history of hip dysplasia when subluxation or dislocation is present is predictable. The long-term outcome is worse than with acetabular dysplasia without subluxation.[13]
  - The onset of symptoms and radiographic deterioration is directly related to the degree of subluxation and dysplasia.
  - Clinical symptoms, typically pain, may antecede the radiographic deterioration by 10 years.
  - If the hip is completely dislocated, limb length discrepancy and back and knee pain are common, whereas painful arthritis correlates with the presence of a false acetabulum and its adverse effect on the femoral head articular cartilage.
- Acetabular dysplasia with no subluxation
  - The natural history of acetabular dysplasia is much less predictable when subluxation or dislocation is absent.[13]
  - During childhood, hips that are well centered improve their acetabular dysplasia, although not always to normal, whereas the hip that is radiologically eccentric typically does not improve.
  - If the center-edge angle in the mature hip is less than 20 degrees, the hip will likely develop arthritis sometime during the patient's lifetime. However, it is difficult to determine how early in life the deterioration will occur.
  - Although hips with acetabular dysplasia can spontaneously improve, this improvement is not predictable or necessarily complete.[10]
  - A hip with a persistently upsloping lateral margin seen on an anteroposterior (AP) radiograph generally develops arthritis by late adulthood.[11]

## PATIENT HISTORY AND PHYSICAL FINDINGS

- Because 75% of DDH occurs in female infants with no other risk factures, clinical examination of all infants is the most important method of detecting hip dysplasia.
- All newborn infants should receive a gentle and focused examination of the hips, including range of motion and Ortolani maneuver.
  - The physical examination of the newborn, rather than imaging studies, should determine the diagnosis of DDH and the need for treatment.
  - An Ortolani-positive hip is dislocated or subluxated and the examiner perceives that the hip partially reduces with abduction. After several months of age, the hip may appear stable on examination but may still be dislocated due to tightening of the soft tissue structures about the hip.
  - The child is examined for any abnormal skin creases (**FIG 3**). Proximal skin creases may indicate a dislocated hip or a short femur. The examiner should also note the

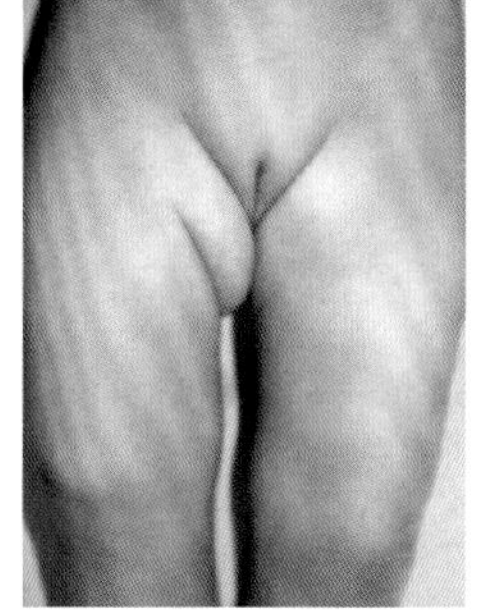

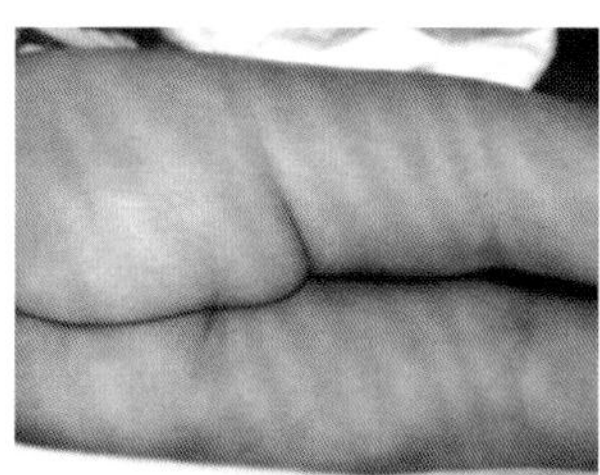

**FIG 3** • **A,B.** Abnormal skin creases.

level of the popliteal skin crease, the position of the knee, and any lateral displacement of the hip.

- A simple, high-pitched and commonly felt "hip click" is not a sign of instability or dislocation.
- Hip instability decreases with time, whereas deformity, such as limited hip abduction, increases with time.
  - The young infant with a dislocated hip may have normal abduction until several months of age. There may be limited abduction in developmental coxa vara. Abduction may appear to be normal if both hips are dislocated.
- The upper extremities, spine, and feet are always inspected to evaluate for possible generalized conditions such as arthrogryposis or neuromuscular conditions.
- In the child of walking age, a delay of walking may be the first indicator that the hip is dislocated.
- Dipping of the pelvis and shoulder (Trendelenburg gait), female profile (pelvic widening from the dislocation), and shortening of the thigh (Galeazzi sign) are classic signs of a dislocated hip in the older child.
  - The Galeazzi test may also be abnormal if the child has a congenital short femur.
  - Additional signs of Trendelenburg gait include side-to-side waddling, indicating weak hip abductors, or the examiner may see lurching, indicating weak hip extensors. The child may stand or walk with hyperlordosis. These are proximal compensations for a hip dislocation and the resulting inadequate muscle strength to support the pelvis.

## IMAGING AND OTHER DIAGNOSTIC STUDIES

- Ultrasound is a useful imaging method up to 6 months of age (**FIG 4A**).
  - The two most common indications for ultrasound imaging are for screening the asymptomatic infant considered to be at high risk for hip dislocation (girls born breech have a 133/1000 risk of DDH) and for following an infant with proven DDH, especially during Pavlik harness treatment.
- The AP radiograph is most useful in infants older than 6 months of age.
  - In children older than 3 years of age, the Shenton line is a reliable indicator of subluxation (**FIG 4B**).
  - The Von Rosen view in abduction and internal rotation shows the ability of the femoral head to reduce.
  - In the adolescent or adult hip, a standing AP pelvis view is obtained with measurement of the center-edge angle, as well as standing false-profile views of each hip joint (**FIG 4C–E**).
  - The normal center-edge angle on the AP pelvic radiograph is greater than 24 degrees.
- Decision analysis model indicates that the most effective way to prevent hip arthritis by age 60 years is to do physical examination screening on the hips of all infants and to use ultrasound selectively on those infants with high risk factors.[5]
- Intraoperative arthrography can show whether the femoral head is fully reducible with no medial pooling of contrast (**FIG 4F**).
  - If the femoral head does not easily reduce and remain stable without excessive hip abduction, an open reduction

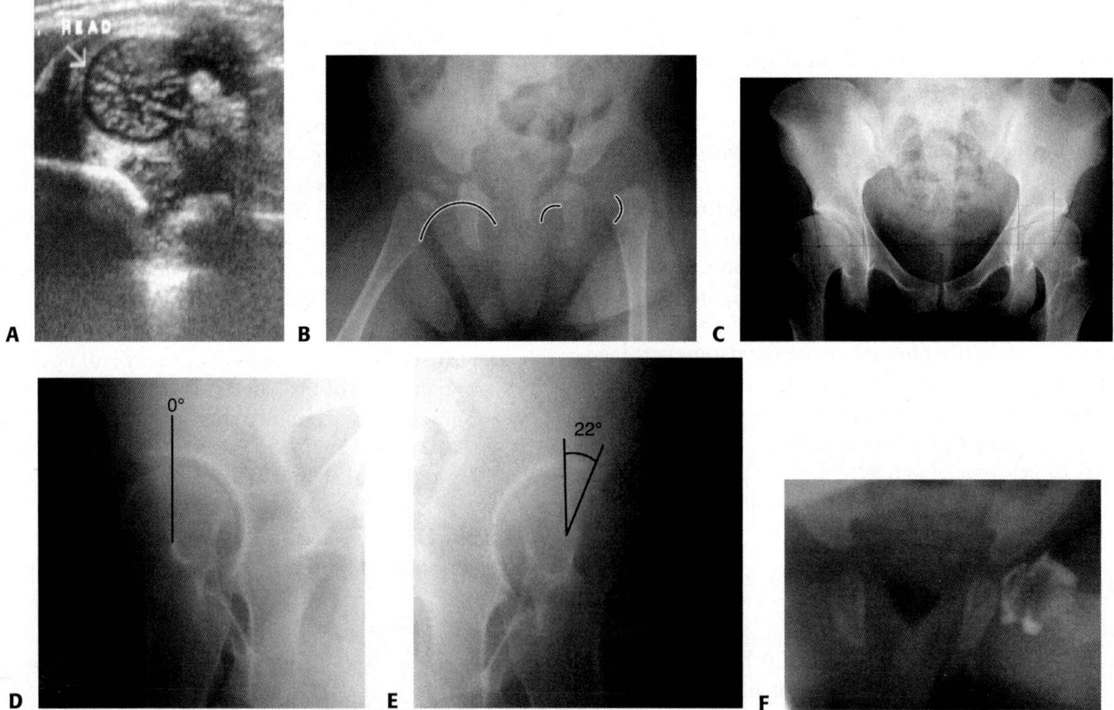


**FIG 4** • **A.** Coronal section ultrasound imaging through the most posterior aspect of the acetabulum. The femoral head is well visualized dislocated from the acetabulum. **B.** Seven-month-old child with a dislocated left hip. The acetabulum is steep. The femoral ossific nucleus is not present. There is a break in the Shenton line on the left and it is normal on the right. **C–E.** Radiographs of young adult with high-grade right acetabular dysplasia. **C.** On the AP pelvic view, the center-edge angle (CEA) on the left is low normal (26 degrees); on the right, it is 10 degrees. The Shenton line is intact, indicating that there is no subluxation. **D,E.** Right hip false-profile views. Right hip CEA is 0 degrees and left hip CEA is 22 degrees. **F.** Left hip intraoperative arthrogram shows concentric reduction. There is no pooling of the intra-articular contrast medially.

is used to address the extra-articular and intra-articular blocks to reduction.
- Computed tomography (CT) scanning is commonly used to evaluate the adequacy of a closed or open reduction after surgery and for preoperative planning of pelvic or femoral osteotomy.
  - However, even a limited CT scan can deliver over 100 times the radiation of daily background or that from a single chest radiograph. If using CT for a child, it is important to child size the peak kilovoltage and milliampere and scan only the indicated area with one scan.[11]
  - For imaging after closed reduction and casting, magnetic resonance imaging (MRI) can replace the use of CT and be accomplished with a limited study and no radiation.[3]

## DIFFERENTIAL DIAGNOSIS

- Septic hip dislocation: This is the most important diagnosis to consider in the young infant.
- Teratologic hip dislocation (arthrogryposis)
- Neuromuscular dislocation (most commonly cerebral palsy and spina bifida)
- Traumatic hip dislocation
- Developmental coxa vara: easy to mistake as DDH before the ossific nucleus is present
- Congenital short femur
- Instability and dysplasia related to underlying condition (Down syndrome, Ehlers-Danlos syndrome, Charcot-Marie-Tooth disease); commonly bilateral

## NONOPERATIVE MANAGEMENT

- The basic principles of treatment are to obtain a concentric, stable reduction while avoiding osteonecrosis; to promote normal growth of the hip; and to achieve normal long-term function.
- The treatment of DDH depends on the age of the child and thus the stage of development of the hip joint.
  - Generally, the earlier that treatment is initiated, the more likely that less invasive treatment will be successful and that a better outcome will result.
- Treatment options range from observation to a Pavlik harness (**FIG 5**) or other brace treatment in the young infant, to closed or open reduction and hip spica casting, pelvic or femoral osteotomies, and salvage procedures in older patients.
- By the time of skeletal maturity, as normal as possible, acetabular anatomy should be restored.[8] Ideally, reconstructive surgery should be performed during early childhood, when the results are believed to be better and the risks acceptable.

## SURGICAL MANAGEMENT

- If the hip remains dislocated or subluxated despite conservative treatment with a Pavlik harness or abduction orthosis, or if a concentric and stable reduction cannot be achieved with closed reduction and casting, open surgical reduction is appropriate.

### Preoperative Planning

- For the infant who has not achieved walking age, an open reduction without associated femoral shortening or pelvic osteotomy is generally sufficient.
- With age and walking, the deformities in and around the hip become more fixed and require a more aggressive surgical approach.
- Prereduction traction is less frequently used than in the past for the infant and is not recommended for the older child.[1]
- Generally, a child older than age 2 to 3 years requires a femoral shortening osteotomy if the femoral head is displaced proximally.[9]
  - Epidural or caudal regional anesthesia may be helpful to supplement the general anesthesia.
  - A type and screen is obtained, but blood transfusion is rarely required.
  - An indwelling bladder catheter is used during the surgery because much of the surgery is intrapelvic.

### Positioning

- A radiolucent table is used in case an intraoperative radiograph will be obtained.
- The child is placed in a semilateral position (**FIG 6**).
- The entire limb is draped free.

### Approach

- Several variations of the medial approach to the hip joint have been described. These are very useful in the infant if the femoral head is not excessively high and for bilateral instability surgery done the same day.

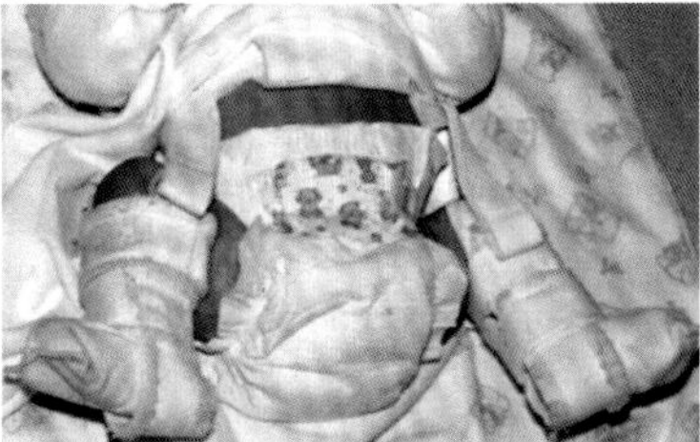

**FIG 5** ● Pavlik harness. This infant is comfortable in the harness; hips and knees are flexed with abduction provided by gravity, not from the lateral straps.

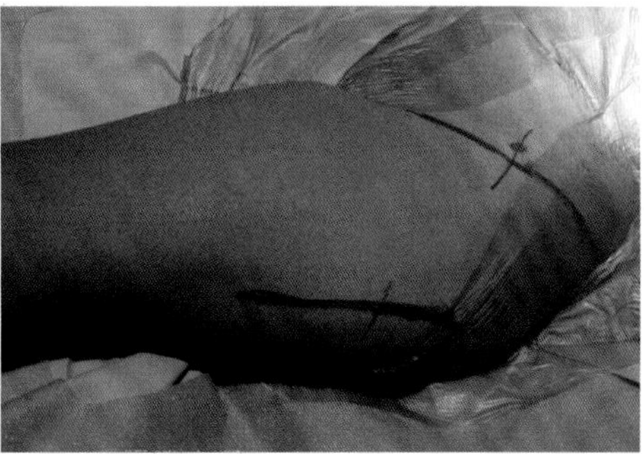

**FIG 6** ● Semilateral position. The anterior hip and lateral thigh incisions are generally parallel when the hip is flexed about 30 degrees.

- For the older infant and child, an anterior approach to the hip joint allows more extensile exposure.
  - The anterior approach is especially useful if there is a false acetabulum with a high dislocation and for fixed dislocations in which the hip capsule is adherent to the hip abductors and pelvic wall.
  - The anterior approach allows for an associated pelvic osteotomy through the same incision.
- The decision to perform a medial approach or an anterior approach to the hip joint will depend on the child's age, the location and severity of the pathology, and the surgeon's experience.



## Anterior Hip Exposure

- A modified anterior Smith-Petersen exposure with the incision placed in the inguinal crease just below the anterior superior iliac spine is cosmetically appealing.
- Sharp dissection is carried deep until no more fat can be identified.
  - This is the deep fascia, which can then be further exposed distally by using a sponge on the fascia.
- If femoral shortening is anticipated, a separate direct lateral approach to the proximal femur is used.
  - Both exposures should be completed before osteotomies are performed because of increased bleeding from the bone.
- The tensor–sartorius internervous interval is easier to identify distally where the muscles are divergent (**TECH FIG 1A**).
- The fascia of the tensor muscle is entered slightly lateral to the fatty interval between the two muscles. The lateral femoral cutaneous nerve is identified and protected.
- Army-Navy retractors are used to separate the tensor and sartorius muscles until the rectus femoris muscle is identified.
  - This dissection is continued proximally and the prow of the pelvis is exposed between the anterior superior and anterior inferior iliac spines.
- The external oblique muscle is gently separated off the iliac crest.
- The iliac crest apophysis is divided exactly in the middle with a single cut using a no. 15 blade down to iliac bone (**TECH FIG 1B**).
- Periosteal elevators are used to expose the inner and outer tables of the iliac crest (**TECH FIG 1C**).
- Laparotomy sponges are used to help dissect deep near the sciatic notch and to pack the surgical site for hemostasis.
  - Perforating vessels into the iliac bone on the inner table are consistently present and require bone wax for hemostasis.
- Smooth Lane retractors are used to further dissect the sciatic notch both medially and laterally.
- The reflected and straight heads of the rectus femoris muscle are identified (**TECH FIG 1D**).

A
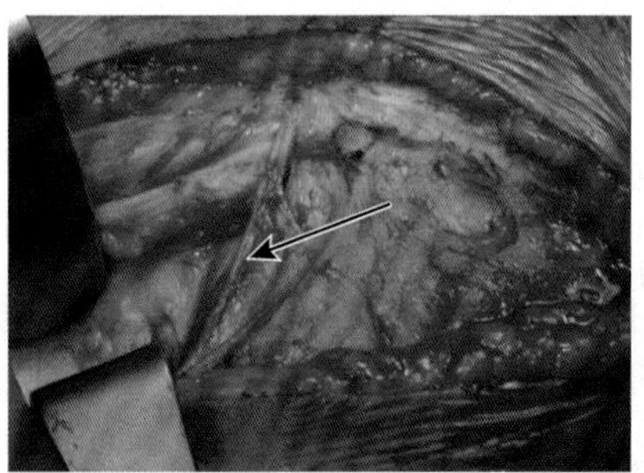
B
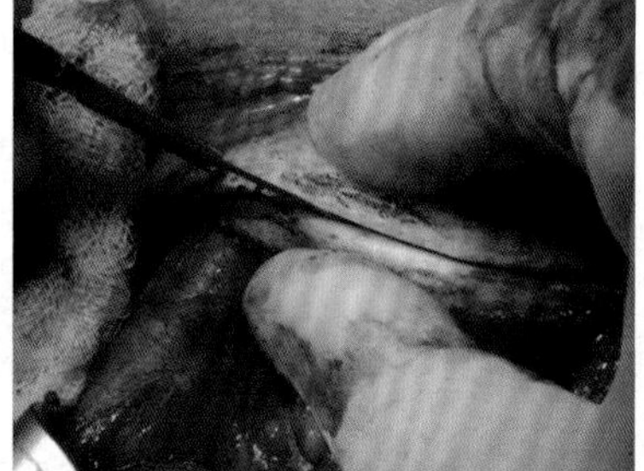
C
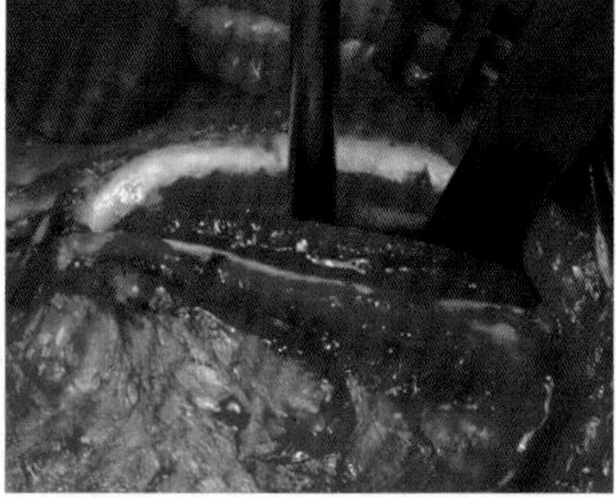
D
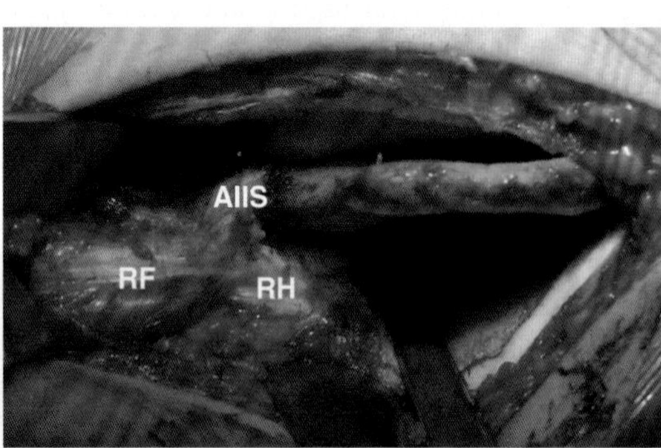

E
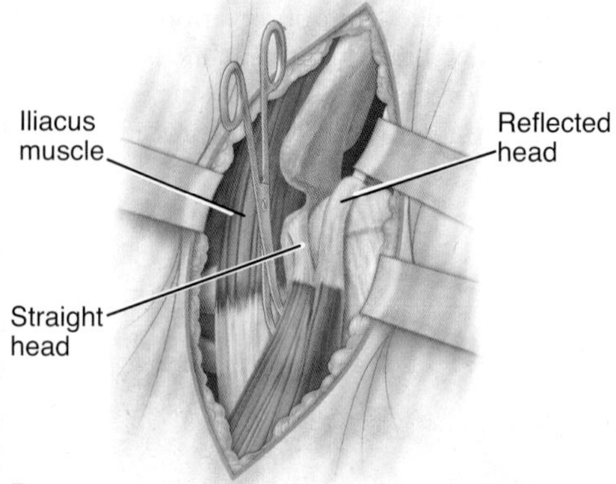


**TECH FIG 1** • **A.** Tensor–sartorius interval. Note the lateral femoral cutaneous nerve (*arrow*). **B.** The external oblique muscle has been detached off the iliac crest apophysis, which is being divided by a no. 15 blade. **C.** Subperiosteal dissection of the iliac inner and outer tables. **D.** Superior view of the left hip (patient's head is to the right) showing the rectus femoris (*RF*), its straight head attachment to the anterior inferior iliac spine (*AIIS*), and the reflected head attaching to the hip capsule (*RH*). **E.** The iliopsoas tendon is identified, dissected distally, and divided at the iliopectineal eminence. *(continued)*

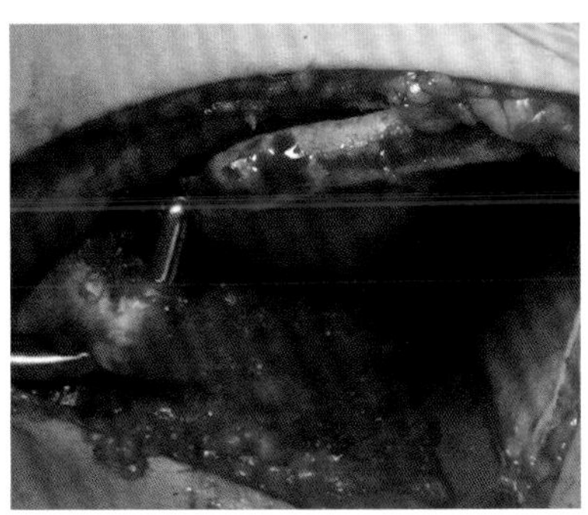
F

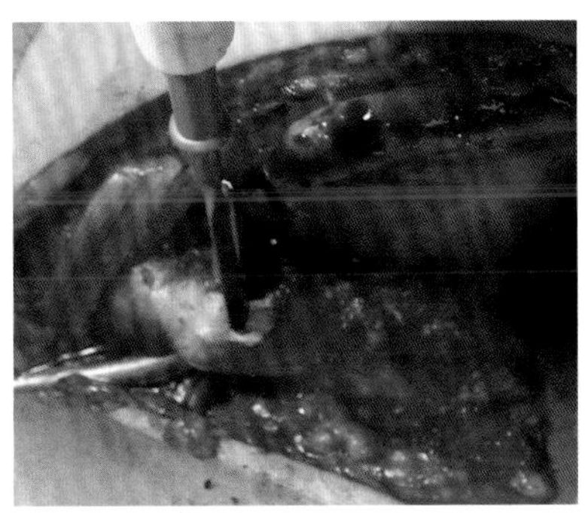
G

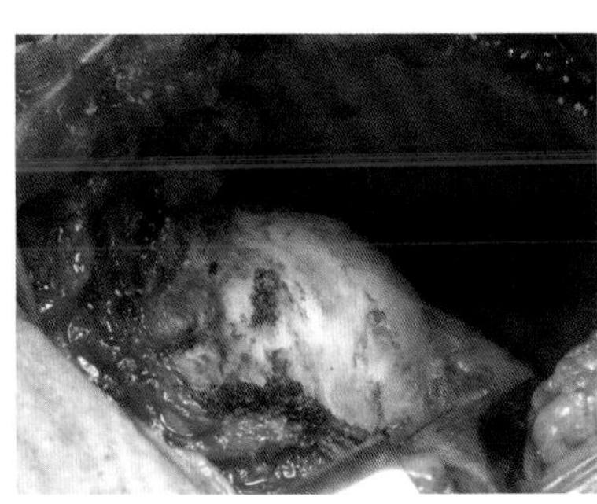
H

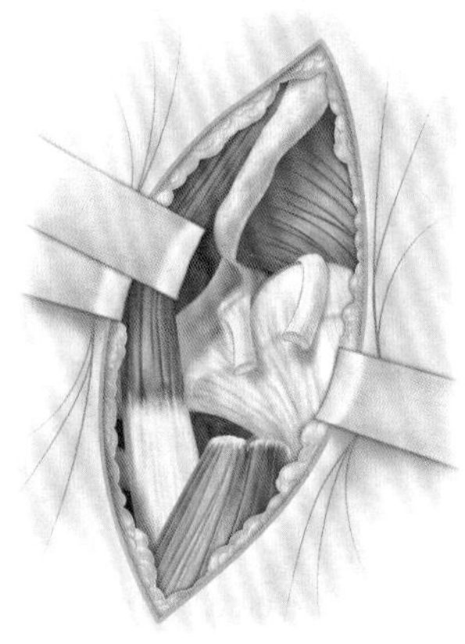
I

**TECH FIG 1** ● *(continued)* The reflected head of the rectus femoris is lifted off the hip capsule (**F**) and divided (**G**). **H.** Deep muscles of the iliacus, rectus femoris, and gluteus medius are reflected off the hip capsule. The capsule must be separated from any false acetabulum on the lateral iliac wall. **I.** The capsule is exposed, particularly the inferior medial aspect.

- It is extremely important for the dissection to continue medially onto the pubis by opening the interval between the iliacus and the rectus femoris muscles (**TECH FIG 1E**).
  - By opening the medial periosteum at the level of the pubis, the iliopsoas tendon is identified, which lies deep on the iliacus muscle.
  - The tendon is followed distally so that the interval between the iliacus muscle and the rectus femoris muscle is separated more deeply.
- The iliopsoas tendon is brought into the superficial surgical site with a right-angled clamp and divided at the level of the iliopectineal groove on the pubis.
- The femoral nerve is close by, superficial and medial to the psoas tendon.
- The reflected and straight heads of the rectus femoris muscle are identified and divided. This allows skeletonization of the femoral head by separating the iliacus, rectus femoris, and hip abductor muscles off the capsule (**TECH FIG 1F–H**).
  - A Cobb elevator is useful for separating these muscles off the hip capsule.
  - It is extremely important to carry the dissection around to the deep inferior medial aspect of the hip capsule (**TECH FIG 1I**).
- With a Kocher clamp, grasp the proximal aspect of the reflected head of the rectus femoris tendon to further expose the capsule. The capsule must be detached from the false acetabulum if present and exposed superiorly and posteriorly.

## Open Reduction

- A T-shaped capsulorrhaphy is made with the redundant proximal limb eventually removed.
  - The incision parallels the acetabular rim but is about a centimeter away so that the labrum is not injured (**TECH FIG 2A**).
- The femoral head is examined for deformity (**TECH FIG 2B**).
- The ligamentum teres is divided off the femoral head (**TECH FIG 2C**).
- The stump of the ligamentum teres is grabbed with a Kocher clamp and it is followed into the depths of the acetabulum.
  - It is essential to visualize the entire acetabulum and the transverse acetabular ligament.
  - The ligamentum teres is removed with Mayo or cartilage scissors at its deep acetabular attachment.
  - Under direct vision, a pituitary rongeur is used to remove the pulvinar tissue that lies within the acetabulum.
  - The transverse acetabular ligament is divided.
- At this point, the femoral head should be reducible.
  - For children older than 2 to 3 years of age, especially if the reduction is tight or unstable, a femoral shortening osteotomy is performed before the capsule is closed.[9]
  - If an acetabular osteotomy is performed, it is also completed before the capsulorrhaphy sutures are tied.
  - An adductor longus and gracilis tenotomy is generally not needed but can be included if these muscles feel excessively tight.

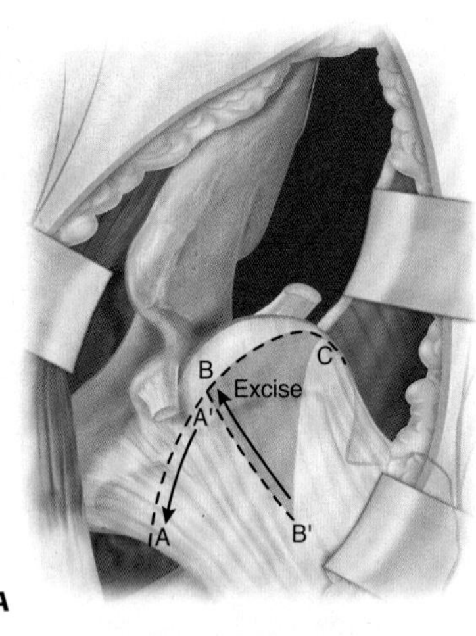


A

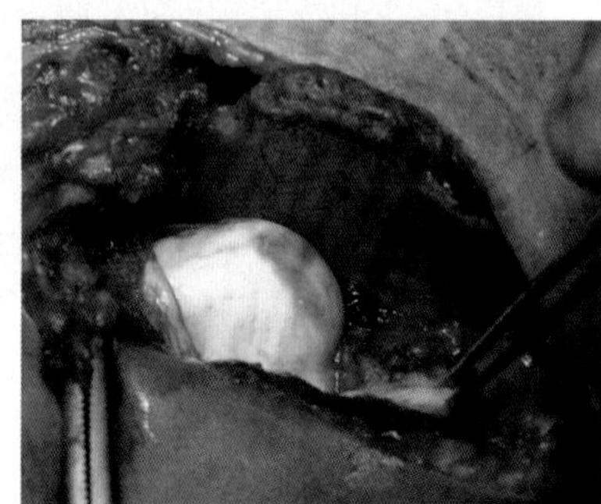

B

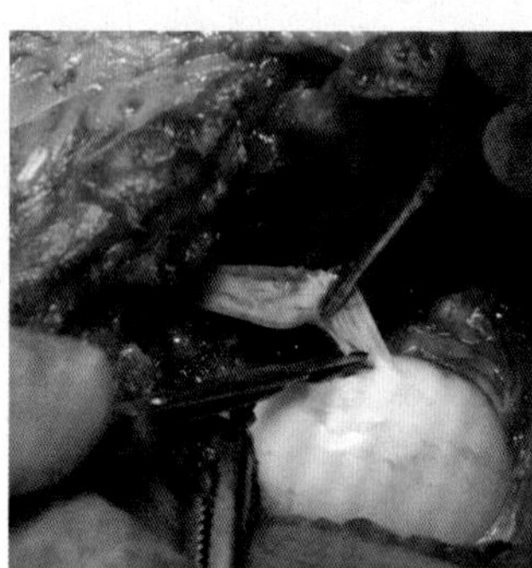

C

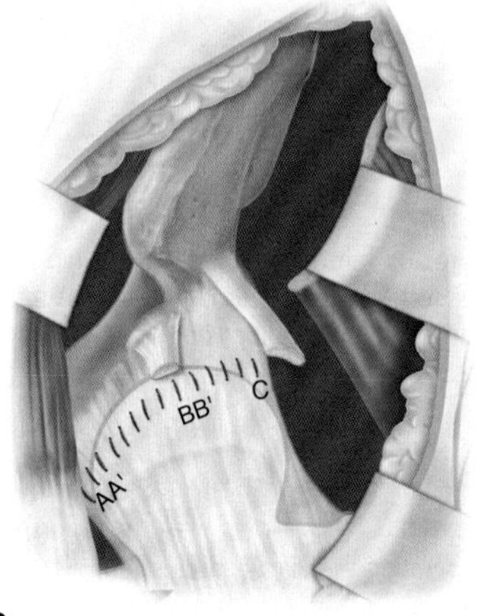


D

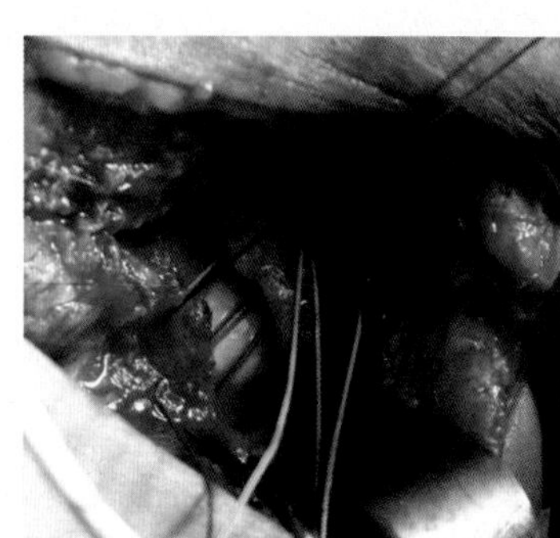

E

**TECH FIG 2** • **A.** A T-shaped capsulorrhaphy is performed. The upper limb is generally excised. **B.** The hip capsule has been opened, exposing the deformed femoral head. **C.** The ligamentum teres is divided off its femoral head attachment. The vascular contribution of the ligamentum teres to the femoral head is minimal. **D.** After any associated femoral and acetabular osteotomies are performed, the capsule is advanced medially. **E.** Nonabsorbable sutures are placed and tied after osteotomies have been completed.

- A capsulorrhaphy is performed by advancing the superolateral capsule to the inferior medial aspect of the capsule on the pubis (**TECH FIG 2D**).
- Nonabsorbable no. 0 sutures are all placed and tagged and then sequentially tied (**TECH FIG 2E**).
- The iliac crest apophysis is reapproximated with heavy suture, and the external oblique muscle is reattached.
- The rectus femoris can be repaired, but the iliopsoas muscles are left divided.
- A surgical drain is not required.
- A one-and-a-half spica cast is applied with the hips in a safe "human" position with no more than 30 degrees of flexion and abduction.

## Proximal Femoral Shortening Osteotomy

- A straight lateral approach to the proximal femur is used.
- The tensor fascia is divided longitudinally.
- The anterior edge of the gluteus medius muscle is identified where it attaches to the greater trochanter.
- Several millimeters of the gluteus medius muscle is detached off the trochanter.
  - This allows palpation of the anterior aspect of the femoral head to estimate the amount of femoral torsion (**TECH FIG 3A**).
- The vastus lateralis muscle is detached off the femur by dividing its proximal attachment in the transverse plane at the trochanteric ridge, leaving enough cartilage attached to the muscle to allow secure fixation during closure (**TECH FIG 3B**).
  - The vastus lateralis muscle should be divided off the posterior intermuscular septum so that the muscle innervation is left completely intact.
- Stiff Steinmann pins are inserted in the proximal and distal femur to ensure that a proper amount of femoral rotation is provided.
- A third pin is placed up the neck of the femur to judge femoral head–neck antetorsion, and a fourth pin is placed just below the lesser trochanter to guide the osteotomy.
- A one-third tubular small fragment plate or a 2.7-mm minifragment dynamic compression plate is generally sufficient in a young child (**TECH FIG 3C**). A 3.5-mm dynamic compression plate is used for an older child.

- The proximal aspect of the plate is fixed loosely.
  - A subtrochanteric osteotomy is believed to be less hazardous to the hip vascularity than an intertrochanteric osteotomy.
  - The femur is shortened by the amount that the cut ends of the femur overlap when the femoral head is reduced (**TECH FIG 3D**).
  - The shortened fragment of femur can be used for holding open a pelvic osteotomy.
- The plate is prebent slightly and is secured with some compression applied.
  - The Steinmann pins are used to judge any rotation that is desired.
  - If excessive femoral torsion was noted, some of this can be judiciously corrected.
- The tension band effect of the vastus lateralis muscle is restored (**TECH FIG 3E**).
- The incision is closed with absorbable suture. No drain is necessary.

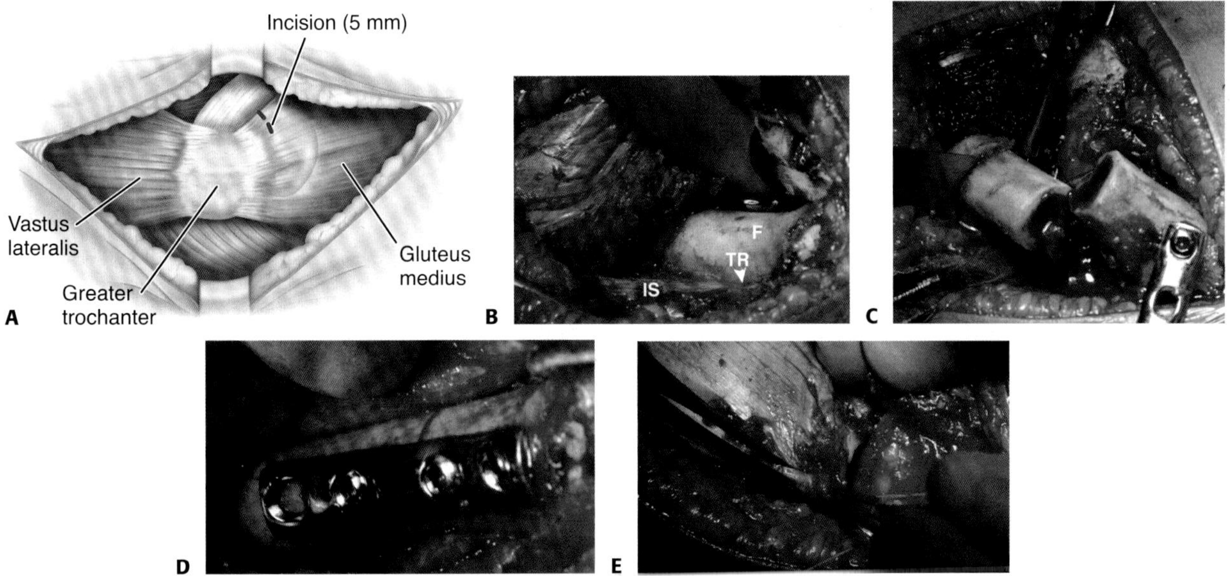


**TECH FIG 3** • **A.** About 5 mm of the most anterior edge of the gluteus medius muscle is detached from the greater trochanter so that the femoral neck can be palpated and visualized (shown on a left hip). **B.** The vastus lateralis muscle is detached from the trochanteric ridge (*TR*) and the posterior intermuscular septum (*IS*) to expose the proximal femur (*F*). **C.** A one-third tubular plate has been attached to the proximal femur, and a 2-cm segment of bone has been removed from the subtrochanteric aspect of the femur. **D.** The femur has been shortened, rotated into less antetorsion, and compressed. **E.** The tension band of the vastus lateralis muscle is reestablished with 0 absorbable suture.

## PEARLS AND PITFALLS

| | |
|---|---|
| **Diagnosis** | ■ A painful dislocated hip in a newborn or young infant could be a septic dislocation.<br>■ Bilateral hip dislocation may be difficult to determine because the hips may be symmetrically dislocated.<br>■ An adolescent with newly diagnosed hip dysplasia, particularly if bilateral, may have an underlying condition such as Charcot-Marie-Tooth disease. |
| **Imaging studies** | ■ Treatment should not be based on a radiology report. The surgeon should personally examine all images.<br>■ An AP pelvis view should be obtained so that the contralateral hip is available for comparison.<br>■ The Shenton line is reliable after age 3 years for indicating subluxation. |
| **Nonoperative treatment** | ■ Pavlik harness treatment should not be extended beyond 3 weeks if it is not working.<br>■ A child should be comfortable in a Pavlik harness or a brace. If not, there may be a risk of nerve palsy or osteonecrosis.<br>■ An inadequate closed reduction or a reduction that requires excessive force or extreme position for stability can result in osteonecrosis. |
| **Operative treatment** | ■ In the anterior approach, the surgeon should always obtain adequate medial exposure and visualize the entire acetabulum.<br>■ Femoral shortening is necessary for a high dislocation if excessive force is required to bring the femoral head into the joint.<br>■ The acetabular labrum should not be resected.<br>■ The older patient may need a simultaneous acetabular osteotomy for stability or because of excessive acetabular dysplasia.<br>■ Patients older than 8 years with a dislocated hip, particularly those with bilateral dislocation, may have excessive deformity to justify reconstructive surgery. |

| | |
|---|---|
| **Postoperative** | ■ The hip should be casted in a safe human position.<br>■ CT or MRI is obtained immediately after surgery to document reduction.<br>■ The surgeon must not accept a postoperative subluxated hip. |
| **Long term** | ■ Operatively treated hips should be followed until skeletal maturity. Late growth arrest may affect the end result.<br>■ Before beginning treatment, the family should be cautioned about the risks of osteonecrosis and the possibility of further surgery.<br>■ Acetabular dysplasia that does not improve with time, particularly when there is subluxation, needs further surgical treatment and osteotomy. |

## POSTOPERATIVE CARE

- A spica cast is applied at the time of surgery.
- A Gore-Tex liner protects the skin from excoriation.
- The cast is removed at 6 weeks.
- A night brace can be used until the acetabulum has remodeled sufficiently.
- Physical therapy is generally not needed.
- Follow-up radiographs are obtained.
  - The acetabulum will remodel the most in the first year after surgery.
  - If the acetabular shape does not normalize within several years, a pelvic osteotomy may be indicated.

## OUTCOMES

- Patients treated with a Pavlik harness may have persistent acetabular dysplasia in adulthood and should be followed until skeletal maturity.
- The younger the age at reduction, the better the final Severin grade at maturity. This in turn predicts the need for total hip arthroplasty in later adulthood.[1]
- About 50% of hips that underwent closed reduction in childhood had residual acetabular dysplasia as adults.[6]
- The best results occur if there is no osteonecrosis, femoral growth disturbance, or residual subluxation.[12]
- Persistent acetabular dysplasia, if present past age 7 years, is associated with a poor late outcome.[4] A persistent upsloping sourcil and a centering discrepancy suggest a need for surgical correction in the younger child.[7]
- Early measurements of the acetabular index (AI) are also predictive for Severin grade at maturity.
  - In particular, an AI of 35 degrees or higher at 5 or more years after reduction has an 80% association with Severin grade III or IV at maturity.[1]

## COMPLICATIONS

- Osteonecrosis
- Late physeal and lateral femoral growth arrest
- Inadequate reduction with persistent subluxation
- Loss of reduction and redislocation
- Stiffness
- Lack of remodeling after reduction
- Infection
- Arthritis

## REFERENCES

1. Albinana J, Dolan LA, Spratt KF, et al. Acetabular dysplasia after treatment for developmental dysplasia of the hip: implications for secondary procedures. J Bone Joint Surg Br 2004;86(6):876–886.
2. Barlow TG. Early diagnosis and treatment of congenital dislocation of the hip. J Bone Joint Surg Br 1962;44(2):292–301.
3. Desai AA, Martus JE, Schoenecker J, et al. Spica MRI after closed reduction for developmental dysplasia of the hip. Pediatr Radiol 2011;41(4):525–529.
4. Kim HT, Kim JI, Yoo CI. Acetabular development after closed reduction of developmental dislocation of the hip. J Pediatr Orthop 2000;20:701–708.
5. Mahan ST, Katz JN, Kim YJ. To screen or not to screen? A decision analysis of the utility of screening for developmental dysplasia of the hip. J Bone Joint Surg Am 2009;91(7):1705–1719.
6. Malvitz TA, Weinstein SL. Closed reduction for congenital dysplasia of the hip. Functional and radiographic results after an average of thirty years. J Bone Joint Surg Am 1994;76(12):1777–1792.
7. Murphy SB, Ganz R, Müller ME. The prognosis in untreated dysplasia of the hip. A study of radiographic factors that predict the outcome. J Bone Joint Surg Am 1995;77(7):985–989.
8. Ponseti IV. Morphology of the acetabulum in congenital dislocation of the hip. Gross, histological and roentgenographic studies. J Bone Joint Surg Am 1978;60(5):586–599.
9. Schoenecker PL, Strecher WB. Congenital dislocation of the hip in children. Comparison of the effects of femoral shortening and of skeletal traction in treatment. J Bone Joint Surg Am 1984;66(1):21–27.
10. Schwend RM, Pratt WB, Fultz JF. Untreated acetabular dysplasia of the hip in the Navajo. A 34-year case series follow-up. Clin Orthop Relat Res 1999;(364):108–116.
11. The Alliance for Radiation Safety in Pediatric Imaging. One size does not fit all . . . so when we image, let's image gently! Available at: http://imagegently.dnnstaging.com/Home.aspx. Accessed March 20, 2014.
12. Weinstein SL. Congenital hip dislocation. Long-range problems, residual signs and symptoms after successful treatment. Clin Orthop Relat Res 1992;(281):69–74.
13. Weinstein SL. Natural history of congenital hip dislocation (CDH) and hip dysplasia. Clin Orthop Relat Res 1987;(225):62–76.

# Medial Approach for Open Reduction of a Developmentally Dislocated Hip

Lori A. Karol and Jeffrey E. Martus

101 CHAPTER

## DEFINITION

- Developmental dislocation of the hip (DDH) occurs in 1.5 babies per 1000 live births. When diagnosed in the newborn period, closed treatment with the Pavlik harness is successful in 95% of dysplastic hips and up to 80% of dislocated hips.
- Closed reduction is indicated when Pavlik harness treatment has failed and when presentation for treatment is delayed past 6 months of age.
- Open reduction is reserved for babies in whom closed reduction either is unobtainable or lacks stability or for those who are diagnosed with a dislocated hip later than 18 to 24 months of age.[16]
- The medial approach for open reduction is used most frequently in the young baby 12 months of age or less in whom an attempted closed reduction under anesthesia has been unsuccessful.

## ANATOMY

- Reduction of a dislocated hip can be impeded by the following:
  - The iliopsoas tendon, which is tautly stretched across the inferior capsule owing to the displacement of the femoral head
  - The inferomedial hip capsule, which becomes constricted
  - The transverse acetabular ligament, which spans the inferior aspect of the horseshoe of the acetabulum and prevents inferomedial seating of the femoral head in the acetabulum
  - The pulvinar, which is fibrofatty tissue occupying the cavity of the true acetabulum
  - The acetabular labrum, which can be infolded and serve as a doorstop blocking a deep and medial reduction
- Anatomic landmarks for the medial approach are as follows:
  - The adductor longus tendon originating on the pubis
  - The pectineus, lying anterior to the adductor brevis (which is deep to the adductor longus)
  - The femoral artery, vein, and nerve, which are located as a bundle anterior to the pectineus muscle
  - The medial femoral circumflex artery, which lies in the interval between the pectineus and the femoral neurovascular bundle and is important for the circulation of the ossific nucleus of the proximal femur

## PATHOGENESIS

- DDH is more common in female babies and is linked with breech presentation, oligohydramnios, and first-born children.
- DDH is associated with congenital knee hyperextension and may be more likely in babies with torticollis, clubfoot, and metatarsus adductus.
- A positive family history is present in a minority of babies with DDH and most likely represents familial hyperlaxity.
- Idiopathic DDH must be differentiated from the teratologic hip dislocation seen in infants with such disorders as arthrogryposis and Larsen syndrome.

## NATURAL HISTORY

- Although research has shown that mild dysplasia, seen on ultrasound imaging of the newborn hip, often resolves spontaneously without treatment, there is significant risk that babies with dislocatable or dislocated hips will progress from unstable hips to fixed dislocations in the absence of treatment.

## PATIENT HISTORY AND PHYSICAL FINDINGS

- The physical examination methods are summarized in the following text. It is very important that the child is relaxed and quiet during the examination.
- Limited abduction during range-of-motion testing may signify a fixed dislocation and merits imaging. Abduction can be symmetric in bilateral dislocations.
- The patient is examined for the Galeazzi sign. Asymmetry is abnormal and may indicate a hip dislocation or a congenital short femur. The apparent femoral lengths will be equal in bilateral dislocations.
- Extra thigh folds may be present in unilateral DDH, but thigh fold asymmetry is usually nonspecific.
- The child is examined for the Ortolani sign. A positive sign represents the reduction of a dislocated hip. It is usually present in the newborn with DDH but disappears as the dislocation becomes fixed.
- A positive Barlow sign represents the ability for a reduced hip to be dislocated because of instability. It disappears as a fixed dislocation develops.
- In addition to a complete examination of each hip, the knees, feet, and upper extremities should be examined for contractures to rule out a teratologic dislocation.
- The spine should be inspected for signs of dysraphism, which may result in a hip dislocation due to muscle imbalance.

## IMAGING AND OTHER DIAGNOSTIC STUDIES

- In infants younger than 4 months of age, ultrasound of the hip is the preferred imaging study.
  - The femoral head, acetabulum, and triradiate cartilage can be identified.
  - The absence of coverage of the femoral head by the bony acetabulum is seen in the dislocated hip, which appears lateralized relative to the pelvis.

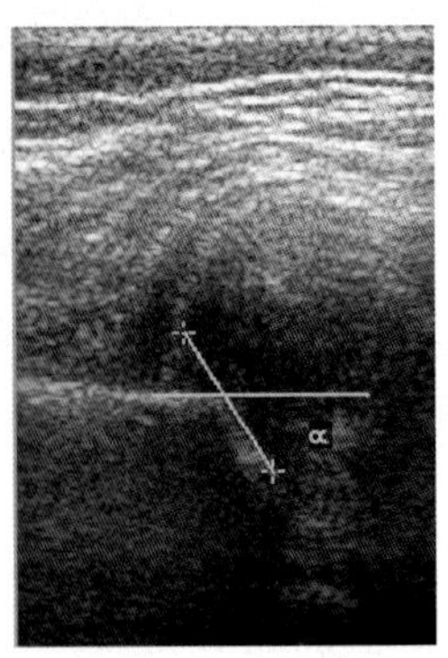


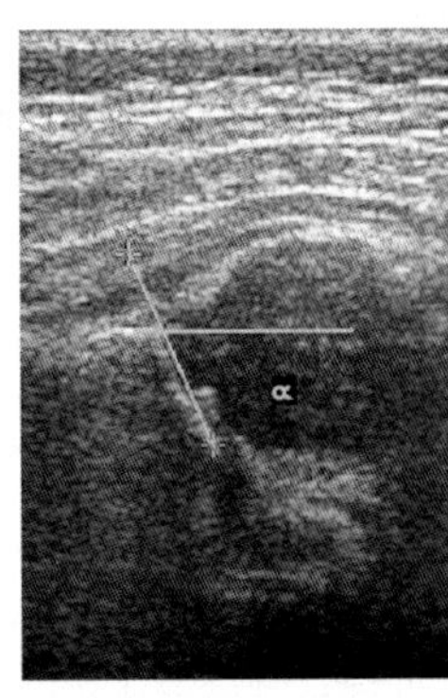


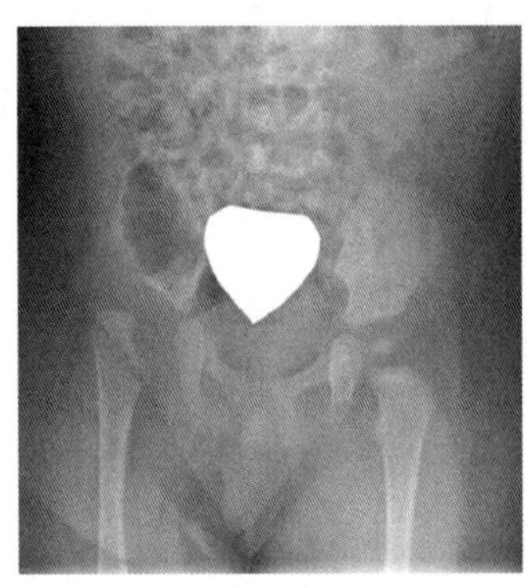


**FIG 1** • **A,B.** Ultrasounds of dislocated right hip with alpha angle of 56 degrees (**A**) and normal left hip with alpha angle of 66 degrees (**B**). **C.** AP pelvis radiograph demonstrating dislocated right hip with small ossific nucleus.

  - The alpha angle, which represents the slope of the bony acetabulum, is decreased (normal is more than 60 degrees), and the beta angle, which represents the cartilaginous acetabulum, is increased (normal is $<55$ degrees) in babies with hip dysplasia and hip dislocation (**FIG 1A,B**).
- In infants 4 months of age and older, an anteroposterior (AP) pelvic radiograph is diagnostic (**FIG 1C**).
  - The line of Shenton, drawn along the inferomedial aspect of the proximal femur and the superior aspect of the obturator foramen, is disrupted.
  - The ossific nucleus may be smaller than the contralateral side or absent altogether.
  - The medial proximal femoral metaphysis lies lateral to the Perkins line (drawn vertically from the lateral aspect of the bony acetabulum).
- The acetabular index, which is the angle subtended by the Hilgenreiner line (a horizontal line drawn through the triradiate cartilages), and a line drawn along the bony acetabulum, is increased.
- A pseudoacetabulum proximal and lateral to the true acetabulum may be present.

## DIFFERENTIAL DIAGNOSIS

- Teratologic hip dislocation (ie, arthrogryposis)
- Neuromuscular dislocation (ie, spina bifida)
- Congenital short femur
- Coxa vara

## NONOPERATIVE MANAGEMENT

- The Pavlik harness is the treatment of choice for infants with hip dysplasia or instability from birth to age 6 months.
- The Pavlik harness is less successful in patients with fixed dislocations but may be attempted for a period not to exceed 4 weeks, following which a reduction must be documented by either sonogram or radiograph.
- There is no role for nonoperative management of an otherwise healthy baby 6 months of age or older with a fixed hip dislocation.

## SURGICAL MANAGEMENT

- Surgical management can be delayed in the very young infant until the baby reaches sufficient size for a safe anesthetic and effective cast immobilization. We favor proceeding with surgical reduction (closed or open) at the age of 6 months in the healthy baby.
- The importance of delaying surgery until the presence of ossification within the femoral head remains controversial.[11] Although some studies report an increased incidence of avascular necrosis when the ossific nucleus is absent, others report an increased number of surgical procedures in children in whom reduction is delayed. We favor proceeding with reduction rather than waiting for ossification.[7]

### Preoperative Planning

- Traction may be used to increase the likelihood of a successful closed reduction, although current trends in the United States show a declining use of preoperative traction.

### Positioning

- The child is positioned supine on a radiolucent operating table.
- The perineum is isolated with adhesive tape.
- Surgical drapes are sutured in place to allow free movement of the extremity.
- Towel clips should be avoided around the groin, as they interfere with fluoroscopic visualization of the hip.

### Approach

- The medial approach to the dislocated hip is best suited to infants younger than 12 months of age, but it has been used by other authors successfully in infants up to 24 months of age.
- The medial approach described by Ludloff[8] accesses the hip in the interval between the pectineus and the adductor brevis.
- We favor the anteromedial approach described by Weinstein[13] and Weinstein and Ponseti,[14] which exposes the hip between the femoral neurovascular bundle anteriorly and the pectineus muscle posteriorly. This interval allows for more direct visualization of the hip capsule and the medial femoral circumflex artery.

## Incision and Initial Dissection

- With the hip flexed and abducted, a transverse incision is made just lateral to the groin crease, centered over the palpable adductor longus tendon (**TECH FIG 1A**).
- The fascia overlying the adductor musculature is opened (**TECH FIG 1B**).
- The adductor longus tendon is isolated and divided (**TECH FIG 1C**). The tendon can be dissected free from the underlying adductor brevis with two blunt retractors.
- The adductor brevis is identified with its overlying anterior branch of the obturator nerve. The pectineus is located anterior to the adductor brevis (**TECH FIG 1D**). Blunt retractors are used to identify the superior border of the pectineus.

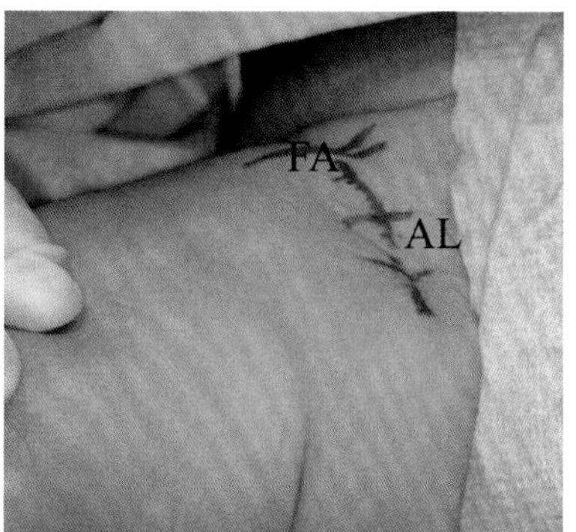


A

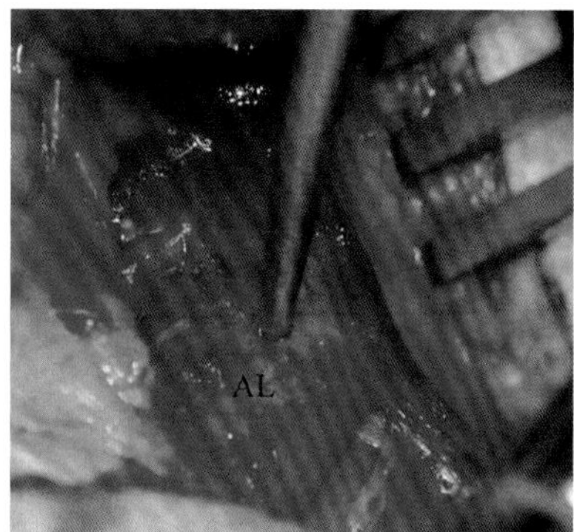


B

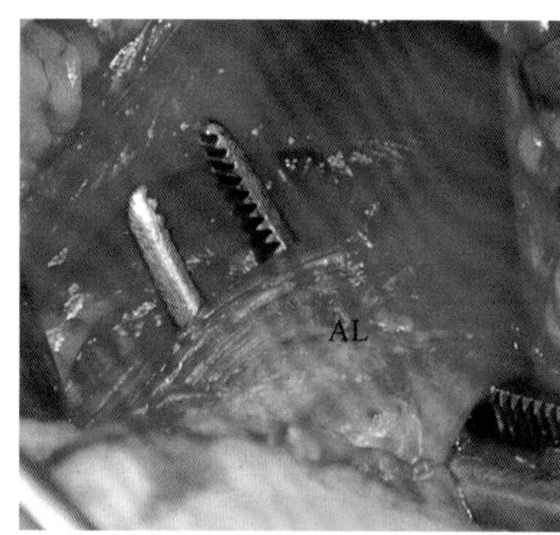


C

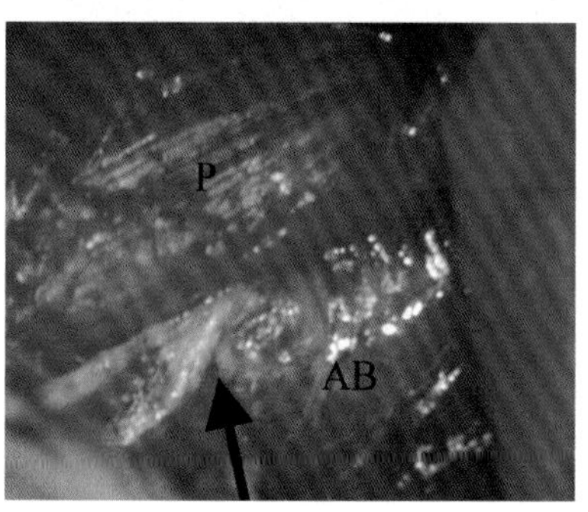


D

**TECH FIG 1** • **A.** Planned transverse incision over the palpable adductor longus tendon (*AL*). The femoral arterial pulse is also noted (*FA*). **B.** The adductor longus after longitudinal incision of the overlying fascia. **C.** The adductor longus is isolated with a right angle clamp and divided. **D.** The adductor longus has been sectioned and retracted distally. *Arrow*, anterior branch of the obturator nerve; *AB*, adductor brevis; *P*, pectineus.

## Deep Dissection

- The femoral neurovascular bundle is retracted gently anteriorly, and the pectineus muscle is retracted posteriorly (**TECH FIG 2A**).
- The iliopsoas tendon can be identified. The surgeon can rotate the hip and feel the insertion site on the small prominence of the lesser trochanter. The psoas tendon is isolated and divided (**TECH FIG 2B**).
- The surgeon carefully identifies the medial femoral circumflex artery as it traverses superior to inferior on the capsule of the hip. If possible, a small vessel loop is passed around the vessel to protect it. Otherwise, visualization of the vessel is maintained throughout the procedure.
- The femoral head is palpated beneath the medial femoral circumflex artery. Kidners are used to bluntly expose the hip capsule (**TECH FIG 2C**).

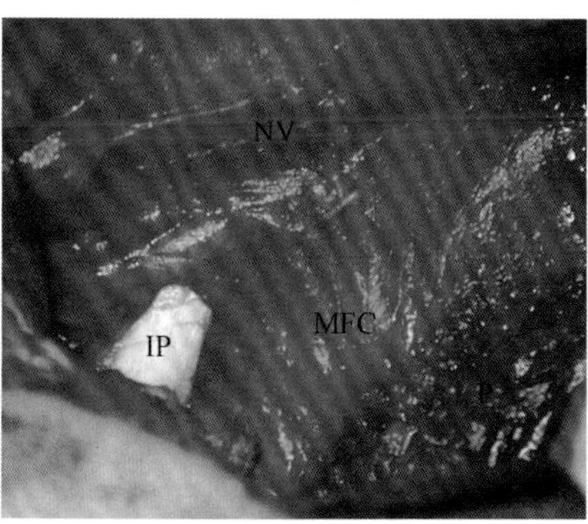


A

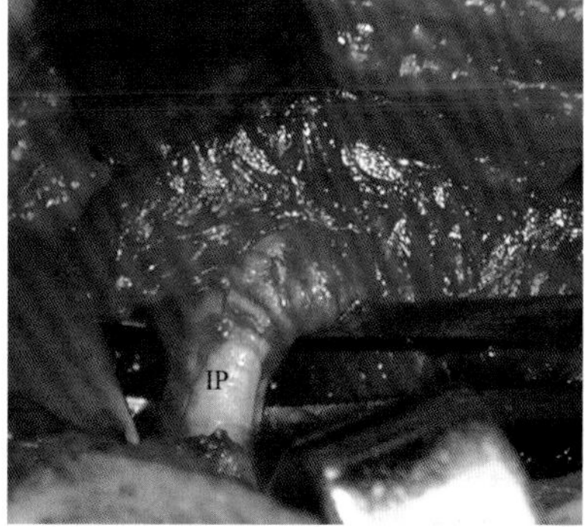


B

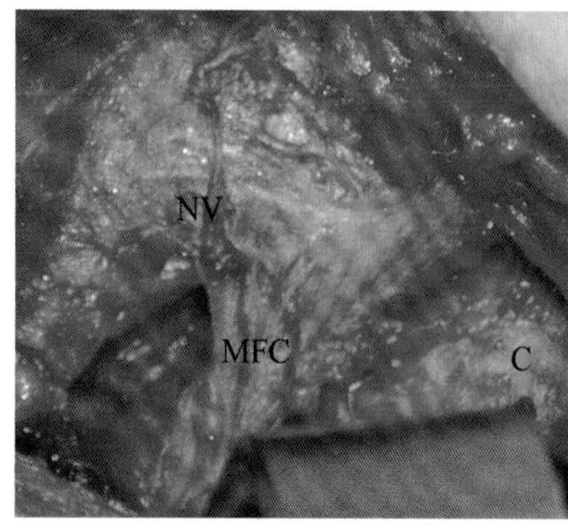


C

**TECH FIG 2** • **A.** The iliopsoas tendon (*IP*) is identified distally after retracting the pectineus posteriorly. **B.** The iliopsoas tendon is isolated with a right angle and divided. **C.** The hip joint capsule (*C*) has been exposed bluntly. *NV*, femoral neurovascular bundle; *MFC*, medial femoral circumflex vessels.

## Capsulotomy and Acetabular Exposure

- The capsule is incised along the rim of the acetabulum using a scalpel.
- The white glistening cartilaginous femoral head is visualized (**TECH FIG 3A**). The hip is rotated to identify the ligamentum teres insertion on the superior aspect of the femoral head (**TECH FIG 3B**) and it is released (**TECH FIG 3C**).
- The stump of the ligamentum is traced into the true acetabulum (**TECH FIG 3D**).
- The incision in the capsule is completed to gain access to the acetabulum.
- The ligamentum teres is excised from the floor of the acetabulum using scissors.
- With a pituitary rongeur, the fibrofatty pulvinar is removed from the acetabulum. The surgeon should take care to preserve the underlying articular cartilage of the acetabulum (**TECH FIG 3E**).
- Acetabular preparation for reduction is completed by releasing (with scissors) the transverse acetabular ligament at the base of the acetabulum.
- The surgeon should not excise or incise the acetabular labrum: It is an important growth center of the acetabulum and should be preserved.

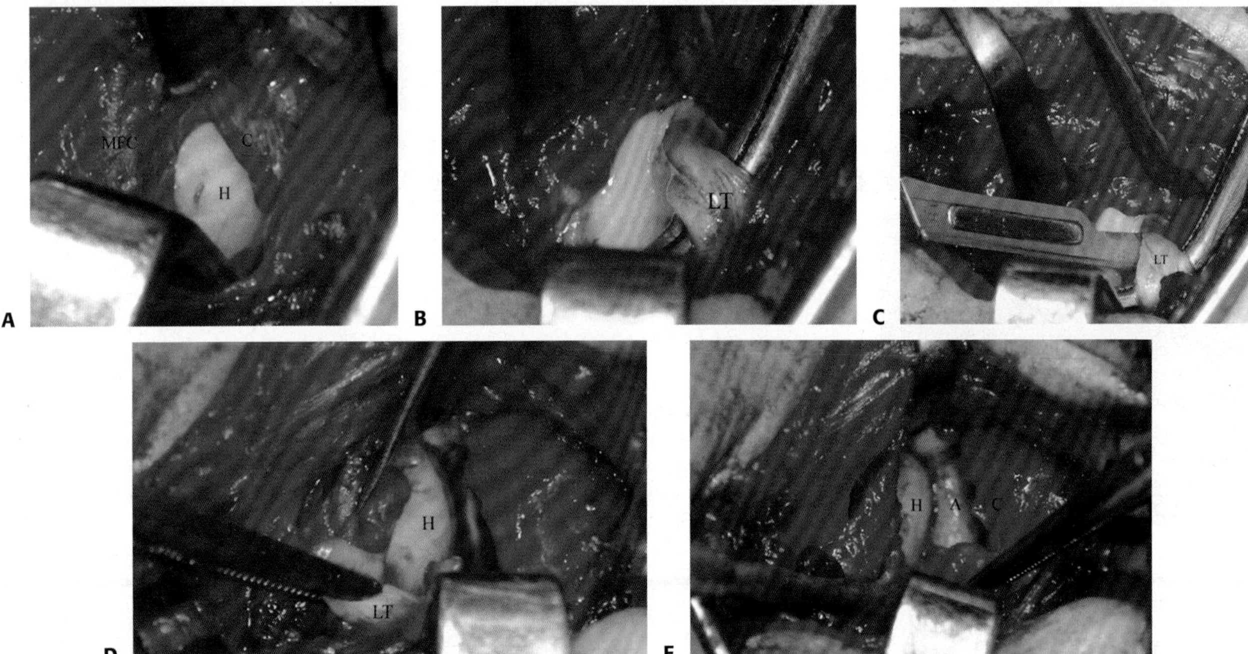


**TECH FIG 3** • **A.** The hip capsule has been incised along the rim of the acetabulum distal to the labrum. **B.** The ligamentum teres (*LT*) is isolated with a right angle clamp. **C.** The ligamentum teres is released sharply from the femoral head. **D.** After release from the femoral head (*H*), the ligamentum teres is grasped with a Kocher and traced into the acetabulum. E. The ligamentum teres and the fibrofatty pulvinar have been excised. *A*, acetabulum; *C*, hip capsule, *MFC*, medial circumflex vessels.

## Hip Reduction and Closure

- The hip is reduced under visualization by abducting the hip and lifting the greater trochanter anteriorly (the Ortolani maneuver). The hip should reduce readily and be quite stable in flexion. It will dislocate posteriorly with adduction. The reduced hip will appear relatively superficial, and the femoral head will be visible in the wound.
- The reduction should be verified fluoroscopically at this point. If it is difficult to assess the reduction because of absence of ossification of the femoral head, a small drop of contrast can be placed in the acetabulum.
- If the hip cannot be reduced, or if the reduction requires undue force to pull the hip into the acetabulum, the surgeon should recheck the capsular incision and the transverse acetabular ligament for completion of release.
- In rare instances, the hip cannot be gently reduced, and femoral shortening through a separate lateral approach is required. In infants younger than 1 year of age who are otherwise normal, this is generally not necessary. A very proximal dislocation with pseudoacetabulum formation may predict the need for femoral shortening. In such instances, anterior open reduction with femoral shortening may be the favored approach.
- From this point onward, the hip must remain flexed to 90 degrees and gently abducted to maintain reduction. An assistant should be assigned to observe the position of the hip.
- The vessel loop is removed from the medial femoral circumflex artery, which has been protected throughout the operation.
- The hip capsule is left open. Capsular reefing (capsulorrhaphy) is not possible via the medial approach to the hip. This is a distinguishing factor from the anterior approach for open reduction.
- The subcutaneous layer and skin are closed. A drain is not necessary.
- The wound is dressed and an occlusive bandage applied to deter contamination from diaper contents.

## Casting

- The anesthetized child is transferred to an infant spica table, and a double-leg spica cast is applied with the hips flexed 90 degrees and gently abducted no greater than 60 degrees (**TECH FIG 4A**).
- The surgeon should take care to cover the posterior aspects of the buttocks and mold beneath the greater trochanters to prevent "falling through" the spica posteriorly (**TECH FIG 4B**).

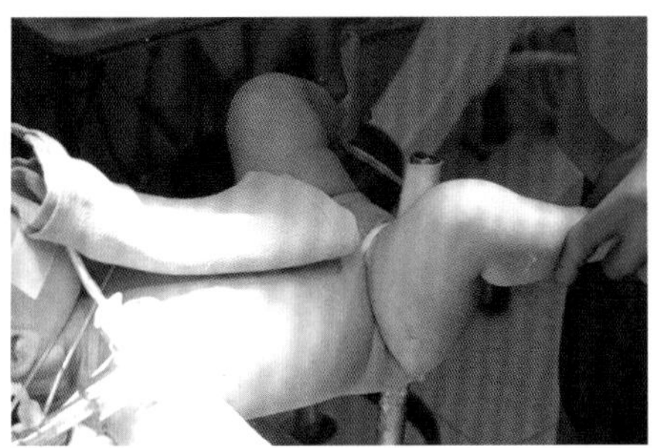

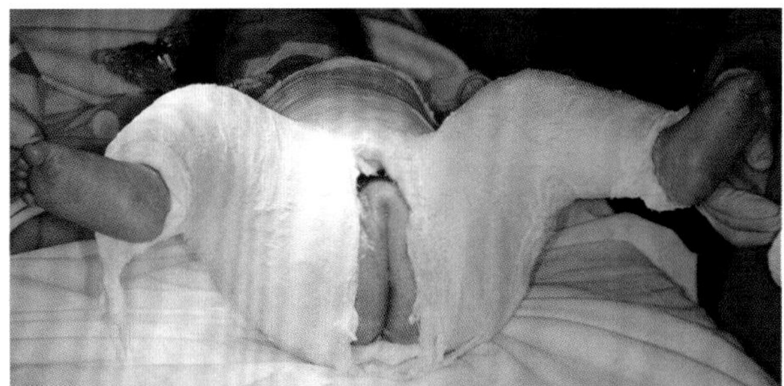

**TECH FIG 4** • **A.** A double-leg spica cast is applied with careful attention to limb position and the maintenance of hip reduction. **B.** The limbs are positioned in 90 degrees of flexion and less than 60 degrees of abduction in the spica cast.

## PEARLS AND PITFALLS

| | |
|---|---|
| **Indications** | ■ Unstable closed reduction or fixed dislocation in an infant younger than 1 year of age. The procedure is still possible to age 2 years but not recommended past the age of 1 year in our center due to inability to perform a capsulorrhaphy and a higher risk of avascular necrosis in the older baby. |
| **Surgical technique** | ■ Drapes are sewn to avoid inability to see the hip on C-arm fluoroscopy.<br>■ The ligamentum teres is used to find the acetabulum.<br>■ The medial femoral circumflex artery is always protected.<br>■ A lighted suction can be invaluable in improving visualization in the small incision.<br>■ If the reduction cannot be assessed easily, a small drop of contrast can be added in the acetabulum, and then the hip is reduced.<br>■ The surgeon should never force a reduction; avascular necrosis may result. |
| **Postoperative care** | ■ The reduction is assessed with either radiographs, limited computed tomography (CT), or magnetic resonance imaging (MRI) once the child is awake.[1,4,5]<br>■ If the hip is dislocated, the cast is removed and reason for redislocation is assessed. |

## POSTOPERATIVE CARE

- A radiograph is taken before waking the child from anesthesia to document the reduced hip within the spica cast (**FIG 2A**).
- A limited CT scan or MRI may be performed within 24 hours after surgery to more clearly visualize the reduced hip after the child moves about in the cast (**FIGS 2B** and **3A–C**).[1,4,5]
- The cast is changed under anesthesia in 6 weeks, and the hip is examined fluoroscopically. At this time, a one-and-a-half spica can be applied.
- On occasion, a third spica will be needed after medial open reduction.
- Bracing with an abduction orthosis after cast removal is prescribed at the discretion of the surgeon.

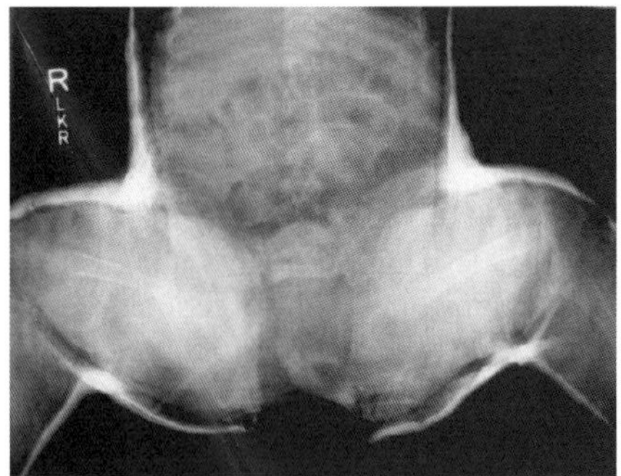


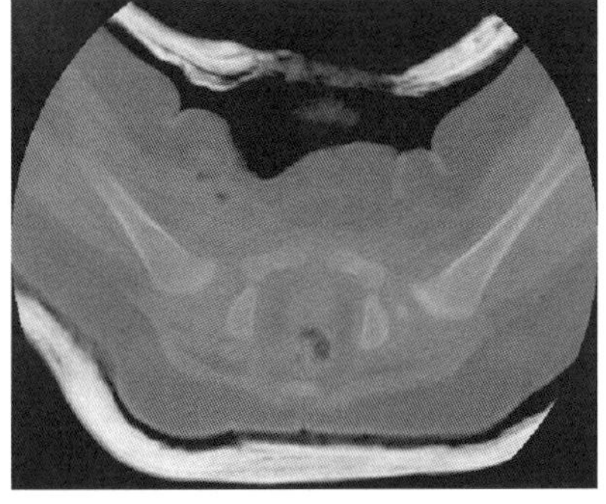

**FIG 2** • **A.** Intraoperative AP pelvis radiograph in the cast to confirm reduction. **B.** Limited CT scan to confirm maintenance of reduction after the child moves about in the cast.

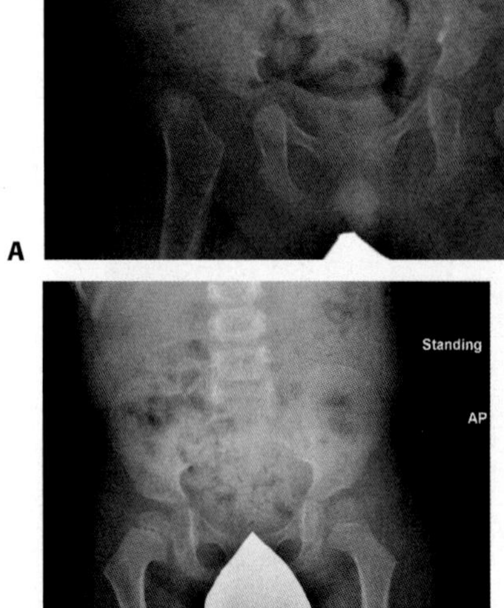


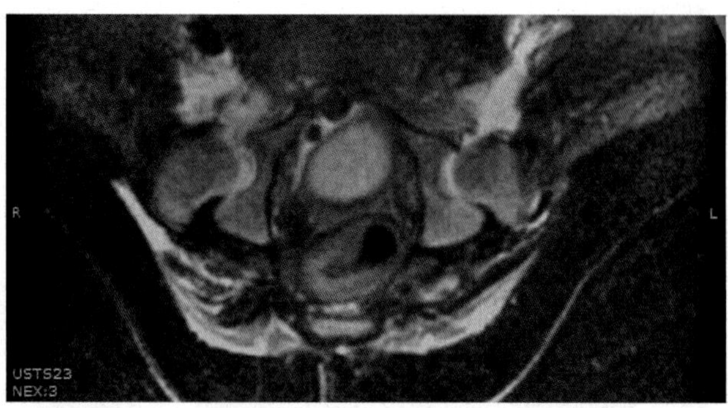


**FIG 3 • A.** Preoperative AP pelvis radiograph of a 6-month-old male with bilateral fixed hip dislocations refractory to Pavlik harness treatment. **B.** Postoperative MRI in spica cast confirming reduction. **C.** Follow-up radiograph 4 years following bilateral medial approach open reductions.

- Periodic radiographs are needed to monitor the growth of the ossific nucleus and the resolution of acetabular dysplasia.

## TECHNICAL VARIATION (LIGAMENTUM TERES TENODESIS)

- Bache et al[2] and Wenger et al[15] have described shortening the ligamentum teres and reattaching the ligamentum via suture to the transverse acetabular ligament site.
- The tenodesis functions to lessen the risk of redislocation.
- Our center does not have experience with ligamentum teres tenodesis.

## ADVANTAGES OF MEDIAL APPROACH

- Dissection is limited so that operative blood loss is minimal, allowing the surgeon to perform bilateral procedures in patients with bilateral hip dislocations.[17]
- Access to the structures blocking reduction of the hip is more direct than in other approaches.
- The ilium is not exposed so there is no tendency toward growth disturbance of the pelvis.

## OUTCOMES

- A satisfactory outcome after medial open reduction of the infant's hip can be expected in about 75% to 87% of children.[3,7,10] Reduction can be nearly universally achieved, and redislocation after a medial open reduction is rare. Owing to the limited dissection, prolonged postoperative stiffness is a rare event.
- When an adverse outcome occurs after medial open reduction, it usually is related to the diagnosis of postoperative avascular necrosis or residual acetabular dysplasia.

### Avascular Necrosis

- Avascular necrosis has been documented in 9% to 43% of hips after medial open reduction.[6,7,10,12] The large discrepancy in rates between series is due to differing criteria for its diagnosis and variation in the length of follow-up.
- The severity of avascular necrosis varies widely between hips that have temporary irregular ossification of the epiphysis (Bucholz-Ogden type I) to complete avascular necrosis with an aspherical femoral head and coxa breva (type IV).
- The presence of type I avascular necrosis does not preclude a successful outcome at skeletal maturity, whereas whole head avascular necrosis dooms the hip to a poor outcome and leg length discrepancy despite multiple surgical procedures.
- Many series do not include the hips with irregular ossification, so it is imperative when comparing complication rates to ascertain which hips were included in the group with postoperative avascular necrosis. Although the published series of medial open reductions vary in the likelihood of avascular necrosis, it is clear that the proximity of the medial femoral circumflex artery to the medial hip capsule places the hip at greater risk for avascular necrosis during this approach compared to the anterior open reduction.
- Because of variation between series in length of follow-up, the rate of type II avascular necrosis ranges widely. Typically, type II avascular necrosis becomes apparent in late childhood and early adolescence, when the proximal femur seems to grow into valgus because of a lateral physeal growth disturbance.[6,10]
  - In series with short-term follow-up, the rate of type II avascular necrosis may be lower than in those where skeletal maturity is achieved. Review of the DDH literature shows that type II avascular necrosis is not specific to the medial approach to the hip, however, as it may also be seen after anterior open reduction and even closed reduction.

### Acetabular Dysplasia

- Persistent acetabular dysplasia may be seen after medial open reduction of the hip. This approach does not facilitate concomitant pelvic osteotomy, unlike the anterior open reduction, in which the iliac crest is exposed. Yet, the optimal age for the medial open reduction (age 1 year or younger) is young enough that the surgeon can expect the majority of patients to experience resolution of their dysplasia with growth.

- Mankey et al[9] found that one-third of babies treated with medial approach open reduction required subsequent pelvic osteotomy for residual acetabular dysplasia.

## COMPLICATIONS

- Redislocation
- Avascular necrosis
- Infection
- Need for future pelvic osteotomy due to persistent acetabular dysplasia

## REFERENCES


1. Atweh LA, Kan JH. Multimodality imaging of developmental dysplasia of the hip. Pediatr Radiol 2013;43:S166–S171.
2. Bache CE, Graham HK, Dickens DR, et al. Ligamentum teres tenodesis in medial approach open reduction for developmental dislocation of the hip. J Pediatr Orthop 2008;28:607–613.
3. Citlak A, Saruhan S, Baki C. Long-term outcome of medial open reduction in developmental dysplasia of hip. Arch Orthop Trauma Surg 2013;133:1203–1209.
4. Gould SW, Grissom LE, Niedzielski A, et al. Protocol for MRI of the hips after spica cast placement. J Pediatr Orthop 2012;32:504–509.
5. Grissom L, Harcke HT, Thacker M. Imaging in the surgical management of developmental dislocation of the hip. Clin Orthop Relat Res 2008;466:791–801.
6. Koizumi W, Moriya H, Tsuchiya K, et al. Ludloff's medial approach for open reduction of congenital dislocation of the hip: a 20-year follow-up. J Bone Joint Surg Br 1996;78(6):924–929.
7. Konigsberg DE, Karol LA, Colby S, et al. Results of medial open reduction of the hip in infants with developmental dislocation of the hip. J Pediatr Orthop 2003;23:1–9.
8. Ludloff K. The open reduction of the congenital hip dislocation by an anterior incision. Am J Orthop Surg 1913;10:438–454.
9. Mankey MG, Arntz CT, Staheli LT. Open reduction through a medial approach for congenital dislocation of the hip. A critical review of the Ludloff approach in sixty-six hips. J Bone Joint Surg Am 1993;75(9):1334–1345.
10. Morcuende JA, Meyer MD, Dolan LA, et al. Long-term outcome after open reduction through an anteromedial approach for congenital dislocation of the hip. J Bone Joint Surg Am 1997;79(6):810–817.
11. Roposch A, Stöhr KK, Dobson M. The effect of the femoral head ossific nucleus in the treatment of developmental dysplasia of the hip. A meta-analysis. J Bone Joint Surg Am 2009;91:911–918.
12. Tumer Y, Ward WT, Grudziak J. Medial open reduction in the treatment of developmental dislocation of the hip. J Pediatr Orthop 1997;17:176–180.
13. Weinstein S. Anteromedial approach to reduction for congenital hip dysplasia. Strategies Orthop Surg 1987;6:2.
14. Weinstein SL, Ponseti IV. Congenital dislocation of the hip. J Bone Joint Surg Am 1979;61(1):119–124.
15. Wenger DR, Mubarak SJ, Henderson PC, et al. Ligamentum teres maintenance and transfer as a stabilizer in open reduction for pediatric hip dislocation: surgical technique and early clinical results. J Child Orthop 2008;2:177–185.
16. Willis RB. Developmental dysplasia of the hip: assessment and treatment before walking age. Instr Course Lect 2001;50:541–545.
17. Zamzam MM, Khoshhal KI, Abak AA, et al. One-stage bilateral open reduction through a medial approach in developmental dysplasia of the hip. J Bone Joint Surg 2009;91:113–118.

CHAPTER 102

# Anterior Drainage of the Septic Hip in Children

Richard M. Schwend

## DEFINITION

- Septic arthritis of the hip affects children of all ages, from the newborn to adolescents. The principles of treatment include early and accurate diagnosis, prompt surgical drainage, appropriate antibiotic coverage, and judicial management of late sequelae. The worse outcomes occur when there has been a marked delay in the diagnosis.

## ANATOMY

- Synovial membrane with its rich blood supply lines the joint capsule.
- Blood supply to the hip is from the medial and lateral femoral circumflex vessels (**FIG 1**).
- Intra-articular retinacular vessels travel up the femoral neck and enter the femoral head. These vessels do not cross the proximal femoral physis.
- Because the proximal femur is an intra-articular metaphysis, primary femoral osteomyelitis in this location can decompress into the hip joint.
- Many muscles that are in close proximity to the hip joint, including iliopsoas, piriformis, and obturator internus and externus, may develop pyomyositis or an abscess; this can mimic septic hip arthritis.

## PATHOGENESIS

- Bacteria can enter the hip joint cavity directly via the hematogenous route to the subsynovial layer of the capsule or indirectly from the proximal femoral metaphysis and occasionally from adjacent acetabular infection.
- Polymorphonuclear cells enter the joint cavity with plasma proteins and inflammatory fluid.
- The resulting tense effusion can increase intracapsular pressure.
- Articular cartilage destruction occurs from proteolytic enzyme degradation from cells of the synovial membrane and from interleukin-1 from monocytes, which releases proteases by chondrocytes and synoviocytes.

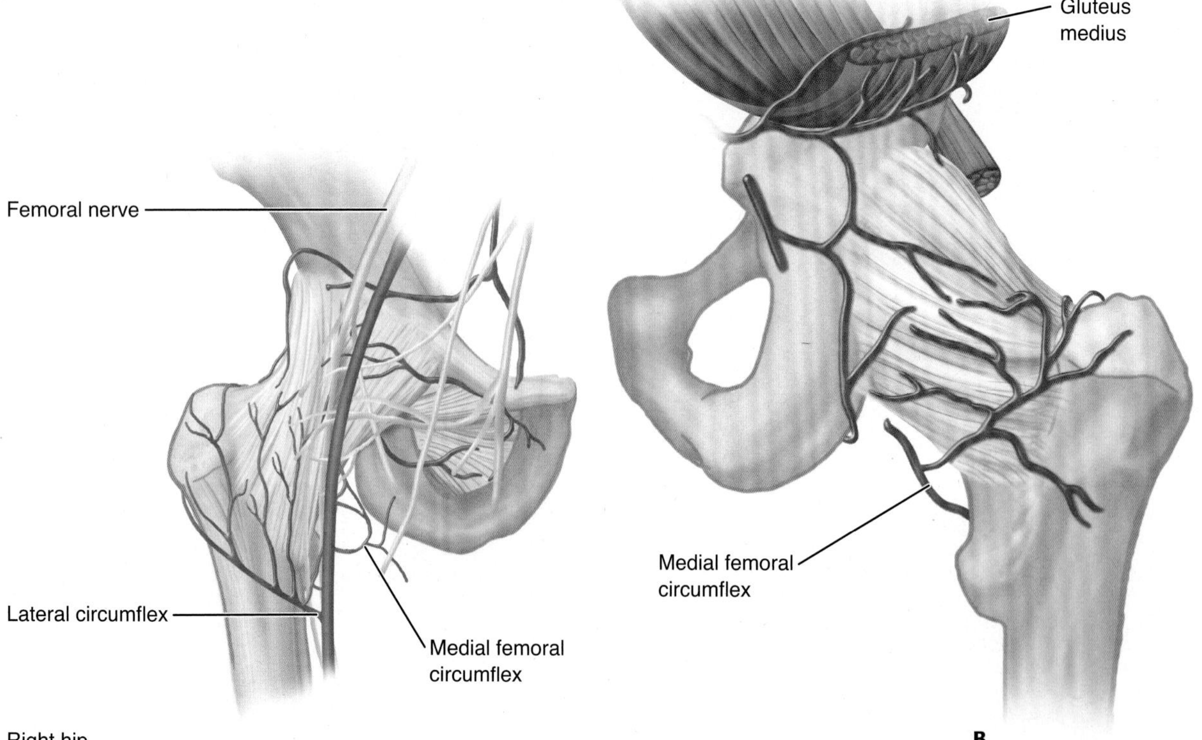


**FIG 1** ● **A.** Anterior hip vascularity. The medial and somewhat the lateral femoral circumflex vessels from the deep femoral artery supply the vascularity to the femoral head. **B.** Posterior hip vascularity. Intracapsular retinacular vessels from the medial circumflex vessel pierce through the capsule and travel up the posterior femoral neck.

- Animal studies show that proteoglycan matrix can be lost by 5 days and collagen by 9 days after an infection starts.[4] Antibiotics do not completely prevent this degradation if treatment is delayed.

## NATURAL HISTORY

- Although most patients have excellent outcomes, the hip joint accounts for about 75% of published reports of poor outcome from septic arthritis.
- Poor results occur more frequently in infants younger than 6 months of age, if there is a delay in treatment of greater than 4 days, and with associated proximal femoral osteomyelitis and infection with *Staphylococcus aureus*.[6]
  - Over the past several decades, there has been an increase in the incidence and the severity of musculoskeletal infections. Commonly, there is a spectrum of infections in which septic arthritis may occur with osteomyelitis, pyomyositis, and deep and superficial abscesses.
  - During this time, there has been an increase in the incidence of methicillin-resistant *Staphylococcus aureus* (MRSA) infections, leading to severe complications such as deep venous thrombosis, septic emboli, and life-threatening multisystem organ failure.[11]
- The most severe sequelae are more often seen in newborns and infants.
- A frequent scenario when there is a poor outcome is the failure to make the diagnosis of septic hip arthritis, either from not recognizing the serious nature of the condition or failure to promptly perform adequate surgical drainage and administer appropriate intravenous antibiotics.

## PATIENT HISTORY AND PHYSICAL FINDINGS

- The history should include a detailed timeline of events leading up to presentation.
- In the most recent prospective studies evaluating clinical predictors for septic hip arthritis, a fever above 38.5° C was the strongest predictor.[1,8,9]
- The severity of pain, particularly pain at rest and night pain, indicates inflammation.
- Associated illnesses and infections, history of trauma to the hip, recent dental procedures, and underlying medical conditions or steroid use may lead to infection in a susceptible host.
- Always ask about recent antibiotic treatment because this may mask many of the findings of septic hip arthritis and change the threshold for obtaining imaging studies and for performing hip aspiration.
- Conduct a visual inspection with the child lying supine on the table, noting whether the hip is in abduction, flexion, and external rotation (**FIG 2**).
  - A septic hip joint assumes this position of least intracapsular pressure.
  - Inspect for skin rash, erythema, warmth, swelling, and tenderness over overlying muscles and the hip joint.
  - The clinician should palpate the pelvis and lower extremities for local swelling and tenderness.
- Examine the child walking. Antalgic limp indicates that the patient is unable to spend much time weight bearing on the hip joint. The child may have mild pain early or the pain may be so severe that the patient is unable to walk.

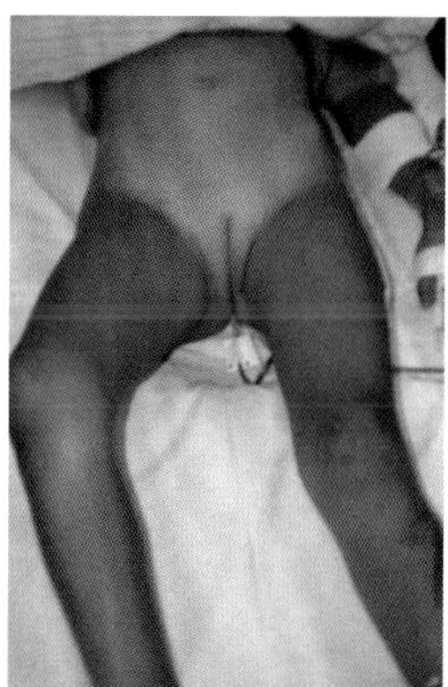

**FIG 2** • Right hip is held in flexion, abduction, and external rotation.

- Observe the hip range of motion. Gradually, there is limited ability to move the hip joint as inflammation and pressure of the hip joint increase. Pain with hip extension and internal rotation suggests involvement of the psoas muscle.
- Inspect and palpate the spine. Septic discitis in a young child can present as refusal to walk and can resemble septic hip arthritis.

## IMAGING AND OTHER DIAGNOSTIC STUDIES

- Imaging and laboratory studies are determined by the clinical evaluation, probability of the findings being septic hip arthritis, and need to exclude other conditions.
- Plain radiographs (**FIG 3A**)
  - Key features include hip abduction, increased soft tissue density, widened medial joint space, osteopenia if the infection is long-standing, and femoral or acetabular osteolytic lesions.
  - A particularly worrisome finding in the neonate is a painful dislocated hip (**FIG 3B**). Bone lesions and destruction are typically delayed 1 to 2 weeks.
- Ultrasound imaging (**FIG 3C**) is performed bilaterally, with images obtained along the axis of the anterior femoral neck. This is very specific for detecting intra-articular fluid in the hip.
- Because the pelvis is deep and difficult to examine, magnetic resonance imaging (MRI) is an extremely useful imaging modality to examine the tissues surrounding the hip joint or within the pelvis (**FIG 3D–F**).
  - It is the preferred imaging technique if the hip joint moves better than would be expected for septic hip arthritis but the patient has symptoms within or near the pelvis suggesting myositis or an abscess.[7,13]
  - MRI is useful if by 48 hours there is an inadequate response to treatment of septic hip arthritis, suggesting persistent hip joint infection, pelvic osteomyelitis, or infection in the muscles near the hip joint.
  - With the changing clinical spectrum of musculoskeletal infections, the severity of infections is increasing. MRI is becoming the preferred imaging modality to provide detailed anatomy, clinical classification, and clarify early surgical decision making.[5]
- A bone scan is not generally recommended. If the patient has a septic hip arthritis, he or she should be in the operating room, not the nuclear medicine department.

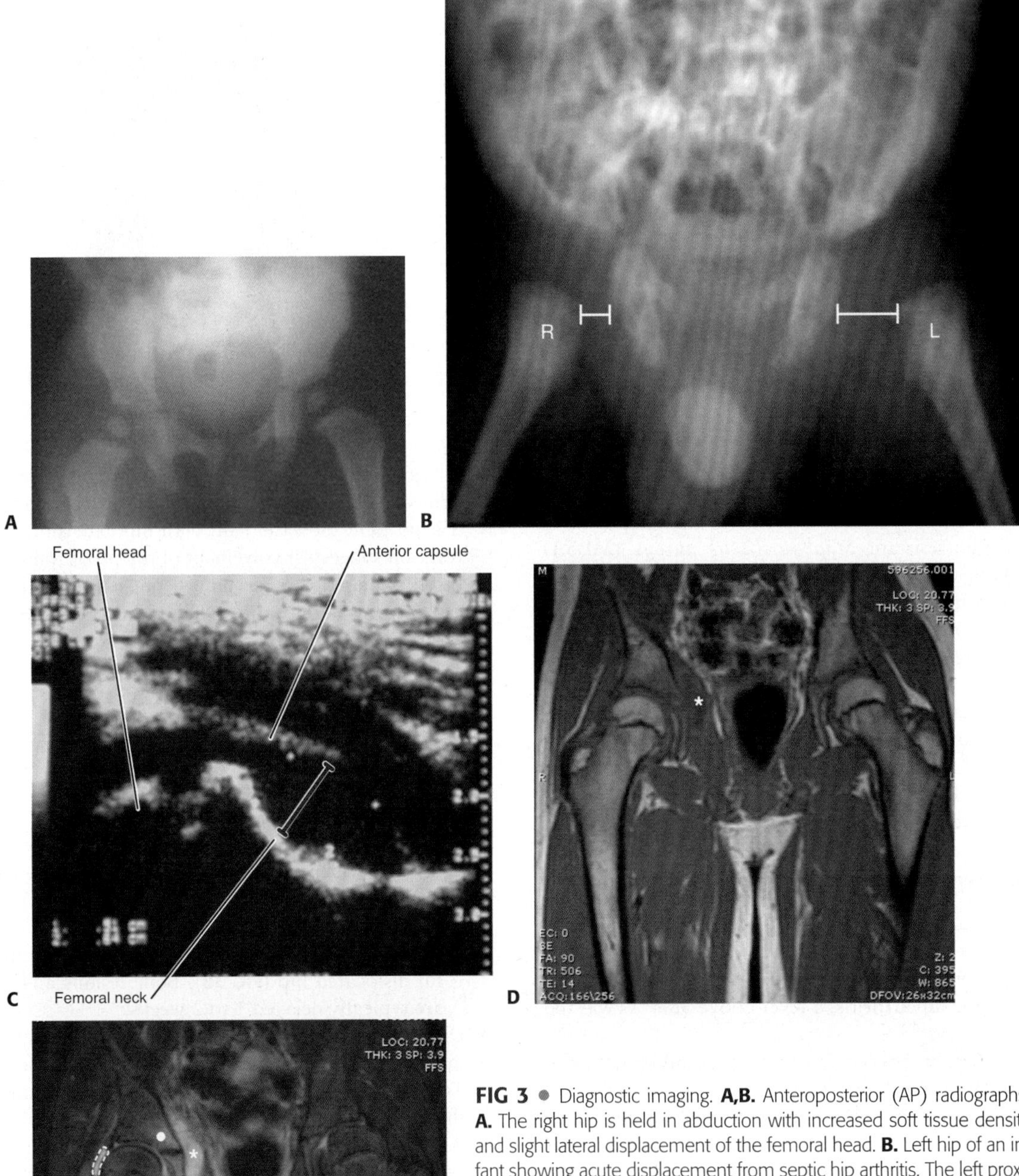


**FIG 3** ● Diagnostic imaging. **A,B.** Anteroposterior (AP) radiographs. **A.** The right hip is held in abduction with increased soft tissue density and slight lateral displacement of the femoral head. **B.** Left hip of an infant showing acute displacement from septic hip arthritis. The left proximal femur is laterally displaced compared with the right. **C.** Ultrasound imaging of hip along axis of the femoral neck. The distance between the femoral neck and head is shown by the *red line*. There is increased intracapsular fluid. **D–F.** MRIs in an 11-year-old boy with fever and pain with internal rotation of the hip. He was limping but able to walk. ESR was 50 mm per hour and CRP level was 5.8 mg/L. The radiograph was normal. **D.** T1-weighted coronal image of pelvis. There is an abscess (*asterisk*) within the obturator internus muscle. **E.** T2-weighted coronal image of pelvis. The abscess (*asterisk*) is more apparent, as is the involvement of the acetabulum (*solid dot*) and small hip joint effusion (*dashed outline*). *(continued)*

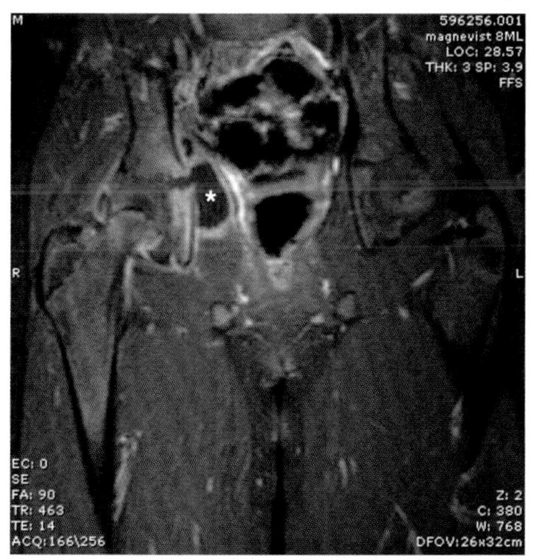


F

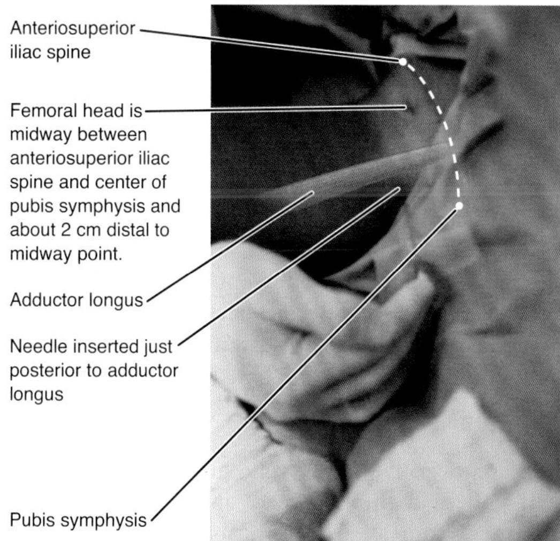


G

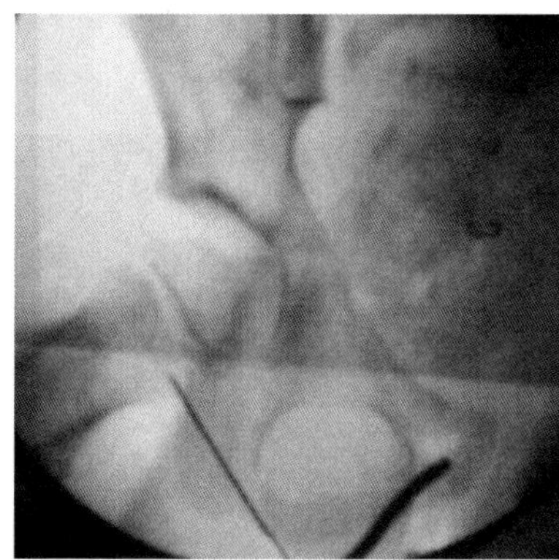

H

**FIG 3** • *(continued)* **F.** T1-weighted coronal image with gadolinium for enhancement. Cavitary nature of the abscess (*asterisk*) is even more apparent. Patient underwent percutaneous interventional radiology catheter drainage on two occasions and received intravenous antibiotics for treatment of this methicillin-sensitive *Staphylococcus aureus* infection. **G,H.** Hip aspiration. **G.** Aspiration of right hip through adductor approach. The large-bore needle is inserted just posterior to the adductor longus and is directed toward the femoral head. **H.** Fluoroscopy image of needle tip at the junction of the femoral head and proximal femoral metaphysis. (**A:** From Sucato DJ, Schwend RM, Gillespie R. Septic arthritis of the hip in children. J Am Acad Orthop Surg 1997;5:249–260; **D–F:** Courtesy of Mark Sinclair, MD, Children's Mercy Hospital, Kansas City, MO.)

- White blood cell (WBC) count is always done but may not always be elevated in septic hip arthritis.
- Blood culture is positive in 40% to 50% of cases.
- Erythrocyte sedimentation rate (ESR) is slow to respond to inflammation.
- In septic hip arthritis, C-reactive protein (CRP) increases and returns to normal earlier with treatment than does the ESR.
  - CRP is a very useful indicator of disease progression and response to therapy.
  - A CRP level above 20 mg/L is an important independent risk factor for the presence of septic hip arthritis.[1]
- Hip aspiration, either under ultrasound guidance in the younger child or with fluoroscopic guidance, is useful if the diagnosis is not clear and there is a reasonable possibility of a septic hip arthritis (**FIG 3G,H**).[9,12]
  - If it is performed under fluoroscopy, the clinicians must always confirm a negative aspiration (dry tap) with an arthrogram to document that the needle was intra-articular.
  - Any fluid obtained is sent to the laboratory for cell count, gram stain, and cultures. WBC above 50,000 cells/mm$^3$ is highly suggestive of septic arthritis; a level below 25,000 is suggestive of reactive arthritis. Gram stain and cultures may be positive in more than 50% of cases.
- Several recent studies have related clinical and laboratory findings to the child's chance of having septic hip arthritis.
  - An oral temperature above 38.5° C has been found to be the best predictor of septic arthritis; an elevated CRP, elevated ESR, non–weight-bearing status, and elevated serum WBC are considered to be other predictive factors.[1]
  - Another prospective study of clinical predictors of septic arthritis has shown that with a combination of fever, non–weight-bearing status, ESR above 40 mm per hour, and serum WBC of more than 12,000 cells/mm$^3$, the probability of hip sepsis was 86%.[8]
  - However, this algorithm has shown lower predictive value when tested at other centers.[7]

## DIFFERENTIAL DIAGNOSIS

- Transient synovitis
- Trauma
- Pelvic or proximal femur osteomyelitis
- Pyomyositis of the adductors, hamstrings, obturator muscles, or piriformis muscles
  - Pericapsular pyomyositis, which can mimic septic hip arthritis, may be more common.[10]
- Langerhans cell histiocytosis
- Leukemia, Ewing sarcoma, metastatic neuroblastoma
- Other forms of arthritis, including Lyme disease, tuberculosis, fungal or chronic childhood arthritis
- Iliopsoas or iliacus abscess
- Appendicitis or ovarian cyst
- Child abuse
- Osteonecrosis of the femoral head and sickle cell disease

## NONOPERATIVE MANAGEMENT

- There is growing interest to apply evidence-based treatment guidelines by multidisciplinary teams to triage and treat children with musculoskeletal infections. This can expedite evaluation, increase the yield of cultured organisms, and improve efficiency of antibiotic treatment.[3]
- Surgical treatment is indicated when septic hip arthritis has been confirmed.
- Nonoperative management is an adjuvant to surgery and includes making an early and specific bacterial diagnosis, administering the correct intravenous antibiotic and dose, and adjusting the antibiotic coverage based on culture and sensitivity results.
- Intravenous antibiotics are converted to oral when the child is clearly recovering (feels well, afebrile, able to walk, minimal pain with hip range of motion, and improving laboratory studies). The duration of antibiotic treatment is generally shorter than for osteomyelitis and depends on the severity of infection and the virulence of the organism.
- A peripherally inserted central catheter (PICC) is used if intravenous antibiotics will be given for several weeks. An infectious disease consultation is helpful for cases with an unusual organism, unusual host, or unusual site of infection.

## SURGICAL MANAGEMENT

- Confirmed septic hip arthritis is a surgical emergency and the hip should be drained without excessive delay.
- If the joint aspiration is performed in the operating room, the arthrotomy can be performed in the same setting.
- The principles of surgical intervention include open arthrotomy, irrigation of purulence, and débridement of dead tissue.

### Preoperative Planning

- Radiolucent table
- An aspiration of the hip is performed before an arthrotomy if the diagnosis is not clear. In children, the hip joint is aspirated with a spinal needle inserted just posterior to the adductor longus tendon and directed toward the femoral head (**FIG 3G,H**).

### Positioning

- Lateral or semilateral position with hip and lower extremity draped free (**FIG 4**).

### Approach

- There are several approaches to draining the pediatric hip, including medial, direct anterior, anterior through a modified Smith-Petersen approach, anterolateral, and posterior.
  - The posterior approach is not recommended because of the femoral head vascularity and potential for posterior hip instability.

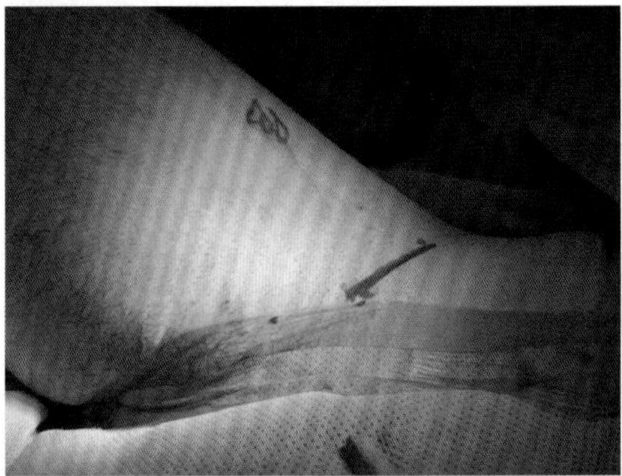

**FIG 4** • Patient is in a semilateral position with the entire hip and lower extremity draped free.

TECHNIQUES

## Modified Smith-Petersen Anterior Approach

- The entire hip and lower extremity is draped free so that the hip joint can be moved through a full range of motion.
- The incision is a modification of the classic Smith-Petersen approach with a cosmetic and limited incision in the groin, centered just below the anterior superior iliac spine (ASIS) (**TECH FIG 1A**).
- Sharp knife dissection is used to the deep fascia. The incision is continued until no more fat is apparent and the deep fascia is exposed.
- A sponge is used to separate the distal flap from the deep fascia.
- There is a small interval of fat between the tensor and sartorius muscles several centimeters distal to the ASIS (**TECH FIG 1B**). The surgeon should incise slightly lateral to the fat on the fascia of the tensor.
- Army-Navy retractors are used to separate this internervous interval until the rectus femoris muscle is visualized.
  - A Kittner sponge is used on the lateral edge of the rectus femoris muscle, and the surgeon dissects along this edge proximally until the reflected head of the rectus femoris muscle is exposed (**TECH FIG 1C**).
  - Just lateral to the reflected head is the hip capsule, which is covered with fat.
- The fat is reflected to expose the hip capsule. The reflected head of the rectus femoris muscle may be divided for better exposure of the hip capsule.
  - It is best to visualize a large area of the hip capsule for better orientation before making an incision into it.
- The capsule is incised with a no. 15 blade.
  - A 3-mm, 45-degree Kerrison rongeur is useful to remove several millimeters of the anterior capsule for continued postoperative decompression (**TECH FIG 1D**).
- The joint is irrigated with saline through a large-bore intravenous catheter placed deep within the joint.
- A suction drain is placed for several days after surgery until there is only minimal drainage.
- The skin is closed loosely with interrupted nylon sutures to allow potential drainage.
  - Closing the deep fascia increases the risk of reaccumulation.

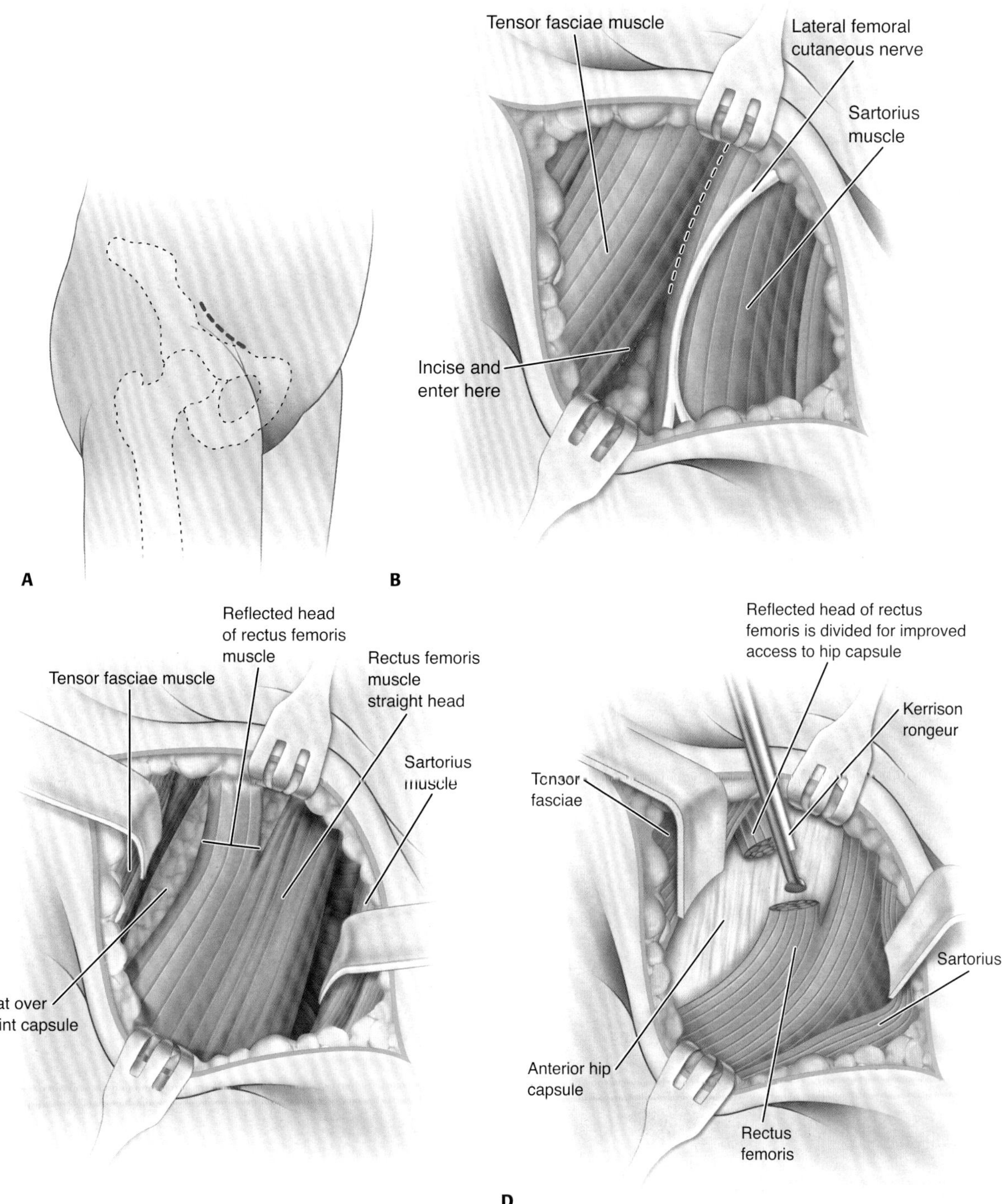


**TECH FIG 1** • Modified Smith-Petersen anterior approach to the right hip. **A.** The incision is placed in the anterior groin crease for best cosmesis. **B.** The tensor–sartorius muscle interval is identified distally where the muscles begin to separate. **C.** The reflected head of the rectus femoris muscle can be released to reveal the underlying hip capsule. **D.** A 45-degree Kerrison rongeur is used to enlarge the anterior hip capsulorrhaphy.

## Direct Anterior Approach

- The direct anterior approach is especially useful when there is infection in the iliopsoas bursa, which needs to be opened along with the hip joint.
  - This is also a direct approach for dividing the psoas tendon over the pelvic brim for a tight tendon, as seen in cerebral palsy, or a snapping hip related to the iliopsoas tendon.
    - It uses a similar incision as the anterior approach, placed just below the ASIS but centered more medially, between the femoral neurovascular bundle and the ASIS.
- Sharp dissection continues to the deep fascia until no further superficial fat is identified.
- A sponge separates both flaps off the deep fascia.
- The medial border of the sartorius muscle is identified. Just medial and slightly deeper is the fascia of the iliacus muscle, which is opened (**TECH FIG 2A**).
- The femoral nerve is identified, reflected medially, and protected (**TECH FIG 2B**). This provides assurance that the femoral artery and vein, which lie medial to the femoral nerve, are out of the field.
- The dissection is continued along the medial border of the iliacus muscle until the iliopectineus eminence of the pubic bone is identified.
- Deep to the iliacus muscle is the large bursa of the iliopsoas (**TECH FIG 2C**). This is opened and the psoas tendon is isolated proximally and distally.
- Deep and lateral to the psoas tendon is the hip capsule.
  - A small elevator is used to visualize the surface of the capsule before entering it with a no. 15 blade.
  - A 3-mm, 45-degree Kerrison rongeur is used to enlarge the capsulotomy.
- The joint is irrigated and a suction drain placed. If this approach is used for infection, the surgeon should not close the deep fascia.

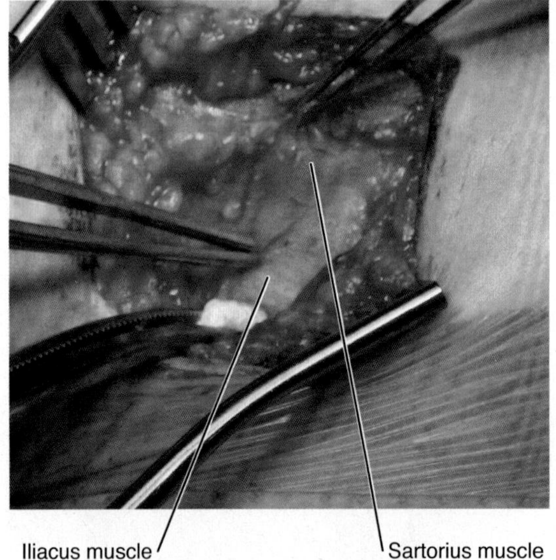

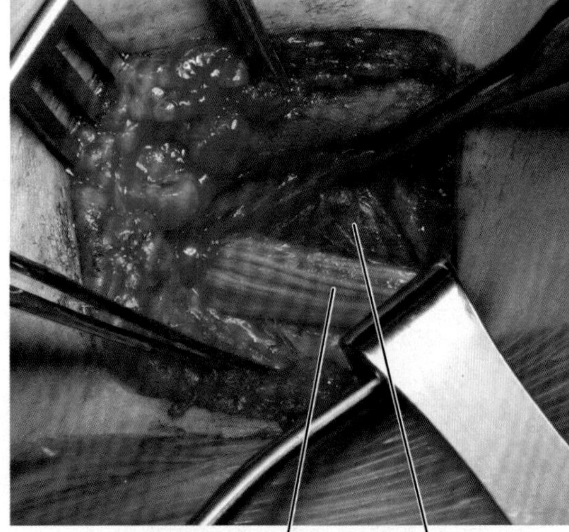


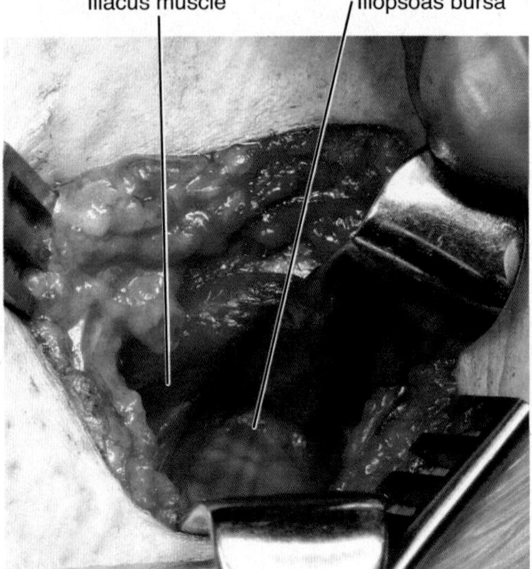


**TECH FIG 2** • Direct anterior approach to the right hip. **A.** The sartorius muscle and the iliacus muscle are covered by deep fascia. **B.** After opening the fascia of the iliacus muscle, the femoral nerve is identified and protected. **C.** The femoral nerve is reflected medially, and the deep medial border of the iliacus muscle is exposed until the iliopsoas bursa is located. The iliopsoas bursa is opened to reveal the iliopsoas tendon.

## Anterior Lateral Approach

- A straight longitudinal incision centered over the greater trochanter is used.
- The tensor fascia is divided longitudinally in line with the skin incision.
- The interval between the most anterior border of the gluteus medius muscle as it attaches to the greater trochanter and the proximal aspect of the vastus lateralis muscle is identified (**TECH FIG 3A**).
- Several millimeters of the gluteus medius attachment to the greater trochanter is released. This allows the examiner to palpate the anterior aspect of the femoral neck, up to the level of the femoral head.
- The gluteus medius muscle is retracted proximally and an incision is made in the anterior capsule (**TECH FIG 3B**). It can be enlarged with the Kerrison rongeur.
- After irrigation and débridement, a drain is left in the hip joint for several days.
- The skin is closed with several interrupted nylon sutures, but the deep fascia should not be closed.

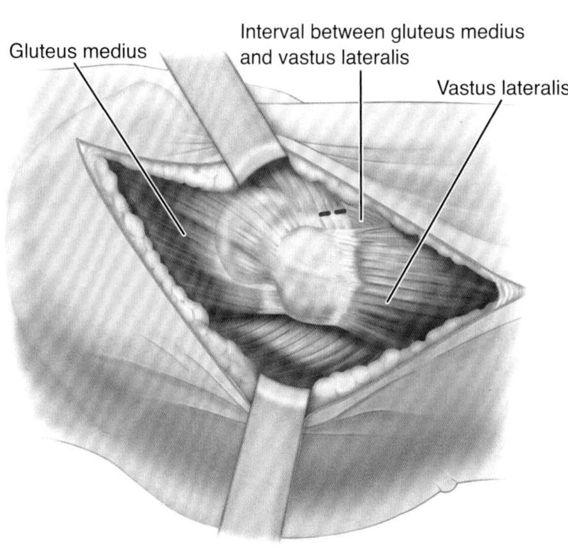


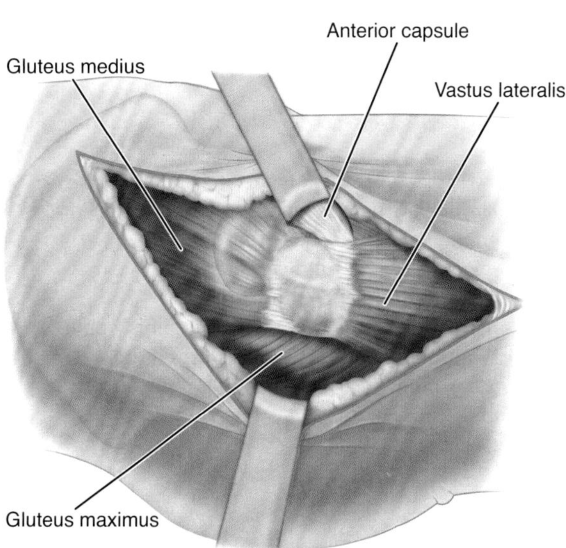


**TECH FIG 3** • **A.** The most anterior fibers of the gluteus medius muscle are divided (*dashed line*) as they insert on the vastus lateralis and greater trochanter. **B.** The gluteus medius muscle is retracted, and the anterior capsule is palpated and visualized.

## PEARLS AND PITFALLS

| | |
|---|---|
| **Newborns and infants** | ■ The child may be systemically ill, with few findings related to the hip.<br>■ In about 70% of cases, there are other sites of infection.<br>■ A painful hip dislocation may be the result of hip joint sepsis.<br>■ Numerous different organisms can be the source of the infection.<br>■ Ultrasound imaging should be obtained and aspiration of both hips should be done if septic hip arthritis is a concern.<br>■ Infants are more likely than older patients to have associated osteomyelitis of the proximal femur. |
| **Be aware of a negative hip aspiration.** | ■ The needle may not be in the hip joint.<br>■ A large-bore needle should be used for joint aspiration.<br>■ A contrast hip arthrogram is done to document intra-articular needle position if there is a question.<br>■ A negative hip aspiration may indicate that the infection is in the acetabulum, proximal femur, or pelvis and has not yet decompressed into the hip joint.<br>■ Pericapsular pyomyositis may have a smaller joint effusion than septic arthritis and be more difficult to obtain fluid on aspiration.[10] |
| **Bone scan** | ■ This test is not necessary to diagnose septic hip arthritis.<br>■ A "cold" bone scan with an area of hypoperfusion indicates poor vascularity and a risk for osteonecrosis; the hip joint should have been drained earlier. |
| **Patient is not responding to treatment.** | ■ The clinician should consider the possibility of coexisting osteomyelitis, seen in 15% of cases.<br>■ Bacteria may be resistant to the selected antibiotic or an inadequate dose is being given.<br>■ Drainage may be inadequate, with reaccumulation of purulence.<br>■ There may be adjacent extension of the infection or abscess.<br>■ There may be unusual host factors such as immune deficiency. |

## POSTOPERATIVE CARE

- A surgical drain is used for several days. It is removed when it is no longer functioning.
- The family needs to understand that repeat drainage is a possibility should symptoms recur or if improvement is inadequate.
- A spica cast is frequently used if the radiograph shows laxity and lateral displacement, especially in the infant.
- Another radiograph is obtained when the antibiotics are discontinued to be sure there is no evidence of osteomyelitis.
- Another radiograph is obtained at 4 to 6 months to document adequate physeal growth.
- In a growing child with a septic joint, the parents should be informed that growth of the bones in that area can be affected.

## OUTCOMES

- In reports of poor results from septic arthritis, 75% involve the hip joint.
- Severe sequelae with a destroyed femoral head are most commonly seen in newborns and infants and are often related to a delay in diagnosis and treatment (**FIG 5**).
- Infants in particular should be followed for several years to document adequate development of the hip joint.
- Simple late reconstruction should focus on maintaining pain-free hip range of motion, realignment procedures if there is a reasonably formed femoral head, and simple procedures to achieve comparable limb lengths.[2]

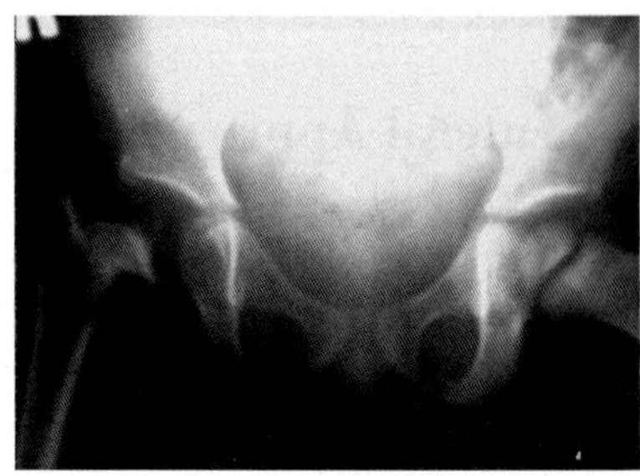

**FIG 5** • This 3-year-old child had septic hip arthritis missed as an infant with a week-long delay in treatment, resulting in osteonecrosis of the right femoral head.

- Complex late reconstruction should rarely be used unless the functional goal can clearly be stated and the procedure has a reasonable chance of meeting that goal.

## COMPLICATIONS

- Avascular necrosis of the hips can lead to complete destruction of the femoral head (**FIG 6**).
- Septic hip dislocation
- Complete separation of the proximal femoral epiphysis
- Proximal femur growth arrest and limb length discrepancy[12]
- Closure of the triradiate cartilage
- Late arthritis

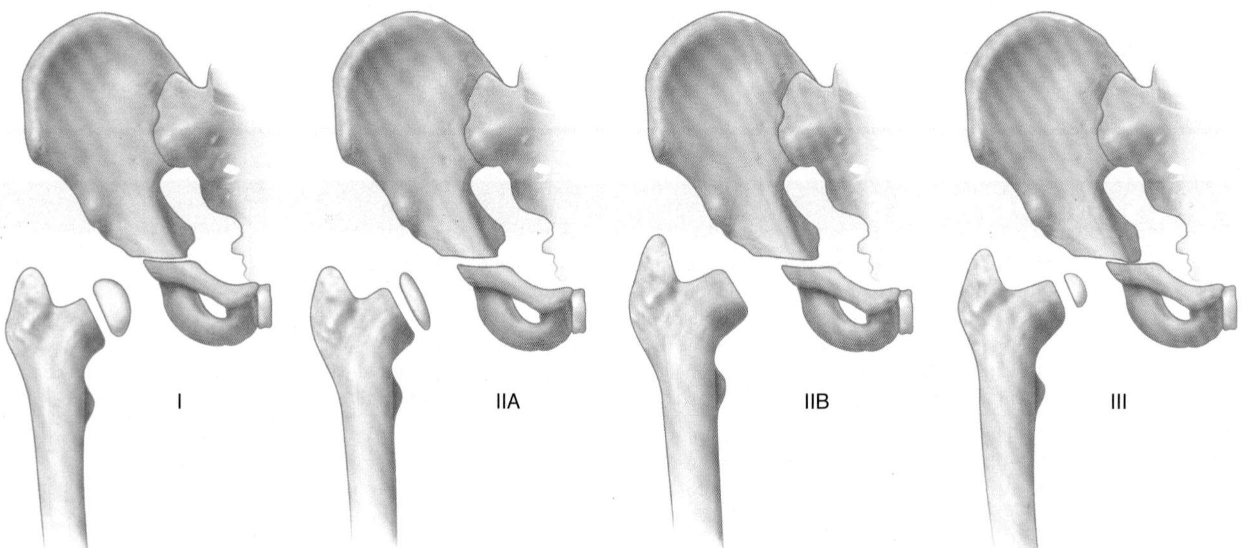


**FIG 6** • Radiographic classification of the sequelae of septic hip as developed by Hunka et al. (From Hunka L, Said SE, MacKenzie DA, et al. Classification and surgical management of the severe sequelae of septic hips in children. Clin Orthop Relat Res 1982;[171]:30–36.) *(continued)*

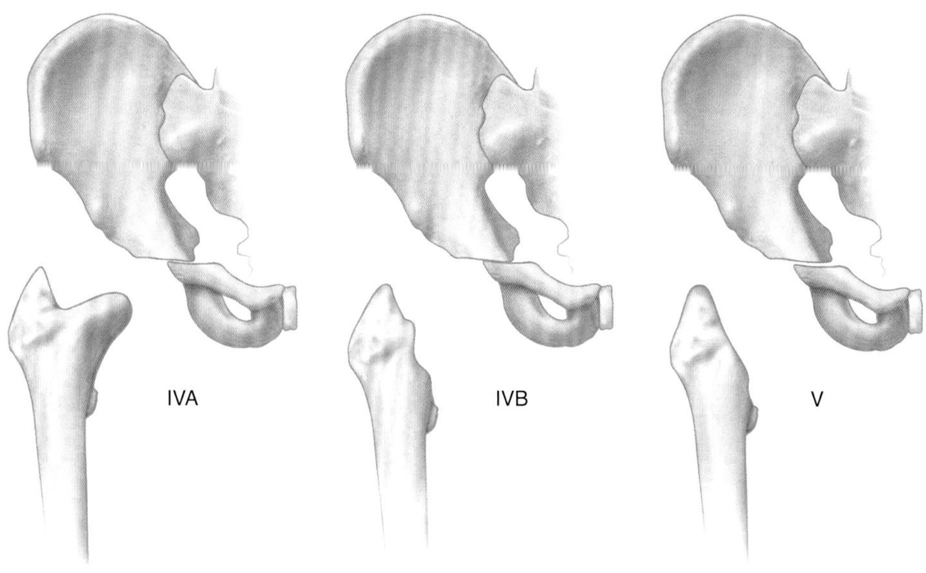


**FIG 6** • *(continued)*

## REFERENCES


1. Caird MS, Flynn JM, Leung YL, et al. Factors distinguishing septic arthritis from transient synovitis of the hip in children: a prospective study. J Bone Joint Surg Am 2006;88(6):1251–1257.
2. Choi IH, Shin YW, Chung CY, et al. Surgical treatment of the severe sequelae of infantile septic arthritis of the hip. Clin Orthop Relat Res 2005;(434):102–109.
3. Copley LA, Kinsler MA, Gheen T, et al. The impact of evidence-based clinical practice guidelines applied by a multidisciplinary team for the care of children with osteomyelitis. J Bone Joint Surg Am 2013;95(8):686–693.
4. Daniel D, Boyer J, Green S, et al. Cartilage destruction in experimentally produced *Staphylococcus aureus* joint infections: in vivo study. Surg Forum 1973;24:479–481.
5. Gafur OA, Copley LA, Hollmig ST, et al. The impact of the current epidemiology of pediatric musculoskeletal infection on evaluation and treatment guidelines. J Pediatr Orthop 2008;28(7):777–785.
6. Gillespie R. Septic arthritis of childhood. Clin Orthop Relat Res 1973;(96):152–159.
7. Karmazyn B, Kleinman MB, Buckwalter K, et al. Acute pyomyositis of the pelvis: the spectrum of clinical presentations and MR findings. Pediatr Radiol 2006;36:338–343.
8. Kocher MS, Mandiga R, Zurakowski D, et al. Validation of a clinical prediction rule for the differentiation between septic arthritis and transient synovitis of the hip in children. J Bone Joint Surg Am 2004; 86-A(8):1629–1635.
9. Luhmann SJ, Jones A, Schootman M, et al. Differentiation between septic arthritis and transient synovitis of the hip in children with clinical prediction algorithms. J Bone Joint Surg Am 2004;86-A(5):956–962.
10. Mignemi ME, Menge TJ, Cole HA, et al. Epidemiology, diagnosis, and treatment of pericapsular pyomyositis of the hip in children. J Pediatr Orthop 2014;34(3):316–325.
11. Morrison MJ, Herman MJ. Hip septic arthritis and other pediatric musculoskeletal infections in the era of methicillin-resistant Staphylococcus aureus. Instr Course Lect 2013;62:405–414.
12. Peters W, Irving J, Letts M. Long-term effects of neonatal bone and joint infection on adjacent growth plates. J Pediatr Orthop 1992;12:806–810.
13. Song KS, Lee SM. Peripelvic infections mimicking septic arthritis of the hip in children: treatment with needle aspiration. J Pediatr Orthop B 2003;12:354–356.

# Innominate Osteotomy of Salter

Simon P. Kelley and John H. Wedge

## DEFINITION

- The Salter innominate osteotomy is commonly performed in conjunction with an open reduction for the dislocated hip in developmental dysplasia of the hip (DDH) after 18 months of age.
- The osteotomy can also be performed to treat acetabular dysplasia in the child with a concentrically reduced hip.[6]

## ANATOMY

- The Salter innominate osteotomy rotates through the symphysis pubis to increase anterior and lateral coverage of the femoral head.
- The center of the hip undergoes slight distal, posterior, and medial displacement in addition to rotation.[4]
- A 30-degree bone wedge inserted in the osteotomy site consistently increases femoral head coverage by 25 degrees anteriorly and 15 degrees laterally.[4]

## PATHOGENESIS

- Acetabular dysplasia is caused by the following:
  - Lack of a reduced, spherical head within the growing acetabulum
  - Abnormal interstitial or appositional growth within the acetabular and triradiate cartilage
  - Abnormal development of the secondary centers of ossification of the ilium, pubis, and ischium
- In the developmentally dislocated hip, the acetabular labrum is flattened, hypertrophied, everted, and is referred to as the *Limbus*.
- Acetabular dysplasia in the infant and young child with DDH is predominantly anterior and lateral.[7]

## NATURAL HISTORY

- The natural history of the dysplastic hip with subluxation is worse than the hip with acetabular dysplasia alone.
- Patients with subluxated dysplastic hips develop pain and disability and radiographic evidence of osteoarthrosis. The age of onset of symptoms depends on the degree of subluxation, with severe subluxation leading to symptoms in the third decade of life.[10]
- Patients with acetabular dysplasia without subluxation develop radiographic evidence of osteoarthrosis in the sixth decade of life and some will develop pain and disability, depending on the degree of dysplasia.[10]

## PATIENT HISTORY AND PHYSICAL FINDINGS

- Patients with developmental hip dislocation may have a positive family history and are usually female and firstborn children.
- There may be a history of breech presentation at birth.
- Children with a dislocated hip usually meet their gross motor milestones within the appropriate timeframe.
- In children with bilateral dislocations, walking is frequently delayed until 16 to 18 months.
- The pertinent physical examination findings in the walking child (the timeframe when this operation is typically performed) are listed in the following text.
- Gluteus medius lurch: Trunk lean over the stance phase leg signifies a positive test, which is a nonspecific sign of hip pathology caused by dislocation, coxa vara, or painful hip conditions.
- Trendelenburg sign: If the pelvis dips away from the affected leg during single-limb stance, the test is positive. Like the gluteus medius lurch, a positive test is a nonspecific sign of hip pathology caused by dislocation, coxa vara, or painful hip conditions.
- Galeazzi sign: Knees at different levels signify a positive test, which indicates unilateral hip dislocation or congenital shortening of the femur.
- Limitation of hip abduction: Normal abduction range of motion is 70 to 80 degrees tested in flexion in the newborn and infant. Asymmetric abduction suggests unilateral hip dysplasia, subluxation, or dislocation. Bilaterally decreased abduction suggests bilateral disease.
- Hamstring tightness test: Normally, the hamstrings will tighten with passive knee extension, and no knee hyperextension should be possible. A positive test implies hip dislocation or flaccid paralysis of the hamstring muscles.
- Inspection of inguinal skin folds: Normal inguinal skin folds are symmetric and stop short of the anal aperture posteriorly. Asymmetric skin folds are a relatively nonspecific finding in the dislocated hip.

## IMAGING AND OTHER DIAGNOSTIC STUDIES

- Standing anteroposterior (AP), supine frog-leg lateral, supine abduction–internal rotation view, and standing false-profile view pelvic radiographs may be used.
  - On the AP film, the acetabular index should be measured to diagnose acetabular dysplasia. Normal values are 35 degrees at birth, 25 degrees at 1 year of age, and 20 degrees at 2 years of age (**FIG 1**).[8]
  - Also on the AP film, Shenton line is inspected for discontinuity, which represents hip subluxation (see **FIG 1**).
- Widening of the acetabular teardrop can be seen with persistent acetabular subluxation due to inadequate loading of the medial acetabular wall.
- A false-profile view of the hip can identify more subtle cases of acetabular dysplasia, particularly in the walking child.
- The abduction–internal rotation view demonstrates the likely position of correction following Salter innominate osteotomy.

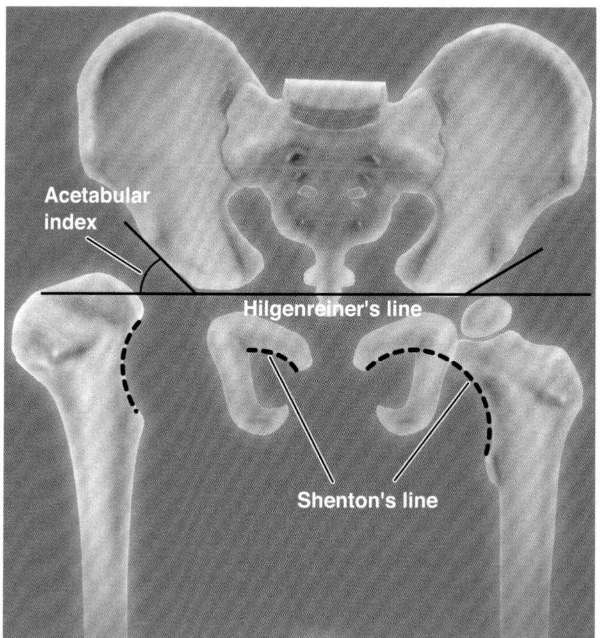


**FIG 1** ● Measurement of the acetabular index and location of Shenton line. This schematic of an AP pelvis radiograph demonstrates a dislocated right hip. Hilgenreiner line is drawn through the top of the triradiate cartilages. A second line is drawn from Hilgenreiner at the inferior edge of the ossified margin of the acetabulum to the lateral edge of the ossified margin of the acetabulum. The angle between these two lines is the acetabular index. Shenton line should be a continuous arc between the medial femoral neck and the superior aspect of the obturator foramen in the normal hip. It is discontinuous in the subluxated or dislocated hip.

- Advanced imaging studies (three-dimensional [3-D] computed tomography [CT] scanning of the acetabulum, magnetic resonance imaging [MRI] of the hip) may be of value in older children to assess acetabular morphology.

## DIFFERENTIAL DIAGNOSIS

- Congenital femoral deficiency
- Developmental coxa vara
- Legg-Calvé-Perthes disease

## NONOPERATIVE MANAGEMENT

- The acetabular index should be observed for improvement over 12 to 18 months after successful closed reduction in the child younger than 18 months of age.
- Indications for a Salter innominate osteotomy include residual acetabular dysplasia with an increased acetabular index, widening of the acetabular teardrop, a broken Shenton line, and adductor tightness on clinical examination.
- A child younger than 18 months old who fails closed reduction can be treated with an isolated open reduction of a dislocated hip and observed for improvement in the acetabular index into the normal range over 12 to 18 months. Salter innominate osteotomy is only indicated as per the criteria stated earlier.

## SURGICAL MANAGEMENT

### Indications

- Age 18 months to 9 years[5]
- Concentric hip reduction on an abduction–internal rotation radiograph (either preoperatively or intraoperatively after an open reduction)[5]
- No or minimal osteoarthrosis of the hip
- At least 100 degrees of hip flexion and 30 degrees of hip abduction
- Anterolateral acetabular dysplasia

### Preoperative Planning

- For the dislocated hip, a closed reduction is attempted.
- If a gentle concentric closed reduction is achieved and the patient is older than 18 months old, a Salter innominate osteotomy including intramuscular psoas lengthening without open hip reduction can be performed.
- An estimation of femoral anteversion with fluoroscopy before patient positioning is used to decide if a concurrent femoral derotational osteotomy is necessary.
- We perform a judicious femoral derotational osteotomy if femoral anteversion is greater than 60 degrees if it is felt that it will enhance stability of the hip.

### Positioning

- The patient is placed supine on the operating table with a gel roll under the ipsilateral hemithorax (but not under the pelvis), raising the affected side into an oblique position.
- The hip is prepared from the midline anterior and posterior, to the inferior rib cage proximally, and the ankle distally (**FIG 2**).

### Approach

- An anterior Smith-Petersen approach to the hip is used (**FIG 3**).
- The oblique incision is centered 1 to 2 cm distal to the anterior superior iliac spine (ASIS).
- No vertical extension is used, as it leads to a poor cosmetic result and does not enhance the exposure.

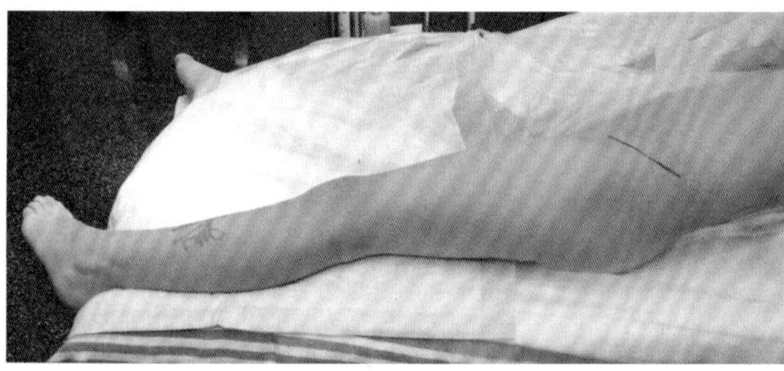

**FIG 2** ● Patient positioning. The patient is placed with a gel roll longitudinally under the left hemithorax, elevating the left hemipelvis. The area of sterile preparation is from the rib cage proximally, the midline anteriorly and posteriorly, and the entire leg distally.

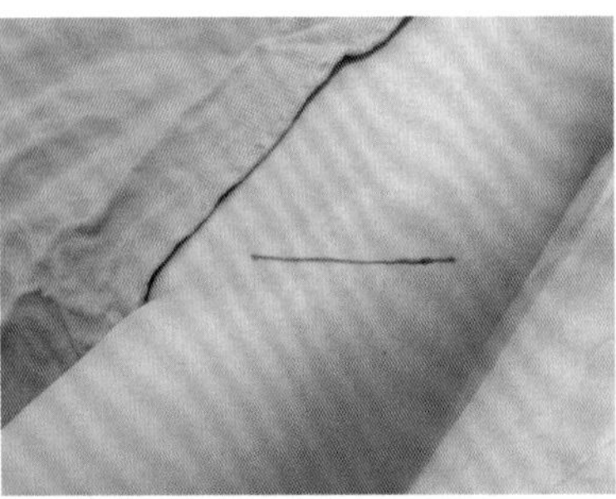

**FIG 3** • Surgical incision. A straight incision is placed obliquely over the anterior aspect of the hip and is centered 2 cm below the ASIS. Proximally, the incision lies distal to the iliac crest. Because the skin is mobile in the child, the incision can be easily moved to complete the exposure of the iliac crest and the anterior aspect of the hip without having it rest directly on the iliac crest. This also allows the incision to lie directly over the hip joint. A vertical distal limb of the incision is unnecessary for exposure and just leaves an unsightly scar.



## Exposure of the Anterior Hip and Ilium

- The exposure of the anterior hip is the same as for an open reduction of the hip in Chapter 87.
- While retracting the external oblique muscle proximal and medial, the iliac apophysis is split with a no. 10 blade scalpel from the midpoint of the iliac crest to the anterior inferior iliac spine (AIIS).
- The inner and outer tables of the ilium are subperiosteally dissected with a broad periosteal elevator to visualize the sciatic notch.
- Sponges are used to facilitate subperiosteal dissection and to achieve hemostasis.
- An intramuscular psoas tendon lengthening is performed at the pelvic brim.
- The rectus femoris tendon is only exposed and divided if exposure for an open reduction of the hip is required.

## Salter Innominate Osteotomy

- Rang retractors are placed subperiosteally in the sciatic notch from the medial and lateral sides.
- The medial retractor is placed on top of the lateral retractor in the notch.
- The Gigli saw is placed into a Kelly clamp and passed through the sciatic notch from medial to lateral (**TECH FIG 1A**).
- Care is taken to push and not pull the Gigli saw through the sciatic notch, as pulling will cause engagement of the saw, and thus preventing its smooth passage.
- The operating room table is lowered, and with hands as wide as possible, the Gigli saw is used to make the osteotomy, exiting just above the AIIS (**TECH FIG 1B,C**).
- It is critical to make the cut perpendicular to the ilium and not the long axis of the patient.

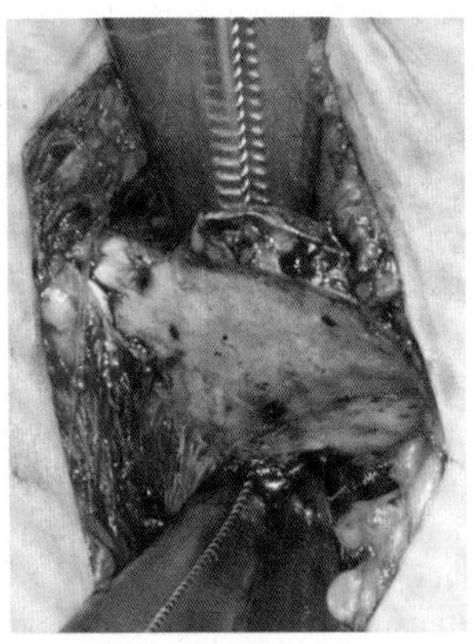

A

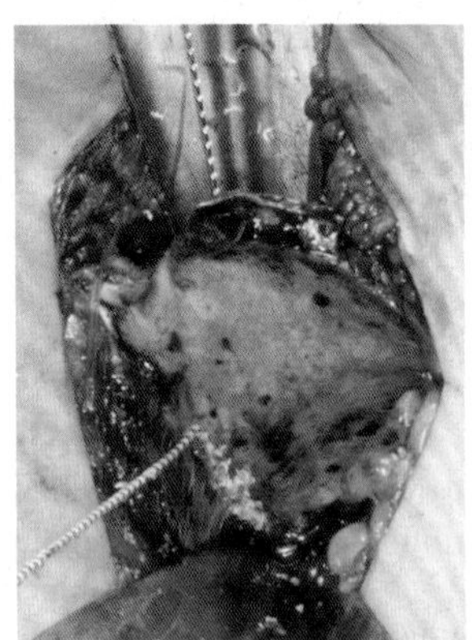

B

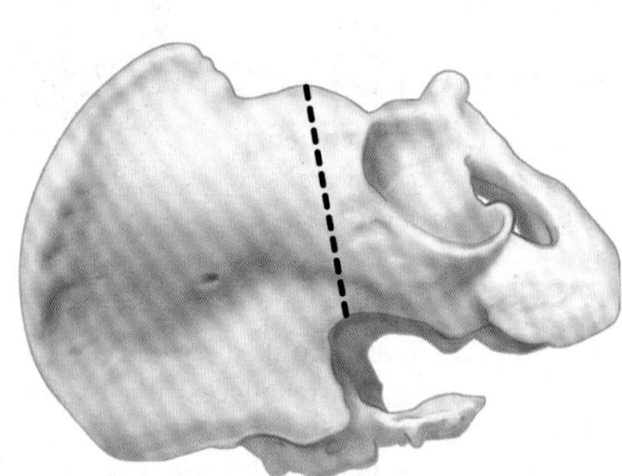

C

**TECH FIG 1** • **A.** Gigli saw on top of Rang retractors placed subperiosteally in the sciatic notch. **B.** The osteotomy is created perpendicular to the plane of the ilium using the Gigli saw from the sciatic notch to the proximal edge of the AIIS. **C.** Location of the Salter innominate osteotomy.

## Harvesting Bone Graft

- The triangular-shaped iliac crest bone graft is grasped with a Kocher clamp and removed with an oscillating saw from lateral to medial, from the AIIS to the iliac tubercle (**TECH FIG 2A,B**).
- The resultant graft is a 30-degree tricortical bone wedge.

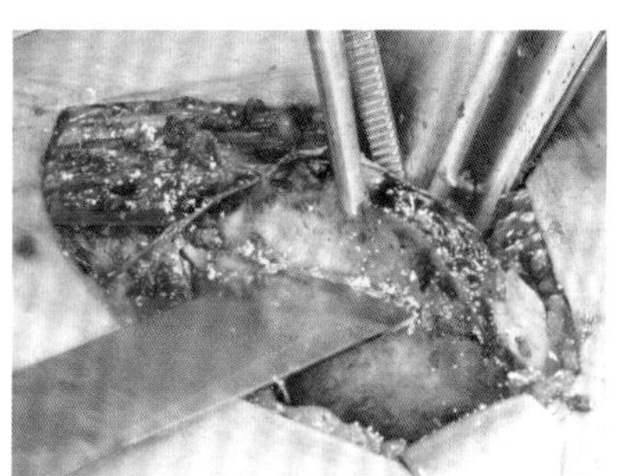
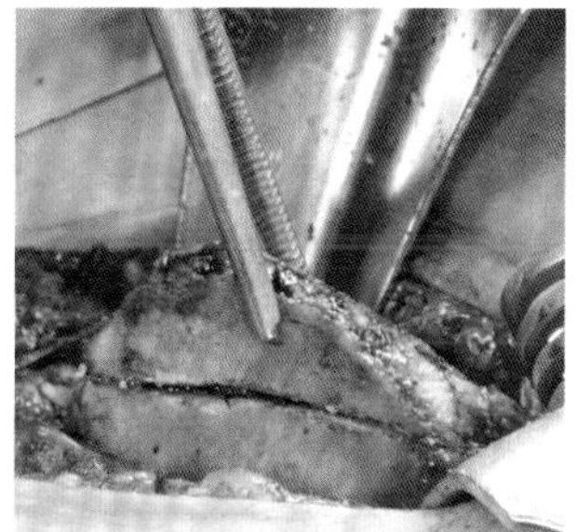

**TECH FIG 2** • **A.** An oscillating saw is used to cut the iliac crest bone graft from the AIIS to the midpoint of the iliac crest. **B.** The iliac crest graft is removed with Kocher clamp.

## Placing the Graft

- A pointed towel clamp is used to hinge the distal fragment in line with the ilium rotating anterolaterally. The distal fragment is pulled anteriorly to prevent posterior displacement, and the posterior part of the osteotomy is kept apposed (**TECH FIG 3A**).
- If done as an isolated procedure, opening the osteotomy site can be facilitated by placing the leg in the figure-4 position.
- The graft is placed in the osteotomy gap concave side medial, with the medial cortex flush with the medial cortex of the proximal and distal fragments (**TECH FIG 3B**).
- The graft is secured with two 2.8- or 3.2-mm threaded Steinmann pins placed from proximal across the graft into the medial and posterior portion of the distal fragment up to the triradiate cartilage (**TECH FIG 3C**).
- Estimating Steinmann pin length: The Steinmann pin can be held along the medial surface of the osteotomy and graft to estimate the depth of pin insertion (**TECH FIG 3D**).
- The acetabulum is palpated (if done with an open reduction) or the hip taken through full range of motion (if done as an isolated procedure) to ensure pins are extra-articular.
- An intraoperative obturator oblique radiograph is taken with the pins in place to ensure they do not enter the triradiate cartilage or the hip joint (**TECH FIG 3E,F**).
- Any prominent graft is trimmed anteriorly.

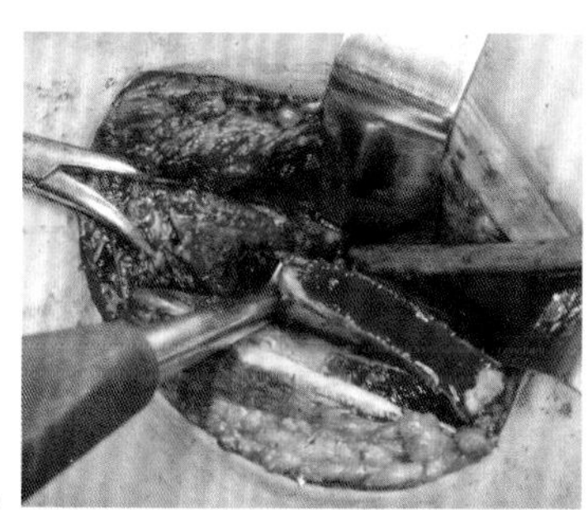
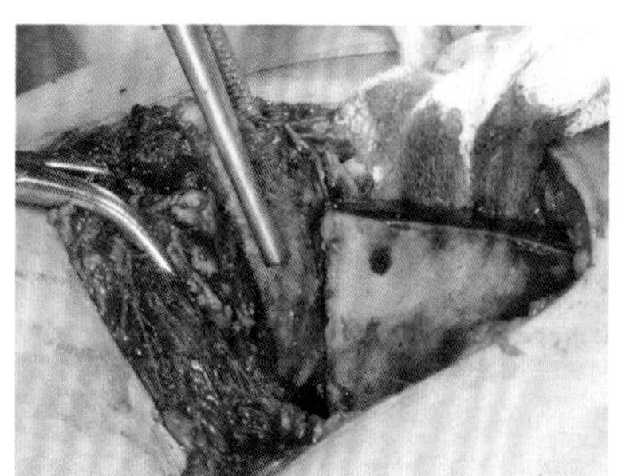
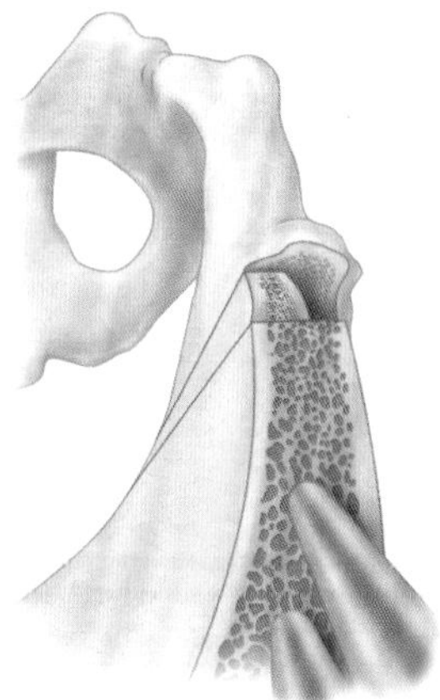

**TECH FIG 3** • **A.** Hinging open the osteotomy. A towel clamp is used to grasp the distal osteotomy fragment only. The proximal fragment is merely stabilized and the distal fragment is pulled in an anterolateral direction in line with the ilium. A spade-shaped elevator may be used to assist with hinging of the osteotomy. **B.** The graft is placed in the osteotomy site biased toward the medial cortex of the ilium. The medial cortex of the proximal fragment, graft, and distal fragment are flush with each other. The proximal, and particularly the distal, osteotomy fragments are wider than the graft, meaning that the lateral cortex of the graft is significantly more medial than the lateral cortices of the proximal and distal fragments. The posterior aspect of the osteotomy should remain closed to allow correct angulation. The graft need not be pushed fully to the apex of the osteotomy, as this may prevent angular correction by the osteotomy and instead just lengthen the ilium. **C.** Two threaded Steinmann pins are drilled from the proximal fragment across the posterior half of the graft to the distal fragment. The pins are placed just deep to the medial cortices. The surgeon is looking from proximal lateral to distal medial along the Steinmann pin path in this figure. *(continued)*

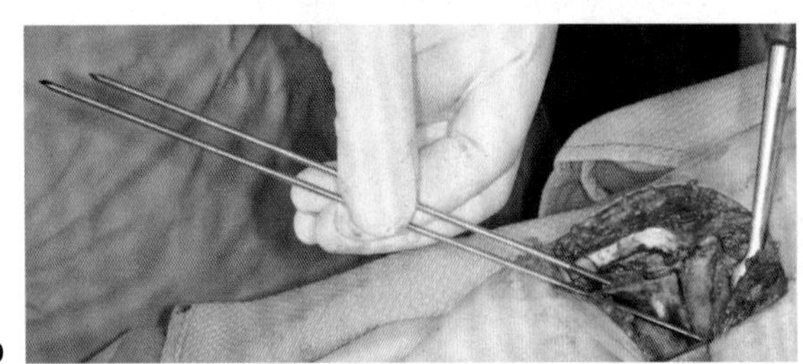

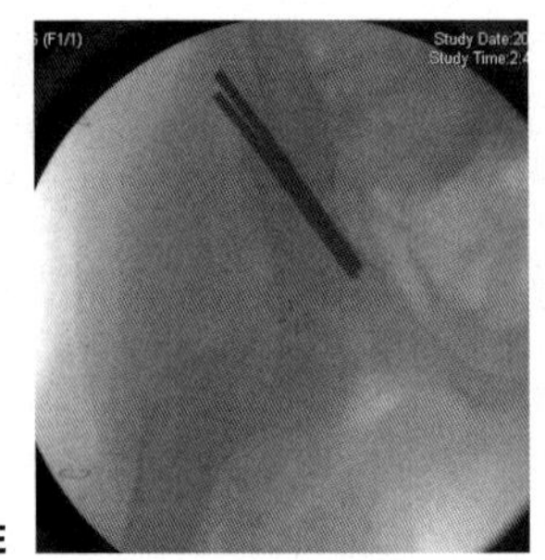

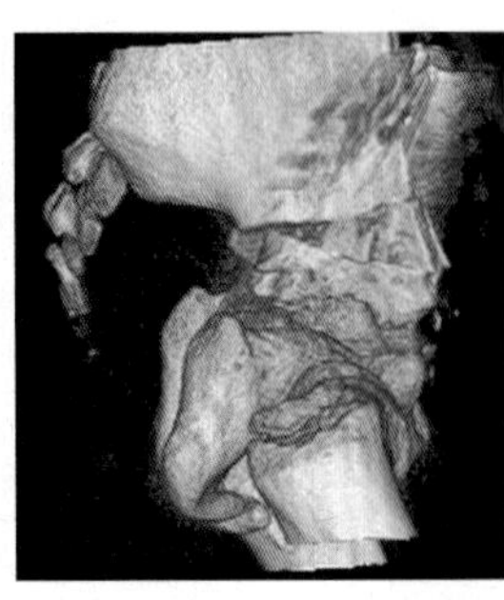

**TECH FIG 3** • *(continued)* **D.** Estimating Steinmann pin length. The Steinmann pin can be held along the medial surface of the osteotomy and graft to estimate the depth of pin insertion. **E.** Intraoperative obturator oblique pelvic radiograph shows the Steinmann pins holding the graft in place and stopping short of the triradiate cartilage. **F.** Reconstructed 3-D CT image to show exact position of graft, with optimally hinged osteotomy with desirable minimal anterior translation of distal fragment.

## Wound Closure

- The iliac apophysis is approximated with a pointed towel clip and closed with absorbable suture in a figure-8 fashion (**TECH FIG 4**).
- The first loop of the figure 8 is circumferential around the entire apophysis, and the second loop captures only the superficial half of the apophysis.
- The pins are cut above the apophysis, coming to lie in the subcutaneous fat, for easy future removal.
- The common head of the rectus femoris tendon is repaired to its insertion if it was divided to facilitate an open reduction.
- Subcutaneous tissue and skin are closed in the standard fashion.

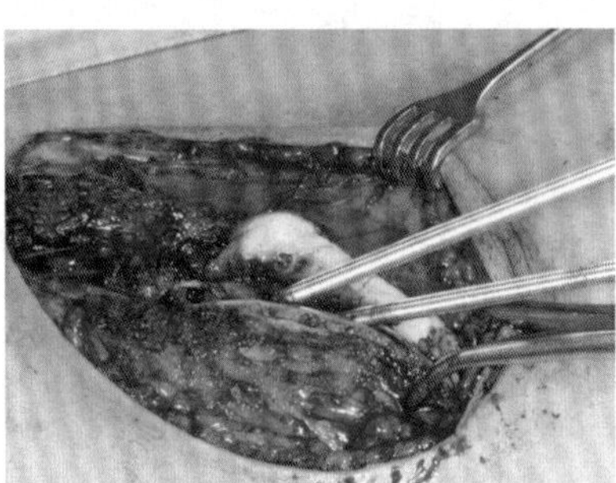

**TECH FIG 4** • The iliac apophysis is approximated with a pointed towel clip and closed with absorbable suture in a figure 8 fashion. Note final position of the two Steinmann pins.

## PEARLS AND PITFALLS

| | |
|---|---|
| **Indications** | ▪ The osteotomy should be performed only for anterior and lateral acetabular deficiency in the concentrically reduced hip.<br>▪ The surgeon should avoid performing the osteotomy in conditions with known posterior hip dysplasia, such as myelomeningocele or cerebral palsy. |
| **Iliac exposure** | ▪ Retracting the external oblique muscle away from the iliac apophysis avoids unnecessary bleeding when cutting it.<br>▪ Raytec sponges placed subperiosteally on the inner and outer tables of the ilium aid in dissection and decrease bleeding. |
| **Performing the osteotomy** | ▪ The AIIS needs to be fully exposed to determine the proper osteotomy exit position.<br>▪ The osteotomy is perpendicular to the ilium not the long axis of the patient. |
| **Opening the osteotomy** | ▪ The osteotomy should be hinged open, pulling the distal fragment anterior and keeping the posterior cortex of the osteotomy opposed. |
| **Fixation problems** | ▪ It is imperative to use intraoperative fluoroscopy to optimize pin position.<br>▪ Intra-articular pin placement should be ruled out by direct palpation if concomitant hip open reduction is being performed or by placing the hip through a full range of motion and feeling and listening for crepitus. |

## POSTOPERATIVE CARE

- The patient is placed in a single-leg hip spica cast with the affected hip in the position of maximal hip stability at 30 degrees of flexion, 20 degrees of abduction, and 20 degrees of internal rotation (**FIG 4**).
- When performed as an isolated procedure or with concomitant open reduction, young children should be immobilized in a single-leg spica cast for about 6 weeks, when early radiographic evidence of healing is evident. No supplementary bracing is typically required.

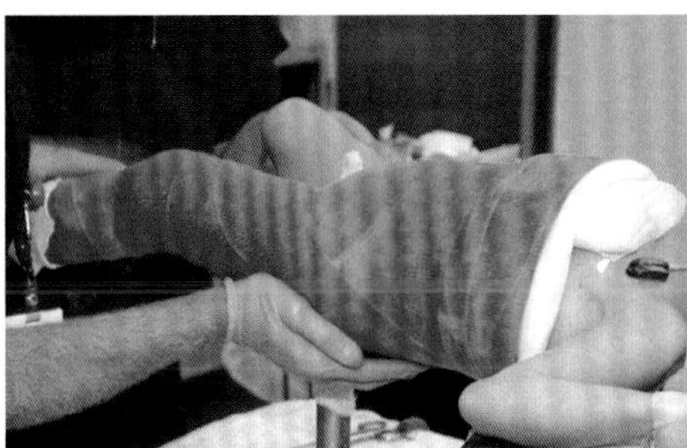

**FIG 4** • The patient is placed in a single-leg hip spica cast with the affected hip in the position of maximal hip stability at 30 degrees of flexion, 20 degrees of abduction, and 20 degrees of internal rotation.

- Children older than the age of 7 years who are reliable may be allowed to use crutches and perform touch-down weight bearing on the affected side without the use of a single-leg spica cast.

## OUTCOMES

- Patients who have undergone an open reduction and Salter innominate osteotomy for late presenting developmentally dislocated hips have good to excellent functional and radiographic outcomes scores at older than 45 years after the index procedure.[9]
- Functional outcomes are best when the acetabular dysplasia is initially corrected to near-normal radiographic values.[1,3]

## COMPLICATIONS

- Neurovascular injury to structures in the sciatic notch
- Lateral femoral cutaneous nerve injury during surgical exposure
- Inadequate correction of acetabular dysplasia due to inadequate patient selection preoperatively or inadequate acetabular rotation intraoperatively[2]
- Injury to the femoral nerve due to prolonged retraction of the psoas muscle or incorrect identification of the psoas tendon during intramuscular tenotomy
- Pin penetration into the hip joint or triradiate cartilage
- Migration of the graft due to inadequate fixation[2]
- Avascular necrosis of the femoral epiphysis[2]
- Growth arrest of the triradiate cartilage

## ACKNOWLEDGMENT

- We thank Richard E. Bowen and Norman Y. Otsuka who wrote this chapter in the first edition.

## REFERENCES

1. Barrett WP, Staheli LT, Chew DE. The effectiveness of the Salter innominate osteotomy in the treatment of congenital dislocation of the hip. J Bone Joint Surg Am 1984;68(1):79–87.
2. Gür E, Sarlak O. The complications of Salter innominate osteotomy in the treatment of congenital dislocation of the hip. Acta Orthop Belg 1990;56:257–261.
3. Macnicol MF, Bertol P. The Salter innominate osteotomy: should it be combined with concurrent open reduction? J Pediatr Orthop B 2005;14:415–421.
4. Rab GT. Biomechanical aspects of Salter osteotomy. Clin Orthop Relat Res 1978;(132):82–87.
5. Salter RB. Innominate osteotomy in treatment of congenital dislocation of the hip. J Bone Joint Surg Br 1961;43-B(3):518–539.
6. Salter RB. Role of innominate osteotomy in the treatment of congenital dislocation and subluxation of the hip in the older child. J Bone Joint Surg Am 1966;48:1413–1439.
7. Sarban S, Ozturk A, Tabur H, et al. Anteversion of the acetabulum and femoral neck in early walking age patients with developmental dysplasia of the hip. J Pediatr Orthop B 2005;14:410–414.
8. Scoles PV, Boyd A, Jones PK. Roentgenographic parameters of the normal infant hip. J Pediatr Orthop 1987;7:656–663.
9. Thomas SR, Wedge JH, Salter RB. Outcome at forty-five years after open reduction and innominate osteotomy for late-presenting developmental dislocation of the hip. J Bone Joint Surg Am 2007;89(11):2341–2350.
10. Weinstein SL. Natural history of congenital hip dislocation (CDH) and hip dysplasia. Clin Orthop Relat Res 1987;(225):62–76.

# 104 CHAPTER Pericapsular Osteotomies of Pemberton and Dega

Tim Schrader and W. Timothy Ward

## DEFINITION

- The Pemberton[7] (**FIG 1**) and Dega[1,2] (**FIG 2**) osteotomies are performed for acetabular dysplasia that is either part of a developmental disorder or an acquired disorder due to muscle imbalance in neuromuscular conditions.
- These are not reorienting procedures such as an innominate osteotomy but rather reshaping procedures that alter the geometry of the acetabulum and its volume.[6,11]
- They are used to increase anterior and lateral acetabular coverage.

## ANATOMY

- The acetabulum develops at the confluence of the growth centers of the ilium, ischium, and pubis.
- Normal growth of the acetabulum requires not only that all of these growth centers remain open and function normally but also that the femoral head remains concentrically reduced and stable within the acetabulum.
- If the growth centers are damaged, either from pathologic conditions or iatrogenically, or if the femoral head is not stable within the acetabulum, normal growth is unlikely to occur and hip dysplasia develops.

## PATHOGENESIS

- Because of an abnormality in the growth centers of the acetabulum, abnormal periosteal growth, or abnormal positioning of the femoral head, the acetabulum does not develop properly.
- Even with a concentric reduction of the femoral head, the prior period of abnormal growth may prevent the acetabulum from achieving a normal configuration at maturity. The older the child is at the time of reduction, the more likely an osteotomy will be necessary to normalize acetabular appearance.

## NATURAL HISTORY

- Many patients with acetabular dysplasia develop subluxation or dislocation of the femoral head. This can lead to early arthritis as an adult.
- The degree of subluxation does not necessarily correlate with the time to onset of symptoms or the degree of arthritic changes.

## PATIENT HISTORY AND PHYSICAL FINDINGS

- Developmental hip dysplasia is a spectrum of pathology that can be diagnosed by physical examination in newborns and young infants if instability of the hip exists but may require ultrasonography or radiographs for diagnosis in cases of dysplasia without clinical instability.

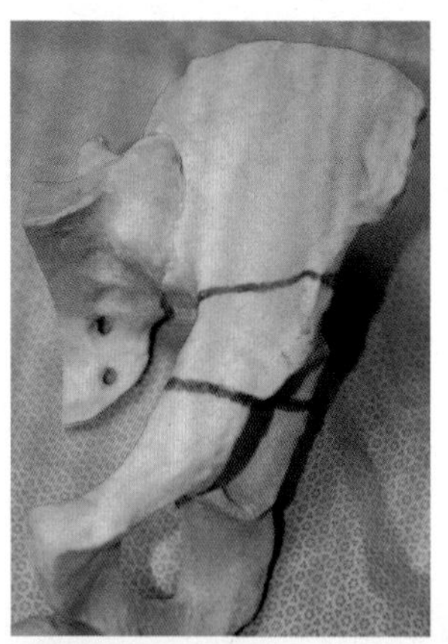
A

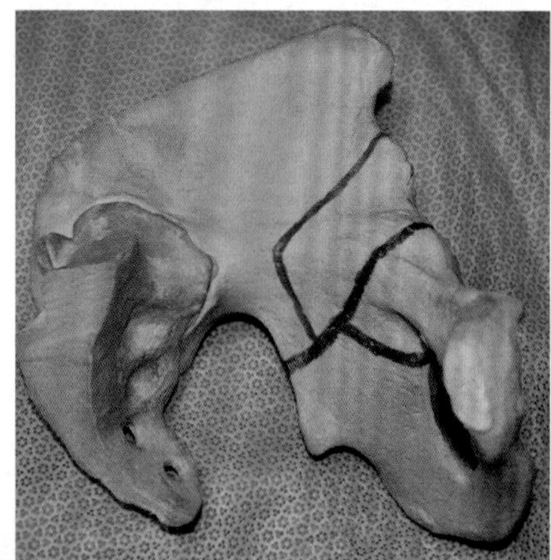
B

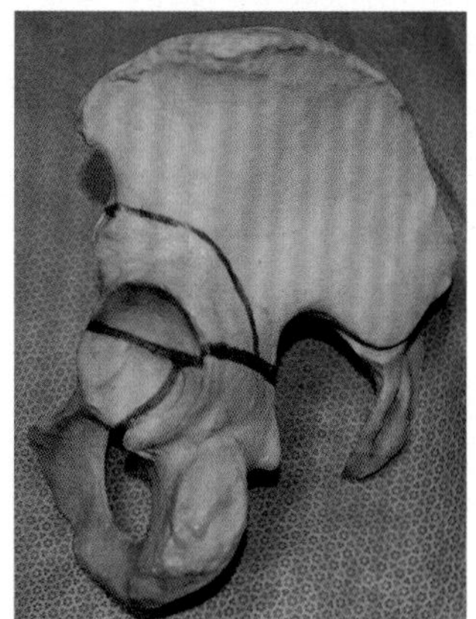
C

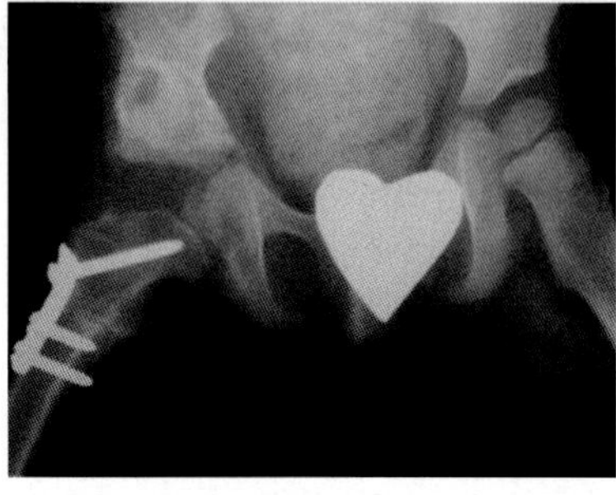
D

**FIG 1** • Pemberton osteotomy depicted on a bone model viewed from anteriorly (**A**), from inside the pelvis medially (**B**), and from outside the pelvis laterally (**C**). The osteotomy starts at the AIIS and extends posteriorly following the insertion of the capsule. It then turns caudally and bisects the posterior column to the level of the triradiate cartilage. **D.** AP radiograph of a Pemberton osteotomy in a 2-year-old child.

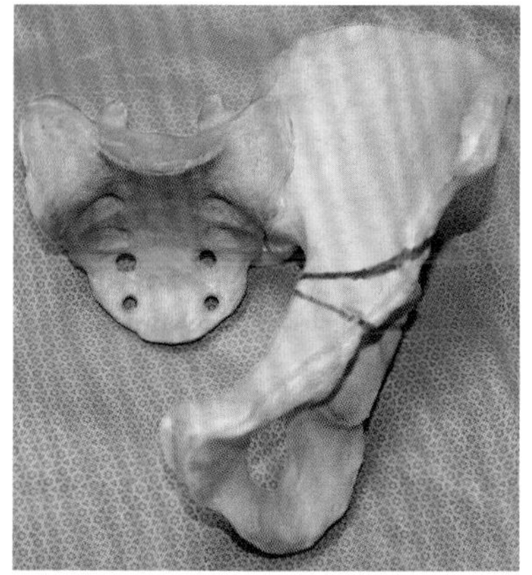
A
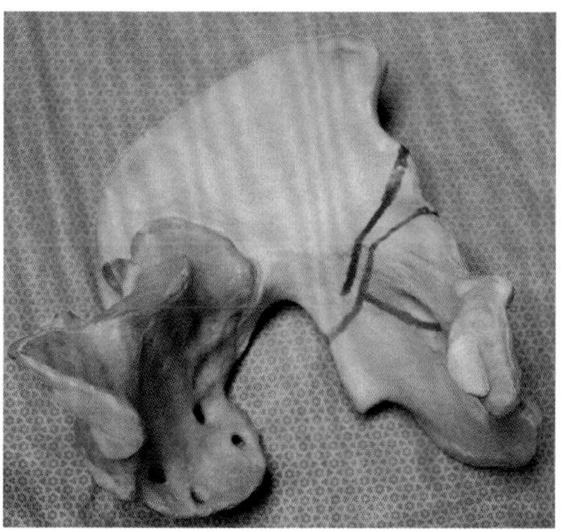
B
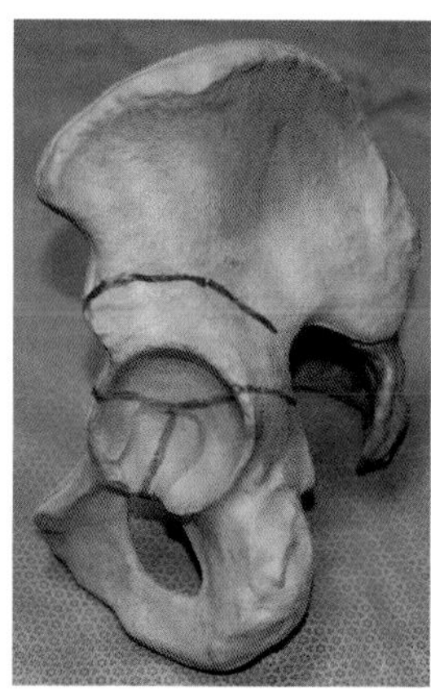
C
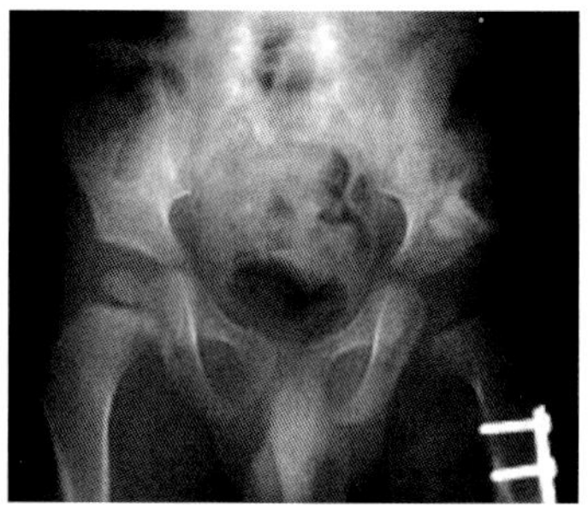
D

**FIG 2** • Dega osteotomy depicted on bone model viewed from anteriorly (**A**), from inside the pelvis medially (**B**), and from outside the pelvis laterally (**C**). As for the Pemberton, the Dega osteotomy starts at the AIIS and extends posteriorly following the insertion of the capsule. However, it then stops about 1 cm from the sciatic notch on the lateral surface. The medial surface is cut just above the horizontal limb of the triradiate cartilage. The more of the medial surface that is left intact, the more lateral coverage the osteotomy provides. **D.** AP radiograph.

- Risk factors include breech position, female, firstborn, and oligohydramnios. Developmental hip dysplasia is associated with other "packaging disorders."
- Patients with a history of hip dysplasia are typically followed with radiographs until adulthood to ensure normal acetabular development.
- Asymptomatic older children without a prior history of developmental hip dysplasia may be diagnosed on incidental radiographs taken for other reasons in cases of mild dysplasia or by history or clinical examination in those children who become symptomatic.
- Symptomatic patients will present in childhood with one or more features including hip pain, limp, limb length discrepancy, or asymmetric hip abduction, particularly those with underlying neuromuscular conditions.
- Routine screening for hip dysplasia using radiographs is widely performed in neuromuscular conditions.
- Examinations and tests to perform include the following:
  - Ortolani test: Positive if a clunk is felt as a dislocated hip reduces.
  - Barlow test: Positive if a clunk is felt as a reduced hip dislocates.
  - Hip abduction: In a normal hip, abduction should be more than 60 degrees and symmetric. This may be the only abnormal sign in infants. A difference of 10 degrees or more is significant.
  - Galeazzi sign: A difference in thigh length is a positive result. A positive Galeazzi sign can indicate a dislocated hip, a short femur, or a congenital hip deformity.
  - Abnormal skin folds can occur in normal children but may alert the pediatrician to an underlying hip problem. This finding is neither highly sensitive nor specific.
  - Limp with ambulation, Trendelenburg sign, or limp associated with limb length discrepancy may be the only abnormal sign in older children.

## IMAGING AND OTHER DIAGNOSTIC STUDIES

- Dynamic hip ultrasound can be used to detect hip dysplasia in very young infants (younger than 6 months of age).
- Plain radiographs, including an anteroposterior (AP) view of the pelvis, frog lateral, and false-profile views, typically can be used to make the diagnosis in older children.
  - Radiographic parameters, including the acetabular index, lateral center–edge angle, anterior center–edge angle, the position of the sourcil, and the line of Shenton, should be evaluated (**FIG 3**).
  - Dislocation is defined by lack of contact between the acetabulum and femoral head.
  - Subluxation is defined by a break in the line of Shenton.
  - Dysplasia is defined by a decrease in the lateral center–edge angle or an increased acetabular index on the AP pelvic radiograph or a decrease in the anterior center–edge angle on the false-profile view.
- An AP pelvic radiograph taken with the legs abducted and internally rotated may show reduction of the femoral head implying that combined pelvic and femoral osteotomy would be expected to increase acetabular coverage.
- A computed tomography (CT) scan, particularly with three-dimensional (3-D) reconstruction can provide a more detailed evaluation of anterior and lateral coverage.

## DIFFERENTIAL DIAGNOSIS

- Slipped capital femoral epiphysis
- Legg-Calvé-Perthes disease
- Congenital coxa vara
- Proximal femoral focal deficiency

## NONOPERATIVE MANAGEMENT

- Infants are typically treated with full-time braces, such as the Pavlik harness.

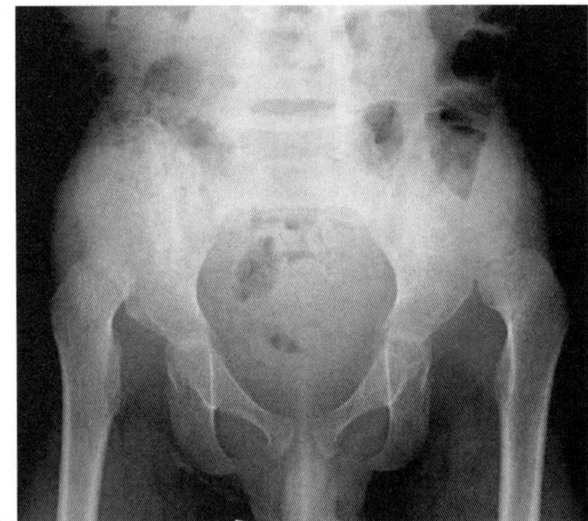

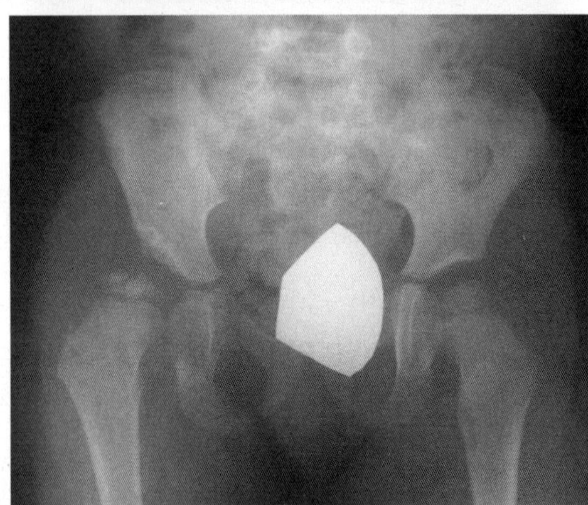

**FIG 3** • **A.** Preoperative AP pelvic radiograph of a child with bilateral hip dislocations. **B.** Preoperative AP pelvic radiographs of a child with right hip dysplasia. This child underwent a closed reduction and adductor tenotomy at 12 months of age. The hip remains subluxated with persistent acetabular dysplasia and did not improve over a year of observation. Changes consistent with avascular necrosis are present in the right femoral epiphysis.

- Young children can be treated with closed reduction and cast immobilization.
- The initial treatment for primary acetabular dysplasia without hip instability or residual acetabular dysplasia following treatment for instability is observation.
  - As long as the acetabular index continues to improve and the hip remains concentrically reduced, observation can be continued.
  - If hip subluxation develops or the acetabular index fails to improve over a 12-month period, operative treatment is indicated.
- Neuromuscular patients with a migration index less than 25% can be observed as long as their abduction remains greater than 45 degrees. Patients with migration indexes over 50% generally will benefit from surgical treatment of their dysplasia, which can include a femoral or pelvic osteotomy.

## SURGICAL MANAGEMENT

- The Pemberton and Dega osteotomies are incomplete transiliac osteotomies used to treat acetabular dysplasia with anterior and lateral deficiencies.
- They are used when more than 10 degrees of acetabular index correction is needed.
- They are also used to increase femoral head coverage during open reduction in a patient with severe acetabular dysplasia.

### Preoperative Planning

- Hip and knee contractures should be carefully evaluated preoperatively so they can be addressed during the surgical procedure.
- With neuromuscular patients, the femoral head may be deformed. An open capsulotomy to look at the articular cartilage may prove to be beneficial.
  - If there is significant articular cartilage damage, particularly laterally from the hip capsule, a resection arthroplasty may be indicated as opposed to a reduction.
- The primary area of acetabular deficiency needs to be determined to plan the osteotomy.
- The triradiate cartilage should be opened because the osteotomy hinges on this cartilage. Generally, this osteotomy can be performed up to about age 10 to 12 years. After this age, hinging is less likely to occur at the triradiate cartilage and moves significantly to the symphysis pubis, resulting in less reshaping and more reorienting of the acetabulum.
- Hip mobility must be good, especially abduction and internal rotation.
- A concentric reduction of the femoral head in the acetabulum before the osteotomy is an absolute prerequisite. This can be assessed preoperatively with an abduction internal rotation hip radiograph or can be assessed intraoperatively after an open reduction or varus proximal femoral osteotomy.

### Positioning

- Patients are positioned supine on a radiolucent table with a bump under the lumbosacral spine to provide about 30 degrees of elevation of the ipsilateral hip (**FIG 4**).
- A fluoroscopic evaluation should be done at this time to ensure adequate radiographic visualization.
- The entire limb is prepared from the lower rib cage to midline.

### Approach

- A standard anterolateral approach using the interval between the tensor fascia lata and sartorius is used.

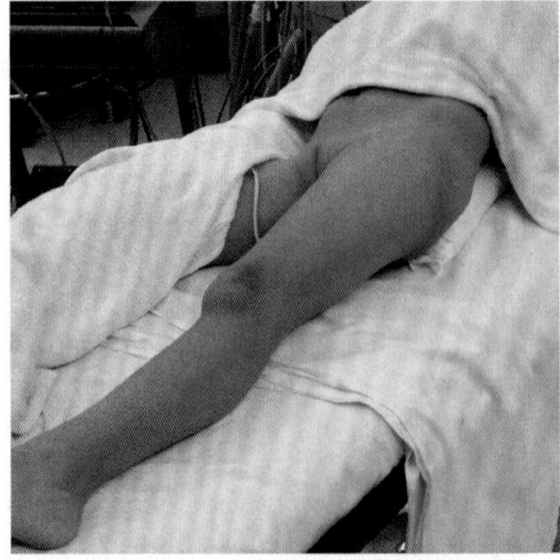

**FIG 4** • Patient positioning. A bump is placed under the lumbosacral area, and the entire lower extremity is draped free.

## Incision and Superficial Exposure for Both Osteotomies

- Two different skin incisions have been described. The choice is determined by the need for concomitant femoral osteotomy but is fundamentally surgeon preference.
  - An anterolateral curvilinear incision starts 1 cm inferior and posterior to the anterior superior iliac spine (ASIS) extending distally over the greater trochanter down the proximal femur. This incision is only used when anterior open reduction and femoral osteotomy is included. It is expansile and provides excellent visualization for all aspects of an open reduction combined with pelvic and femoral osteotomy (**TECH FIG 1A**).
  - Alternatively, a "bikini" oblique incision can be used, particularly if Dega or Pemberton osteotomy is done in isolation. This incision is more cosmetically appealing than the anterolateral curvilinear incision if the pelvic osteotomy is done in isolation. A separate additional lateral incision is used if femoral osteotomy is planned (**TECH FIG 1B,C**).
- The skin incision is deepened to expose the iliac crest and the interval between the sartorius and tensor fascia lata.
- The deep fascia is incised just lateral to the tensor fascia lata muscle to avoid injury to the lateral femoral cutaneous nerve, and the sartorius muscle is released from its origin on the ASIS.
- The tensor–sartorius interval is deepened until the straight head of the rectus femoris is encountered at its origin on the anterior inferior iliac spine (AIIS). The straight head is generally released at its origin if concomitant anterior open reduction is done but can be left intact if only a pelvic osteotomy is done. If released, it is repaired during closure.

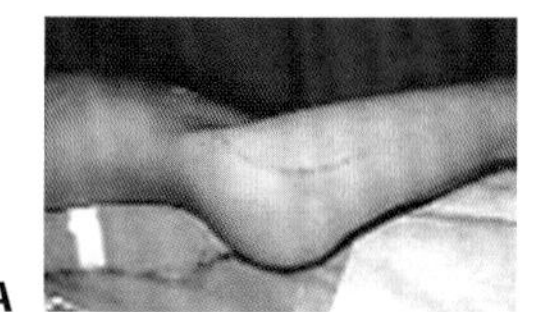
A
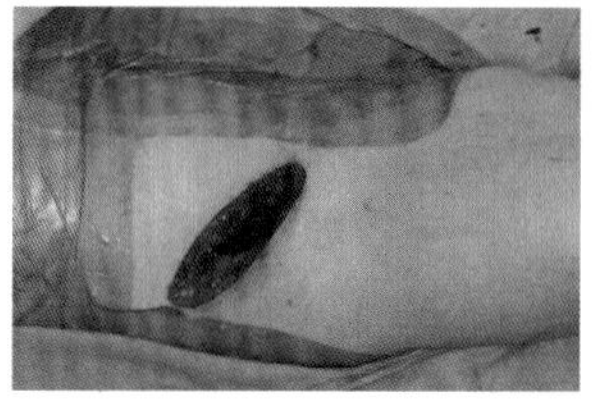
B
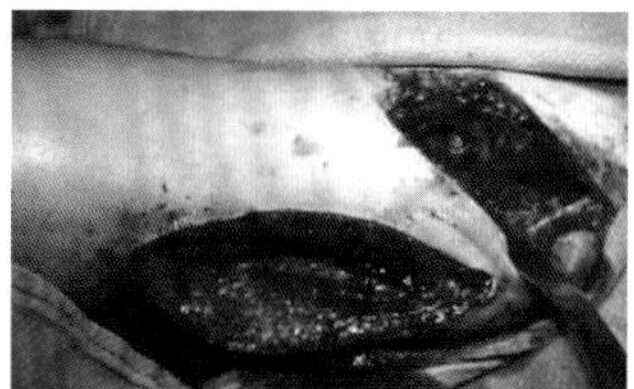
C

**TECH FIG 1** • Skin incisions. **A.** An anterolateral curvilinear incision starts 1 cm inferior and posterior to the ASIS extending distally over the greater trochanter down the proximal femur. **B,C.** The more limited bikini incision provides plenty of exposure for the pelvic osteotomy, leaves an unassuming scar, and can be combined with a lateral incision for concurrent femoral osteotomies.

## Pemberton Osteotomy

### Deep Exposure

- The exposure is important in this osteotomy. Before any cuts are made, the surgeon should be able to clearly see the inner and outer portions of the iliac wing to the sciatic notch posteriorly and the entire hip capsule anteriorly.
- The outer table of the ilium can be exposed either by splitting the iliac apophysis or by dissecting just below the apophysis, in which case, the apophysis is then taken off as an entire piece to minimize injury to this growth area.
- The outer and inner tables are exposed in a subperiosteal fashion to the sciatic notch.
- Chandler retractors are placed into the sciatic notch from medial and lateral to protect the neurovascular bundle (**TECH FIG 2**).
- The reflected head of the rectus is then released and followed posteriorly. It acts as a guide to the border of the hip capsule.

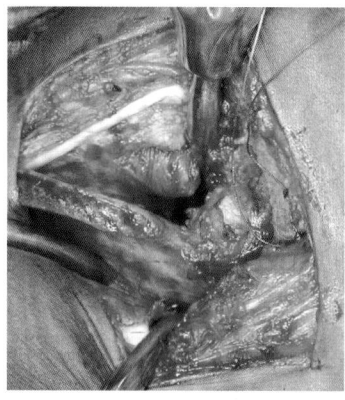

**TECH FIG 2** • Deep exposure. The medial and lateral portions of the iliac wing have been exposed by splitting the apophysis. The Chandler retractors are in the sciatic notch. The capsule has been exposed. The direct head of the rectus is tagged with the suture.

### Creating the Osteotomy

- The first cut is made on the outer table starting 1 to 1.5 cm above the AIIS and extending posteriorly and parallel to the joint capsule.
- About 0.5 to 1 cm from the sciatic notch, the osteotome should be turned and directed distally down the ischium to the level of the ischial limb of the triradiate cartilage (**TECH FIG 3A**).
  - The last portion of this cut is made in a blind fashion with fluoroscopic guidance, and care must be taken to avoid cutting into the sciatic notch, the hip joint, or the triradiate cartilage.
- The osteotome should remain midway between the capsular attachment and the sciatic notch, splitting the posterior column in half to the level of the triradiate cartilage.
- The inner cut is started at the same point as the outer cut on the anterior surface, and the cut is generally at the same level as the outer cut running parallel to it (**TECH FIG 3B**).

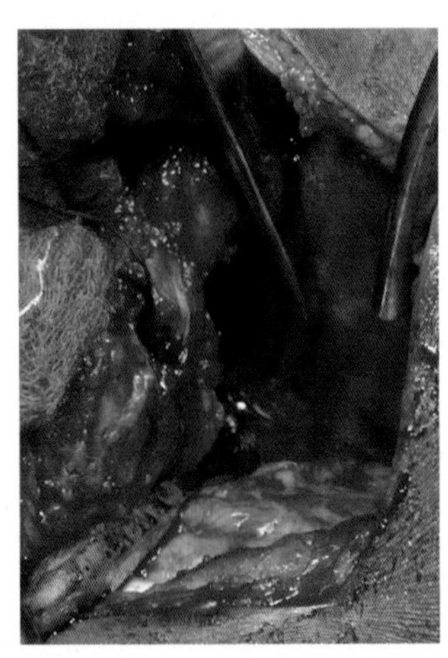

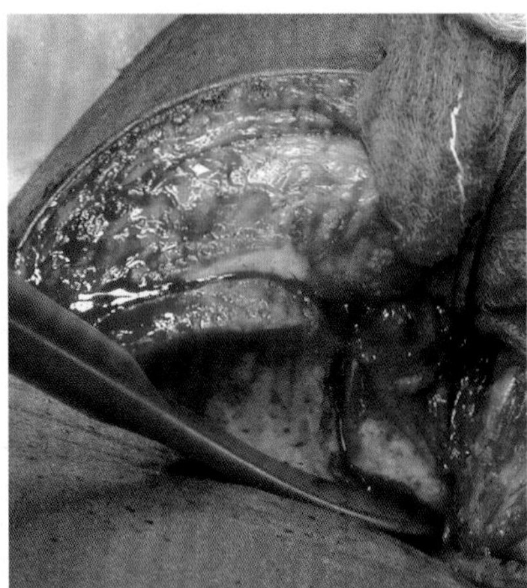

**TECH FIG 3** • **A.** Lateral wall cut. The Chandler retractor is in the sciatic notch and the osteotome is used to cut the lateral cortex. The cut has started between the ASIS and AIIS and is extending parallel to the joint. The posterior portion of this osteotomy will be made in a blind fashion. **B.** Medial wall cut. The Chandler retractor is in the sciatic notch, and the osteotome is used to cut the medial cortex. The cut has started at the same location as the lateral wall cut, between the ASIS and the AIIS, and is extending in the same direction as the lateral wall cut.

## Osteotomy Variation

- If more lateral coverage is needed, the inner cut is moved more distal and shortened to make a more oblique osteotomy.
- This changes the fulcrum of rotation from straight posterior to more posteromedial, giving more lateral coverage as the fragment is levered downward (**TECH FIG 4**).

## Separating the Bone

- A special curved osteotome (**TECH FIG 5A**) is inserted into the osteotomy to connect the two cuts. This osteotome is advanced by hand.
- Once the osteotome is at the level of the triradiate cartilage (**TECH FIG 5B**), the acetabular roof is gently levered down (**TECH FIG 5C**).

## Graft Placement and Closure

- Once the roof is in the desired position (usually an opening of 1 to 2 cm anteriorly), bone wedges are placed in the opening to hold the osteotomy open. Allograft or a wedge of the ASIS can be used.[5]
- An autograft wedge of the ASIS can be harvested with a straight cut of the ilium (**TECH FIG 6A**).
- The graft is usually placed from anterior to posterior. A gouge may be used to make a trough in the iliac wing and the acetabular fragment for the graft to rest in (**TECH FIG 6B**).
  - Internal fixation is usually not necessary.
- The apophysis and muscles are then reattached with suture, and the skin is closed in routine fashion.
- A hip spica cast is then applied (**TECH FIG 6C**).

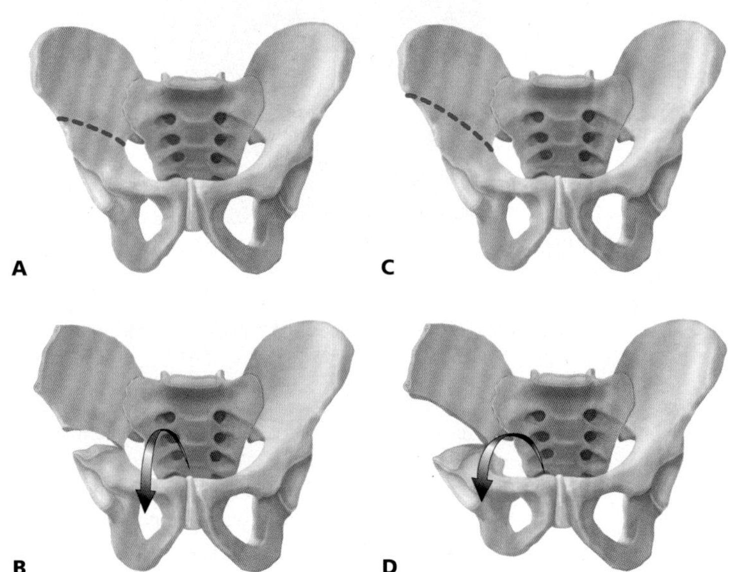

**TECH FIG 4** • Variations in the Pemberton osteotomy. The inner and outer iliac wing cuts determine the amount of coverage based on their direction. **A,B.** If more anterior coverage is required, then the inner cut is more transverse. **C,D.** If more lateral coverage is required, then the osteotomy is inclined laterally and both cuts begin a little farther away from the capsule.

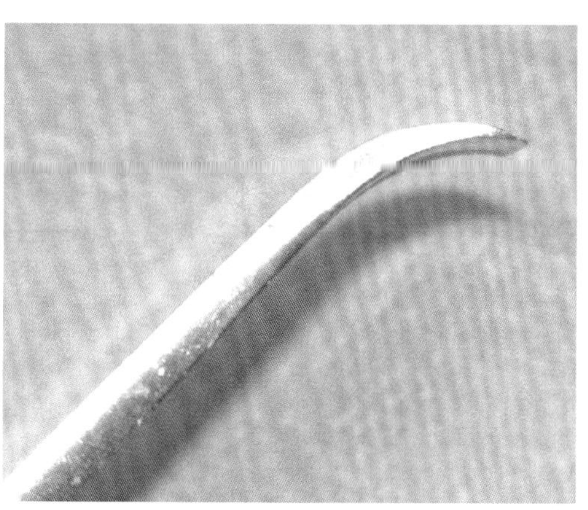

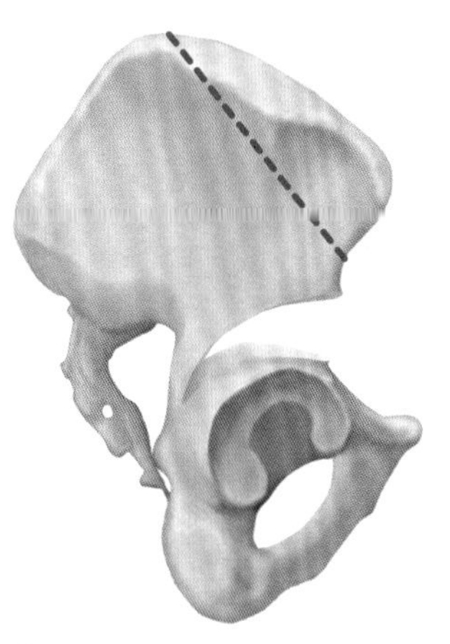

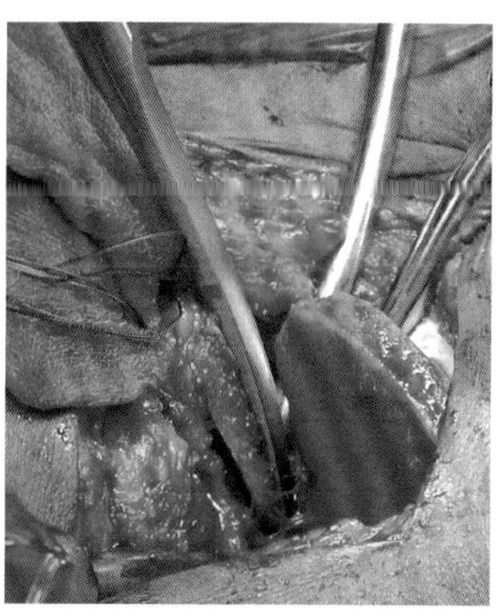

**TECH FIG 5** ● **A.** Pemberton osteotome. The special curved Pemberton osteotome is necessary to connect the inner and outer wall cuts and make the sharp posterior curve. **B.** Connecting the cuts. A special curved osteotome is necessary to make the sharp curve of the osteotomy posteriorly. The osteotome is advanced by hand, connecting the inner and outer wall cuts made previously. The osteotome is advanced to the level of the triradiate cartilage. The *dotted line* represents the ASIS autograft fragment that can be used to hold the osteotomy open. **C.** Levering down the osteotomy. The osteotomy is levered downward with the osteotome. A lamina spreader can also be used with caution. In this patient, a femoral shortening osteotomy and open reduction have been performed and sutures are in place allowing for a capsulorrhaphy once Pemberton osteotomy has been completed.

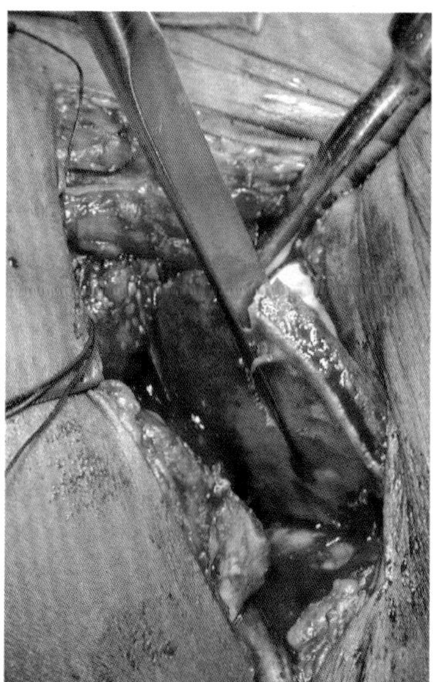

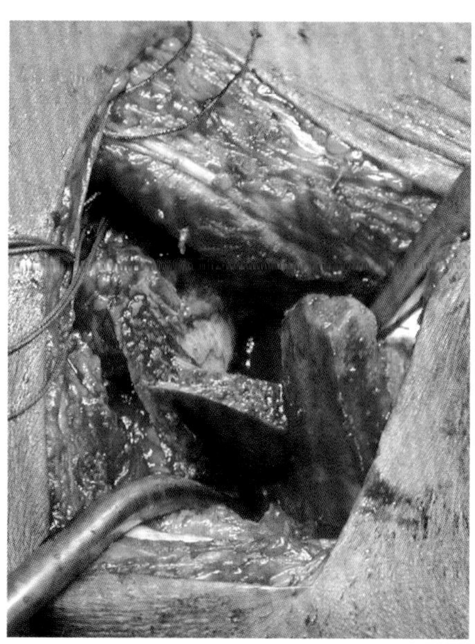

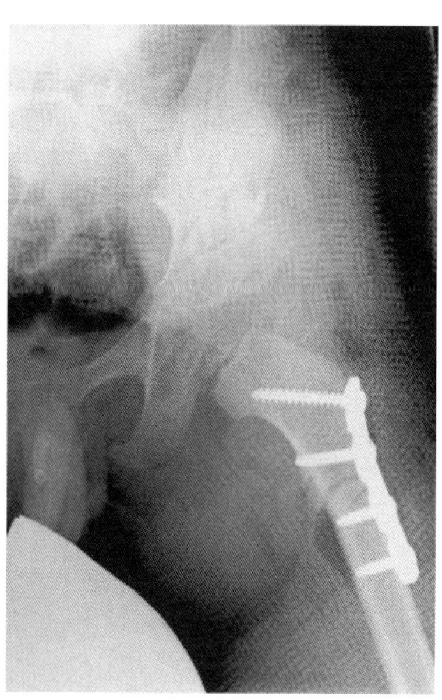

**TECH FIG 6** ● **A.** ASIS autograft bone wedge. An osteotome is used to harvest the ASIS autograft bone wedge. The height of the wedge is determined by the amount the osteotomy will be levered downward. **B.** Graft placement. An autograft bone wedge from the ASIS or an allograft wedge can be used. The graft is inserted in an anterior to posterior direction and should be stable after it is impacted. Internal fixation is seldom necessary. **C.** AP postoperative pelvic radiograph of a left Pemberton osteotomy in a spica cast. An open reduction, capsulorrhaphy, and femoral shortening osteotomy have also been performed.

## Dega Osteotomy

### Exposure

- The abductor muscles are reflected off of the lateral cortex of the ilium just distal to the iliac apophysis. The apophysis itself is neither split nor taken off of the ilium in order to maintain normal apophyseal growth.
- The outer table is exposed subperiosteally back to the sciatic notch. A blunt adult size Hohmann retractor is inserted into the notch laterally to provide visualization of the notch during the osteotomy.
  - Neither the muscles nor the periosteum is dissected off of the inner wall of the ilium. Their preservation is thought to aid in bone graft consolidation (**TECH FIG 7**).

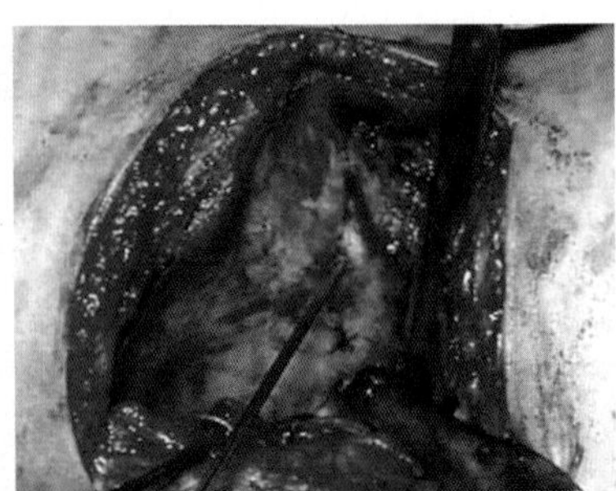

**TECH FIG 7** • Intraoperative photo of a right hip with the patient's head to the left showing complete exposure of the lateral ilium, Hohmann retractor in the notch posteriorly, guidewire at the superior aspect of the osteotomy, and *x* mark where osteotomy will end 1 cm in front of notch. It is essential to clearly see the notch during use of the chisel to make the bone cut and to lever open the osteotomy.

## Creating the Osteotomy

- A curvilinear osteotomy is performed on the outer wall starting just above the AIIS to end at a point 1 to 1.5 cm in front of the sciatic notch. The exact level of the osteotomy on the ilium is determined by the steepness of the acetabulum and is usually about 1 to 2 cm above the capsular insertion.
- A guidewire is inserted at the most cephalad portion of the osteotomy directed to exit just above the horizontal limb of the triradiate cartilage. The guidewire is placed under radiographic guidance and adjusted as needed to end at the triradiate cartilage. A line is drawn on the ilium, based on the guidewire, and serves as the directional guide for the chisel as the osteotomy is made (**TECH FIG 8A–D**).
- A straight 0.25- or 0.5-inch (0.64- or 1.3-cm) osteotome is used to cut the ilium obliquely medially and inferiorly in line with the guidewire to exit through the inner wall above the iliopubic and ilioischial limbs of the triradiate cartilage but leaving the sciatic notch and posterior one-third of the inner cortex intact to act as a fulcrum for rotation (**TECH FIG 8E,F**).
- The cortex is levered down with a wide osteotome to provide the desired coverage. A small laminar spreader is also useful for this maneuver (**TECH FIG 8H–I**).
- The amount of lateral and anterior coverage is determined by how much of the medial inner cortical wall is left intact.
  - If more of the medial wall is left intact, then fulcrum of rotation will move more anterior and more lateral coverage will be obtained (**TECH FIG 9A,B**).
  - If more of the medial wall is cut, the fulcrum of rotation will move posteriorly and more anterior coverage will be obtained (**TECH FIG 9C,D**).

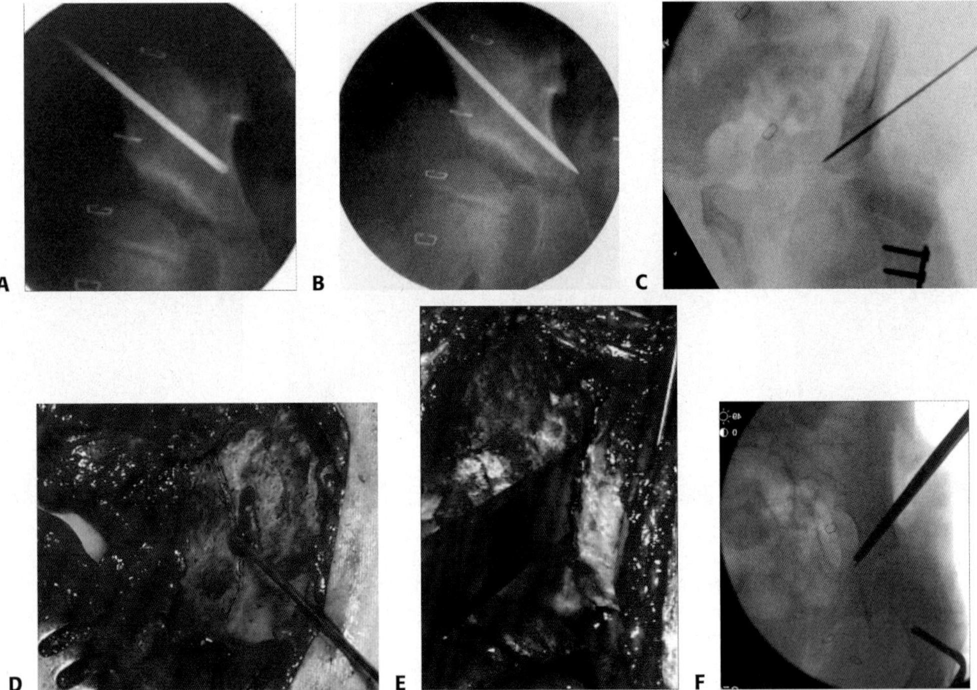

**TECH FIG 8** • **A–D.** Guidewire placement. **A.** Intraoperative fluoroscopy image showing that initial placement of guidewire is too superior. **B.** The guidewire is redirected more obliquely to end at the correct point just above the triradiate cartilage. **C.** Another example of proper guidewire placement ending just above the triradiate cartilage. **D.** Guidewire placement and osteotomy mapping line on outer ilium. (This is the left hip and the patient's head is to the right.) The guidewire is always placed at the most cephalic point of the osteotomy and verified to be in the correct plane by C-arm fluoroscopy. The mapping line is then drawn off of the guidewire. A curvilinear osteotomy is performed on the outer wall starting just above the AIIS to a point 1 to 1.5 cm in front of the sciatic notch. **E.** Right hip with ½-inch osteotome in osteotomy plane. The guidewire is removed once the correct plane of the osteotomy has been created. The progression of the osteotomy is checked by fluoroscopy but can be visualized grossly. **F.** Intraoperative fluoroscopy showing correct orientation of the chisel prior to removal of the guidewire. *(continued)*

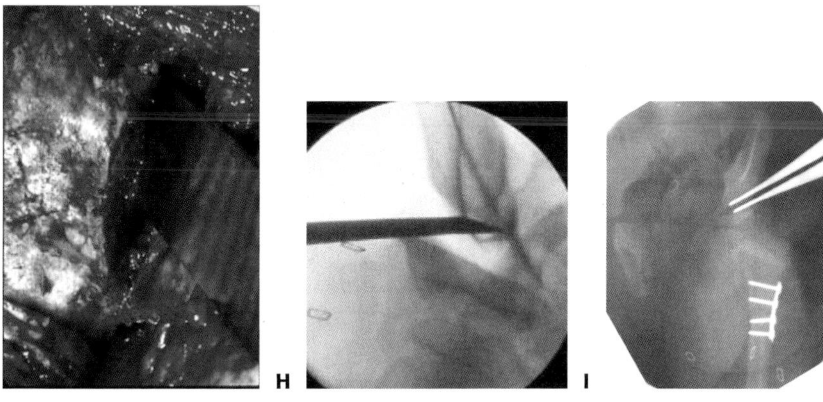

**TECH FIG 8** • *(continued)* **G.** Right hip with osteotome levering open the osteotomy. Note the intact posterior sciatic notch at bottom of picture, which acts as a fulcrum for rotation and provides recoil for graft stability. **H.** Intraoperative fluoroscopic view showing osteotomy levered open by osteotome. **I.** Separate example of a small lamina spreader used to open the osteotomy.

## Graft Placement and Closure

- Triangular or trapezoidal bone wedges, either autogenous or allograft, are used to hold the osteotomy open. Autograft wedges are harvested from a concurrent femoral shortening osteotomy or from the iliac crest. When larger grafts are required, a freeze-dried fibular allograft works well (**TECH FIG 10A–D**).
- The wedges are inserted in a manner that places the largest graft where the most coverage is desired. Smaller grafts are then added as needed to fill the defect (**TECH FIG 10E–G**).
- The grafts are stable and internal fixation is not necessary because of the inherent recoil at the osteotomy site produced by the intact sciatic notch.
- The apophysis and muscles are then reattached with suture, and the skin is closed in routine fashion.
- A hip spica cast is then applied.

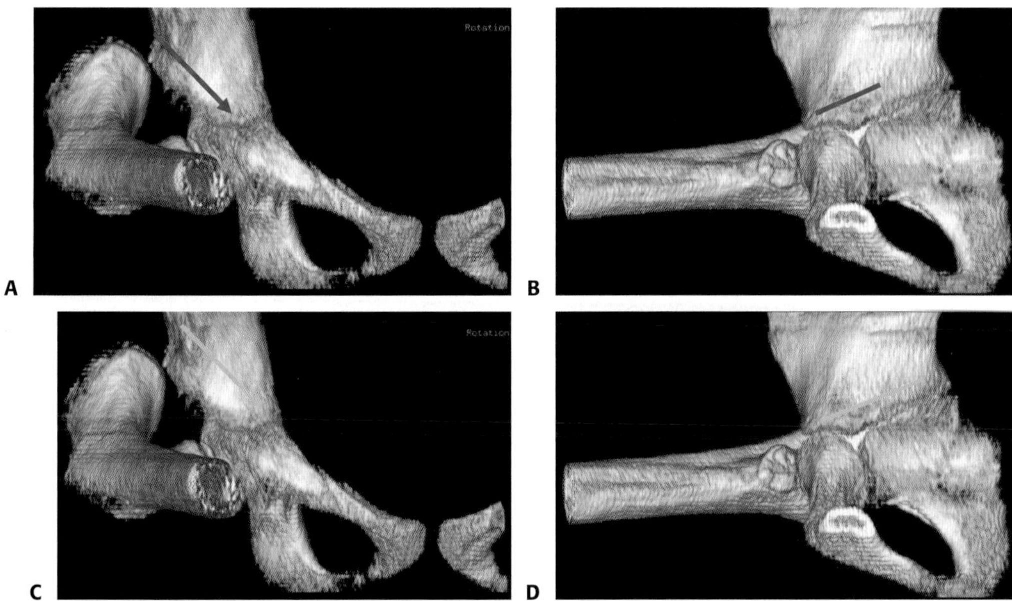


**TECH FIG 9** • 3-D CT preoperative reconstruction. Viewed from anterior oblique direction, the *blue arrow* denotes the direction of osteotomy so that the anterior end point of the osteotomy on the inner wall leaves the posterior two-thirds of the inner cortex intact. Lateral coverage is optimized (**A**). Viewed from inner pelvis, the *blue line* denotes the amount of inner cortex that is cut when lateral coverage is emphasized (**B**); when more anterior coverage is desired, more of the inner cortex is cut. *Green arrow* points toward a more posterior end point on the anterior view (**C**); when viewed from the inner side, *green line* marks the extent of inner cortical cut when anterior coverage is emphasized (**D**).

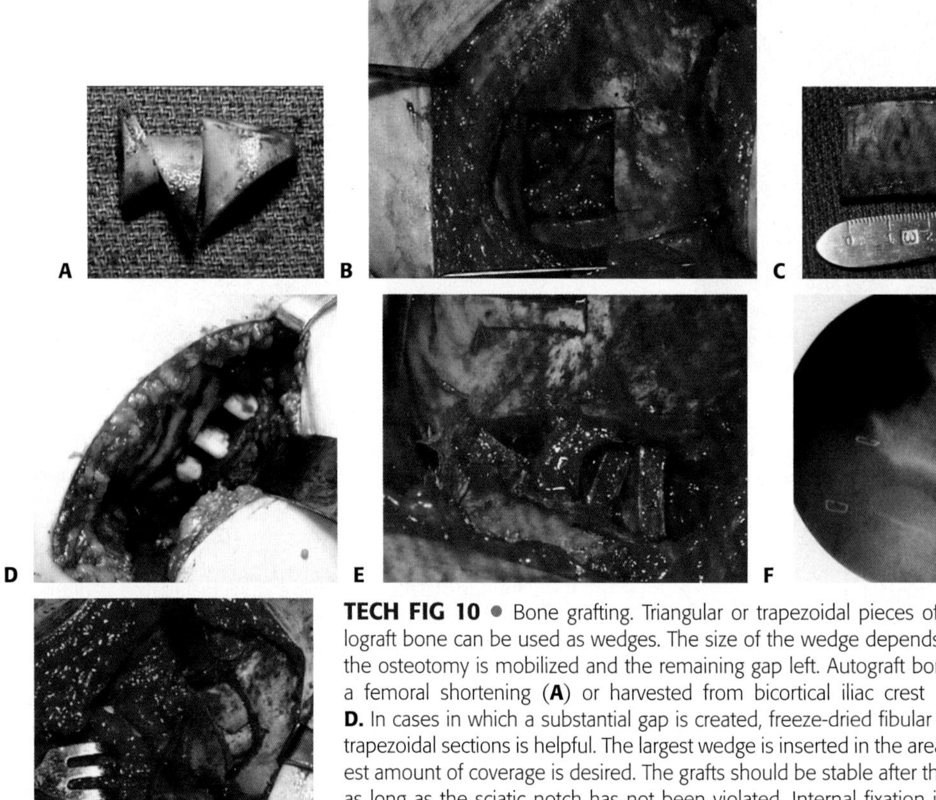

**TECH FIG 10** • Bone grafting. Triangular or trapezoidal pieces of autograft or allograft bone can be used as wedges. The size of the wedge depends on the amount the osteotomy is mobilized and the remaining gap left. Autograft bone wedges from a femoral shortening (**A**) or harvested from bicortical iliac crest (**B,C**) are used. **D.** In cases in which a substantial gap is created, freeze-dried fibular allograft cut into trapezoidal sections is helpful. The largest wedge is inserted in the area where the largest amount of coverage is desired. The grafts should be stable after they are impacted as long as the sciatic notch has not been violated. Internal fixation is not necessary. **E–G.** Examples of other grafts. **E.** Right hip with head at top showing three stable trapezoidal bicortical iliac crest grafts. **F.** Corresponding intraoperative fluoroscopic image of the grafts. **G.** Use of femoral autograft.

## PEARLS AND PITFALLS

| | |
|---|---|
| **Inadequate exposure of sciatic notch** | ▪ For the Dega, if the sciatic notch is not exposed, a Hohmann retractor not inserted in the notch, and the osteotomy is not stopped at least 1 cm short of the notch, disruption can occur resulting in instability at the graft site and inability to reshape the acetabulum. |
| **Need lateral coverage** | ▪ For the Dega, the osteotomy should be more of an oblique osteotomy starting higher on the ilium and the length of the inner wall cut should be much less than the length of the outer cut. This allows the osteotomy to rotate around a more medial fulcrum, giving more lateral coverage. |
| **Need anterior coverage** | ▪ For the Pemberton, the inner and outer wall cuts should be on the same level and the two cuts should be about the same length. For the Dega osteotomy, the inner cut might be slightly shorter (no less than 75% of the length of the outer cut). These considerations allow either osteotomy to rotate around a more posterior fulcrum, giving more anterior coverage. |
| **Graft loosening** | ▪ A gouge can be used to make a trough for the graft.<br>▪ Pemberton: The stability of the graft is tested with a Kocher clamp. If it is unstable, then the osteotomy is secured with a temporary Kirschner wire. The Kirschner wire must remain extra-articular.<br>▪ Dega: The largest graft is placed in the area that needs the most coverage. The outer cortex of the graft should be buried below the outer cortex of the ilium. |
| **Entry into the acetabulum** | ▪ Without careful fluoroscopic guidance, the osteotome can be directed into the acetabular cartilage, causing significant damage. |
| **Excessive anterior coverage** | ▪ In a patient with prolonged subluxation or significant retroversion, the anterior coverage may subsequently leave the posterior acetabulum more unstable. |

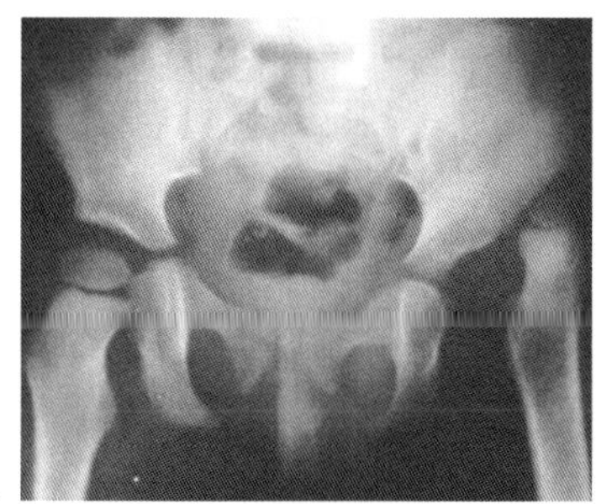
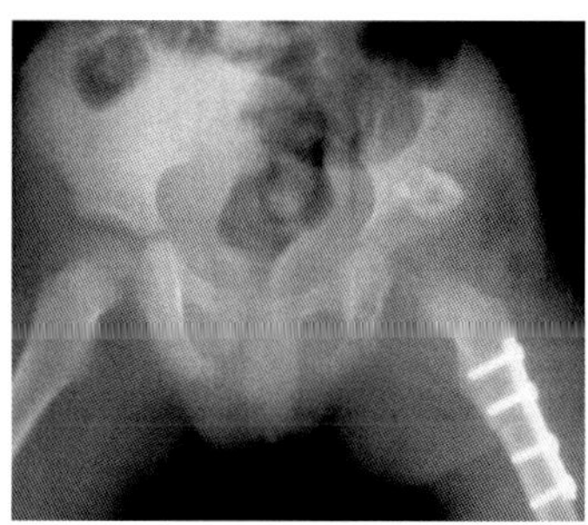
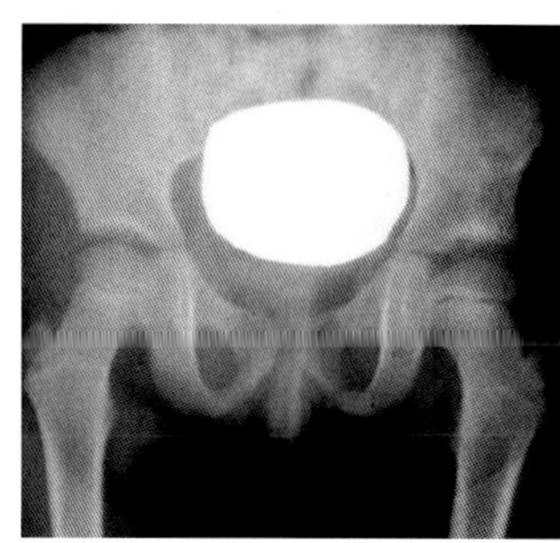

**FIG 5** ● Example of Dega osteotomy done in conjunction with anterior open reduction and femoral shortening in a toddler. **A.** Preoperative radiograph showing complete dislocation. **B.** Immediate postoperative radiograph following open reduction, femoral shortening, and Dega pelvic osteotomy. **C.** Three-year follow-up showing very satisfactory coverage.

## POSTOPERATIVE CARE

- Patients are almost exclusively treated with a hip spica cast for 6 to 12 weeks. If this is a staged procedure, the patient should be left in half of the spica cast while the second procedure is being done.
- Radiographs are obtained to make sure graft displacement has not occurred.
- Once good radiographic healing has been demonstrated, progressive weight bearing over 4 weeks can be started.
- Children are followed until maturity to detect avascular necrosis and ensure adequate acetabular coverage.
- Physical therapy is typically not needed to regain mobility after immobilization.

## OUTCOMES

- The Pemberton osteotomy provides excellent long-term acetabular correction in children, particularly those younger than age 4 years.[3,7,8,12,13]
  - The osteotomy has also been effective in patients with neuromuscular dysplasia.[10]
- The Dega osteotomy has been successfully used in the treatment of developmental dysplasia of the hip and neuromuscular dysplasia (**FIG 5**).
  - Several studies have found excellent results in younger children (younger than age 6 years), with results in older children less reliable.[4,9]

## COMPLICATIONS

- Stiffness
- Subluxation or dislocation
- Late recurrence of dysplasia either femoral or acetabular
- Closure of triradiate cartilage
- Chondrolysis
- Avascular necrosis of the femoral head

## REFERENCES


1. Dega W. Osteotomis trans-iliakalna w leczeniu wrodzonej dysplazji biodra. Chir Narzadow Ruchu Ortho Pol 1974;39:601–613.
2. Dega W, Krol J, Polakowski L. Surgical treatment of congenital dislocation of the hip in children; a one-stage procedure. J Bone Joint Surg Am 1959;41-A(5):920–934.
3. Faciszewski T, Kiefer GN, Coleman SS. Pemberton osteotomy for residual acetabular dysplasia in children who have congenital dislocation of the hip. J Bone Joint Surg Am 1993;75(5):643–649.
4. Grudziak JS, Ward WT. Dega osteotomy for the treatment of congenital dysplasia of the hip. J Bone Joint Surg Am 2001;83-A(6): 845–854.
5. Kessler JI, Stevens PM, Smith JT, et al. Use of allografts in Pemberton osteotomies. J Pediatr Orthop 2001;21:468–473.
6. Ozgur AF, Aksoy MC, Kandemir U, et al. Does Dega osteotomy increase acetabular volume in developmental dysplasia of the hip? J Pediatr Orthop B 2006;15:83–86.
7. Pemberton PA. Pericapsular osteotomy of the ilium for the treatment of congenital subluxation and dislocation of the hip. J Bone Joint Surg Am 1965;47:65–86.
8. Pemberton PA. Pericapsular osteotomy of the ilium for the treatment of congenitally dislocated hip. Clin Orthop Relat Res 1974;(98):41–54.
9. Reichel H, Hein W. Dega acetabuloplasty combined with intertrochanteric osteotomies. Clin Orthop Relat Res 1996;(323): 234–242.
10. Shea KG, Coleman SS, Carroll K, et al. Pemberton pericapsular osteotomy to treat a dysplastic hip in cerebral palsy. J Bone Joint Surg Am 1997;79(9):1342–1351.
11. Slomczykowski M, Mackenzie WG, Stern G, et al. Acetabular volume. J Pediatr Orthop 1998;18:657–661.
12. Vedantam R, Capelli AM, Schoenecker PL. Pemberton osteotomy for the treatment of developmental dysplasia of the hip in older children. J Pediatr Orthop 1998;18:254–258.
13. Wada A, Fujii T, Takamura K, et al. Pemberton osteotomy for developmental dysplasia of the hip in older children. J Pediatr Orthop 2003;23:508–513.

# 105 CHAPTER Labral Support (Shelf) Procedure for Perthes Disease

J. Richard Bowen

## DEFINITION

- The labral support (shelf) procedure has been used in patients with Legg-Calvé-Perthes disease (or Perthes disease) in Waldenström stages of necrosis or fragmentation in which the femoral head shows deformity or is at risk for deformity[6,12] (**FIG 1**).
- The concept of the labral support (shelf) procedure in patients with Perthes disease includes the following steps[6,12]:
  - Eliminating hinge subluxation and improving femoral head coverage by reducing the necrotic femoral epiphysis into the acetabulum (containment therapy)
    - Maintaining containment of the necrotic femoral epiphysis in the acetabulum during bony maturation of the labral support shelf—(usually, maturation is acceptable after 6 weeks of casting and an additional month of daytime crutch walking and nighttime abduction bracing)
    - Long-term containment is necessary until reossification of the lateral aspect of the femoral epiphysis. A mature labral support (shelf) will usually maintain long-term containment; however, any loss of containment necessitates its restoration.

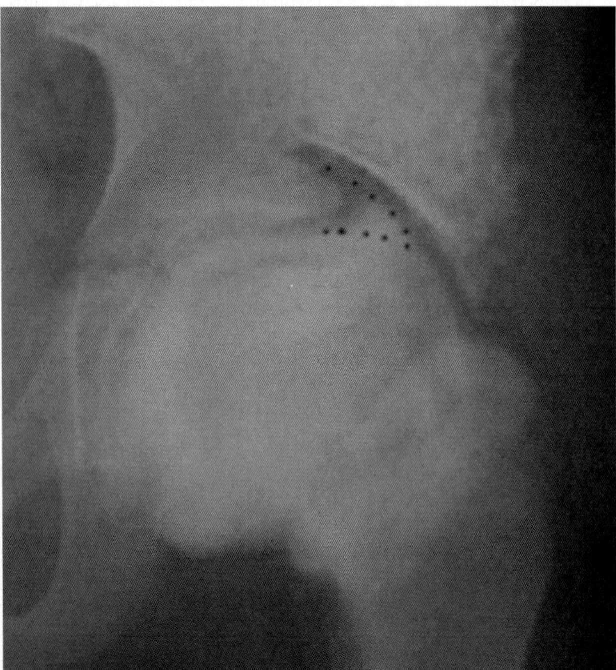

**FIG 1** • Anteroposterior (AP) radiograph of an arthrogram demonstrates a labral support (shelf) in a patient with Perthes disease. The shelf supports the labrum and enlarges the acetabulum to prevent subluxation of the femoral epiphysis.

  - Supporting the labrum and preventing deformity of the acetabulum (femoroacetabular impingement)
  - Preparing for the (labral support) shelf to reabsorb after reossification of the femoral head
  - Stimulating overgrowth of the acetabulum and remodeling of the femoral head
- The labral support (shelf ) procedure has not been effective as a reconstructive procedure to restore sphericity of a deformed femoral head in the Waldenström stages of reossification and remodeling.[12]

## ANATOMY

- The posterior branch lateral femoral cutaneous nerve
  - The lateral femoral cutaneous nerve arises from divisions of the second and third lumbar nerves and courses the lateral border of the psoas muscle, crosses the iliacus muscle obliquely, passes under the inguinal ligament, and divides into an anterior and posterior branch.
  - The posterior branch traverses beneath the sartorius muscle and exits the fascia lata about 1 to 2 cm below the anterior superior iliac spine.
  - The nerve supplies sensation to the skin anterolaterally from the level of the greater trochanter to the middle thigh.
  - The medial aspect of the bikini skin incision used in the labral support (shelf) procedure is very near the posterior branch of the lateral femoral cutaneous, which requires protection.
- The labrum is located at the lateral rim of the acetabulum and has acetabular cartilage medially and fibrocartilage and fibrous tissue laterally.
  - The labrum growth plate contributes depth to the acetabulum and must not be damaged while performing the labral support (shelf).
  - In the adult, the average width of the acetabular labrum is 5.3 mm (standard deviation 2.6 mm).
  - The labrum is wider superiorly and anteriorly than posteriorly.
  - The average surface area of the acetabulum without the labrum is 28.8 $cm^2$ and with the labrum is 36.8 $cm^2$.

## PATHOGENESIS

- Perthes disease is a condition of the immature hip caused by necrosis of the epiphysis and the growth plate of the proximal capital area of the femur.
  - The necrotic tissue is gradually resorbed and replaced by new bone.
  - During the process, the epiphysis may become deformed and the growth of the proximal femur retarded.
- Typically, the age at onset of symptoms is between 4 and 8 years but may occur in children from 2 years to maturity.

- There is a male predominance of 4:1, and the condition occurs bilaterally in up to 17% of cases.
- Factors with the greatest prognostic significance in Perthes disease are the following:
  - Age at onset of the disease (younger than 6 years of age at onset have much better outcomes than at older ages and onset after 11 years of age have the poorest outcomes)[27]
  - Degree of necrosis of the capital epiphysis (poorer outcomes occur with total or near-total necrosis of the femoral epiphysis)[3,4]
  - Premature capital physeal growth plate closure[1,2]
  - Persistent stiffness of the hip, with deformity of the femoral head (impingement)
- At maturity, the hip may be normal or may have one of four patterns of deformity: coxa magna, coxa breva, coxa irregularis (impingement), and osteochondritis dissecans.
- In adulthood, patients with irregular (incongruent) hips can develop impingement with progressive degenerative joint disease.
  - About 50% of all patients with Perthes disease have severe degenerative arthritis by the sixth and seventh decades of life.[15–17,23]

## NATURAL HISTORY

- Waldenström[25,26] described four sequential stages of Perthes disease in childhood (later modified to the following): necrosis, fragmentation (resorption), reossification, and remodeling.
- The stage of necrosis begins with an infarction of the capital femoral epiphysis and lasts about 6 months.
  - After the infarction, the child is usually asymptomatic, but a subchondral fracture subsequently develops in the necrotic bone and the hip becomes irritable[22] (**FIG 2**).
  - A mild effusion develops and the femoral heal begins to lateralize in the acetabulum.
  - The hip becomes painful and adduction–flexion–external rotation contractures develop.
- The first radiographic sign of removal of necrotic bone begins the fragmentation stage (resorption).
  - Gradually, revascularization of the epiphysis begins, usually at the anterolateral area of the epiphysis.

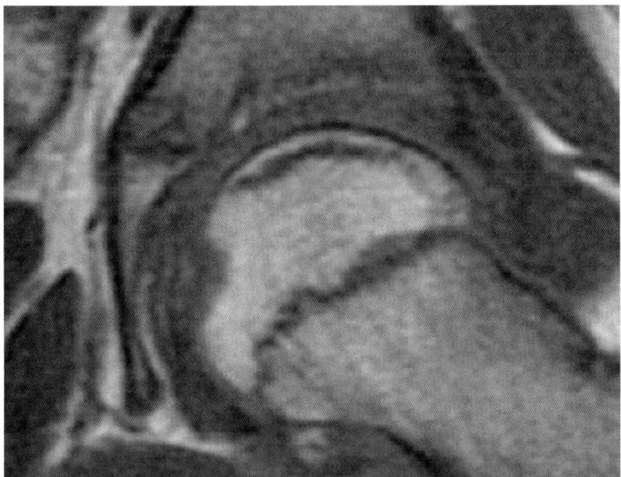

**FIG 2** • Computed tomography of the hip of a patient with Perthes disease showing necrotic bone in the epiphysis and a subchondral fracture.

**Table 1 Lateral Pillar Classification**

| Group | Loss of Height of the Lateral Column of the Femoral Epiphysis | Prognosis |
|---|---|---|
| A | None | Favorable |
| B | ≤50% of the original height | Intermediate |
| C | >50% | Poor |

From Herring JA, Neustadt JB, Williams JJ, et al. The lateral pillar classification of Legg-Calve-Perthes disease. J Pediatr Orthop 1992;12:143–150; Herring JA, Kim HT, Browne R. Legg-Calve-Perthes' disease. Part I: classification of radiographs with use of the modified lateral pillar and Stulberg classifications. J Bone Joint Surg Am 2004;86-A(10):2103–2120.

  - Over the ensuing months, the necrotic bone is removed, and the epiphysis may begin to deform, subluxate, and impinge on the margin of the acetabulum (hinged subluxation).
  - During the fragmentation stage, the height of the lateral pillar of the femoral epiphysis correlates with outcome and predicts the chance of developing arthritis in adulthood (Table 1).[10]
- The first radiographic signs of new bone formation indicate the reossification stage.
  - About 12 to 14 months after the initial infarction, new bone begins forming in the epiphysis, usually at the anterolateral margin.
  - Once the anterolateral column of the epiphysis has reossified, further epiphyseal deformity does not typically occur.[24]
  - Reossification continues until the entire epiphysis is healed, which may take up to about 4 years.
- The remodeling stage extends from the end of reossification until skeletal maturity.
  - The femoral epiphysis may improve in sphericity with continued growth.
  - Premature closure of the physis may cause limb shortening or deformity of the femoral neck.
- Common deformities of the hip following Perthes disease include coxa magna, coxa breva (premature physeal closure), coxa irregularis (asphericity and incongruence of the hip with acetabular–femoral impingement), and osteochondral loose bodies.[8,27]
- Stulberg et al[23] classified hips into five groups that predict development of arthritis in adulthood (Table 2).

**Table 2 Stulberg Classification of Hips in Perthes Disease**

| Group | Description | Prognosis |
|---|---|---|
| I | Normal | Excellent |
| II | Loss of height in the femoral neck and the femoral epiphysis remains spherical | Excellent |
| III | Elliptical femoral epiphysis | Arthritis in late adulthood |
| IV | Femoral head flattening and a congruent acetabulum | Early arthritis |
| V | Flattened femoral head and an incongruent acetabulum | Early arthritis |

From Stulberg SD, Cooperman DR, Wallensten R. The natural history of Legg-Calve-Perthes disease. J Bone Joint Surg Am 1981;63(7):1095–1108.

## PATIENT HISTORY AND PHYSICAL FINDINGS

- Perthes disease may present in children as an acute or chronic ache, which is commonly felt in the area of the hip, thigh, or knee. There is often an associated limp and hip stiffness.
- The ache is mild and usually presents immediately after getting up in the morning and after extended exercise, but it does not prevent walking.
- An antalgic limp is observed in the first few weeks of the disease, and then the gait may become a stiff pattern with flexion and adduction hip contractures.
- The flexion–adduction hip contracture results in an apparent limb shortening, with dipping of the pelvis and a short stride length during ambulation.
- Muscle atrophy is often observed at the buttock, thigh, and knee.
- Additional clinical signs that may be seen include a positive Thomas test (hip flexion contracture) and a positive logroll test (loss of internal rotation of the hip).
- Growth in height is decreased during the early stages but returns to normal after healing.

## IMAGING AND OTHER DIAGNOSTIC STUDIES

- The diagnosis is typically confirmed by anteroposterior and frog-leg lateral radiographs.
- Early in the disease (Waldenström stage of necrosis), radiographs show the following:
  - Increased inferomedial joint space
  - Lateral displacement of the femoral head[19]
  - Subchondral fracture[22]
  - Increased epiphyseal density
  - A small proximal epiphysis of the femur
- During the Waldenström stage of resorption (fragmentation), there is a gradual removal of the sclerotic necrotic bone and the femoral epiphysis may deform.
  - As healing progresses with reossification, the epiphysis returns to a normal density and the femoral neck widens.
  - The proximal femoral physis may close prematurely.[2]
- If the radiograph is not diagnostic, a bone scan or magnetic resonance imaging usually confirms the bone necrosis.
  - The bone scan shows a cold area in the femoral epiphysis in the early stage of necrosis.
    - With early revascularization (fragmentation stage of Waldenström), the scan will show the vascular ingrowth before radiographs.
  - Magnetic resonance imaging clearly demonstrates the necrotic epiphysis in the early stage of the disease; however, marrow edema should not be confused with the area of necrosis.
    - In the early stage, synovitis is observed, collapse and deformity of the cartilage of the epiphysis is usually clearly visible, and the degree of hinged subluxation (impingement) can be determined (**FIG 3**).[18]
  - In the fragmentation and reossification phases, vascular ingrowth is clearly visible.
- Computed tomography shows bone well and is most helpful to evaluate hip incongruity during the late stages of remodeling and during young adulthood.
- Skeletal hand bone age is decreased during the first year of the disease.

## DIFFERENTIAL DIAGNOSIS

- Toxic synovitis (irritable hip syndrome)
- Infection, such as Lyme disease or tuberculosis

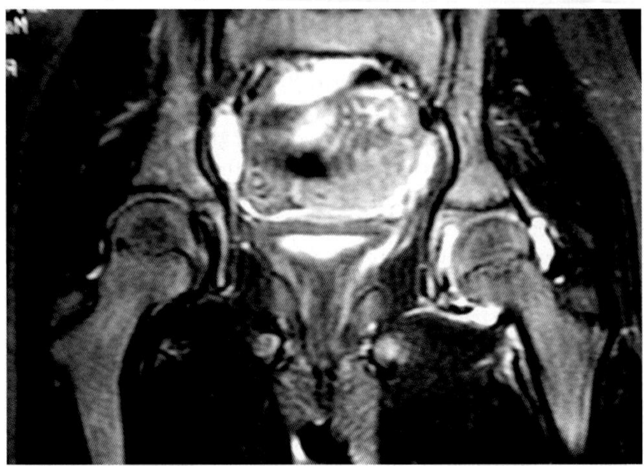

**FIG 3** • Magnetic resonance image of the hip of a patient with Perthes disease showing lateral subluxation, synovitis, and acetabular–femoral impingement (hinged subluxation).

- Avascular necrosis of known etiology such as sickle cell disease, hemoglobinopathies, Gaucher disease, trauma, and steroid bone necrosis
- Arthritis, such as rheumatic fever
- Multiple epiphyseal dysplasia
- Tumors, such as chondroblastoma, leukemia, and lymphoma
- Slipped femoral epiphysis (preslip stage)

## NONOPERATIVE MANAGEMENT

- Children younger than 6 years of age without severe collapse of the femoral epiphysis have a good prognosis and do not require operative treatment.[1]
  - Their pain can be treated with nonnarcotic analgesic medications and protected weight bearing.
  - Hip stiffness can be managed with physical therapy that emphasizes hip abduction, internal rotation, and extension and bracing.
- Children with necrosis involving less than 50% of the femoral epiphysis often have a good prognosis and operative treatment is often not necessary.
  - Children older than 11 years of age may be an exception in that a femoral epiphyseal deformity may develop (segmental collapse) even with less than 50% involvement.[9,21,27]

## SURGICAL MANAGEMENT

- Indications are controversial, but guidelines include the following:
  - Necrosis of over 50% of the proximal capital femoral epiphysis
  - Age 6 to 11 years: Younger children often heal well without operations, whereas adolescents poorly remodel the femoral deformity.
  - Waldenström stages of necrosis or fragmentation. Ideally, the operation should be performed before substantial deformity occurs to the capital femoral epiphysis.
  - Mild subluxation of the hip with femoroacetabular impingement
- Other possible indications
  - Children older than 11 years of age with mild femoral epiphyseal collapse: These older children do not have adequate remaining growth to remodel the femoral epiphysis.

- Children younger than 6 years of age with marked collapse of the femoral epiphysis: Typically, children younger than 6 years of age heal well without treatment, but in severe cases, treatment may be indicated.
- Patients with collapse of the epiphysis and hinged impingement: This operation may allow remodeling, but the outcome is less predictable.
- Contraindications
  - Subluxation that cannot be reduced into the acetabulum
  - Most children younger than 6 years of age (these patients heal well without treatment)
  - Necrosis less than 50% of the proximal capital femoral epiphysis (these cases typically heal well without treatment)
  - Children who are too old to achieve acetabular overgrowth: Children older than 11 years of age may get less benefit.

## Positioning

- The patient is placed in the supine position with the involved hip elevated by a longitudinal roll under the shoulder and back.
- The roll should not extend down to the hip area.
- The entire leg and hip is prepared and draped sterile to the anterior midline, to the posterior midline, and to the inferior rib line superiorly.

## Approach

- The approach for the labral support procedure is between the tensor fascia lata muscle and the sartorius and rectus femoris muscles.
- The dissection continues at the level of the anterior inferior iliac spine, beneath the origin of the gluteus minimus muscle (inferior gluteal line of ilium).
- The triangular interval is developed: the iliac wing medially, the hip capsule inferiorly, and the gluteus minimus laterally.
- With this approach, the origins of the abductor muscles are not elevated from the iliac wing, which we believe preserves the strength of hip abduction.
- The reflected tendon of the rectus muscle is retracted laterally and then used to secure the bone graft of the labral support shelf.[20]

TECHNIQUES

## Arthrography

- Arthrography is performed to verify reduction of the subluxation and femoroacetabular impingement.
- With the arthrographic dye in the hip joint, the degree of femoral epiphyseal deformity and subluxation is observed with the image intensifier.
- The leg is then abducted and the area of hinge abduction is observed.
  - In many cases, the deformed femoral head will press against the lateral margin of the labrum and block the reduction of the femoral head into the acetabulum (**TECH FIG 1A–C**).
- The arthrographic dye will pool in the medial–inferior joint, and with additional attempted abduction of the leg, the lateral margin of the labrum will deform upward.
  - In these cases, an adductor muscle tenotomy is then performed through a medial adductor incision.
- Afterward, the leg is again abducted to determine if the hinged abduction has been corrected (ie, reduction of the weight-bearing surface of the femoral epiphysis within the acetabulum).
- The hip is considered to be reduced if the deformed part of the femoral head (weight-bearing area) is under the lateral margin of the acetabulum (contained within the acetabulum), the medial dye pool is reduced, and the lateral margin of the labrum is not deformed.

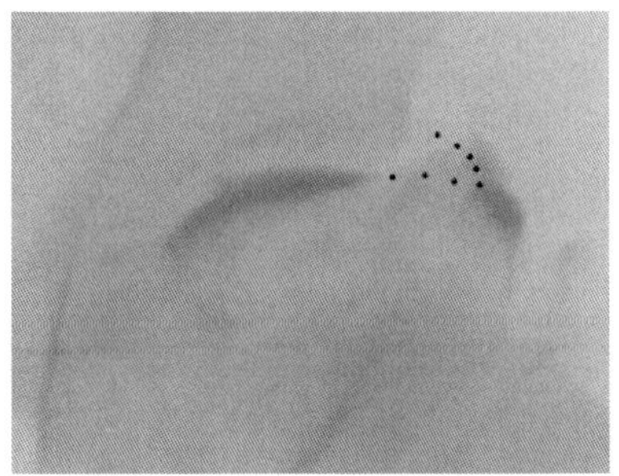

A

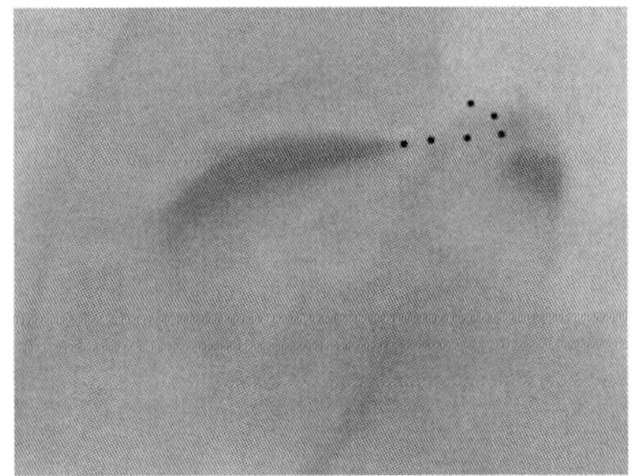

B

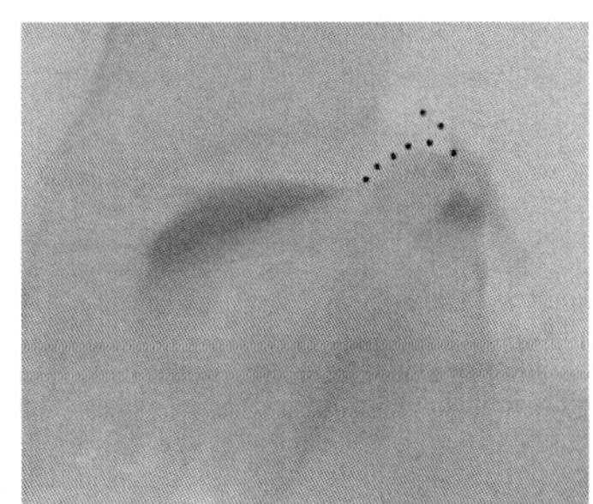

C

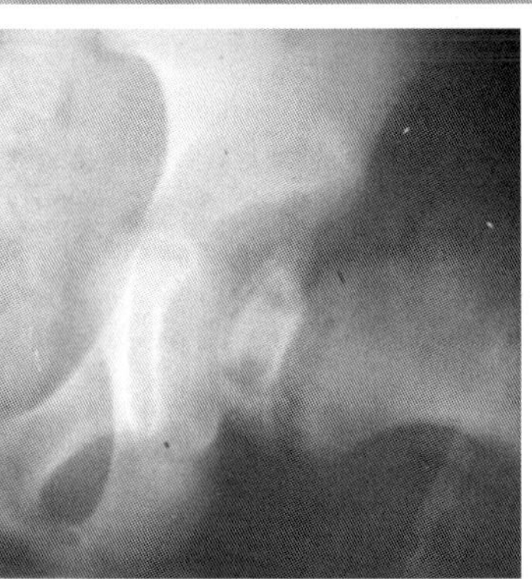

D

**TECH FIG 1** ● **A–C.** Arthrograms of the hip of a patient with Perthes disease in which the leg is progressively abducted. The abnormal femoral head deforms the labrum with progressive abduction of the leg. **D.** AP radiograph of the hip of a patient with Perthes disease in which the femoral epiphysis is contained within the acetabulum as the leg is placed in abduction.

- If the hip reduces (**TECH FIG 1D**), proceed with the shelf procedure as described in the following section.
- If the reduction is incomplete, a capsulotomy of the inferior aspect of the hip capsule can be performed through the same incision as used for the adductor muscle tenotomy. Then, the hip can again be tested to determine reduction.
- If hip reduction cannot be obtained, it is recommended that the procedure be terminated and, postoperatively, the leg be placed in skin traction or a bilateral broomstick cast until a gradual hip reduction can be obtained.
  - This is achieved by the patient's legs being progressively abducted in the ensuing postoperative days until complete reduction is accomplished.
  - The patient then returns to the operating room for continuation of the labral support shelf procedure.

## Incision and Superficial Dissection

- The incision starts at a point 1 cm inferior to the anterior superior iliac crest and extends laterally along the skin lines of Langer for about 3 cm (**TECH FIG 2**).
- The dissection continues with a Cobb periosteal elevator between the tensor fascia lata muscle and the sartorius and rectus femoris muscles.
  - The superior origins of the abductor muscles are not elevated from the outer wall of the iliac crest. Maintaining the abductor muscles attached to the outer wall of the iliac wing improves postoperative hip abduction power.
- With the periosteal elevator, a subperiosteal plane along the outer iliac wing about 3 cm wide is then developed beneath the gluteus medius and minimus muscles just above the hip. The image intensifier is useful to direct the periosteal elevator at a level of about 1 cm above the lateral margin of the acetabulum.

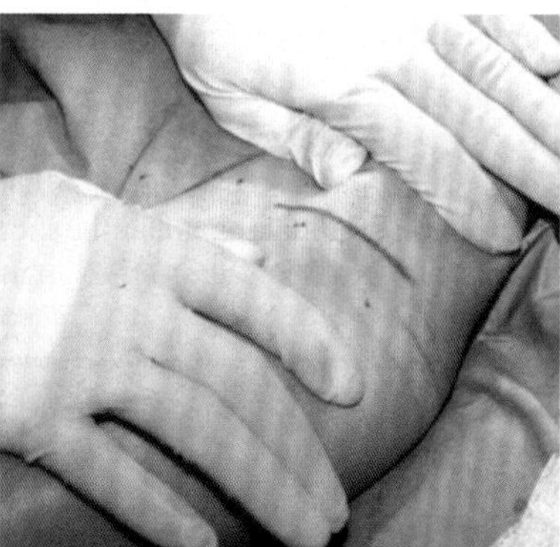

**TECH FIG 2** • The bikini skin incision.

## Deep Dissection

- An arthroscope is helpful for visualization during the remainder of the procedure.
- The subperiosteal plane is developed further along the outer iliac wing over the hip capsule from the anterior inferior iliac spine toward the sciatic notch.
  - Caution is taken not to injure the labral growth cartilage of the acetabular margin.
- The tendon of the reflected head of the rectus femoris, which is adherent to the hip capsule, is retracted laterally and preserved to be used later to support the bony shelf.
- The capsule is exposed with a periosteal elevator: anteriorly to the level of the anterior iliac spine, posteriorly to the sciatic notch, and laterally about 2 cm.
  - While exposing the capsule, do not injure the lateral growth plate of the acetabulum. (The capsule may be thickened, but it is never thinned.)

## Trough Creation and Graft Collection

- The level for the buttress shelf along the ilium is identified as about 3 mm above the labral growth plate of the acetabular rim. This corresponds to the superomedial margin of the hip capsule insertion into the ilium, a position that is verified with fluoroscopy by a metal marker (**TECH FIG 3A**).
- A trough is then developed at this level, as described by Staheli,[20] by making a series of 1-cm deep holes at the edge of the acetabulum using a 5/32-inch drill (**TECH FIG 3B**).
  - The holes should be directed upwardly about 20 degrees and extended posteriorly and anteriorly sufficiently to provide the needed coverage.
  - Care must be taken not to damage the cartilaginous margin of the acetabular growth plate.
- An osteotome, narrow rongeur, or power burr (or a combination) is used to connect the holes to make a trough that is about 1 cm deep and angled cephalad about 15 degrees. The floor of the trough is the subchondral bone of the acetabulum and should be level with the capsule (**TECH FIG 3C**).
- Autogenous bone graft is obtained from the previously exposed outer wall of the iliac wing, which is just superior to the trough and beneath the gluteus medius muscle.
  - The graft is typically about 1 × 1 × 1.5 cm and is cut into three longitudinal strips.

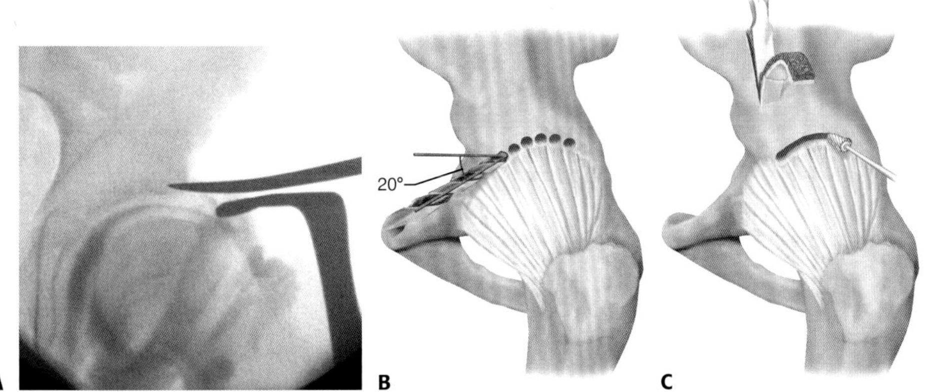


**TECH FIG 3** • **A.** Intraoperative anteroposterior (AP) fluoroscopy image with the level of the labral support (shelf) identified with a medal marker. The proper level is just above the cartilaginous labral growth area. **B.** To begin creation of the trough, a line of upwardly inclined, 1-cm deep holes is made where the rectus femoris tendon (now reflected) attaches to the acetabular margin. **C.** The holes are connected using a burr, osteotome, or narrow rongeur to create a slightly angled 1-cm deep trough. An osteotome is then used to collect strips of cancellous and corticocancellous bone for the outer wall of the iliac wing.

## Creation of the Shelf

- Several absorbable sutures (usually three) are placed through the outer fibers of the hip capsule to be used later to secure the pieces of bone graft to the capsule.
- The leg is then placed in about 45 degrees of abduction and the deformed femoral head is again reduced into the acetabulum (contained), and this position is verified by the image intensifier. Caution: The femoral head must be contained within the acetabulum with no hinged subluxation, no deformity of the lateral labrum, and no impingement.
- The leg is held in abduction of 45 degrees, flexion of 15 degrees, and neutral rotation through the remainder of the procedure (and as the spica cast is applied).
- Autogenous bone graft is placed over the capsule, with the strips of bone inserted medially in the trough and laterally under the reflected head of the rectus femoris tendon, and the sutures are tied around the strips of graft to hold them snugly to the capsule (**TECH FIG 4A**).
- The reflected head of the rectus femoris tendon is placed over the lateral aspect of the graft to add additional support.
- About 30 to 60 mL of donor allograft bone may be added above the labral support (shelf) to create a buttress for additional support (**TECH FIG 4B**).
- The graft will appear extensive when visualized by the image intensifier.
  - The purpose of the shelf is to support the labrum and prevent the hip from anterolateral subluxation during reossification of the lateral column of the femoral epiphysis.
  - Remember: The shelf is expected to resorb in about 3 years because it is not expected to be weight bearing but only to act as a buttress with support of the acetabular labrum.
- The leg is held in abduction (as described earlier) with the femoral head in the reduced position as the incision is closed in layers.
- The patient is placed in a one-and-one-half hip spica cast with the involved leg in abduction of 45 degrees, flexion of 15 degrees, and neutral rotation.

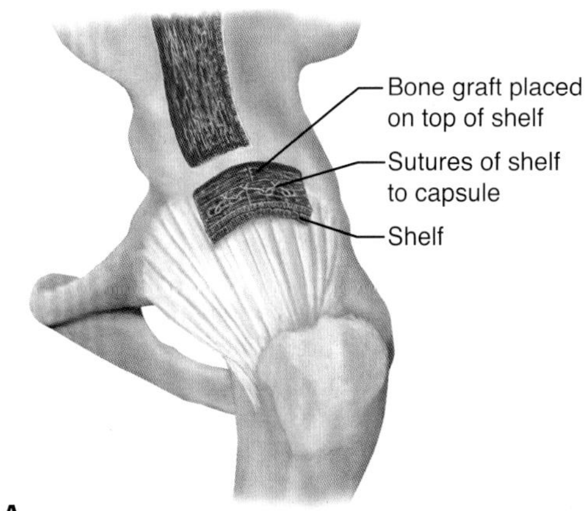


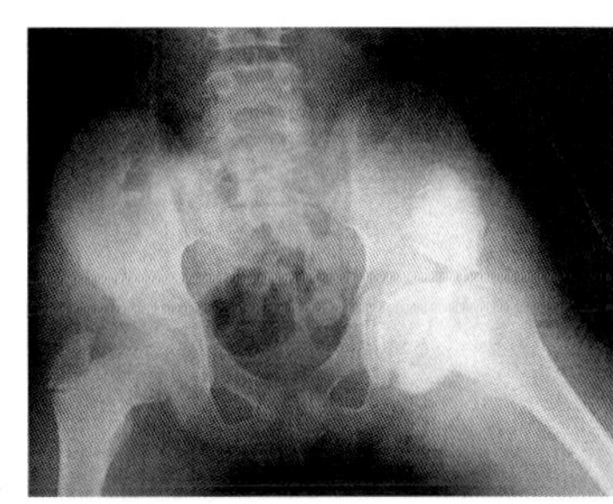


**TECH FIG 4** • **A.** Two layers of autogenous bone graft strips are placed over the capsule, one with the strips inserted lengthwise and the other with the pieces laid side by side widthwise. The strips of bone are inserted medially in the trough and laterally under the reflected head of the rectus femoris tendon. Strong, nonabsorbable sutures are used to anchor the graft into the capsule, and additional morselized bone graft is placed on top of the created shelf. **B.** Anteroposterior (AP) arthrogram of the hip of a patient with Perthes disease in whom the femoral epiphysis and labrum is supported by a labral support (shelf) procedure.

## PEARLS AND PITFALLS

| | |
|---|---|
| **Small procedure without internal fixation** | ■ An arthroscope is helpful to visualize the dissection and placement of the labral support (shelf). |
| **Walking in the cast** | ■ Children can walk in the cast as soon as the postoperative pain resolves. |
| **No permanent deformity** | ■ The procedure does not cause a permanent deformity of the femur or acetabulum, and there is no impingement from the graft because the labral shelf resorbs in about 3 years postoperatively. |
| **Containment of the hip** | ■ The femoral head must be contained within the acetabulum with no hinged subluxation, no deformity of the lateral labrum, and no impingement. |
| **Do not damage the labral growth plate of the acetabulum.** | ■ The buttress shelf is placed on the outer iliac wing above the labral growth plate of the acetabulum. The graft functions only as a buttress to prevent resubluxation of the femoral epiphysis until the lateral column reossifies. The graft is not expected to be weight bearing and is expected to resorb after about 3 years. |
| **Hip motion** | ■ Maintain good hip abduction after cast removal. |

## POSTOPERATIVE CARE

- The cast, subsequent abduction contracture, and an abduction hip pillow at night offer initial containment. Later, the labral support (shelf) acts as a buttress for the labrum to prevent resubluxation and hinging of the hip until the lateral column of femoral epiphysis reossifies.
- The cast is maintained for 6 weeks, and the child is allowed to walk in the cast as soon as postoperative pain resolves.
- When the cast is removed, the patient is allowed daytime walking with "toe-touch" crutch weight bearing and nighttime abduction bracing for an additional 4 weeks and then allowed full ambulation without support.
- An abduction contracture of the hip is expected to persist additionally for about 6 weeks after cast removal.
- During the month after cast removal, an abduction bracing is used at night.
- Exercises of the hip are encouraged to maintain flexion, extension, and abduction; adduction is not encouraged for at least 6 to 8 weeks after the cast is removed.
- Abduction exercises of the hip to maintain at least 45 degrees abduction are continued until reossification of the lateral column of the femoral head.
- Long-term containment is necessary until reossification of the lateral aspect of the femoral epiphysis. A mature labral support (shelf) procedure will usually maintain long-term containment; however, any loss of containment necessitates its restoration.

## OUTCOMES

- Domzalski et al[6] reported the results of 49 consecutive patients treated by the labral support (shelf) procedure for Perthes disease.
  - The procedure has a combined effect to prevent subluxation, to stimulate additional growth of the lateral rim of the acetabulum in a vertical dimension, and to provide temporary osseous containment until the shelf resorbs with time in a manner that is beneficial for preventing impingement of the femoral neck and greater trochanter on the shelf (**FIG 4**).
- Willett et al[28] reported the results of 20 children treated by a lateral shelf acetabuloplasty and recommended its use in children older than 8 years of age with Perthes disease of Catterall groups II, III, and IV.
- Van der Heyden and van Tongerloo[29] reported on 25 patients with Perthes disease who were treated by a shelf procedure and had good or excellent results.
- Kadhim et al[12] performed a meta-analysis of observational studies and concluded the shelf arthroplasty to be a satisfactory containment method during the early stages of necrosis and fragmentation but to be unsatisfactory for reconstruction during the stages of reossification and remodeling.
- Other authors have also reported encouraging results with similar labral support (shelf) procedures,[5,7,9,11,13,14,21,27] but to my knowledge, there has been no controlled, prospective, and randomized study comparing this procedure to other methods of treatment.

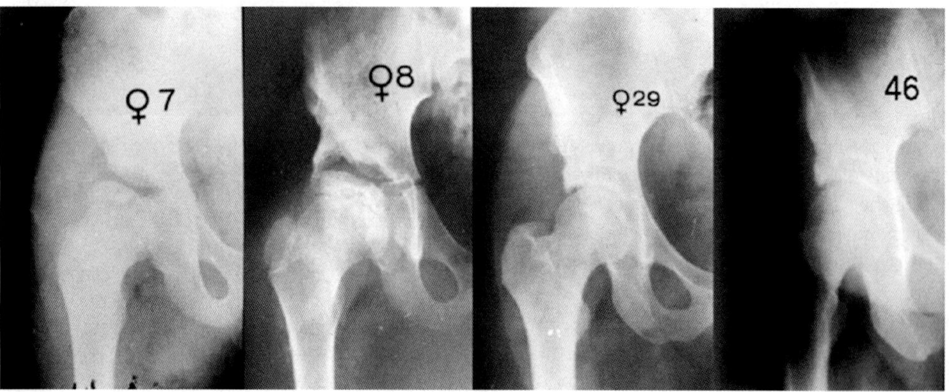


**FIG 4** ● Anteroposterior (AP) radiographs of the hip of a patient with Perthes disease in whom the deformed femoral head was treated by a labral support (shelf) procedure. There is remodeling of the femoral epiphysis, widening of the acetabulum, and resolution of the shelf.

## COMPLICATIONS

- Loss of containment for the necrotic femoral epiphysis before bony maturation of the labral shelf support (usually maturation is acceptable after 6 weeks of casting and an additional month of daytime crutch walking and nighttime abduction bracing)
- Infection
- Injury of the labral growth cartilage, which prevents growth stimulation of the acetabulum
- Displacement of the labral support (shelf) bone graft
- Improper placement of the labral support (shelf)
- Neurovascular injury
- Cast problems

## REFERENCES


1. Bowen JR, Foster BK, Wein BK, et al. Legg-Calve-Perthes disease in patients under six years of age. Orthop Trans 1981;5:446.
2. Bowen JR, Schreiber FC, Foster BK, et al. Premature femoral neck physeal closure in Perthes' disease. Clin Orthop Relat Res 1982;(171):24–29.
3. Catterall A. Adolescent hip pain after Perthes' disease. Clin Orthop Relat Res 1986;(209):65–69.
4. Catterall A. Legg-Calve-Perthes syndrome. Clin Orthop Relat Res 1981;(158):41–52.
5. Daly K, Bruce C, Catterall A. Lateral shelf acetabuloplasty in Perthes' disease. A review of the end growth. J Bone Joint Surg Br 1999; 81(3):380–384.
6. Domzalski ME, Glutting J, Bowen JR, et al. Lateral acetabular growth stimulation following a labral support procedure in Legg-Calve-Perthes disease. J Bone Joint Surg Am 2006;88(7):1458–1466.
7. Gill AB. Plastic construction of an acetabulum in congenital dislocation of the hip: the shelf operation. J Bone Joint Surg 1935;17:48–59.
8. Grzegorzewski A, Synder M, Koztowski P, et al. The role of the acetabulum in Perthes disease. J Pediatr Orthop Am 2006;26:316–321.
9. Herring JA, Kim HT, Browne R. Legg-Calve-Perthes' disease. Part I: classification of radiographs with use of the modified lateral pillar and Stulberg classifications. J Bone Joint Surg Am 2004;86-A(10): 2103–2120.
10. Herring JA, Neustadt JB, Williams JJ, et al. The lateral pillar classification of Legg-Calve-Perthes disease. J Pediatr Orthop 1992;12:143–150.
11. Heyman CH. Long-term results following a bone-shelf operation for congenital and some other dislocations of the hip in children. J Bone Joint Surg Am 1963;45:1113–1146.
12. Kadhim M, Holmes L, Bowen JR. The role of shelf arthroplasty in early and late stages of Perthes disease: a meta-analysis of observational studies. J Child Orthop 2012;6:379–390.
13. Kruse MRW, Guille JT, Bowen JR. Shelf arthroplasty in patients who have Legg-Calve-Perthes disease. J Bone Joint Surg Am 1991; 73(9):1338–1347.
14. Love BR, Stevens PM, Williams PF. A long-term review of shelf arthroplasty. J Bone Joint Surg Br 1980;62-B(3):321–325.
15. McAndrew MP, Weinstein SL. A long-term follow-up of Legg-Calve-Perthes disease. J Bone Joint Surg Am 1984;66(6):860–869.
16. Mose K. Methods of measuring in Legg-Calve-Perthes with special regard to the prognosis. Clin Orthop Relat Res 1980;(150):103–109.
17. Mose K, Hjorth J, Ulfeldt M, et al. Legg-Calve-Perthes disease. The late occurrence of coxarthrosis. Acta Orthop Scand Suppl 1977;169:1–39.
18. Quain S, Catterall A. Hinge abduction of the hip: diagnosis and treatment. J Bone Joint Surg Br 1986;68(1):61–64.
19. Richards BS, Coleman SS. Subluxation of the femoral head in coxa plana. J Bone Joint Surg Am 1987;69(9):1312–1318.
20. Staheli LT. Slotted acetabular augmentation. J Pediatr Orthop 1981;1: 321–327.
21. Salter RB. The present status of surgical treatment of Legg-Perthes Disease. J Bone Joint Surg Am 1984;66(6):961–966.
22. Salter RB, Thompson GH. Legg-Calve-Perthes disease. The prognostic significance of the subchondral fracture and a two-group classification of the femoral head involvement. J Bone Joint Surg Am 1984; 66(4):479–489.
23. Stulberg SD, Cooperman DR, Wallensten R. The natural history of Legg-Calve-Perthes disease. J Bone Joint Surg Am 1981;63(7): 1095–1108.
24. Thompson G, Westin GW. Legg-Calve-Perthes disease: results of discontinuing treatment in the early reossification stage. Clin Orthop Relat Res 1979;139:70–80.
25. Waldenström H. The first stage of coxa plana. Acta Orthop Scand 1934;5:1–34.
26. Waldenström H. The first stage of coxa plana. J Bone Joint Surg 1938;20: 559–566.
27. Wang L, Bowen JR, Puniak MA, et al. An evaluation of various methods of treatment for Legg-Calve-Perthes disease. Clin Orthop Relat Res 1995;(314):225–233.
28. Willett K, Hudson I, Cattarall A. Lateral shelf acetabuloplasty: an operation for older children with Perthes' disease. J Pediatr Orthop 1991;12:563–568.
29. van der Heyden AM, van Tongerloo RB. Shelf operation in Perthes disease. J Bone Joint Surg Br 1981;63B:282.

# Triple Innominate Osteotomy

Dennis R. Wenger, Maya E. Pring, and Vidyadhar V. Upasani

## DEFINITION

- Triple innominate osteotomy (TIO) is a surgical procedure that includes osteotomy of the ilium, ischium, and pubis, allowing rotation of the acetabulum around the femoral head (**FIG 1**). This greater freedom of rotation allows it to be used in more severe cases where the Salter innominate osteotomy would not provide enough rotation to cover the femoral head.
- Because the procedure does not damage the triradiate cartilage, it can be used in skeletally immature patients without the risk of disrupting acetabular growth. The volume of the acetabulum remains constant, but the weight-bearing surface is reoriented to improve femoral head coverage.
- TIO is most commonly used for correction of acetabular dysplasia. Dysplasia may be a primary disorder or result from incomplete treatment of developmental dysplasia of the hip (DDH).[5] It is also seen as a result of neuromuscular conditions such as cerebral palsy, myelomeningocele, Down syndrome, Charcot-Marie-Tooth syndrome, etc.
- TIO can also be used to improve coverage/containment of a malformed femoral head and for a combination of acetabular and femoral head deformities such as in patients with Legg-Calvé-Perthes disease[19] (Perthes disease), avascular necrosis (AVN), epiphyseal dysplasia, or an irregular femoral head resulting from a previous septic hip.
- The TIO has the advantage of maintaining hyaline cartilage contact between the femoral head and acetabulum.[17] This is in contrast to other procedures sometimes used to correct severe hip dysplasia/instability (shelf procedure, Chiari osteotomy) which must rely on fibrocartilage to maintain a joint surface.

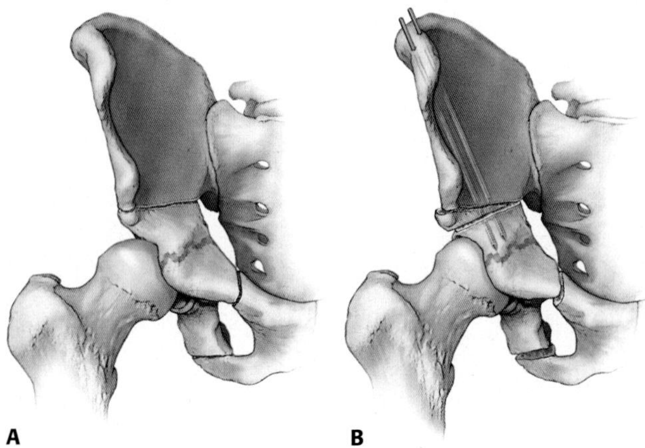


**FIG 1** • **A.** 3-D representation of the iliac, ischial and pubic osteotomies. **B.** TIO allows rotation of the entire acetabulum around the femoral head without damage to the triradiate cartilage in the skeletally immature child.

## ANATOMY

- The acetabulum is formed by the ilium, ischium, and pubis, which in the immature pelvis are joined by the triradiate growth cartilage. This complex, triflanged growth center allows the acetabulum to grow properly, providing a deep, stable hip joint.
- The femoral head should be covered by the roof of the acetabulum. The center–edge angle of Wiberg (angle between a line from the center of the femoral head to the lateral edge of the acetabular roof and a vertical line drawn through the center of the femoral head) should be greater than 25 degrees.[20]
- Lateral subluxation of the femoral head can be measured as the percent of the femoral head not covered by the acetabulum.
- The acetabulum should be concave with a transverse sourcil ("eyebrow"—French) above the femoral head. Patients with hip dysplasia frequently have a very flat acetabulum with an up-turned sourcil. This results in shear forces on the joint that leads to early degenerative joint disease.
- The normal hip joint has a spherical femoral head that is congruent with a well-formed acetabulum. Sphericity of the femoral head can be measured with Mose templates (concentric circles). Deformity in Perthes or AVN can be measured as a percentage of the femoral head (lateral pillar) that has collapsed when compared to the contralateral side.[7] Conditions that change femoral head sphericity lead to abnormal hip development and increased wear patterns within the joint.

## PATHOGENESIS

- Hip dysplasia: Many factors play a role in the etiology of hip dysplasia. The high concordance between twins and studies noting that babies with parents or siblings with dysplasia have a much higher DDH incidence than the general population confirm a genetic component. Mechanical factors also contribute to the risk for dysplasia. First babies and babies that are large have a higher risk thought to be secondary to inadequate space in the uterus during development. There also appears to be a hormonal component, as females and babies with increased joint laxity are at greater risk of hip dysplasia.
- Legg-Calvé-Perthes disease: The etiology of Perthes disease remains obscure and can be thought of as idiopathic AVN of the hip in childhood. Some have postulated a deficiency in protein C leading to a hypercoagulable state with thrombosis triggered by prothrombotic insults.[11]
- As most Perthes patients have a delayed bone age, some have suggested that Perthes may represent a form of epiphyseal

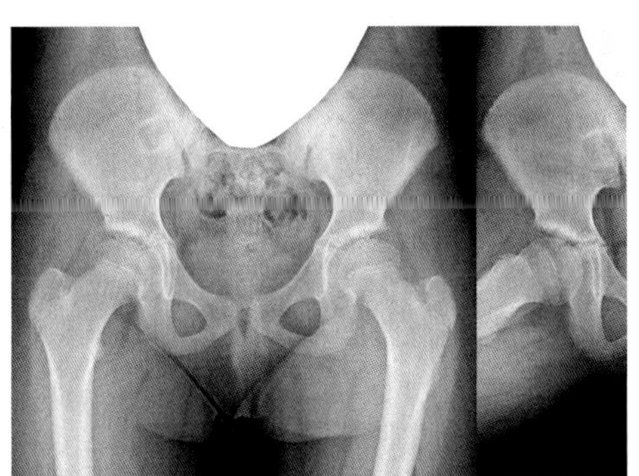

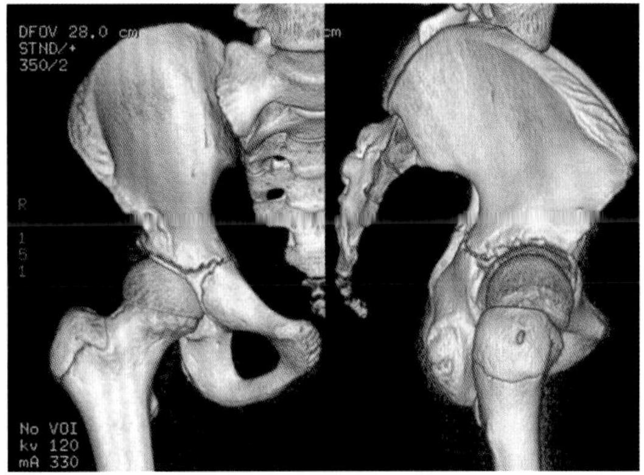


**FIG 2** • **A.** AP and frog view of the pelvis in a 10-year-old girl with bilateral hip dysplasia. She was most symptomatic on the right. **B.** AP and lateral image of 3-D CT study of the right hip.

dysplasia. Delayed skeletal maturation, is a routine finding in a typical Perthes case. The delay in maturation of the femoral head preossific nucleus may not adequately protect the vessels that ascend the femoral neck to the epiphysis, predisposing to AVN.

## NATURAL HISTORY

- Hip dysplasia
  - Untreated hip dysplasia is the leading cause of premature hip arthritis that results in early total hip replacement.
  - Abnormal sheer stresses on the hip lead to early osteoarthritis, and the more severe the dysplasia, the more likely the development of arthritis (**FIG 2**).
- Legg-Calvé-Perthes disease
  - The natural history for younger patients (younger than age 8 years at onset) and patients with milder disease (Herring A classification) is more benign with little long-term disability.
  - Children who are older at onset and who have more severe disease (Herring B or C classification) are more likely to develop femoral head deformity which predisposes to early osteoarthritis.

## PATIENT HISTORY AND PHYSICAL FINDINGS

- Hip dysplasia
  - Hip dysplasia is often asymptomatic in childhood and adolescence. Patients may have decreased abduction on examination or pain with internal rotation of the hip.
  - When symptoms are present, they are likely due to increased shear stresses, labral damage, and later to osteoarthritis. The pain is usually groin pain rather than lateral or trochanteric pain.
- Legg-Calvé-Perthes disease
  - Perthes may present as hip or knee pain. Early pain may be episodic.
  - Patients with severe disease may have subluxation and more severe pain. A Trendelenburg gait is often noticed.
  - Decreased abduction can be mild or severe. A marked loss of abduction with the hip in the fully extended position (pelvis rotates rather than hip abducting) suggests hinge abduction and is a bad prognostic sign.

## IMAGING AND OTHER DIAGNOSTIC STUDIES

- Plain radiographs: Anteroposterior (AP) and frog lateral views provide two orthogonal views of the femoral head. However, to get two views of the acetabulum, a false-profile x-ray should be taken in addition to the AP view (**FIG 3A**). Always image both hips (to allow comparison).
- We advise a surgeon performed arthrogram to evaluate the hip deformity and to assess for hinge abduction as well as the desired limb position following surgical correction (**FIG 3B**).
- Three-dimensional (3-D) computed tomography (CT) scans with reconstructions provide a better understanding of pathologic bony anatomy.[2]
- Magnetic resonance imaging (MRI) with arthrogram helps to evaluate the labrum and joint space (**FIG 3C**).

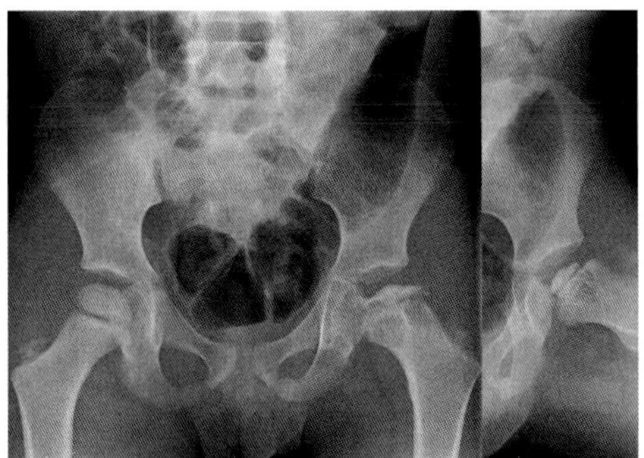

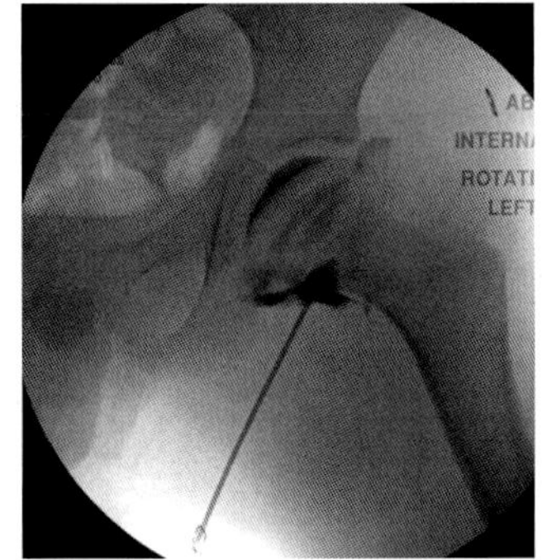

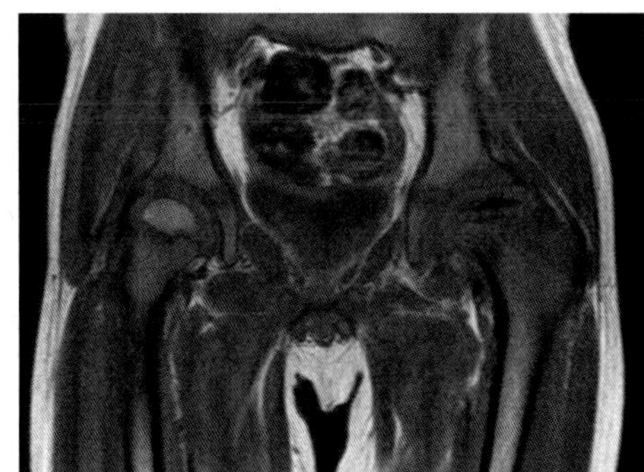

**FIG 3** • **A.** AP and frog view of a 7-year-old boy with severe left Legg-Calvé-Perthes disease with subluxation and lateral extrusion despite prior attempts to treat with conservative methods including Petrie casts. **B.** Dynamic arthrogram of left hip showing femoral head deformity. **C.** MRI study of pelvis showing marked femoral head extrusion of the left hip.

## DIFFERENTIAL DIAGNOSIS

- Hip dysplasia
  - DDH
  - Dysplasia secondary to neuromuscular disease (cerebral palsy, myelomeningocele, Charcot-Marie-Tooth disease, etc.)
  - Dysplasia, subluxation secondary to syndromes (Down syndrome)
- Legg-Calvé-Perthes disease
  - AVN secondary to Perthes disease
  - AVN secondary to steroid use, chemotherapy, metabolic disruption, infection, sickle cell disease
  - Epiphyseal dysplasia with poor femoral head coverage

## NONOPERATIVE MANAGEMENT

- Hip dysplasia
  - From infancy to childhood (up to 18 months of age), if the hip is located within a dysplastic acetabulum, a Pavlik harness or abduction orthosis can be worn to treat the dysplasia.[3]
  - From age 18 months to 5 years, abduction bracing has not been found to predictably improve dysplasia, although nighttime brace use is occasionally recommended. Most advise monitoring during this period with hope that the acetabular growth centers will mature and correct the dysplasia.[14]
  - Older children with hip dysplasia are typically asymptomatic until the hip begins to have degenerative changes or a labral tear. Anti-inflammatory medications and activity modification can be used to decrease pain, but these do not correct the underlying problem, and by masking symptoms may delay surgical correction.
- Legg-Calvé-Perthes disease
  - Children younger than 8 years and patients with hips classified as Herring A can be treated conservatively with predictable results. Conservative treatment includes activity modification and observation, abduction exercises, abduction bracing, and percutaneous adductor longus lengthening followed by Petrie casting (**FIG 4**) or bracing to maintain abduction.

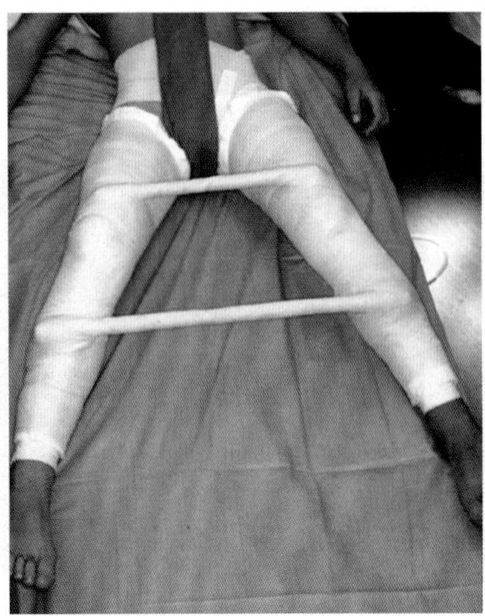

**FIG 4** • Petrie casts, which provide containment of the femoral head, are often used in patients with Perthes disease in preparation for TIO.

  - Older children and those with Herring B and C hips require prolonged Petrie casting or bracing (rarely practiced) or surgical containment.

## SURGICAL MANAGEMENT

- Hip dysplasia
  - Dysplasia before age 4 years is treated nonoperatively unless the hip is dislocated and requires open reduction or the dysplasia is very severe.
  - Patients aged 4 to 10 years can be treated with an acetabular redirecting osteotomy[16] or an osteotomy that bends through the triradiate cartilage.[12]
  - From the age of about 10 years until triradiate cartilage closure, a TIO is preferred for correction of dysplasia. Once the triradiate cartilage closes, TIO can still be performed but a periacetabular osteotomy may be preferred because the posterior column remains intact, providing greater stability and earlier weight bearing.[4]
- Legg-Calvé-Perthes disease
  - Children older than age 6 to 8 years or with more severe disease can be treated with a variety of surgical procedures aimed at containing the capital femoral epiphysis during the early fragmentation phase when the biologically plastic femoral head is at risk for subluxation, hinge abduction, and the development of permanent femoral head deformity. The simplest surgical treatment is adductor lengthening followed by Petrie casting or bracing. This can be used alone for very mild cases or in preparation for containment surgery.
  - Formal containment procedures include varus proximal femoral osteotomy designed to direct the capital femoral epiphysis into the acetabulum. A Salter innominate osteotomy can also be performed, but Rab[15] has clarified that the degree of acetabular rotation achieved with the Salter procedure is often not enough to cover the femoral head in more severe Perthes disease. A combined femoral and Salter procedure may be a better choice.
  - TIO, which rotates the entire acetabulum around the femoral head, allows containment in more severe cases[18] while avoiding the problems of femoral osteotomy (limp, limb shortening). A shelf (labral support) osteotomy or Chiari procedure may be a better choice for a severely deformed femoral head that cannot be congruently centered in the acetabulum.

### Preoperative Planning

- Hip dysplasia
  - Radiographs and a 3-D CT scan (if available) helps to better understand the nature and location of the acetabular deficiency.
    - Typical dysplasia patients have an anterolateral deficiency.
    - Children with neuromuscular disorders such as cerebral palsy, due to muscle imbalance around the hip joint and flexion contracture, often have a posterior deficiency.[8]
  - Once the amount and direction of dysplasia has been determined, acetabular rotation can be planned.
    - One should avoid overrotating the acetabulum, as this can cause anterolateral impingement.
    - Also, external rotation of the acetabulum should be avoided to prevent the creation of acetabular retroversion (which in itself can predispose to hip arthritis).

- Legg-Calvé-Perthes disease
  - A preoperative dynamic arthrogram provides information about how to best contain the femoral head. We perform an arthrogram and percutaneous adductor lengthening followed by Petrie casting (for 6 weeks) prior to definitive containment surgery.

**Positioning**

- The patient is positioned supine on a radiolucent table (**FIG 5**). A Foley catheter can be considered to minimize any risk for bladder injury with the pubic ramus cut.
- A sandbag bolster is placed under the trunk to tip the patient toward the opposite side giving better exposure of the hip laterally. Avoid placing the bolster directly behind the pelvis because it often distorts the image intensifier views.
- The leg is draped free, and the abdomen is prepped past the midline medially, to just below the nipple level superiorly, and around the buttock posteriorly. The ischial tuberosity must be kept in the surgical field.
- The C-arm and screen of the image intensifier are positioned to allow a clear view for the surgeon.

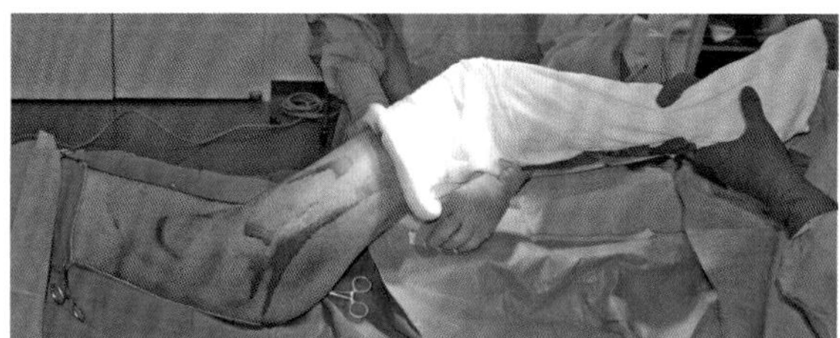

**FIG 5** • Patient position on operating table for TIO.

TECHNIQUES

## Exposure

- TIO (**TECH FIG 1A**) is generally performed through two incisions, one anterolateral and a second medial incision in the adductor (groin) area. However, three smaller incisions can be considered to allow a more precise exposure for each osteotomy cut, especially in larger patients.
- The first incision is below the iliac crest as for a Salter osteotomy (**TECH FIG 1B**). The second incision is distal to the groin crease, slightly below the superior pubic ramus, lateral to the adductor longus tendon origin, and medial to the femoral neurovascular bundle. The pubic osteotomy is performed through this medial incision with the ischial osteotomy also possible with posterior extension of the incision.

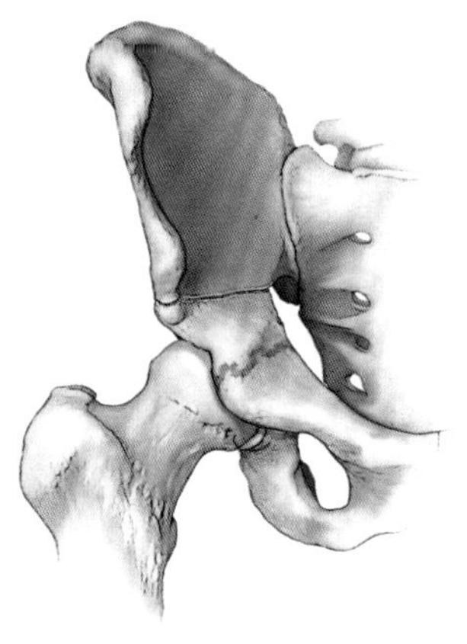

A

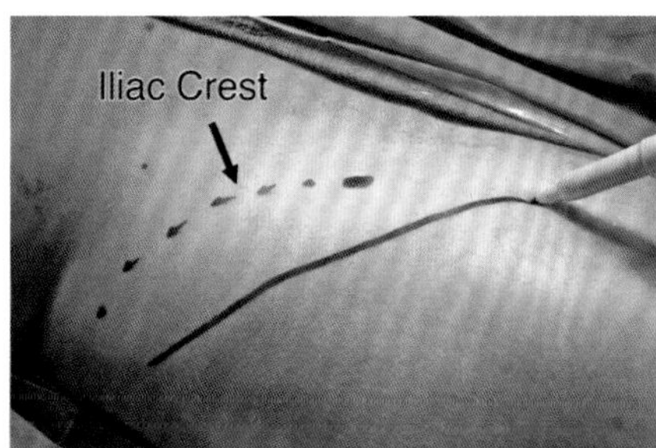


B

**TECH FIG 1** • **A.** The first cut is the iliac cut. **B.** Lateral view of the right hip showing that the incision is made just below the iliac crest, as for a Salter osteotomy.

## Making the Bony Cuts

### Iliac Osteotomy

- After making the anterolateral incision (**TECH FIG 2A**), the cartilaginous iliac crest apophysis is split, starting at the anterior superior iliac spine (ASIS) and continuing posteriorly for 6 to 8 cm. With care, this cartilage splitting can be carried anteriorly down to the anterior inferior iliac spine (AIIS).
- Both sides of the iliac wing are exposed subperiosteally down to the sciatic notch using a Cobb periosteal elevator. Specially designed Rang retractors (Jantek Engineering, Inc., Paso Robles, CA) can be placed in the sciatic notch to improve exposure (**TECH FIG 2B**) and a Gigli flexible wire saw passed through the notch (**TECH FIG 2C**).
- The iliac osteotomy is then performed by bringing the Gigli saw anteriorly through the ilium, exiting at a point just above the AIIS. In older, larger patients, we make this cut slightly more proximal than in a Salter osteotomy, which allows room to place a temporary Schanz screw to guide the acetabular segment.

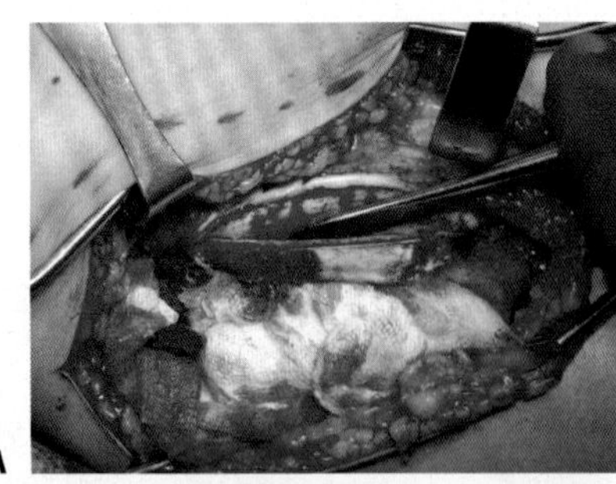

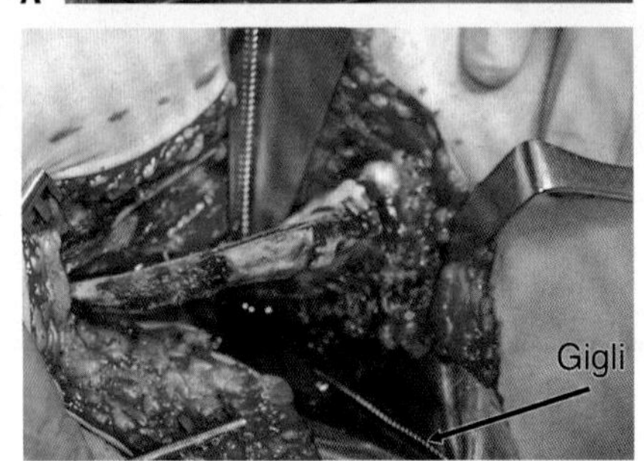


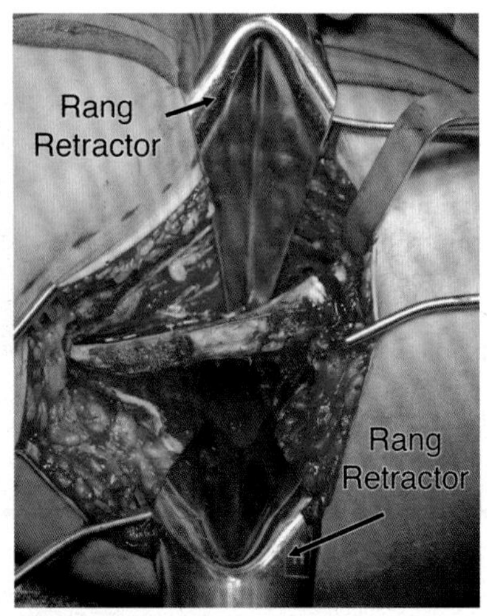


**TECH FIG 2** • Lateral view of the right hip. **A.** The iliac crest apophysis is split to expose the medial and lateral aspects of the ilium down to the sciatic notch. **B.** Rang retractors are placed in the sciatic notch to facilitate passing the Gigli saw. **C.** A Gigli saw is passed through the sciatic notch and is brought through the ilium to create the osteotomy.

## Psoas Intramuscular Lengthening at the Pelvic Brim

- At the distal end of the Salter incision, the structures are retracted on the medial side of the pelvic brim. The iliopsoas muscle is identified and rotated to expose the psoas tendon which lies posteriorly and medially in relation to the muscle mass of the iliopsoas.
  - Because the femoral nerve lies just anterior to the psoas muscle, care should be taken to be certain that you have identified the psoas tendon. A right angle hemostat can then be placed around the tendon and the tendon is sectioned leaving the muscle belly intact. This allows an intramuscular lengthening.
- The Salter incision can now be packed with a damp sponge and the wound edges pulled together with a towel clip, whereas the other osteotomies are completed.

## Pubic Osteotomy

- Earlier descriptions of TIO technique advised that the superior pubic ramus be cut from the anterolateral Salter incision.
  - We initially used this but then changed to performing the pubic cut through the medial incision which makes exposure easy, avoiding risk to the neurovascular bundle due to overretraction with the anterolateral approach (**TECH FIG 3A**).
- A 4-cm transverse incision (parallel to the inguinal ligament) is made just lateral to the adductor longus origin and 2 cm distal to the groin crease.
  - This incision can then be extended medially and distally to allow subsequent exposure of the ischium (**TECH FIG 3B**).
- The pectineus muscle is identified just lateral to the adductor longus origin and is partially elevated off of the superior pubic ramus (**TECH FIG 3C**). The saphenous vein, which often crosses the field, should be identified and retracted laterally. The pubic

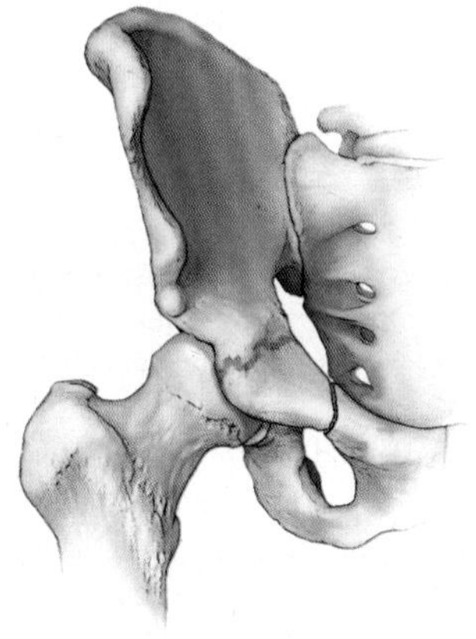

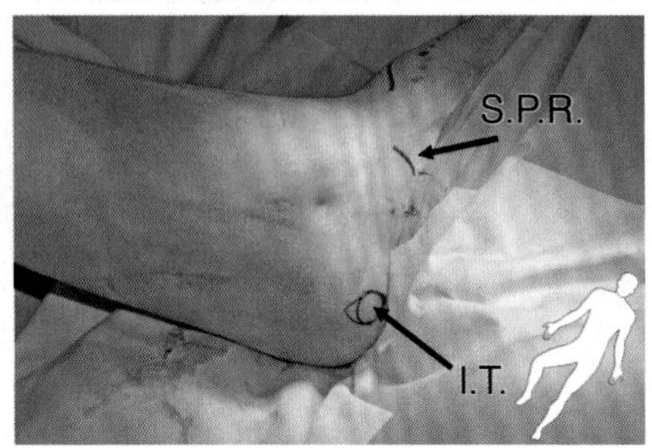


**TECH FIG 3** • **A.** The second cut is the superior pubic ramus cut. **B,C.** Medial views of the right groin area. **B.** The incision for the pubic cut is made distal to the groin crease. *S.P.R.*, superior pubic ramus; *I.T.*, ischial tuberosity. *(continued)*

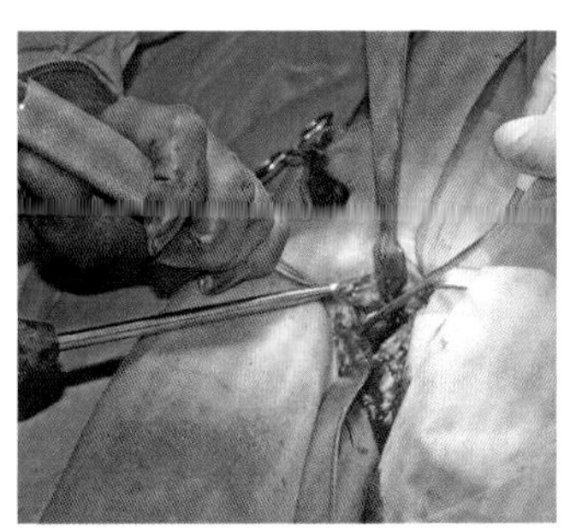
C

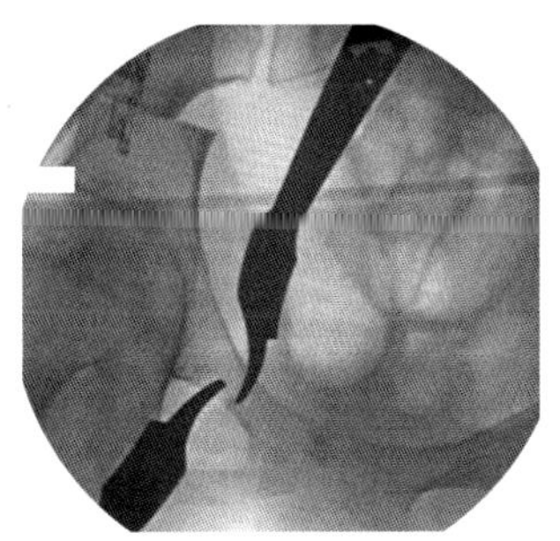
D

**TECH FIG 3** • *(continued)* **C.** After elevating the medial border of the pectineus off the pubic ramus, Hohmann retractors are placed above and below the pubis extraperiosteally. **D.** Intraoperative radiograph showing appropriate site for pubic osteotomy.

ramus is identified, and Hohmann retractors are placed above and below the pubis extraperiosteally.
  - Those new to the operation might be advised to begin with a subperiosteal approach to the pubic ramus.
- Use fluoroscopy to confirm your retractor placement before making the osteotomy. The closer you are to the acetabulum, the easier it will be to rotate the acetabulum (**TECH FIG 3D**).
- Once position is confirmed, one can use a narrow rongeur or osteotome to make the pubic cut.
  - The cut can be angled slightly to allow subsequent superomedial acetabular displacement.
  - If a rongeur is used (the safest method), the bits of excised bone should be maintained and returned to the osteotomy site to avoid the risk for pseudarthrosis.

## Ischial Osteotomy

- The 3-D nature of the ascending ischium, buried deeply in muscle, is not easy to comprehend.
  - When first performing this procedure, you should have a skeletal model of the pelvis in the operating room and the circulating nurse should hold it for you to inspect as needed (**TECH FIG 4A**).

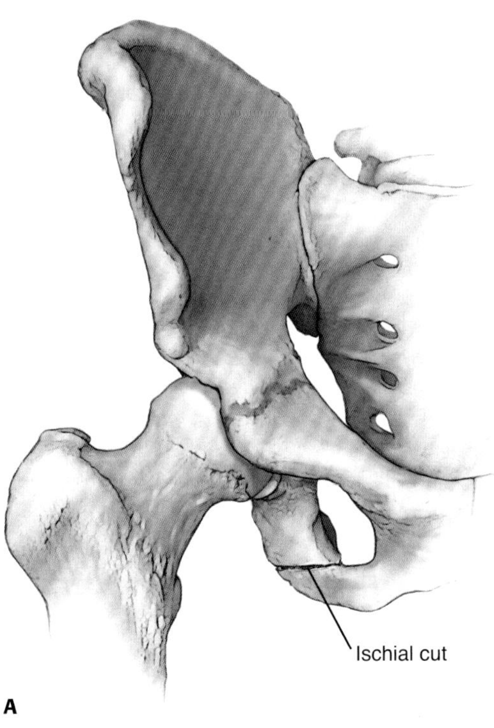

A

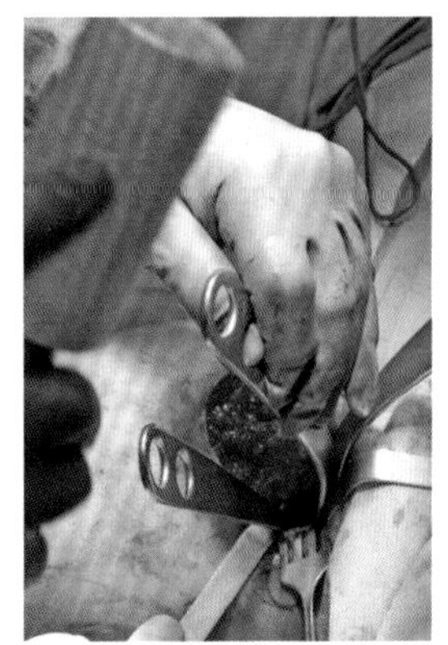
B

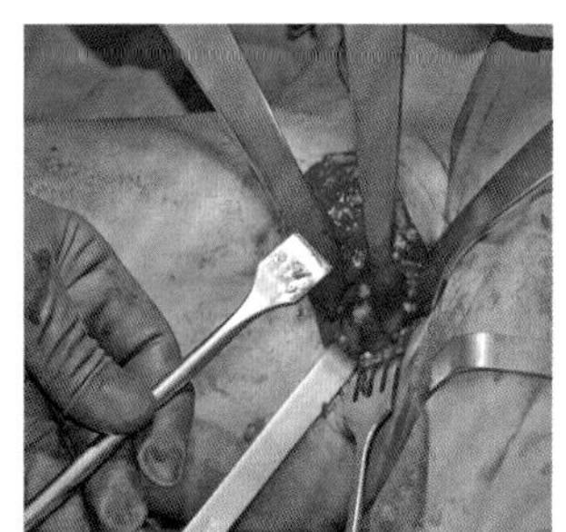
C

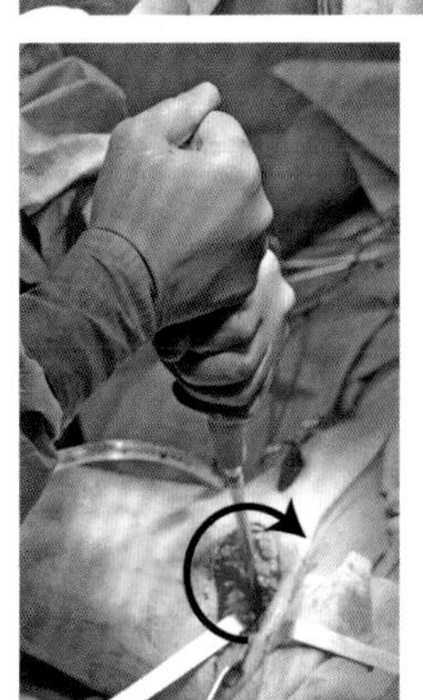
D

**TECH FIG 4** • **A.** The third cut is the ischial cut. **B–D.** Medial views of the right ischial exposure. **B.** Two Hohmann retractors are placed around the ischium. Tapping the retractors with a mallet helps to get them positioned. **C.** A third sharp Hohmann is driven into the ischium in the proximal end of the wound (just below the acetabulum) to help with retraction. The osteotome can then be introduced. **D.** When the osteotome enters the posterior cortex, it is rotated medially to displace the ischium. *(continued)*

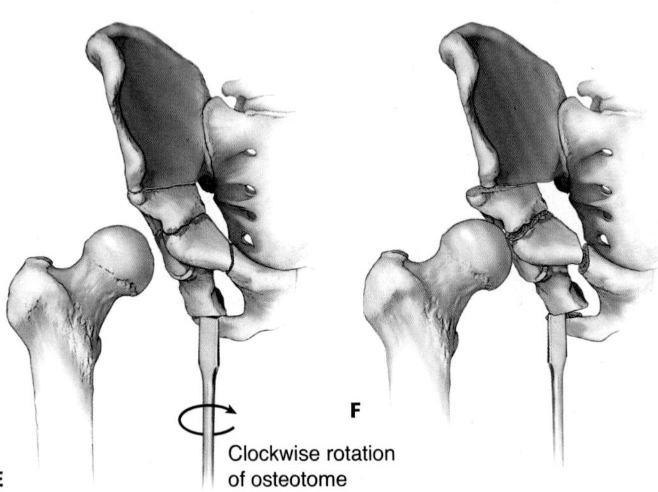


**TECH FIG 4** • *(continued)* **E,F.** Illustrations of the effective rotational maneuver described in **D**. In this right hip, after the ischium has been completely cut, the osteotome is rotated in a clockwise manner medially to displace the iliac bone just below the acetabulum. This aids in placing the femoral head in an ideal biomechanical circumstance when performing TIO.

- The proximity of the ischial spine to the sciatic nerve must be appreciated. After full exposure of the ischium, external rotation of the femur may help to avoid injury to the sciatic nerve during the ischial osteotomy.
- Through the adductor incision, blunt dissection is carried out subcutaneously down to the ischial spine (**TECH FIG 4B**).
- The electrocautery is used to take down the posterior portion of the adductor magnus muscle origin just anterior and medial to the proximal origin of the hamstrings.
- The ischial tuberosity is identified, and an initial sharp Hohmann retractor is placed inside the obturator foramen. A Cobb elevator is used to clear the ischium up to its origin just below the acetabulum.
- Blunt Hohmann retractors are then placed extraperiosteally around the ischium with one retractor in the obturator foramen and the other lateral to the ischium.
  - Using a mallet to tap a blunt Hohmann into these spaces makes it easier (helps to safely elevate the thick periosteum and tendon origins). (This is a very deep exposure and the neophyte will be surprised at the depth of the ascending ischium.)
- Finally, a third Hohmann retractor (sharp) is driven into the ischial bone just below the acetabulum to allow easier superior retraction (**TECH FIG 4C**). Thus, a total of three Hohmann retractors—one medial, one lateral, and a sharp-tipped—tapped into the bone proximally.
  - Fluoroscopy is used to check position. The ischial cut should be just below but not in the acetabulum (about 1 cm below the lower end of the "teardrop").
- Once position is confirmed, a rongeur can be used to start the osteotomy creating a groove for the osteotome to prevent the osteotome from slipping.
  - A long, straight osteotome is then inserted and used to complete the osteotomy.
- To confirm completion and begin displacement of the osteotomy, the large wooden handle of the osteotome is used to radically rotate the acetabular segment medially before the osteotome is withdrawn.
  - This begins the desired medial displacement of the ischium (**TECH FIG 4D**).
  - Using a very long (approximately 20 inch) wooden handled osteotome makes this essential rotational maneuver easier (**TECH FIG 4E,F**).

TECHNIQUES

## Rotation of the Acetabulum

- The packing sponges are now removed from the Salter incision.
- A temporary Schanz screw is placed in the acetabular segment just above the hip joint to use as a handle to guide acetabular positioning (**TECH FIG 5A**).
- A long ballpoint pusher is placed in the superior pubic ramus just lateral to the pubic cut and impacted into the bone via the medial incision (**TECH FIG 5B**).
  - This is pushed upward and inward, whereas the Schanz screw is levered downward and laterally to rotate the entire acetabulum around the femoral head (**TECH FIG 5C**).
  - A Cobb elevator is placed posteriorly in the Salter (iliac) cut and rotated to encourage lateral positioning of the acetabular fragment in the coronal plane.
- A wedge of bone is removed from the iliac crest using an oscillating saw. The base of the wedge should be fashioned to fit tightly in the gap of the iliac osteotomy (**TECH FIG 5D**).
  - This triangular graft needs to be only about half as large as in a Salter osteotomy for the same size patient because a good deal of the rotation should have occurred through the pubic and ischial cuts (**TECH FIG 5E**).

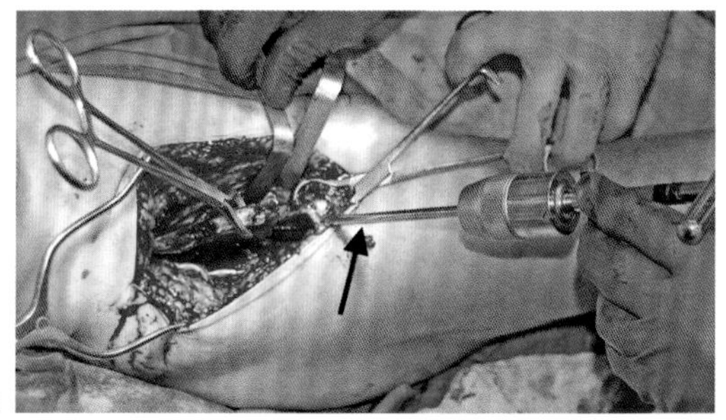
A

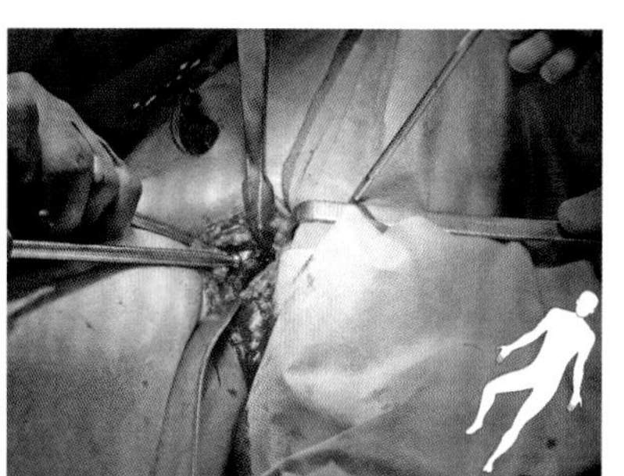
B

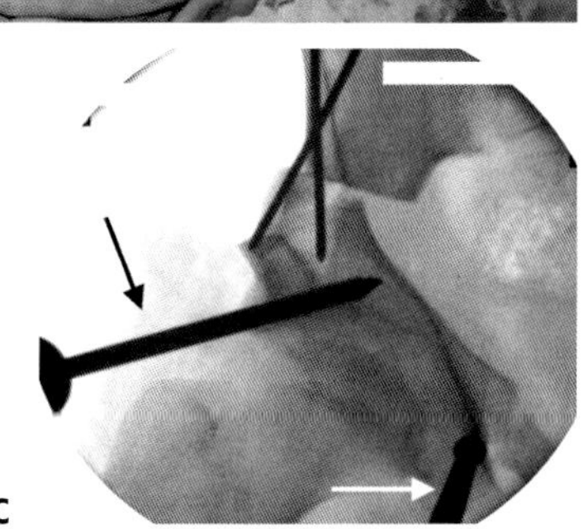
C

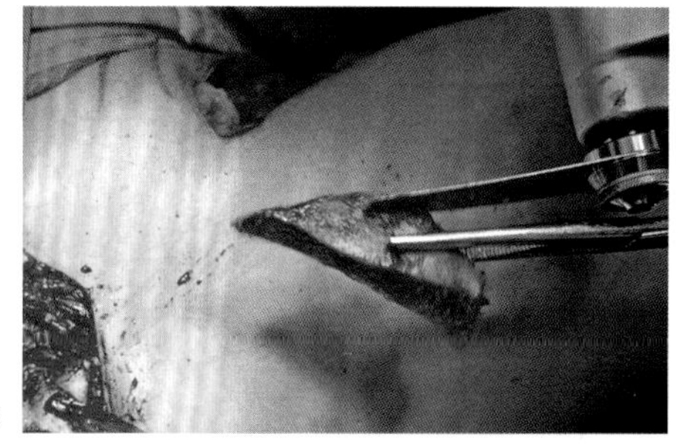
D

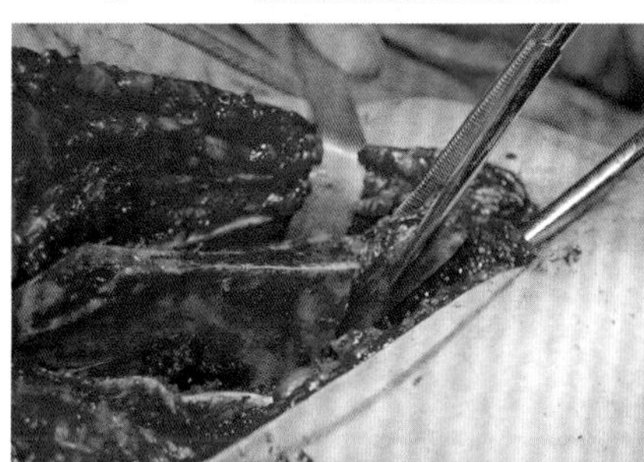
E

**TECH FIG 5** • **A**. Lateral view of the right hip. A Schanz screw is placed just above the hip (*arrow*); it can be used as a lever to help rotate the acetabulum. **B.** A ballpoint pusher can be used to push the pubic portion upward and inward, whereas the Schanz screw levers the superior acetabulum anterolaterally. **C.** Fluoroscopic image showing ballpoint pusher (*white arrow*) and Schanz screw (*black arrow*). **D,E.** Lateral views show bone graft taken from the iliac crest and fashioned to fit into the iliac osteotomy.

## Temporary Fixation

- The osteotomy is first fixed with temporary smooth K-wires.
- Acetabular position is checked with fluoroscopy to confirm the amount of coverage that has been obtained (**TECH FIG 6A**).
- Be careful not to overrotate anteriorly (producing anterior impingement), which is indicated by a crossover sign and an overly prominent ischial spine on the radiograph (**TECH FIG 6B**).
- A well-performed TIO (**TECH FIG 6C**) should have these x-ray features:
  - Ilium: The acetabular segment should be positioned 8 to 10 mm lateral to the inner wall of the ilium above.
  - Pubis: The acetabular segment should be displaced slightly superior and medial.
  - Approximately 50% step-off of the ischial cut with the proximal portion moving superomedially.
  - Teardrop angled about 20 degrees (vertical prior to rotation)
  - The ischial spine should be only a little (if any) more prominent than on the opposite side.
  - Sourcil: in a transverse position

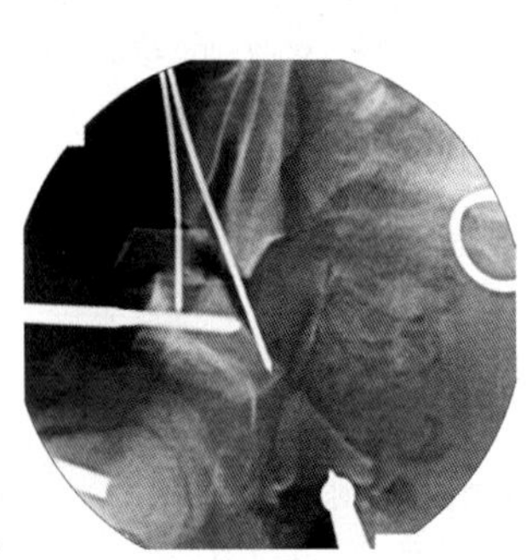

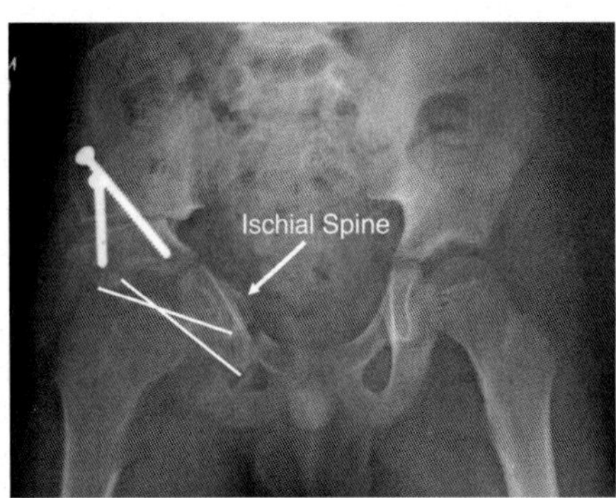


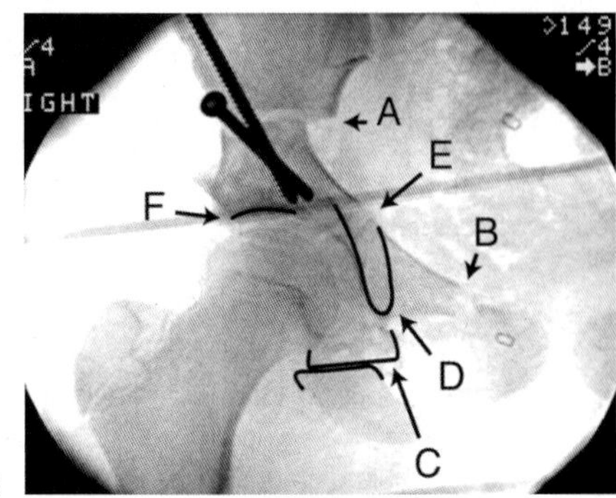


**TECH FIG 6** • **A.** The osteotomy is temporarily fixed using smooth K-wires to confirm position with fluoroscopy before final screw fixation. **B.** This acetabulum has been rotated too far anteriorly and laterally. Note the prominent ischial spine and crossover sign. **C.** Radiographic features of an ideal TIO. *A:* The acetabular segment of the ilium should be positioned 8 to 10 mm lateral to the inner wall of the ilium above. *B:* The acetabular segment of the pubis should be displaced slightly superior and medial. *C:* About 50% step-off of the ischial cut with the proximal segment displaced medially. *D:* Teardrop is angled about 20 degrees (vertical before rotation). *E:* The ischial spine should be only a little (in any) more prominent than on the opposite side. *F:* The sourcil is in a transverse position.

## Fixation

- 4.5-mm fully threaded screws can be inserted from the iliac crest across the bone graft and into the superior acetabular bone.
- Using fully threaded screws minimizes the tendency for loss of correction which can occur when a partially threaded screw is tightened too much, overcompressing the graft and pulling the acetabular edge upward. Instead, the screws should stabilize and maintain some distraction.[21]
- We use two or three screws to adequately fix the acetabular fragment. Threaded K-wires can be used in smaller patients where the bone may not be thick (strong) enough to hold the 4.5-mm screw.
- In older, larger patients, we often place an additional single screw from medial to lateral across the pubic osteotomy to prevent further rotation of the acetabular fragment or nonunion of the pubis (**TECH FIG 7**).
- Any remaining bone graft fragments can be packed into the pubic and ischial osteotomies to prevent nonunion.

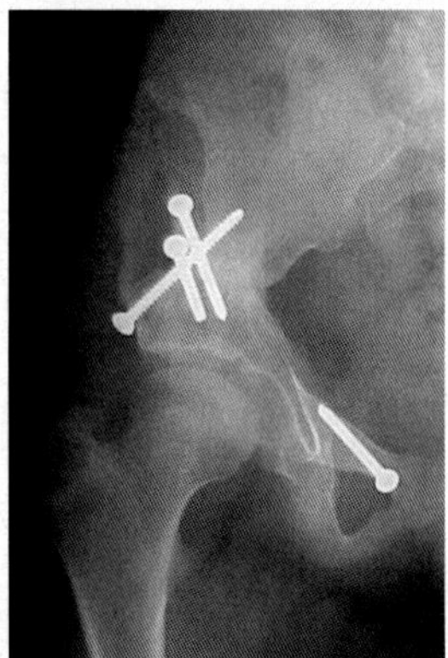

**TECH FIG 7** • Supplementation of the iliac screw fixation with a pubic fixation screw.

## Wound Closure

- After thorough irrigation, the iliac crest apophysis is reapproximated and closed with a running absorbable suture.
- Hemovac drains are placed in the Salter, pubic, and ischial incisions.
- The incisions are then closed in layers with absorbable suture followed by sterile dressings. In most cases, a single hip spica is applied.
- If both iliac and pubic fixation is secure in a cooperative patient, we sometimes use no formal postoperative immobilization.

## PEARLS AND PITFALLS

| | |
|---|---|
| **Preoperative arthrogram** | ■ A dynamic arthrogram is the best way to determine hip joint function, mobility, and stability. The study also allows visualization of the labrum and possible impingement of the femoral neck on the labrum or acetabulum. |
| **Pubic osteotomy** | ■ Performing the pubic osteotomy through the medial incision makes exposure easier and avoids risk to the neurovascular bundle due to overretraction with the anterolateral approach.<br>■ Extraperiosteal exposure of the pubis allows easier periosteal sectioning because the periosteum is strong in this area and may prevent movement of the pubic segment. Care must be taken to avoid the obturator nerve which courses just below the superior pubic ramus. |
| **Ischial osteotomy** | ■ When trying to palpate the ischium, the femur should be internally rotated to avoid erroneously palpating the greater trochanter which can be in close proximity to the ischium. Once the bony prominences have been identified, external rotation of the femur should protect the sciatic nerve during the ischial osteotomy.<br>■ To confirm completion of the ischial osteotomy, the osteotome is used to radically rotate the acetabular segment medially. This begins the desired medial displacement of the ischial segment that is attached to the acetabulum. |
| **Rotation of the acetabular fragment** | ■ Care must be taken to not externally rotate the acetabular fragment (this is easy to do in a triple osteotomy and will cause undesired acetabular retroversion). A temporary Schanz screw can help to control acetabular position. To avoid undesirable external rotation, Salter's advice was that "even after the osteotomy is performed the anterior superior and anterior inferior iliac spines should remain aligned." |
| **Fixation of the osteotomy** | ■ Fully threaded screws should be used to stabilize the acetabular fragment and maintain some distraction. This minimizes the tendency for loss of correction which can occur when a partially threaded screw is tightened too much, overcompressing the graft and pulling the acetabular edge upward. |

## POSTOPERATIVE CARE

- The single-leg spica cast is maintained for 4 to 6 weeks followed by partial weight bearing with crutches for an additional 4 weeks. If adequate bone healing is noted on x-ray, activity can then be advanced as tolerated.
- Physical therapy may be useful for regaining abductor strength and motion.
- The fixation screws can be removed 6 to 12 months postoperatively is desired.

## OUTCOMES

- As TIO is most commonly used for late juveniles, adolescents, and young adults, very long-term follow-up studies are required to evaluate function over a lifetime, with 30 to 60 years of follow-up. Unfortunately, these long-term studies have not yet been done. There are several studies that look at short- to medium-term results.
- Guille et al[6] reported more than 10-year follow up of 11 patients ages 11 to 16 years with symptomatic hip dysplasia treated with TIO, 10 hips improved radiographically, 8 improved functionally, 1 required a total hip arthroplasty.
- Faciszewski et al[1] followed 56 hips in 44 patients that underwent TIO for 2 to 12 years.
  - Improvement in pain and function was considered good in 53 hips.
  - Three hips were considered failures.[1]
- Peters et al[13] evaluated 60 hips in 50 patients who underwent TIO.
  - At average 9-year follow-up, 12 (20%) hips had been converted to total hip arthroplasty and 4 (7%) hips had incapacitating pain.
  - Radiographically, there was significant improvement in the center–edge angle of Wiberg and the acetabular angle of Sharp.
  - There also was a statistically significant relationship between failure of the osteotomy and severity of preexisting hip arthrosis.[13]
- In patients with acetabular dysplasia, indications and outcomes are better understood. Application of TIO for patients with femoral deformity (Perthes, AVN, epiphyseal dysplasia) has a shorter track record but appears to provide clear benefit in properly selected cases.[9,10]

## COMPLICATIONS

- Pubic or ischial osteotomy nonunion
- Overcorrection of the acetabular fragment resulting in iatrogenic impingement
- Retroversion of the acetabular fragment
- Sciatic or obturator nerve injury
- Loss of fixation or correction

## REFERENCES

1. Faciszewski T, Coleman SS, Biddulph G. Triple innominate osteotomy for acetabular dysplasia. J Pediatr Orthop 1993;13:426–430.
2. Frick SL, Kim SS, Wenger DR. Pre- and postoperative three-dimensional computed tomography analysis of triple innominate osteotomy for hip dysplasia. J Pediatr Orthop 2000;20:116–123.
3. Gans I, Flynn JM, Sankar WN. Abduction bracing for residual acetabular dysplasia in infantile DDH. J Pediatr Orthop 2013;33:714–718.
4. Ganz R, Klaue K, Vinh TS, et al. A new periacetabular osteotomy for the treatment of hip dysplasias: technique and preliminary results. Clin Orthop Relat Res 1988;(232):26–36.
5. Gillingham BL, Sanchez AA, Wenger DR. Pelvic osteotomies for the treatment of hip dysplasia in children and young adults. J Am Acad Orthop Surg 1999;7:325–337.
6. Guille JT, Forlin E, Kumar SJ, et al. Triple osteotomy of the innominate bone in treatment of developmental dysplasia of the hip. J Pediatr Orthop 1992;12:718–721.
7. Herring JA, Kim HT, Browne R. Legg-Calve-Perthes disease. Part II: prospective multicenter study of the effect of treatment on outcome. J Bone Joint Surg Am 2004;86-A:2121–2134.

8. Kim HT, Wenger DR. The morphology of residual acetabular deficiency in childhood hip dysplasia: three-dimensional computed tomographic analysis. J Pediatr Orthop 1997;17:637–647.
9. Kumar D, Bache CE, O'Hara JN. Interlocking triple pelvic osteotomy in severe Legg-Calve-Perthes disease. J Pediatr Orthop 2002;22:464–470.
10. Kumar SJ, MacEwen GD, Jaykumar AS. Triple osteotomy of the innominate bone for the treatment of congenital hip dysplasia. J Pediatr Orthop 1986;6:393–398.
11. Mehta JS, Conybeare ME, Hinves BL, et al. Protein C levels in patients with Legg-Calve-Perthes disease: is it a true deficiency? J Pediatr Orthop 2006;26:200–203.
12. Pemberton PA. Pericapsular osteotomy of the ilium for the treatment of congenitally dislocated hips. Clin Orthop Relat Res 1974;(98):41–54.
13. Peters CL, Fukushima BW, Park TK, et al. Triple innominate osteotomy in young adults for the treatment of acetabular dysplasia: a 9-year follow-up study. Orthopedics 2001;24:565–569.
14. Ponseti IV. Growth and development of the acetabulum in the normal child. Anatomical, histological, and roentgenographic studies. J Bone Joint Surg Am 1978;60:575–585.
15. Rab GT. Containment of the hip: a theoretical comparison of osteotomies. Clin Orthop Relat Res 1981;(154):191–196.
16. Salter RB, Dubos JP. The first fifteen year's personal experience with innominate osteotomy in the treatment of congenital dislocation and subluxation of the hip. Clin Orthop Relat Res 1974;(98):72–103.
17. Steel HH. Triple osteotomy of the innominate bone. J Bone Joint Surg Am 1973;55:343–350.
18. Wenger DR, Pandya NK. Advanced containment methods for the treatment of Perthes disease: Salter plus varus osteotomy and triple pelvic osteotomy. J Pediatr Orthop 2011;31(2 suppl):S198–S205.
19. Wenger DR, Pring ME, Hosalkar HS, et al. Advanced containment methods for Legg-Calve-Perthes disease: results of triple pelvic osteotomy. J Pediatr Orthop 2010;30:749–757.
20. Wiberg G. Shelf operation in congenital dysplasia of the acetabulum and in subluxation and dislocation of the hip. J Bone Joint Surg Am 1953;35:65–80.
21. Yassir W, Mahar A, Aminian A, et al. A comparison of the fixation stability of multiple screw constructs for two types of pelvic osteotomies. J Pediatr Orthop 2005;25:14–17.

# Chiari Medial Displacement Osteotomy of the Pelvis

**Travis H. Matheney and Brian Snyder**

## DEFINITION

- The Chiari osteotomy is primarily a "salvage" osteotomy for acetabular dysplasia in the painful, unstable hip.
- It is generally reserved for hips where a congruous reduction is not possible because of arthrosis or femoral head asphericity that prevents use of one of the more standard rotational osteotomies.[1,4,5]
- It is a single pericapsular osteotomy through the iliac (innominate) bone of the pelvis with medialization of the acetabulum and hip joint to improve posterior and lateral coverage. The ilium forms a shelf over the dysplastic, subluxated hip (**FIG 1**).
- The goals are improved femoral head coverage, a stable articulation, and metaplastic transformation of the hip capsule to fibrocartilage to create a stable, pain-free hip.
- Contraindications include severe arthrosis, age older than 45 years (relative, where arthroplasty may be a better option), and significant proximal migration of the femoral head (may prevent adequate coverage by thinner proximal ilium).[5]

## ANATOMY

- Developmental acetabular dysplasia most commonly involves deficiency of the anterior and anterolateral acetabulum.
- In cases of spastic hip dysplasia, the lateral and posterolateral acetabulum is most often deficient.
- The location of acetabular deficiency must be considered when planning the shape and orientation of the osteotomy and positioning of the iliac shelf over the hip joint.
- Femoral head deformity may include coxa breva, coxa magna, or coxa plana.
- In cases of trochanteric overgrowth, simultaneous advancement of the greater trochanter may provide improved abductor mechanics (although the risk of heterotopic ossification may be slightly increased).
- This osteotomy may not provide adequate coverage in cases of high dislocation and in the pelvis in patients with advanced neurologic conditions (eg, myelomeningocele, where the ilium is very thin above the acetabulum). Therefore, careful

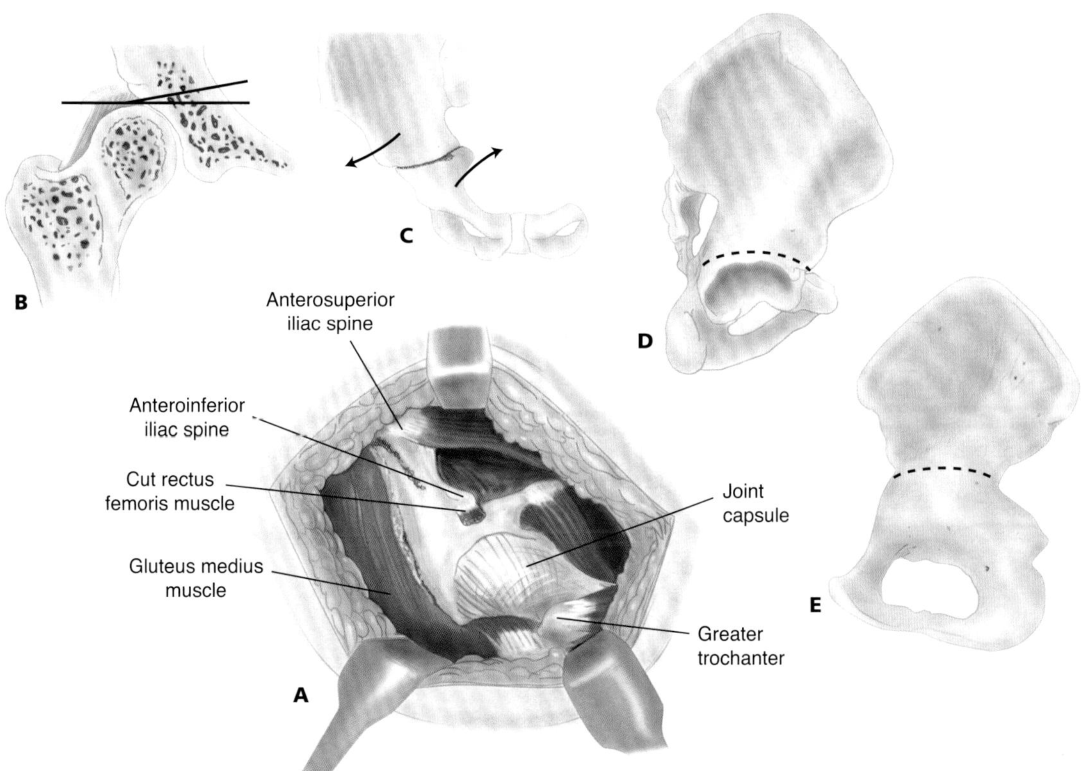


**FIG 1** • Concept and steps of the Chiari osteotomy. **A.** The view required to properly perform the osteotomy. **B.** The proper placement of the osteotomy in the coronal plane is at the superior border of the acetabulum, just above the capsule and angled upward 10 to 15 degrees. **C.** The acetabular fragment is displaced medially, hinging on the symphysis pubis. **D.** The proposed osteotomy (*dotted line*) as seen from the lateral projection. **E.** The line of the osteotomy as seen from the inside view of the pelvis. It is above the triradiate cartilage.

consideration of the available periacetabular bone stock should be made before considering the Chiari osteotomy.
- The need for additional bone graft to supplement posterior, lateral, and (especially) anterior coverage is common.
- This procedure does not require concentric reduction of the femoral head into the acetabulum.
- It has the advantage of medializing the femoral head and decreasing the force across the hip joint by increasing the surface area of coverage.
- Lateralizing the ilium to form a shelf causes obligatory shortening of the gluteal muscle length and abductor moment arm that weakens the muscle and contributes to postoperative Trendelenburg limp. However, advancing the greater trochanter can restore the resting length of the gluteus medius. Delp et al[3] found that decreasing the obliquity of the supra-acetabular osteotomy may decrease the effect on the abductor lever arm.

## PATHOGENESIS

- The causes of advanced hip disease requiring salvage surgery are many and include late diagnosis of developmental dysplasia of the hip (DDH), spastic or neuromuscular hip dysplasia, failed prior hip procedures (reduction, periacetabular osteotomy), and acetabular trauma.
- Femoral head conditions that can lead to incomplete or incongruous femoral head coverage include primary malformation, secondary avascular necrosis, slipped capital femoral epiphysis, epiphyseal–metaphyseal dysplasia, and secondary malformation from long-standing subluxation or impingement.

## NATURAL HISTORY

- Because this osteotomy is used as a salvage procedure for many hip diseases, it can be used to treat any of the several conditions that result in progressive, painful arthrosis and instability.
- The threshold of acetabular dysplasia required to induce arthrosis is incompletely understood. However, when assessing lateral uncovering, Murphy et al[6] found that a lateral center-edge angle less than 16 degrees on an anteroposterior (AP) view of the pelvis correlated with a significantly increased risk of requiring arthroplasty by age 65 years.
- Spastic hip dysplasia can lead to progressive subluxation and painful dislocation in 30% to 50% of cases. It is more common in nonambulatory patients.

## PATIENT HISTORY AND PHYSICAL FINDINGS

- Key portions of the history include the following:
  - Personal or family history of or treatment for DDH
  - History of other hip disorders, including Legg-Calvé-Perthes disease
  - Trauma
  - Skeletal dysplasias
  - History of cerebral palsy
  - Birth order and weight
  - Description of pain and mechanical symptoms, including location, duration, activity limitation, giving way, clicking, catching, and popping
- The physical examination should include gait, limb length, assistive devices, and strength.
- Specific hip tests include the following:
  - Trendelenburg test: demonstrates weakness in abductors
  - Anterior apprehension test with extension and external rotation of the hip: A positive result is a subjective noting of "apprehension" or instability by the patient.
  - Gluteus medius and maximus strength
  - Anterior impingement test (pain with passive hip flexion, adduction, and internal rotation): test of anterior labral pathology, not just a tear
  - "Bicycle test" for abductor fatigability of the hip while lying in the contralateral decubitus position
  - Range of motion: It is important to test internal and external rotation at multiple degrees of flexion, as femoral head and acetabular deformities vary. This can often aid in determining where the pathologic articulation is located.
  - Galeazzi sign: demonstrates hip subluxation or dislocation
- The Chiari osteotomy can increase abduction. It does not always significantly improve range of motion in other planes, and therefore preoperative flexion to 90 degrees, full (or near full) extension, and at least 10 to 20 degrees of adduction are requirements.
- Gait is assessed preoperatively. It is important to discern whether any limp is antalgic, due to abductor weakness or instability. The Chiari osteotomy classically can improve antalgia and instability. However, the patient should understand that abductor weakness may not be improved.

## IMAGING AND OTHER DIAGNOSTIC STUDIES

- Radiography should include weight-bearing AP views of bilateral hips, false profile of hips, and AP of hips in maximal abduction and internal rotation (**FIG 2**). These studies allow assessment of lateral and anterior coverage of the femoral head as well as congruency of the hip joint. Also noted will be the presence of hinge abduction.
- Computed tomography (CT) scan with three-dimensional reconstruction may help in preoperatively assessing the amount and direction of acetabular deficiency.

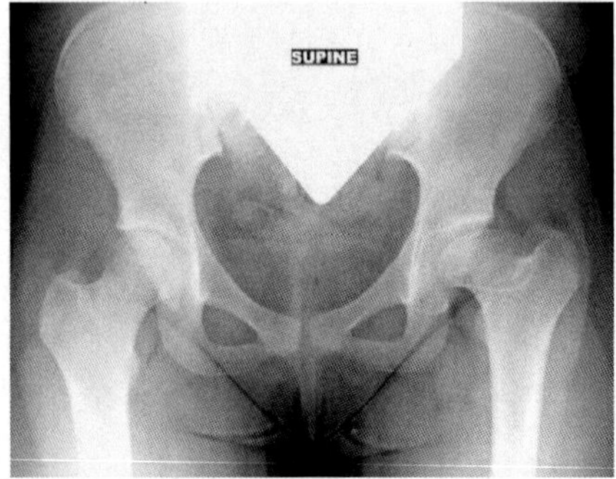


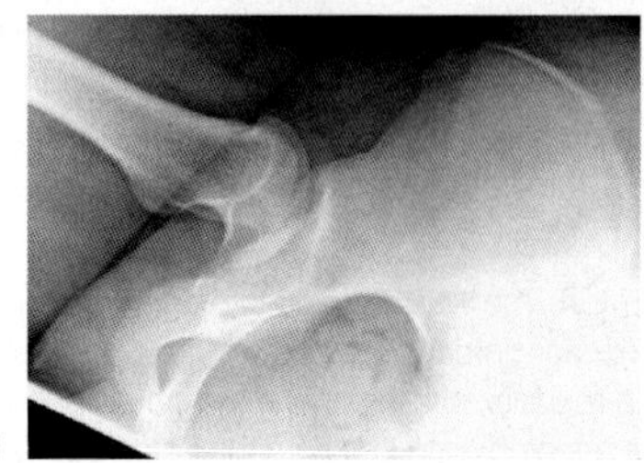

**FIG 2** • **A.** AP radiograph of bilateral hips and pelvis of patient with right hip with Legg-Calvé-Perthes disease. **B.** Frog-leg lateral radiograph of left hip with Legg-Calvé-Perthes disease.

- Magnetic resonance imaging (MRI) of involved hips with radial sequences centered at the femoral head can also help with preoperative assessment of articular and labral cartilage.

## DIFFERENTIAL DIAGNOSIS

- DDH
- Spastic hip dysplasia
- Legg-Calvé-Perthes disease, avascular necrosis
- Multiple or spondyloepiphyseal dysplasia
- Posttraumatic hip or femoral dysplasia

## NONOPERATIVE MANAGEMENT

- The patient being considered for Chiari osteotomy usually presents with pain and arthrosis.
- Activity and job modification and weight loss may be of benefit in delaying or mitigating the onset of arthritic symptoms.
- Physical therapy may be of some benefit in increasing range of motion and strength. To date, there are no data to suggest that a specific physical therapy regimen can stop the onset of arthritis in the dysplastic hip.

## SURGICAL MANAGEMENT

- Hip adductor tenotomy, lengthening, or Botox can be used in an attempt to delay the onset of spastic hip dysplasia (if performed before age 4 to 6 years) and if hip abduction is less than 45 degrees with hips flexed and extended.
- This is especially important if a varus intertrochanteric osteotomy is being performed simultaneously.
- Painful, unstable, moderate to severe dysplasia with incongruent articulation with or without femoral head deformity often requires surgical correction.
- Additional options to Chiari include arthrodesis, shelf procedures, and arthroplasty.

### Preoperative Planning

- A complete physical examination is performed and radiographs are obtained.
- In the case of marked proximal migration, preoperative traction for 2 to 3 weeks may improve the position of the femoral head relative to the acetabulum, thereby increasing proximal ilial fragment coverage after osteotomy.

### Positioning

- The patient is placed supine on a radiolucent table with a rolled blanket bump under the operative hip. Without a bump, it can be difficult to visualize the posterior column adequately enough to complete the osteotomy along the posterior wall.
- All other bony prominences are carefully padded.
- A Foley catheter is placed and prophylactic antibiotics are administered.
- The use of epidural anesthesia depends on patient and surgeon preferences.
- The extremity is prepared free proximally to the costophrenic margin, including the groin and buttock regions.

### Approach

- The ilioinguinal approach begins along the iliac crest and continues medially for about 10 cm.
- The iliofemoral approach is less cosmetic but can aid in visualization in larger patients and can allow combined pelvic and femoral procedures to be done through one incision.

TECHNIQUES

## Exposure

- The skin incision begins laterally 1 to 1.5 cm below the iliac crest, extending distally to 1.5 cm below the anterior superior iliac spine and then posteriorly over the lateral thigh or medially across the groin to 1.5 to 2 cm medial to the anterior superior iliac spine (ilioinguinal approach; **TECH FIG 1A**).
- The tensor fascia lata (TFL) compartment is entered just lateral to its intermuscular septum with the sartorius muscle, which is retracted medially.
- The TFL muscle belly is bluntly dissected off the intermuscular septum and dissection is carried proximally to the ilium. This allows visualization of the anterior ilium and easy continuation of subperiosteal exposure of the ilium (**TECH FIG 1B**).
- Although the lateral femoral cutaneous nerve is not routinely visualized or isolated, it may be encountered underneath the fascia in the interval between the sartorius and the TFL. Therefore, care should be taken when retracting the medial structures during this dissection, the procedure, and closure of the interval.
- The iliac apophysis is split (in younger patients) or subperiosteally dissected (in skeletally mature patients) to allow subperiosteal exposure of the inner and outer tables of the ilium. A moist sponge is packed along the inner table to provide retraction and hemostasis.
- The outer table of the ilium is subperiosteally cleared of abductor musculature. This is carried out until a firm end point is reached, usually indicating that the surgeon has reached the indirect head of the rectus femoris.
- Expose the anterior and superior aspects of the hip joint capsule. Identify the rectus femoris, release the indirect head at its bifurcation from the direct head, and follow it posteriorly. Incise the periosteum of the outer ilium along the border of the indirect head of the rectus and carefully dissect it off the hip capsule. This will allow you to strip the abductor minimus capsular insertion from medial to lateral off the superior capsule.
- A pseudoacetabulum may be present; it can feel like the capsular edge during the initial approach. Intraoperative fluoroscopy will help to discern when you have reached the edge of the true acetabulum if there is any question.
- Although Chiari originally described a semi-blind osteotomy, it is important to have excellent visualization of the superior hip capsule from the anterior ilium to the greater sciatic notch and along the posterior wall of the acetabulum to the ischial spine. Placement of the osteotomy must be at the capsular edge of the acetabulum (**TECH FIG 1C**).

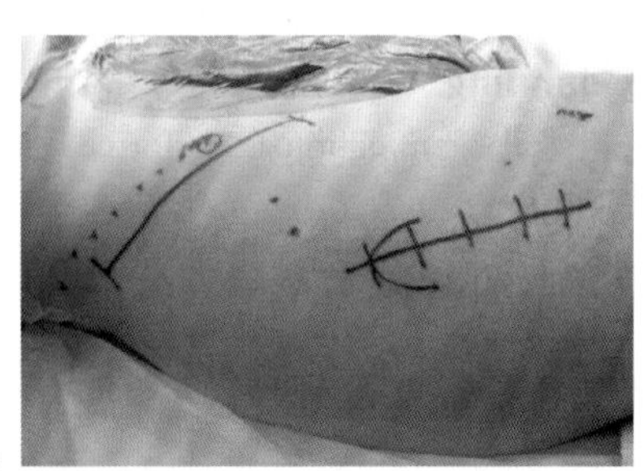

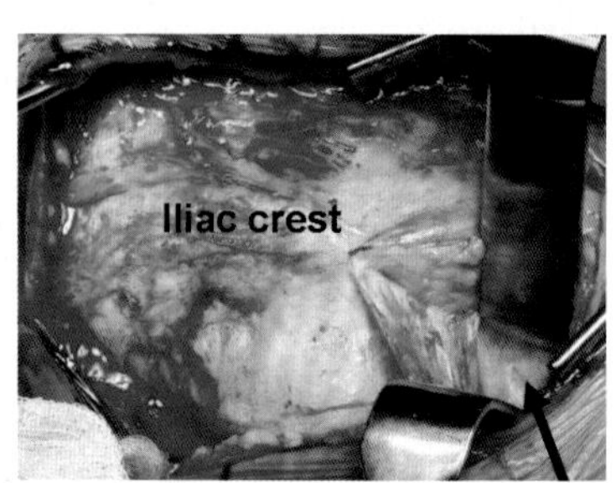


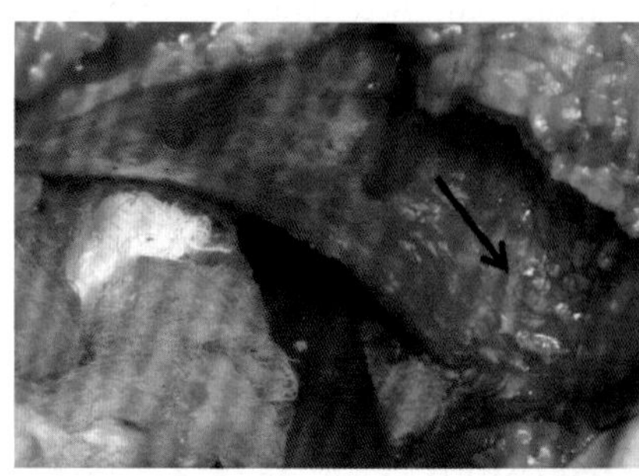

**TECH FIG 1** • **A.** Planned incisions for both the ilioinguinal approach and the direct lateral approach to the proximal femur for additional intertrochanteric osteotomy. **B.** Ilioinguinal approach. Shown are the iliac crest and the direct head of the rectus femoris (*arrow*) deep to the TFL compartment (TFL retracted posteriorly). **C.** The outer table of the ilium is exposed. A Lane bone lever placed subperiosteally into the greater sciatic notch allows excellent visualization of the acetabular rim (*arrow*) all the way to the ischial spine.

## Osteotomy

- Once the exposure is complete, a variety of methods may be used to create the osteotomy.
- The supra-acetabular osteotomy is a curvilinear cut from the anterior ilium, along the capsular edge of the acetabulum, and posterior to the greater sciatic notch. We use a modification advocated by Hall that simply makes a concerted effort to create a dome osteotomy by curving the osteotomy distally when aiming for the notch to maximize the posterior coverage.
- The osteotomy starts at the capsular margin and is aimed proximal and medial at an angle of about 10 to 15 degrees (see **FIG 1A**). This facilitates "sliding down" of the ilium over the hip joint capsule. When properly completed, the cut

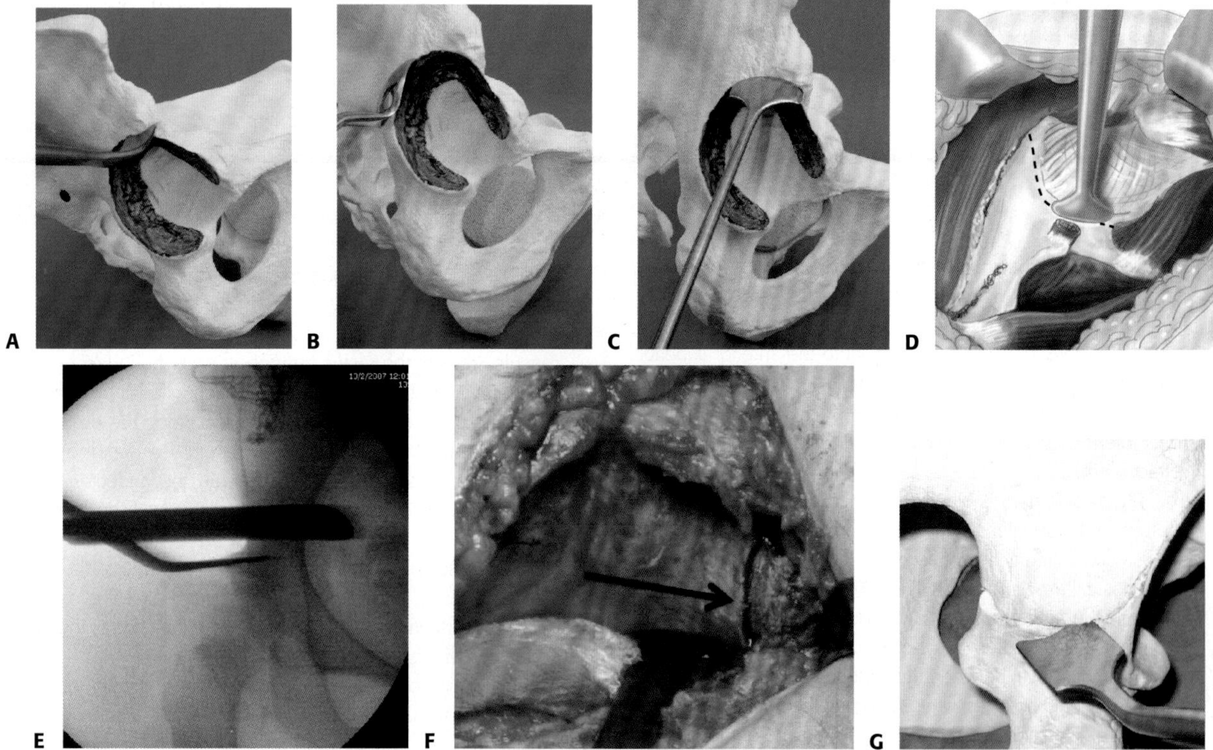

**TECH FIG 2** • **A–C.** Bone models demonstrate the planned supra-acetabular osteotomy using a combination of curved and dome-shaped osteotomes. **D.** Scoring the inner table of the ilium along the projected course of the osteotomy minimizes splintering. **E.** AP fluoroscopic view of the right hip during osteotomy. The osteotome enters at the edge of the acetabulum and is directed upward at an angle of about 10 to 15 degrees. **F.** The completed supra-acetabular osteotomy (*arrow*). **G.** Bone model representation of the posterior aspect of the osteotomy. Note the attempt to continue the osteotomy posterior to just above the ischial spine.

surface of the ilium will lie in direct contact with the hip capsule and will be in continuity with the lateral bony edge of the acetabulum.

## Chiari Conventional Method

- A Gigli saw is passed through the greater sciatic notch while protecting its contents and is used in a posterior to anterior direction.
- We find that as the starting point is crucial, it is helpful to notch the posterior column in the sciatic notch and the outer table of the ilium to create a track for the Gigli.

## Authors' Preferred Method

- We prefer a combination of curved and dome-shaped osteotomes used under fluoroscopic guidance to create the osteotomy.
- It is often helpful to score the inner table of the ilium along the projected course of the osteotomy to minimize splintering of the inner table (**TECH FIG 2A–F**).
- To maximize the amount of posterior coverage, an attempt is made to continue the osteotomy at the acetabular rim as far distal and posterior as possible.
  - This is carried out only to a level just above the ischial spine (**TECH FIG 2G**).

# Acetabular Displacement

- The hip is abducted and pushed medially to displace the distal fragment (**TECH FIG 3A,B**).
- The amount of displacement required is somewhat dependent on the amount of coverage required. One hundred percent displacement is possible and often necessary. In particular, when posterior coverage is required, the ilium is displaced posteriorly over the sciatic notch; take care to prevent compression or entrapment of the sciatic nerve (**TECH FIG 3C**).

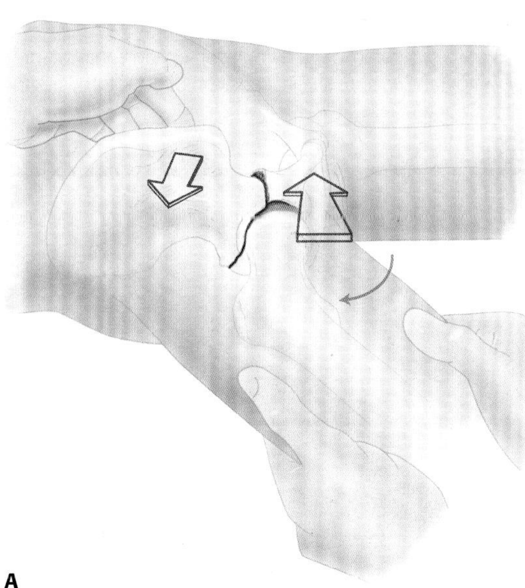

A

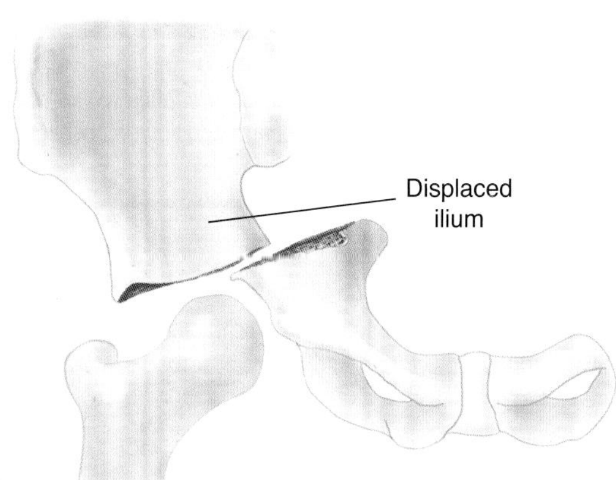


B

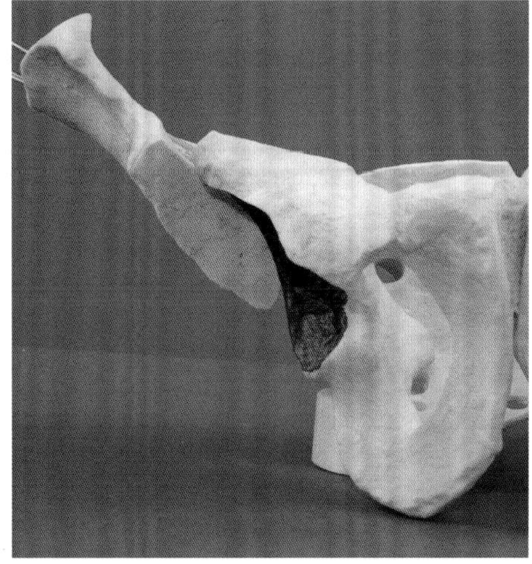

C

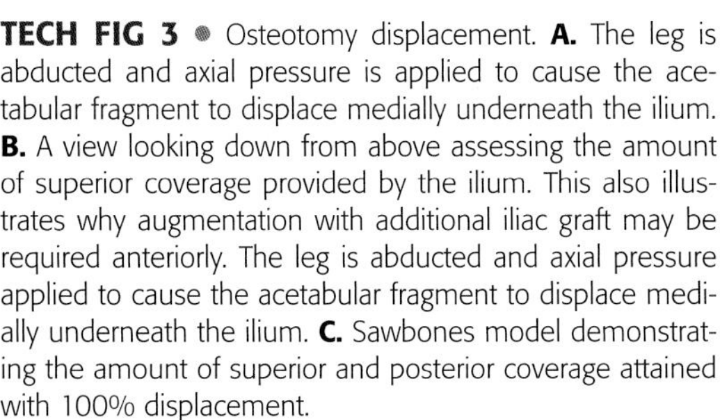

**TECH FIG 3** • Osteotomy displacement. **A.** The leg is abducted and axial pressure is applied to cause the acetabular fragment to displace medially underneath the ilium. **B.** A view looking down from above assessing the amount of superior coverage provided by the ilium. This also illustrates why augmentation with additional iliac graft may be required anteriorly. The leg is abducted and axial pressure applied to cause the acetabular fragment to displace medially underneath the ilium. **C.** Sawbones model demonstrating the amount of superior and posterior coverage attained with 100% displacement.

## Osteotomy Fixation

- The osteotomy is fixed in place with 3.5- or 4.5-mm cortical screws placed either along the iliac crest or along the outer table of the ilium under fluoroscopic guidance directed into the posterior column of the ischium (**TECH FIG 4A,B**).
- If additional coverage is required (especially anterior), a corticocancellous graft is excised from the inner table of the ilium using a saw or osteotome (**TECH FIG 4C**). This fragment is interposed between the hip capsule and the transposed ilium now forming part of the roof of the acetabulum (**TECH FIG 4D**).
- Bone graft may also be placed medially over the distal acetabular fragment to facilitate bony healing.
- Stable reduction through range of motion is confirmed by fluoroscopy before wound closure.
  - It is important to verify in multiple planes of projection that no screw impinges on the hip joint.

A 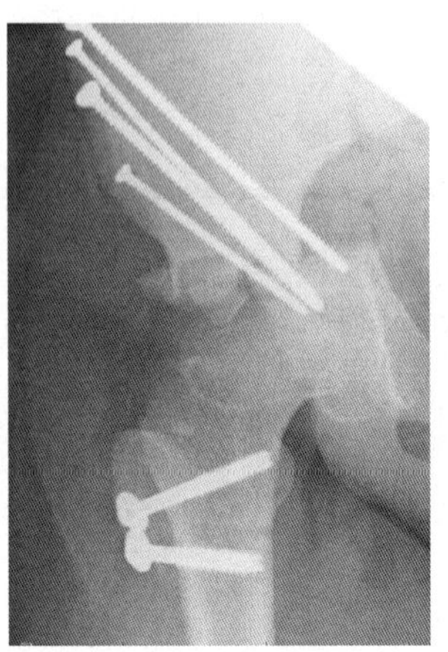

B 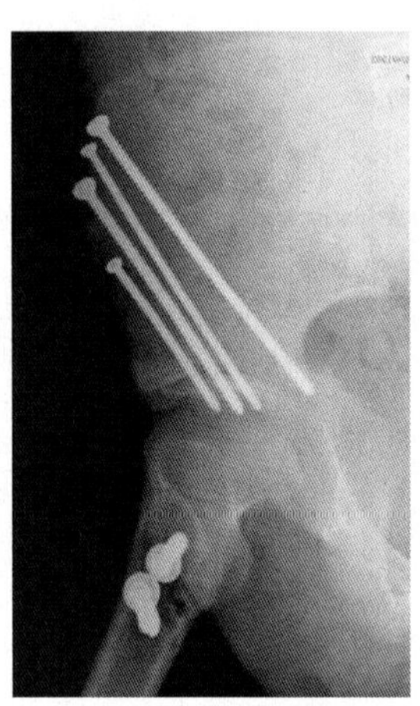

C 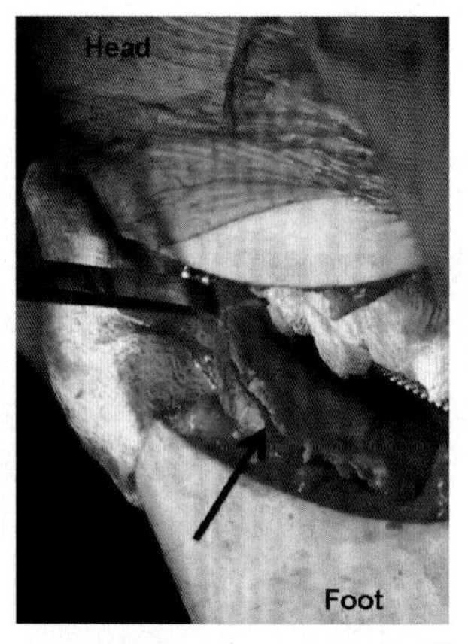


D 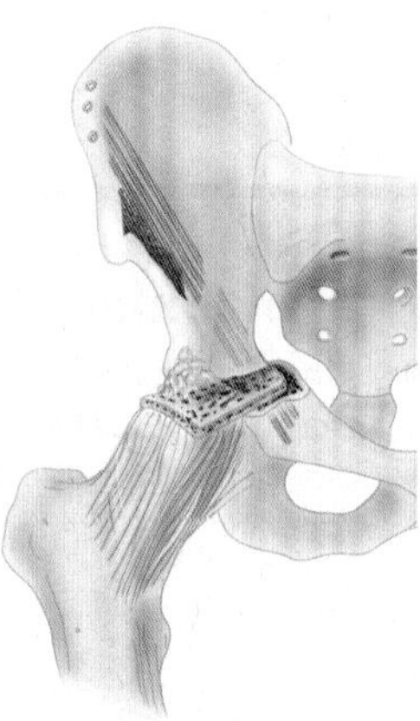

**TECH FIG 4** • **A,B.** AP and frog-leg lateral views of the right hip after fixation of the osteotomy and completion of additional intertrochanteric osteotomy. **C.** Inner table of the ilium is taken for additional anterior coverage autograft (*arrow*). **D.** Final position of osteotomy fragments, iliac crest graft between ilium and hip capsule, and additional cancellous graft placed above.

## Wound Closure

- Drains can be used at the surgeon's discretion.
- The iliac apophysis is closed with heavy, absorbable, interrupted sutures.
- The remainder of the wound is closed in layers.

## PEARLS AND PITFALLS

| | |
|---|---|
| **Indications** | ■ Proper patient selection. Severe arthrosis or proximal migration may be incompletely managed by Chiari osteotomy. Care should be taken when considering this procedure in young patients or in patients with neuromuscular disease as they may have insufficient thickness of ilium to provide adequate coverage. |
| **Osteotomy** | ■ Curving the osteotomy distally and posteriorly toward the sciatic notch maximizes posterior coverage. The more dome-like the osteotomy, the more anterior coverage is afforded. The posterior osteotomy may follow the posterior acetabulum as far distally as the ischial spine. Then it must be carried posteriorly to the notch, exiting proximal to the sacrospinous ligament. Again, the contents of the sciatic notch must be carefully protected by subperiosteal placement of retractors. |
| **Screw fixation** | ■ Screws are placed at the iliac crest for fixation. However, with increased displacement, it may be necessary to start the screws along the outer table of the ilium. They are directed into the posterior column of the ischium under fluoroscopic guidance. |
| **Additional coverage** | ■ A corticocancellous segment of the inner table of the ilium is used as bone graft for augmenting deficient (especially anterior) coverage. |
| **Sciatic nerve** | ■ Careful subperiosteal dissection of the sciatic notch will help to protect the neurovascular contents. We recommend palpation of the posterior edge of the osteotomy after displacement to confirm that there is no soft tissue (sciatic nerve) entrapment. |

## POSTOPERATIVE CARE

- Patients are kept toe-touch weight bearing for 6 weeks.
- Range of motion is allowed from full extension to 70 degrees of flexion.
- Therapy is allowed for gentle passive range of motion within these limits for 6 weeks.
- Weight bearing is advanced with evidence of radiographic healing.
- If trochanteric advancement was performed, active abduction is limited for 6 weeks.
- Patients who have a neuromuscular condition with spasticity or underwent tendon lengthenings in the same surgery are placed in either bilateral long-leg casts held in abduction by a connector bar or knee immobilizers and abduction foam pillow.
- Neuromuscular patients will stay in the immobilization for 3 weeks. After 3 weeks, patients come out of immobilization for gentle passive range of motion and bathing for an additional 3 weeks.

## OUTCOMES

- In general, reported outcomes with follow-up from 11 to 34 years are good to excellent for pain relief.[1,2,4,5,7,8]
- Outcomes are better for younger patients with mobile hips (at least 90 degrees of flexion) and adequate corrected coverage.

## COMPLICATIONS

- Sciatic neurapraxia from sciatic nerve entrapment or injury during osteotomy or neurapraxia of the lateral femoral cutaneous nerve
- Incomplete correction and resubluxation
- Heterotopic ossification
- Infection

## REFERENCES

1. Bailey TE Jr, Hall JE. Chiari medial displacement osteotomy. J Pediatr Orthop 1985;5:635–641.
2. Debnath UK, Guha AR, Karlakki S, et al. Combined femoral and Chiari osteotomies for reconstruction of the painful subluxation or dislocation of the hip in cerebral palsy. A long-term outcome study. J Bone Joint Surg Br 2006;88(10):1373–1378.
3. Delp SL, Bleck EE, Zajac FE, et al. Biomechanical analysis of the Chiari pelvic osteotomy. Preserving hip abductor strength. Clin Orthop Relat Res 1990;(254):189–198.
4. Ito H, Matsuno T, Minami A. Chiari pelvic osteotomy for advanced osteoarthritis in patients with hip dysplasia. J Bone Joint Surg Am 2004;86-A(7):1439–1445.
5. Migaud H, Chantelot C, Giraud F, et al. Long-term survivorship of hip shelf arthroplasty and Chiari osteotomy in adults. Clin Orthop Relat Res 2004;(418):81–86.
6. Murphy SB, Ganz R, Müller M. The prognosis in untreated dysplasia of the hip. A study of radiographic factors that predict the outcome. J Bone Joint Surg 1995;77(7):985–989.
7. Ohashi H, Hirohashi K, Yamano Y. Factors influencing the outcome of Chiari pelvic osteotomy: a long-term follow-up. J Bone Joint Surg Br 2000;82(4):517–525.
8. Windhager R, Pongracz N, Schönecker W, et al. Chiari osteotomy for congenital dislocation and subluxation of the hip. Results after 20 to 34 years follow-up. J Bone Joint Surg Br 1991;73(6):890–895.

# Bernese Periacetabular Osteotomy

Travis H. Matheney and Michael B. Millis

## DEFINITION

- Hip dysplasia is the most common etiology of coxarthrosis, often leading to arthroplasty long before joint replacement can be considered a lifetime solution.[3]
- Surgical realignment of the congruous dysplastic acetabulum can improve or eliminate symptoms for years, sometimes indefinitely, in a majority of appropriately selected patients, even in those with some degree of preoperative arthrosis.[1,3,4,6–8]
- Age limits for this procedure are adolescence (closed triradiate cartilage) to an indefinite upper age limit (limited by preoperative arthrosis and other considerations that might make arthroplasty a better choice).

## ANATOMY

- The acetabulum lies between the anterior and posterior columns of the pelvis.
- The most common area of acetabular deficiency in developmental dysplasia of the hip (DDH) is anterior and lateral.
- The Bernese periacetabular osteotomy (PAO) differs from the triple osteotomy primarily by maintaining the integrity of the posterior column of the pelvis.
- The Bernese PAO uses up to five steps to divide the acetabular fragment from the remainder of the pelvis, allowing multiplanar reorientation.
- Important bony landmarks include the following:
  - Iliopectineal eminence (which marks the medialmost extent of the acetabulum)
  - Infracotyloid groove (just distal to the acetabulum, where the obturator externus tendon lies; this is the site of the anterior ischial osteotomy)
  - Anterior superior iliac spine (ASIS)
  - Apex of the greater sciatic notch
  - Ischial spine
- The posterior column is triangular and thickest just posterior to the acetabulum; it becomes much thinner closer to the sciatic notch. For this reason, the optimal plane for the posterior column is angled obliquely to the medial cortex and perpendicular to the lateral cortex of the ischium–posterior column.

## PATHOGENESIS

- Genetic and developmental causes exist for "developmental dysplasia."
- Neuromuscular: Charcot-Marie-Tooth disease and spastic diplegia
- Posttraumatic: injuries to the triradiate cartilage and aggressive excision of the limbus in the infant hip

## NATURAL HISTORY

- There is a clear correlation between acetabular dysplasia and osteoarthrosis of the hip.
- The more severe the acetabular dysplasia and any subluxation, the earlier the onset of symptoms from arthrosis.
- Murphy et al[5] found that every patient with a lateral center-edge angle less than 16 degrees developed osteoarthritis by age 65 years.

## PATIENT HISTORY AND PHYSICAL FINDINGS

- Key portions of the history include the following:
  - Personal or family history or treatment of DDH
  - History of other hip disorders, including Legg-Calvé-Perthes
  - Trauma
  - Skeletal dysplasias
  - History of cerebral palsy
  - Birth order and weight
  - Description of pain or mechanical symptoms, including location, duration, activity limitation, giving way, "clicking," "catching," and "popping"
- Physical examination should include gait, limb length, assistive devices, and strength.
- Specific hip tests include the following:
  - Trendelenburg test: demonstrates weakness in abductors
  - Anterior apprehension test: A positive result is a subjective noting of "apprehension" or instability by the patient.
  - Anterior impingement test (pain with passive hip flexion, adduction, and internal rotation): test of anterior labral pathology, not just a tear
  - Bicycle test for abductor fatigability
- Range of motion (ROM): Dysplastic hips may demonstrate a relative increase in flexion due to anterior acetabular uncoverage. Decreased ROM with pain may indicate arthrosis.

## IMAGING AND OTHER DIAGNOSTIC STUDIES

- Radiography includes weight-bearing anteroposterior (AP) views of bilateral hips (**FIG 1A**), false profile of hips (**FIG 1B**), and AP views of the hips in maximal abduction and internal rotation (von Rosen view; **FIG 1C**). These studies allow assessment of lateral and anterior coverage of the femoral head as well as congruency of the hip joint. Additionally noted will be the presence of hinge abduction, which is a relative contraindication to PAO.
- Radiographic parameters include the following:
  - Lateral center-edge angle of Wiberg measured from AP view of the hip (lower limits of normal about 25 degrees; see **FIG 1A**)

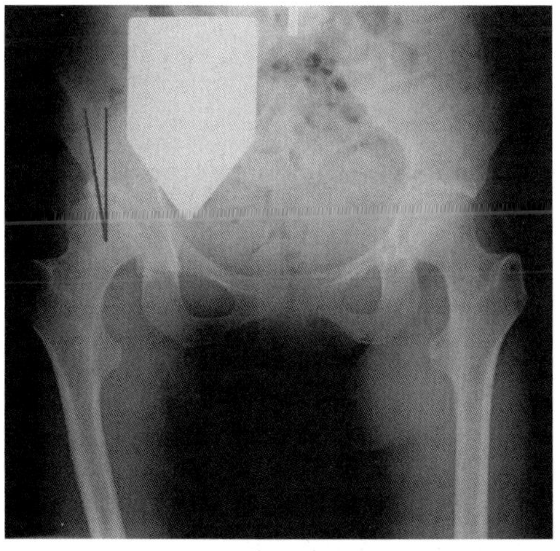
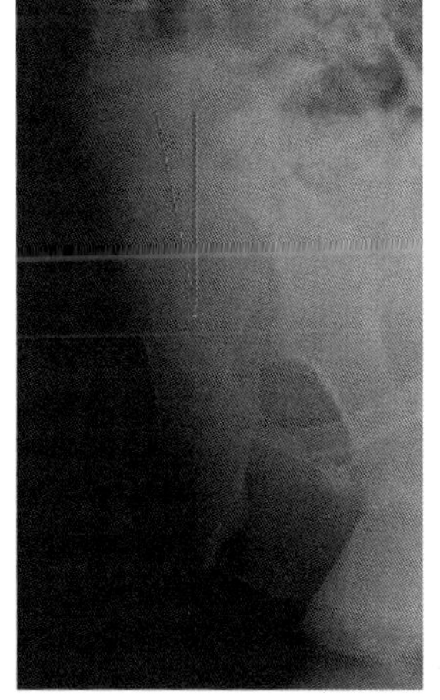
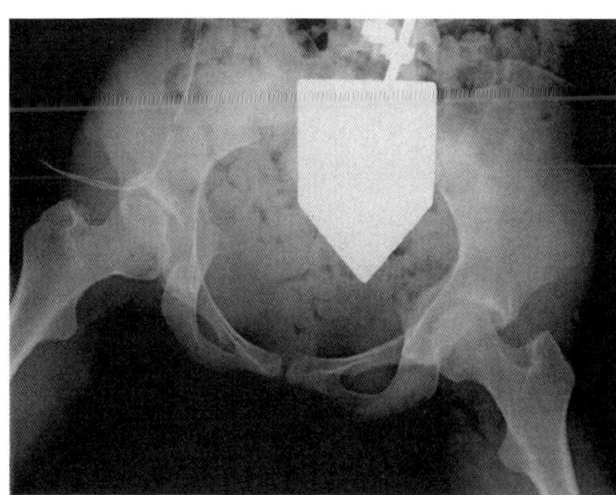
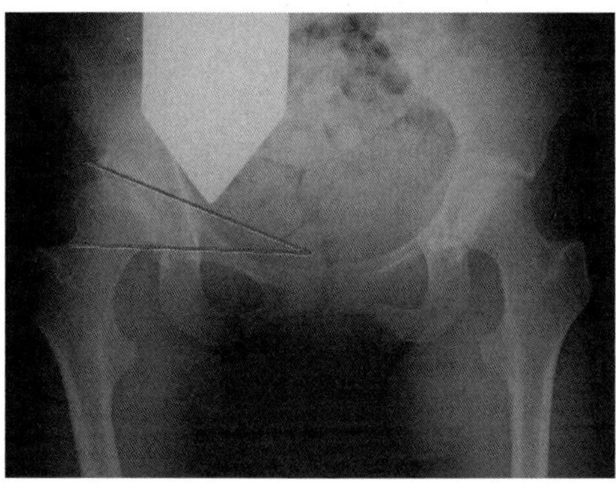

**FIG 1** • **A.** AP view of pelvis and hips. Lateral center-edge angle of Wiberg is marked on right hip. **B.** False-profile view of right hip. Anterior center-edge angle of Lequesne and de Seze is marked. The anterior edge is marked to the edge of the sourcil. **C.** Von Rosen AP view of pelvis with hips in maximal abduction and internal rotation. This is used to assess congruency and mimic the appearance of the hip after reorienting acetabular osteotomy. **D.** AP view of pelvis and hips. The Tönnis acetabular roof angle is marked on the right hip.

  - Anterior center-edge angle of Lequesne and de Seze (lower limits of normal 20 degrees measured on the false-profile view; see **FIG 1B**)
  - Tönnis acetabular roof angle measured on the AP view of the hip (upper limits of normal 10 to 15 degrees; **FIG 1D**)
  - Crossover sign (anterior wall shadow crossing posterior wall shadow on AP view of the pelvis)
  - Assessment of the line of Shenton for breaks indicative of femoral head subluxation
- Computed tomography (CT) scan of both hips with three-dimensional reconstruction as well as with axial slices through the femoral condyles may be of assistance in preoperatively assessing the amount and direction of correction required as well as the potential need for proximal femoral osteotomy.
- Magnetic resonance imaging (MRI) of involved hips with radial sequences centered at the femoral head allows assessment of articular and labral cartilage.
  - Delayed gadolinium-enhanced MRI of cartilage (dGEMRIC) is a recently developed technique that assesses the mechanical damage to the articular cartilage. It has been demonstrated to be a better preoperative predictor than plain radiographs in determining outcome after PAO.[2]

## NONOPERATIVE MANAGEMENT

- Activity and job modification may be of benefit in delaying or mitigating arthritic symptoms.
- Physical therapy may be of some benefit in increasing ROM and strength. To date, there are no data to suggest that a specific therapy regimen can affect the onset of arthritis in the dysplastic hip.

## SURGICAL MANAGEMENT

- Indication: symptomatic, congruous acetabular dysplasia (closed triradiate cartilage) with lateral and anterior center-edge angles 18 degrees or less
- Contraindications: Tönnis osteoarthrosis grade 2 or more (subchondral cysts, significant joint space narrowing), severe limitation of motion secondary to arthrosis, active joint infection

### Preoperative Planning

- Radiographs and MRI are evaluated to assess the following:
  - Degree and character of dysplasia
  - Amount and direction of correction required to normalize the Tönnis acetabular roof angle (0 to 10 degrees), correct subluxation, and improve mechanical stability
- Proximal femoral deformity may also require treatment at time of PAO.
- Presence of acetabular articular or labral lesions (seen on MRI) should also be taken into consideration, as treatment either arthroscopically (before the osteotomy) or intraoperatively through limited arthrotomy may be required for best long-term results.
  - Isolated treatment of a labral lesion in the presence of acetabular dysplasia is contraindicated. Simultaneous acetabular realignment must be considered.
  - The torn acetabular labrum is usually associated with other structural abnormality within the hip (femoroacetabular impingement or DDH), which may also require correction for best results.[9]

- Partial weight-bearing technique is taught preoperatively in preparation for postoperative mobilization.
- For perioperative pain management, we recommended considering either epidural or lumbar plexus catheter placement preoperatively as well as multimodal perioperative analgesia. Catheters are removed the morning of postoperative day 1 or 2.

## Positioning

- The patient is positioned supine on a radiolucent table.
- The operative extremity is prepared and draped free up to the costal margin; the surgeon should be certain to prepare and drape posteriorly to at least the posterior third of the ilium and medially to the umbilicus.

## Approach

- The standard longitudinal anterior Smith-Petersen incision and approach to the hip provides the appropriate access (**FIG 2A**).
- As an alternative, an ilioinguinal (bikini) incision may be used followed by a similar deep approach (**FIG 2B**). This incision typically provides a better cosmetic result but can limit access for the anterior ischial osteotomy. Therefore, we recommend the standard anterior incision for larger and more muscular patients.

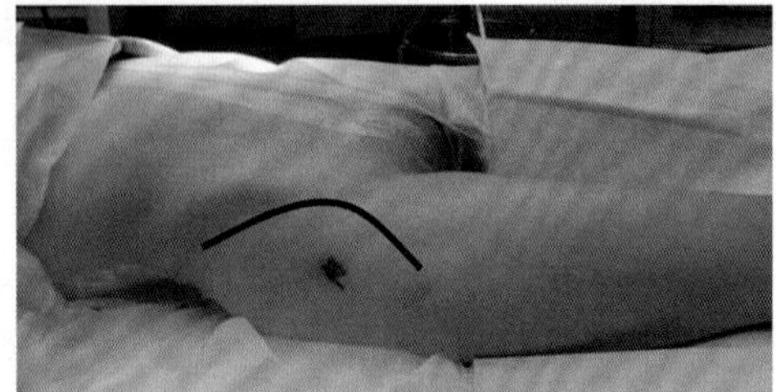
A

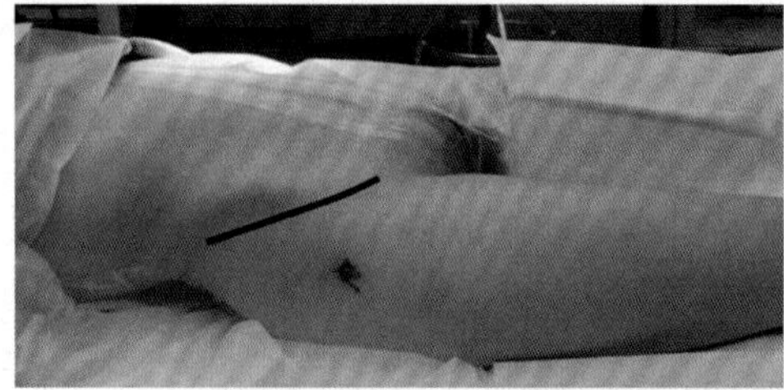
B

**FIG 2** • **A.** Hip with traditional Smith-Petersen incision marked. **B.** Hip with bikini-type incision marked.

TECHNIQUES

## Superficial Dissection

- The skin is incised into subcutaneous tissue.
- The fascia over the external oblique and gluteus medius is identified and incised posterior to the ASIS, and the plane between the two muscles is developed to expose the periosteum over the iliac crest.
- The periosteum is sharply divided over the iliac crest and subperiosteal dissection carried out over the inner table of the ilium. This space is packed with sponges for hemostasis.
- Entry into the tensor fascia lata–sartorius interval is initially accomplished via the compartment of the proximal tensor fascia lata to avoid injury to the lateral femoral cutaneous nerve. The tensor fascia lata is bluntly elevated off the intermuscular septum and the compartment floor is identified proximally until the anterior ilium is palpated.
- Once hemostasis is attained, the ASIS is predrilled with a 2.5-mm drill and the anterior 1- × 1- × 1-cm portion is osteotomized to facilitate the medial dissection and later repair.
    - Alternatively, the sartorius can be taken off with just a thin wafer of bone that will be sewn back in place at the end instead of with a screw.
- Subperiosteal dissection is continued to the anterior inferior iliac spine (AIIS).

## Deep Dissection

- Before proceeding with the deep dissection, it is important to have determined preoperatively whether there is intra-articular pathology that will require performing an arthrotomy to address. Examples include labral tear, perilabral cyst, and femoral head–neck cam lesion. If so, the rectus femoris generally is detached (see in the following text). If however, no intra-articular work is needed, the rectus tendon can be left intact.
- Flexion and adduction of the hip facilitates the deep intrapelvic and superior ramus dissection.
- The reflected head of the rectus femoris is divided at its junction with the direct head (**TECH FIG 1A,B**).
- The direct head and underlying capsular iliacus are elevated as a unit and reflected distally and medially off the underlying joint capsule.
- If one is performing a rectus femoris-sparing PAO, identifying the interval between the capsular portion of the iliacus and the rectus femoris can be a challenge. To assist with this, it is recommended to start within the pelvis dissecting underneath the iliacus there, then following it over the pelvic brim onto the capsule.
- The iliacus, sartorius, and abdominal contents are reflected medially.
- The psoas sheath is opened longitudinally, and the psoas tendon is retracted medially to allow access to the superior pubic ramus medial to the iliopectineal eminence.
- The interval between the medial joint capsule and the iliopsoas tendon is created and sequentially dilated using the tip of a long-handled Mayo scissor, then further by Lane bone levers, with the tips of each palpating the anterior ischium at the infracotyloid groove.
    - Proper placement of the scissor and bone levers can be confirmed with the image intensifier (**TECH FIG 1C,D**).

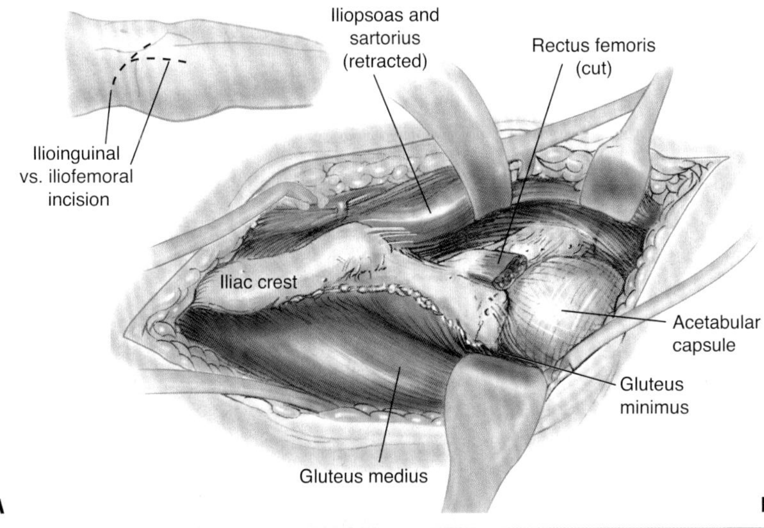


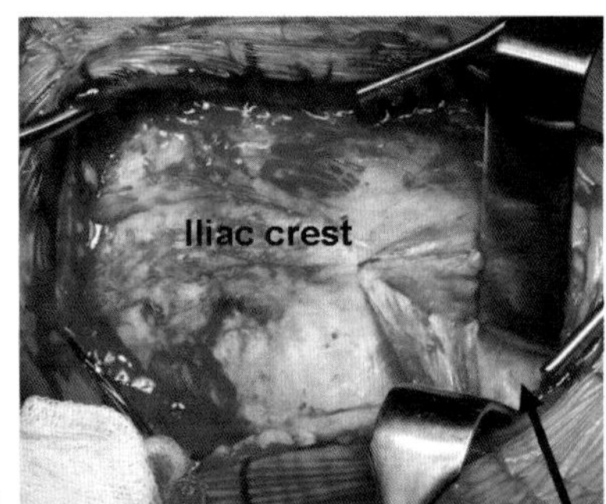


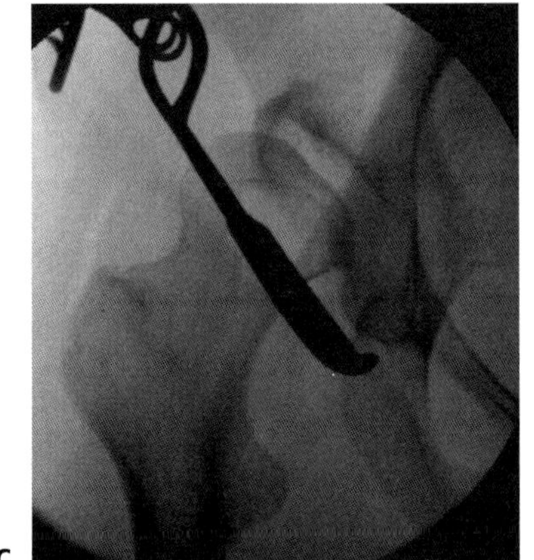


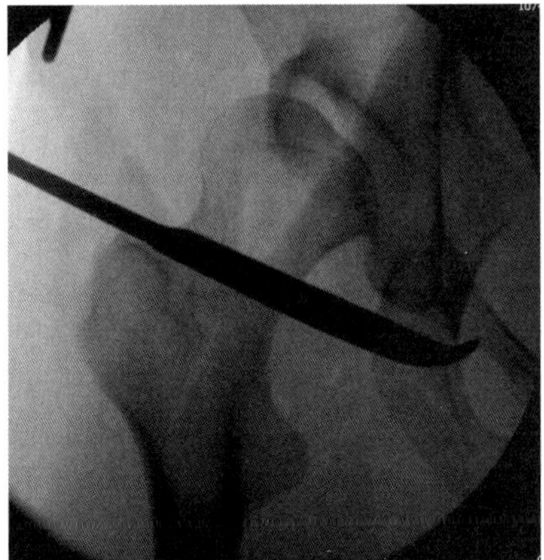


**TECH FIG 1** • **A.** Deep dissection through anterior hip interval. The direct and indirect heads of the rectus femoris have been cut. **B.** Surgical exposure of the anterior hip capsule (*arrow*). The iliac crest is marked in the left half of the wound before subperiosteal dissection of the iliacus. **C,D.** Intraoperative fluoroscopic AP views of the right hip. Lane bone lever is used to first palpate the outer and inner aspects of the anterior ischium.

## Osteotomies

### Anterior Ischial Osteotomy

- Before performing the first osteotomy, it is recommended that one confirms with the anesthesia team that the patient is no longer paralyzed. Without paralytic, direct contact of the sciatic or obturator nerves during any of the osteotomies will elicit a muscular response, warning the surgeon of that they may be in harms way.
- With the hip flexed 45 degrees and slightly adducted, a 30-degree forked, angled bone chisel (Synthes USA, West Chester, PA; in 15- or 20-mm blade widths) is carefully inserted through the previously created interval between the medial capsule and psoas tendon to place its tip in contact with the superior portion of the infracotyloid groove of the anterior ischium, just superior to the obturator externus tendon (**TECH FIG 2A–C**).
- Staying proximal to the obturator externus tendon helps to protect the nearby medial femoral circumflex artery. The medial and lateral aspects of the ischium should be gently palpated with the chisel. Proper chisel placement (about 1 cm below the inferior acetabular lip) is confirmed on AP and oblique projections with the image intensifier (**TECH FIG 2D**).
- The osteotome is impacted in a posterior direction to a depth of 15 to 20 mm and through both medial and lateral cortices of the ischium (**TECH FIG 2E**).
- Care should be taken not to drive the osteotome too deeply out the lateral cortex, as the sciatic nerve is nearby.

### Superior Pubic Ramus Osteotomy

- The hip is kept flexed and adducted to relax the anterior soft tissues.
- The psoas tendon and medial structures are gently retracted medially (**TECH FIG 3A**).
- After circumferential subperiosteal dissection of the ramus, either a spiked Hohmann retractor or a large-gauge Kirschner wire may be impacted into the superior aspect of the ramus at least 1 cm medial to the iliopectineal eminence (**TECH FIG 3B**).
- Blunt Hohmann retractors, Rang retractors, or Lane bone levers are placed anteriorly and posteriorly as well as inferior to the ramus to protect the obturator nerve and artery.
- The osteotomy is perpendicular to the long axis of the ramus when viewed from above but oblique from distal medial to proximal lateral when viewed from the front and may be carried out either by passing a Gigli saw around the ramus and sawing upward away from the retractors or by impacting a straight osteotome just lateral to the spiked Hohmann or Kirschner wire. In the former method, the Gigli saw is passed with the aid of a Satinsky vascular clamp.
  - The key to this osteotomy is to *stay medial* to the iliopectineal eminence and avoid entering the medial acetabulum (**TECH FIG 3C**).

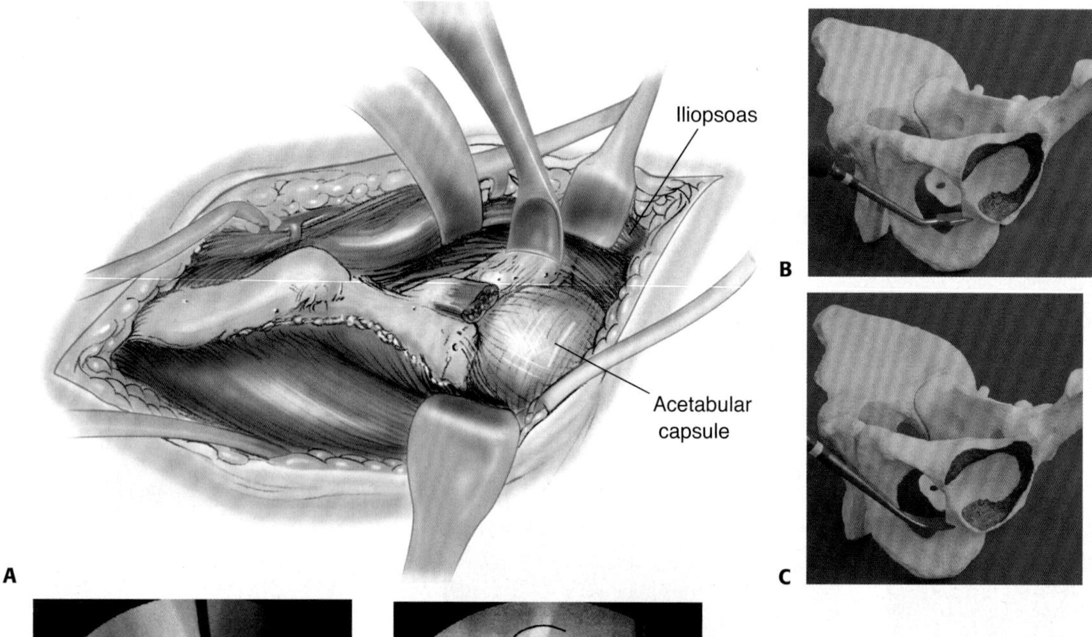


D E

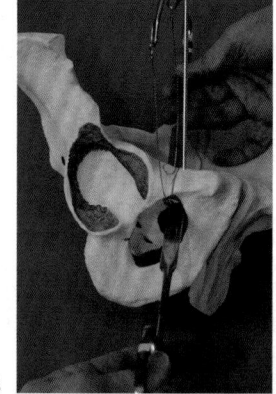

**TECH FIG 2** • **A.** Surgical exposure and placement of osteotome for ischial cut. The osteotome is placed medial to the joint capsule and lateral to the iliopsoas. **B,C.** Bone models demonstrating the planned position of the osteotome for the ischial cut: Ganz angled chisel (**B**) and Mast curved chisel (**C**). **D,E.** Intraoperative fluoroscopic AP view of right hip with Ganz 30-degree osteotome (**D**) at the anterior ischium and false-profile view of right hip with Mast curved chisel (**E**) seated into anterior ischium. The sciatic notch and ischial spine are outlined in *black*. Proper direction of this cut should also be confirmed on fluoroscopic false-profile view.

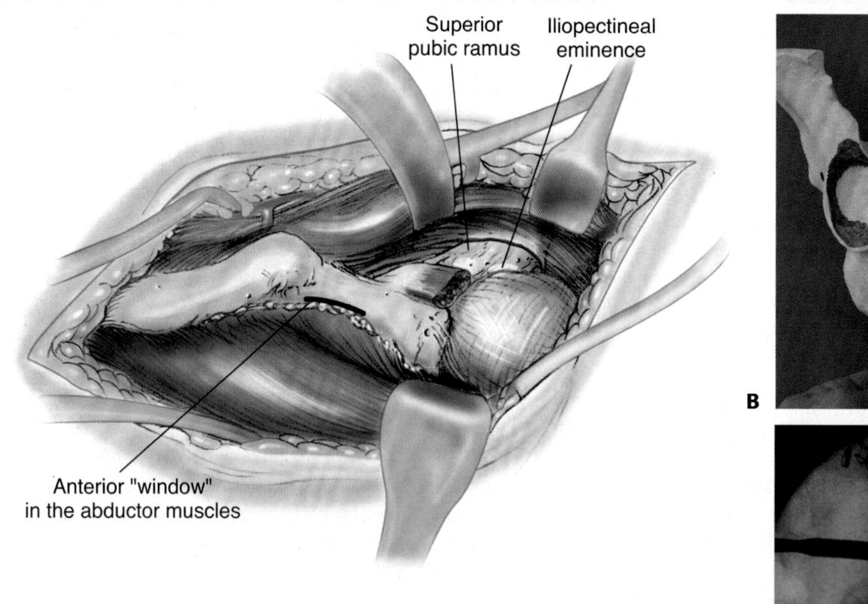


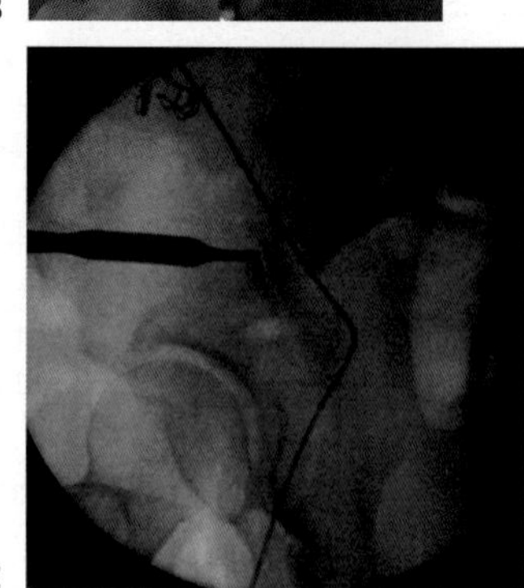


**TECH FIG 3** • **A.** Anterior approach. The superior pubic ramus is exposed and the iliopsoas is retracted medially. **B.** Bone model demonstrating the superior ramus osteotomy. The Lane bone levers are placed on either side of the ramus and a Kirschner wire is placed as a retractor. The iliopectineal eminence is marked with a *circle*. **C.** Intraoperative fluoroscopic false-profile view of hip. A small Hohmann retractor is placed under the abductors aiming toward the apex of the sciatic notch.

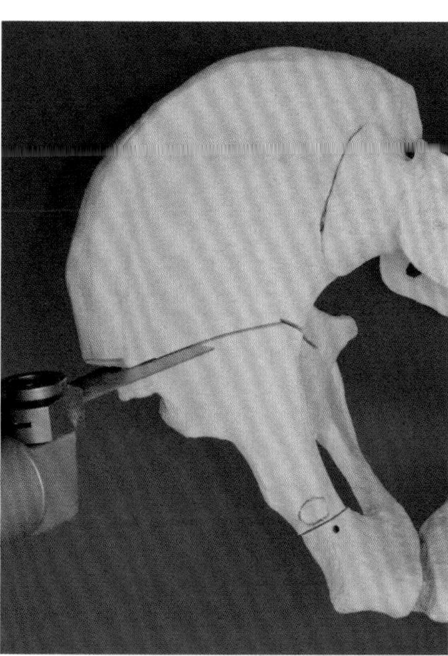

**TECH FIG 4** ● Bone model demonstrating the saw cut of the ilium aiming toward a point about 1 cm above the iliopectineal line.

- Arthrotomy and intracapsular inspection: At a point before all osteotomies are completed, an arthrotomy may be performed to identify and treat intra-articular lesions such as a torn labrum or impingement lesions of the femoral head and neck.
  - This is closed loosely with simple, interrupted absorbable suture before proceeding with the remainder of the osteotomies.

## Supra-acetabular Iliac Osteotomy

- A 1.5- to 2-mm subperiosteal window is started beneath the anterior abductors just distal to the ASIS without disturbing the abductor origin.
- The leg is slightly abducted and extended to allow atraumatic subperiosteal dissection using a narrow elevator posteriorly toward, but not into, the apex of the greater sciatic notch.
- A narrow, long, spiked Hohmann retractor is placed in this window. Correct placement is confirmed with image intensifier; in the lateral projection, the spike of the Hohmann should point toward the apex of the sciatic notch (**TECH FIG 3C**).
- The iliacus and abdominal contents are retracted medially with a reverse Hohmann with its tip on the quadrilateral surface.
- Under direct vision, the iliac osteotomy is performed with an oscillating saw and cooling irrigation in line with the Hohmann retractor until reaching a point about 1 cm above the iliopectineal line (well anterior to the notch). This end point of the iliac saw cut represents the posterosuperior corner of the PAO. This corner is also the starting point of the posterior column osteotomy, which will be midway between the sciatic notch and posterior acetabulum (**TECH FIG 4**).
- At this point, a single Schanz screw on T-handled chuck is inserted into the acetabular fragment distal and parallel to the iliac saw cut, well above the dome of the acetabulum, into a hole predrilled with a 3.2-mm drill.

## Posterior Column Osteotomy

- The leg is once again flexed and adducted to relax the medial soft tissues.
- A reverse blunt Hohmann retractor is placed medially with the tip on the ischial spine. Dissection into the sciatic notch is neither necessary nor recommended.
- The osteotomy is made through the medial cortex with a long, straight 1.5-cm osteotome. It extends from the posterior end of the iliac saw cut, passing over the iliopectineal line, through the medial quadrilateral plate, parallel to the anterior edge of the sciatic notch on iliac oblique fluoroscopy, and is directed toward the ischial spine (**TECH FIG 5A**).
- This osteotomy must extend at least 4 cm below the iliopectineal line to avoid entry into the acetabulum when completing the

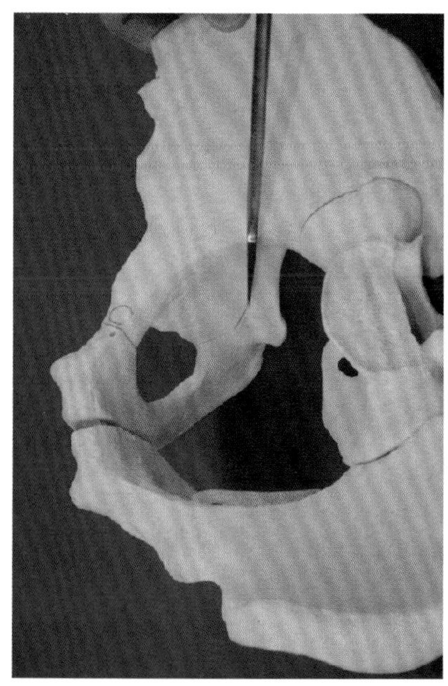
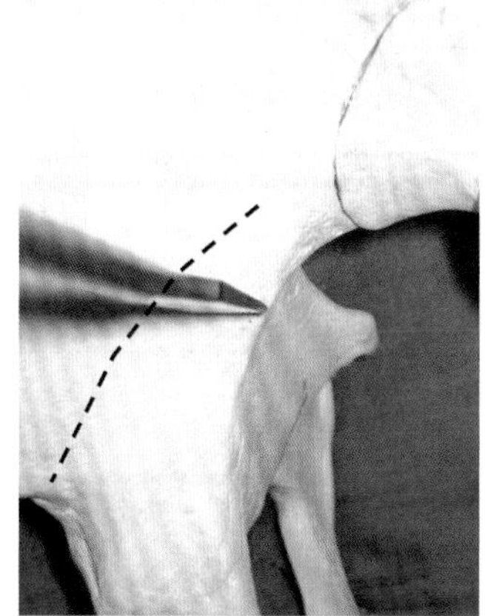
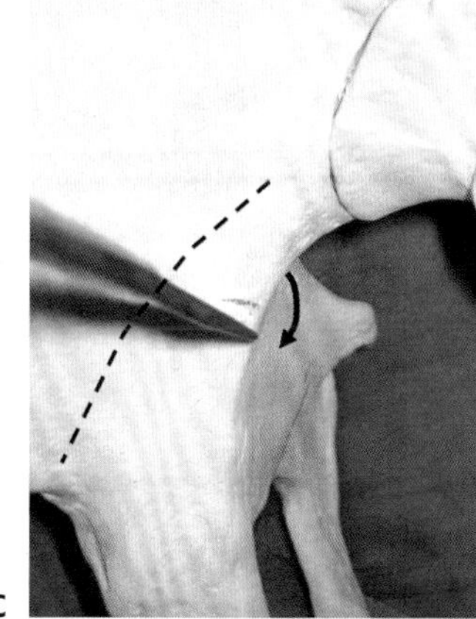

A B C

**TECH FIG 5** ● **A.** Bone model demonstrating the division of the posterior column. **B,C.** The incorrect (**B**) and the correct (**C**) angles of the osteotome for division of the posterior column. The *dotted line* indicates the relative position of the acetabulum and lateral aspect of the ischium. The proper angle of the osteotome is *away* from the sciatic notch about 10 to 15 degrees. *(continued)*

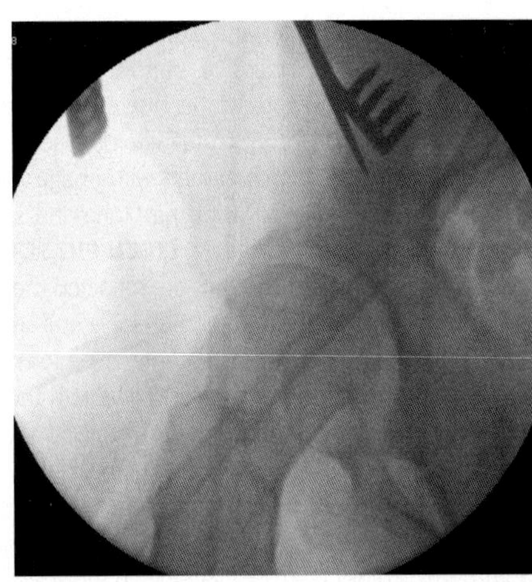

**TECH FIG 5** • *(continued)* **D.** Intraoperative fluoroscopic false-profile view of the right hip. Division of the posterior column is performed here. The borders of the osteotomy (acetabulum anteriorly and sciatic notch posteriorly) should be clearly visible to avoid intra-articular or intranotch extension of the osteotomy.

final (posteroinferior) infra-acetabular osteotomy. This posterior cut is made first through the medial, then second through the lateral wall of the ischium.

- The ischium is wider here than at its anterior extent. If pictured from above, it resembles a triangle with the narrower apex at the anterior edge of the sciatic notch. Therefore, the surgeon should not place the osteotome perpendicular to the medial quadrilateral plate. Instead, the free medial edge of the osteotome should be tipped 10 to 15 degrees *away* from the sciatic notch to create a more true coronal plane osteotomy, perpendicular to the *lateral* cortex of the posterior column (**TECH FIG 5B,C**).

- Correct angulation and positioning are once again confirmed by the image intensifier (**TECH FIG 5D**).
  - If your initial anterior ischial osteotomy was placed sufficiently deep, it is possible to have this osteotomy propagate into your anterior osteotomy and potentially avoid the need for the "completion" osteotomy described in the next step.

## Completion Osteotomy

- The final osteotomy is a completion osteotomy of the posteroinferomedial corner of quadrilateral plate connecting the anterior and posterior ischial cuts.
- A 30-degree long-handled chisel is used to connect these two prior osteotomies (**TECH FIG 6**).
- A key point: The blade is placed to connect the prior cuts, and the osteotome face should *not* be more than 50 degrees off the quadrilateral plate. This will prevent accidentally aiming anteriorly into the acetabulum.

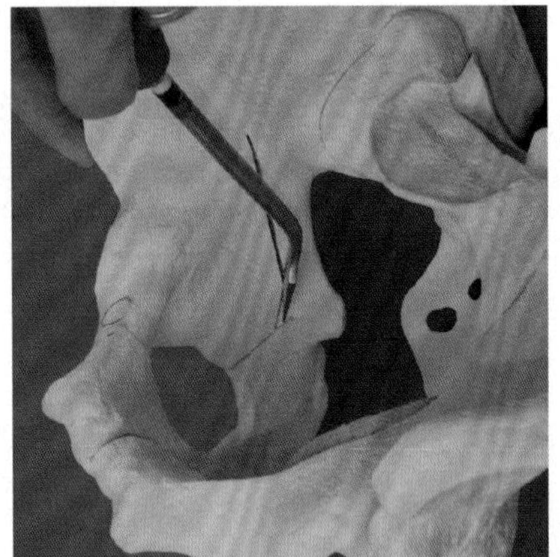

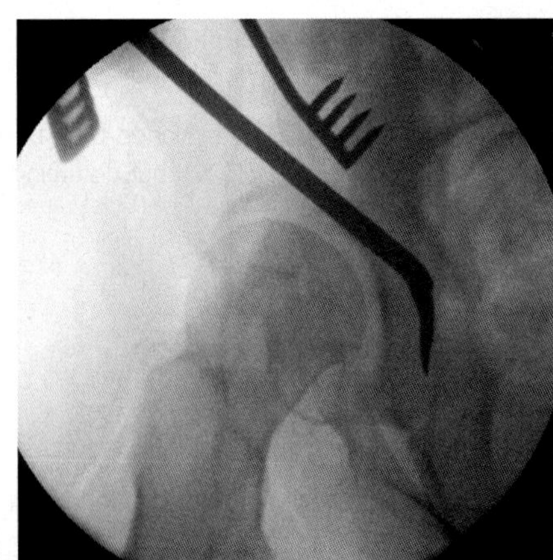

**TECH FIG 6** • **A.** Bone model of right pelvis demonstrating the final cut with a bent osteotome to connect the anterior ischial and posterior column osteotomies. **B.** Intraoperative fluoroscopic false-profile view showing proper positioning of the osteotome.

# Acetabular Displacement

- A 1-inch straight Lambotte chisel is placed into the supra-acetabular iliac saw cut to both confirm completion of the lateral cortex osteotomy and protect the cancellous bone above the acetabulum during displacement.
- The tines of a Weber bone clamp are placed onto the superior ramus portion of the acetabular fragment in such a way as to place its handle anterior and in contact with the Schanz screw (**TECH FIG 7A**).
- A lamina spreader is placed into the iliac osteotomy between the posterosuperior intact ilium and the Lambotte chisel anteriorly.
- While gently opening the lamina spreader, the Schanz screw and Weber clamp are used to mobilize the acetabular fragment. It is important to ascertain whether the posterior and anterior osteotomies are complete; otherwise, the fragment will not

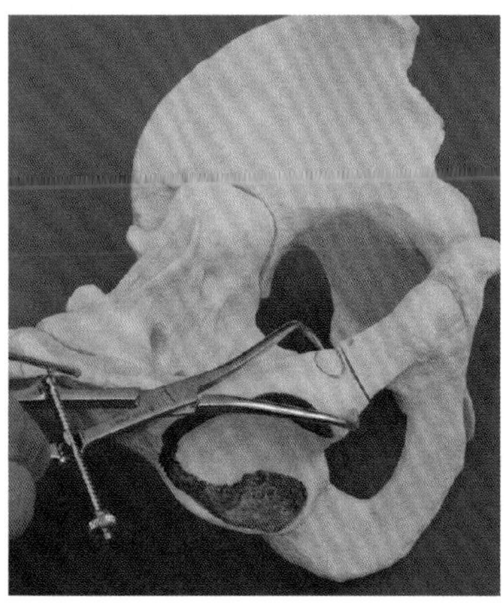
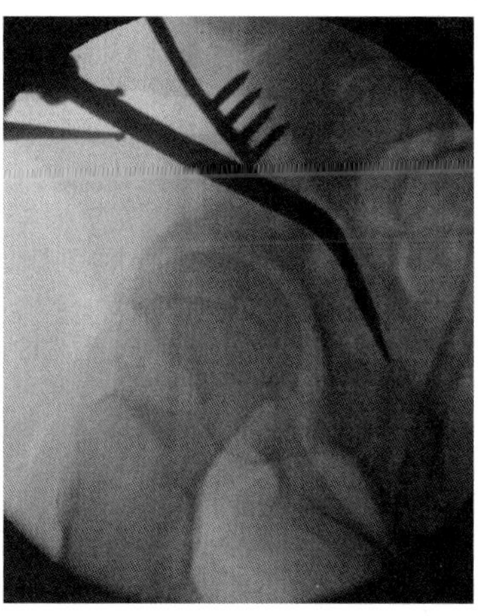
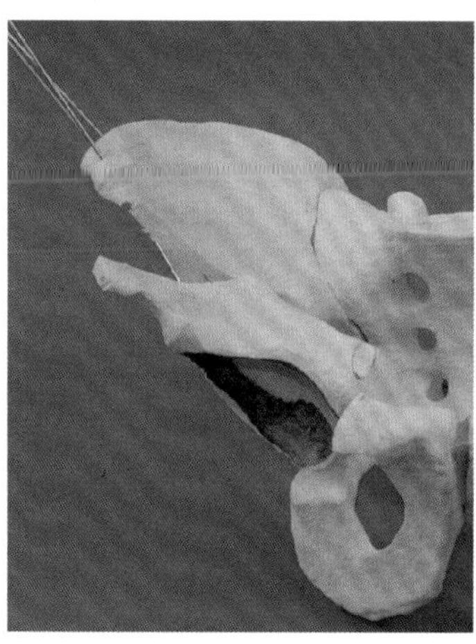

**TECH FIG 7** • **A.** Bone model showing placement of Schanz screw (*far left*) and large bone-holding clamp for manipulation of acetabular fragment. The bone clamp is placed anterior to the Schanz screw. **B.** Intraoperative fluoroscopic false-profile view of right hip. Seen here is displacement of the acetabular fragment with a lamina spreader (*top*) and use of an angled chisel from medial to lateral to find areas where the osteotomies are not complete. **C.** Sawbones model showing acetabular fragment placement. The posteroinferior corner of the fragment is impacted into the superior iliac wing and its prominent anterior spike is roughly in line with the intact iliac crest.

freely rotate and the common outcome will be distal and lateral displacement as you hinge on the lateral, intact cortices. These cuts can be inspected with a narrow or broad 30-degree chisel (**TECH FIG 7B**).

- Once the fragment is completely free, it may be positioned to obtain the desired correction. As previously noted, the most common deficiency is anterior and lateral. Therefore, the most commonly used maneuvers are to lift the acetabular fragment slightly toward the ceiling, creating an initial displacement, followed by a three-step movement of lateral, distal, and internal rotation.
  - When performed properly, the posteroinferior corner of the acetabular fragment should be impacted slightly into the superior intact iliac cut and the prominent superior tip of the acetabular fragment should be roughly in line with the superior intact iliac crest (**TECH FIG 7C**).
- The radiographic "teardrop" and its relation to the femoral head after fragment positioning should be elevated and tilted laterally commensurate with the amount of lateral correction.
  - It is commonly necessary to medialize the acetabular fragment a little once the desired anterolateral coverage is obtained to recreate the proper position of the femoral head in relation to the medial pelvis. This will maintain proper biomechanical position of the femur in relation to the pelvis.

## Acetabular Fixation

- Once the desired acetabular position is obtained, 3/32- or 7/64-inch smooth Kirschner wires (the approximate diameter of a 2.5- and 3.5-mm drill bits) are placed proximal to distal through the ilium and into the fragment in a divergent pattern.
- At this point, we perform a final fragment position check in the AP and false-profile views (**TECH FIG 8A,B**).
  - Importantly, in the false-profile view, we check the anterior femoral head coverage in full extension and at 100 degrees of flexion (**TECH FIG 8C**). In the former view, the sourcil should be roughly horizontal, the femoral head should be well covered, and the line of Shenton should be intact. The false-profile view is to confirm that we have neither overcovered the femoral head nor created impingement from a femoral-sided deformity.
  - If there is less than 90 degrees of flexion on palpation or radiograph, it may be necessary to either reposition the fragment or address femoral-sided deformity.
- The Kirschner wires are measured for depth and length and then replaced with either 3.5- or 4.5-mm cortical screws.
- The image intensifier is used to confirm extra-articular placement of all screws (**TECH FIG 8D,E**).
- An additional "home-run" screw may be placed anterior to posterior from the AIIS posteriorly into the inferior ilium if required for stability (especially in patients who are ligamentously lax or have a neuromuscular condition or poor bone quality). We prefer not to use this screw unless necessary, as it is our practice to remove these screws once bony healing is confirmed for screw head irritation or in case MRI is to be performed at a later point.
- The anterior iliac prominence of the acetabular fragment is trimmed and used for bone graft.
- Gelfoam may be placed along osteotomy sites to assist with hemostasis.

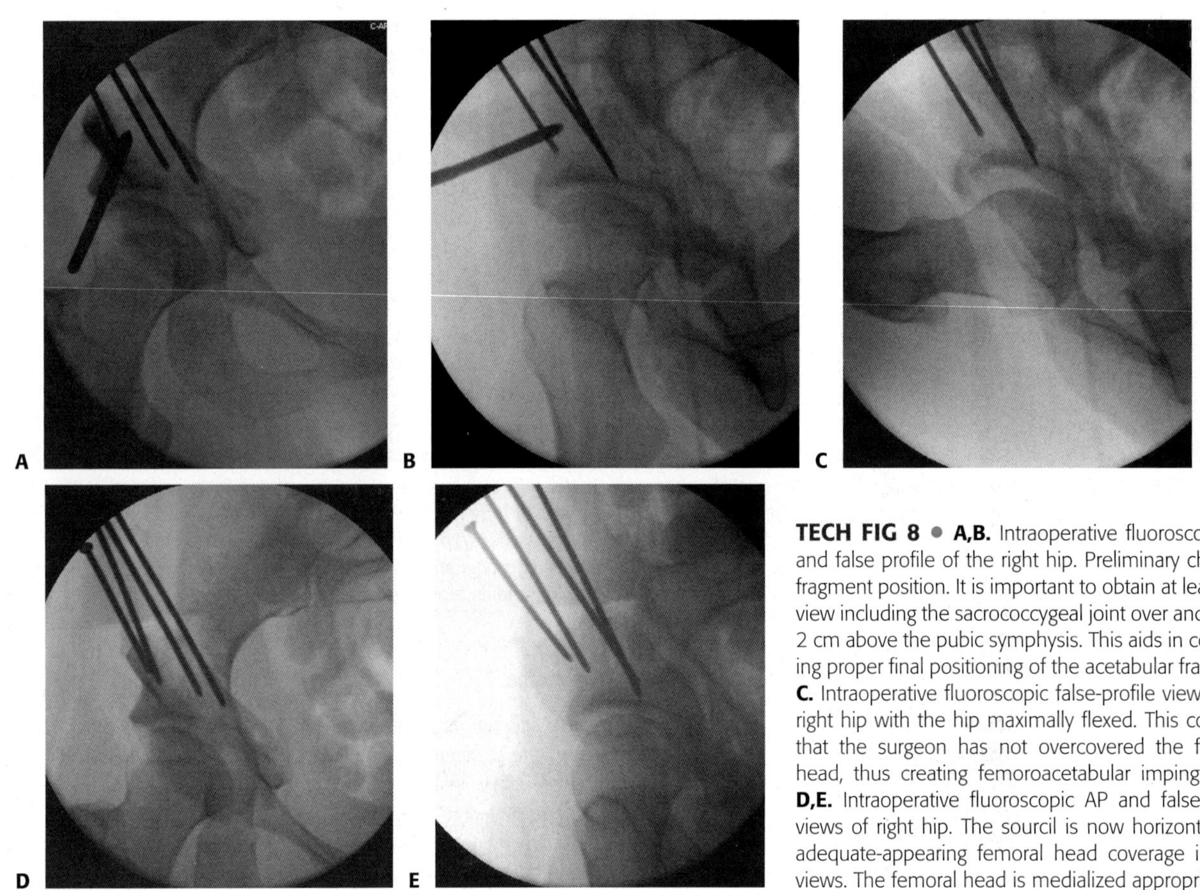

**TECH FIG 8 • A,B.** Intraoperative fluoroscopic AP and false profile of the right hip. Preliminary check of fragment position. It is important to obtain at least one view including the sacrococcygeal joint over and about 2 cm above the pubic symphysis. This aids in confirming proper final positioning of the acetabular fragment. **C.** Intraoperative fluoroscopic false-profile view of the right hip with the hip maximally flexed. This confirms that the surgeon has not overcovered the femoral head, thus creating femoroacetabular impingement. **D,E.** Intraoperative fluoroscopic AP and false-profile views of right hip. The sourcil is now horizontal with adequate-appearing femoral head coverage in both views. The femoral head is medialized appropriately.

## Wound Closure

- All sponges are removed, and wounds are irrigated copiously.
- Suction drains are placed under the iliacus.
- The ASIS osteotomy (if performed) is reattached either by using a 3.5-mm, partially threaded cancellous screw and washer or by being sewn back with heavy, absorbable suture passed through the thinner wafer.
- Careful attention is paid to proper, tight closure over the iliac crest. This is accomplished by predrilling holes in the iliac crest to facilitate passage of heavy, absorbable sutures to reattach the abductor, iliacus, and external oblique musculature.
- The remainder of the wound is closed in layers.

## PEARLS AND PITFALLS

| | |
|---|---|
| **Patient selection** | ■ Appropriate patient selection is paramount.<br>■ Risk factors for failure include older age, poor congruency, decreased joint space (<2 mm), and advanced arthrosis.<br>■ Presence of a labral tear preoperatively may also be an indicator of degeneration, more than may be apparent on plain radiographs. |
| **Pubic osteotomy** | ■ The hip should be flexed 40–50 degrees for making the pubis osteotomy, which takes tension off the iliopsoas and improves access to the brim of the pelvis. |
| **Ischial osteotomy** | ■ If the medial joint is entered while attempting to gain access for the ischial cut, the surgeon can open the psoas sheath and try a second approach dissecting through the floor of the sheath. This technique can be helpful in reestablishing an extra-articular dissection to the ischium.<br>■ Straying too medial risks injury to the neurovascular bundle. |

| | |
|---|---|
| **Iliac osteotomy** | ■ In general, given true supine positioning of the pelvis and patient, the iliac wing osteotomy will be roughly directed perpendicular to the floor. This sighting technique gives a second visual reference, which, in combination with intraoperative imaging, will aid in proper positioning of the osteotomy. |
| **Incomplete osteotomies** | ■ Connecting the inferior ischial (infracotyloid) osteotomy and the posterior ischial cuts may require a medial to lateral osteotome cut through their medial junction. This is most commonly necessary when the lateral portion of these osteotomies is incomplete and the finding is an inability to freely move the acetabular fragment at the initial completion of all planned osteotomies. |
| **Schanz screw placement** | ■ The Schanz pin (screw) should be placed nearly in line with and 1–1.5 cm below the iliac wing osteotomy. In poorer quality bone, it may be necessary to place the screw closer to the acetabular subchondral bone. Additionally, the acetabular fragment should be mobilized by using both the Schanz pin and the bone clamp holding the pubic portion of the free fragment. |

## POSTOPERATIVE CARE

- Partial weight bearing is reviewed by a physical therapist.
  - Out-of-bed mobilization is permitted on the first postoperative day if a lumbar plexus block is used; day 2 or 3 if an epidural catheter is used.
- Weight bearing is progressed from partial to full, typically by 4 to 6 weeks with radiographic healing and return of abductor strength.
- ROM is limited to 90 degrees of flexion; 10 degrees from full extension; and 10 degrees of adduction, abduction, and rotation for the first 4 to 6 weeks.
- Resistive exercises are avoided for 3 months.
- Patients older than 16 years are given either low-molecular-weight heparin or warfarin for 4 to 6 weeks.
- Nonsteroidal anti-inflammatories are avoided.

## OUTCOMES

- Outcomes are generally good to excellent in the appropriately selected patient.
- Hips with minimal arthrosis (more than 2 mm of joint space and no significant subchondral changes) in younger (younger than 35 years old) patients have demonstrated significant improvement in Harris hip and Merle D'Aubigne scores that can last at least 20 years.[1,3,4,6–8]
- Hips with moderate to advanced arthrosis in older patients can still show significant improvement in symptoms. However, their symptom relief may be shorter lived, requiring conversion to either a surface replacement or total hip arthroplasty.

## COMPLICATIONS

- Sciatic or lateral femoral cutaneous nerve palsy
- Postoperative wound hematoma requiring return to operating room
- Wound infection
- Nonunion of pubic ramus
- Heterotopic ossification
- Vascular injury
- Intra-articular osteotomy
- Malalignment of fragment leading to insufficient correction or overcorrection

## REFERENCES


1. Clohisy JC, Barrett SE, Gordon JE, et al. Periacetabular osteotomy for the treatment of severe acetabular dysplasia. J Bone Joint Surg Am 2005;87(2):254–259.
2. Cunnigham T, Jessel R, Zurakowski D, et al. Delayed gadolinium-enhanced magnetic resonance imaging of cartilage to predict early failure of Bernese periacetabular osteotomy for hip dysplasia. J Bone Joint Surg Am 2006;88(7):1540–1548.
3. Ganz R, Leunig M, Leunig-Ganz K, et al. The etiology of osteoarthritis of the hip: an integrated mechanical concept. Clin Orthop Relat Res 2008;466:264–272.
4. Millis MB, Kim YJ. Rationale of osteotomy and related procedures for hip preservation: a review. Clin Orthop Relat Res 2002;(405):108–121.
5. Murphy SB, Ganz R, Muller M. The prognosis in untreated dysplasia of the hip. A study of radiographic factors that predict the outcome. J Bone Joint Surg Am 1995;77(7):985–989.
6. Peters CL, Erickson JA, Hines JL. Early results of the Bernese periacetabular osteotomy: the learning curve at an academic medical center. J Bone Joint Surg Am 2006;88(9):1920–1926.
7. Steppacher SD, Tannast M, Ganz R, et al. Mean 20-year followup of Bernese periacetabular osteotomy. Clin Orthop Relat Res 2008;466:1633–1644.
8. Trousdale RT, Ekkernkamp A, Ganz R. Periacetabular and intertrochanteric osteotomy for the treatment of osteoarthrosis in dysplastic hips. J Bone Joint Surg Am 1995;77(1):73–85.
9. Wenger DE, Kendell KR, Miner MR, et al. Acetabular labral tears rarely occur in the absence of bony abnormalities. Clin Orthop Relat Res 2004;(426):145–150.

# Surgical Dislocation of the Hip

**Farshad Adib and Young-Jo Kim**

## DEFINITION

- Surgical dislocation of the hip can be done safely to treat a number of conditions, including femoroacetabular impingement (FAI), labral tears, chondral injuries, reduction of femoral neck fractures, femoral head, acetabular fractures, excision of tumors, reduction of acute severe slipped capital femoral epiphysis (SCFE), or any condition that requires wide complete access to the hip joint.[14,15]
- There is little morbidity associated with this procedure, and avascular necrosis of the femoral head is a rare complication.[5]
- This technique allows functional assessment of motion intraoperatively which is the most critical step in the treatment of FAI. Majority of reoperations after FAI treatment is due to under- or overcorrection.[4]
- Also, surgical hip dislocation approach is comprehensive enough to assess and treat extra-articular impingement at the same time.[16]

## ANATOMY

- The blood supply to the femoral head is mainly from the medial femoral circumflex artery (MFCA) (**FIG 1A**).[17]
- The intact external rotator muscles, most notably the obturator externus muscle, protect the MFCA during the dislocation (**FIG 1B**).[7]

## PATHOGENESIS

- In FAI, anatomic deformity leads to abnormal contact between the proximal femur and the acetabular rim at the terminal extent of motion. This repetitive collision damages the soft tissue structures within the joint.[3]
- In cam impingement, an abnormal prominence on the femoral neck passes into the hip beneath the labrum and mechanically damages the labrum and cartilage of the acetabulum.
- Pincer impingement occurs with overcoverage of the acetabular rim impinging on the anterior femoral neck or head–neck junction with terminal flexion.
  - Both cam and pincer impingement can, and frequently do, coexist.
- The early chondral and labral lesions that occur in physically active adolescents and young adults can progress and result in degenerative joint disease of the hip.
- Causes of FAI can be idiopathic, secondary to an SCFE, anterior overcoverage of the hip with a retroverted acetabulum, residual deformity from Perthes disease, or posttraumatic changes.

## NATURAL HISTORY

- A pistol grip deformity of the femoral head has been associated with early arthrosis of the hip.[9]
- End-stage osteoarthrosis of the hip, once thought to be mainly idiopathic, is now believed to be a result of mild deformities similar to those caused by childhood diseases of the hip such as developmental hip dysplasia, SCFE, and Legg-Calvé-Perthes.[1]

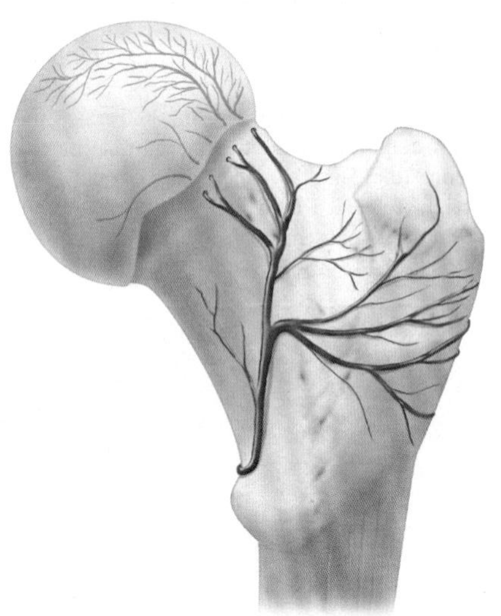


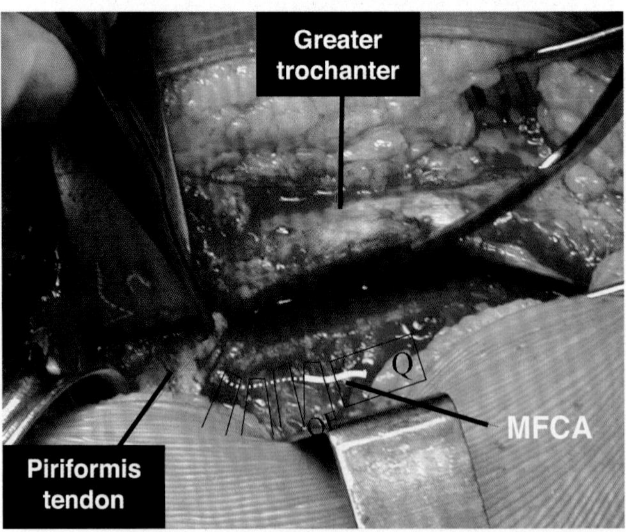


**FIG 1** • **A.** Vascular anatomy of the femoral head. Note the proximity of the terminal branches of the MFCA to the insertion of the piriformis tendon. **B.** Intraoperative photograph showing the path of the MFCA over and behind the intact short external rotators, including the quadratus femoris (*Q*) and the obturator externus (*OE*).

## PATIENT HISTORY AND PHYSICAL FINDINGS

- FAI usually presents in active adolescents or young adults with slow onset groin pain, which may be exacerbated by athletic activities.
- Many patients have difficulty sitting for long periods and adjust their seating posture to decrease lumbar lordosis to allow less flexion at the hips. Frequently, they complain of difficulty getting into or out of a car.
- There can be a family history of hip pain, early arthrosis, or hip arthroplasty.
- Patients may walk with an antalgic gait, favoring the side of impingement. A foot progression angle externally rotated may indicate a chronic SCFE or femoral retroversion.
- The impingement test, if positive, shows reproducible groin pain with internal rotation, which is relieved with external rotation.
- The physical examination should include both flexion and internal rotation range-of-motion tests.
  - Patients with impingement will have less than 90 degrees of true hip flexion.
  - Patients with impingement will have less internal rotation in flexion than extension and may have a compensatory external rotation of the hip as it is flexed.
- Radiographic findings of FAI are common in the normal, healthy population; therefore, it is paramount that good clinical–radiographic correlation be done. Additionally, other causes of hip pain such as osteoid osteoma, stress fracture, osteonecrosis are ruled out.

## IMAGING AND OTHER DIAGNOSTIC STUDIES

- Plain radiographs should include an anteroposterior (AP) view of the pelvis and a lateral view of the hip (**FIG 2A,B**).

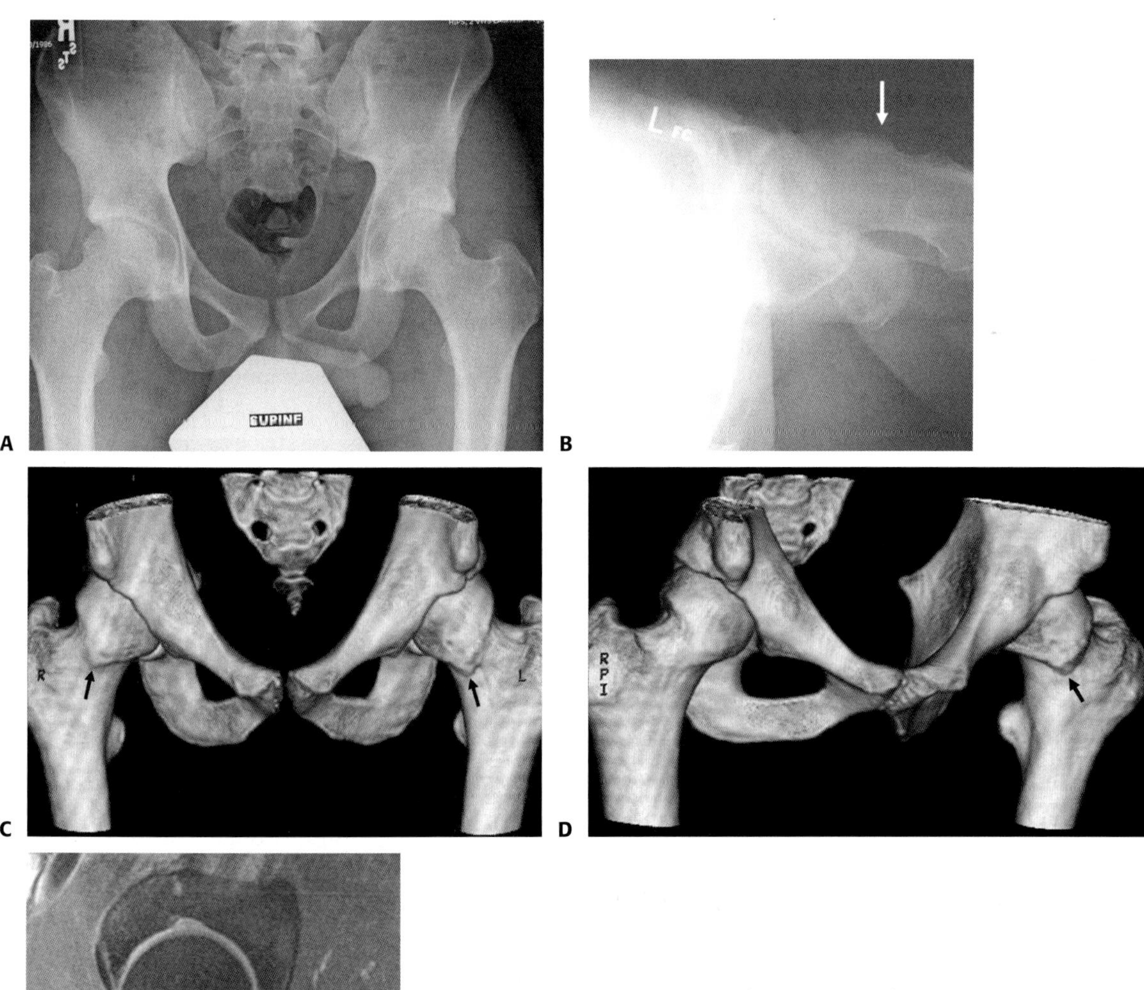


**FIG 2** • AP pelvis (**A**) and true lateral (**B**) radiographs which show the lack of femoral head–neck offset anteriorly (*arrow* in **B**) that is causing cam impingement. 3-D reconstructions of the same pelvis from an AP (**C**) and a slightly left rotated (**D**) perspective. The large "bumps" (*arrows*) obscuring the anterior femoral head–neck junction account for the lack of offset appreciated in **B**. **E.** T1-weighted sagittal magnetic resonance imaging (MRI) showing a large anterior osteophyte (*arrow*).

The maximal deformity of the head–neck junction in FAI could be localized best by the 45-degree Dunn view.[10]

- Computed tomography (CT) scans with two- and three-dimensional (3-D) reconstructions are helpful for preoperative planning and detecting subtle femoral head–neck junction prominence (**FIG 2C,D**).
- Magnetic resonance imaging can further delineate the labral and cartilage pathology (**FIG 2E**). If the study is performed with gadolinium and high-resolution sagittal oblique or radial sequences, labral pathology can be detected.

## DIFFERENTIAL DIAGNOSIS

- FAI
- Labral tear
- Hip dysplasia
- SCFE
- Acetabular retroversion

## NONOPERATIVE MANAGEMENT

- Nonoperative management includes cessation of aggravating activities and symptomatic treatment using nonsteroidal anti-inflammatories.
- Physical therapy to strengthen the hip musculature does not address the mechanical impingement of FAI but may have a role in affecting pelvic inclination.

## SURGICAL MANAGEMENT

- Hip pathology may be addressed through hip arthroscopy. However, it may be difficult to dynamically assess hip mechanics before and after débridement.
- Femoral head–neck osteoplasty may be performed through an anterior approach to the hip without a surgical dislocation. However, the articular cartilage of the acetabulum and most of the femoral head cannot be evaluated with this limited approach.

### Preoperative Planning

- All imaging studies are reviewed.
- The lack of femoral head–neck offset is best appreciated on the 45-degree Dunn lateral view of the hip (see **FIG 2A,B**) or on the radial reformats of CT or magnetic resonance (MR) scans around the femoral neck axis or 3-D reconstruction of a CT scan.
- A CT scan that includes cuts through the distal femoral condyles may be used to accurately measure the amount of femoral version.[11]
- After general anesthesia is administered, the patient's hips are examined. The amount of true hip flexion and internal and external rotation with the hip extended and hip flexed are noted and compared to the preoperative assessment.

### Positioning

- The patient is placed in the full lateral position, secured on a pegboard. A flat-top cushion (with a half-moon–shaped cutout for the down leg) placed beneath the operative side helps to stabilize the leg during the approach (**FIG 3A–C**).
- A hip drape with a sterile side bag is used, which will capture the leg during the dislocation maneuver (**FIG 3D**).

A
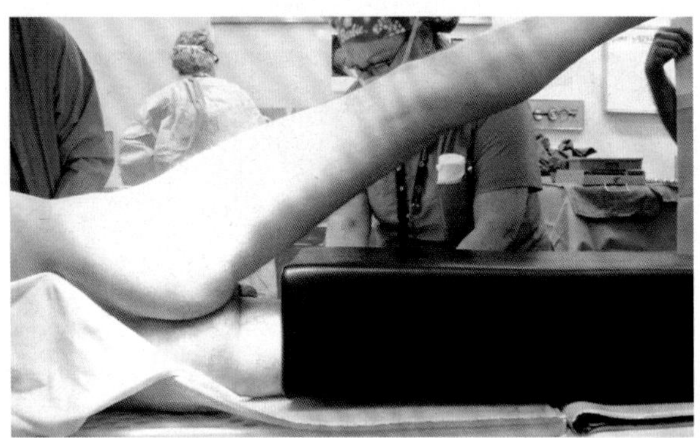
B
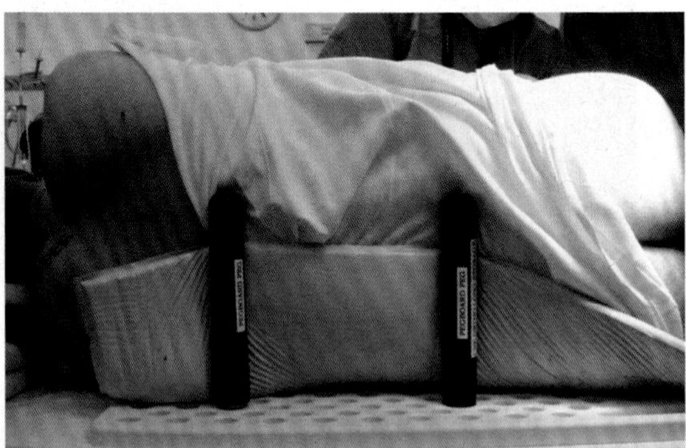
C
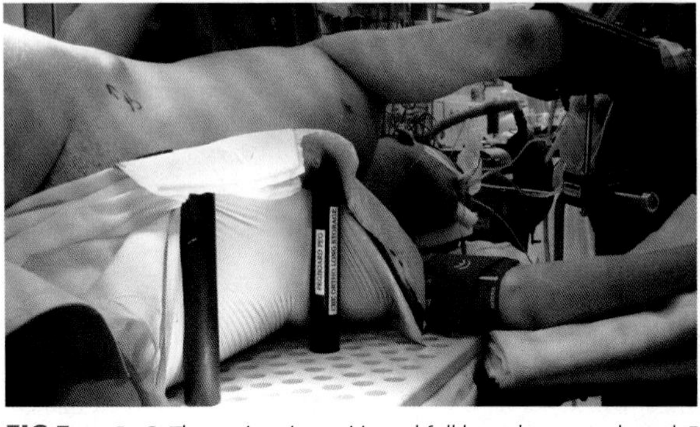
D
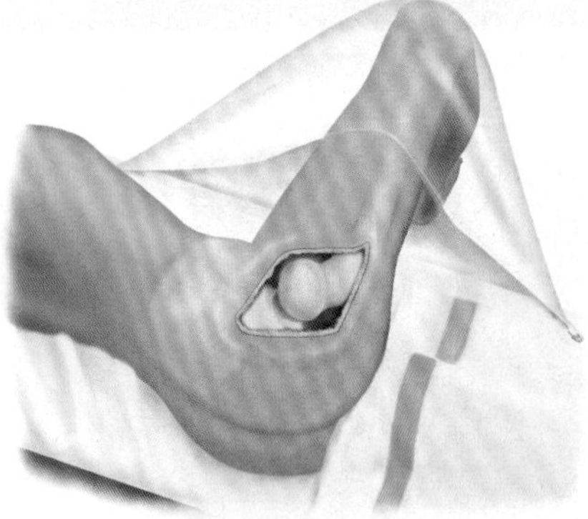

**FIG 3** • **A–C.** The patient is positioned full lateral on a pegboard. Before patient preparation, the surgeon should ensure that the leg can be flexed and adducted fully and is not blocked by the anteroinferior peg. **D.** Position of the leg in the sterile leg holder after dislocation. The hip is flexed, adducted, and externally rotated.

## Approach

- The approach consists of an anterior dislocation through a Kocher-Langenbeck or a Gibson approach with a trochanteric flip osteotomy (**FIG 4A,B**).
- A Kocher-Langenbeck incision is followed by splitting the gluteus maximus muscle.
- The abductors and gluteus maximus muscles can be spared by performing a Gibson approach, which proceeds between the gluteus medius and maximus (**FIG 4C,D**).[8]
  - The Gibson approach may result in less hip extensor dysfunction but may make anterior exposure more difficult.
- A Z-shaped capsulotomy is made to allow entry to the hip joint while protecting the deep branch of the MFCA (**FIG 4E**).[5]

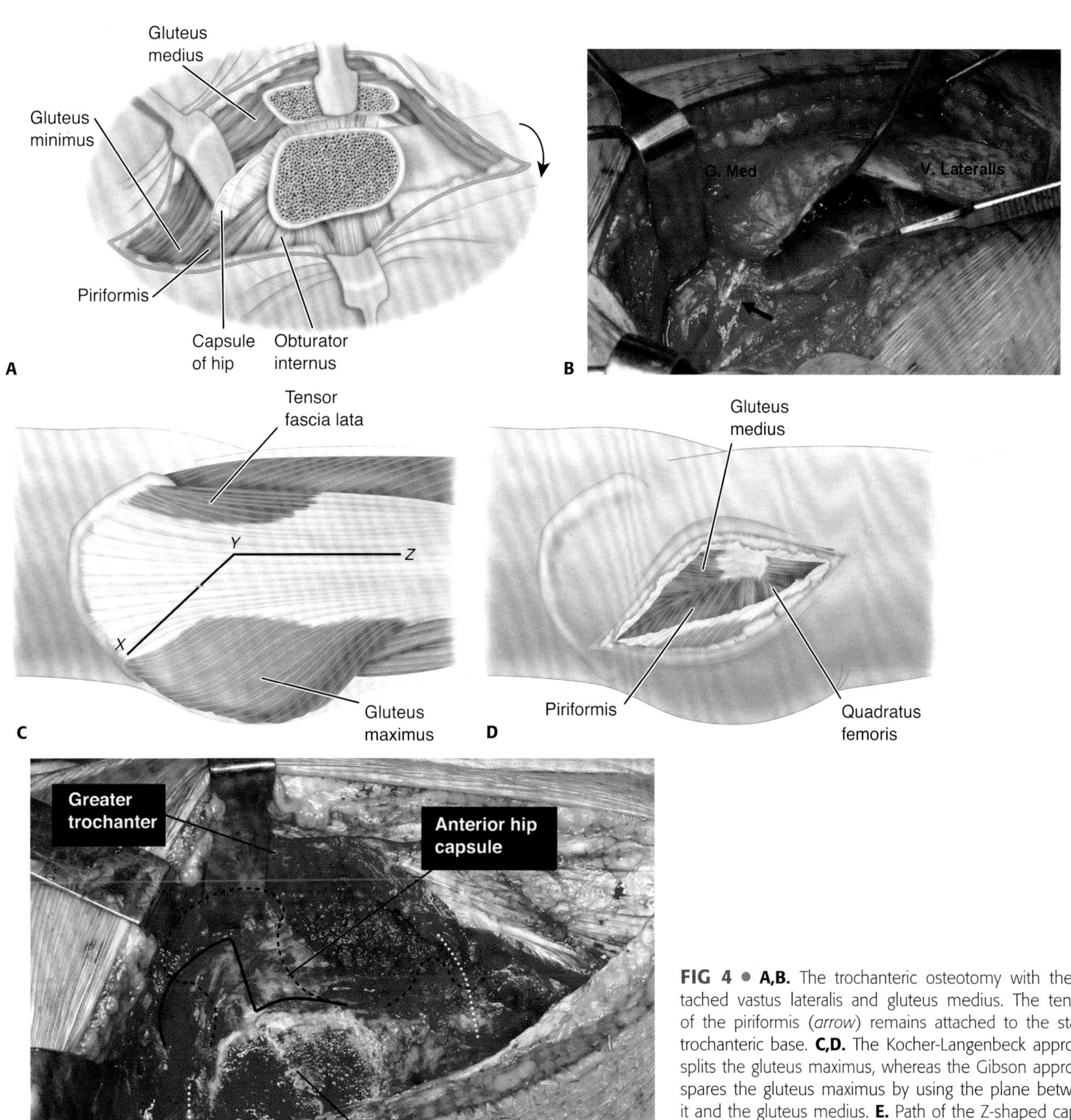


**FIG 4** • **A,B.** The trochanteric osteotomy with the attached vastus lateralis and gluteus medius. The tendon of the piriformis (*arrow*) remains attached to the stable trochanteric base. **C,D.** The Kocher-Langenbeck approach splits the gluteus maximus, whereas the Gibson approach spares the gluteus maximus by using the plane between it and the gluteus medius. **E.** Path of the Z-shaped capsulotomy (*solid line*). The limb along the posterior aspect of the acetabulum protects the entry of the terminal branches of the MFCA (*white dashed line*) and allows access to the hip joint and femoral head (*black dashed line*).

## Surgical Hip Dislocation by a Transtrochanteric Approach

### Approach to Hip Capsule

- A longitudinal lateral incision is made, centered over the junction between the anterior and middle thirds of the greater trochanter (**TECH FIG 1A**).
- The fascia lata is split distally in line with the incision. The proximal dissection progresses through the interval between the anterior edge of the gluteus maximus and the tensor (**TECH FIG 1B**).
- The proximal 4 to 5 cm of fascia of the vastus lateralis is incised, and the vastus muscle fibers are reflected anteriorly.
- The gluteus maximus, along with the fascia of the gluteus medius, which is left on the undersurface of the gluteus

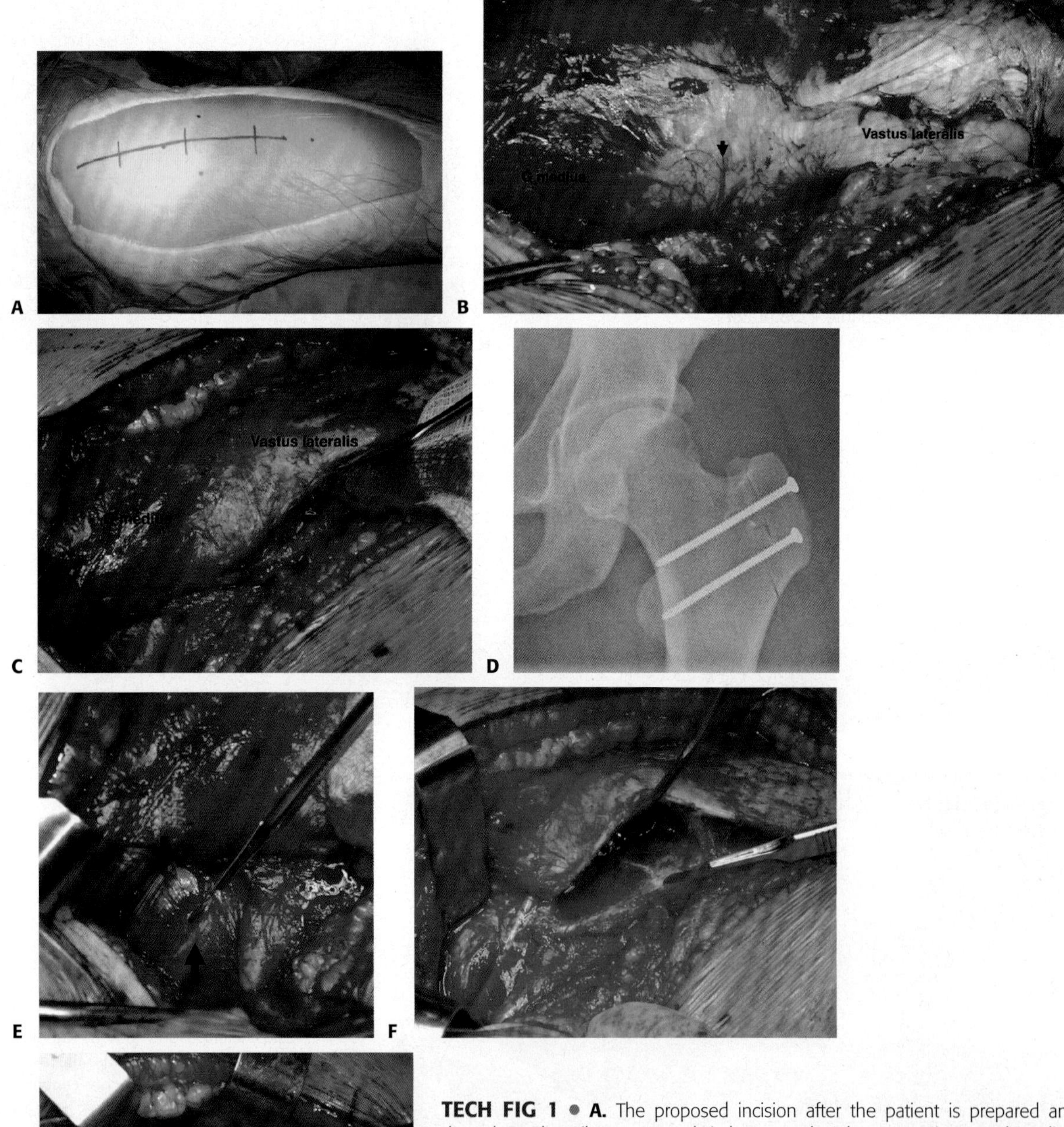


**TECH FIG 1** • **A.** The proposed incision after the patient is prepared and draped. **B.** The Gibson approach is between the gluteus maximus and medius. Note the trochanteric branches of the MFCA on the greater trochanter (*black arrow*). **C.** The trochanteric osteotomy is made with an oscillating saw. **D.** A step cut osteotomy provides improved stability and healing of the trochanteric osteotomy. **E.** The fascia over the piriformis tendon (*bottom arrow*) is divided to develop the interval between it and the capsular minimus (*top arrow*). **F.** A 1- to 1.5-cm trochanteric wafer is lifted anteriorly with the gluteus medius and vastus lateralis left attached. **G.** The anterior capsule is completely exposed before the arthrotomy is made.

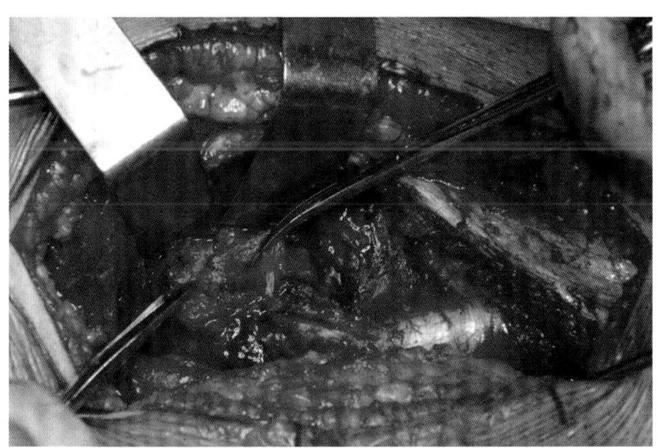

**TECH FIG 2** • The longitudinal limb of the capsulotomy is first made. This will allow visualization and prevent inadvertent cutting of the labrum while the posterior limb of the capsulotomy is made.

maximus for protection, is reflected posteriorly to expose the gluteus medius and insertion.

- A 1- to 1.5-cm thick trochanteric osteotomy is made with an oscillating saw, leaving the piriformis tendon and short external rotators intact on the remaining base of the greater trochanter (**TECH FIG 1C**).
- A trochanteric step cut can be performed using two saw blades 6 mm apart if a relative neck lengthening is not planned. This provides excellent stability of the trochanteric osteotomy with lower rates of trochanteric delayed union (**TECH FIG 1D**).
- The fascia overlying the piriformis tendon is incised to identify the tendon and the interval between the piriformis and capsular minimus muscles (**TECH FIG 1E**).
- The trochanteric wafer is next reflected and flipped anteriorly with its attached sleeve of vastus lateralis and the gluteus medius (**TECH FIG 1F**).
- The capsular minimus is elevated in an anterior direction off the hip capsule by carefully dissecting in the interval between the posterior edge of the capsular minimus and the piriformis tendon (**TECH FIG 1G**).
  - An assistant may use a right angled retractor to assist with the exposure of the capsule.
  - Progressive hip flexion, external rotation, and adduction further aid the exposure.
- The hip capsule is exposed up to the rim of the acetabulum.

## Hip Arthrotomy and Dislocation

- A Z-shaped capsulotomy is then performed, with the longitudinal arm of the Z in line with the anterior neck of the femur (**TECH FIG 2**).
  - The distal arm of the capsulotomy extends anteriorly well proximal to the lesser trochanter.
  - The proximal arm is extended posteriorly along the acetabular rim, just distal to the labrum and well proximal to the retinacular branches of the MFCA entering the capsule posteriorly to supply the femoral head.
- Depending on the pathology, the hip is brought through a range of motion to determine areas of impingement in a dynamic fashion.
- The leg is then placed in the sterile side bag, flexed, externally rotated, and adducted while the hip is subluxated anteriorly through the arthrotomy.
  - A bone hook placed around the anterior femoral neck may be needed to subluxate the hip.
  - The ligamentum teres is then divided using curved meniscus scissors to allow full dislocation of the hip.

## Dynamic Assessment and Osteoplasty

- The entire femoral head and acetabulum can now be assessed for chondral flaps or labral tears, which can be repaired using suture anchors spaced about 7 to 10 mm apart or débrided.
- The aspherical segment of the femoral head at the head–neck junction can be resected using a quarter-inch osteotome and rongeur (**TECH FIG 3A,B**).
- After reestablishing sphericity of the femoral head, the hip is reduced and the results of the débridement are assessed by bringing the hip through a range of motion and confirming the relief of impingement and improvement in range of motion.
- Intraoperative fluoroscopy showing a lateral of the hip in 90 degrees of flexion will determine if the femoral head–neck offset has been reestablished (**TECH FIG 3C**).

## Osteotomy Fixation

- The trochanteric wafer is reduced and held in position with a towel clip.
- Three 3.5-mm small fragment screws are placed to secure the trochanter. Fluoroscopy confirms reduction and fixation of the osteotomy (**TECH FIG 4**).

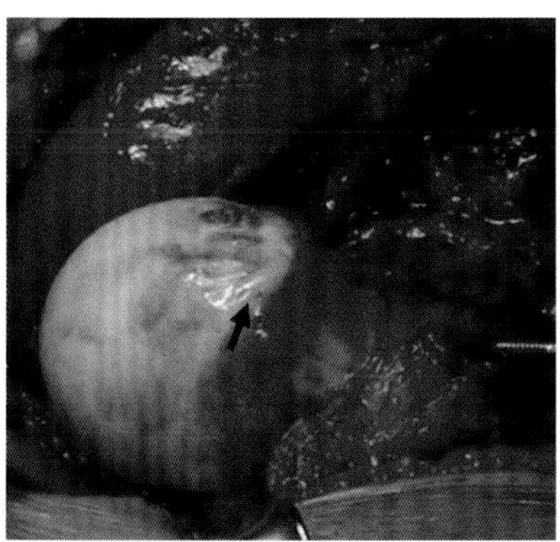
A

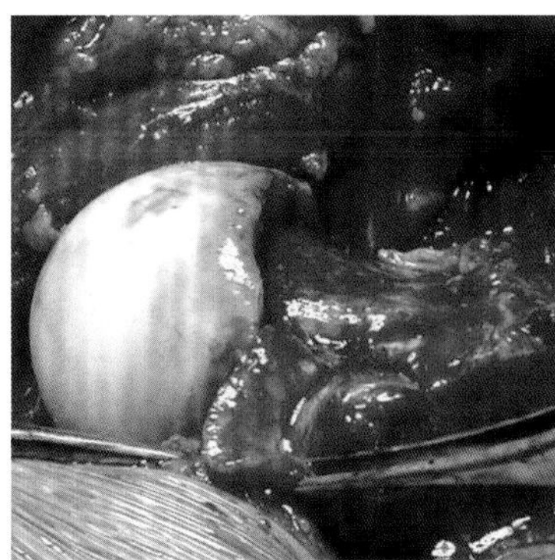
B

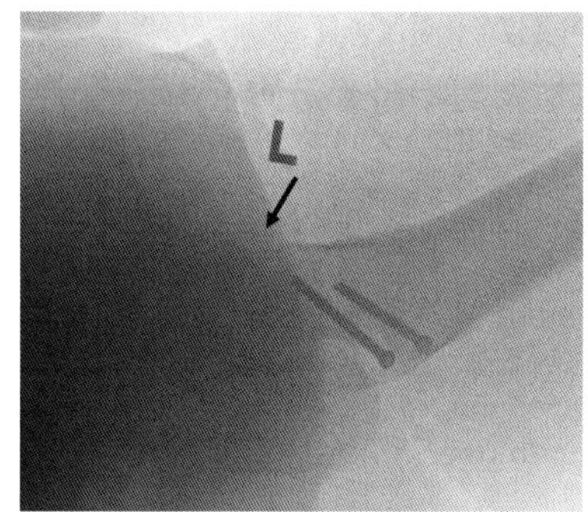

C

**TECH FIG 3** • **A.** The hips have been dislocated, and the lack of femoral head–neck offset as well as the cartilage damage is readily apparent (*black arrow*). **B.** The femoral head–neck offset has been restored, eliminating the cam-type FAI. **C.** The *black arrow* shows the restoration of the femoral head–neck offset (compare with **FIG 2B**).

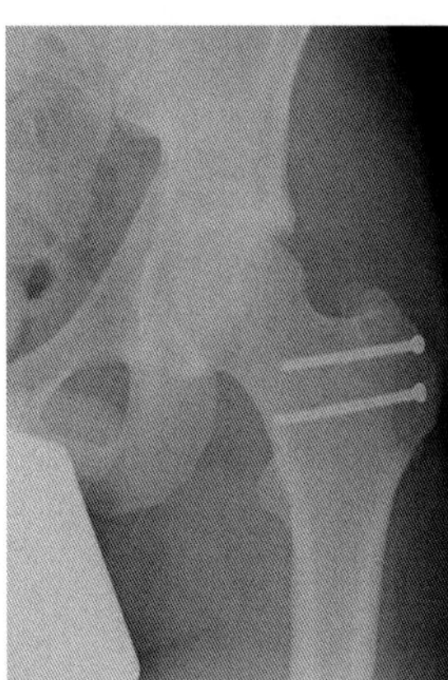

**TECH FIG 4** • The trochanteric osteotomy is fixed with two or three 3.5-mm screws.

- Alternatively, 4.0-mm cannulated screws or 4.5-mm cortical screws may be used for trochanteric fixation.

## Closure

- The Z-shaped capsulotomy is loosely repaired using absorbable 2-0 suture (**TECH FIG 5**).

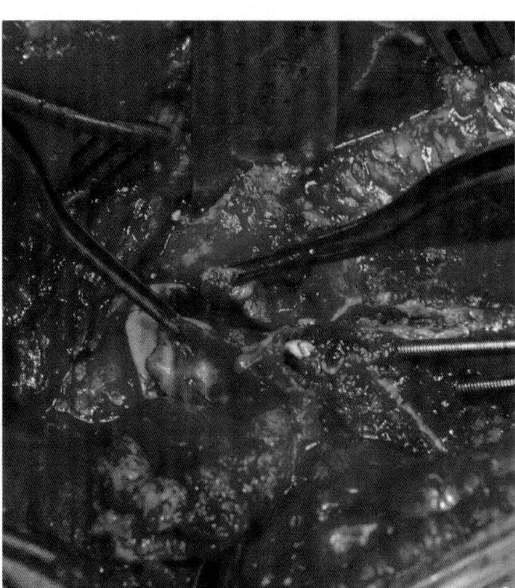

**TECH FIG 5** • The Z-shaped capsulotomy is loosely reapproximated with absorbable suture.

- The fascia of the vastus lateralis is closed with a running absorbable suture. The fascia lata and the fascia between the tensor and gluteus maximus are reapproximated.
- Skin is closed in routine fashion.

## PEARLS AND PITFALLS

| | |
|---|---|
| **Indications** | ■ A complete history and physical examination should be performed.<br>■ All associated pathology should be addressed. |
| **Approach** | ■ Exposure may be easier when the gluteus maximus is split as opposed to the Gibson approach. |
| **Trochanteric osteotomy** | ■ A small muscular cuff of gluteus medius may be left on the stable trochanteric base so the blood supply from the MFCA is not disrupted.<br>■ After scoring the greater trochanter, the full thickness of the trochanter should first be cut anteriorly to safely assess the size of the wafer. |
| **Heterotopic ossification** | ■ If a large portion of capsular minimus is left on the capsule during the dissection, the patient may develop heterotopic ossification. |
| **Femoral neck fracture** | ■ Aggressive resection of the bone at the femoral head–neck junction can weaken the bone and theoretically cause a fracture during relocation or dislocation of the hip. |

## POSTOPERATIVE CARE

- The hip is held flexed and in neutral rotation by placing two pillows under the leg and one under the greater trochanter.
- The patient is placed in a continuous passive motion machine for 6 hours a day, set from 30 to 80 degrees of flexion.
- Prophylaxis for deep venous thrombosis is individualized; however, all patients should be started on mechanical compression devices immediately.
- After the epidural is removed (if used), out-of-bed ambulation is permitted with one-sixth body weight partial weight bearing.
- Range-of-motion exercises are started, but care is taken to protect the greater trochanter osteotomy by limiting adduction to midline and avoiding resisted abduction exercises for 6 weeks.
- Some patients may benefit from heterotopic ossification prophylaxis using indomethacin.
- AP view of the pelvis or hip and true lateral hip radiographs are obtained 6 weeks postoperatively. Weight bearing is increased to full, and hip strengthening exercises are prescribed.

## OUTCOMES

- Ganz et al[6] has performed over 1200 surgical hip dislocations with no cases of osteonecrosis reported.
- Generally, outcomes are excellent if the correct pathology is addressed in a joint without significant preexisting arthrosis.
- In a clinical assessment in adults by Murphy et al[12] using the Merle d'Aubigné scale, hip scores improved significantly.

- Almost 80% of patients were satisfied with results of surgical dislocation approach treatment for FAI at midterm.[13]

## COMPLICATIONS

- Avascular necrosis of the femoral head can occur if care is not taken to follow the technique and to preserve the retinacular vessels.
- Femoral neck fracture if the femoral head–neck junction is aggressively débrided.
- Sciatic or femoral nerve neurapraxia
- Greater trochanteric nonunion
- Heterotopic ossification
- Repeat labral tear
- Continued arthrosis of the joint
- Painful postoperative joint adhesions[2]

## REFERENCES


1. Aronson J. Osteoarthritis of the young adult hip: etiology and treatment. Instruct Course Lect 1986;35:119–128.
2. Beck M. Groin pain after open FAI surgery: the role of intraarticular adhesions. Clin Orthop Relat Res 2009;467:769–774.
3. Clohisy JC, Kim YJ. Femoroacetabular impingement research symposium. J Am Acad Orthop Surg 2013;21(suppl 1):vi–viii.
4. Clohisy JC, Nepple JJ, Larson CM, et al. Persistent structural disease is the most common cause of repeat hip preservation surgery. Clin Orthop Relat Res 2013;471(12):3788–3794.
5. Ganz R, Gill T, Gautier E, et al. Surgical dislocation of the adult hip. J Bone Joint Surg Br 2001;83(8):1119–1124.
6. Ganz R, Parvizi J, Beck M, et al. Femoroacetabular impingement: a cause for osteoarthritis of the hip. Clin Orthop Relat Res 2003;(417):112–120.
7. Gautier E, Ganz K, Krügel N, et al. Anatomy of the medial femoral circumflex artery and its surgical implications. J Bone Joint Surg Br 2000;82(5):679–683.
8. Gibson A. Posterior exposure of the hip joint. J Bone Joint Surg Br 1950;32-B(2):183–186.
9. Goodman DA, Feighan JE, Smith AD, et al. Subclinical slipped capital femoral epiphysis. Relationship to osteoarthrosis of the hip. J Bone Joint Surg Am 1997;79(10):1489–1497.
10. Meyer DC, Beck M, Ellis T, et al. Comparison of six radiographic projections to assess femoral head/neck asphericity. Clin Orthop Relat Res 2006;445:181–185.
11. Murphy SB, Simon SR, Kijewski PK, et al. Femoral anteversion. J Bone Joint Surg Am 1987;69(8):1169–1176.
12. Murphy S, Tannast M, Kim YJ, et al. Debridement of the adult hip for femoroacetabular impingement: indications and preliminary clinical results. Clin Orthop Relat Res 2004;(429):178–181.
13. Naal FD, Miozzari HH, Schär M, et al. Midterm results of surgical hip dislocation for the treatment of femoroacetabular impingement. Am J Sports Med 2012;40:1501–1510.
14. Spencer S, Millis M, Kim YJ. Early results of treatment for hip impingement syndrome in slipped capital femoral epiphysis and pistol grip deformity of the femoral head-neck junction using the surgical dislocation technique. J Pediatr Orthop 2006;26:281–285.
15. Tannast M, Krüger A, Mack PW, et al. Surgical dislocation of the hip for the fixation of acetabular fractures. J Bone Joint Surg Br 2010;92(6):842–852.
16. Tibor LM, Sink EL. Pros and cons of surgical hip dislocation for the treatment of femoroacetabular impingement. J Pediatr Orthop 2013;33(suppl 1):S131–S136.
17. Trueta J, Harrison MH. The normal vascular anatomy of the femoral head in adult man. J Bone Joint Surg Br 1953;35-B(3):442–461.

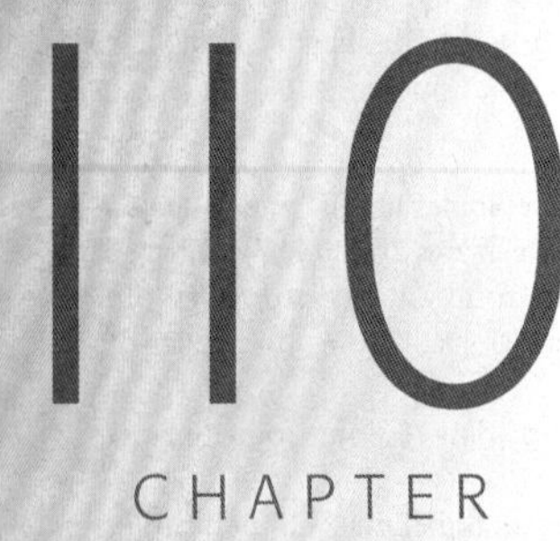

# Valgus Osteotomy of the Proximal Femur

Wudbhav N. Sankar

## DEFINITION

- Valgus osteotomy of the proximal femur can be performed for a number of different conditions including (among others) congenital or acquired coxa vara, fracture nonunion, avascular necrosis (AVN), or Legg-Calvé-Perthes disease (LCPD).
- Coxa vara is a deformity of the proximal femur associated with a neck–shaft angle of less than 110 degrees.[11] It can be congenital or developmental in origin.
- Femoral neck fracture nonunions can result (in part) from a vertically oriented fracture plane. A valgus osteotomy can improve mechanical loading at the fracture site and aid in fracture healing.
- AVN of the femoral head typically affects the anterosuperior region of the femoral head while sparing the medial and posterior regions. In certain cases, a valgus osteotomy (with flexion) can rotate better parts of the femoral head into the weight-bearing zone.
- In LCPD, valgus osteotomy can help those hips in which the primary goal of containment is no longer possible owing to hinge abduction. Under these circumstances, a valgus osteotomy can relieve the hinging and improve congruency of the joint.

## ANATOMY

- Valgus osteotomy creates an apex medial angulation in the proximal femur.
- In doing so, the medial aspects of the femoral head are rotated more centrally into the joint and, correspondingly, the lateral aspects of the head are rotated away from the joint.
- Adding flexion or extension at the osteotomy site similarly rotates the posterior (flexion) or anterior (extension) aspects of the femoral head into the joint.
- Valgus osteotomy increases a patient's effective hip abduction by the amount of correction and similarly reduces the patient's adduction by an equivalent amount.
- Length of the limb is increased by a valgus correction, which can be useful in cases of mild limb shortening (eg, LCPD).
- Valgus correction moves the greater trochanter distally, which improves abductor mechanics.

## PATHOGENESIS

- The pathogenesis of the deformity to be treated by valgus osteotomy is specific to the underlying condition.
- The exact cause of developmental coxa vara is unknown, but one theory postulates that the varus deformity is due to a primary ossification defect in the medial femoral neck that results in a more vertical physis. The physiologic shearing stresses that occur during weight bearing fatigue the dystrophic bone in the medial femoral neck, resulting in progressive varus.[7]
- AVN of the femoral head is the final common pathway of a spectrum of disease processes that disrupt circulation to the femoral head including embolism from deep sea diving, alcohol use, corticosteroid use, hemoglobinopathies, chemotherapy, LCPD, and traumatic injuries to the hip.[1]
- Hinge abduction in LCPD can result from fragmentation and extrusion of the epiphysis, which can create coxa magna and/or a ridge of lateral bone. As a result, the lateral aspect of the deformed femoral head may impinge on the acetabulum with attempted abduction. Continued abduction creates a lateral hinge, which pulls the inferomedial portion of the head away from the acetabulum.[8]

## NATURAL HISTORY

- As described by Weinstein et al,[11] the most reliable factor for progression of coxa vara is the Hilgenreiner–epiphyseal angle (HEA), measured between the line of Hilgenreiner and a line parallel to the proximal femoral physis (**FIG 1**).
  - Patients with HEAs more than 60 degrees will invariably progress, whereas those between 45 and 60 degrees have a less defined prognosis and must be followed for progression of varus deformity or increased symptoms.
- AVN of femoral head typically results in progressive collapse, pain, and stiffness often necessitating total hip arthroplasty.[1]
- At maturity, patients with LCPD and unrelieved hinge abduction would generally be classified as Stulberg category IV

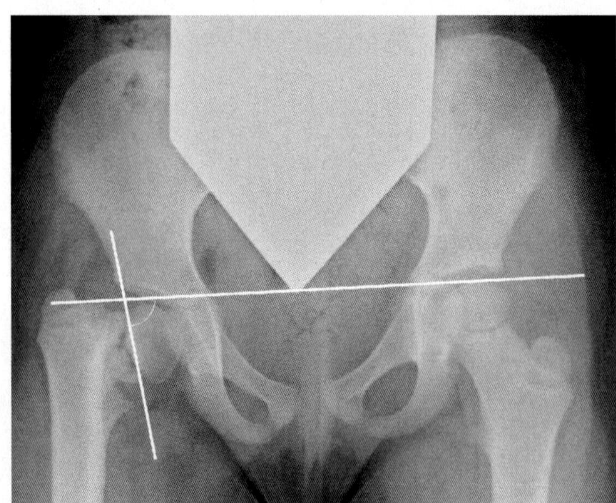

**FIG 1** • AP radiograph of the pelvis demonstrates the classic appearance of developmental coxa vara on the right side. The HEA is formed by crossing Hilgenreiner line with a line parallel to the proximal femoral physis. This angle is thought to be the best predictor of progression and postoperative recurrence.

(flattened femoral head with congruent acetabulum) or category V (flattened femoral head with a round acetabulum), both of which have been found to be associated with early-onset osteoarthritis.[10]

## PATIENT HISTORY AND PHYSICAL FINDINGS

- History and physical findings are specific to the underlying condition.
- Typically, patients who would benefit from a valgus osteotomy have pain with ambulation that is relieved by rest.
- There is generally 1 to 2 cm of limb shortening.
- Abductor weakness often causes a Trendelenburg gait.
- Limited abduction is common, and occasionally, patients have frank adduction contractures.

## IMAGING AND OTHER DIAGNOSTIC STUDIES

- Plain radiographs are generally diagnostic for the conditions that may require a valgus osteotomy.
- Anteroposterior (AP) x-rays of the hip in coxa vara will demonstrate a reduced neck–shaft angle and a wider more vertically oriented proximal femoral physis. Classically, a triangular metaphyseal fragment will be seen in the inferior neck surrounded by physis, giving an inverted Y pattern[11] (see **FIG 1**).
- Femoral neck nonunions typically result in medial collapse and varus deformity. Subtle nonunions can be confirmed by computed tomography (CT) scan.
- On the AP view, AVN typically results in sclerosis and/or collapse of the lateral and superior regions of the femoral head. On the frog view, the anterior head is more commonly affected.
- Hinge abduction in LCPD is best diagnosed using dynamic arthrography. Although pooling of dye medially is often considered diagnostic for hinge abduction, this can simply reflect an area of flattening of the epiphysis. It is most accurate to determine whether the lateral edge of the femoral head is able to rotate underneath the lip of the acetabulum and labrum with abduction (**FIG 2**). Congruency is generally improved when the hip is adducted.
  - The arthrogram should also be studied in AP and lateral projections with abduction, adduction, and internal and external rotation to determine the position that maximizes congruency and relieves impingement.

## DIFFERENTIAL DIAGNOSIS

- Congenital or acquired coxa vara
- Femoral neck nonunion
- AVN
- LCPD with hinge abduction or poor congruency
- Pathologic bone condition causing progressive varus deformity (eg, fibrous dysplasia, osteogenesis imperfecta, renal osteodystrophy)

## NONOPERATIVE MANAGEMENT

- Mild forms of coxa vara, precollapse AVN, and early-stage LCPD may be managed conservatively.
- Depending on the circumstance, short courses of anti-inflammatory medications, protected weight bearing, and/or activity modification can be helpful.
- In LCPD, if hinge abduction is seen on radiographs but the patient is symptom-free, an osteotomy can still improve the prognosis. In that scenario, it would be reasonable to wait until the patient is symptomatic before proceeding with surgery.

## SURGICAL MANAGEMENT

- The valgus osteotomy is indicated for unacceptable varus deformity, fracture nonunion, and certain cases of AVN among others.
- In LCPD, valgus osteotomy is considered a salvage operation for late cases in which the femoral head has developed a lateral ridge that can no longer be brought under the acetabulum (hinge abduction) or to improve congruency of an aspherical hip (**FIG 3**).

### Preoperative Planning

- Clinically or radiographically assess limb lengths to determine if concomitant shortening is necessary.
- Carefully evaluate preoperative range of motion including flexion, extension, and rotation.
- Specifically evaluate a patient's adduction and abduction prior to surgery to guide the amount of correction. Keep in

A

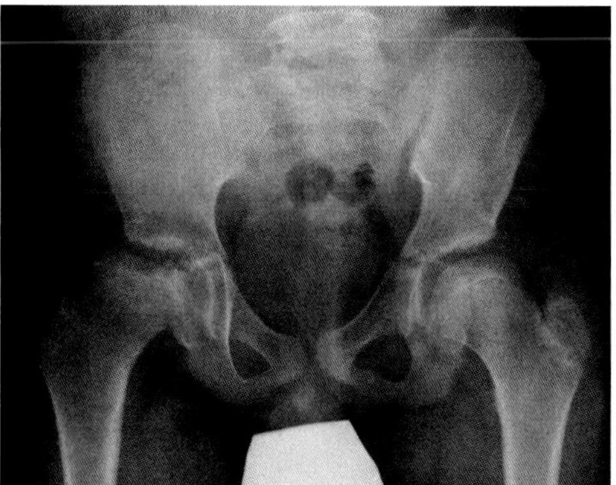

B

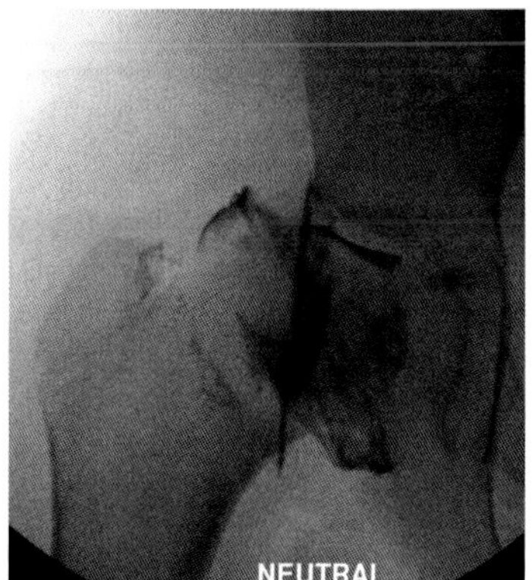


C

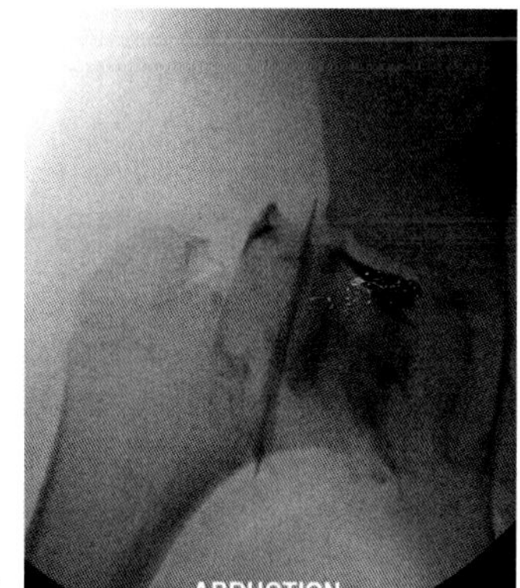


**FIG 2** • **A.** AP radiograph of the pelvis demonstrates bilateral Perthes disease, worse on the right. **B.** Arthrogram of the right hip in neutral demonstrates poor congruence and a lateral ridge on the femoral head. **C.** As the hip is brought into abduction, the lateral aspect of the femoral head impinges on the edge of the acetabulum causing pooling of dye medially (hinge abduction). The head does not truly slip underneath the labrum/lateral aspect of the cartilaginous acetabulum in this position.

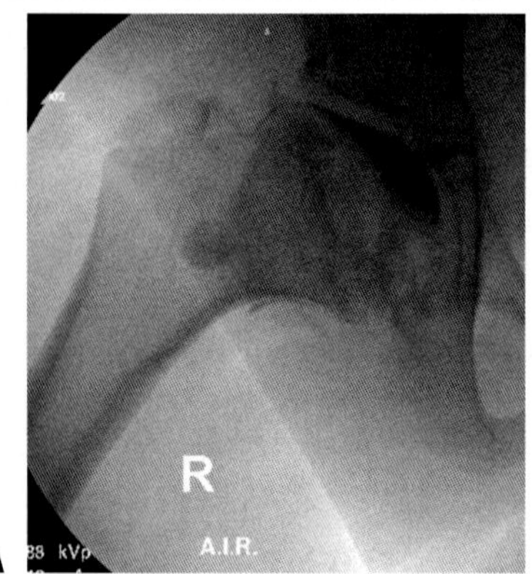


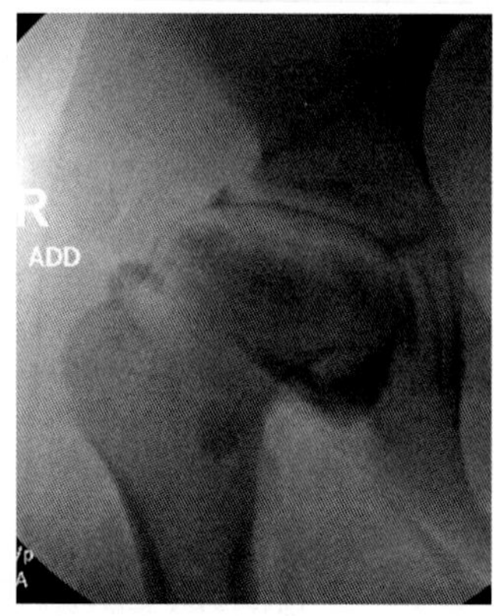


**FIG 3** • **A.** Arthrogram of the hip in a patient with healed LCPD. Note the poor congruence in the neutral position. **B.** Congruence is improved when the hip is adducted.

mind that adduction will be decreased and abduction will be increased by the amount of osteotomy correction. Generally, it is preferable to achieve at least 20 degrees of abduction after surgery.

- If an arthrogram was performed, it should be reviewed carefully. In cases of hinge abduction, extension, flexion, or rotation may be required in addition to valgus to fully relieve impingement and maximize congruency.
- Review preoperative AP and frog lateral radiographs to determine the native neck–shaft angle and size of bone.
- Based on range-of-motion measurements and preoperative radiographs, one should determine the desired amount of valgus correction.
- Implant choice is critical as the placement and shape of the implant, rather than the saw cut, will determine the final position of the osteotomy.
- The author prefers a 130-degree nonoffset blade plate, which lateralizes the femoral shaft and preserves head–shaft offset (**FIG 4A**).
  - Using a standard blade plate or proximal femoral locking plate can medialize the femoral shaft excessively such that the limb resembles a "post" without any physiologic offset (**FIG 4B**).
- Depending on the size and weight of the patient, both 3.5- and 4.5-mm plate options exist for one particular manufacturer (Orthopediatrics, Warsaw, IN). The width of the 3.5-mm blade plate system is 11 mm. The width of the 4.5-mm blade plate system is 14 mm.
- The blade plate should occupy 50% to 75% of the width of the femoral neck on the lateral projection for optimum strength.
- To calculate the angle for insertion of the blade plate relative to the femoral shaft, the angle of the planned correction is subtracted from 130 degrees.
  - Example: For a desired 20 degrees of valgus correction, the blade is inserted at 110 degrees from the shaft. With the blade at 110 degrees, the shaft must come into 20 degrees of valgus to accommodate a 130-degree fixed-angle blade plate.

## Positioning

- The patient is placed supine on a radiolucent surgical table with a small bump under the ipsilateral pelvis to facilitate access to the lateral femur. Too large of a bump can distort orthogonal imaging.
- The surgeon should check that sufficient AP and frog lateral radiographs can be obtained.
- The entire limb should be draped free to allow manipulation of the limb during surgery.

## Approach

- The standard lateral approach to the proximal femur is used.

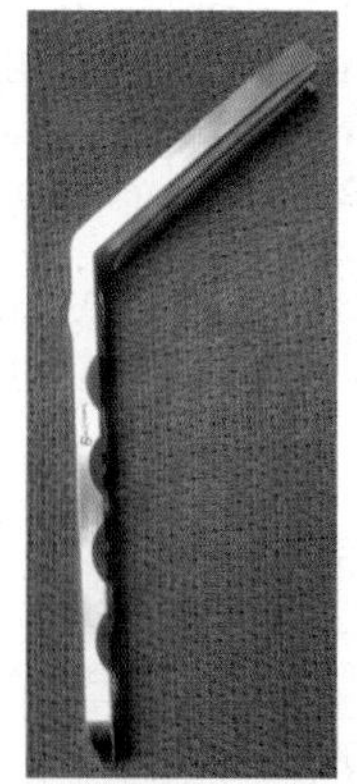

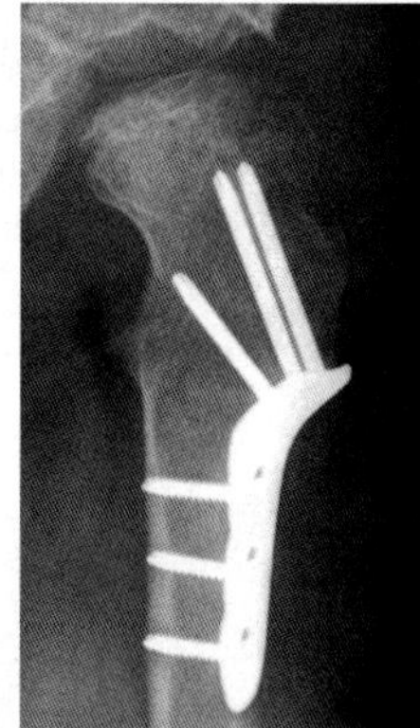

**FIG 4** • **A.** A 130-degree nonoffset blade plate. **B.** AP of the left hip demonstrates a valgus osteotomy for a patient with LCPD using a proximal femoral locking plate designed for valgus correction. Note that the shaft is medialized excessively such that the limb resembles a post without any physiologic offset.

## Exposure

- Skin incision is made in line with the proximal femur starting a few centimeter proximal to the vastus ridge and extending distally approximately 10 to 12 cm depending on the size of the patient and the intended implant.
- The fascia lata is split in line with the fibers over the palpated lateral border of the femur.
- The vastus lateralis fascia is incised longitudinally about 5 to 10 mm anterior to the intermuscular septum and is elevated atraumatically from the femur. Perforating vessels are identified and cauterized.
- Proximally, the fascia of the vastus lateralis is opened anteriorly with the electrocautery along the vastus ridge, creating an L shape (**TECH FIG 1A**).
- The periosteum is incised along the anterolateral femur, and subperiosteal dissection is performed circumferentially just proximal to the level of the lesser trochanter. The exposure should be extended sufficiently distal to allow shortening of the bone (if necessary) and application of the plate (**TECH FIG 1B**).

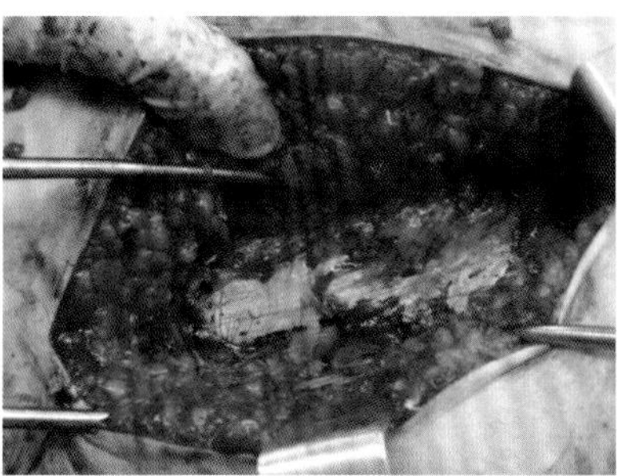

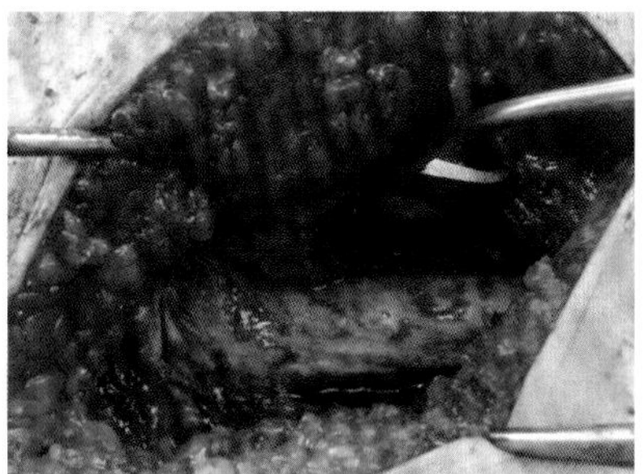

**TECH FIG 1 • A.** The vastus lateralis is opened in an L fashion (*purple*) with the vertical limb along the vastus ridge and the posterior limb 5 mm anterior to the posterior border of the muscle. **B.** The lateral femur is exposed in a subperiosteal fashion circumferentially.

## Valgus Osteotomy of the Femur Using a Cannulated Blade Plate

### Guidewire Placement

- In a cannulated blade plate system, the guidewire establishes the position of the chisel which in turn dictates the position and trajectory of the blade. Therefore, precise placement is critical.
- To provide a reference, a standard Kirschner (K) wire is inserted perpendicular to the femoral shaft at the intended osteotomy site (usually at the proximal aspect of the lesser trochanter).
- The entry site for the cannulated blade plate guidewire is proximal to the osteotomy site at a distance specified by the implant design. This typically ends up being just distal to the vastus ridge and trochanteric apophysis. The entry site should be centered on the lateral aspect of the femur in the sagittal plane (**TECH FIG 2A**).
- Using a triangle template to guide the trajectory (chosen based on the amount of intended correction), the guidewire is inserted into the femoral neck.
  - To use the previous example, if a 20-degree correction is desired and a 130-degree implant is being used, the guidewire should be placed 110 degrees from the shaft. A 110-degree angle with the shaft corresponds to a 20-degree angle compared to the perpendicular K-wire (90 + 20). Therefore, a 20-degree triangle is used to confirm the angle between the wires (**TECH FIG 2B,C**).
- In the lateral plane, the wire should parallel the proposed track of the blade plate (ie, centered in the femoral neck) (**TECH FIG 2D**).
- The guidewire is advanced short of the physis, and length is measured.
- The guidewire should be inserted bit further than the intended blade plate depth to prevent dislodgement during chisel placement.

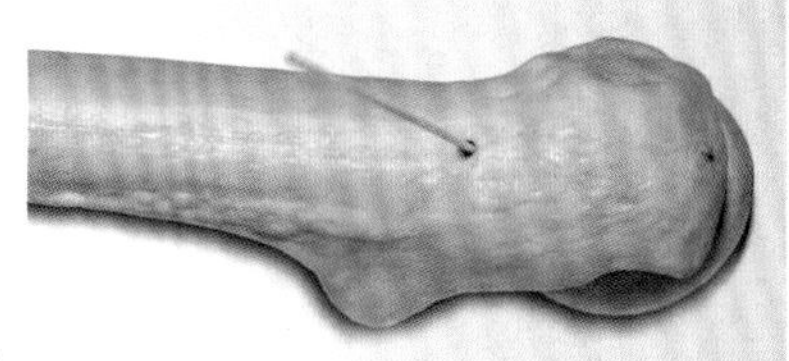

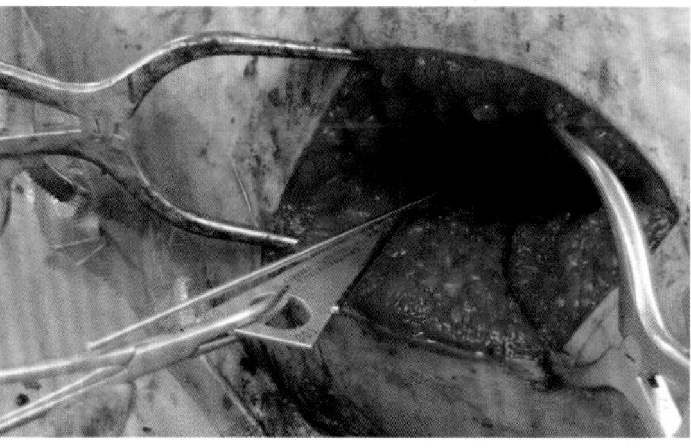

**TECH FIG 2 • A.** In the sagittal plane, the guidewire entry site is in the midpoint of the femur. A reference K-wire is inserted perpendicular to the femoral shaft. Depending on the amount of desired correction, the guidewire for the cannulated blade plate is then inserted up the femoral neck at a specific angle to the first K-wire. **B.** A triangle is used to judge the angle between the K-wires. *(continued)*

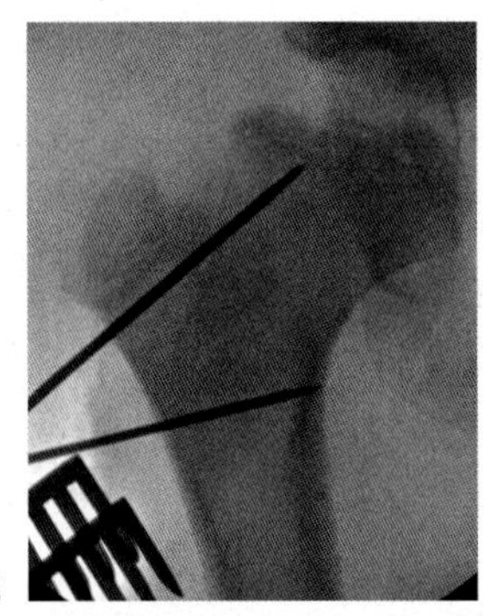

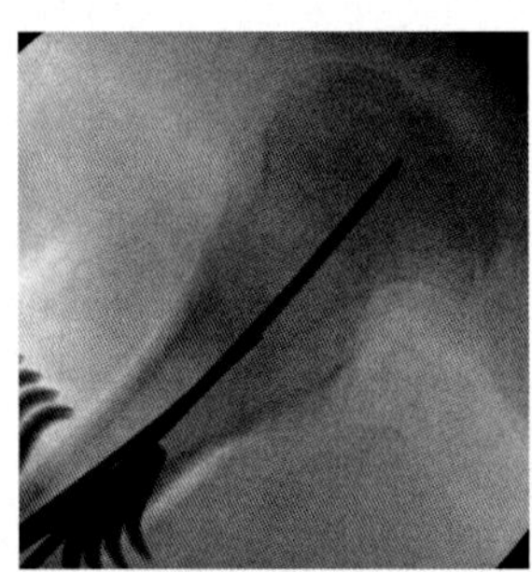

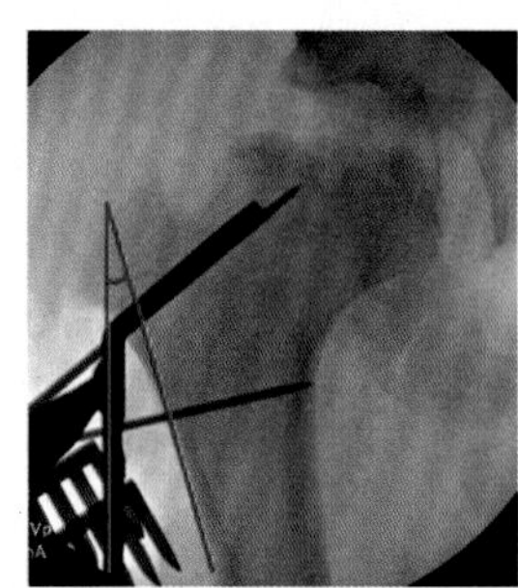

**TECH FIG 2** • *(continued)* **C.** The angle between the two wires can also be confirmed using the C-arm. **D.** The position of the guidewire is confirmed in the frog lateral view. **E.** As a double check to confirm that the guidewire that was just placed will result in the desired correction, the 130-degree blade plate is laid over the skin of the patient in line with the guidewire and imaged using the C-arm. The angle created between the lateral aspect of the femoral shaft and the shaft of the plate will be the amount of correction.

- As a double check to confirm that the guidewire that was just placed will result in the desired correction, the 130-degree blade plate is laid over the skin of the patient in line with the guidewire and imaged using the C-arm. The angle created between the lateral aspect of the femoral shaft and the shaft of the plate will be the amount of correction. This can be estimated visually or measured using a goniometer (**TECH FIG 2E**).

## Chisel Insertion

- The cannulated chisel is now inserted over the guidewire (**TECH FIG 3A**).
- For pure valgus, the chisel is rotated so that it is perpendicular to the lateral shaft of the femur.
- To add extension or flexion, the chisel is rotated posteriorly or anteriorly from perpendicular, respectively. The desired amount of flexion or extension should be marked on the bone (**TECH FIG 3B,C**).
  - A guide arm that can be slid over the chisel is helpful to visualize the amount of flexion or extension.
- The chisel should be frequently backed out a bit during insertion (using a slap hammer) to prevent incarceration.
- The path of the chisel is checked periodically with fluoroscopy.
- The chisel is backed up to loosen it before making the osteotomy. The surgeon should verify it has actually backed up by checking the depth measurement or by taking a C-arm image.

## Making the Osteotomy

- Prior to making the cut, the bone is scored longitudinally with electrocautery or a saw across the osteotomy site, or K-wires can be placed proximal and distal to the osteotomy site to assess rotation after the osteotomy has been performed (see **TECH FIG 3A**).
- A transverse osteotomy is made using an oscillating saw at the site of the original, perpendicularly directed K-wire (generally at the proximal aspect of the lesser trochanter). The K-wire can be left in place to help guide the saw cut so that it is perpendicular to the femoral shaft or the trajectory can be confirmed using the C-arm.
  - A single transverse cut is the simplest means of performing the osteotomy and generally heals quite well, but it does

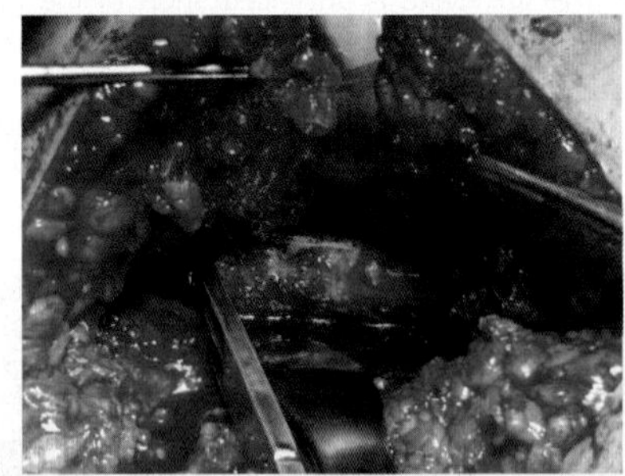

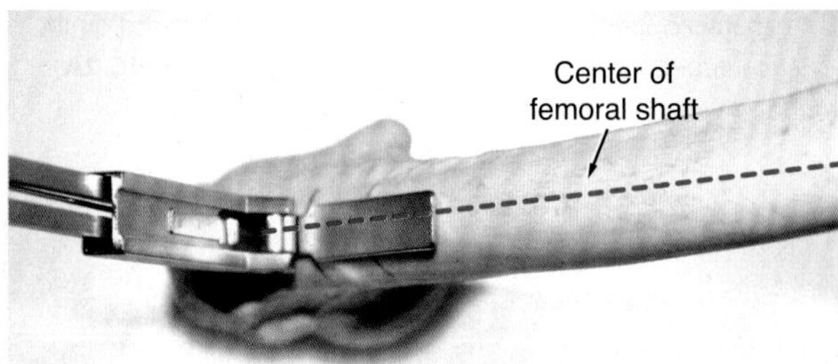


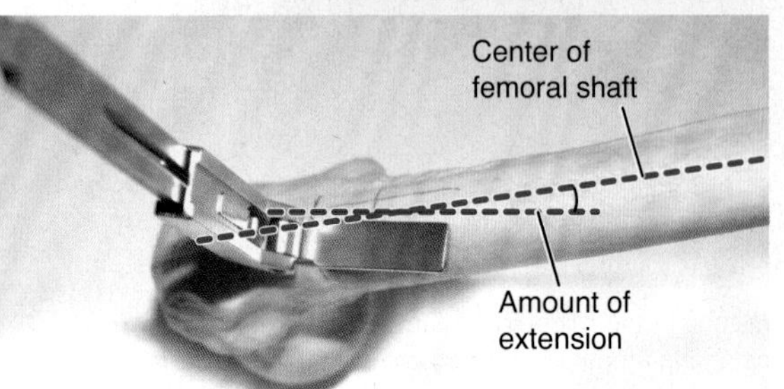


**TECH FIG 3** • **A.** The cannulated chisel is now inserted over the guidewire. Prior to making the cut, the bone is scored longitudinally with a saw to assess rotation after the osteotomy has been performed. **B.** A guide arm can be slipped over the chisel. Placing this arm in line with the shaft will produce pure valgus. **C.** Rotating the guide arm posteriorly will add extension to the osteotomy (conversely, rotating the arm anteriorly will add flexion).

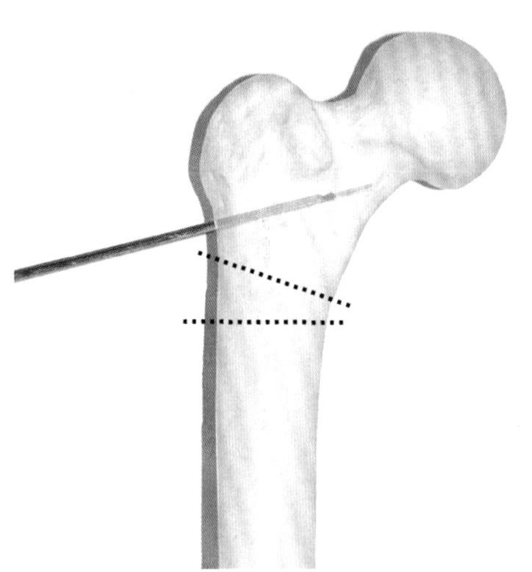

**TECH FIG 4** • An alternative technique is to perform a closing wedge osteotomy using two cuts.

not provide the maximum surface area for osteotomy healing.
  - If better apposition is desired, a step cut can be made in the lateral cortex or a wedge can be removed (**TECH FIG 4**).
- Hohmann or other retractors can be placed around the femur subperiosteally to protect soft tissue structures during the osteotomy.
- If the femur needs to be shortened, the distal fragment can be delivered out of the wound. This allows the surgeon to measure, mark, and cut the bone as needed.

## Blade Plate Placement

- A bone tenaculum clamp is now placed around the greater trochanter to provide control of the proximal fragment.
- The chisel is removed, and the cannulated blade plate is inserted over the guidewire. The exchange should be done quickly to minimize the chance that the proper rotation is lost.
- The blade plate should be inserted by hand initially to prevent deviation from the desired path. It can then be impacted into place using a mallet.
- A frog lateral view should be obtained during blade plate insertion to be sure that it is following the guidewire.
- Once impacted fully, the shaft of the femur is reduced to the side plate and secured with a bone reduction clamp (**TECH FIG 5A**).
- Rotation is confirmed using the previously placed orientation line or K-wires.
- The side plate is secured to the femur using standard techniques with the initial screws inserted in compression (**TECH FIG 5B**).
- In certain implant systems (Orthopediatrics), an additional locking screw can be placed through the shoulder of the plate into the proximal fragment.

## Closure

- The vastus lateralis is repaired using interrupted absorbable sutures at the vastus ridge followed by a running suture along its posterior border.
- The fascia lata is closed in a watertight fashion using interrupted heavy absorbable suture (eg, no. 1 Vicryl), followed by layered closure of the dermis (2-0 Vicryl) and the subcuticular layer (4-0 Monocryl).

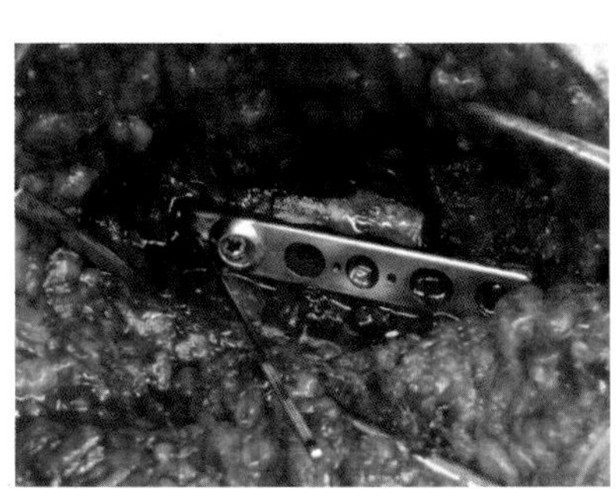

A

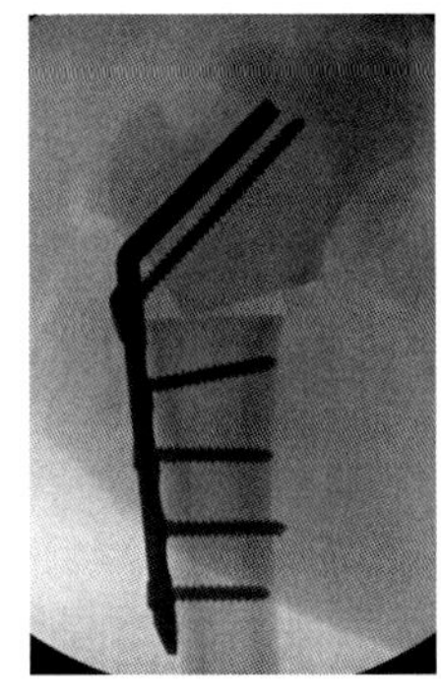

B

**TECH FIG 5** • **A.** Once the blade is impacted fully, the shaft of the femur is reduced to the side plate. **B.** Final AP fluoroscopic view after valgus osteotomy. Note the lateralization of the femoral shaft.

## PEARLS AND PITFALLS

| | |
|---|---|
| **Chisel incarceration** | ■ This can be prevented by frequently backing the chisel out.<br>■ The surgeon should be sure it really backs up. Check the markings or confirm using C-arm. It is easy to be deceived. |
| **Loss of guidewire** | ■ This happens when the chisel is inserted past the end of the guidewire.<br>■ The surgeon should check with a radiograph while removing the chisel to verify the guidewire is staying in place. |
| **Inaccurate correction** | ■ Meticulous preoperative planning, wire insertion, and use of triangle guides can prevent errors.<br>■ Double-check guidewire placement by obtaining a C-arm image with the blade plate laid over the patient's skin in line with the wire. The angle between the shaft of the plate and the lateral femur will be your correction. |
| **Avoiding implant cutout** | ■ The femoral shaft should be brought to the blade plate as much as possible. Excessive torque on the blade plate should be avoided.<br>■ The blade can break out of the proximal fragment, especially if insufficient distance was maintained between the bottom of the chisel and the osteotomy.<br>■ Shortening of the femur can reduce the tension from valgus correction. |

## POSTOPERATIVE CARE

- Patients are made toe-touch weight bearing with crutches. Younger patients and those who are expected to be noncompliant with crutches and activity limitations can be placed in a single-leg spica cast. Weight bearing is generally advanced at 4 to 6 weeks based on radiographic healing of the osteotomy.
- Elective hardware removal is controversial. I prefer hardware removal 1 year postoperatively or after bony union is obtained in patients in whom the likelihood of future surgery, including joint arthroplasty, is high. This is particularly true of younger patients who can develop bone growth over their implants.

## OUTCOMES

- Coxa vara
  - If adequate valgus is achieved, the triangular defect will spontaneously close by 3 to 6 months after surgery in nearly all patients.
  - Between 50% and 89% of operated hips sustain a premature closure of the proximal femoral physis, which occurs 1 to 2 years postoperatively and has not been found to correlate with patient age, surgical trauma, or degree of valgus.[6,9]
  - Recurrence has been reported in 30% to 70% of patients, although correction of the HEA to less than 38 degrees has been shown to have a 95% success rate.[4]
  - These patients must be monitored for recurrent varus deformity or significant leg length discrepancy that may require further surgical intervention.
- Femoral neck nonunion
  - One study reported an 86% union rate at a mean of 20 weeks following valgus osteotomy for femoral neck nonunion in young patients.[5]
- AVN
  - One series reported improved hip function (based on Harris Hip Score) in six patients treated with valgus osteotomy for posttraumatic AVN.[3]
  - Comparison of magnetic resonance imaging (MRI) scans before and after valgus correction demonstrated resorption of the necrotic segment of the femoral head and its remodeling in all six patients with segmental osteonecrosis.[3]
- LCPD/hinge abduction
  - Three recent publications[2,8,12] reported subjectively satisfactory results (by varying standards) in 66% to 94% of patients at 5 to 10 years of follow-up. Average Iowa hip scores ranged from 86 to 93. Further hip surgery had been performed on 10% to 20% of patients.
  - Two of the three recent articles noted no significant changes in the Sharp angle and percent coverage.[2,8] One study noted a significant difference in the percent coverage and superior joint space.[12]
  - Bankes et al[2] reported two factors associated with favorable remodeling, both concerning the timing of surgery: when the osteotomies were carried out during the healing phase of Perthes disease and when they were carried out in patients with open triradiate cartilages.

## COMPLICATIONS

- Nonunion is rare in otherwise healthy patients.
- Hardware failure most commonly occurs via the blade plate breaking out of the proximal fragment when too small of a bone bridge was preserved.
- Infection

## ACKNOWLEDGMENTS

- Thank you to Ellen M. Raney, Michael B. Millis, and Joshua A. Strassberg for their work on previous related chapters from the first edition.

## REFERENCES

1. Assouline-Dayan Y, Chang C, Greenspan A, et al. Pathogenesis and natural history of osteonecrosis. Semin Arthritis Rheum 2002;32(2):94–124.
2. Bankes MJ, Catterall A, Hashemi-Nejad A. Valgus extension osteotomy for 'hinge abduction' in Perthes' disease: results at maturity and factors influencing radiographic outcome. J Bone Joint Surg Br 2000;82(4):548–554.
3. Bartonicek J, Vavra J, Bartoska R, et al. Operative treatment of avascular necrosis of the femoral head after proximal femur fractures in adolescents. Int Orthop 2012;36(1):149–157.
4. Carroll K, Coleman S, Stevens P. Coxa vara: surgical outcomes of valgus osteotomy. J Pediatr Orthop 1997;17:220–224.
5. Ghosh B, Bhattacharjya B, Banerjee K, et al. Management of the nonunited neck femur fracture by valgus osteotomy—a viable alternative. J Indian Med Assoc 2012;110(11):819–820.
6. Kehl D, LaGrone M, Lovell W. Developmental coxa vara. Orthop Trans 1983;7:475.
7. Pylkkanen P. Coxa vara infantum. Acta Orthop Scand 1960;48(suppl 48):1–120.
8. Raney EM, Grogan DP, Hurley ME, et al. The role of proximal femoral valgus osteotomy in Legg-Calve-Perthes disease. Orthopedics 2002;25:513–517.
9. Schmidt TL, Kalamchi A. The fate of the capital femoral physis and acetabular development in developmental coxa vara. J Pediatr Orthop 1982;2(5):534–538.
10. Stulberg SD, Cooperman DR, Wallensten R. The natural history of Legg-Calve-Perthes disease. J Bone Joint Surg Am 1981;63:1095–1108.
11. Weinstein JN, Kuo KN, Millar EA. Congenital coxa vara. A retrospective review. J Pediatr Orthop 1984;4:70–77.
12. Yoo WJ, Choi IH, Chung CY, et al. Valgus femoral osteotomy for hinge abduction in Perthes' disease: decision-making and outcomes. J Bone Joint Surg Br 2004;86:726–730.

# Percutaneous In Situ Cannulated Screw Fixation of the Slipped Capital Femoral Epiphysis

Richard S. Davidson and Michelle S. Caird

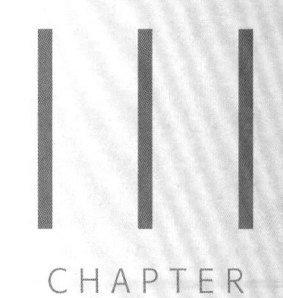


## DEFINITION

- Slipped capital femoral epiphysis (SCFE) is a common hip disorder in adolescents in which the neck and femur displace anterolaterally (most commonly into varus and extension) with respect to the proximal femoral epiphysis.
- SCFE can be classified as stable or unstable. A child with a stable SCFE has pain and a possible limp but is able to ambulate with or without walking aids, whereas a child with an unstable SCFE is unable to ambulate even with crutches. A stable slip has a nearly 0% risk of osteonecrosis, but an unstable slip has risk of osteonecrosis somewhere between 10 and 50%.[10]
- SCFEs have also been described by duration of symptoms as chronic (>3 weeks of symptoms), acute (<3 weeks of symptoms) or acute on chronic (long-standing mild symptoms with an increase in symptoms of >3 weeks' duration). This latter classification correlates less well with the risks of avascular necrosis (AVN) and chondrolysis.

## ANATOMY

- The proximal femoral physis and epiphysis are located within the hip capsule. Although the proximal physis provides length and shape to the femoral neck, most SCFEs occur in adolescence, when little growth remains at this growth plate.
- The blood supply to the proximal femoral epiphysis comes from the medial femoral circumflex artery, which travels along the femoral neck. From the circumflex arise the lateral epiphyseal vessels, which enter the epiphysis posterosuperiorly. Small contributions come from the vessels of the round ligament and the posterior inferior epiphyseal vessels off the medial femoral circumflex artery. Injury to this tenuous capsular blood supply can result in osteonecrosis.

## PATHOGENESIS

- In SCFE, the epiphysis stays within the acetabulum while the neck and distal femur slip (most commonly into extension and varus).
- SCFE occurs more commonly in boys than girls (60% of patients are boys). Most patients (up to 75%) are adolescents (boys 13.5 years, girls 12.0 years on average). Most patients are obese and in the 90th to 95th weight percentile for age. SCFE occurs bilaterally in about 25% of patients.[9]
- Biochemical factors likely play a role. Hormonal changes that occur during adolescent growth influence the strength of the physis.[4]
- Biomechanical factors also likely play a role. The physis in SCFE is subjected to higher shear force. The physis is more oblique during adolescence and in obese children; both factors increase shear in normal activities. The proximal femur is relatively retroverted in many cases of SCFE, which also increases the shear force on the physis. The reinforcing perichondral ring of the proximal physis also weakens with age until growth plate closure.
- If the physis of an SCFE patient is studied histologically, it looks widened, with abnormal chondrocyte maturation and endochondral ossification. The slip occurs mainly through the hypertrophic zone of the physis.[6]
- Patients younger than age 10 years should be evaluated for an underlying endocrine abnormality, including hypothyroidism, renal osteodystrophy, and panhypopituitarism.[11]

## NATURAL HISTORY

- The natural history of untreated SCFE and the ultimate outcome are difficult to predict, although it is widely accepted in adult reconstructive circles that most cases of degenerative hip arthritis are secondary to an underlying structural cause, such as SCFE. The risk of progression exists while the physis remains open. The slip severity increases with the duration of symptoms.[7]
- The development of degenerative joint disease is related to the severity of the slip.[3]

## PATIENT HISTORY AND PHYSICAL FINDINGS

- Physical examination methods include the following:
  - The resting position of the knee and foot is observed with the patient lying supine and it is compared to the other side. Excessive external rotation is a result of the slip.
  - Hip range of motion (ROM) between affected and normal sides (for stable SCFE only) is compared. Because of the slip, the affected side has decreased flexion, abduction, and internal rotation of the hip. There may be guarding with ROM.
  - In SCFE that presents with knee pain, passive knee ROM is normal and effusion is absent.
  - In stable SCFE, the patient has an antalgic gait. The foot may be externally rotated. In unstable SCFE, the patient is unable to bear weight at all on the affected side.
- Patients complain of hip or groin pain, thigh pain, or knee pain, which may be exertional and usually occurs without a history of trauma.
- The patient may have a limp (stable slip) or frank inability to ambulate (unstable slip).
- Examination of the hip can reveal an externally rotated foot and knee, guarding of the hip with ROM, and decreased flexion and internal rotation of the hip.
- Findings on the knee examination are normal.

## IMAGING AND OTHER DIAGNOSTIC STUDIES

- Plain radiographs of the pelvis, including anteroposterior (AP) and frog-leg lateral views, should be obtained in any pediatric patient with hip, thigh, or knee pain.
- A widened physis on AP or lateral views can be an early sign of SCFE.
- The Klein line, which can demonstrate SCFE, is drawn along the superior neck of the femur, on the AP view. In a normal hip, this line should touch at least some part of the epiphysis, but in SCFE, it will not cross the epiphysis (**FIG 1**).
- The metaphyseal blanch sign of Steel is a crescent-shaped double density along the medial femoral neck where the slipped epiphysis overlaps the metaphysis on the radiograph.
- Images of the contralateral hip should be scrutinized for evidence of bilateral SCFE. If present, both sides should be treated.
- The severity of an SCFE can be described by displacement relative to the width of the metaphysis[7]:
  - Mild: less than one-third the width
  - Moderate: one-third to half the width
  - Severe: more than half the width
- Another method of describing slip severity is measuring the difference between the epiphyseal shaft angle on each side[16]:
  - Mild: less than 30 degrees
  - Moderate: 30 to 50 degrees
  - Severe: 50 degrees or greater
- If the patient is younger than 10 years of age, underlying endocrine abnormalities should be investigated with laboratory studies, including thyroid function tests and basic chemistries.

## DIFFERENTIAL DIAGNOSIS

- SCFE
- Legg-Perthes disease
- Hip labral tear
- Femoral neck stress fracture
- Septic arthritis of the hip
- Knee derangement
- Greater trochanteric bursitis

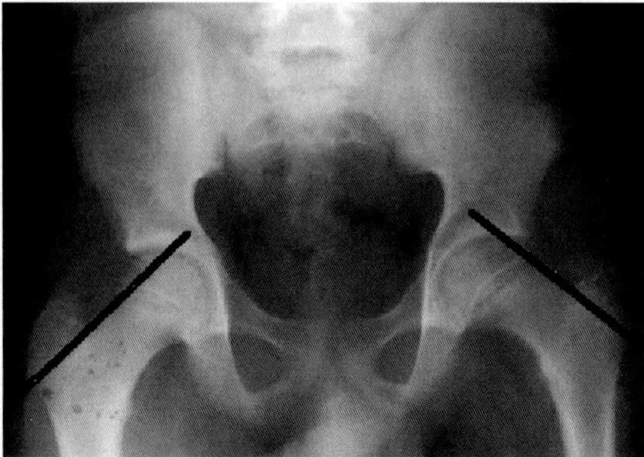

**FIG 1** • An AP radiograph of the pelvis shows the Klein line drawn on the left hip. The line does not cross the epiphysis, indicating the SCFE. (Copyright Richard S. Davidson, MD.)

## NONOPERATIVE MANAGEMENT

- Immobilization in a spica cast was the historical treatment but is no longer recommended for SCFE.
- Once SCFE is identified in any patient with an open physis, management is surgical to avoid further slippage and the possible development of femoral head AVN.

## SURGICAL MANAGEMENT

- When SCFE is identified in a patient with an open physis, surgical management with percutaneous in situ cannulated screw fixation should be undertaken on an urgent basis if the slip is stable or on an emergent basis if unstable.[2] There is a fair amount of evidence that the risk of AVN in *unstable* SCFE can be reduced if the hip is decompressed in some manner within 24 hours.[5]
- Before surgery, the patient should remain strictly non–weight bearing on the affected leg to prevent conversion of a stable SCFE to an unstable SCFE.
- In unstable SCFE, purposeful reduction of the displacement is controversial. Both open and closed reduction techniques have been associated with osteonecrosis, but the unstable slip itself may be the more likely cause of osteonecrosis.[1,13,19]
  - Because of the risk of contralateral slip, prophylactic pinning of the contralateral hip can be considered and discussed with the patient and family, especially if the patient is younger than age 10 years or has an endocrine abnormality.[8,14,15]

### Preoperative Planning

- All imaging studies are reviewed. The plain films of the contralateral hip should be scrutinized for evidence of early or clinically silent slip.
- Laboratory studies should be reviewed in patients younger than 10 years of age.

### Positioning

- We place the patient supine on the radiolucent operating room (OR) table with the entire affected leg prepared and draped free to the umbilicus. The ipsilateral arm is padded and positioned across the chest.
- The fluoroscopy monitor is placed at the patient's head and the C-arm unit is positioned for AP views of the hip from the contralateral side of the operating table. The hip is flexed 90 degrees and abducted 45 degrees to obtain lateral views. Not using a fracture table allows multiple views to be sure that the guide pin and the bone screws do not penetrate the femoral head.
- Some surgeons prefer to perform in situ screw fixation on a fracture table.

### Approach

- In situ cannulated screw fixation of SCFE involves percutaneous placement of the guidewire into the central third of the epiphysis perpendicular to the physis. In most cases, this involves a small incision on the anterolateral thigh. This is followed by drilling and placement of the screw over the guidewire. Some screws are self-tapping and self-drilling.
- Careful examination of spot fluoroscopy images ensures that the screw tip is within the femoral head, as detailed in the Techniques section.

## Guidewire Placement

- The goal of guidewire placement is to place the tip of the wire perpendicular to the physis in the middle third of the epiphysis, about 3 mm from the subchondral bone. Spacing of the screw threads can be measured (usually 1 mm) and compared on the image intensification screen as a ruler. For the most common SCFE (varus slip), the starting point is on the anterior neck to place the wire properly in the middle of the epiphysis.

### Determining the Course of the Guidewire

- Under image guidance (AP view with the image machine placed vertical), the hip is internally and externally rotated until the neck appears to be its longest. At this position of rotation, the femoral neck is horizontal to the operating table and perpendicular to the image beam (**TECH FIG 1A**).
- A guidewire is placed on the anterior hip and image intensification is used to align the point of the wire over the center of the femoral head. The guidewire is then aligned along the neck (**TECH FIG 1B**). The skin is marked at the tip to identify the position of the center of the femoral head.
  - The marker then follows the guidewire laterally to the lateral aspect of the femur. This line represents the course along which the guide pin for the bone screw will follow in the AP image (**TECH FIG 1C**). The marked line is drawn with a pen (**TECH FIG 1D**).

### Determining the Entry Point along the Femoral Neck

- Although we know that the femoral neck is following this marked line, the position of the femoral head in the sagittal plane is determined by flexing the hip 90 degrees and abducting the hip 45 degrees for the frog-leg lateral view. A line is drawn on the image as a diameter of the femoral head, and then a line is drawn perpendicular to the diameter at its center representing the desired path of the bone screw in the sagittal plane (**TECH FIG 2A**). The angle this line makes with the femoral neck tells the position of the femoral head with respect to the end of the femoral neck. The position at which this line crosses the femoral neck line also defines the entry point for the guide pin along the femoral neck (**TECH FIG 2B,C**). The degree of slip of the epiphysis posteriorly with respect to the neck is estimated.
- Having taken the steps earlier, the surgeon has now determined how to make the femoral neck horizontal to the operating table and perpendicular to the image beam and has determined the angle that the femoral head is with respect to the end of the femoral neck and the entry point on the anterolateral neck for the guide pin and screw.

### Determining the Skin Entry Site

- The final issue for the surgeon to determine is where to enter the skin. The skin is like a circle around the hip. The mark for the center of the femoral head is at 90 degrees and the lateral (palpable) femoral shaft is at 0 degree (**TECH FIG 3A**). If the head–neck angle measured is, for example, 30 degrees, the entry point on the skin should be 30 degrees from the lateral palpable femoral shaft toward the femoral head.
  - Helpful hint: This position can be obtained by taking a length of suture that goes from the femoral head mark to the lateral femur mark (representing 90 degrees) and dividing it into thirds (30 degrees). The surgeon then measures from the lateral femoral shaft (0-degree mark)

A 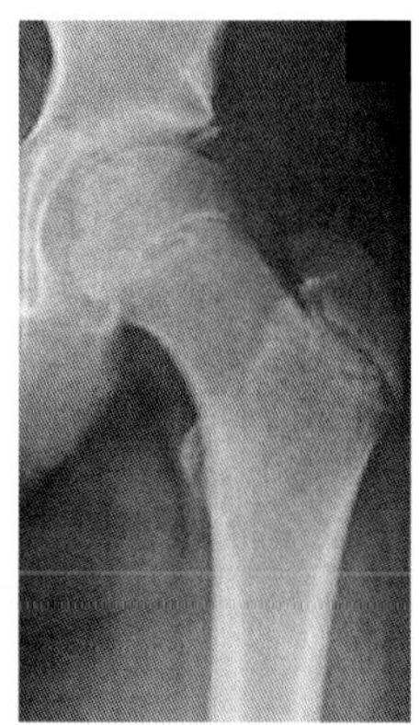

B 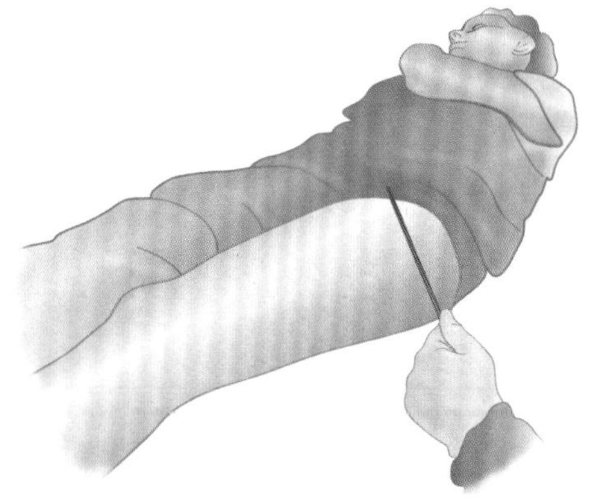

C 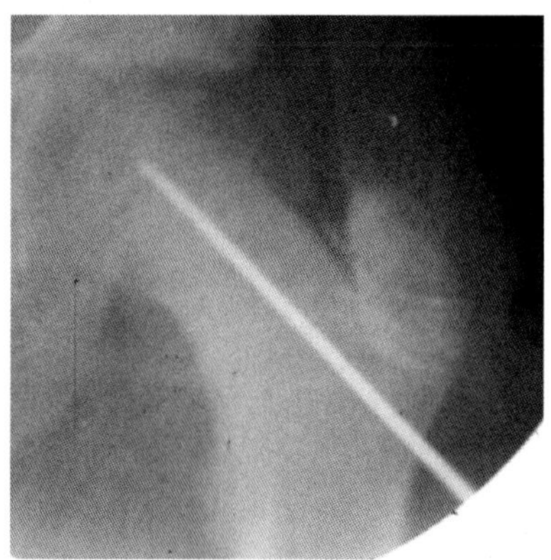

D 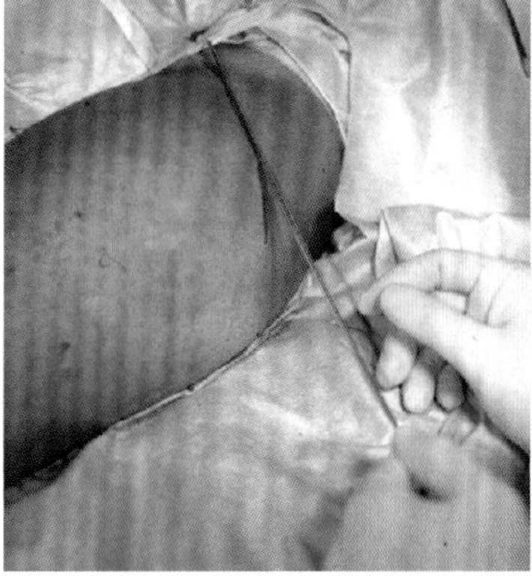

**TECH FIG 1** • Patient is supine on the operating table. **A.** The image intensifier is set for an AP view and an image is obtained. The hip to be operated on is rotated internally and externally until the length of the neck appears longest. The femoral neck is now horizontal. This position is maintained. **B.** A long guidewire is placed on the patient at the hip with the point centered on the center of the femoral head and the guidewire over the center of the neck. **C.** This is confirmed with an image view. **D.** An OR pen is used to mark the skin with this line. The femoral shaft is palpated laterally on this line; this point is marked as 0 degree. The point over the femoral head is marked as 90 degrees. (**A,C:** Copyright Richard S. Davidson, MD.)

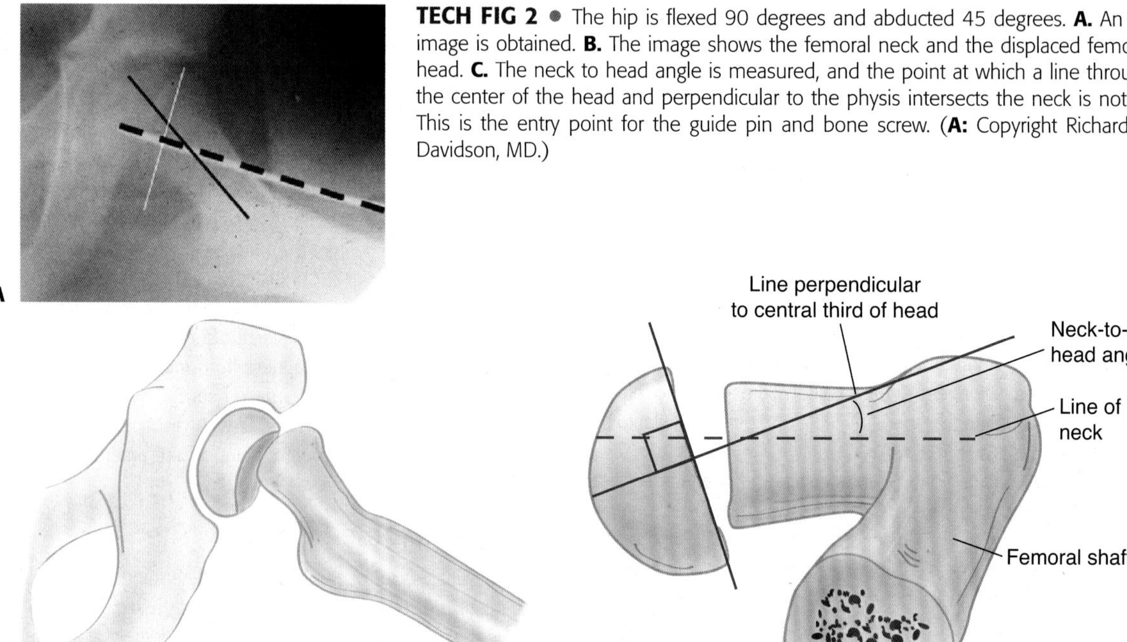


**TECH FIG 2** • The hip is flexed 90 degrees and abducted 45 degrees. **A.** An AP image is obtained. **B.** The image shows the femoral neck and the displaced femoral head. **C.** The neck to head angle is measured, and the point at which a line through the center of the head and perpendicular to the physis intersects the neck is noted. This is the entry point for the guide pin and bone screw. (**A:** Copyright Richard S. Davidson, MD.)

toward the head along the drawn line. A 1-cm incision is made through skin and spread with a hemostat down to bone along the drawn line but at an angle of 30 degrees toward the horizontal (ie, the head–neck angle) (**TECH FIG 3B**).

- The guide pin should enter the incision in line with the drawn line and at an angle of 30 degrees to the horizontal (**TECH FIG 3C**). The point of the guide pin should be positioned on the anterolateral femoral neck where the entry was estimated earlier.

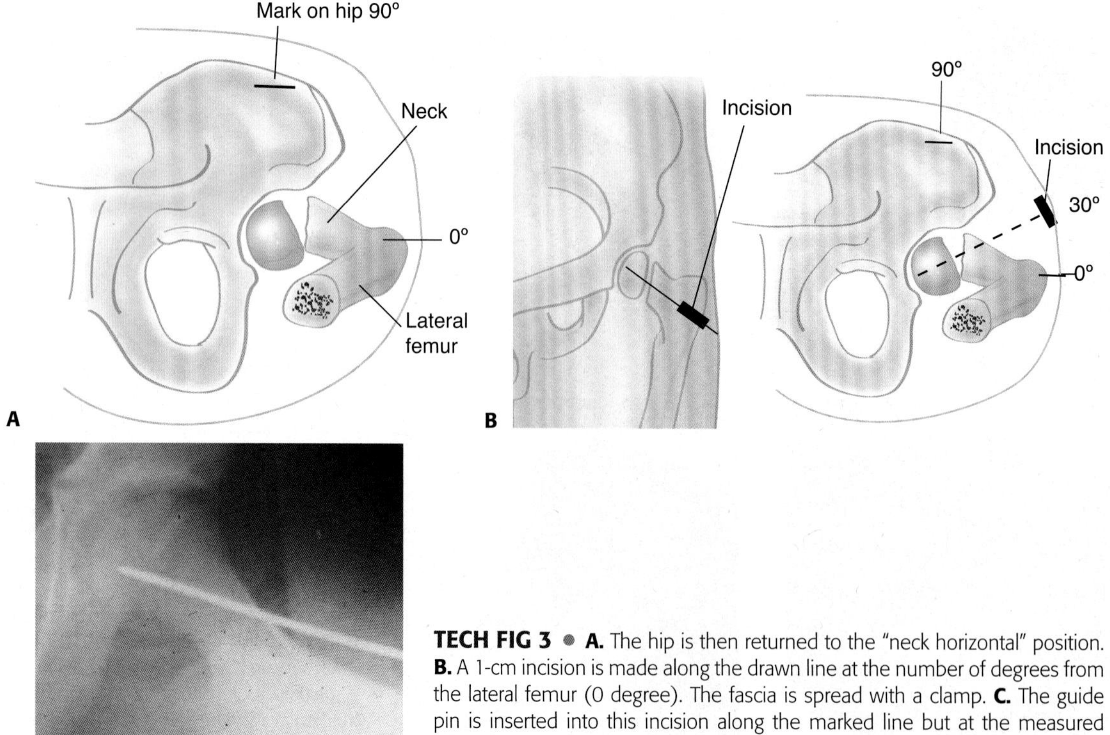


**TECH FIG 3** • **A.** The hip is then returned to the "neck horizontal" position. **B.** A 1-cm incision is made along the drawn line at the number of degrees from the lateral femur (0 degree). The fascia is spread with a clamp. **C.** The guide pin is inserted into this incision along the marked line but at the measured neck–head angle. The level of insertion at the neck is at the point observed in **TECH FIG 2C**. (**C:** Copyright Richard S. Davidson, MD.)

### Inserting the Guidewire

- The guide pin is drilled part-way into the femoral neck and the hip is rotated to assess the guide pin trajectory on the lateral view. In obese patients, it is easy to inadvertently bend the guidewire from the pressure of the soft tissues. This can be minimized by extending the incision a bit and by using the cannulated depth gauge to help protect the wire. When satisfactory, the guide pin is advanced to within 3 mm of the articular surface and measured, and a bone screw is chosen. Multiple image views should confirm the guide pin position before inserting the bone screw to avoid stress risers from too many holes in the bone.
  - Helpful hint: The surgeon can rotate the hip to prevent bending of the guide pin while flexing to get multiple views.
- The chosen bone screw is inserted to within 3 mm of the articular surface.
  - Helpful hint: If the end of the guide pin is threaded, the bone screw may advance the guide pin through the articular surface. The hip must *not* be moved because of the risk of breaking off the end of the guide pin in the hip joint. Instead, the surgeon can retract the guide pin partially into the bone screw and then continue to advance the bone screw to the appropriate position. Again, multiple views are obtained to ensure that the bone screw does not penetrate the articular surface.

## Drilling and Cannulated Screw Placement

- The guidewire is measured with the cannulated depth gauge to determine desired screw length.
- The cannulated drill is drilled over the guidewire. Care is taken to keep the drill colinear with the guidewire to avoid binding. The drill should stop 1 or 2 mm before the tip of the guidewire to keep the guidewire in place.
- The bone is tapped with the cannulated tap over the guidewire.
- The 6.5- to 7.5-mm cannulated screw is placed over the guidewire.
- The guidewire is removed.

## Radiographic Evaluation

- Radiographic evaluation (**TECH FIG 4**) ensures good screw position to minimize risk of complications.
- Spot fluoroscopic AP and frog-leg lateral views are used to make sure that four or five threads of the screw are within the epiphysis to decrease the risk of slip progression.
- The approach and withdraw technique allows evaluation of the screw tip to ensure that it remains within the femoral head. With live fluoroscopy, the hip is ranged from internal to external rotation at varying degrees of flexion and the screw tip is observed to approach and withdraw from the subchondral bone. The closest point is observed and the screw should remain within the femoral head.[12]

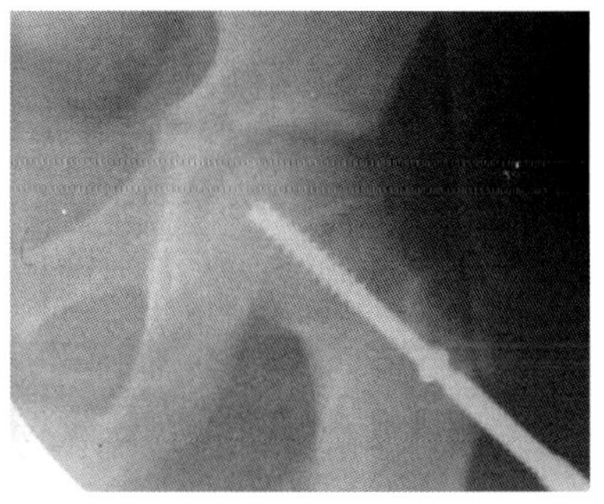
A

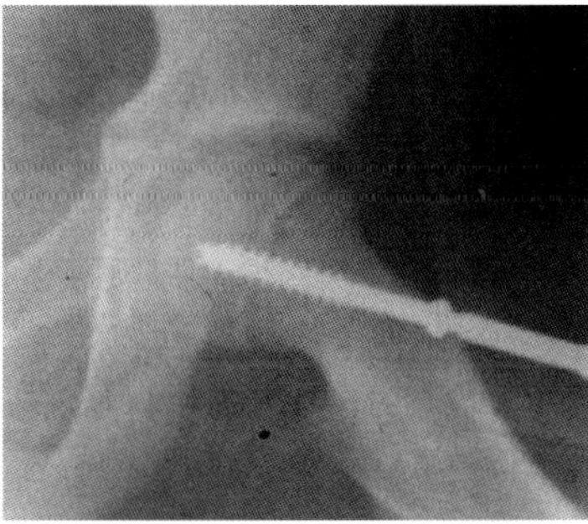
B

**TECH FIG 4** • Radiographic evaluation of the threads across the physis on the AP (**A**) and frog-leg lateral (**B**) views. (Copyright Richard S. Davidson, MD.)

## PEARLS AND PITFALLS

| | |
|---|---|
| **Guidewire placement** | ▪ In general, the larger the slip, the more proximal the starting point along the anterior neck.<br>▪ The guidewire should be placed into the center of the epiphysis parallel to the physis to obtain maximum fixation, like the handle of an umbrella. |
| **Guidewire bending** | ▪ When the hip is moved from resting position to frog-leg lateral position or back again, the pin can bend from pressure of the soft tissues. This can be minimized by using a 1- to 2-cm incision and by using the cannulated depth gauge to protect the pin. |
| **Guidewire pullout** | ▪ Drilling should stop 1–2 mm before the end of the guidewire to keep it seated in bone. The surgeon should check spot fluoroscopy as the drill is backed out to make sure the guidewire remains in place.<br>▪ The guidewire should be gently tapped back into place if it begins to pull out. |
| **Guidewire binding** | ▪ During drilling, tapping, or screw placement, the instrument can bind the guidewire and cause unwanted advancement of the guidewire.<br>▪ The cannulated instrument must remain perfectly colinear with the guidewire during advancement.<br>▪ The surgeon should check spot fluoroscopy to make sure the guidewire is not advancing. |

## POSTOPERATIVE CARE

- No immobilization is recommended. Patients should remain non–weight bearing or touch-down weight bearing on crutches on the affected leg for about 6 weeks to allow healing.
- Patients are gradually allowed to return to activities after 6 weeks.
- If the SCFE and fixation were unilateral, patients and families must be made aware of symptoms to watch for that could indicate slipping in the other hip, such as hip, thigh, or knee pain.
- Patients should be followed at regular intervals until the proximal femoral physis closes completely on radiographs.

## OUTCOMES

- Outcomes of SCFE treatment are related to the severity of slip and the development of complications. The best long-term results are seen with in situ screw fixation.[3] In patients with mild and moderate SCFE treated with in situ screw fixation, results are good to excellent.

## COMPLICATIONS

- Chondrolysis is articular cartilage necrosis of the femoral head that causes hip pain and limited motion.
  - It has been associated with SCFE and its treatment, and the incidence has decreased with modern treatment techniques of in situ screw fixation.
  - Risk factors include unrecognized pin or screw penetration, spica cast treatment, more severe slips, and female sex. The joint space appears narrowed to less than 3 mm on radiographs, and treatment involves revision of prominent hardware, limited weight bearing until symptoms improve, physical therapy, and nonsteroidal anti-inflammatories. Overall, patients may have cartilage recovery and good midterm functional outcomes.[18]
- Osteonecrosis is a difficult and often debilitating complication associated with SCFE and its treatment. It involves the death and possible collapse (**FIG 2**) of the epiphysis because of disruption of its blood supply. Patients present with groin, thigh, or knee pain and limited hip motion.
  - Risk factors for osteonecrosis are unstable SCFE, pins in the posterosuperior quadrant of the epiphysis, an increased number of pins, and severe displacement.[17] A stable slip has a nearly 0% risk of osteonecrosis, but an unstable slip can have as high as a 50% risk of osteonecrosis.[10]
  - Treatment involves removal of prominent hardware if the physis has closed, limited weight bearing until healing, symptomatic management, and later reconstructive procedures.
- Further slippage after in situ fixation occurs most frequently with improper screw placement outside of the desired middle third of the epiphysis and insufficient thread purchase into the epiphysis.

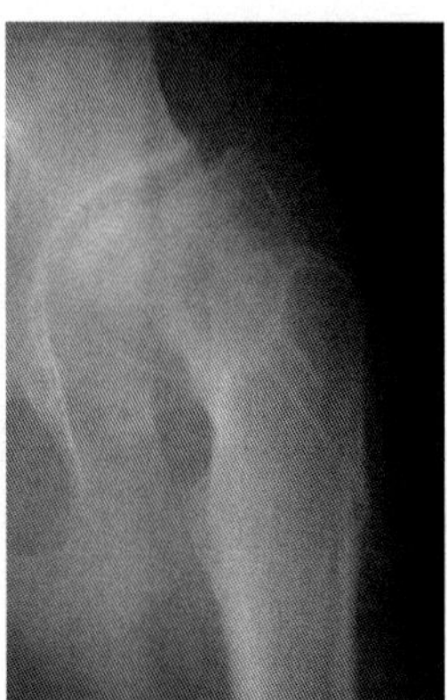

**FIG 2** • Osteonecrosis and collapse of the femoral head in a severe case of SCFE. The in situ fixation had become prominent and has been removed. (Copyright Richard S. Davidson, MD.)

## REFERENCES


1. Alves C, Steele M, Narayanan U, et al. Open reduction and internal fixation of unstable slipped capital femoral epiphysis by means of surgical dislocation does not decrease the rate of avascular necrosis: a preliminary study. J Child Orthop 2012;6:277–283.
2. Aronson DD, Carlson WE. Slipped capital femoral epiphysis. A prospective study of fixation with a single screw. J Bone Joint Surg Am 1992;74(6):810–819.
3. Carney BT, Weinstein SL. Natural history of untreated chronic slipped capital femoral epiphysis. Clin Orthop Relat Res 1996;(322):43–47.
4. Harris WR. The endocrine basis for slipping of the femoral epiphysis. J Bone Joint Surg Br 1950;32-B(1):5–11.
5. Herrera-Soto JA, Duffy MF, Birnbaum MA, et al. Increased intracapsular pressures after unstable slipped capital femoral epiphysis. J Pediatr Orthop 2008;28:723–728.
6. Ippolito E, Mickelson MR, Ponseti IV. A histochemical study of slipped capital femoral epiphysis. J Bone Joint Surg Am 1981;63(7):1109–1113.

7. Jacobs B. Diagnosis and natural history of slipped capital femoral epiphysis. Instr Course Lect 1972;21:167–173.
8. Kocher MS, Bishop JA, Hresko MT, et al. Prophylactic pinning of the contralateral hip after unilateral slipped capital femoral epiphysis. J Bone Joint Surg Am 2004;86:2658–2665.
9. Loder RT. The demographics of slipped capital femoral epiphysis. An international multicenter study. Clin Orthop Relat Res 1996;(322):8–27.
10. Loder RT, Richards BS, Shapiro PS, et al. Acute slipped capital femoral epiphysis: the importance of physeal stability. J Bone Joint Surg Am 1993;75(8):1134–1140.
11. Loder RT, Whittenberg B, DeSilva G. Slipped capital femoral epiphysis associated with endocrine disorders. J Pediatr Orthop 1995;15:349–356.
12. Moseley C. The “approach–withdraw phenomenon” in the pinning of slipped capital femoral epiphysis. Orthop Trans 1985;9:497.
13. Rhoad RC, Davidson RS, Heyman S, et al. Pretreatment bone scan in SCFE: a predictor of ischemia and avascular necrosis. J Pediatr Orthop 1999;19:164–168.
14. Sankar WN, Novais EN, Lee C, et al. What are the risks of prophylactic pinning to prevent contralateral slipped capital femoral epiphysis? Clin Orthop Relat Res 2013;471:2118–2123.
15. Schultz WR, Weinstein JN, Weinstein SL, et al. Prophylactic pinning of the contralateral hip in slipped capital femoral epiphysis: evaluation of long-term outcome for the contralateral hip with use of decision analysis. J Bone Joint Surg Am 2002;84:1305–1314.
16. Southwick WO. Osteotomy through the lesser trochanter for slipped capital femoral epiphysis. J Bone Joint Surg Am 1967;49(5):807–835.
17. Tokmakova KP, Stanton RP, Mason DE. Factors influencing the development of osteonecrosis in patients treated for slipped capital femoral epiphysis. J Bone Joint Surg Am 2003;85-A(5):798–801.
18. Vrettos BC, Hoffman EB. Chondrolysis in slipped upper femoral epiphysis. Long-term study of the aetiology and natural history. J Bone Joint Surg Br 1993;75(6):956–961.
19. Zaltz I, Baca G, Clohisy JC. Unstable SCFE: review of treatment modalities and prevalence of osteonecrosis. Clin Orthop Relat Res 2013;471:2192–2198.

# Flexion Intertrochanteric Osteotomy for Severe Slipped Capital Femoral Epiphysis

Young-Jo Kim

## DEFINITION

- Pistol grip deformity after slipped capital femoral epiphysis (SCFE) can cause anterior impingement leading to pain, cartilage and labral damage, and eventual osteoarthritis.[1,2,8]
- Realignment of the proximal femur, as well as restoration of the anterior head–neck offset, has been shown to improve hip clinical outcomes.[7]
- This technique can be used to correct anterior impingement after an SCFE that has healed with residual posterior displacement.
- The first part of the procedure is a surgical hip dislocation approach with femoral head–neck osteoplasty.
- If additional deformity correction is needed, the flexion intertrochanteric osteotomy is performed.

## PATHOGENESIS

- The true etiology of SCFE is unclear. However, because it occurs mainly in adolescent boys (80%), hormonal factors are thought to be involved.
- Additionally, the orientation of the growth plate becomes more vertical in adolescents compared to the juvenile hip, leading to increased shear stress across the physis.
- The transition from juvenile to adolescent is a period of rapid weight gain, leading to the stereotypical obese body habitus in the SCFE patient.

## NATURAL HISTORY

- Undetected SCFEs can lead to hip arthrosis. Murray[4] suggests that up to 40% of hips with degenerative arthritis have a "tilt deformity" or other deformities that may be due to an undetected subclinical SCFE or other developmental problems.
- A review by Aronson[1] found that 15% to 20% of patients with SCFE had painful osteoarthritis by age 50 years. Additionally, 11% of patients with end-stage osteoarthritis had an SCFE.

## PATIENT HISTORY AND PHYSICAL FINDINGS

- Patients will complain of insidious-onset groin or knee pain that may have previously been diagnosed as a sprain.
  - They may walk with a limp, but typically they walk with an externally rotated foot progression angle, which may indicate chronic SCFE or femoral retroversion.
  - Pain is elicited with hip flexion, adduction, and internal rotation stress (impingement test).
  - The physical examination should include flexion and internal rotation range-of-motion tests. Normal, physiologic hip flexion needed for activities of daily living is at least 90 degrees.
  - Patients with a chronic SCFE and anterior impingement will have less than 90 degrees of true hip flexion.
  - Patients with impingement secondary to SCFE will have less internal rotation in flexion than extension and may have a compensatory external rotation of the hip as it is flexed (obligate external rotation).

## IMAGING AND OTHER DIAGNOSTIC STUDIES

- Plain radiographs include an anteroposterior (AP) and frog-leg lateral views of the pelvis or the involved hip (**FIG 1A,B**).
- Computed tomography (CT) scans with two- and three-dimensional reconstructions are helpful for preoperative planning (**FIG 1C,D**).

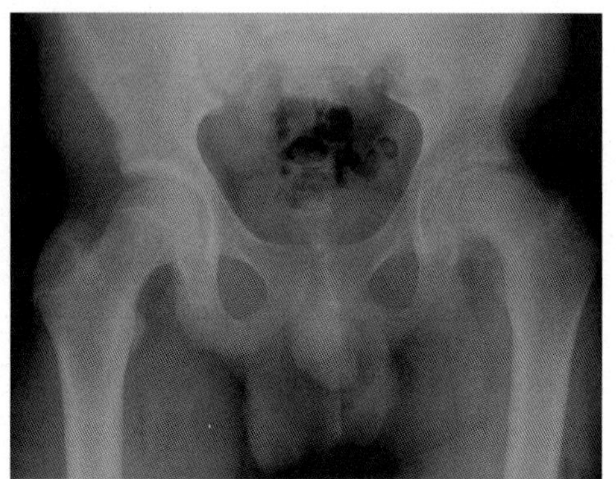
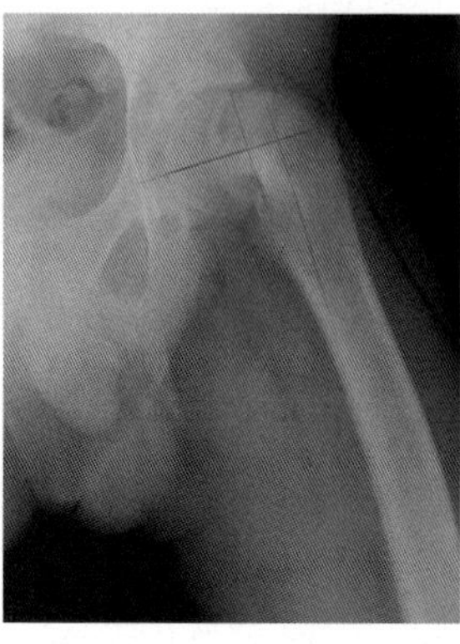

**FIG 1** • Preoperative AP (**A**) and frog-leg lateral (**B**) radiographs of the left hip demonstrate a chronic, stable severe SCFE with greater than 70 degrees of posterior slippage. *(continued)*

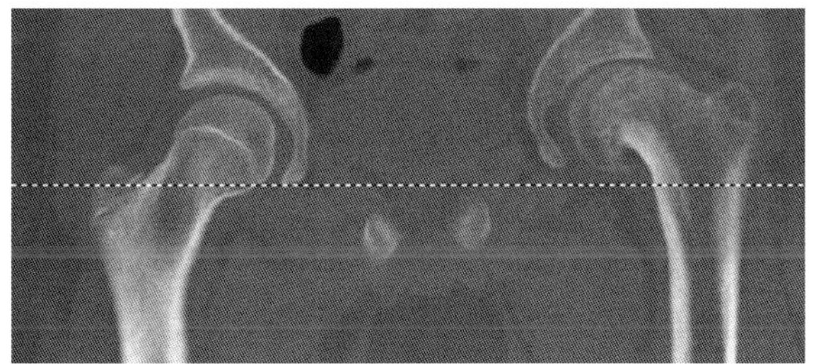

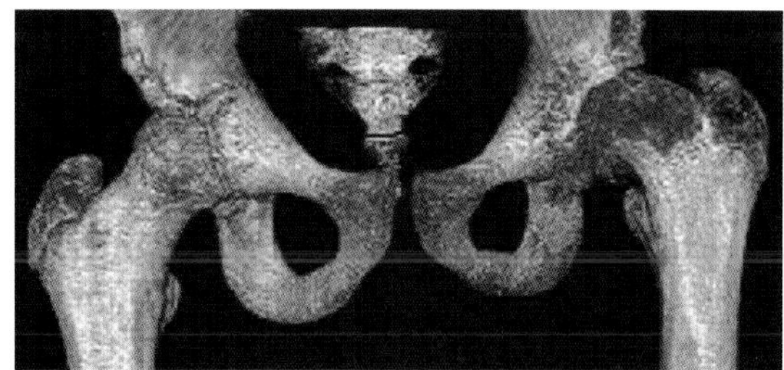

FIG 1 • *(continued)* Preoperative two-dimensional (**C**) and three-dimensional (**D**) CT reconstructions further define the severity of the deformity.

## DIFFERENTIAL DIAGNOSIS

- Femoral or acetabular retroversion
- Idiopathic femoroacetabular impingement

## NONOPERATIVE MANAGEMENT

- Nonoperative management includes cessation of aggravating activities and symptomatic treatment using nonsteroidal anti-inflammatories.
- Physical therapy to strengthen the hip musculature does not address the mechanical impingement associated with an SCFE.
- All SCFE should be stabilized surgically. Nonoperative management if for impingement symptoms.

## SURGICAL MANAGEMENT

- A chronic slip may be pinned in situ to prevent continued slippage. Remodeling of the SCFE deformity has been described in long-term follow-up studies.
- Corrective osteotomies have been described through the femoral neck at the growth plate (cuneiform), at the base of the femoral neck, or intertrochantic or subtrochanteric.[6]

### Preoperative Planning

- The anterior head–shaft angle is measured on the AP pelvis radiograph on both the affected and normal sides. The difference is the amount of varus deformity on the slip side that can be addressed with a valgus-producing intertrochanteric osteotomy (**FIG 2A**).
- The lateral head–shaft angle is measured on the frog-leg lateral view in a manner similar to that used on the AP view. The difference is the amount of posterior deformity present that is corrected with a flexion-producing intertrochanteric osteotomy (**FIG 2B**).

### Positioning

- Because the first part of the procedure is done through a surgical hip dislocation, the patient is placed in the full lateral position secured on a pegboard, as shown in Chapter 109, Figure 3. A flat-top cushion placed beneath the operative side is helpful to stabilize the leg during the approach.
  - A hip drape with a sterile side bag is used, which will capture the leg during the dislocation maneuver.

### Approach

- The incision from the surgical hip dislocation is extended slightly distal, along the lateral aspect of the thigh, in line with the femoral shaft.
- The lateral approach to the proximal third of the femur is required for the intertrochanteric osteotomy.

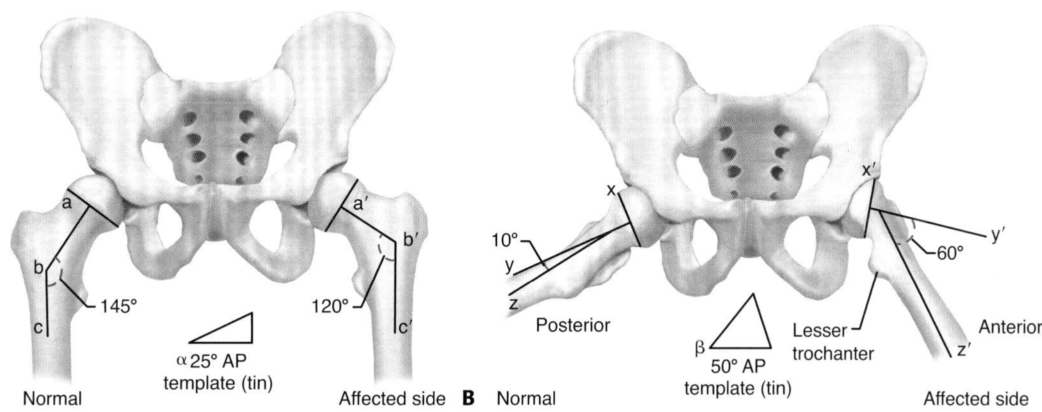


FIG 2 • Methods for determining the anterior head–shaft angle (**A**) and the lateral head–shaft angle (**B**). **A.** The difference in the angle determines the anterior osteotomy template. **B.** The posterior angulation of the affected side determines the angle of the lateral osteotomy template.

## Approach to Proximal Femur

- The longitudinal incision from the surgical hip dislocation can be extended distally, in line with the lateral shaft of the femur (**TECH FIG 1A**).
- The vastus lateralis, supplied by the femoral nerve, is reflected anteriorly from the vastus ridge distally (**TECH FIG 1B**).
- Several perforating vessels from the profunda femoris artery to the vastus lateralis should be identified and coagulated before they are avulsed by blunt dissection.
- The anterolateral aspect of the femoral shaft is then exposed subperiosteally, and the lesser trochanter is identified.

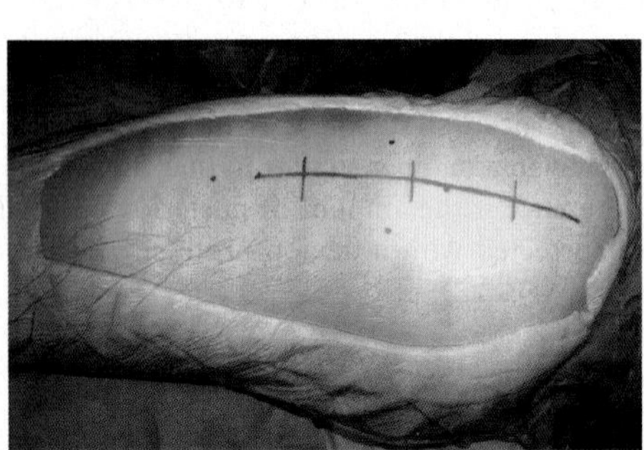

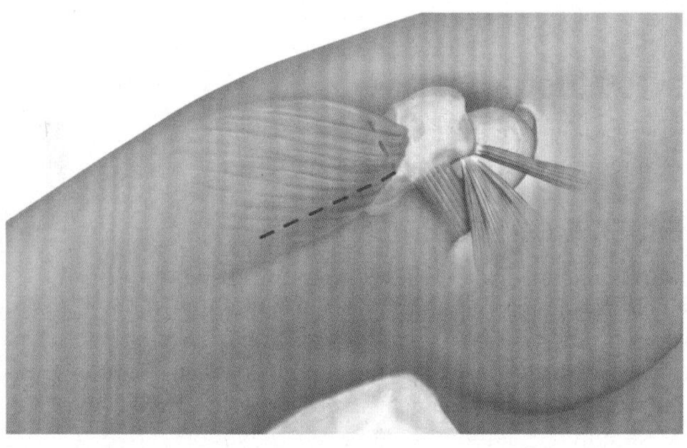

**TECH FIG 1** • **A.** The proposed incision after the patient is prepared and draped. **B.** Approach to the intertrochanteric region of the femur. The vastus lateralis is reflected anteriorly from its origin at the vastus ridge.

## Planning the Osteotomy

- A 2-0 Kirschner wire is placed just above the level of the lesser trochanter, beginning in the lateral cortex of the proximal femur. This is placed parallel to the floor in the axial plane and perpendicular to the shaft of the femur in the coronal plane. This is the reference for the level of the osteotomy.
- A second Kirschner wire is placed 3 cm proximal to the first. This is placed parallel to the first guidewire in the axial plane. In the coronal plane, the Kirschner wire is placed with an appropriate amount of valgus, determined from the anterior head–shaft angle difference on preoperative radiographs. In the Imhauser technique, addition of a valgus osteotomy is not necessary, hence, a pure flexion osteotomy is performed. This will act as the guidewire for the seating chisel for the blade plate.

## Creating the Slot for the Blade Plate

- The seating chisel is directed parallel to the most proximal guide pin with the appropriate amount of flexion, as determined on the frog-leg lateral head–shaft angle difference.
- A slot for the blade plate should now be made in the trochanteric fragment to allow for anatomic fixation of the trochanter after the osteotomy.
- The blade plate chisel is placed into the proximal fragment after preparation of the trochanteric flip fragment and before cutting the intertrochanteric osteotomy (**TECH FIG 2**).

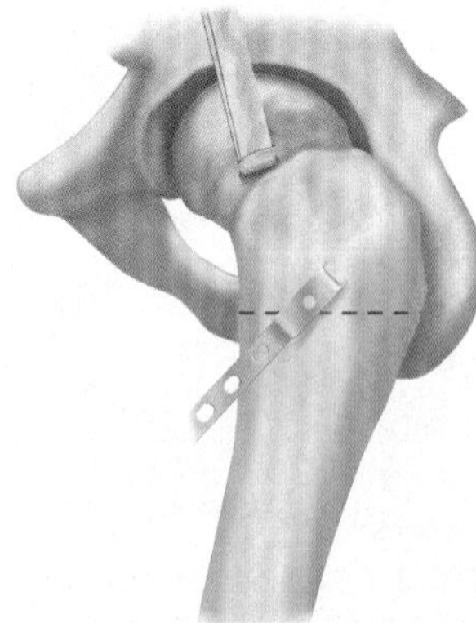

**TECH FIG 2** • The blade plate is impacted into the proximal fragment through a slot created in the trochanteric wafer. The amount of flexion is based on the preoperative lateral head–shaft angle measurement.

## Osteotomy

- Before osteotomy, a rotational reference mark is made at the level of the osteotomy on both the proximal and distal fragments.
- Using an oscillating saw, the proximal femur is cut using the distal Kirschner wire as a guide. The cut should be made perpendicular to the shaft of the femur.

## Blade Plate Placement

- The seating chisel is removed and the blade plate is impacted into the proximal fragment.
- The osteotomy is provisionally reduced and held with a Verbrugge clamp.
- Often, the distal fragment will need to be internally rotated to match the hip rotation of the normal side.
- After confirming reduction using an image intensifier, the plate is fixed to the shaft of the femur in standard fashion (**TECH FIG 3**).

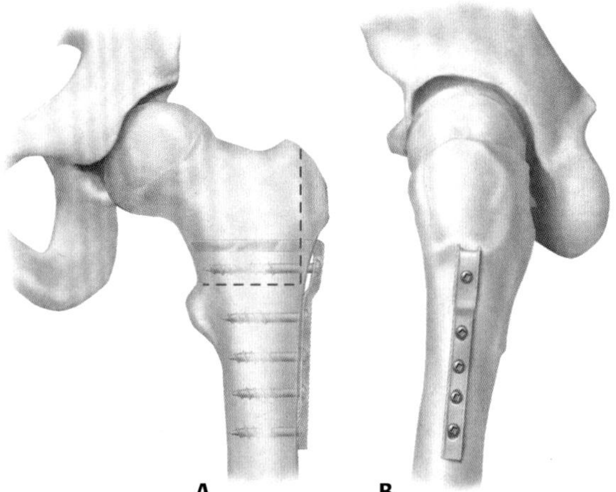


**TECH FIG 3** • After the osteotomy, the distal fragment is reduced to the blade plate (**A**) and secured in standard fashion (**B**).

## Closure

- The vastus lateralis fascia is closed with 2-0 absorbable running suture.
- The iliotibial band is closed using a running no. 1 absorbable suture.
- Skin is closed in routine fashion.

## PEARLS AND PITFALLS

| | |
|---|---|
| **Indications** | ▪ A complete history and physical examination should be performed.<br>▪ All associated pathology should be addressed. |
| **Osteotomy planning** | ▪ Southwick's technique advises against needing a flexion osteotomy of greater than 60 degrees. If there is greater than 60 degrees of posterior slippage, the femoral head–neck osteoplasty performed through a surgical hip dislocation can reduce the amount of flexion needed to relieve anterior impingement. |
| **Seating chisel removal** | ▪ After fully inserting the seating chisel, the surgeon should remove and replace it by hand before making the osteotomy. This will allow easy removal after the proximal fragment is less stable. |
| **Reduction of osteotomy** | ▪ Control of the proximal fragment is gained with a Weber bone-holding clamp instead of using the inserted blade plate for fragment manipulation, which could weaken the fixation. |
| **Nonunion** | ▪ Any areas that lack bone-to-bone contact require bone graft. |

## POSTOPERATIVE CARE

- The hip is held flexed and in neutral rotation by placing two pillows under the leg and one under the greater trochanter.
- The patient is placed in a continuous passive motion machine for 6 hours a day, set from 30 to 80 degrees of flexion.
- Prophylaxis for deep venous thrombosis is individualized; however, all patients should be started on mechanical compression devices immediately.
- After the epidural is removed, out-of-bed ambulation is permitted with one-sixth body weight partial weight bearing.

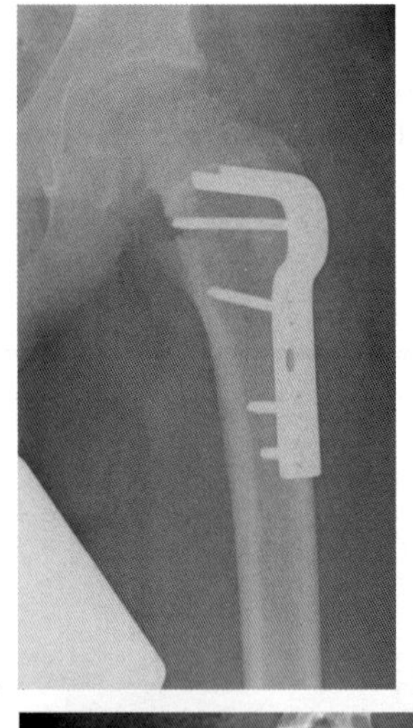
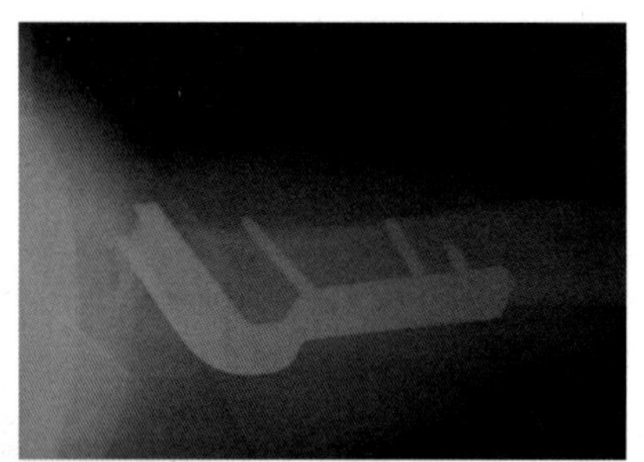
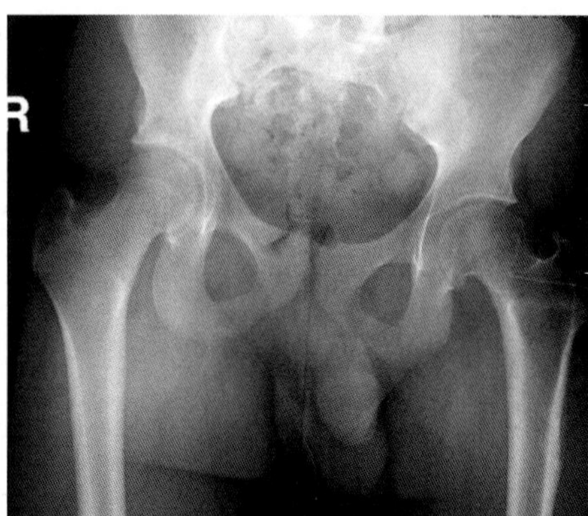

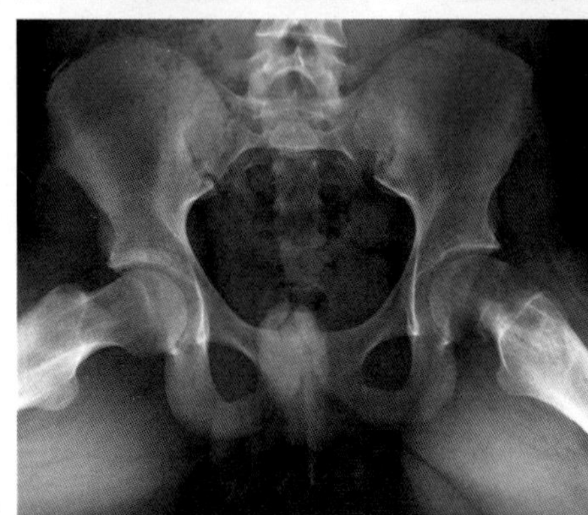

A B C D

**FIG 3** • Postoperative AP (**A**) and true lateral (**B**) radiographs demonstrate the correction of most of the SCFE deformity. AP (**C**) and frog-leg lateral (**D**) radiographs of the pelvis 4 months after removal of hardware. The patient has no symptoms.

- Range-of-motion exercises are started, but care is taken to protect the greater trochanter osteotomy by limiting adduction to midline and avoiding resisted abduction exercises for 6 weeks.
- AP and true lateral hip radiographs are obtained to evaluate healing of the osteotomy (**FIG 3A,B**).
- Prominent hardware may be removed after 6 months if radiographic evidence of a healed osteotomy is seen (**FIG 3C,D**).

## OUTCOMES

- In Southwick's original article,[6] where he treated the deformity with a proximal femoral osteotomy without surgical hip dislocation, out of 28 hips (26 patients) with at least 5 years of follow-up, 21 were rated as excellent, 5 as good, and 2 as fair.
- In patients who had both osteoplasty and an intertrochanteric osteotomy, Western Ontario and McMaster Universities (WOMAC) pain and function scores improved in four of six patients.[7]
- Internal rotation in flexion improved from −20 to +10 degrees.[7]
- Long-term results of flexion osteotomy for SCFE shows 55% to 77% good to excellent results at ~20 year follow-up.[3,5]

## COMPLICATIONS

- Avascular necrosis of the femoral head can occur if care is not taken to follow the technique and to preserve the retinacular vessels.
- Nonunion of the greater trochanteric osteotomy or the intertrochanteric osteotomy
- Sciatic or femoral nerve neurapraxia
- Heterotopic ossification

## REFERENCES


1. Aronson J. Osteoarthritis of the young adult hip: etiology and treatment. Instr Course Lect 1986;35:119–128.
2. Goodman DA, Feighan JE, Smith AD, et al. Subclinical slipped capital femoral epiphysis: relationship to arthrosis of the hip. J Bone Joint Surg Am 1997;79(10):1489–1497.
3. Kartenbender K, Cordier W, Katthagen BD. Long-term follow-up study after corrective Imhäuser osteotomy for severe slipped capital femoral epiphysis. J Pediatr Ortho 2000;20:749–756.
4. Murray RO. The aetiology of primary osteoarthrosis of the hip. Br J Radiol 1965;38:810–824.
5. Schai PA, Exner GU, Hänsch O. Prevention of secondary coxarthrosis in slipped capital femoral epiphysis: a long-term follow-up study after corrective intertrochanteric osteotomy. J Pediatr Orthop B 1996;5:135–143.
6. Southwick WO. Osteotomy through the lesser trochanter for slipped capital femoral epiphysis. J Bone Joint Surg Am 1987;49(5):807–835.
7. Spencer S, Millis M, Kim Y. Early results of treatment for hip impingement syndrome in slipped capital femoral epiphysis and pistol grip deformity of the femoral head-neck junction using the surgical dislocation technique. J Pediatr Orthop 2006;26:281–285.
8. Wenger DR, Kishan S, Pring ME. Impingement and childhood hip disease. J Pediatr Orthop B 2006;15:233–243.

113

CHAPTER

# Modified Dunn Procedure for Slipped Capital Femoral Epiphysis

Wudbhav N. Sankar

## DEFINITION

- The modified Dunn procedure is an open realignment of the capital femoral epiphysis performed through a surgical dislocation approach.[18]
- Like the original Dunn osteotomy, the modified Dunn corrects a slipped capital femoral epiphysis (SCFE) at the site of maximal deformity (ie, the physis).[4]
- The procedure can be performed on both unstable SCFEs and stable SCFEs.

## ANATOMY

- The main source of perfusion to the femoral epiphysis is the medial femoral circumflex artery (MFCA) (**FIG 1**).
- The deep branch of the MFCA runs posterior to the obturator externus and perforates the hip capsule just distal to the piriformis and proximal to the superior gemellus.[5]
- It ends in two to four retinacular branches that enter the superior aspect of the femoral head.
- The intact external rotator muscles, especially the obturator externus, protect the MFCA during surgical dislocation of the hip.
- To safely reduce a SCFE, which typically displaces posterior and inferior to the neck, tension must be minimized on the retinacular vessels.[18]

## PATHOGENESIS

- The pathogenesis of a SCFE is well discussed in Chapter 111.
- The posteroinferior translation of the epiphysis relative to the femoral neck alters the resting position of the femoral head within the acetabulum.
- This altered position combined with the residual offset of the metaphysis can dramatically affect the motion of the hip joint.
- With flexion and internal rotation, the metaphyseal prominence can either enter the joint potentially causing damage to the acetabular cartilage or abut against the acetabular rim and the labrum[13] (**FIG 2**).
- In situ fixation, while effective for preventing further slippage, does not correct the deformity associated with SCFE.

## NATURAL HISTORY

- Historically, the long-term outcome after in situ screw fixation has generally been considered to be good.[1,2]
- Recent studies, however, have established an association between the residual proximal femoral metaphyseal deformity left by in situ treatment and the development of femoroacetabular impingement, lost hip motion, and premature osteoarthritis.[6,9,11,17]
- Increasing slip severity has been associated with poorer outcome.[3]

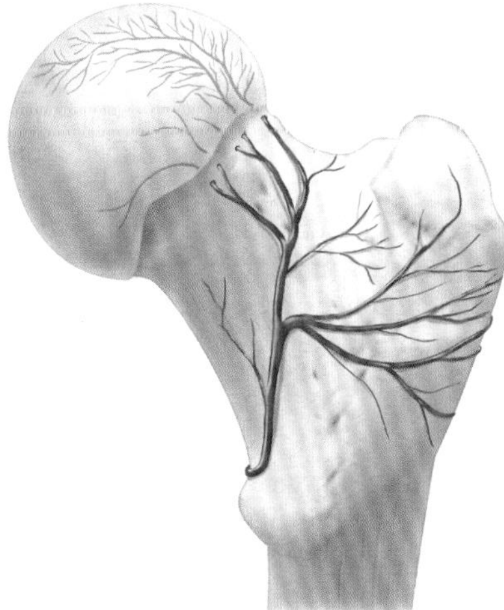

**FIG 1** • Posterior view of the vascular anatomy of the proximal femur. Note the proximity of the terminal branches of the MFCA to the insertion of the piriformis tendon.

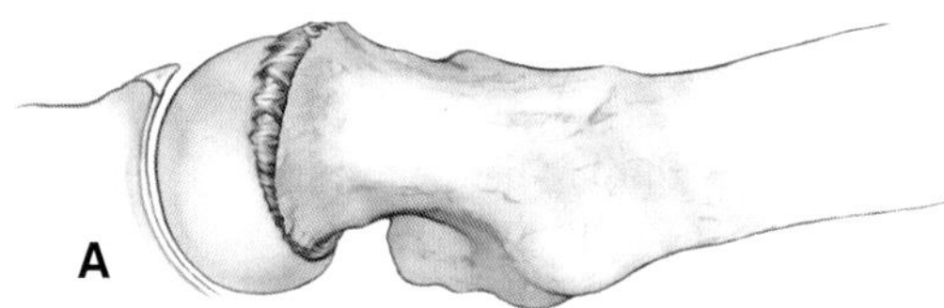


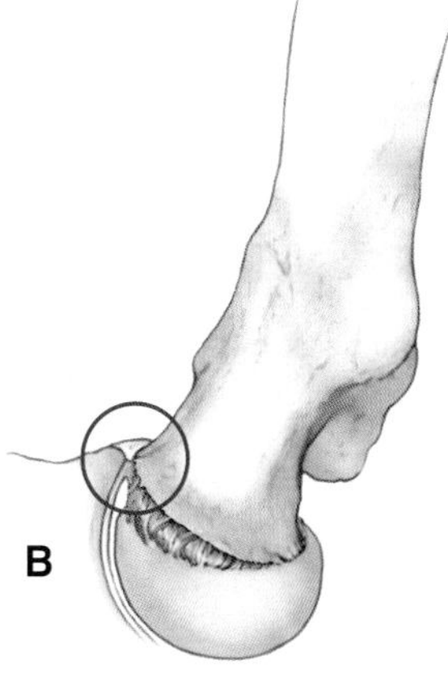


**FIG 2** • Clinical implication of a residual SCFE deformity: With flexion and internal rotation, the metaphyseal prominence can either enter the joint potentially causing damage to the acetabular cartilage (**A**) or abut against the acetabular rim and the labrum (**B**).

## PATIENT HISTORY AND PHYSICAL FINDINGS

- Patients with an unstable SCFE usually present acutely with an abrupt onset of symptoms.
  - Pain is intense and can be elicited even with simple logrolling of the affected extremity.
  - By definition, patients with unstable SCFE are unable to ambulate with or without walking aids.[10]
  - Further forced range of motion (ROM) of the affected hip is discouraged to minimize the risk of additional trauma to the femoral head blood supply.
- Patients with severe, stable SCFE can present with variable duration of symptoms.
  - Patients complain of hip or groin pain, thigh pain, or knee pain and usually occurs without a history of trauma.
  - By definition, patients are able to ambulate with or without walking aids and typically present with an antalgic gait and an external foot progression angle.[10]
  - Hip flexion, abduction, and internal rotation in the flexed position will be markedly decreased in a severe SCFE as a result of femoroacetabular impingement.
  - Many patients will also demonstrate obligate external rotation which is forced external rotation that results from passive hip flexion.

## IMAGING AND OTHER DIAGNOSTIC STUDIES

- Plain radiographs of the pelvis, including anteroposterior (AP) and frog-leg lateral views, should be obtained in any pediatric patient with hip, thigh, or knee pain and are generally diagnostic of a SCFE.
  - The femoral epiphysis is typically displaced posterior (on the frog view) and slightly inferior (on the AP view) in relation to the femoral neck.
- A widened physis on AP or lateral views can be an early sign of SCFE.
- The severity of a SCFE can be described by displacement relative to the width of the metaphysis:
  - Mild: less than one-third the width
  - Moderate: one-third to half the width
  - Severe: more than half the width
- Another method of describing slip severity is measuring the difference between the epiphyseal shaft angle on each side[16]:
  - Mild: less than 30 degrees
  - Moderate: 30 to 50 degrees
  - Severe: 50 degrees or greater
- In cases with delayed presentation in which the modified Dunn is being considered, computed tomography (CT) scan can be used to more accurately assess the degree of displacement and the amount of physeal closure.
- In certain patients with unstable SCFEs who present late, bone scan or contrast magnetic resonance imaging (MRI) can be used to assess the perfusion to the epiphysis.

## DIFFERENTIAL DIAGNOSIS

- SCFE
- Legg-Calvé-Perthes disease
- Hip labral tear
- Femoral neck fracture
- Septic arthritis of the hip
- Knee derangement
- Greater trochanteric bursitis

## NONOPERATIVE MANAGEMENT

- Immobilization in a spica cast was the historical treatment but is no longer recommended for SCFE.
- Once SCFE is identified in any patient with an open physis, management is surgical to avoid further slippage and the possible development of femoral head avascular necrosis (AVN).

## SURGICAL MANAGEMENT

- The modified Dunn procedure is indicated for unstable SCFEs and for certain stable SCFEs in which the residual deformity that would be left by in situ fixation is deemed unacceptable.
- It is most easily performed when the physis is still open.
- The modified Dunn procedure is a technically demanding procedure that requires familiarity with the surgical dislocation approach and the development of the retinacular flap.
- Alternative techniques for treating unstable SCFEs include (1) positional reduction followed by percutaneous screw fixation (with at least two screws) and capsular decompression[7] or (2) gentle manual open reduction performed via an anterolateral approach followed by Kirschner wire (K-wire) or screw fixation.[12]
- Alternative techniques for treating severe stable SCFEs include in situ fixation followed by osteoplasty of the femoral head–neck junction and/or proximal femoral osteotomy.

### Preoperative Planning

- All imaging studies are reviewed.
- Both AP and frog views should be reviewed for the presence of posteroinferior callus. This finding implies some chronicity to the SCFE and its removal is necessary to achieve an anatomic reduction.
- Pure displacement (ie, angulation or translation) can be corrected via the modified Dunn, but some chronic changes such as femoral neck retroversion are more difficult to address.
- In chronic and severe stable SCFEs, CT scans can be used to assess the status of the physis and determine the indication for the modified Dunn procedure.
- The contralateral hip should be evaluated both clinically and radiographically to determine whether a SCFE is present.
- In younger patients, and those with endocrinopathies, prophylactic percutaneous screw fixation of the normal side should be considered. This can be done in the supine position before commencing with the modified Dunn procedure (see Chap. 111).
- Timing of surgery for an unstable SCFE is somewhat controversial. For cases that present overnight, the author prefers performing the modified Dunn procedure the next morning with an appropriately skilled surgical team.

### Positioning

- As with a standard surgical dislocation of the hip (see Chap. 109), the patient is placed in full lateral position, secured on a pegboard. A flat-top cushion (with cutout for the down leg) supports the operative extremity during the procedure (**FIG 3**).
- A hip drape with a sterile side bag is used, which will capture the leg during the dislocation maneuver.

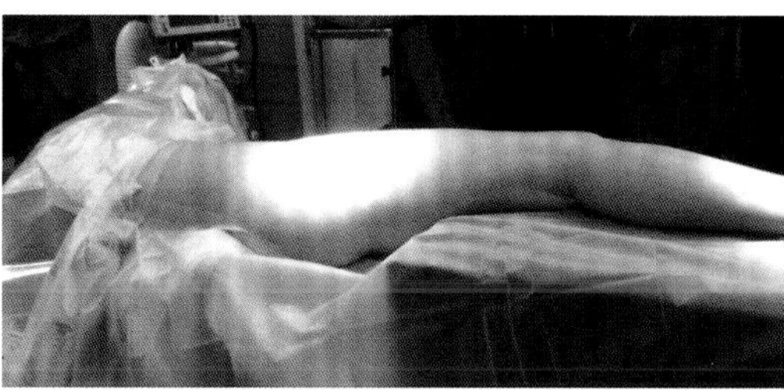

**FIG 3** • As with a standard surgical dislocation of the hip, the modified Dunn procedure is performed with the patient placed in full lateral position, secured on a pegboard. A flat-top cushion (with cutout for the down leg) supports the operative extremity during the procedure.

## Approach

- As with other surgical dislocations of the hip, the Kocher-Langenbeck or Gibson approach may be used.
- The Kocher-Langenbeck incision is followed by splitting of the gluteus maximus muscle. In obese patients, this approach does facilitate anterior exposure.
- The abductors and gluteus maximus muscles can be spared by performing a Gibson approach, which proceeds between the gluteus medius and maximus. This results in less hip extensor dysfunction but may make anterior exposure more difficult especially in obese patients.



## Exposure

- For a detailed description of the surgical dislocation approach please refer to Chapter 109. The following technique for the modified Dunn procedure begins after the hip capsule has been fully exposed.

## Hip Arthrotomy, Provisional Fixation, and Dislocation

- A Z-shaped capsulotomy is performed, with the longitudinal arm of the Z in line with the anterior neck of the femur (**TECH FIG 1A**).
  - The inferior limb extends along the intertrochanteric line toward but proximal to the lesser trochanter. A cuff of capsular tissue should be left for later repair.
  - Superior limb extends along the acetabular rim posteriorly toward the piriformis tendon. Care should be taken not to injure the labrum (**TECH FIG 1B**).
- It is helpful to tag the corners of the capsulotomy to help distinguish this layer from the retinacular flap which will be developed later in the procedure.

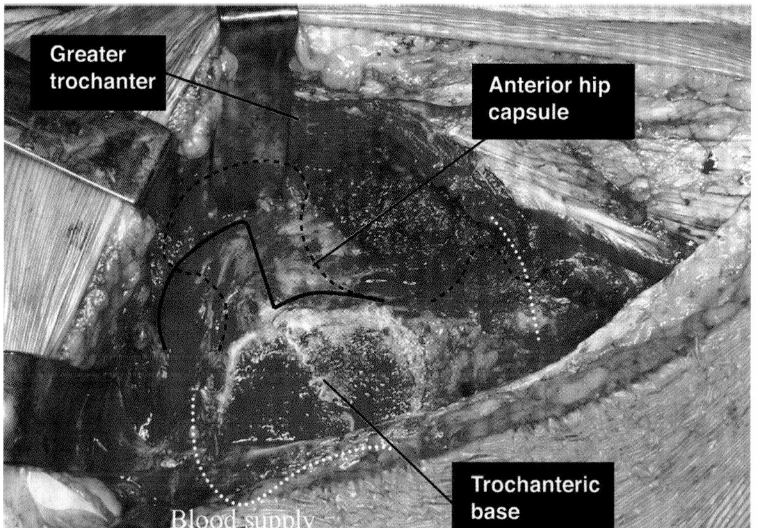


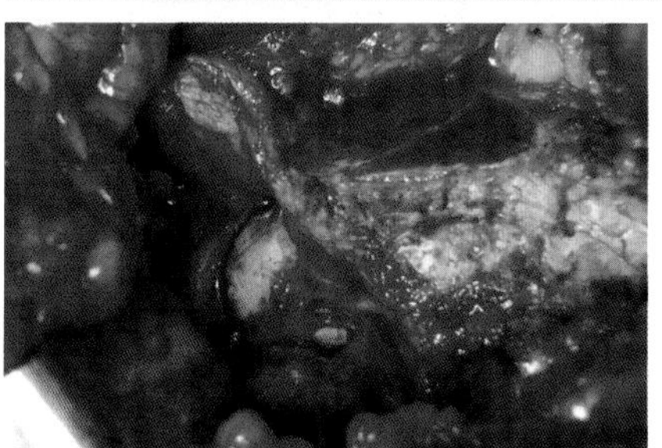


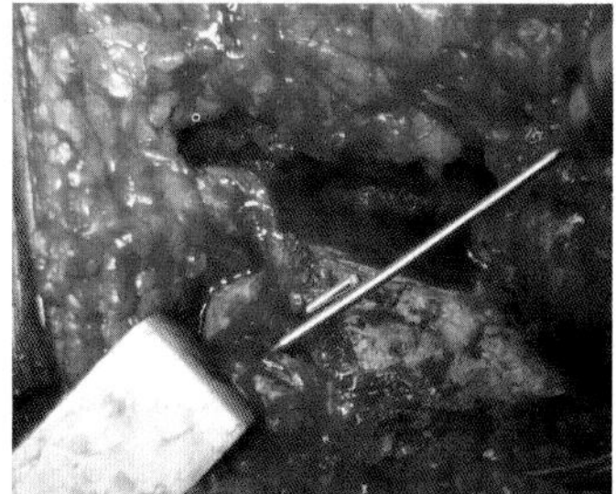


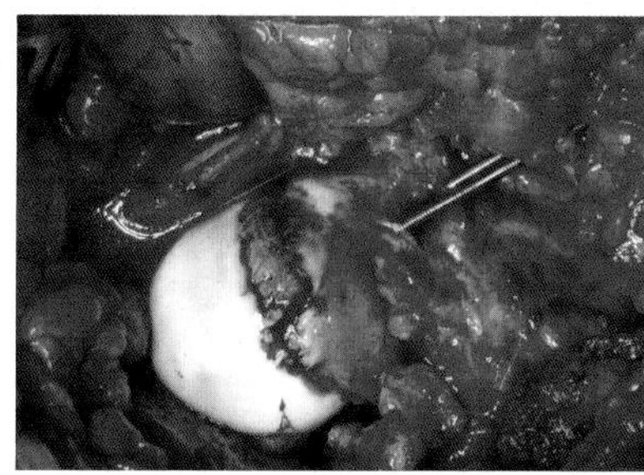


**TECH FIG 1** • **A.** Path of the Z-shaped capsulotomy (*solid line*). The limb along the posterior aspect of the acetabulum protects the entry of the terminal branches of the MFCA (*white dashed line*) and allows access to the hip joint and the femoral head (*black dashed line*). **B.** Z-shaped capsulotomy. **C.** For unstable SCFEs, threaded K-wires are used to provisionally pin the epiphysis in situ in order to allow the hip to be dislocated without endangering the retinacular vessels. **D.** Once the hip is dislocated, the full SCFE deformity can be assessed. In this unstable SCFE, note the tearing of the periosteum.

- At this point, the hip should be gently manipulated to assess the intraoperative stability of the slip and the acuity of the injury.
  - Unstable slips characteristically have torn periosteum anteriorly with the epiphysis clearly disengaged from the metaphysis.
  - Stable slips move as a single unit.
- For unstable SCFEs, one to two threaded K-wires are used to provisionally pin the epiphysis in situ to allow the hip to be dislocated without endangering the retinacular vessels (**TECH FIG 1C**).
  - The wires are cut with approximately 2 cm out of bone to keep the fixation out of the way but still allow later removal.
- A bone hook is placed around the neck.
- The limb is then gently flexed, adducted, and externally rotated, and the bone hook is used to subluxate the hip. Curved scissors are inserted into the joint, and the ligamentum teres is transected to allow full dislocation of the hip.
- The full SCFE deformity can now be assessed. It is important to evaluate the acetabulum as well for chondral or labral pathology (**TECH FIG 1D**).

## Retinacular Flap

- The retinacular flap is best developed with the hip located.
- The periosteum is split longitudinally on the femur distal to the trochanteric osteotomy site, and a periosteal elevator is used to start the periosteal flap posteriorly (**TECH FIG 2A**).
- Similarly, the periosteum on the anterior neck can be split in line with the capsulotomy and elevated.
- To reduce tension on the retinacular flap and allow the epiphysis to be safely mobilized, the posterosuperior third of the trochanteric base needs to be removed.
- The apophyseal cartilage in skeletally immature patients provides a useful landmark for the extent of trochanteric resection.
- The original technique uses an osteotome to perform the osteotomy (at the site of apophyseal cartilage) followed by careful peeling of the freed trochanteric fragment from the periosteal flap[18] (**TECH FIG 2B,C**).
- Alternatively, the subperiosteal flap can be carefully extended proximally around the tip of the greater trochanter and a Kerrison rongeur or standard rongeur can be used to "nibble" back the trochanteric base (**TECH FIG 2D**).
- As the trochanteric base is trimmed, the periosteal flap can be extended to the base of the femoral neck (**TECH FIG 2E**).

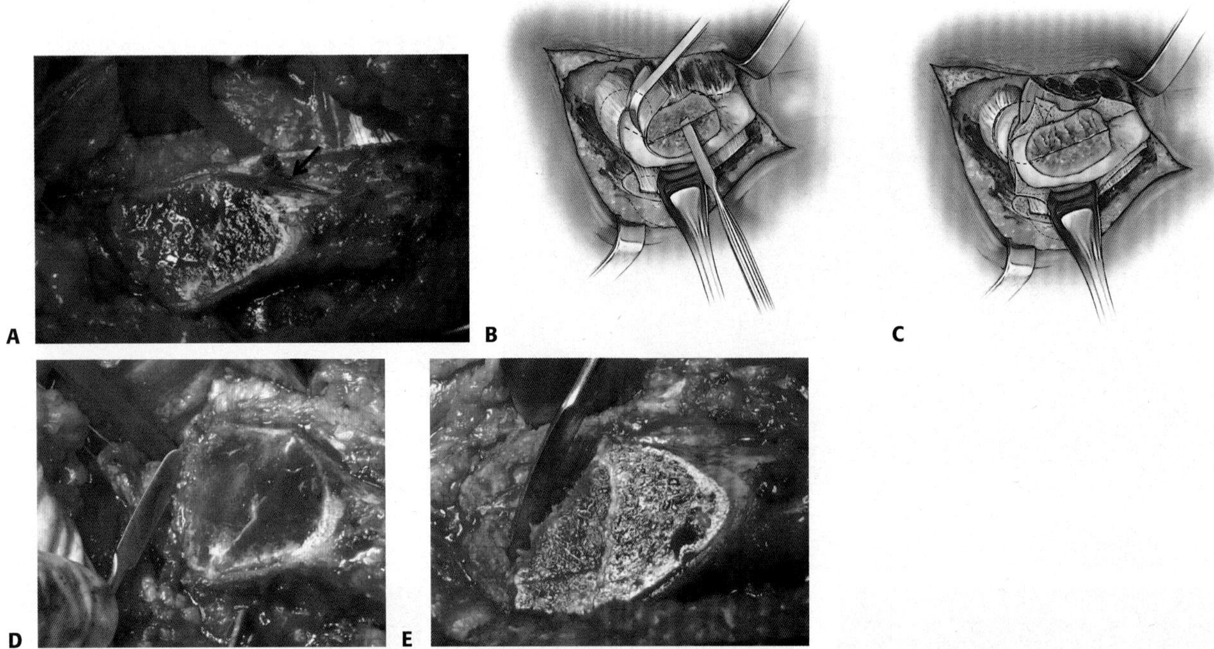

**TECH FIG 2** • **A.** To develop the retinacular flap, the periosteum is first split longitudinally on the femur distal to the trochanteric osteotomy site and a periosteal elevator is used to elevate the periosteal flap posteriorly (*arrow*). **B,C.** The posterosuperior segment of the stable trochanter can be removed with an osteotome and peeled from the periosteal sleeve to allow access to the posterior periosteum of the femoral neck for further subperiosteal dissection. **D.** One technique for developing the retinacular flap involves careful elevation of the periosteal sleeve proximally around the tip of the greater trochanter; a Kerrison rongeur or standard rongeur can then be used to nibble back the trochanteric base. **E.** As the trochanteric base is trimmed, the periosteal flap can be extended to the base of the femoral neck. (*Note*: up is posterior on all panels.)

## Mobilization of the Epiphysis

- The hip is dislocated to complete the retinacular flap.
- The periosteum over the anterior neck is split and elevated over the superior neck and the piriformis fossa to connect to the previously created periosteal sleeve (**TECH FIG 3A**).
- A sponge can be placed inside the acetabulum to prevent the femoral head from falling posteriorly as it is mobilized.
- While manually stabilizing the epiphysis, the provisional K-wires are removed.
- In unstable SCFEs, a small elevator placed into the slip site should be sufficient to mobilize the epiphysis. The remaining adhesions to the retinacular flap can be addressed (**TECH FIG 3B**).
- In stable SCFEs, the physis should be localized and an elevator or osteotome used to separate the epiphysis from the metaphysis.
- Once the epiphysis has been freed, any residual physis should be curetted to facilitate bone healing.

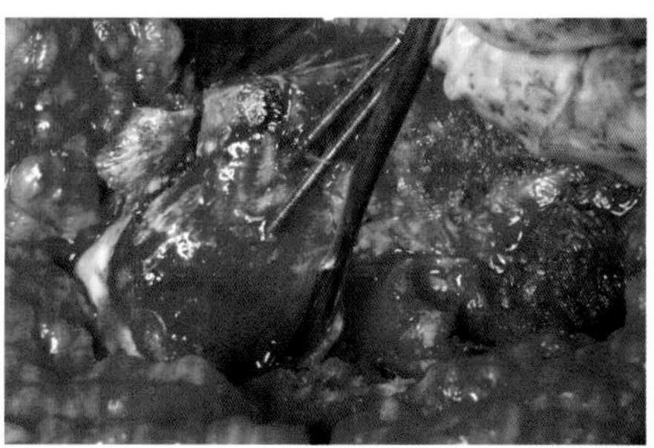

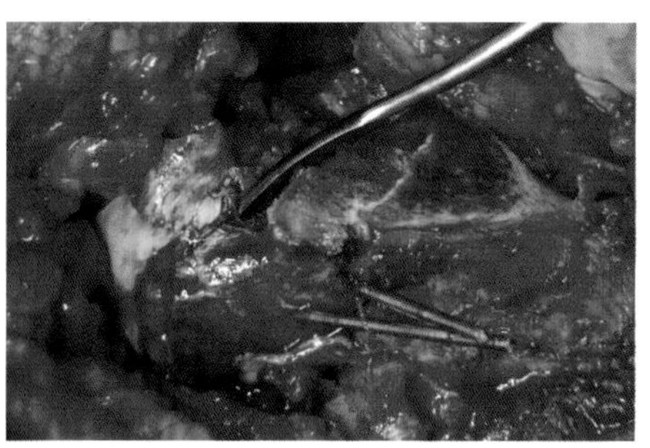

**TECH FIG 3** • **A.** With the hip dislocated, the periosteum is elevated over the anterior neck as well as superiorly into the piriformis fossa to connect to the previously created periosteal sleeve. **B.** In unstable SCFEs, a small elevator placed into the slip site should be sufficient to mobilize the epiphysis. The remaining adhesions to the retinacular flap can be released.

## Reducing the Epiphysis

- The fully exposed metaphysis/neck should be inspected for signs of chronic callus. This is typically located posterior and inferior. Removing this with an osteotome and rongeur helps facilitate epiphyseal reduction (**TECH FIG 4A**).
- The end of the neck should be trimmed slightly to provide a fresh bony surface for healing. Excessive shortening should be avoided as this can create postoperative instability (**TECH FIG 4B**).
- The epiphysis can now be manually reduced. There should be minimal tension on the retinacular flap during this maneuver. If excessive tension persists, the retinacular flap should be extended and the epiphysis and metaphysis should be revisited to be sure that all callus has been removed (**TECH FIG 4C**).

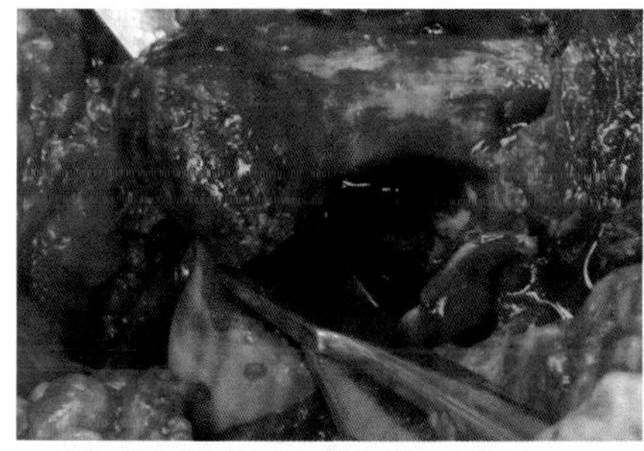

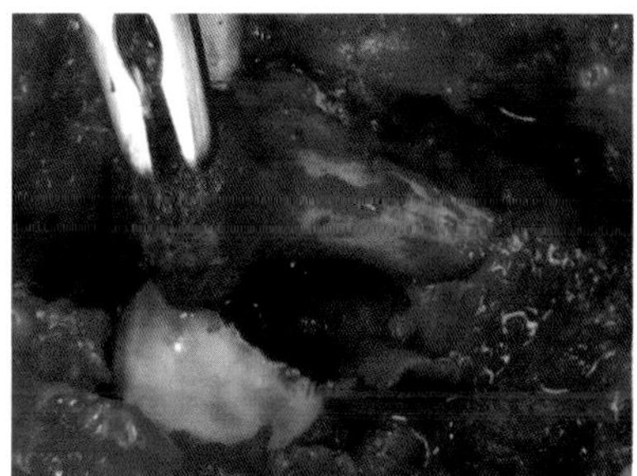

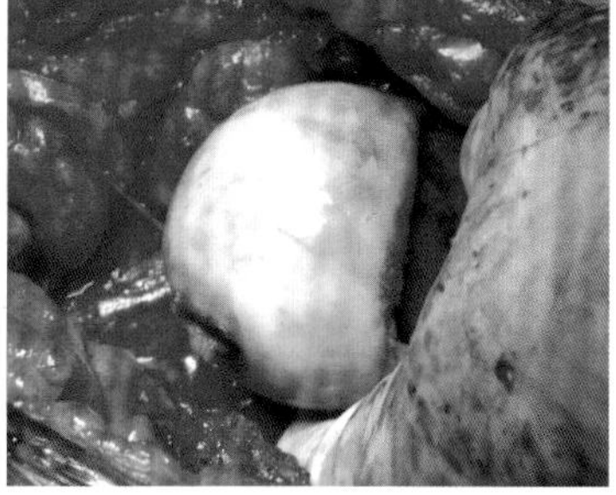

**TECH FIG 4** • **A.** The fully exposed metaphysis/neck should be inspected for signs of chronic callus. This is typically located posterior and inferior. Removing this with an osteotome and/or rongeur helps facilitate epiphyseal reduction. **B.** The end of the neck should be trimmed slightly to provide a fresh bony surface for healing. Excessive shortening should be avoided, as this can create postoperative instability. **C.** The epiphysis can now be manually reduced.

## Epiphyseal Fixation

- Initial fixation is achieved by inserting a threaded K-wire from proximal to distal through the fovea and exiting out the anterolateral femur (**TECH FIG 5A**).
- The hip is carefully relocated to allow assessment of reduction and placement of definitive fixation.
- To confirm adequate epiphyseal reduction, the C-arm can be brought underneath the table and rotated to provide an AP view of the hip. The limb can be manually frogged to achieve a lateral view of the proximal femur.
- If the reduction is acceptable, definitive fixation for the epiphysis should be placed distal or anterior to the trochanteric base to facilitate later removal if necessary.
- The author prefers using two 6.5-mm cannulated screws to minimize the risk of implant failure; however, two or three solid 4.5-mm screws or multiple threaded K-wires can also be used.[14]
- Implant position can be checked using the C-arm (**TECH FIG 5B,C**).
- The initial threaded K-wire can now be removed if desired.

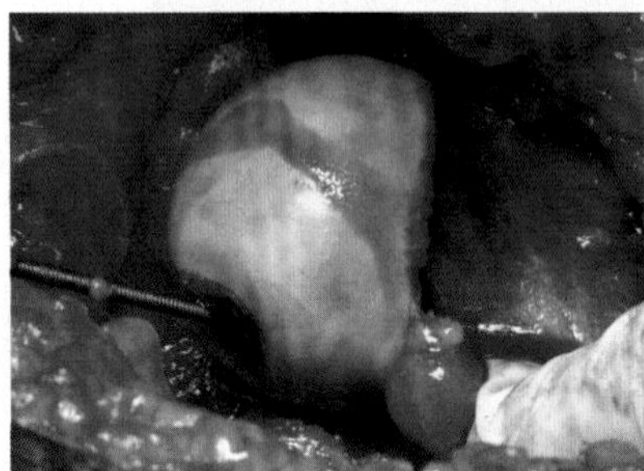
A

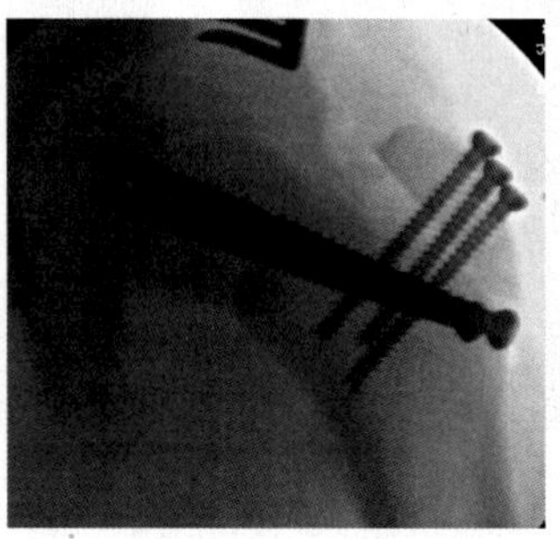
B

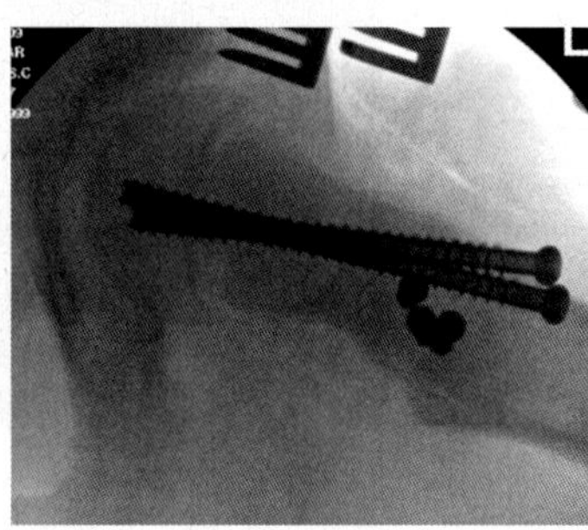
C

**TECH FIG 5** • **A.** Provisional fixation is achieved by inserting a threaded K-wire from proximal to distal through the fovea and exiting out the anterolateral femur. **B,C.** AP and frog lateral fluoroscopic views demonstrating implant position (for both epiphyseal and trochanteric fixation).

## Monitoring Perfusion

- Perfusion of the epiphysis can be monitored periodically throughout the case (eg, during development of the retinacular flap, after epiphyseal reduction, etc.) by placing a small 1.5-mm drill hole into the anterior head away from the weight-bearing surface. Fresh bleeding should be visualized from the head.
- A more objective means of perfusion monitoring involves placement of an intracranial pressure catheter into the small drill hole. A discrete waveform should be visualized (**TECH FIG 6**).
- If perfusion is lost after epiphyseal reduction, the tension on the retinacular flap should be checked. If necessary, the flap should be extended, the neck slightly shortened, and the epiphysis rereduced in a tension-free manner.

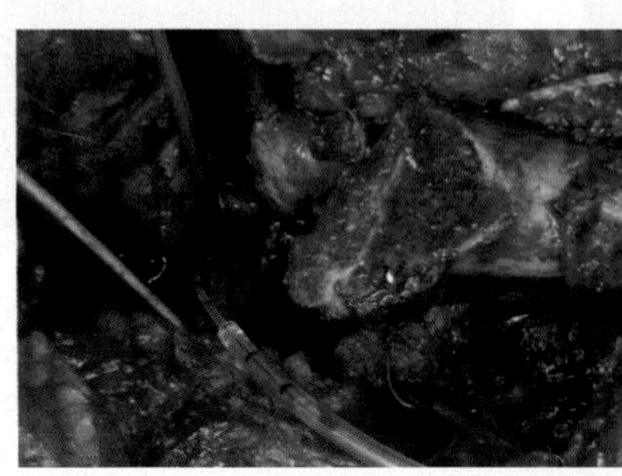
A

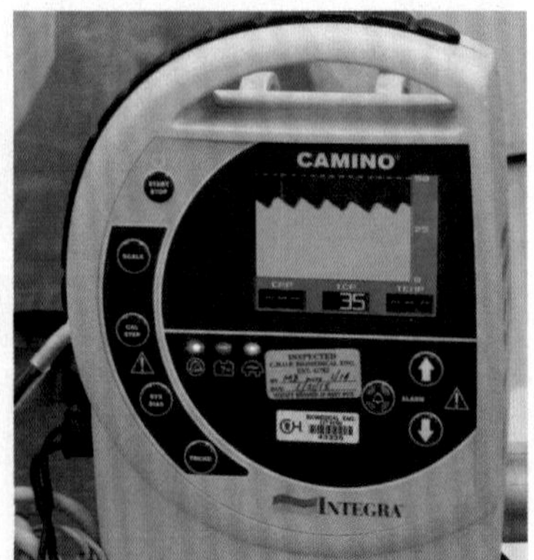

B

**TECH FIG 6** • **A.** Perfusion can be monitored by placing an intracranial pressure catheter into a small drill hole. **B.** A discrete waveform should be visualized.

## Deep Closure

- A few tacking sutures can be placed loosely in the anterior periosteum; but in general, the retinacular flap should not be repaired to avoid causing unnecessary tension.
- The capsule is loosely approximated with interrupted heavy (no. 1) absorbable sutures. Again, it is important to avoid creating unnecessary tension on the retinacular flap (**TECH FIG 7**).

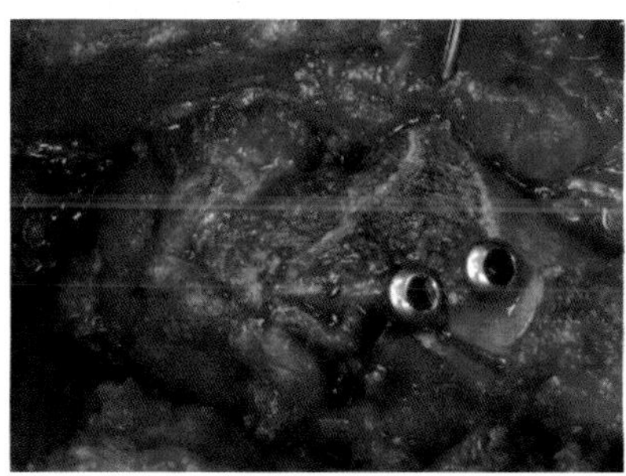

**TECH FIG 7** • The capsule should be loosely approximated.

## Trochanteric Osteotomy Fixation

- The trochanteric wafer is reduced to the same or slightly distal position and held in place using a ball spike probe.
- Three guidewires for a 4.5-mm cannulated screw system are inserted across the osteotomy site aiming slightly distal (toward the lesser trochanter) (**TECH FIG 8**).
- The reduction of the osteotomy and the wires can be confirmed with the C-arm.
- The wires are then measured and overdrilled. Fully threaded 4.5-mm cannulated screws are used to facilitate later removal if necessary.
- Alternatively, solid 3.5- or 4.5-mm screws can be used.

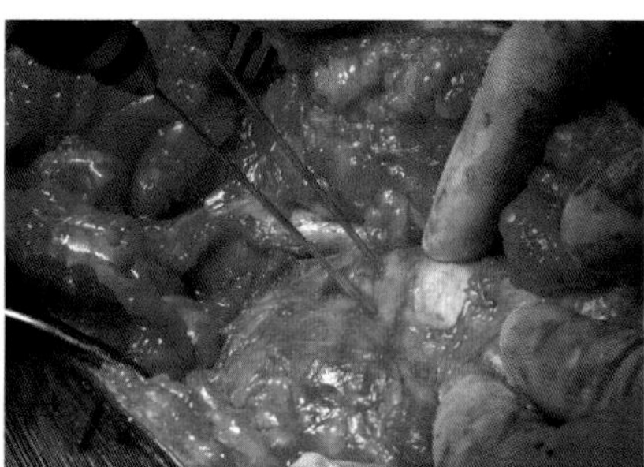

**TECH FIG 8** • Placement of guidewires for trochanteric fixation with 4.5-mm cannulated screws.

## Closure

- The vastus lateralis is repaired using a running absorbable suture (eg, 2-0 Vicryl).
- The fascia lata is closed in a watertight fashion using interrupted heavy absorbable suture (eg, no. 1 Vicryl), followed by layered closure of the dermis (2-0 Vicryl) and the subcuticular layer (4-0 Monocryl).

## PEARLS AND PITFALLS

| | |
|---|---|
| **Difficulty distinguishing capsule from retinacular flap during closure** | ▪ This can be prevented by tagging the capsule after performing the Z-shaped capsulotomy. |
| **Excessive tension on retinacular flap during mobilization of the epiphysis** | ▪ This happens if the flap has not been developed distal enough. |
| **Excessive tension on retinacular flap during reduction of the epiphysis** | ▪ This can be prevented by being sure the flap is developed distal enough, by trimming posteroinferior callus from the neck, and by shortening the neck slightly. |
| **Implant failure** | ▪ One study suggests that using larger implants (eg, 6.5-mm cannulated screws) for epiphyseal fixation may minimize the risk of hardware breakage.[14] |
| **Tension on the retinacular flap during closure** | ▪ This can be avoided by not repairing the retinacular flap and by loosely approximating the capsule. |
| **AVN** | ▪ The risk of this complication is best minimized by meticulous surgical technique and frequent monitoring of epiphyseal perfusion. |

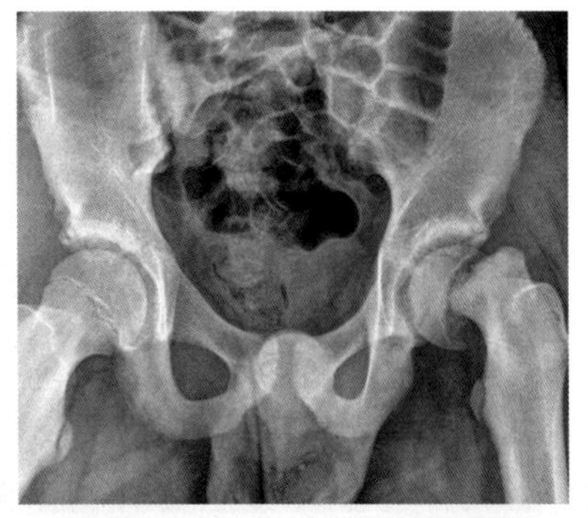

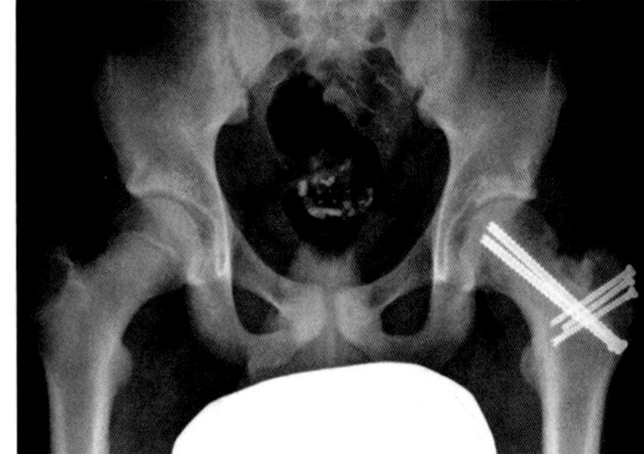

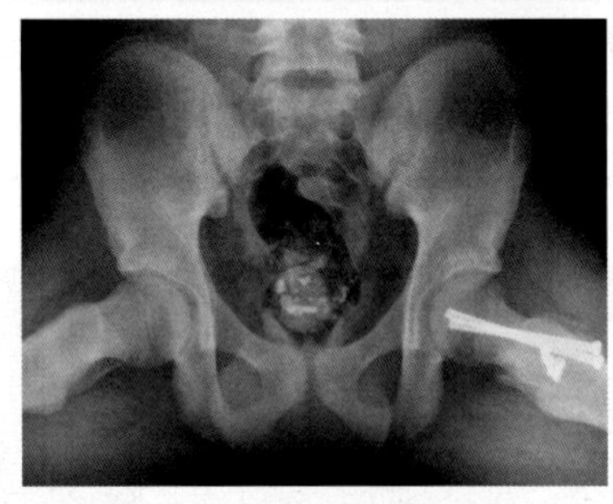

**FIG 4** • **A.** Preoperative AP view of the hip reveals a severe left unstable SCFE. **B,C.** Postoperative AP and frog-leg lateral views, respectively, of the pelvis 18 months later demonstrate a well-reduced epiphysis with no signs of AVN.

## POSTOPERATIVE CARE

- Patients are made toe-touch weight bearing with crutches. Weight bearing is generally advanced around 8 weeks based on early radiographic signs of healing at the physis.
- Physical therapy is then initiated for gait training and abductor strengthening.
- If radiographic healing progresses as expected, patients are generally cleared for sports around 6 months after surgery.
- After the immediate postoperative period, patients are followed every 2 to 3 months for at least a year with AP and frog lateral radiographs to monitor for the development of osteonecrosis.

## OUTCOMES

- The initial series describing the modified Dunn procedure consisted of 40 patients followed for a minimum of 1 year and 3 years from two institutions.[18] The authors reported excellent functional outcomes, improved ROM, near-anatomic slip angles, and no cases of AVN.
- Two additional follow-up studies have also reported excellent functional scores and anatomic radiographic results following the modified Dunn procedure in both stable and unstable SCFEs.
  - One series of 23 patients reported excellent clinical and radiographic outcomes in 21 patients. The poor outcomes occurred in 2 patients who developed osteonecrosis and osteoarthritis.[15]
  - Another series of 30 SCFEs reported near-anatomic reduction in all cases. Twenty-eight patients had excellent clinical outcomes with one patient developing AVN. Failure of implants requiring revision surgery occurred in four hips.[8]
- A multicenter study of 27 unstable SCFEs treated with the modified Dunn procedure demonstrated higher rates of AVN (26%) and failed epiphyseal fixation (15%) than previous reports.[14] Patients that did not develop osteonecrosis had excellent clinical and radiographic results (**FIG 4**).

## COMPLICATIONS

- Chondrolysis
- AVN (more common with unstable SCFEs)
- Nonunion
- Failed epiphyseal fixation

## REFERENCES


1. Boyer DW, Mickelson MR, Ponseti IV. Slipped capital femoral epiphysis. Long-term follow-up study of one hundred and twenty-one patients. J Bone Joint Surg Am 1981;63(1):85–95.
2. Carney BT, Weinstein SL, Noble J. Long-term follow-up of slipped capital femoral epiphysis. J Bone Joint Surg Am 1991;73(5):667–674.
3. Castañeda P, Ponce C, Villareal G, et al. The natural history of osteoarthritis after a slipped capital femoral epiphysis/the pistol grip deformity. J Pediatr Orthop 2013;33(suppl 1):S76–S82.
4. Dunn DM. The treatment of adolescent slipping of the upper femoral epiphysis. J Bone Joint Surg Br 1964;46:621–629.
5. Gautier E, Ganz K, Krugel N, et al. Anatomy of the medial femoral circumflex artery and its surgical implications. J Bone Joint Surg Br 2000;82(5):679–683.
6. Goodman DA, Feighan JE, Smith AD, et al. Subclinical slipped capital femoral epiphysis. Relationship to osteoarthrosis of the hip. J Bone Joint Surg Am 1997;79(10):1489–1497.
7. Gordon JE, Abrahams MS, Dobbs MB, et al. Early reduction, arthrotomy, and cannulated screw fixation in unstable slipped capital femoral epiphysis treatment. J Pediatr Orthop 2002;22(3):352–358.
8. Huber H, Dora C, Ramseier LE, et al. Adolescent slipped capital femoral epiphysis treated by a modified Dunn osteotomy with surgical hip dislocation. J Bone Joint Surg Br 2011;93(6):833–838.
9. Leunig M, Casillas MM, Hamlet M, et al. Slipped capital femoral epiphysis: early mechanical damage to the acetabular cartilage by a prominent femoral metaphysis. Acta Orthop Scand 2000;71(4):370–375.

10. Loder RT, Richards BS, Shapiro PS, et al. Acute slipped capital femoral epiphysis: the importance of physeal stability. J Bone Joint Surg Am 1993;75(8):1134–1140.
11. Mamisch TC, Kim YJ, Richolt JA, et al. Femoral morphology due to impingement influences the range of motion in slipped capital femoral epiphysis. Clin Orthop Relat Res 2009;467(3):692–698.
12. Parsch K, Weller S, Parsch D. Open reduction and smooth Kirschner wire fixation for unstable slipped capital femoral epiphysis. J Pediatr Orthop 2009;29(1):1–8.
13. Rab GT. The geometry of slipped capital femoral epiphysis: implications for movement, impingement, and corrective osteotomy. J Pediatr Orthop 1999;19(4):41–424.
14. Sankar WN, Vanderhave KL, Matheney T, et al. The modified Dunn procedure for unstable slipped capital femoral epiphysis: a multicenter perspective. J Bone Joint Surg Am 2013;95(7):585–591.
15. Slongo T, Kakaty D, Krause F, et al. Treatment of slipped capital femoral epiphysis with a modified Dunn procedure. J Bone Joint Surg Am 2010;92(18):2898–2908.
16. Southwick WO. Osteotomy through the lesser trochanter for slipped capital femoral epiphysis. J Bone Joint Surg Am 1967;49(5):807–835.
17. Tannast M, Goricki D, Beck M, et al. Hip damage occurs at the zone of femoroacetabular impingement. Clin Orthop Relat Res 2008;466(2):273–280.
18. Ziebarth K, Zilkens C, Spencer S, et al. Capital realignment for moderate and severe SCFE using a modified Dunn procedure. Clin Orthop Relat Res 2009;467(3):704–716.

# CHAPTER 114 Treatment of Anterior Femoroacetabular Impingement through Mini-Open Anterior Approach

Diana Bitar and Javad Parvizi

## DEFINITION

- Femoroacetabular impingement (FAI) is a mechanical hip disorder defined as abnormal abutment between the femoral head or the femoral head–neck junction and the acetabulum. It was initially described as a distinct physiologic entity by Myers et al,[28] who noted abnormal contact between the femoral neck and the acetabular rim in a cohort of patients undergoing periacetabular osteotomy (PAO) to correct hip dysplasia.
- One of the earlier descriptions of this condition was by Smith-Petersen[35] in 1936, when a case of malum coxae senilis was described. The case in that original article resembled what we now describe as FAI. Another description of this condition came in 1970s when the term *pistol grip deformity* was introduced. The latter was a description of aberrant morphologic features of the femoral head and neck on anteroposterior (AP) radiographs of patients with early idiopathic hip osteoarthritis (OA).[24]
- FAI can be anterior or posterior, with anterior abnormalities being more frequent. The estimated prevalence of FAI in the general population is 10% to 15%[38] and is increasingly being recognized as a cause of hip pain in young, active individuals. Repetitive anterolateral impingement produces acetabular articular cartilage delamination, labral disease, and eventually secondary OA. Establishment of a correlation between clinical picture, physical findings, suggestive radiographic structural abnormalities, and positive magnetic resonance angiogram (MRA) is crucial for diagnosis and appropriate treatment of this condition.

## ANATOMY

- Establishing an accurate diagnosis and selecting the optimal surgical treatment strategy relies on a thorough understanding of the pathoanatomy of hip impingement disorders.
- Two different structural impingement types have been described:
  - Femoral-based abnormality (ie, cam impingement) is more common in the young, athletic male[16] (M:F ratio = 14:1).[38] Cam is a term applied to an eccentric prominence in a rotating mechanism which converts rotary motion into linear motion.[26]
  - Acetabular-based abnormality (ie, pincer impingement) is seen more commonly in athletic middle-aged women (M:F ratio = 1:3).[38] Pincer comes from the French word meaning "to pinch" (**FIG 1**).[1,13,23]
- It is important to note that most FAI cases are likely to be a combination of cam and pincer impingement. In this state, both the proximal femur and the acetabulum present with distorted structural characteristics. Isolated cam or pincer deformities are rare; in 86% of cases, a combined deformity is present.[38] In one study of 149 hips with FAI lesions, only 26 hips presented with an isolated cam lesion and 16 hips presented with an isolated pincer lesion.[1]
- Cam-type impingement syndrome can be primary (reduced femoral head–neck offset or an aspherical femoral head) with abnormal physeal development or secondary to previous pathologies (eg, slipped capital femoral epiphysis [SCFE], Perthes abnormalities, developmental dysplasia of the hip [DDH], or as a result of a prior trauma to the proximal femur and/or acetabulum).
- Morphologically, cam lesions can result from an osseous bump or from angular deformities of the proximal femur (eg, femoral retrotorsion or coxa vara). The osseous bump location further divides cam lesions into lateral-based prominence (pistol grip) or anterosuperior-based prominence, which is only detected on lateral radiographic views of the hip. Cam impingement owing to femoral angular deformities is uncommon.
- Pincer-type impingement syndrome consists of an overcoverage abnormality, which can be focal or global. Focal overcoverage can be anterior (acetabular retroversion with or without a deficient posterior wall) or posterior (prominent

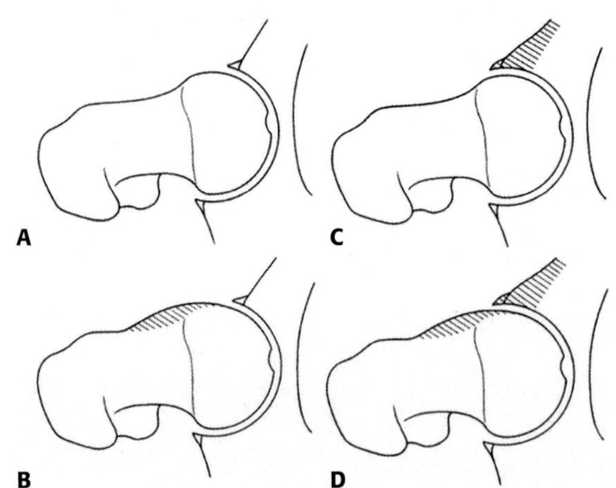


**FIG 1** • The factors causing FAI are shown. Reduced clearance during joint motion leads to repetitive abutment between the proximal femur and the anterior acetabular rim. **A.** Normal clearance of the hip. **B.** Reduced femoral head and neck offset. **C.** Excessive overcoverage of the femoral head by the acetabulum. **D.** Combination of reduced head and neck offset and excessive anterior over coverage can be seen.

posterior wall). Global overcoverage consists of concentric deepening of the acetabulum (acetabular dome breaching the pelvic brim) which presents as coxa profunda or protrusio acetabuli, with the latter being the most severe form.

## PATHOGENESIS

- If left untreated, the process of FAI is likely to lead to hip joint degeneration.[13,23,39] Mechanical impingement is most noticeable with hip flexion alone or hip flexion combined with internal rotation.
- In pincer impingement, a linear contact occurs between the acetabular overcovering rim with a labrum, which acts like a bumper.[1] The head–neck junction, with the maximal impact force tangential to the joint surface,[38] leads to a full tear of the labrum, which is the first structure to fail in this situation. Sustained mechanical abutment results in degeneration of the labrum with intrasubstance ganglion formation; ossification of the injured labrum leads to further deepening of the acetabulum and worsening of the overcoverage.[24]
- In cam impingement, a jamming of the aspherical head portion (shear stress) into the acetabulum occurs, with the maximal impact force perpendicular to the joint surface, leading to an undersurface tear of the labrum fibrocartilaginous separation,[38] which more accurately should be called *separation of the acetabular cartilage from the labrum*.[1]
- Based on this pathophysiology, the typical location of femoral cartilage damage is circumferential in pincer impingement with contrecoup lesion and is localized between 11 o'clock and 3 o'clock positions in cam impingement.[38] A contrecoup lesion is acetabular cartilaginous damage in the opposite part of the femoroacetabular abutment. It is seen in one-third of all cases of pincer impingement and is associated with slight joint subluxation.[38] Therefore, the cartilaginous lesions are more benign in pincer impingement than those seen in cam impingement with an average depth of 4 mm in the former and 11 mm in the latter.[1,38]

## ETIOLOGY

### Genetics

- Numerous studies conducted on family members, especially sets of twins, have demonstrated a genetic component to OA, which is mostly seen in Caucasians. Furthermore, it has been shown that genetic factors are largely responsible for variations in hip and acetabular morphology and cartilage thickness.[26]
- Based on one genetic study, cam deformity tends to be more prevalent in the family members of affected patients than pincer deformity. There is a relative risk of 2.8 and 2, respectively, that a sibling will have the same abnormal anatomy. Likewise, a positive family history increases the risk of bilateralism of the deformity.[18]

### Geographical Variation

- FAI is more prevalent in the Western world where the majority of hip OA, previously labeled primary OA, is currently considered to be the consequence of abnormal hip joint anatomy.
- In contrast, in a retrospective study of 946 primary total hip arthroplasty (THA) conducted in Japan, Takeyama et al[37] identified FAI as an underlying pathology in only six hips.

### Underlying Hip Pathologies

- In some cases, FAI is secondary to childhood hip disorders such as SCFE, DDH, Legg-Calvé-Perthes disease, or femoral neck fracture complicated by malunion.
  - In one study that followed patients for 15 years, those formerly treated for SCFE subsequently displayed signs of FAI.[18]
  - As reported by Eijer et al,[9] previous femoral neck fractures may result in secondary FAI, specially if the reduction is not completely anatomic.
  - Snow et al[36] reported four cases of anterior cam impingement which occurred after an asymptomatic period following reossification of the femoral head in Legg-Calvé-Perthes disease.

## NATURAL HISTORY

- Because FAI is a newly identified condition, the natural history of its development has not been clearly defined in the literature. However, there is an association between morphologic deformities and secondary OA of the hip.
- Not all patients with FAI will progress to end-stage disease that requires intervention. It is estimated that one-third of patients with mild OA in the presence of FAI will take more than 10 years to develop end-stage OA, if at all.[26]
- Symptomatic impingement disorders most likely progress to secondary OA, making surgical treatment a rational option.
- Close observation and follow-up or prompt and timely conservative surgical treatment should be tailored to each case, taking into consideration clinical presentation, radiographic findings, family history, and especially, the rate of disease progression. Clinicians should be aware that delay of surgical correction may lead to chondral damage and disease progression to a stage where joint preservation procedures may be of little benefit.[26]

## PATIENT HISTORY AND PHYSICAL FINDINGS

### History

- FAI usually affects active young adults and begins with slow onset of activity-related anterior inguinal (groin) pain that is often preceded by a minor traumatic event.[24]
- Associated lateral (trochanteric) and posterior hip (gluteal) pain is common but the pain is most commonly felt in the groin (83% of cases).[26] The pain is often manifested after sitting for a prolonged period.[24]
- In the early stages of the disease, the pain or aching is intermittent and could be aggravated by excessive physical demands on the hip, such as prolonged walking or high-demand athletic activities, including running, cutting, pivoting, and repetitive hip flexion.
- Labral disease or unstable articular cartilage flaps[3] may cause mechanical symptoms of locking and catching. Anterior FAI is almost always associated with labral tears,[5] which are rarely isolated and most likely indicate underlying bony pathologies. Acetabular labral tears should be considered in active patients with a history of groin pain that is exacerbated by activity without radiologic evidence or other hip pathology.[3]
- Stiffness is common, with reductions in the range of hip flexion, adduction, and internal rotation in particular,[26] whereas overall hip function is almost unaffected.[24]

- After inquiring about the overall performance of the patient (including age, activity level, and comorbidities), a detailed hip-focused history should be conducted to determine any trauma, childhood hip disease, previous surgeries and treatments as well as the impact of hip pain on quality of life.

## Physical Examination

- After assessment of overall health and body habitus, the hip clinical examination should be done with great care because it provides the most reliable diagnostic information. Physical findings will dictate further tests and necessary management.
- Observation of sitting posture, gait, palpation of the hip, abductor strength testing, careful hip range-of-motion (ROM) assessment, and specific provocative tests should be performed.
  - Anterior FAI commonly provokes discomfort/pain in an upright sitting position, which involves hip flexion greater than 90 degrees.
  - The gait pattern over short distances and abductor strength are usually normal in the early stages of the disease. A limp, secondary to mild abductor weakness, and positive Trendelenburg test may develop as labral disease and joint degeneration progress.
- Hip ROM testing should be performed carefully with stabilization of the pelvis to accurately define motion end points. Passive flexion is often limited to approximately 90 degrees and reduced compared with the contralateral hip. Internal rotation may be severely restricted to just a few degrees. Hip discomfort is often reproduced at the end points of passive motion.
- Surgical scars from any previous procedures are inspected to aid in planning of any subsequent surgery. When in doubt, infection should be ruled out.
- The anterior impingement test and Patrick test are sensitive maneuvers to detect intrinsic hip disease and usually reproduce hip symptoms in patients with anterior FAI.
  - The anterior impingement test, also known as the *flexion, adduction*, and *internal rotation test*, is performed by flexing the patient's hip to 90 degrees, adducting and internally rotating it simultaneously.
  - Patrick test, which is also known as the *flexion, abduction*, and *external rotation test*, is performed by crossing the examined limb on the other in a figure-of-four (the ipsilateral heel resting on the contralateral knee) and by applying downward pressure to the knee. If pain is elicited on the ipsilateral side anteriorly, it is suggestive of a hip joint disorder on the same side. If pain is elicited on the contralateral side posteriorly around the sacroiliac joint, it is suggestive of pain caused by dysfunction in that joint.
  - Moreover, the distance from the ipsilateral knee to the bed should be noted. The test is positive if this distance is greater than the corresponding measurement on the opposite side, if the contralateral hip is considered normal.[26]
- For posterior FAI, an impingement test (performed in the prone position) is considered positive if forced external rotation in full extension is reproducibly painful. Posterior impingement results from focal acetabular overcoverage (pincer); it is manifested radiographically by a posterior wall sign where the too prominent posterior acetabular wall runs lateral to the femoral head center (normally, the posterior rim runs approximately through the femoral head center).[38]
- A posterior impingement test can also be positive in anterior FAI when the disease progresses and posteroinferior traction osteophytes develop, producing clinical symptoms of posterior impingement in extension.
- The Drehman sign is positive if hip flexion produces unavoidable passive external rotation of the hip.[38]
- Logroll test is also a useful provocative test in patients with FAI. With the patient in supine position and with the hip and knee in full extension, the foot on the affected extremity is externally rotated. Positive sign is present if this maneuver results in pain in the anterior hip of the rotated extremity.

# IMAGING AND OTHER DIAGNOSTIC STUDIES

- Investigation of FAI requires a combination of roentgenographic examination and more sophisticated cross-sectional studies, such as magnetic resonance imaging (MRI)/MRA and sometimes a computed tomography (CT) scan.

## Roentgenography

- Is the first-line investigation and ideally may include five views: a supine AP view of the pelvis, an axial cross-table lateral view (surgical profile of Arcelin and Danelius-Miller view), a frog-leg lateral view, a false profile (Lequesne view), and a Dunn-Rippstein view in 45 or 90 degrees of flexion.[4,27,31]
- The AP and axial cross-table views are crucial and should be taken with the legs in 15 degrees of internal rotation to adjust for femoral antetorsion and fully expose the femoral neck length.
- Obtaining an AP view in the supine position allows for a direct comparison with intraoperative and immediate postoperative roentgenograms.[38] Standing AP views are important to accurately evaluate and follow joint space narrowing and to apply coxometric measurements.
- The AP view of the pelvis mainly detects pincer lesions and laterally based cam lesions (pistol grip). Anterosuperior cam lesion can be missed on AP views and should be investigated on at least one, if not all, of the three lateral views (**FIG 2**).
- Lequesne view (false profile) is not used for diagnosing FAI because it does not show the relationship between the anterior and posterior acetabular walls. However, it is more likely used for the diagnosis of early joint degeneration in the posteroinferior part of the acetabulum, which is a relative contraindication for joint-preserving surgery.[38] The Lequesne view should be included in a thorough radiologic evaluation to exclude associated mild hip dysplasia because it highlights anterior femoral head coverage (anterior center-edge angle of Lequesne) (**FIG 3**). Attention should be paid to radiographs where the pelvic tilt, rotation, and inclination are seen. X-ray beam centralization should be taken into consideration for correct interpretation of the radiologic hip parameters. The film-focus distance is different for each view: It should be 120 cm in AP and cross-table views but 102 cm in Dunn, frog-leg, and Lequesne views.[38]
- The structural parameters of the hip are assessed on all radiographic views (**FIGS 4** and **5**).

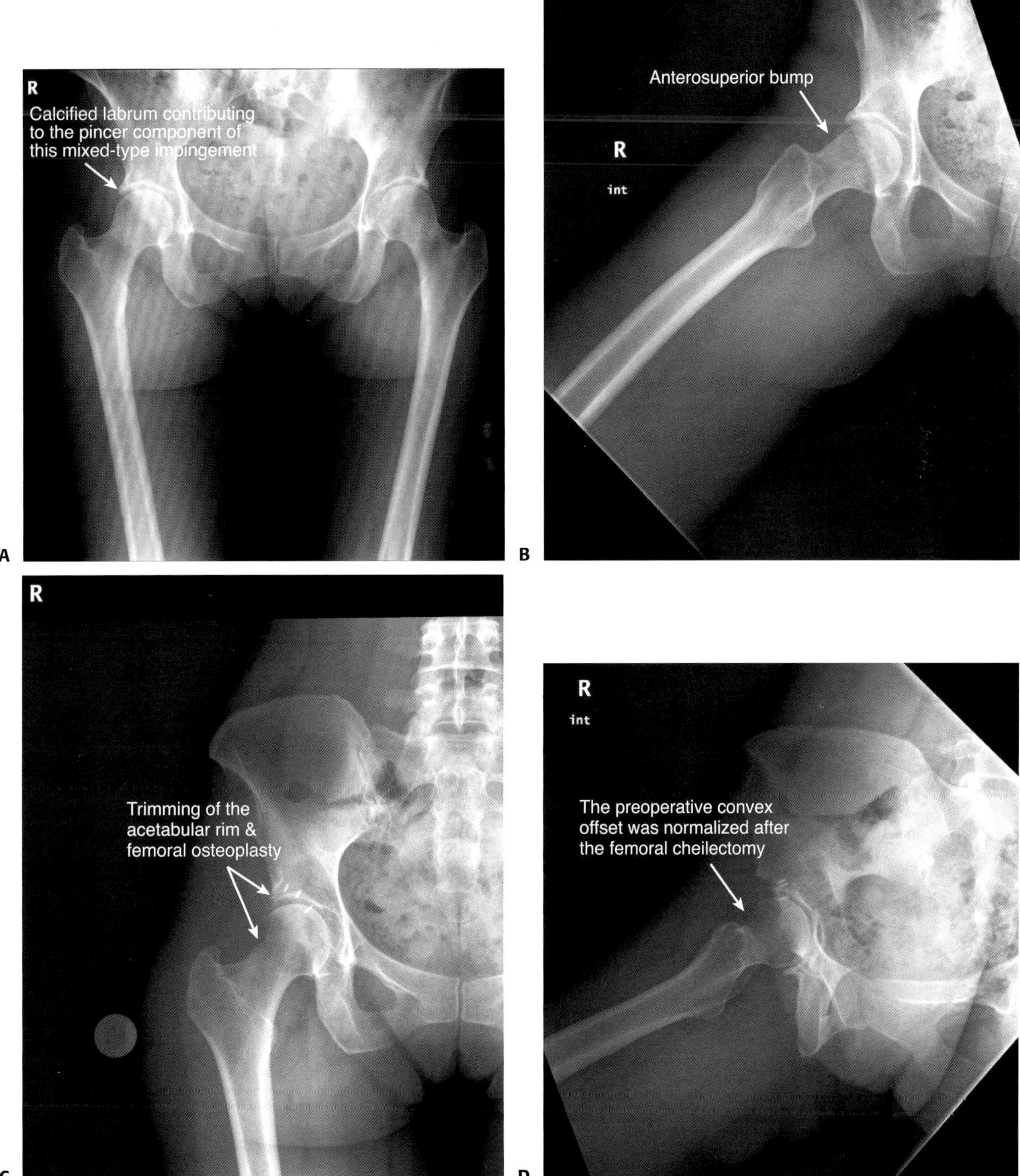


**FIG 2** • **A.** AP pelvis view of 34-year-old female complaining of 1-year duration of right hip groin pain, noticed after a minor motor vehicle accident. This view shows a calcified labrum posteriorly and laterally, a finding that was confirmed on the MRA. Note the relatively normal head–neck junction on this view. **B.** Frog-leg lateral view of the right hip shows an anterosuperior prominence responsible for decreased offset, contributing to impingement during hip flexion and internal rotation. **C,D.** AP and lateral views of the right hip after femoroacetabular osteoplasty through mini-open direct anterior approach, showing the trimmed acetabular rim, reattached superolateral labrum, and femoral bump osteoplasty.

- AP view of the pelvis can identify the following:
  - Lateral cam lesion, which is a pistol grip deformity that has a prominent, convex head–neck junction with reduced head–neck offset[26] and an aspherical femoral head (alpha angle measurement)
  - Acetabular depth, where the acetabular fossa location is noted relative to the Kohler line to look for general acetabular overcoverage. Normally, the fossa is lateral to the Kohler line; coxa profunda is noted when the fossa is medial to this line and protrusio acetabuli when the medial aspect of the

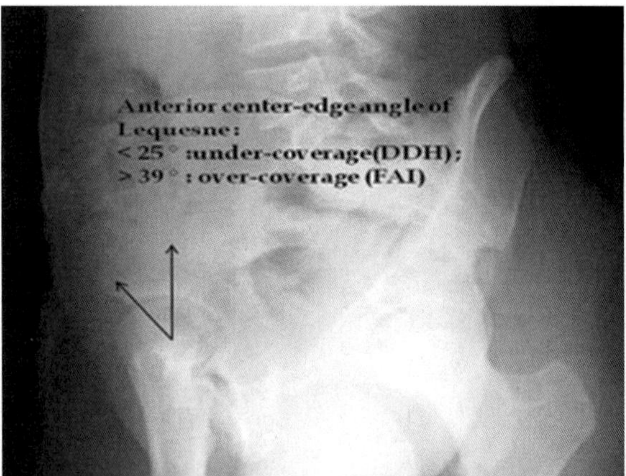


**FIG 3** • False profile of the angle of Lequesne, which measures the anterior coverage of the femoral head. The anterior center-edge angle is measured between the vertical line passing through the femoral head center and the line connecting the femoral head center to the anterior sourcil edge.

femoral head is medial to this line. Acetabular version: look for the following:

- The crossover sign or figure-of-eight sign (first described by Reynolds)[26] in anterior acetabular overcoverage (ie, acetabular retroversion)
- The prominent wall sign in posterior acetabular overcoverage. Normally, the posterior wall passes approximately through the femoral head center.

- Often, with so-called acetabular retroversion, the ischial spine is abnormally prominent into the true pelvis medially.[38] Acetabular inclination is quantified by the Tönnis

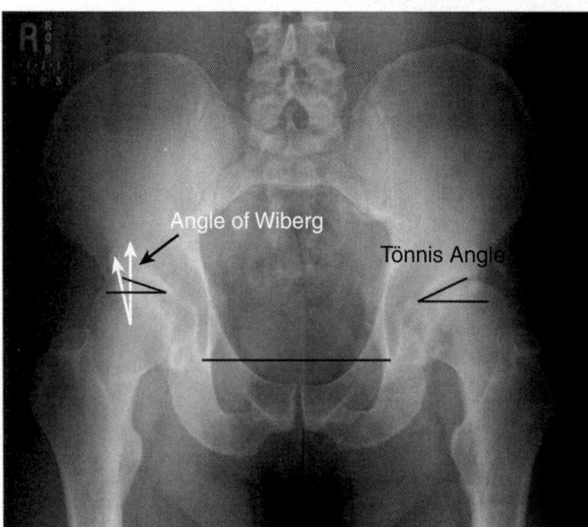


**FIG 4** • Pelvis AP view of a 43-year-old gentleman complaining of bilateral groin pain. The *black lines* represent the Tönnis angle, which measures 25 degrees bilaterally in this case; it is the angle between the horizontal line (in reference to the bi-tear drop line) and the line joining the medial edge to the lateral edge of the acetabular sourcil. The *white arrows* depict the LCE angle of Wiberg, measured between the vertical line passing through the femoral head center and the line joining this center to the lateral sourcil edge; it measures 7 degrees on the left side and 10 degrees on the right. These values are consistent with bilateral hip dysplasia with coxa valga (femoral neck–shaft angle measuring 160 degrees on the right side and 152 degrees on the left).

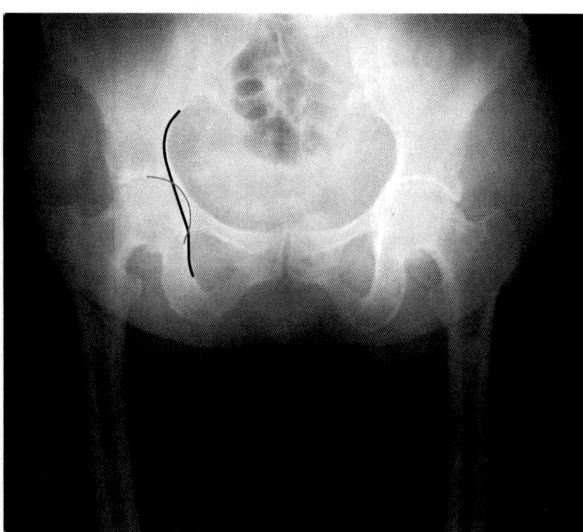

**FIG 5** • AP pelvis view of 57-year-old lady complaining of long-standing left hip pain. It shows right hip coxa profunda where the acetabular fossa is medial to the Kohler line and left hip protrusio acetabuli where the femoral head is medial to this line. The *thick line* depicts the ilioischial line (Kohler line) and the *thin line* designs the acetabular fossa. Advanced bilateral OA is noted on this x-ray, making left THA option undisputable.

angle (acetabular index and acetabular roof angle), which is normally 10 degrees or slightly less.

- Other coxometric measurements noted on the AP view that quantify acetabular depth include the following:
  - The lateral center-edge (LCE) of Wiberg: normally varies between 25 and 39 degrees[38]
  - The femoral head extrusion index, where the uncovered horizontal portion of the femoral head is quantified, should not exceed 20% to 25%.
- The lateral views are examined to assess the following (**FIG 6**):
  - Femoral head sphericity: either by gross visual inspection or using the Mose template. Asphericity can be quantified by measuring the alpha angle of Nötzli (abnormal if >50 degrees in women and >68 degrees in men[38]). However, this angle measurement is subject to poor intraobserver reliability, with 30% of reliability based on an MRI study.[23]
    - The triangle index has better reproducibility than the alpha angle because it is constructed using clear geometric landmarks and is more independent from femoral rotation.[38]
  - Femoral head–neck offset is normally 11.6 ± 0.7 mm.[8] Generally, a value inferior to 10 mm is a strong indicator of cam impingement. The offset ratio (femoral offset divided by femoral head diameter) can also be deduced where a value inferior to 0.17 is considered abnormal.[21] Indentation sign on the femoral head in pincer impingement.[38]
- These projections best visualize the anterior and anterolateral femoral head–neck deformity that characterizes cam impingement disease.
- Joint space narrowing, periarticular cysts, and labral ossification are also noted on AP and lateral views.
- The alpha angle and head–neck offset can be measured on the AP view only in the case of pistol grip deformity. Both AP and lateral views should be scrutinized for abnormal morphologic features consistent with FAI.

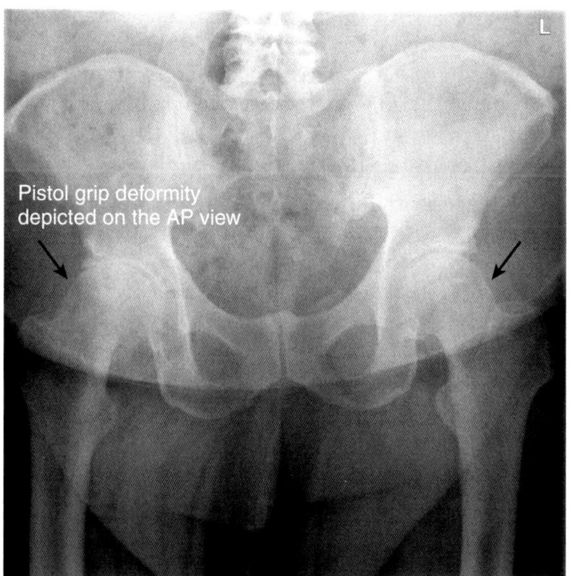


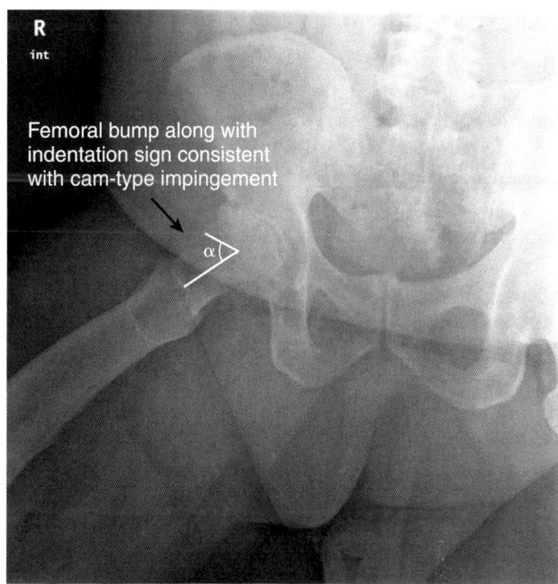


**FIG 6** • AP and frog-leg lateral views of the hip of a 60-year-old man complaining of right hip pain. The roentgenograms shows advanced right hip OA with underlying etiology of a cam-type impingement. The anterolateral femoral osseous bump is noted on both hips, which is quantified by the alpha angle, calculated between the femoral neck axis and the line connecting the femoral head center to the point of beginning of the asphericity on the anterior femoral head contour. It measures 66 degrees on the right hip.

- Secondary changes in impingement can include labral ossification, acetabular stress fracture, and herniation pits (defined as radiolucencies surrounded by a sclerotic margin and located in the anterosuperior quadrant of the femoral neck).

### Magnetic Resonance Angiogram

- MRA of the hip has been increasingly used in recent years for all patients with suspected impingement and associated intra-articular diseases.
  - The contour of the femoral head–neck junction,[19] labral disease,[7] and associated articular cartilage disease (especially in the posteroinferior joint) are better visualized on the MRA. The alpha angle and head–neck offset can be measured more accurately this way.
  - MRI also excludes other uncommon disorders such as stress fracture, osteonecrosis of the femoral head, neoplasm, infection, and synovial diseases.
- The sensitivity of an MRA is estimated to be 90% with a specificity of 91%.[11]
- Kassarjian et al[22] reported that in 88% of cases of symptomatic cam-type impingement, MRA detects a triad of abnormal head–neck morphology, anterosuperior cartilage abnormality, and anterosuperior labral abnormality.
- Using gadolinium-enhanced MRA, Nötzli et al[29] produced the first quantitative study of femoral head asphericity, describing the alpha angle and reporting that values of greater than 55 degrees on average are indicative of FAI.
- MRA is the most reliable technique to detect intra-articular lesions and should be performed in conjunction with x-rays whenever FAI is suspected.

### Computed Tomography Scan

- It is the best investigation tool for bone characterization and can be useful in defining the extent of osseous impingement lesions. It shows in detail the contour of the femoral head–neck junction and the exact morphology of the femoral bump and complements other radiologic modalities.
- Alpha angles can be quantified using three-dimensional (3-D) reconstruction of CT scan. The beta angle (the angle at which the posterior aspect of the femoral head becomes aspherical) can also be measured.[26]
- All coxometric measurements (such as acetabular version) can be assessed thoroughly on CT images, confirming the roentgenographic findings.

## DIFFERENTIAL DIAGNOSIS

- Differential diagnosis of FAI is mainly that of groin pain and other pathologies, including multiple hip disorders and pathologies of the adjacent bony and soft tissue structures.
- Mild hip dysplasia (joint instability) is the first and most important diagnosis to rule out. Usually, most dysplastic hips have excessive acetabular anteversion; however, as stated by Li and Ganz,[25] one in six dysplastic hips have some degree of retroversion. This finding should be noted preoperatively to avoid impingement worsening following routine anterior repositioning at the time of PAO.
- Isolated intra-articular hip disease (such as villonodular synovitis, chondrocalcinosis, isolated labral tear, chondral disease, and loose body) could explain hip pain in the absence of an impingement deformity.[3]
- Extra-articular hip disorders (such as sacroiliac joint disorders, tendinitis, and bursitis) or referred pain (lumbar spine diseases, inguinal hernia, and symptomatic femoral artery aneurysm) should not be overlooked.
- In cases where multiple disorders coexist or overlap, a diagnostic hip injection can be performed in order to confirm that the hip joint is the pain generator, with complete or near-complete pain relief indicating an intra-articular hip pathology.

## Conservative Treatment

- Nonoperative measures to treat FAI have not been documented in the literature. However, this option should always be considered first. Conservative treatment may help and should be applied as a first-line treatment in symptomatic hips, especially those with mild and intermittent symptoms, before surgery is considered. Treatment may include activity restrictions, hydrotherapy, anti-inflammatory medicines, and intra-articular cortisone injections. The severity of the clinical picture will dictate the eventual therapeutic modalities.
- Physical therapy, emphasizing the improvement of passive hip ROM or stretching, is counterproductive and should be avoided because it will irritate the hip and subsequently worsen the pain by sustaining and evolving articular surface damage.
- Anti-inflammatory medicines may be appropriate to relieve acute-onset pain but may also mask the symptoms of an underlying destructive process.[23] These medications should be prescribed with caution and administered for a short period of time, given their side effects and taking into consideration symptoms necessitating an extended course of analgesics.
- Activity restriction or cessation may alleviate symptoms in some patients. Athletes involved in repetitive hip flexion activities may experience significant relief of discomfort if they refrain from their sport. Although conservative measures are likely to be temporarily successful in some patients, those with a high activity level and athletic ambitions usually have low compliance.[23]

# SURGICAL MANAGEMENT

- Recognition of the detrimental effect of FAI has led to the development of novel joint-preserving techniques[24] aimed at restoring normal structural configurations of the proximal femur and/or acetabulum, interrupting the advancement of osseous morphology, and preventing the development of end-stage OA.
- Corrective surgery can be performed via several modalities, including a mini-open anterior approach, surgical dislocation of the hip,[12] combined hip arthroscopy and limited open decompression,[5] and arthroscopic decompression alone.[15]
- Selection of the adequate treatment option depends on multiple factors but is mainly dictated by the type and severity of the underlying abnormal anatomy.
- Open surgical dislocation of the hip with trochanteric flip osteotomy to perform osteochondroplasty, initially described by Ganz et al[12] in 2001, was the mainstay of early surgical management of FAI before the encouraging results of less invasive techniques were published.[26]
- Independently of the chosen technique, the primary goal of surgery is to address osseous structural impingement lesions and associated soft tissue intra-articular injuries (eg, labrum or articular cartilage). Many studies have demonstrated more favorable clinical, radiologic, and functional outcomes with labral repair compared to labral débridement in selected cases.[2,10,23,32]
- Surgical dislocation of the hip is reserved for less common cases with nonfocal (global) impingement problems or severe deformities such as advanced nonfocal femoral head deformity encountered in Legg-Calvé-Perthes disease or circumferential pincer impingement where the posterior acetabular rim cannot be exposed via the minimally invasive anterior approach or arthroscopy.
- For hips with focal cam-type FAI, the mini-open anterior surgical approach may provide excellent exposure, allowing appropriate correction of the osseous pathology on both sides of the joint while being a minimally invasive procedure.

## Preoperative Planning

- The patient's history and physical examination findings should be reviewed shortly before proceeding with the surgery, with specific attention drawn to preoperative hip ROM, especially flexion and internal rotation, because these clinical parameters should improve after recontouring of the anterolateral femoral head–neck junction.
- Preoperative radiographic studies (x-rays, MRA, and CT scan if obtained) are reevaluated. The size and location of the impingement lesion or lesions are determined, as well as the status of the acetabular labrum and articular cartilage, and are correlated with intraoperative findings.
- It is of utmost importance to determine the type (cam, pincer, or a combined cam-pincer) and subtype of the impingement lesion (focal or global, femoral bump or angular deformity) because the characteristics of the specific deformity will dictate the surgical decision making:
  - On the acetabular side, the focal or global overcoverage can be corrected by resection osteoplasty of the excessive acetabular brim or by a reverse PAO to reorient a retroverted acetabulum.[24] The presence or absence of posterior overcoverage (as detected by the posterior wall sign) as well as the status of the acetabular articular cartilage determines which of these options is elected[24]; a reverse PAO is preferred if the posterior wall is deficient or the acetabular cartilage is injured.
  - On the femoral side, an osseous bump is nearly always the culprit lesion in reducing the clearance of the femoral neck during flexion; it can be corrected by resection osteoplasty.
- Although infrequent, proximal femur reorientation osteotomies can be done to address the FAI lesion such as femoral neck lengthening with trochanteric advancement or flexion-valgus intertrochanteric osteotomy (in case of decreased anteversion or varus position of the femoral neck).[24]
- In our practice, osteochondroplasty of the femoral head–neck junction and/or acetabular brim via mini-open anterior approach of the hip is used for the treatment of anterior cam-type impingement and associated intra-articular lesions.

## Positioning

- Spinal or general anesthesia can be administered. However, regional anesthesia resulting in optimal muscle relaxation is preferred to facilitate joint distraction.
- The patient is positioned supine on a regular operating table. We prefer manual distraction of the joint while assessing the central compartment of the hip to minimize the risk of osteonecrosis of femoral head, which is correlated with the duration and force of traction applied through a fracture table.
- The hip region from the umbilicus to the upper thigh is scrubbed and draped. The whole leg is also scrubbed and draped free to allow unrestricted ROM of the hip during the procedure, a crucial surgical time for the assessment of the adequacy of the osteoplasty.

## Techniques of Mini-Open Osteochondroplasty through the Direct Anterior Approach

### Surgical Approach (Hueter Approach or Smith-Petersen Approach)

- A 3- to 4-cm incision is made extending from the lateral aspect of the anterior superior iliac spine heading distally toward the lateral side of the patella (**TECH FIG 1A**).
- This approach is a muscle-splitting approach, which dissects the interval between the sartorius (innervated by the femoral nerve) and the tensor fascia lata (TFL) (innervated by the superior gluteal nerve). We avoid developing this interval to protect the lateral femoral cutaneous nerve (LFCN) of the thigh.
- The dissection is carried through the subcutaneous tissue to the perimysium of the TFL muscle. The subcutaneous dissection is performed slightly lateral to the sartorius–tensor interval. The gap between the sartorius and the TFL can be easily identified and avoided by externally rotating the lower extremity to stretch the sartorius, making it more prominent.
- The fascia of the tensor muscle is incised over the muscle belly (**TECH FIG 1B**), and the TFL muscle is reflected downward and laterally. The medial soft tissue flap, including the tensor perimysium and the sartorius, is reflected upward and medially. The underlying rectus tendon is exposed.
- The original deep dissection of this approach involves an internervous passage between the rectus femoris (innervated by the femoral nerve) and the gluteus medius (innervated by the superior gluteal nerve). We do not dissect this interval; instead, we medially retract the rectus femoris without division of any of its insertions to avoid weakness of hip flexion.
- After medial retraction of the rectus, the soft tissue and iliocapsularis muscle fibers (iliacus minor, which originates from the

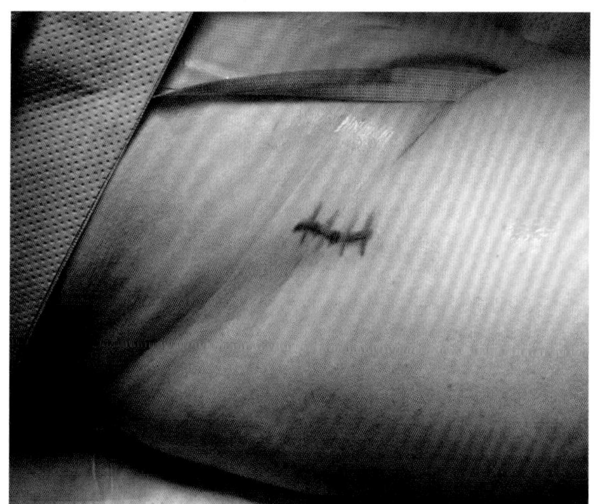

A

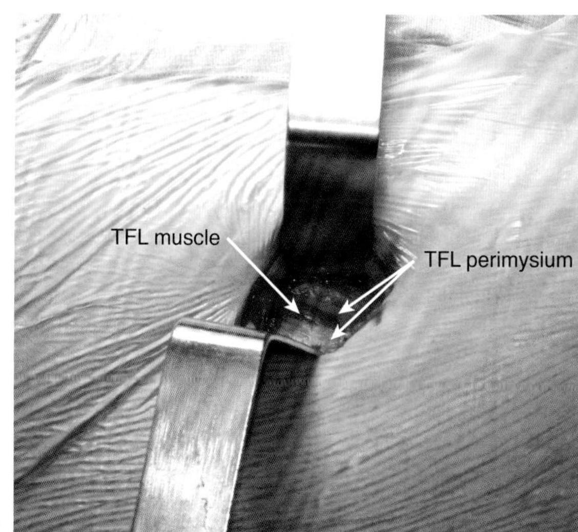


B

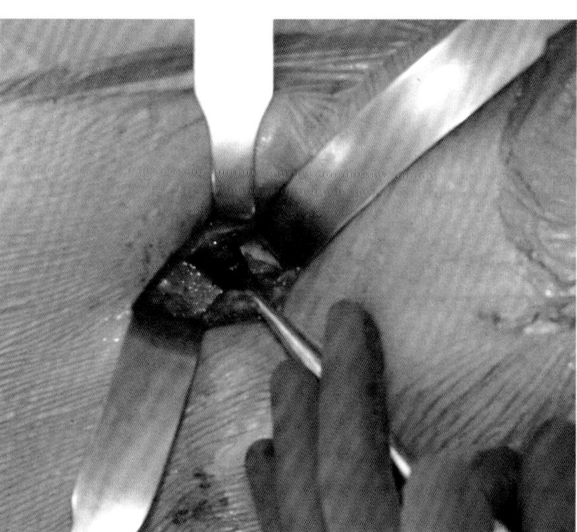

C

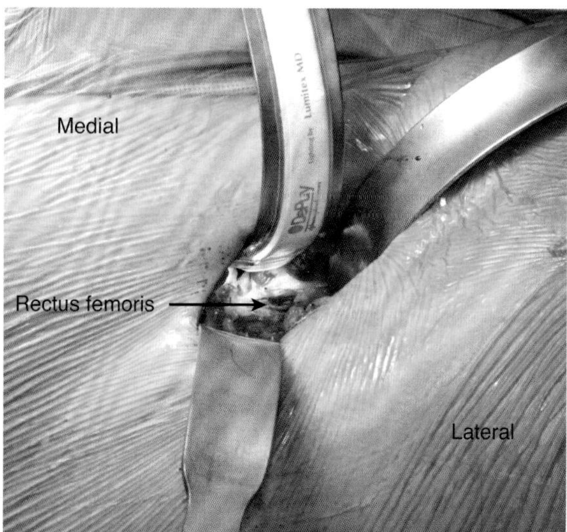


D

**TECH FIG 1** • Mini-open anterior approach. **A.** Laterally to the ASIS, a 3-cm incision is drawn heading distally toward the lateral side of the patella. **B.** The TFL perimysium is opened, exposing the TFL muscle belly. **C.** Stripping of the pericapsular fat pad and the iliocapsularis muscle fibers using a Cobb elevator. **D.** Exposure of the rectus femoris after extra-articular placement of three curved retractors; the TFL and sartorius muscles are retracted laterally and medially, respectively, using two blunt-tipped retractors. A sharp-tipped retractor equipped with source light is placed proximally to the AIIS and medially to the origin of the rectus femoris. *(continued)*

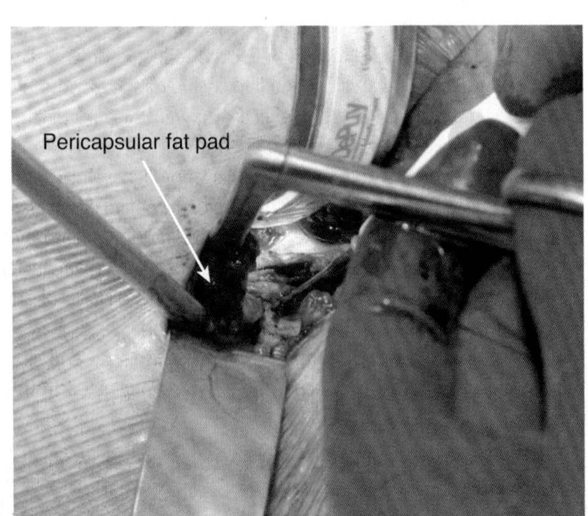


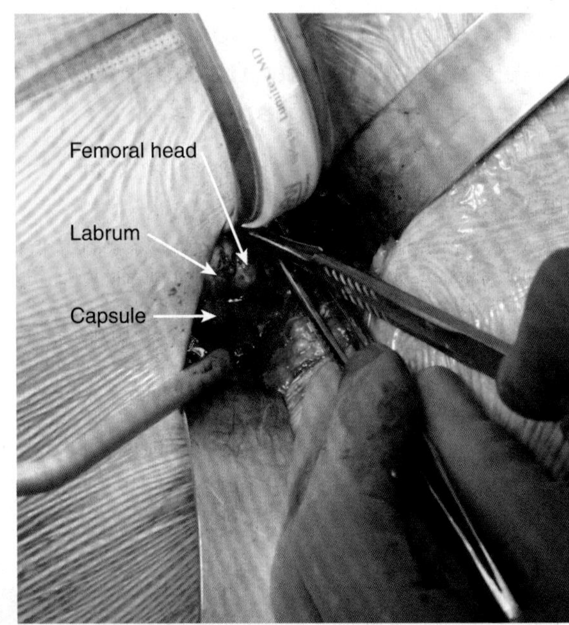


**E** **F**

**TECH FIG 1** • *(continued)* **E.** Excision of the pericapsular fat pad using Bovie cautery. **F.** I-shaped capsulotomy is performed with scalpel blade.

anterior inferior iliac spine [AIIS] and inserts into the iliofemoral ligament) are stripped from the anterior hip capsule using a Cobb elevator (**TECH FIG 1C**).

- Blunt-tipped curved retractors are placed, one laterally around the capsule overlying the neck of the femur and one medially retracting the sartorius and rectus muscles to expose the medial capsule of the femoral neck. At this point, the ascending branch of the lateral femoral circumflex artery is ligated or electrocoagulated if it crosses the surgical field.
- A third sharp-tipped retractor with a light source is placed at the upper part of the AIIS and under the rectus femoris; the hip should be flexed during placement of this retractor (**TECH FIG 1D**).

- The pericapsular fat pad is grasped with a pituitary instrument and completely excised, giving perfect visualization of the capsule (**TECH FIG 1E**). The capsule can be stretched and more easily identified by adducting and externally rotating the leg. An "I"-shaped capsulotomy is performed starting with the longitudinal limb (**TECH FIG 1F**), and the retractors are moved to the intra-articular space to reflect the medial and lateral capsular flaps, providing ample access to the femoral head and neck.
- Our mini-invasive anterior approach, which does not detach any muscle insertion, provides excellent access to the joint, which can be inspected with specific attention drawn to the femoral head–neck junction.

## Femoral Head–Neck Reshaping Osteoplasty

- Based on the preoperative roentgenograms, after adequate exposure of the joint, a thorough assessment of the ROM is done to locate the FAI lesion. This step is crucial in the decision-making process for treatment of FAI.[23] The femoral head–neck junction should be inspected while the hip is brought into full and extreme motion. Although impingement in flexion and internal rotation is by far the most common, impingement also may occur in flexion–adduction, flexion–abduction, and rarely in extension and external rotation.[23]
- The lower extremity should be brought up into a figure-of-four position to provide adequate visualization of the posteromedial head–neck junction.
- The extent of the femoral bump, the presence of labral tear, and cartilaginous lesions are assessed and documented.
  - There is usually a clear delineation between the normal area of white femoral articular cartilage and the area of the femoral head afflicted with the impingement. The area of FAI (femoral bump) is convex shaped and may be covered by diseased hyaline cartilage, which presents as obvious wear and abnormal creases (indentation sign) created by repetitive contact with the acetabular rim. The femoral bump is often red or blue in appearance, in contrast to the untarnished white hyaline cartilage of the femoral head.[23]
  - The labrum should be carefully examined for evidence of tear and/or degeneration. A nerve hook is used to palpate the articular surface of the labrum[6] to reveal any tear concealed by the integrity of the capsular aspect of the labrum. Every effort should be made to repair an injured labrum[6,23]; resection should be reserved only for ossification, attrition, or extensive degeneration and scarring.
  - The central compartment of the hip is inspected and palpated by applying a manual traction to the extremity; with the arthrotomy done, minimal traction is sufficient to allow adequate subluxation of the hip and visualization of the weight-bearing dome region of the acetabulum.[6] To adequately palpate the cartilage using a hook, the joint subluxation can be maintained and optimized by inserting a smooth Cobb retractor into the joint. Any cartilaginous lesion should be noted and addressed either with conservative débridement, resection of the unstable

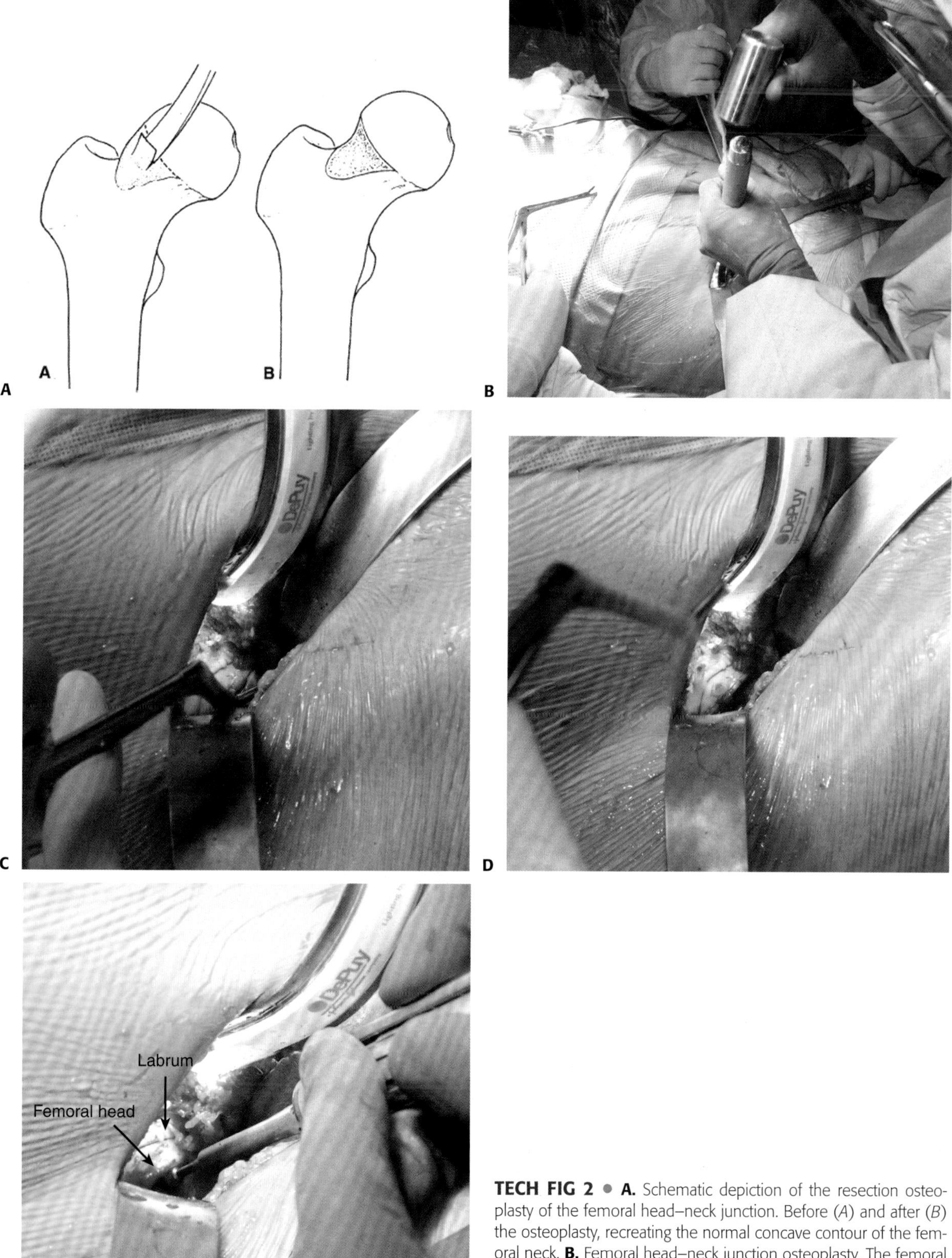


**TECH FIG 2** • **A.** Schematic depiction of the resection osteoplasty of the femoral head–neck junction. Before (*A*) and after (*B*) the osteoplasty, recreating the normal concave contour of the femoral neck. **B.** Femoral head–neck junction osteoplasty. The femoral osteoplasty is started with an osteotome. Note the cephalocaudal orientation of the osteotome. **C,D.** Removal of the osteotomized bump. **E.** A high-speed pneumatic burr is used to fine-tune the femoral reshaping. *(continued)*

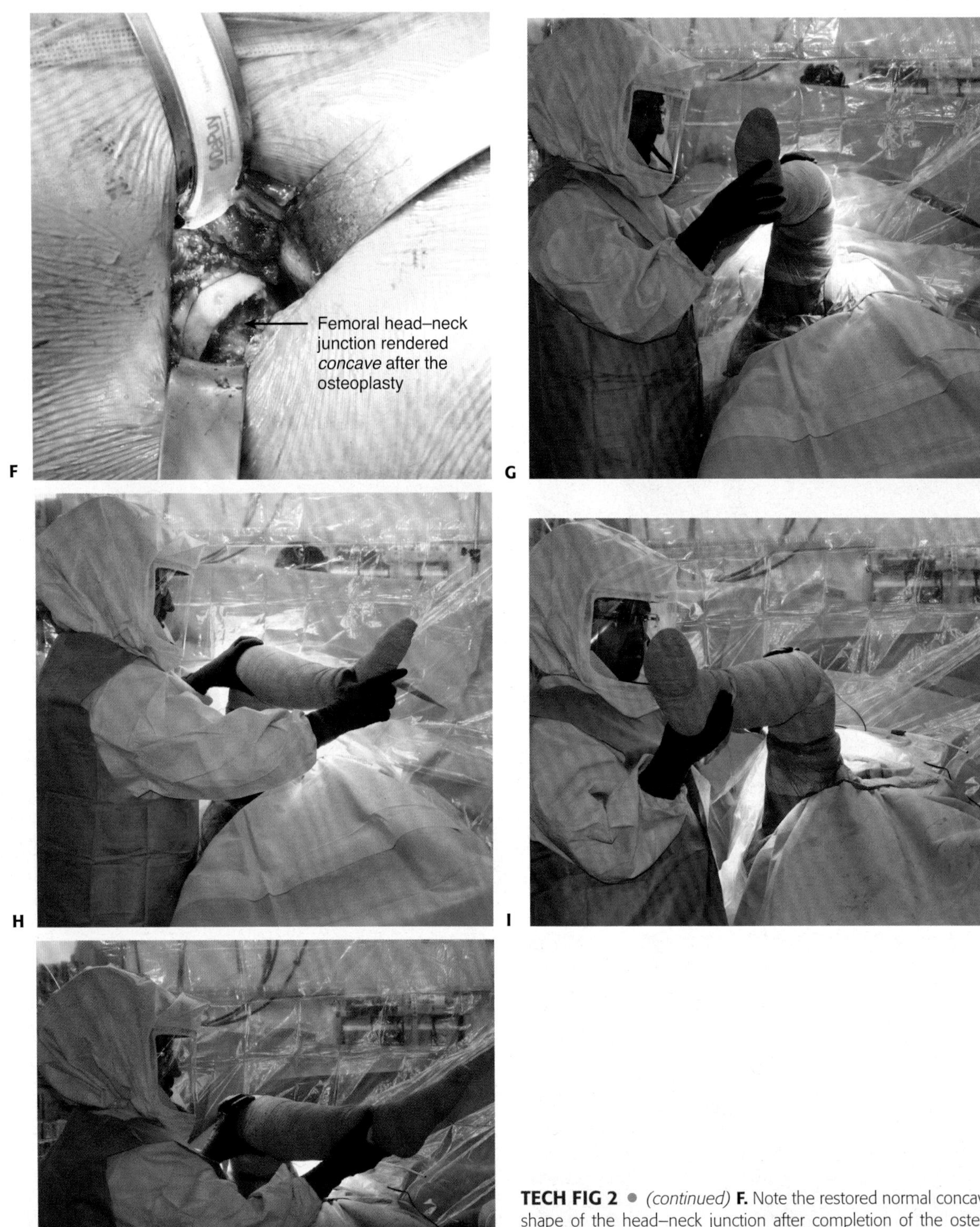


**TECH FIG 2** • *(continued)* **F.** Note the restored normal concave shape of the head–neck junction after completion of the osteoplasty. **G.** ROM before and after the osteoplasty. Extremely limited internal rotation of the hip (<5 degrees) before the osteoplasty. **H.** Preoperative external rotation. **I,J.** Note the remarkable improvement of ROM after completion of the femoral osteoplasty, especially internal rotation, which increased about 30 degrees.

displaced cartilage flap (which can be responsible for clicking and catching), or microfracture of a full-thickness Outerbridge IV lesion, exposing the underlying subchondral bone.

- With the mini-open anterior approach, 60% to 70% of the acetabular cavity can be adequately visualized; the only portion that cannot be exposed is the posteroinferior part of the socket, which can be alternatively palpated by a blunt-tipped nerve hook.[6]
- The osteochondroplasty of the neck can be performed using a combination of osteotomes (**TECH FIG 2A**) (half- and quarter-inch curved osteotomes) and pneumatic burr (**TECH FIG 2B**). The femoral bump is located in the anterosuperior region and has a characteristic bluish-reddish discoloration. During this fundamental surgical step, the articular cartilage of the femoral head is protected by releasing the manual traction, allowing the head to re-sit inside the acetabulum.[6] If the socket contributes to the impingement lesions, it should be trimmed before proceeding with the femoral osteoplasty.
- The reshaping of the femoral head–neck junction should begin proximal to the impingement site (**TECH FIG 2B**) and tapered distally in a near circumferential manner, avoiding the superior portion of the neck where the posterosuperior retinacular vessels enter the bone[23]; these vessels are the terminal branches of the medial femoral circumflex artery.[14]
- The femoral cheilectomy should proceed in a stepwise manner, resecting at once a small bony sleeve. The adequacy of the resection is dynamically assessed perioperatively by bringing the hip into full ROM. The visualization of the lateral neck is maximized by internal rotation of the hip. The posteroinferior part of the neck is reached by placing the leg in a figure-of-four position.[6]
- If direct visualization and the palpation of the femoral head–neck junction detect residual impingement, the osteoplasty is incrementally refined until it is deemed to be adequate. Ultimately, it should be smoothly beveled inferiorly to prevent notching of the femoral neck.
- The extent of bone removal, as well as its depth (which ranges from 5 to 10 mm), is determined by the recreation of the normal smooth concave contour of the head–neck junction and achievement of impingement-free ROM.[6] In severe cases, the resection may expand to cover more than 180 degrees of the femoral head–neck circumference.
- After completion of the femoral head recontouring, the hip motion should improve at least 10 to 15 degrees in flexion and at least 15 to 20 degrees in internal rotation (**TECH FIG 2C**), with the concave femoral neck remaining free of abutment with the acetabular brim.[23]
- Fluoroscopic examination can be performed after completion of the cheilectomy, especially at the beginning of the procedure to confirm establishment of head sphericity and adequate osteochondral resection, with special attention paid to match the preoperative views based on the obturator foramen and the ischial tuberosity.
- AP and frog-leg lateral views should be obtained to better visualize the anterolateral head–neck junction. Varying degrees of flexion and internal–external rotation permit excellent assessment of the osteochondroplasty. In our practice, where FAI surgical correction is routine, we do not use perioperative fluoroscopic control.

## Acetabular Rim Trimming by Resection Osteoplasty

- Whether to address the acetabular rim in the treatment of FAI is governed by two essential factors: the existence of anterior focal overcoverage and the condition of the acetabular articular cartilage and the labrum. Taking both factors into consideration will dictate the nature of treatment that should be done on the acetabular side: limited rim osteoplasty versus reverse PAO. If acetabular trimming is deemed necessary to restore normal hip morphology, it should be done before the femoral reshaping.
- Acetabular trimming necessitates full exposure of the bony acetabular ridge (**TECH FIG 3B**); for this purpose, the acetabular labrum must be carefully mobilized. As stated previously, resection of the labrum is done when it is ossified or when it is afflicted with attrition or excessive scarring. If required, the excision of the labrum should be as conservative as possible and limited to the injured area only. Otherwise, a healthy labrum with firm substance or minimally damaged (linear tears) should be preserved and repaired.
- If a focal anterior overcoverage contributes to FAI (acetabular retroversion with a positive crossover sign), a resection osteoplasty of the anterosuperior rim should be performed.
  - Before the osteoplasty of the rim is accomplished, the labrum, if not torn, is detached cautiously from the anterosuperior acetabular rim using a sharp blade[23] while preserving its continuity with the uninvolved normal segment.
- Once the bony lip of the acetabulum is adequately exposed, a 10-mm curved osteotome or 5-mm high-speed burr is used to trim the overhanging part of the brim (between 2 and 5 mm).[6,23] As for the femoral osteoplasty, the acetabular trimming should be carried out in a stepwise manner until the overcoverage has been entirely resected (**TECH FIG 3B**).
- The amount of rim resection is determined by the magnitude of the anterior overcoverage and extent of the chondral lesion as detected intraoperatively where the area of cartilage damage should be included in the trimming, but excessive (>1 cm) resection should be avoided at all costs to prevent any iatrogenic instability. Roughly 1 mm of resected acetabular edge corresponds to 2 to 3 degrees of correction of the Wiberg angle.
- After completion of the acetabular osteoplasty, the labrum is reattached with anchored sutures to the underlying cancellous acetabular rim, which is trimmed down to bleeding bone.[6] Three to four anchors are needed to reattach the labrum, and if the acetabular rim is analogous to a clock face, there should be an interval of 1 hour between the two anchors, with 6 hours located at the transverse ligament level.
- In cases where the acetabular retroversion is coexistent with a deficient posterior wall (running medial to the femoral head center) or at least lack of posterior overcoverage[23] (posterior wall passing through the head center), a reverse PAO should be done after confirming the integrity of the acetabular articular cartilage through MRA. Routine arthrotomy of the hip should always be done at the time of PAO to evaluate the labrum and the articular cartilage for the presence of lesions and to ensure impingement-free hip ROM. However, describing the PAO surgical technique is beyond the scope of this chapter.

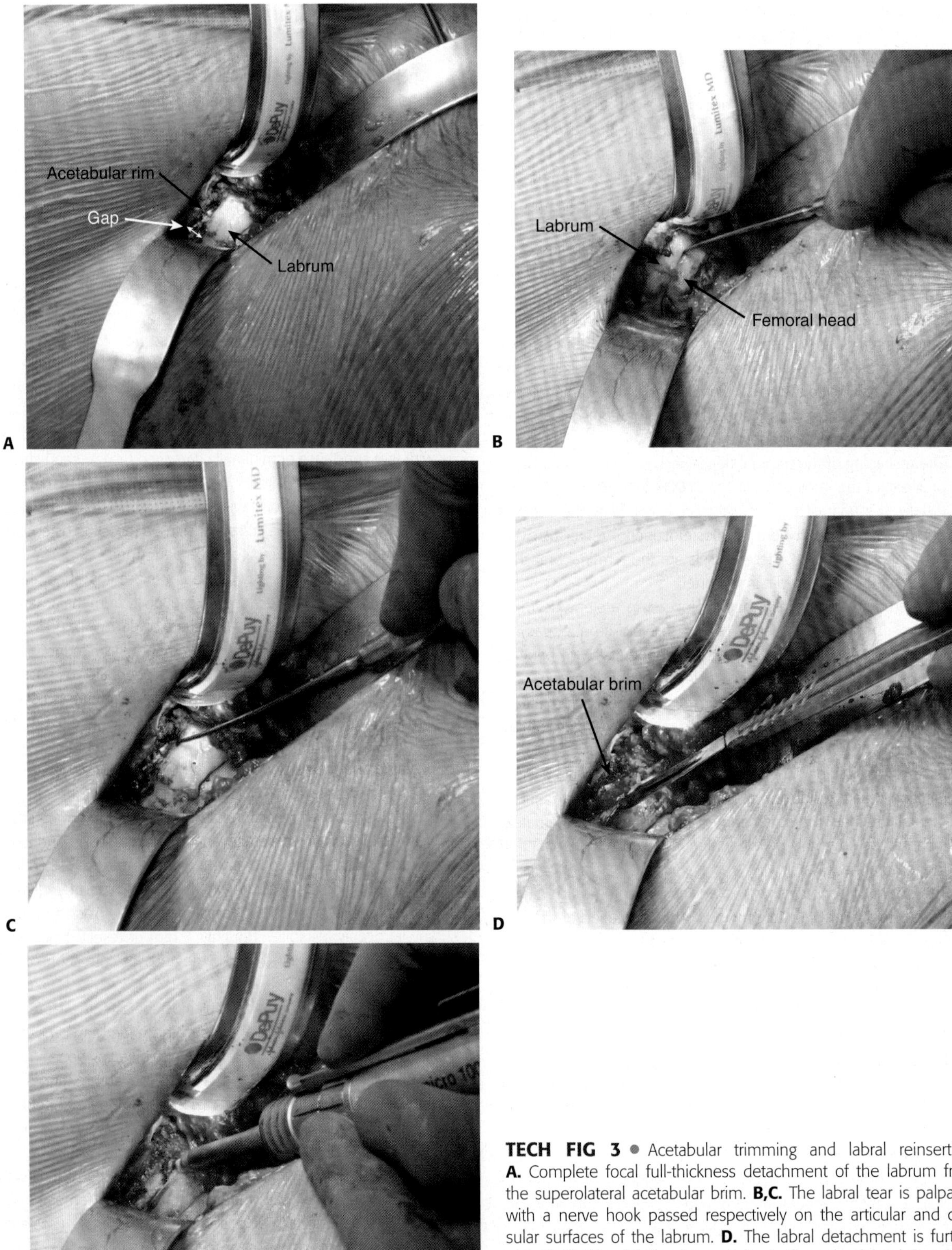


**TECH FIG 3** • Acetabular trimming and labral reinsertion. **A.** Complete focal full-thickness detachment of the labrum from the superolateral acetabular brim. **B,C.** The labral tear is palpated with a nerve hook passed respectively on the articular and capsular surfaces of the labrum. **D.** The labral detachment is further extended with a blade, giving access to the anterolateral rim of the acetabulum. **E.** Trimming of the overhanging acetabular edge using a 5-mm high-speed burr. *(continued)*

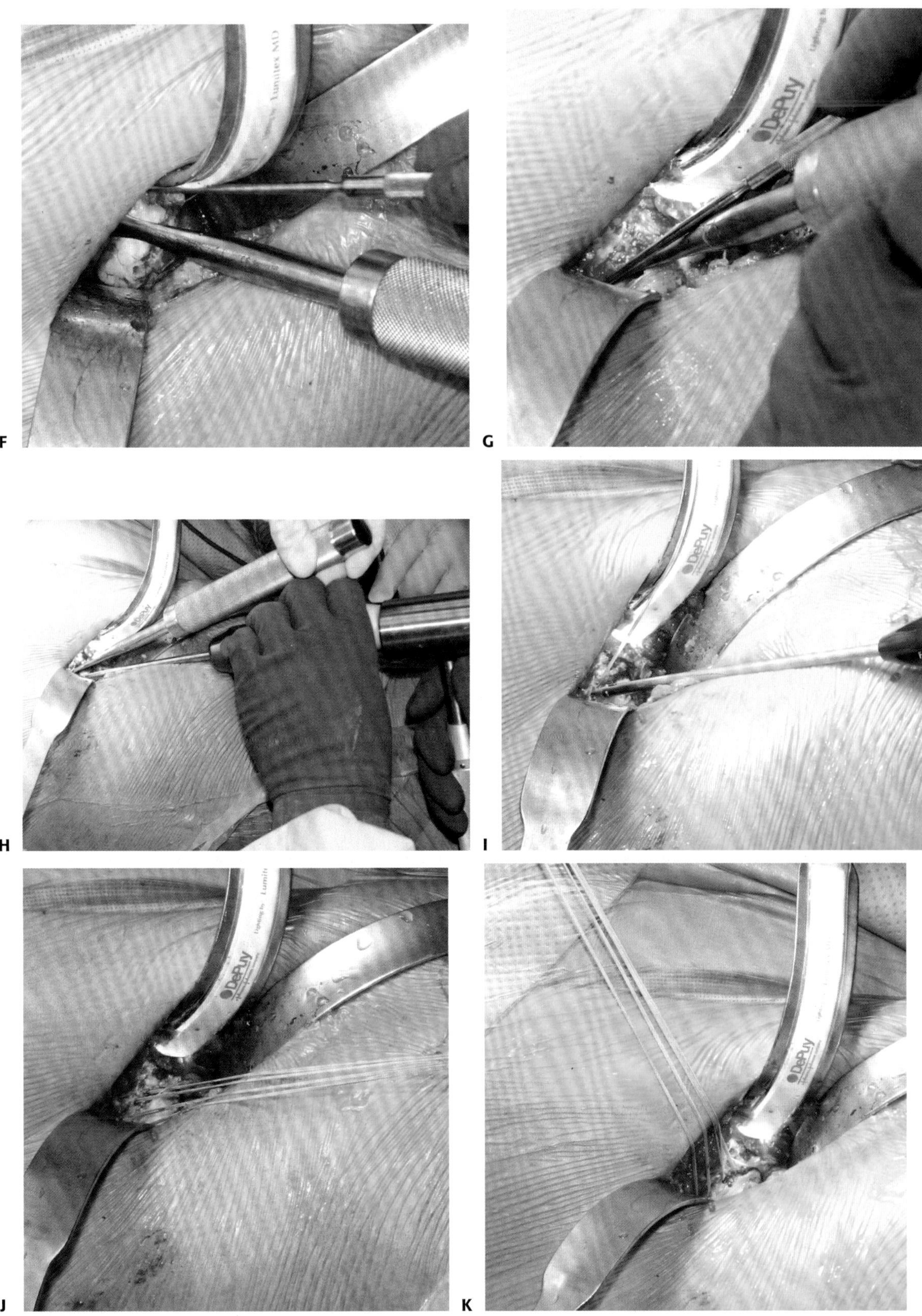

**TECH FIG 3** • *(continued)* **F,G.** The cartilage of the central compartment is circumferentially palpated with the hook, whereas a Cobb retractor is placed inside the joint to maintain and enhance the femoroacetabular subluxation conferred by the manual traction. **H.** Microfracture is realized in the acetabular zone of full-thickness cartilaginous loss. **I–K.** Nonabsorbable suture anchors are inserted into the trimmed and revived acetabular rim; in this case, four anchors were used. *(continued)*

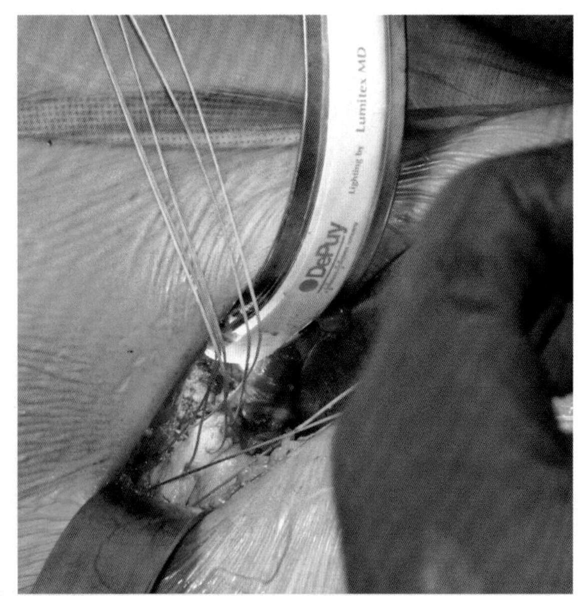

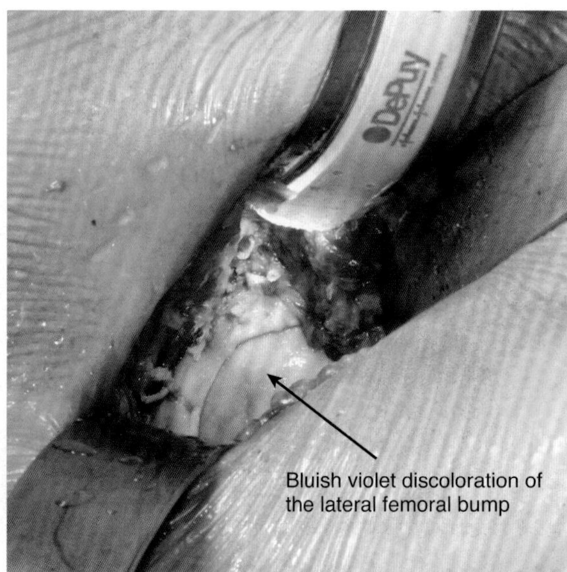


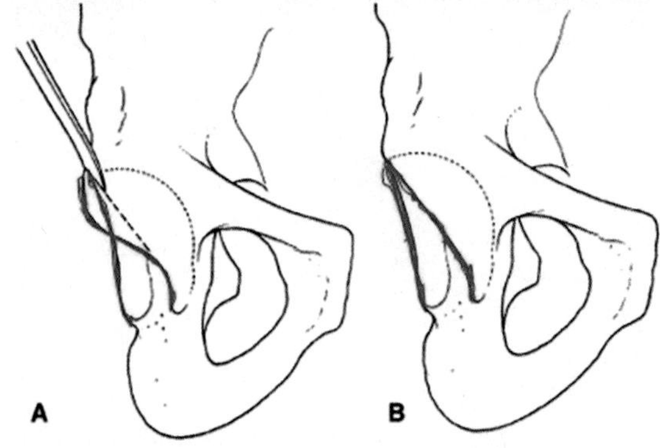

**TECH FIG 3** • *(continued)* **L.** Equidistant passage of the sutures through the labral substance, taking good and stable bites. **M.** The sutures are tied, reattaching the labrum to its acetabular rim and reproducing its sealing effect. **N.** Resection osteoplasty of the excessive anterior rim of the acetabulum. Before (*A*) and after (*B*) the osteoplasty, removing the site of anterior impingement. Note the preoperative crossover sign, which disappeared after achievement of the trimming.

## Closure

- After copious irrigation of the hip joint, bone wax is applied to the areas of bone resection on the femoral neck. After a final check of the hip ROM, a meticulous capsulorrhaphy is performed.[6]
- The capsular flaps are reapproximated loosely with an absorbable running suture. Tight closure of the capsule should be avoided because this may compromise the blood supply of the femoral head by placing excessive tension on the retinacular vessels.[23] Only the longitudinal limb of the capsulotomy needs to be closed.
- The fascia, subcutaneous tissue, and skin are closed in standard fashion (**TECH FIG 4**).

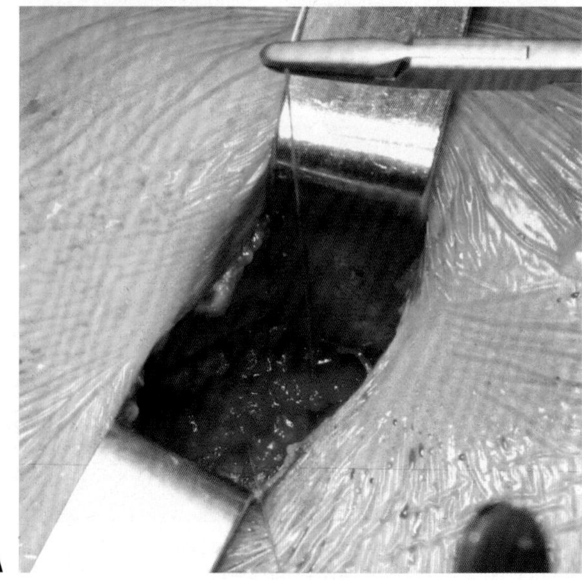

**TECH FIG 4** • Closure. **A.** Capsulorrhaphy is performed by closing the longitudinal capsular limb. *(continued)*

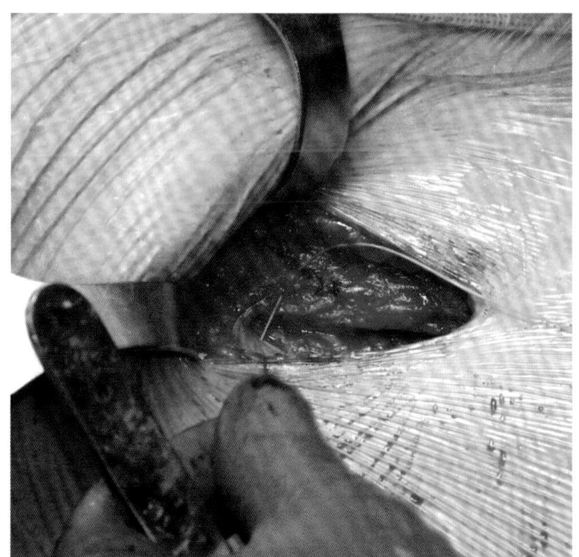

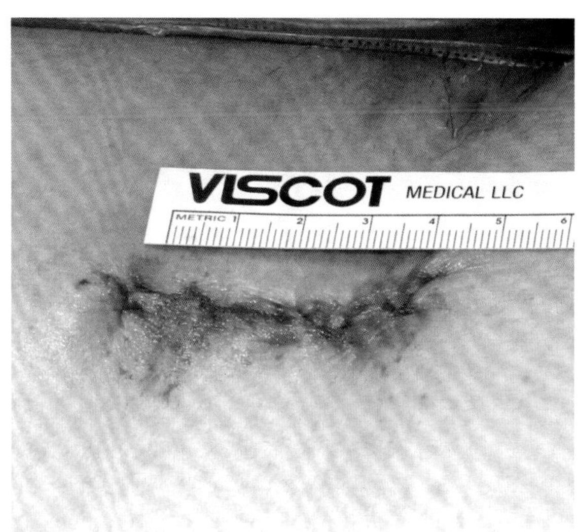


**TECH FIG 4** • *(continued)* **B.** Closure of the TFL perimysium with absorbable running suture. **C.** Incision length of 4 cm.

## PEARLS AND PITFALLS

| | |
|---|---|
| **Indications** | ▪ Ideal surgical candidates are young (younger than 50 years old), have symptomatic FAI that has failed all conservative means, are well-conditioned, or have no or mild secondary cartilaginous damage.<br>▪ Every aspect of the clinical picture should be taken into consideration to make a definitive diagnosis of anterior FAI.<br>▪ The type of impingement disease should be accurately classified to exclude a coexistent hip dysplasia.<br>▪ The surgical strategy presented here is primarily used for the treatment of anterior cam-type deformities. For severe and global deformities, hip dislocation is a valuable option and should be considered. |
| **Articular cartilage and labrum** | ▪ Cartilaginous lesions of the anterior and superolateral acetabular rim are common in both types of impingement.[23]<br>▪ Articular flaps should be débrided back to stable articular cartilage.<br>▪ Microfracture of the acetabular rim disease should be performed for full-thickness cartilage defects.<br>▪ In rare cases where the labrum is revealed to be completely normal, it should not be detached from the acetabular rim. |
| **Limited open osteochondroplasty** | ▪ The sartorius–tensor muscle interval should not be developed in order to avoid damaging the LFCN.<br>▪ None of the rectus femoris heads should be released.<br>▪ For mixed FAI cases, the acetabular trimming and labral reinsertion should be performed first in order to accurately judge the adequacy of femoral recontouring back into a normalized acetabular socket.<br>▪ The posteroinferior acetabular rim can be reached and, if needed, trimmed by placing the lower limb in a figure-of-four position (**FIG 7**).<br>▪ A combination of curved osteotomes and pneumatic burr facilitates the osteoplasty through this surgical approach.<br>▪ Perioperative dynamic examination of the hip and palpation through the arthrotomy ensures complete resection of the impinging structures. |
| **Postoperative rehabilitation** | ▪ Partial weight bearing should be continued for 6 weeks postoperatively to minimize the risk of iatrogenic femoral neck fracture.<br>▪ Excessive therapy within the first 2 months after surgery should be avoided because it can hamper the rehabilitation process.<br>▪ Emphasis should be on gentle ROM within the patient's comfort zone and gentle, progressive strengthening as tolerated by the patient. |

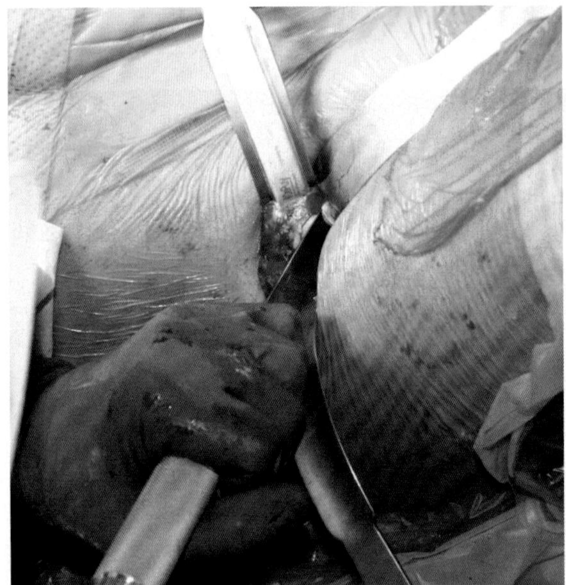

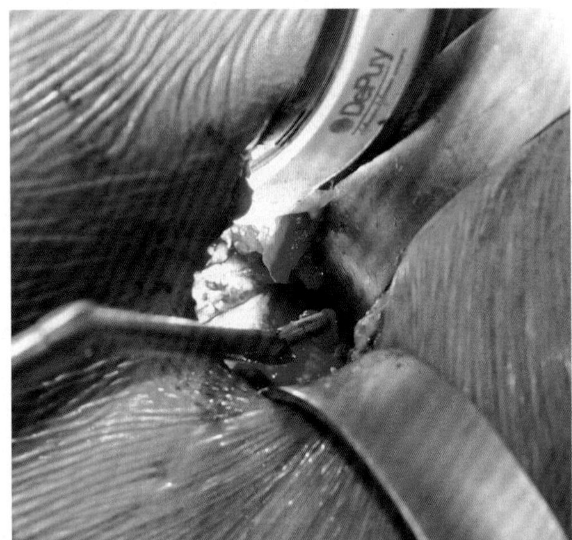


**FIG 7** • Posteroinferior acetabular rim resection. **A,B.** By placing the lower limb in a figure-of-four position, the posteroinferior aspect of the medial acetabular brim can be reached and osteotomized.

## POSTOPERATIVE CARE

- The patients are usually hospitalized for 24 hours and postoperative radiographs are obtained to verify the adequate recontouring of the femoral head–neck junction and to document the integrity of the femoral neck (see **FIG 2**). Postoperative films should be compared to the preoperative films, avoiding any pelvic tilt or malrotation.
- Pharmaceutical deep venous thrombosis prophylaxis is treated with aspirin, one tablet of 325 mg administered two times a day for 6 weeks.
- Heterotopic ossification (HO) risk can be minimized with prophylactic administration of anti-inflammatory medications for 6 weeks: celecoxib (400 mg/day) or indomethacin (75 mg/day). The mini-open anterior approach involves little surgical dissection and avoids any muscular detachment, decreasing the risk of HO with minimal blood loss. Copious irrigation of the joint also reduces the risk of HO development.
- The rehabilitation program consists of touchdown partial weight bearing using crutches for 6 weeks to decrease the risk of femoral neck stress fracture, and then progresses gradually to full weight bearing. During this period, hip flexion is limited to 70 degrees.
- To prevent adhesions between the capsule and the osteotomized zone of the femoral neck, continuous passive motion (no more than 70 degrees of hip flexion) can be used for 4 to 6 hours per day for 1 or 2 weeks postoperatively.[23]
- Formal physical therapy can be started 6 weeks after surgery. The rehabilitation should consist of a gentle ROM program and progressive strengthening within the patient's comfort zone. Because the surgical technique does not involve trochanteric osteotomy, abduction strengthening can be initiated early in the postoperative period.
- The patient may return to normal daily activities (such as walking, ascending or descending stairs, and riding a stationary bicycle) as tolerated 4 to 6 weeks after surgery and may return to full activity once ROM and strength are restored and pain reduced, typically 4 to 6 months postoperatively.

## OUTCOMES

- Because FAI has gained significant interest only during the last decade, only a small number of studies have been published documenting the clinical outcome of conservative surgical treatment.[2,10,15,32] Good midterm results have been reported using various surgical approaches for treatment of FAI, including surgical dislocation, arthroscopy, combined arthroscopy, and limited open and direct anterior mini-open approaches.[30]
- As surgical dislocation of the hip was the mainstay of treatment for FAI, several studies evaluated this particular surgical option, providing early- to midterm clinical outcomes which are promising.[2,10,32,40] Despite its ease of performance and relatively good clinical outcome, dislocation carries a risk of developing complications, mainly HO[12] (37%) and greater trochanter malunion (up to 20%).[40]
- In addition, although there were no reported cases of avascular necrosis (AVN), in the initial description of the procedure, laser Doppler flowmetry showed transient changes in head perfusion during the procedure, which returned to baseline after reduction of the joint.[5] Dislocation also requires the rupture or division of the ligamentum teres with loss of its proprioceptive nerve fibers, the consequences of which are currently unknown.[5]
- Arthroscopic osteochondroplasty has certain potential disadvantages, including the risk of inadequate exposure of the anterolateral head–neck junction, entrapment of bony debris within the joint, increasing the risk of HO, and the possibility of inadequate osseous débridement, leading to failed procedure.
- The mini-open anterior approach combine the advantages of arthroscopic decompression and open surgical dislocation while avoiding the main drawbacks of these two techniques:
  - Similar to hip arthroscopy, no traction is required, and the mini-open procedure carries less risk of neural damage and scuffing of the femoral head cartilage.

- It is a minimally invasive approach that avoids hip dislocation and the need for trochanteric osteotomy, which is top on the list of complications (trochanteric malunion) associated with this surgical method.
- It provides a wide and comprehensive view of all the compartments of the hip, which can be suboptimal in the technically demanding arthroscopic-only procedure, allowing adequate care for chondral and labral lesions.

- Our experience with the mini-open anterior approach has been encouraging when applied to appropriately indicated impingement cases. Analysis of 293 consecutive cases performed in 265 patients between January 2006 and February 2011 revealed good to excellent clinical outcomes; 156 hips (149 patients) achieved a minimum of 2-year follow-up. Out of these, 11 hips underwent THA and 1 hip underwent resurfacing due to degenerative joint disease at an average of 1.4 years postoperatively.[30]
- Despite the auspicious outcome of this technique, it may not be advocated for more advanced disease with posterior impingement lesions or for hips that have circumferential lesions of the femoral head where surgical dislocation, as described by Ganz et al,[12] seems to be more accommodating.

## COMPLICATIONS

### General Complications

- As with any surgical procedure, this less invasive intervention carries a risk for general complications not directly related to the surgical technique; the most relevant are the following:
  - Infection
  - Deep venous thrombosis
- The relatively short operative time and young age of the patients, along with the fast recovery following the procedure, indicates that the likelihood of developing these complications is exceedingly small.

### Specific Complications Related to the Surgical Technique

- The rate and nature of complications associated with the surgical treatment of FAI differ according to the type of surgical procedure performed. The mini-open approach nullifies the risk of trochanteric malunion observed with the surgical dislocation technique and reduces significantly the risk of articular cartilage scuffing, which can occur in hip arthroscopy, especially if the instruments are introduced before obtaining sufficient hip distraction of 8 to 10 mm.
- Neurovascular injury
  - The LFCN is at greatest risk of injury through the mini-open approach.[6] If the interval between the TFL and the sartorius is dissected, the fascia of the latter should be avoided because the LFCN runs over it. Dissection of this interval is not mandatory to provide wide access to the hip joint.
  - This approach does not carry the risk of neurologic damage associated with the arthroscopy where
    - Excessive hip flexion can injure the sciatic nerve.
    - An inadequately padded perineal post can compress the pudendal nerve.
  - Transient neurapraxia has been reported with the use of excessive traction applied during hip arthroscopy.
  - The femoral artery and nerve can be injured through both the arthroscopic and open approaches. Following anatomic landmarks carefully during the mini-open anterior approach spares these vital structures.
- HO
  - Copious irrigation of the joint after the cheilectomy is completed and before proceeding with the capsulorrhaphy decreases the risk of HO. This risk is higher with the purely arthroscopic technique where osteochondroplasty is performed with a high-speed burr, yielding osseous debris; in this case, high-flow hip irrigation along with continuous suction should be used all the time.
  - In addition to profuse irrigation, prophylactic use of indomethacin minimizes the risk of HO development.
- Femoral neck fracture
  - Removing more bone proximally than distally on the head–neck junction can create an apple-bite[20] defect instead of the normal concave-shape junction; this defect can get wedged into the acetabular dome during hip flexion, breaking the suction seal of the labrum and increasing the risk of postoperative femoral neck fracture.
  - In contrast, incomplete reshaping of the head–neck junction is probably more frequent with the purely arthroscopic technique, which has a long learning curve. Several publications have stated that the main reasons for hip arthroscopy revision are inadequate remodeling of FAI deformities.[17]
  - The technique described here provides an excellent visualization of the hip and is associated with lesser risk of failure due to inadequate osteoplasty. However, recurrence of the osseous bump can still occur with any technique used to treat FAI; applications of bone wax on the bleeding reshaped bony cuts reduce the risk of bump reappearance.
- AVN of the femoral head
  - The risk of AVN following hip arthroscopy was theoretical until the results of two cases were published in the literature.[33,34] It is believed that femoral head osteonecrosis may develop secondary to a combination of increased intra-articular pressure and traction.
  - A constant and reliable landmark to identify the hip blood supply arthroscopically is the lateral synovial fold.[17]
  - Because no traction is needed during the mini-open approach, it can be hypothesized that the risk of AVN is less with this procedure, but special care needs to be taken to avoid the zone of the femoral neck where the retinacular vessels run. Because FAI treatment through hip dislocation has not been shown to increase the risk of AVN,[12] this risk is small after cheilectomy through an anterior approach, sparing the need for hip dislocation.
  - In our large series of patients operated on using the mini-open anterior approach, postoperative complications included one neuroma (0.6%) that required excision, one subtrochanteric hip fracture (0.6%) that required open reduction and internal fixation, one repeat labral tear (0.6%) that underwent arthroscopic débridement, and one case of persistent trochanteric bursitis (0.6%) that required iliotibial band lengthening/greater trochanteric bursa excision.[30]

## REFERENCES


1. Beck M, Kalhor M, Leunig M, et al. Hip morphology influences the pattern of damage to the acetabular cartilage: femoroacetabular impingement as a cause of early osteoarthritis of the hip. J Bone Joint Surg Br 2005;87:1012–1018.
2. Beck M, Leunig M, Parvizi J, et al. Anterior femoroacetabular impingement: part II. Midterm results of surgical treatment. Clin Orthop Relat Res 2004;(418):67–73.
3. Burnett RS, Della Rocca GJ, Prather H, et al. Clinical presentation of patients with tears of the acetabular labrum. J Bone Joint Surg Am 2006; 88:1448–1457.
4. Clohisy JC, Keeney JA, Schoenecker PL. Preliminary assessment and treatment guidelines for hip disorders in young adults. Clin Orthop Relat Res 2005;441:168–179.
5. Clohisy JC, McClure JT. Treatment of anterior femoroacetabular impingement with combined hip arthroscopy and limited anterior decompression. Iowa Orthop J 2005;25:164–171.
6. Cohen SB, Huang R, Ciccotti MG, et al. Treatment of femoroacetabular impingement in athletes using a mini-direct anterior approach. Am J Sports Med 2012;40:1620–1627.
7. Czerny C, Hofmann S, Neuhold A, et al. Lesions of the acetabular labrum: accuracy of MR imaging and MR arthrography in detection and staging. Radiology 1996;200:225–230.
8. Eijer H, Leunig M, Mohamed N, et al. Cross table lateral radiographs for screening of anterior femoral head neck offset in patients with femoro acetabular impingement. Hip Int 2001;11:37–41.
9. Eijer H, Myers SR, Ganz R. Anterior femoroacetabular impingement after femoral neck fractures. J Orthop Trauma 2001;15(7):475–481.
10. Espinosa N, Rothenfluh DA, Beck M, et al. Treatment of femoroacetabular impingement: preliminary results of labral fixation. J Bone Joint Surg Am 2006;88:925–935.
11. Ferguson TA, Matta J. Anterior femoroacetabular impingement: a clinical presentation. Sports Med Arthrosc 2002;10:134–140.
12. Ganz R, Gill TJ, Gautier E, et al. Surgical dislocation of the adult hip: a technique with full access to the femoral head and acetabulum without the risk of avascular necrosis. J Bone Joint Surg Br 2001;83: 1119–1124.
13. Ganz R, Parvizi J, Beck M, et al. Femoroacetabular impingement: a cause for osteoarthritis of the hip. Clin Orthop Relat Res 2003;417:112–120.
14. Gautier E, Ganz K, Krügel N, et al. Anatomy of the medial femoral circumflex artery and its surgical implications. J Bone Joint Surg Br 2000;82:679–683.
15. Guanche CA, Bare AA. Arthroscopic treatment of femoroacetabular impingement. Arthroscopy 2006;22:95–106.
16. Hack K, Di Primio GD, Rakhra K, et al. Prevalence of cam-type femoroacetabular impingement morphology in asymptomatic volunteers. J Bone Joint Surg Am 2010;92(14):2436–2444.
17. Ilizaliturri VM Jr. Complications of arthroscopic femoroacetabular impingement treatment: a review. Clin Orthop Relat Res 2009;467: 760–768.
18. Imam S, Khanduja V. Current concepts in the diagnosis and management of femoroacetabular impingement. Int Orthop 2011;35:1427–1435.
19. Ito K, Minka MA II, Leunig M, et al. Femoroacetabular impingement and the cam-effect. An MRI-based quantitative anatomical study of the femoral head-neck offset. J Bone Joint Surg Br 2001;83:171–176.
20. Jackson T, Stake CE, Trenga AP, et al. Arthroscopic technique for treatment of femoroacetabular impingement. Arthrosc Tech 2013;2(1): e55–e59.
21. Kappe T, Kocak T, Bieger R, et al. Radiographic risk factors for labral lesions in femoroacetabular impingement. Clin Orthop Relat Res 2011;469(11):3241–3247.
22. Kassarjian A, Yoon LS, Belzile E, et al. Triad of MR arthrographic findings in patients with cam-type femoroacetabular impingement. Radiology 2005;236:588–592.
23. Lavigne M, Parvizi J, Beck M, et al. Anterior femoroacetabular impingement: part I. Techniques of joint preserving surgery. Clin Orthop Relat Res 2004;418:61–66.
24. Leunig M, Parvizi J, Ganz R. Nonarthroplasty surgical treatment of hip osteoarthritis. Instr Course Lect 2006;55:159–166.
25. Li PL, Ganz R. Morphologic features of congenital acetabular dysplasia: one in six is retroverted. Clin Orthop Relat Res 2003;(416): 245–253.
26. Macfarlane RJ, Haddad FS. The diagnosis and management of femoro-acetabular impingement. Ann R Coll Surg Engl 2010;92: 363–367.
27. Meyer DC, Beck M, Ellis T, et al. Comparison of six radiographic projections to assess femoral head/neck asphericity. Clin Orthop Relat Res 2006;445:181–185.
28. Myers SR, Eijer H, Ganz R. Anterior femoroacetabular impingement after periacetabular osteotomy. Clin Orthop Relat Res 1999;(363): 93–99.
29. Nötzli HP, Wyss TF, Stoecklin CH, et al. The contour of the femoral head-neck junction as a predictor for the risk of anterior impingement. J Bone Joint Surg Br 2002;84(4):556–560.
30. Parvizi J, Huang R, Diaz-Ledezma C, et al. Mini-open femoroacetabular osteoplasty: how do these patients do? J Arthroplasty 2012;27 (8 suppl):122–125.
31. Peelle MW, Della Rocca GJ, Maloney WJ, et al. Acetabular and femoral radiographic abnormalities associated with labral tears. Clin Orthop Relat Res 2005;441:327–333.
32. Peters CL, Erickson JA. Treatment of femoroacetabular impingement with surgical dislocation and debridement in young adults. J Bone Joint Surg Am 2006;88:1735–1741.
33. Sampson TG. Complications of hip arthroscopy. Clin Sports Med 2001;20:831–835.
34. Scher DL, Belmont PJ Jr, Owens BD. Osteonecrosis of the femoral head after hip arthroscopy. Clin Orthop Relat Res 2010;468: 3121–3125.
35. Smith-Petersen MN. The classic: treatment of malum coxae senilis, old slipped upper femoral epiphysis, intrapelvic protrusion of the acetabulum, and coxa plana by means of acetabuloplasty. J Bone Joint Surg 1936;18:869–880.
36. Snow SW, Keret D, Scarangella S, et al. Anterior impingement of the femoral head: a late phenomenon of Legg-Calvé-Perthes' disease. J Pediatr Orthop 1993;13(3):286–289.
37. Takeyama A, Naito M, Shiramizu K, et al. Prevalence of femoroacetabular impingement in Asian patients with osteoarthritis of the hip. Int Orthop 2009;33(5):1229–1232.
38. Tannast M, Siebenrock K. Conventional radiographs to assess femoroacetabular impingement. Instr Course Lect 2009;58:203–212.
39. Tanzer M, Noiseux N. Osseous abnormalities and early osteoarthritis: the role of hip impingement. Clin Orthop Relat Res 2004;429: 170–177.
40. Yun HH, Shon WY, Yun JY. Treatment of femoroacetabular impingement with surgical dislocation. Clin Orthop Surg 2009;1:146–154.

# Hip Arthroscopy

John P. Salvo and Daniel P. Woods

## DEFINITION

- Hip arthroscopy is a minimally invasive technique to address a variety of painful hip conditions in the athletic and prearthritic population.
- A surge in technologic development since the mid-1990s has allowed surgeons to effectively and reliably treat a variety of painful hip conditions arthroscopically.
- The outcomes of hip arthroscopic techniques are equivocal to traditional, more invasive open techniques.[2]
- There is a tremendous learning curve when compared to knee and shoulder arthroscopy.

## ANATOMY

- The hip is a constrained ball-and-socket joint, with the femoral head (ball) articulating with the acetabulum (socket) of the pelvis (**FIG 1**).
- The labrum is a pad of fibrocartilage attached to the acetabulum that deepens the acetabulum and provides stability to the

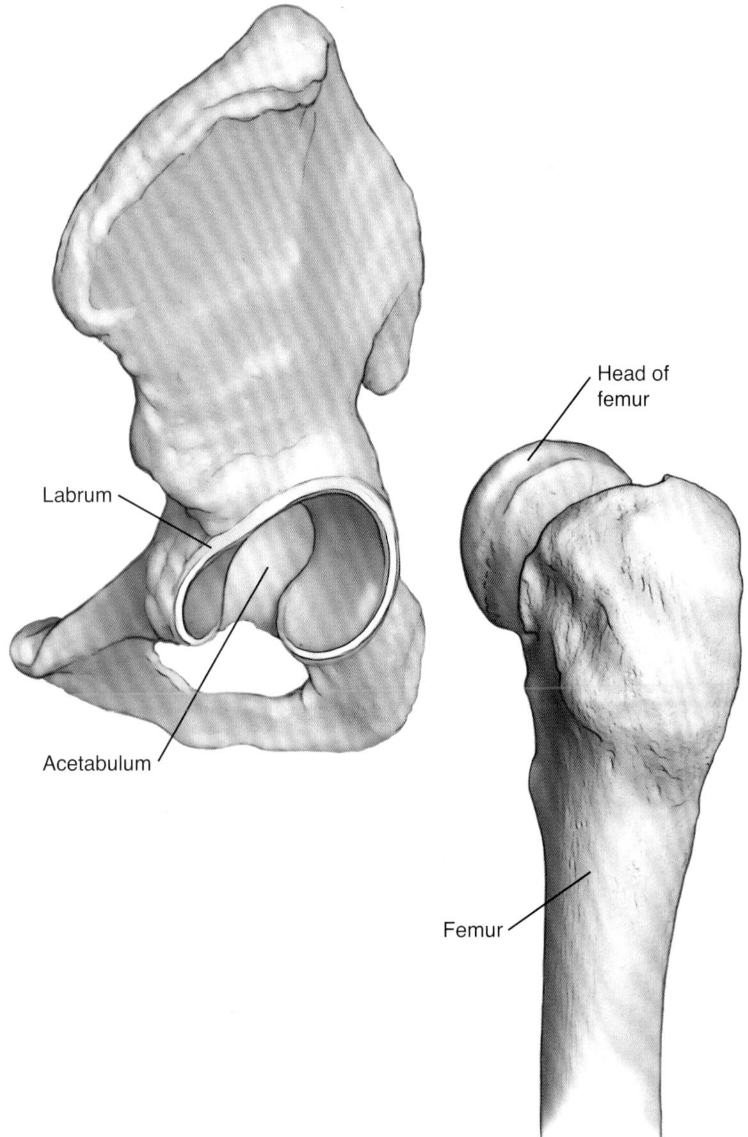


**FIG 1** • Picture represents the bony and soft tissue anatomy of the hip joint. Femoral head, acetabulum, articular cartilage, and labrum are shown.

hip as well as a "suction-seal" effect around the femoral head, providing a secure environment for the articular cartilage and synovial fluid[6] (**FIG 2**).

- The alignment and shape of the hip is critical when determining the etiology of hip pain and thus proper treatment.
- Femoroacetabular impingement (FAI) refers to a bony over-constraint of the joint either from the femur (cam) or acetabulum (pincer) or both (combined)[11] (**FIGS 3** and **4**)
- Dysplasia refers to a shallow acetabulum, undercoverage of the femoral head, or both[12] (**FIG 5**).

## PATHOGENESIS

- Hip and groin pain in athletic and prearthritic population has a wide variety of etiologies:
  - Labral tear
  - FAI
  - Loose bodies
  - Osteoarthritis
  - Core muscle injury (also known as *sports hernia*)
- Labral tear is the most common cause of hip pain and dysfunction in this population.
- Labral tears are usually secondary to FAI or dysplasia or both.

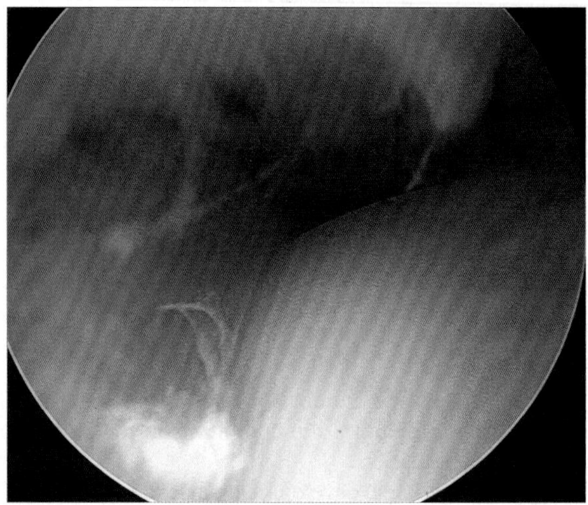

**FIG 2** • Arthroscopic picture showing the femoral head (*right*) and the labrum (*left*) and the suction-seal effect of a normal labrum with the hip off traction.

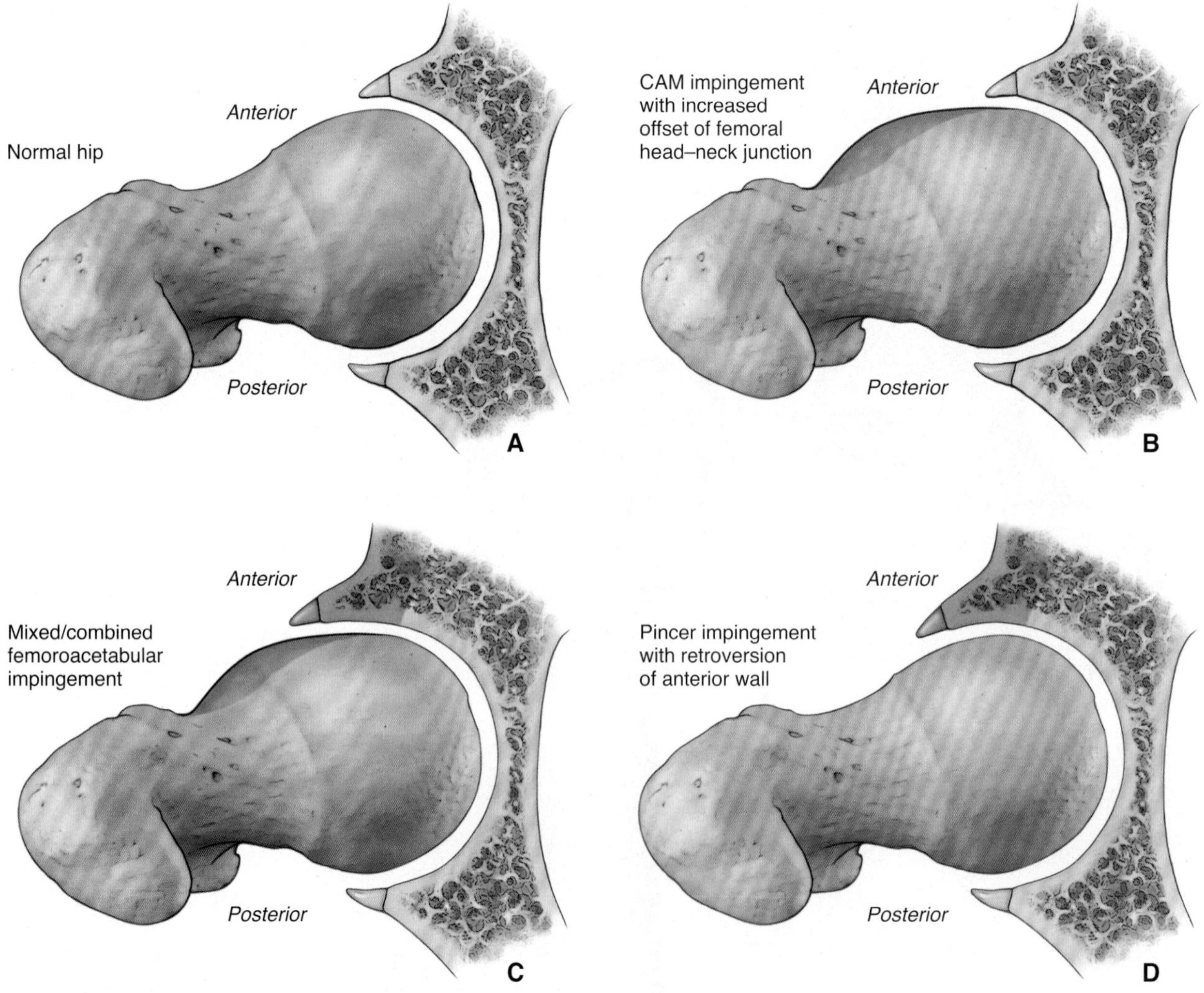

Normal hip
Anterior
Posterior
A

CAM impingement with increased offset of femoral head–neck junction
Anterior
Posterior
B

Mixed/combined femoroacetabular impingement
Anterior
Posterior
C

Pincer impingement with retroversion of anterior wall
Anterior
Posterior
D

**FIG 3** • FAI. Schematic diagram shows views of a normal hip, cam impingement with increased offset of femoral head–neck junction, pincer impingement with retroversion of anterior wall, and mixed/combined FAI.

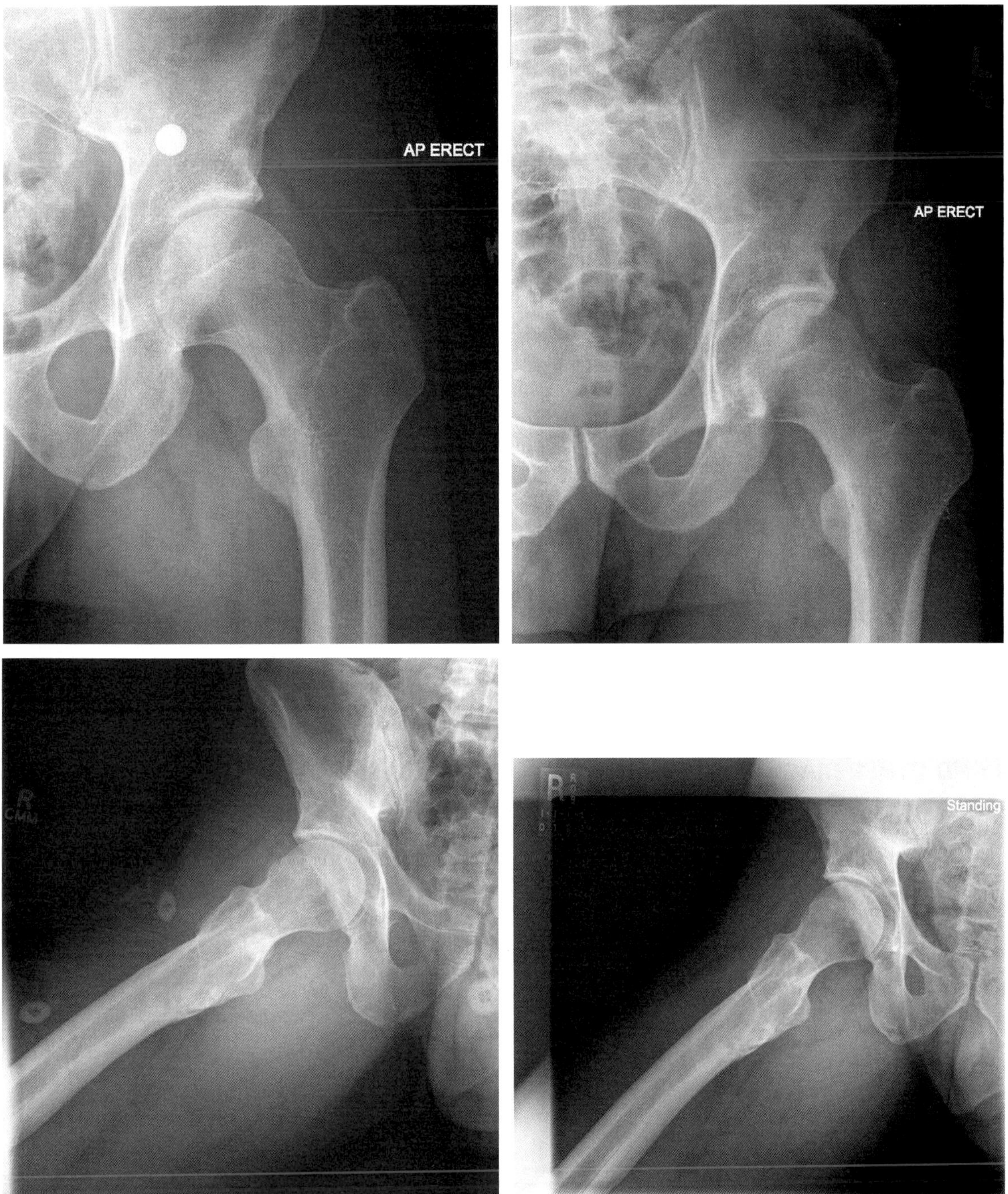


**FIG 4** • X-rays preoperative weight-bearing views AP and lateral of hip with mixed FAI. Postoperative AP and lateral views after femoroplasty and acetabuloplasty.

- If left unchecked, FAI may lead to early development of degenerative joint disease.[7]

## NATURAL HISTORY

- Labral tear
  - If left untreated, labral tears can lead to continued pain and dysfunction as well as damage to the adjacent articular cartilage.
- FAI
  - If left untreated, many believe that FAI is a precursor to arthritis.
  - If treated at the appropriate time before irreversible articular cartilage damage occurs, the hip may be preserved.
- Loose bodies
  - If left untreated, loose bodies will lead to articular cartilage damage and continued pain and dysfunction.[9]
- Snapping hip
  - In general, snapping hip will cause no damage to the hip joint proper; but if left untreated, it can lead to continued pain and dysfunction.
  - Internal snapping hip can impinge on the anterior labrum, leading to tears in this area.

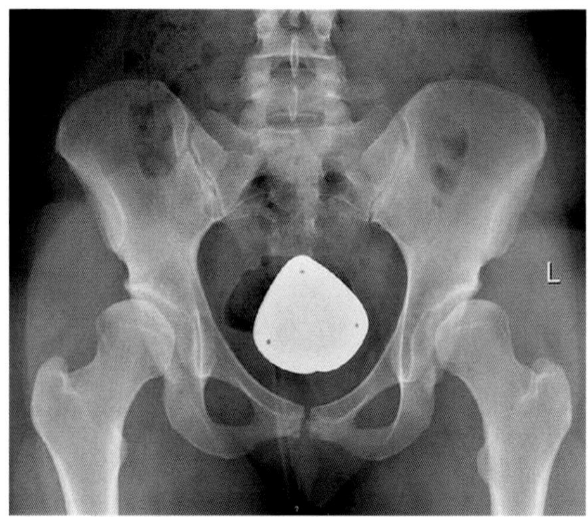


**FIG 5** ● X-ray of hip with acetabular dysplasia with decreased center-edge angle and lack of coverage of femoral head.

## PATIENT HISTORY AND PHYSICAL FINDINGS

- A thorough and focused physical examination is essential.
- Observe gait, manual motor testing, palpation of bony prominences and tendons, range of motion (ROM), and provocative maneuvers for reproducing pain and symptoms.
- Perform the examination on the asymptomatic hip first to assess the ROM and stability of the normal hip when possible.

## IMAGING AND OTHER DIAGNOSTIC STUDIES

- Weight-bearing x-rays (anteroposterior [AP] pelvis, frog lateral, false profile, and Dunn 45-degree views)[10]
- High resolution magnetic resonance imaging (MRI). Direct MRI arthrogram allows injection of lidocaine to determine if pain is generated from hip.
- Computed tomography (CT) scan allows the best detailed determination of FAI and alignment (dysplasia or version) and allows for detailed preoperative planning for decompression of FAI.[10]

## DIFFERENTIAL DIAGNOSIS

- Labral tear
- FAI
- Loose bodies
- Synovitis
- Snapping hip
- Articular cartilage disease
- Arthritis

## NONOPERATIVE MANAGEMENT

- Nonoperative management is always the first step in the treatment of painful hip conditions in the athletic and prearthritic population.
- Activity modification; physical therapy aimed at restoring strength, motion, and balance; and nonsteroidal anti-inflammatory drugs or other medications are the mainstays of nonoperative treatment.[11]
- The success of treatment depends on the etiology of the hip pain and the patient's activity level (college or professional athlete or "weekend warrior") and age.

## SURGICAL MANAGEMENT

- The vast majority of patients treated with hip arthroscopy have a combination of labral tear and FAI.
- The goal of surgical treatment is to repair the labrum, treat any articular cartilage injury, and restore the normal biomechanics of the hip joint (ie, decompressing the FAI).

### Preoperative Planning

- Weight-bearing x-rays (AP pelvis, frog lateral, false profile, and Dunn 45-degree views)
- Be sure to determine that the pain generates from the hip joint and is not referred (lumbar spine or sacroiliac joint) or from muscular pathology (core muscle injury or sports hernia).
- Be wary of other pathology such as dysplasia, connective tissue disorders, or myofascial pain syndrome.
- Make sure all appropriate equipment and personnel (eg, radiology technician) are available.

### Positioning

- Distraction is required for hip arthroscopy as well as fluoroscopic visualization of the joint in all planes.
- Place the patient in the supine or lateral position on either a fracture table or commercially available distraction table to allow appropriate distraction of the hip (**FIG 6**).
- A well-padded perineal post, preferably with a lateralized post, should be used to allow distraction in the plane of the femoral neck.

### Approach

- Standard portals (**FIG 7**)
  - Anterolateral
  - Anterior
  - Midanterior
  - Posterolateral
- Accessory portals
  - Modified anterior
  - Proximal midanterior
  - Distal lateral portal
  - Proximal lateral portal

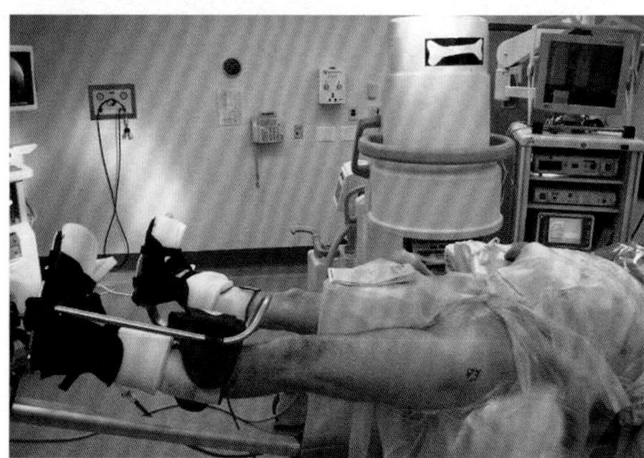

**FIG 6** ● Patient positioned supine on a hip distractor attached to operating room (OR) table. Full access for C-arm is noted.

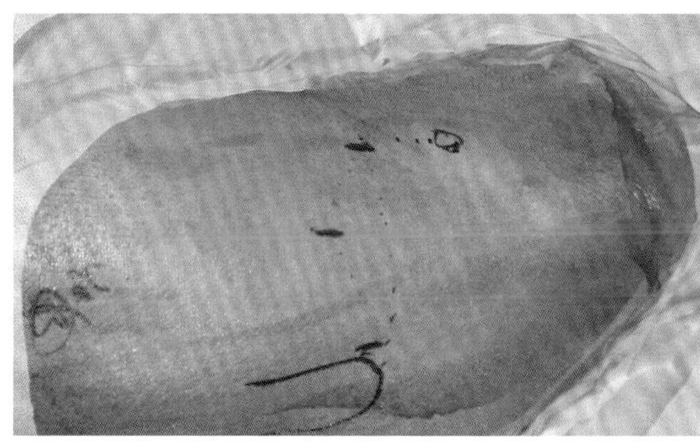

**FIG 7** • Portals. Left hip demonstrating anterolateral, anterior, midanterior, and posterolateral portals.



## Positioning

- Allow free access around the hip with fluoroscopic access as well (see **FIG 6**).
- Use fluoroscopy to confirm appropriate distraction (**TECH FIG 1**).
- If appropriate distraction cannot be easily obtained, place a needle in the hip under sterile conditions to release the negative intra-articular pressure of the joint and allow distraction.[3]

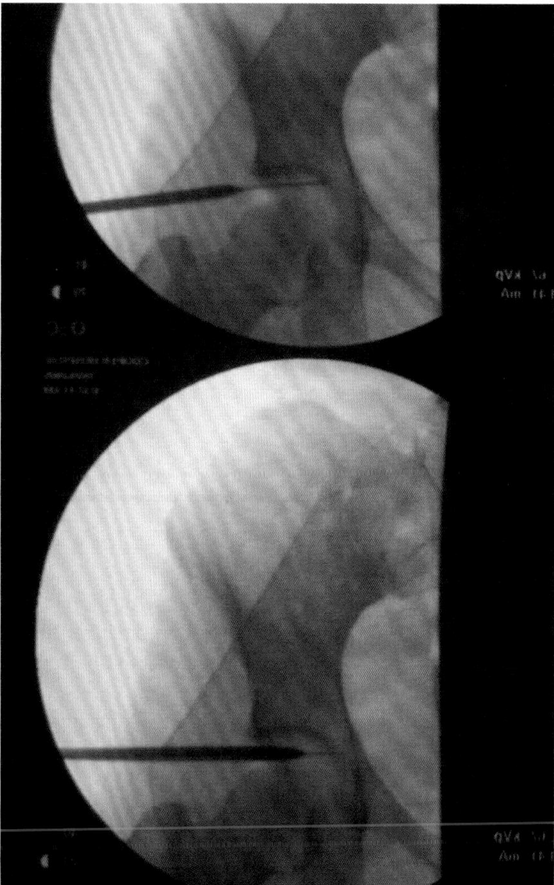

**TECH FIG 1** • Fluoroscopic pictures of a right hip. Views show initial distraction of the hip followed by aeration of the capsule. Portals are created over flexible Nitinol guidewires with a metal cannula.

## Portals

- Anterolateral (see **FIG 7**)
  - Initial portal established under fluoroscopic guidance
  - Start needle 1 to 2 cm proximal and 1 to 2 cm anterior to the tip of greater trochanter at a sufficient angle to enter the hip joint without damaging the cartilage.[3,5]
    - Removing the obturator from the needle releases the negative intra-articular pressure of the joint and allows increased distraction with the same amount of traction.
    - Some surgeons inject the hip with 20 to 40 mL of sterile saline prior to placing the guidewire through the needle.
  - After placing needle in hip, flexible guidewire is placed for creation of the portal.
  - Place cannula with gentle steady pressure and be careful not to bend or break the pin.
    - Use fluoroscopy as you are creating this portal.

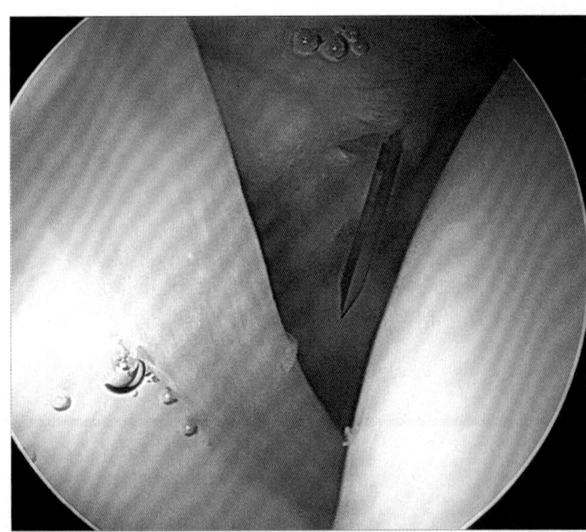

**TECH FIG 2** • Capsulotomies are created using a banana or beaver blade to connect portals. Exercise care with the blade to prevent iatrogenic cartilage damage.

- Anterior
  - Consists of the intersection of sagittal line from anterior superior iliac spine distal and line from tip of greater trochanter[3,5]
  - Placed after triangulation when viewing from the anterolateral portal
  - Most use a modified anterior portal, which is 2 cm more lateral than a standard anterior portal.
  - After establishing the anterior portal and performing appropriate capsulotomies (see next step), view initial anterolateral portal from anterior portal and complete capsulotomy.
- Capsulotomies
  - After entering the joint, perform capsulotomy with a banana blade or beaver blade under arthroscopic visualization (**TECH FIG 2**; **Video 1**).
  - Capsulotomies are required to allow sufficient movement of instruments in the hip.
  - Horizontal capsulotomy connecting the anterolateral and midanterior or modified anterior portal is generally required.
    - Try to keep a proximal flap of cartilage in case you want to close the horizontal capsulotomy at the end of the case.
  - "T capsulotomy" can be used for access to peripheral compartment for large cam lesions.
    - Must be repaired at the end of the case.
- Midanterior
  - Approximately 45-degree angle between anterolateral and anterior portals and starting distal[1,3]
  - Used for anchor placement or for access to peripheral compartment
  - Used for T capsulotomy when performed
- Accessory
  - See description of portal creation discussed earlier.
  - The steps are same for establishment of accessory portals.

## Diagnostic Arthroscopy

- Perform a complete diagnostic arthroscopy of the hip in the same order as a routine arthroscopy (the order of structures inspected does not matter, but it is important to be consistent in your method).
- Perform diagnostic arthroscopy of the central compartment and complete repairs before removing traction and going on to the peripheral compartment.
- Inspect all structures in the central compartment with traction and peripheral compartment after traction released (list is not complete or comprehensive):
  - Central compartment (**TECH FIG 3A**)
    - Labrum, articular cartilage acetabulum, ligamentum teres, articular cartilage femoral head, and loose bodies
  - Peripheral compartment (**TECH FIG 3B**)
    - Medial synovial fold, medial head-neck, middle head-neck, lateral head-neck, labrum, lateral synovial fold, lateral gutter, and medial gutter
- Other areas are listed below but not covered in detail in this chapter:
  - Peritrochanteric space
  - Subgluteal space
  - Iliopsoas tendon

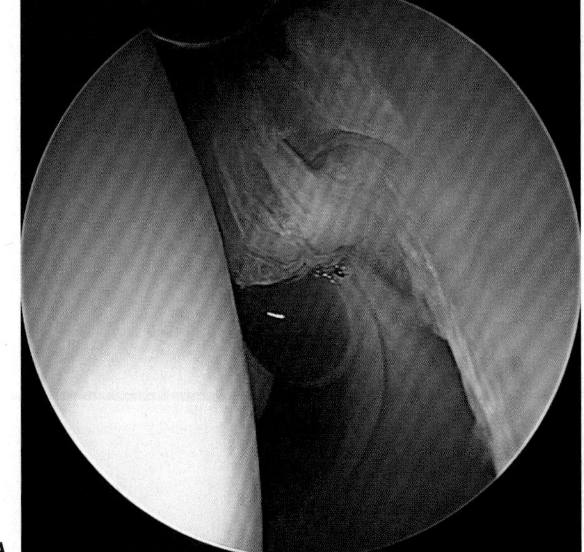

**A**

**TECH FIG 3** • **A.** Central compartment. Labrum with tear, femoral head, acetabulum with tear of articular cartilage. *(continued)*

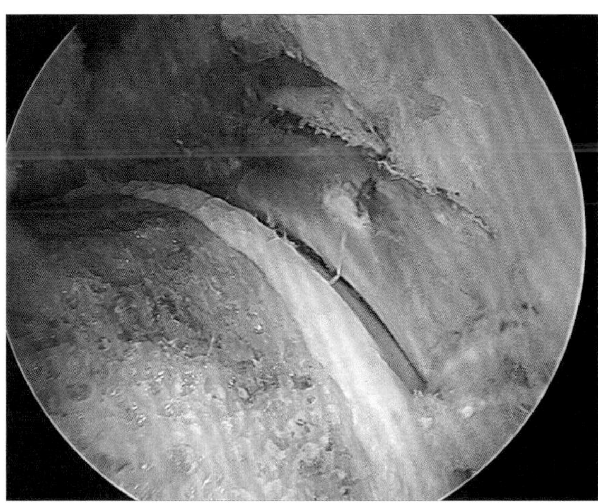

**TECH FIG 3** • *(continued)* **B.** View of anterolateral portal of peripheral compartment post labral repair and femoroplasty.

## Labral Repair or Débridement (Video 2)

- We prefer to repair the labrum to reestablish the suction-seal effect (**TECH FIG 4A**).
- If débridement is required, use a combination of shaver and radiofrequency device to remove pathologic tissue while preserving as much healthy and stable tissue as possible.
- Remove loose bodies, chondroplasty, and microfracture as indicated.
- Repair
  - Suture anchors or knotless device (according to surgeon preference)
  - The goal is to repair labrum to the edge of the articular margin of the acetabulum to restore the anatomy and the suction-seal effect of the labrum (**TECH FIG 4A**).
  - Vertical mattress or base stitch should be used when possible (tissue quality and size) because it gives the best restoration of the labral anatomy[8] (**TECH FIG 4B**).

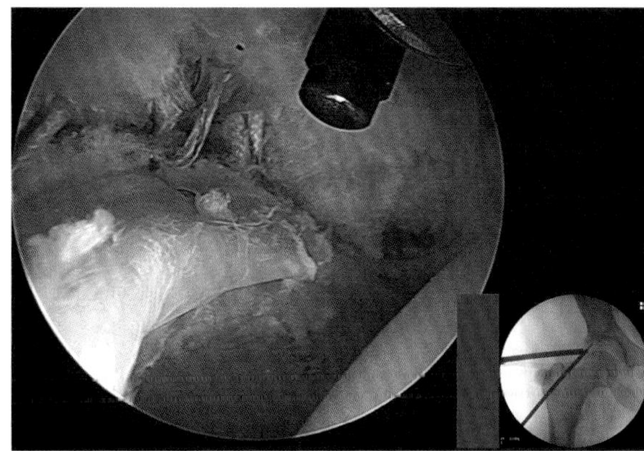

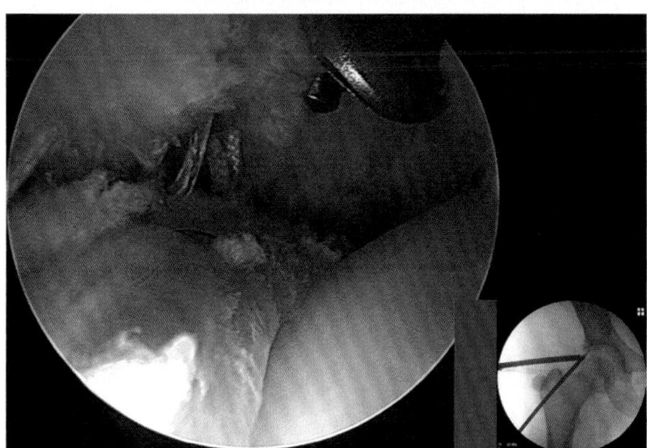

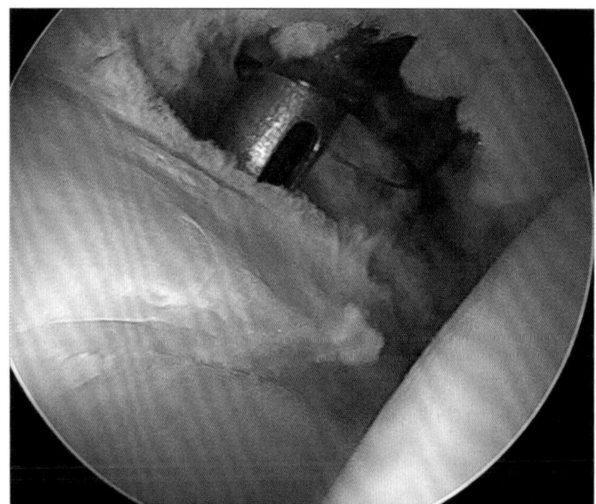

**TECH FIG 4** • **A.** View from anterolateral portal after labral repair. Traction is removed and restoration of the suction-seal effect of the labrum is shown. **B.** Labral repair with vertical mattress base stitch restoring the labrochondral junction. Vertical mattress stitch avoids blunting of the labrum. **C.** Drill guide is placed from the midanterior portal at the edge of the acetabular rim. Care is taken not to medialize the labrum and also not to penetrate the subchondral plate.

- Elevate and mobilize labrum off acetabulum and try to preserve the labrocartilaginous junction.
- Perform acetabuloplasty/rim trimming when indicated or decorticate acetabular rim to provide a healing surface for labral repair.[8]
- Place anchors through the midanterior portal at a 30- to 45-degree angle relative to the edge of the acetabulum (**TECH FIG 4C**).
- Place anchors from anterior (medial) to anterolateral while viewing from anterolateral portal.
- Pass a single arm of suture under labrum at labrocartilagenous junction and retrieve the same suture through the labrum to create a vertical mattress stitch.
    - You may do a single pass around labrum in a "wrap around" fashion as well.
- Pass-retrieve-tie, move to next anchor, and repeat.
- Keep knots off articular surface (**TECH FIG 4B; Video 3**).

## Acetabuloplasty/Rim Trimming

- Typically done as noted earlier during labral repair while under traction
- May also perform acetabuloplasty without labral detachment or repair
- Follow preoperative plan regarding location and amount of acetabulum to trim.
- Round burr (side cutting) or flat-top burr (end and side cutting) (**TECH FIG 5**)
    - Use combination of arthroscopic elevators, rasps, shaver, and a radiofrequency device to clear acetabular rim of periosteal coverage.
    - Use fluoroscopy to help guide resection (it is critical to obtain true AP of hip to allow appropriate resection).
- Can take down to edge of articular cartilage damage in small defects
- Preserve the labrum while performing acetabuloplasty.
- Exercise caution with resection to prevent overresection and subsequent iatrogenic instability.

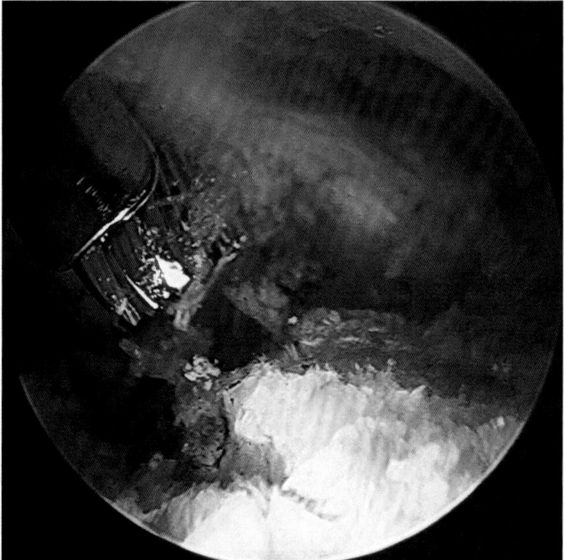

**TECH FIG 5** • Arthroscopic view through anterolateral portal with flat-top burr performing acetabuloplasty. Femoral head on left and burr is on acetabular rim.

## Femoroplasty

- Careful preoperative planning for location and amount of femoral resection for femoroplasty (**Video 4**)
- Allows access to peripheral compartment after completion of work in the central compartment and removal of traction
- Initially assess peripheral compartment through the capsulotomies.
- Flex hip to approximately 45 degrees and slight abduction to relax the capsule and allow access to peripheral compartment and head–neck junction.[4]
- Can access further lateral with internal rotation of the leg
- Begin with assessment and localizing the cam lesion and confirming access arthroscopically (**TECH FIG 6A**).
- Begin resection proximally with round burr slightly into the articular margin (usually in line with physeal scar but not always) (**TECH FIG 6B**).
- Work from anterior to anterolateral to lateral and proximal to distal, setting a proximal template and contouring distally in a gentle progression to the femoral neck.[4]
- Switch between anterolateral, midanterior, and anterior portals for viewing and working, depending on the area to be resected.
- Perform a dynamic examination at the end of femoroplasty, putting the hip in the impingement position to confirm resolution of the bony conflict.
- May need to perform a T capsulotomy to access large lesions or distal and lateral
    - Close the "T" with side-to-side sutures at end of femoroplasty (**Video 5**).

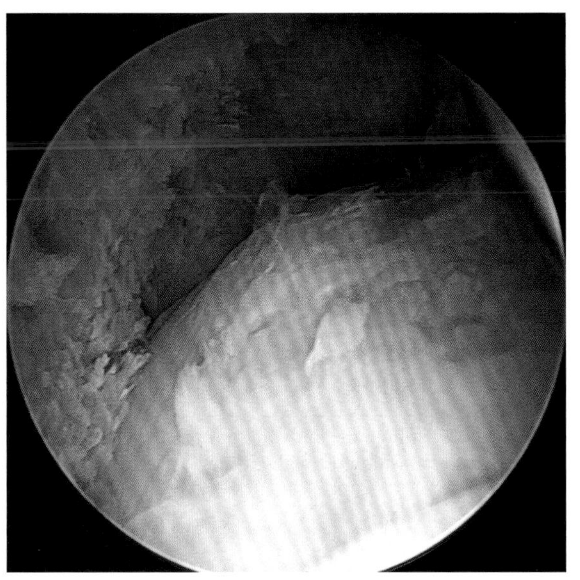

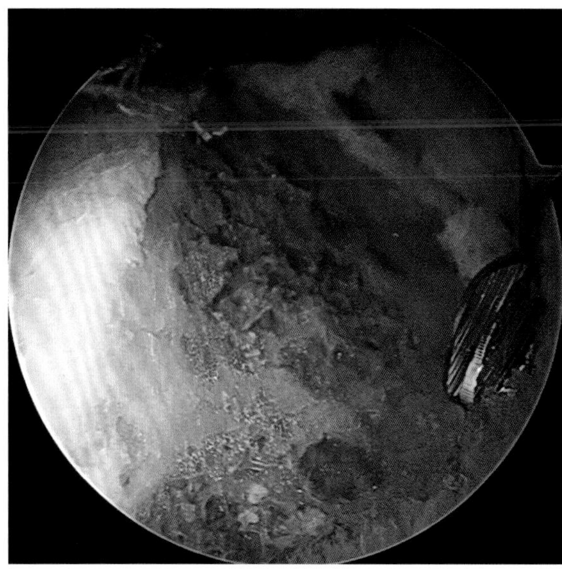

**TECH FIG 6** • **A.** Arthroscopic view of cam lesion through anterolateral portal prior to femoroplasty. **B.** Arthroscopic view through anterolateral portal after femoroplasty showing resection of the cam lesion.

## Loose Bodies

- Loose bodies that form in the hip can be located in the central and peripheral compartments.
- Removal of all loose bodies from central compartment typically requires use of the posterolateral portal.[9]
- Thorough examination of peripheral compartment is needed to remove all loose bodies.

## Microfracture

- Typically used for acetabular cartilaginous defects
- Use curettes and a shaver to stabilize the edges of cartilage and remove calcified layers of cartilage in area of microfracture.
- Various angle picks are available.
  - However, you must be careful with the angle to avoid cutting off the acetabulum.

## Iliopsoas Snapping (Internal Coxa Saltans)

- The iliopsoas tendon may snap or pop over the femoral head or iliopectineal line, causing pain.
- Tendon release can be done transcapsular at the level of the joint in the central compartment or extracapsular at the lesser trochanter.
- A radiofrequency device or beaver blade is used for release.

## PEARLS AND PITFALLS

| | |
|---|---|
| Confirm appropriate joint distraction prior to prep and drape and then release; replace traction after prep and drape. This will allow you to minimize traction time. | ■ After completion of work in the central compartment, remove traction and check status of labral repair viewing through the capsulotomy. |
| After placing initial needle into hip for anterolateral portal, remove under fluoroscopy and replace to ensure that it does not penetrate the labrum. | ■ View the peripheral compartment through the capsulotomy after flexion and slight abduction of the hip and confirm full access to cam lesion for femoroplasty. |
| Use fluoroscopy judiciously as needed, especially early in the learning curve, until you are comfortable with portal and instrument placement. | ■ If it is difficult to access the full cam lesion, then perform a T capsulotomy through the midanterior portal. This must be repaired with side-to-side stitches at the end of the procedure. |
| When placing anchors, get close to the edge of acetabulum without penetrating subchondral bone to prevent medialization of the labrum. Keep angle of drill guide at 30–45 degrees, relative to the acetabulum. | ■ Put hip through dynamic examination while viewing arthroscopically via anterolateral and anterior portals at the end of femoroplasty to confirm resection of the cam and resolution of the bony conflict. |
| Expose rim fully to allow appropriate anchor placement on edge of rim. | ■ Place all anchors through the midanterior portal and then pass sutures in vertical mattress fashion through labrum. |

## POSTOPERATIVE CARE

- Outpatient procedure and discharge with crutches and a hip brace
- Continuous passive motion is to be performed at home during the first week to 10 days.
- For labral débridement with or without FAI, crutches for 1 to 2 weeks.
- For labral repair, crutches and protected weight bearing for 2 to 4 weeks.
- Begin physical therapy 1 week after surgery.
- Advance to formal physical therapy and home programs throughout the recovery period.

## OUTCOMES

- Multiple studies have reported good to excellent outcomes for hip arthroscopy used to treat FAI.
- A systematic review showed that 10 of 12 studies reported good to excellent outcomes in 75% or more of patients treated with hip arthroscopy.
- One of the keys to successful outcome is the stage of arthritis at the index surgery.

## COMPLICATIONS

- Complication rates reported in the literature are low.
- Iatrogenic
  - Cartilage damage from cannulas or instrumentation
  - Damage from misplacement of anchors
  - Iatrogenic instability (overresection of acetabulum or capsular insufficiency or both)
- Neurologic
  - Positioning: perineal numbness/pudendal nerve
  - Traction: sciatic nerve
  - Portals: lateral femoral cutaneous nerve
  - Regional pain syndrome
- Procedure
  - Iatrogenic injury
  - Failure of fixation
  - Medialization of labrum with repair
- Postoperative
  - Deep vein thrombosis/blood clot
  - Fracture: overzealous resection of femoral neck for cam
- Other
  - Avascular necrosis
  - Stiffness

## REFERENCES


1. Alwattar BJ, Bharam S. Hip arthroscopy portals. Op Tech Sports Med 2011:19(2):74–80.
2. Botser IB, Smith TW, Naser R, et al. Open surgical dislocation vs. arthroscopy for femoroacetabular impingement: a comparison of clinical outcomes. Arthroscopy 2011;27:270–278.
3. Byrd JW. Hip arthroscopy: applications and technique. J Am Acad Orthop Surg 2006:14(7):433–444.
4. Byrd JW, Jones KS. Arthroscopic femoroplasty in the management of cam-type femoroacetabular impingement. Clin Ortho Relat Res 2009;3:739–746.
5. Byrd JW, Pappas JN, Pedley MJ. Hip arthroscopy: an anatomic study of portal placement and relationship to the extra-articular structures. Arthroscopy 1995;12:603–612.
6. Fergunson SJ, Bryant JT, Ganz R, et al. The acetabular labrum seal: a poroelastic finite element model. Clin Biomech 2000;15:463–468.
7. Ito K, Leunig M, Keller I, et al. Impingement-induced damage of the acetabular labrum: a possible initiator of hip arthrosis. Eighth Annual Meeting, European Orthopaedic Research Society, 1998:55.
8. Kelly BT, Weiland DE, Schenker ML, et al. Arthroscopic labral repair in the hip: Surgical technique and review of the literature. Arthroscopy 2005;21:1496–1504.
9. Krebs VE. The role of hip arthroscopy in the treatment of synovial disorders and loose bodies. Clin Ortho Relat Res 2003;406:48–59.
10. Nepple JJ, Prather H, Trousdale RT, et al. Diagnostic imaging of femoroacetabular impingement. J Am Acad Orthop Surg 2013;21: S16–S19.
11. Parvizi J, Leunig M, Ganz R. Femoroacetabular impingement. J Am Acad Orthop Surg 2007;15:561–570.
12. Sanchez-Sotolo J, Trousdale RT, Berry DJ, et al. Surgical treatment of developmental dysplasia of the hip in adults: I. Nonarthroplasty options. J Am Acad Orthop Surg 2002;10:321–333.

# Triple Arthrodesis

R. Justin Mistovich, David A. Spiegel, and James J. McCarthy

## DEFINITION

- Triple arthrodesis involves fusion of the talocalcaneal, calcaneocuboid, and talonavicular joints. The procedure is most commonly indicated for salvage in severe, rigid deformities of the hindfoot which are unresponsive to less invasive methods of treatment.
- This procedure is typically considered in adolescents but has been reported in children as young as 8 years of age.

## ANATOMY

- Joints of the hindfoot: the ankle, subtalar, talonavicular, and the calcaneocuboid joints
- Ankle joint motion: plantarflexion and dorsiflexion. Dorsiflexion is associated with outward deviation of the foot, whereas plantarflexion is associated with inward deviation.
- Subtalar (talocalcaneal) joint components: anterior, middle, and a posterior facet. The anterior and middle facets are confluent in a subset of patients. Although there is considerable variation, this joint is usually oriented 23 degrees medially in the transverse plane and 42 degrees dorsally in the sagittal plane. The subtalar joint thus functions as a hinge along an inclined axis and serves as the linkage between the ankle and the distal articulations of the foot. During the gait cycle, the subtalar joint is everted at heel strike and then inverts progressively until push off.
- The transverse tarsal joints: These include the talonavicular and calcaneocuboid joints. When the calcaneus is everted, these joints become parallel, and there is greater flexibility at the articulation. This aids in shock absorption during initial contact and early stance phase. In contrast, the transverse tarsal joints become nonparallel and more rigid when the calcaneus is inverted. Functionally, the calcaneus becomes inverted during late stance phase, which locks the transverse tarsal joints and provides a rigid lever for push off.
- Muscles crossing the ankle and subtalar joints:
  - Ankle plantarflexors: gastrocnemius and soleus, tibialis posterior, flexor digitorum longus, flexor hallucis longus
  - Ankle dorsiflexors: tibialis anterior, extensor digitorum longus, extensor hallucis longus
  - Subtalar inverters: tibialis anterior and posterior, flexor digitorum longus, flexor hallucis longus
  - Subtalar everters: peroneus longus, brevis, tertius, extensor digitorum longus, extensor hallucis longus

## PATHOGENESIS

- Congenital conditions causing foot deformities: clubfoot, vertical talus, tarsal coalition
- Neuromuscular diseases causing foot deformities: cerebral palsy, polio, myelomeningocele, hereditary motor and sensory neuropathies. The etiology involves muscle weakness and/or imbalance.
- The most common deformities are equinovarus, equinovalgus, and cavovarus. Calcaneovalgus, calcaneovarus, calcaneocavus, and equinocavus may also be seen. This spectrum of deformities may result from soft tissue contractures, from bony malalignment, or from both.
- Although some deformities have a structural component at birth, the majority develop gradually, are initially flexible, and only become fixed or rigid over time. Although a loss of passive motion may result from contracture of the soft tissue elements, progressive adaptive changes in the osteocartilaginous structures subsequently result in fixed bony malalignment.
- Causes of equinovarus deformity: This deformity is present at birth in a congenital clubfoot. Although the etiology/pathogenesis of congenital clubfoot remains debated, it is most likely multifactorial. Equinovarus deformity may result from spastic muscle imbalance in patients with cerebral palsy (most often spastic hemiplegia) or flaccid muscle imbalance in poliomyelitis. The pathogenesis in neuromuscular diseases involves muscle imbalance (strong inversion/plantarflexion and weak eversion/dorsiflexion).
- Causes of equinovalgus deformity: This deformity is most common in patients with a congenital vertical talus or cerebral palsy (most commonly spastic diplegia).
- A valgus deformity of the hindfoot is common in patients with a tarsal coalition.
- Pathogenesis of the cavovarus foot: This deformity is most commonly associated with hereditary motor and sensory neuropathies (Charcot-Marie-Tooth) and results from muscle imbalance. Weakness of the tibialis anterior relative to the peroneus longus is associated with plantarflexion of the first ray. This results in forefoot valgus, a deformity which is initially flexible. Over time, a contracture of the plantar fascia and neighboring intrinsic muscle groups develops. To compensate for forefoot valgus, the hindfoot aligns in varus during stance phase. Over time, both the forefoot valgus and the hindfoot varus become rigid. The hindfoot also appears to be in equinus due to plantarflexion of the midfoot on the hindfoot. A common mistake is to assume that the equinus occurs at the ankle and to perform a tendo Achilles lengthening.

## NATURAL HISTORY

- The natural history depends on the underlying disease process. Deformities associated with the neuromuscular diseases will usually progress (and become rigid) over time and will often recur despite treatment due to the underlying disease process.

## PATIENT HISTORY AND PHYSICAL FINDINGS

- Patients present with an abnormality or change in appearance of the foot, gait disturbance, pain in the region of the hindfoot, difficulties with shoe wear, or more than one of these. Although the deformities treated by triple arthrodesis may be diagnosed from birth to adolescence, and have often been treated previously, we focus on the older child or adolescent.
- The history focuses on the presence of symptoms including functional limitations, cosmetic concerns, shoe wear, and on the family history (similar deformities, neuromuscular diseases) and previous treatment.
- A detailed history is especially important in children of walking age, as a foot deformity may be the first clue to the presence of an underlying neuromuscular problem. Although unilateral foot deformities may be seen with tethering of the spinal cord (or other problems such as a spinal cord tumor), bilateral deformities may be the initial finding in patients with a hereditary motor and sensory neuropathy.
- The location and character of pain should be determined, in addition to the activities which produce discomfort.
- A comprehensive physical examination is required. The spine should be examined to rule out any deformity or evidence of an underlying dysraphic condition, and a careful neurologic examination should be performed. The extremities are evaluated for alignment, limb lengths, and range of motion. Observational gait analysis should be performed. The shoes should be inspected for patterns of wear, which indicate weight distribution during stance phase.
- The physical examination of the foot and ankle: Focus on the skin, identifying the presence and location of callosities and points of tenderness. Examine the overall appearance in both the weight bearing and non–weight bearing positions, visualizing the relationship between the forefoot and hindfoot. Check the range of motion of the hindfoot joints. Perform a complete neuromuscular assessment.
- Tests to perform during the physical examination include the following:
  - Range of motion at the ankle joint (plantarflexion and dorsiflexion) to diagnose and determine the magnitude of equinus contracture
  - Range of motion at the subtalar joint (inversion and eversion), which quantifies motion at the subtalar joint. Generally, the amount of inversion is twice the amount of eversion. The total range is 20 to 60 degrees.
  - Range of motion at the transverse tarsal joints
  - Relationship between forefoot and hindfoot alignment, which identifies any coexisting deformity of the forefoot, either varus (dorsiflexion of the medial column relative to the lateral column) or valgus (plantarflexion of the medial column relative to the lateral column)
  - Coleman block test, which determines if hindfoot varus is flexible or rigid
  - Manual muscle testing, which assesses relative strengths of motor units across the ankle and subtalar joints. This helps to diagnose muscle imbalance and to plan tendon transfers if appropriate.

## IMAGING AND OTHER DIAGNOSTIC STUDIES

- Imaging studies complement the history and physical examination, and plain radiographs, specifically in a weight-bearing position are required in all cases. In addition to a standing anteroposterior (AP) and lateral radiograph of the foot, a standing AP of the ankle should be obtained to determine whether the deformity affects the ankle joint, the subtalar joint, or both locations. Other imaging modalities such as a computed tomography (CT) scan or magnetic resonance imaging (MRI) may be required in selected cases.
- Plain radiographs are used to evaluate bone and joint morphology, and measuring the angular relationships between the tarsal bones (or segments of the foot) help to further define both the location and the magnitude of deformities.
- On the standing AP radiograph, measurements include the talocalcaneal (Kite) angle (10 to 56 degrees) and the talo–first metatarsal angle (range −10 to +30 degrees). For the AP talocalcaneal angle, values less than 20 degrees suggest hindfoot varus, whereas an angle greater than 40 to 50 degrees suggests hindfoot valgus. For the talo–first metatarsal angle, values less than −10 degrees indicate forefoot varus and values greater than +30 degrees indicate forefoot valgus.
- On the standing lateral radiograph of the foot, measurements include the lateral talocalcaneal angle, the tibiocalcaneal angle, and the talo–first metatarsal angle. For the lateral talocalcaneal angle (range 25 to 55 degrees), values greater than 55 degrees indicate hindfoot valgus or calcaneus, whereas values less than 25 to 30 degrees indicate hindfoot varus or equinus deformities. For the tibiocalcaneal angle (55 to 95 degrees), values greater than 95 degrees suggest equinus, whereas those below 55 degrees are suggestive of calcaneus. For the talo–first metatarsal, or Meary angle (0 to 20 degrees), values greater than 20 degrees indicate midfoot equinus (cavus), whereas values less than 0 degree indicate midfoot dorsiflexion (midfoot break). The angle of the calcaneus relative to the horizontal axis (calcaneal pitch) is increased with calcaneus or calcaneocavus or with cavovarus deformities.

## DIFFERENTIAL DIAGNOSIS

- Equinovarus: congenital clubfoot, poliomyelitis or other flaccid weakness/paralysis, spastic hemiplegia
- Equinovalgus: congenital vertical talus, spastic diplegia or quadriplegia, tarsal coalition, flexible flatfoot with tight tendo Achilles
- Cavovarus: hereditary motor and sensory neuropathies, poliomyelitis or other flaccid weakness/paralysis, myelomeningocele

## NONOPERATIVE MANAGEMENT

- The goals of nonoperative treatment are to achieve and/or maintain mobility and normal alignment. The specific treatments are based on the underlying disease process.
- Options include physical therapy, injection of botulinum A toxin, serial casting, and orthoses.
- Physical therapy is directed toward improving range of motion and improving strength.
- Serial casting may help to improve range of motion.
- Botulinum toxin injections result in a chemical denervation of the muscle group lasting for 3 to 8 months. Botox has been used most frequently in patients with cerebral palsy to decrease spasticity and reduce dynamic muscle imbalance. Such treatment may prevent or delay the need for surgical intervention in patients with spastic equinovarus or equinovalgus.

- Orthoses may be used to maintain alignment during ambulation or as a nighttime splint to prevent the development of contractures. The deformity should be passively correctable. Foot orthoses such as the University of California Biomechanics Laboratory (UCBL) may help to control varus/valgus alignment of the hindfoot during ambulation. An ankle-foot orthosis improves prepositioning of the foot during swing phase, provides stability during stance phase, and can be used as a night splint.

## SURGICAL MANAGEMENT

- Surgical treatment is offered when nonoperative measures have failed to alleviate the symptoms. Triple arthrodesis is a salvage procedure or "last resort" for rigid deformities in older patients, many of whom have been previously treated by both nonoperative and operative strategies.
- The procedure often requires removal of bony wedges. As such, careful preoperative planning is required to determine the appropriate size and location of these wedges. Triple arthrodesis shortens the foot, which may be cosmetically objectionable especially when the deformity is unilateral.
- Arthrodesis transfers additional stresses to neighboring joints, which may result in degenerative changes and pain. Although there are reports of the procedure being successful in children as young as 8 years of age, it has been suggested that surgery should be delayed until the foot has reached adult proportions. One recent study concluded that growth rates were no different in those children treated before or after 11 years of age.[14]
- The deformity should be of sufficient severity that soft tissue releases and osteotomies would be unlikely to achieve correction or when painful degenerative changes are observed in the joints of the hindfoot. Indications include the recurrent or neglected clubfoot, cavovarus associated with Charcot-Marie-Tooth disease, and severe equinovalgus deformities in patients with spastic diplegia.
- The goal of surgery is to achieve a plantigrade foot by restoring the anatomic relationships between the affected bones and/or regions of the foot and to relieve pain.
- Additional procedures may be required. An equinus deformity of the ankle will require a lengthening of the tendo Achilles at the time of triple arthrodesis. In patients with neuromuscular diseases, lengthening or transfer of tendons may be required to restore muscle balance and prevent further deformity. Recurrence of deformity may occur when coexisting muscle imbalance has not been treated.[4,27]
- A hindfoot arthrodesis should be avoided in patients with insensate feet, such as myelomeningocele.
- Although triple arthrodesis has been performed without fixation, or with minimal fixation such as Kirschner wires or staples, fixation with staples or screws reduces the chances of correction loss and pseudarthrosis.
- Biomechanical studies have demonstrated no significant difference in stability when comparing fixation with staples versus cannulated screws.[17,18]

### Preoperative Planning

- Weight-bearing radiographs are used to evaluate the relationships between the tarsal bones, to identify any morphologic abnormalities and/or degenerative changes, and to identify the location of the deformity. These radiographs help to plan the location of wedge resections.

### Positioning

- The patient is placed in the supine position.

### Approach

- Several skin incisions have been described for triple arthrodesis, and the specific choice depends on the type of deformity and the previous experience of the surgeon. These include the single lateral or anterolateral approach, the medial approach, and a combined lateral and medial approach.
- The lateral approach (Ollier) is used in triple arthrodesis for neglected clubfoot (**FIG 1**).
- A medial approach has been used for the calcaneovalgus foot, especially if previous incision or surgery has made lateral aspect tenuous.
- The Lambrinudi procedure is used for severe equinus deformity. A double-incision approach is used to do triple arthrodesis when no significant deformity is present.

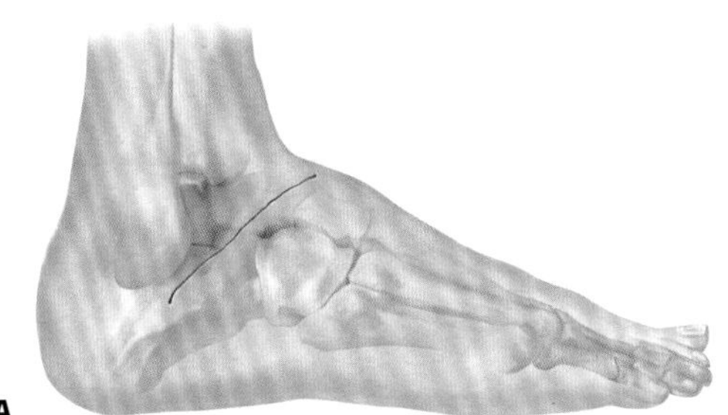


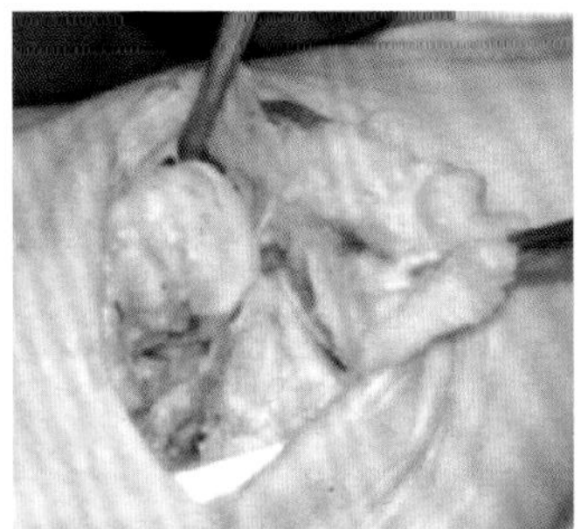


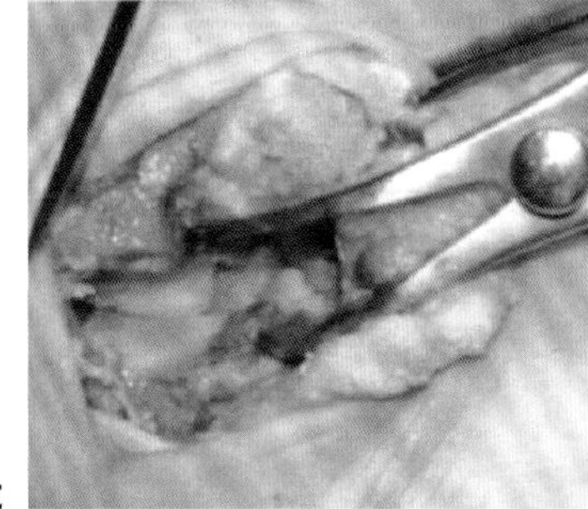


**FIG 1** • The lateral approach is used most frequently. **A.** The skin incision extends from distal to the fibular malleolus across the sinus tarsi. **B.** All three joints can be visualized after dissection of the subcutaneous tissues, elevation of the extensor digitorum brevis off the anterior process of the calcaneus, and opening of the joint capsules. **C.** Placement of a laminar spreader may facilitate visualization of the posterior facet of the subtalar joint.

## Triple Arthrodesis for the Neglected Clubfoot (Modified Lambrinudi Procedure)

- There are several unique features associated with the neglected clubfoot in adolescents which require special attention when performing a triple arthrodesis.[8,20]
- A lengthening of the tendo Achilles is required and is performed as the first step.
- The main components are hindfoot equinus and varus, midfoot cavus, and forefoot adduction.
- In contrast to other equinovarus deformities, there is always significant obliquity of the calcaneocuboid joint, which requires a specially oriented lateral wedge excision of that joint.
- The foot is typically severely plantarflexed and this component of the deformity comes from both hindfoot equinus and midfoot cavus.
- An aggressive resection of the talar head is commonly required to correct the midfoot cavus and bring the forepart of the foot to a plantigrade position.
- The skin incision is started 1 cm distal to tip of fibula. It is curved dorsolaterally and extends to the lateral border of talonavicular joint.
- After spreading the subcutaneous tissues, the extensor tendons are retracted medially and the sural nerve and peroneal tendons are mobilized and protected (**TECH FIG 1**).
- The extensor digitorum brevis is elevated off its origin and reflected distally, exposing the sinus tarsi, the calcaneocuboid joint, and the lateral aspect of the talonavicular joint.
- Soft tissues are cleared from the sinus tarsi, which promotes visualization of the facets of subtalar joint. The anterior and middle facets will be confluent in a subset of cases.
- The first step of the procedure is a calcaneocuboid resection. This involves removing a lateral wedge to shorten the lateral border of the foot (**TECH FIGS 2** and **3A**). One unique feature of the neglected clubfoot is the obliquity at the calcaneocuboid joint. An osteotome or oscillating saw is used to make a cut transverse to the long axis of the calcaneus. The second cut removes the joint surface of the cuboid and should be conservative (several millimeters). The majority of this wedge resection comes from the calcaneus.
- The second step involves resecting a portion of the head and neck of the talus (**TECH FIG 3B**). The cut begins at the superior margin of the articular surface of the talus and extends in a proximal and plantar direction through the inferior portion of the talar neck. This cut is oriented perpendicular to the long axis of the tibia. This essentially removes the entire talar head and a portion of the talar neck.
- The third step (**TECH FIG 3C**) completes the wedge resection and lies along the anterior surface of the calcaneus, parallel to long axis of forefoot in sagittal plane. Completion of this sagittal-oriented wedge resection facilitates dorsiflexion of the forepart of the foot in order to achieve a plantigrade position (correction of midfoot cavus).
- The fourth step involves a conservative resection of the articular surface of navicular. A notch is made in the inferior articular surface of navicular to accept the anterior portion of the talus.
- With the surfaces of talus and calcaneus apposed, the anterior end of talus is pushed into the notch under the navicular while abducting the forefoot (**TECH FIG 3D**).

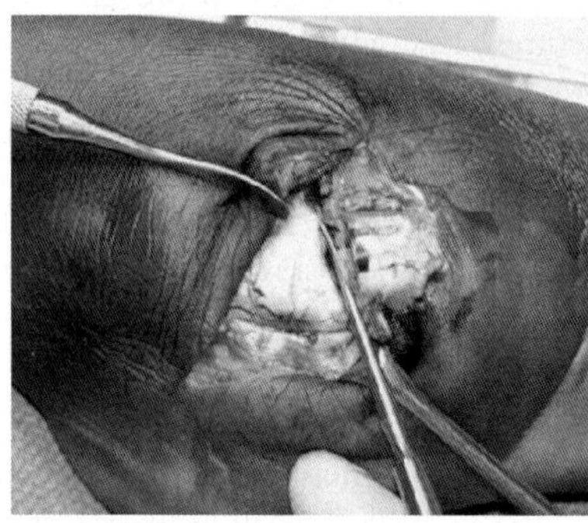

**TECH FIG 1** • Lateral exposure. (From Penny JN. The neglected clubfoot. Tech Orthop 2005;7:19–24.)

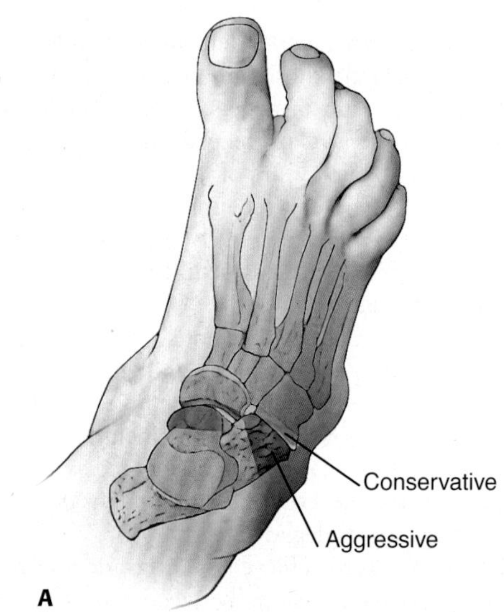


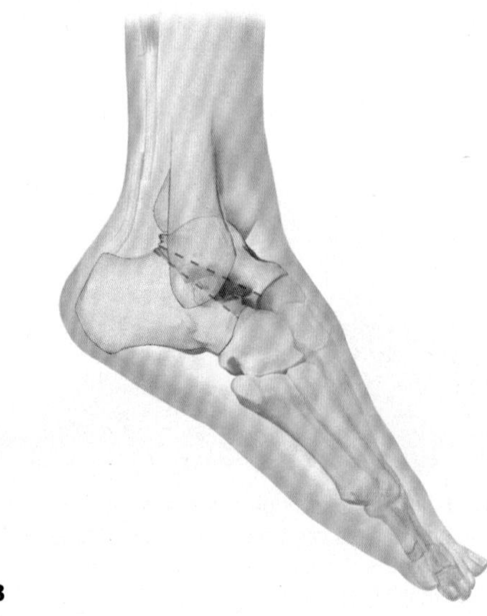


**TECH FIG 2** • **A.** The bony segments are removed to correct the neglected clubfoot. **B.** Conservative resection is shown in *blue*.

- With forefoot abduction, heel varus usually corrects. It is not usually necessary to cut lateral-based wedge to correct heel varus.
- Fixation of the joints is achieved with Kirschner wires, staples, or screws (**TECH FIG 3E**).

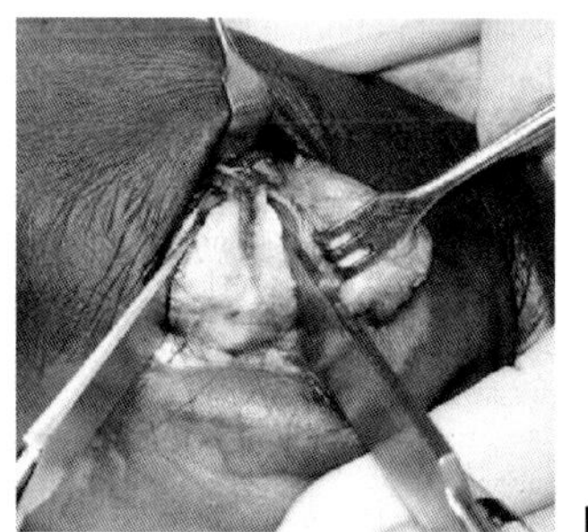
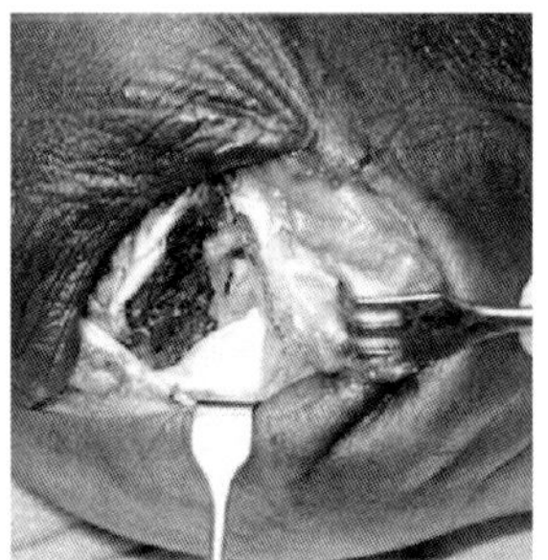
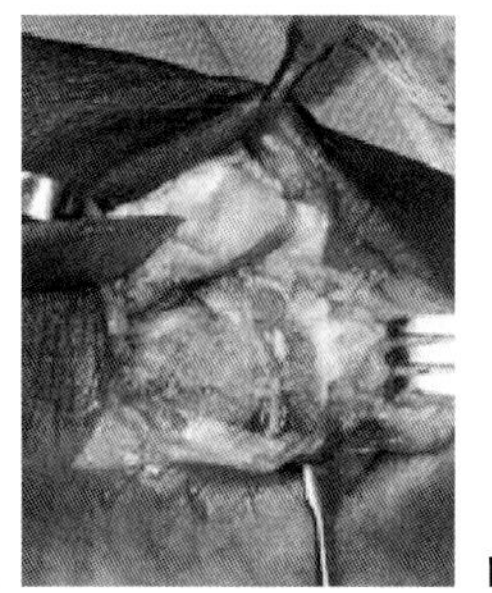
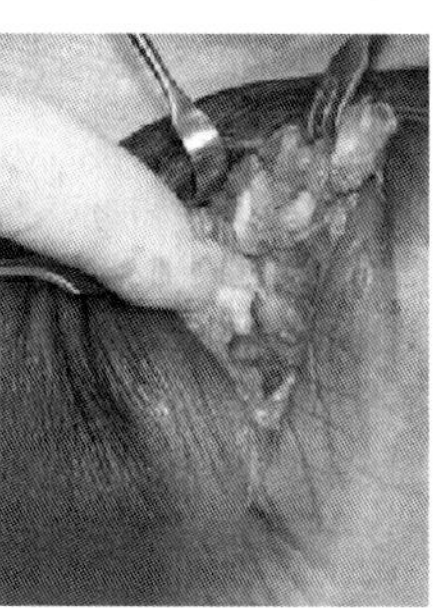
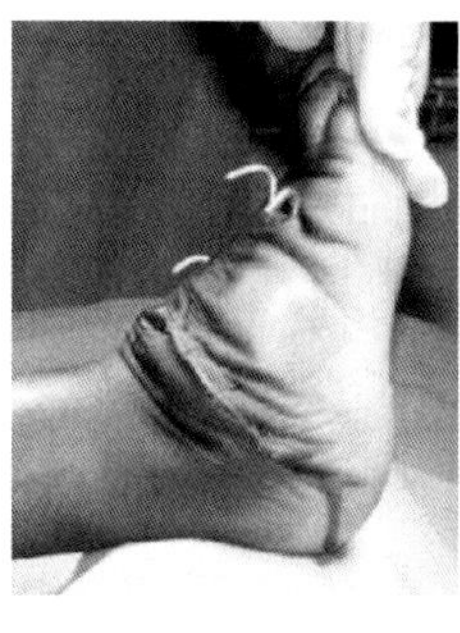

**TECH FIG 3** • **A.** Wedge resection of the calcaneocuboid joint. **B.** Wedge resection of the anterior process of the calcaneus. **C.** Excision of the head and neck of the talus back to the posterior facet of the subtalar joint. **D.** The anterior talus is placed into a notch in the navicular. **E.** The joint is pinned with the foot in a corrected position. The heel varus corrects with the subtalar joint resection. (From Penny JN. The neglected clubfoot. Tech Orthop 2005;7:19–24.)

## Lambrinudi Triple Arthrodesis

- The incision begins 1 cm distal to the tip of the fibula, curves dorsolaterally, and extends to the lateral border of the talonavicular joint.[8]
- The extensor tendons are retracted medially, whereas the peroneal tendons are mobilized and protected. The extensor digitorum brevis is reflected distally, exposing the sinus tarsi, calcaneocuboid joint, and the lateral aspect of the talonavicular joint.
- The sinus tarsi is cleared of soft tissue to expose the anterior, middle, and posterior facets of the subtalar joints.
- Sequential osteotomies are made with a broad osteotome or power saw (**TECH FIG 4A**).
- The first osteotomy is made along the inferior part of the talus perpendicular to long axis of tibia in both planes.
- The second osteotomy is made along the superior part of calcaneus parallel to the sole of foot in both the longitudinal and transverse planes.
- The third cut is made at distal end of calcaneus at right angle to long axis of calcaneus.
- The final cut is made along the proximal end of the cuboid at right angle to longitudinal axis of forefoot.
- A groove is fashioned in the inferior proximal part of the navicular to accept the anterior end of the talus.
- The osteotomized surfaces are approximated and held with staples (**TECH FIG 4B**).
- The extensor digitorum is lightly sutured back into place, and the subcutaneous tissue and skin edges are reapproximated.

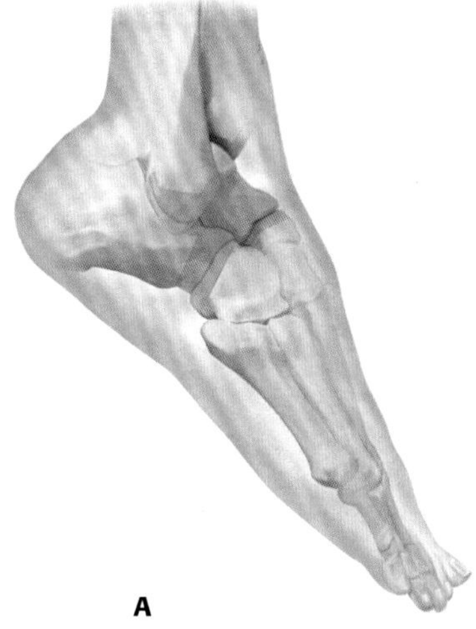
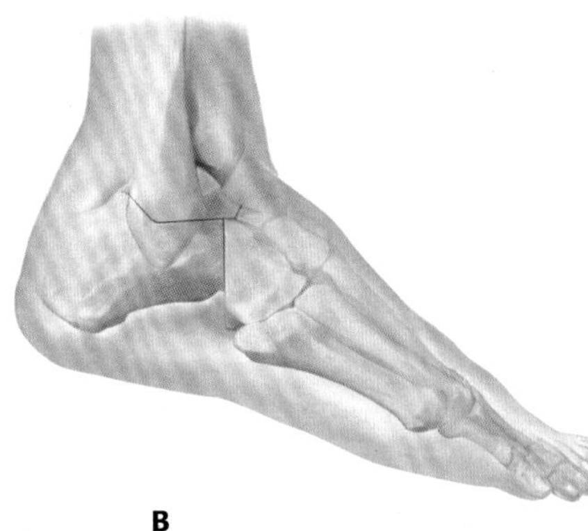

**TECH FIG 4** • Lambrinudi technique. **A.** The *shaded area* represents the bone to be removed. **B.** Realignment of the foot is achieved after removal of bony wedges.

## Triple Arthrodesis Using Single Medial Incision

- A 2-cm longitudinal incision is made over peroneal tendons 10 cm above the level of ankle joint, and both tendons are delivered using a mosquito clamp and divided sharply.[13]
- An 8-cm medial longitudinal incision extends from undersurface of the posterior medial malleolus across the talonavicular joint.
- The talonavicular joint is exposed, and the tibialis posterior tendon is released from its insertion. The talonavicular capsule is released. Flexor digitorum longus tendon, flexor hallucis tendon, and neurovascular bundle are protected by retractor.
- The talocalcaneal interosseous ligament is divided, and the anterior, middle, and posterior facets of subtalar joint are visualized.
- The subtalar and talonavicular joint surfaces are denuded and prepared.
- The calcaneocuboid joint capsule and bifurcate ligaments are released sharply, and a lamina spreader is inserted to facilitate removal of the joint surfaces.
- Fixation of the subtalar joint is achieved with a single 6.5-mm cannulated screw from the posterior calcaneus into the talar body.
- The talonavicular and calcaneocuboid joints are realigned and stabilized with 5-mm cannulated screws.

## Beak Triple Arthrodesis for Severe Cavus Deformity

- A lateral approach is employed, as outlined in the sections discussed earlier (**TECH FIG 5A**).[24]
- The articular cartilage of subtalar and calcaneocuboid joints is denuded.
- The talar neck is osteotomized from inferior to superior forming a beak superiorly. The soft tissues structures on the superior aspect of the talus anterior to ankle are left undisturbed.
- The dorsal cortex of the navicular is excised.
- The forefoot is displaced plantarward and the navicular is locked beneath the remaining part of the talar head and neck.
- Stability can be maintained while plaster is applied by slight upward pressure under the forefoot (**TECH FIG 5B**). A staple may be used for fixation.

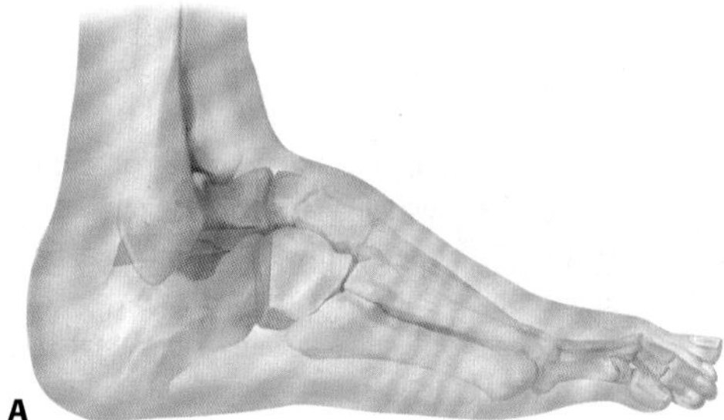


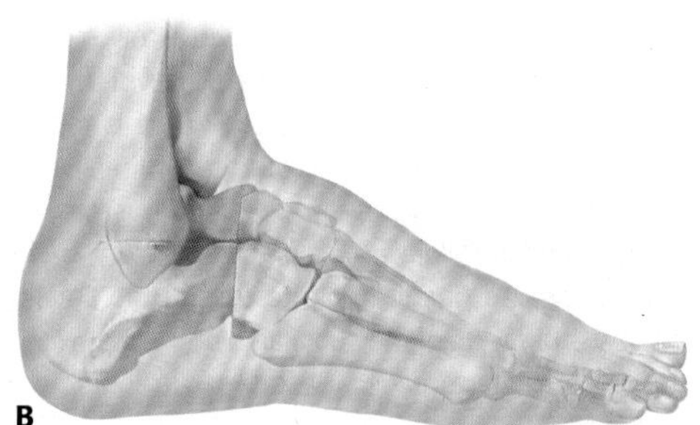


**TECH FIG 5** • Beak triple arthrodesis technique. **A.** Wedges to be removed. **B.** Final alignment after correction.

## Inlay Grafting Method for Valgus Deformity

- This technique obviates the need for a medially based closing wedge osteotomy for valgus deformity of the hindfoot.[28]
- An exposure is used, as described previously.
- The joint surfaces are removed, and the hindfoot is realigned and stabilized with two Kirschner wires.[5] An inlay graft is taken from the tibia and placed into a rectangular trough created across the talonavicular, calcaneocuboid, and anterior subtalar joints. The posterior subtalar joint is then denuded and local bone graft is placed.[21]
- A cast is applied, and the Kirschner wires are removed (**TECH FIG 6**).

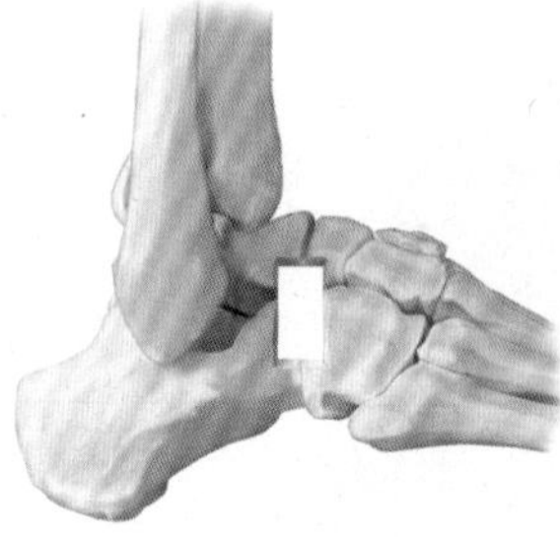

**TECH FIG 6** • Modified Williams and Menelaus' inlay grafting technique.

## PEARLS AND PITFALLS

| | |
|---|---|
| **Preoperative planning** | ■ Weight-bearing radiographs should always be obtained. |
| **Soft tissue handling** | ■ Gentle soft tissue handling should limit the incidence of wound complications. |
| **Bone graft** | ■ Local bone graft is sufficient. |
| **Screw fixation of the subtalar joint** | ■ Placing the screw from the calcaneus into the talus (rather than vice versa) may decrease incidence of avascular necrosis. |

## POSTOPERATIVE CARE

- The limb is typically immobilized in a short- or long-leg cast for at least 6 weeks, and weight bearing is permitted after 6 weeks.
- An ankle–foot orthosis may be required in patients with a neuromuscular diagnosis.

## OUTCOMES

- Most studies have included mixed populations. With both children and adults, a variety of diagnoses at early to mid-range follow-up, and variable objective and subjective criteria to assess outcome, it is difficult to draw entirely accurate conclusions. Overall though, successful results have been reported in the majority of patients, with patient satisfaction in the range of 50% to 95%.[7,22,23,26] Rates of union are 89% to 95%.[10,13,23] In general, poor outcomes have been associated with residual deformity and/or pseudarthrosis. Outcomes seem to be similar when comparing children and adults. The results vary somewhat based on the underlying diagnosis and to deteriorate with longer term follow-up.
- The majority of patients have difficulty walking on uneven surfaces. Instrumented motion analysis studies have revealed an increase in ipsilateral knee flexion during stance phase (including push-off) and a loss of ankle plantarflexion during push-off.[2,29] Power generation at the ankle is decreased up to 45%.[2,29]
- Degenerative changes are common in the surrounding joints at long-term follow-up, but do not imply the presence of pain or a deterioration in results. Chronic pain is seen in a subset of cases.
- In cerebral palsy, Ireland and Hoffer[12] found excellent results in all patients at 4.5-year follow-up. Tenuta et al[25] found that 80% of patients were satisfied at 18 years follow-up, although 25% had occasional pain and 14% had persistent pain. Lack of satisfaction was correlated with residual deformity and/or pain.
- The results in patients with cavovarus feet due to Charcot-Marie-Tooth are less predictable. At 12-year follow-up, Wukich and Bowen[30] observed excellent/good results in 88%, with 15% pseudarthrosis and degenerative changes in 64%. At 21-year follow-up, Wetmore and Drennan[27] found excellent or good results in only 24%, with recurrence in nearly 50% because of progressive weakness/muscle imbalance. Twenty percent required conversion to a pantalar arthrodesis for ankle pain associated with degenerative changes.
- With flaccid neuromuscular imbalance (polio), the results have been adequate in most patients, provided that adequate muscle balance has been achieved in addition to the arthrodesis.[4] Crego and McCarroll[4] found recurrence in 20% of patients, mostly due to persistent muscle imbalance.

## COMPLICATIONS

- Injury to neurovascular or tendinous structures. The medial neurovascular bundle and flexor hallucis longus tendon must be protected during resection of posterior facet of the subtalar joint
- Wound infection
- Wound breakdown or skin necrosis
- Pseudarthrosis of one or more joints (6% to 23%), most commonly the talonavicular[3,6,8,9,11,15,16,19,22,23,27,28]
- Residual deformity
- Recurrent deformity may be observed in patients with progressive neuromuscular disease (Charcot-Marie-Tooth) or persistent muscle imbalance (polio, cerebral palsy).[4,27]
- Degenerative changes are commonly observed at longer term follow-up (longest study is 44 years) and result from increased stress transmission to the neighboring joints. These changes may be observed in both the midfoot (54% to 99%[1,22,30]) and/or the ankle joint (24% to 100% at 44 years[22,25,30]).
- Pain from persistent malalignment, degenerative changes, or avascular necrosis of the talus
- Difficulties with shoe wear
- Need for orthotic support or an assistive device for ambulation

## REFERENCES


1. Angus PD, Cowell HR. Triple arthrodesis. A critical long-term review. J Bone Joint Surg Br 1986;68(2):260–265.
2. Beischer AD, Brodsky JW, Pollo FE, et al. Functional outcome and gait analysis after triple or double arthrodesis. Foot Ankle Int 1999;20:545–553.
3. Bernau A. Long-term results following Lambrinudi triple arthrodesis. J Bone Joint Surg Am 1977;59(4):473–479.
4. Crego CH, McCarroll HR. Recurrent deformities in stabilized paralytic feet. A report of 1100 consecutive stabilizations in poliomyelitis. J Bone Joint Surg Am 1938;20(3):609–620.
5. El-Batouty MM, Aly ES, el-Lakkany MR, et al. Triple arthrodesis for paralytic valgus—a modified technique. J Bone Joint Surg Br 1988;70(3):493.
6. Galindo MJ Jr, Siff SJ, Butler JE, et al. Triple arthrodesis in young children: a salvage procedure after failed release in severely affected feet. Foot Ankle 1987;7:319–325.
7. Graves SC, Mann RA, Graves KO. Triple arthrodesis in older adults. Results after long-term follow-up. J Bone Joint Surg Am 1993;75:355–362.
8. Hall JE, Calvert PT. Lambrinudi triple arthrodesis: a review with particular reference to the technique of operation. J Pediatr Orthop 1987;7:19–24.
9. Hersh A, Fuchs LA. Treatment of the uncorrected clubfoot by triple arthrodesis. Orthop Clin North Am 1973;4:103–115.
10. Hill NA, Wilson HJ, Chevres F, et al. Triple arthrodesis in the young child. Clin Orthop Relat Res 1970;70:187–190.
11. Hoke JW, Lovell WW. Hoke triple arthrodesis. J Bone Joint Surg Am 1978;60(6):795–798.

12. Ireland ML, Hoffer M. Triple arthrodesis for children with spastic cerebral palsy. Dev Med Child Neurol 1985;27:623–627.
13. Jeng CL, Vora AM, Myerson MS. The medial approach to triple arthrodesis. Indications and technique for management of rigid valgus deformities in high-risk patients. Foot Ankle Clin 2005;10:515–521.
14. Kuhns CA, Zeegen EN, Kono M, et al. Growth rates in skeletally immature feet after triple arthrodesis. J Pediatr Orthop 2003;23: 488–492.
15. Mann DC, Hsu JD. Triple arthrodesis in the treatment of fixed cavovarus deformity in adolescent patients with Charcot-Marie-Tooth disease. Foot Ankle 1992;13:1–6.
16. Mann RM, Coughlin MJ, eds. Surgery of the Foot and Ankle, ed 6. St. Louis: Mosby, 1993:13–28.
17. Meyer MS, Alvarez BE, Njus GO, et al. Triple arthrodesis: a biomechanical evaluation of screw versus staple fixation. Foot Ankle Int 1996;17:764–767.
18. Payette CR, Sage RA, Gonzalez JV, et al. Triple arthrodesis stabilization: a quantitative analysis of screw versus staple fixation in fresh cadaveric matched-pair specimens. J Foot Ankle Surg 1998;37:472–480.
19. Pell RF IV, Myerson MS, Schon LC. Clinical outcome after primary triple arthrodesis. J Bone Joint Surg Am 2000;82(1):47–57.
20. Penny JN. The neglected clubfoot. Tech Orthop 2005;7:19–24.
21. Rosenfeld PF, Budgen SA, Saxby TS. Triple arthrodesis: is bone grafting necessary? The results in 100 consecutive cases. J Bone Joint Surg Br 2005;87(2):175–178.
22. Saltzman CL, Fehrle MJ, Cooper RR, et al. Triple arthrodesis: twenty-five and forty-four-year average follow-up of the same patients. J Bone Joint Surg Am 1999;81(10):1391–1402.
23. Sangeorzan BJ, Smith D, Veith R, et al. Triple arthrodesis using internal fixation in treatment of adult foot disorders. Clin Orthop Relat Res 1993;(294):299–307.
24. Siffert RS, del Torto U. "Beak" triple arthrodesis for severe cavus deformity. Clin Orthop Relat Res 1983;(181):64–67.
25. Tenuta J, Shelton YA, Miller F. Long-term follow-up of triple arthrodesis in patients with cerebral palsy. J Pediatr Orthop 1993;13: 713–716.
26. Vlachou M, Dimitriadis D. Results of triple arthrodesis in children and adolescents. Acta Orthop Belg 2009;75(3):380–388.
27. Wetmore RS, Drennan JC. Long-term results of triple arthrodesis in Charcot-Marie-Tooth disease. J Bone Joint Surg Am 1989;71(3): 417–422.
28. Williams PF, Menelaus MB. Triple arthrodesis by inlay grafting—a method suitable for the undeformed or valgus foot. J Bone Joint Surg Br 1977;59(3):333–336.
29. Wu WL, Huang PJ, Lin CJ, et al. Lower extremity kinematics and kinetics during level walking and stair climbing in subjects with triple arthrodesis or subtalar fusion. Gait Posture 2005;21:263–270.
30. Wukich DK, Bowen JR. A long-term study of triple arthrodesis for correction of pes cavovarus in Charcot-Marie-Tooth disease. J Pediatr Orthop 1989;9:433–437.

# Calcaneal Lengthening Osteotomy for the Treatment of Hindfoot Valgus Deformity

Vincent S. Mosca

## DEFINITION

- Valgus deformity of the hindfoot exists when the calcaneus is angled away from the midline of the body in relationship to the talus.
- Eversion is a more specific and appropriate term for the hindfoot valgus deformity that is seen in congenital and developmental flatfoot and skewfoot deformities.
  - Valgus deformity of the hindfoot, which is often perhaps inappropriately referred to as *pronation*, is one component of eversion of the subtalar joint.
  - The other, and more important, components of eversion are external rotation and dorsiflexion of the calcaneus (acetabulum pedis) in relation to the plantarflexed talus.
- *Flatfoot* is the term used to describe a weight-bearing foot shape in which the hindfoot is in valgus alignment, the midfoot sags in a plantar direction with reversal of the longitudinal arch, the forefoot is supinated in relation to the hindfoot, and the foot points in an externally rotated direction from the knee.
- There is no agreement on strict clinical or radiographic criteria for defining a flatfoot. Therefore, the point beyond which a foot with a low-normal arch becomes defined as a flatfoot is unknown.
- There are three recognized types of flatfoot: flexible (hypermobile) flatfoot, flexible (hypermobile) flatfoot with a short Achilles tendon, and rigid flatfoot.
- Valgus deformity of the hindfoot is also seen in skewfoot, congenital oblique talus, and congenital vertical talus.

## ANATOMY

- Acetabulum pedis is a term that was coined by Scarpa over 200 years ago to describe and compare the subtalar joint with the hip joint because of certain similarities that exist between them. It is a cup like structure consisting of the navicular, spring ligament, and anterior end of the calcaneus that rotates around the talus following the oblique axis of the subtalar joint.
- The axis of the subtalar joint is not in any of the standard planes of motion of the body. In the transverse plane, the subtalar axis deviates about 23 degrees medial to the long axis of the foot. In the sagittal plane, the axis deviates about 41 degrees dorsal from horizontal. The summation of the angles creates an oblique axis for the subtalar joint that produces downward and inward motion during inversion and upward and outward motion during eversion.
- Eversion of the acetabulum pedis results in loss of support for, and plantarflexion of, the talus. Although the calcaneus dorsiflexes "upward" in relation to the talus, it becomes plantarflexed in relation to the weight-bearing axis of the tibia. The navicular also dorsiflexes upward at the talonavicular joint as the focal point for the midfoot sag. "Outward" motion of the acetabulum pedis creates the external rotation of the rest of the foot in relation to the talus and tibia that is manifest as a positive thigh–foot angle and an out-toeing gait. Convexity of the plantar–medial border of the foot is also a manifestation of outward motion of the acetabulum pedis, reflecting the dorsolateral positioning of the navicular on the head of the talus. These altered relationships create a real, or apparent, shortening of the lateral column (or border) of the foot relative to the medial column.
- A flatfoot combines valgus deformity of the hindfoot with supination deformity of the forefoot to create a low or absent longitudinal arch (**FIG 1**). These are rotationally opposite deformities.
- The forefoot in a flatfoot is supinated in relation to the pronated/valgus hindfoot. Were it not, forefoot weight bearing would occur solely on the first metatarsal with the fifth metatarsal off the ground.
- In a skewfoot, the forefoot is supinated in relation to the pronated/valgus hindfoot but pronated in relation to the midfoot. The midfoot is adducted in relation to the hindfoot.
- The shapes of the bones and the laxity of the ligaments of the foot determine the height of the longitudinal arch. The muscles maintain balance, accommodate the foot to uneven terrain, protect the ligaments from unusual stresses, and propel the body forward.
- The intrinsic muscles are the principal stabilizers of the foot during propulsion. Greater intrinsic muscle activity is required to stabilize the transverse tarsal and subtalar joints in a flatfooted individual than in an individual with an average height longitudinal arch.

## PATHOGENESIS

- Based on clinical and radiographic studies, flatfoot is ubiquitous in infants and children and is seen in over 20% of adults. The arch increases in height in most children through normal growth and development during the first decade of life. The arch decreases in height in most of those older children and adolescents who have a rigid flatfoot, a condition affecting about 2% to 5% of the population that is most often associated with a tarsal coalition.
- Flexibility (hypermobility) in a flexible flatfoot refers to the motion in the subtalar joint. There is full excursion of the Achilles tendon in this class of flatfoot. It is the normal congenital foot shape seen in almost all babies and accounts for about two-thirds of the 23% of flatfooted adults. It is the normal contour of a strong and stable foot, not the cause of disability.

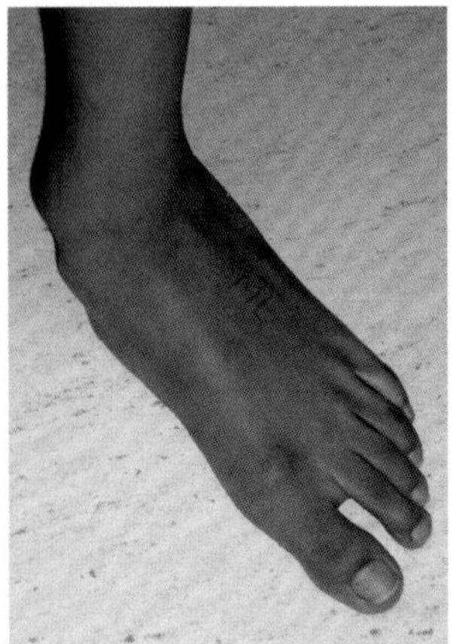

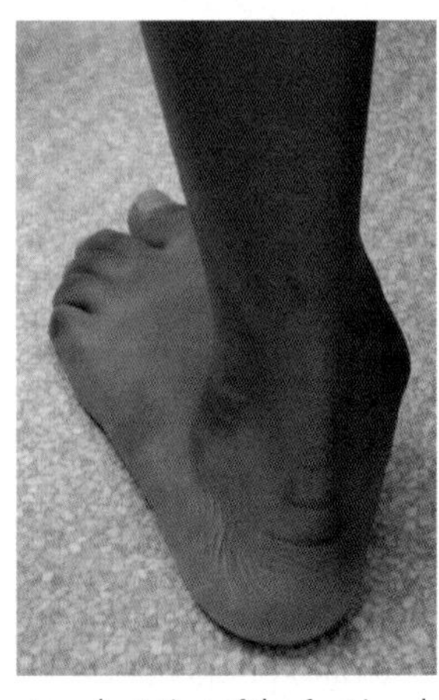

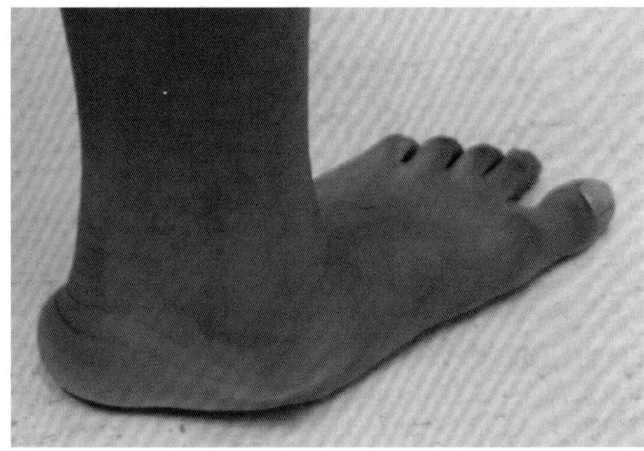

**FIG 1** • Flatfoot. **A.** Top view shows outward rotation of the foot in relation to the lower extremity. The patella is facing forward in this image. **B.** Back view shows valgus alignment of the hindfoot and "too many toes" seen laterally. **C.** Medial view shows depression of the longitudinal arch and a convex medial border of the foot. (From Mosca VS. Calcaneal lengthening osteotomy for valgus deformity of the hindfoot. In: Tolo V, Skaggs D, eds. Master Techniques in Orthopaedic Surgery: Pediatric Orthopaedics. Philadelphia: Lippincott Williams & Wilkins, 2008:263–276.)

- A flexible flatfoot with a short Achilles tendon has the same flexibility in the subtalar joint as a flexible flatfoot but has limited ankle dorsiflexion owing to contracture of the Achilles tendon. This entity accounts for about one-fourth of the 23% of flatfooted adults and often causes pain with callus formation under the head of the talus. The age or point at which the Achilles tendon contracture develops is unknown.
  - A contracted Achilles tendon prevents normal dorsiflexion of the talus in the ankle joint during the late midstance phase of the gait cycle. The dorsiflexion stress is shifted to the subtalar joint complex where, as a feature of eversion, the acetabulum pedis dorsiflexes in relation to the talus and also in relation to the tibia. The talus remains rigidly plantarflexed. The soft tissues under the head of the talus are subjected to excessive direct axial loading and shear stresses.
  - These stresses create callus formation and pain at that site.
  - Pain may also be experienced in the sinus tarsi region because of impingement of the beak of the calcaneus with the lateral process of the talus at the extreme range of eversion.
- Rigidity in a rigid flatfoot refers to the restriction of motion in the subtalar joint. This type of flatfoot accounts for about 9% of the 23% of flatfooted adults. It is usually associated with a tarsal coalition and is, therefore, developmental rather than congenital.
  - The longitudinal arch gradually lowers to a flatfoot shape in these feet in late childhood, generally after the age of 8 years. This is the time at which the fibrous coalition begins undergoing metaplasia to cartilage and eventually to bone. Tarsal coalitions cause pain in less than 25% of cases. A coalition may be associated with an Achilles tendon contracture. The frequency of that association is not known.
- Valgus deformity of the hindfoot is one of the segmental deformities in a congenital skewfoot, a condition for which the incidence, natural history, and even an objective definition are not known. Skewfoot also exists as an iatrogenic deformity, typically seen in a surgically treated clubfoot. Congenital and acquired skewfoot may be associated with an Achilles tendon contracture, thereby increasing its risk for creating pain in the same way that a flexible flatfoot with a short Achilles tendon may cause pain. The frequency of that association is not known.

## NATURAL HISTORY

- Flatfoot is a poorly defined foot shape found in most children and over 20% of adults. For most, it is an anatomic variation from average that does not cause pain or other disability.
- The longitudinal arch develops spontaneously in most children during the first decade of life.
- Flexible flatfoot with a short Achilles tendon often causes pain with callus formation under the head of the talus and/or pain in the sinus tarsi area.
- The age or point at which the Achilles tendon contracture develops is unknown.
- Rigid flatfoot causes pain in less than 25% of cases, although it causes restriction of subtalar motion in all.
- Skewfoot is a poorly defined foot shape for which the natural history is not known. Review of the literature would suggest that most are, and remain, asymptomatic throughout life.

## PATIENT HISTORY AND PHYSICAL FINDINGS

- Children with flexible flatfoot are rarely symptomatic, although they may experience nonspecific leg or foot aches after strenuous activities or at the end of the day. Older children and adolescents with flexible flatfoot with a short Achilles tendon will often experience pain, tenderness, and callus formation under the head of the plantarflexed talus in the midfoot or in the sinus tarsi area or at both sites. About 25% of children and adolescents with a tarsal coalition report activity-related pain that may be located in the sinus tarsi area, along the medial hindfoot and/or under the head of the talus.
- Commonly, parents seek consultation for their child with a painless flatfoot because of concerns regarding the appearance of the foot, the child's uneven shoe wear, or concerns about the potential for future disability. Such concerns about future disability are based on unsubstantiated claims

by generations of health care providers that flatfoot is a deformity that requires treatment to prevent pain and disability.

- Evaluation of the child's foot should begin with a screening evaluation of the entire musculoskeletal system. The general examination includes assessment of ligament laxity, torsional and angular variations of the lower extremities, and the walking pattern. Their interrelationships are important to keep in mind during evaluation of the foot because all of these features, including the shape of the foot, change as the child grows.
- Assessment of the foot begins with the recognition that a flatfoot is not a single segment deformity. It is a multisegment combination of deformities that includes a valgus/eversion deformity of the hindfoot and a supination deformity of the forefoot on the hindfoot. There is a lateral rotational deformity as well, which is a component of eversion. The axis of the subtalar joint is in an oblique plane, such that eversion creates valgus, external rotation, and dorsiflexion of the so-called acetabulum pedis around the talus.
- The foot must be evaluated in weight bearing and non–weight bearing.
  - In weight bearing, the clinician should note the valgus alignment of the hindfoot, the depression of the longitudinal arch, and the outward rotation of the foot in relation to the sagittal plane of the tibia, which is perpendicular to the flexion–extension plane of the knee.
- The flexibility of the flatfoot pertains to the mobility of the subtalar joint. A flexible flatfoot has free and supple subtalar joint motion. A rigid flatfoot has restriction of motion in that joint.
  - Flexibility of the subtalar joint can be assessed manually. With the hindfoot cupped in one hand and the forefoot held (for better foot control) in the other hand, the subtalar joint is inverted and everted around its oblique axis of motion using the hand that is cupping the hindfoot (**FIG 2**). It is important to ensure that the apparent motion is occurring in the subtalar joint and that it is not false motion through hypermobile Chopart joints.

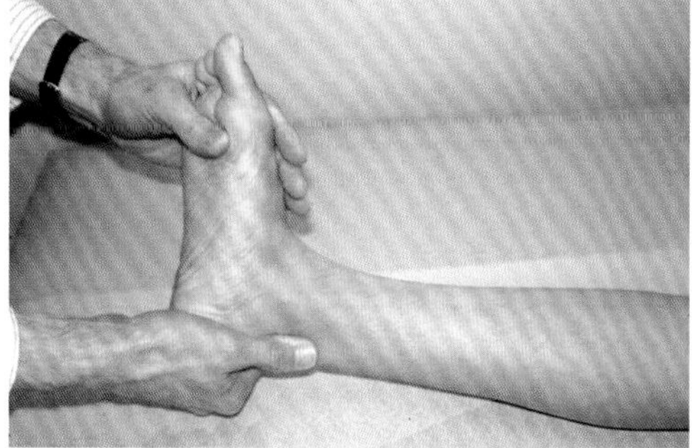

**FIG 2** • Inversion and eversion of the subtalar joint is assessed by manually moving the acetabulum pedis back and forth along the axis of the subtalar joint. Forefoot supination can be appreciated when the hindfoot is inverted to neutral. While maintaining subtalar joint neutrality, the ankle is dorsiflexed with the knee first flexed and then extended to assess the excursion of the soleus and the gastrocnemius, respectively. (From Mosca VS. Flexible flatfoot and skewfoot. In: McCarthy J, Drennan J, eds. The Child's Foot and Ankle, ed 2. Philadelphia: Lippincott Williams & Wilkins, 2010:136.)

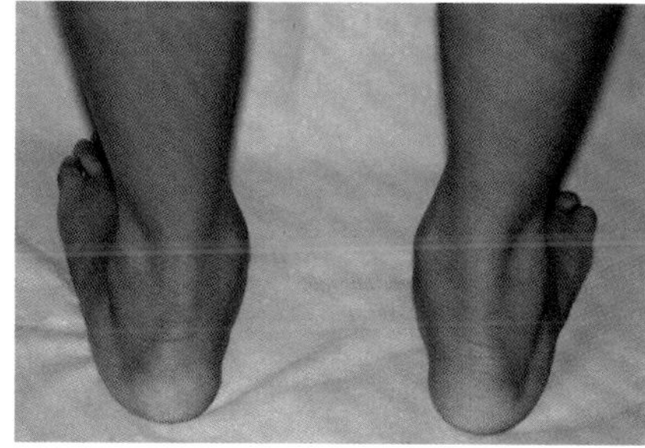

A

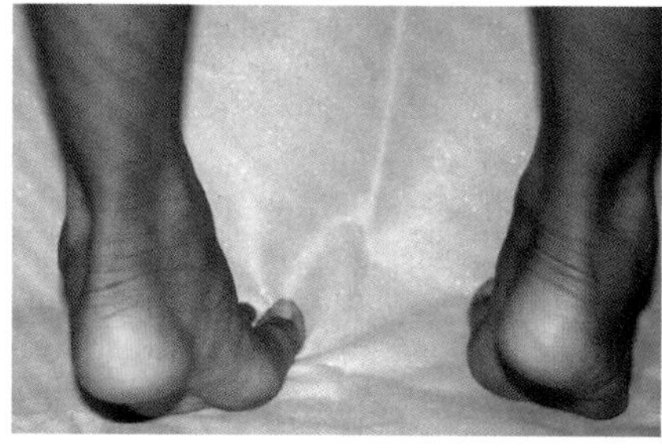

B

**FIG 3** • **A,B.** With toe standing, the heel vagus converts to varus and the longitudinal arch elevates in a flexible flatfoot. (From Mosca VS. Flexible flatfoot and skewfoot. In: McCarthy J, Drennan J, eds. The Child's Foot and Ankle, ed 2. Philadelphia: Lippincott Williams & Wilkins, 2010:136.)

  - Flexibility of the subtalar joint can also be assessed dynamically in weight bearing. The arch elevates and the hindfoot corrects from valgus to varus in a flexible flatfoot during toe standing (**FIG 3**) and with the Jack toe raise test (see Exam Table for Pediatrics: Lower Extremities). These two maneuvers take advantage of the windlass action of the plantar fascia to mobilize the subtalar joint into inversion and create a longitudinal arch.
- Supination of the forefoot is revealed when the hindfoot is passively inverted to neutral alignment (see **FIG 2**).
- Dorsiflexion of the ankle joint, as assessed by excursion of the Achilles tendon, is important yet difficult to evaluate accurately. A component of subtalar joint eversion is dorsiflexion of the calcaneus in relation to the talus. Therefore, the subtalar joint must be held inverted to the neutral position to isolate and assess the motion of the talus in the ankle joint.
- The Silfverskiöld test is used to differentiate ankle joint dorsiflexion from subtalar joint dorsiflexion (see "Flexibility of the Achilles tendon and the Gastrocnemius Tendon" in Exam Table for Pediatrics: Lower Extremities).
  - With the subtalar joint inverted to neutral, the knee is flexed to 90 degrees. The ankle is maximally dorsiflexed without allowing the subtalar joint to evert. The degree of dorsiflexion is measured as the angle between the lateral border of the foot and the anterior shaft of the tibia. The knee is then extended while maintaining subtalar neutral, even if it creates plantar flexion of the ankle. The degree of ankle dorsiflexion is once again measured.
  - It is normal for the ankle to dorsiflex at least 10 degrees above neutral with the knee extended and even further with the knee flexed. The entire triceps surae (gastrocnemius and soleus) is contracted if the ankle does not dorsiflex at least 10 degrees above neutral with the knee flexed or extended. The gastrocnemius is selectively contracted if the ankle dorsiflexes at least 10 degrees above neutral with the knee flexed but not when it is extended.

## IMAGING AND OTHER DIAGNOSTIC STUDIES

- Radiographs reveal the static anatomic relationships between bones. They should not be used, in and of themselves, as an indication for treatment.
- Radiographs of the flatfoot are not necessary for diagnosis. They may be indicated for the assessment of pain or decreased flexibility and for surgical planning.
  - Weight-bearing anteroposterior (AP), lateral, medial oblique, and axial (or Harris) views are appropriate for those indications (**FIG 4**).
  - The lateral oblique (nonstandard) view is helpful for the identification of an accessory navicular that could be the cause of a painful medial prominence in the midfoot that is not the head of the talus.
- An AP ankle radiograph is useful to determine whether any of the hindfoot valgus deformity is in the tibiotalar joint.
- A computed tomography (CT) scan in all three planes and with three-dimensional (3-D) reconstruction is the imaging modality of choice for assessment of a rigid flatfoot, particularly when there is a high degree of suspicion for a subtalar tarsal coalition. The published criteria for operative management of a subtalar tarsal coalition are based on CT scan findings.
- A bone scan can help with the assessment of atypical pain in a flatfoot.
- A magnetic resonance imaging (MRI) may be indicated if these other imaging studies fail to reveal the etiology for atypical pain in a flatfoot. An MRI scan is not the imaging study of choice for evaluation of a tarsal coalition.

## DIFFERENTIAL DIAGNOSIS

- Flexible (hypermobile) flatfoot
- Flexible (hypermobile) flatfoot with short Achilles tendon
- Rigid flatfoot
- Congenital oblique talus
- Congenital vertical talus
- Skewfoot
- Pauciarticular juvenile rheumatoid arthritis affecting the subtalar joint
- Peroneal spastic flatfoot

## NONOPERATIVE MANAGEMENT

- Flexible flatfoot is a normal foot shape and not the cause of pain or functional disability in most individuals. Therefore, treatment must be applied only to those who have symptoms. "Prophylactic" treatment, even if nonoperative, cannot be justified, based on the literature.
  - Some children with flexible flatfoot have activity-related pain or pain at night in the leg or foot. The pain is usually nonlocalized and it is believed to represent an overuse muscle fatigue syndrome. This is consistent with the finding that flatfooted individuals demonstrate greater intrinsic muscle activity than normal.
  - Both over-the-counter and molded shoe inserts have been shown to relieve or diminish symptoms in physiologic flexible flatfeet and to increase the useful life of shoes without a simultaneous permanent increase in the height of the arch.
- Children, adolescents, and adults with flexible flatfoot, as well as skewfoot, with a short Achilles tendon will often experience pain with weight bearing and callosities under the head of the plantarflexed talus. Some additionally experience pain in the sinus tarsi area.
  - The contracted Achilles tendon prevents normal dorsiflexion of the ankle joint during the midstance phase of gait. The dorsiflexion stress is shifted to the subtalar joint complex, which dorsiflexes as a component of eversion. The talus remains rigidly plantarflexed in the ankle joint, thereby subjecting the soft tissues under the head of the talus to painful excessive direct axial loading and shear stress. The forceful external rotation component of eversion causes the beak of the calcaneus to impinge on the lateral process of the talus, thereby creating pain in the sinus tarsi.
- Both firm and hard arch supports concentrate pressures under the head of the talus in children with flatfeet and skewfeet. For those with short Achilles tendons, the pressures and pain are exaggerated because the talus cannot dorsiflex. Arch supports (particularly firm or hard arch supports) are, therefore, contraindicated in this condition.
- An aggressive stretching program for the Achilles tendon, performed with the subtalar joint inverted, may relieve symptoms but is challenging to carry out effectively.

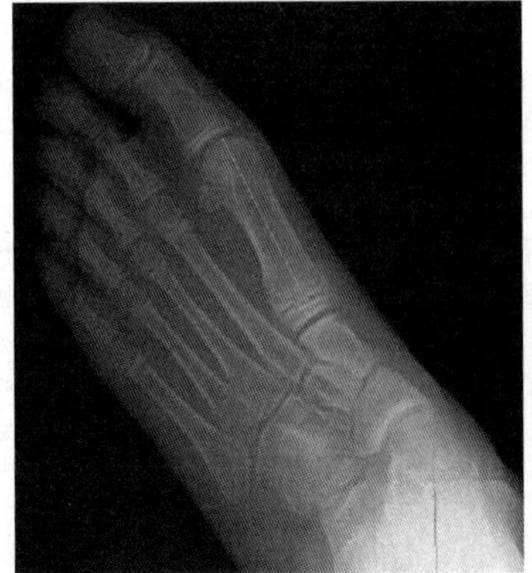

A

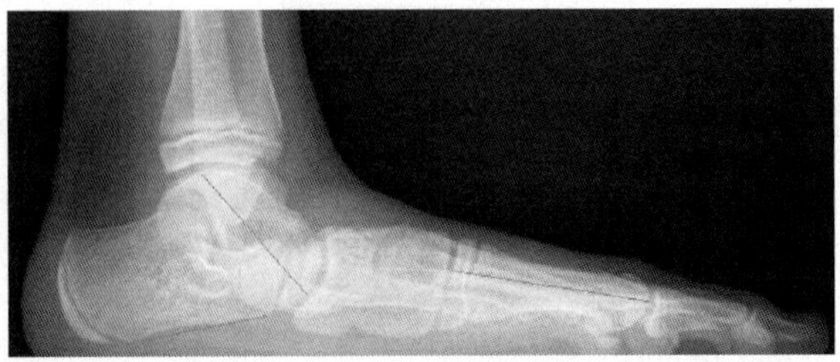

B

**FIG 4** • Standing radiographs of a flatfoot. **A.** AP image demonstrates the external rotation component of eversion or valgus of the subtalar joint. **B.** The lateral image reveals plantarflexion of the talus, sag at the talonavicular joint, and a low calcaneal pitch. (From the private collection of Vincent Mosca, MD.)

    - It is difficult to almost impossible to stretch a contracted Achilles tendon when it is associated with a flexible flatfoot. The subtalar joint must be inverted and held in neutral alignment for the Achilles to stretch. Otherwise, the apparent Achilles tendon stretch will merely create further eversion/valgus stretch in the subtalar joint.
- Children with rigid flatfoot due to a tarsal coalition may experience pain at the site of the coalition or at adjacent mobile joints. They may also experience pain under the head of the talus and/or in the sinus tarsi, symptoms identical to those experienced by children with flexible flatfoot with a short Achilles tendon. The feet with tarsal coalitions and these site-specific symptoms are usually associated with Achilles tendon contractures.
    - Both firm and hard arch supports are contraindicated in rigid flatfeet, whether or not the Achilles tendon is contracted, although the latter further justifies the contraindication. The subtalar joint cannot invert, so there will be concentrated pressure and exaggerated pain under the head of the talus with the use of these devices.

## SURGICAL MANAGEMENT

### Indications and Contraindications

- The calcaneal lengthening osteotomy is indicated for the flexible flatfoot, or skewfoot, with a short Achilles tendon when prolonged attempts at nonoperative treatment fail to relieve the pain under the head of the plantarflexed talus and/or in the sinus tarsi area.
- It is also indicated for a painful flatfoot associated with a talocalcaneal tarsal coalition in which the persistent symptoms are at least in part due to the hindfoot valgus deformity. Concurrent or staged resection of the coalition may be necessary. In other cases, the calcaneal lengthening osteotomy is a stand-alone procedure.
- This procedure is not indicated to change the shape of a pain-free flexible flatfoot or skewfoot.
- Surgery should not be performed in young children with flexible flatfeet or skewfeet who have nonlocalized, activity-related aching foot pain or nighttime pain in the lower extremities.
- Surgery should not be carried out for incongruous signs or symptoms. In such situations, the flatfoot or skewfoot may be an incidental finding and not the cause of the symptoms.
- Finally, the calcaneal lengthening osteotomy is contraindicated in the iatrogenic flatfoot created by overcorrection of a clubfoot in which the talonavicular joint is well aligned and the thigh–foot angle is neutral despite the valgus alignment of the hindfoot.
- It must be stressed that the calcaneal lengthening osteotomy does not correct a flatfoot or a skewfoot. It corrects all components of hindfoot valgus/eversion deformity at the site of deformity. The coincident forefoot and ankle deformities must be corrected concurrently with the appropriate procedures, which are included in the following text for completeness.

### Preoperative Planning

- The clinician should discuss with the family the risks and complications of allograft versus autograft for the required tricortical (bicortical) iliac crest bone graft as well as the possible need for a medial cuneiform plantar-based closing wedge osteotomy.
    - The need for this additional procedure can only be accurately determined intraoperatively after correction of the hindfoot and lengthening of the heel cord.
- Discussion about staged versus concurrent correction of bilateral deformities should include issues relating to the need for strict non–weight bearing on the operated foot or feet for 8 weeks. Most adolescents choose the correction of one foot at a time, with correction of the other foot 6 months later. This interval allows adequate rehabilitation for the operated foot to function comfortably while non–weight bearing on the second foot.

### Positioning

- The patient is placed in the supine position with a folded towel under the ipsilateral buttock and prepared from iliac crest to toes. A sterile tourniquet is included if using autograft. If using allograft, only the lower extremity is prepared and a nonsterile tourniquet is used.
- Special equipment includes a narrow sagittal saw, smooth Steinmann pins, straight osteotomes, laminar spreader with smooth teeth, Joker elevators and narrow Crego retractors, and a mini-fluoroscope.

### Approach

- A modified Ollier incision is made over the sinus tarsi in a Langer skin line for the calcaneal lengthening osteotomy. The superficial peroneal and sural nerves are protected.
- A longitudinal incision along the medial aspect of the midfoot and hindfoot is used for the medial soft tissue plications and for the medial cuneiform osteotomy, if it is required.
- The Achilles tendon can be lengthened through a longitudinal incision on the posteromedial surface of the ankle, half the distance between the tendon and the tibia.
- If an isolated gastrocnemius recession is needed, it can be performed through a longitudinal incision along the posteromedial aspect of the leg about half the distance from the knee to the ankle.

## Calcaneal Osteotomy Exposure and Lateral Soft Tissue Releases

- Make a modified Ollier incision over the sinus tarsi in a Langer skin line from the superficial peroneal nerve to the sural nerve (**TECH FIG 1A**).
- Elevate the soft tissues from the sinus tarsi. Avoid exposure of, or injury to, the capsule of the calcaneocuboid joint.
- Release the peroneus longus and the peroneus brevis from their tendon sheaths on the lateral surface of the calcaneus (**TECH FIG 1B**).
- Resect the tendon sheath septum between the tendons and, if large, the peroneal tubercle. Z-lengthen the peroneus brevis tendon. Do not lengthen the peroneus longus (**TECH FIG 1C**).
- Divide the aponeurosis of the abductor digiti minimi transversely approximately 2 cm proximal to the calcaneocuboid joint (**TECH FIG 1C**).
- Identify the interval between the anterior and middle facets of the subtalar joint with a Freer elevator. Insert it into the sinus tarsi perpendicular to the lateral cortex of the calcaneus at the level of the isthmus (ie, the lowest point of the dorsal cortex of the calcaneus proximal to the beak and distal to the posterior facet) (**TECH FIG 1D**). The middle facet will be encountered.
- Slowly angle the Freer distally until it falls into the interval between the anterior and middle facets (**TECH FIG 1E**).
- Confirm that the Freer is in the interval using fluoroscopy (**TECH FIG 1F**).
- Replace the Freer with a curved Joker elevator. Place a second Joker elevator around the plantar aspect of the calcaneus in an extraperiosteal plane in line with the dorsal Joker.
- Remove the Jokers and prepare the exposures for the other procedures before performing the calcaneal osteotomy.

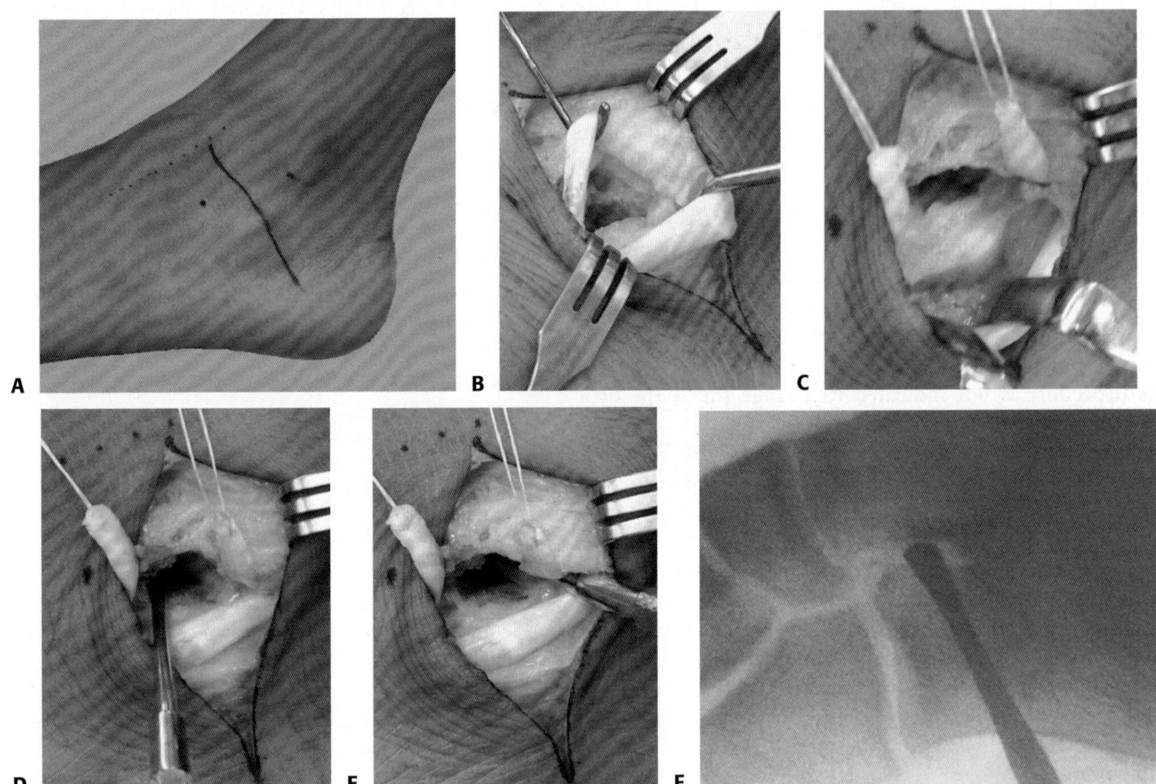


**TECH FIG 1** • **A.** Modified Ollier incision marked in a Langer skin line halfway between the tip of the lateral malleolus and the beak of the calcaneus (*two dots*) and extending from the superficial peroneal nerve (*dotted line*) to the sural nerve. **B.** The peroneus brevis (*above*) and the peroneus longus (*below*) have been released from their tendon sheaths. **C.** The soft tissue contents have been elevated from the isthmus of the calcaneus. The peroneus brevis is lengthened, and the peroneus longus is retracted. The aponeurosis of the abductor digiti minimi is exposed for release. **D–F.** Finding the interval between the anterior and middle facets of the subtalar joint. **D.** A Freer elevator is inserted perpendicular to the lateral border of the calcaneus just proximal to the beak of the calcaneus. It makes contact with the middle facet. **E.** The Freer is rotated distally until the tip falls into the interval between the anterior and middle facets. **F.** This is confirmed with the mini-fluoroscope. (From Mosca VS. Calcaneal lengthening osteotomy for valgus deformity of the hindfoot. In: Tolo V, Skaggs D, eds. Master Techniques in Orthopaedic Surgery: Pediatric Orthopaedics. Philadelphia: Lippincott Williams & Wilkins, 2008:263–276.)

## Medial Soft Tissue Plication Exposure and Preparation

- Make a longitudinal incision along the medial border of the foot starting at a point just distal to the medial malleolus and continuing to the base of the first metatarsal.
- Release the tibialis posterior from its tendon sheath. Cut the tendon in a Z fashion, releasing its dorsal half from the navicular (**TECH FIG 2A**). The stump of tendon remaining attached to the navicular contains the plantar half of the fibers.
- Incise the talonavicular joint capsule around the medial side from dorsal lateral to plantar lateral, including the spring ligament.
- Resect a 3- to 5-mm wide strip of redundant capsule from the medial and plantar aspects of this tissue (**TECH FIG 2B**).

A 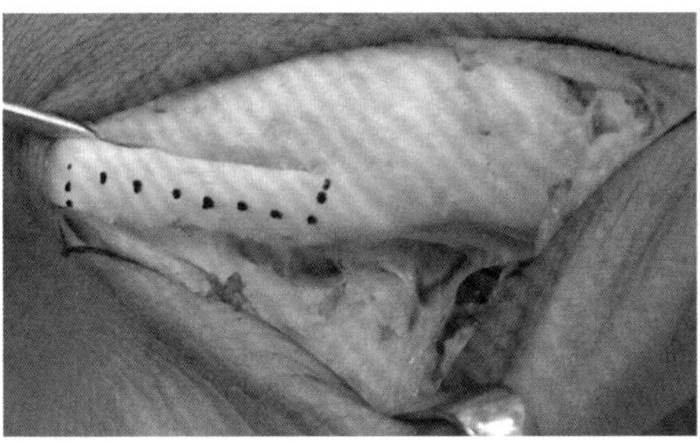

B 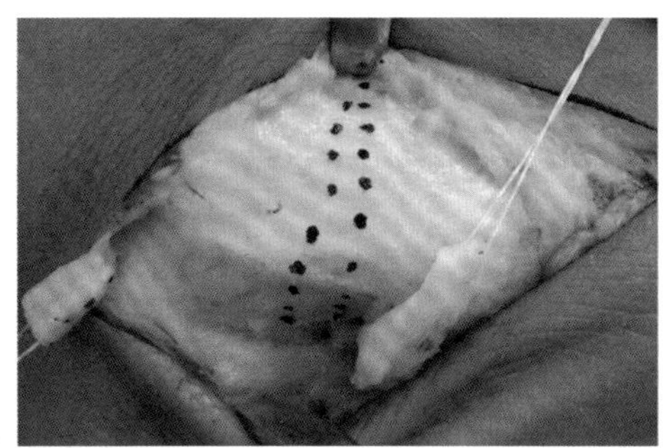

**TECH FIG 2** • **A.** The tibialis posterior is cut in a Z fashion, releasing the dorsal slip from the navicular. **B.** The talonavicular joint capsule is released from dorsolateral to plantar lateral, including release of the spring ligament. A 3- to 5-mm wide strip of redundant capsule is resected from its plantar–medial aspect. (From Mosca VS. Calcaneal lengthening osteotomy for valgus deformity of the hindfoot. In: Tolo V, Skaggs D, eds. Master Techniques in Orthopaedic Surgery: Pediatric Orthopaedics. Philadelphia: Lippincott Williams & Wilkins, 2008:263–276.)

## Achilles Tendon or Gastrocnemius Lengthening

- Assess the equinus contracture by the Silfverskiöld test with the subtalar joint inverted to neutral and the knee both flexed and extended.
- Perform a gastrocnemius recession if 10 degrees of dorsiflexion can be achieved with the knee flexed but not with it extended.
- Perform an open or percutaneous Achilles tendon lengthening if 10 degrees of dorsiflexion cannot be obtained even with the knee flexed (**TECH FIG 3**).

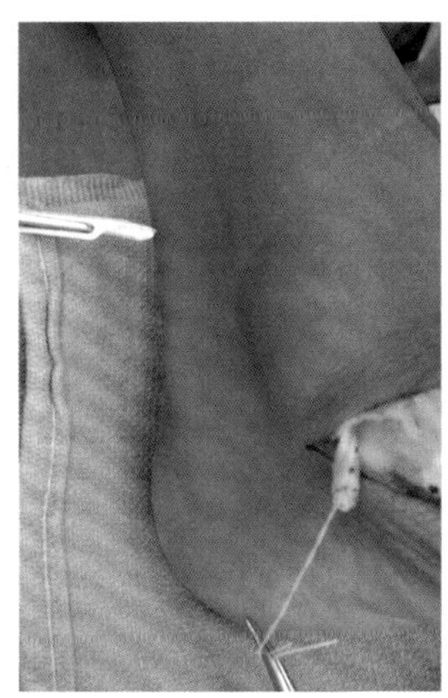

**TECH FIG 3** • The Achilles tendon or the gastrocnemius tendon is lengthened based on the results of the Silfverskiöld test. (From Mosca VS. Calcaneal lengthening osteotomy for valgus deformity of the hindfoot. In: Tolo V, Skaggs D, eds. Master Techniques in Orthopaedic Surgery: Pediatric Orthopaedics. Philadelphia: Lippincott Williams & Wilkins, 2008 :263–276.)

## Calcaneal Osteotomy and Bone Graft Interposition

- Replace the Joker elevators, or Crego retractors, both dorsal and plantar to the isthmus of the calcaneus, meeting in the interval between the anterior and middle facets of the subtalar joint.
- Perform an osteotomy of the calcaneus using a sagittal saw or osteotome (**TECH FIG 4A**).
  - It is an oblique osteotomy from posterolateral to anteromedial that starts about 2 cm proximal to the calcaneocuboid joint at the lowest point of the calcaneus where the beak of the calcaneus meets the posterior facet/lateral process of the talus (ie, the critical angle of Gissane) and exits between the anterior and middle facets (**TECH FIG 4B**).
  - It is a complete osteotomy through the medial cortex. Cut the plantar periosteum and long plantar ligament (not the plantar fascia) under direct vision if necessary (ie, if these soft tissues resist distraction of the bone fragments).
- Insert a 2-mm smooth Steinmann pin retrograde from the dorsum of the foot passing through the cuboid, across the center of the calcaneocuboid joint, and stopping at the osteotomy (**TECH FIG 4C,D**).
  - This is performed with the foot in the original deformed (everted) position before the osteotomy is distracted. By so doing, the pes acetabulum (navicular, spring ligament,

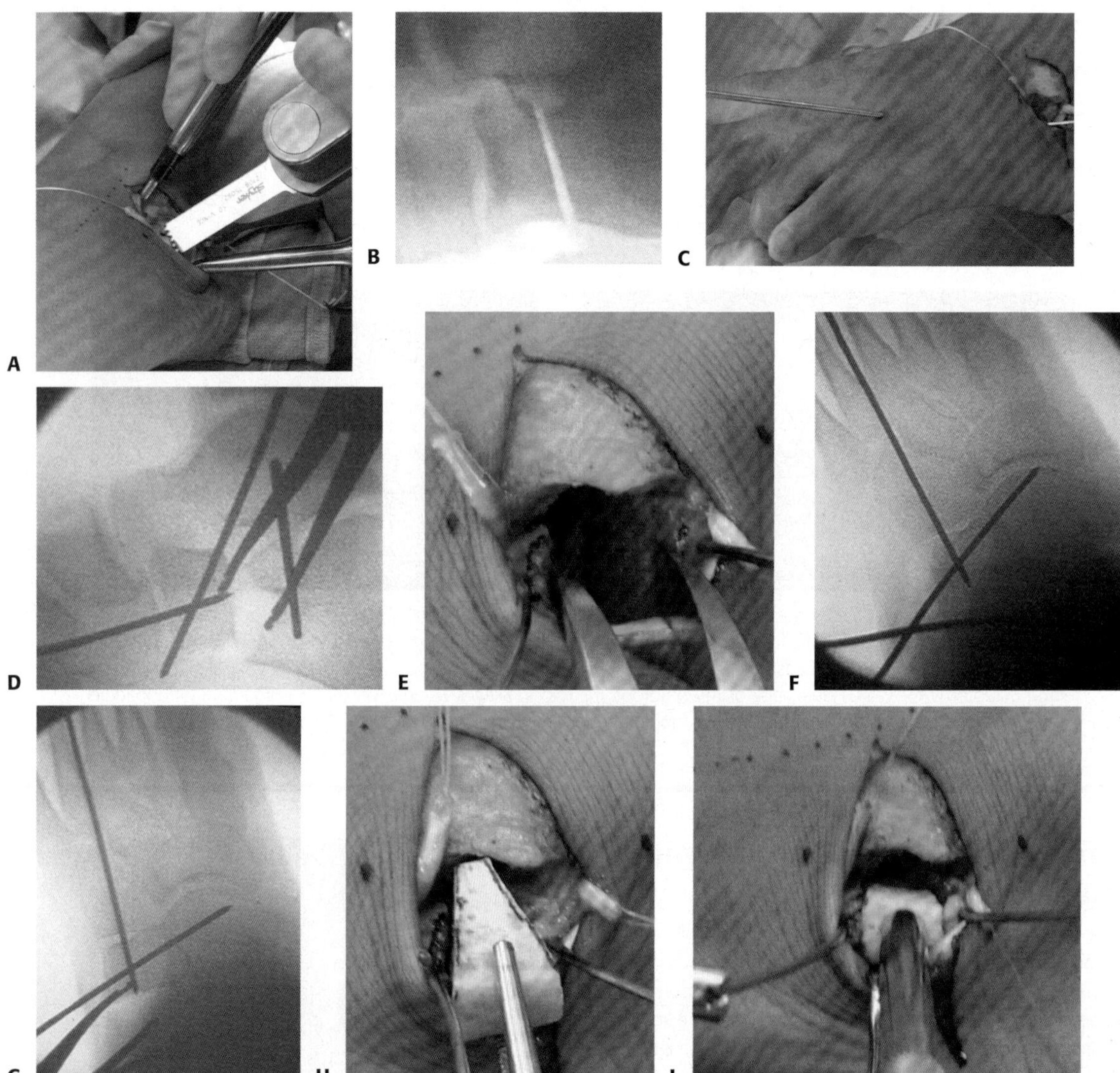

**TECH FIG 4** • **A.** With Joker and Crego retractors surrounding the isthmus of the calcaneus and meeting in the interval between the anterior and middle facets, the osteotomy is performed with a sagittal saw in line with the retractors. **B.** Fluoroscopic appearance of the osteotomy in the proper location. **C.** With the foot in the original flat and everted position, a 2-mm smooth wire is inserted retrograde from the dorsum of the foot through the middle of the calcaneocuboid joint, stopping at the osteotomy. **D.** Position of the wire at the calcaneocuboid joint is confirmed with fluoroscopy. **E.** Steinmann pins in the posterior and anterior calcaneal fragments can be used as joysticks to distract the osteotomy during graft insertion. The lamina spreader is used to determine the necessary graft size. **F,G.** Fluoroscopy can help confirm the required graft size by showing, with the lamina spreader opened, when the talonavicular joint is aligned and the talus and first metatarsal axes are colinear. **H.** The tricortical iliac crest bone graft is frequently 11 to 15 mm in lateral length and 3 to 5 mm in medial length. The cortical surfaces are aligned with the dorsal, lateral, and plantar cortical surfaces of the calcaneus. **I.** The graft is impacted and usually inherently stable. Nevertheless, the 2-mm Steinmann pin can be advanced retrograde through the graft and into the posterior calcaneal fragment for additional stability. (From Mosca VS. Calcaneal lengthening osteotomy for valgus deformity of the hindfoot. In: Tolo V, Skaggs D, eds. Master Techniques in Orthopaedic Surgery: Pediatric Orthopaedics. Philadelphia: Lippincott Williams & Wilkins, 2008 :263–276.)

anterior facet of calcaneus) will be maintained intact, and the distal fragment of the calcaneus will not subluxate dorsally on the cuboid during distraction of the osteotomy.

- Insert a 0.062-inch smooth Steinmann pin from lateral to medial in both of the calcaneal fragments immediately adjacent to the osteotomy. These will be used as joysticks to distract the osteotomy at the time of graft insertion.
- Place a smooth-toothed lamina spreader in the osteotomy and distract maximally, trying to avoid crushing the bone (**TECH FIG 4E**).
- Assess deformity correction of the hindfoot clinically and using mini-fluoroscopy. The deformity is corrected when the axes of the talus and first metatarsal are colinear in both the AP and lateral planes (**TECH FIG 4F,G**).
- Measure the distance between the lateral cortical margins of the calcaneal fragments. This is the lateral length dimension of the trapezoidal iliac crest graft that will be obtained either from the child's iliac crest or from the bone bank.
  - The trapezoid should taper to a medial length dimension of 20% to 30% of the lateral length (**TECH FIG 4H**).

- The calcaneal lengthening osteotomy is a distraction wedge rather than a simple opening wedge, as the center of rotation for angular deformity correction is within the talar head rather than the medial cortex of the calcaneus.
- Remove the laminar spreader, and use the Steinmann pin joysticks to distract the calcaneal fragments.
- Insert and impact the graft with the cortical surfaces aligned from posterior to anterior in the long axis of the foot (**TECH FIG 4I**). This will place the cancellous bone of the graft in direct contact with the cancellous bone of the calcaneal fragments.
- Advance the previously inserted 2-mm Steinmann pin retrograde through the graft and into the posterior calcaneal fragment. Bend the pin at its insertion site on the dorsum of the foot for ease of retrieval in the clinic.
  - No additional fixation is required. In fact, were the pin not needed to prevent subluxation at the calcaneocuboid joint, no graft fixation would be needed.
- Repair the peroneus brevis tendon with an absorbable suture after a 5- to 7-mm lengthening.

## Medial Soft Tissue Plication

- Plicate the talonavicular joint capsule plantar medially but not dorsally (**TECH FIG 5A**).
- Advance the proximal slip of the tibialis posterior tendon about 5 to 7 mm through a slit in the distal stump of the tendon. Repair this Pulvertaft weave with an absorbable suture material (**TECH FIG 5B,C**).

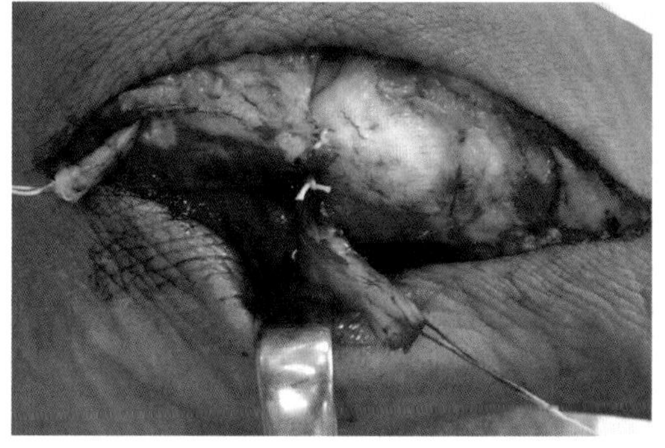

A

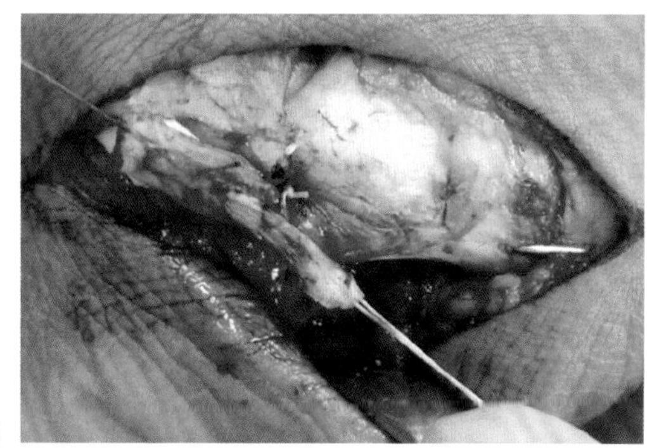

B

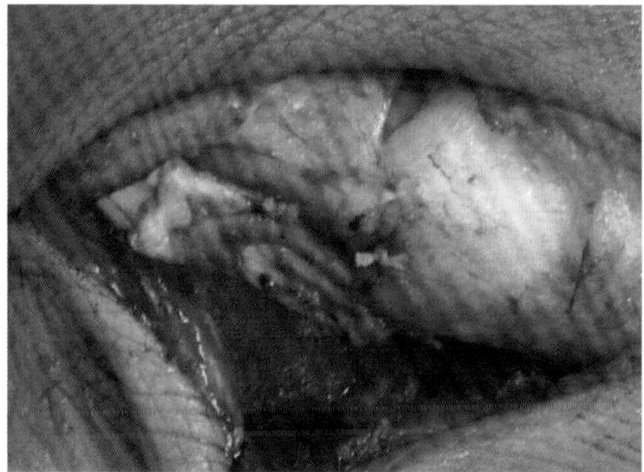

C

**TECH FIG 5** • **A.** The plantar and medial aspects of the talonavicular joint capsule are repaired side to side with large-gauge dissolving suture material; the redundant capsule has already been resected. **B,C.** The proximal slip of the tibialis posterior is advanced distally through a slit in the distal stump of the tendon and repaired with large-gauge dissolving sutures. (From Mosca VS. Calcaneal lengthening osteotomy for valgus deformity of the hindfoot. In: Tolo V, Skaggs D, eds. Master Techniques in Orthopaedic Surgery: Pediatric Orthopaedics. Philadelphia: Lippincott Williams & Wilkins, 2008:263–276.)

## Medial Cuneiform Osteotomy

- Assess the forefoot for structural supination deformity by holding the heel with the ankle in neutral dorsiflexion and viewing in line with the axis of the foot from toes to heel.
- Visualize the plane of the metatarsal heads in relation to the long axis of the tibia (**TECH FIG 6A**).
- Also, assess the dorsal–plantar mobility of the first metatarsal–medial cuneiform joint.
  - A plantarflexion osteotomy of the medial forefoot–midfoot is required if the metatarsals are supinated.
- A plantar-based closing wedge osteotomy in the midportion of the medial cuneiform is an effective procedure to correct this deformity (**TECH FIG 6B**). The plantar base of the resected wedge generally measures 4 to 7 mm in length.
- The osteotomy is closed and internally fixed with a 0.062-inch smooth wire staple inserted from plantar to dorsal.
- Check to ensure correction of the forefoot deformity (**TECH FIG 6C**).

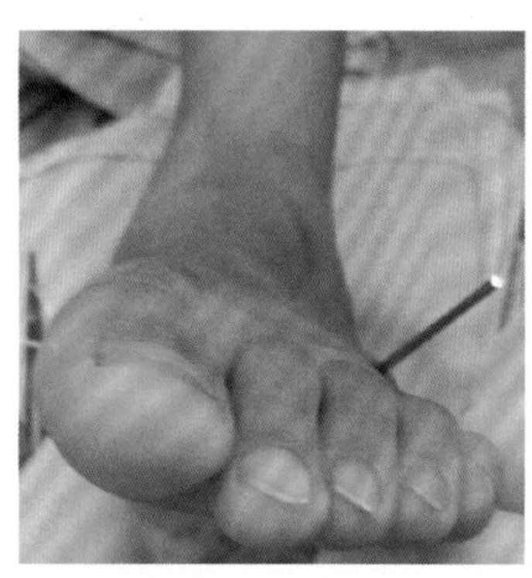
A

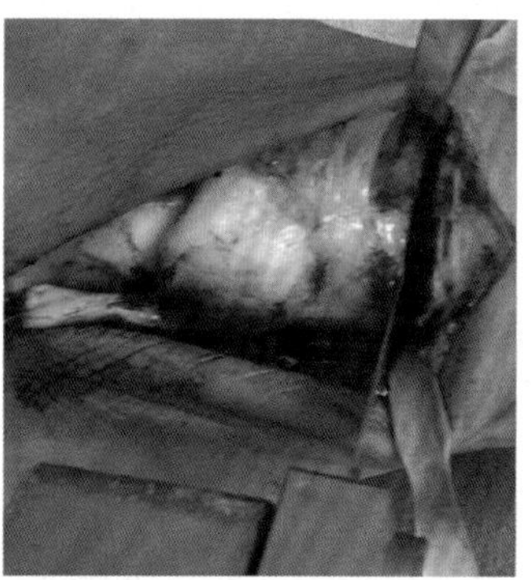
B

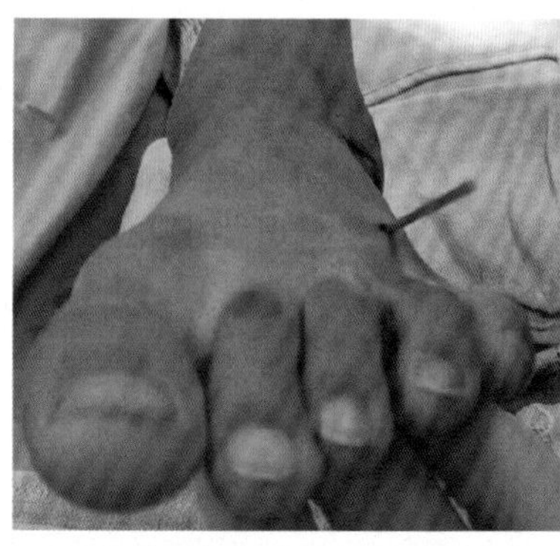
C

**TECH FIG 6** • **A.** The rotational alignment of the forefoot is assessed after correction of the hindfoot deformity and the heel cord contracture. If, as in this case, the forefoot is supinated, an osteotomy of the forefoot is required. **B.** A medial cuneiform plantar-based closing wedge osteotomy will correct the supination deformity of the forefoot. **C.** Forefoot deformity has been corrected. (From Mosca VS. Calcaneal lengthening osteotomy for valgus deformity of the hindfoot. In: Tolo V, Skaggs D, eds. Master Techniques in Orthopaedic Surgery: Pediatric Orthopaedics. Philadelphia: Lippincott Williams & Wilkins, 2008:263–276.)

## PEARLS AND PITFALLS

| | |
|---|---|
| **Indications** | ▪ Flexible flatfoot is a normal foot shape that rarely causes pain or disability. Associated contracture of the Achilles or gastrocnemius tendon may cause activity-related pain under the medial midfoot and/or in the sinus tarsi. The absolute indication for surgery is pain that interferes with the enjoyment of desired activities and cannot be relieved by prolonged attempts at nonoperative management. |
| **Calcaneal osteotomy location** | ▪ The surgeon should try to find the interval between the anterior and middle facets of the subtalar joint to create an extra-articular osteotomy, although only about 60% of individuals have separate facets. |
| **Lateral soft tissue management** | ▪ The surgeon lengthens the peroneus brevis and the aponeurosis of the abductor digiti minimi to facilitate distraction of the bone fragments. However, the peroneus longus is not lengthened because it is the plantarflexor of the medial forefoot. Lengthening the lateral bony column of the foot results in a relative shortening of the peroneus longus, which, in turn, plantarflexes the medial forefoot to help correct the supination deformity. |
| **Calcaneocuboid joint protection** | ▪ Inadvertent subluxation of the calcaneocuboid joint when the calcaneal osteotomy is distracted can be prevented by inserting a retrograde smooth Steinmann pin across the middle of the joint before the fragments are distracted. |
| **Forefoot supination deformity** | ▪ The surgeon must not ignore the forefoot deformity. It is assessed intraoperatively after correction of the hindfoot deformity. Significant uncorrected residual forefoot supination deformity will create a bipod, rather than the normal tripod, foot shape with lack of support under the first metatarsal head. If untreated, this may lead to recurrence of valgus deformity of the hindfoot. A plantar-based closing wedge osteotomy of the medial cuneiform is performed to correct structural forefoot supination deformity if identified. |
| **Achilles or gastrocnemius contracture** | ▪ This is the deformity that changed a normal flexible flatfoot into a painful flatfoot. The contracted tendon should be lengthened. |

## POSTOPERATIVE CARE

- The incisions are closed with absorbable sutures.
- A well-padded, short-leg, non–weight-bearing cast is applied and bivalved to allow for swelling overnight.
- Radiographs in the cast are obtained (**FIG 5**).
- The patient is discharged from the hospital the following day after the bivalved cast is overwrapped with cast material.
- The patient is immobilized in a below-knee cast and is not permitted to bear weight on the operated extremity for 8 weeks.
- At 6 weeks, the cast is removed to obtain simulated standing AP and lateral radiographs and to remove the Steinmann pin. Another below-the-knee, non–weight-bearing cast is applied.
- Upon removal of this cast 2 weeks later, final simulated standing AP and lateral radiographs are obtained.
- Over-the-counter arch supports are used indefinitely.
- Physical therapy is rarely needed.

## OUTCOMES

- The calcaneal lengthening osteotomy has the best reported long-term results of any procedure that has been used to correct flatfoot deformity.
- It has been shown to correct all components of even severe valgus–eversion deformity of the hindfoot, restore function of the subtalar complex, relieve symptoms, and, at least

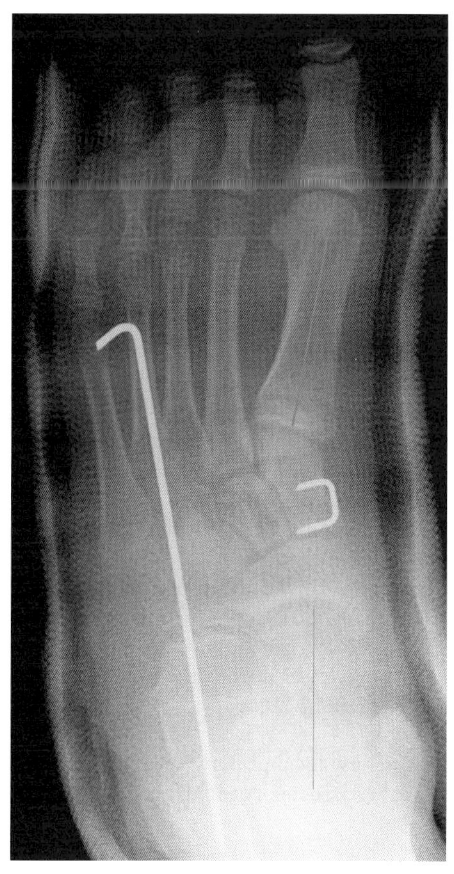

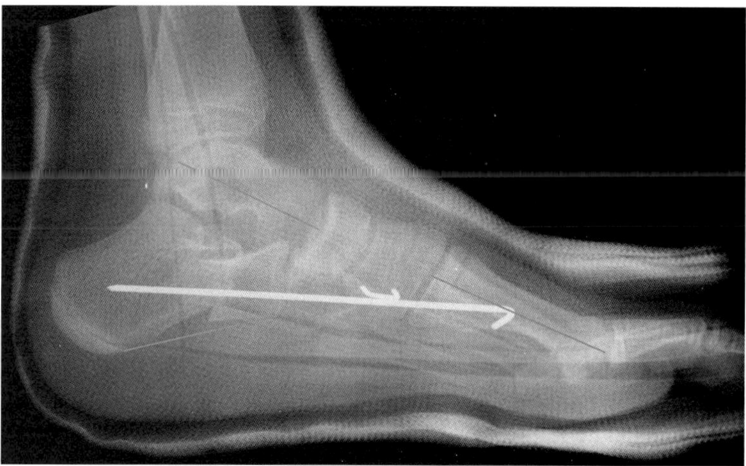

**FIG 5** • Final radiographs in the bivalved cast. **A.** On the AP view, note the correction of the external rotation deformity at the talonavicular joint as also assessed by the talo–first metatarsal angle. **B.** The lateral view demonstrates dorsiflexion of the talus, alignment at the talonavicular joint, correction of the talo–first metatarsal angle, and normalization of the calcaneal pitch. (From Mosca VS. Calcaneal lengthening osteotomy for valgus deformity of the hindfoot. In: Tolo V, Skaggs D, eds. Master Techniques in Orthopaedic Surgery: Pediatric Orthopaedics. Philadelphia: Lippincott Williams & Wilkins, 2008:263–276.)

theoretically, protect the ankle and midtarsal joints from early degenerative arthrosis by avoiding arthrodesis.

## COMPLICATIONS

- Subluxation of the calcaneocuboid joint may occur when the calcaneal osteotomy is distracted. This can be avoided by lengthening the peroneus brevis, releasing the aponeurosis of the abductor digiti minimi, releasing the plantar calcaneal periosteum and long plantar ligament (*not* the plantar fascia), and pinning the calcaneocuboid joint in a retrograde fashion before the osteotomy is distracted.
- Deformity correction may be incomplete. This can be avoided by performing the procedures exactly as described earlier and by releasing the entire dorsal talonavicular joint capsule. The surgeon should use a graft that is large enough to make the axes of the talus and the first metatarsal colinear in both planes. This is confirmed with intraoperative imaging, such as mini-fluoroscopy.
- Persistent equinus can be avoided by lengthening the contracted Achilles tendon or gastrocnemius tendon.
- Persistent supination deformity of the forefoot on the hindfoot can be avoided by identifying it after the calcaneal lengthening and heel cord lengthening. It is treated with a medial cuneiform plantar-based closing wedge osteotomy.
- Recurrence of hindfoot deformity can be avoided by performing all steps of the procedure exactly as described and by concurrent correction of forefoot supination and equinus deformities.[1–6]

## REFERENCES


1. Evans D. Calcaneo-valgus deformity. J Bone Joint Surg Br 1975;57(3):270–278.
2. Mosca VS. Calcaneal lengthening for valgus deformity of the hindfoot. Results in children who had severe, symptomatic flatfoot and skewfoot. J Bone Joint Surg Am 1995;77(4):500–512.
3. Mosca VS. Calcaneal lengthening osteotomy for valgus deformity of the hindfoot. In: Tolo V, Skaggs D, eds. Master Techniques in Orthopaedic Surgery: Pediatric Orthopaedics. Philadelphia: Lippincott Williams & Wilkins, 2008:263–276.
4. Mosca VS. Flexible flatfoot and skewfoot. In: McCarthy J, Drennan J, eds. The Child's Foot and Ankle, ed 2. Philadelphia: Lippincott Williams & Wilkins, 2010:136.
5. Mosca VS. Principles and Management of Pediatric Foot and Ankle Deformities and Malformations. Philadelphia: Wolters Kluwer Health/Lippincott Williams & Wilkins, 2014.
6. Mosca VS. The foot. In: Morrissy RT, Weinstein SL, eds. Lovell and Winter's Pediatric Orthopedics, ed 7. Philadelphia: Lippincott Williams & Wilkins, 2014:1388.

# Open Lengthening of the Achilles Tendon

Anna V. Cuomo, Norman Y. Otsuka, and Richard E. Bowen

## DEFINITION

- Shortening of the Achilles tendon, gastrocsoleus complex (triceps surae), or both results in an equinus (plantarflexed) position of the calcaneus relative to the tibia.
- An equinus deformity is either congenital or acquired and can be dynamic or rigid.
  - A dynamic deformity will correct with passive manipulation.
  - A rigid, or fixed, deformity does not correct.
- Achilles or gastrocsoleus contracture often occurs in combination with other soft tissue contractures.

## ANATOMY

- The two heads of the gastrocnemius originate on the posterior aspect of the medial and lateral condyles of the distal femur.
  - The muscle fibers terminate at the muscle–tendon junction at the midcalf.
  - From here, the Achilles tendon is joined by tendon fibers from the posterior aspect of the soleus as the tendon courses distally.
- The tendon is broad proximally and then becomes rounded at the midsection when it undergoes a 90-degree internal rotation before its insertion on the posterosuperior third of the calcaneus.
  - The rotation causes the medial fibers of the midtendon to insert on the posterior portion of the calcaneus (**FIG 1**).

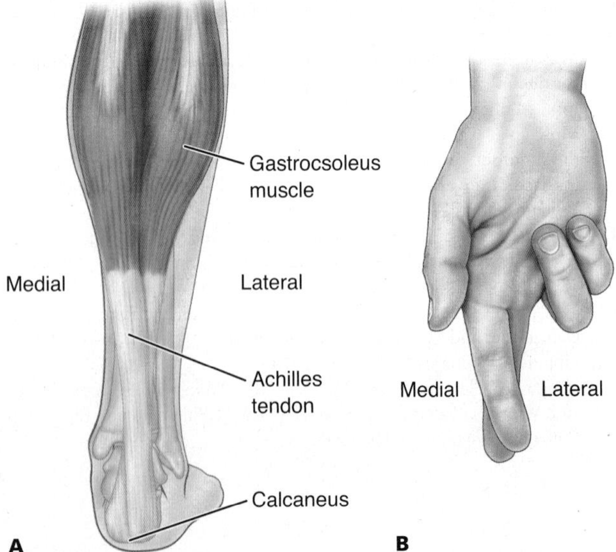


**FIG 1** • **A.** Posterior view of Achilles tendon, demonstrating 90-degree rotation of tendon fibers from posterior to medial and anterior to lateral. **B.** This can be easily remembered because it is a similar alignment to a crossed index and middle finger.

  - The insertion footprint is delta-shaped, and a small portion of the fibers course distally to meet the origin of the plantar fascia.
- The blood supply of the Achilles tendon is limited.
  - The proximal portion is supplied by branches from within the gastrocnemius muscle.
  - The distal portion is supplied by branches from the tendon–bone interface.
  - There is no true synovial sheath. Instead, the surrounding paratenon, comprising loose connective tissue, supplies the rest of the blood supply via branches from the posterior tibial artery and, to a lesser degree, the peroneal artery.[2]
- There are two synovial bursae at the Achilles tendon insertion site.
  - One is subcutaneous, located between the skin and tendon, and the other is deep, located between the tendon and the calcaneus.

## PATHOGENESIS

- The pathogenesis of congenital equinus is poorly understood and it is often associated with other limb deformities such as clubfoot or congenital vertical talus.
- Acquired equinus deformity secondary to cerebral palsy results from muscle spasticity or imbalance, leading to subsequent contracture of the Achilles tendon and gastrocsoleus complex.
  - Muscle imbalance and spasticity in spastic diplegic cerebral palsy often results in equinoplanovalgus deformity.
  - Muscle imbalance and spasticity in spastic hemiplegic cerebral palsy often results in equinus or equinovarus deformity.
- Compensatory balance mechanisms to help maintain ambulation in patients with Duchenne muscular dystrophy also may result in equinus deformity.
- Posttraumatic equinus can also be a result of severe burns and posterior scar contracture, postburn positioning, anterior leg muscle loss, or continued tibial growth in a rigid scar.[3]
- Talocrural and subtalar capsular adhesions and an abnormal tibiotalar articulation may also contribute to loss of dorsiflexion and equinus deformity.[7]

## NATURAL HISTORY

- Fixed equinus deformity will not correct spontaneously and requires prescribed stretching, surgical intervention, or both.[4]
- Equinus associated with cerebral palsy is progressive. Despite both conservative and surgical treatments, the deformity can recur due to persistent spasticity, muscle imbalance, or limb growth.
- Equinus deformity results in abnormal gait because of altered ankle range of motion and decreased ankle plantarflexion

moment during terminal stance. It can result in chronic pain, poorly fitting footwear, callosities on the plantar forefoot, and possible skin ulceration in patients with altered sensation.

## PATIENT HISTORY AND PHYSICAL FINDINGS

- Birth history may reveal gestational or perinatal complications, such as traumatic brain injury or global hypoxic events, which are risk factors for cerebral palsy.
- Family history may reveal a heritable neuromuscular disease or idiopathic toe walking.
- A delay in gross motor milestones may suggest the presence of a static neurologic disorder such as cerebral palsy, whereas regression of gross motor function may suggest a progressive neuromuscular disease such as muscular dystrophy or Rett syndrome.
  - The age of equinus deformity onset will depend on the type and severity of the underlying condition.
- Posttraumatic equinus, particularly a burn, should prompt questions regarding severity of the soft tissue loss, type of treatment, period of immobilization, and current problems with skin ulceration to assess the severity of scarring and overlying skin quality. Electrical burns can have extensive internal scarring well beyond the involvement of the overlying skin.
- Physical examination should include a thorough examination of the entire lower extremities to look for associated deformities at the hip, knee, hindfoot, and forefoot.
- The patient is examined supine on the examination table. It is important that the table has a hard surface so as not to mask any other contractures. The alignment and passive range of motion of the lumbosacral spine, pelvis, hips, and knees must also be tested because equinus may be a functional compensation for coexistent contractures.[9]
  - Ankle range of motion: Absence of dorsiflexion beyond neutral is ankle equinus.
  - Silfverskiöld test: A positive test indicates isolated gastrocnemius contracture. This is present if ankle equinus is present with the knee extended but improves with knee flexion.
  - Palpation of Achilles tendon: A tight tendon suggests spasticity of the gastrocsoleus complex or contracture of the Achilles tendon. Absence of a taut Achilles tendon with maximum dorsiflexion suggests tibiotalar joint deformity or a contracted posterior tibiotalar capsule.
  - Palpation of posterior tibial and peroneal tendons: Taut tendons suggest additional contracture or spasticity of the involved musculotendinous units contributing to the ankle equinus contracture.
  - Ankle clonus: More than two beats of clonus is abnormal and indicates gastrocsoleus spasticity or an upper motor neuron lesion.
  - Examination of the forefoot is important because isolated severe forefoot equinus may give a clinical appearance of hindfoot equinus. Lateral foot standing radiographs may be indicated if the physical examination is not clear. This is a common finding in the hereditary motor and sensory neuropathies.
- If the child is ambulatory, the clinician should observe the gait in a hallway or large area where the patient can both walk and run.
  - Socks, shoes, and clothing that extend below the knee are removed.
  - Hindfoot alignment is best observed from behind.
  - The foot progression angle (axis of the foot to the axis of progression) and any associated coronal plane abnormalities, such as scissoring (excessive hip adduction during gait), knee progression angle, and pelvic rotation, are best observed from the front.
  - Ankle equinus and any associated sagittal plane abnormalities, such as a crouch gait (hip and/or knee flexion contracture) or a stiff-knee gait (decreased knee range of motion during swing phase), are best observed from the side.
    - In mild equinus, the normal heel-to-toe gait of the plantargrade foot will be replaced with early lift-off during stance. Subtle deformity in patients with cerebral palsy is often unmasked by asking the patient to run. In severe equinus, the heel will not make contact during heel strike.
    - Equinovarus or equinoplanovalgus deformity will cause initial contact during gait to occur on either the lateral or medial border of the foot, respectively. There may be a callus or foot pain at the area of initial contact.
- Associated muscle spasticity or contracture in cerebral palsy should be diagnosed with the appropriate physical examination maneuvers described in the relevant chapters.

## IMAGING AND OTHER DIAGNOSTIC STUDIES

- Anteroposterior (AP) and lateral weight-bearing radiographs of the affected ankle should be obtained.
  - Ossification centers of the talus, calcaneus, and cuboid are present at infancy. The navicular does not appear until age 3 to 4 years.
  - Equinus deformity will result in a decreased lateral tibiocalcaneal angle. Normal values range from 25 to 60 degrees. It can be difficult to measure this angle in young children with a partially ossified calcaneus.
  - Although usually associated with hindfoot varus, equinus deformity can also result in a decreased lateral talocalcaneal angle (intersection of a line through the longitudinal axis of the talus and a line along the plantar surface of the calcaneus; **FIG 2**). The normal range is 25 to 55 degrees.
  - Bony abnormalities, such as a flattened talar dome or anterior talar neck and anterior distal tibial osteophytes, can also contribute to ankle equinus.

## DIFFERENTIAL DIAGNOSIS

- Congenital equinus
  - Talipes equinovarus (clubfoot)
  - Planovalgus
  - Congenital vertical talus
  - Arthrogryposis
  - Tibial longitudinal deficiency
- Acquired equinus
  - Neuromuscular

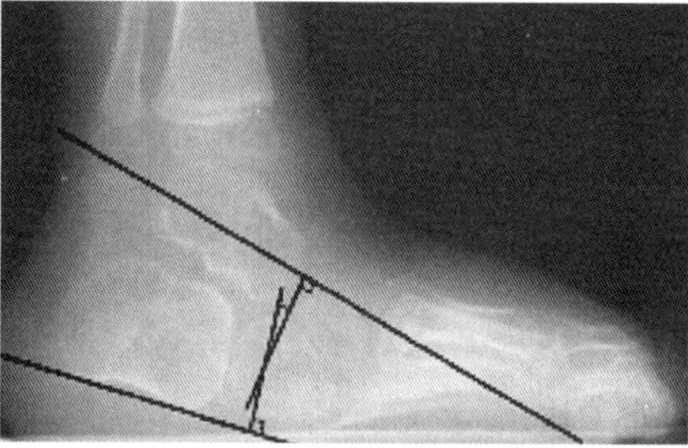

**FIG 2** • Measurement of the lateral talocalcaneal angle. The normal range of 25 to 55 degrees is decreased in equinus.

- Cerebral palsy
- Myelomeningocele
- Hereditary motor and sensory neuropathies
- Spinal muscular atrophy
- Sacral agenesis
- Rett syndrome or other genetic neuromuscular diseases

- Posttraumatic
  - Posterior scar contracture
  - Posttrauma positioning
  - Anterior leg muscle loss
  - Continued tibial growth in a rigid scar
- Other
  - Idiopathic toe walking
  - Juvenile arthropathy
  - Autism

## NONOPERATIVE MANAGEMENT

- Many children with equinus deformity secondary to a contracture of the Achilles tendon or gastrocsoleus complex can be successfully managed with nonoperative treatment.
  - This is typically performed with serial casting for 3 to 6 weeks or more to achieve neutral sagittal alignment.
  - The success of nonoperative management depends on the age of the patient, the severity of the deformity, and the cause of the equinus.
- In patients with equinus and cerebral palsy, early surgery may have an unpredictable outcome, with high rates of recurrence.
  - For this reason, surgery is often delayed with nonoperative treatments until after age 6 years.
- Physical therapy for Achilles tendon stretching helps correct and maintain correction of equinus deformity.
  - The efficacy of stretching is likely dependent on the duration and frequency of stretching.
- Use of an ankle–foot orthosis (AFO) in patients with cerebral palsy and dynamic equinus is a useful adjunct to nonsurgical management.
- Botulinum toxin A (BtA) has been shown to be at least as effective as serial casting, with fewer side effects and more prolonged benefit.[1]
  - Serial casting and physical therapy are recommended as an adjunct to BtA injections.
- Oral medications for muscle relaxation, such as baclofen, diazepam, dantrolene sodium, and tizanidine, can be helpful in selected patients with cerebral palsy if generalized reduction in tone is desired.

## SURGICAL MANAGEMENT

- Indications for surgical management include fixed ankle equinus that exists with the knee flexed as well as extended and that also interferes with normal gait.
  - Clinical difficulties may include pain with weight bearing, toe walking, callosities on the plantar forefoot, poorly fitting orthoses, or plantar midfoot pain.
- Surgical management of fixed ankle equinus in knee extension that disappears in knee flexion should consist of surgery to the gastrocnemius fascia alone.
- Especially in patients with cerebral palsy, surgical management of ankle equinus should include concurrent treatment of all pelvic and lower extremity deformities, particularly hamstring contractures.[6]

### Preoperative Planning

- The quality of the overlying skin will be crucial for successful wound healing and should be considered during the preoperative planning phase.
  - Inadequate skin elasticity may require incomplete correction and staged surgery or staged casting in the postoperative period.
  - In severe posttraumatic cases, tissue loss and significant scarring may require additional tissue transfer procedures.
- In cerebral palsy patients with severe spasticity, examination under anesthesia can help determine if equinus deformity is dynamic or fixed because paralytic medications during anesthesia eliminate spasticity.

### Positioning

- The patient can be positioned either prone or supine.
  - The prone position allows improved access to the tibiotalar and subtalar joint capsules but requires careful padding to the hips and knees (**FIG 3**).
  - We prefer the supine position for patients undergoing isolated tendo Achilles lengthening.
- A thigh tourniquet can be used.
- The leg is prepared sterilely from the tourniquet distally.
  - If other concurrent soft tissue tendon lengthenings are to be performed, the patient is positioned and prepared according to the additional procedures.

### Approach

- To avoid postoperative wound complications, a longitudinal incision along the anteromedial border of the Achilles tendon is recommended.
  - This decreases the risk of wound dehiscence because the thinnest portion of the overlying skin is directly posterior to the tendon and should remain intact.
  - For sliding procedures, a modified approach that exposes only the transected portion of the tendon can also be performed.
- The open sliding Achilles lengthening technique, first described by White,[10] is performed with partial transections at the (1) proximal and medial and (2) distal and anterior portions of the tendon. The 90-degree rotation of the tendon fibers between the transected areas maintains continuity of the tendon fibers as the tendon is lengthened (**FIG 4A**).
- Another (percutaneous) method of a sliding Achilles lengthening was described by Hoke.[5] It involves three longitudinal incisions. The first is made in the midsubstance of the tendon at its calcaneal insertion, and the scalpel blade is turned medially to cut the medial half of the tendon. The second is then made one-half to one inch (1–2 cm) more proximal, and the lateral half is cut. The third is made one-half to one

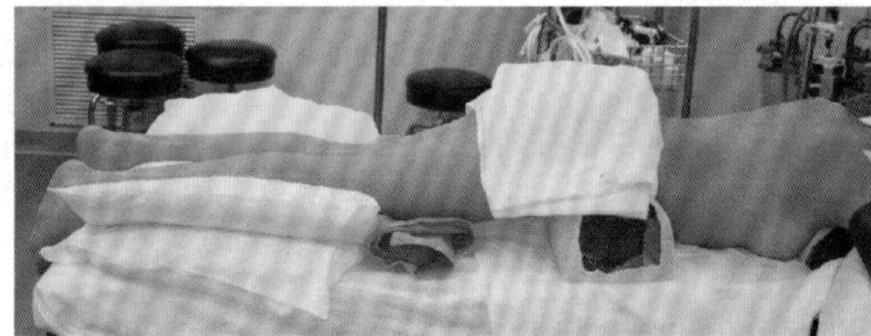

**FIG 3** • Prone positioning of patient on table with appropriate hip and knee padding during anesthesia.

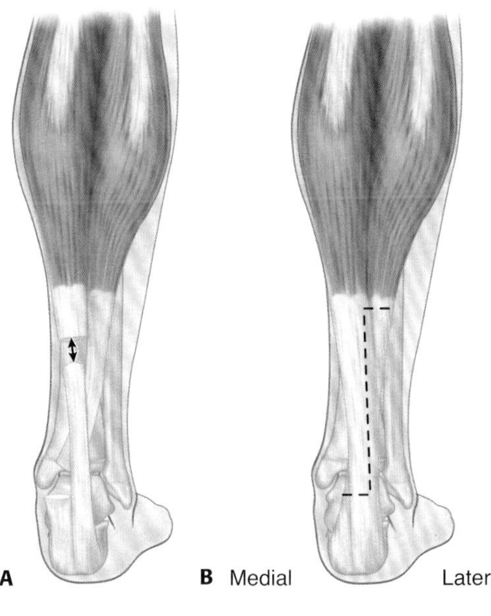


inch (1–2 cm) from the second incision, and the medial half is cut. After half of the tendon has been cut in each of these three spots, gentle pressure is applied to the foot. This allows the fibers of the cut tendon to slide over each other and the Achilles tendon is gently lengthened.

- The modified open sliding Achilles lengthening technique decreases the size of the skin incision but uses the same technique of a sliding Achilles lengthening.
- The open Achilles Z-lengthening procedure uses the same incision and closure as the modified approach. Here, the entire tendon is divided in a Z-fashion (**FIG 4B**), and the two sides or ends of the tendon are sutured to each other.

**FIG 4** • **A.** Posterior view of Achilles tendon demonstrating distal anterior and proximal medial transections and subsequent sliding of attached tendon fibers during dorsiflexion. **B.** Posterior view of planned Achilles tendon sectioning to achieve Z-lengthening.



## Open Sliding Achilles Lengthening

- The skin incision is made along the anteromedial border of the Achilles tendon.
  - The skin incision begins just proximal to the calcaneal insertion (**TECH FIG 1A**) and continues proximally to the proximal extent of the tendon.
- Sharply divide the subcutaneous fat in line with the incision. There are no neurovascular structures at risk, and the incision can be directed deeply until the paratenon sheath surrounding the tendon has been fully incised.
  - It is helpful to maintain the attachment of the paratenon to the subcutaneous fat to preserve the blood supply of the surrounding tissues and avoid postoperative wound complications.
- Insert a new blade, cutting edge directed inferiorly, just proximal to the calcaneus in the coronal plane between the

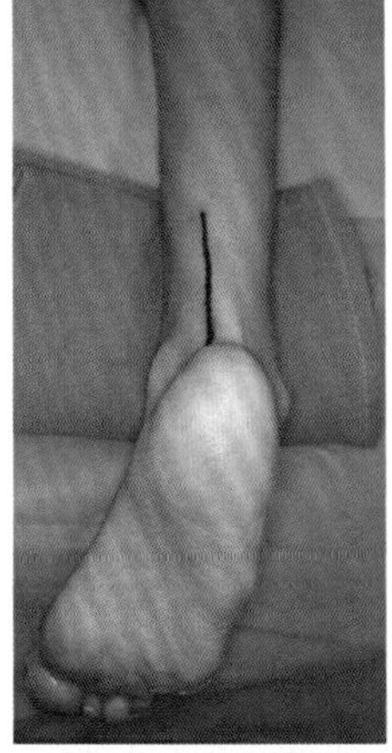
A

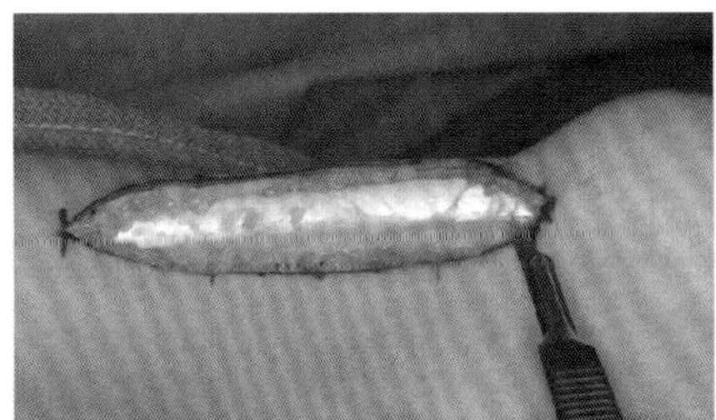
B

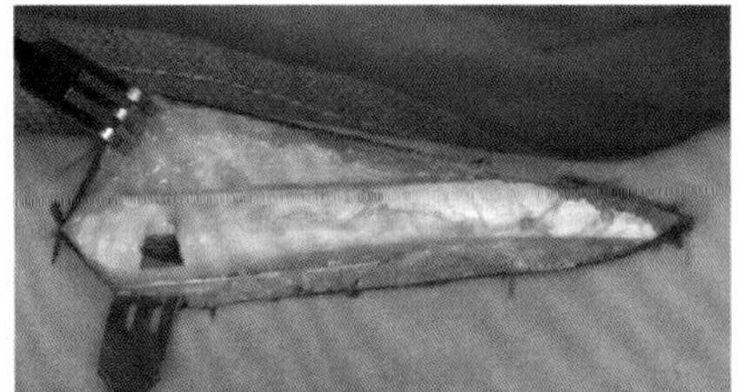
C

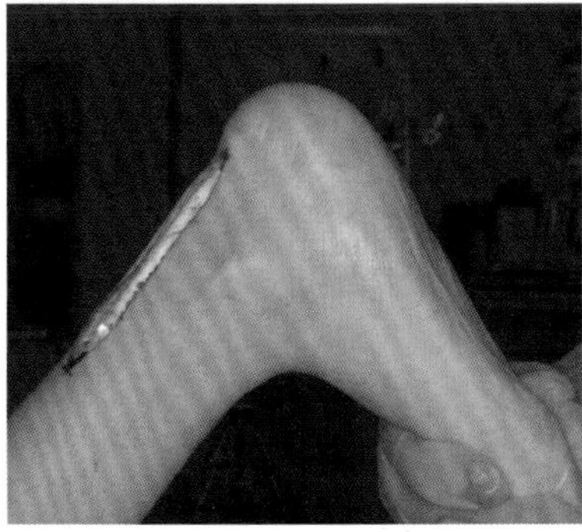
D

**TECH FIG 1** • **A.** Planned incision along anteromedial border of tendon. **B.** Full exposure of the tendon has been achieved, and the blade, cutting edge directed inferiorly, is inserted into the tendon in the coronal plane, dividing the anterior two-thirds and posterior one-third of the tendon. **C.** The medial two-thirds of the proximal Achilles tendon has been transected, and the ankle has been dorsiflexed to separate the tendon fibers. **D.** The ankle is dorsiflexed to the desired position.

anterior two-thirds and posterior one-third of the distal tendon (**TECH FIG 1B**).
  - Rotate the blade so the cutting edge is anterior and divide the anterior two-thirds of the tendon transversely.
- Identify the most proximal portion of the tendon that has been exposed.
  - Transversely divide the medial two-thirds of the tendon, taking care to avoid any underlying muscle fibers of the soleus (**TECH FIG 1C**).
- Slowly dorsiflex the foot with firm pressure to cause the divided portions of the tendon to slide past one another until 10 degrees of dorsiflexion is achieved (**TECH FIG 1D**).
- Maintain the desired correction of alignment while closing the wound to allow even distribution of any new tension of the surrounding tissues.
  - Avoid overtensioning, which presents as complete blanching of the skin; it may lead to skin necrosis.
- Using fine absorbable suture, loosely approximate the subcutaneous fat with several simple interrupted sutures. Then run the suture in the subcuticular tissue to close the skin.
- Although a long-leg cast can be used, the authors prefer a short-leg cast with the ankle and subtalar joints in neutral positioning.

## Modified Open Sliding Achilles Lengthening

- Identify the anteromedial border of the Achilles tendon as described previously and, with a pen, draw the length of incision as if planning a fully open procedure.
  - This helps ensure alignment of the two incisions and avoids gaping of the wound after dorsiflexion and subsequent uneven tensioning of the skin.
  - Using a skin blade, create two short longitudinal incisions at the distal and proximal ends of the drawn line (**TECH FIG 2**).
- As previously described, sharply dissect the overlying tissues to reach the Achilles tendon at the proximal and distal incisions and partially divide the tendon at each area of exposure.
- As for the original open lengthening technique, slowly dorsiflex the foot with gentle pressure to cause the divided portions of the tendon to slide past one another until 10 degrees of dorsiflexion is achieved.
- Close the subcutaneous tissues and skin and apply a short- or long-leg cast as described previously.

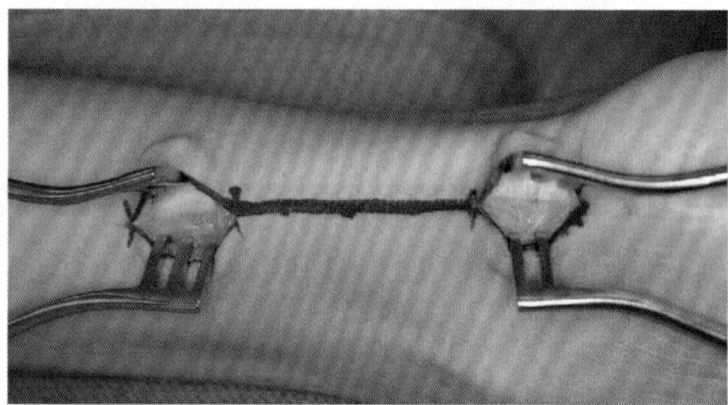

**TECH FIG 2** • The incision is marked as if planning for an extensive exposure, except only the most proximal and distal 2 cm are used to expose the medial aspect of the Achilles tendon.

## Open Achilles Z-Lengthening

- Once the entire tendon has been exposed through the anteromedial approach, gently retract the most distal and medial tissues anteriorly to protect the underlying neurovascular structures.
- Align a new no. 15 blade longitudinally with the tendon fibers at the midpoint of the tendon in the sagittal plane. Introduce the blade deeply into the tendon until there is a discernable release in resistance, signifying complete transection through the tendon.
  - Alternately, a small osteotome may be introduced along the anterior border of the tendon, and the blade can be carried safely through the entire tendon until metal-on-metal contact.
- Carry the incision distally until the calcaneal insertion is reached (**TECH FIG 3A**).
- Without removing the blade, rotate the blade medially 90 degrees and with a slight sawing motion, transversely divide the medial portion of the tendon.
- Once this is achieved, retraction of the medial structures can be safely released.
- Return the blade to the proximal starting point and extend the division proximally until an adequate portion of the tendon is involved.
  - This is usually about two-thirds of the Achilles tendon but will ultimately depend on the desired lengthening and overlap between the two ends.
  - Take care to stay along the midline of the tendon.
- Complete the proximal division of the tendon laterally in this transverse plane (**TECH FIG 3B**).
- The entire tendon should now be divided in a Z-fashion (**TECH FIG 3C**).
- Dorsiflex the ankle to neutral. Under moderate tension, reapproximate the tendon with a braided nonabsorbable suture.
  - A side-to-side repair can be performed with multiple interrupted simple or vertical mattress sutures (**TECH FIG 3D**).
  - Alternately, the overlapping ends of the tendon can be excised for approximation of the ends. Multiple intratendinous and epitendon suture techniques are acceptable for reapproximation. The intratendinous technique reduces exposed suture and diminishes inflammatory reaction around the suture and is recommended. The simplest of these is the modified Kessler suture (locking loops of the core suture; **TECH FIG 3E**).
- Apply either a long- or short-leg cast as discussed earlier.

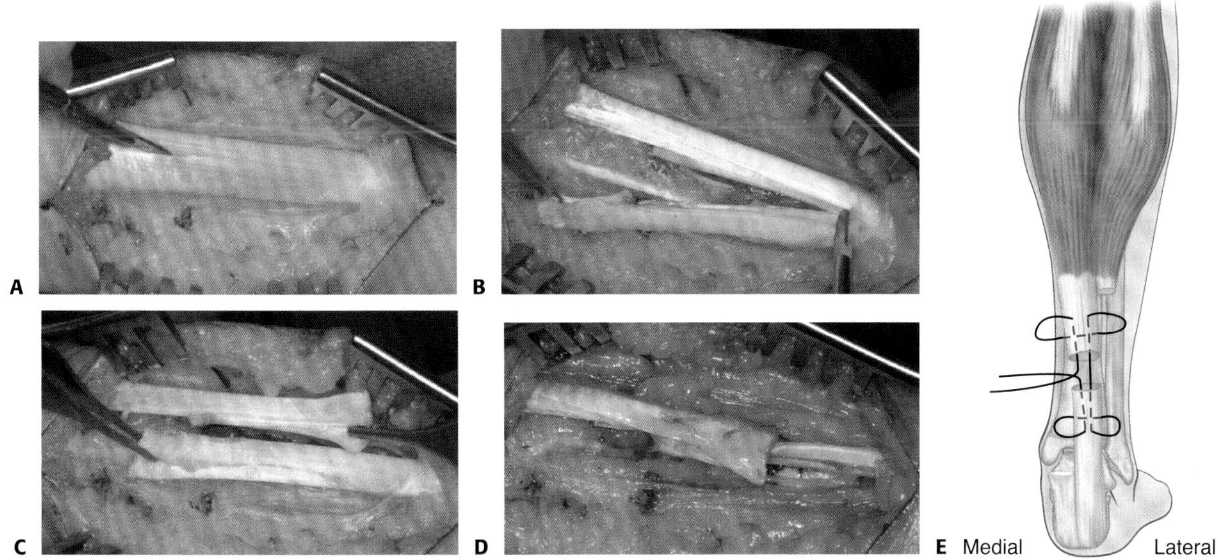


**TECH FIG 3** • **A.** Full exposure of the Achilles tendon has been achieved, and the initial transection in the sagittal plane, dividing the medial and lateral halves of the tendon, has been performed with a blade. **B.** The entire tendon is exposed and is being transected in a Z-fashion. **C.** The ankle is dorsiflexed to the appropriate position, and the overlapping tendon is noted. **D.** The desired amount of overlapping tendon has been joined with vertical mattress sutures. **E.** Alternately, the tendons can be reapproximated end to end. After Z-lengthening, the remaining overlapping tendon has been removed and the ends of the tendon are joined with a nonabsorbable suture and a modified Kessler repair.

## PEARLS AND PITFALLS

| | |
|---|---|
| **Failure to address coexistent contractures** | ▪ All associated joint contractures, particularly in cerebral palsy, should be addressed to achieve optimal surgical results. |
| **Surgical indications** | ▪ Patients with a positive Silfverskiöld test should not be treated with an Achilles lengthening. |
| **Overlengthening** | ▪ In an open Z-lengthening, repairing the tendon with the ankle in dorsiflexion or under inadequate tension can lead to overlengthening.<br>▪ In a sliding lengthening, dorsiflexing the ankle beyond 10 degrees can lead to overlengthening. |
| **Wound healing problems** | ▪ The paratenon should not be dissected free from the overlying subcutaneous tissue posteriorly.<br>▪ Posterior skin contractures should be treated intraoperatively with tissue transfer procedures or postoperatively with undercorrection and serial casting. |
| **Inadequate correction** | ▪ Severe equinus deformity often requires a concurrent release of the posterior subtalar and tibiotalar joint capsules, lengthening of the posterior tibial and peroneal tendons, or both.<br>▪ Failure to extend the Z-lengthening incision to the most proximal portion of the tendon can lead to insufficient length of tendon at repair and therefore to undercorrection.<br>▪ In a sliding lengthening, failure to dorsiflex the ankle to 10 degrees with the knee extended and the subtalar joint inverted can result in undercorrection. |
| **Revision surgery** | ▪ The normal 90-degree spiral architecture of the tendon is altered with surgery, and an open Z-lengthening procedure is indicated for revision surgery. |

## POSTOPERATIVE CARE

- Adequate pain control in the acute postoperative setting is imperative. This is both to promote the child's comfort and to reduce additional muscle spasms, which may alter the desired surgical correction.
  - Because children with neuromuscular diseases may have significant communicative barriers, pain should be presumed to be present and should be treated with both morphine derivatives and muscle relaxants.
- The limb should be elevated as much as possible for 2 or 3 days until acute swelling resolves.
- The child can then become ambulatory and weight bearing as tolerated if a sliding tendon lengthening was performed.
- Patients undergoing open Z-lengthening should remain non–weight bearing in a cast until tendon healing is sufficient (6 weeks).
- Once the cast is permanently removed, the child needs postoperative physical therapy or use of an AFO, as dictated by the diagnosis.

## OUTCOMES

- Surgical lengthening results in gains in dorsiflexion, from a preoperative average of 25 degrees of plantarflexion to 8 degrees of dorsiflexion, without significant changes in the arc range of motion.
- Correction is maintained in 80% to 90% of patients for at least 7 years postoperatively.[4]

## COMPLICATIONS

- Calcaneovalgus deformity occurs in less than 2% of open Achilles tendon lengthenings.
- Recurrent deformity is common in neuromuscular diseases owing to continued spasticity and normal longitudinal tibial growth.
  - After surgical correction, 18% of children with diplegia and 41% of those with hemiplegia will experience recurrence.
  - Ambulatory patients maintain correction better than nonambulatory patients.
  - Recurrence is also more frequent in children 4 years or younger.[8]
- Wound dehiscence and necrosis are infrequent and the incidence is not well reported.
  - These can be devastating, however, and should remain a matter of concern as potential complications.

## REFERENCES

1. Ackman JD, Russman BS, Thomas SS, et al. Comparing botulinum toxin A with casting for treatment of dynamic equinus in children with cerebral palsy. Dev Med Child Neurol 2005;47:620–627.
2. Ahmed IM, Lagopoulos M, McConnell P, et al. Blood supply of the Achilles tendon. J Orthop Res 1998;16:591–596.
3. Carmichael KD, Maxwell SC, Calhoun JH. Recurrence rates of burn contracture ankle equinus and other foot deformities in children treated with Ilizarov fixation. J Pediatr Orthop 2005;25:523–528.
4. Damron TA, Greenwald TA, Breed AL. Chronologic outcome of surgical tendoachilles lengthening and natural history of gastroc-soleus contracture in cerebral palsy. A two-part study. Clin Orthop Relat Res 1994;(301):249–255.
5. Hoke M. An operation for stabilizing paralytic feet. J Orthop Surg 1921;3:494–507.
6. Karol LA. Surgical management of the lower extremity in ambulatory children with cerebral palsy. J Am Acad Orthop Surg 2004;12: 196–203.
7. Mary P, Damsin JP, Carlioz H. Correction of equinus in clubfoot: the contribution of arthrography. J Pediatr Orthop 2004;24:312–316.
8. Rattey TE, Leahey L, Hyndman J, et al. Recurrence after Achilles tendon lengthening in cerebral palsy. J Pediatr Orthop 1993;13: 184–187.
9. Rome K. Ankle joint dorsiflexion measurement studies. A review of the literature. J Am Podiatr Med Assoc 1996;86:205–211.
10. White WJ. Torsion of the Achilles tendon: its surgical significance. Arch Surg Am 1943;46:784.

# Split Posterior Tibial Tendon Transfer

CHAPTER 119

David A. Spiegel and James J. McCarthy

## DEFINITION

- The equinovarus deformity involves hindfoot equinus and varus and results from imbalance between inversion (tibialis posterior, tibialis anterior, or both) and eversion of the foot.
- The deformity may interfere with ambulation, orthotic wear, or both.
- Split tendon transfers are used in patients with spastic muscle imbalance to prevent overcorrection or production of the opposite deformity, usually in children with cerebral palsy who have spastic hemiplegia.[1] The procedure weakens a deforming force while augmenting a weakened muscle. In contrast, patients with a flaccid equinovarus deformity, due to poliomyelitis or other causes, are typically treated by transfer of an entire muscle(s) to augment the strength of selected muscle groups.

## ANATOMY

- The tibialis posterior muscle originates from the posterolateral aspect of the tibia, the interosseous membrane, and the medial fibula.
  - Although the main insertion is into the tuberosity of the navicular, fibers also insert onto the cuneiforms, the second through fourth metatarsals, the cuboid, and the sustentaculum tali.
- The gastrocnemius muscle originates from the posterior surface of the distal femur, and its tendon blends with the tendon of the soleus muscle to form the Achilles tendon, which then inserts on the posterior tuberosity of the calcaneus.
- The soleus muscle takes origin from the posterior portion of the upper third of the fibula, the fibrous arch between the tibia and the fibula, and the posterior aspect of the tibia. The broad tendinous portion along the posterior aspect of the soleus joins with the gastrocnemius tendon to form the Achilles tendon.

## PATHOGENESIS

- The deformity results from muscle imbalance between plantarflexion–inversion (strong) and dorsiflexion–eversion (weak). Spasticity of the tibialis posterior, the tibialis anterior, or both may be responsible for the imbalance.

## NATURAL HISTORY

- The deformity is initially dynamic, with a full range of motion on physical examination.
  - A myostatic contracture often develops over time, evidenced by the inability to achieve a full passive range of motion.
  - Tethering of growth may subsequently result in structural bony deformities such as hindfoot varus.
- The equinovarus deformity may result in pathologic changes in both the stance and swing phases of gait, including impaired clearance during swing phase, inability to preposition the foot in terminal swing, and loss of stability during stance phase.

## PATIENT HISTORY AND PHYSICAL FINDINGS

- Patients present with progressive gait disturbance, with or without pain, and may have difficulty wearing orthotics.
- Pain is due to the abnormal stress distribution on the plantar surface of the foot and is commonly experienced over the distal fifth metatarsal and the lateral border of the foot. Calluses may be observed laterally.
- Recurrent ankle sprains may occur as the hindfoot rolls into varus. This may also be associated with a tarsal coalition.
- In addition to a comprehensive neurologic examination, examination of the spine and both extremities, the physical examination focuses on observational gait analysis, the presence of and degree of spasticity in the individual muscle groups, the range of motion (active and passive) of the foot and ankle, and the selectivity of motor control.
- Observational gait analysis focuses on the alignment of the foot and ankle during both the swing and stance phases of gait.
  - During swing phase, the foot is inverted and plantarflexed, which impairs clearance.
  - The inability to maintain the foot in neutral plantarflexion–dorsiflexion during midswing may be due to muscle weakness (tibialis anterior), muscle spasticity (tibialis anterior or posterior, gastrocsoleus), or a fixed equinovarus deformity.
  - There is inadequate prepositioning of the foot for weight acceptance during terminal swing.
  - Initial contact often occurs over the lateral forefoot (no heel contact), or over the lateral border of the foot, and the foot rolls into varus, which interferes with stability during stance phase.
  - The equinovarus deformity may also contribute to intoeing (internal foot progression angle).
- The presence and degree of spasticity should be documented.
  - The most common system for grading is the modified Ashworth scale. Each muscle is tested by gentle stretch; for example, spasticity of the tibialis posterior is assessed by everting the foot, whereas the gastrocsoleus complex is assessed by dorsiflexion.
  - The strength of individual muscle groups should be graded if possible.
- Testing the passive range of motion determines whether the deformity is dynamic (full passive range of motion) or whether there is a myostatic component (restriction of passive range of motion).
  - Although bench examination provides a useful estimate of motion, an examination under anesthesia provides the

most accurate evaluation, as spasticity is eliminated. Such an examination is always performed at the time of surgery to finalize the treatment plan, as a full passive range of motion is a prerequisite for a tendon transfer.

- For patients with an equinovarus deformity, the examination focuses on the degree of passive eversion and dorsiflexion. Equinus contracture is often limited to the gastrocnemius muscle but may also involve the soleus muscle.
- The Silfverskiöld test evaluates the contribution of each component of the gastrocsoleus complex to an equinus contracture, and the amount (in degrees) of passive dorsiflexion is quantified with the knee both flexed and extended. The degree of passive dorsiflexion with the knee extended indicates the absolute magnitude of contracture from the gastrocnemius and soleus. Flexion of the knee relaxes the gastrocnemius muscle and allows the contribution of the soleus to be quantified.

- Selectivity of motor control is commonly impaired in children with cerebral palsy and is tested by asking the patient to contract an isolated muscle group against resistance. This is graded as normal if the patient can isolate the individual muscle and no "overflow" movement is observed in other muscle groups of the same limb. Most commonly, movements of more than one muscle group, or the entire limb, are elicited when testing individual muscle groups.

## IMAGING AND OTHER DIAGNOSTIC STUDIES

- Although imaging studies are not routinely obtained, plain radiographs of the foot may be helpful in the presence of a fixed deformity.
  - Weight-bearing anteroposterior (AP) and lateral views are reviewed, and a Harris heel view may be considered to evaluate the degree of hindfoot varus in the weight-bearing position.
- Instrumented motion analysis (gait analysis) is used in many centers to assist with surgical decision making.
  - Slow-motion video is an important component of the assessment and supplements the findings on observational gait analysis.
  - Dynamic electromyelography (EMG) monitors the electrical activity of the tibialis posterior and tibialis anterior throughout the gait cycle, determining whether individual muscles act out of phase or whether they are continuously active throughout the gait cycle.[13] Although a surface electrode may be used to assess the tibialis anterior, monitoring of the tibialis posterior requires insertion of a fine needle electrode.
  - One study determined that the deformity was due to the tibialis posterior in 33%, the tibialis anterior in 34%, or both (31%).[9]
  - Findings on pedobarography include increased pressure across the lateral midfoot, decreased pressure on the heel at the time of initial contact, and increased pressure on the lateral border of the foot throughout stance phase.

## NONOPERATIVE MANAGEMENT

- Specific aspects within a comprehensive physical therapy program include stretching exercises to maintain or improve range of motion and strengthening exercises to reduce dynamic muscle imbalance.
- An ankle–foot orthosis is often required to maintain alignment of the ankle and hindfoot during ambulation.
  - The orthotic facilitates clearance during swing phase by maintaining the foot in a neutral position, prepositions the foot for initial contact with the ground, and promotes stability during stance phase.
- Night splinting may help to prevent myostatic contracture.
- Injection of botulinum toxin A (Botox or Dysport) into the tibialis posterior, the gastrocsoleus, or both results in a reversible chemical denervation that decreases spasticity for about 3 to 6 months.
  - In addition to reducing dynamic muscle imbalance, a temporary reduction in spasticity may facilitate stretching exercises, improve bracing tolerance, and delay the need for surgical intervention.

## SURGICAL MANAGEMENT

- Surgical treatment of the spastic equinovarus foot is offered when the deformity impairs ambulation, interferes with bracing, or both.
- The goal of tendon transfer is to balance the muscle forces across the hindfoot to maintain a neutral position during the swing and stance phases of gait. A split tendon transfer is preferred as transfer of the entire tendon is associated with a significant risk of overcorrection.
- A normal passive range of motion is a prerequisite. In the presence of fixed soft tissue or bony deformity, concomitant muscle lengthening, with or without osteotomy, may be required to restore motion and alignment.
- Although an instrumented motion analysis with dynamic EMG will enable the treating surgeon to identify whether the tibialis posterior, the tibialis anterior, or both is/are contributing to the deformity, this technology is not always available. The clinical indications suggested for split tibialis posterior tendon surgery include hindfoot varus during both the stance and swing phases of gait. In contrast, overactivity of the tibialis anterior typically produces varus/supination of the midfoot/forefoot during swing phase.
- It has been suggested that the procedure be delayed until at least 4 to 6 years of age, and one recent report suggested that consideration should be given to delaying split tendon transfer beyond the age of 8 years if possible as there may be a greater risk of recurrence.[2]
- Lengthening of the tibialis posterior muscle may be considered in milder deformities, especially in young patients. Techniques include a distal Z-lengthening or a proximal intramuscular recession. Recognize that it may be very difficult to perform a split tendon transfer if a Z-lengthening has been performed previously.
- Several techniques have been described for split tibialis posterior transfer.
  - The most common involves transferring the split tendon (posterior to the tibia and fibula) to the peroneus brevis, either at its insertion or just behind the lateral malleolus. This approach focuses on balancing inversion–eversion but does not address dorsiflexion weakness (**FIG 1**).
  - An alternate technique, which may be considered when there is inadequate active dorsiflexion, involves anterior transfer of the split tendon through the interosseous membrane to the peroneus brevis (**FIG 2A,B**) or the lateral cuneiform (**FIG 2C**).

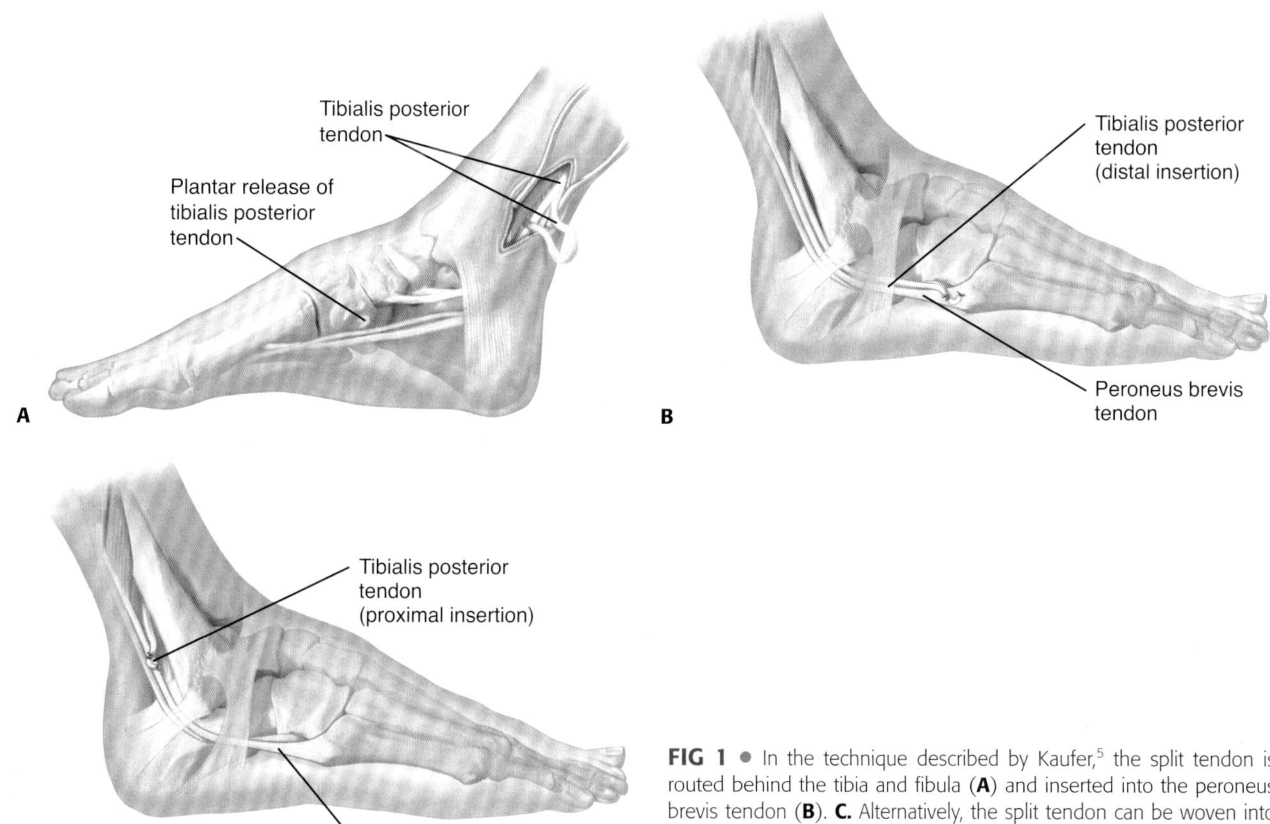


**FIG 1** ● In the technique described by Kaufer,[5] the split tendon is routed behind the tibia and fibula (**A**) and inserted into the peroneus brevis tendon (**B**). **C.** Alternatively, the split tendon can be woven into the peroneus brevis just behind the lateral malleolus. This approach is easier and works as well when the tendon is not long enough.

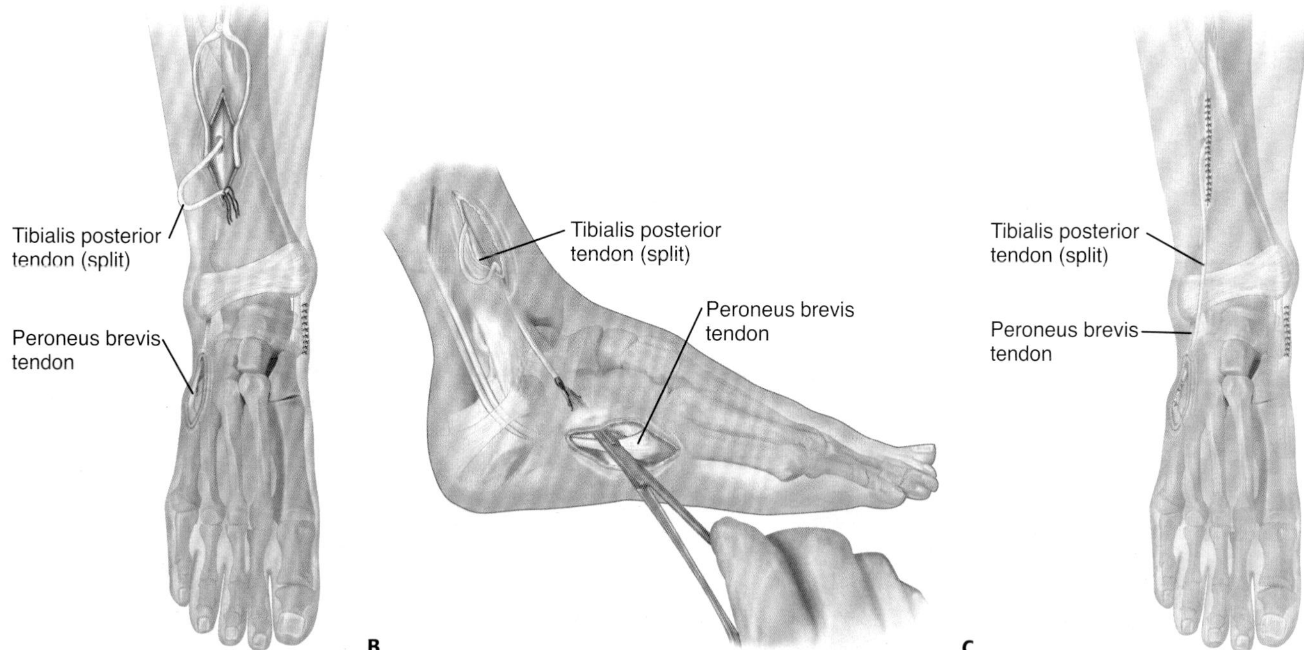


**FIG 2** ● In the technique described by Mulier et al,[11] the split tendon is passed through the interosseous membrane (**A**) and through a subcutaneous tunnel to insert into the peroneus brevis tendon (**B**). **C.** Saji et al[16] transferred the split tendon through the interosseous membrane into the lateral cuneiform.

- Biomechanical investigations using cadaveric specimens have studied the technical aspects of the split tendon transfer.[15]
  - Moran et al[10] found that all routing variations reduce the ability of the tibialis posterior to invert the hindfoot, that there was no difference between attaching the tendon proximally or distally into the peroneus brevis, and that transfer through the interosseous membrane reduced the ability to plantarflex the foot. Calculation of muscle moment arms across the subtalar joint suggested that adequate results could be achieved over a wide range of tensioning.
- Other procedures are commonly performed in concert with a split tibialis posterior tendon transfer.
  - Lengthening of the tendo Achilles (gastrocnemius with or without the soleus) is required in most cases of spastic equinovarus deformity. Depending on the degree of myostatic contracture, this can be achieved with either a recession technique (Vulpius, Baker) or a tendinous lengthening (open Z-plasty, percutaneous or open sliding lengthening).
  - Fixed varus deformity of the hindfoot requires a calcaneal osteotomy, either a lateral closing wedge osteotomy (Dwyer) or a sliding lateral displacement osteotomy of the calcaneus. Options for fixation include a staple, a Steinmann pin, or a screw.
  - Older patients with a severe fixed equinovarus deformity may require a triple arthrodesis.
  - A subset of patients may also have tibial torsion of a degree that warrants surgery. Consideration should be given to staging the procedures, as one study suggested that tibial derotational osteotomy should not be performed at the time of tendon transfer because of the increased risk of failure of the tendon transfer.
  - In some cases, both the tibialis anterior and the tibialis posterior will be found to be responsible for the deformity. Options for this group of patients, depending on the age and clinical circumstances, include (1) split tibialis anterior tendon transfer with concomitant intramuscular lengthening of the tibialis posterior or (2) split tendon transfers of both the tibialis anterior and the tibialis posterior.

## Preoperative Planning

- The indications for surgery are based on the physical examination, with or without an instrumented motion analysis study.
- An examination under anesthesia (eliminates spasticity) is performed to assess the range of motion and finalize the surgical plan. A prerequisite for tendon transfer is that full passive mobility be present (or achievable), and occasionally, other soft tissue and/or bony procedures are required in additional to the tendon transfer. Concomitant lengthening of the gastrocsoleus complex is frequently required.

## Positioning

- The patient is placed supine.

## Approach

- Either three or four incisions are employed for split tibialis posterior tendon transfer.
- The tendon must be released from its insertion, tunneled either anteriorly (through the interosseous membrane) or posteriorly behind the tibia and fibula, and then attached to either the peroneus brevis or lateral cuneiform.

TECHNIQUES

## Split Tibialis Tendon Transfer to Peroneus Brevis (after Kaufer)

- A longitudinal incision is made over the insertion of the tibialis posterior on the navicular, and the sheath is opened (**TECH FIG 1A**).
  - The plantar half of the tendon is released and the tendon is split longitudinally (**TECH FIG 1B,C**).
- A second incision is made just posterior to the medial malleolus, extending proximally for 4 cm (**TECH FIG 1D,E**).
  - The sheath of the tibialis posterior is split longitudinally, and the free end of the tendon is delivered into this wound.
  - The longitudinal split in the tendon is extended proximally to the musculotendinous junction.
- The third longitudinal incision is made about 2 cm proximal to the tip of the lateral malleolus and extends proximally (**TECH FIG 1F,G**).
  - The peroneal tendon sheath is incised longitudinally.
  - The split tendon is then passed posterior to the tibia and fibula, and anterior to the neurovascular bundle, into the third incision. The split tibialis posterior tendon can be sutured into the peroneus brevis tendon at this level (see **FIG 1C**) or can be transferred distally, which requires a fourth incision.

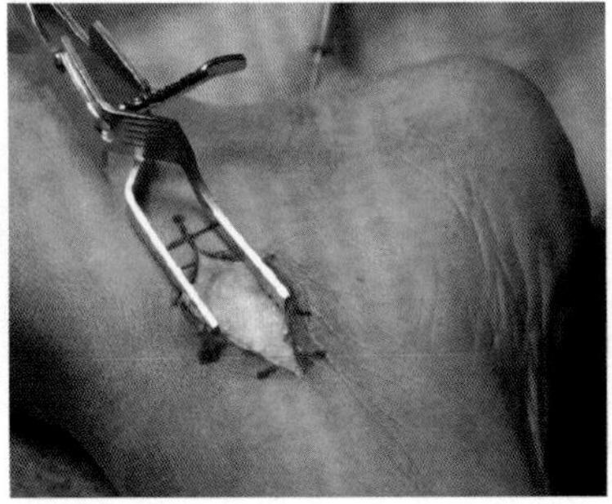
A

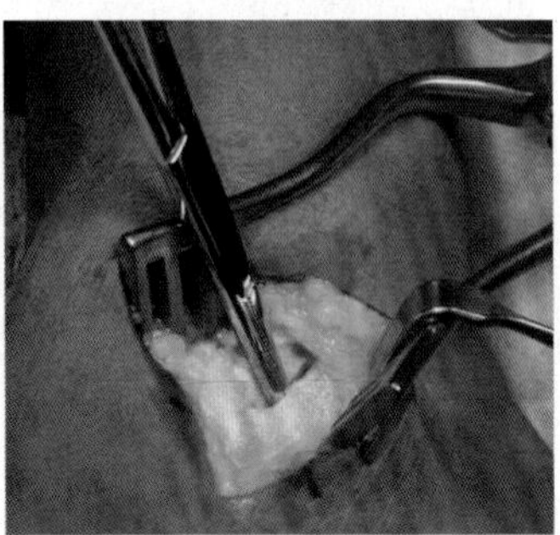
B

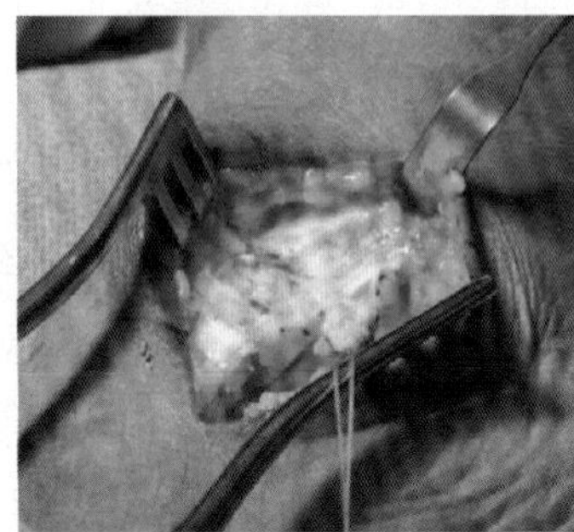
C

**TECH FIG 1** • **A.** A longitudinal incision is made over the insertion of the tibialis posterior. **B.** The tibialis posterior tendon is then dissected free at its insertion, and half of the tendon is released, most often from the plantar surface. **C.** The distal end of the tendon is tagged with a running locked suture, and the division in the tendon is developed proximally as far as possible. *(continued)*

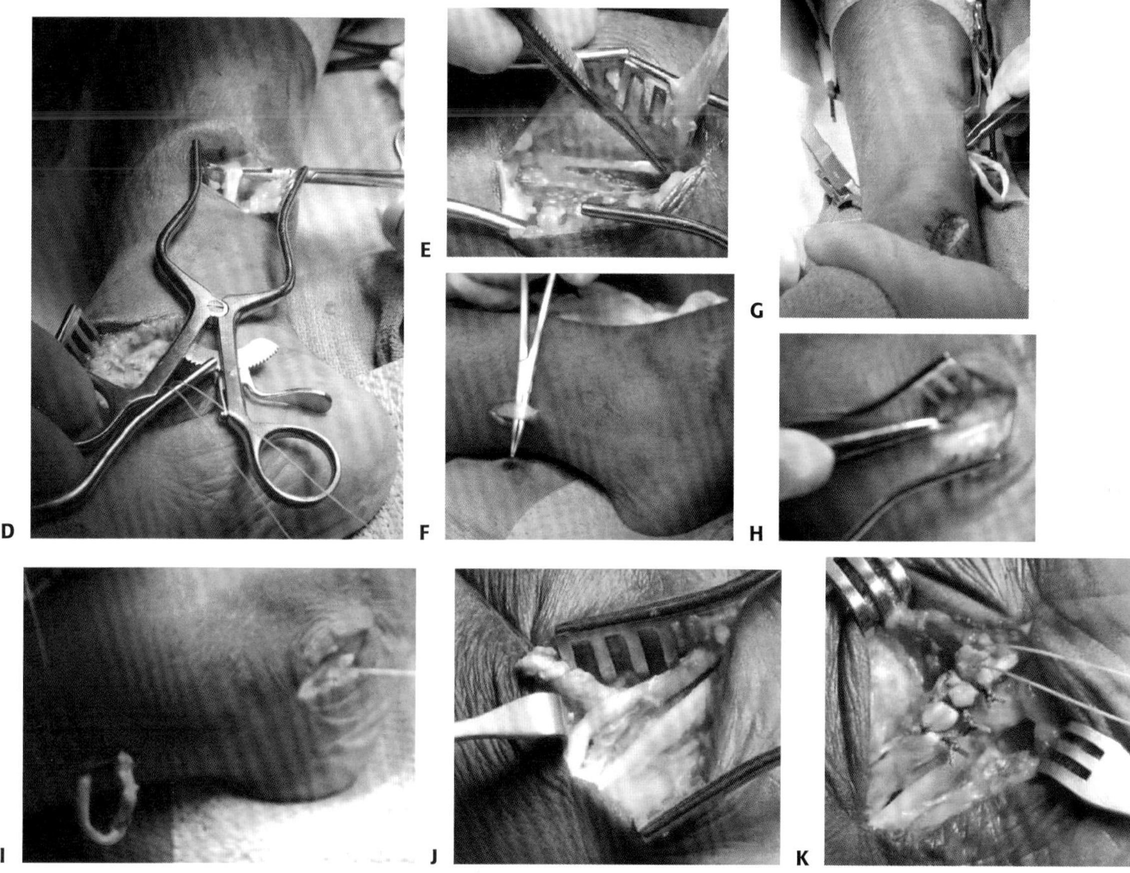

**TECH FIG 1** • *(continued)* **D.** A second incision is made just posterior to the medial border of the tibia, proximal to the medial malleolus. The fascia is divided longitudinally, and the tibialis posterior muscle is identified. **E.** The suture ends are delivered from distal to proximal through the tendon sheath, and the split tendon is brought out from the second incision. **F.** A short longitudinal incision is then made over the lateral side of the leg, posterior to the fibula, across from the medial incision. **G.** The split tendon is then passed from medial to lateral along the posterior border of the tibia and the fibula, anterior to the neurovascular bundle. The tendon is delivered through the lateral wound. **H.** The fourth incision is distal and just behind the fibular malleolus. The peroneal sheath is incised longitudinally. **I.** The split tendon is brought through the sheath from the more proximal incision through this distal incision. **J,K.** The tibialis posterior tendon is then woven through small longitudinal splits in the peroneus brevis and anchored with nonabsorbable suture.

- The fourth longitudinal incision is made distal to the lateral malleolus, overlying the insertion of the peroneus brevis into the fifth metatarsal base (**TECH FIG 1H**).
  - The split tibialis posterior tendon is then passed through the sheath, along the peroneus brevis, into the distal incision (**TECH FIG 1I**).
  - The tendon is woven through the peroneus brevis and secured with nonabsorbable sutures (**TECH FIG 1J,K**).
  - The foot is held in a neutral position.
- A weight-bearing, long-leg cast with the knee extended and the foot at neutral is worn for 4 weeks, and then a short-leg, weight-bearing cast is worn for 4 additional weeks.
- No bracing is required if the patient is able to actively dorsiflex the foot to neutral. If not, an ankle–foot orthosis is recommended.

## Split Tibialis Tendon Transfer through the Interosseous Membrane to the Lateral Cuneiform (after Saji)

- A medial approach extends from 5 cm proximal to the medial malleolus to the insertion of the tibialis posterior tendon on the navicular.
- The anterior (dorsal) half of the tendon is released and split up to the musculotendinous junction, preserving the retinaculum.
- A 2-cm incision is made anteriorly, and a window is made in the interosseous membrane just proximal to the syndesmotic ligament.
- The split tendon is passed anteriorly through the interosseous membrane.

- A 2-cm incision is made over the lateral cuneiform, and the split tendon is delivered subcutaneously and then passed through a drill hole in the lateral cuneiform.
  - The tendon is secured over a button on the plantar surface of the foot, with the foot held in a neutral position.
- The patient is placed in a below-knee cast with the foot in slight valgus and neutral dorsiflexion–plantarflexion.
  - Weight bearing is allowed after 3 weeks, and a brace is worn for 6 to 12 months.

## Split Tibialis Tendon Transfer through the Interosseous Membrane to the Peroneus Brevis (after Mulier)

- A longitudinal incision is made at the insertion of the tibialis posterior, and the plantar half of the tendon is released from the navicular. The muscle is split longitudinally as described previously.
- A second incision is made proximally, and the tendon is delivered through this incision and split up to the musculotendinous junction.
- The third incision is made anteriorly, and the tendon is delivered through a window in the interosseous membrane (just above the anterior inferior syndesmotic ligament).
- The fourth incision is made over the distal insertion of the peroneus brevis tendon, and the tibialis posterior is passed through a subcutaneous tunnel and woven into the distal peroneus brevis with nonabsorbable suture.
- A long-leg cast is used for 3 weeks and then a short-leg cast (weight bearing as tolerated) for an additional 3 weeks.

## PEARLS AND PITFALLS

| | |
|---|---|
| **Define etiology of equinovarus preoperatively** | ▪ Dynamic EMG may help to determine which muscle is responsible (tibialis posterior, tibialis anterior, or both). |
| **Achieve full range of passive motion** | ▪ The patient may need additional procedures such as osteotomy to restore alignment and motion. |
| **Avoid overcorrection** | ▪ The transfer should be tensioned with the hindfoot at neutral to slight valgus.<br>▪ Concomitant tibial derotational osteotomy should not be performed at the same time. |
| **Avoid recurrence** | ▪ The surgeon should consider waiting after 6–8 years of age to perform the procedure. |

## POSTOPERATIVE CARE

- Casting is recommended for 6 to 8 weeks, and options include a long-leg cast for 3 to 4 weeks, followed by a short-leg cast (weight bearing as tolerated) for 3 to 4 weeks,[3,11] versus a short-leg cast for 6 weeks.[16] The hindfoot is kept in neutral to slight valgus.
- Physical therapy is advised when the cast is removed.
- Weight bearing is typically delayed for 6 weeks, and an ankle–foot orthosis is worn after the cast is removed. Therapy focuses on range of motion and strengthening.
- An ankle–foot orthosis is commonly recommended for up to 6 months after removal of the cast and may be required over the long term to facilitate clearance if active dorsiflexion is inadequate.

## OUTCOMES

- Several authors have reported short- to midterm results after transfer behind the tibia and fibula to the peroneus brevis.[3–8,12]
- The long-term results after this procedure have been the subject of two studies.[2,17–19]
  - In one study,[2] 25% developed recurrent equinus, and treatment failure was observed in 44% (14 with more than 10 degrees varus, 25 with more than 10 degrees valgus). Results were inferior in diplegics and quadriplegics, patients younger than 8 years of age, and those who had not achieved a community level of ambulation. A host of variables, including persistent spasticity, may result in progressive deformity through growth and development, especially in children with more profound degrees of neuromuscular involvement.
  - In the second study, involving the 38 feet treated by the Green technique[3] followed for an average of 10 years, 89.5% had a good or excellent result.[18] The mean age at surgery was 10.8 years. The 4 feet graded as failures all had recurrence of equinovarus, which was felt to be due to technical errors.
- The technique involving split tibialis posterior transfer through the interosseous membrane has been the subject of two reports, in which 44 patients were studied at short- to midterm follow-up.[11,16]
  - Forty-one of these had an excellent or good result, and the three poor results were due to overcorrection (one) and undercorrection (two).
  - The transfer helped to restore active dorsiflexion in most of the patients, eliminating the need for orthotics.

## COMPLICATIONS

- Although immediate complications are uncommon (wound infection, pull-out of the transferred tendon, undercorrection or overcorrection), late complications are more common and relate to the effects of many variables in a growing child with spasticity and persistent neuromuscular imbalance.

- Recurrent deformity results from persistent muscle imbalance, pull-out of the tibialis posterior from the peroneus brevis, insufficient tension when suturing the tibialis posterior tendon, or other variables associated with growth.[14]
- Overcorrection into valgus is most common in younger children and in patients treated by concurrent tibial derotational osteotomy.

## REFERENCES

1. Barto PS, Supinski RS, Skinner SR. Dynamic EMG findings in varus hindfoot deformity and spastic cerebral palsy. Dev Med Child Neurol 1984;26:88–93.
2. Chang CH, Albarracin JP, Lipton GE, et al. Long-term followup of surgery for equinovarus foot deformity in children with cerebral palsy. J Pediatr Orthop 2002;22:792–799.
3. Green NE, Griffin PP, Shiavi R. Split posterior tibial-tendon transfer is spastic cerebral palsy. J Bone Joint Surg Am 1983;65(6):748–754.
4. Kagaya H, Yamada S, Nagasawa T, et al. Split posterior tibial tendon transfer for varus deformity of hindfoot. Clin Orthop Relat Res 1996;(323):254–260.
5. Kaufer H. Split tendon transfer. Orthop Trans 1977;191:1.
6. Kling TF, Kaufer H, Hensinger RN. Split posterior tibial tendon transfers in children with spastic cerebral paralysis and equinovarus deformity. J Bone Joint Surg Am 1985;67(2):186–194.
7. Liggio FJ, Kruse R. Split tibialis posterior tendon transfer with concomitant distal tibial derotational osteotomy in children with cerebral palsy. J Pediatr Orthop 2001;21:95–101.
8. Medina PA, Karpman RR, Yeong AT. Split posterior tibial tendon transfer for spastic equinovarus foot deformity. Foot Ankle 1989;10:65–67.
9. Michlitsch MG, Rethlefsen SA, Kay RM. The contributions of anterior and posterior tibialis dysfunction to varus foot deformity in patients with cerebral palsy. J Bone Joint Surg Am 2006;88(8):1764–1768.
10. Moran MF, Sanders JO, Sharkey NA, et al. Effect of attachment site and routing variations in split tendon transfer of the tibialis posterior. J Pediatr Orthop 2004;24:298–303.
11. Mulier T, Moens P, Molenaers G, et al. Split posterior tibial tendon transfer through the interosseous membrane in spastic equinovarus deformity. Foot Ankle Int 1995;16:754–759.
12. O'Byrne JM, Kennedy A, Jenkinson A, et al. Split tibialis posterior tendon transfer in the treatment of spastic equinovarus foot. J Pediatr Orthop 1997;17:481–485.
13. Perry J, Hoffer MM. Preoperative and postoperative dynamic electromyography as an aid in planning tendon transfers in children with cerebral palsy. J Bone Joint Surg Am 1977;59(4):531–537.
14. Piazza SJ, Adamson RL, Moran MF, et al. Effects of tensioning errors in split transfers of tibialis anterior and posterior tendons. J Bone Joint Surg Am 2003;85-A(8):858–865.
15. Piazza SJ, Adamson RL, Sanders JO, et al. Changes in muscle moment arms following split tendon transfer of tibialis anterior and tibialis posterior. Gait Posture 2001;14:271–278.
16. Saji MJ, Upadhyay SS, Hsu LC, et al. Split tibialis posterior transfer for equinovarus deformity in cerebral palsy. J Bone Joint Surg Br 1993;75(3):489–501.
17. Synder M, Kumar SJ, Stecyk MD. Split tibialis posterior tendon transfer and tendo-Achilles lengthening for spastic equinovarus feet. J Pediatr Orthop 1993;13:20–23.
18. Vlachou M, Beris A, Dimitriadis D. Split tibialis posterior tendon transfer for correction of spastic equinovarus hindfoot deformity. Acta Orthop Belg 2010;76:651–657.
19. Vlachou M, Dimitriadis D. Split tendon transfers for the correction of spastic varus foot deformity: a case series study. J Foot Ankle Res 2010;3:28.

120 CHAPTER

# Surgical Correction of Juvenile Bunion

**B. David Horn**

## DEFINITION

- Adolescent bunion is a multifactorial, complex deformity consisting of medial deviation of the first metatarsal (metatarsus primus varus), lateral deviation of the great toe through the first metatarsophalangeal joint (hallux valgus), and enlarged medial eminence of the distal first metatarsal.[2–4,6]
- Other findings include contracted lateral and lax medial soft tissues of the first metatarsophalangeal joint, lateral subluxation of the sesamoids, pronation of the great toe, plantar subluxation of the abductor hallucis muscle, and generalized ligamentous laxity, flexible pes planus, and gastrocnemius contracture.

## ANATOMY

- Metatarsus primus varus resulting in increased intermetatarsal (IM) angle[2,3]
- Obliquity of the medial cuneiform–first metatarsal joint[2,3]
- Medial prominence of the first metatarsal head
- Valgus angulation through the first metatarsophalangeal joint[2,3]
- Minimal or no deformity through the first interphalangeal joint
- Lateral translation of sesamoids
- Plantar–lateral positioning of the abductor hallucis with unopposed pull of the adductor hallucis muscle
- Lateral subluxation of the extensor hallucis longus and flexor hallucis longus tendons
- Pronation (internal rotation) of the first toe
- Differs from an adult bunion
  - Physis of the first metatarsal and proximal phalanx are located proximally (this limits ability to perform proximal osteotomies in skeletally immature patients).
  - The first metatarsophalangeal joint does not have osteoarthrosis.
  - The medial eminence is less prominent in adolescent bunions than in adult bunions.

## PATHOGENESIS

- Multiple theories exist; it is difficult to differentiate primary findings from secondary ones.[2,3,6]
- Extrinsic and intrinsic factors contribute to formation of adolescent bunions.
- Intrinsic
  - Metatarsus primus varus
  - Obliquity of the medial cuneiform–first metatarsal joint
  - Long first metatarsal
  - Ligamentous laxity
  - Heel cord contracture causes foot pronation, which in turn places a valgus force on the hallux while walking
- Extrinsic
  - Shoe wear, particularly those with a narrow toe and elevated heel

## NATURAL HISTORY

- Natural history is believed to be favorable. Most patients with adolescent bunions can be treated nonoperatively.[2,5]

## PATIENT HISTORY AND PHYSICAL FINDINGS

- Patients typically present in late childhood or adolescence.[2,3]
- Complaints about appearance of foot
- Complaints of pain over the medial exostosis or about the first metatarsophalangeal joint
- Pain is exacerbated by shoe wear.
- Complaints about finding shoes that are comfortable
- Physical examination[2,3]
  - Areas of tenderness: first metatarsophalangeal joint, medial prominence
  - Alignment when standing and walking
  - Mobility of first metatarsophalangeal joint
  - Skin condition: the clinician should search for calluses, areas of irritation
  - Foot and ankle range of motion
- Careful neurologic examination

## IMAGING AND OTHER DIAGNOSTIC STUDIES

- Standing anteroposterior (AP), lateral, and oblique radiographs should be obtained if surgical correction is being contemplated.[1,2]
- Measurements on the AP radiograph[1,2] (**FIG 1**)
  - IM angle: Normal is 9 degrees or less.
    - IM angle usually is 12 to 18 degrees in adolescent bunion.
  - Hallux valgus angle: Normal is 16 degrees or less.
    - Less than 25 degrees indicates mild deformity.
    - Twenty-five to 40 degrees is moderate deformity.
    - More than 40 degrees is severe.
    - Most adolescent bunions are mild to moderate.
  - Distal metatarsal articular angle: Normal is 15 degrees or less.
  - Proximal phalangeal articular angle: Normal is 5 degrees of valgus.

## DIFFERENTIAL DIAGNOSIS

- Hallux valgus interphalangeus

## NONOPERATIVE MANAGEMENT

- Initial treatment is nonoperative.[2,4]
- Proper-fitting shoes
- Achilles tendon/calf muscle stretching if there is a heel cord/gastrocnemius contracture
- Orthotics may be useful when there is also ligamentous laxity and pes planus.

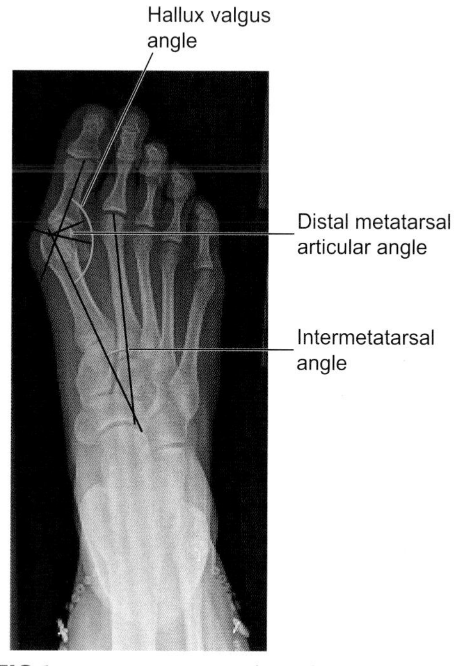


**FIG 1** ● Measurements made on the AP radiograph.

## SURGICAL MANAGEMENT

- Surgery should be reserved for patients with persistent symptoms despite adequate nonoperative care.[2–5]
- Goals are to decrease pain and to restore the alignment of the first ray, with respect to both the second ray and the joints of the ray itself.[2–5]
- If feasible, surgery is delayed until early adolescence, as recurrence rates are higher in younger children.
- Patients and their families should be carefully counseled regarding postoperative expectations, particularly the risk of recurrence.
- The surgical plan needs to factor in the age of the patient and address the unique characteristics of each deformity.
- Multiple procedures have been described, including hemiepiphysiodesis of the lateral first metatarsal physis, distal osteotomies, scarf osteotomies, and proximal osteotomies.[2–5]
- For "typical" adolescent bunion (IM angle 12 to 18 degrees, hallux valgus angle <40 degrees), surgery generally consists of a distal soft tissue procedure, excision of the medial prominence, and corrective osteotomy.
- In older adolescents, where the physis of the first metatarsal is closed, the corrective osteotomy can be performed proximally.
- If the physis of the first metatarsal is open, a first metatarsal neck osteotomy has been described (Mitchell procedure).

### Preoperative Planning

- The surgeon should review the patient's radiographs to determine IM angle and hallux valgus angle.[2–4]

### Positioning

- The patient is positioned supine.
- A tourniquet is used.

### Approach

- A dorsomedial incision is made starting just distal to the first metatarsophalangeal joint and extending proximally for 5 to 6 cm.
- The surgeon should avoid injury to the dorsal medial sensory nerve.

TECHNIQUES

## Mitchell Bunionectomy (Stevens Modification)

- Expose the medial first metatarsophalangeal joint.
- Make a distally based Y-shaped incision in the capsule and periosteum. The stem of the Y is over the metatarsal, whereas the upper portion of the Y is formed distally.
  - The joint and medial eminence are then exposed.
- A medial release of the first metatarsophalangeal joint is performed. Leave the lateral portion of the joint intact to avoid disrupting the blood supply to the head of the first metatarsal.
- The first cut involves removing the prominent medial eminence with an osteotome, starting distally at the sagittal groove (groove of Clark).
- The second cut is made at the distal metaphyseal–diaphyseal junction of the first metatarsal. This should be perpendicular to the shaft of the first metatarsal and extend two-thirds the width of the shaft of the first metatarsal (**TECH FIG 1A**).
- The third, proximal cut is made about 2 to 3 mm proximal to the first cut and is created completely across the first metatarsal. The cut is oriented perpendicular to the shaft of the second metatarsal when viewed from the dorsum of the foot and is angled (when viewed from the medial aspect of the first metatarsal) to create a small plantar-based wedge (**TECH FIG 1B**). This ensures that the distal fragment does not dorsiflex during reduction of the osteotomy.
- The interposed bone is removed.
- The osteotomy is reduced and pinned with two smooth 0.062-inch Kirschner wires (**TECH FIG 1C**).
- The prominence of the distal portion of the metatarsal shaft is smoothed off with a rongeur, and a capsulorrhaphy is performed with absorbable sutures.
- Sterile dressings are applied, and the toe is splinted in neutral to slight plantarflexion. A short-leg cast is usually applied over the dressing for additional protection.

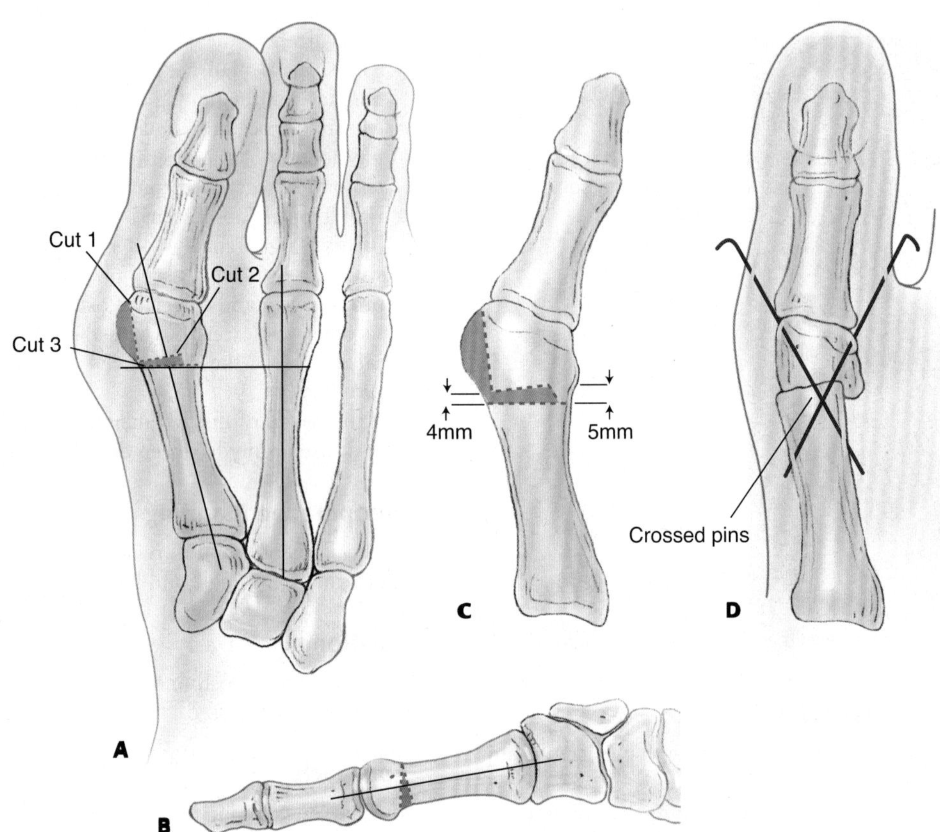


**TECH FIG 1** • **A.** Bone cuts required to perform a modified Mitchell osteotomy. The medial prominence is excised first (*cut 1*). The first cut of the osteotomy is performed two-thirds of the way through the first metatarsal at the junction of the metaphysis and diaphysis and is oriented perpendicular to the long axis of the first metatarsal (*cut 2*). The second bone cut (*cut 3*) is made completely through the bone and completes the osteotomy. It should be made 2 to 4 mm proximal to the first cut and is perpendicular to the long axis of the second metatarsal. **B.** When seen from the medial side, the osteotomy should be oriented so that a small plantar-based wedge is produced. This helps avoid dorsiflexion of the distal fragment when the osteotomy is reduced. **C,D.** The osteotomy is reduced and stabilized with a 0.062-inch smooth Kirschner wire.

## PEARLS AND PITFALLS

| | |
|---|---|
| **Approach** | ▪ The surgeon should identify and protect the dorsal sensory nerve. |
| **Osteotomy** | ▪ The surgeon should avoid resecting more than about 3 mm of bone to prevent shortening of the first metatarsal. |
| **Proximal osteotomy** | ▪ It should create a slight plantar-based wedge with the distal cut to avoid dorsiflexion of the osteotomy. |

## POSTOPERATIVE CARE

- The toe is splinted in slight flexion.
- The dressing is covered with a cast.
- Weight bearing is allowed as tolerated.
- Pins are removed in 6 weeks.

## OUTCOMES

- Most studies report 65% to 85% good to excellent results with the Mitchell osteotomy.[1–4]
- The modified Mitchell osteotomy (described earlier) produces 81% satisfactory results, with no cases of malunion, nonunion, avascular necrosis of the first metatarsal head, infection, or transfer metatarsalgia.[3,4]
- Sixty percent good to excellent results are reported in younger patients.

## COMPLICATIONS

- Infection
- Neurovascular injury
- Inadequate fixation of the osteotomy
- Malunion or nonunion of the osteotomy
- Avascular necrosis of the first metatarsal head

- Transfer metatarsalgia
- Recurrence
- Stiffness of the first metatarsophalangeal joint
- Hallux varus (overcorrection)
- Pronation
- Pain

## REFERENCES


1. Davids JR, McBrayer D, Blackhurst DW. Juvenile hallux valgus deformity: surgical management by lateral hemiepiphyseodesis of the great toe metatarsal. J Pediatr Orthop 2007;27:826–830.
2. Farrar NG, Duncan N, Ahmed N, et al. Scarf osteotomy in the management of symptomatic adolescent hallux valgus. J Child Orthop 2012;6:153–157.
3. Kuo CH, Huang PJ, Cheng YM, et al. Modified Mitchell osteotomy for hallux valgus. Foot Ankle Int 1998;19:585–589.
4. McDonald MG, Stevens DB. Modified Mitchell bunionectomy for management of adolescent hallux valgus. Clin Orthop Relat Res 1996;(332):163–169.
5. Mitchell CL, Fleming JL, Allen R, et al. Osteotomy-bunionectomy for hallux valgus. J Bone Joint Surg Am 1958;40-A(1):41–58.
6. Weiner BK, Weiner DS, Mirkopulos N. Mitchell osteotomy for adolescent hallux valgus. J Pediatr Orthop 1997;17:781–784.

# Butler Procedure for Overlapping Fifth Toe

B. David Horn

## DEFINITION

- Overlapping fifth toe is a congenital condition where the fifth toe is rotated and overrides the fourth toe.[1–3]
- It is frequently bilateral.
- Males are affected as frequently as females.

## ANATOMY

- There are seven main components:
  - The fifth toe may be smaller than normal.
  - The fifth toe is adducted toward the fourth toe.
  - The fifth metatarsophalangeal joint has a dorsiflexion contracture.
  - The phalanges of the fifth toe are rotated laterally.
  - The fifth extensor digitorum longus tendon is shortened.
  - The fifth metatarsophalangeal joint is dislocated dorsally.
  - The skin in the fourth web space is contracted.

## PATHOGENESIS

- The exact pathogenesis is unknown, but the condition is believed to be secondary to a congenital contracture of the fifth extensor digitorum longus tendon.[1]

## NATURAL HISTORY

- This condition rarely causes pain or difficulty in shoe wear in children younger than 10 years of age.
- In older children and adolescents, there will be painful dorsal callosities about 50% of the time.
- There may also be difficulty in finding shoes that fit appropriately in older children and adolescents.
- Parents are frequently concerned about the cosmetic appearance of the foot.

## PATIENT HISTORY AND PHYSICAL FINDINGS

- The fifth toe will be dorsiflexed, adducted, and laterally rotated. It will not be passively correctable into a neutral position (**FIG 1A,B**).
- A careful neurovascular examination should be performed and documented.

## IMAGING AND OTHER DIAGNOSTIC STUDIES

- Plain anteroposterior (AP), lateral, and oblique radiographs may be obtained and will demonstrate a dorsolaterally subluxated fifth metatarsophalangeal joint.

## NONOPERATIVE MANAGEMENT

- Conservative treatment (eg, stretching, splinting, taping) is ineffective in the treatment of this condition.[1,2]

## SURGICAL MANAGEMENT

- Surgery is indicated when nonoperative treatment fails, such as failure to find comfortable shoes or when there is intractable pain from shoes.

### Positioning

- The patient is supine, preferably with a bolster beneath the ipsilateral hemipelvis to make the lateral foot more accessible.
- A tourniquet should be used during the procedure.

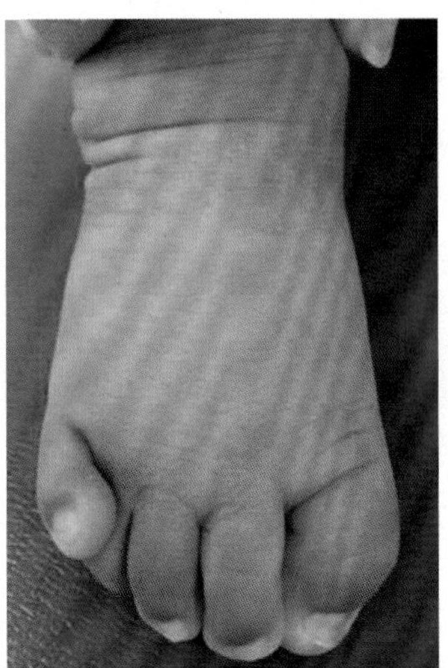


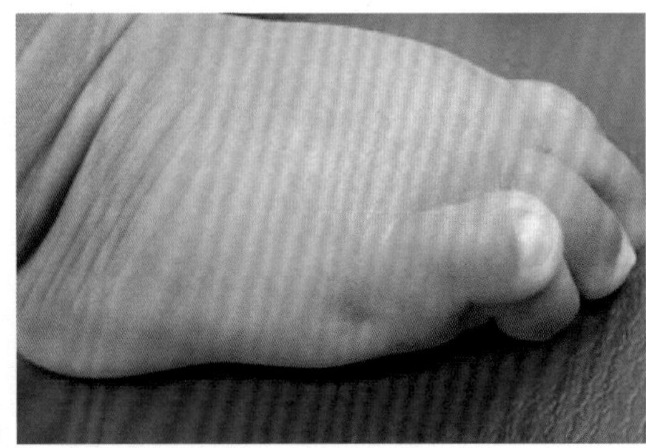


**FIG 1** • **A,B.** Frontal and lateral image of overlapping fifth toe. (Picture courtesy of Richard Davidson, MD.)

## Butler Procedure for Overlapping Fifth Toe

- A dorsal racquet incision is made about the toe with a second handle to the racquet added on the plantar aspect of the toe (**TECH FIG 1A**).
- The plantar handle should be slightly longer than the dorsal handle and directed slightly laterally.
- The skin flaps are elevated and the tight extensor tendon is exposed.
- Care should be taken to identify and protect the neurovascular bundles (**TECH FIG 1B**).
- The extensor tendon is lengthened, and a dorsomedial release of the fifth metatarsophalangeal joint is performed. If needed, the plantar aspect of the fifth metatarsophalangeal joint may be dissected off the metatarsal head and divided to increase joint mobility (**TECH FIG 1C**).
- The toe should freely move plantarward and laterally into its corrected position (**TECH FIG 1D**).
  - There should be no tension on the toe, and the toe should rest within the plantar handle of the racquet incision.
- Interrupted sutures are then used to hold the toe reduced in place (**TECH FIG 1E**).
- A cast or hard-soled shoe can be used postoperatively.

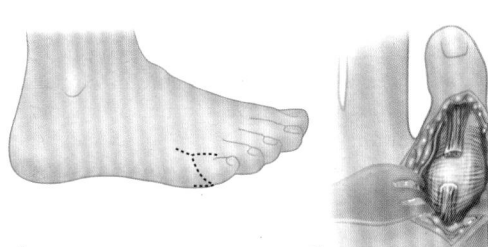

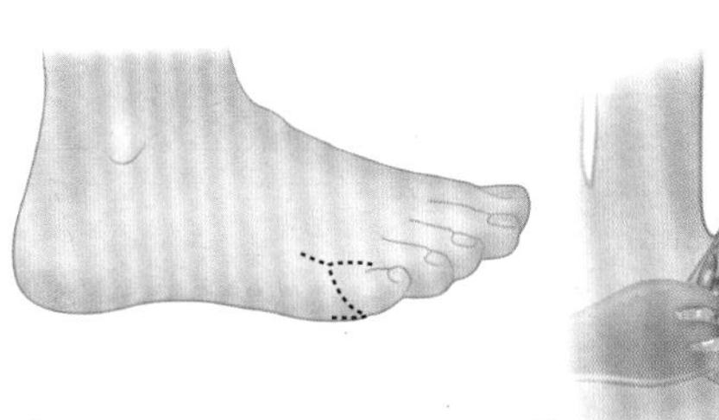

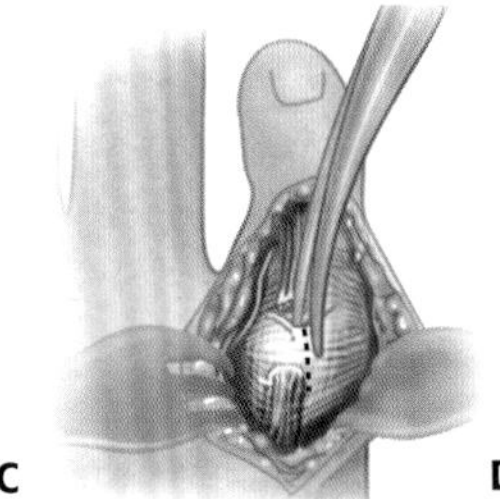

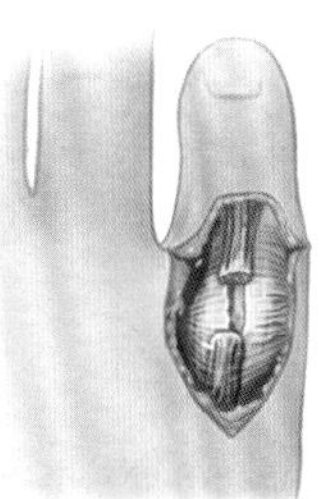

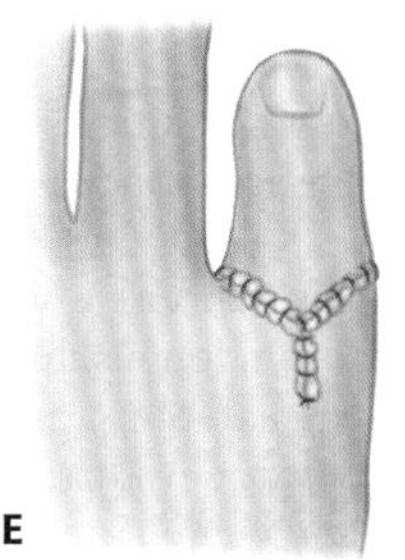

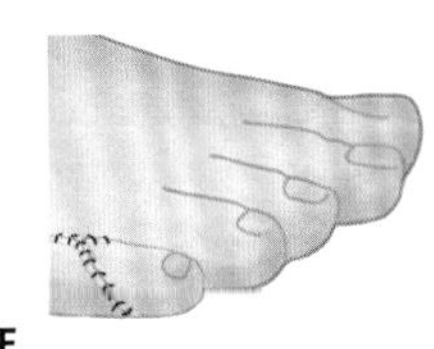


**TECH FIG 1** • **A.** A racquet incision with plantar and dorsal extensions is used. **B.** Deep dissection is performed, preserving the neurovascular bundles. An extensor tenotomy is performed. **C.** A capsular release is performed. **D.** The toe should now reside in its corrected position. **E,F.** The incisions are closed with interrupted sutures. They help provide stability to the reconstruction.

## PEARLS AND PITFALLS

| | |
|---|---|
| **Incomplete release of soft tissues** | ■ The surgeon should assess the plantar capsule for tightness as well as the dorsal capsule. |
| **Neurovascular compromise** | ■ The neurovascular bundles should be protected during the procedure, and traction on the fifth toe is avoided. Circumferential dressings about the toe are avoided. |

## POSTOPERATIVE CARE

- Postoperative care includes sterile dressings and allowing mobilization and weight bearing as tolerated.

## OUTCOMES

- This procedure has a high patient satisfaction rate (about 90%) in various studies.
- Black et al[1] reported 94% good to excellent results.

## COMPLICATIONS

- Incomplete correction
- Neurovascular compromise
- Scar contracture
- Infection

## REFERENCES


1. Black GB, Grogan DP, Bobechko WP. Butler arthroplasty for correction of the adducted fifth toe: a retrospective study of 36 operations between 1968 and 1982. J Pediatr Orthop 1985;5:439–441.
2. Cockin J. Butler's operation for an over-riding fifth toe. J Bone Joint Surg Br 1968;50(1):78–81.
3. De Boeck H. Butler's operation for congenital overriding of the fifth toe. Retrospective 1- to 7-year study of 23 cases. Acta Orthop Scand 1993;64:343–344.

CHAPTER 122

# Surgical Treatment of Cavus Foot

Richard M. Schwend and Brad Olney

## DEFINITION

- A cavus foot deformity in children develops from muscle imbalance that leads to forefoot pronation in relation to the hindfoot. When well established, it is readily recognizable by an abnormally high medial arch that persists with weight bearing (**FIG 1**).
- Commonly a result of hereditary sensory motor neuropathy (HSMN), it is frequently difficult to determine the underlying cause.

## ANATOMY

- The plantar fascia is an extensive fibrous structure that spans the foot between the medial aspect of the calcaneal tuberosity and the transverse metatarsal ligaments at the metatarsal heads (**FIG 2**). It stabilizes the arch of the foot and protects the underlying neurovascular structures from injury.
- During the gait cycle, the plantar fascia assists in the dynamic changes of the arch.
  - At heel strike, there is forefoot supination and heel inversion, whereas eccentric contraction of the quadriceps muscles absorbs much of the energy.
  - During midstance, there is unlocking of the midtarsal joints with hindfoot pronation and internal tibia rotation.
  - At toe off, the plantar fascia helps lock the midtarsal joints to assist the foot to be a rigid lever for forward propulsion.
- This is termed the *windlass effect*, when passive dorsiflexion at the metatarsophalangeal joints tightens the plantar fascia, leading to elevation of the medial arch and tarsal joint stability (**FIG 3**).

## PATHOGENESIS

- In progressive conditions such as HSMN, there is muscle imbalance with weakness of the intrinsic, tibialis anterior, and peroneus brevis muscles. This can lead to a relative overpull of the peroneus longus and posterior tibialis muscles.
  - Clinical muscle testing shows that although both peroneal muscles are weak, the larger peroneus longus muscle retains relatively more strength. Differential peroneal nerve compression at the proximal fibula is postulated to cause relative sparing of the peroneus longus innervation.[5]
- Computed tomography (CT) imaging studies in Charcot-Marie-Tooth disease, a major category of HSMN, showed early foot intrinsic muscle atrophy with sparing of the abductor hallucis and involvement of the peroneus brevis, peroneus longus, and flexor hallucis longus muscles.[13]
- Magnetic resonance imaging (MRI) studies have shown dominance in the size of the peroneus longus muscle versus the tibialis anterior.[16]
- The muscle imbalance and intrinsic muscle weakness lead to an unopposed extensor digitorum longus, hyperextension of the lesser toe metatarsophalangeal joints, and phalangeal joint flexion by the long and short toe flexors.
  - There is an exaggeration of the windlass effect with claw toe deformities.

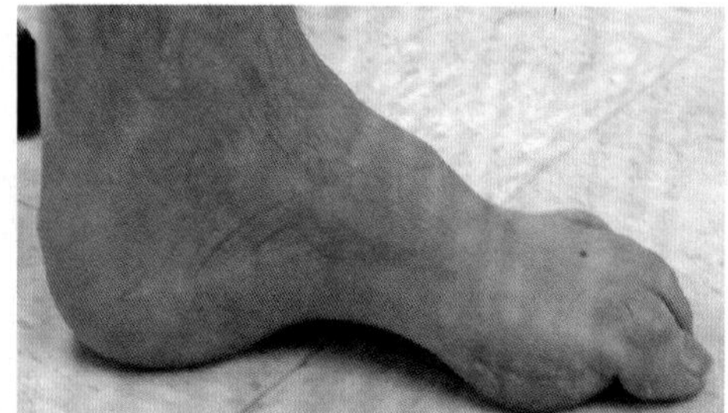

**FIG 1** • A 17-year-old girl with HSMN type 1A. Cavus right foot deformity with high arch, plantar crease, apex of deformity at the midfoot, and claw toes.

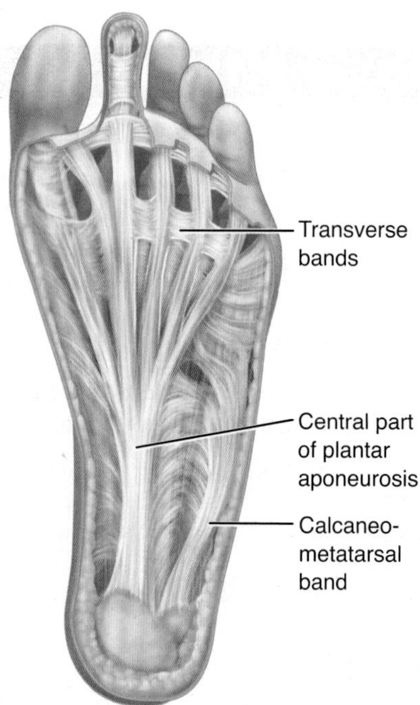


**FIG 2** • Plantar view of plantar fascia.

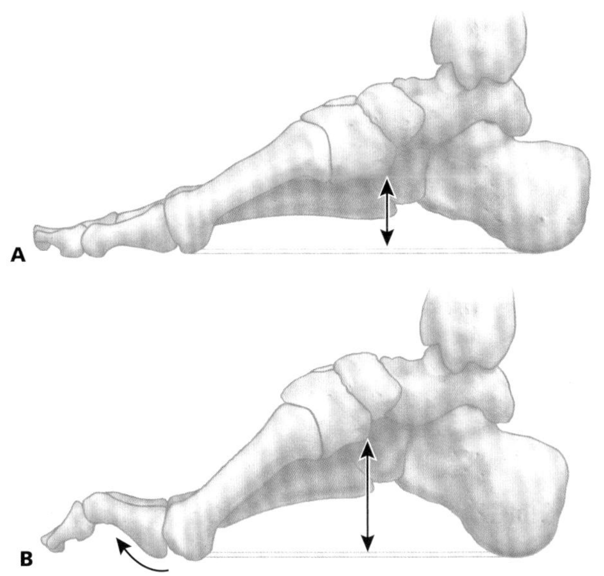


**FIG 3** ● **A,B.** Windlass effect. The foot is an arch. If the plantar tissues tighten and become shorter, the fixed length of the arch forces it to become taller.

- The first metatarsal becomes even more plantarflexed by the action of the peroneus longus and with time becomes fixed in this position.
- The plantar aspect of the foot assumes a tripod position, resulting in hindfoot varus (**FIG 4**).
- The cavus foot remains a rigid lever throughout stance phase, leading to increased stress and lack of shock absorption, pain, and callosities.

## NATURAL HISTORY

- Cavus foot is rarely present at birth but develops with time.
- The natural history depends on the underlying diagnosis. The underlying cause affects the outcome, so determination of cause is essential. An underlying diagnosis can be found in the brain, spinal cord, peripheral nerves, or the foot itself.
- Cavus foot deformity can be either progressive or nonprogressive.
- Cavus foot deformity involves either a dorsiflexion deformity of the calcaneus or a forefoot plantarflexion deformity.
- The most common cause of progressive bilateral cavus foot deformity is HSMN. HSMN is a group of progressive peripheral nerve diseases and has a heterogeneous genetic classification.
  - Charcot-Marie-Tooth disease involves types I and II HSMN, with HSMN IA the most common type seen in 60% of patients with HSMN.
    - HSMN type I has myelin degeneration, type II is the axonal degeneration form, and type III (Dejerine-Sottas disease) is more severe and presents in infancy.
    - There are more than 17 different genetic loci determined for Charcot-Marie-Tooth disease.
    - The prognosis for these progressive conditions is less favorable than for the nonprogressive disorders.
  - The natural history of HSMN is related to the underlying type.
    - Progression of muscle involvement begins initially in the intrinsic muscles, followed by the anterior compartment, the peroneal muscles, and then the posterior muscles.[14]

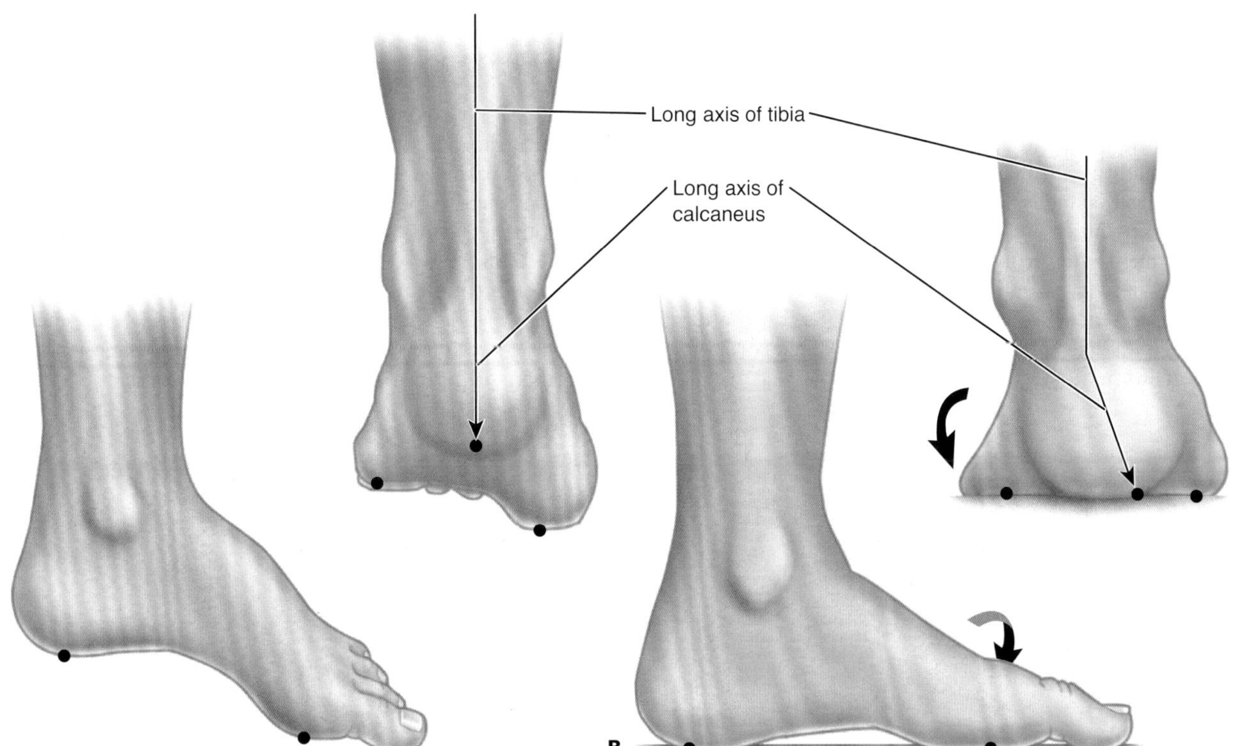


**FIG 4** ● **A,B.** Tripod effect. Weight bearing is shared between the heel and medial and lateral columns of the forefoot. If the medial column is in plantarflexion, the heel is forced into varus with weight bearing.

- The foot can assume a cavovarus, calcaneocavus deformity, or even a valgus deformity and may have more unilateral severity (HSMN type III).[4]
- Associated hip dysplasia may be asymptomatic or may present with symptoms. Acetabular dysplasia may be the first indicator of HSMN.[3]
- In progressive conditions that are left untreated, a flexible and correctable foot may become rigid with structural bony changes. This can lead to inability to participate in athletics and pain and difficulty with shoe wear and normal walking. Treatment is recommended when the foot is still flexible.

- Unilateral cavus foot can have a number of causes. The idiopathic variety may be progressive, with an unpredictable natural history.
- Patients with nonprogressive conditions, as seen in cerebral palsy or spinal cord disorders, may fare better but still can have long-term problems with athletics, metatarsalgia, plantar fasciitis, and iliotibial band syndrome.[9]
- Calcaneocavus deformity is often seen with nonprogressive conditions such as spina bifida or clubfoot deformity with an overlengthened heel cord. Problems include heel pain or heel pad ulceration if sensation is deficient and weak or no push-off or crouch gait if not braced.

## PATIENT HISTORY AND PHYSICAL FINDINGS

- The physical examination is used to determine the underlying diagnosis and to determine characteristics of the cavus foot deformity that would indicate surgical correction is needed.
- Physical examination should include observation of the spine and its range of motion. Skin changes, scoliosis, or kyphosis may represent an underlying spinal cord abnormality.
- The upper extremities are evaluated for intrinsic muscle wasting and weakness. Atrophy or weakness in the hand suggests HSMN.
- The clinician evaluates hip range of motion and looks for Trendelenburg gait. Bilateral hip dysplasia newly diagnosed in a teenager is highly suggestive of HSMN.
- Lower extremities are evaluated for size, muscle strength, and firmness and tenderness along the course of major nerves. Bilateral calf atrophy is seen with spina bifida and may be present in severe HSMN. Unilateral atrophy may be seen with diastematomyelia, tethered spinal cord, or split cord malformation.
- A neurologic examination is performed. Patients with HSMN may have decreased sensation to light touch, position sense, or vibration. There may be obvious weakness of the anterior tibialis muscle, preventing ability to heel walk. Deep tendon reflexes may be decreased or absent in HSMN and Friedreich ataxia.
- The foot is examined for deformity (cavus, cavovarus, or calcaneocavus). Bilateral deformity is typical for HSMN. Unilateral deformity may be present with a structural abnormality. The clinician locates the apex of the midfoot deformity and determines whether the foot is rigid or flexible. The hindfoot is rarely in equinus.
- The Coleman block test is performed (**FIG 5**).
- The toes are examined for any deformities. Cavus foot may not have associated toe abnormality. Rigid claw toe abnormality requires surgical treatment.

## IMAGING AND OTHER DIAGNOSTIC STUDIES

- Bilateral standing anteroposterior (AP) and lateral radiographs are standard.
  - On the lateral weight-bearing radiograph, the clinician should determine the calcaneal pitch; greater than 30 degrees indicates chronic gastrocnemius–soleus weakness (**FIG 6A**).
  - The Meary angle, the angle between the shaft of the first metatarsal and the axis of the talus, is normally 0 degree.
  - Ankle equinus, forefoot equinus, the amount of cavus, and the apex of the midfoot deformity are determined.
- With the foot positioned for the Coleman block test, a lateral radiograph of the foot can document the degree of hindfoot correction.[1]
- In the patient with known or possible HSMN, a standing AP pelvis view is obtained to screen for the presence of hip dysplasia.[17]
- Standing full-length posteroanterior and lateral spine radiographs are obtained when a spinal abnormality is suspected or if the underlying diagnosis is in question.
- MRI of the entire brainstem and cervical, thoracic, and lumbar spine is performed when a spinal cord tumor, syrinx, tethered cord, or Chiari I malformation is of concern (**FIG 6B,C**).
- Nerve conduction and electromyelographic (EMG) studies may be done to evaluate for HMSN. In HMSN type I, motor nerve conduction is markedly slowed. In HMSN type II, there is near-normal motor nerve conduction but EMG

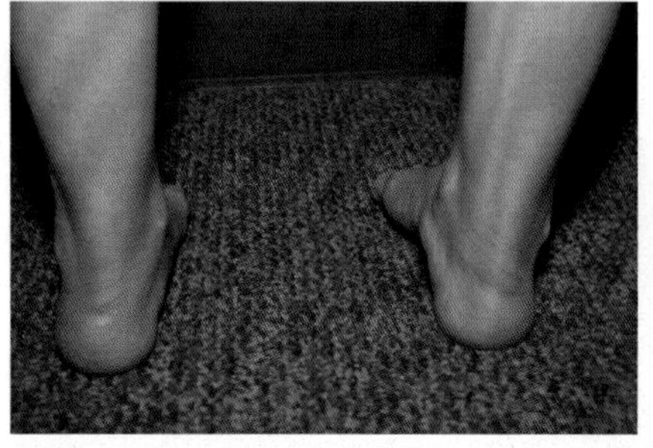


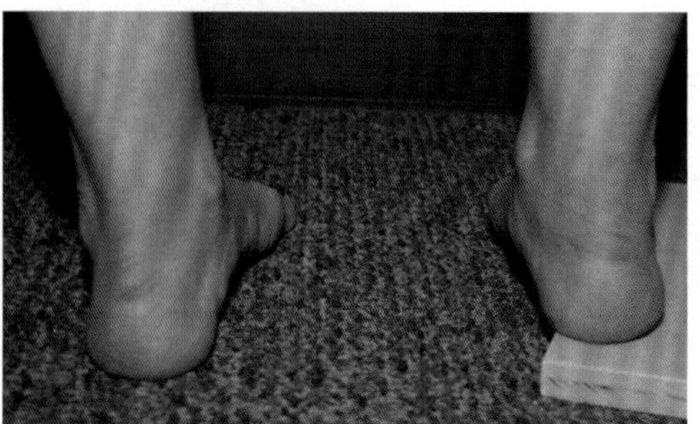


**FIG 5** • **A,B.** In the Coleman block test, the patient bears weight with the lateral border of the foot on a 2-cm block while the first metatarsal is allowed to drop down off the edge of the block. If hindfoot varus corrects to neutral position, the hindfoot is flexible and the medial forefoot is the source of hindfoot varus.

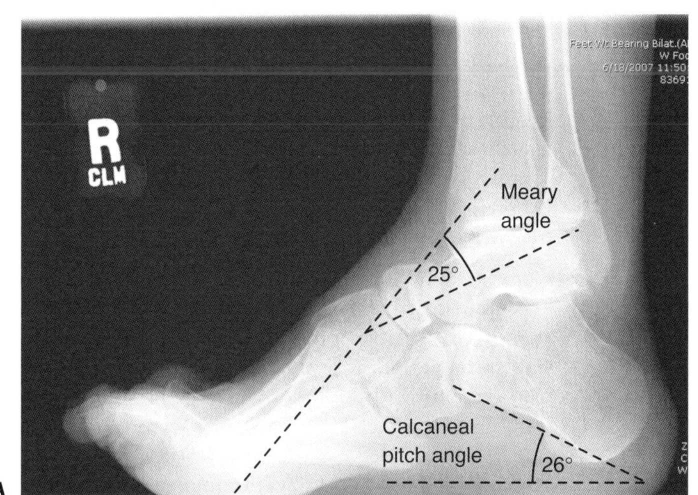


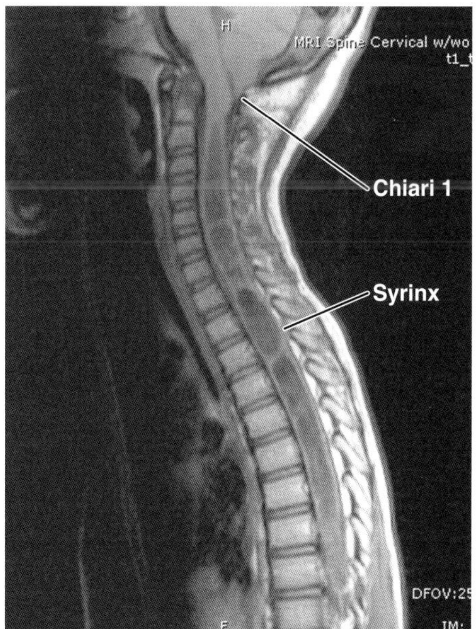


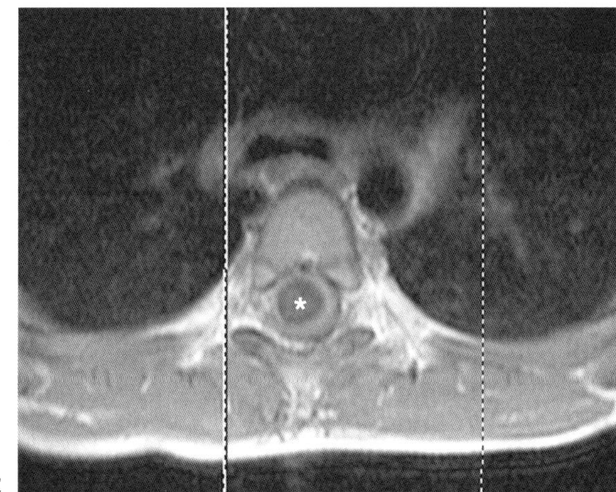


**FIG 6** ● **A.** A 15-year-old boy with HSMN type 1A with severe bilateral cavus foot deformity. Lateral standing radiograph of right foot. The Meary angle, measured between the axis of the talus and the first metatarsal, is 25 degrees, but it should be 0 degrees. The calcaneal pitch angle, measured between the horizontal and the plantar aspect of the calcaneus, is 26 degrees but should be less than 20 degrees. **B.** A 5-year-old girl with 28-degree right thoracic scoliosis. MRI T1-weighted sagittal view of large cervical thoracic syrinx with Chiari I malformation at foramen magnum. **C.** MRI T1-weighted axial view showing large central cord syrinx (*asterisk*).

evidence of denervation. Molecular DNA testing of peripheral blood may be used for diagnosing HSMN; therefore, sural nerve biopsy is generally not necessary.

## DIFFERENTIAL DIAGNOSIS

- Hemiplegic cerebral palsy
- Spastic diplegic cerebral palsy with calcaneocavus foot deformity if the Achilles tendon has been overlengthened
- Friedreich ataxia
- Myelodysplasia
- Chiari I malformation with syringomyelia and scoliosis
- Diastematomyelia and split cord malformation
- Poliomyelitis
- Spinal cord tumors
- Guillain-Barré syndrome
- Peripheral nerves: HSMN types I and II
- Sciatic nerve injury
- Peripheral nerve tumor
- Silent compartment syndrome after tibia or foot fracture
- Residual deformity of clubfoot
- Idiopathic
- Subtalar tarsal coalition (rare)
- Severe limb length discrepancy leading to a fixed equinus gait

## NONOPERATIVE MANAGEMENT

- Nonoperative management is appropriate for mild or nonprogressive deformity.
  - Inserts that support the lateral forefoot and eliminate hindfoot inversion may be helpful.
  - Gel heel cups and replacing worn athletic shoes assist the stiff foot in energy absorption.
  - Extra-depth shoes and orthotics that unload pressure points may help in more advanced cases.

## SURGICAL MANAGEMENT

- Surgical treatment is necessary for more severe nonprogressive cases or for progressive cases. The functional goal is to correct the cavus deformity and to obtain a mobile, plantigrade, and well-balanced foot while avoiding common pitfalls. Treatment is best performed when the foot is still flexible. Staged procedures, correcting deformity first and balancing muscles at a later stage, may be safer for the foot.[12]

- Specific principles for surgical decision making include the following:
  - Surgical management is usually needed when there is an identified functional problem or progression of the deformity. For progressive cavus deformity, it is better to use simple procedures early.
  - Plantar fascia release is the initial procedure of choice in young children with nonprogressive deformity. We prefer to do this through a medial plantar incision with postoperative serial corrective casting used to gain further correction. Plantar fascia release is generally done with other procedures.
  - The surgeon can correct any underlying muscle imbalance with tendon transfers or lengthening or by bony correction of the lever arm that the muscles work through.
  - In a more rigid deformity, a forefoot osteotomy is used to correct the pronated medial forefoot.
    - The goal is to correct the fixed deformity while preserving joint mobility. The site of the osteotomy is determined by the location of the deformity apex. The most common are first metatarsal dorsal closing, medial cuneiform plantar opening, and midfoot wedge osteotomies. If the fixed cavus deformity on the medial side of the foot is severe enough, the first metatarsal dorsal osteotomy can be combined with the medial cuneiform plantar opening osteotomy.[11]
    - For marked and rigid forefoot equinus (**FIG 7**), a more extensive midfoot osteotomy is used; this is typically needed during the patient's second decade of life.[20]
- Calcaneal osteotomy is used if the Coleman block test indicates a fixed heel varus. We recommend a slide osteotomy through a lateral approach, although a lateral closing wedge alone or combined with the slide may also be used for more correction. Tendon transfers are frequently required to achieve a balanced foot. These may involve a transfer of the relatively strong posterior tibialis tendon to the dorsum of the foot,[1] a Jones procedure in which the extensor hallucis tendon is transferred to the neck of the first metatarsal with fusion of the great toe interphalangeal (IP) joint, a split or complete anterior tibialis tendon transfer if the muscle has preserved strength, or a transfer of the peroneus longus to the peroneus brevis.[21]

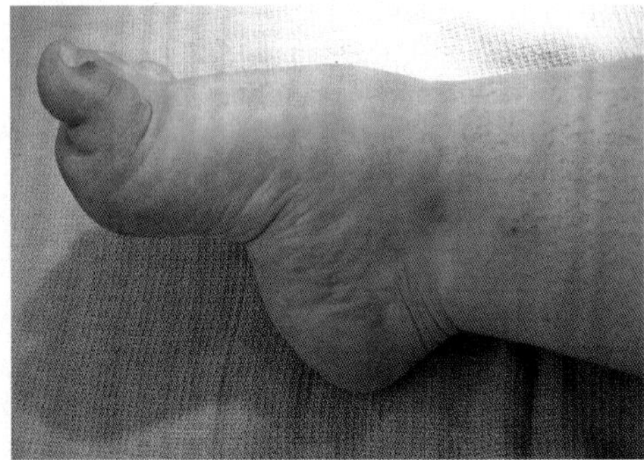

**FIG 7** • An 18-year-old girl with HSMN type 1A with marked cavus and fixed midfoot deformity and shortening. Owing to her age and the degree of rigid deformity, a midfoot osteotomy is required.

- Calcaneal cavus deformity may need a posterior sliding calcaneal osteotomy to increase the calcaneal lever arm. We prefer this to be a crescent-shaped cut. A plantar fascia release facilitates posterior sliding of the distal fragment.
- Triple arthrodesis is used as a salvage procedure for rigid hindfoot deformity. We are reluctant to recommend this for a foot with sensory deficit because the long-term outcome when this procedure is used is poor.[19] With a triple arthrodesis, tendon transfers may still be necessary to maintain a balanced foot.

## Preoperative Planning

- Intraoperative epidural anesthesia may be continued in the postoperative period.
- Preoperative antibiotics are given.
- A tourniquet allows optimal visualization of the operative site.
- In patients with HSMN, the surgeon must be very careful about tourniquet use because the sciatic and femoral nerves in the thigh are very sensitive to the pressure and time effects of the tourniquet. We recommend the minimal pressure needed and less than 1 hour of inflation time.

## Positioning

- The patient is positioned supine on a radiolucent imaging table.

## Approach

- A combination of surgical procedures may be needed to fully correct the foot deformity.
  - For most deformities, an extensive plantar release is used.
  - As the extensor hallucis longus muscle function may be spared in HSMN, the Jones procedure is useful for the child with a plantarflexed medial column and dynamic great toe hyperextension during swing phase. It is generally combined with a medial or midfoot osteotomy.
  - For more extensive and rigid deformity, an osteotomy may be needed. A younger patient may require only an osteotomy of the proximal first metatarsal or first cuneiform. A midfoot wedge osteotomy is useful for the rigid midfoot deformity in an adolescent or young adult when the midfoot does not sufficiently correct after the plantar fascia release. If the lateral and medial aspects of the midfoot are in equinus, an osteotomy across the entire midfoot will more reliably correct the deformity than a medial column osteotomy.
- An alternative to the dorsal closing midfoot osteotomy is a technique where the deformity is corrected by excising the navicular and doing a dorsal closing osteotomy of the cuboid. The excision of the navicular is done through a medial incision and the dorsal closing osteotomy of the cuboid is done through a lateral incision. The advantage of this technique is that it does not fuse any joints in the midfoot. It does correct the deformity and the articular surface of the cuneiforms now articulates with the head of the talus.[10]
  - The lateral calcaneal slide osteotomy is used to correct fixed hindfoot varus that does not correct with the Coleman block test.
    - Advantages include use of a simple single cut with control of the amount of correction needed.
  - The posterior slide calcaneal osteotomy is useful in the calcaneocavus foot with a high calcaneal pitch angle.

- Incisions should be longitudinal and placed over the areas of relevant pathology (**FIG 8**).
- A cavus foot is short and will be lengthened in the course of treatment. It may be safer to obtain some of the correction with postoperative corrective casts rather than doing all of the correction at the initial surgery.

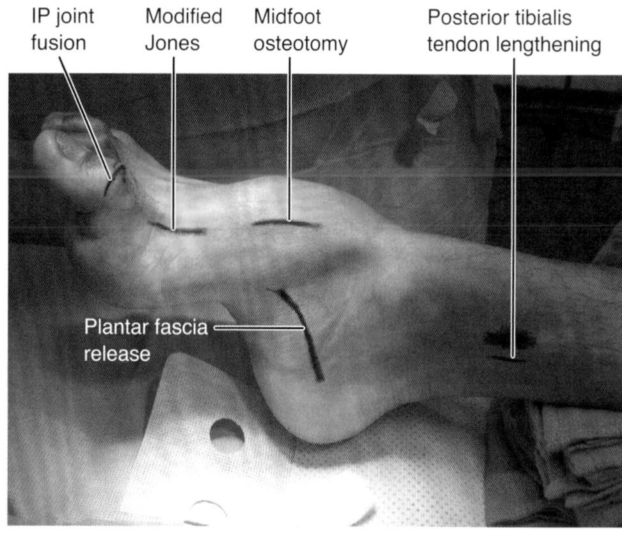


**FIG 8** ● Cavus deformities typically require a combination of procedures. For this right foot, incisions for an extensive plantar medial release, modified Jones procedure, midfoot osteotomy, and posterior tibialis tendon lengthening are drawn. The midfoot osteotomy is at the apex of the deformity.



## Plantar Release

- A longitudinal incision is made medially over the plantar fascia. Sharp knife dissection is used through the skin and subcutaneous fat (**TECH FIG 1A**).
- The abductor hallucis is the first structure identified and is released off its deep fascia (**TECH FIG 1B**).
- The fascia deep to the abductor hallucis is next exposed. The posterior tibial nerve and artery are identified proximally and followed distally by releasing the overlying fascia. Note the division of the posterior tibial nerve into its plantar medial and lateral branches.
- Posterior to the neurovascular bundle, the plantar fascia is exposed as it attaches to the medial tubercle of the calcaneus.
- The flexor digitorum brevis, quadratus plantae, and abductor digiti quinti muscles are released at their proximal origins with Mayo scissors.
- Capsulotomies of the medial talonavicular and subtalar joints may be needed if superficial release is not adequate to achieve correction.[2]
- Severe cases may need posterior tibialis tendon lengthening or transfer.
- The incision is loosely closed with interrupted sutures. By widely spacing the sutures, blood can drain and not cause excessive postoperative pressure.
- In severe cases, serial casting may be necessary after the release.

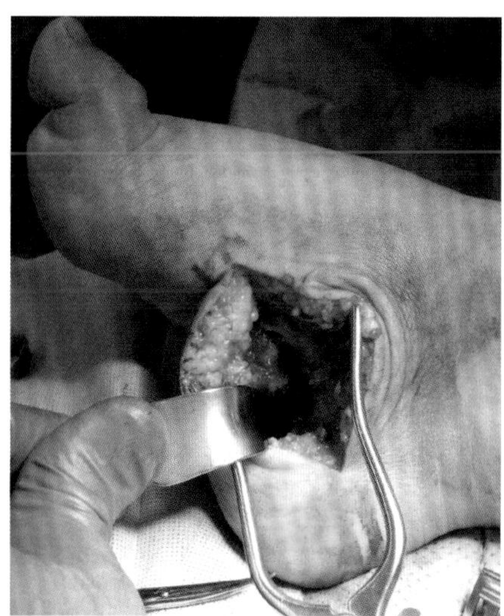


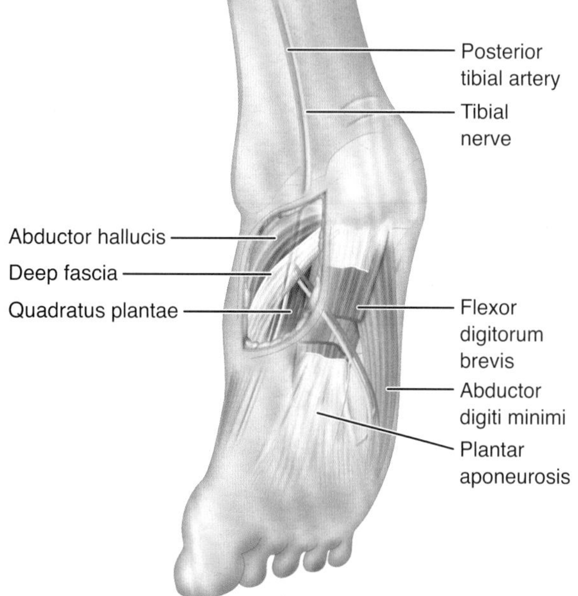


**TECH FIG 1** ● **A.** Plantar medial incision. Because the foot will be lengthened, the incision should be placed longitudinally and gentle sharp dissection used. **B.** The abductor hallucis muscle has been dissected off its deeper fascia, and the plantar aponeurosis and muscles have been isolated posterior to the neurovascular bundle.

## Medial Column Osteotomy

- A plantar medial release should also be performed if an osteotomy is required.
- A stiff forefoot, an older patient, or painful forefoot calluses indicate the need for an osteotomy.
- Depending on the apex of the deformity, the osteotomy can be performed on the medial cuneiform or the first metatarsal. In a younger child, it may be safer to avoid the proximal metatarsal physis and perform a medial cuneiform osteotomy.
- The osteotomy can be performed either as a first metatarsal dorsal-based closing wedge osteotomy or as a medial cuneiform plantar-based open wedge.
  - The first metatarsal dorsal closing wedge osteotomy does not require a bone graft, has one bony surface to heal, and can be held closed with a single screw. However, it may shorten the metatarsal slightly.
  - The first cuneiform plantar open wedge osteotomy requires only a single cut, the amount of correction can be fine-tuned after the bone has been cut, and it does not shorten the foot, but a bone graft is required to hold it open, typically a freeze-dried allograft.
- For a proximal, dorsal-based oblique closing wedge first metatarsal osteotomy, a longitudinal incision is made directly over the proximal metatarsal; be careful to protect the dorsal digital nerve (**TECH FIG 2A,B**).
- Subperiosteal dissection of the proximal metatarsal is performed; be careful to leave the plantar periosteum and soft tissue intact.
- Two small-diameter Steinmann pins are drilled at the site of the bone cuts, converging at the plantar apex. The apex of the correction is quite proximal and plantar. A bony and soft tissue posterior hinge is left intact so that the osteotomy is an incomplete closing wedge.

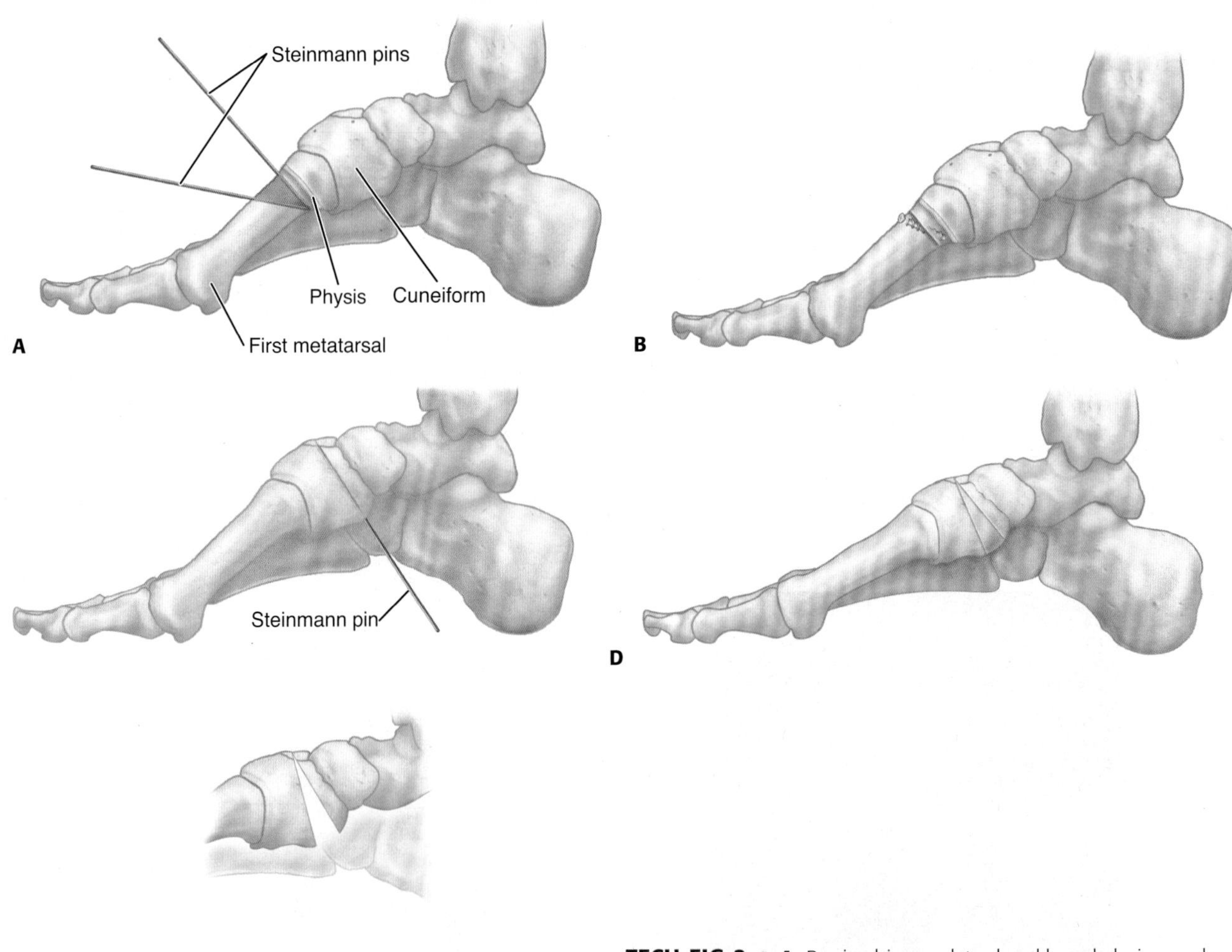


**TECH FIG 2** • **A.** Proximal incomplete dorsal-based closing wedge osteotomy of proximal metatarsal. The plantar aspect of the metatarsal and soft tissues are left intact to act as a hinge to allow closure of the osteotomy. Steinmann pins are placed to accurately guide the bony cuts. **B.** The plantar hinge remains intact for proper closure. A screw or percutaneous pin holds the osteotomy closed. **C.** Plantar opening wedge osteotomy of the medial cuneiform. **D.** The dorsal hinge must remain intact. A triangular bone graft is inserted in the plantar aspect. Fixation is with a single screw, percutaneous wire, or suture on the plantar surface.

- A small oscillating saw is used to make the bone cuts. The wires are used to guide the cuts toward the plantar apex. A small osteotome and pituitary rongeur may be used to remove some of the bone at the apex.
- When sufficient bone has been removed from the apex, the cut ends can be slowly closed together while maintaining integrity of the bony hinge. A wire, screw, or dorsal plate can be used to secure the corrected osteotomy.
- In a younger child with an open metatarsal physis or when the deformity apex is at the medial cuneiform, the opening wedge osteotomy can be performed at this level (**TECH FIG 2C,D**).

## Modified Jones Procedure

- Two incisions are used, a dorsal transverse incision over the great toe IP joint and a longitudinal incision over the distal first metatarsal (**TECH FIG 3**).

### Interphalangeal Joint Fusion

- Through the transverse incision over the IP joint, the incision is carried down to the extensor hallucis tendon.
- The tendon is transected at the level of the IP joint, and the IP joint capsule is incised transversely.
- Continue with the no. 15 blade to expose the articular distal aspect of the proximal phalanx.
- A rongeur is used to remove the articular cartilage and some of the subchondral cortical bone on both sides of the IP joint. Only a minimal amount of bone is removed.
- A cannulated 4.0-mm screw is used for fixation. This is placed by retrograde insertion of a guidewire through the center of the distal phalanx, exiting distally just plantar to the nail.
- The IP joint is then reduced in a neutral position, and the screw is inserted; be careful to provide compression at the IP joint.
  - Proper length places the tip of the screw into the proximal aspect of the proximal phalanx.

### Transfer of the Extensor Hallucis Tendon to the Metatarsal Neck

- A longitudinal skin incision is made over the distal first metatarsal.
- The extensor hallucis tendon is identified and isolated distally until its cut end can be pulled into the incision.
- A 0 suture whipstitch is placed into the distal tendon.
- Subperiosteal exposure of the distal metatarsal allows a transverse drill hole to be made in the metatarsal neck.
  - The drill diameter is roughly the diameter of the extensor hallucis longus tendon.
  - A wire or suture passer aids passage of the extensor hallucis longus tendon through the hole.
- After the medial column or midfoot osteotomy is secured, the end of the extensor hallucis longus tendon is secured to itself (**TECH FIG 4**).

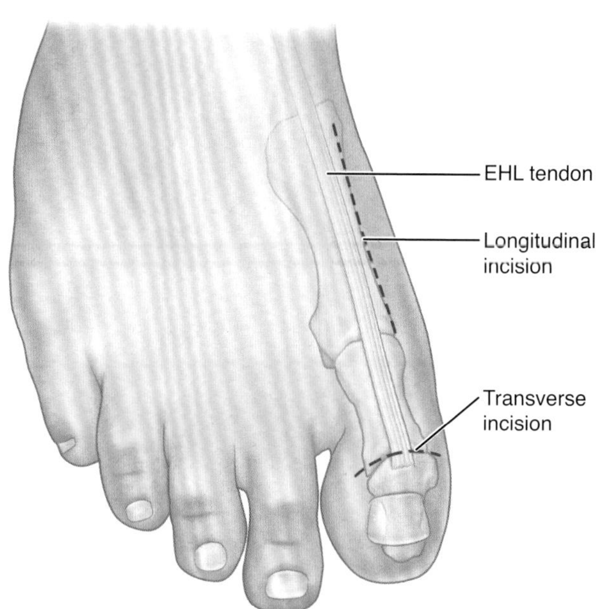


**TECH FIG 3** • Two incisions are used: one transverse over the IP joint and the other longitudinal along the distal first metatarsal.

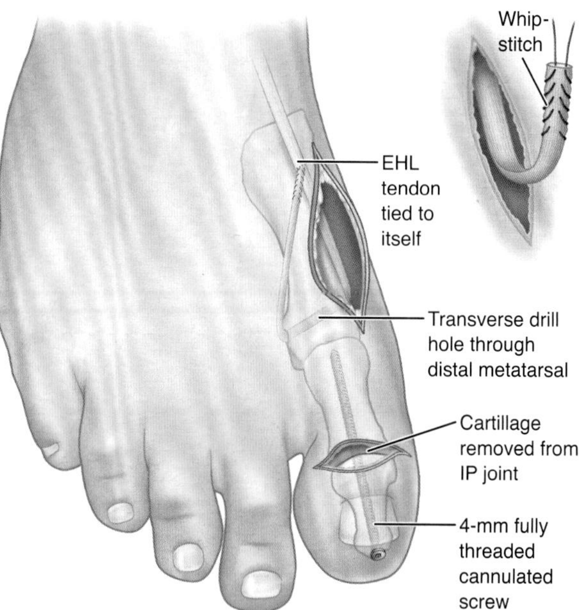


**TECH FIG 4** • After denuding the IP joint articular cartilage, a 4.0-mm screw transfixes this joint. A whipstitch is placed into the cut end of the extensor hallucis longus tendon (*inset*) and the tendon is passed through a transverse drill hole and sutured to itself.

## Midfoot Osteotomy

- The osteotomy is placed at the apex of the deformity, which should be proximal to any plantar calluses (**TECH FIG 5A,B**).
  - Too distal placement results in a rocker bottom residual deformity.
  - If the deformity is severe, a triple arthrodesis may be needed to bring the forefoot into a plantigrade position.
- Muscle balancing procedures will still be required because the foot will further deform with time if imbalance remains.
  - Several types of osteotomies have been described.[6,7,20]
  - We recommend a simple procedure that uses a truncated wedge placed at the apex of the deformity.
  - Once cut, the distal fragment may be laterally rotated to compensate for excessive medial column flexion.
- A long, single dorsomedial skin incision is used at the apex of the deformity.
  - It is more effective to place the osteotomy proximally so that correction is achieved at the level of the deformity; it is generally at the navicular cuneiform joint.
- The Hohmann retractors are placed dorsal and plantar, with the entire midfoot exposed (**TECH FIG 5C**).
- Smooth Steinmann pins are inserted to define the proximal and distal aspects of the osteotomies. The osteotomy is cut with the oscillating saw and completed with osteotomes and rongeurs. A dorsal-based wedge of bone is removed; it can be a triangle for moderate deformities or a truncated trapezoid for more significant deformities.
- Fixation is with two threaded Steinmann pins, which are removed in 4 to 6 weeks.
- The incision is loosely closed with interrupted sutures.
- The foot is casted for 6 weeks with toe-touch weight bearing. Because of the potential for nonunion, an additional 6 weeks of weight-bearing casting should be considered.

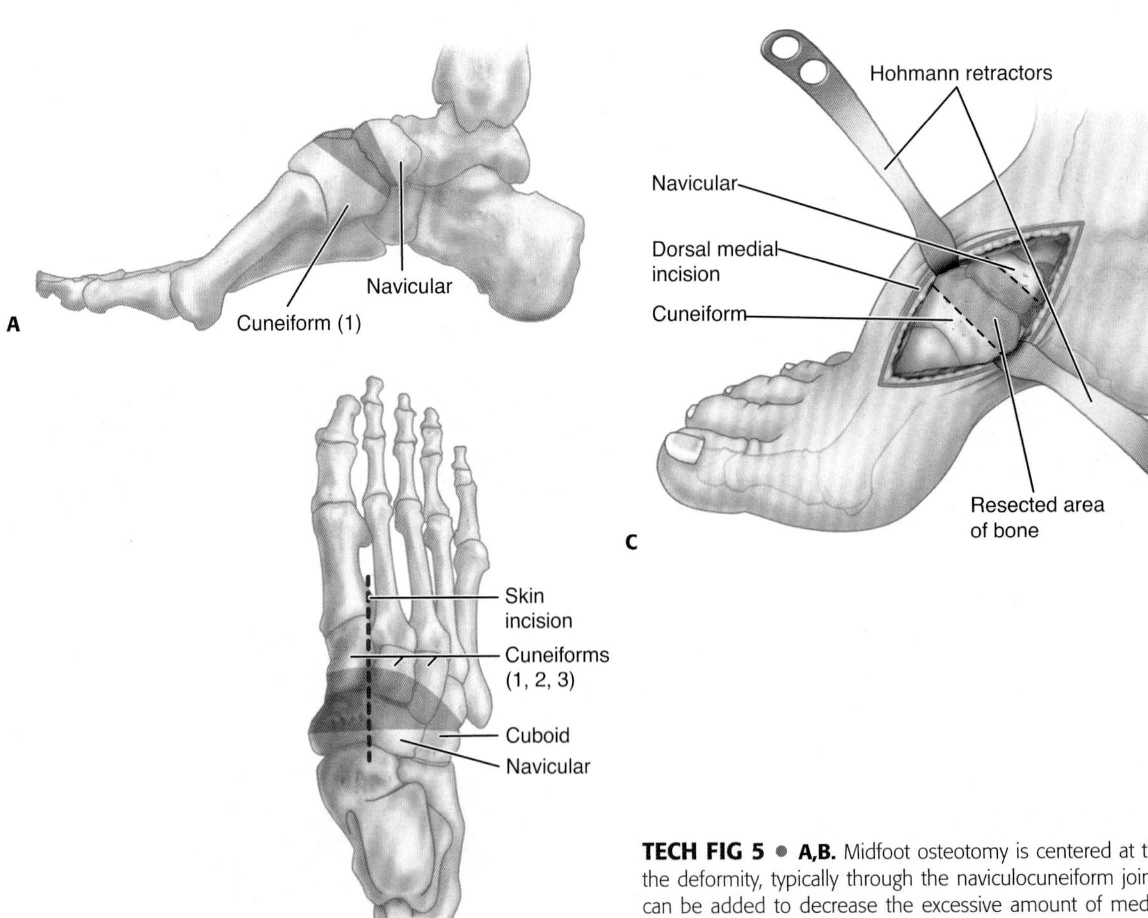


**TECH FIG 5** • **A,B.** Midfoot osteotomy is centered at the apex of the deformity, typically through the naviculocuneiform joint. Rotation can be added to decrease the excessive amount of medial column plantarflexion. **C.** Neurovascular structures are protected with two Hohmann retractors.

## Calcaneal Osteotomies

### Lateral Calcaneal Slide Osteotomy

- The incision is placed lateral to the calcaneus, parallel to the peroneal tendons.
- The peroneal tendons are reflected proximally to gain access to the lateral aspect of the calcaneus tubercle.
- A sharp Hohmann retractor is placed just anterior to the Achilles insertion and another is placed plantar and distal.
  - Fluoroscopy can be used to check the orientation of the osteotomy by the position of the retractors (**TECH FIG 6A**).
- A 1-inch osteotome or saw is used to make the osteotomy across the calcaneus to the opposite cortex. A smooth lamina spreader is used to distract the fragments, and the medial cortex can be freed up with a pituitary rongeur and a Cobb elevator.
- The calcaneal tubercle with the heel is then slid medially about 50% of its width. The correct position is for the heel to be underneath and in line with the tibial shaft (**TECH FIG 6B**). A laterally based wedge can also be removed if more correction is needed.
- A large threaded Steinmann pin is placed in the sinus tarsi and directed toward the most posteroinferior aspect of the tubercle (**TECH FIG 6C**).
- The pin is removed in the clinic in 3 weeks. A cast is used for a total of 6 weeks.

### Posterior Slide Calcaneal Osteotomy

- A lateral approach to the calcaneus is used, similar to the lateral slide osteotomy.
- Hohmann retractors are placed for protection and orientation.
- An oblique straight cut may be used, but we prefer a curved cut using a Chiari chisel (**TECH FIG 7**).
- Once cut, the distal calcaneal fragment is slid posterior and transfixed with a threaded Steinmann pin.
- Because the bone may continue to bleed, loose interrupted suture closure and a bulky dressing are used.
- The pin is removed in 3 weeks, and the foot is casted for a total of 6 weeks.

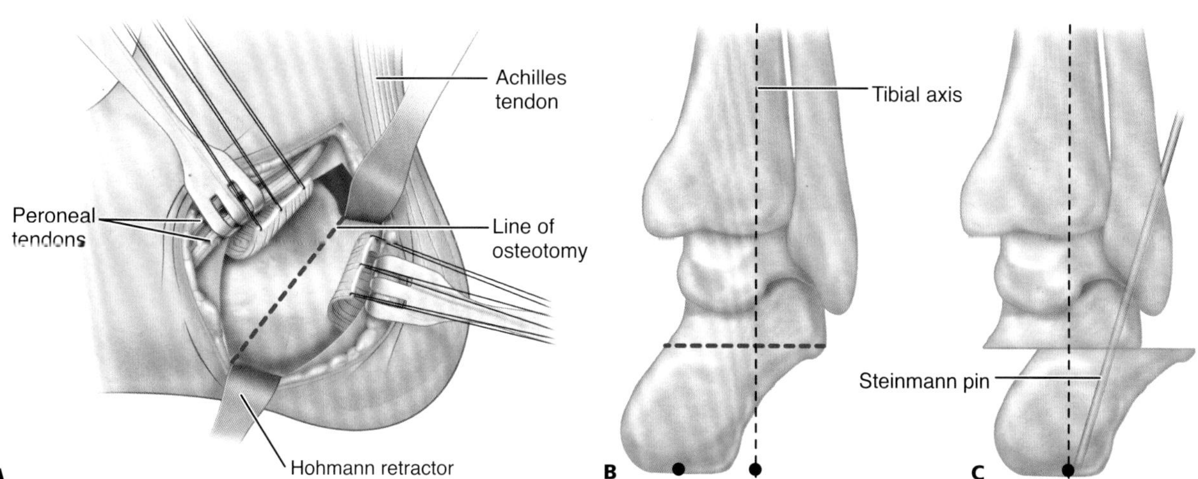


**TECH FIG 6** • **A.** Lateral exposure of the calcaneus for calcaneal slide osteotomy. The peroneal tendon sheath is divided and the tendons are reflected proximally. One Hohmann retractor is placed anterior to the Achilles tendon insertion and a second is placed distally on the plantar aspect of the calcaneus. **B.** Posterior view of the foot showing the lateral slide calcaneal osteotomy. **C.** The distal tubercle with the heel pad is positioned underneath the tibia. Fixation is with a threaded Steinmann pin for 3 weeks.

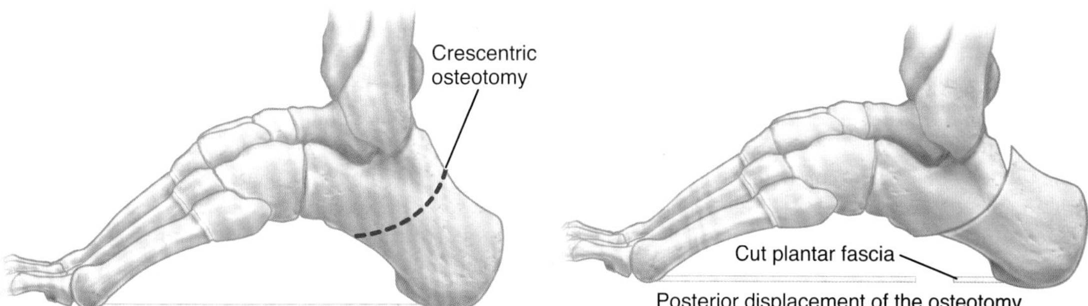


**TECH FIG 7** • Crescent-shaped calcaneal osteotomy allows posterior positioning of the calcaneus to improve the lever arm function of the gastrocnemius–soleus muscles and to decrease the point pressure on the heel.

## PEARLS AND PITFALLS

| | |
|---|---|
| **Failure to diagnose underlying spine condition** | ■ A child presenting with a foot problem must always have the spine examined.<br>■ A markedly small foot or calf may be a sign of a split cord malformation or diastematomyelia. |
| **Failure to diagnose a structural lesion of a major nerve** | ■ The clinician must examine the entire lower limbs along the course of major nerves to detect a localized peripheral nerve tumor or site of nerve compression. |
| **Failure to diagnose HSMN** | ■ Bilateral cavus may be subtle.<br>■ The clinician should always ask about a family history of cavus feet or peripheral neuropathy.<br>■ Sometimes, there is not an established diagnosis of HSMN in the family. In these cases, the family members may need to be examined.<br>■ The hand and foot intrinsics are examined.<br>■ HSMN may initially present as bilateral adolescent hip dysplasia. |
| **Missing a diagnosis with a very treatable lesion** | ■ Several conditions may cause a cavus foot deformity. Subtalar coalition generally causes a rigid valgus hindfoot deformity but may cause a spastic hindfoot varus (**FIG 9**). |
| **Insufficient surgical procedure** | ■ With adolescence, severe cavus deformities often require a more extensive midfoot osteotomy to correct the deformity. |
| **Severe idiopathic cavus foot deformity often requires repeat surgical procedures** | ■ The family should be warned that further surgical procedures may be necessary with time as the child grows and the deformity changes. |

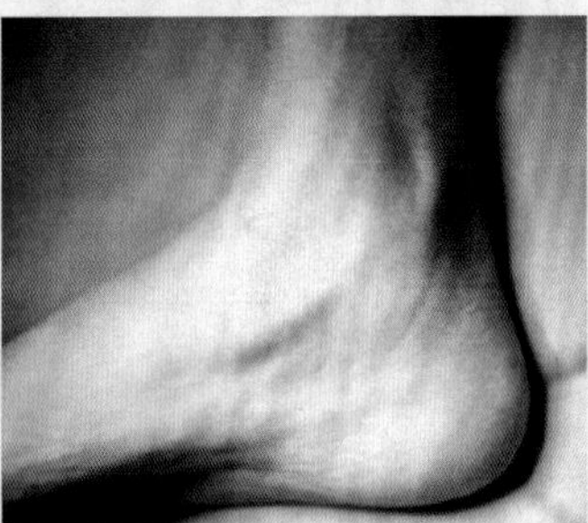

**FIG 9** • Spastic hindfoot varus.

## POSTOPERATIVE CARE

- After a plantar release, the foot should be wrapped with soft, bulky cotton and casted with minimal external correction.
- At 2 weeks, the sutures are removed and gentle correction is obtained. This may require serial casting for up to 6 weeks.
- After a midfoot or forefoot osteotomy, weight bearing is restricted until the osteotomy has healed, generally about 6 weeks.

## OUTCOMES

- Long-term outcome studies are limited for progressive conditions such as HSMN.[15]
- One study demonstrated that patients with Charcot-Marie-Tooth disease that had a first metatarsal osteotomy and soft tissue procedures had lower rates of degenerative changes and lower rates of reoperations when compared with patients treated with a triple arthrodesis.[18] This study seemed to confirm that patients treated with procedures that attempt to rebalance the foot and keep a mobile foot have a better outcome than those treated with an arthrodesis.
- Triple arthrodesis for progressive cavus deformity has a poor long-term outcome. Results are further compromised by technical problems at the time of surgery as well as from undercorrection and overcorrection.
- Most patients with a progressive cavus deformity and a triple arthrodesis performed as a teenager had significant foot problems by their 30s.[19]
- Nonprogressive deformities such as spastic cavovarus with equinus can be surgically balanced with acceptable results.
- Progressive deformities may require several surgeries during childhood followed by a triple arthrodesis at maturity. The patient and family should be warned about this possibility.

## COMPLICATIONS

- Femoral or sciatic nerve injury from tourniquet. This can occur with excessive pressure or time on the tourniquet or even with minimal time and pressure. The tourniquet time should be under 1 hour, using minimal pressure needed for visualization.
- Plantar medial incision dehiscence if excessive correction is attempted at the time of surgery
- Pressure sores in patients with HSMN
- Surgical correction of midfoot deformity distal to the apex may result in a rocker bottom foot deformity.
- Nonunion of the midfoot osteotomy[8]
- Persistent midfoot cavus if the deformity is too severe for a medial column or midfoot osteotomy
- Persistent hindfoot varus if deformity is fixed and a calcaneal osteotomy is not performed

## REFERENCES


1. Azmaipairashvili Z, Riddle EC, Scavina M, et al. Correction of cavovarus foot deformity in Charcot-Marie-Tooth disease. J Pediatr Orthop 2005;25:360–365.
2. Bradley GW, Coleman SS. Treatment of the calcaneocavus foot deformity. J Bone Joint Surg Am 1981;63(7):1159–1166.
3. Fuller JE, DeLuca PA. Acetabular dysplasia and Charcot-Marie-Tooth disease in a family. A report of four cases. J Bone Joint Surg Am 1995;77(7):1087–1091.
4. Ghanem I, Zeller R, Seringe R. The foot in hereditary motor and sensory neuropathies in children [in French]. Rev Chir Orthop Reparatrice Appar Mot 1996;82:152–160.
5. Guyton GP. Peroneal nerve branching suggests compression palsy in the deformities of Charcot-Marie Tooth disease. Clin Orthop Relat Res 2006;451:167–170.
6. Jahss MH. Evaluation of the cavus foot for orthopedic treatment. Clin Orthop Relat Res 1983;(181):52–63.
7. Japas LM. Surgical treatment of pes cavus by tarsal V-osteotomy. Preliminary report. J Bone Joint Surg Am 1968;50(5):927–944.
8. Levitt RL, Canale ST, Cooke AJ, et al. The role of foot surgery in progressive neuromuscular disorders in children. J Bone Joint Surg Am 1973;55(7):1396–1410.
9. Lutter LD. Cavus foot in runners. Foot Ankle 1981;1:225–228.
10. Mubarak SJ, Dimeglio A. Navicular excision and cuboid closing wedge for severe cavovarus foot deformities: a salvage procedures. J Pediatr Orthop 2011;31(5):551–556.
11. Mubarak SJ, Van Valin SE. Osteotomies of the foot for cavus deformities in children. J Pediatr Orthop 2009;29(3):294–299.
12. Paulos L, Coleman SS, Samuelson KM. Pes cavovarus. Review of a surgical approach using selective soft-tissue procedures. J Bone Joint Surg Am 1980;62(6):942–953.
13. Price AE, Maisel R, Drennan JC. Computed tomographic analysis of pes cavus. J Pediatr Orthop 1993;13:646–653.
14. Sabir M, Lyttle D. Pathogenesis of pes cavus in Charcot-Marie-Tooth disease. Clin Orthop Relat Res 1983;(175):173–178.
15. Schwend RM, Drennan JC. Cavus foot deformity in children. J Am Acad Orthop Surg 2003;11:201–211.
16. Tynan MC, Klenerman L, Helliwell TR, et al. Investigation of muscle imbalance in the leg in symptomatic forefoot pes cavus: a multidisciplinary study. Foot Ankle 1992;13:489–501.
17. Walker JL, Nelson KR, Heavilon JA, et al. Hip abnormalities in children with Charcot-Marie-Tooth disease. J Pediatr Orthop 1994;14:54–59.
18. Ward CM, Dolan LA, Bennett DL, et al. Long-term results of reconstruction for treatment of a flexible cavovarus foot in Charcot-Marie-Tooth disease. J Bone Join Surg Am 2008;90(12):2631–2642.
19. Wetmore RS, Drennan JC. Long-term results of triple arthrodesis in Charcot-Marie-Tooth disease. J Bone Joint Surg Am 1989;71(3):417–422.
20. Wilcox PG, Weiner DS. The Akron midtarsal dome osteotomy in the treatment of rigid pes cavus: a preliminary review. J Pediatr Orthop 1985;5:333–338.
21. Younger ASE, Hansen ST Jr. Adult cavovarus foot. J Am Acad Orthop Surg 2005;13:302–315.

CHAPTER 123

# Resection of Calcaneonavicular Coalition

David Scher

## DEFINITION

- A calcaneonavicular coalition is an abnormal connection between the calcaneus and the navicular.
- This extra connection between the tarsal bones typically limits subtalar motion.
- The major consequence of this condition is a rigid flatfoot that may be painful.

## ANATOMY

- The coalition typically occurs between the anterior process of the calcaneus and the most lateral aspect of the navicular (**FIG 1**).
- The connection may comprise bone, cartilage, or fibrous tissue (bony, cartilaginous, or fibrous coalitions, respectively).

## PATHOGENESIS

- The cause of calcaneonavicular coalitions remains unknown.
- It has been hypothesized that coalitions may result from failure of segmentation of the individual tarsal bones during fetal development.[1]
- Symptoms typically develop in later childhood, usually between 8 and 12 years old, for calcaneonavicular coalitions.[5]
- It is theorized that the reason for the delayed onset of symptoms, despite presumed presence from birth, is that the coalition ossifies over time, making it more rigid and more likely to limit subtalar motion.[5]
- The pain from a calcaneonavicular coalition may arise from altered kinematics of the foot due to local limitation of motion.
  - Alternatively, micromotion through adjacent portions of the coalition may make it painful, akin to a fracture nonunion.
  - It has also been suggested that a fracture through a previously solid coalition could render it painful.

## NATURAL HISTORY

- Many people with calcaneonavicular coalitions are probably pain-free, although they may have a rigid flatfoot, with loss of the longitudinal arch and valgus alignment of the heel.[6]
- If pain develops in a child with a calcaneonavicular coalition, it usually does so between ages 8 and 12 years.

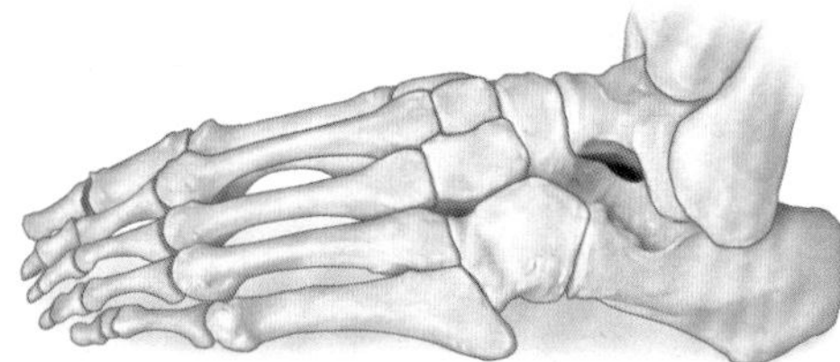

**FIG 1** • A complete bony calcaneonavicular coalition.

## PATIENT HISTORY AND PHYSICAL FINDINGS

- Patients present with complaints of foot pain exacerbated by activity, typically localized to the lateral aspect of the foot, just distal to the sinus tarsi, in the region of the anterior process of the calcaneus. They may complain of medial foot and ankle pain or pain at the distal tip of the fibula as well.
- There may be a history of progressive out-toeing and loss of arch height due to an increase in the planovalgus position of the foot.
- Patients may also relate difficulty walking on uneven surfaces, presumably due to decreased subtalar motion.
- The physician should observe the patient's gait; he or she may walk with an antalgic gait on the affected side (decreased stance phase) and an out-toeing gait.
- The physician should examine the patient's foot alignment. The heel may be in valgus alignment with the forefoot abducted.
- The physician should examine the rigidity of the patient's flatfoot. A flexible flatfoot has restoration of the arch upon toe-rise, whereas a rigid flatfoot has no arch restoration. A rigid flatfoot is a sign of decreased subtalar motion and may indicate a tarsal coalition.
- The physician should palpate over the anterior process of the calcaneus and just distal to the anterior process. Point tenderness is suggestive of a painful calcaneonavicular coalition.
- The physician should examine the range of motion of the foot. Decreased subtalar motion can be a sign of a tarsal coalition. Also, pain with maximal plantarflexion may also indicate a calcaneonavicular coalition.

## IMAGING AND OTHER DIAGNOSTIC STUDIES

- Plain radiographs, including anteroposterior (AP), lateral, and oblique views, should be obtained to visualize the coalition.
  - A calcaneonavicular coalition is best seen on the oblique view (inversion oblique) (**FIG 2**).
  - A prominent anterior process of the calcaneus, the "anteater nose" sign, may be seen on the lateral view.[4]
  - Standing AP and lateral views can be included to assess foot alignment.
- A Harris axial view or Saltzman hindfoot alignment view can be obtained to assess heel alignment.
- A computed tomography (CT) or magnetic resonance imaging (MRI) scan should be obtained to rule out a concurrent talocalcaneal coalition or the presence of arthritis in adjacent joints. CT or MRI may also be useful if the diagnosis is in question.

## DIFFERENTIAL DIAGNOSIS

- Flexible flatfoot
- Subtalar arthritis
- Other tarsal coalition (talocalcaneal or other less common ones)

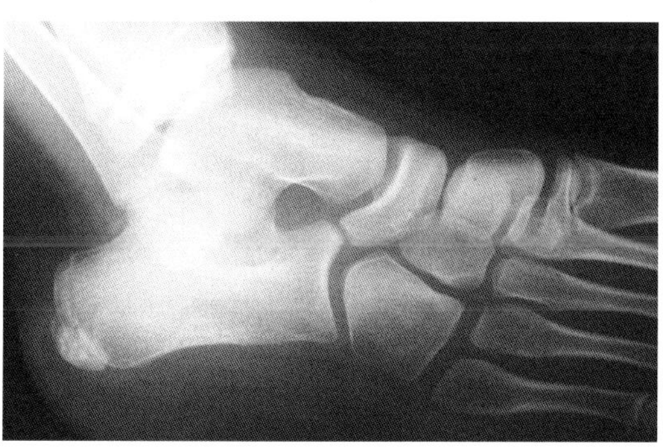

**FIG 2** ● Oblique radiograph depicting a cartilaginous calcaneonavicular coalition.

- Tumor or infection involving the subtalar joint
- Idiopathic rigid flatfoot

## NONOPERATIVE MANAGEMENT

- Nonoperative management is an option for all patients with a painful calcaneonavicular coalition at first presentation.
- Painless coalitions need no treatment.
- Initial treatment for painful coalitions may consist of activity modification, anti-inflammatory medication, or immobilization in a short-leg walking cast for 4 to 6 weeks.

## SURGICAL MANAGEMENT

- The indication for surgical management is persistence of pain despite nonoperative management.
- The main goals of treatment are elimination of pain and restoration of function.
- Restoration of subtalar motion is a secondary goal.
- Restoration of arch height is unlikely after resection.

### Preoperative Planning

- All imaging studies are reviewed.
- An examination of subtalar motion may be performed under anesthesia to serve as a comparison to the examination immediately after resection.

### Positioning

- The patient is positioned supine with a bump under the hip of the operative side to slightly internally rotate the leg.
- If subcutaneous fat autograft is to be used as an interposition material after resection, the limb should be prepared up to the buttocks and a sterile tourniquet should be used (**FIG 3**).
- Alternatively, an Esmarch tourniquet may be used just proximal to the ankle.

### Approach

- The approach involves exposure and resection of the entire coalition.
- A graft material is interposed between the ends of the resected bone consisting of local muscle (extensor digitorum brevis) or autologous fat.

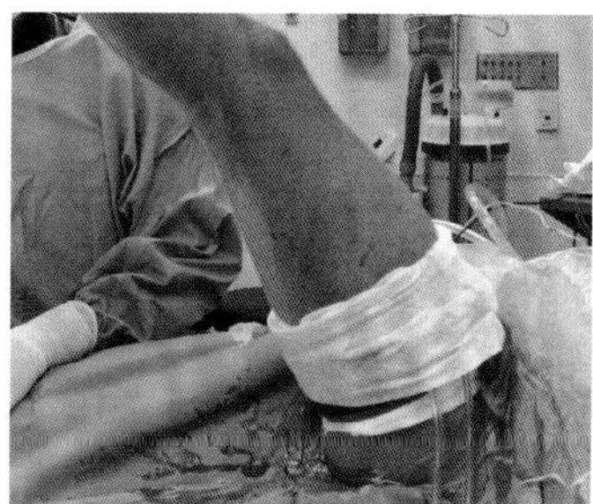

**FIG 3** ● A sterile tourniquet is used with sufficient room proximal to it for harvesting of fat graft.

TECHNIQUES

## Incision and Dissection

- The procedure can be done under tourniquet control if desired.
- An oblique incision is made along the lateral side of the foot between the extensor tendons and the peroneal tendons, directly overlying the anterior process of the calcaneus (**TECH FIG 1A**).
- The skin and subcutaneous tissue are incised sharply, taking care not to undermine the tissues. Look for branches of the superficial peroneal and sural nerves (**TECH FIG 1B**).
- The extensor digitorum brevis is exposed and followed proximally to its origin at the sinus tarsi (**TECH FIG 1C,D**).
- Fibrofatty tissue within the sinus tarsi is exposed.
- This fibrofatty tissue is incised and reflected distally along with the attached origin of the extensor digitorum brevis, exposing the anterior process of the calcaneus and the calcaneonavicular coalition (**TECH FIG 1E**).
- Fluoroscopic confirmation of the coalition is obtained by placing a surgical instrument or needle directly over it (**TECH FIG 1F**).

A

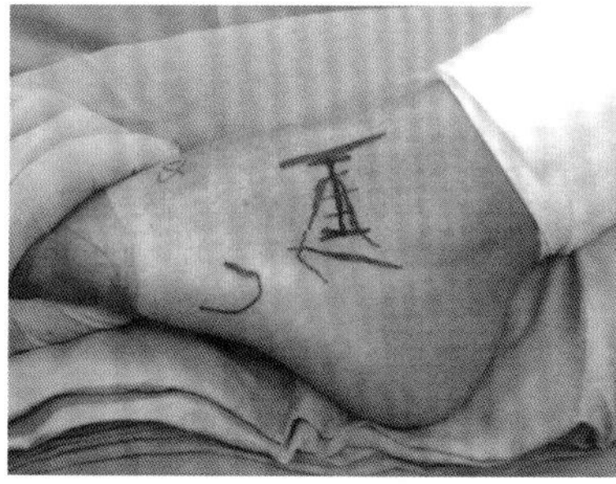

B

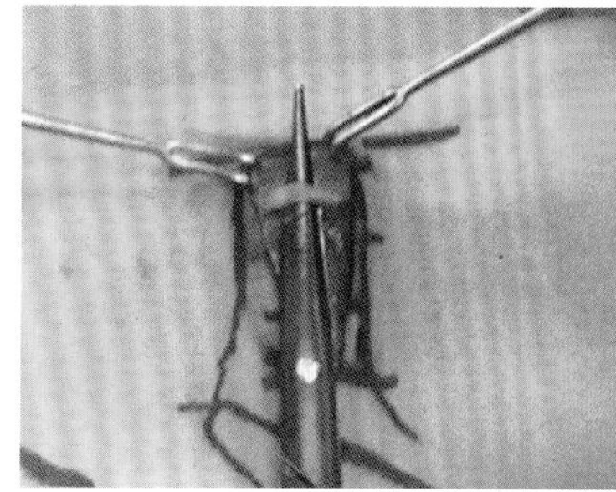

**TECH FIG 1** ● **A.** The incision lies between the extensor tendons and peroneal tendons. **B.** A branch of the superficial peroneal nerve is identified and protected. *(continued)*

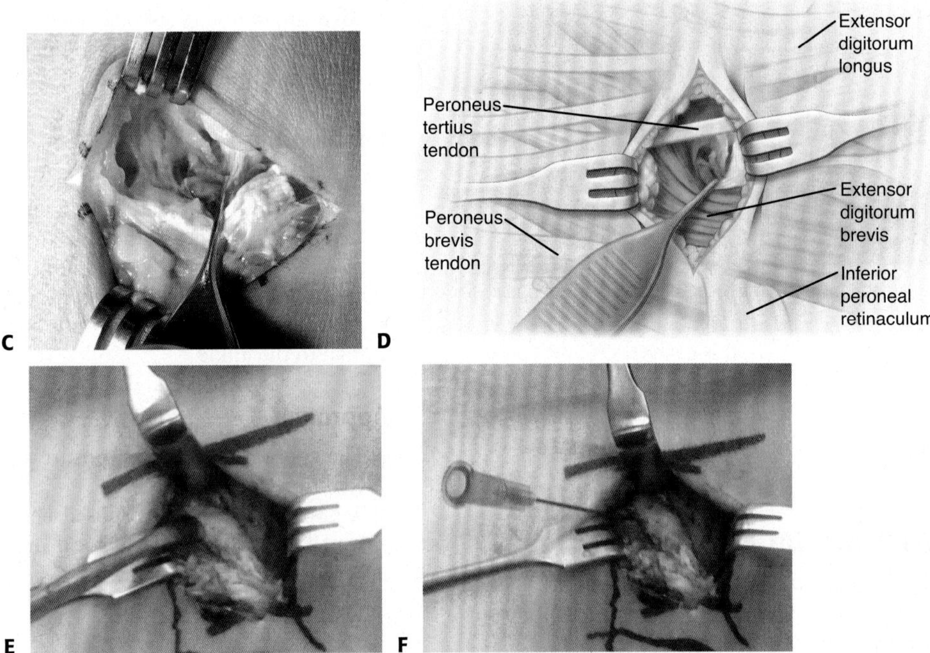


**TECH FIG 1** • *(continued)* **C,D.** The extensor digitorum brevis is identified and reflected distally. **E.** The tip of the freer points to the cartilaginous coalition. **F.** A hypodermic needle is inserted into the coalition and its location is confirmed fluoroscopically.

## Resection of the Calcaneonavicular Coalition

- The extensor digitorum brevis is retracted distally and any remaining fibrofatty tissue from the sinus tarsi is retracted proximally.
- A small osteotome is used to remove a trapezoidal piece of bone (**TECH FIG 2A–C**).
- The first cut is made in the region of what would be the middle of the anterior process of the calcaneus. This cut should be inclined about 40 to 60 degrees from the vertical relative to the plantar surface of the foot and directed medially toward the lateral aspect of the navicular, deep within the wound.
- The next cut is made at the most lateral aspect of the navicular, directed toward nearly the same point as the first cut.
- The ends of these two cuts should not meet, as the goal is to resect a trapezoidal piece and not a triangular piece. The bone may be removed in "piecemeal" fashion, using straight, pituitary and Kerrison rongeurs, and need not be removed as one.

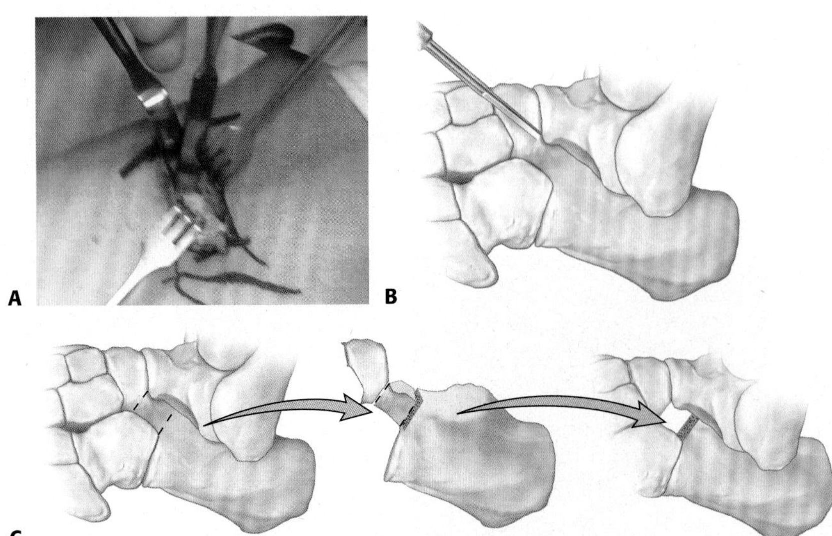


**TECH FIG 2** • **A–C.** The coalition is resected with a small osteotome. When performing the medial cut, care is taken to avoid damaging the adjacent articular surface of the talar head. The piece of bone removed is trapezoidal in shape, not triangular. *(continued)*

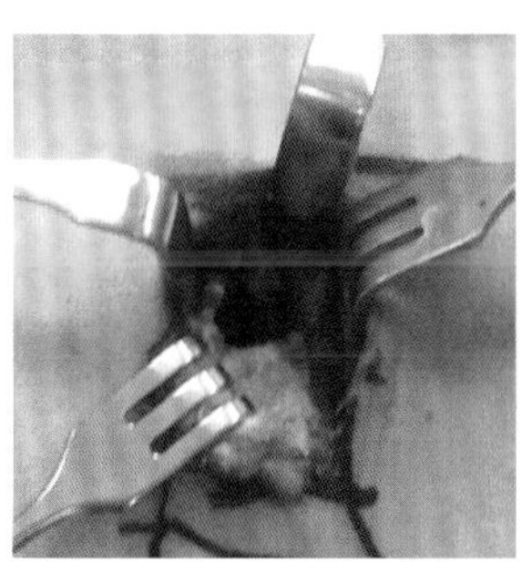

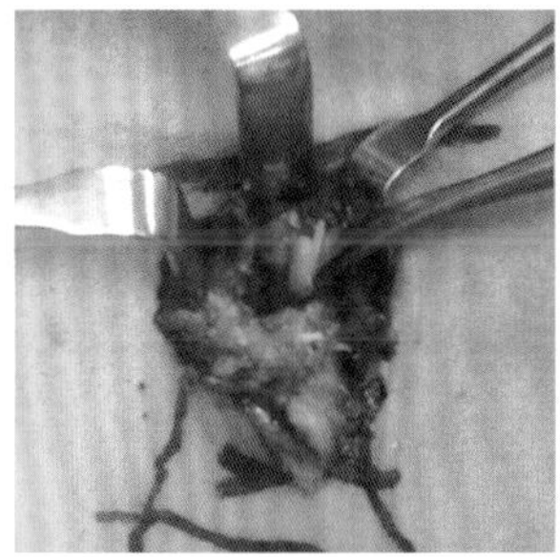

**TECH FIG 2** • *(continued)* **D.** Remaining bone is removed. **E.** Bone wax is applied to cut bone surfaces.

- When making these cuts, especially the medial one, care must be taken to avoid injuring the articular cartilage of the talar head, which lies directly medial and proximal to the osteotome.
- Attention must also be paid to removing sufficient bone so that there is a visible space between the calcaneus and navicular, which is confirmed fluoroscopically on the inversion view. After resection, the lateral edge of the navicular should line up with the lateral aspect of the talar neck and the medial edge of the anterior process of the calcaneus should line up with the medial edge of the cuboid.
- Remaining bone is removed as necessary with rongeurs (**TECH FIG 2D**).
- Bone wax is placed over the exposed cut bone surfaces (**TECH FIG 2E**).

## Interposition of Fat Graft

- A piece of subcutaneous fat can be taken from just beneath the buttock crease. Use of this donor site allows for a cosmetic incision with minimal donor site morbidity. There is always abundant fat in this location and there are no neurovascular structures at risk during this dissection.
- A transverse incision is made at the base of the buttocks while an assistant elevates the limb (**TECH FIG 3A**).
- A piece of subcutaneous fat about 2 cm in diameter is removed and placed directly into the gap that has been created (**TECH FIG 3B–E**).

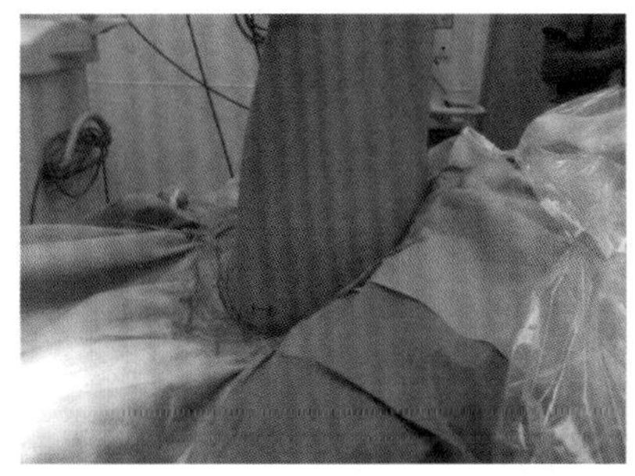

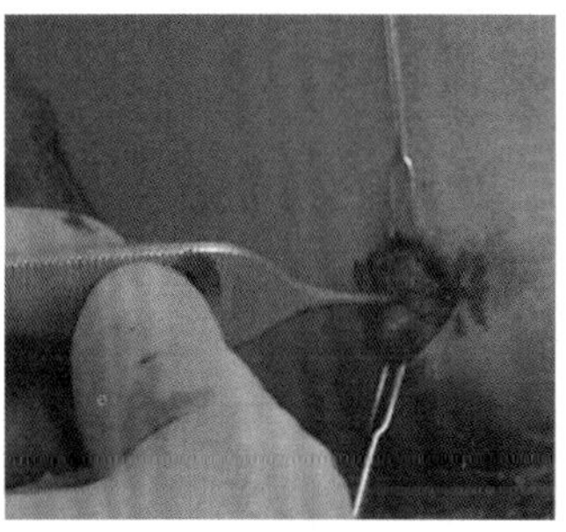

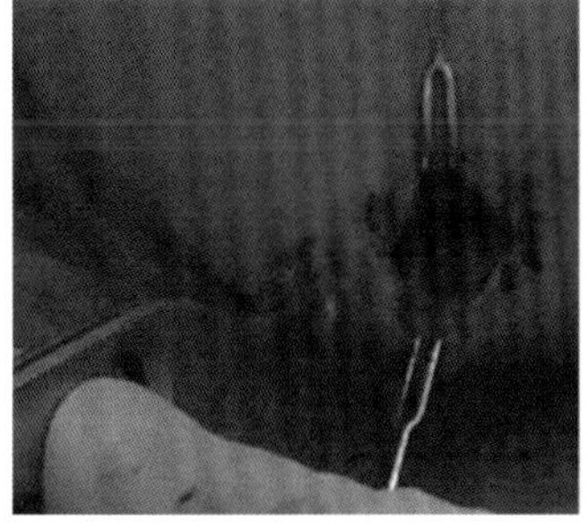

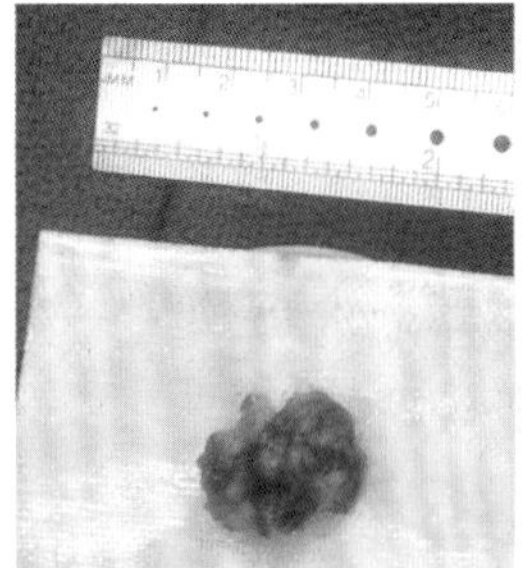

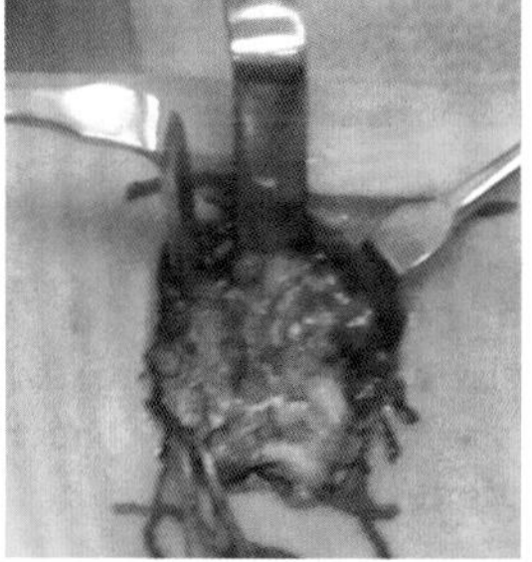

**TECH FIG 3** • **A.** The incision to harvest the fat autograft is marked on the skin just proximal to the gluteal crease. **B–E.** A piece of subcutaneous fat is harvested and placed into the defect created by excision of the coalition.

TECHNIQUES

## Interposition of Peroneus Brevis Muscle (Alternative Technique)

- After the coalition has been resected, heavy absorbable sutures are woven through the proximal end of the peroneus brevis that had been detached from its origin.
- The ends of the sutures are passed through Keith needles.
- The Keith needles are passed through the space that has been created in the depth of the wound to exit the medial side of the foot.
- The needles are passed through a piece of sterile felt and a button and the sutures are sewn over the button, drawing the muscle into the gap where the calcaneonavicular coalition was previously (**TECH FIG 4**).

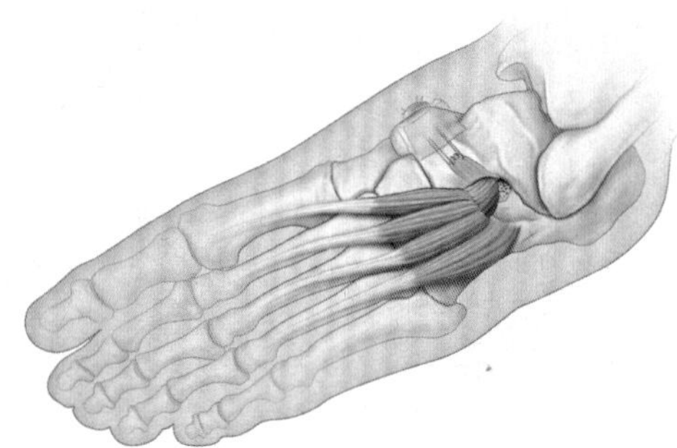

**TECH FIG 4** • Absorbable sutures are passed through the proximal edge of the extensor digitorum brevis and the ends are passed into the space created by the resection and out the medial side of the foot. They are then tied over felt and a button.

## Wound Closure

- The tourniquet is released and hemostasis is obtained.
- If fat was used as graft material, the extensor digitorum brevis is sewn back down anatomically to its origin with absorbable suture.
- Subcutaneous tissue and skin are closed in standard fashion.

## PEARLS AND PITFALLS

| | |
|---|---|
| **Approach** | ▪ The surgeon should avoid undermining the skin to prevent wound complications.<br>▪ The surgeon should take care to avoid injuring branches of the superficial peroneal or sural nerves. |
| **Coalition resection** | ▪ To prevent bone regrowth, the surgeon should ensure adequate bone is removed so that there is a visible gap between the calcaneus and navicular.<br>▪ The surgeon should be cognizant of the local anatomy, specifically the location of the head of the talus, to avoid damaging the talus when making cuts. |
| **Graft harvesting and placement** | ▪ When using fat graft, sufficient fat should be removed to fill the defect created by the resection. |

## POSTOPERATIVE CARE

- The patient is placed in a cast or splint for 2 to 3 weeks to allow the graft to consolidate and the wound to heal.
- Progressive weight bearing is allowed after cast removal, and range-of-motion exercises are performed to address subtalar motion.

## OUTCOMES

- Better than 90% good or excellent results have been reported in most series.[2]
- Poor results with persistent pain are attributed to failure to resect adequate bone or the presence of concurrent arthritis in the midfoot or hindfoot.[3]

## COMPLICATIONS

- Failure to resect adequate bone
- Injury to adjacent articular cartilage
- Wound healing complications
- Recurrence of the coalition

## REFERENCES

1. Harris RI, Beath T. Etiology of peroneal spastic flat foot. J Bone Joint Surg Br 1948;30-B(4):624–634.
2. Gonzalez P, Kumar SJ. Calcaneonavicular coalition treated by resection and interposition of the extensor digitorum brevis muscle. J Bone Joint Surg Am 1990;72(1):71–77.
3. Moyes ST, Crawfurd EJ, Aichroth PM. The interposition of extensor digitorum brevis in the resection of calcaneonavicular bars. J Pediatr Orthop 1994;14:387–388.
4. Oestreich AE, Mize WA, Crawford AH, et al. The "anteater nose": a direct sign of calcaneonavicular coalition on the lateral radiograph. J Pediatr Orthop 1987;7:709–711.
5. Stormont DM, Peterson HA. The relative incidence of tarsal coalition. Clin Orthop Relat Res 1983;(181):28–36.
6. Varner KE, Michelson JD. Tarsal coalition in adults. Foot Ankle Int 2000;21:669–672.

# Excision of Talocalcaneal Coalition

David Scher

124 CHAPTER

## DEFINITION

- A talocalcaneal coalition is an abnormal connection between the talus and the calcaneus that limits subtalar motion.
- As is the case for calcaneonavicular coalitions, which are described in the prior chapter, talocalcaneal coalitions typically result in a rigid flatfoot that is sometimes painful.

## ANATOMY

- Talocalcaneal coalitions occur within the subtalar joint, most commonly involving the middle facet.[9]
- These connections can be bony, cartilaginous, or fibrous and can involve any amount of the joint.
- The size of the coalition is described with respect to the percentage of the entire subtalar joint that is coalesced.[9]

## PATHOGENESIS

- Like calcaneonavicular coalitions, the cause of talocalcaneal coalitions remains unknown, but they may be the result of failure of segmentation during fetal development.[1]
- Although they are presumed to be congenital in nature, symptoms typically do not appear until early adolescence, ages 12 to 16 years.[7,10]
- It is unclear why some coalitions become painful. One theory suggests the possibility of altered talar joint kinematics placing additional stress on adjacent joints. Another is the development of microfractures or stress fractures through the coalition over time, rendering them painful.[1]

## NATURAL HISTORY

- Most talocalcaneal coalitions are asymptomatic.[6]
- They may result in the development of a rigid flatfoot, characterized by valgus alignment of the heel, abduction of the forefoot, loss of the arch, and failure of the arch to reconstitute on toe-rise or when non–weight bearing.
- Pain secondary to talocalcaneal coalitions usually develops between 12 and 16 years of age.[7,10]

## PATIENT HISTORY AND PHYSICAL FINDINGS

- Patients typically describe pain in the foot that is activity related; it is exacerbated by walking on uneven surfaces and relieved by rest.
- This pain may be generalized to the midfoot and hindfoot or can be specifically localized to the medial aspect of the hindfoot and ankle.
- Patients may also complain of lateral pain at the tip of the fibula.
- There may be a history of progressively worsening out-toeing or loss of the arch.
- The clinician should observe the patient's gait for an antalgic pattern and torsional alignment, with specific attention to foot position during stance.
- The patient's foot alignment is examined; the heel may be in valgus alignment with the forefoot abducted.
- The rigidity of the flatfoot is observed. Flexible flatfoot has a restoration of the arch on toe-rise; rigid flatfoot has no arch restoration. A rigid flatfoot is a sign of decreased subtalar motion and may indicate a tarsal coalition.
- The physician should test for subtalar motion. The test is not specific for talocalcaneal coalition but is indicative of some process within the subtalar joint.
- The physician should palpate over the medial aspect of the hindfoot, just plantar to the medial malleolus, in the region of the sustentaculum tali. Tenderness in this region may be indicative of a middle facet talocalcaneal coalition.

## IMAGING AND OTHER DIAGNOSTIC STUDIES

- Plain radiographs should be obtained in an attempt to identify the coalition and assess foot alignment. These should include anteroposterior (AP), lateral, oblique, and Harris axial views (**FIG 1A,B**).
  - A talocalcaneal coalition is best seen on the Harris axial view, but it may be difficult to obtain the exact orientation to adequately visualize the middle facet.
  - On the lateral view, there may be a continuous C-shaped line along the talar dome and into the posterior facet (C-sign).[8]
  - On the AP and oblique view, one may identify other concurrent coalitions.
- Standing AP and lateral radiographs and a Saltzman hindfoot alignment view can be useful for assessing foot alignment, especially hindfoot valgus.
- A computed tomography (CT) or magnetic resonance imaging (MRI) scan is mandatory to clearly visualize the coalition and determine the percentage of the subtalar joint that is involved (**FIG 1C**).[9]
- An MRI may be useful if the diagnosis is equivocal and a cartilaginous or fibrous coalition is suspected.

## DIFFERENTIAL DIAGNOSIS

- Flexible flatfoot
- Subtalar arthritis
- Other tarsal coalition (calcaneonavicular or less common ones)

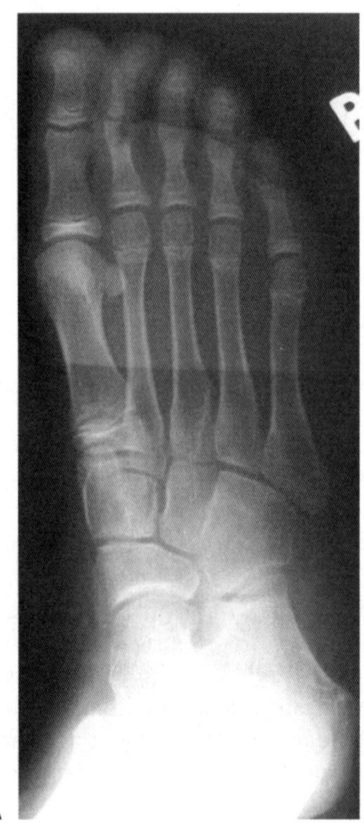

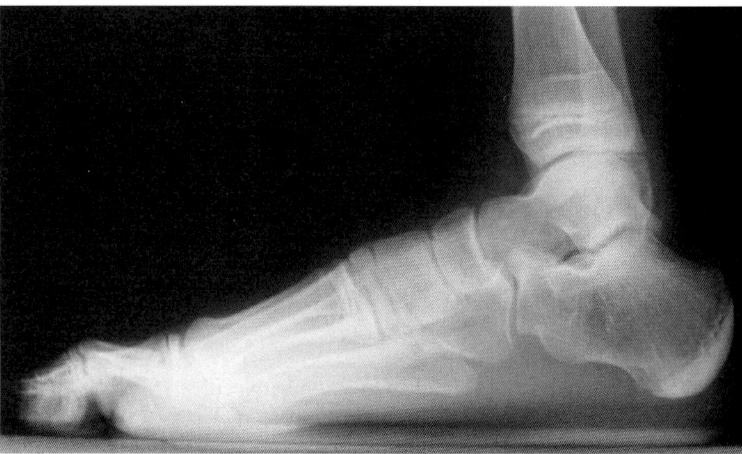

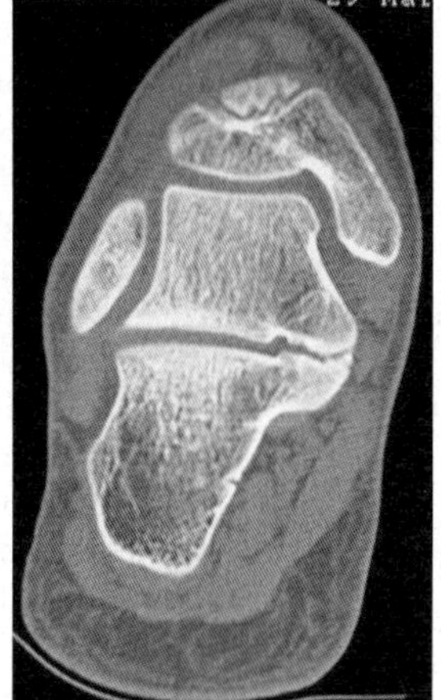

**FIG 1** • **A.** The oblique radiograph confirms the absence of a concurrent calcaneonavicular tarsal coalition. **B.** On the lateral radiograph, a C-sign is visible as a confluent line around the posterior margin of the talar body and the posterior aspect of the calcaneus just beneath the posterior facet of the subtalar joint. This sign is often associated with a talocalcaneal tarsal coalition. **C.** CT scanning can be used to visualize the coalition and determine the percentage of the subtalar joint that is involved.

- Tumor or infection involving the subtalar joint
- Idiopathic rigid flatfoot

## NONOPERATIVE MANAGEMENT

- Nonoperative management is indicated for all patients with talocalcaneal coalition at first presentation.
- Painless coalitions need no treatment.
- The initial treatment for painful talocalcaneal coalitions is activity modification, anti-inflammatory medication, or immobilization in a short-leg walking cast.

## SURGICAL MANAGEMENT

- The indication for surgical management is persistence of pain despite nonoperative management.
- The main goals of treatment are, primarily, elimination of pain and restoration of function.
- Restoration of subtalar motion is a secondary goal.
- Restoration of arch height is unlikely following excision of a talocalcaneal coalition.

### Preoperative Planning

- All imaging studies are reviewed.
- An examination of subtalar motion may be performed under anesthesia to compare to the motion obtained after excision of the coalition.

### Positioning

- The patient is positioned supine on the operating table.
- Generally, the leg assumes an external rotation posture at rest so that the medial ankle and hindfoot are easily accessible. If this is not the case, then a small bump can be placed beneath the opposite hip.
- A tourniquet is placed on the upper thigh or an Esmarch tourniquet may be used just proximal to the ankle.

### Approach

- The approach involves identification of the entire coalition with delineation of the normal cartilage on either side.
- The bone representing the coalition is exposed, and subcutaneous fat or a portion of the flexor hallucis longus is interposed.

## Incision and Dissection

- The procedure can be done under tourniquet control, if desired.
- A straight horizontal incision is made along the medial aspect of the hindfoot centered over the sustentaculum tali.
  - The incision should extend from the location of the neurovascular bundle to the prominence of the navicular tuberosity (**TECH FIG 1A**). For harvesting of fat graft from the retrocalcaneal space, it is sometimes useful to extend the incision more posteriorly.
- If any fibers of the abductor hallucis are encountered, they are retracted plantarly.
- The tibialis posterior tendon is identified dorsally (**TECH FIG 1B**).
- The flexor digitorum longus tendon is identified and its sheath is opened along the length of the incision (**TECH FIG 1C**).
- The neurovascular bundle is identified just posterior to the flexor digitorum longus.
- The flexor hallucis longus tendon sheath can be opened if it is to be used as interposition material. If autologous fat graft is to be used, then this step is unnecessary.
- The Achilles tendon is then identified at the most posterior aspect of the wound.
- At this point, all of the critical anatomic structures have been identified and the coalition can now be exposed.

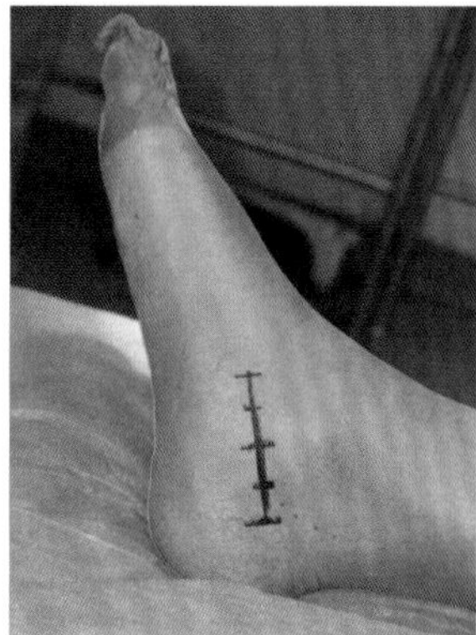
A

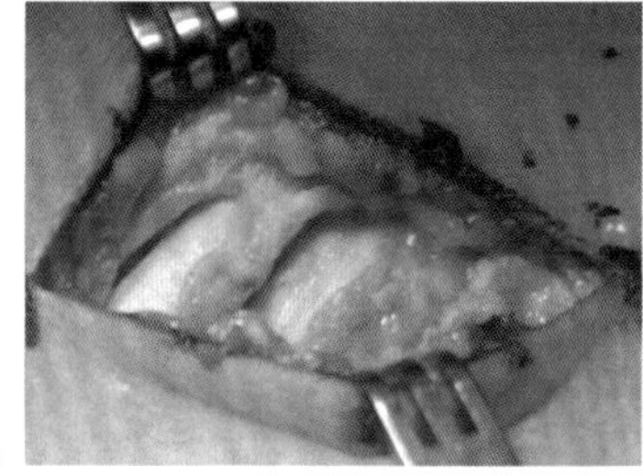
B

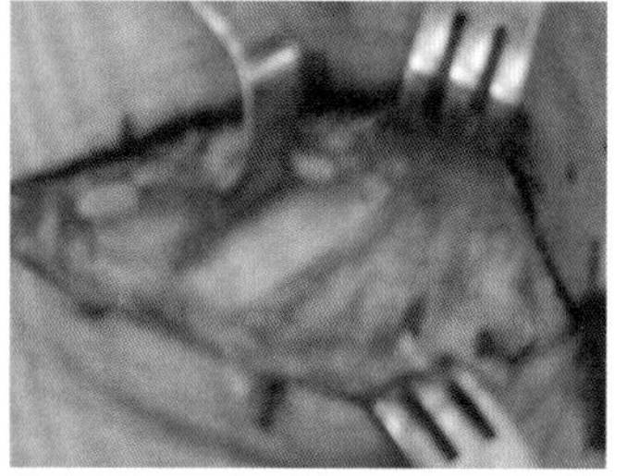
C

**TECH FIG 1** • **A.** Incision marked on the skin. **B.** The posterior tibial tendon (superior) and flexor digitorum longus tendon (inferior). **C.** The neurovascular bundle is seen directly posterior to the posterior tibial tendon.

## Exposure of the Talocalcaneal Coalition

- The talocalcaneal coalition lies just dorsal to the sustentaculum tali and deep to the sheath of the flexor digitorum longus.
- While retracting the flexor digitorum longus tendon plantarly, palpate the sustentaculum tali.
- The coalition lies deep to the medial portion of the sheath of the flexor digitorum longus and periosteum.
- The medial aspect of the flexor digitorum longus sheath, along with the periosteum just deep to it, should be incised slightly dorsal to the prominence of the sustentaculum tali, taking care to maintain an adequate layer to be used later for closure (**TECH FIG 2A,B**).
- Because the normal joint in this area is now obscured by the coalition, it is often difficult to determine the appropriate level for bone resection without first identifying some normal joint space.
  - If this is the case, the dissection may be carried posteriorly and anteriorly to identify the posterior and anterior facets of the subtalar joint, respectively, so that the normal articular cartilage in these areas can be identified.
  - The posterior facet can be identified by retracting the neurovascular bundle posteriorly and dissecting deep to it.
  - The anterior facet is identified just proximal to the talonavicular joint and plantar to the talar neck.
  - Occasionally, a stripe of cartilage can be identified traversing through the center of the coalition. In these cases, resection may proceed directly to this level.
- Next, while retracting the flexor digitorum longus plantarly and the tibialis posterior dorsally, the bone is resected between the two previously identified areas of normal articular cartilage.
  - This can be accomplished with a high-speed burr, rongeurs, and curettes (**TECH FIG 2C**).
- Resection of bone is continued until normal articular cartilage is encountered deep within the wound, lateral to the coalition as well as anterior and posterior to it (**TECH FIG 2D–F**).
- Careful attention to the preoperative imaging studies (namely CT scan and possibly MRI) will aid in estimating how far lateral the dissection should continue.
- Take care to resect bone from known to unknown areas, as it is possible to drift dorsal or plantar into the body of the talus or calcaneus, consequently missing the coalition.
- Once the entire coalition has been resected, the foot should be inverted and everted, demonstrating an improvement in subtalar motion.
  - It should be possible at this point to see clear space from the posterior facet to the anterior facet with supple motion through the joint.
- Apply a thin layer of bone wax to the exposed bony surfaces to minimize bleeding and theoretically decrease the risk of recurrence of the coalition.

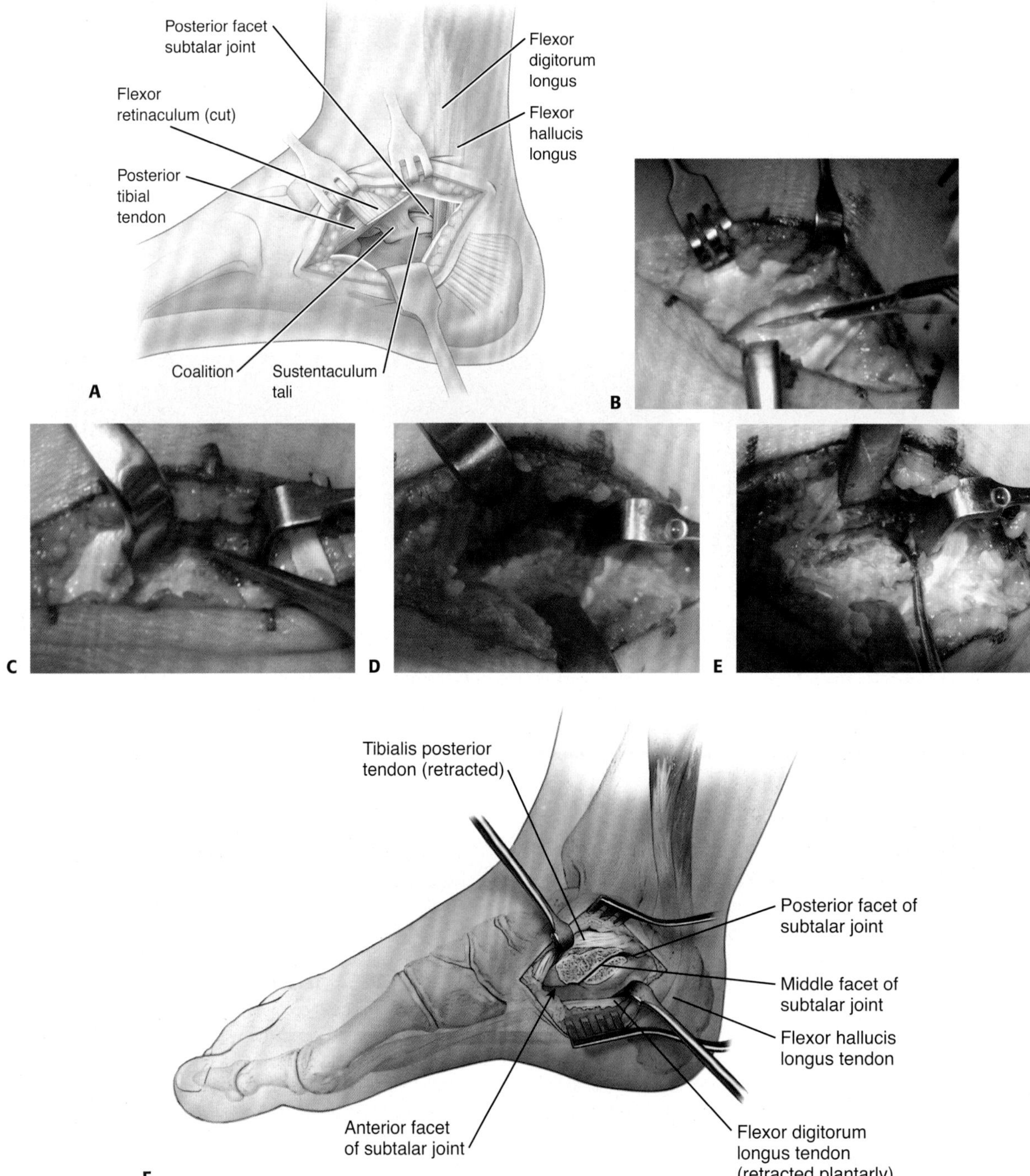


**TECH FIG 2** • **A,B.** The medial aspect of the sheath of the flexor digitorum longus and the periosteum overlying the talus are incised. **C.** The posterior facet is visualized (just posterior to the curette) and the coalition is entered with a curette. **D–F.** The coalition has been removed and there is a visible gap between the talus (superior) and calcaneus (inferior). Just beyond the excised bone, normal articular cartilage can be seen.

## Interposition of Fat Graft

- Next, to retrieve fat graft, the neurovascular bundle is retracted anteriorly, exposing the retrocalcaneal fat between the Achilles tendon and the calcaneus (**TECH FIG 3A**).
  - If there is insufficient fat in this area, fat autograft can be harvested from the buttock instead.
- A piece of fat about 1 cm in diameter is excised from the area.
- This fat is interposed into the space from where the coalition was resected (**TECH FIG 3B,C**).
- The layer of tissue composed of periosteum and flexor digitorum longus sheath is then repaired over this fat with absorbable sutures helping to secure it in place (**TECH FIG 3D**).

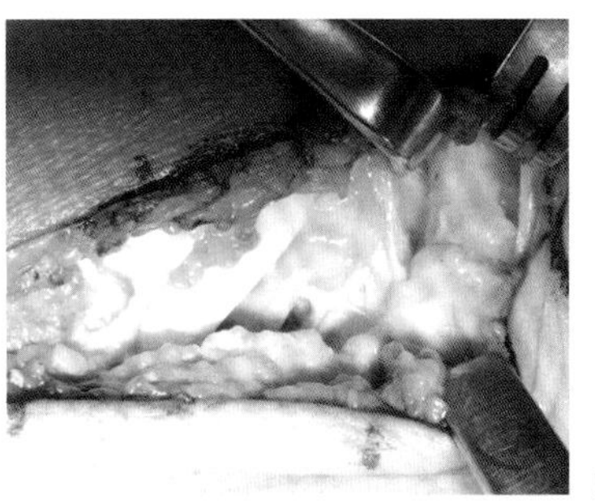
A

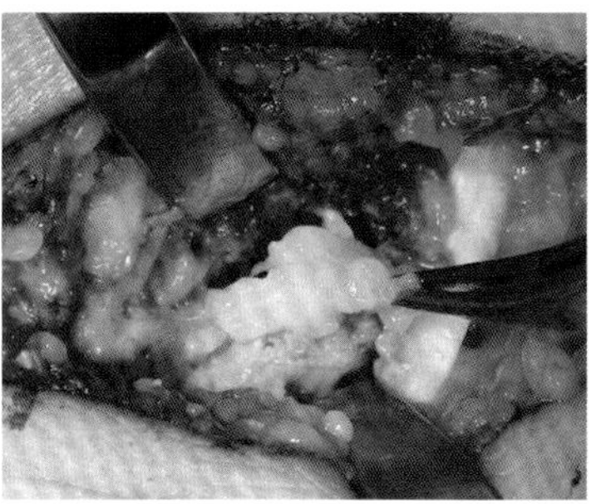
B

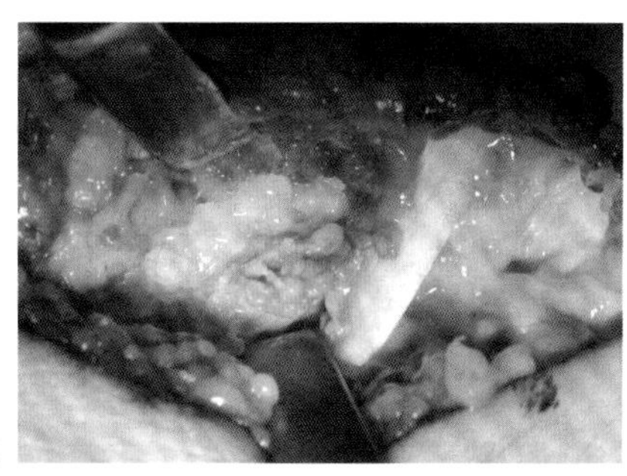
C

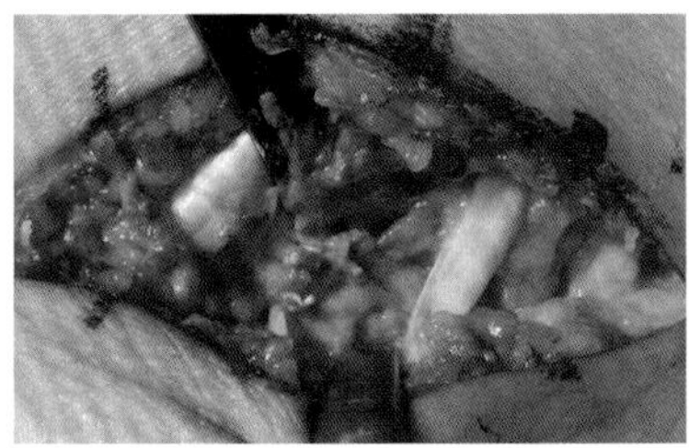
D

**TECH FIG 3** • **A.** Retrocalcaneal fat is exposed between the Achilles tendon and the neurovascular bundle and harvested for the graft. **B–D.** The graft is inserted into the area of the resected coalition, and the periosteum is closed over the graft.

## Interposition of a Portion of the Flexor Hallucis Longus Tendon (Alternative Technique)

- As an alternative to autologous fat graft, half of the flexor hallucis longus tendon may be interposed.[3,6]
- After completely resecting the coalition and confirming adequate motion of the subtalar joint, the flexor hallucis longus tendon is exposed by opening its sheath just inferior to the sustentaculum tali, if this has not been done during the surgical approach.
- The flexor hallucis longus lies in a groove directly inferior to the sustentaculum tali.
- The flexor hallucis is then split longitudinally but left in continuity along its length.
- The superior half of the tendon is then placed in the gap that has been created where the coalition was resected.
- Care is taken to ensure that the length of tendon that is split is sufficiently long so that the motion of the flexor hallucis longus is not restricted.
  - This is accomplished by moving the interphalangeal joint of the great toe through a range of motion and confirming that motion is not restricted.
- The periosteum from the talus is then sutured to the periosteum from the sustentaculum to prevent the tendon from slipping out of place.

## Wound Closure

- The tourniquet is released and hemostasis is obtained.
- The tendon sheaths of the flexor digitorum and tibialis posterior are closed with fine absorbable sutures.
- Subcutaneous tissue and skin are closed in standard fashion.

## PEARLS AND PITFALLS

| | |
|---|---|
| **Indications** | ■ The preoperative CT scan should be carefully assessed for the extent of the coalition and the presence of subtalar arthritis. Excision of the coalition is contraindicated if greater than 50% of the joint surface is coalesced or in the presence of subtalar arthritis.<br>■ Hindfoot alignment is determined clinically and radiographically to assess for hindfoot valgus. Excessive valgus has been associated with poor outcomes. |
| **Approach** | ■ The incision should be long enough to allow adequate identification of normal subtalar joint.<br>■ The periosteum and medial sheath of the flexor digitorum longus are preserved to secure the graft. |
| **Excision of coalition** | ■ The surgeon should identify normal articular cartilage posterior and anterior to the coalition so that the level of resection can be identified.<br>■ Bone is resected from the area where the normal joint can be seen toward the center of the coalition.<br>■ It is possible to resect bone into the body of the talus or calcaneus, missing the coalition, if careful attention is not paid to the level of resection. |
| **Closure** | ■ The periosteum and medial sheath of the flexor digitorum longus tendon are repaired to prevent extrusion of the graft. |

## POSTOPERATIVE CARE

- A splint or short-leg cast is applied.
- The foot is immobilized and the patient should remain non–weight bearing for 2 to 3 weeks to allow for wound healing and consolidation of the graft.
- After that, progressive weight bearing and gentle range-of-motion exercises are initiated, focusing on restoring subtalar motion.

## OUTCOMES

- Most series report better than 85% good to excellent results.[3,6,7,9]
- Poor results, characterized by persistent pain, have generally been associated with coalitions of more than 50% of the joint surface, subtalar arthritis, or severe valgus alignment of the heel in excess of 21 degrees.[4,9,11]
- There may be a role for deformity correction in cases of severe planovalgus with ongoing pain despite complete resection of the coalition or, in some cases concurrently, at the same time as coalition excision.[5]
- A long-term study of functional outcomes in patients with tarsal coalitions found those with talocalcaneal coalitions entailing over 50% surface area and those with more than 16 degrees of hindfoot valgus did as well as those with less than 50% surface area and less than 16 degrees of valgus. Also, outcomes were both favorable and comparable between talocalcaneal and calcaneonavicular coalitions.[2]

## COMPLICATIONS

- Failure to adequately resect the coalition
- Recurrence of the coalition
- Residual pain or stiffness due to preexisting subtalar arthritis or severe malalignment

## REFERENCES


1. Harris RI, Beath T. Etiology of peroneal spastic flat foot. J Bone Joint Surg Br 1948;30:624–634.
2. Khoshbin A, Law PW, Caspi L, et al. Long-term functional outcomes of resected tarsal coalitions. Foot Ankle Int 2013;34:1370–1375.
3. Kumar ST, Guille JT, Lee MS, et al. Osseous and non-osseous coalition of the middle facet of the talocalcaneal joint. J Bone Joint Surg Am 1992;74:529–535.
4. Luhmann SJ, Schoenecker PL. Symptomatic talocalcaneal coalition resection: indications and results. J Pediatr Orthop 1998;18: 748–754.
5. Mosca VS, Bevan WP. Talocalcaneal tarsal coalitions and the calcaneal lengthening osteotomy: the role of deformity correction. J Bone Joint Surg Am 2012;94:1584–1594.
6. Olney BW, Asher MA. Excision of symptomatic coalition of the middle facet of the talocalcaneal joint. J Bone Joint Surg Am 1987;69: 539–544.
7. Raikin S, Cooperman DR, Thompson GH. Interposition of the split flexor hallucis longus tendon after resection of a coalition of the middle facet of the talocalcaneal joint. J Bone Joint Surg Am 1999;81: 11–19.
8. Sakellariou A, Sallomi D, Janzen DL, et al. Talocalcaneal coalition: diagnosis with the C-sign on lateral radiographs of the ankle. J Bone Joint Surg Br 2000;82:574–578.
9. Scranton PE Jr. Treatment of symptomatic talocalcaneal coalition. J Bone Joint Surg Am 1987;69:533–539.
10. Stormont DM, Peterson HA. The relative incidence of tarsal coalition. Clin Orthop Relat Res 1983;(181):28–36.
11. Wilde PH, Torode IP, Dickens DR, et al. Resection for symptomatic talocalcaneal coalition. J Bone Joint Surg Br 1994;76(5): 797–801.

# Ponseti Casting

Blaise Nemeth and Kenneth J. Noonan

125 CHAPTER

## DEFINITION

- Clubfoot, also known as *congenital talipes equinovarus*, occurs in approximately 1 in 1000 live births.
- The clubfoot contains four identifiable components that are easily remembered using the acronym CAVE (cavus, adductus, varus, and equinus). Idiopathic clubfoot contains each of the four components to varying degrees.
  - The so-called postural clubfoot is held by the infant in an equinovarus position, but all components are nearly completely correctable with gentle manipulation and resolve over time without intervention.
- A small proportion of clubfeet are teratologic, occurring as part of other neuromuscular diseases, such as Larsen syndrome, any of the arthrogryposis syndromes, and spina bifida.
- The complex clubfoot, a severe type of idiopathic clubfoot, has a tighter hindfoot and plantar structures.
- In 1948, Dr. Ignacio Ponseti began manipulating clubfeet through serial casting, completely correcting the clubfoot deformity. The principles of Ponseti casting lay in gently stretching the soft tissue structures and gradually inducing remolding of the primarily cartilaginous bones of the hindfoot during immobilization.
  - For the definitive publication on clubfoot and the Ponseti technique, the reader is referred to Dr. Ponseti's book.[7]
  - The success of the treatment protocol that bears his name has been borne out through over 30 years of follow-up, establishing it as the standard for initial treatment of clubfoot.[1]
  - In 2006, Dr. Ponseti published a modification to his original casting technique that addresses the specific deformities characteristic of the complex clubfoot.[8]

## ANATOMY

- The Achilles and posterior tibialis tendons, as well as the posterior and medial ligaments of the foot between the calcaneus, talus, and navicular, are thickened and fibrotic.[7]
- The clubfoot contains a number of changes in bony alignment and shape (**FIG 1**).
  - Relative to normal foot anatomy, the first ray is plantarflexed, generating the cavus deformity. By comparison, all rays are plantarflexed in the complex clubfoot, resulting in full-foot cavus.
  - The navicular is medially displaced on the talus, and the cuboid is medially displaced on the calcaneus as part of the adductus deformity. The medial corners of the head of the talus and the anterior calcaneus are flattened.
  - The calcaneus is inverted under the talus, creating the hindfoot varus, while also being in equinus and elevated in the fat pad of the heel.
- In children with unilateral clubfoot, the affected foot usually is smaller, as is the lower leg, relative to the unaffected side.
- Up to 85% of clubfeet have an insufficient or absent anterior tibial artery.[6]

## NATURAL HISTORY

- The exact cause of the fibrotic changes in clubfoot is unknown. Recently, candidate genes have been identified in familial clubfoot, including *Pitx1* and *Tbx4*.[3]
- Left uncorrected the weight-bearing surface in a clubfoot becomes the dorsolateral surface.
  - Thick callosities develop, and the positioning of the foot creates significant functional disability.

## PATIENT HISTORY AND PHYSICAL FINDINGS

- Clubfoot may be identified on prenatal ultrasound as early as 12 to 13 weeks (**FIG 2**).
  - Half or more of fetuses with clubfeet identified on second trimester ultrasounds are found to have other anomalies (most commonly cardiac, neurologic, and/or urogenital) or are syndromic/teratologic.[9]
  - The exact sensitivity and specificity of prenatal ultrasound are unknown. False positives are rare on 20-week ultrasounds but may be as high as 40% during the third trimester (when false negatives are rare).[9] Cases not found on prenatal ultrasound are readily identifiable at birth.

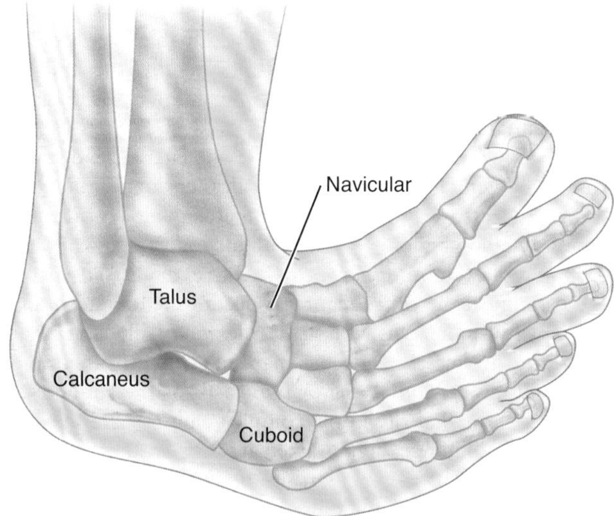


**FIG 1** • Anatomic alignment in neonatal clubfoot. Note the medial displacement of the navicular and cuboid, the inversion and internal rotation of the calcaneus under the talus, and equinus of the talus and calcaneus.

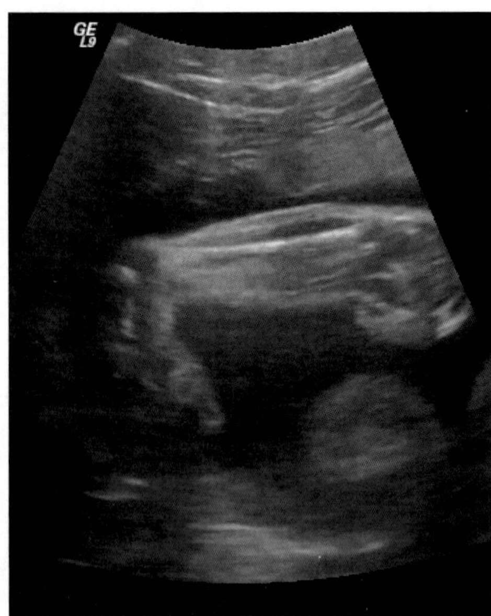


**FIG 2** • Ultrasound at 20 weeks of a child born with clubfoot.

- All children with clubfeet should be examined for other findings that may suggest a syndromic or neuromuscular association, such as other contractures or joint dislocations (especially hip dislocation), cutaneous lesions, spinal abnormalities, and abnormal facial features.
- The clubfoot is easily identified by the combined deformities of cavus, adductus, varus, and equinus.
  - Consider complex clubfoot if a deep midfoot crease and cavus extend transversely across the entire plantar aspect of the foot, and the foot appears short and broad.
- The ability to abduct or dorsiflex the foot completely on examination suggests etiologies other than idiopathic clubfoot, such as isolated metatarsus adductus, neuromuscular disease, or focal anatomic abnormalities.
- The fat pad of the heel will feel empty upon palpation due to equinus positioning of the calcaneus. This is especially dramatic in the complex clubfoot.
- The lateral head of the talus is easily palpable over the dorsolateral surface of the foot. More laterally, the anterior calcaneal tuberosity is also palpable. Care must be taken in differentiating these two structures because Ponseti casting necessitates stabilizing the foot over the lateral head of the talus, allowing free motion of the calcaneus under the talus, whereas pressure at the calcaneal tuberosity blocks calcaneal rotation, allowing only forefoot abduction.
- The complex clubfoot has a crease that extends transversely across almost the entire plantar aspect of the foot accompanied by full-foot cavus with plantarflexion of all metatarsals. Also, the heel crease is deeper than that of most other clubfeet. During the initial one or two casts, as the adductus is corrected, the first ray in the complex clubfoot becomes retracted, if not noticeably retracted at presentation. The cavus also persists, with all metatarsals remaining plantarflexed.
- It is important to examine the clubfoot before each casting to evaluate for the adjustments that must be made during casting to correct residual deformities or to identify and modify casting for a complex clubfoot.
  - A number of classification systems have been introduced as an attempt to predict outcome, but the ability of these systems to evaluate correction, predict recurrence and final function is still unclear.[5]
  - The degree of dorsiflexion and abduction, and the distance of the navicular anterior to the medial malleolus, provide other objective measurements of deformity and correction.
- Some children are born with one or both feet held in an equinovarus deformity at birth that is nearly completely correctable on examination. Nearly complete dorsiflexion (more than 20 degrees) is present, although abduction may be slightly limited. The calcaneus is also readily palpable in the fat pad of the heel. These feet may be thought of as "postural" in nature, and most will resolve spontaneously or with parental stretching over 1 to 2 months.
  - If persistent, one or two casts usually correct the deformity, and Achilles tenotomy is rarely required. Feet corrected with casting may require maintenance in a foot abduction orthosis.

## IMAGING AND OTHER DIAGNOSTIC STUDIES

- Clinical examination is sufficient to diagnose the congenital clubfoot.
- Plain radiographs at birth are not helpful in diagnosing clubfoot because the ossific nuclei of the talus and calcaneus are spherical, so orientation and relationship are not discernible, and the other tarsal bones are unossified.
- Once full abduction is obtained by casting, if dorsiflexion of more than 10 degrees is present, forced dorsiflexion lateral films are helpful in differentiating midfoot breach, producing apparent dorsiflexion, from true dorsiflexion occurring at the ankle, obviating the need for a percutaneous Achilles tenotomy (**FIG 3**).

## DIFFERENTIAL DIAGNOSIS

- Metatarsus adductus
- Neurologic equinovarus or cavovarus deformity
  - Both deformities may be differentiated from clubfoot by absence of the other components of clubfoot.
- Teratologic or syndromic clubfeet (including neuromuscular disorders)
  - Clubfoot deformity may be more difficult to correct and tends to recur.
- Postural clubfoot
- Complex clubfoot

## NONOPERATIVE MANAGEMENT

- Ponseti casting of the idiopathic clubfoot involves a specific sequence of corrective maneuvers that correct the deformities of the clubfoot in combination.
  - Each manipulation is maintained with a plaster cast.
- Ponseti casting ideally begins during infancy, although good results are achievable through toddlerhood. Casting in older children can also produce good results or at least reduce the amount of surgery required for complete correction.
  - An open tendo Achilles lengthening may be more appropriate than a percutaneous tenotomy in children older than 2 years old.

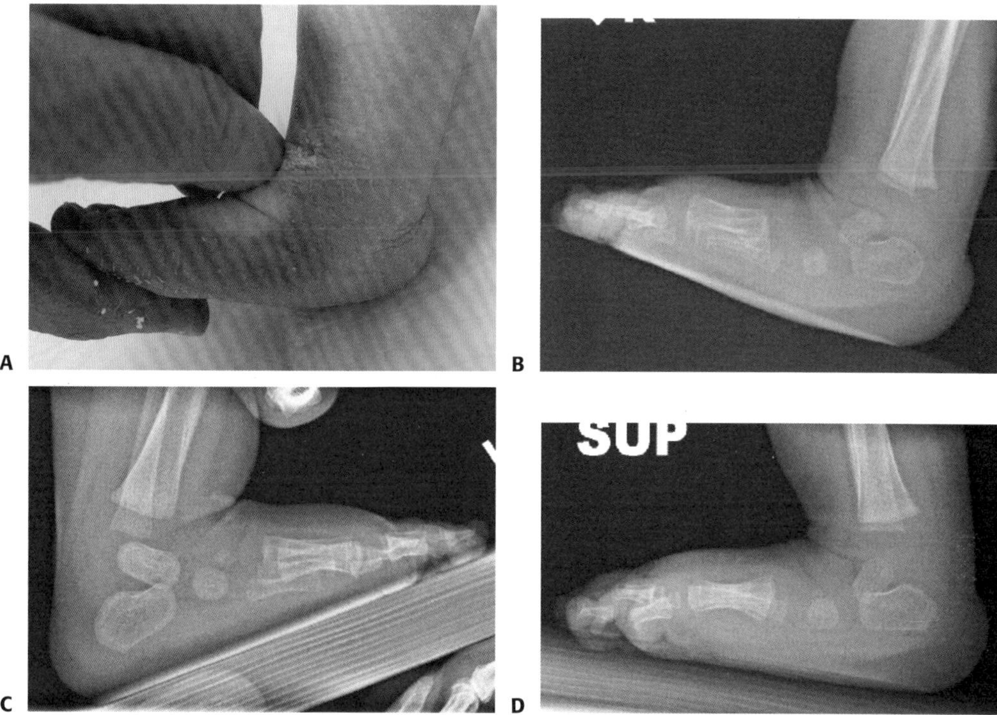


**FIG 3** • **A.** Dorsiflexion of right clubfoot after five corrective casts, before tenotomy. Dorsiflexion of 10 degrees would appear to be sufficient to avoid Achilles tenotomy. **B.** Forced dorsiflexion lateral radiograph of same foot. Dorsiflexion of the metatarsals relative to the axis of the talus reveals midfoot breach as the source of clinical dorsiflexion. The calcaneus is still in equinus (relative to the tibial axis) and a percutaneous Achilles tenotomy is required to complete the correction. **C.** Forced dorsiflexion lateral radiograph of the left (uninvolved) foot. The calcaneus is dorsiflexed and the axis of the first metatarsal is almost parallel to the axis of the talus. **D.** Forced dorsiflexion lateral radiograph of the right foot 3 weeks after the percutaneous Achilles tenotomy. Now, the calcaneus is dorsiflexed relative to the tibial axis and in comparison to the pretenotomy radiograph (**B**).

- Long-leg casts should always be used to prevent cast slippage and maintain rotational control of the lower leg.
  - Initially, applying a short-leg cast allows focused attention on maintaining foot position and molding before extending the cast above the knee.
  - Padding should be minimal, and plaster is preferable for its ability to be molded precisely to the contours of the foot and ankle.
- Four to six casts should correct the cavus, adductus, and varus deformities. If correction is not achieved in eight casts or the child pulls back in the casts (**FIG 4A**), the possibility of an unrecognized complex clubfoot or improper casting technique should be considered.
- Casting is facilitated by the child being relaxed and calm. Feeding the infant during casting assists in this.
  - For breast-fed infants, it is helpful if the family introduces, and uses once daily, a bottle so the child may feed during casting. If a bottle is not tolerated, other calming measures may be necessary.
  - For older children, music, television, or playing with toys often proves helpful, as does casting with the child sitting upright or on the parent's lap.
- Before leaving the clinic, the toes should be checked to make sure they are pink and well perfused.
  - Some toes will become reddish-purple as the casts cool (appearing much like the acrocyanosis present at birth) but will become pink if the child is bundled and monitored over 1 hour or so (**FIG 4B,C**).
  - Toes that become more purple and dusky indicate that the cast is too tight and should be reapplied.
- Casts are changed every 5 to 7 days. The final cast, following percutaneous Achilles tenotomy, is left in place for 3 weeks.
- Almost all clubfeet will require a percutaneous Achilles tenotomy to correct the residual equinus deformity once the other components are corrected.
- Once complete correction is obtained, correction must be maintained by placing the feet in a foot abduction orthosis (**FIG 5A–D**).
  - Constructs include straight last shoes, soft ankle–foot orthoses (AFO), or rigid AFOs mounted on rigid or articulating bars (see Postoperative Care).

## SURGICAL MANAGEMENT

- Percutaneous Achilles tenotomy is required in almost all idiopathic clubfeet to correct the residual equinus.
- About 20% of patients require anterior tibialis tendon transfer at 3 to 4 years old to correct recurrent or persistent dynamic varus deformity (see Chap. 116).

### Preoperative Planning

- Degree of dorsiflexion
  - If dorsiflexion is less than 10 degrees, a percutaneous Achilles tenotomy is required to correct the residual equinus.

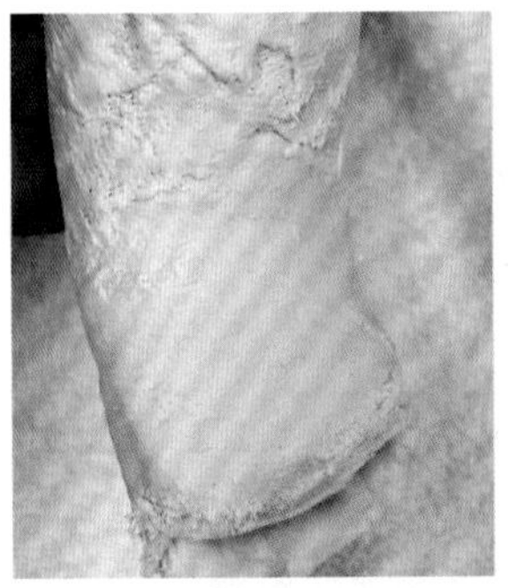
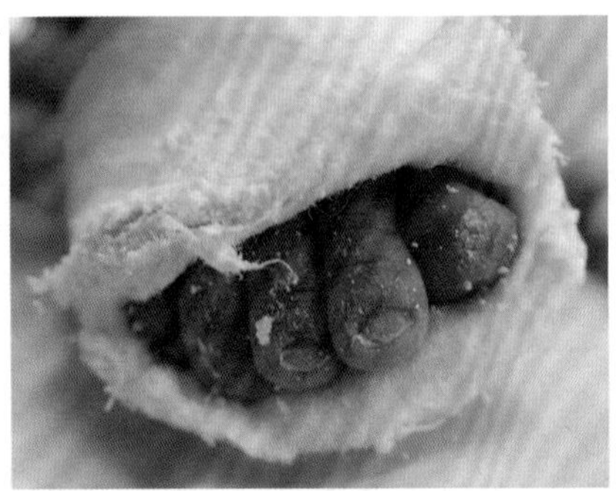
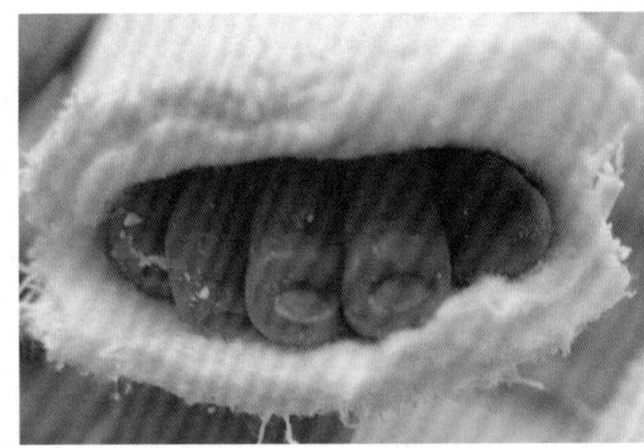

**FIG 4** • **A.** A complex clubfoot that has pulled back in the cast. The cast was originally trimmed to the base of the toes. The heel is elevated in the cast and the toes are no longer visible. **B.** Purple discoloration of toes after application of the first cast, as the cast begins to cool. **C.** One hour later, the cast temperature has stabilized and the toes are pink.

- If dorsiflexion is more than 10 degrees, forced dorsiflexion lateral foot radiographs help to differentiate midfoot dorsiflexion, with residual calcaneal equinus, from true dorsiflexion occurring at the hindfoot (see **FIG 3**).
- Location
  - The risk of anesthesia must be balanced against the perceived pain and duration of the procedure as well as the degree of sedation necessary for safe performance of the procedure and optimizing posttenotomy casting. Approximately half of pediatric orthopedists report performing the percutaneous tenotomy under general anesthesia or conscious sedation.[10]
  - Local analgesia, with 1% lidocaine, affords the opportunity to perform the tenotomy in the clinic setting and avoids any potential risk of general anesthesia.

## Positioning

- The child should be supine on the table with the contralateral leg held out of the way by the parent or an assistant during tenotomy and casting.

## Approach

- A medial approach is used to remain posterior to medial neurovascular bundle.

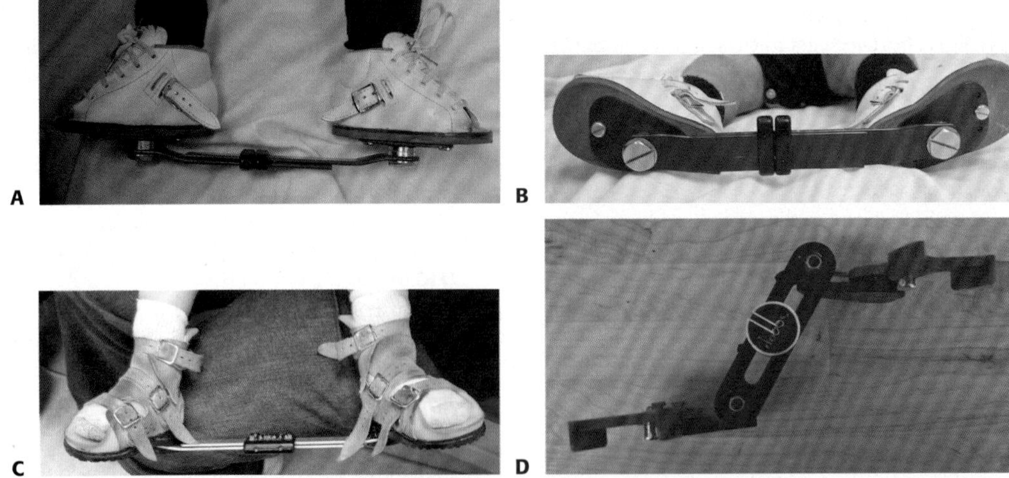

**FIG 5** • The foot abduction orthosis. **A.** Straight last shoes attached to a solid bar. **B.** Heels of the orthoses should be placed at shoulder width with the buckles along the medial aspect of the shoe to ease application. Feet should be positioned in 60 to 70 degrees of abduction in cases of bilateral clubfoot. **C.** A soft AFO on a solid bar. **D.** A hinged bar to which straight last shoes or AFOs may be attached.

## Casting

### Stretching

- Before casting, the foot should be stretched in the same manner as used for immobilization during casting (**TECH FIG 1A,B**).
  - The thumb of the examiner's contralateral hand (eg, the left hand when manipulating the right foot) should be placed over the head of the talus, and the index finger of the other hand should lie along the medial aspect of the first ray with the second through fourth fingers under the plantar aspects of the forefoot.
  - The calcaneocuboid joint should be avoided, so as not to block subtalar motion.
- The first casting should focus on elevation of the first ray to correct the cavus deformity (**TECH FIG 1C**).
  - This places the forefoot in supination, locking the midfoot and aligning the forefoot with the hindfoot, allowing for correction of the hindfoot deformities during later abduction maneuvers.
  - Some of the adductus may also be corrected during the first casting.

### Lower Leg Cast Application

- A thin layer of cotton padding should be applied.
  - The padding is wrapped three times around the toes distally, then extended proximally over the foot and lower leg to pad with no more than two layers of padding.
  - The foot should be held in the position to be casted throughout (**TECH FIG 2A**). The popliteal fossa should be avoided proximally.
- A thin layer of plaster is applied over the foot and lower leg.
  - The plaster may be applied more loosely over the toes but should be snug over the hindfoot and ankle to immobilize the foot properly and allow for precise molding (**TECH FIG 2B**).
  - Avoid making the cast too snug so as to impair venous return or apply unnecessary pressure on the fat pad of the heel.
- The lower leg cast should be precisely molded around the malleoli and above the calcaneus posteriorly.
  - Do not apply pressure over the fat pad of the heel.
  - Throughout, the foot should be held in the position of correction, but the fingers should be in fairly constant motion to prevent pressure spots within the minimally padded cast.

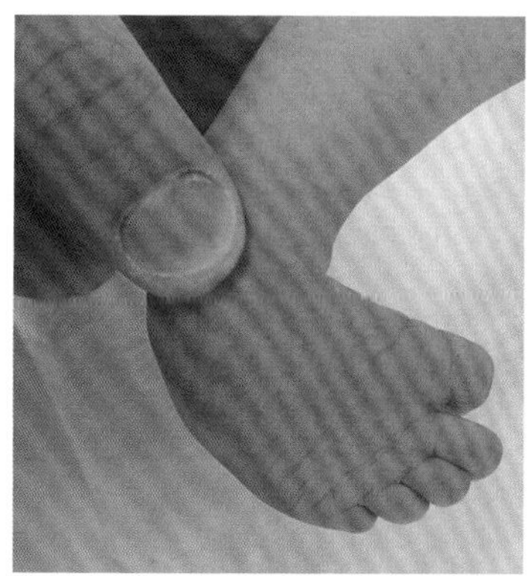
A

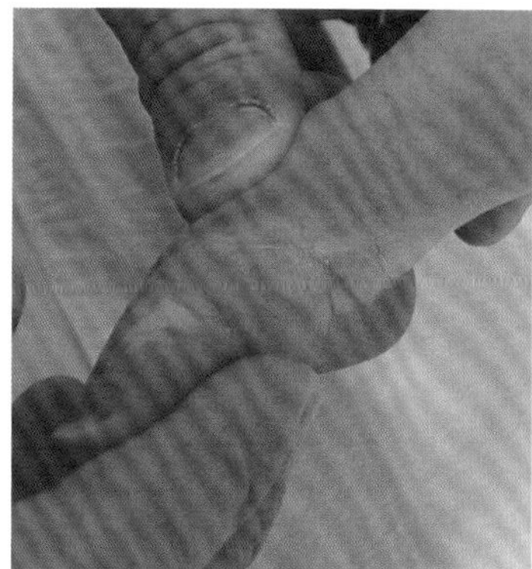
B

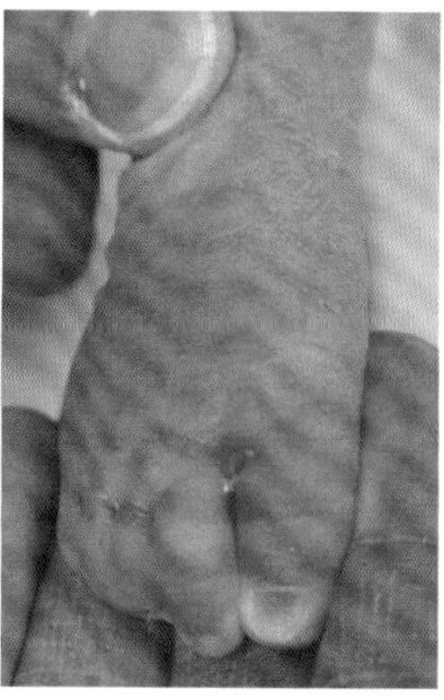
C

**TECH FIG 1** • **A.** The thumb should be placed over the lateral head of the talus, just anterior to the lateral malleolus, during all corrective maneuvers, including during stretching and casting. **B.** The fingers of the opposite hand are placed under the metatarsals of the foot to keep all rays aligned. The index finger is placed slightly more medially on the first ray to provide an abduction force to the forefoot. **C.** The first casting corrects the cavus deformity by elevation of the first ray, bringing it into alignment with the other rays. The metatarsus adductus also improves as a result of the first cast.

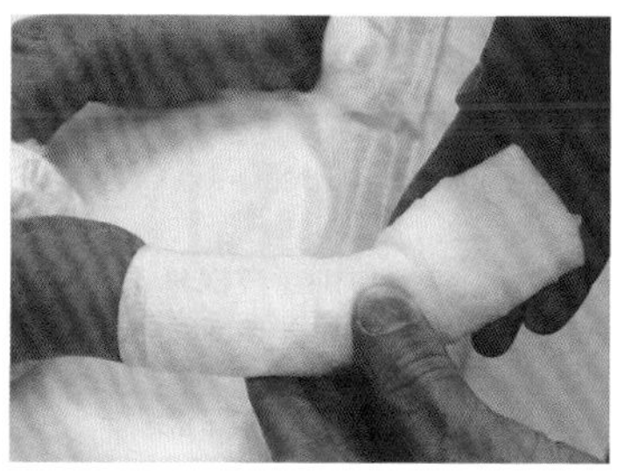
A

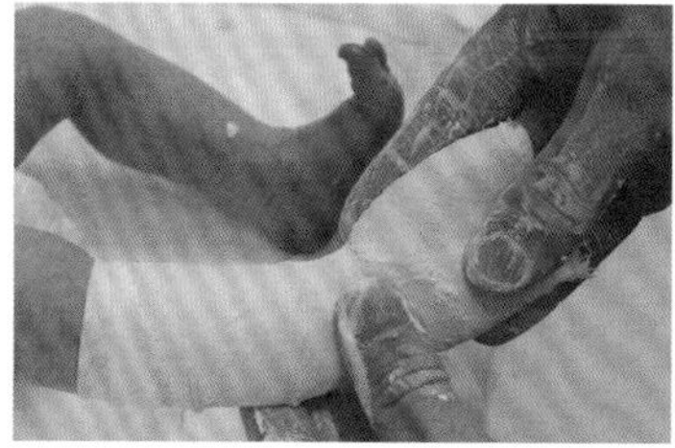
B

**TECH FIG 2** • **A.** The foot should be held in the position of correction. Casting of the lower leg begins with two layers of cotton padding. **B.** A thin amount of plaster is applied and the foot is held in position while the plaster sets. The thumb provides counterpressure over the lateral head of the talus as the foot is abducted. The cast is molded above the calcaneus and around the malleoli; the fingers should remain in constant motion to prevent pressure spots.

## Completing the Cast

- Once the lower leg cast has set, padding should be applied over the rest of the leg up to the groin, again in no more than two or three layers.
  - The knee should be held at 90 degrees, and the lower leg should be in slight external rotation.
  - Padding should be minimized in the popliteal fossa to prevent impingement of the neurovascular structures. The padding should be wrapped three to five times over the proximal thigh to pad adequately.
  - Plaster should then be wrapped over the short-leg cast above the ankle and extended proximally over the padded knee and thigh to the groin. A plaster splint of three or four layers of plaster roll should be placed over the knee from the proximal thigh to the middle of the shin to strengthen the cast against knee extension while minimizing bulk in the popliteal fossa. The plaster is then wrapped distally to incorporate the splint, ending once the lower leg cast has been adequately incorporated.
  - The knee should be molded while held at 90 degrees with the lower leg in slight external rotation until set (**TECH FIG 3A**). Rolling the plaster at the proximal edge of the cast before the plaster sets up completely helps minimize chafing of the thigh.

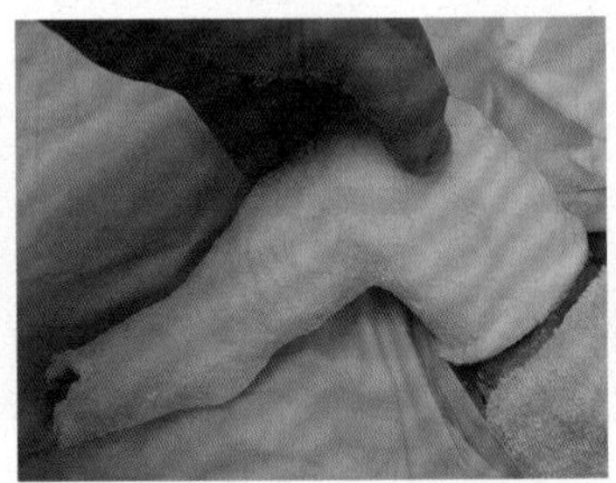

A

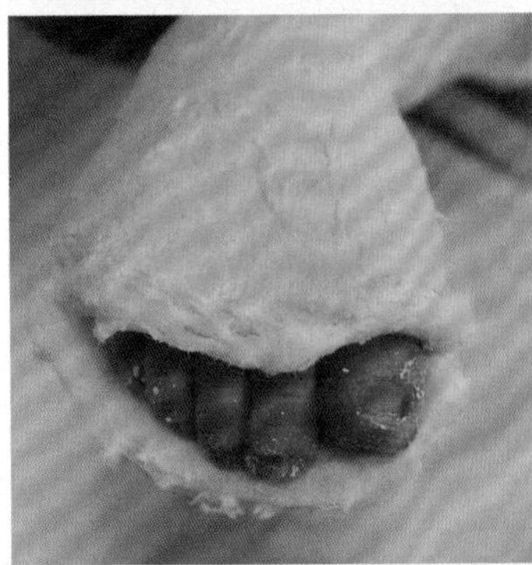

B

**TECH FIG 3** • **A.** Padding and plaster are applied up to the proximal thigh, incorporating the short-leg cast into a long-leg cast. The knee is flexed to 90 degrees. The proximal margin of the cast is rolled to decrease skin irritation. **B.** The distal end of the cast is trimmed to the web space of the toes dorsally, revealing pink, well-perfused digits.

- The cast should be trimmed distally to expose the toes. The practitioner should confirm that they are pink and well perfused (**TECH FIG 3B**) before the child is sent home.
  - Trimming the plaster over the dorsal aspect too far proximally, beyond the web space, may create a tourniquet effect over the forefoot.
  - Parents should be instructed on signs and symptoms of cast problems before discharge.

## Cast Changes and Follow-Up

- Casts are typically changed every 7 days, although they may be changed as frequently as every 5 days; up to 2 weeks may be tolerated if necessary to accommodate conflicts preventing weekly cast changes.
- Casts should not be removed until just before recasting.
  - Casts can be soaked by the family before coming to the office, then removed with a plaster knife in the clinic.
  - Alternatively, dry casts may be removed with a cast saw, using extreme caution.
  - Having the parents remove the casts the night before results in varied degrees of recurrence overnight and prolongs casting.
- After the first casting, the cavus deformity should be nearly, or completely, corrected. If not, adopt complex casting modifications.
  - Abduction may be increased.
  - Stretching is performed with the forefoot in supination, maintaining alignment of all rays, abducting the foot under the talus, again stabilizing the talus laterally.
- The foot is then casted in the newly maintained position, just to where the foot may be comfortably corrected without significant resistance.
  - Trying to overabduct the foot during a single casting results in intolerance as the foot tries to return to its position of comfort and in the worst cases results in pressure sores or vascular compromise of the soft tissues along the medial foot. A keen sense of touch and patience are essential.
  - Each subsequent manipulation results in increased abduction of the forefoot and correction of the hindfoot varus (**TECH FIG 4A–D**).
  - Throughout, the forefoot should remain in neutral (appearing supinated due to the hindfoot varus) and the hindfoot in equinus (**TECH FIG 4E**).
  - Dorsiflexion of the calcaneus remains blocked under the neck of the talus until approximately 25 degrees of abduction has been obtained. Dorsiflexion before that point results in midfoot breach (see **FIG 3**).
  - Subsequent eversion of the calcaneus will bring the forefoot and hindfoot into more neutral positions, and dorsiflexion may be obtained by percutaneous Achilles tenotomy.
- Once abduction of 70 degrees is obtained (**TECH FIG 4F**), correction of the remaining equinus deformity may occur.
  - Overabduction to 70 degrees is necessary to accommodate some of the inevitable recurrence, without allowing progression beyond a normal position that would require recorrection.

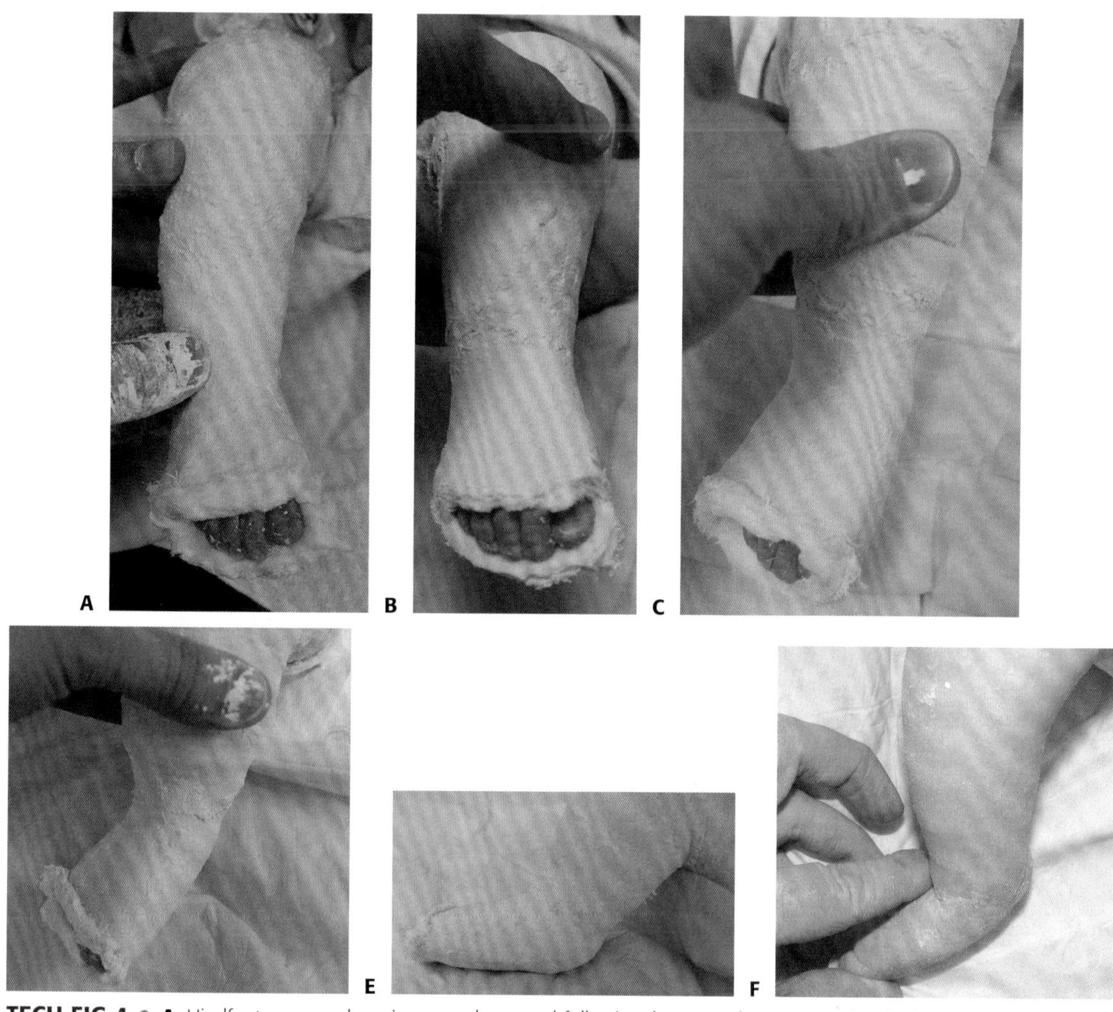

**TECH FIG 4** • **A.** Hindfoot varus and equinus are decreased following the second cast. **B.** By the third cast, the foot is in line with the leg. **C.** By the fourth casting, the foot is abducted 20 degrees and held in this position with the cast. **D.** With the fifth cast, the foot is now held at 45 degrees of abduction. **E.** Prior to the tenotomy, the foot remains in plantarflexion throughout abduction. **F.** After removal of the fifth cast, the foot can be abducted 70 degrees and is ready for percutaneous Achilles tenotomy. The amount of dorsiflexion in this foot is seen in **FIG 3**.

## Complex Clubfoot

- The complex clubfoot may not be immediately recognizable at presentation.
- Correction usually begins using the standard maneuvers, elevating the first ray with the first cast and continuing abduction with the second cast.
  - Within one or two casts, the foot begins to clearly demonstrate a deviation from the expected correction as the cavus persists and evolves, involving plantarflexion of all metatarsals, and the first ray becomes retracted.
  - At this point, the technique must be modified.
- In the complex clubfoot, the tight plantar intrinsics and toe flexors induce full-foot cavus. This is exacerbated by the tight hindfoot structures, which also limit correction of the varus to just beyond neutral.
  - As a result, the casting technique must be modified not only to correct these features but also to decrease the propensity for pulling out of even long-leg casts.
- Lateral counterpressure still occurs at the lateral head and neck of the talus, but stabilization of the fibula should also occur.
  - The index finger of the contralateral hand (eg, the examiner's left hand when manipulating a patient's right clubfoot) should be flexed at the proximal interphalangeal joint and placed posterior to the distal fibula.
  - The thumb of the same hand is placed just anterior to the lateral malleolus along the neck of the talus.
- As the foot begins to approach neutral, the full-foot cavus, along with the dramatic equinus, can pose significant casting difficulties and make the foot prone to pulling back in, or out of, the cast.
- After applying cotton padding, a posterior splint of three or four layers of plaster should be applied under the plantar surface of the foot, extending from beyond the tips of the toes proximally over the posterior lower leg.
  - As in the upper leg portion of the traditional cast, the posterior splint about the foot strengthens the plantar portion of the cast against the forceful plantarflexion of the

complex clubfoot without increasing bulk over the anterior ankle, which may impede molding and immobilization.
- Then, a thin layer of plaster may be wrapped in the usual manner to encompass the foot and lower leg. A minimal amount of plaster should be used because precise molding is even more important for the complex clubfoot.
- The pads of the thumbs of both hands are placed under the forefoot, with the pads of the index fingers placed over the dorsal surface of the talar neck, anterior to the medial and lateral malleoli, with the middle fingers posterior to the malleoli. The forefoot is then forcefully dorsiflexed against the counterpressure over the dorsal talar neck, enough to produce blanching of the digits (**TECH FIG 5A**).
- Further counterpressure to dorsiflexion is applied over the anterior thigh above the flexed knee.
- Upon release of dorsiflexion pressure after setting of the cast, the slight relaxation of the cast should result in revascularization of the digits and pink coloration (**TECH FIG 5B**). If not, the cast should be removed and reapplied.

- On extending the cast up over the lower leg, the knee should be flexed to 110 degrees to minimize the ability to pull out of the cast. An anterior plaster splint over the thigh and knee should be used just as in the traditional technique.
- Tenotomy occurs once the cavus and adductus deformities are corrected and about 40 degrees of abduction is obtained.
  - Attempting to abduct the complex clubfoot beyond 40 degrees results in no further hindfoot correction and only overabducts the forefoot, creating deformity and making immobilization of the foot in the cast more difficult.

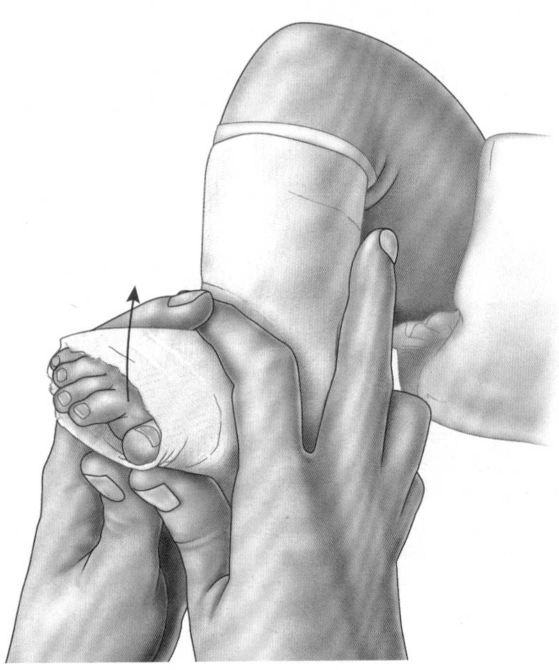
A

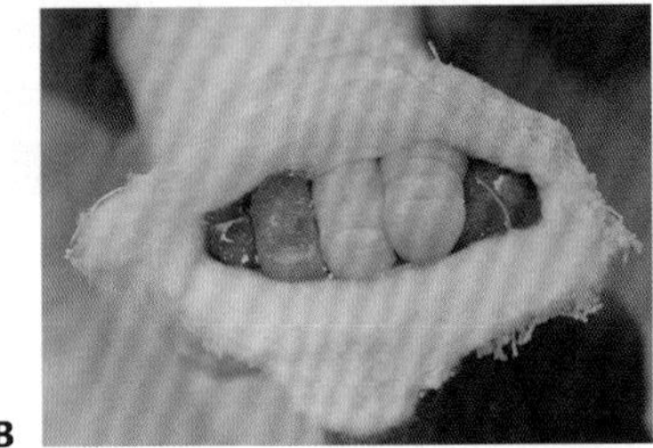
B

**TECH FIG 5** • **A.** When casting the complex clubfoot, to correct the full-foot cavus, a dorsiflexion force is applied to dorsiflex the forefoot and stretch the midfoot. The fat pads of both thumbs are placed under the heads of the metatarsals, with the index fingers over the dorsal aspect of the talar neck; the middle fingers are placed behind the malleoli to help mold the cast. **B.** When dorsiflexing the complex clubfoot during initial castings (before tenotomy), the toes should blanch. When dorsiflexion pressure is released, the slight relaxation of the cast results in reperfusion of the digits. In this case, blood flow returned initially to the first, fourth, and fifth digits; the second and third became pink a few moments later.

## Percutaneous Achilles Tenotomy

- The tenotomy should occur 1 to 1.5 cm above the insertion of the Achilles on the posterior tuberosity of the calcaneus.
  - In many feet, this is 1 to 1.5 cm above the posterior heel crease.
  - Performing the tenotomy too low results in damage to the posterior calcaneal tuberosity.
- For procedures in the clinic, local anesthesia must be used.
  - A small amount of 1% lidocaine may be injected locally adjacent to the tendon at the site of blade insertion before the procedure, taking care not to inject so much as to obscure the Achilles tendon to identification by palpation necessary for the procedure (**TECH FIG 6A**).
- Whether performed in the operating room or clinic, sterile technique should be observed using skin preparation, sterile gloves, and draping and sterile equipment.
- An assistant should hold the foot in maximal dorsiflexion to increase tension on the Achilles tendon, making it more easily palpable and able to be transected (**TECH FIG 6B**).
  - A second assistant should hold the contralateral leg and foot out of the field.
- A thin, sharp scalpel should be used to perform the tenotomy. Cataract surgical blades (5100 or 5400 Beaver blades) are well suited for this procedure, although a no. 11 blade is also acceptable. One of two techniques may be used to insert the blade:
  - The blade of the scalpel may be inserted perpendicular to the skin, anterior to the Achilles tendon, from the medial side, with the blade itself oriented parallel to the longitudinal axis of the tendon. The blade must be advanced far enough to pass beyond the lateral side of the tendon so that complete transection occurs. Once advanced far enough, the blade may be rotated in place, orienting the blade perpendicular to the tendon (**TECH FIG 6C**).

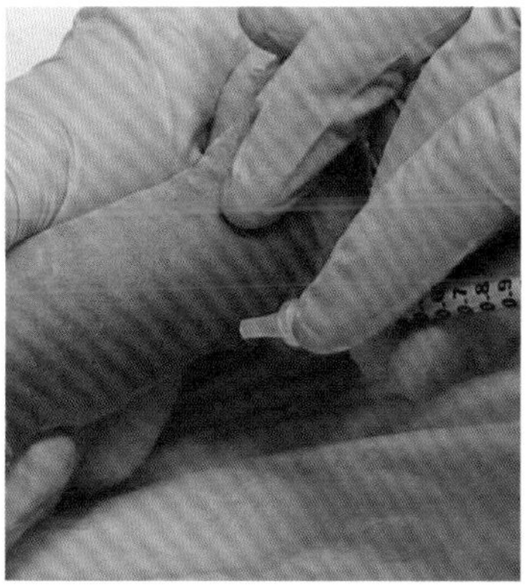

A 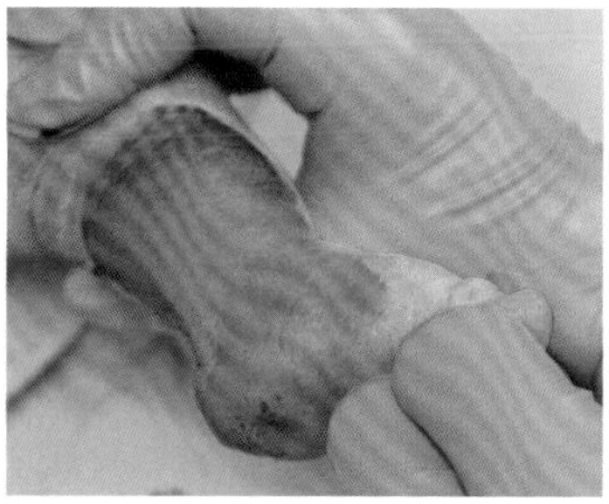 B

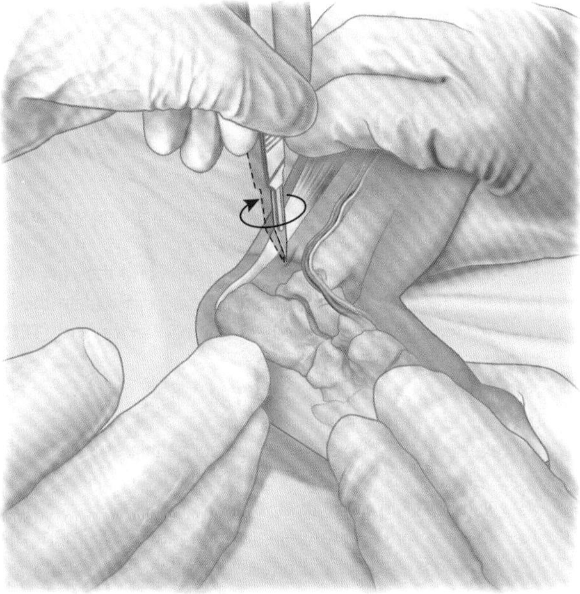

C 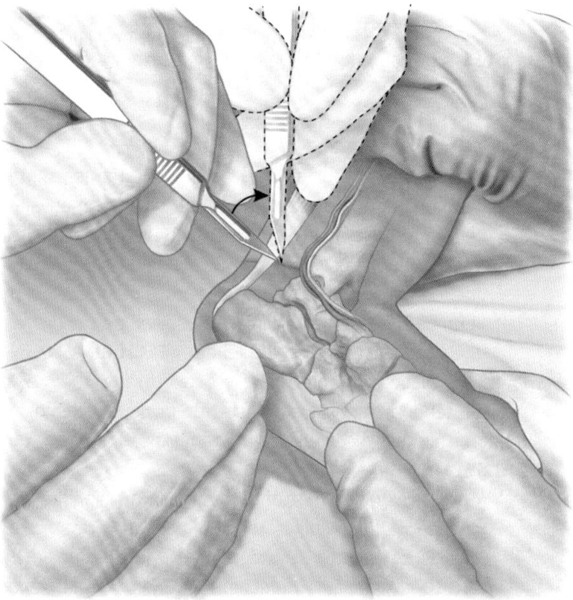 D

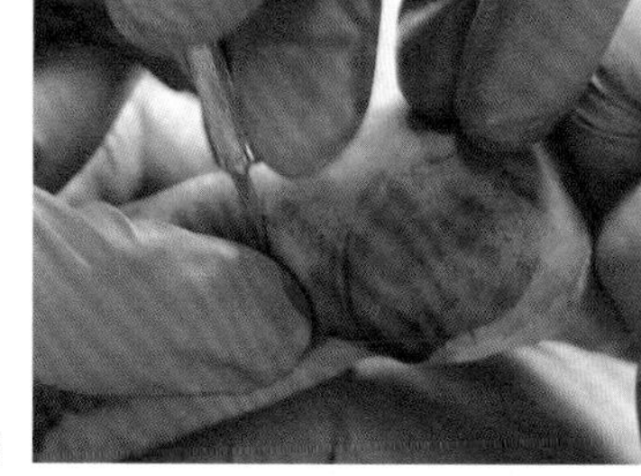

E

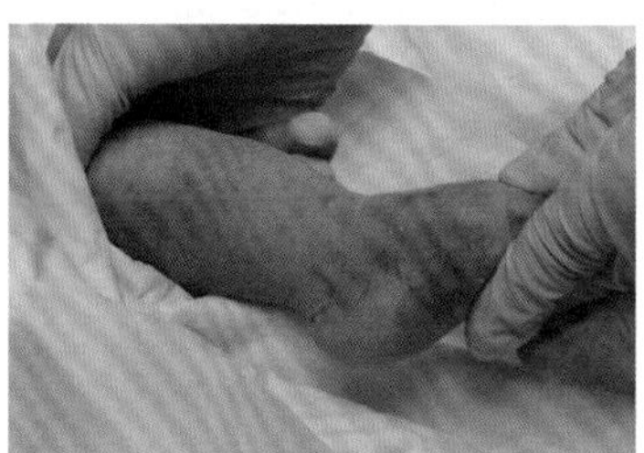

F

**TECH FIG 6** • **A.** Local anesthesia for percutaneous Achilles tenotomy of the left foot. Lidocaine is injected 1 to 1.5 cm above the insertion of the Achilles tendon on the calcaneus, which in this case occurs at the level of the hindfoot crease. **B.** An assistant dorsiflexes the left foot, applying tension to the Achilles tendon, making it easier to palpate and transect with the scalpel. **C.** One of the two techniques used to insert the scalpel blade and transect the tendon. (The illustration is of the left foot.) The handle of the scalpel is perpendicular to the skin over the medial heel cord, with the blade parallel to the axis of the tendon. Once the tip of the blade has been advanced beyond the lateral edge of the tendon, the blade is turned perpendicular to the tendon (*arrow*). **D.** The second of the two techniques for blade insertion. (The illustration is of the left foot.) The handle and the blade are advanced at a 45-degree angle to the skin, with the sharp edge of the blade oriented perpendicular to the tendon. Once advanced deeply enough for the tip to be beyond the lateral edge of the tendon, the handle is swung anteriorly to bring the blade into contact with the tendon (*arrow*). The handle is now perpendicular to the skin. **E.** Transection of the Achilles tendon of the left foot. Pressure is applied with the contralateral thumb, pressing the tendon onto the blade, resulting in tendon transection. The level of the tenotomy is 1 cm above the posterior heel crease. **F.** The foot is in plantarflexion before the tenotomy. *(continued)*

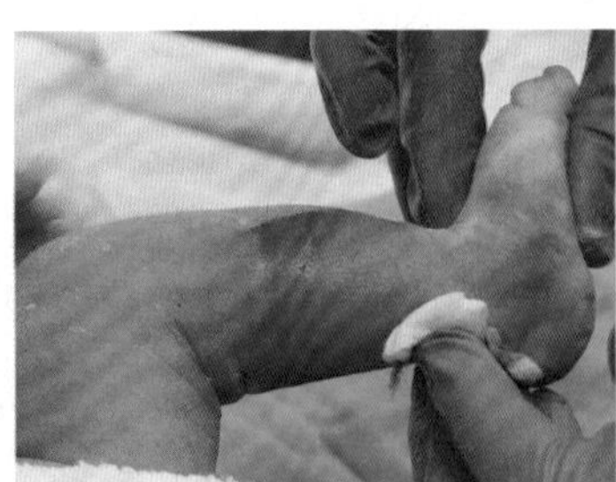

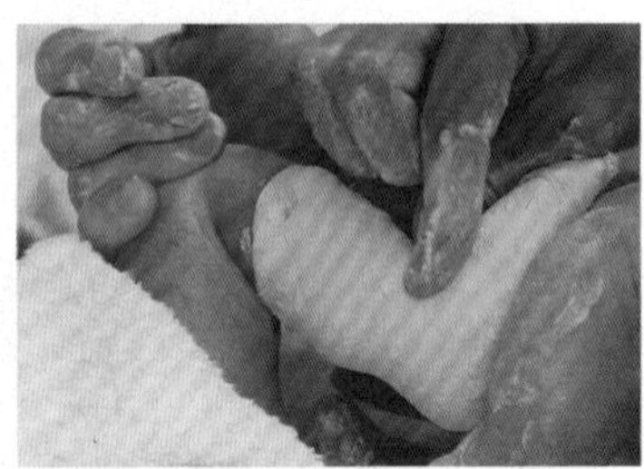

**TECH FIG 6** • *(continued)* **G.** After the tenotomy, 30 degrees of dorsiflexion is obtained. In extreme dorsiflexion, the digits blanch, presumably due to impingement of the posterior tibial artery. Decreasing dorsiflexion just a few degrees resulted in reperfusion. **H.** During application and molding of the short-leg cast, the foot should be held in maximum dorsiflexion and abduction. An assistant provides counterpressure above the knee. Dorsiflexion pressure is applied only over the plantar aspect of the midfoot and forefoot, and the heel remains untouched while the cast is molded around the ankle with the fingers of the other hand.

  - Alternatively, the blade may be advanced anterior to the tendon at a 45-degree angle to the skin, again advancing the tip of the blade deep enough to pass the lateral side of the tendon but with the blade oriented perpendicular to the tendon from the outset. The handle of the scalpel may then be lifted ventrally, bringing the blade perpendicular to the skin, resting against the tendon (**TECH FIG 6D**).
- Once the blade is oriented perpendicular to the fibers of the Achilles tendon, the safest maneuver involves pressing the tendon onto the blade using the contralateral thumb (**TECH FIG 6E**).
  - Complete transection often results in a palpable "pop," release of the Achilles tendon, and an immediate increase of 15 to 20 degrees of dorsiflexion (**TECH FIG 6F**). A palpable defect in the tendon confirms complete transection.
  - If incomplete transection occurs, the tendon should be revisited, adjusting blade position as necessary, to complete the release.
    - Care should be taken not to pull the blade through the tendon lest laceration of the overlying skin occur once the resistance of the tendon disappears following transection.
- The skin prep (Betadine or chlorhexidine) should be cleansed from the skin to prevent burns to the neonatal skin, and pressure should be applied to the incision site to stop all bleeding before cast application.
- The foot should now be held in the new position of maximum dorsiflexion and abduction.
- In some cases, the increased dorsiflexion will cause spasm of the solitary posterior tibial artery, constricting it and resulting in blanching of the digits (**TECH FIG 6G**). Slight relaxation of dorsiflexion should result in reperfusion. The foot should be casted at the position of maximum dorsiflexion that still allows perfusion of the digits.

## Casting

- The lower leg is wrapped with sterile cotton in the usual manner, accommodating the increased dorsiflexion.
- The plaster is applied in the usual manner, and the cast must be molded well at the anterior ankle to accommodate the increased dorsiflexion and prevent pulling back in the cast (**TECH FIG 6H**).
- For the complex clubfoot, the posterior plaster splint should be used in the short-leg cast.
- On release of dorsiflexion pressure after setting of the cast, the slight relaxation of the cast should result in revascularization.
  - If revascularization does not occur, the cast may need to be removed and reapplied. Although maximum dorsiflexion is prevented because of vascular compromise, what is gained is usually sufficient for adequate correction without the need for a second tenotomy or later recorrection.
- Extension of the cast above the thigh as a long-leg cast should occur with the knee in the usual 90 degrees of flexion, first with padding (**TECH FIG 7A**) and then with plaster, holding the lower leg in slight external rotation (**TECH FIG 7B**).
  - The complex clubfoot should have the knee flexed at 110 degrees.
  - An anterior knee splint should be used in both cases.
- The posttenotomy cast should be left on for 3 weeks before removal to allow tendon healing.
- Frequently, blood seeps through the cast and becomes visible, and parents should be alerted to this.
  - Persistent bleeding, resulting in a spot above the heel larger than a quarter in size, may signify injury to vascular structures on the lateral aspect of the foot, rarely requiring any intervention other than further assessment.[2]
- When the cast is removed, complete correction should have been obtained (**TECH FIG 7C,D**).

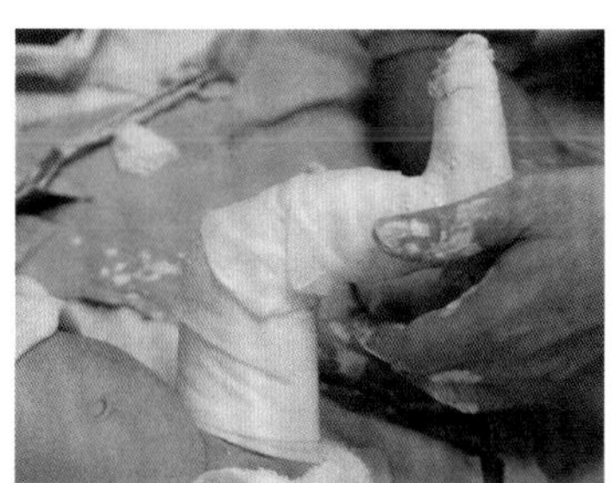
A

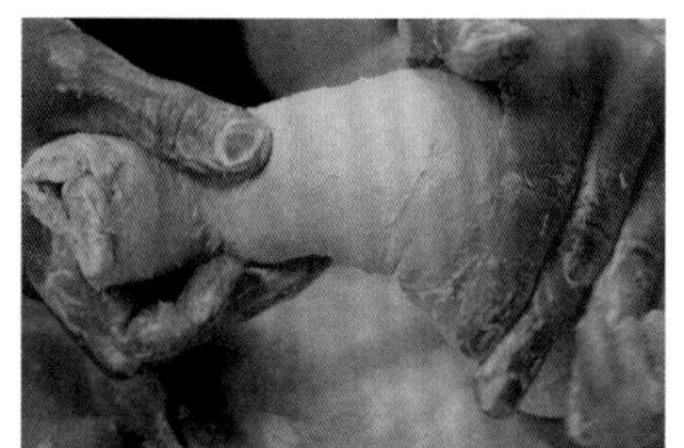
B

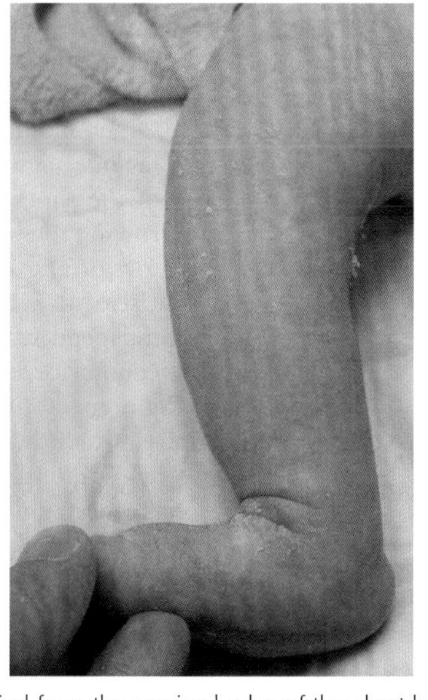
C

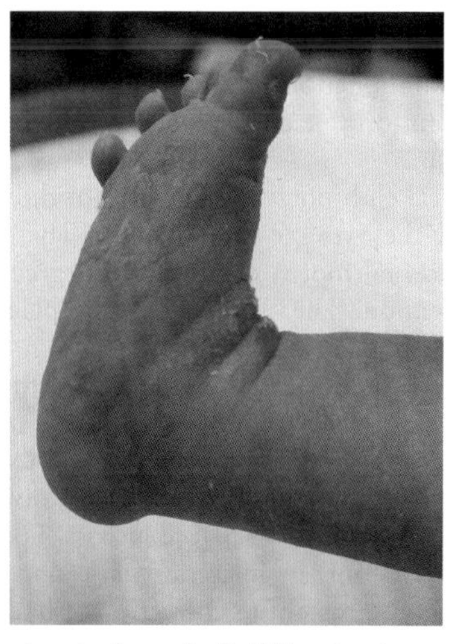
D

**TECH FIG 7** • **A.** Cotton padding is applied from the proximal edge of the short-leg cast up to the groin. **B.** With extension to the long-leg cast, the lower leg is held in slight external rotation, and the knee is held at 90 degrees of flexion. The foot is now in maximum dorsiflexion and abduction. **C,D.** Three weeks after tenotomy, after the final cast is removed, complete correction is obtained. **C.** The foot abducts 70 degrees. **D.** The foot actively dorsiflexes 20 degrees.

## PEARLS AND PITFALLS

| | |
|---|---|
| **Failure to correct the cavus deformity with initial casting** | ■ Failure to elevate the first ray will result in worsening cavus during abduction, and only the forefoot will abduct. The hindfoot varus will fail to correct. The foot will then pull back in the cast. The same deformities will occur in the complex clubfoot if the full-foot cavus is not corrected before or during early abduction. |
| **Toes turn purple after cast application (see FIG 4).** | ■ Some neonatal feet have poor vascular control and will turn purple as the cast cools. Do not be too hasty to remove the cast. Bundle the child, elevate the feet, and recheck every 15 minutes for four times. As the cast dries, the toes should become pink (see **FIG 4**). Increasing purplish discoloration indicates a cast that is too tight and should be removed and reapplied. |
| **An older child who resists casting** | ■ A child who fights casting prevents good molding, and too much motion may prevent the cast from setting up in the desired position. A quiet room with music may relax the child. Likewise, entertaining the child with a toy may distract him or her. Feeding may also be helpful. Older children often do better if sitting slightly upright, propped against a pillow, or even in a parent's lap. |
| **Child pulling out of foot abduction orthosis** | ■ Add padding in the heel, above the posterior calcaneal tuberosity, use a shoe with a heel cutout, or both (see **FIG 5C**). If the child has a strong propensity for toe curling, try a Plastazote plate under the toes to keep them extended. For persistent intolerance, try using only the strap without the tongue. Switching to a different brace may be beneficial (see **FIG 5D**). |
| **Child cries while in casts or in bar and shoes** | ■ Make sure the toes are well perfused. Discomfort for 24 hours after the first casting or tenotomy is common and easily relieved with acetaminophen. The child should be seen and the cast might need to be removed if discomfort persists for greater than 48 hours.<br>■ If the child is in an orthosis, examine the feet for sores. If the orthosis is removed whenever crying occurs, the child may associate crying with subsequent bar removal. Feet may be hyperesthetic after casting: massage during diaper changes and other times out of the orthosis accelerates desensitization. |
| **Recurrence** | ■ Monitor for decreases in abduction and dorsiflexion.<br>■ Treating an early identified, minimal recurrence with stretching by the parents with every diaper change may prevent progression. Later or more marked recurrence should be treated with recasting and possibly a second percutaneous tenotomy. For recurrence in older children, an open Achilles tendon lengthening may be more appropriate for feet with minimal dorsiflexion. For residual dynamic varus, a transfer of the anterior tibialis tendon may be necessary (see Chap. 116). |

## POSTOPERATIVE CARE

- After removal of the posttenotomy cast, the child should immediately be placed in a foot abduction orthosis. Acceptable constructs include straight last shoes or AFOs connected to a solid or articulated bar (see **FIG 5A–D**).
- In the case of bilateral corrected clubfeet, both shoes should be placed in abduction/external rotation on the bar to the degree of comfortable correction, typically 60 to 70 degrees (see **FIG 5A,B**).
- For unilateral clubfoot, only the shoe of the affected foot is placed near the extreme of abduction. The shoe of the uninvolved, normal foot is placed at 30 degrees of abduction/external rotation. The shoes should be placed at shoulder width on the bar.
- Mounting the shoes on the bar such that the buckle of the anterior ankle strap is on the medial aspect of the foot eases application of the orthosis (see **FIG 5A** and **C**).
- In cases of unilateral clubfoot, application of the orthosis is easier if the affected foot is placed into its shoe first, followed by the normal foot. In bilateral cases, one foot is usually "tighter" (more resistant to correction or had less correction from the tenotomy) and this is the one that should be placed in the orthosis first.
- The anterior ankle strap secures the foot in the shoe and should be tightened sufficiently to prevent pulling the foot out of the shoe. Additional straps or laces should be tightened just enough to keep the shoe or orthosis in place on the foot.
- Only a single, thin pair of socks should be worn with the shoes. For the first 1 or 2 days, two socks may be used to prevent blisters (much like the double sock method used by runners), but thereafter only one pair should be used.
  - Thick, well-padded socks prevent adequate securing of the foot and make it easier to pull the foot out of the shoe.
- For the first week, the orthosis and socks should be removed with every diaper change to inspect the feet for evidence of developing pressure sores.
  - Red spots that do not disappear within 5 minutes signal a potential problem spot and require refitting of the shoes with Plastazote or repositioning on the bar.
  - Care should be taken to remove the orthosis when the child is calm to prevent the child from associating crying with subsequent removal, resulting in persistent resistance to orthosis wear with unrelenting crying.
- After casting, the leg and foot are hyperesthetic.
  - Massaging the leg, initially deeply and progressing to light touch, with each diaper change during the first week helps with desensitization.
  - The lower leg may also develop intermittent purple discoloration when dependent to gravity after casting. This usually resolves over the first month out of casts.
- After the first week, the orthosis should be worn full time, but it may be removed once daily for bathing and a short period of play (1 to 2 hours).
  - Full-time wear continues for 3 to 4 months to maintain correction.
  - Tighter feet, or those more difficult to correct, may benefit from periodic stretching in dorsiflexion and abduction whenever the orthosis is removed.
- If the foot is not secured in the shoe or sores develop, adjustments to the shoe may be necessary.
  - If necessary, pads or pressure saddles on the tongue distribute pressure and/or restrict pulling the foot out of the shoe.
  - In some cases, the tongue provides an obstruction to secure the foot, and removing the tongue may actually improve the ability of the strap to secure the foot.
  - Other modifications that may help prevent pulling out include slightly decreasing the degree of external rotation of the shoes (no less than 45 degrees), widening or narrowing the bar or placement of Plastazote pads under the toes or above the calcaneus.
  - Use of an articulated bar allows the child to move each leg independently and decreases the ability to use one leg as a counterforce to pulling with the contralateral foot.
- Children should be reexamined in and out of the orthosis after 1 month, then 2 months later.
- After 3 months of full-time wear and maintenance of full correction, children wear the orthosis for 16 hours per day, primarily at nighttime and during naps.
  - Children should be examined every 3 to 6 months, depending on the level of concern regarding recurrence, until bar and shoe wear is complete.
- Any episodes of recurrence warrant recasting as soon as identified.
  - Casting is performed in the usual manner to obtain complete correction again.
  - Casting is usually sufficient to correct the recurrence. Rarely, a repeat percutaneous tenotomy is necessary for more severe recurrence. Once complete correction is again obtained, orthosis wear occurs for 3 months full time before resuming part-time wear.
- Straight last shoes may be worn until the child's toes curl over the edge of the shoe. Then the next appropriate size should be fitted and attached to the bar which may need to be widened to maintain shoulder width positioning of the heels.
- Part-time wear continues until the child is 4 years old, when orthosis wear may be discontinued. Children should be monitored for recurrence, which occurs rarely after 4 years old.
- Complex clubfeet almost always pull out of standard straight last shoes. A variety of newer bar-and-shoe constructs have been developed to address the limitations of traditional foot abduction bracing (see **FIG 5C,D**).

## OUTCOMES

- A corrected clubfoot tends to recur to its original position, requiring maintenance of correction in the orthosis. Noncompliance with bar-and-shoe wear increases the likelihood of recurrence to more than 80%. Compliance is increased with close follow-up and explicit discussions with the family and all caregivers.[4]
- Twenty percent to 50% of corrected clubfeet will require anterior tibialis tendon transfer to correct dynamic varus present during ambulation (see Chap. 116).

## COMPLICATIONS

- Cast sores, cast saw burns
- Prolonged casting or pulling back in the cast due to improper technique, unrecognized clubfoot, or failure to modify casting for complex clubfoot
- Overabduction from unrecognized complex clubfoot or overabduction in foot abduction orthosis (beyond degree of correction)

- Posterior tibial artery impingement
- Peroneal artery or lesser saphenous vein laceration during tenotomy[2]
- Pulling back in cast from poor cast molding, unrecognized complex clubfoot, or not enough knee flexion in long-leg cast if complex clubfoot
- Recurrence due to incomplete correction or lack of orthosis wear

## REFERENCES


1. Cooper DM, Dietz FR. Treatment of idiopathic clubfoot. A thirty-year follow-up note. J Bone Joint Surg Am 1995;77(10):1477–1489.
2. Dobbs MB, Gordon JE, Walton T, et al. Bleeding complications following percutaneous tendo Achilles tenotomy in the treatment of clubfoot deformity. J Pediatr Orthop 2004;24:353–357.
3. Dobbs MB, Gurnett CA. Genetics of clubfoot. J Pediatr Orthop B 2012;21:7–9.
4. Dobbs MB, Rudzki JR, Purcell DB, et al. Factors predictive of outcome after use of the Ponseti method for the treatment of idiopathic clubfeet. J Bone Joint Surg Am 2004;86-A(1):22–27.
5. Flynn JM, Donohoe M, Mackenzie WG. An independent assessment of two clubfoot-classification systems. J Pediatr Orthop 1998;18: 323–327.
6. Greider TD, Siff SJ, Gerson P, et al. Arteriography in club foot. J Bone Joint Surg Am 1982;64(6):837–840.
7. Ponseti IV. Congenital Clubfoot: Fundamentals of Treatment. New York: Oxford University Press, 1996.
8. Ponseti IV, Zhivkov M, Davis N, et al. Treatment of the complex idiopathic clubfoot. Clin Orthop Relat Res 2006;451:171–176.
9. Treadwell MC, Stanitski CL, King M. Prenatal sonographic diagnosis of clubfoot: implications for patient counseling. J Pediatr Orthop 1999;19:8–10.
10. Zionts LE, Sangiorgio SN, Ebramzadeh E, et al. The current management of idiopathic clubfoot revisited: results of a survey of the POSNA membership. J Pediatr Orthop 2012;32:515–520.

# 126 CHAPTER

# Posteromedial and Posterolateral Release for the Treatment of Resistant Clubfoot

Richard S. Davidson

## DEFINITION

- Clubfoot, or talipes equinovarus, is a congenital or acquired deformity in which the foot is stiffly positioned in hindfoot equinus and varus and forefoot varus, supination, and plantarflexion.[8]
- When the deformity is not corrected, the patient limps, bearing weight on the lateral forefoot. This can limit ambulation and lead to foot and ankle pain, abnormal calluses, and ulcers and infections.[2]
- The deformity may present as an isolated or syndromic birth defect. Clubfoot has been documented in conjunction with diagnoses of polio, spina bifida, cerebral palsy as well as other disorders.[6]

## ANATOMY

- Clubfoot deformity begins as soft tissue imbalance and contractures altering the positions predominantly of the talus, calcaneus, and navicular as well as their corresponding articulations.[6]
- The displacement of these bones differs, producing varying amounts of four different positional deformities: cavus, adductus, varus, and equinus.[3]
- Eventually, the abnormal forces and positions lead to plantarflexion and medialization of the talar neck.[6]
- Weakness and underdevelopment of the foot and calf result to varying degrees.[5]
- Although radiographic measurements are hard to reproduce, the anteroposterior (AP) and lateral talocalcaneal angles are reduced from about 28 degrees to about 5 degrees in children with clubfoot.[6]

## PATHOGENESIS

- The exact cause of clubfoot remains unknown. Many theories can be found in the literature. The cause is probably multifactorial and includes some extent of the following[2,5–7]:
  - Primary germ plasma defect: Initial investigations into multiple cases of clubfoot speculate that the consistent bony deformity is caused by primary bone dysplasia.
  - Uterine restriction: A reduced amount of amniotic fluid causes limited fetal foot movement and, incidentally, clubfoot.
  - Bone–joint hypothesis: The cause of the deformity is abnormalities in the ossification of the bones of the foot.
  - Connective tissue hypothesis: Degeneration in the connective tissues of the skeletally immature foot causes clubfoot.
  - Vascular hypothesis: Muscle wasting has been documented in most children with idiopathic congenital talipes equinovarus. Type 1 fiber predominance and grouping also coincides with most cases of clubfoot.
  - Neurologic complication: Clubfoot is seen in conjunction with a long list of neurologic disorders, including spina bifida, anencephaly, hydrocephaly, and so forth.
  - Developmental arrest hypothesis: Due to a noted similarity between clubfeet and the embryonic foot at the beginning of the second month of fetal development, it has been suggested that the maturation of the fetal foot was arrested while under genetic control.
  - Genetics: This is the most probable cause, as agreed on by many physicians; a family history of talipes equinovarus has been documented in a majority of the reported cases.

## NATURAL HISTORY

- The overall incidence of talipes equinovarus is about one per thousand live births but varies with sex and race: It is more commonly seen in boys, and there is a high frequency of affected children in Polynesian cultures.[7]
- Untreated, the deformity leads to limping, abnormal calluses due to weight bearing on the lateral forefoot, atrophy and hypoplasia due to disuse, and pain.
- Research has been extensive regarding the appropriate approach to treating clubfoot, but few long-term comparative studies exist. Although in the past century extensive surgery predominated, it is now believed that extensive surgical techniques are necessary in fewer than 5% of cases.
- Currently, the most popular treatment of clubfoot follows Ponseti method, which was not generally accepted until his review article of 1992 in which he demonstrated results similar to those of more extensive surgery with fewer complications. The technique has gained such popularity that most pediatric orthopaedists throughout the world are employing Ponseti basic principles of manipulation, casting, and minimal operative treatment of the clubfoot.

## PATIENT HISTORY AND PHYSICAL FINDINGS

- The deformity of clubfoot is identified at birth as unilateral or bilateral hindfoot equinus and varus and midfoot supination, varus, and equinus.
  - To perform the examination, the leg is extended at the knee and the foot is then dorsiflexed. The foot-to-tibia angle is measured to assess the amount of equinus in the frontal plane and the amount of heel varus in the sagittal plane.
  - The dorsolateral aspect of the midfoot is palpated to locate the talar head. The forefoot is then manipulated to determine if the forefoot can be reduced onto the talar head.
  - The lateral rotation of the foot–thigh angle can be assessed by flexing the knee and ankle to 90 degrees and gently laterally rotating the foot. The angle is measured.
  - These examinations do not determine a classification but rather the stiffness of the foot and the amount of improvement attained with serial casting and surgical intervention.

- The clinician should investigate associated anomalies, such as spina bifida, spasticity, muscular dystrophy, arthrogryposis, and so forth. By understanding the cause, the likelihood of treatment success can be predicted.
- The clinician should observe the shape and size of the foot. The clubfoot is generally shorter and wider than a normal foot.
  - Examination reveals equinus and varus of the ankle and midfoot. Creases or clefts are seen at the midfoot and ankle. Calf atrophy is expected, particularly in the older child (**FIG 1A–C**).
  - Treatment may be altered depending on the presentation of the clubfoot.
- Range of motion: equinus
  - Ankle motion (dorsiflexion and plantarflexion) is assessed in both knee extension and flexion. The os calcis may remain in equinus (by palpation) even though the heel pad appears to come out of equinus (by observation) (**FIG 1D,E**). This is the so-called empty heel pad sign.
  - Therefore, the foot may "look" as if the equinus is corrected, but the physician must palpate it to know for sure.
- Range of motion: subtalar joint
  - Range of motion is difficult to measure. The resting alignment of the heel to the talus is usually varus in the untreated clubfoot and 5 to 10 degrees of valgus in the corrected foot. The clinician looks at the sole of the foot to observe midfoot varus. The sole is manipulated to see how flexible it is (**FIG 1F,G**).
  - Overcorrection of the heel into valgus can lead to painful pronation. Residual varus of the lateral border of the foot may be due to subtalar rotation, varus of the calcaneus, medialization of the cuboid on the calcaneus, or varus deformity of the metatarsals. Correction may be required at the site of deformity.
- Range of motion: forefoot on the talar head
  - The foot is palpated dorsolaterally at the lateral midfoot. It usually is lined up with the patella, although plantarflexed. Manipulation is used to reduce the forefoot (**FIG 1H**).
- The more difficult it is to reduce the forefoot onto the talar head, the stiffer the deformity.
- Forefoot supination
  - The clinician observes that the forefoot of the clubfoot appears supinated with respect to the tibia. However, supination relates to the position of the forefoot to the hindfoot (**FIG 1I,J**).
  - If the forefoot appears 30 degrees supinated to the tibia and there is 30 degrees varus to the hindfoot varus, then

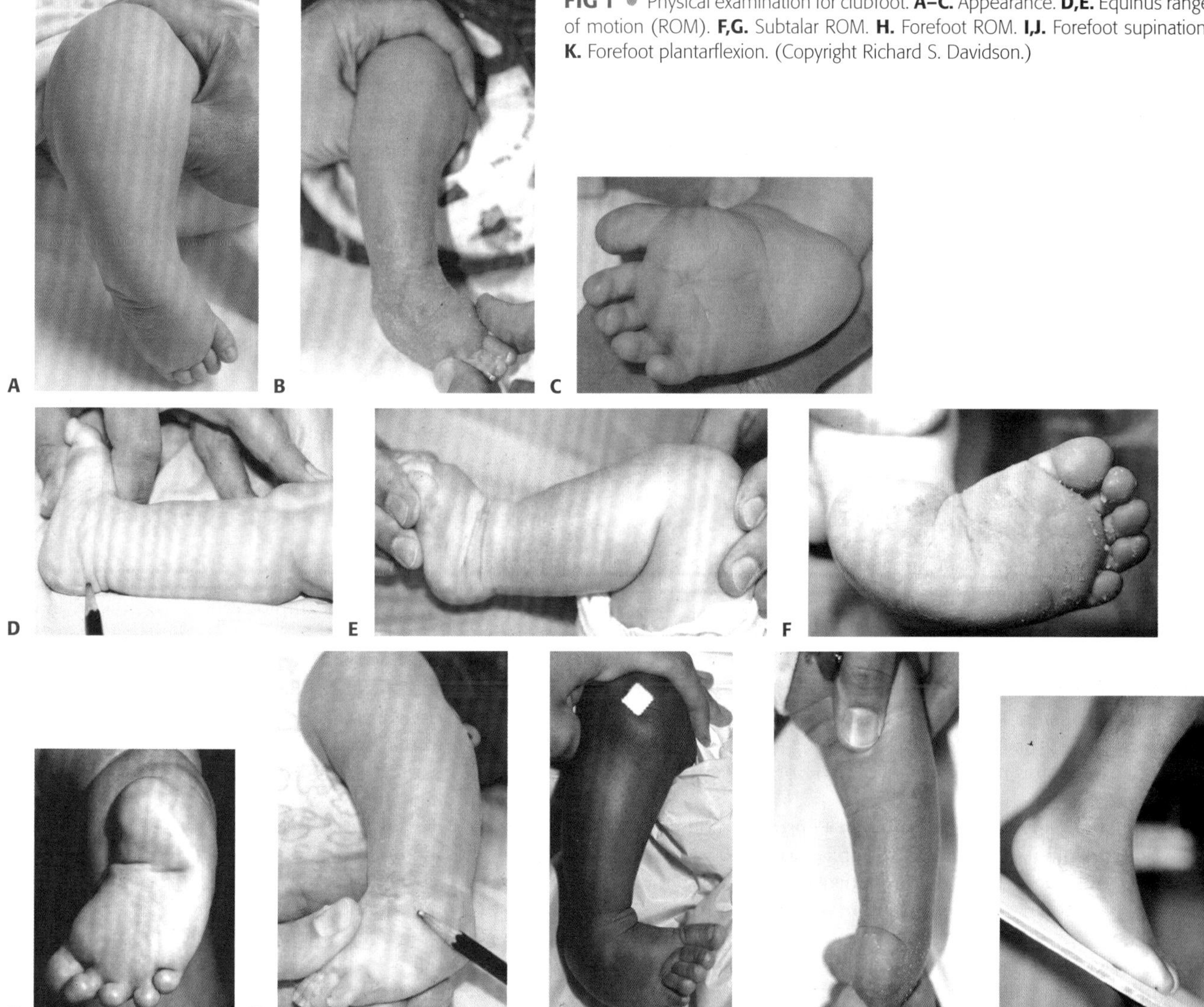

**FIG 1** • Physical examination for clubfoot. **A–C.** Appearance. **D,E.** Equinus range of motion (ROM). **F,G.** Subtalar ROM. **H.** Forefoot ROM. **I,J.** Forefoot supination. **K.** Forefoot plantarflexion. (Copyright Richard S. Davidson.)

the deformity is hindfoot varus and not supination, that is, the forefoot is properly aligned to the hindfoot and there is no supination.
- It is important to know where this deformity is. Errors in this assessment may lead the surgeon to overcorrect the midfoot or surgically create a pronation deformity.

- Forefoot plantarflexion
  - The physician begins with palpation of the medial column from the first metatarsal to the talar head. Plantarflexion of the forefoot on the hindfoot is measured.
  - In the operated foot, the physician checks for dorsolateral subluxation or dislocation of the navicular on the talar head (**FIG 1K**).
  - Deformity must be corrected where it is. This assessment, in conjunction with radiographs, will help to assess its location in the soft tissues, the ankle, the bone, or the joints (such as subluxation of the talonavicular joint).

## IMAGING AND OTHER DIAGNOSTIC STUDIES

- Sonograms may be used to diagnose clubfoot prenatally.[5] Although no prenatal treatment is available, many parents want to know the diagnosis of clubfoot so they can learn about the natural history and treatment options available to them.
- The prenatal ultrasonographic diagnosis of clubfoot may be made if the bones of the lower leg are in the same plane as the plantar surface of the fetal foot. To ensure a correct diagnosis, images in which the leg is extended away from the wall of the uterus should be obtained.[5]
  - This deformity may be seen as early as 12 or 13 weeks.[5]
- Plain radiographic images in the newborn period add little to the physical examination. Films are not reproducible and contribute little to the management.
- With older children, radiographs may be necessary to treat the deformity effectively, as they can identify fixed individual bone deformities such as flat-top talus, varus deformity of the calcaneus, or dorsolateral subluxation of a triangular navicular on the talar head.[6]
- The most common images used are those of the talocalcaneal angle in both the AP and lateral planes. Both must be obtained while bearing weight or simulated weight bearing on the affected foot.[6]

## DIFFERENTIAL DIAGNOSIS

- Identifying the underlying cause is often helpful. Examination should be complete to identify spinal dysraphisms, syndromes, cerebral palsy, spina bifida, and so forth.

## NONOPERATIVE MANAGEMENT

- Most would claim that extensive surgical techniques are necessary in less than 5% of cases.
- Two of the major techniques preferred for nonoperative treatment:
  - Optimal for very young patients, the Ponseti method uses weekly manipulations and cast applications to treat the deformity. About 90% of the patients treated with the Ponseti method will need posterior releases, and about 30% will require additional surgical and nonsurgical (repeat casting) management after age 2 years, including repeat posterior release, posteromedial release, and complete subtalar release.
  - Also used predominantly in newborns, the French method incorporates daily manipulation and stimulation of the foot muscles with nonelastic adhesive strapping to correct clubfoot.
- There will always be the recalcitrant clubfoot that resists methods such as the Ponseti technique. These cases usually fall into the "arthrogrypotic" or "teratologic" category and should be treated with the releases described in the following text. About 1 in 15 idiopathic clubfeet have rigid equinus, midfoot (metatarsal ) plantarflexion, a deep heel crease at the posterior ankle, a transverse midsole or midfoot crease, and a short hyperextended hallux. These feet may not be apparent until after one to three casts. They have been called *complex idiopathic clubfoot* and are more difficult to treat. Treatment of complex idiopathic clubfoot required up to five additional casts: first to correct the forefoot plantarflexion then to abduct the forefoot at the midfoot, laterally rotating the anterior tuberosity of the calcaneus under the head of the talus. Recurrence of deformity is more common in this type.[4]

## SURGICAL MANAGEMENT

- All authors agree that the goal of surgical treatment is first to release enough of the tight structures to bring the foot into an anatomically correct position without tension.
- Many will add that muscles should be balanced to help maintain the anatomic position.

### Preoperative Planning

- The age of the child will play an important role in what must be done to restore anatomic alignment. Generally, soft tissue releases are adequate from age 2 months to 4 years and in some cases to age 6 years. By the age of 4 years, many of the clubfeet are beginning to show bony deformity, which will block correction after soft tissue releases alone.
- The choice of operative procedure depends on not only the age of the patient but also the degree of rigidity, the deformities present, and the extent of correction by previous treatment.[7]

### Positioning

- The child is placed on the operating table in the prone position.
- The patient is supported using bolsters underneath the shoulders and waist.
- The legs are kept free and the knee is fully extended.

### Approach

- Surgical release should begin posteriorly and then continue medially. These areas should reveal the tightest structures in an equinovarus foot.
- As recommended by Henri Bensahel, often, the "à la carte" approach is used in which intraoperative evaluation leads the surgeon to release any and all tight structures. The surgeon must be prepared to do as little or as much as needed to accomplish anatomic realignment.
- For each of the soft tissue releases described in Techniques section, it is important to evaluate each foot after each step of the surgical release to determine if the anatomy is corrected or if additional release is necessary.
  - The goal is to do as little or as much of a release as will place the foot in a corrected position without force.
  - Lengthening tendons and then capsules and ligaments at each location will minimize scarring and stiffness.

## Incision

### Turco Posteromedial Incision

- The Turco incision allows for access to the medial and posterior portions of the foot (**TECH FIG 1**).
- The technique begins with a medial incision at the first metatarsal–medial cuneiform joint.
- The cut is extended proximally until it is just distal to the tip of the medial malleolus.
- Care is taken to curve the incision in a vertical direction, up the calf to expose the Achilles tendon.
- To reach the lateral side, the subtalar joint must be opened like a book or a separate lateral incision must be made.

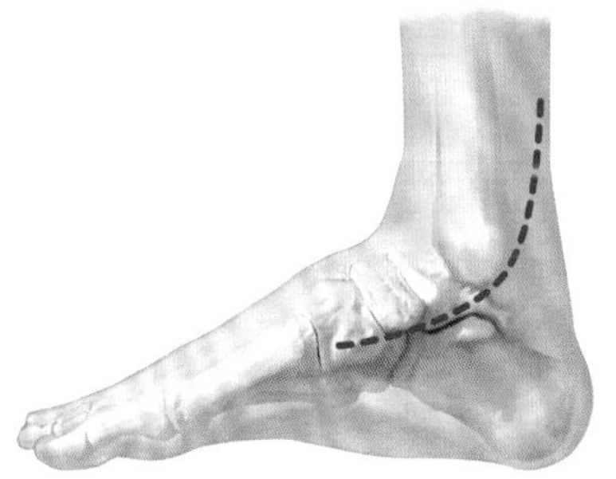

**TECH FIG 1** • The medial Turco incision.

### Carroll Medial and Posterolateral Incisions

- The Carroll types of incisions allow medial or more posterolateral access (**TECH FIG 2**).
- For the medial incision, a triangle is cut that is demarcated by the center of the os calcis, the front of the medial malleolus, and the base of the first metatarsal.
- The incision is made parallel with the base of the triangle, then curved proximal-plantar, and then curved distally over the dorsum of the foot.
- For the posterolateral incision, an oblique incision is created that runs from the midline of the distal posterior calf to a point between the tendo Achilles and the lateral malleolus.
- A lateral incision may be required to reach the lateral talonavicular joint.

### Cincinnati Incision (Author's Preferred Incision)

- The Cincinnati incision provides the most extensive access to the foot, including medial, posterior, and lateral access (**TECH FIG 3**).
- The incision begins medially over the talonavicular joint, extending posteriorly at the level of the subtalar joint. It is continued distally to the talonavicular joint laterally and may be extended distally on both the medial and lateral sides.
- The Cincinnati incision is most easily performed with the patient prone. Flexing the knee provides excellent access to the Achilles tendon for Z-lengthening.
- For severely deformed feet (equinus), closure may be difficult.

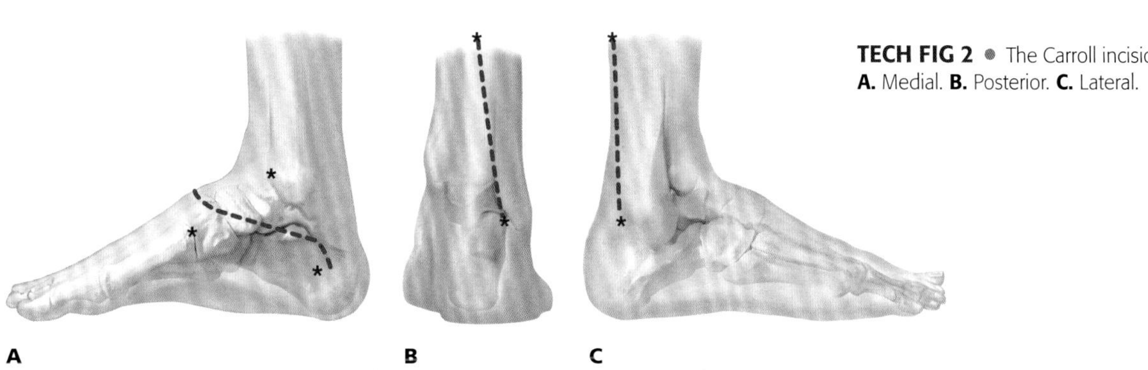


**TECH FIG 2** • The Carroll incision. **A.** Medial. **B.** Posterior. **C.** Lateral.

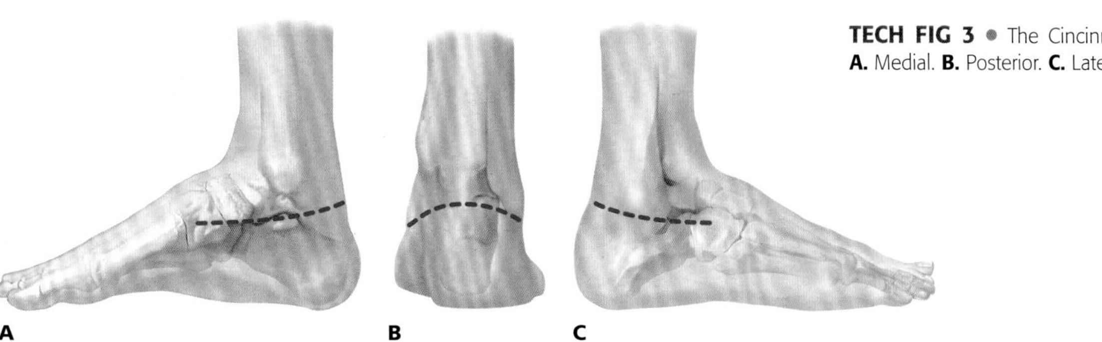


**TECH FIG 3** • The Cincinnati incision. **A.** Medial. **B.** Posterior. **C.** Lateral.

## Posterior Soft Tissue Release

- In the exsanguinated prone foot, the posterior portion of the Cincinnati incision is made from the distal tip of the medial malleolus around the posterior ankle to the distal tip of the lateral malleolus.
- The Achilles tendon sheath is incised to expose the Achilles tendon. In a child younger than 18 months, the tendon can be lengthened by tenotomy, but in the older child, it should be lengthened by Z-lengthening.
- To facilitate visualization for a Z-lengthening of the Achilles through the Cincinnati incision, the knee is flexed in the prone patient. With the Cincinnati incision, the surgeon is looking at the plantar aspect of the foot and through the incision and tendon extending up the calf.
- The Achilles tendon is lengthened in Z-plasty fashion, releasing the insertion of the distal half of the tendon at the medial side of the calcaneus to reduce the varus force. Fibrotic bands and tendon sheath should also be released.
- If the Achilles lengthening is not sufficient to restore the anatomy, the posterior aspects of the subtalar and ankle joints are sequentially released.
- The first step is to identify and protect the sural nerve and vessels laterally and the posterior tibial neurovascular bundle medially. The flexor hallucis is then identified posteromedially and protected. The peroneal tendons are also identified and protected (**TECH FIG 4**).
- The ankle capsule is noted and incised from the posteromedial to the posterolateral corners to allow dorsiflexion of the talus in the mortise.
- The subtalar joint is found and incised posteriorly, then medially and laterally to the interosseous ligament. The fibulotalar and fibulocalcaneal ligaments can be released as needed.
- This release should allow the ankle joint to dorsiflex at least 20 degrees. If the hallux is tightly flexed, the flexor hallucis can be lengthened through this incision by Z-lengthening.

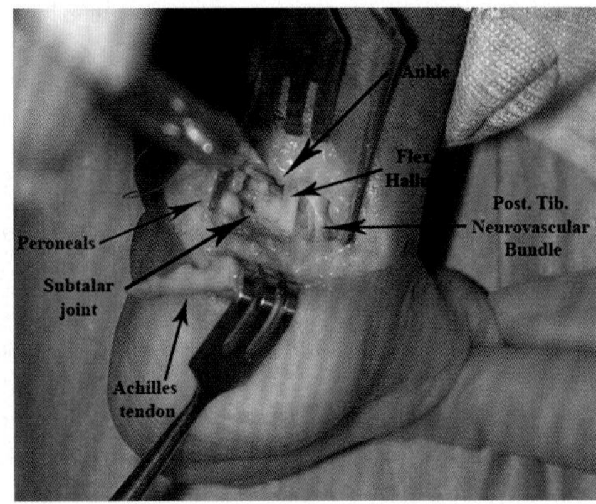


**TECH FIG 4** • Posterior portion of the Cincinnati incision. The Achilles tendon has been cut for lengthening and retracted. (Copyright Richard S. Davidson.)

## Medial Soft Tissue Release

- Medial release is undertaken if the posterior release as described earlier does not correct the anatomy.
- First, the posterior portion of the Cincinnati incision is extended medially to the medial aspect of the navicular.
- The posterior tibial neurovascular bundle is protected while releasing any thickened fascia as well as the flexor hallucis, which may have been lengthened through the posterior part of the incision.
- The posterior tibial tendon is located just distal to the flexor digitorum tendon and is lengthened using a Z-plasty as necessary.
- The abductor hallucis muscle is lengthened proximally or distally. The flexor digitorum tendon is identified just anterior to the posterior tibial neurovascular bundle and lengthened in notch fashion as necessary (**TECH FIG 5**).
- Deciding whether to lengthen the anterior tibialis tendon can be difficult. If the anterior tibialis tendon appears contracted on anatomic correction, it should be lengthened in a Z-lengthening. Occasionally, the anterior tibialis tendon remains overactive and will need to be lengthened at a future time.
- A helpful hint for the lengthening of the tendons on the medial side of the foot: Each of the ends of the lengthened tendons should be tagged with suture, which is then held in a color-coded bulldog clamp. Each group of the proximal and distal sets of clamps can then be held in proper order by a safety pin. This will avoid confusion when it is time to repair the tendons after anatomic realignment of the foot is accomplished.
- Release of the plantar fascia has been recommended in the past but is currently avoided because it can contribute to later pes planovalgus. Do not release the plantar fascia in cases of rocker-bottom deformity during the casting.
- Care should be taken to avoid injury to the medial plantar vessels and nerve.
- If lengthening of these tendons does not permit anatomic alignment, follow this addendum:
  - Identify and release the talonavicular joint. The navicular is medially displaced on the talar head, making the talonavicular joint obliquely, rather than transversely, oriented.
  - Follow the distal stump of the Z-plasty–lengthened posterior tibial tendon to its insertion on the navicular.
  - The capsule is released medially, plantarly, and dorsally and as far laterally as can be reached safely. Be careful not

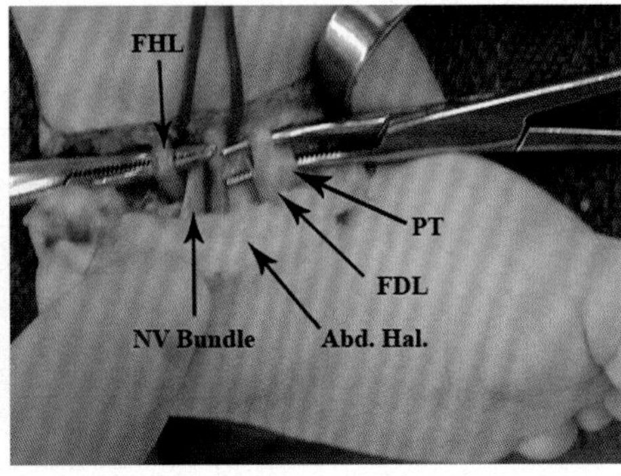


**TECH FIG 5** • Medial portion of Cincinnati incision, superficial. (Copyright Richard S. Davidson.)

to cut the talar neck, as this may lead to avascular necrosis or growth disturbances.

- Release the subtalar capsule from the talonavicular joint to the interosseous ligament medially, including the spring ligament. Be careful not to damage the deep deltoid ligament. A Freer elevator placed into the ankle joint posteriorly can help identify the ankle and subtalar joints.
- Reach the medial aspect of the calcaneocuboid joint by carefully dissecting the soft tissues from the plantar aspect of the talar neck. Release of this capsule will allow a wedge opening of the calcaneocuboid joint to straighten the lateral column. Another landmark to the calcaneocuboid joint from the medial side of the foot is the peroneus longus tendon crossing from lateral to plantar.
- Many authors have described release of the interosseous ligament through this incision. It is important to preserve this ligament as a pivot axis and to preserve its associated blood supply to the talus.

## Lateral Soft Tissue Release

- A problem often occurs when the calcaneus has rotated under the talus on the interosseous membrane and is tethered by a stiff, fibrotic lateral capsule. If the above posterior and medial releases do not permit anatomic alignment, a lateral release may be needed.
- The posterior portion of the Cincinnati incision, made for the posterior release, is extended laterally at the level of the subtalar joint to the talonavicular joint.
- The extensor digitorum brevis is identified over the sinus tarsi. Its plantar edge is divided from the lateral calcaneus and the muscle is elevated to expose the sinus tarsi and neck and head of the talus.
- The lateral capsule of the talonavicular joint is exposed and released. A circumferential release of the talonavicular joint is thus completed (**TECH FIG 6**).
- The beak of the calcaneus is then palpated. From the lateral aspect of the talonavicular joint, cut the lateral subtalar capsule, between the beak of the calcaneus and the talar neck, proximally to the interosseous ligament, completing circumferential release of the subtalar capsule.

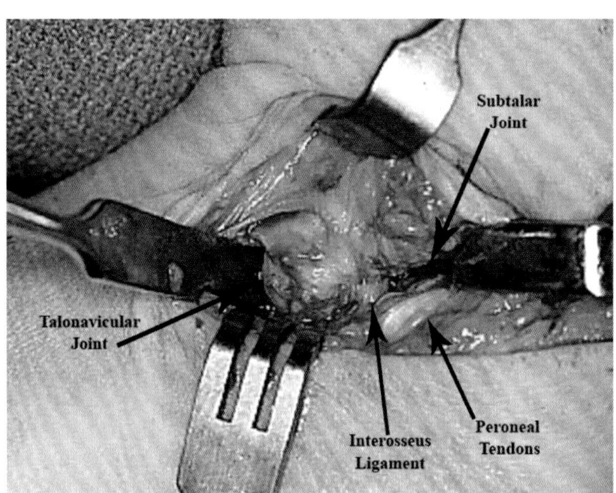


**TECH FIG 6** • Lateral portion of the Cincinnati incision showing the lateral structures. (Copyright Richard S. Davidson.)

## Realignment of the Bones of the Foot

- Once the appropriate soft tissues have been released, the foot can be realigned.
- A finger is placed over the talar head dorsolaterally while the foot is laterally rotated in slight supination. This is similar to the Ponseti manipulation.
- A Freer elevator can be placed in the ankle joint in line with the dome of the talus (axis of the talus). The foot should be rotated until the first metatarsal is just lateral to the talar dome axis.
- This maneuver should correct the lateral border to straight and the heel into slight valgus and reduce the talar head under the navicular (the navicular should be slightly proud to palpation as in normal feet), without wedging open the subtalar joint (**TECH FIG 7**).

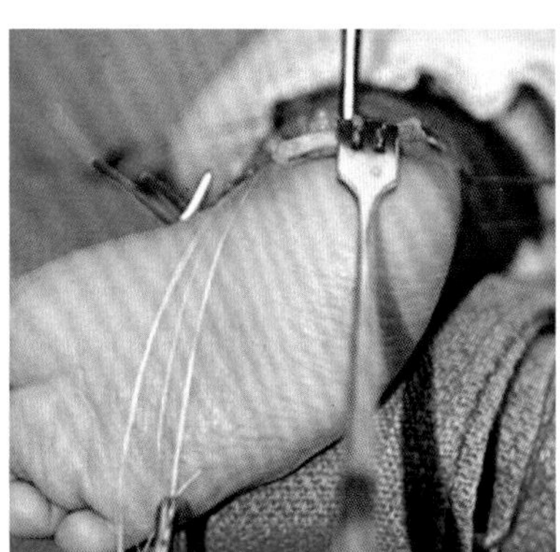

A

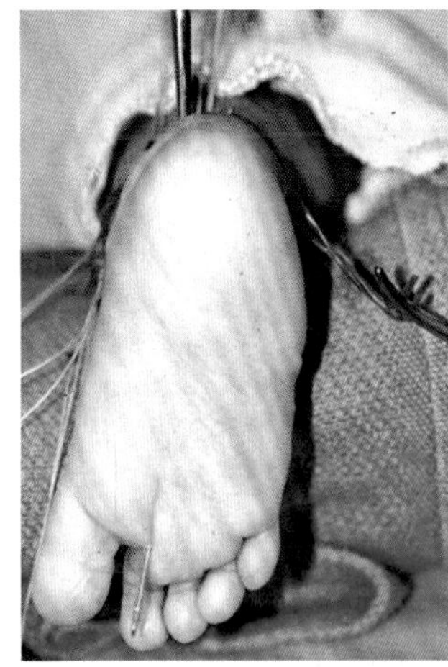

B

**TECH FIG 7** • **A.** Subtalar rotation of the foot. The Freer elevator is in the ankle joint and demonstrates the alignment of the ankle joint. The foot is medially rotated through the subtalar joint. **B.** The reduced foot is held in place with a pin through the talonavicular joint. Heel is in slight valgus. (Copyright Richard S. Davidson.)

## Fixation

- Holding the foot in the anatomically corrected position until the capsules and tendons heal is best done with a 0.062-inch Kirschner wire, which is passed from the posteromedial talus through the center of the head and into the navicular and the medial cuneiform and out the first web space (**TECH FIG 8A**).
- Intraoperative radiographic images should be obtained at this point to confirm that all components of the reduction have been obtained (**TECH FIG 8B,C**).
- All of the joints should be congruous. Wedged-open joints may indicate incomplete release of bone deformity, requiring osteotomy.
- Proper reduction should result in near-normal motion of the ankle. The fixation pin restricts the foot motion.
- If division of the interosseous ligament has been performed (rarely needed in the author's experience), a second pin should be placed from the calcaneus into the talus to maintain the alignment of the subtalar joint.

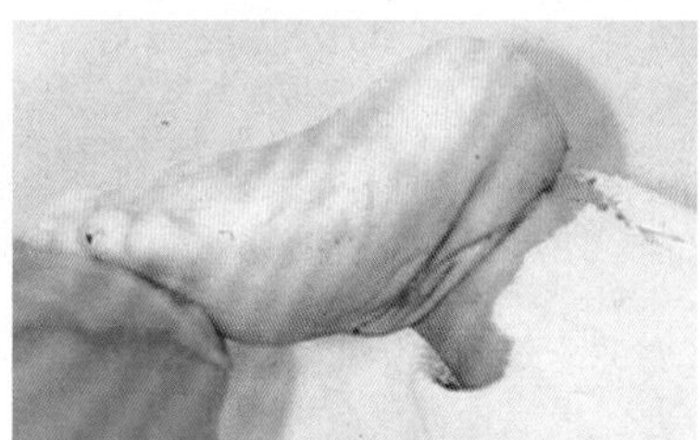
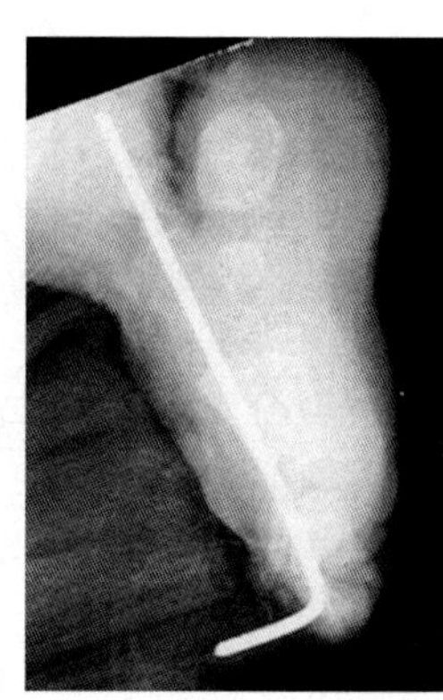
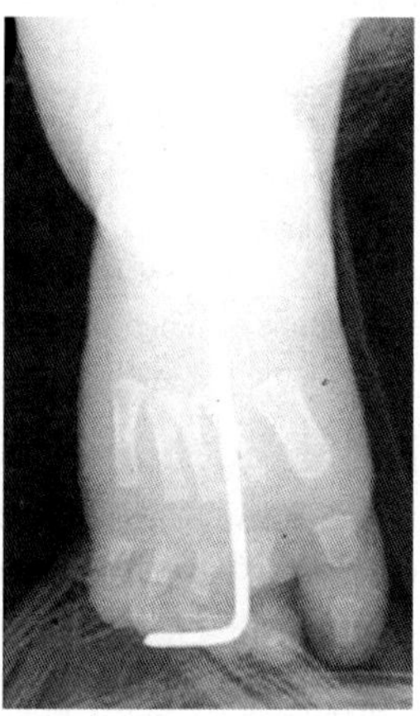

A B C

**TECH FIG 8** • **A.** The foot of a prone patient positioned for posteroanterior (PA) and lateral intraoperative radiographs. **B,C.** AP and lateral intraoperative radiographs with internal fixation. On the lateral view (**B**), the talus points into the first metatarsal, and on the AP view (**C**), the talus points just medial to the first metatarsal. (Copyright Richard S. Davidson.)

## Repair of Tendons

- Once the foot is anatomically aligned, the tendons are repaired with the foot at 90 degrees to the tibia. Bunnell-type stitches are used for end-to-end repair of tendons and four to six simple stitches in a side-to-side pattern of 2-0 or 3-0 Vicryl suture for Z-plasty–type lengthening of tendons.
- Do not repair the tendons until the bones have been realigned anatomically. Repairing the tendons at too short a length will result in rapid recurrence.
- Capsules and ligaments should not be repaired surgically. They will heal.

## PEARLS AND PITFALLS

| | |
|---|---|
| **Medial release** | ▪ Failure to lengthen flexor hallucis longus, flexor digitorum longus, and peroneus longus tendon may lead to failure to adequately rotate the subtalar joint or to rapid recurrence of deformity. The preservation or repair of the tendon sheaths is not of value. As long as all the tethers and blocks to motion are removed, a flexible foot and ankle can result. |
| **Fixation** | ▪ The surgeon should not overreduce the talonavicular joint. Lateral overcorrection will cause valgus dorsal overcorrection. This later will cause dorsolateral subluxation with cavus and metatarsus adductus; incomplete medial and plantar reduction will cause incomplete correction of equinovarus. Plantarflexion of the first metatarsal from the axis of the talus can cause permanent forefoot plantarflexion, supination, and hindfoot varus. |
| **Additional bone issues** | ▪ Severe, stiffly deformed clubfeet may develop bone deformity, which can prevent adequate anatomic correction with soft tissue release alone. Posterior soft tissue release will do little for ankle stiffness due to flat-top talus. The surgeon should always obtain radiographs preoperatively for these severely deformed stiff feet. Metatarsal and talar neck osteotomies are rarely indicated in the young child. |
| **Turco incision** | ▪ Scar contracture may cause recurrence of equinovarus deformity. |
| **Problems with correction** | ▪ Overcorrection can lead to valgus deformity; failure to correct the deformity after such releases is likely due to scarring of the lateral structures, which blocks derotation of the subtalar joint. |

## POSTOPERATIVE CARE

- During the first postoperative week, a Jones-type dressing is preferred to allow for swelling in children younger than 6 months of age. Bulky dressings and casts are recommended for children older than 6 months.
- Non–weight-bearing casts protect the tendon repair for 6 weeks.
- Ponseti-type casting will help maintain the alignment. Casts should be changed at 1 week and continue for 3 months.
- Braces are helpful for prolonged periods, if recurrence occurs or underlying neuromuscular disease has been identified.
- After incisions, wound closure and positioning in equinus for 2 weeks allows healing and can be followed by serial casting to stretch the soft tissues to dorsiflex the ankle.
- Pins may be removed after 4 to 6 weeks.
- Muscle balancing is better left for a later time, after rehabilitation from extensive surgical release.

## OUTCOMES

- As noted previously, surgery is usually necessary only with the most resistant forms of clubfoot.
- Successful results can be obtained in 52% to 91% of cases, enabling most children to participate in normal activities.[5]
- Stiffness, recurrence, and weakness are common, and no treatment known today can correct the underlying neuromuscular causes.
- The incidence of a poor outcome is higher in children who have surgery before 6 months of age. Waiting to treat young patients may be beneficial because it allows for growth of the anatomy as well as time to fully evaluate the case.[1]
- These children should be referred to centers with the most experience.

## COMPLICATIONS

- The challenges that this deformity presents ultimately may lead to a variety of complications[1]:
  - Skin slough and wound dehiscence
  - Neurovascular complication
  - Physeal damage
  - Osteonecrosis of the talus
  - Aseptic necrosis of the navicular
  - Failure to achieve or loss of correction
  - Overcorrection or undercorrection
  - Hindfoot valgus
  - Forefoot abduction or adduction
  - Calcaneus deformity
  - Pes planus
  - Persistent equinus
  - Heel varus
  - Dorsal forefoot subluxation with apparent cavus
  - Skew foot
  - Dorsal bunion
  - Claw toes
  - Anesthetic foot
  - Sinus tarsi syndrome
  - Restricted motion
  - Reduced calf girth and foot size
  - Recurrence of the deformity
- Neuromuscular abnormalities, growth disturbances, and simple muscular or mechanical imbalance can lead to recurrence or overcorrection throughout the growth period. Stretching, bracing, casting, and even additional surgery may be needed.

## REFERENCES


1. Crawford AH, Gupta AK. Clubfoot controversies: complications and causes for failure. Instr Course Lect 1996;45:339–346.
2. Miedzybrodzka Z. Congenital talipes equinovarus (clubfoot): a disorder of the foot but not the hand. J Anat 2003;202:37–42.
3. Noonan KJ, Richards BS. Nonsurgical management of idiopathic clubfoot. J Am Acad Orthop Surg 2003;11:392–402.
4. Ponseti IV, Zhivkov M, Davis N, et al. Treatment of the complex idiopathic clubfoot. Clin Orthop Relat Res 2006;451:171–176.
5. Rochon M, Eddleman K. Controversial ultrasound findings. Obstet Gynecol Clin North Am 2004;31:61–99.
6. Roye DP Jr, Roye BD. Idiopathic congenital talipes equinovarus. J Am Acad Orthop Surg 2002;10(4):239–248.
7. Tachdjian MO. The Child's Foot. Philadelphia: WB Saunders, 1985:139–239.
8. Turco VJ. Current Problems in Orthopaedics: Clubfoot. Hartford, CT: Churchill Livingstone, 1981:xi–xii.

# Anterior Tibialis Transfer for Residual Clubfoot Deformity

CHAPTER 127

Kenneth J. Noonan

## DEFINITION

- The incidence of residual deformity in congenital clubfoot ranges from 26.6% to 50%, regardless of the initial treatment provided.[2]
- The disparity in the reported incidence is due to varying severity of clubfoot deformity, different methods of treatment, and, in part, differing definitions of residual deformity.
- Residual deformities include isolated equinus, cavus, metatarsus adductus, hindfoot varus, forefoot supination, and combinations of the above.
- Dynamic forefoot adduction and supination can be observed after clubfoot treatment with or without soft tissue releases.
- Dynamic forefoot supination deformity results from muscle imbalance. Anatomic imbalances can be due to primary absence or weakness of the anterior tibialis or peroneal muscles or as a result of neurologic abnormalities in the central nervous system or the peroneal nerve. Functional muscle imbalance can result from residual medial displacement of the navicular on the head of the talus. In this case, because its insertion is medially displaced, the anterior tibialis becomes a forefoot supinator instead of a dorsiflexor (**FIG 1**).
- The aim of treatment is to correct any fixed deformity and to rebalance the muscles of the foot, thereby correcting dynamic deformity and improving foot alignment.

## ANATOMY

- The anterior tibialis muscle originates from the upper two-thirds of the tibia.
- The anterior tibialis tendon fibers rotate 90 degrees from the musculotendinous junction to its insertion on the medial cuneiform and first metatarsal.
  - Medial rotation begins proximally, so the most medial muscle fibers proximally rotate to the posterior surface of the tendon near the midpoint and continue to rotate so that their final insertion is as the distal–lateral fibers on the first metatarsal.
  - Meanwhile, the most lateral muscle fibers proximally rotate to the anterior surface at the midpoint and continue distally to insert on the cuneiform as the proximal–medial fibers (**FIG 2**).[4]

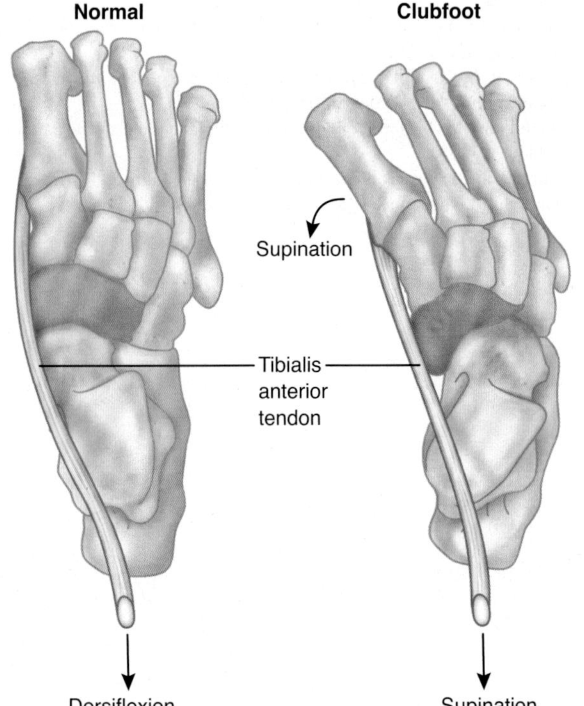


**FIG 1** • Normal foot versus supinated foot. Medial subluxation of the navicular, the medial cuneiform, and the first metatarsal results in supination deformity as the line of pull of the tibialis anterior tendon directs the foot into supination instead of dorsiflexion.

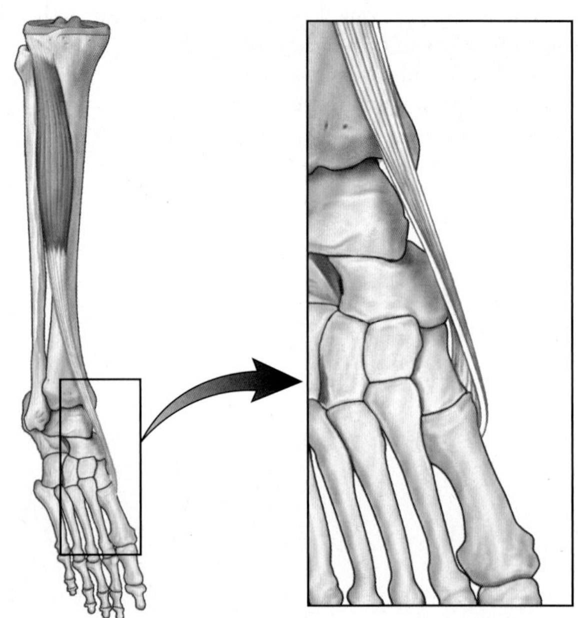

**FIG 2** • Anatomy of the tibialis anterior muscle–tendon. The anterior tibialis tendon fibers rotate 90 degrees from their musculotendinous junction to their insertion on the medial cuneiform and the first metatarsal such that the proximal–medial insertional fibers on the cuneiform begin as the lateral fibers at the musculotendinous junction (see window).

- The anterior tibialis muscle is active in two important stages of the gait cycle; it concentrically fires during the initiation of swing phase and keeps the foot dorsiflexed during early swing phase and then it relaxes. The anterior tibialis muscle then fires eccentrically as the foot is lowered to the floor from heel strike to foot flat in stance phase.
- As a dorsiflexor, the anterior tibialis muscle opposes gravity and the strong gastrocsoleus complex. Importantly, the anterior tibialis muscle may also be a supinator of the forefoot in the face of peroneal longus weakness or medial displacement of the insertion.
- There are important bony abnormalities associated with residual clubfoot deformity.
  - The subtalar joint may have an absent anterior facet and small, narrow medial and posterior facets, resulting in restricted subtalar motion. In this setting, the calcaneus does not slide fully into valgus with casting such that the navicular remains medially displaced.
  - The navicular itself is wedge-shaped and is medially displaced along with the cuneiforms and metatarsals.[10] With medial displacement of its insertion, the biomechanical advantage favors the action of the anterior tibialis muscle as a strong supinator over its role as a dorsiflexor (**FIG 3**).

## PATHOGENESIS

- The cause of residual clubfoot deformity may be incomplete correction or recurrence of deformity as part of the natural history of the resistant clubfoot.
- Electromyographic and magnetic resonance imaging (MRI) studies have demonstrated that the peroneal muscle group can be absent, smaller, and relatively weaker, thus increasing the supinator action of the tibialis anterior muscle.[1,3]
- Medial subluxation of the navicular is considered an important factor influencing both the appearance of the foot and the lateral rotation of the ankle.[9]
- In addition to the bony abnormalities associated with clubfeet, anatomic variations from the customary insertion of the anterior tibialis muscle into adjacent areas of the first metatarsal and medial cuneiform occur in 10% of pathologic specimens.
  - In these variants, the distal anterior tibialis muscle inserts more medially than normal, optimizing the force vector for supination.[8]

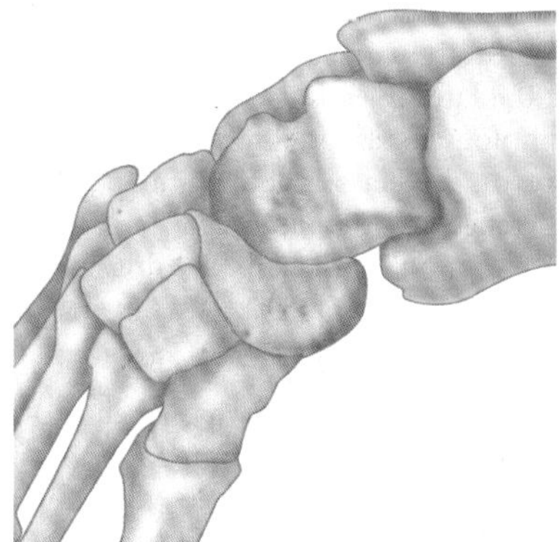

**FIG 3** • Bony abnormalities associated with residual clubfoot deformity. The navicular is wedge-shaped and is medially displaced along with the cuneiforms and metatarsals.

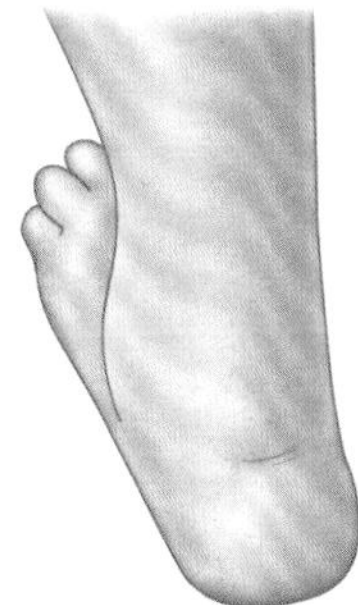
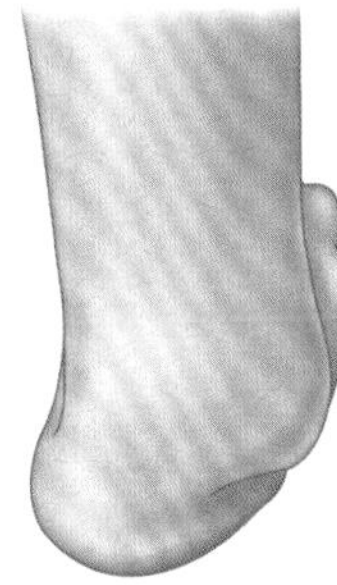

**FIG 4** • Hindfoot varus. When untreated, residual deformity may become stiff. When fixed inversion deformity is combined with residual equinus deformity, hindfoot varus occurs.

## NATURAL HISTORY

- Residual deformities are usually encountered within the first year after initial treatment and generally before the age of 5 years, even in congenital clubfeet that had been fully corrected since the first month of life.
- Residual forefoot adduction and supination are common deformities after nonoperative treatment and can also be seen after initial operative repair. They can result from undercorrection at the time of the primary intervention.[13]
- Correction of resistant congenital clubfoot often requires more than one surgery, not because of a "failed initial intervention," but because the dynamic muscle imbalances may not be fully manifest at the time of the initial intervention. Thus, the need for an additional operation can be perceived as part of the natural history of congenital clubfoot.[12]
- If left untreated, the dynamic deformity may become stiff and the foot tends to invert.
  - When inversion deformity is combined with residual equinus deformity, hindfoot varus may recur (**FIG 4**).

## PATIENT HISTORY AND PHYSICAL FINDINGS

- Residual deformity is more likely in patients who have clubfoot as a result of myelomeningocele or other neuromuscular syndromes and genetic disorders such as Larsen syndrome. Therefore, it is important to consider neurologic causes, such as tethered cord, when confronted with residual deformity.
- Recurrent deformity may be found in children with only four toes on the affected foot, as these individuals may have absence of the peroneal muscle group (similar to that seen in fibular hemimelia), thus leaving them prone to recurrence.
- Recurrent deformity may be suspected prior to treatment in newborns with curled toes and no active toe dorsiflexion when scratching the plantar aspect of the foot. In those infants that have been treated with the Ponseti method, later recurrence may be heralded by scratching the bottom of the foot that leads to more supination than dorsiflexion.
- One of the first clinical signs of recurrence is a dynamic inversion of the foot with slight equinus. Equinus may be difficult to quantify, as midfoot breech will often accommodate and hide the hindfoot equinus (**FIG 5**).
- Residual deformity most frequently occurs in severe or atypical cases, which are often associated with a small calf size. These children may also have short, fat feet with a deep plantar crease that extends from the medial border

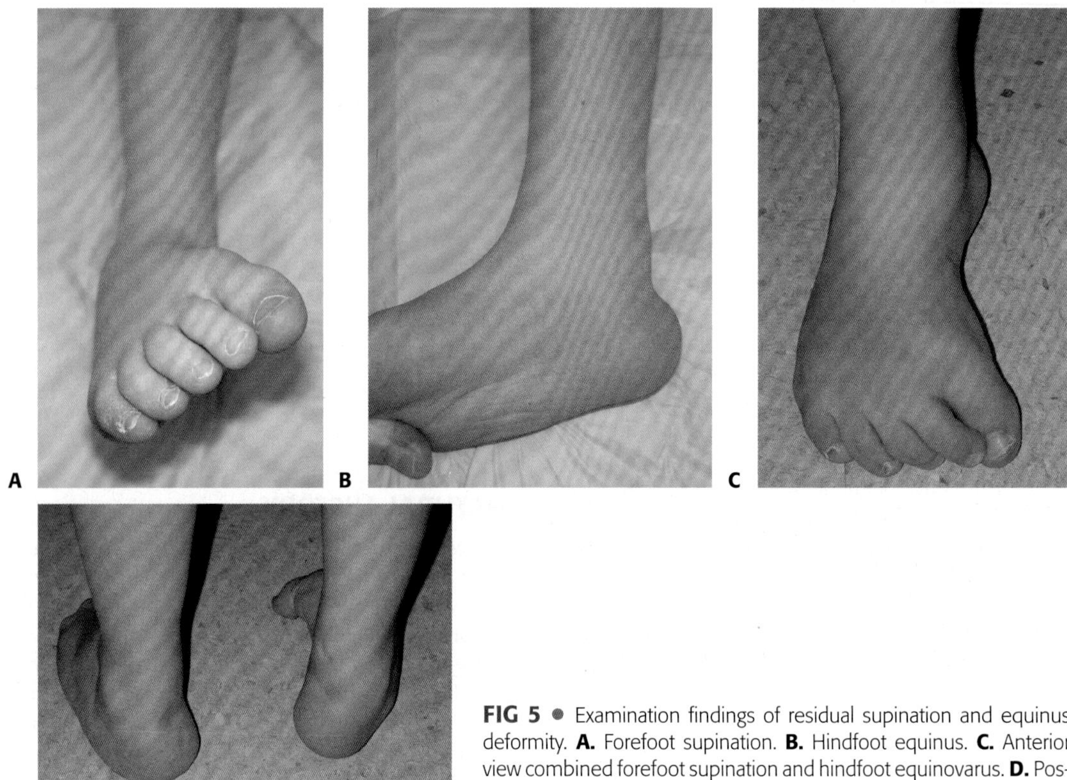

**FIG 5** ● Examination findings of residual supination and equinus deformity. **A.** Forefoot supination. **B.** Hindfoot equinus. **C.** Anterior view combined forefoot supination and hindfoot equinovarus. **D.** Posterior view combined forefoot supination and hindfoot equinovarus.

to the lateral border of the foot and a shortened first ray. These findings are consistent with severe or atypical clubfeet (often termed *complex clubfoot*) that have a propensity for residual deformity.

- In maximum pronation or maximum supination, the navicular–medial malleolar distance is decreased compared to the normal foot. In fact, the medial malleolus can be difficult to delineate because it is in contact with the navicular. The navicular malleolar distance demonstrates the extent of medial subluxation.
- It is important to examine gait when possible.
  - During examination of gait, the clinician should identify whether the tibialis anterior is a dynamic supinator; this is best observed in swing phase when no antagonist muscles contract.
  - This finding will confirm the appropriateness of surgery.
- The strength of the tibialis anterior is tested. With dynamic supination deformity, the supinator action of the anterior tibialis muscle will overpower the dorsiflexor action, thus demonstrating the appropriateness of surgery. In addition, good power is needed for a successful transfer.
- The clinician should evaluate for other deformities, such as equinus, cavus, varus, adductus, and tibial torsion.
- Range of motion of the ankle is examined. Transfer will work only as long as there is no fixed contracture of the ankle or heel cord.

## IMAGING AND OTHER DIAGNOSTIC STUDIES

- Anteroposterior (AP) and lateral radiographs may be helpful to study and quantify various deformities.
- AP radiographs will demonstrate medial deviation of the metatarsals, which can indicate residual medial displacement of navicular, which is yet to ossify (**FIG 6**).
  - On an AP radiograph of normal feet, the line drawn through the long axis of the talus should point to the first metatarsal, whereas the line drawn through the long axis of the calcaneus should point toward the fourth metatarsal.
    - In clubfeet, these lines become more parallel, depicting "stacking" of the talus and calcaneus.
  - Forced maximum dorsiflexion lateral radiographs may reveal hindfoot equinus with midfoot breech.
    - Stacking of the metatarsals on the lateral radiograph identifies the presence of residual forefoot supination (a decreased talocalcaneal angle).
- Ultrasound evaluation of the foot is not done routinely. However, experimental studies have demonstrated that this technique is capable of documenting the location of the navicular in relationship to the head of the talus. The navicular is subluxated plantarward and medially on the head of the talus.
- Similarly, MRI can be performed to completely identify the relationships of the cartilaginous bones and the size and presence of the lateral leg muscles.
  - This technology is rarely clinically used, as orthopaedists are aware of the classic deformities that are associated with recurrence and the increased risk of general anesthesia for a childhood MRI scan may not be justified.

## DIFFERENTIAL DIAGNOSIS

- Residual deformities in clubfoot may be due to unrecognized tarsal coalitions or other conditions in syndromic clubfoot, severe, or complex clubfeet.
- Unexpected and rapid recurrent deformity in children with previously corrected feet and with known myelomeningocele may be a result of continued neurologic involvement, such as tethering of the spinal cord.

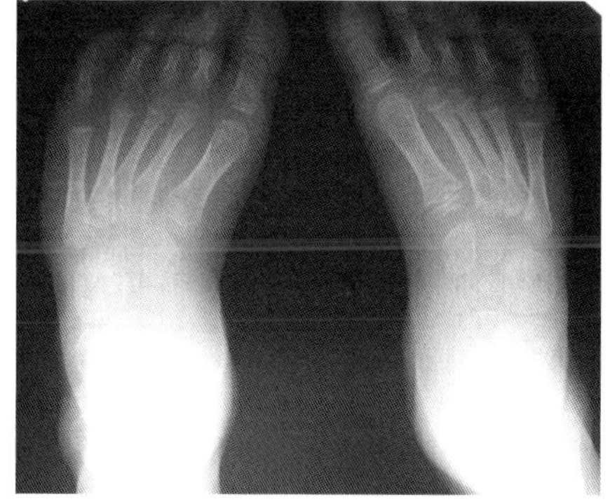
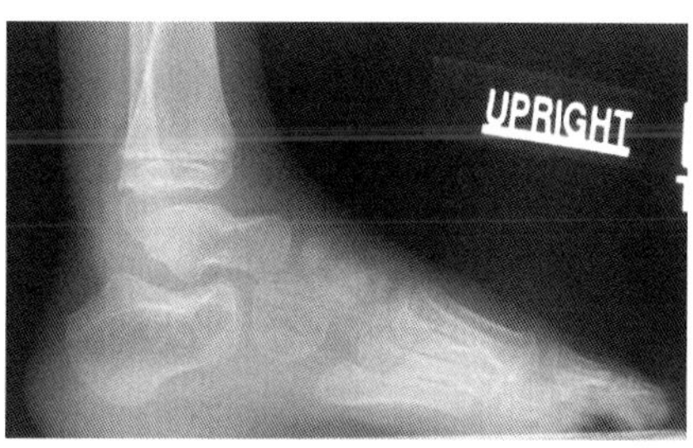

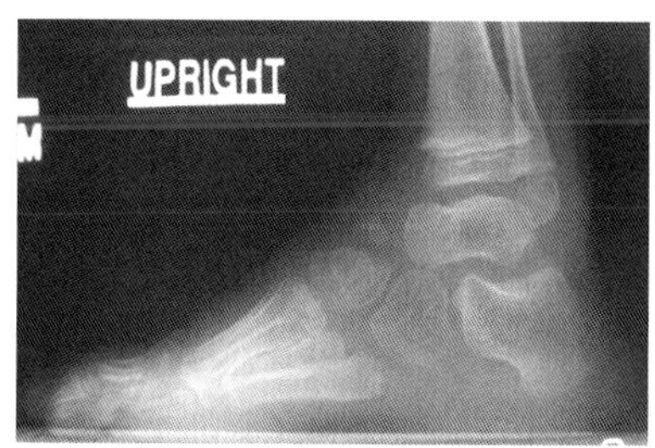


A B C

**FIG 6** ● Weight-bearing AP and lateral radiographs of feet shown in **FIG 5**. **A.** The long axes of the talus and calcaneus are somewhat parallel rather than divergent. The metatarsals appear adducted in relation to the talus. **B,C.** The long axis of the talus and calcaneus appear somewhat parallel rather than divergent on the lateral view of the right foot. The axes of the talus and the first metatarsal do not form a straight line, as opposed to a normal foot. This degree of divergence from this linear alignment represents intrinsic deformity of the clubfoot. The metatarsals are stacked on the weight-bearing lateral views.

## NONOPERATIVE MANAGEMENT

- Treatment of residual deformity depends on the location, severity, and age of the child.
- Recasting and repeat tenotomy may be considered in children younger than 18 months of age who have residual deformity.
  - Most residual deformities at this age can be treated by manipulation, followed by application of a toe-to-groin plaster cast with the feet in a fully corrected position for 2 weeks. Most of these patients have residual equinus that requires progressive dorsiflexion at each casting session.
  - After 2 weeks, the casts are removed and reapplied.
  - Usually, three casting sessions are required, for a total of 6 weeks.
  - Thereafter, abduction bracing is reinstituted. Several different abduction orthosis are commercially available and if one system is not well accepted, another maybe better tolerated.
  - In larger children, ankle–foot orthoses (AFOs) may also be used to prevent recurrence.
- Physiotherapy may also be used in patients with residual deformity. The therapist must be familiar with techniques to manipulate residual forefoot adductus and stretch the posterior contracture without producing or accentuating midfoot breech. In older children and in patients with midfoot breech, it can be difficult to effectively stretch any hindfoot equinus contracture.
- With residual equinus contracture, abduction bracing is difficult.
  - Unbraceable posterior contracture can then lead to recurrent metatarsus adduction and forefoot supination. Thus, a repeat percutaneous heel cord tenotomy and casting may be required.

## SURGICAL MANAGEMENT

- In children more than 2 to 3 years of age, and who failed conservative measures to correct deformity, it may be preferable to correct any residual deformity using soft tissue lengthenings or transfers with or without bony procedures.
- As the anterior tibialis acts as a supinator, lateral transfer of the anterior tibialis tendon is often necessary to correct dynamic supination deformity.
- The optimal age for lateral transfer of the anterior tibialis tendon varies from case to case. Important factors are the rapidity of recurrence, the strength of the anterior tibialis muscle, the presence of fixed forefoot deformity, or the presence of concurrent equinus deformity or cavus and the desired location to transfer the tendon.
  - Ponseti advocated transferring the tendon completely into the lateral cuneiform as such the surgery should be performed after the lateral cuneiform ossification center appears (2 to 4 years of age). Although some surgeons have successfully transferred tendons into cartilage anlage, this chapter outlines transfer of the tendon into the ossified cuneiform.
  - Alternatively, some surgeons have advocated transfer of the anterior tibialis tendon into the peroneus tertius, half of the peroneus brevis, or occasionally into metatarsals. In general, insertion of the tendon along an axis drawn along the third metatarsal will promote foot dorsiflexion.
  - The split anterior tibialis tendon transfer (SPLATT) of Hoffer et al[6] is rarely used in idiopathic clubfeet but is an excellent method for correcting dynamic supination deformity as a result of spasticity associated with disorders such as cerebral palsy. This method may have some use in children with mild, flexible forefoot supination who require surgery for other deformity.

### Preoperative Planning for Transfer into the Lateral Cuneiform

- Feet with residual deformity should be extensively evaluated by clinical and radiographic assessment before surgical planning. Each foot should be treated individually, as no single treatment plan is appropriate for all feet.
  - Associated deformities must be identified. For example, an anterior tibialis transfer will function poorly in the face of a fixed equinus contracture. In this case, it will be necessary to correct equinus deformity with a heel cord tenotomy or lengthening or posterior release.
  - Residual varus deformity may indicate the need for an opening wedge or sliding calcaneal osteotomy.
  - Persistent metatarsus adductus may necessitate midfoot osteotomies in order for the lateral border of the foot to be reduced.

- Anterior tibialis tendon transfer does not correct restricted subtalar motion.
- It is important to confirm that the ossific nucleus of the lateral cuneiform is present in order to place the anterior tibialis tendon into an appropriate anchor site.

## Positioning

- The patient is placed in the supine position on a standard operating table or the legs draped over a hand table.
  - Either positioning is done in a way to ensure good fluoroscopic images.
- A well-padded, thigh-high tourniquet should be placed before preparing and draping the patient.

## Approach

- A medial incision is based over the insertion of the anterior tibialis tendon.
- From this incision, the surgeon may be able to perform an opening wedge osteotomy of the medial cuneiform if indicated.
- Once the anterior tibialis tendon is detached, a lateral incision is based over the lateral cuneiform.
- Fluoroscopic imaging can assist in planning this incision.
- The lateral incision may need to be longer and more laterally based should the surgeon decide to perform a cuboid closing wedge osteotomy at the same time.

TECHNIQUES

## Full Anterior Tibialis Tendon Transfer to the Lateral Cuneiform[5,11]

### Approach

- A 4-cm long dorsal–medial longitudinal skin incision is made over the course of the anterior tibialis tendon from the inferior margin of the ankle retinaculum (the superior limb of the inferior extensor retinaculum) to its palpable distal insertion based over the medial cuneiform (**TECH FIG 1**).
- Dissection is carried down through subcutaneous tissues and the inferior limb of the inferior extensor retinaculum to expose the tendon sheath.
  - The anterior tibialis tendon sheath is incised sharply and opened as far distally as possible and then proximally to just short of the ankle retinaculum.
- A hemostat is placed under the anterior tibialis tendon to help expose the insertion.
  - This broad extensive insertion is detached as far distally as possible to gain maximum length of tendon for the transfer.
  - It is critical to obtain as much length as possible.

### Transferring the Tendon

- Once the tendon is freed and detached distally, a strong absorbable suture (eg, 1-0 Vicryl) is woven in a Bunnell-type fashion through the anterior tibialis tendon.
  - Care is taken to weave the suture in a fashion that does not lead to a bulbous end, thus making the tendon difficult to deliver to the lateral wound and subsequently pass into the lateral cuneiform.
  - Occasionally, the loose ends of the tendon insertion are trimmed or incorporated with a 3-0 absorbable suture to facilitate passage and anchoring.
- By pulling on the suture, the tendon is gently pulled distally while the soft tissue attachments to the tendon are freed up to, but not beyond, the ankle retinaculum.
  - To avoid bowstringing of the tendon, it is important not to release the ankle retinaculum.
- A dorsal–lateral longitudinal incision, 1.5 to 2 cm long, is made over the lateral cuneiform.
  - The lateral cuneiform is identified just proximal to the base of the third metatarsal.

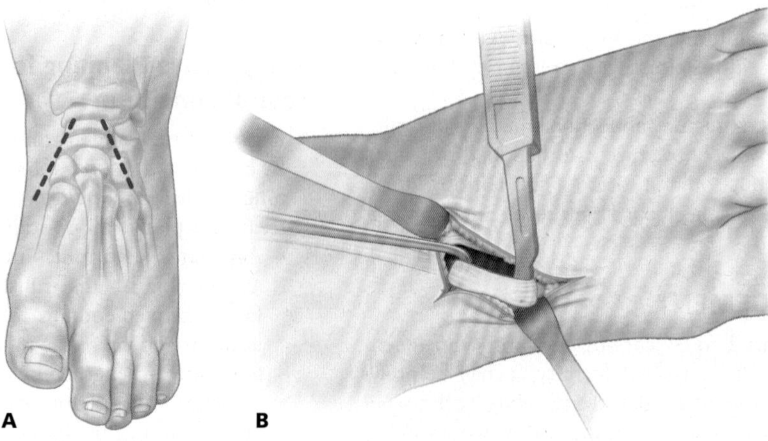


**TECH FIG 1** • **A.** Two incisions are made. **B.** The medial incision is made over the course of the tibialis anterior tendon. The surgeon frees the tendon from its broad insertion as far distally as possible and proceeds proximally as far as the ankle retinaculum.

- Dissection is carried down through subcutaneous tissues to the toe extensors.
  - To expose the lateral cuneiform, the toe extensors are retracted medially and the extensor digitorum brevis muscle is retracted laterally.
- A cruciate periosteal incision is made directly over the lateral cuneiform, carefully avoiding the adjacent joint articulations.
  - In young children, a Keith needle is used to fluoroscopically locate the center of the ossific nucleus.
  - In older children, a small periosteal elevator is used to elevate the periosteal flaps off the lateral cuneiform.
  - Occasionally, these flaps may be sutured into the transferred tendon, thus supplementing fixation. In young children, however, it may be difficult and futile to elevate perichondrium from the predominantly cartilaginous bone.
- A blunt hemostat is then passed from the lateral incision over the lateral cuneiform and under the extensor tendons to the point where the anterior tibialis tendon passes beneath the ankle retinaculum.
- Use the hemostat to develop a tract for the transfer of the anterior tibialis tendon.
- The hemostat is passed into this same tract into the medial wound to grasp the suture ends and bring the anterior tibialis tendon into the lateral wound (**TECH FIG 2**).
  - Ensure that the available length of the tendon will reach the proposed transfer site into the lateral cuneiform.

## Attaching the Transferred Tendon

- A drill bit is selected to be slightly larger than the diameter of the sutured anterior tibialis tendon end.
  - Once the bit is selected, make a hole directly in the center of the lateral cuneiform, drilling just through the plantar aspect of the bone (dorsal to plantar while aiming for the arch of the foot).
- The suture ends of the tendon are threaded onto Keith needles (**TECH FIG 3A**).
- While the foot is maximally dorsiflexed and everted, the suture needles are passed through the lateral cuneiform drill hole and out through the plantar aspect of the foot, guiding the tendon through the drill hole.
- The tendon is confirmed to easily and reproducibly slide into its new insertion.
  - This is a critical step: Be certain that the tendon reliably enters the anchoring hole after the skin is closed when the foot is dorsiflexed and when the suture is tensioned. Smooth passage of the tendon into the third cuneiform may be facilitated by a drop or two of sterile mineral oil.
- The suture needles on the plantar aspect of the foot are passed through a nonadhesive dressing (eg, Adaptic) and a sterile felt pad.
- At this time, it is advisable to irrigate and close all other associated wounds, leaving the lateral recipient wound for last.
  - This way, the surgeon can ensure that the anterior tibialis is in the intended position just before dressing and cast application.
- The periosteum of the lateral cuneiform is sutured with two interrupted absorbable sutures to the transferred anterior tibialis tendon while it is pulled into the recipient site (**TECH FIG 3B**).
- The lateral wound is irrigated and closed in layers while the foot is held in a dorsiflexed position, thus ensuring that the anterior tibialis remains in the hole and the continuity of the periosteal sutures is preserved.
- Sterile dressings are applied while an assistant simultaneously maintains the foot dorsiflexed with tension on the suture.
- The distal foot and ankle portion of a toe-to-groin cast is applied while ensuring that the suture ends of the tendon are in tension.
- In the past, we have tied the button over the felt underneath the cast. However, a high rate of pressure sores has led us to consider alternative fixation.
  - After the cast is hardened, the suture is tied over a button on the exterior of the plantar aspect of the cast (**TECH FIG 3C**).
  - To prevent plantar pressure sores, make sure the plaster is sufficiently hardened.
  - Commercially available suture anchors can also be used to facilitate fixation of the tendon.
- Some surgeons will perform the exact procedure except transfer the whole tendon into the cuboid. These surgeons choose this

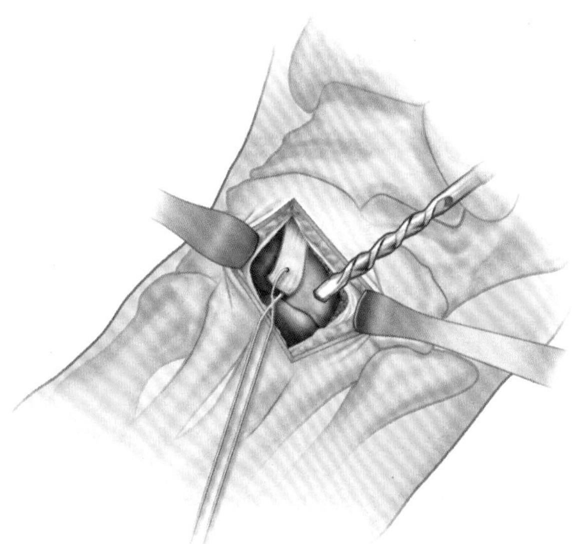

**TECH FIG 2** • The freed anterior tibialis tendon is brought into the lateral wound.

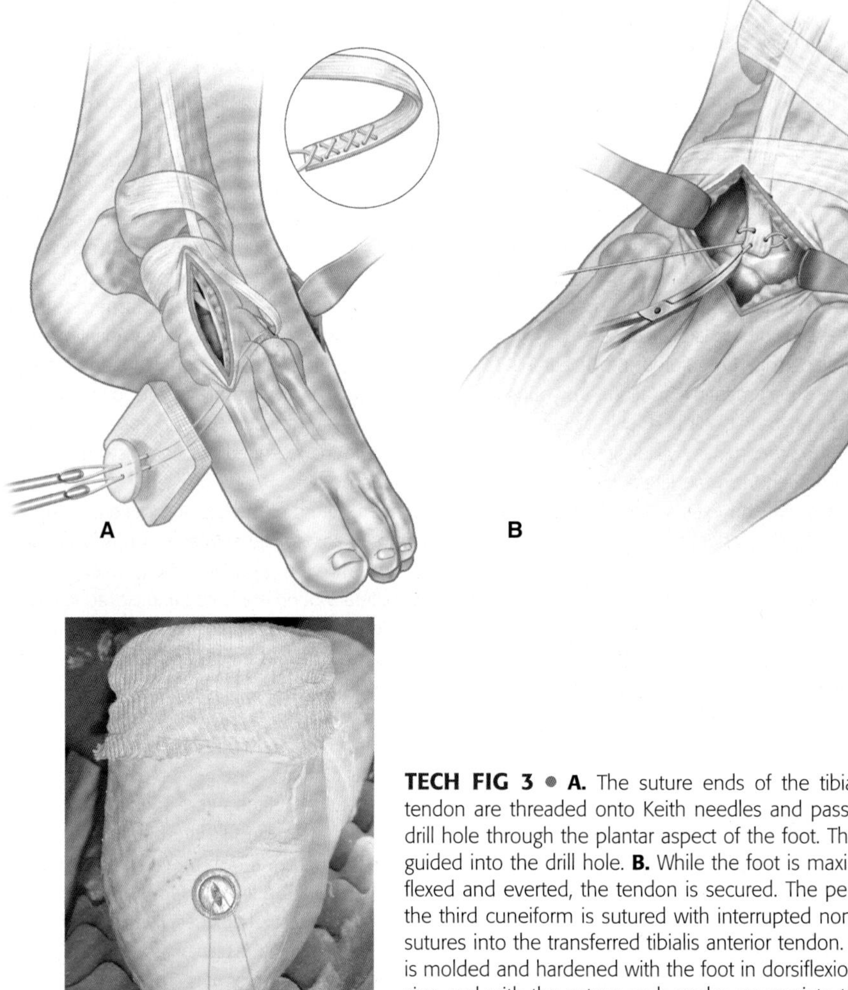


**TECH FIG 3 • A.** The suture ends of the tibialis anterior tendon are threaded onto Keith needles and passed into the drill hole through the plantar aspect of the foot. The tendon is guided into the drill hole. **B.** While the foot is maximally dorsiflexed and everted, the tendon is secured. The periosteum of the third cuneiform is sutured with interrupted nonabsorbable sutures into the transferred tibialis anterior tendon. **C.** The cast is molded and hardened with the foot in dorsiflexion and eversion and with the suture ends under appropriate tension. The suture is tied over a button on the exterior of the hardened cast to prevent plantar pressure sores.

insertion site if the foot has a concurrent fixed forefoot deformity and mild hindfoot varus that they choose not to correct.
  - We prefer to correct the fixed deformity and transfer the anterior tibialis into the lateral cuneiform, as we fear overcorrection from the more lateral insertion into the cuboid.
- Some surgeons add a third incision at the anterior distal tibia directly over the anterior tibialis tendon and just lateral to the tibial crest. The tendon can be easily palpated. The tendon sheath is incised here and the freed distal tendon end is pulled with a hemostat into this incision. From this incision, the freed distal tendon end is eventually pulled into the lateral incision for attachment.

## Split Anterior Tibialis Tendon Transfer

### Approach

- A 4-cm long dorsal–medial skin incision is made over the course of the anterior tibialis tendon from the inferior margin of the ankle retinaculum (the superior limb of the inferior extensor retinaculum) to its palpable distal insertion based over the medial cuneiform.
- Dissection is carried down through subcutaneous tissues and the inferior limb of the inferior extensor retinaculum to expose the tendon sheath.
  - The anterior tibialis tendon sheath is incised sharply and opened as far distally as possible and then proximally to just short of the ankle retinaculum.
- The lateral half of the anterior tibialis tendon insertion is detached as far distally as possible to gain maximum length of tendon for the transfer.
  - A strong absorbable suture (eg, 1-0 Vicryl) is woven in a Bunnell-type fashion through the lateral half of the anterior tibialis tendon.

### Transferring the Tendon

- The suture is grasped and pulled, allowing the lateral tendon to be gently dissected proximally but not beyond the ankle retinaculum.
  - To avoid bowstringing of the tendon, it is important not to release the ankle retinaculum.
- A dorsal–lateral longitudinal incision, 1.5 to 2 cm long, is made over the cuboid in line with the fourth metatarsal axis.

- Dissection is carried down through subcutaneous tissues to the toe extensors.
- To expose the cuboid, the toe extensors are retracted medially.
- A cruciate periosteal incision is made directly over the cuboid, carefully avoiding the adjacent joint articulations.
- An appropriate drill hole is then made in the cuboid, drilling dorsal to plantar in line with the fourth metatarsal axis and through the plantar aspect of the bone.
- A blunt hemostat is then passed from the incision over the cuboid under the extensor tendons to the point where the split anterior tibialis tendon passes beneath the ankle retinaculum.
  - Use the hemostat to develop a tract for the transfer of the anterior tibialis tendon.
- The hemostat is passed into this same tract into the medial wound to grasp the suture ends and bring the split anterior tibialis tendon into the lateral wound.
- The suture ends of the tendon are threaded onto Keith needles.

## Fixation of the Tendon to Bone

- While the foot is maximally dorsiflexed and everted, the suture needles are passed through the cuboid drill hole and out through the plantar aspect of the foot, guiding the tendon through the drill hole.
- The tendon is confirmed to easily and reproducibly slide into its new insertion.
- The suture needles are passed through a nonadhesive dressing (eg, Adaptic) and a sterile felt pad.
- The periosteum of the cuboid is sutured with two interrupted absorbable sutures to the transferred split anterior tibialis tendon.
- The wounds are irrigated and closed in layers.
- Sterile dressings are applied while ensuring that the felt pad is flush with the plantar skin and the suture ends of the tendon are at hand.
- Alternative fixation may include use of suture anchor into the cuboid or transfer of the lateral half of the tendon into half of the peroneus brevis tendon or the peroneus tertius tendon prior to its insertion into base of the fifth metatarsal.[9]
- With the standard technique described earlier, the most medial muscle fibers proximally are the ones attached to the laterally transferred split tendon, resulting in a proximal crossing over as the split tendon is laterally transferred.
  - Fennell and Phillips[4] suggest releasing the proximal medial insertion on the cuneiform instead of the distal lateral insertion on the first metatarsal to avoid this proximal crossing over, allowing for a more direct line of pull of the muscle on the transferred tendon.

## PEARLS AND PITFALLS

| | |
|---|---|
| **Indications** | ■ Anterior tibialis transfer will work only as long as there is no fixed contracture. Flexibility of the foot is the main condition for a successful surgical result because the surgical procedure is based on the dynamic muscle imbalance of the forefoot. |
| **Positioning** | ■ Use of a tourniquet at 200–250 mm Hg will allow easier surgery. |
| **Tendon harvest** | ■ Too short a tendon can make transfer difficult, so the surgeon should obtain as much length as possible.<br>■ Bowstringing and weakness by inadvertently cutting the extensor retinaculum should be avoided.<br>■ The surgeon should attach a suture to the released tendon to allow ease of handling and passing. This will also keep the tendon from fraying as it exits the donor site. |
| **Tendon fixation** | ■ It may be difficult to locate the lateral cuneiform in small children. Therefore, intraoperative fluoroscopy should be available.<br>■ An absorbable suture is used to hold the tendon as it usually dissolves and weakens by 6 weeks.<br>■ Alternative forms of fixation may be considered in older children with large bones, such as a suture anchor (**FIG 7**).<br>■ Overcorrection can be avoided with insertion of the full tendon transfer along the third metatarsal axis. For the split tendon transfer, the optimal site for insertion to obtain maximal dorsiflexion in biomechanical studies is along the fourth metatarsal axis.[7]<br>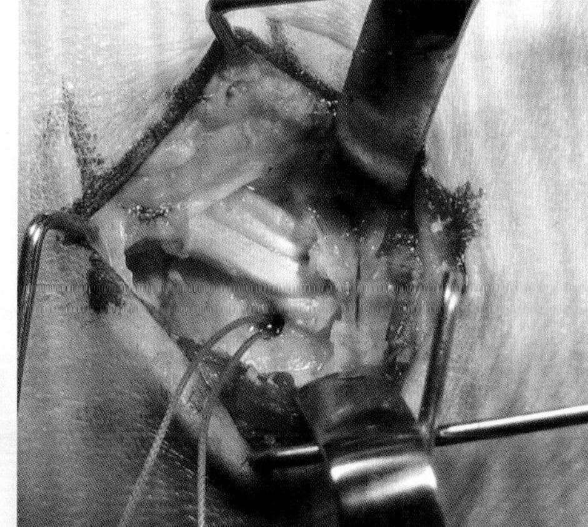<br>**FIG 7** • Intraoperative photo of lateral (recipient) wound. Alternative forms of fixation may be considered in older children with large bones, such as a suture anchor. |
| **Wound closure** | ■ All wounds are closed except the recipient site to be sure that the transferred tendon stays in the tunnel. Also, the foot is kept in maximum dorsiflexion during final wound closure and casting. A well-trained assistant is paramount. |
| **Cast management** | ■ Pressure sores on the bottom of the foot can result from too much tension on the button. Therefore, it should be placed on the exterior of the cast.<br>■ Swelling and pressure sores may result if extensive and lengthy procedures are done. In these cases, prophylactic dorsal splitting of the cast in the operating room is important. |

## POSTOPERATIVE CARE

- In patients younger than 5 years of age and those who may be noncompliant, a toe-to-groin bent-knee cast is maintained with the patient non–weight bearing for about 6 weeks.
  - At 6 weeks, the button and suture are removed and the patient is allowed to begin walking.
- In older children, a short-leg cast for an initial 6 weeks is maintained.
  - At 6 weeks, the button is removed and patient is placed in a short-leg walking cast for an additional 3 weeks to ensure healing and to avoid tendon rupture.
- Clinical and radiographic assessment of outcomes is performed at the end of healing. Plain radiographs (standing AP and lateral foot radiographs) are usually sufficient. Computed tomography (CT) examination may be obtained if indicated (**FIG 8**).
- A nighttime stretching AFO is often recommended for use in those children with residual Achilles contracture that required reduction. This may be needed for a year or so.

## OUTCOMES

- Successful surgery will be noted by correction of the supination deformity and conversion of the anterior tibialis into the primary dorsiflexor of the foot. Clinical examination of the foot during active dorsiflexion demonstrates the new insertion site of the anterior tibialis tendon.
- Twenty-seven previously treated clubfeet in 25 patients were retrospectively evaluated after tibialis anterior tendon transfer to correct residual dynamic supination deformity.[1] All showed active contraction of the transferred tibialis anterior tendon. There was no case of overcorrection.

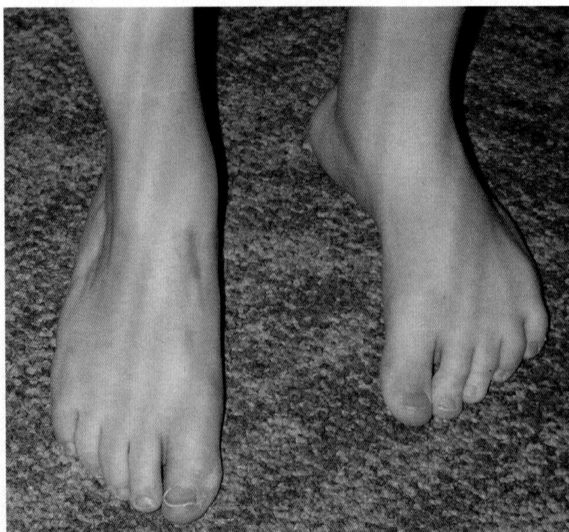

**FIG 8** • Postoperative clinical photograph of patient in **FIG 5**. Foot alignment is restored after full-thickness anterior tibialis tendon transfer in the right foot. The left foot is shown as comparison.

- Clinical and radiographic improvement in both forefoot adduction and supination was demonstrated in 71 cases of residual dynamic congenital clubfoot deformity treated by full and split anterior tendon transfer, with an increase in the eversion strength of the tibialis anterior muscle.[8]
- Farsetti et al[2] confirmed the findings of multiple studies, demonstrating that transfer of the anterior tibial tendon to the lateral cuneiform underneath the extensor retinaculum corrects and stabilizes relapsing clubfeet by restoring normal function of foot dorsiflexion–eversion. In their two series of patients reviewed at the end of skeletal growth, none of the operated patients had further relapse.

## COMPLICATIONS

- Undercorrection
- Cast sores
- Wound infection
- Loosening of the transferred tendon
- Rupture of the transferred tendon
- Bowstring at the anterior ankle joint resulting in weakness and a cosmetic deformity
- Loss of dorsiflexion force
- Overcorrection

## REFERENCES

1. Ezra E, Hayek S, Gilai AN, et al. Tibialis anterior tendon transfer for residual dynamic supination deformity in treated clubfeet. J Pediatr Orthop B 2000;9:207–211.
2. Farsetti P, Caterini R, Mancini F, et al. Anterior tibial tendon transfer in relapsing congenital clubfoot. J Pediatr Orthop 2006;26:83–90.
3. Feldbrin A, Gilai AN, Ezra E, et al. Muscle imbalances in the etiology of idiopathic clubfoot: an EMG study. J Bone Joint Surg Br 1995;77(4):596–601.
4. Fennell CW, Phillips P III. Redefining the anatomy of the anterior tibialis tendon. Foot Ankle Int 1994;15:396–399.
5. Garceau GJ. Anterior tibial tendon transposition in recurrent congenital clubfoot. J Bone Joint Surg 1940;22:932–936.
6. Hoffer MM, Reiswig JA, Garrett AM, et al. The split anterior tibial tendon transfer in the treatment of spastic varus hindfoot of childhood. Orthop Clin North Am 1974;5:31–38.
7. Hui JP, Goh JH, Lee EH. Biomechanical study of tibialis anterior tendon transfer. Clin Orthop Relat Res 1998;(349):249–255.
8. Kay RM. Lower extremity surgery in children with cerebral palsy. In: Tolo V, Skaggs D, eds. Master Techniques in Orthopaedic Surgery: Pediatrics. Philadelphia: Lippincott Williams & Wilkins, 2008.
9. Kuo KN. Anterior tibial tendon transfer. In: Tolo V, Skaggs D, eds. Master Techniques in Orthopaedic Surgery: Pediatrics. Philadelphia: Lippincott Williams & Wilkins, 2008.
10. Kuo KN, Hennigan SP, Hastings ME. Anterior tibial tendon transfer in residual dynamic clubfoot deformity. J Pediatr Orthop 2001;21:35–41.
11. Main BJ, Crider RJ. An analysis of residual deformity in clubfeet submitted to early operation. J Bone Joint Surg Br 1978;60:536–543.
12. Ponseti IV, El-Khoury GY, Ippolito E, et al. A radiographic study of skeletal deformities in treated clubfeet. Clin Orthop Relat Res 1981;(160):30–31.
13. Ponseti IV, Smoley EN. Congenital clubfoot: the results of treatment. J Bone Joint Surg Am 1963;45A:261–344.

# Treatment of Vertical Talus

Matthew B. Dobbs

128

CHAPTER

## DEFINITION

- Congenital vertical talus is a rare foot deformity that presents at birth as a rigid flatfoot deformity.
- Although the exact incidence of vertical talus is unknown, it has an estimated prevalence of 1 in 10,000 live births.
- It is associated with neuromuscular disorders or genetic syndromes in half of all cases, whereas the remainder occurs as isolated deformities.
- Of the 50% of cases of vertical talus that are isolated, almost 20% of these have a positive family history of other members affected with vertical talus.

## ANATOMY

- The hindfoot is in marked equinus and valgus caused by contracture of the tendo Achilles and the posterolateral ankle and subtalar joint capsules.[6,12]
- The midfoot and forefoot are dorsiflexed and abducted relative to the hindfoot due to contractures of the tibialis anterior tendon, extensor digitorum longus, extensor hallucis brevis, peroneus tertius, extensor hallucis longus tendons, and the dorsal aspect of the talonavicular capsule.
- The navicular is dorsally and laterally dislocated on the head of the talus resulting in the development of a hypoplastic and wedge-shaped navicular.
- The talar head and neck are flattened and medially deviated.
- The extreme plantarflexion of the talus results in attenuation of the calcaneonavicular or spring ligament and a rocker bottom appearance of the foot where the sole is convex and deep creases are seen in the dorsolateral aspect of the foot.
- The calcaneus is plantarflexed, leading often to dorsolateral subluxation or frank dorsal dislocation of the cuboid on the calcaneus.
- The posterior tibial tendon is usually subluxed anteriorly over the medial malleolus, whereas the peroneus longus and brevis may be subluxed over the lateral malleolus; the subluxed tendons may then function as ankle dorsiflexors rather than plantarflexors.

## PATHOGENESIS

- With a host of different genetic and neuromuscular etiologies for vertical talus, it is likely that the pathophysiologic basis for its development is heterogeneous in nature.
- Genetic factors play a significant role not only in syndromic cases but in many isolated cases as well.[17,19]
- The most common gene mutations identified to date for isolated vertical talus are in the *HOXD10* gene, encoding a homeobox transcription factor gene expressed in early limb development and the *GDF5* (cartilage-derived morphogenetic protein-1) gene.[8,9]
- Some neurologic cases present with significant muscle imbalances that can explain the resulting clinical deformity.
- Congenital muscle abnormalities are responsible in other patients as supported by abnormal skeletal muscle biopsies.
- Magnetic resonance angiography in this patient population demonstrates vascular insufficiencies in the lower limb that may be an etiologic factor.

## NATURAL HISTORY

- Left untreated, the deformities present in vertical talus worsen with weight bearing as secondary adaptive changes occur in the tarsal bones.
- Painful callosities develop along the plantar medial border of the foot around the prominent and unreduced talar head.
- Heel strike does not occur, shoe wear becomes difficult, and pain develops.

## PATIENT HISTORY AND PHYSICAL FINDINGS

- Hindfoot equinus, hindfoot valgus, forefoot abduction, and forefoot dorsiflexion are present in all patients with vertical talus in the newborn period, but the deformities vary in severity resulting in many patients not being diagnosed correctly at birth (**FIG 1**).
- In congenital vertical talus, the plantar surface of the foot is convex, creating a rocker bottom appearance.
- There are deep creases on the dorsolateral aspect of the foot.
- The forefoot dorsiflexion results in a palpable gap dorsally where the navicular and talar head would normally be articulating.
- The presence of active dorsiflexion and plantarflexion of the toes is recorded as absent, slight, or definitive. This should be recorded for the great toe alone as well as the lesser toes as a separate group.

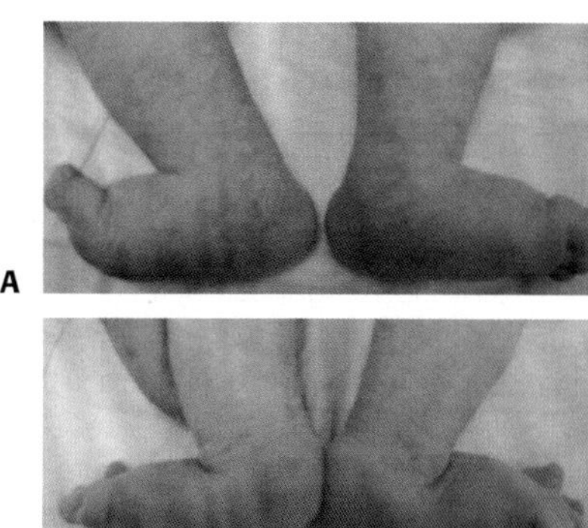

**FIG 1** • **A.** Convex plantar surface of the feet associated with bilateral congenital vertical talus. **B.** View from behind illustrating the deep creases on the dorsolateral aspect of the feet.

- Slight or absent ability to move the toes with stimulation correlates, in our experience, with vertical talus deformities that are more rigid and less responsive to treatment.
- In addition to examining the feet, the physician should look for the presence of a sacral dimple which may signify a central nervous system anomaly.

## IMAGING AND OTHER DIAGNOSTIC STUDIES

- Standard radiographs in evaluation of vertical talus include an anteroposterior radiograph of the foot and three laterals of the foot: maximal dorsiflexion, maximal plantarflexion, and neutral (standing for older children).
- The maximal plantarflexion lateral radiograph is the most critical film because a lateral talar axis–first metatarsal base angle (TAMBA) of greater than 35 degrees is pathognomonic for the disorder (**FIG 2**).
  - Values below 35 degrees do not rule out a vertical talus, however. In such cases, to differentiate a more flexible vertical talus from an oblique talus, the presence or absence of hindfoot equinus must be documented. If equinus is present, then the deformity is rigid and warrants treatment in the same manner as those vertical tali with a TAMBA angle of more than 35 degrees.
- The forced dorsiflexion lateral demonstrates persistent rigid hindfoot equinus.
- The anteroposterior radiograph demonstrates an increased talocalcaneal angle indicative of hindfoot valgus.

## DIFFERENTIAL DIAGNOSIS

- Oblique talus
- Calcaneovalgus foot
- Posteromedial bow of the tibia

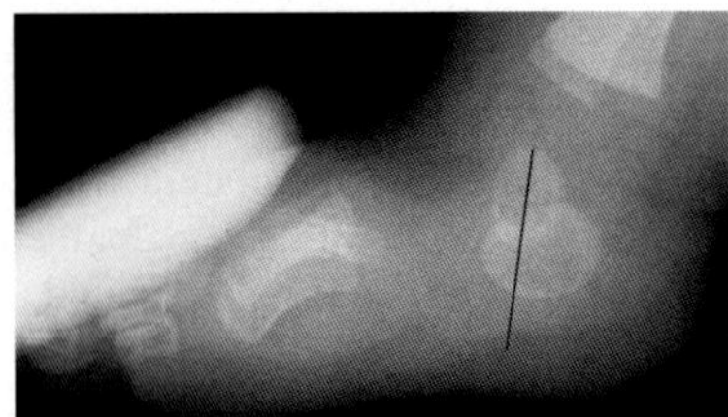

**FIG 2** • Plantarflexion lateral radiograph of the left foot of the patient in **FIG 1**, demonstrating the lack of reduction of the talonavicular joint.

## NONOPERATIVE MANAGEMENT

- Older casting techniques were not successful in correcting vertical talus deformities.
- With the advent of new casting technique,[1,10,11] focused on the functional anatomy of the subtalar joint, excellent correction can be achieved leaving the need for only a minimally invasive surgery to stabilize the reduction.

## SURGICAL MANAGEMENT

- Correction of all rigid vertical tali should be considered due to the unfavorable natural history.
- The use of the Dobbs method of serial manipulation and casting followed by temporary Kirschner wire stabilization of the talonavicular joint and a tendo Achilles tenotomy has provided a new treatment strategy that avoids more extensive soft tissue release surgery while providing excellent correction and preserving ankle and subtalar mobility.[1–5,7,10,13–15,20]
- Treatment should be initiated in the first 2 months of life if possible.
- The goals are to provide flexible feet that are plantigrade and functional.
- For syndromic and/or severely involved neuromuscular patients, careful consideration should be given to child's overall health and ambulatory potential before proceeding with treatment.

### Preoperative Planning

- The treatment process starting with serial casting should not be initiated with premature infants still in hospital and of low birth weight. These very small patients are difficult to fit into braces which are required to prevent relapse after correction is achieved.
- The age of the patient is important in preoperative planning as a tibialis anterior tendon transfer to neck of talus should be considered for those patients older than 2 years at time of treatment.
- Neural axis imaging should be performed for those patients in which abnormalities are present, suggestive of spinal pathology.

### Positioning

- Patient is positioned supine on radiolucent table.
- Nonsterile tourniquet is placed on proximal thigh.

TECHNIQUES

## Dobbs Method Part 1: Serial Manipulation

- The method of correction is based on a thorough understanding of the subtalar joint and the ability of the treating physician to accurately localize the head of the talus on the plantar medial aspect of the midfoot.
- The head of the talus is the fulcrum and the point around which the rest of the foot will be manipulated.
- All components of the deformity are corrected simultaneously with the exception of the hindfoot equinus, which is corrected last.
- The manipulations are gentle in nature and consist of stretching the foot into plantarflexion and adduction with one hand while counterpressure is applied with the thumb of the opposite hand gently pushing the talus dorsally and laterally (**TECH FIG 1**).
- It is essential not to touch the calcaneus during manipulations, as this can prevent the calcaneus from correcting from a valgus to a varus position.
- Manipulations are done weekly in the clinic and are gentle in nature. The head of the talus is palpated with the thumb of the examiner, and once identified, direct pressure is placed with the thumb on the head of the talus in a plantar and lateral direction while the examiner using the other hand brings the foot into plantarflexion and adduction.
- Ideally, an assistant is present during the manipulations as well to provide a counterfulcrum by applying gentle traction underneath the knee in the direction of the head of the patient. This allows

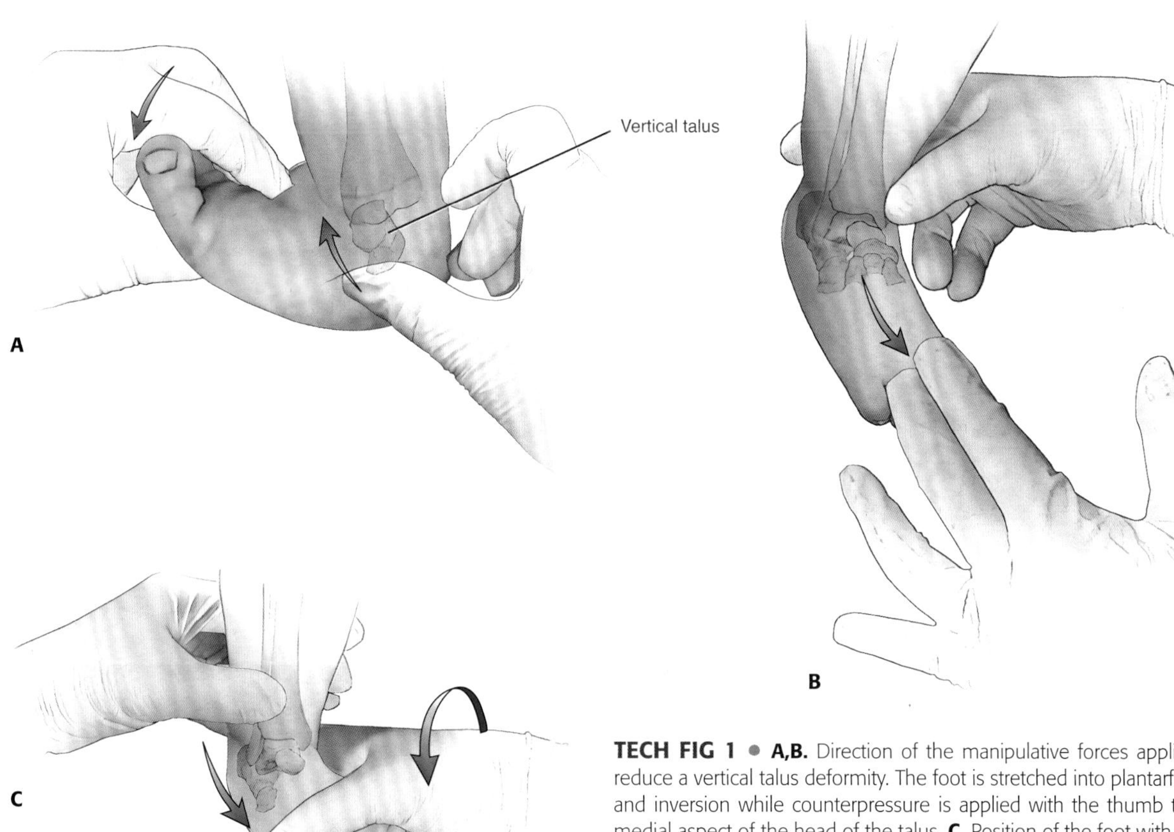


**TECH FIG 1** ● **A,B.** Direction of the manipulative forces applied to reduce a vertical talus deformity. The foot is stretched into plantarflexion and inversion while counterpressure is applied with the thumb to the medial aspect of the head of the talus. **C.** Position of the foot with maximum hindfoot varus and forefoot adduction before pinning of the talonavicular joint and lengthening of the Achilles tendon. The foot is also placed in maximum plantarflexion to ensure adequate stretching of the contracted dorsolateral tendons, joint capsules, and skin (not shown).

the physician to effectively plantarflex the foot without pulling the patient down the examination table.

- After a minute or two of manipulations, a long-leg plaster cast is applied to hold the foot in the position achieved with stretching.
- The cast is applied in two sections with the short-leg portion applied first to allow the treating physician to make the appropriate molds.
- Once the plaster has been applied, the treating physician then molds carefully around the talar head, the malleoli, and above the calcaneus posteriorly.
- Once the plaster has set, the dorsum of the toes are exposed just enough to be able to assess circulation while leaving enough plaster dorsally to stretch the toes into plantarflexion.
- The cast is then extended above the knee, with the knee in 90 degrees of flexion.
- Casting and manipulations are repeated weekly in the clinic for an average of 5 to 6 weeks using the same manipulative technique but gaining more correction each time.
- The skilled physician can palpate when the talonavicular joint is reduced and visualize when the heel has corrected into varus.
- The position of the foot when the talonavicular joint is fully reduced is an extreme clubfoot position. This position is critical to achieve to adequately stretch the contracture dorsolateral soft tissues.

## Dobbs Method Part 2: Limited Surgery and Percutaneous Stabilization

- When reduction is achieved, the patient is scheduled for the operating room for stabilization of the talonavicular joint with a Kirschner wire followed by a percutaneous tendo Achilles tenotomy.
- In the operating room under tourniquet control and in the supine position, a small 1-cm incision is made dorsomedially over the talonavicular joint. This allows the surgeon, without opening the joint capsule in most cases, to ensure the talonavicular joint is reduced and aids in Kirschner wire placement.
- If the joint is not completely reduced, a small capsulotomy is made in the anterior subtalar joint which allows the placement of an elevator to gently complete the reduction.

- Once the talonavicular joint is reduced, a smooth 0.062-mm Kirschner wire is placed in a retrograde manner across the joint under direct visualization and confirmed radiographically.
- Care should be taken under radiographic visualization to ensure the anteroposterior talocalcaneal angle has been reduced as well correcting the hindfoot valgus.
- The wire is buried to prevent it from backing out.
- Once the talonavicular joint is stabilized, a tenotomy is done of the tendo Achilles to correct residual equinus.
- A long-leg cast is applied with the ankle and forefoot in a neutral position.

## One-Stage Extensive Soft Tissue Release

- Patient is positioned supine on a radiolucent table and tourniquet is placed on the proximal thigh.
- An extensive dorsolateral approach is used to perform a talonavicular capsulotomy and lengthening of the tibialis anterior tendon, extensor digitorum longus, and peroneal tendons.[16,18,21–23]
- Capsulotomies of the subtalar joint both medially and laterally.
- A posterior incision is performed next to lengthen the Achilles tendon and release the posterior subtalar and ankle joints.
- The talonavicular joint is then reduced and held with a Kirschner wire.
- The calcaneocuboid joint is released if subluxation of this joint is still present. This is also held reduced with a Kirschner wire.

## PEARLS AND PITFALLS

| | |
|---|---|
| **Localizing the talar head** | ■ The talar head in vertical talus is located plantar medially and can be difficult to palpate in an infant's foot. If the distal medial calcaneus is used as the fulcrum instead of the head of the talus, the correction will not be achieved. |
| **Importance of equinovarus** | ■ A position of maximal equinovarus (clinically looks like clubfoot) must be achieved in the last cast prior to pin fixation of the talonavicular joint. This is analogous to achieving 70 degrees of external rotation in the final clubfoot cast using the Ponseti method.<br>■ Failure to do so will result in an incomplete reduction of the talonavicular joint and a failure to adequately stretch the contracted dorsolateral soft tissue structures placing the patient at a higher risk of early relapse. |
| **Treatment timing** | ■ Begin treatment in the newborn stage if possible. Just as for clubfoot casting, treatment should be initiated at young age to take advantage of the more pliable soft tissues. |
| **Approach** | ■ In some stiffer syndromic patients in whom gaining maximal equinovarus positioning is difficult, a small dorsolateral incision is made rather than the dorsomedial incision to allow access to the tighter anterolateral subtalar joint capsule to complete reduction.<br>■ Approaching the anteromedial subtalar joint capsule in this group of patients may not be enough to gain complete reduction of the talonavicular joint—the anterolateral subtalar joint is more contracted in this patient group and release at this level gives better results. |
| **Tendon transfer** | ■ For patients older than 2 years at time of treatment, adding transfer of the tibialis anterior tendon to the neck of the talus should be considered to minimize risk of relapse.<br>■ The tendon is sutured directly into the neck of the talus and approached through the same dorsomedial skin incision used for pin placement. |
| **Casting** | ■ Do not touch the calcaneus at all during the serial casting portion of treatment or it will be blocked from correction from valgus to varus.<br>■ This is the same principle followed in the Ponseti method where touching the calcaneus prevents it from correcting from varus to valgus. |
| **Avoiding relapse** | ■ Use shoe and bar dynamic bracing as prescribed to minimize risk of relapse. Failure to do so result in increased risk of relapse. |

## POSTOPERATIVE CARE

- The cast is changed 2 weeks postoperatively to manipulate the ankle to 10 degrees of dorsiflexion.
- The pin is removed in the operating room at 6 weeks from the index procedure.
- The patient is placed in a dynamic shoe and bar brace system, which they are to wear 23 hours a day for 2 months and then at nighttime for 2 years to prevent relapse (**FIG 3**).
- The shoes on the brace are set pointing ahead to stretch the peroneal tendons. The dynamic bar allows active motion at the knees and ankles and also encourages active plantarflexion stretching of the dorsolateral soft tissues.
- Follow-up is at 1 month after initiating brace wear and then every 3 months for the first 2 years. After that, follow-up is yearly for several years and then every 2 years until the age of 8 years.

## OUTCOMES

- Treatment with the Dobbs method has been shown in multiple studies from around the world to allow excellent clinical and radiographic (**FIG 4**) correction in by isolated and nonisolated (syndromic and neuromuscular) cases.
- A recent study comparing the Dobbs method with traditional extensive soft tissue release surgery demonstrated that while both methods achieve good radiographic correction, the Dobbs method provides superior clinical and functional results as measured in better subtalar and ankle range of motion and less pain with growth.

## COMPLICATIONS

- Dobbs method
  - Skin complications from casting
  - Kirschner wire back out from soft cartilaginous structures
  - Difficulties with postoperative bracing
- Extensive soft tissue release
  - Avascular necrosis of talus
  - Wound dehiscence
  - Undercorrection
  - Overcorrection
  - Ankle and subtalar joint stiffness
  - Vascular and neurologic injuries

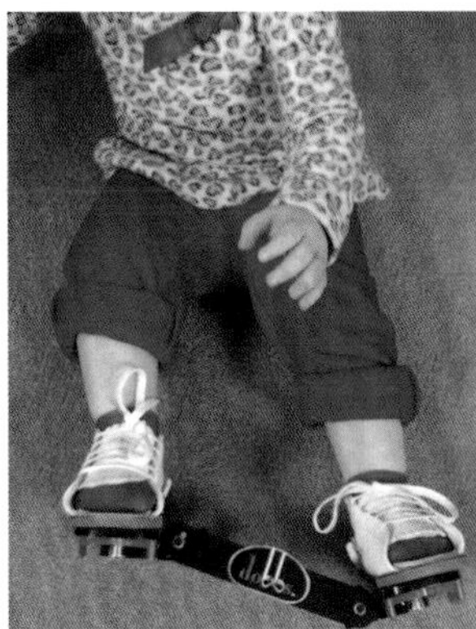

**FIG 3** • Dynamic shoe and bar system used to maintain correction of the vertical talus that was achieved with casting and minimally invasive surgery.

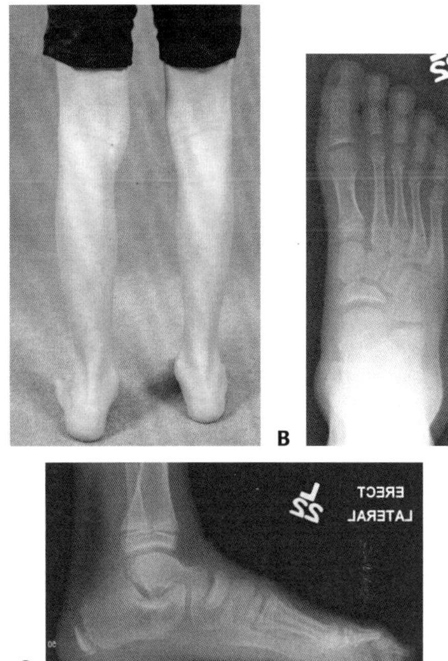


**FIG 4** • **A.** Clinical photograph of patient with bilateral vertical talus 10 years after correction with the Dobbs method. **B,C.** Anteroposterior and lateral radiographs, respectively, of the patient's left foot, demonstrating maintenance of excellent correction.

## REFERENCES

1. Alaee F, Boehm S, Dobbs MB. A new approach to the treatment of congenital vertical talus. J Child Orthop 2007;1:165–174.
2. Aslani H, Sadigi A, Tabrizi A, et al. Primary outcomes of the congenital vertical talus correction using the Dobbs method of serial casting and limited surgery. J Child Orthop 2012;6:307–311.
3. Aydin A, Atmaca H, Müezzinoglu US. Bilateral congenital vertical talus with severe lower extremity external rotational deformity: treated by reverse Ponseti technique. Foot 2012;22:252–254.
4. Bhaskar A. Congenital vertical talus: treatment by reverse Ponseti technique. Indian J Orthop 2008;42:347–350.
5. Chalayon O, Adams A, Dobbs MB. Minimally invasive approach for the treatment of non-isolated congenital vertical talus. J Bone Joint Surg Am 2012;94:e73.
6. Coleman SS, Stelling FH III, Jarrett J. Pathomechanics and treatment of congenital vertical talus. Clin Orthop Relat Res 1970;70:62–72.
7. David MG. Simultaneous correction of congenital vertical talus and talipes equinovarus using the Ponseti method. J Foot Ankle Surg 2011;50:494–497.
8. Dobbs MB, Gurnett CA, Pierce B, et al. HOXD10 M319K mutation in a family with isolated congenital vertical talus. J Orthop Res 2006;24:448–453.
9. Dobbs MB, Gurnett CA, Robarge J, et al. Variable hand and foot abnormalities in family with congenital vertical talus and CDMP-1 gene mutation. J Orthop Res 2005;23:1490–144.
10. Dobbs MB, Purcell DB, Nunley R, et al. Early results of a new method of treatment for idiopathic congenital vertical talus. J Bone Joint Surg Am 2006;88:1192–1200.
11. Dobbs MB, Purcell DB, Nunley R, et al. Early results of a new method of treatment for idiopathic congenital vertical talus. Surgical technique. J Bone Joint Surg Am 2007;89(suppl 2, pt 1):111–121.
12. Drennan JC. Congenital vertical talus. Instr Course Lect 1996;45:315–322.
13. Eberhardt O, Fernandez FF, Wirth T. Treatment of vertical talus with the Dobbs method [in German]. Z Orthop Unfall 2011;149:219–224.

14. Eberhardt O, Fernandez FF, Wirth T. The talar axis-first metatarsal base angle in CVT treatment: a comparison of idiopathic and non-idiopathic cases treated with the Dobbs method. J Child Orthop 2012;6:491–496.
15. Eberhardt O,Wirth T, Fernandez FF. Minimally invasive treatment of congenital foot deformities in infants: new findings and midterm-results [in German]. Orthopade 2013;42:1001–1007.
16. Hamanishi C. Congenital vertical talus: classification with 69 cases and new measurement system. J Pediatr Orthop 1984;4:318–326.
17. Kruse L, Gurnett CA, Hootnick D, et al. Magnetic resonance angiography in clubfoot and vertical talus: a feasibility study. Clin Orthop Relat Res 2009;467:1250–1255.
18. Mathew PG, Sponer P, Karpas K, et al. Mid-term results of one-stage surgical correction of congenital vertical talus. Bratisl Lek Listy 2009;110:390–393.
19. Merrill LJ, Gurnett CA, Connolly AM, et al. Skeletal muscle abnormalities and genetic factors related to vertical talus. Clin Orthop Relat Res 2011;469:1167–1174.
20. Rodriguez N, Choung DJ, Dobbs MB. Rigid pediatric pes planovalgus: conservative and surgical treatment options. Clin Podiatr Med Surg 2010;27:79–92.
21. Seimon LP. Surgical correction of congenital vertical talus under the age of 2 years. J Pediatr Orthop 1987;7:405–411.
22. Stricker SJ, Rosen E. Early one-stage reconstruction of congenital vertical talus. Foot Ankle Int 1997;18:535–543.
23. Zorer G, Bagatur AE, Dogan A. Single stage surgical correction of congenital vertical talus by complete subtalar release and peritalar reduction by using the Cincinnati incision. J Pediatr Orthop B 2002;11:60–67.

# Exam Table for Pediatric Orthopaedic Surgery

| Examination | Technique | Illustration | Grading & Significance |
|---|---|---|---|
| **Upper Extremities/Hand, Wrist, and Elbow** | | | |
| **Abductor pollicis brevis muscle test** | Abduction of thumb against resistance with palpation of thenar muscle | 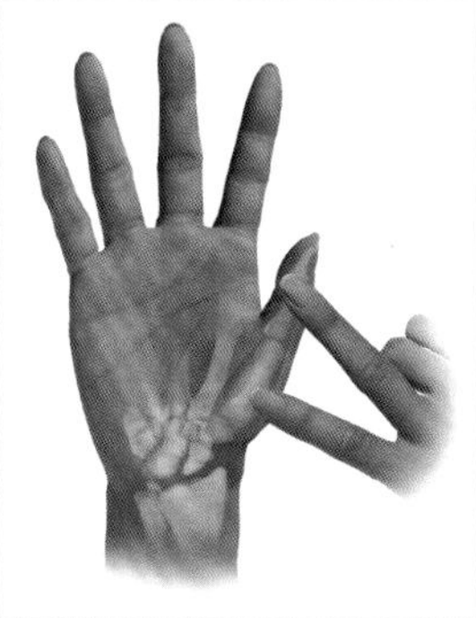 | MRC grading. If weak, the surgeon should consider a median nerve lesion. |
| **Advancing Tinel sign** | Percussion along course of a nerve in a distal to proximal direction | 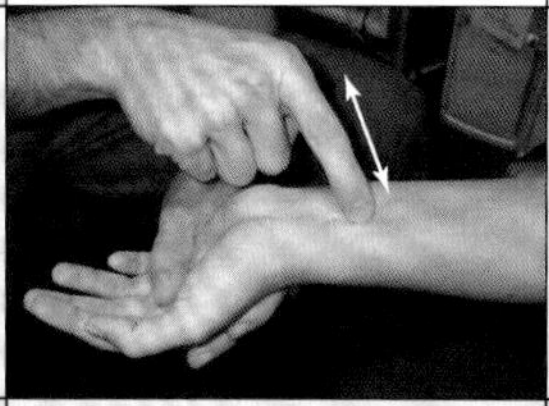 | During percussion, the patient notes a tingling sensation in the sensory distribution of the nerve. Detects regenerating (unmyelinated) axons. Serial progression of a Tinel sign distally is useful to monitor axon progression after nerve repair or injury. |
| **Allen test** | The patient is asked to actively open and close the hand to create blanching in the palm. With the hand tightly closed, the examiner occludes the radial and ulnar arteries. The examiner releases one artery and watches for reperfusion and then repeats, releasing the other artery. | 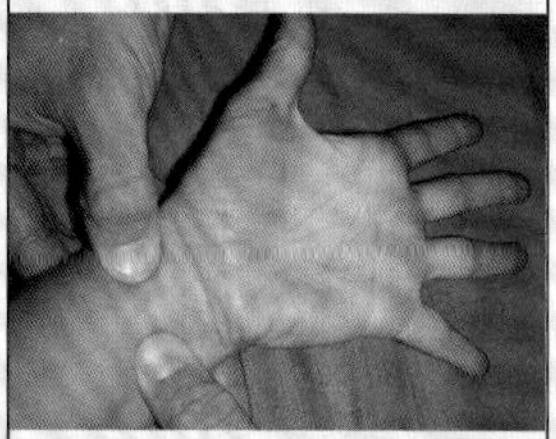 | Reperfusion should occur within a few seconds. If it does not, then that artery does not provide good flow to the hand. If, for example, the radial artery is dominant (ie, the ulnar artery does not reperfuse the hand), then injury to this vessel during the procedure could lead to ischemia of the hand. |
| **Anatomic snuffbox palpation** | The examiner palpates the anatomic snuffbox between the first and third extensor compartment tendons while moving the wrist from radial to ulnar deviation. | 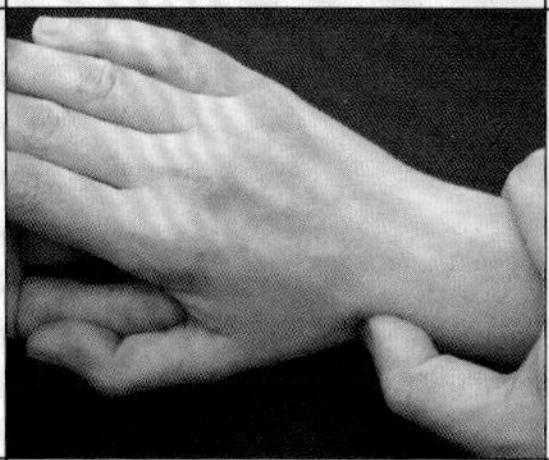 | Pain at the articular–nonarticular junction of the scaphoid may be the result of periscaphoid synovitis, scaphoid instability, radial styloid arthrosis, or scaphoid fracture or nonunion. |
| **Boyes oblique retinacular ligament tightness test** | The examiner passively extends the proximal interphalangeal (PIP) joint and evaluates distal interphalangeal (DIP) motion. Tightness of the oblique retinacular ligaments of Landsmeer is evaluated by assessing the relative degree of resistance to active and passive DIP joint flexion with the PIP joint held in maximum extension by the examiner. | 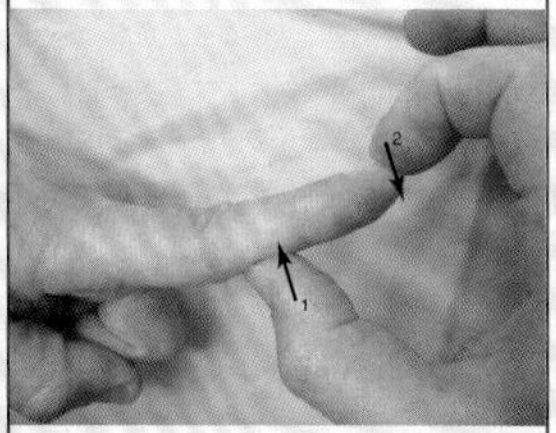 | In a positive test, passive extension of the PIP joint will result in extension of the DIP joint. Increased resistance to active and passive DIP joint flexion with the PIP joint held in extension signifies relative tightness of the oblique retinacular ligaments (ORLs) of Landsmeer, signifying a potential subacute or chronic central slip injury. Continued shortening of the ORLs will result in a boutonnière deformity. |

(continued)

| Examination | Technique | Illustration | Grading & Significance |
|---|---|---|---|
| **Bunnell intrinsic tightness test** | While holding the metacarpophalangeal (MCP) joint in extension, the examiner assesses the degree of resistance to passive PIP joint flexion. The test is repeated with the MCP joint held in flexion. | 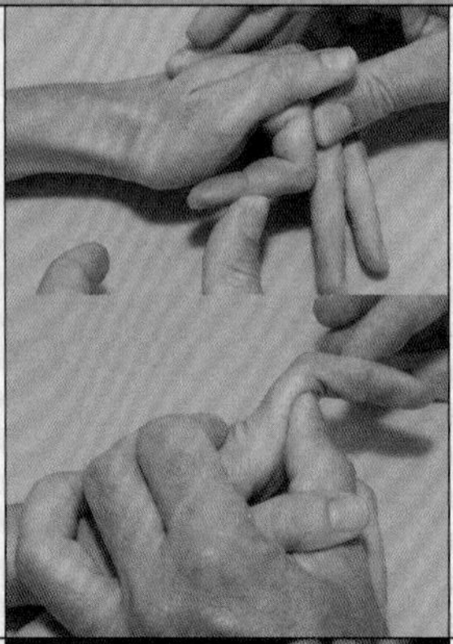 | Intrinsic tightness results in limited passive flexion of the PIP joint when the MCP joint is held extended. Extrinsic tightness results in limited PIP joint passive flexion when the MCP joint is held flexed. |
| **Carpal supination reduction test** | The examiner applies dorsally directed pressure to the volar aspect of the supinated ulnar carpus. | 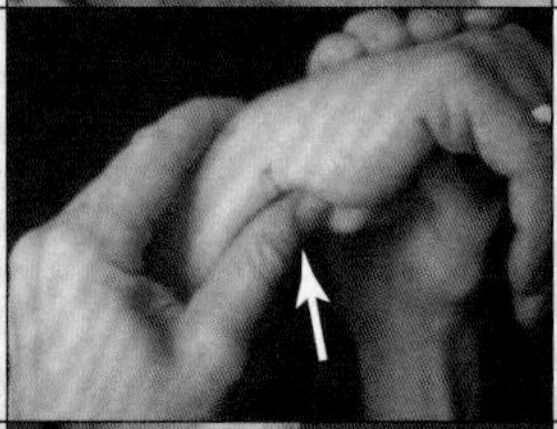 | The ulnar carpus will be supinated and the distal ulna prominent, signifying an ulnar extrinsic ligament injury. Reduction is noted visually after application of the force. |
| **Carpal tunnel compression test** | The examiner applies direct compression to the median nerve at the level of the carpal tunnel for 60 seconds or until symptomatic. | 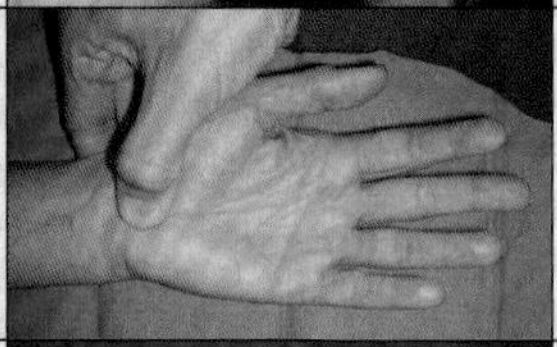 | Reproduction of symptoms in the median nerve distribution is consistent with carpal tunnel syndrome. |
| **Carpometacarpal (CMC) distraction test** | The examiner distracts the thumb and palpates the CMC joint. | 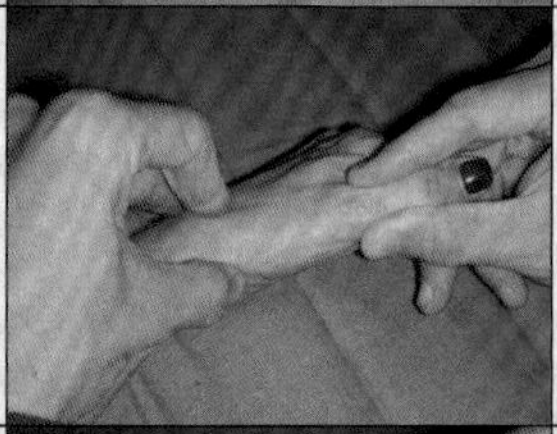 | Reproduction of pain confirms the CMC joint as a site of disease or inflammation. |
| **CMC grind test** | The examiner axially compresses the thumb and applies flexion, extension, circumduction, and rotation. | 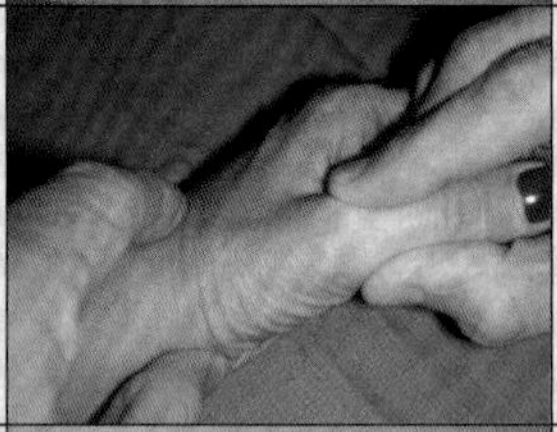 | Usually crepitus is appreciated starting with stage II disease, but it is more predictable in stage III or IV disease. A positive test is suggestive of degenerative thumb CMC joint disease. |
| **Cross-finger test** | The patient is asked to cross the long and index fingers. | 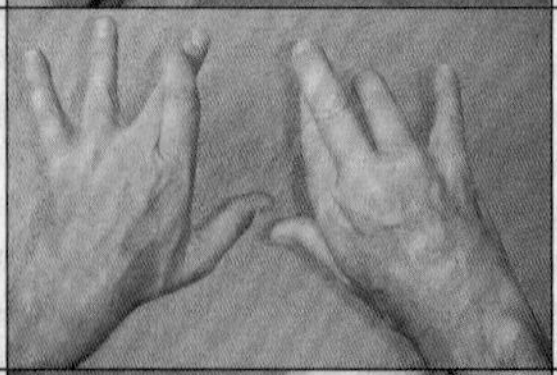 | The test is positive if the patient cannot cross the fingers. This test demonstrates weakness of dorsal and palmar interossei. |
| **Cubital tunnel Tinel sign** | The ulnar nerve is percussed around the elbow. | 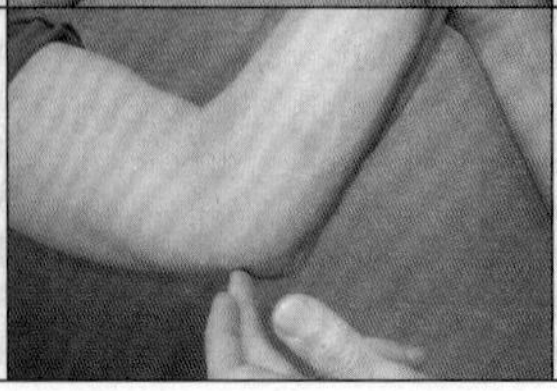 | A positive test results in radiating paresthesias into the ulnar nerve distribution of the hand. This test may not be specific for ulnar nerve pathology. |

| Examination | Technique | Illustration | Grading & Significance |
|---|---|---|---|
| **Distal radioulnar joint (DRUJ) compression test** | The examiner compresses the ulnar head against the sigmoid notch while holding the patient's mid-forearm and passively rotating. | 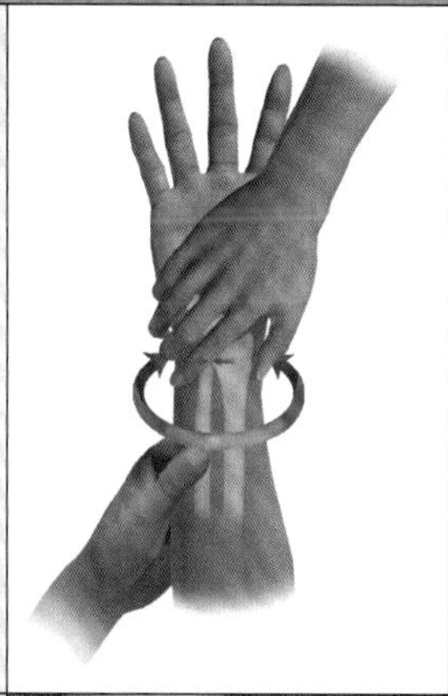 | Positive or negative. A positive test is exacerbation of pain, which suggests arthritis or instability; dorsal or palmar subluxation may be noted. |
| **DRUJ press test** | With both wrists pronated, the patient rises from a chair using the affected hand and wrist or pushes downward on a tabletop. | 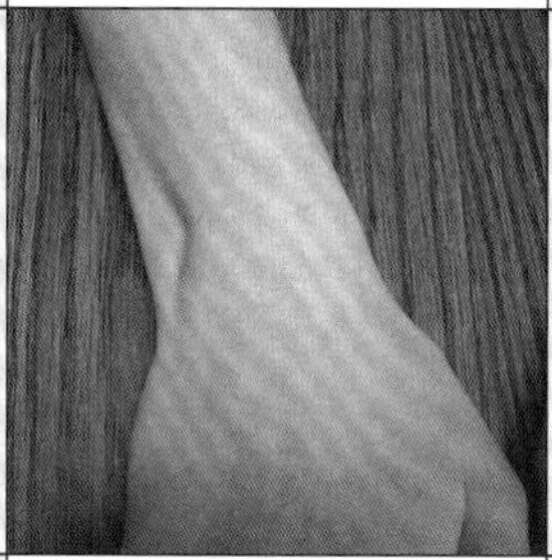 | Increased depression of the ulnar head on the affected side results in a "dimple sign" indicating instability. Pain without increased ulnar head depression may indicate a triangular fibrocartilage complex tear. |
| **DRUJ stability test** | With the elbow flexed 90 degrees, the examiner grasps the radius over its distal third with one hand and holds the ulna head between the index finger and thumb with the other hand. The examiner displaces the ulna volarly and dorsally in neutral rotation, full supination, and full pronation. The sides are compared. | 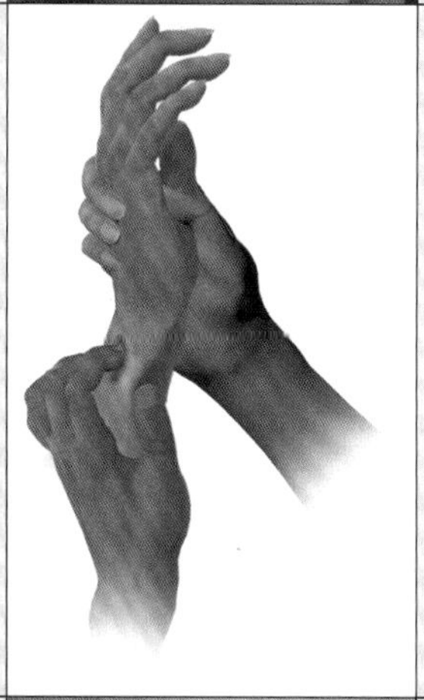 | Substantially less stability than is noted on the opposite side or pain at extremes of rotation may correlate with symptomatic DRUJ instability related to triangular fibrocartilage complex or ligamentous instability. Palpable crepitus at the DRUJ may be indicative of DRUJ arthrosis. Instability Grading Scale. 0. normal; about 1 cm of motion in neutral, no motion at extremes of rotation I: <0.5 cm of motion at extremes. Firm endpoint. II: >0.5 cm of motion at extremes with soft endpoint but no dislocation III: reduced joint before stress with dislocation of the DRUJ at extremes IV: dislocated joint. "Mushy" feeling with stressing joint. |
| **Effusion** | The examiner palpates the anconeus triangle (radial head [RH], lateral epicondyle [L], and olecranon tip [O]) and lateral gutter, noting prominence of lateral epicondyle, gutter effusion, or subcutaneous atrophy from prior corticosteroid injections. | 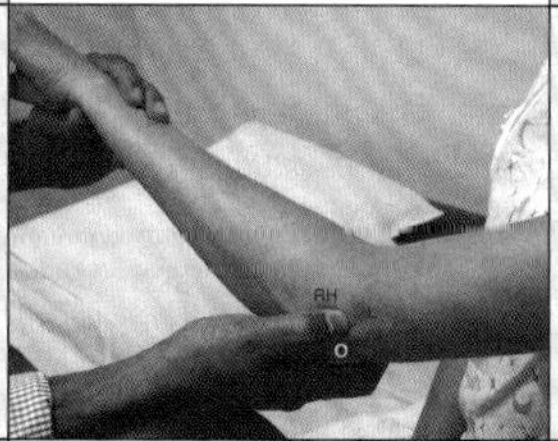 | It is difficult to estimate the amount of fluid, but the presence of an effusion should be noted and may represent hemarthrosis due to intra-articular fracture, radiocapitellar wear, or ligamentous disruption. In acute injuries an effusion should be present; in more chronic situations it may be absent. |
| **Elbow drawer test** | With the patient in prone position, the humerus is stabilized with one arm while a distraction force is placed on the forearm to sublux the ulnohumeral joint. | 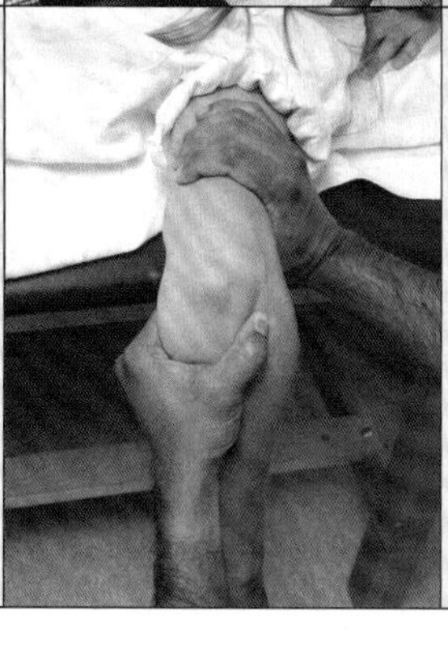 | A positive test reveals ulnohumeral subluxation. |

(continued)

| Examination | Technique | Illustration | Grading & Significance |
|---|---|---|---|
| **Elbow flexion test** | The elbow is fully flexed with the forearm supinated for 60 seconds or until symptoms develop. | 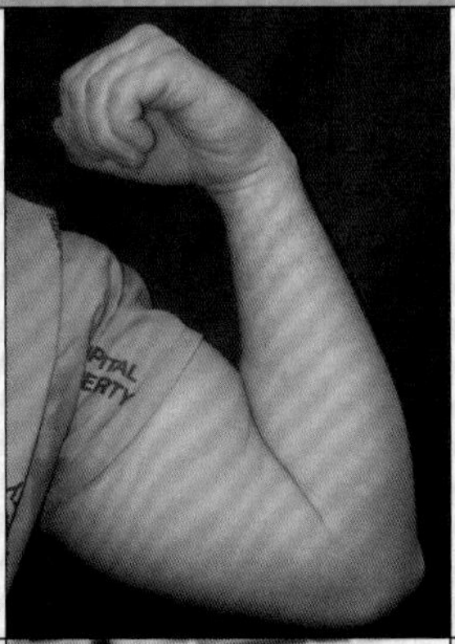 | The test is positive for cubital tunnel syndrome if the patient's symptoms are reproduced in the ulnar nerve distribution while holding this position. |
| **Elsen test** | The patient's injured PIP joint is flexed 90 degrees over the edge of a table. The patient is asked to actively extend the PIP joint against resistance. The examiner palpates for active middle phalanx extension and simultaneous extension rigidity of the DIP joint. | 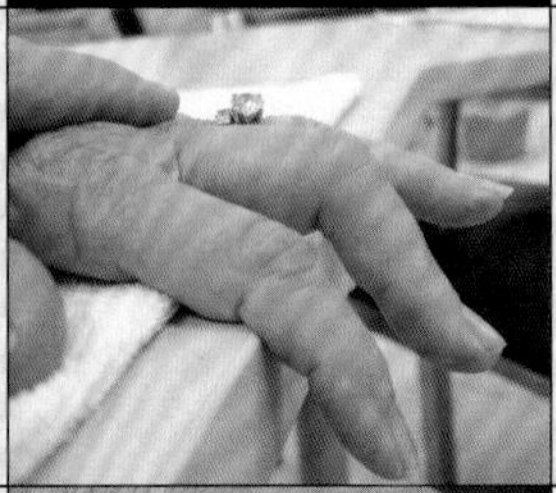 | A positive test is consistent with a complete central slip disruption at any time frame. No extension force is felt associated with the middle phalanx but DIP joint rigidity is readily perceived secondary to the effects of the lateral bands. This test will not necessarily detect a partial central slip injury. |
| **Extensor apparatus examination** | The examiner observes and palpates the extensor tendon and sagittal bands at MCP and PIP. | 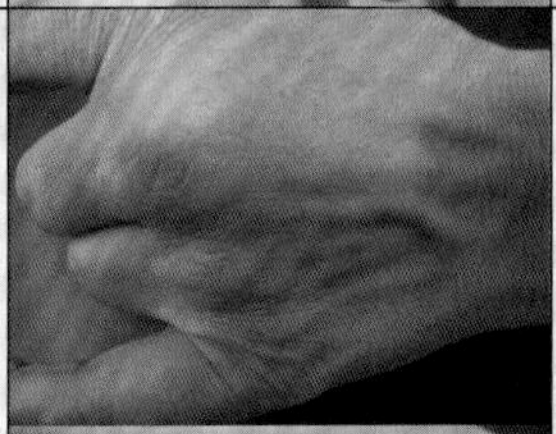 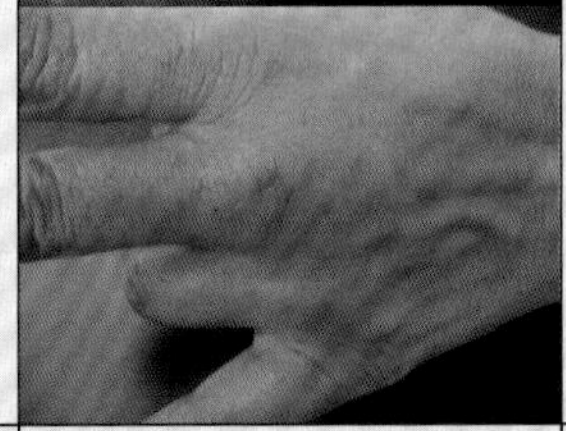 | The examiner should look for:<br>1. Tenderness adjacent to MCP<br>2. Tendon subluxation at MCP<br>3. Swan-neck deformity<br><br>Rules out extensor mechanism abnormalities, which may cause overlapping signs or symptoms. |
| **Extensor carpi ulnaris (ECU) subluxation test** | The patient is asked to ulnarly deviate the wrist while actively pronating and supinating. The examiner palpates the ECU tendon at and just proximal to the ulnar groove with the patient's wrist in supination, mild flexion, and ulnar deviation. The sides are compared. | 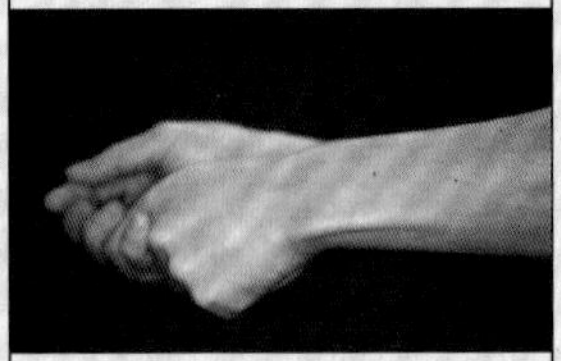 | Passively subluxatable versus actively subluxatable. Click versus no click. Pain with subluxation versus no significant pain with subluxation. If the tendon dislocates with passive supination, palmar flexion, and ulnar deviation the ECU is grossly unstable. If the addition of ECU contraction is required for frank dislocation, some inherent stability remains. Pain with subluxation is a critical finding when contemplating surgical treatment. |
| **Flexor digitorum profundus (FDP) examination** | The patient is asked to flex the DIP with the PIP joint blocked in extension. | 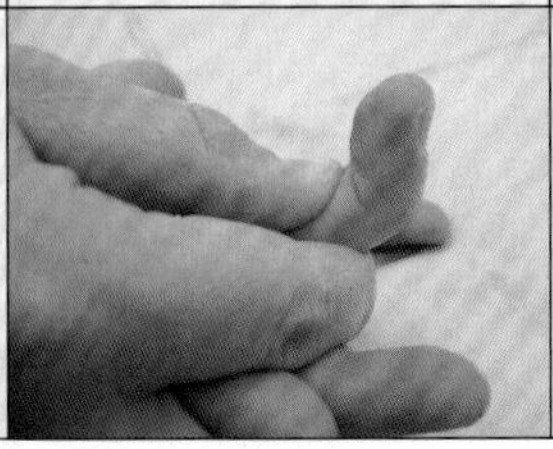 | FDP function present or absent. Loss of active DIP flexion suggests disruption or loss of FDP function. |

| Examination | Technique | Illustration | Grading & Significance |
|---|---|---|---|
| **Flexor digitorum superficialis (FDS) examination** | The patient is asked to flex the finger with the adjacent digits held in extension. | | FDS function present or absent. Loss of active PIP flexion suggests disruption or loss of FDS function. |
| **Finger cascade** | The examiner observes the position of the fingers with the patient at rest. | | Loss of the normal cascade suggests disruption or loss of function of the flexor tendons. |
| **Finkelstein maneuver** | With palpation along the first dorsal compartment, the thumb is flexed and the wrist is ulnarly deviated. | | Pain indicates DeQuervain tenosynovitis. |
| **Flexor tendon contracture** | The wrist and metacarpophalangeal joints are extended, and the examiner assesses extension of the interphalangeal joints. | | With flexor tendon contracture there will be limited extension of the interphalangeal joints. |
| **Foveal sign** | The examiner palpates the ulnocarpal joint in the interval between the ulnar styloid and the flexor carpi ulnaris tendon. | | Pain is indicative of triangular fibrocartilage complex pathology. |
| **Froment sign** | The patient is asked to pinch a piece of paper between the index and thumb. Then the examiner attempts to pull the paper out. Both hands are tested simultaneously. | | Positive if paper is held only by flexing the thumb interphalangeal joint. This results from recruitment of the flexor pollicis longus and paralysis of the adductor pollicis, usually from an ulnar nerve disorder. |

*(continued)*

| Examination | Technique | Illustration | Grading & Significance |
| --- | --- | --- | --- |
| **Grip strength** | The Jamar Dynometer can be used to objectively measure grip strength. The patient's elbow is placed in 90 degrees of flexion and the forearm and wrist in neutral. The recorded value is the average of three maximal attempts with the dynamometer set on the third station. | 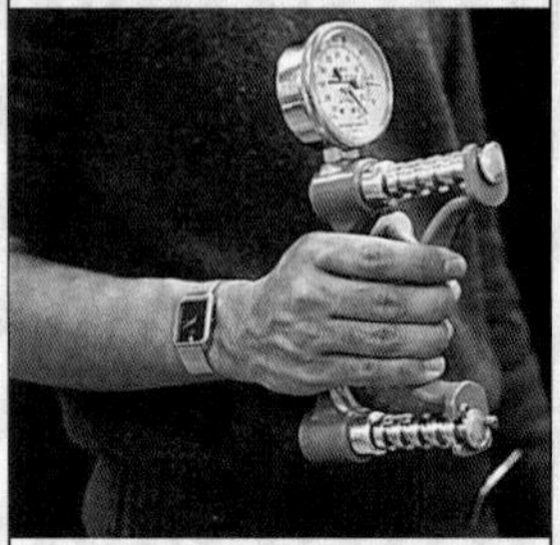 | Findings are compared to the contralateral side. Decreased strength in association with physical findings can be indicative of wrist pathology. The presence of pain in the central aspect of the wrist with attempted grip has been associated with scapholunate ligament disruption. Mean grip strength for males is 103 to 104 for the dominant extremity and 92 to 99 for the non-dominant extremity. Mean grip strength for females is 62 to 63 for the dominant extremity and 53 to 55 for the non-dominant extremity. |
| **Lichtman midcarpal shift test** | With the hand pronated and the forearm stabilized, the examiner positions the wrist in 15 degrees ulnar deviation. The examiner grabs the patient's hand and exerts palmar pressure on the distal capitate. The examiner axially loads and ulnarly deviates the wrist. The procedure is repeated for radial deviation. | 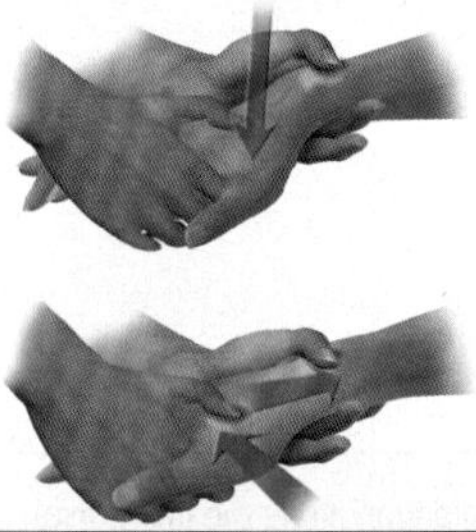 | No characteristic clunk to severe clunk with pain. Midcarpal instability. |
| **Love pin test** | The head of a pin or paperclip is gently pressed against the tender area to localize the pain. | 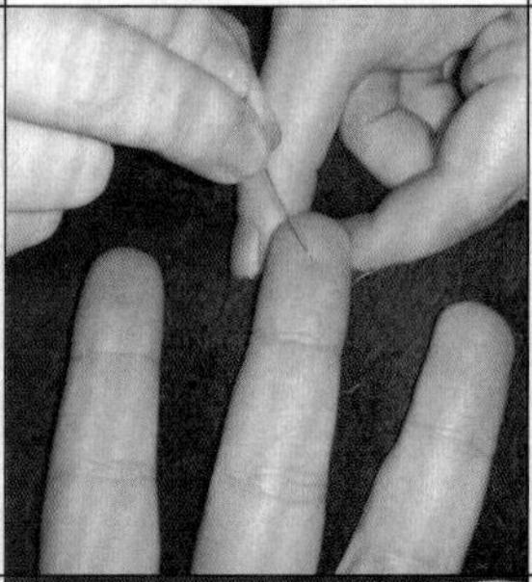 | Locates a glomus tumor. In subungual tumors, the pin is placed on the nail plate at various locations to find the tumor. |
| **Lunotriquetral (LT) compression test** | Compression is applied in the ulnar snuffbox to give a radially directed force across the LT joint. | 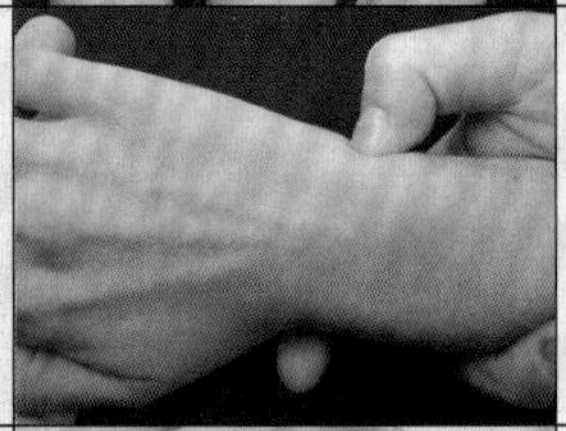 | Pain with this maneuver may indicate pathology at the LT or triquetral hamate joints. |
| **Lumbrical muscle contracture** | An intrinsic tightness test is performed with the fingers radially or ulnarly deviated. Alternatively, the test can be performed with the DIP joint flexed as well as the PIP joint. | 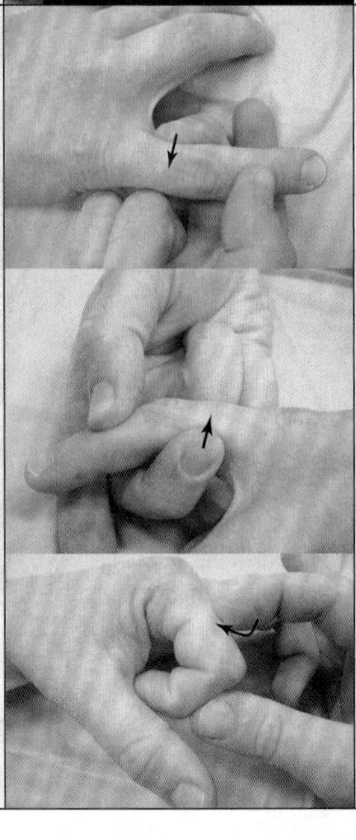 | With lumbrical contracture, there is less passive flexion of the PIP joint with the finger deviated or with the DIP joint flexed in comparison to intrinsic testing. If present, this suggests lumbrical muscle contracture as part of the pathology. |

| Examination | Technique | Illustration | Grading & Significance |
|---|---|---|---|
| **LT ballottement (Reagan) test** | The examiner secures the lunate between the thumb and index finger of one hand and the pisotriquetral unit with the other hand. Anterior and posterior stress is applied across the LT joint. | | The test is positive if increased anteroposterior laxity and pain are present. Pain and instability are indicative of LT ligament tear or arthrosis. |
| **LT shear (Kleinman) test** | The forearm is placed in neutral rotation and the elbow on the examination table. The examiner's contralateral thumb is placed over the dorsum of the lunate. With the lunate supported, the examiner's ipsilateral thumb loads the pisotriquetral joint from the palmar aspect, creating a shear force at the LT joint. |  | Positive with pain, crepitance, and abnormal mobility of the LT joint |
| **LT Shuck test** | The examiner stabilizes the pisotriquetral joint while passively ulnarly and radially deviating the wrist. Findings are compared with the contralateral wrist. | | In a positive test the patient experiences a painful click as the lunate and triquetrum slide abnormally. It signifies a LT ligament injury. |
| **Medial collateral ligament shear test** | Patient places the contralateral arm under the injured elbow and grasps the thumb of the symptomatic extremity. With the elbow maximally flexed the patient applies a valgus load to the elbow as he or she brings it out into extension. | | A positive test will localize pain to the medial elbow, suggesting an incompetent ulnar collateral ligament. |
| **Metacarpophalangeal (MCP) and proximal interphalangeal (PIP) joint instability testing** | The individual MCP or PIP joints are tested by the examiner grasping the patient's finger and then applying a valgus and then a varus stress with the joint extended and flexed. The resultant motion is compared to the contralateral side. Differences in laxity indicate ligamentous instability. | | Grade 1: No difference in joint line opening compared to the contralateral joint<br>Grade 2: Notable opening of the joint line compared to the contralateral joint, but a solid "endpoint" is reached<br>Grade 3: Complete opening of the radial or lateral joint line with valgus or varus stress. No endpoint can be discerned. Attempts at hyperextension of the digit at the PIP of the MCP joints can identify volar plate instability and the propensity of the digit to subluxate or dislocate. |
| **Mill test** | With the elbow flexed, the forearm slightly pronated, and the wrist slightly extended, the patient actively supinates against resistance. | | Pain either at the epicondyle or radiating distally along the extensor carpi radialis brevis represents a positive test. Increasing strain in an inflamed or degenerative tendon causes pain. |

*(continued)*

| Examination | Technique | Illustration | Grading & Significance |
|---|---|---|---|
| **Palpation of LT interval** | The LT joint is deeply palpated dorsally and slightly distal to the site of the 4–5 arthroscopy portal. | 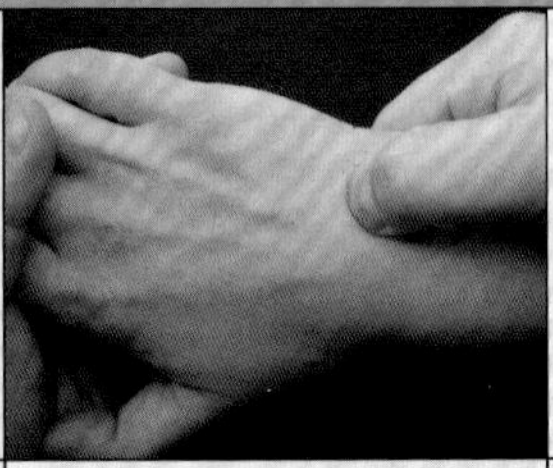 | Point tenderness indicates LT interosseous ligament injury or triangular fibrocartilage complex pathology. |
| **Palpation of scapholunate (SL) interval** | The SL joint is deeply palpated dorsally and 1.5 cm distal to the tubercle of Lister (slightly distal to the 3–4 arthroscopy portal). Alternatively, the examiner palpates the third metacarpal, moving proximally until a depression is felt. Just proximal to this cavity is the SL joint, which is palpable between the second and fourth dorsal extensor compartments. | 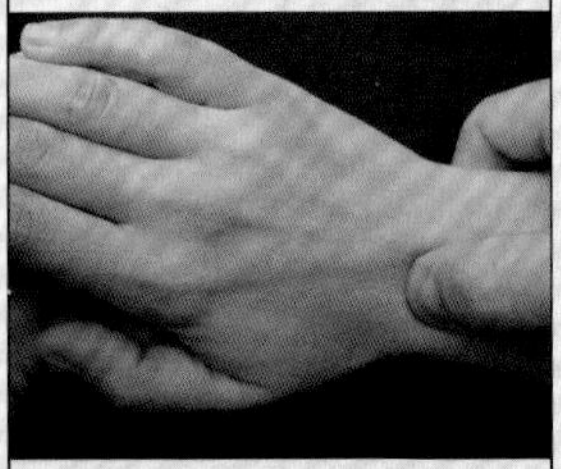 | Point tenderness may indicate SL interosseous ligament injury, scaphoid injury, ganglion cyst, or Kienbock disease. |
| **Phalen test** | The patient's wrist is placed in maximum flexion and the elbow in extension for 60 seconds or until symptomatic. | 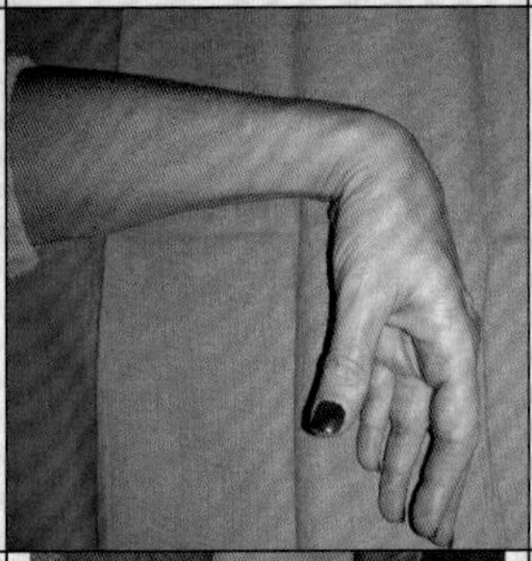 | Reproduction of symptoms in the median nerve distribution indicates carpal tunnel syndrome. |
| **Piano key sign** | The radius is stabilized with one hand. The ulna is passively translated dorsally and volarly with the opposite hand. This test is performed in pronation, neutral, and supination, and findings are compared to the opposite side. | 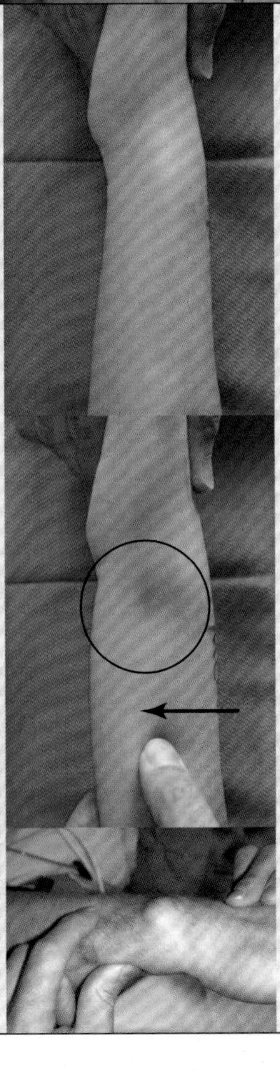 | A positive result is characterized by painful laxity in the affected wrist compared with the contralateral wrist, suggesting DRUJ synovitis related to instability. "Winging" is associated with loss of structural support at the DRUJ and may indicate a complete peripheral tear of the triangular fibrocartilage complex. Depression and rebounding of the ulnar head is a positive finding. |

| Examination | Technique | Illustration | Grading & Significance |
|---|---|---|---|
| **Pisotriquetral shear test** | The examiner's thumb is placed over the pisiform and a circular grinding motion and dorsally directed pressure are applied. | 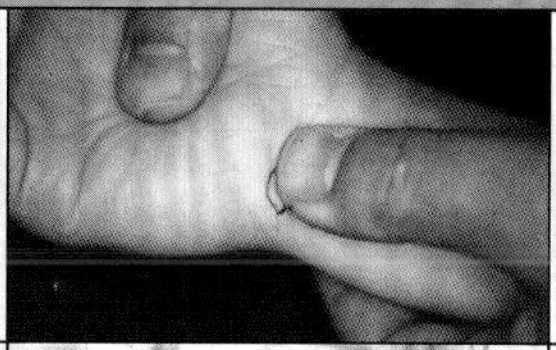 | Crepitus and pain over pisotriquetral joint. Pisotriquetral arthritis. |
| **Prone pivot-shift test** | Placing the patient prone with the arm hanging over the table stabilizes the humerus and leaves one of the examiner's hands free to palpate the radial head. | 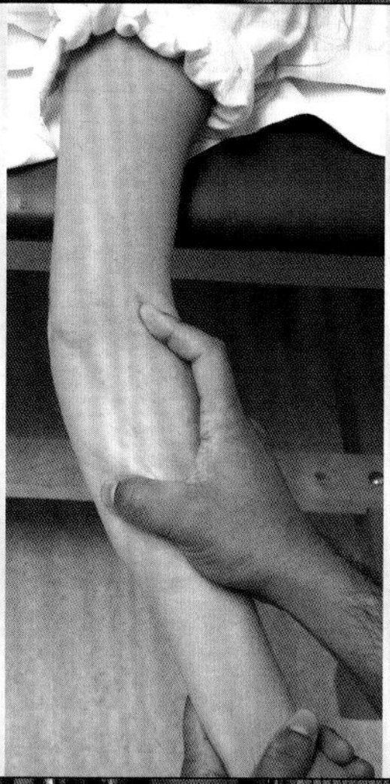 | A positive test reveals radial head or ulnohumeral subluxation. Same as pivotshift test. |
| **Push-off test** | From a seated position the patient attempts to push off from the armrests. Pain or apprehension is suggestive of lateral ligamentous insufficiency. | 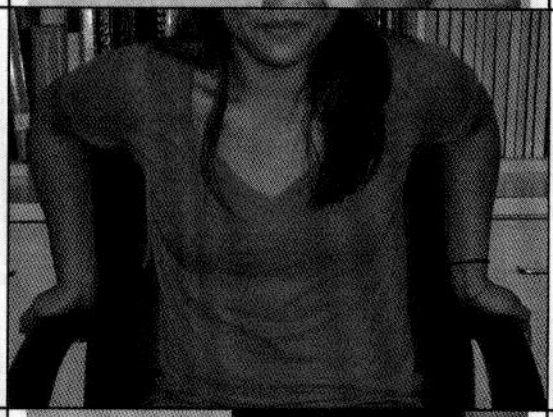 | A positive test will reproduce the patient's symptoms of apprehension during supination and not pronation. Inability to complete the push-up is a positive test. A positive test indicates a posterolateral rotatory insufficiency. |
| **Range of motion (ROM), elbow** | Active and passive ROM (flexion–extension of the elbow, rotation of the forearm) is compared to the uninjured side. Palpable and auditory crepitus should be noted. | 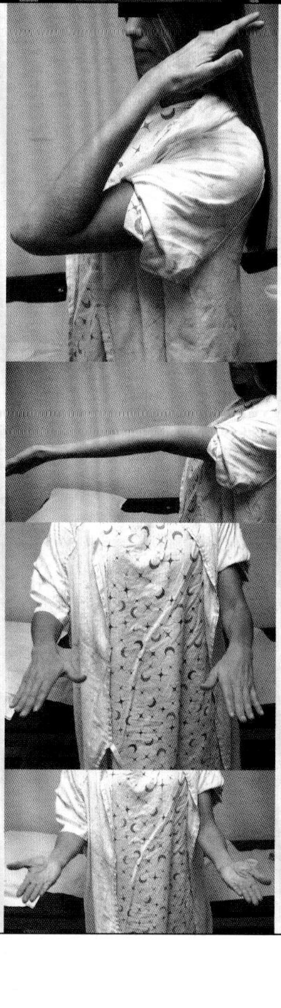 | Normal values: 0 to 145 degrees of flexion–extension, 85 degrees of supination, and 80 degrees of pronation. The examiner should check for perching on the lateral view. Locking of the elbow could represent loose bodies. Stiffness may indicate intrinsic capsular contracture. |

*(continued)*

| Examination | Technique | Illustration | Grading & Significance |
|---|---|---|---|
| **Scaphoid ballottement test** | The scaphoid is grasped with one hand and the lunate with the other. The scaphoid is then balloted anteroposteriorly. Anteroposterior translation is compared to the contralateral side. | | Pain and increased anteroposterior laxity are highly suggestive of SL instability. |
| **Scaphoid shift test (Watson)** | Dorsally directed pressure is exerted on the patient's volar scaphoid tuberosity (distal pole) by the examiner's ipsilateral thumb while the wrist is passively moved from ulnar to radial deviation by the examiner's contralateral hand. The distal pole of the scaphoid is stabilized with the wrist in ulnar deviation, and then the examiner passively radially deviates the wrist. Next the pressure on the distal pole is removed and the examiner feels for relocation of the scaphoid into the scaphoid facet of the distal radius. Findings are compared with the contralateral wrist. | | The scaphoid normally flexes as the wrist goes from ulnar to radial deviation. The examiner's thumb prevents scaphoid flexion and in scapholunate dissociation, the proximal scaphoid pole subluxates dorsally out of the scaphoid fossa, causing pain. When the thumb is released from the distal pole of the scaphoid, there may be a palpable or audible clunk, signifying spontaneous reduction of the scaphoid back into the scaphoid fossa. This clunk may be present in 11% of asymptomatic wrists. It is the presence of pain along with the clunk that is diagnostic for scapholunate ligament disruption. If only pain is present and no clunk is felt, a sprain or a partial tear of the scapholunate ligament is likely. This test is not terribly specific and may be positive in patients with hyperlaxity, synovitis, occult ganglia, and radioscaphoid impingement or arthritis |
| **Squeeze test** | Deep palpation of interosseous membrane and distal radioulnar joint | | This test screens for potential longitudinal instability. |
| **Supination test (Ouellette)** | With the forearm mildly pronated, the examiner uses their contralateral hand to stabilize the distal ulna and their ipsilateral hand to secure the pisotriquetral unit and with that hand exert a supination force on the ulnar carpus along with compression across the ulnocarpal joint. The examiner listens for clicks and clunks. | | Pain, instability and the presence of clicks or clunks are compared to the contralateral wrist. Graded from stable to unstable. The examiner should note the presence of clicks and clunks in both wrists. Abnormal supination of carpus in relation to the forearm. |
| **Supine lateral pivot-shift test** | Patient is supine, with arm extended overhead and supinated. The examiner stabilizes the humerus with one hand and applies a valgus force with the other as the elbow is taken from extension to flexion. | | When the elbow is slightly flexed the radial head can be palpated to subluxate or frankly dislocate; as the elbow flexes past 40 degrees, it will relocate, often with a palpable clunk. This test is difficult to perform on an awake patient; often apprehension will be felt and the patient will not allow the test to continue. Examination under anesthesia may be required. |

| Examination | Technique | Illustration | Grading & Significance |
|---|---|---|---|
| **Table-top relocation test** | The symptomatic hand/arm is placed on the lateral edge of a table. The patient is asked to perform push-up with the elbow pointing laterally. The maneuver is repeated with the examiner's thumb stabilizing the radial head during press-up. The maneuver is once again repeated without the examiner's thumb in place. | 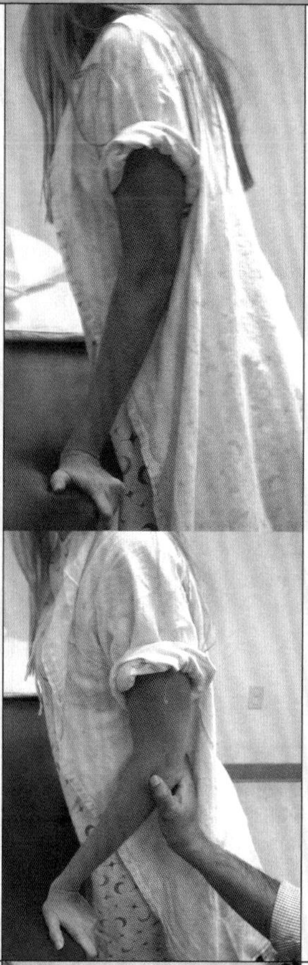 | A positive test elicits pain or apprehension as the elbow reaches 40 degrees. |
| **Thompson test** | With the elbow extended, the wrist in slight extension, and the digits in a fist, the patient extends the wrist against the examiner. | 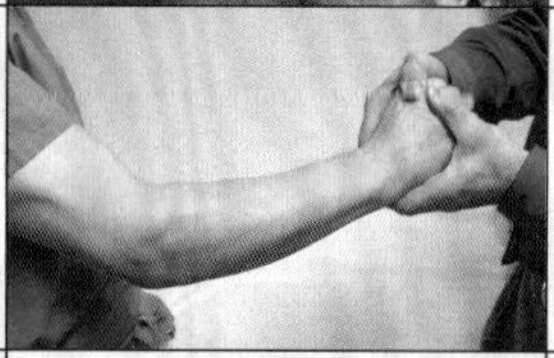 | Pain either at the lateral epicondyle or radiating distally along the extensor carpi radialis brevis is indicative of inflamed or degenerative tendon. |
| **Thumb MCP joint collateral ligament stability test** | The metacarpal is stabilized between the examiner's thumb and index finger of one hand and the proximal phalanx is stabilized between the examiner's thumb and index finger of the other hand. Radially or ulnarly directed forces are applied with the joint flexed 30 to 35 degrees and with the joint extended. Findings are compared with the uninjured thumb. Use of a digital block is sometimes helpful to obtain an accurate assessment. | 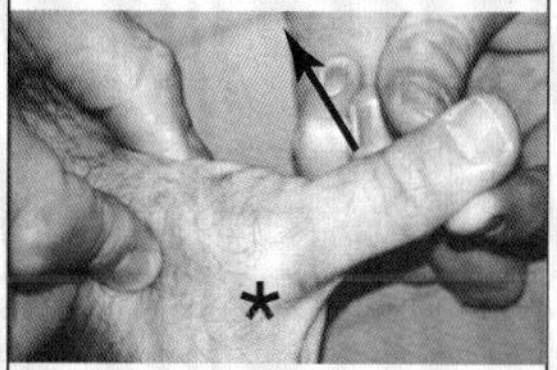 | Grade 0: No significant instability<br>Grade 1, Mild: <25 degrees of opening<br>Grade 2, Moderate: <30 degrees of difference versus the contralateral thumb<br>Grade 3, Severe: Gross instability, without a solid endpoint in both flexion and extension. Consistent with a complete disruption of the proper and accessory collateral ligaments. Severe collateral ligament injury is uncommon in conjunction with volar plate instability but must be recognized and treated where indicated. |
| **Tinel's test** | Percussion of the ulnar nerve proximal to or across the cubital tunnel | 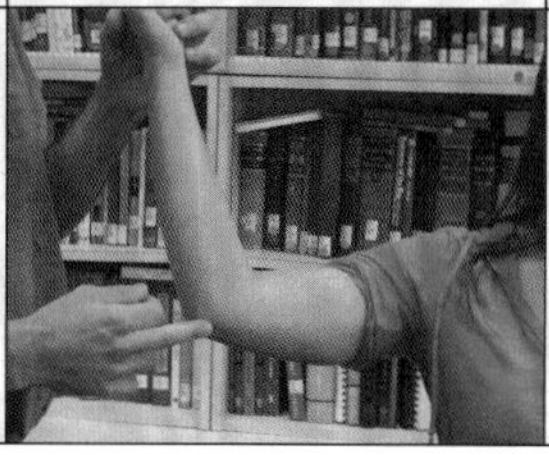 | A positive test elicits pain at the site of percussion and paresthesias in an ulnar nerve distribution distally, which indicates ulnar neuropathy at the elbow. |

*(continued)*

| Examination | Technique | Illustration | Grading & Significance |
|---|---|---|---|
| **Trigger digit evaluation** | A digit is placed along the volar aspect of the thumb or finger, proximal to the MP joint, and the patient is asked to flex and extend the digit. | 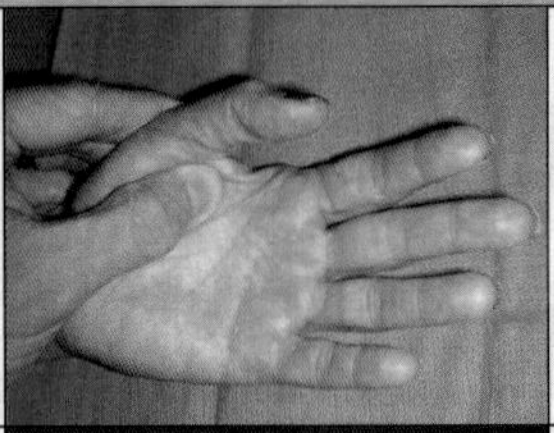 | Reproduction of pain, triggering, or locking of the thumb indicates trigger thumb as a cause. |
| **Ulnocarpal (triangular fibrocartilage complex) compression test** | The examiner ulnarly deviates, pronates, and axially loads the wrist. Passive pronation and supination may be added. | 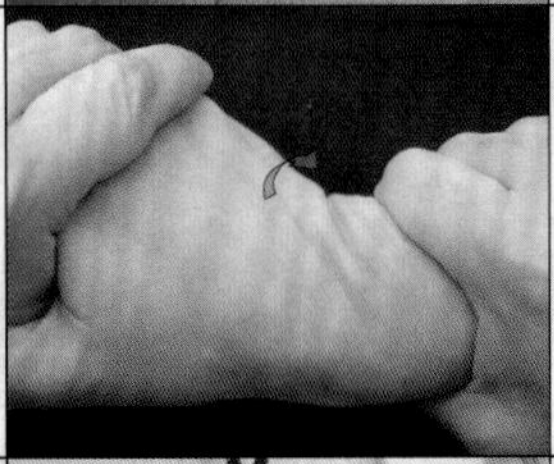 | A click or snap reproducing pain and symptoms is a positive test and consistent with triangular fibrocartilage complex, LT, and midcarpal pathology. This maneuver will also be painful if ulna impaction syndrome is present. |
| **Valgus stress test** | The examiner stabilizes the humerus and stresses the lateral ulnar collateral ligament in slight flexion. | 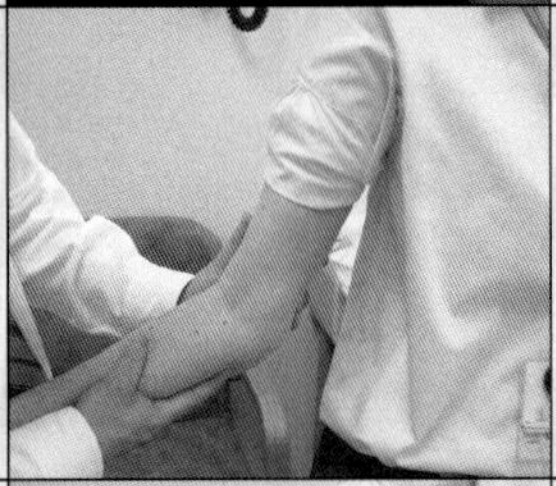 | A positive test indicates injury to the lateral ulnar collateral ligament. |
| **Varus stress test** | Stabilize the humerus and stress the elbow in supination and slight flexion. | 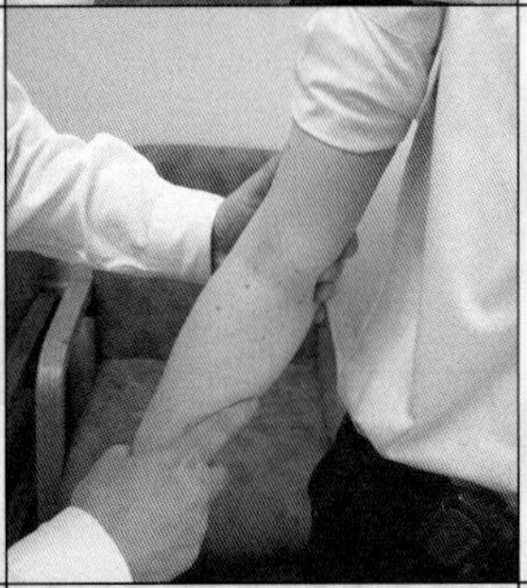 | A positive test indicates injury to the anterior band of the medial collateral ligament. |
| **Volar plate stability** | The metacarpal is stabilized between the examiner's thumb and index finger of one hand and the proximal phalanx is stabilized between the examiner's thumb and index finger of other hand. Hyperextension force is applied. | 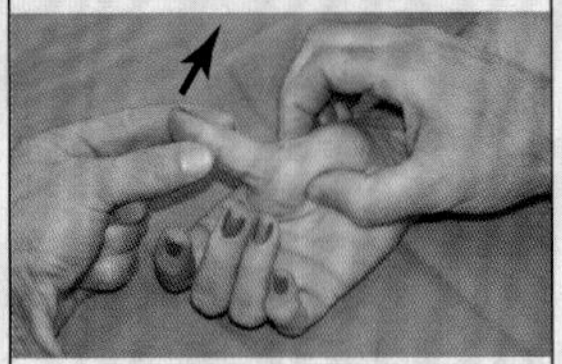 | 0 = No hyperextension; 1 = Mild, definite endpoint; 2 = moderate, soft endpoint; 3 = severe, gross instability. Volar instability must be recognized and treated appropriately to maximize outcomes. |
| **Wartenberg sign** | The patient is asked to extend the fingers. | 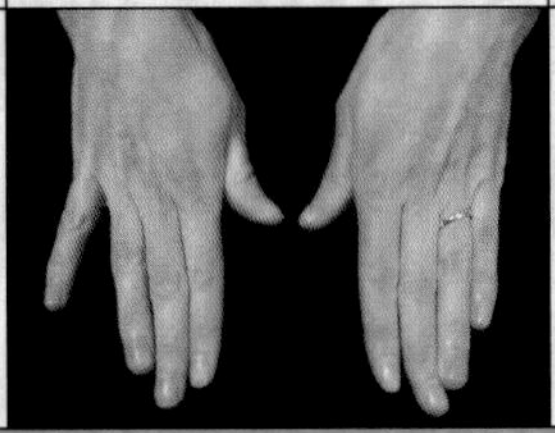 | The sign is considered positive if the small finger assumes an abducted posture with finger extension. This sign is the result of palmar interossei weakness resulting in unopposed ulnar pull of the extensor digiti quinti. |
| **Shoulder** | | | |
| **Abduction strength testing** | The arm is placed in 90 degrees abduction in the scapular plane. The patient is asked to resist downward force. | 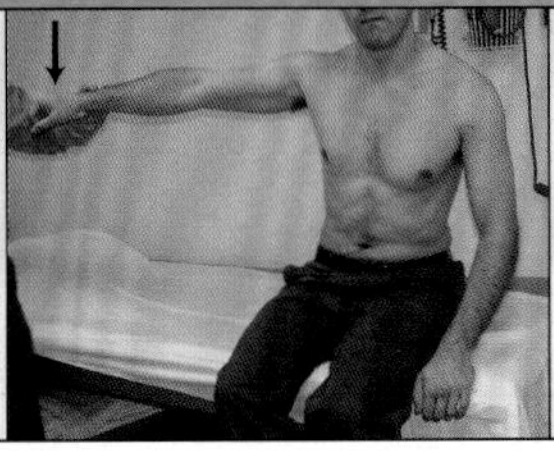 | Tests deltoid muscle strength: full strength, decreased strength, or unable to maintain position against gravity. Weak deltoid suggests less postoperative active range of motion secondary to inadequate strength. |

| Examination | Technique | Illustration | Grading & Significance |
|---|---|---|---|
| **Active forward flexion** | Patient attempts to actively bring the arm forward above his or her head. | 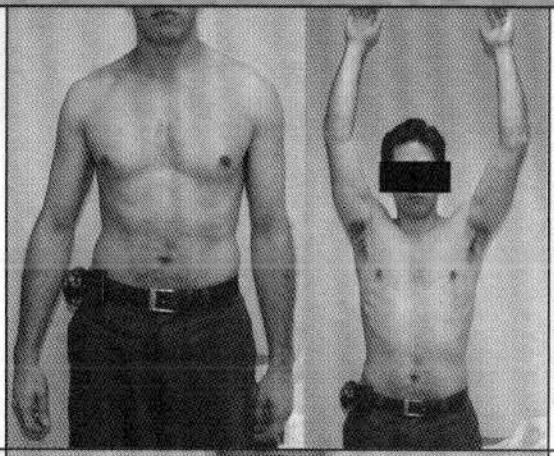 | Normal active flexion is 170–180 degrees. Limited active forward flexion is indicative of possible large rotator cuff tear. Patients with function at or above shoulder level are more likely to have improved active forward flexion postoperatively. |
| **Active external rotation** | With arms at the patient's side and the elbows flexed to 90 degrees, the patient is asked to maximally externally rotate the arms. | 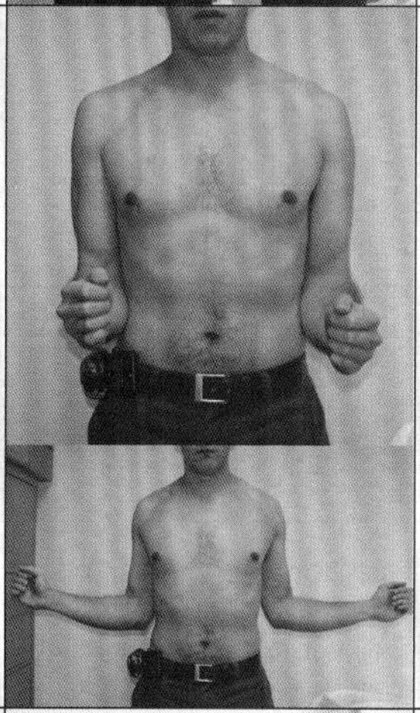 | Less active external rotation on the affected side. Decreased external rotation on affected side indicates partial or complete loss of infraspinatus function due to tear involvement or muscle dysfunction. |
| **Active radiocapitellar compression test** | Forearm pronation and supination with the elbow in full extension is performed. | 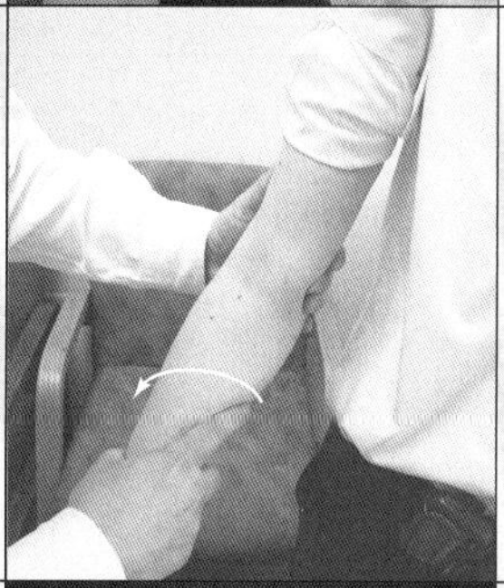 | Most clinicians just grade this as none, mild, moderate, or significant pain. This test loads the radiocapitellar joint in pronation. Pain on pronation that is reduced in supination may be present in osteochondritis dissecans. |
| **Anterior interosseous nerve** | "OK" sign (flexion of distal interphalangeal of index and interphalangeal of thumb herald flexor digitorum profundus and flexor pollicis longus function of these digits) | 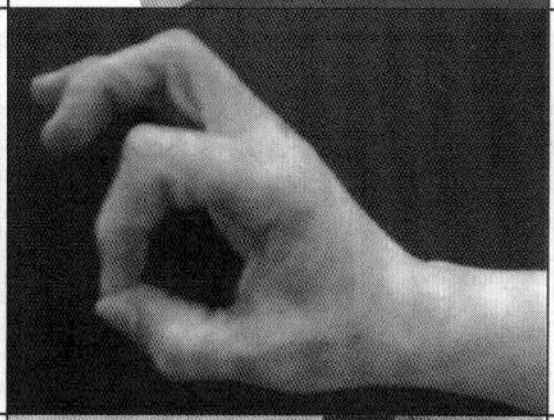 | Motor branch only (it has no cutaneous innervation, only articular). Isolated palsy has been reported secondary to constrictive dressings and after proximal ulna fracture. |
| **Anterior load and shift test** | The patient is positioned supine with the arm in 20 degrees abduction, 20 degrees flexion, and neutral rotation. With axial load to reduce the humeral head, an anterior force is applied to the arm. | 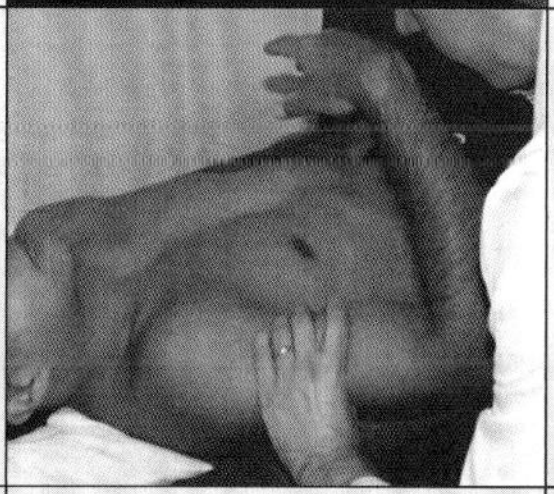 | 0 = no translation; 1+ = to the anterior rim; 2+ = over the rim but spontaneously reduces; 3+ = dislocation of the humeral head that locks over the anterior rim. Indicates anterior instability. |
| **Apprehension test** | The arm is placed in 90 degrees of abduction. The arm is slowly brought into external rotation and extension. | 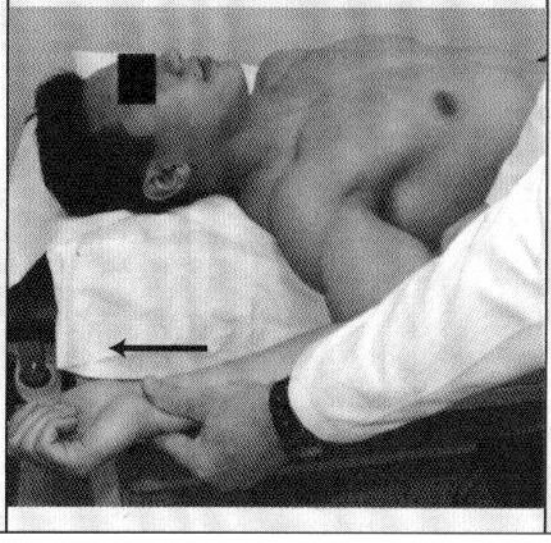 | Apprehension, not simply pain, is required for a positive apprehension test. The apprehension test has a sensitivity of 72% and specificity of 96% for anterior instability. Positive anterior apprehension can be associated with anterior labral injuries. Patient feels a sensation of instability with the arm in the at-risk position. Sensation of pain suggests internal impingement, not instability. |

*(continued)*

| Examination | Technique | Illustration | Grading & Significance |
|---|---|---|---|
| **Bear hug test** | The hand of the affected side is placed on the opposite shoulder with the fingers extended and the elbow elevated forward. The patient resists as the examiner attempts to lift the hand off the shoulder. | 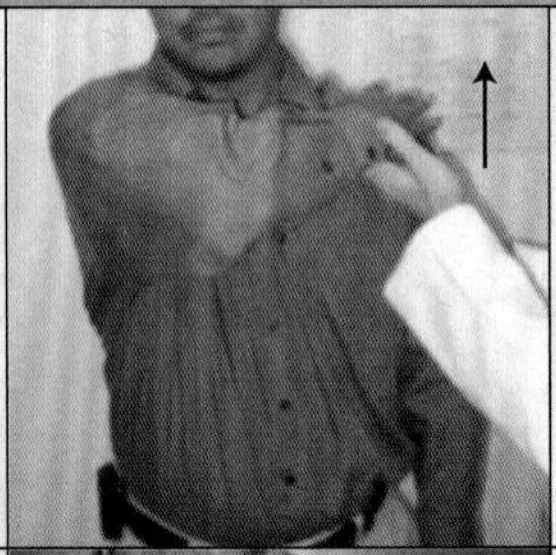 | If the examiner can lift the hand off the shoulder, then the patient likely has a partial or complete tear of the upper subscapularis tendon. This is perhaps the most sensitive test for a subscapularis tear. |
| **Belly press test (Napoleon test)** | The patient is asked to keep the palm of his or her hand on the abdomen with the wrist extended and the shoulder flexed and in maximal internal rotation while the examiner attempts to forcefully pull the patient's hand off the abdomen. | 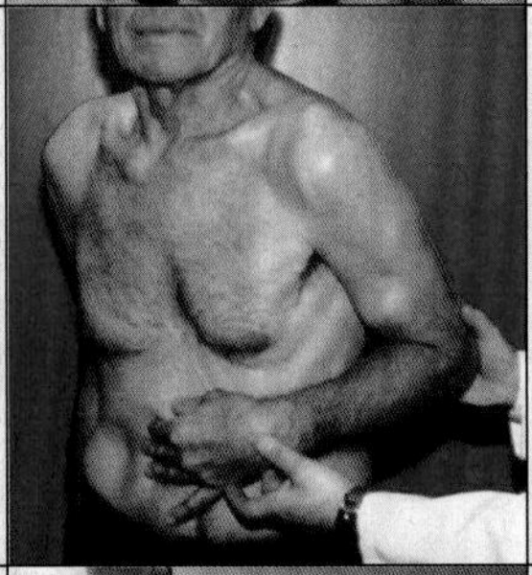 | A positive belly-press test occurs when the patient must flex the wrist and extend the arm to maintain the palm on the abdomen. This indicates subscapularis muscle weakness or tear. |
| **Biceps resistance test (Speed's test)** | With the patient's arm at 90 degrees of forward elevation, a downward force is applied to the arm while the patient tries to resist that force. | 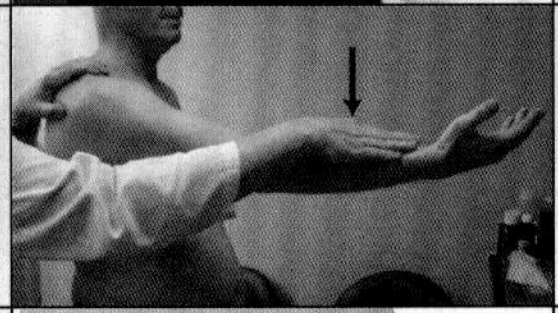 | A positive test is pain along the tendon of the long head of the biceps. Pain during this maneuver indicates involvement of the long head of the biceps tendon. |
| **Capitellum tenderness** | Examiner's thumb pushes against the posterior capitellum while taking the elbow through a range of motion of flexion to extension. | 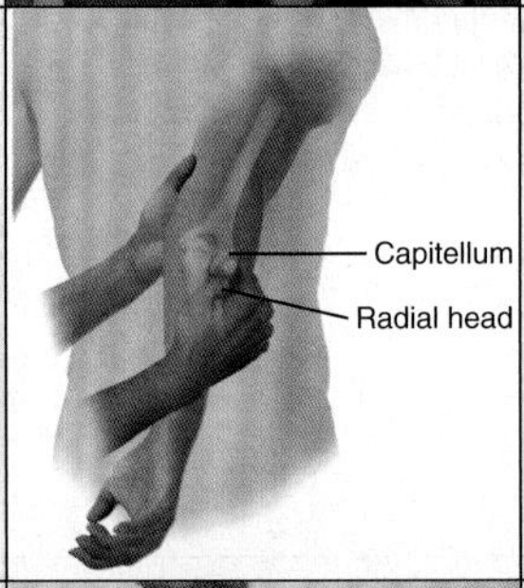  | Most clinicians just grade this as none, mild, moderate, or significant pain. Tenderness may be present with osteochondritis dissecans. |
| **Coracoid impingement** | The arm is forward flexed to 90 degrees, internally rotated, and adducted. | 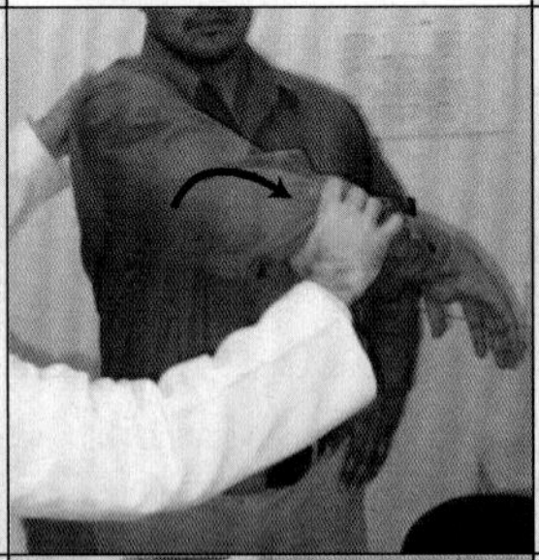 | Reproduction of pain or a painful click indicates a positive test. A positive test is indicative of impingement of the coracoid onto the subscapularis. |
| **Effusion** | The examiner palpates the posterolateral gutter of the elbow and ballotes the soft tissue. | 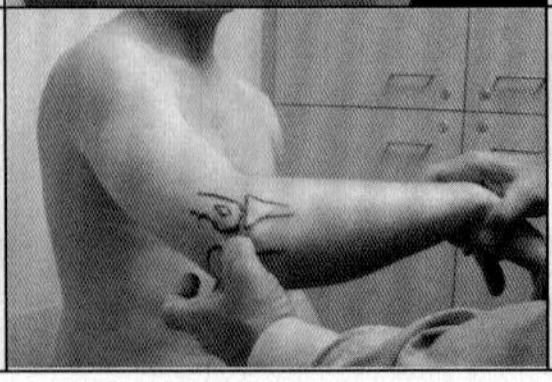 | Most clinicians simply grade as none, mild, moderate, large. Normally, fluid is not present. Effusion indicates intra-articular irritation and may be consistent with a loose or unstable osteochondritis dissecans lesion or loose body. |

| Examination | Technique | Illustration | Grading & Significance |
|---|---|---|---|
| **External rotation lag sign** | Arm is passively placed in maximal external rotation and then released. Patient is asked to maintain the arm in external rotation. | 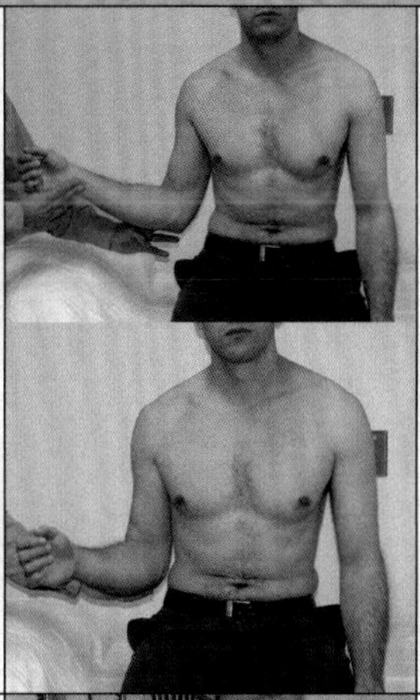 | Inability to maintain maximal external rotation (≥20 degree lag sign) suggests the tear extends well into the infraspinatus. |
| **External rotation strength testing** | Arm is placed in maximal external rotation and patient is asked to resist internal rotation force. | 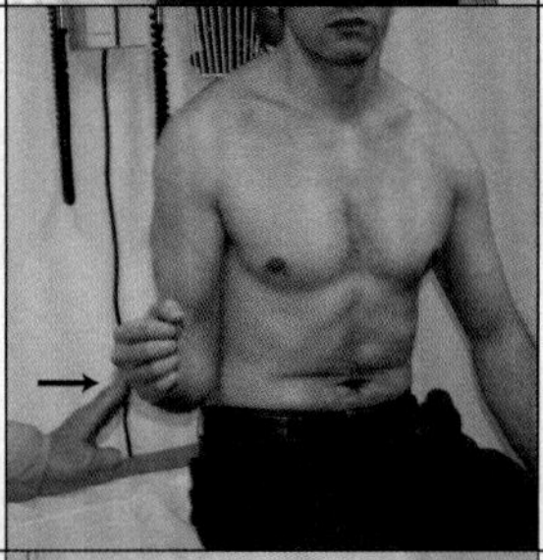 | Full-strength resistance suggests no infraspinatus tear involvement. Weakness suggests progressive infraspinatus involvement or dysfunction. |
| **Hawkins sign** | The examiner forward flexes the shoulder to 90 degrees and then passively internally rotates the shoulder. | 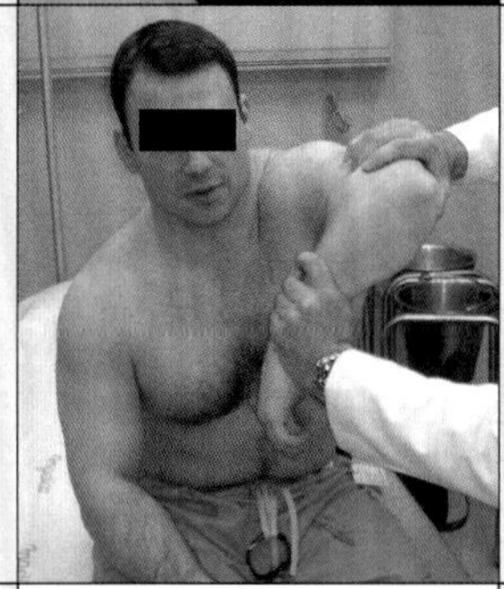 | Presence or absence of pain. This maneuver compresses the supraspinatus tendon against the coracoacromial ligament, reproducing the pain of impingement. High sensitivity but low specificity. |
| **Hornblower sign** | Arm is positioned in 90 degrees of abduction with the elbow flexed to 90 degrees and the shoulder in neutral rotation. External rotation of the shoulder to a position of full abduction–external rotation is performed and weakness or inability to achieve full external rotation is noted. | 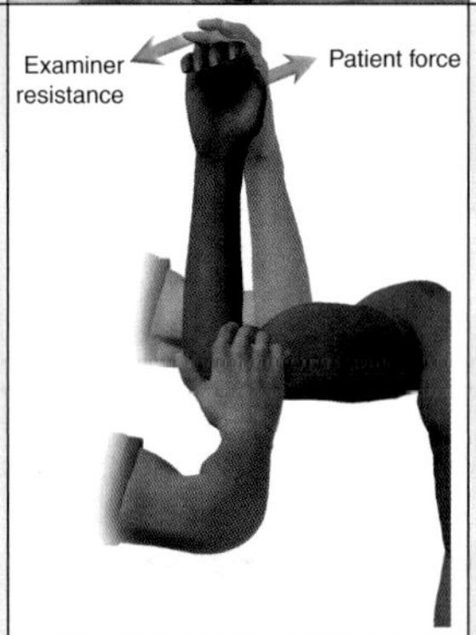  | Ability to fully externally rotate in an abducted position indicates good teres minor function. Weakness or inability to achieve full external rotation in abducted position indicates teres minor dysfunction or tearing. |
| **Impingement sign** | With the patient upright, the examiner fixes the scapula to prevent it from moving and then brings the arm into full forward elevation with some force. | 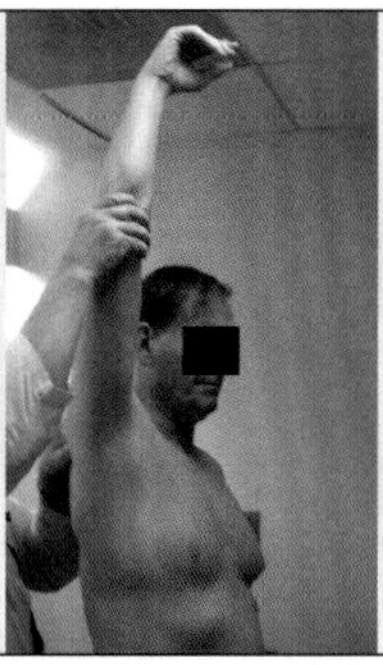 | A positive test is pain during this maneuver. Forcing the fully forward elevated arm against the fixed scapula helps to localize the finding to the rotator cuff. |

*(continued)*

| Examination | Technique | Illustration | Grading & Significance |
|---|---|---|---|
| **Jobes sign ("empty can" test)** | Arm is placed in 90 degrees of elevation in the scapular plane with the hand in the thumbs-down position. Manual resistance is provided by the examiner to elevation and weakness or pain is recorded. | 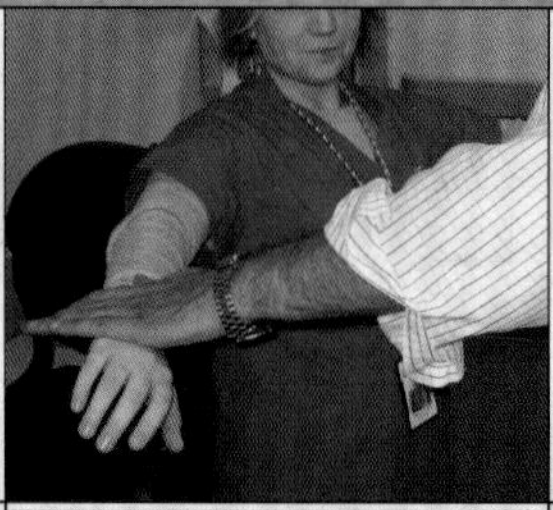 | Weakness or pain represents dysfunction of the supraspinatus tendon. |
| **Kim test** | With the patient seated, the arm is placed in 90 degrees of abduction and the elbow and hand are supported by the examiner. An axial and upward elevating force of 45 degrees is applied to the distal arm while an inferior and posterior force is applied to the proximal arm. | 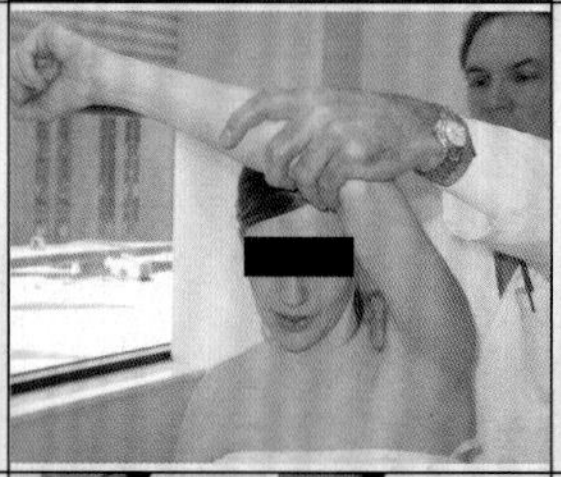 | A sudden onset of posterior shoulder pain is considered a positive test result. A positive Kim test is suggestive of a posterior inferior labral tear or subluxation. |
| **Lift-off test** | Patient places the dorsum of the hand against the lumbar region of the back and attempts to lift the hand from the back and hold it. | 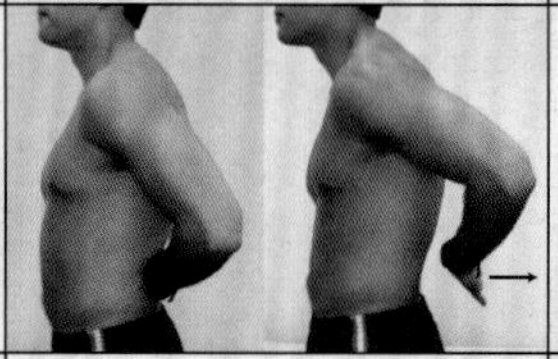 | Inability to lift the hand from the back is a positive result. Indicates subscapularis muscle weakness or tear. |
| **Load and shift test** | If the right shoulder is examined, the examiner's left hand grasps the humeral shaft with the fingers anterior and the thumb posterior. The examiner's right hand grasps the forearm and positions the arm in the plane of the scapula in 40 to 60 degrees of abduction and neutral rotation. An axial load is applied to the humerus through the forearm and the examiner's left hand displaces the humeral head anteriorly. The degree of displacement of the humeral head on the glenoid rim is noted. | 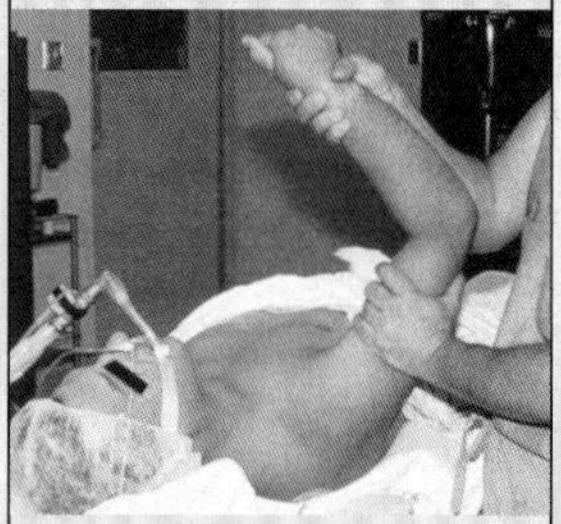 | Grade 0: Little or no movement<br>Grade 1: Shift to edge of glenoid<br>Grade 2: Shift over edge of glenoid but spontaneously reduces<br>Grade 3: Shift over edge of glenoid but does not spontaneously relocate<br><br>This is difficult to perform in the awake patient in clinic but sensitive when the patient is under anesthesia. |
| **Median nerve** | Rock (pronated fist with flexor pollicis longus function as well as flexor digitorum profundus function to index and long) | 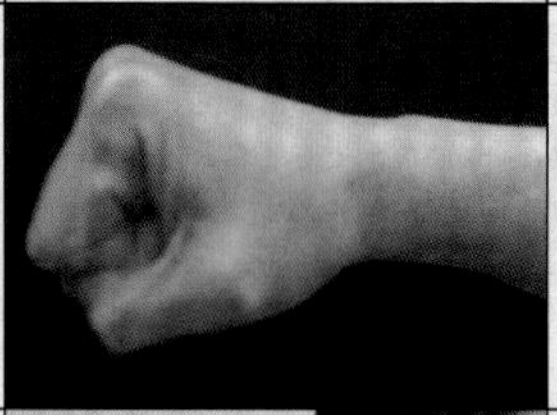 | Autonomous zone is palmar tip index finger. Most commonly injured nerve after closed or open forearm shaft fractures. |
| **Milking maneuver** | With forearm fully supinated, elbow is placed in greater than 90 degrees of flexion. The examiner pulls on the patient's thumb. | 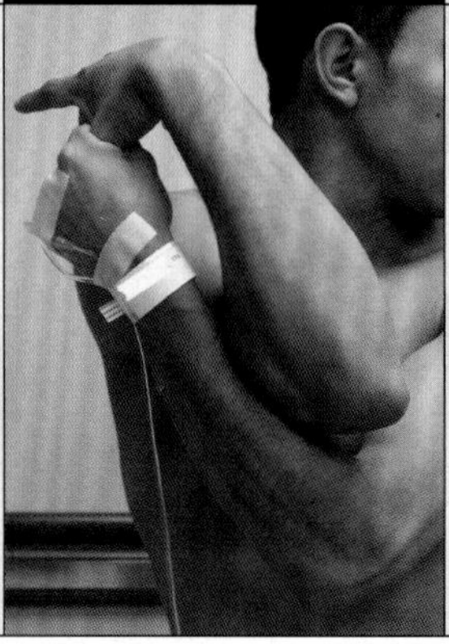 | Maneuver eliciting pain, apprehension, or instability is indicative of ulnar collateral ligament (UCL) insufficiency. Posterior bundle of anterior band of UCL. |

| Examination | Technique | Illustration | Grading & Significance |
|---|---|---|---|
| **Miniaci bony apprehension test** | The arm is placed in approximately 45 degrees of abduction. With external rotation, there is development of apprehension. | 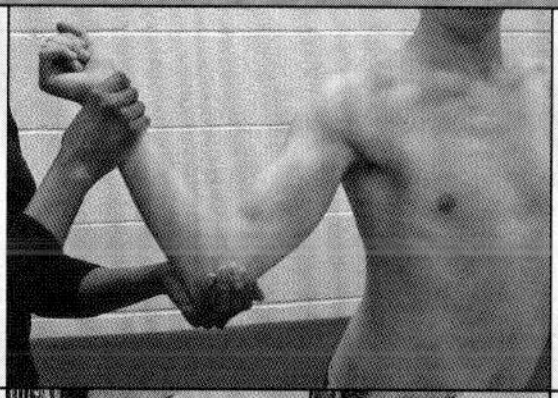 | Apprehension with lower degrees of abduction indicates a significant and symptomatic bony contribution to the instability. |
| **Modified belly press** | With palm on abdomen, the patient is asked to bring the elbow forward, in front of the plane of the body. | 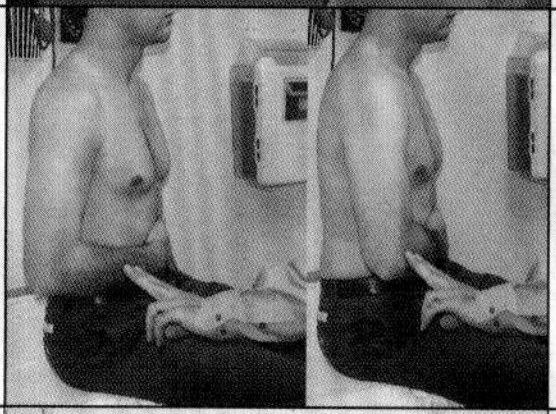 | Inability to perform action demonstrates dysfunctional or torn subscapularis tendon and a higher rate of clinical failure with muscle transfer. |
| **Neer impingement sign** | Passive elevation of the arm while stabilizing the scapula | 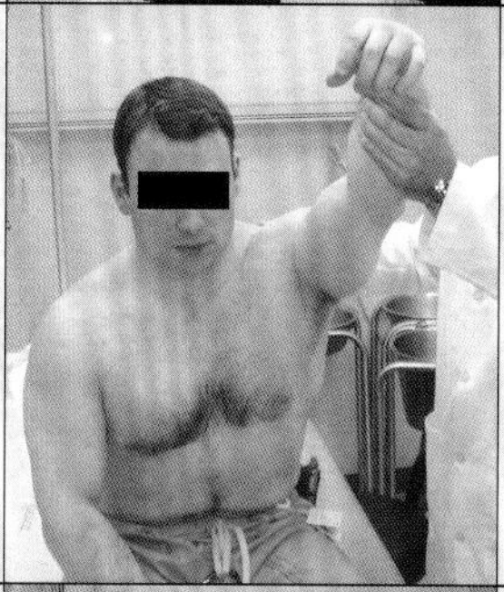 | Presence or absence of pain or facial grimace. This maneuver compresses the critical area of the supraspinatus tendon against the anterior inferior acromion, reproducing impingement pain. The pain will resolve following subacromial lidocaine injection. |
| **Painful abduction arc** | The patient is asked to abduct the arm in the coronal plane. | 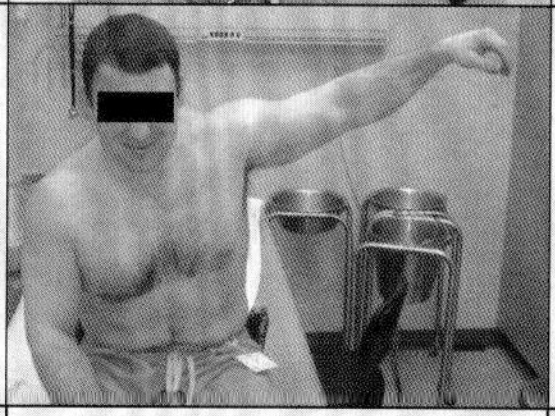 | Abduction is compared to the contralateral side. Pain from 60 to 120 degrees (maximally at 90) suggests impingement. Patients may externally rotate at 90 degrees to clear the greater tuberosity from the acromion and increase motion. |
| **Palm-down abduction test** | With the scapula stabilized by the examiner, the arm is internally rotated and then elevated forcibly in the plane of the scapula. | 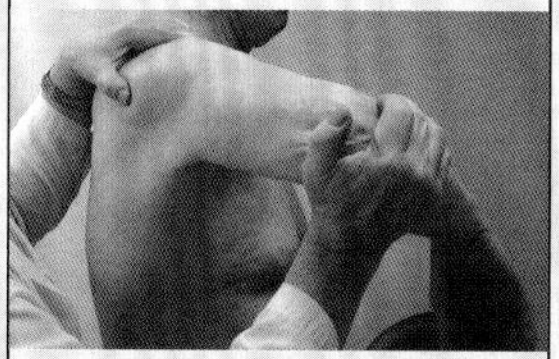 | A positive test produces pain with the maneuver. By internally rotating the arm, the supra- and anterior infraspinatus tendons are placed directly under the coracoacromial arch. Elevating the arm in the scapular plane when it is in internal rotation compresses these tendons against the undersurface of the acromion. |
| **Radial nerve (really posterior interosseous nerve in the forearm)** | Paper (extension of fingers and wrist well above a zero-degree wrist position) | 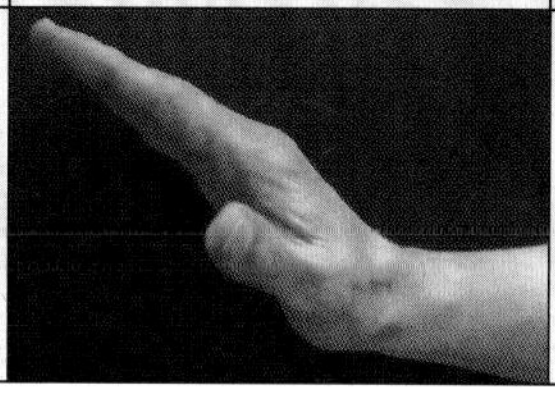 | Autonomous zone is dorsal web space between thumb and index. Risk of iatrogenic injury during surgical exposure of proximal radial shaft. |

*(continued)*

| Examination | Technique | Illustration | Grading & Significance |
|---|---|---|---|
| **Range of motion (ROM)** | The examiner observes active and passive ROM for forward elevation (20 to 30 degrees in sagittal plane), external rotation and internal rotation (both at side and 90 degrees of abduction). | 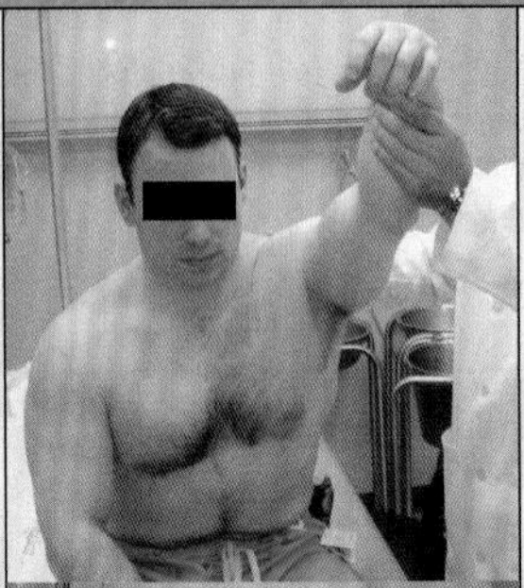 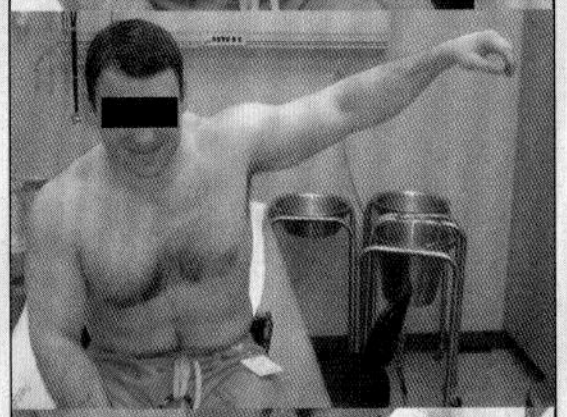 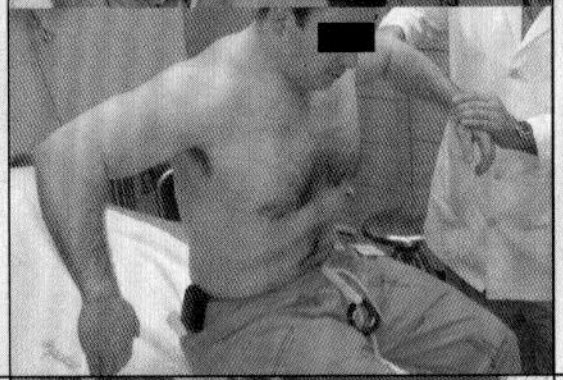 | Average normal ROM: forward flexion 180 degrees, abduction 180 degrees, adduction 50 degrees, internal rotation at the side 80 degrees, external rotation at the side 90 degrees. Loss of ROM may indicate adhesive capsulitis, rotator cuff pathology (tendinitis or rotator cuff tear), degenerative changes. ROM is compared to contralateral side. Patients with impingement may have limited internal rotation from posterior capsular tightness. Active motion is typically more painful than passive motion, especially in descending phase of elevation. |
| **Resisted external rotation in adduction** | Arm is placed in full adduction, elbows are bent at 90 degrees, and the shoulder is internally rotated 20 to 30 degrees. Manual resistance is provided by the examiner to external rotation, and weakness is recorded. | 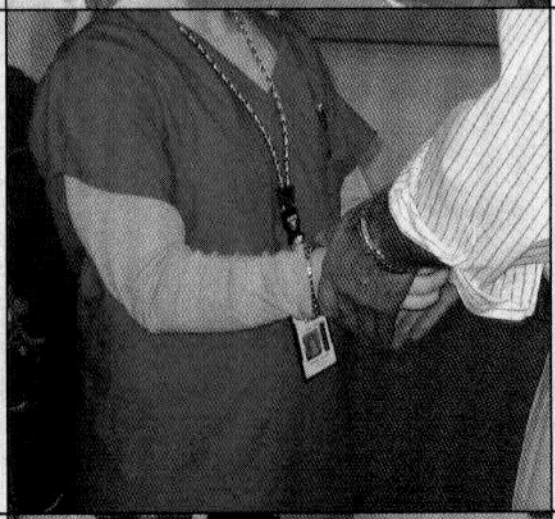 | Weakness represents dysfunction or tearing of the infraspinatus tendon. |
| **Scapula stabilization test** | When winging is observed, a hand is placed to stabilize the scapula in a reduced position, and the patient then elevates the arm. | 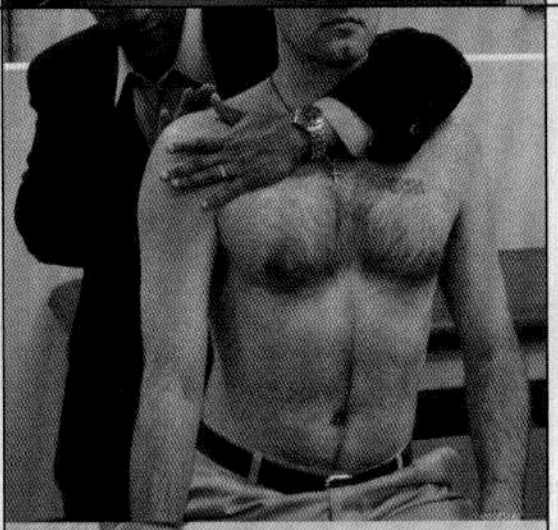 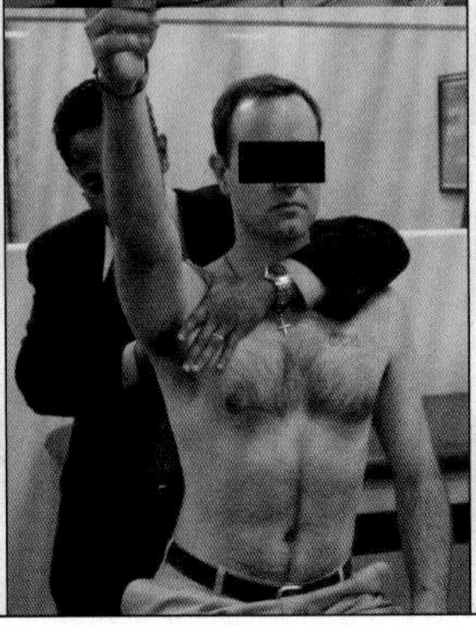 | The examiner should assess for fixed scapula winging versus reducible winging as well as improvement in arm elevation and comfort with the scapula reduced. This is crucial in determining fixed versus reducible winging. |

| Examination | Technique | Illustration | Grading & Significance |
|---|---|---|---|
| **Selective injection with local anesthetic and corticosteroid** | The involved arm is placed on the back to lift the scapula off the chest wall. The injection is given in the scapulothoracic bursa under the superomedial border of the scapula. | 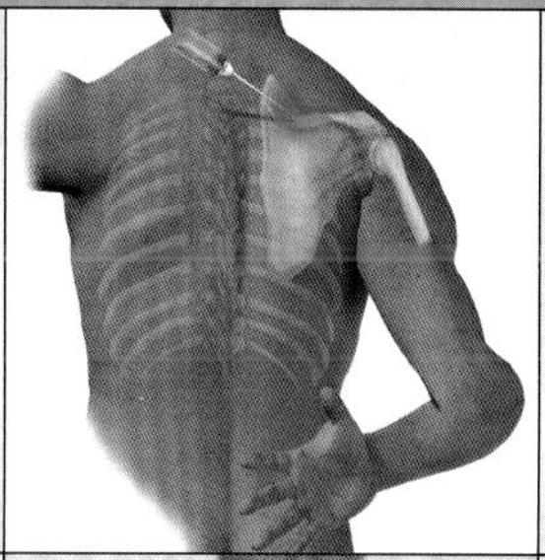 | Significant pain relief or elimination of the pain confirms the diagnosis. |
| **Speed's test** | The arm is abducted to 90 degrees and brought forward 45 degrees while the forearm is supinated and the elbow extended. The patient then resists a downward force. | 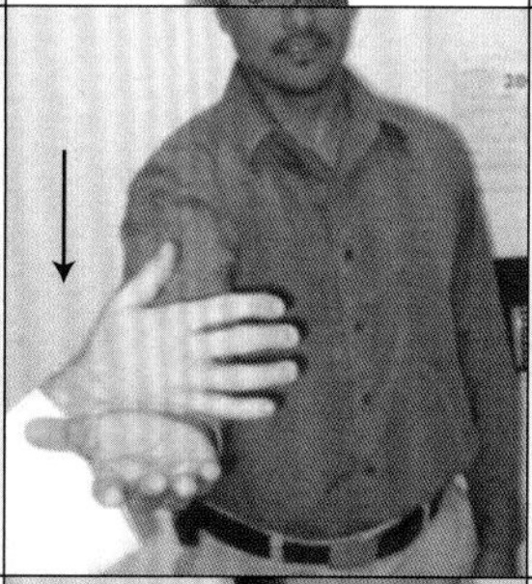 | If the maneuver produces pain or tenderness, the test is positive. A positive test may indicate bicipital pathology, although the test is not specific. |
| **Sulcus sign** | An inferior force is applied to the arm at the side. | 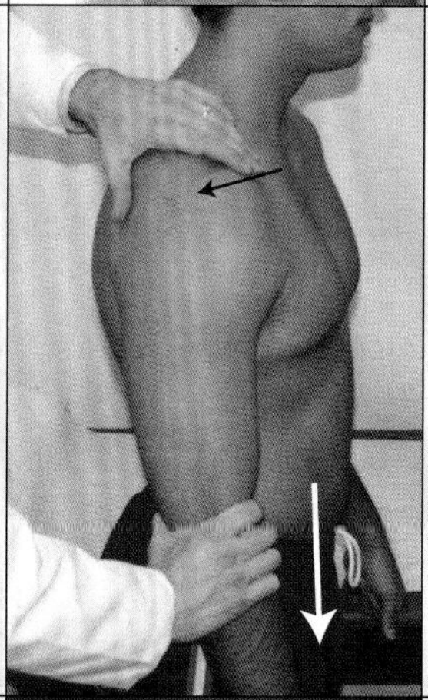 | 0 = no translation; 1+ = <1 cm; 2+ = 1–2 cm; 3+ = >3 cm. Indicates an inferior component of instability. |
| **Ulnar nerve** | Scissors (adducted thumb, abducted fingers, and flexor digitorum profundus function to ring and pinky) | 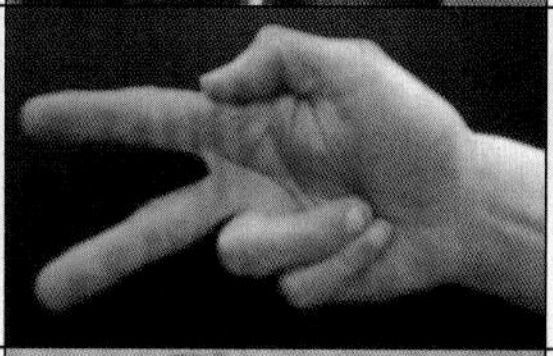 | Autonomous zone is palmar tip pinky finger. Most common iatrogenic nerve injury after internal fixation of forearm shaft fractures. |
| **Wall push-up** | The patient is asked to perform a wall push-up by placing the hands at shoulder level on a wall and doing a push-up. | 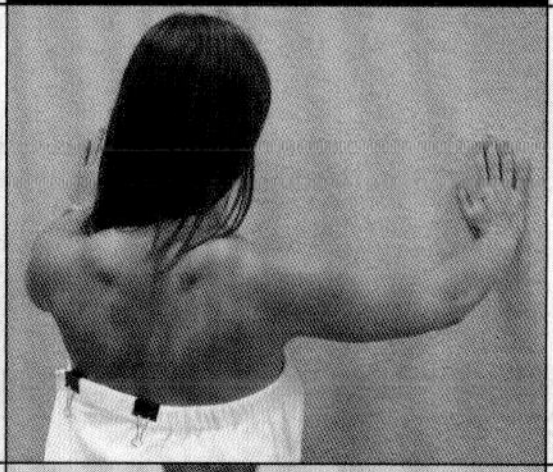 | The scapula is carefully evaluated for signs and severity of medial or lateral translation. |
| **Yergason test** | The elbow is flexed to 90 degrees. The patient attempts to supinate the arm from a pronated position while the examiner resists. | 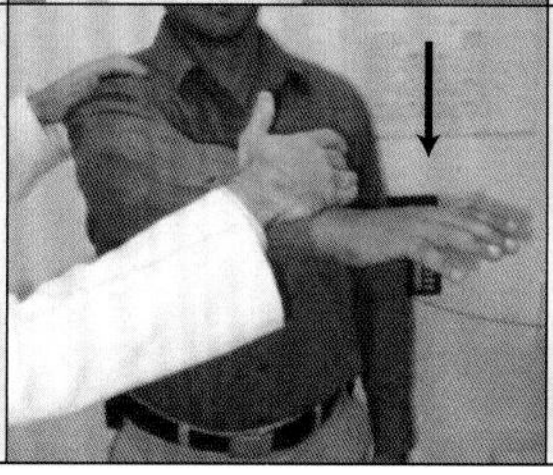 | The patient will experience pain as the biceps tendon subluxes out of the groove with a positive test. A positive test indicates biceps instability. |

*(continued)*

| Examination | Technique | Illustration | Grading & Significance |
|---|---|---|---|
| **Spine** | | | |
| **Adams forward bend test** | Examiner sits or stands behind patient. With the patient's feet together and knees straight, he or she is asked to bend forward at the waist while letting the arms hang free. Abnormalities in vertebral rotation become apparent as an asymmetrical rib hump, prominence, or fullness. | 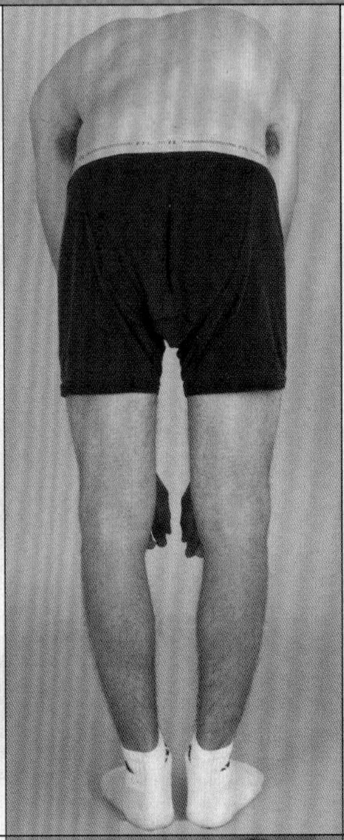 | The rotational deformity of the thoracic and lumbar spine can be graded using a scoliometer. The rotational deformity seen in scoliosis can be very prominent and the most obvious deformity seen by the patient and family. Characterizes the axial-plane deformity seen in scoliosis. |
| **Adson test** | Examiner stands behind the patient, radial pulse is palpated with the arm relaxed at the side. The arm is then abducted, extended, and externally rotated. Have patient take a deep breath and turn head to the side being tested. Evaluate pulse again. | 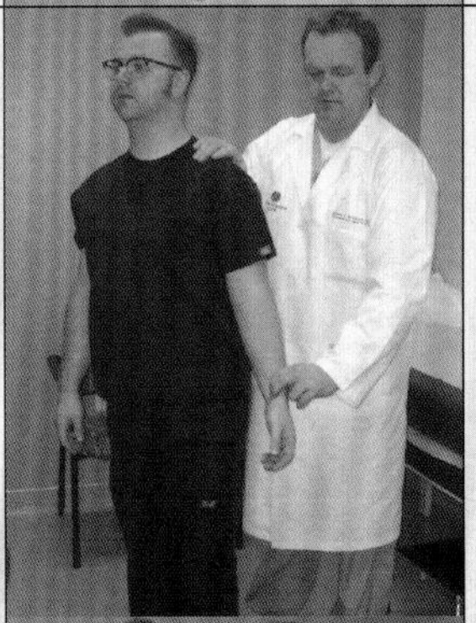 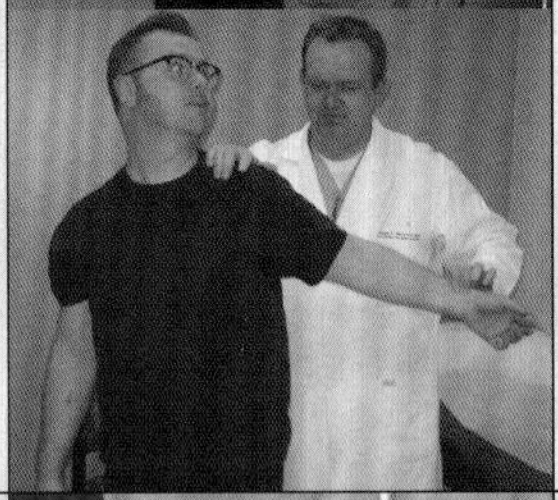 | Diminution or absence of the radial pulse. A positive Adson test indicates compression of the subclavian artery by a cervical rib or tight scalene muscle. This test is used to rule out thoracic outlet syndrome. |
| **Altered sensation evaluation** | Sensation can be assessed by light touch, pin prick, pain and temperature sensation. | 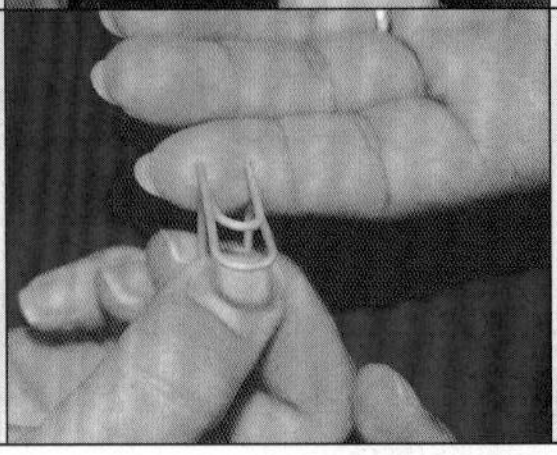 | Normal, decreased, or increased. Can aid in diagnosis of nerve root or spinal cord level. |

| Examination | Technique | Illustration | Grading & Significance |
|---|---|---|---|
| **Babinski reflex test** | The outside of the plantar aspect of the foot is stimulated, beginning at the heel and going forward to the base of the great toe. The Babinski sign is manifest by the upturning of the big toe and by fanning of the other toes. | 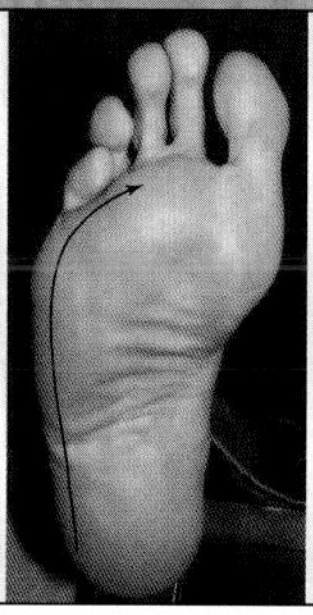 | A positive Babinski sign is an upper motor neuron sign and may indicate the presence of cervical or thoracic myelopathy. |
| **Biceps, wrist extension exam for C-spine nerve root syndrome** | Patient flexes elbow and extends wrist against examiner's resistance; sensation lateral forearm and radial two digits | 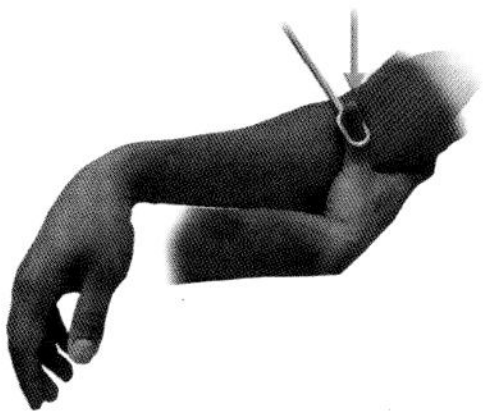 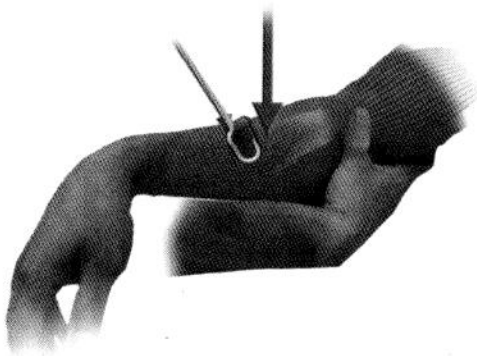 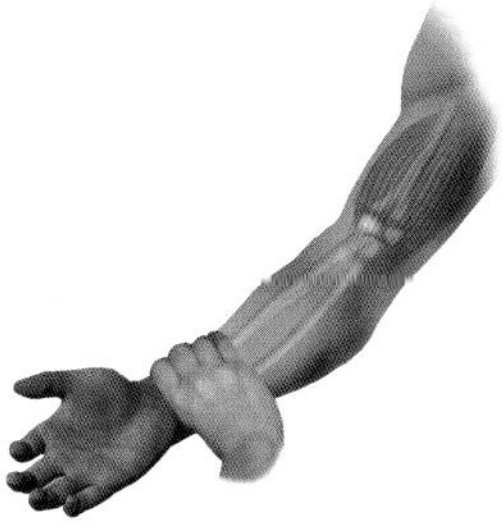 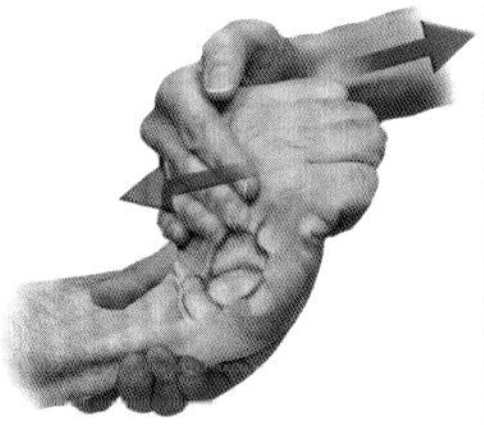 | Muscle strength graded 0–5. Deficits reveal abnormal function of C6 nerve root. |
| **Clavicle (shoulder) asymmetry** | The examiner observes and palpates the vertical relationship of the right and left acromion with the patient standing. | 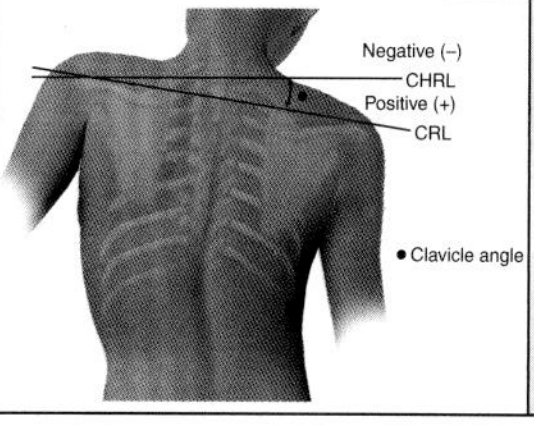 Negative (−) CHRL Positive (+) CRL • Clavicle angle | Vertical discrepancy is measured in centimeters. Shoulder asymmetry may occur with certain patterns of scoliosis. |

*(continued)*

| Examination | Technique | Illustration | Grading & Significance |
|---|---|---|---|
| **Coronal balance** | Posterior observation of the patient standing. The examiner drops a plumb line from the occiput and measures deviation at the sacrum. | 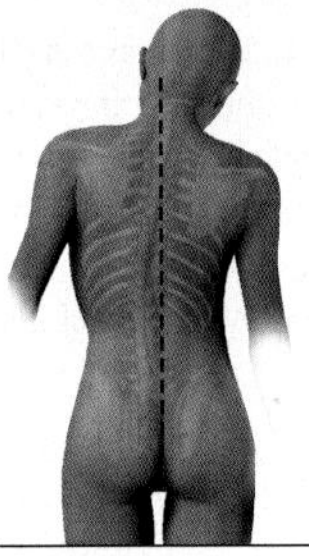 | Leftward or rightward shift in centimeters. Centered posture is biomechanically and cosmetically desirable. |
| **Deltoid exam for C-spine nerve root syndrome** | Patient abducts arm against examiner's resistance; sensation tested in deltoid region and along lateral arm | 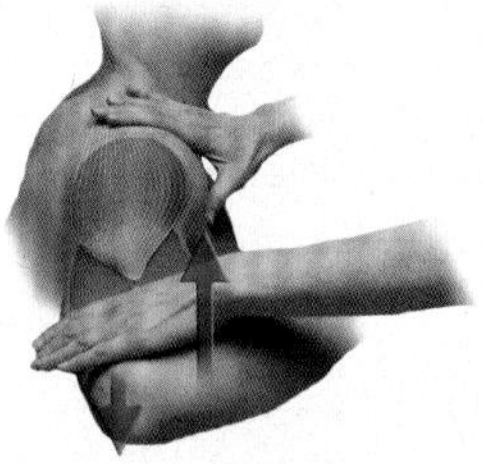 | Muscle strength graded 0–5. Deficits reveal abnormal function of C5 nerve root. |
| **Finger abduction exam for C-spine nerve root syndrome** | Sensation to medial arm; motor to interossei | 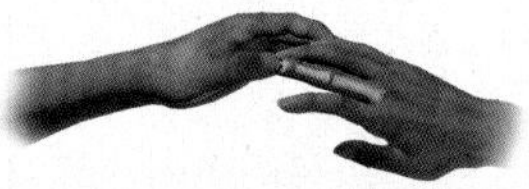 | Muscle strength graded 0–5. Deficits reveal abnormal function of T1 nerve root. |
| **Finger escape sign (ulnar escape sign)** | Performed with eyes closed, fingers adducted. Observe hands while patient is asked to maintain adducted finger position. | 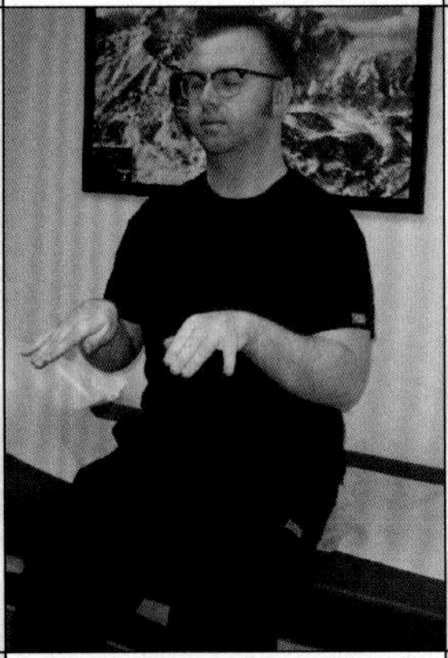 | Abduction of the small finger indicates intrinsic muscle weakness associated with cervical myelopathy. |
| **Handgrip exam for C-spine nerve root syndrome** | Sensation to medial forearm and ulnar two digits; motor to finger flexors–grip | 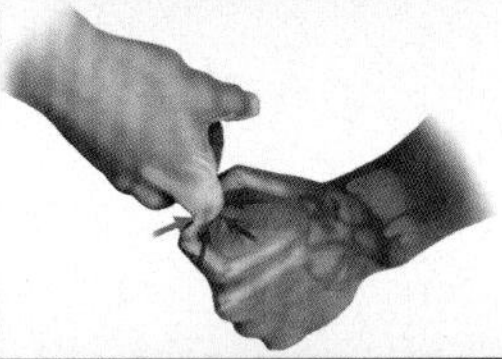 | Muscle strength graded 0–5. Deficits reveal abnormal function of C8 nerve root. |
| **Hawkins modified impingement sign** | Forward flexion of the humerus with internal rotation | 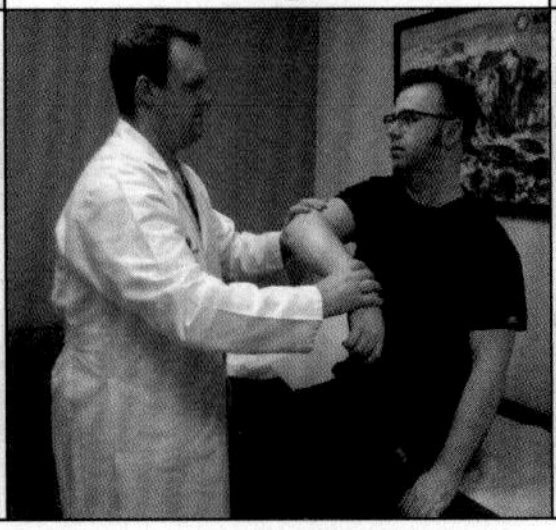 | This test rotates the greater tuberosity under the coracoacromial ligament, and a painful response at anterolateral corner of the acromion is indicative of impingement syndrome. |

| Examination | Technique | Illustration | Grading & Significance |
|---|---|---|---|
| **Hip flexion contractures** | One hip is maximally flexed with the pelvis stabilized in order to evaluate a flexion contracture on the opposite side. | 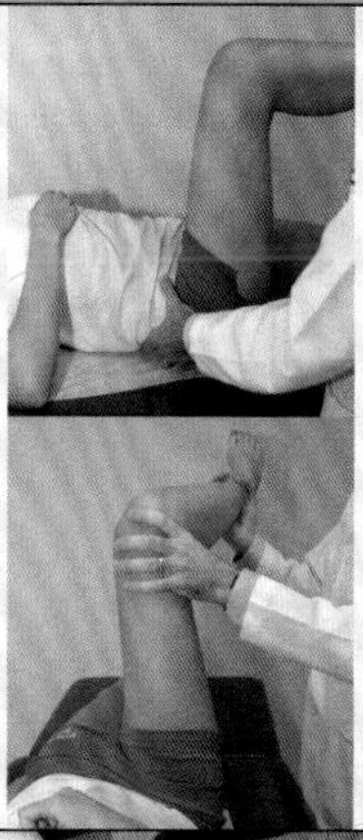 | Measured in degrees. Longstanding sagittal plane deformities, as well as neurogenic claudication, may result in hip and knee flexion contractures. |
| **Hoffman reflex** | Elicited by taking the middle finger and flipping the distal phalanx. | 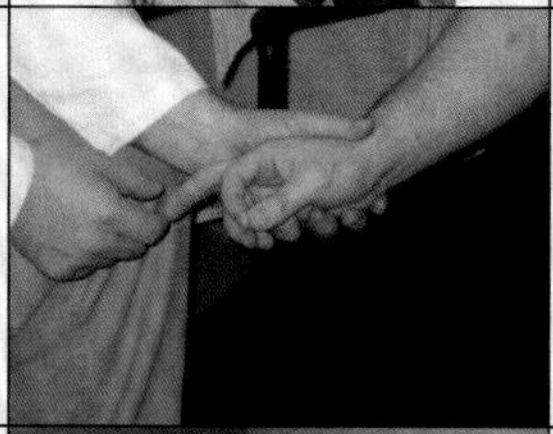 | Pincer response between thumb and forefinger has a correlation with cervical spondylotic myelopathy. May be a normal variant. Comparison with contralateral side showing asymmetry may be a better indicator of myelopathy. |
| **Impingement sign** | With patient seated and examiner's hand on scapula to prevent rotation, the affected arm is forward flexed causing greater tuberosity to contact the acromion. | 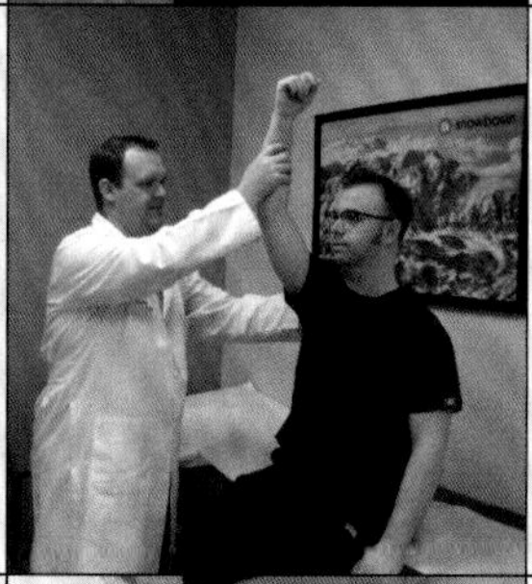 | Pain at the anterolateral acromion indicates a positive result. |
| **Inverted radial reflex** | This reflex is demonstrated by tapping the brachioradialis tendon. | 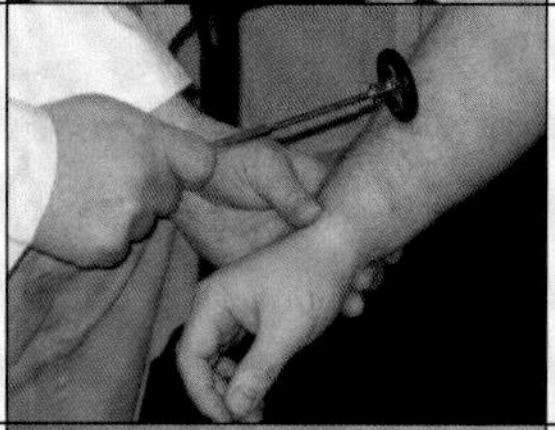 | A diminished normal reflex is noted along with a reflex contraction of the finger flexors. Abnormal reflex denotes peripheral compression of the C6 nerve root. Compression at C6 allows pathologic upper motor neuron response. |
| **Lhermitte phenomenon** | Flexion and/or extension in sagittal plane. The test is generally positive at the extremes of flexion and/or extension. | 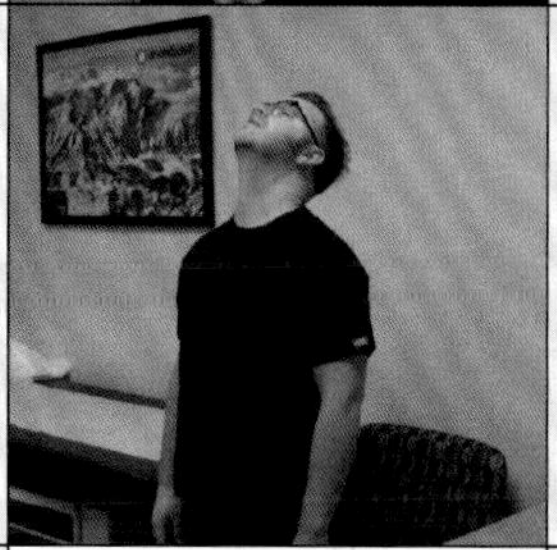 | Positive test causes shock-like sensation running down the spine. Pain in extension suggests spondylotic myelopathy, whereas symptoms in flexion are more suggestive of posttraumatic or iatrogenic kyphosis. |
| **Pelvic obliquity** | The examiner observes and palpates the vertical relationship of the right and left iliac crests. | 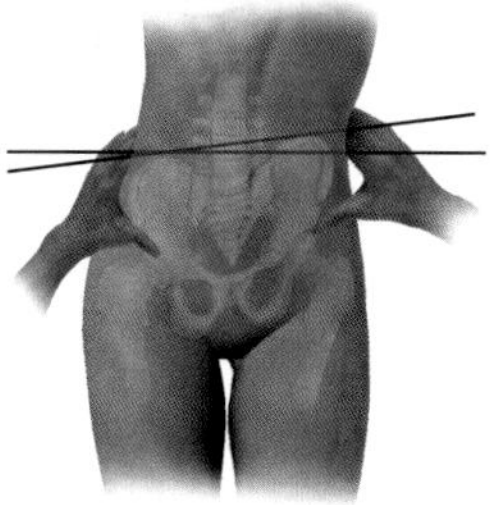 | Vertical difference between posterior superior iliac spines (PSIS) in centimeters. Pelvic obliquity may be a primary or compensatory mechanism with spinal deformity. |

*(continued)*

| Examination | Technique | Illustration | Grading & Significance |
|---|---|---|---|
| **Scapular and shoulder asymmetry** | Examiner sits or stands behind patient and notes presence of scapular asymmetry in terms of size and contour and shoulder asymmetry in terms of height. | 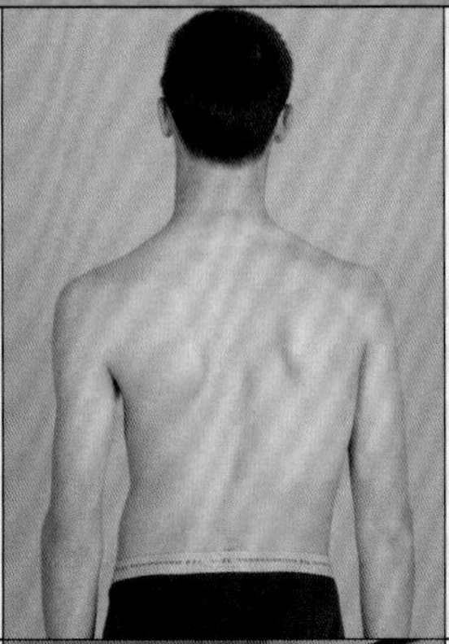 | Important to point out to parents as this is not always corrected by surgery |
| **Spurling test** | Ipsilateral axial rotation, extension, axial compression | 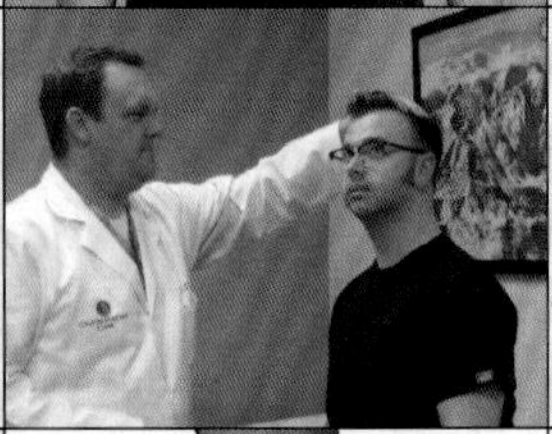 | Reproduces radicular symptoms when compressive pathology is present. Dermatomal distribution of pain should correlate with level of pathology. |
| **Thumb excursion test** | The base of the chest is encircled from the back by the examiner's hands, with the fingers just anterior to the anterior axillary line. The tips of the thumbs are positioned so that they are equidistant from the spine. The patient takes a deep breath, and the distance that each thumb tip moves laterally away from the spine is graded. | 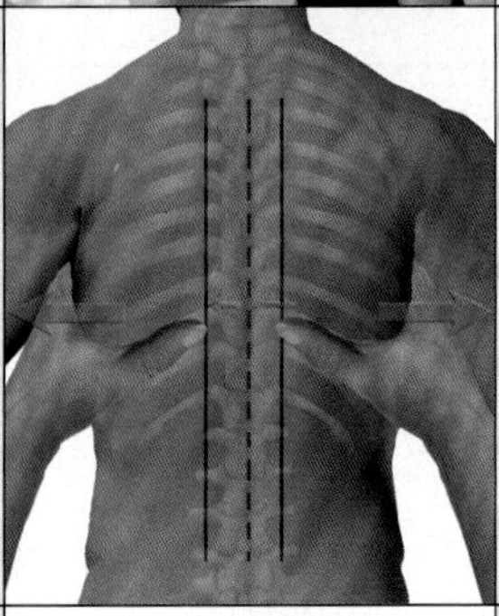 | No movement is classified as +0; 0.5 cm or less of excursion as +1; 0.5 to 1 cm as +2; and >1 cm as +3. The higher the grade, the greater the clinical secondary breathing mechanism in the respective hemithorax. |
| **Triceps and wrist flexion exam for C-spine nerve root syndrome** | Patient extends elbow and flexes wrist; sensation to middle finger | 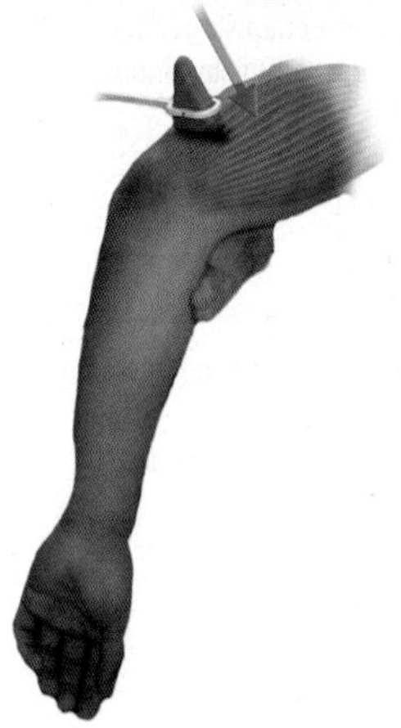 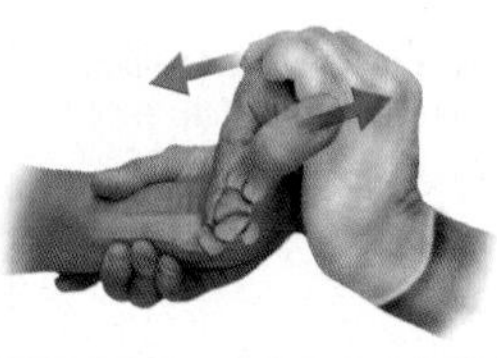 | Muscle strength graded 0–5. Deficits reveal abnormal function of C7 nerve root. |

| Examination | Technique | Illustration | Grading & Significance |
|---|---|---|---|
| **Trunk shift** | Examiner sits or stands behind patient. A C7 plumb line is used to evaluate for truncal shift. | 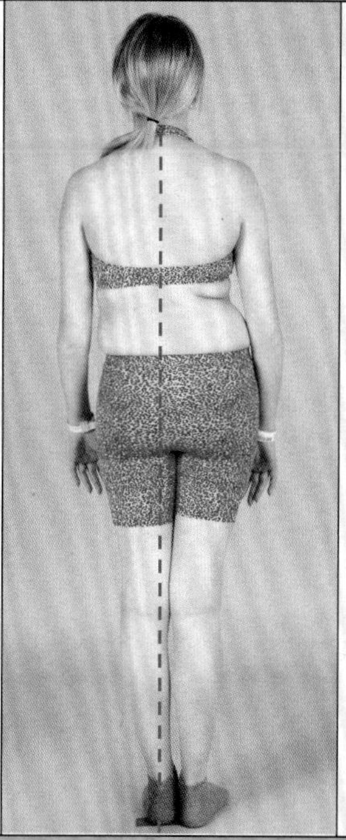 | Trunk shift is graded based on the number of centimeters that the plumb line, dropped from C7 spinous process, deviated from the midline. For example, if the plumb line fell 3 cm to the left, then the patient would have a leftward trunk shift of 3 cm. |
| **Hip/Pelvis** | | | |
| **Apprehension test** | The hip is externally rotated in an (over-) extended position. | 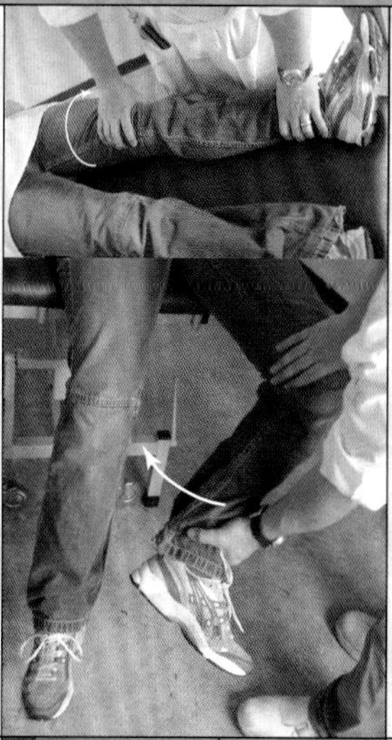 | Test is positive if the patient complains about the feeling of imminent joint luxation. Indicates an insufficient coverage of the femoral head. |
| **Arc of rotation, hip** | This is performed in the prone position, starting with the knee flexed to 90 degrees. Starting with the hip in neutral rotation, the hip is internally rotated and externally rotated. | 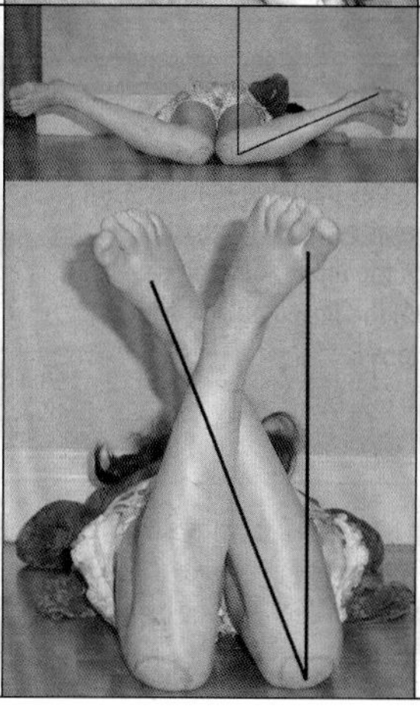 | The arcs of internal and external rotation from the midline are measured in degrees with a goniometer. Normal arc of rotation is age-dependent. External rotation usually exceeds internal rotation. When the arc of internal rotation exceeds the arc of external rotation, the presence of increased anteversion can be inferred. |

*(continued)*

| Examination | Technique | Illustration | Grading & Significance |
|---|---|---|---|
| **Barlow maneuver** | The examiner's hand is on the proximal femur, fingers over the greater trochanter, and the leg is in a flexed position. The leg is adducted with gentle posterior pressure to see if the hip can be dislocated. | | Positive or negative. Positive Barlow sign represents the ability for a reduced hip to be dislocated due to instability. Disappears as fixed dislocation develops. |
| **Gait** | Legs should be exposed. Gait is observed with and without the use of walking aids. | | Trendelenburg gait suggests abductor weakness or hip discomfort. Coxalgic gait suggests hip pain of any cause. Stiff hip gait may be present with hypertrophic osteoarthritis. Short limb gait may be present with developmental dysplasia of the hip. No limp is normal. A slight abductor lurch or antalgic gait is abnormal. Intra-articular hip disease (labral tear or chondral flap) can produce an early limp. As secondary osteoarthritis progresses, a limp is common. The examiner should look for varus thrust. Painful total hip arthroplasty may result in shortened stance phase or stride length, or abnormal pelvic rotation. May confirm hip pathology or indicate extrinsic source of pain. May raise concern regarding hip abductor function that can limit success of revision. Pain or muscle weakness may cause limp. Trunk may shift over affected hip. |
| **Galeazzi sign** | On a flat surface, the thigh lengths are assessed with the knees flexed. The examiner flexes the hips to 90 degrees and notes the height of the knees. | | Positive if there is a difference in thigh length. A positive Galeazzi sign can indicate a dislocated hip, a short femur, or a congenital hip deformity. The apparent femoral lengths will be equal in bilateral dislocations. |
| **Hip abduction** | On a flat surface, the patient's hips are flexed to 90 degrees and abducted and the anterior superior iliac spines palpated to make sure the pelvis remains level. Abduction of the hips should be checked in both the flexed and extended positions. | | In a normal hip, abduction should be >60 degrees and symmetric. May be the only abnormal sign in infants. A difference of 10 degrees or more is significant.<br><br>Decreased hip abduction is the most common physical finding in patients with hip pathology. A marked loss of abduction in extension is particularly important in Perthes disease, suggesting hinge abduction. |
| **Hip abductor strength** | In the lateral decubitus position, the patient is asked to elevate the limb and the examiner applies manual resistance. | | Graded using traditional manual muscle testing five-point scale. May indicate abductor weakness, trochanteric bursitis, abductor avulsion, or loose femoral component. |

| Examination | Technique | Illustration | Grading & Significance |
|---|---|---|---|
| **Ortolani sign** | With a hand on the proximal femur, fingers over the greater trochanter, and the leg in a flexed position, the examiner abducts the leg with gentle traction to see if the hip can be reduced.<br><br>The hip is flexed 90 degrees. The hip is abducted gently with the thumb on the medial femoral condyle and the third finger on the greater trochanter. The examiner lifts with the third finger and feels for a "clunk." | 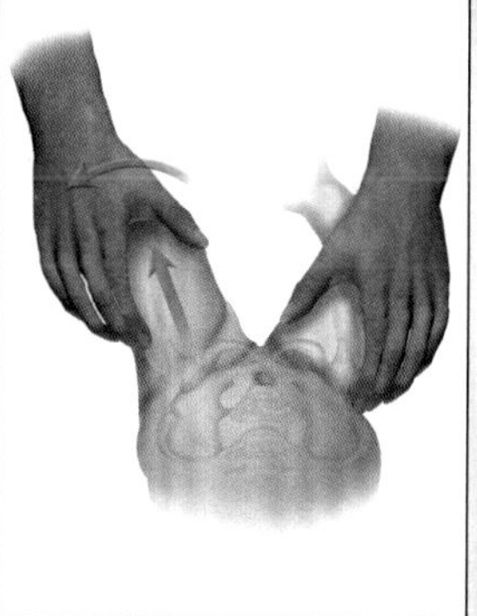 | Positive or negative. A positive Ortolani sign represents the reduction of a dislocated hip. Usually present in the newborn with developmental dysplasia of the hip, but disappears as the dislocation becomes fixed.<br><br>The test is positive if a clunk is felt as a dislocated hip reduces. |
| **Pelvic obliquity** | Examiner sits or stands behind patient. Fingers are placed on the iliac crests and the thumbs are placed on the posterior superior iliac spines. Presence of asymmetry is noted. | 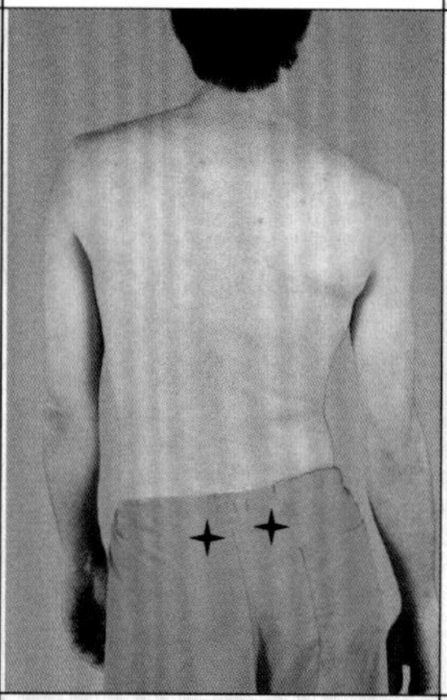 | Can indicate a possible leg-length discrepancy that can mimic a lumbar scoliosis |
| **Range of motion (ROM), hip** | Abduction–adduction and flexion ROM is examined in the supine position. Fixed flexion deformity of the hip is measured. Hip internal rotation–external rotation is measured in prone position, together with the thigh–foot angle. Muscle length tests include popliteal angle (hamstring length) and prone knee bend (rectus femoris muscle length). | 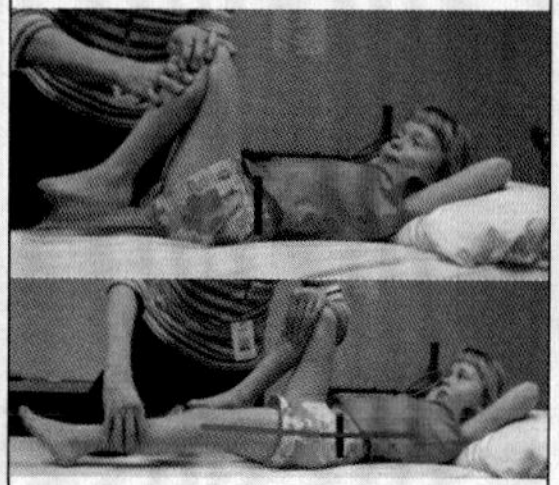 | ROM is measured and contractures are identified and quantified in degrees. A popliteal angle >0 degrees and prone knee bend less than supine knee bend indicates tightness of hamstring and rectus femoris muscles, respectively. Contractures need to be treated in preparation for lengthening. Lengthening of rectus femoris and hamstring muscles is recommended for positive muscle tightness.<br><br>Normal extension range of motion is from 10 degrees beyond horizontal. Maximum flexion is limited by the abdomen and the trunk. Normal walking function requires 7 degrees extension beyond neutral pelvic position. Therefore, even small contractures limit functional range of motion, shorten step length, and induce compensatory movements.<br><br>Restricted ROM can indicate a joint abnormality, capsular contracture, or spasticity of the internal or external rotators of the hip. Excessive ROM indicates relative ligamentous laxity. Shifted ROM (eg, excessive internal ROM) indicates excessive femoral anteversion. |

*(continued)*

| Examination | Technique | Illustration | Grading & Significance |
|---|---|---|---|
| **Lower Extremities** | | | |
| **Abduction external rotation test** | The hip is passively forced into maximal abduction with external rotation. | 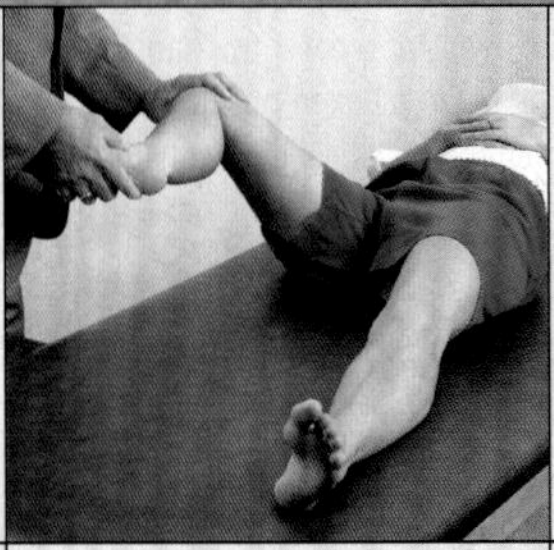 | May create symptoms associated with posterior joint pathology by compression, or anterior pathology by anterior translation of the femoral head. |
| **Apley grind test** | With the patient prone, the knee is flexed to 90 degrees and the anterior thigh is fixed against the examining table. The foot and leg are then pulled upward to distract the joint and rotated to place rotational strain on the ligaments. Next, with the knee in the same position, the foot and leg are pressed downward and rotated as the joint is slowly flexed and extended. | 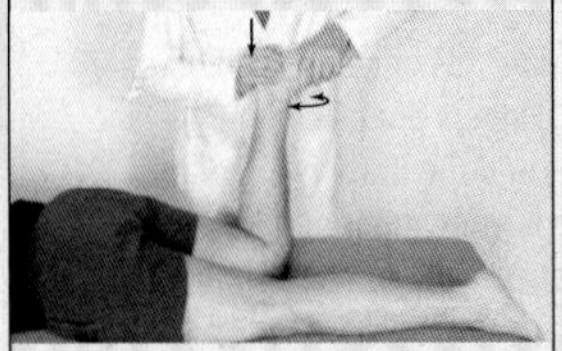 | When the ligaments have been torn, pulling the leg upward and rotating it usually are painful. When the foot and leg are pressed downward and rotated, popping and pain localized to the joint line usually indicate a torn meniscus. |
| **Anterior compression of the iliopsoas tendon** | Firm digital pressure over the anterior hip capsule may block the snapping. | 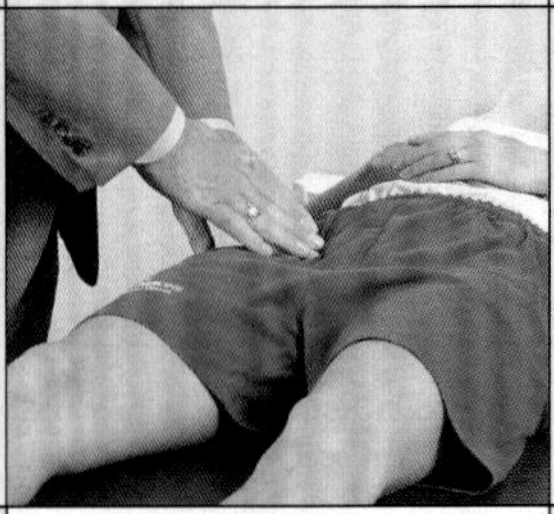 | Applying pressure to block the snapping of the tendon substantiates the diagnosis. However, often this maneuver is uncomfortable and not well tolerated by the patient. |
| **Anterior drawer test** | The patient is examined in the supine position with the knee flexed 90 degrees. The leg is held below the joint line and the tibia is pulled forward. | 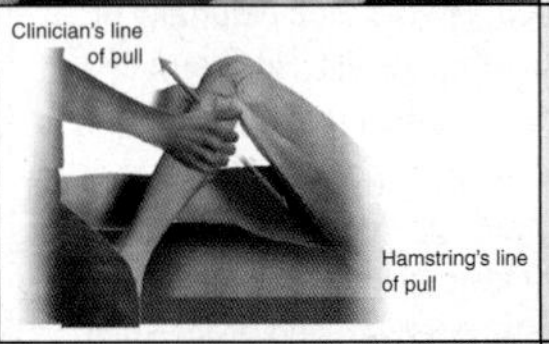 Clinician's line of pull<br>Hamstring's line of pull | Positive examination indicates knee joint laxity. Not as sensitive as the Lachman in testing for anterior cruciate ligament deficiency. |
| **C sign** | Patient cups hand above greater trochanter, gripping fingers into groin. | 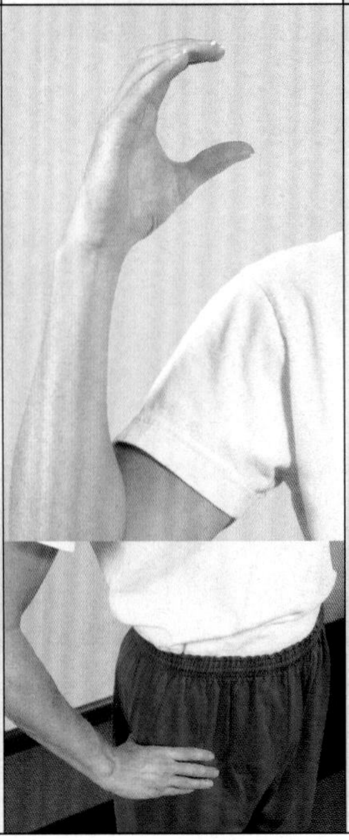 | Common observation with patients describing interior hip pain. |

| Examination | Technique | Illustration | Grading & Significance |
|---|---|---|---|
| **Collateral ligament laxity** | Varus or valgus stress with the knee in full extension as well as 30 degrees of flexion | | Normal = symmetric to the opposite side; Mild = 1 to 3 mm of increased laxity from the opposite side; Moderate = 3 to 5 mm; Severe = 5 mm or more difference. In children varus instability may be due to accommodation of the large discoid lateral meniscus. |
| **Dial test** | With the patient in prone position, the tibia is externally rotated at 30 and 90 degrees. The foot-to-thigh angle is compared between the two legs. | | Difference of more than 10 degrees at 30 degrees is consistent with injury to posterolateral corner (PLC). Difference of more than 10 degrees at 90 degrees is consistent with injury to PLC and posterior cruciate ligament. |
| **Flexibility of the Achilles tendon and the gastrocnemius tendon (Silfverskiold Test)** | The knee is flexed to 90 degrees. The subtalar joint is inverted to neutral. The ankle is maximally dorsiflexed without allowing the subtalar joint to evert. The degree of dorsiflexion is measured. The knee is extended while maintaining subtalar neutral, even if it creates plantarflexion of the ankle. Once again the degree of ankle dorsiflexion is measured. | | The degree of ankle dorsiflexion is measured with the knee both flexed and extended. It is normal for the ankle to dorsiflex at least 10 degrees above neutral with the knee extended, and even further with the knee flexed. The entire triceps surae (gastrocnemius and soleus) is contracted if the ankle does not dorsiflex at least 10 degrees above neutral with the knee flexed or extended. The gastrocnemius is selectively contracted if the ankle dorsiflexes at least 10 degrees above neutral with the knee flexed but not extended.<br><br>Image from the private collection of Vincent Mosca MD. |
| **Gait** | Legs should be exposed. Gait is observed with and without the use of walking aids. | | Trendelenburg gait suggests abductor weakness or hip discomfort. Coxalgic gait suggests hip pain of any cause. Stiff hip gait may be present with hypertrophic osteoarthritis. Short limb gait may be present with developmental dysplasia of the hip. No limp is normal. A slight abductor lurch or antalgic gait is abnormal. Intra-articular hip disease (labral tear or chondral flap) can produce an early limp. As secondary osteoarthritis progresses, a limp is common. The examiner should look for varus thrust. Painful total hip arthroplasty may result in shortened stance phase or stride length, or abnormal pelvic rotation. May confirm hip pathology or indicate extrinsic source of pain. May raise concern regarding hip abductor function that can limit success of revision. Pain or muscle weakness may cause limp. Trunk may shift over affected hip. |

*(continued)*

| Examination | Technique | Illustration | Grading & Significance |
|---|---|---|---|
| **Hamstring strength** | Patient lies prone. Patient attempts knee flexion against resistance. | 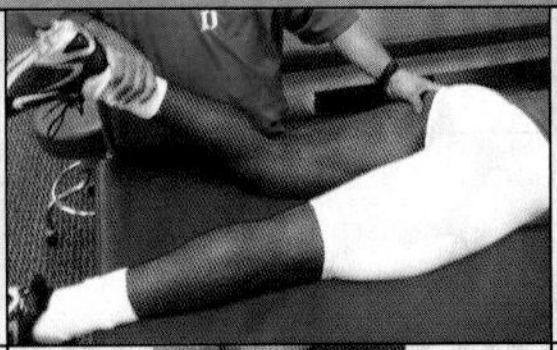 | Mild: minimal loss of strength; moderate: clear loss of strength; severe: complete loss of strength. Severe injury implies proximal avulsion. |
| **Heel strike** | Light blows of the fist or heel of hand to the heel of the injured leg | 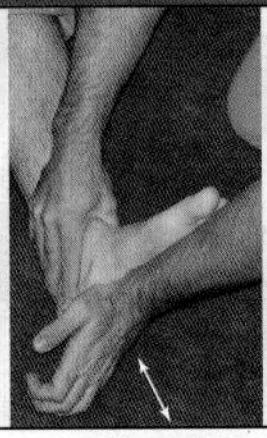 | Groin pain that did not exist at rest implies hip fracture. |
| **Iliac wing compression** | The examiner can test for stability of the pelvic ring by placing the palms of the hands on the outside of the iliac wings and pushing the two wings together. | 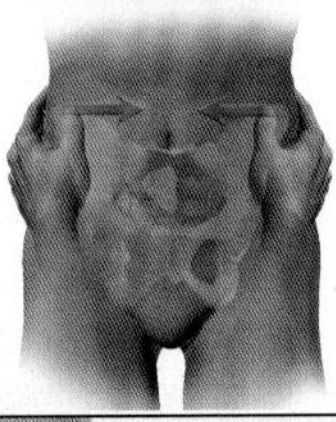 | This should be avoided if radiology demonstrates displacement. |
| **Impingement test** | The hip is passively forced into maximal flexion, adduction, and internal rotation. | 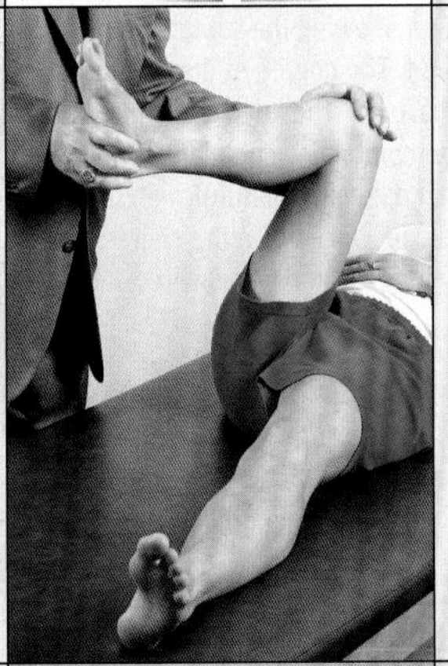 | A more sensitive test for detecting hip joint irritability. This is associated with impingement findings but is positive with most sources of hip pathology. |
| **Inspection for Effusion** | The examiner palpates and performs ballottement of the patella. Smaller effusions can be detected by compressing fluid from the suprapatellar pouch. | 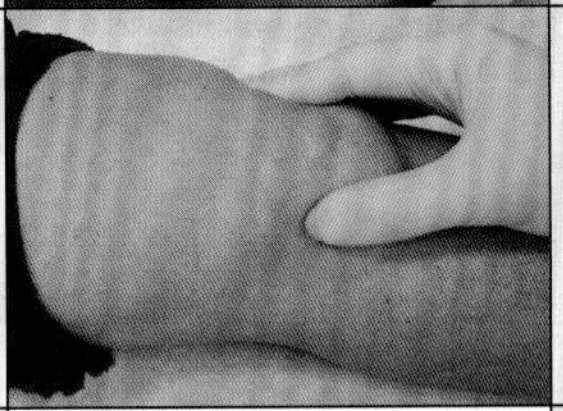 | Trace, mild, moderate, or large. Presence of an effusion is indirect evidence of intra-articular injury. Most commonly graded subjectively as mild, moderate, or larger. New onset of effusion after injury localizes injury to within the capsule of the knee. |
| **Lachman Test** | The test is performed with the knee in slight flexion (between 20 and 30 degrees). The examiner grasps the thigh above the patella and uses the other hand to grasp the leg. The tibia is pulled forward while the other hand restrains the patient's thigh. | 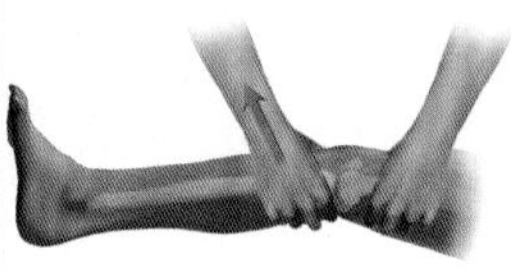 | A positive examination indicates deficiency of the anterior cruciate ligament complex. The test has greater sensitivity and specificity for anterior cruciate ligament tears. |

| Examination | Technique | Illustration | Grading & Significance |
|---|---|---|---|
| **Leg length, apparent** | With patient supine, the distance from the umbilicus to each medial malleolus is measured. | 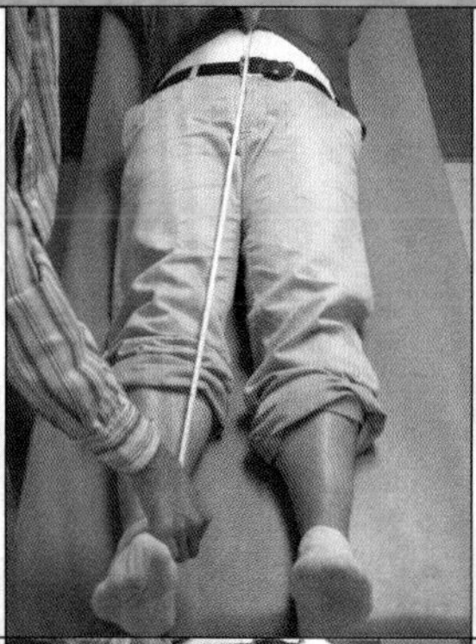 | Values may be affected by atrophy, obesity, or asymmetric positioning of the legs. May indicate abductor or adductor contractures, or pelvic obliquity due to scoliosis. |
| **Leg length, true** | With the patient supine with feet 15 to 20 cm apart, the examiner measures the distance from the anterior superior iliac spines to the medial malleolus of each leg. In obese patients with poor pelvic landmarks, the examiner should line up the medial malleoli to get an approximation of leg lengths. It is important to assess the patient while standing and to observe for pelvic obliquity and scoliosis. | 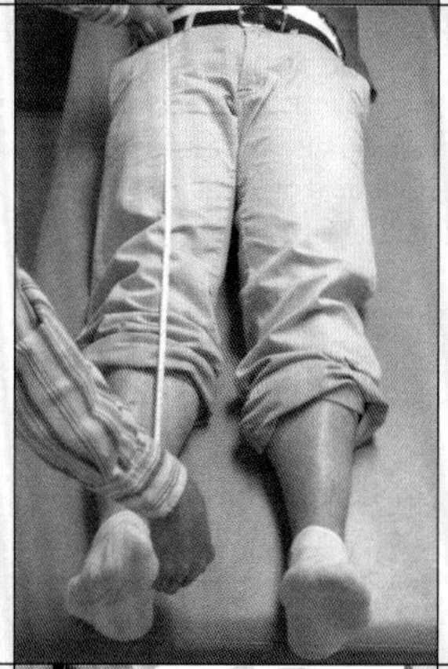 | A slight difference of $<1$ cm is considered normal but may be symptomatic in some patients. Progressive leg-length discrepancy suggests implant subsidence. Adduction contracture may cause apparent shortening when supine, but may elevate the hemipelvis when standing. Pelvic tilt from spinal deformity may contribute to functional leg-length inequality. |
| **Log roll test** | With the patient supine, the affected leg is simply rolled back and forth. | 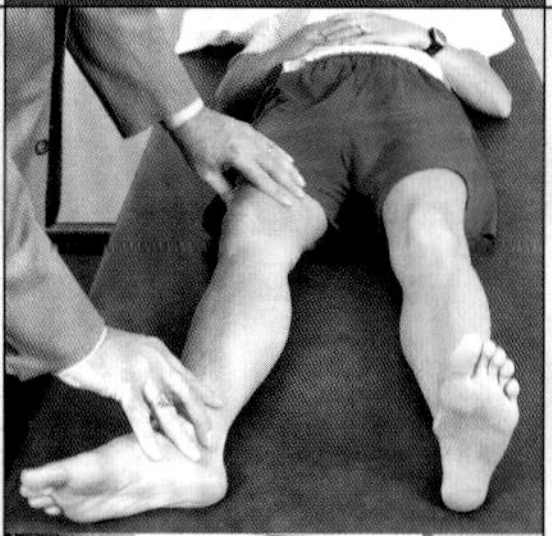 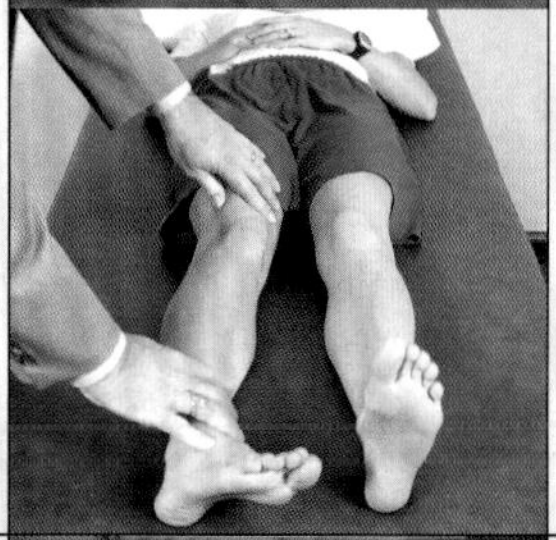 | Most specific test for hip joint pathology since femoral head is being rotated in relation to the acetabulum and capsule without stressing any of the extra-articular structures |
| **Lower extremity rotation** | In a patient with a suspected femoral neck fracture, gentle internal and external rotation at the leg is all that is needed to elicit pain. | 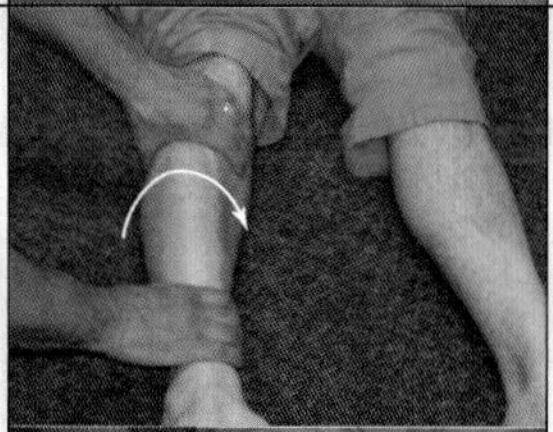 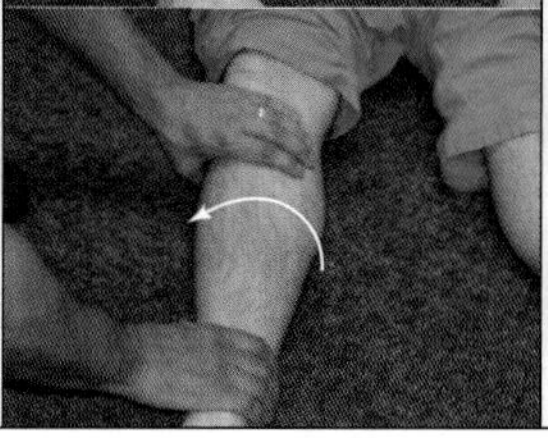 | Pain in the groin is concerning for femoral neck fracture but may also be caused by fractures of the anterior pelvic ring. |

(continued)

| Examination | Technique | Illustration | Grading & Significance |
|---|---|---|---|
| **McMurry test** | With the patient supine and the knee acutely and forcibly flexed, the examiner can check the medial meniscus by palpating the postero-medial margin of the joint with one hand while grasping the foot with the other hand. Keeping the knee completely flexed, the leg is externally rotated as far as possible and then the knee is slowly extended. As the femur passes over a tear in the meniscus, a click may be heard or felt. The lateral meniscus is checked by palpating the posterolateral margin of the joint, internally rotating the leg as far as possible, and slowly extending the knee while listening and feeling for a click. With the knee maximally flexed, it is extended to 90 degrees while applying internal rotation and valgus force to the foot and ankle. Repeat with external rotation and varus force. | 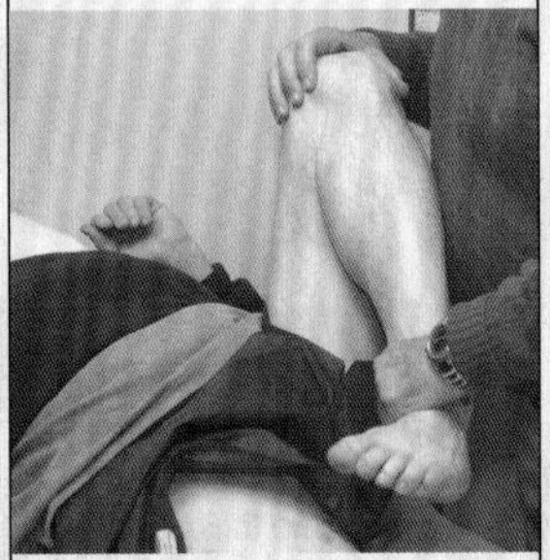 | A click produced by the McMurray test usually is caused by a posterior peripheral tear of the meniscus and occurs between complete flexion of the knee and 90 degrees. Popping, which occurs with greater degrees of extension when definitely localized to the joint line, suggests a tear of the middle and anterior portions of the meniscus. Thus, the position of the knee when the click occurs may help locate the lesion. A positive McMurray click localized to the joint line is additional evidence that the meniscus is torn; a negative McMurray test does not rule out a tear. A palpable or audible pop in combination with pain is considered positive. Results are variable, but a positive McMurray test is indicative of a meniscus lesion and not a chondral lesion. |
| **Midfoot joint palpation** | Direct palpation of each of midfoot joints, particularly the medial column of the foot | 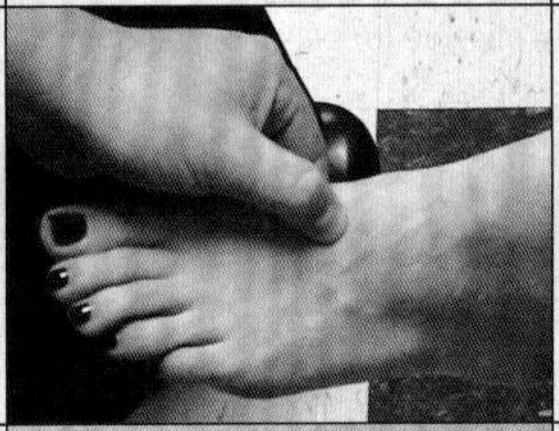 | Presence or absence of pain. The presence of pain at the midfoot with palpation suggests a Lisfranc injury. |
| **Midfoot stability** | Gentle passive dorsiflexion and plantarflexion of each of the metatarsal heads; gentle passive abduction and adduction through the forefoot | 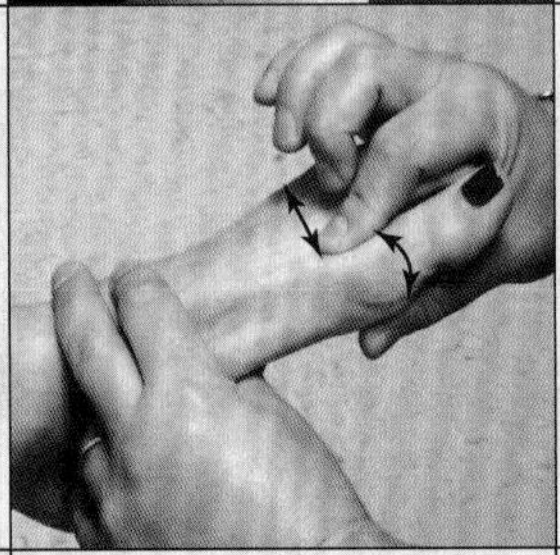 | Presence or absence of pain. The presence of pain at the tarsometatarsal joint region with passive forefoot range of motion suggests a Lisfranc injury. |
| **Ober test** | Patient is placed in lateral decubitus position, with the down hip and knee flexed for stability. The examiner flexes the other hip to 90 degrees and then abducts the hip fully and extends the hip past neutral with the knee in 90 degrees of flexion. The hip and knee are allowed to adduct while the hip is held in neutral rotation. | 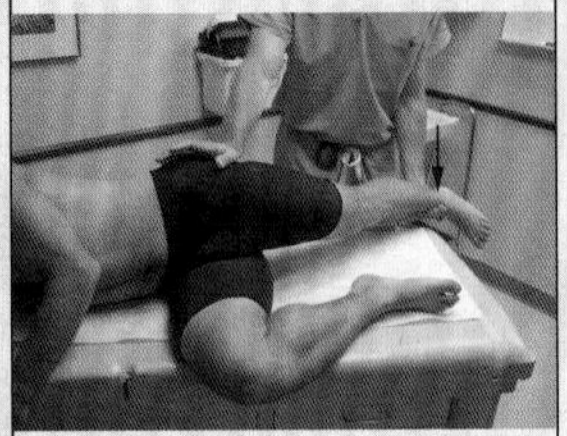 | The test is positive when the upper knee remains in the abducted position after the hip is passively extended and abducted and then adducted with the knee flexed. Used to evaluate iliotibial band tightness. If, when the hip and knee are allowed to adduct while the hip is held in neutral rotation, the knee adducts past midline, the hip abductors are not tight; if the knee does not reach to midline, then the hip abductors are tight. |
| **Passive adductors stretch** | The subject lies supine. The examiner either abducts the leg or places the leg in a figure 4 position. | 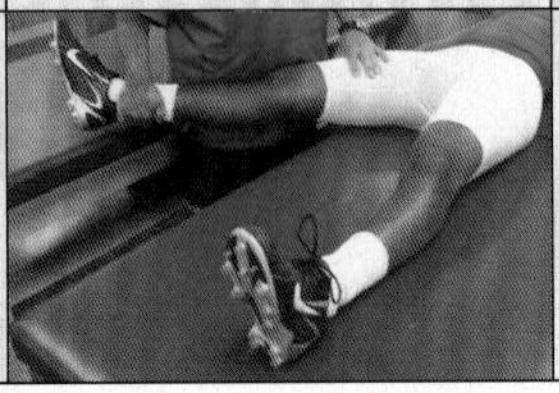 | The presence or absence of pain is noted. Pain localized to the adductor implies adductor-related groin pain. |

| Examination | Technique | Illustration | Grading & Significance |
|---|---|---|---|
| **Passive hamstring stretch** | Patient performs a hurdler's stretch. | | Apparent hamstring flexibility is compared to the uninjured side. An obvious increase in apparent hamstring flexibility of injured extremity implies proximal avulsion. |
| **Patrick test (Faber test)** | Patient is supine on examination table and placed such that one half of the buttock is off the table while the ipsilateral leg is placed in a figure 4 position on the other (extended) knee. The pelvis is stabilized with one of the examiner's hands and a downward force is applied to the flexed knee with the examiner's other hand. | | Pain may be felt with the downward stress on the flexed knee. Pain in the posterior pelvis may be considered positive for the pain coming from the sacroiliac (SI) joint. Indicative of SI abnormalities or iliopsoas spasm. |
| **Pelvic instability: external rotation** | Legs are positioned flexed, abducted, and externally rotated. Hands are placed on the iliac crests and an AP force is applied. | | Palpable widening of the pelvis or increased sacroiliac joint space or symphyseal widening is seen on simultaneous fluoroscopic images with the C-arm. |
| **Pelvic instability: internal rotation** | Legs are positioned extended and internally rotated. Hands are positioned lateral to iliac crests and a lateral-to-medial compressive force is applied. | | Palpable instability of the pelvis or a decrease in sacroiliac joint space or symphyseal diastasis is seen on simultaneous C-arm images. |
| **Pelvic instability: vertical instability** | Legs are positioned extended. While one extremity is supported at the heel, traction is applied to the other. | | A visual change in leg-length discrepancy can be seen in some cases. Otherwise, simultaneous C-arm images may disclose one acetabulum or iliac crest at a different level than the other. |
| **Patellar palpation** | The patella, quadriceps tendon, and patellar tendon are palpated for defects. The examiner notes inferior or superior patellar displacement in comparison to the unaffected side. |  | Patella baja is an inferiorly displaced patella seen with quadriceps tendon rupture; patella alta is a high-riding patella associated with patellar tendon rupture. The placement of the patella and palpation of defects with the patella, quadriceps tendon, or patellar tendon can help differentiate between patellar fracture and ligamentous extensor disruption. |

*(continued)*

| Examination | Technique | Illustration | Grading & Significance |
|---|---|---|---|
| **Patellar stability** | The examiner flexes the knee and palpates the alignment of the patella to the notch in flexion. Tracking of the patella is assessed from 0 to 90 degrees. The examiner attempts to push the thumb into the intercondylar notch. | 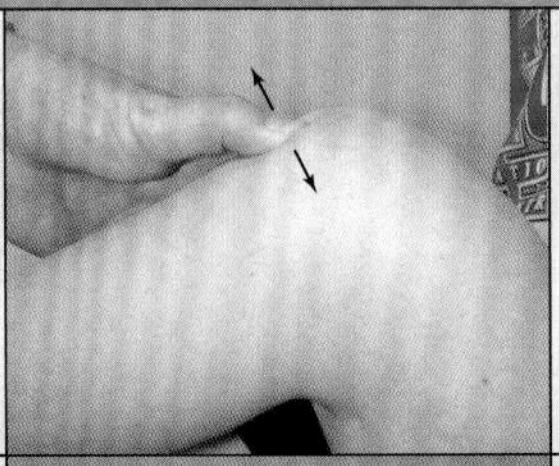 | If the examiner's thumb is able to palpate the intercondylar notch with the patient's knee flexed, this denotes lateral subluxation or dislocation of the patella. Patellar instability is common and can be an indication of lateral rotatory instability of the knee and contracture of the iliotibial band. |
| **Popliteal angles** | With the patient supine, the hip is flexed to 90 degrees, ensuring that the contralateral leg lays flat. The examiner extends the leg at the knee and measures the angle the leg makes with perpendicular to ground. | 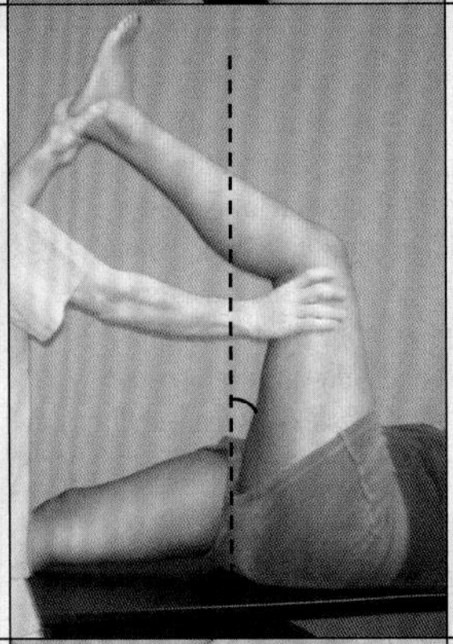 | >40 degrees indicates significant hamstring tightness. Most common neurologic finding in patients with spondylolisthesis. |
| **Posterior drawer test** | With knee in 70 to 90 degrees of flexion, a posterior-directed force is applied to the proximal tibia. | 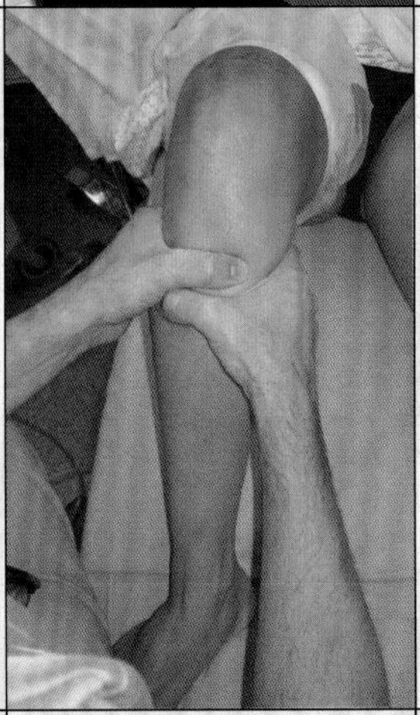 | 0 = no abnormal translation; 1 = 1 to 5 mm; 2 = 6 to 10 mm (but medial tibial plateau [MTP] not beyond medial femoral condyle [MFC]); 3 = >10 mm, or translation of MTP beyond MFC.<br>When compared to contralateral knee, may be indicative of posterior cruciate ligament-deficient knee. |
| **Posterior impingement test** | The hip is extended, externally rotated, and adducted. This can be tested in the supine or prone position. | 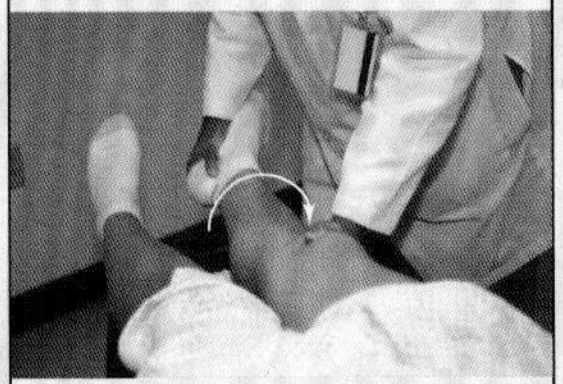 | Pain perceived posteriorly in the buttock corresponds to a positive impingement test. The absence of pain indicates a negative test. Normal internal rotation is considered to be about 15 to 20 degrees. In femoroacetabular impingement, internal rotation is decreased.<br><br>Normal test is no pain. Positive test is groin or buttock pain that reproduces symptoms. Uncommonly, patients have associated structural posterior impingement. The posterior impingement test assists in identifying the presence of associated posterior disease. |

| Examination | Technique | Illustration | Grading & Significance |
|---|---|---|---|
| **Prone rectus femoris test (also known as the Duncan-Ely test)** | The child is placed on the examination table in the prone position, with the hip and knee in full extension and the ankle in a relaxed plantigrade position. The examiner places one hand on the posterior aspect of the pelvis. The other hand is placed about the ankle and the knee is flexed slowly and then rapidly. If the examiner feels the pelvis rise from the examination table when the knee is flexed slowly, then the slow rectus test is noted to be positive. If the examiner notes a catch or sudden increase in resistance to motion as the knee is flexed rapidly, then the fast rectus test is noted to be positive. | 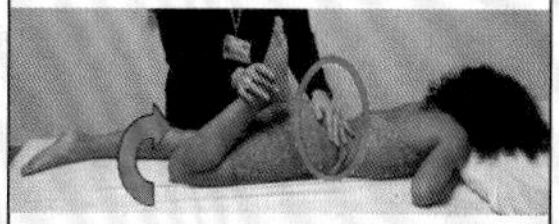 | A positive slow rectus test indicates fixed shortening of the rectus femoris muscle. A apositive fast rectus test indicates spasticity of the rectus femoris muscle. |
| **ROM, hip** | The hip is flexed to its maximum extent and the examiner records the degrees of flexion. The hip is then flexed to 90 degrees and passively internally and externally rotated. | 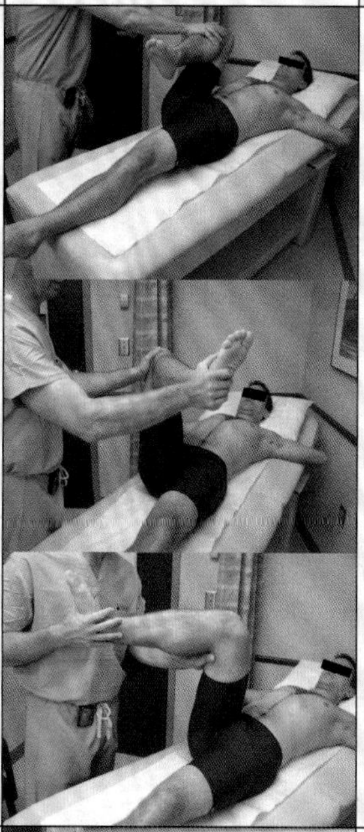 | Loss of motion is often associated with arthritis. |
| **ROM, knee** | Flexion and extension knee ROM is examined in supine and prone positions. | 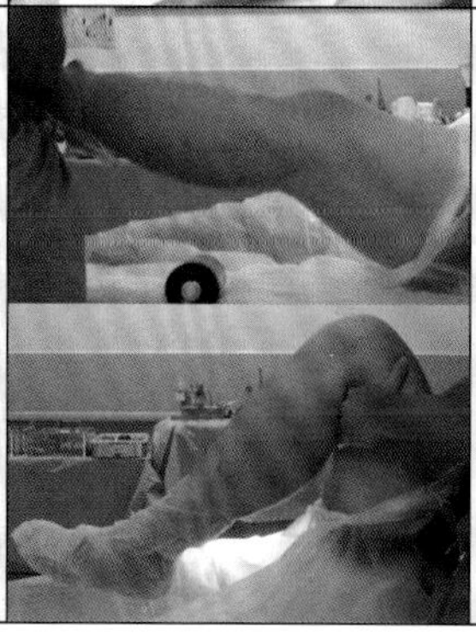 | Normal range of motion is 0 degrees (full extension) to 135 degrees (full flexion). Loss of extension indicates a posterior capsular contracture; loss of flexion could be due to quadriceps contracture and especially rectus femoris spasticity or contracture if the knee is flexed in the prone position. Normal upright walking requires full knee extension range of motion. |

*(continued)*

| Examination | Technique | Illustration | Grading & Significance |
|---|---|---|---|
| **Sensory examination** | Sensation to light touch distally should be evaluated in every patient with injuries, with altered sensation in the first web space potentially leading to the diagnosis of extensor retinaculum syndrome. Sensation to light touch is tested along the length of the entire lower extremity. | 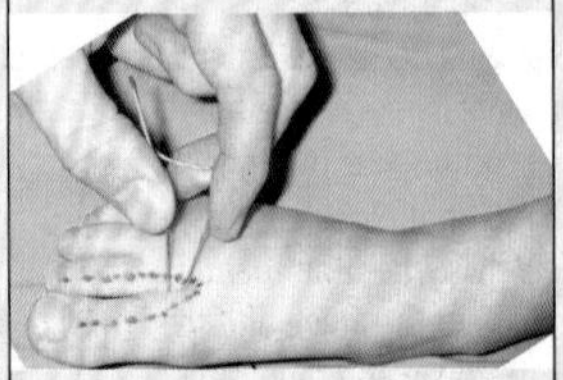 | Sensation to light touch should first be determined. Subjective symmetry should be assessed against the contralateral side. If there is a deficit, although not as sensitive as with the hand examination, two-point discrimination can be quantified. Establishing preoperative deficits is critical in their postoperative management and aids in establishing the need to release the extensor retinacular compartment. |
| **Squeeze test** | Supine subject actively attempts adduction by squeezing legs against resistance provided by examiner. | 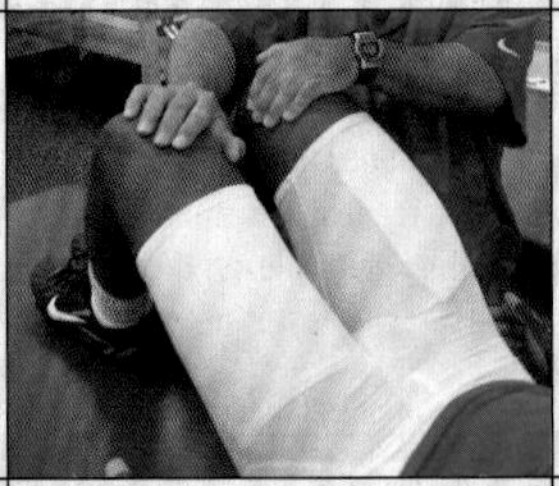 | The presence or absence of pain is noted. Strength is graded as mild (minimal loss of strength); moderate (clear loss of strength); or severe (complete loss of strength). Pain with or without a strength deficit implies adductor-related groin pain. |
| **Straight-leg raise** | The subject is supine, with the hip and knee in full extension, and the ankle in neutral, plantigrade alignment. The examiner holds the foot and ankle and slowly elevates the leg, allowing the hip to flex but maintaining the knee in full extension. The hip is flexed until resistance is met and the pelvis starts to tilt posteriorly or the knee begins to flex. The angle between the elevated leg and the horizontal table top is measured with a goniometer. | 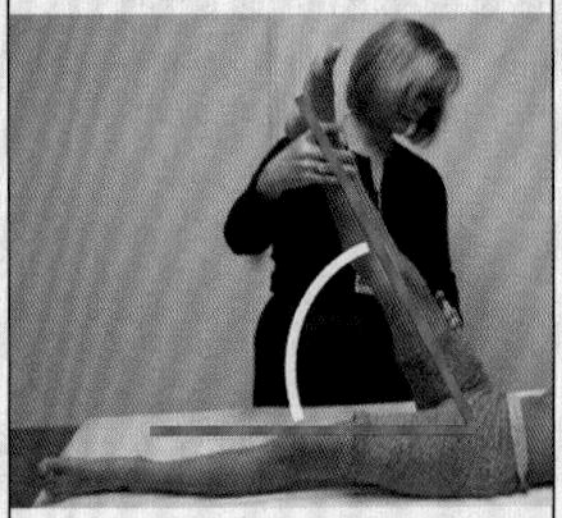 | A straight-leg raise of 60 degrees or less is indicative of shortening of the medial hamstrings. |
| **Toe raise test** | With the individual standing, the examiner passively dorsiflexes the hallux. | 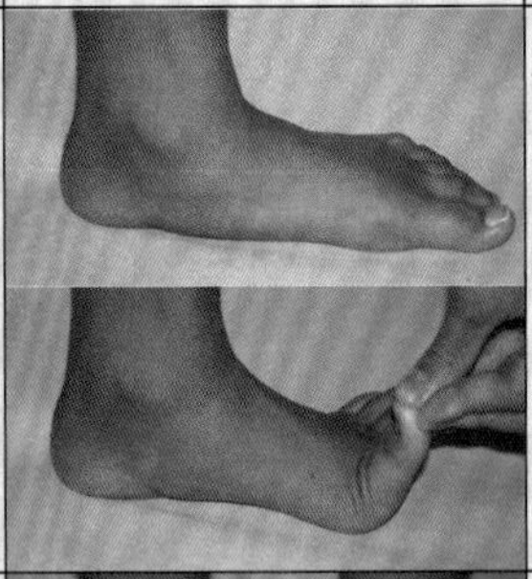 | The examiner should note the reversal of the flat arch to an elevated arch. The longitudinal arch will elevate and the hindfoot valgus will correct to neutral in a flexible flatfoot.<br><br>Image from the private collection of Vincent Mosca MD. |
| **Toe standing test** | The patient is asked to elevate the heels and stand on the toes (ball of the foot). | 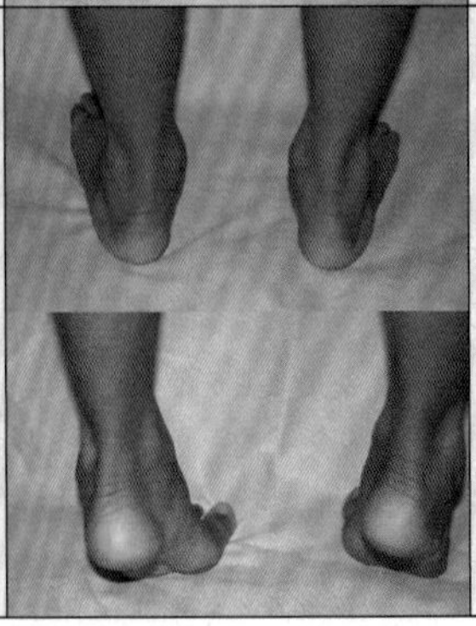 | The examiner should note the reversal of the flat arch to an elevated arch. The longitudinal arch will elevate and the hindfoot valgus will correct to neutral in a flexible flatfoot.<br><br>Image from the private collection of Vincent Mosca MD. |

| Examination | Technique | Illustration | Grading & Significance |
|---|---|---|---|
| **Trendelenburg test** | Observing from behind, the examiner asks the patient to stand on one foot and then the other (for up to 15 seconds). In the figure, the child has right dysplasia. When she stands on her left hip, the right hemipelvis elevates (suggesting normal left hip mechanics). When she stands on the abnormal right hip, the left hemipelvis drops (suggesting poor right hip mechanics). | 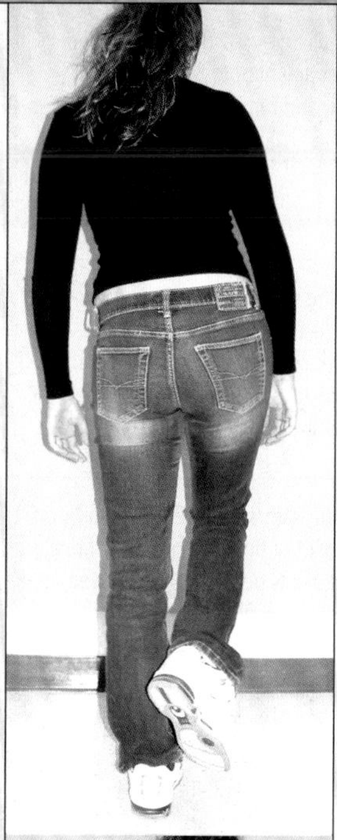 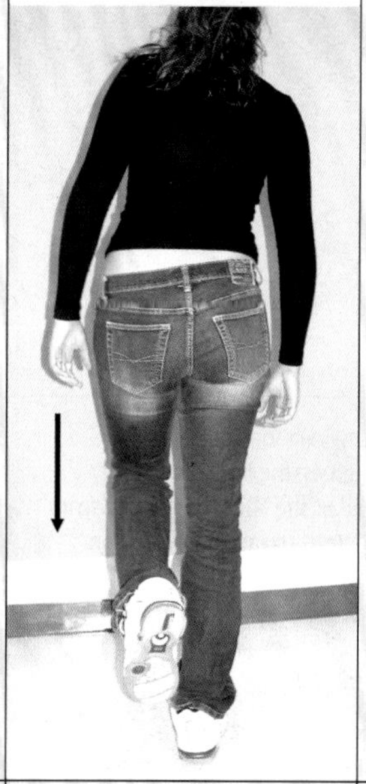 | Tilting of pelvis down toward the non-stance leg is a positive sign, which signifies abductor weakness. |
| **Trochanteric prominence angle test** | This is performed in the prone position, starting with the knee flexed to 90 degrees and the hip in neutral rotation. The hip is internally rotated while palpating the prominence of the greater trochanter. When the greater trochanter is maximally prominent laterally, the femoral neck axis is assumed to be horizontal, and the angle by which the tibia was rotated out (hip rotated in) from the initial upright position provides an estimate of the femoral anteversion. | 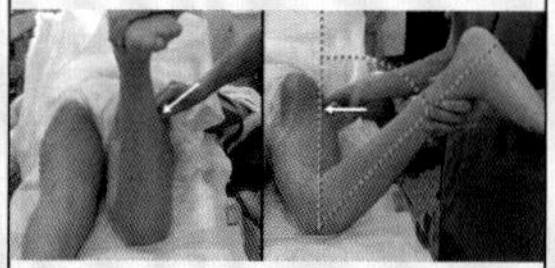 | Anteversion in degrees is measured using a goniometer. Normal range of anteversion is age-dependent; in adults it is typically 10 to 20 degrees. |

*(continued)*

| Examination | Technique | Illustration | Grading & Significance |
|---|---|---|---|
| **Varus and valgus laxity** | A valgus and varus force is applied to the knee in both 30 degrees of flexion and full extension. | 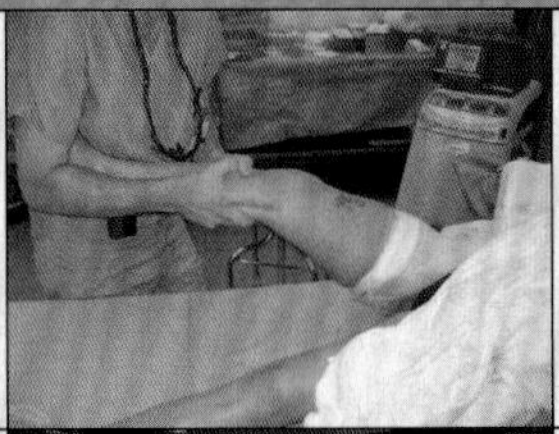 | Classically, displacement of <5 mm is considered a grade I injury, 5 to 10 mm a grade II injury, and >10 mm a grade III injury. Opening in full extension implies a combined injury to the collateral ligament and at least one cruciate ligament. |
| **Varus recurvatum test** | With the patient supine, the examiner lifts both feet by the big toes and watches for varus angulation, hyperextension, and external rotation of the tibia. | 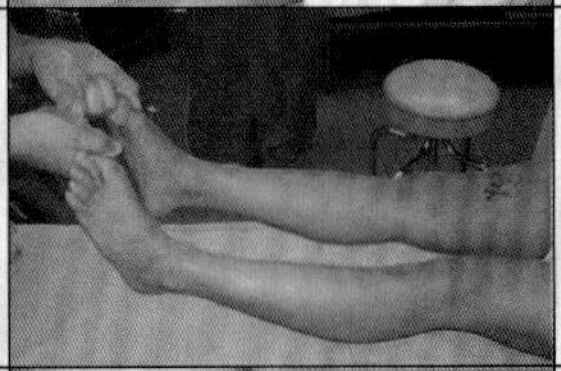 | Suggestive of posterolateral rotatory instability of the knee. |
| **Vascular examination** | Vascular status may be assessed by palpation of both the posterior tibial and dorsalis pedis arteries, as well as capillary refill. If no pulses are palpable, Doppler studies should be obtained. | 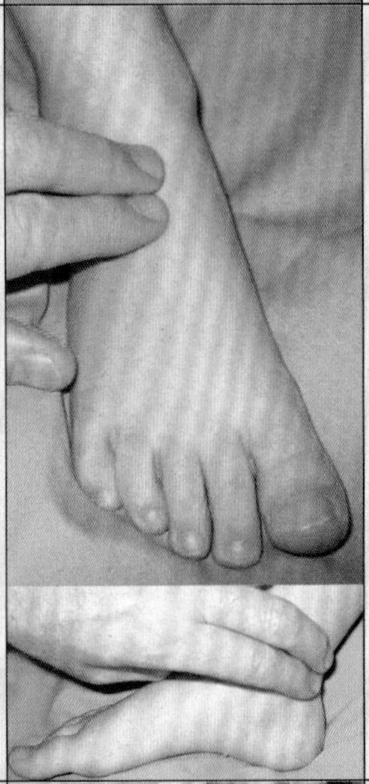 | Palpable pulses can be classified is several ways, from descriptive terms to numerical values. Capillary refill is classified in terms of time. Vascular status is key to the ultimate viability of the extremity. If deficits are found the fracture should be immediately reduced. If a deficit is still present after reduction a vascular study may be considered versus immediate operative exploration to evaluate for transient spasm or vascular injury. |
| **Wilson test** | Starting with the knee flexed to 90 degrees, the tibia is internally rotated as the knee is extended from 90 degrees toward full extension. | 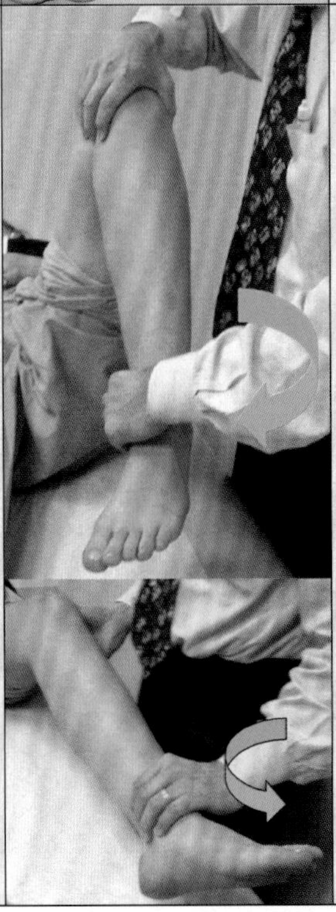 | In a positive test pain is elicited over the anterior aspect of the medial femoral condyle. A weakness of the Wilson test is the lack of sensitivity. |

| Examination | Technique | Illustration | Grading & Significance |
|---|---|---|---|
| **Foot and Ankle** | | | |
| **Achilles tendon rupture: Active plantarflexion test** | With the patient supine, active plantarflexion power is tested. | | Positive: Weak plantarflexion power graded 1 to 5<br>Poorly sensitive and unreliable, as powerful plantarflexion may still be possible due to the action of other ankle plantarflexors. |
| **Achilles tendon rupture: Knee flexion test** | While prone, the patient actively flexes the knee. The examiner observes foot position and compares it with the other side. | | Positive: Foot falls into neutral or dorsiflexion.<br>Negative: Foot maintains plantarflexion posture. Less reliable test; may be difficult to perform due to acute pain. 88% sensitive. |
| **Achilles tendon rupture: Palpable gap test** | Gentle palpation of the tendon reveals a defect at the rupture site. | | Gap present or absent. Gap present indicates complete Achilles rupture with separation of the ruptured ends. More reliable when done early after rupture; 73% sensitive. |
| **Achilles tendon rupture: Thompson or Simmonds test** | With the patient in prone position, the examiner squeezed the calf at the gastrocsoleus muscle level. Limited ankle plantarflexion occurs (as compared to the unaffected side). | | Positive test if ruptured, demonstrating limited ankle plantarflexion. Not as reliable in chronic ruptures as it is in acute ruptures due to formation of "pseudo tendon" scar between ruptured ends. |
| **Ankle instability: Anterior drawer test** | The patient sits on the edge of the examination table with the legs dangling and the feet in a few degrees of plantarflexion. The examiner places one hand on the anterior aspect of the tibia and grasps the calcaneus with the palm of the other hand. The examiner then pulls the calcaneus anteriorly while pushing the tibia posteriorly. This tests the anterior talofibular ligament. To test the calcaneofibular ligament, the same maneuver is performed with the ankle in a dorsiflexed position. | | Typically, anterior drawer is increased when the foot is externally rotated (vs. internally rotated); this is a highly sensitive test for medial ankle instability. The examiner should look for a difference of 3 to 5mm in the relationship between the lateral talus and the anterior aspect of the fibula. On side-to-side comparison the unstable side will have a greater degree of translation. Indicates an insufficient anterior talofibular ligament. |
| **Ankle instability: Suction sign test** | Anterior drawer test as described above. | | As the heel is delivered from the back of the ankle in an unstable ankle, a dimpling will occur in the region just anterior and inferior to the tip of the fibula as a vacuum is created by the talus sliding out from the mortise. |

*(continued)*

| Examination | Technique | Illustration | Grading & Significance |
|---|---|---|---|
| **Distal tarsal tunnel test** | The examiner palpates for medial hindfoot tenderness (plus or minus swelling) at the "soft spot"—the distal edge of the abductor hallucis muscle about 5 cm anterior to the posterior of the heel at the intersection of the plantar and medial skin. | 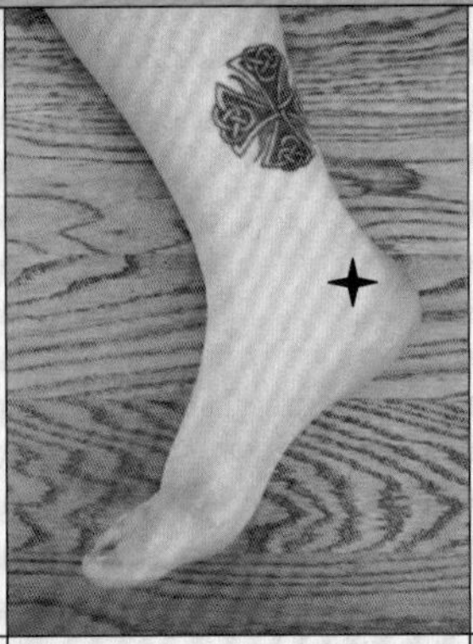 | Tenderness corresponds with the course of the lateral plantar nerve and its first branch and is associated with nerve entrapment or neuritis. |
| **Equinus contracture** | The hindfoot is held in neutral position and the midfoot is aligned by internal rotation of the navicular. Then the forefoot is placed into pronation and the medial ray is held firm. Then the examiner manipulates the foot into dorsiflexion with the knee extended as well as with the knee flexed. | 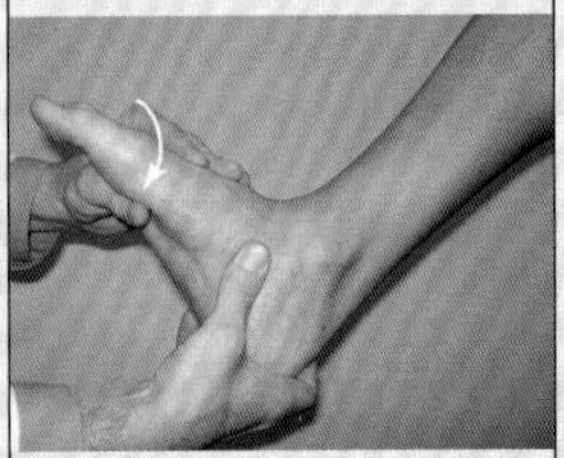 | With knee extended: isolated gastrocnemius contracture when unable to achieve neutral dorsiflexion. Gastrocsoleus contracture is present when the examiner cannot get the ankle to neutral with the knee flexed. May need to perform a gastrocnemius recession or Achilles lengthening procedure concomitantly when there is 5 degrees of equinus in the ankle. |
| **Equinus contracture: Silfverskiold test** | With the patient sitting, the ankle is maximally dorsiflexed with the knee extended and the foot held in a neutral position. The knee is then flexed and the ankle dorsiflexed again. | 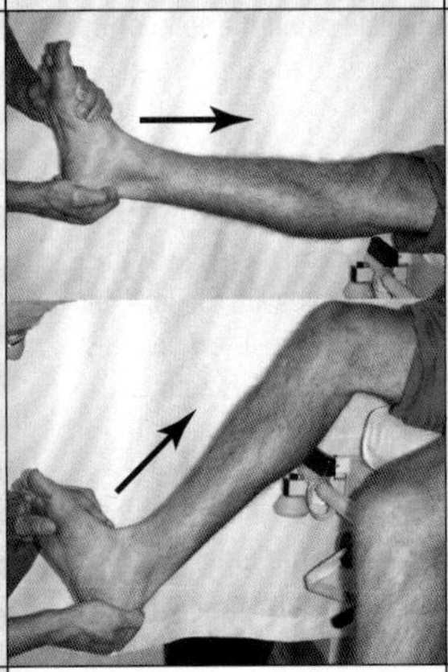 | Positive: When the foot is held in equinus correcting to above neutral with the knee flexed; indicates a tight Achilles tendon within the gastrocnemius muscle. The deformity may aggravate an unstable ankle. |
| **First MTP joint grind test** | The examiner grinds the MTP joint with an axially directed force. | 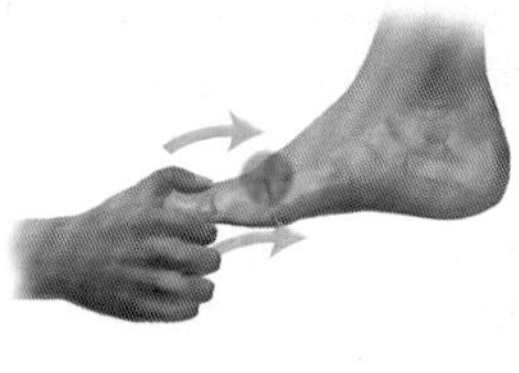 | Pain at MTP joint associated with osteochondral lesion or severe degeneration. Usually not symptomatic in mild cases. If this test causes severe pain, one may consider imaging studies.<br>Not normally painful unless an osteochondral defect is present or degeneration is advanced. If painful, then arthrodesis is indicated. |
| **First MTP joint hypertension test to distinguish hallux rigidus from sesamoid pathology** | The big toe is hyperextended. | 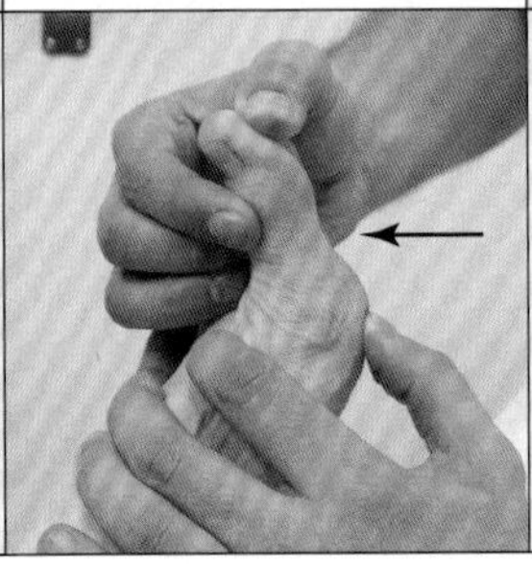 | The examiner must discern between rising pain at the plantar (sesamoid) or dorsal (hallux rigidus) aspect of the MTP joint. High specificity with appropriate history, but otherwise not specific. |

| Examination | Technique | Illustration | Grading & Significance |
|---|---|---|---|
| **First tarsometatarsal hypermobility test (perspective 1)** | The examiner grasps the lesser metatarsal heads with one hand and passively plantarflexes and dorsiflexes the first metatarsal with the other hand. | | Hypermobility has been defined as an elevation of 5 to 8 mm above the level of the second metatarsal, but the diagnosis of hypermobility is often more subjective. Hypermobility at the tarsometatarsal joint creates a valgus moment at the MTP joint that may contribute to failure of distal hallux valgus correction. |
| **First tarsometatarsal joint excursion (perspective 2)** | One hand is placed with the thumb and index finger located plantar and dorsal to the first metatarsal head and the opposite thumb and index finger placed plantar and dorsal to the second metatarsal hand. The first ray is then dorsiflexed and plantarflexed to end range of motion and the intervals between the thumb and index finger of both hands are noted and measured. | | The normal first ray excursion is 10 mm (5 mm of dorsiflexion and 5 mm of plantarflexion). Hypermobility can be defined as total excursion $>$15 mm. Hypermobility of the first ray is significant when contemplating a surgical procedure for the hallux valgus deformity. If hypermobility is present, a first tarsometatarsal joint fusion may be more appropriate. |
| **Fixed forefoot varus** | The calcaneus is held in a neutral position (out of valgus) and any fixed elevation of the first ray relative to the fifth is noted. | | The severity of deformity is noted in degrees. Fixed forefoot varus must be accounted for in any treatment algorithm and is usually the first component of the deformity to become rigid. |
| **Flexor hallucis longus tenosynovitis** | The pain is produced with active–passive motion of the hallux while a thumb palpates the tendon for tenderness and crepitus. | | The presence of flexor hallucis longus tenosynovitis should be documented and treated accordingly. |
| **Forced dorsiflexion of the first MTP joint** | The examiner gradually increases dorsiflexion of the first MTP joint. | | Pain is associated with impingement of the base of the proximal phalanx and metatarsal head. The amount of dorsiflexion obtained is measured as well. Maximum extension is characteristically limited and pain is sometimes present. Also, the osteophytic ridge can be best palpated in the dorsolateral portion of the joint. Pain associated with stretching of the extensor hallucis longus, capsule, and inflamed synovium; often occurs earlier in the disease process. Maximal flexion is sometimes limited, but pain is best brought out. Tenderness is commonly identified in the dorsolateral aspect of the joint. |

*(continued)*

| Examination | Technique | Illustration | Grading & Significance |
|---|---|---|---|
| **Lesser MTP joint pushup test** | With the patient seated and knee flexed, the examiner dorsiflexes the ankle to neutral by applying pressure under the metatarsal heads. The correction of the toe deformity with this manuver is noted. | 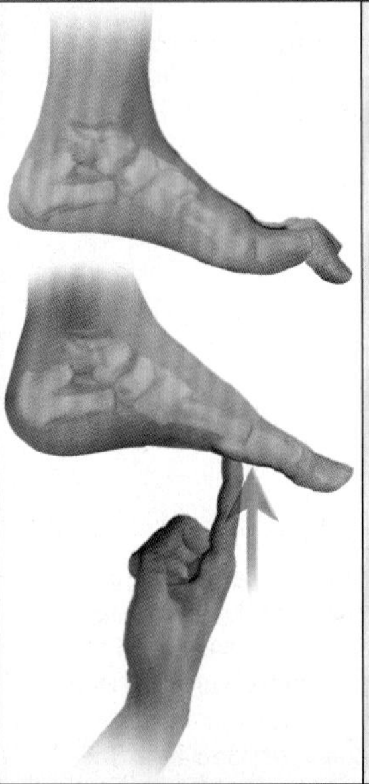 | If the deformity is flexible, with the pushup test the MTP joint will flex to its normal position. If not, it will remain extended defining a fixed deformity. Semiflexible deformities are those that correct partially with the pushup test. A flexible deformity is amenable to soft tissue procedures, including tendon transfers. Fixed deformities will need extensive procedures, including osteotomies.<br><br>This test is also useful in the operating room to assess residual MTP joint contracture after the hammertoe has been corrected at the proximal interphalangeal joint. Residual MTP joint contracture necessitates additional surgical correction at the MTP joint, such as extensor tendon lengthening, capsular release, or collateral ligament release. |
| **Lesser MTP joint stability test** | The metatarsal bone and the proximal phalanx are stabilized and stress is placed in a dorsoplantar direction, attempting to subluxate the joint. | 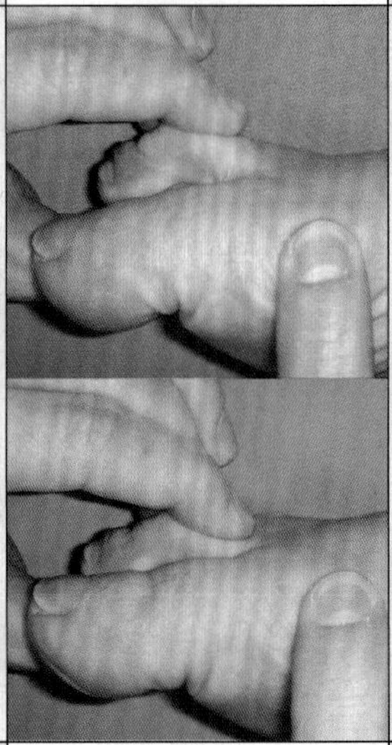 | Stage 0: no laxity to dorsal translation; stage 1: the base of the proximal phalanx can be subluxated with the dorsal stress; stage 2: the proximal phalangeal base can be dislocated and relocated; stage 3: the base of the proximal phalanx is fixed in a dislocated position. For the initial stages (0, 1, 2) a tendon transfer associated with a dorsal MTP soft tissue release will stabilize the deformity. For fixed MTP dislocations a bone-shortening procedure should be added to the soft tissue procedures. |
| **Lesser toe manipulation test** | Gentle manual straightening of the toe to assess the ability of the toe to correct to neutral. | 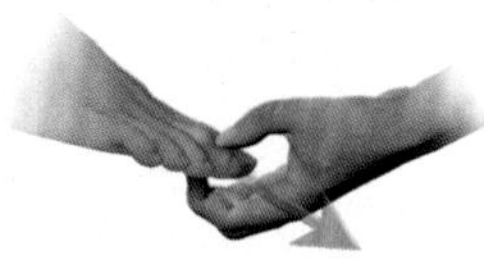 | If the toe completely corrects to neutral it is considered a flexible deformity. If the toe does not completely correct, it is considered a fixed deformity. A flexible deformity can be addressed with a soft tissue procedure such as a flexor-to-extensor tendon transfer. A fixed deformity will require bone resection for surgical correction. |
| **MTP joint vertical Lachman test** | The examiner stabilizes the hallux metatarsal with the thumb and index finger of one hand while attempting to translate the proximal phalanx in a dorsal–plantar direction with the thumb and index finger of the other hand. | 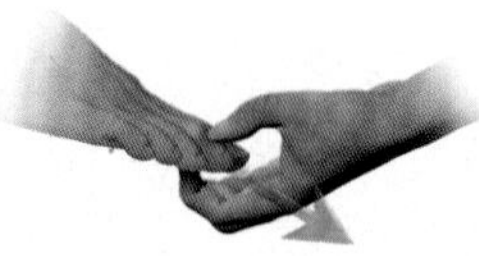 | A positive test is any laxity greater than the contralateral side. |

| Examination | Technique | Illustration | Grading & Significance |
|---|---|---|---|
| **Mulder test for Morton's neuroma** | With the patient prone and the knee flexed 90 degrees, the examiner deeply palpates the plantar aspect web space with the index finger. Maintaining this pressure, the examiner gently squeezes the forefoot. | 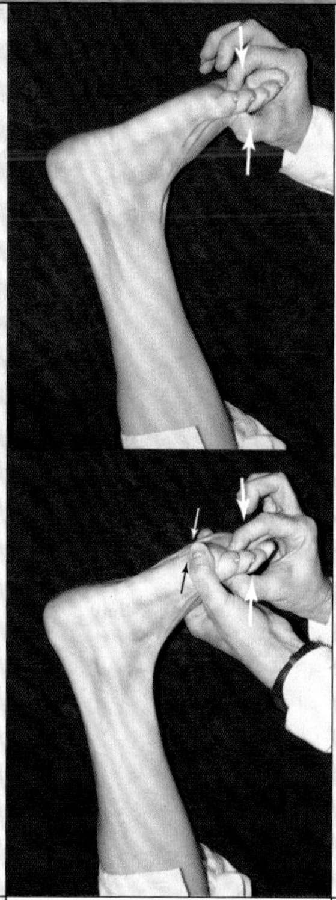 | Palpable "click" and reproduction of symptoms help confirm the diagnosis. |
| **Percussion test for neuralgia** | Percussion over the dorsomedial hallucal nerve or terminal hallucal branch of the deep peroneal nerve in the first web space. | 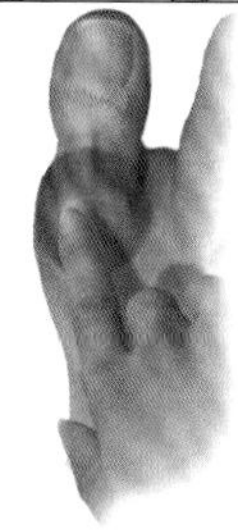 | Hypesthesias or radiating symptoms can occur in the terminal nerve branches because of compression from synovitis or dorsal osteophytes.<br><br>Most clinicians simply note a positive or negative percussion test. Large dorsal osteophytes may compress the dorsal medial or lateral digital nerve. |
| **Posterior ankle impingement: Maquirriain** | In the seated position (90 degrees hip flexion, 90 degrees knee flexion, neutral ankle position), the subject is asked to slide both feet forward while maintaining full contact on the floor. Limited ankle plantarflexion or posterior ankle pain will be evidenced by the inability to maintain forefoot contact. | 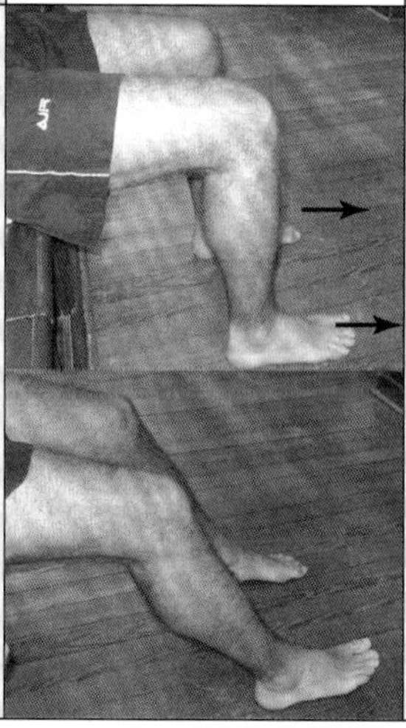 | Negative: symmetric motion; positive: asymmetric motion due to posterior ankle pain or limited ankle plantarflexion. In this office test the examiner should try to reproduce typical painful motion of posterior ankle impingement syndrome in closed position. It also allows the examiner to estimate the passive ROM limitation. |

*(continued)*

| Examination | Technique | Illustration | Grading & Significance |
|---|---|---|---|
| **Posterior ankle impingement: Passive forced plantarflexion test (perspective 1)** | With the patient in prone position with both feet out of the table, the physician performs a forced plantarflexion maneouver. Limitation of range of motion can also be estimated. | 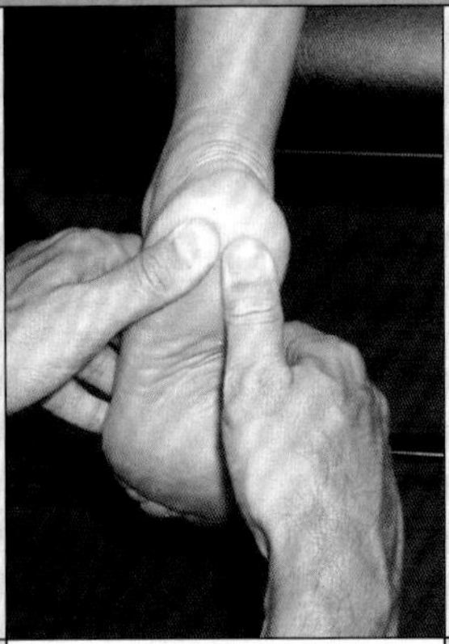 | Discomfort; posterior ankle pain. Normal ankle ROM is 18 degrees dorsiflexion and 48 degrees plantarflexion. In this office test the examiner should try to reproduce typical painful motion of posterior ankle impingement syndrome. It also allows the examiner to estimate the passive ROM limitation. |
| **Posterior ankle impingement: Passive forced plantarflexion test (perspective 2)** | The ankle is passively flexed while the subtalar joint is held in neutral position. The opposite thumb and index finger are used to palpate the retromalleolar regions for any crepitus. | 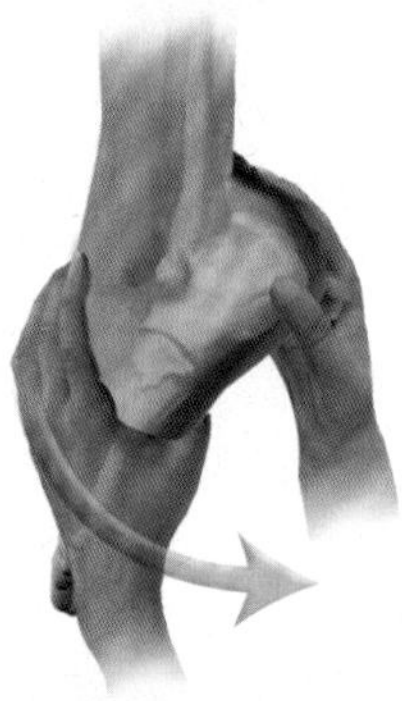 | Sharp pain or crepitus is produced at full plantarflexion with a positive test. |
| **Tibiotalar joint line palpation** | Digital palpation of medial joint line with simultaneous application of valgus force. | 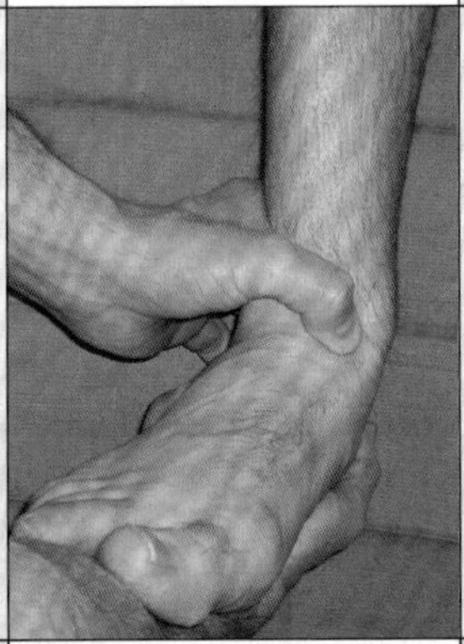 | Valgus tilt present or absent. Presence of valgus tilt indicates insufficiency of deltoid ligament. |
| **Toe palpation** | The examiner palpates the distal and proximal interphalangeal joints and the MTP joint for points of maximal tenderness. | 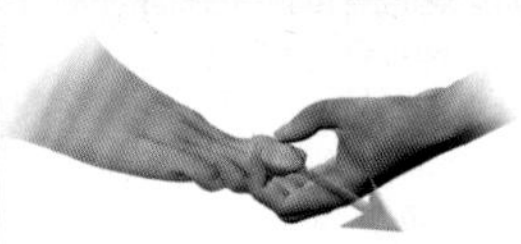 | The proximal interphalangeal joint should be the area of maximal tenderness, but the tip of the toe may be painful as well. |
| **Windlass mechanism test** | The examiner palpates the affected versus unaffected plantar fascia while recreating the windlass mechanism (by combining passive ankle dorsiflexion and 1–5 MTP joint dorsiflexion). | 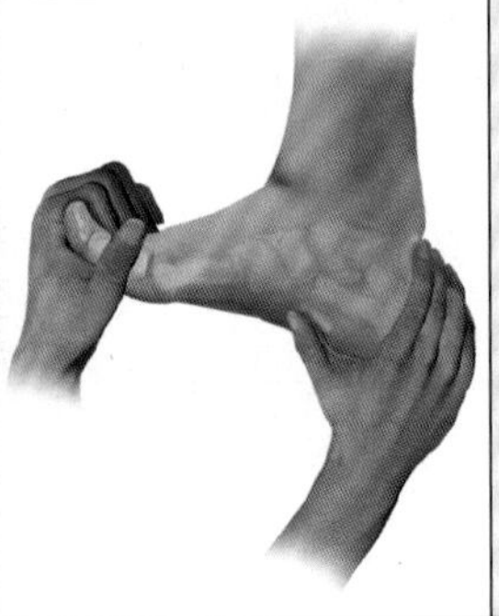 | Less firm or tense plantar fascia compared to the opposite side indicates chronic attenuation or incompetence of the plantar fascia. |

| Examination | Technique | Illustration | Grading & Significance |
|---|---|---|---|
| **Digital purchase: Paper pull-out test** | A thin strip of paper is placed under the affected toe pulp. The examiner attempts to pull the paper strip out while the patient attempts to resist with toe pressure against the ground. | 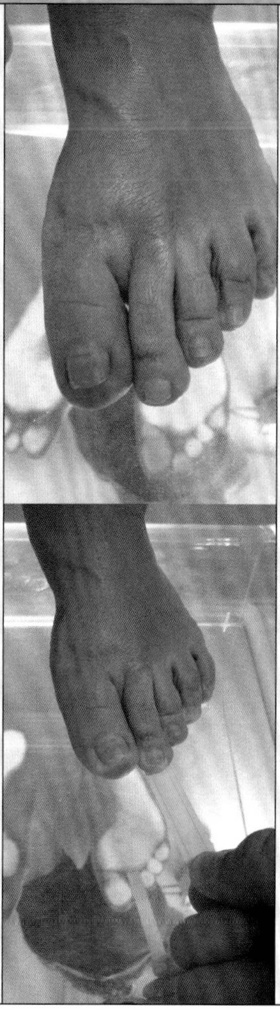 | The test is considered positive when there is no toe purchase present; it is considered reduced when the purchase is present but not powerful enough to resist the paper strip to being pulled out and is considered negative when the toe is able to prevent the paper strip to being pulled out |

# Index

Page numbers followed by *f* and *t* indicate figures and tables, respectively.

## D

## T

## W



## Z